CLINICAL PROCEDURES

in Emergency Medicine

James R. Roberts, M.D.
Assistant Professor
Department of Emergency Medicine
University of Cincinnati,
College of Medicine

Jerris R. Hedges, M.D.
Assistant Professor
Department of Emergency Medicine
University of Cincinnati,
College of Medicine

W. B. Saunders Company **1985**

PHILADELPHIA   LONDON   TORONTO   MEXICO CITY   RIO DE JANEIRO   SYDNEY   TOKYO

W. B. Saunders Company: West Washington Square
Philadelphia, PA 19105

1 St. Anne's Road
Eastbourne, East Sussex BN21 3UN, England

1 Goldthorne Avenue
Toronto, Ontario M8Z 5T9, Canada

Apartado 26370—Cedro 512
Mexico 4, D.F., Mexico

Rua Coronel Cabrita, 8
Sao Cristovao Caixa Postal 21176
Rio de Janeiro, Brazil

9 Waltham Street
Artarmon, N.S.W. 2064, Australia

Ichibancho, Central Bldg., 22-1 Ichibancho
Chiyoda-Ku, Tokyo 102, Japan

Library of Congress Cataloging in Publication Data

Roberts, James R., 1946–

Clinical procedures in emergency medicine.

1. Emergency medicine.   I. Hedges, Jerris R.
   II. Title.   [DNLM: 1. Emergencies.   2. Emergency medicine—Methods. WB 105 C641]

RC86.7.R58   1985   616'.025   83-8658

ISBN 0–7216–7606–5

Clinical Procedures in Emergency Medicine   ISBN 0–7216–7606–5

Last digit is the print number: 9   8   7   6   5   4   3   2   1

To Lydia and Susan

CONTRIBUTORS

TOM I. ABELSON, M.D.
Assistant Clinical Professor of Otolaryngology, Case Western Reserve University School of Medicine, Cleveland, Ohio; Assistant Otolaryngologist, University Hospitals of Cleveland, Cleveland, Ohio; Staff Otolaryngologist, Mt. Sinai Medical Center and Hillcrest Hospital, Cleveland, Ohio; Consulting Staff, Veterans Administration Hospital of Cleveland, Cleveland, Ohio; Adjunct Staff, Department of Otolaryngology and Communicative Disorders, The Cleveland Clinic Foundation, Cleveland, Ohio.

JAMES T. AMSTERDAM, D.M.D., M.D.
Assistant Professor of Emergency Medicine; Assistant Professor of Surgery (Oral Surgery and Dentistry), University of Cincinnati College of Medicine and Hospital, Cincinnati, Ohio; Clinical Instructor of Surgery (Dental Medicine), Medical College of Pennsylvania, Philadelphia, Pennsylvania.

PAUL B. BAKER, M.D.
Clinical Fellow, Division of Emergency Medicine, University of Cincinnati Medical Center, Cincinnati, Ohio.

WILLIAM BARKER, M.D.
Department of Emergency Medicine, The Fairfax Hospital, Falls Church, Virginia

RICHARD C. BARNETT, M.D.
Associate Clinical Professor of Family and Community Medicine, University of California, San Francisco Medical School, San Francisco, California; Director, Family Practice Program at Community Hospital of Souvura County, California.

DAVID H. BARR, M.D.
Attending Ophthalmologist, Northgate, Cabrini, and Group Health Hospitals, Seattle, Washington.

ROBERT L. BARTLETT, M.D.
Associate Educational Director and Director of Research, Department of Emergency Medicine, Richland Memorial Hospital, Columbia, South Carolina; Clinical Instructor of Surgery, Medical University of South Carolina, Charleston, South Carolina.

GEORGES C. BENJAMIN, M.D.
Assistant Professor of Medicine, Uniformed Services University of the Health Sciences, Bethesda, Maryland; Chief, Emergency Medical Services, Walter Reed Army Medical Center, Washington, D.C.

JONATHAN L. BENUMOF, M.D.
Professor of Anesthesia, University of California, San Diego School of Medicine, San Diego, California; Professor of Anesthesiology, University Hospital, San Diego, California.

RICHARD E. BERGER, M.D.
Associate Professor, Department of Urology, University of Washington, Seattle, Washington; Attending Urologist, University Hospital, Seattle, Washington; Chief of Urology, Harborview Hospital, Seattle, Washington; Attending Urologist, Seattle Veterans Administration Hospital, Seattle, Washington; Children's Orthopedic Hospital, Seattle, Washington.

GARRETT E. BERGMAN, M.D.
Associate Professor of Pediatrics, Medical College of Pennsylvania, Philadelphia, Pennsylvania; Attending Pediatrician, Hospital of the Medical College of Pennsylvania, Philadelphia, Pennsylvania; Associate

Staff Pediatrician, St. Christopher's Hospital for Children, Philadelphia, Pennsylvania.

G. RICHARD BRAEN, M.D.
Director, Emergency Department, Newton-Wellesley Hospital, Newton, Massachusetts.

FRANK P. BRANCATO, Ph.D.
Retired Scientist, Director USPHS and Chief, Department of Microbiology, Seattle USPHS Hospital, Seattle, Washington; Affiliate Associate Professor of Microbiology, University of Washington, Seattle, Washington; Consultant, Seattle Veterans' Hospital, Providence Medical Center, Pacific Medical Center, Seattle, Washington.

CHARLES O. BRANTIGAN, M.D.,
F.A.C.S., F.C.C.P.
Associate Clinical Professor of Surgery, University of Colorado Medical Center, Denver, Colorado; Director, Noninvasive Vascular Lab, Presbyterian Medical Center, Denver, Colorado.

MICHAEL L. CALLAHAM, M.D.
Clinical Associate Professor, University of California, San Francisco, San Francisco, California; Chief, Division of Emergency Medicine, University of California at San Francisco, San Francisco, California.

LEVON M. CAPAN, M.D.
Associate Professor of Clinical Anesthesiology, New York University Medical Center, New York, New York.

NISHA CHANDRA, M.D.
Assistant Professor of Medicine, Johns Hopkins School of Medicine, Baltimore, Maryland; Coronary Care Unit Director, Baltimore City Hospitals, Baltimore, Maryland.

JOSEPH E. CLINTON, M.D., F.A.C.E.P.
Senior Associate Physician, Assistant Chief of Emergency Medicine, and Residency Director, Emergency Medicine, Hennepin County Medical Center, Minneapolis, Minnesota.

SAMUEL TIMOTHY COLERIDGE, D.O.
Assistant Clinical Professor of Surgery, Texas Tech University Health Sciences Cen-

ter, School of Medicine, El Paso, Texas; Chief, Emergency Medical Services, William Beaumont Army Medical Center, El Paso, Texas.

WILLIAM C. DALSEY, M.D.
Chief Resident, Department of Emergency Medicine, University of Cincinnati, Cincinnati, Ohio.

RICHARD DAVISON, M.D.
Associate Professor, Department of Medicine, and Section Chief, Critical Care Medicine, Department of Medicine, Northwestern University Medical School, Chicago, Illinois; Director, Medical Intensive Care Facilities, Northwestern Memorial Hospital, Chicago, Illinois.

THOM DICK, EMT-P
Lecturer, University of California, San Diego, San Diego, California; Paramedic, Hartson Ambulance Service, San Diego, California; Associate Editor, Journal of Emergency Medical Services.

LYNNETTE A. DOAN, M.D.
Assistant Professor of Surgery, University of Florida, Jacksonville, Florida; Faculty, Department of Emergency Medicine, University Hospital of Jacksonville, Jacksonville, Florida.

ALICE M. DONAHUE, R.N., M.S.N.
Supervisor, Emergency Department, Sacred Heart Hospital, Norristown, Pennsylvania.

STEVEN C. DRONEN, M.D., F.A.C.E.P.
Assistant Professor of Emergency Medicine, University of Cincinnati College of Medicine, Cincinnati, Ohio; Staff Physician, University of Cincinnati Hospital, Cincinnati, Ohio.

DAVID J. DULA, M.D.
Associate, Emergency Medicine, Geisinger Medical Center, Danville, Pennsylvania.

WILLIAM DURSTON, M.D.
Assistant Chief of Emergency Medicine, Kaiser Foundation Hospital, Sacramento, California.

MICHAEL E. ERVIN, M.D.
Associate Clinical Professor, Wright State

University School of Medicine, Dayton, Ohio; Director, Emergency and Trauma Center, Miami Valley Hospital, Dayton, Ohio.

THOMAS G. FROHLICH, M.D.
Chief Resident, Veterans Administration Hospital Medical Center, Chicago, Illinois.

KENNETH FRUMKIN, M.D., Ph.D.,
Major, Medical Corps, U.S. Army
Chief, Department of Emergency Medicine, Madigan Army Medical Center, Tacoma, Washington.

STEPHEN GAZAK, M.D.
Staff Physician, Department of Emergency Medicine, Methodist Hospital, Philadelphia, Pennsylvania.

JONATHAN M. GLAUSER, M.D.
Director, Residency Program in Emergency Medicine and Director, Department of Emergency Medical Services, Mt. Sinai Medical Center, Cleveland, Ohio.

MICHAEL I. GREENBERG, M.D., F.A.C.E.P.
Clinical Assistant Professor of Emergency Medicine, Medical College of Pennsylvania, Philadelphia, Pennsylvania; Chief of Emergency Medicine, Sacred Heart Hospital, Norristown, Pennsylvania.

BARRY H. HENDLER, D.D.S., M.D.
Associate Professor of Medicine and Surgery and Director of Oral and Maxillofacial Surgery, Medical College of Pennsylvania, Philadelphia, Pennsylvania; Acting Chairman, Oral and Maxillofacial Surgery, University of Pennsylvania School of Dental Medicine and Affiliated Hospitals, Philadelphia, Pennsylvania; Attending Physician, Oral and Maxillofacial Surgery, Holy Redeemer Hospital, Philadelphia, Pennsylvania.

GEOFFREY E. HERTER, M.D.
Chief Resident in Urology, Yale University School of Medicine, New Haven, Connecticut.

MARY ANN HOWLAND, Pharm.D.
Associate Professor of Clinical Pharmacology, St. John's University, Jamaica, New York; Clinical Consultant, New York Poison Center, New York, New York

KENNETH V. ISERSON, M.D., F.A.C.E.P.
Residency Director and Assistant Professor, Section of Emergency Medicine, Department of Surgery, Arizona Health Sciences Center, Tucson, Arizona.

STEVEN M. JOYCE, M.D.
Assistant Professor of Surgery, Section of Emergency Medicine, University of Arizona, Health Sciences Center, Tucson, Arizona.

ROBERT L. KATZ, M.D., F.A.C.S.
Associate Clinical Professor of Surgery and Acting Chairman, Division of Otolaryngology, Case Western Reserve University, Cleveland, Ohio; Surgeon, Case Western Reserve University Hospitals of Cleveland, Cleveland, Ohio.

SEUNG K. KIM, M.D.
Acting Assistant Professor of Surgery, Division of Plastic Surgery, Stanford University School of Medicine, Stanford, California; Attending Plastic Surgeon, Stanford University Medical Center, Stanford, California.

ROBERT KNOPP, M.D.
Assistant Clinical Professor of Family and Community Medicine, University of California, San Francisco, San Francisco, California; Chief of Emergency Medicine, Valley Medical Center, Fresno, California.

JON C. KOOIKER, M.D.
Clinical Assistant Professor of Medicine (Neurology), University of Washington School of Medicine, Seattle, Washington; Attending Neurologist, Department of Medicine, St. Peter Hospital, Olympia, Washington.

MARC KOBERNICK, M.D.
Clinical Assistant Professor of Emergency Medicine, University of Arizona College of Medicine, Tucson, Arizona; Attending Emergency Physician, University of Arizona Health Sciences Center and Kino Community Hospital, Tucson, Arizona.

RICHARD L. LAMMERS, M.D.
Clinical Professor of Family and Community Medicine, University of California, San Francisco, San Francisco, California; Assistant Chief of Emergency Medicine, Valley Medical Center of Fresno, Fresno, California.

ROBERT G. R. LANG, M.D., F.R.C.S.(C)
Attending Neurosurgeon, St. Peter Hospital, Olympia, Washington.

JAMES A. LEMONS, M.D.
Professor of Pediatrics, Indiana University School of Medicine, Indianapolis, Indiana; Neonatologist, Section of Neonatal-Perinatal Medicine, James Whitcomb Riley Hospital for Children, Indianapolis, Indiana.

JOHN L. LYMAN, M.D.
Assistant Professor of Emergency Medicine, Wright State University School of Medicine, Dayton, Ohio.

WILLIAM L. MORRISSEY, M.D.
Professor of Medicine, and Associate Professor of Emergency Medicine, Medical College of Pennsylvania, Philadelphia, Pennsylvania; Chief, Division of Pulmonary and Critical Care Medicine; Medical Director, Medical Intensive Care Unit; and Medical Director, Respiratory Care Services and Pulmonary Function Laboratory, Medical College of Pennsylvania Hospital, Philadelphia, Pennsylvania.

DAVID H. NEUSTADT, M.D.
Clinical Professor of Medicine, University of Louisville School of Medicine, Louisville, Kentucky; Medical Consultant, Veterans Administration, Jewish Hospital, Louisville, Kentucky.

WILLIAM L. NEWMEYER, M.D.
Associate Clinical Professor of Surgery, University of California, San Francisco, San Francisco, California; Active Staff, St. Francis Hospital, San Francisco, California; Courtesy Staff, French Hospital, Children's Hospital, St. Lukes Hospital, and Presbyterian Hospital, San Francisco, and Seton Medical Center, Daly City, California; Consultant, San Francisco General Hospital, University of California Hospitals, and Veterans' Administration Hospital, Martinez, California.

KEVIN M. O'KEEFFE, M.D.
Clinical Attending, Department of Emergency Medicine, Madigan Medical Center, Tacoma, Washington; Emergency Physician, Northgate Hospital, Seattle, Washington.

EDWARD J. OTTEN, M.D.
Assistant Professor of Emergency Medicine, University of Cincinnati College of Medicine, Cincinnati, Ohio; Attending Physician, University Hospital, Cincinnati, Ohio, and Booth Hospital, Florence, Kentucky.

KATIE P. PATEL, M.D.
Associate Professor of Anesthesiology, New York University Medical Center, Department of Anesthesiology, New York, New York.

THOMAS B. PURCELL, M.D.
Adjunct Assistant Professor, Department of Medicine, University of California, Los Angeles, Los Angeles, California; Residency Director, Department of Emergency Medicine, Kern Medical Center, Bakersfield, California.

ELAENA QUATTROCCHI, B.S., R.P.H.
Graduate School of Pharmacy, St. John's University, Jamaica, New York.

LOREN H. REX, D.O.
Associate Clinical Professor, Department of Biomechanics, Michigan State University, College of Osteopathic Medicine, East Lansing, Michigan.

STEPHEN N. ROGERS, M.D.
Research Fellow, Department of Anesthesiology, University of California, San Diego, San Diego, California.

LOUIS F. ROSE, D.D.S., M.D.
Professor of Medicine and Surgery, Chief of Dental Medicine, Medical College of Pennsylvania, Philadelphia, Pennsylvania; Professor of Periodontics, University of Pennsylvania School of Dental Medicine, Philadelphia, Pennsylvania; Chief of Dental Medicine and Chairman of the Medical Board, Hospital of the Medical College of Pennsylvania, Philadelphia, Pennsylvania; Attending Physician, Graduate Hospital, Albert Einstein Medical Center, Philadelphia, Pennsylvania.

DAVID S. ROSS, M.D.
Assistant Professor of Emergency Medicine, University of Cincinnati, College of Medicine, Cincinnati, Ohio; Director, Department of Emergency Medicine, Booth Hospital, Florence, Kentucky; Attending Physician, University Hospital, Cincinnati, Ohio.

ERNEST RUIZ, M.D.
Chief of Service, Department of Emergency Medicine, Hennepin County Medical Center, Minneapolis, Minnesota; Assistant Professor of Surgery, University of Minnesota, Minneapolis, Minnesota.

ALFRED SACCHETTI, M.D.
Assistant Director, Department of Emergency Medicine, Methodist Hospital, Philadelphia, Pennsylvania.

MARTIN SCHIFF, Jr., M.D.
Clinical Professor of Surgery/Urology, Yale University School of Medicine, New Haven, Connecticut; Attending Physician, Yale-New Haven Hospital, New Haven, Connecticut; Consultant, West Haven VA Hospital, West Haven, Connecticut, and Waterbury Hospital, Waterbury, Connecticut.

RICHARD L. SCHREINER, M.D.
Professor of Pediatrics, Indiana University School of Medicine, Indianapolis, Indiana; Director, Section of Neonatal-Perinatal Medicine, James Whitcomb Riley Hospital for Children, Indianapolis, Indiana.

MATTHEW H. SMITH, M.D.
Instructor in Medicine, Medical College of Pennsylvania, Philadelphia, Pennsylvania; Attending Physician, John F. Kennedy Hospital, Edison, New Jersey, Raritan Bay Health Center, Perth Amboy, New Jersey, Rahway Hospital, Rahway, New Jersey, and Roosevelt Hospital, Edison, New Jersey.

ANDERS E. SOLA, M.D.
Clinical Assistant Professor, Department of Anesthesiology, Pain Service, School of Medicine, University of Washington, Seattle, Washington; Attending Physician, Northgate General Hospital, Seattle, Washington.

THOMAS STAIR, M.D.
Assistant Professor of Emergency Medicine, Georgetown University School of Medicine, Washington, D.C.; Residency Director, Emergency Department, Georgetown University Hospital, Washington, D.C.

SCOTT SYVERUD, M.D.
Chief Resident, Department of Emergency Medicine, University of Cincinnati, Ohio

DAN TANDBERG, M.D.
Assistant Professor, Division of Emergency Medicine, University of New Mexico School of Medicine, Albuquerque, New Mexico; Medical Director, New Mexico Poison, Drug Information, and Medical Crisis Center, Albuquerque, New Mexico.

ALEXANDER T. TROTT, M.D.
Assistant Professor of Emergency Medicine, Department of Emergency Medicine, University of Cincinnati College of Medicine; Attending Physician, Division of Emergency Medicine, University Hospital, Cincinnati, Ohio, and Booth Hospital, Florence, Kentucky.

WILLIAM G. TROUTMAN, Pharm.D.
Associate Professor, College of Pharmacy, University of New Mexico, Albuquerque, New Mexico; Director, New Mexico Poison, Drug Information, and Medical Crisis Center, Albuquerque, New Mexico.

HERMAN TURNDORF, M.D.
Professor and Chairman, Department of Anesthesiology, New York University Medical Center, New York, New York.

DAVID E. VAN RYN, M.D.
Attending Emergency Physician, Department of Emergency Medicine, Elkhart General Hospital, Elkhart, Indiana; Goshen Community Hospital, Goshen, Indiana.

LARS VISTNES, M.D.
Professor of Surgery and Chairman, Division of Plastic Surgery, Stanford University School of Medicine, Stanford, California; Attending Plastic Surgeon, Stanford University Medical Center, Stanford, California.

J. THOMAS WARD, Jr., M.D.
Clinical Instructor, Department of Internal Medicine, University of Texas Health Science Center at Dallas, Dallas, Texas; Emergency Department Staff Physician, Plano General Hospital, Plano, Texas; Attending Medical Staff, Parkland Memorial Hospital, Plano, Texas.

TODD M. WARDEN, M.D.
Assistant Director, Department of Emergency Medicine, Methodist Hospital, Philadelphia, Pennsylvania.

THOMAS R. WEBER, M.D.
Associate Professor of Pediatric Surgery, Indiana University School of Medicine, Indianapolis, Indiana; Attending Surgeon, James Whitcomb Riley Hospital for Children, Indianapolis, Indiana.

TERRY M. WILLIAMS, M.D.
Attending Physician, Emergency Medicine, Valley Medical Center, Fresno, California; Emergency Services Physician, Kaiser Hospital, Sacramento, California.

WILLIAM J. WITT, M.D.
Assistant Clinical Professor of Otolaryngology, Case Western Reserve University School of Medicine, Cleveland, Ohio; Assistant Otolaryngologist, University Hospitals, Cleveland, Ohio; Staff Otolaryngologist, Mountain Medical Center and Hillcrest Hospital, Cleveland, Ohio.

STEVEN R. WYTE, M.D.
Formerly Associate Clinical Professor, University of California, San Diego, California; Aurora Community Hospital, Denver, Colorado.

GARY P. YOUNG, M.D.
Emergency Medical Residency, Faculty, Highland General Hospital, Oakland, California; Emergency Department Faculty, University of California, San Francisco, San Francisco, California.

IVAN ZBARASCHUK, M.D., M.A.
Chief of Surgery, Good Samaritan Hospital, Puyallup, Washington.

FOREWORD

The emergency physician has a unique responsibility to utilize and apply his or her skills at all times for all people (young and old, friendly and hostile, and rich and poor). No other health providers are always there. In emergency medicine, our responsibilities have grown and our horizons as emergency physicians have been expanded because of our commitment to people. We have built a system that creates a caring environment from the home to the street and on to the hospital; we have built a system that integrates firemen, policemen, paramedics, nurses, clerks, students, pharmacists, and physicians into the caring service. Roberts and Hedges' text, *Clinical Procedures in Emergency Medicine,* takes another step in the pursuit of excellence in the provision of that care. If we are prepared with the basic skills and the rationale for their use, as defined by Roberts and Hedges, we will all have the potential to provide the type of care that our patients seek.

The last 10 to 15 years in the history of emergency medicine have seen a remarkably rapid evolution in care. We have often been criticized in medicine for our inability to change our ways of thinking, but emergency physicians cannot be criticized in this area. We have broached our responsibilities in a new area, created new relationships, and developed new habits of thought. In the past, we have also been criticized for not looking at our techniques and technology effectively. But the wisdom we have developed over the last several years in emergency medicine has advanced rapidly enough to benefit from the techniques and technologies defined in *Clinical Procedures in Emergency Medicine.* This text is an example of the tremendous progress in thought and technology that marks the success of emergency medicine in America today.

The rapid growth of prehospital care, the ever-increasing access to emergency care, and the evident excitement that emergency medicine has brought have led to the development of a new type of physician in the Emergency Department. This text defines the true extent of academic emergency medicine. From it, one can readily see the enormous task to which each clinician is dedicated.

In emergency medicine, as in many other fields, physicians have felt a need to specialize in a particular aspect of care. Many of these chapters are written by individuals with highly specialized knowledge. Several other groups of authors and editors have attempted to define the diseases and the problems that the emergency physician must handle. Above all, this text defines the technology in emergency medicine. The editors have chosen those techniques whose mastery is a necessity for all of us who consider ourselves emergency physicians.

This text offers an appreciation and understanding of the technology of emergency medicine that should guide emergency physicians in their performance of these tasks. The authors and editors understand the body of facts with regard to these techniques and have effectively organized the material, both inspiring the reader to excellence in these techniques and attempting to define their significance.

This text fills a void in medical practice. We all believe in correct diagnosis, appropriate advice, reassurance, and effective treatment. Treatment in the Emergency Department and for emergency problems has rarely been well defined. This text precisely defines those critical procedures that must be performed in the Emergency Department and the rigorous approach and attention to detail that will allow clinicians to feel at ease with them.

The emergency physician who is trained by knowledge of these techniques can develop the requisite technical skills combined with the warmth and humanity essential to rendering concerned, committed, and compassionate Emergency Department care. Knowledge of these skills and their indications, as well as of their risks and benefits, will allow emergency physicians to achieve a high level of service and research. These skills form a true foundation for excellence in the care of the seriously ill and injured.

Although there are few physicians other than emergency physicians who will use all the technology, there are many others who can and will use this book. The techniques are well defined, well illustrated, and well referenced by clinicians who obviously use them daily. This effort is unique with respect to its depth, and this most comprehensive clinical procedures text available will be useful for all of us in our attempt to improve the delivery of care.

LEWIS GOLDFRANK, M.D.
Director, Emergency Medical Services,
Bellevue Hospital Center and New York University Medical Center,
and Associate Professor of Clinical Medicine,
New York University School of Medicine

PREFACE

Emergency medicine is a procedure-oriented specialty. Indeed, the decision-making processes that go into the performance of clinical procedures represent a major aspect of clinical emergency medicine. Most standard textbooks discuss clinical procedures only briefly and provide little information regarding the thought processes involved in the decision to use a given method. Technique manuals are often more like cookbooks, with sparse text and inadequate illustrations. Alternative techniques may be overlooked in favor of each particular author's preferred method. This textbook offers the reader the clinical rationale for the procedures, alternative methods where appropriate, and potential complications with advice on how to avoid them.

The concept for this book originated over ten years ago, when the editors began to practice the new specialty of emergency medicine and attempted to teach residents the basic procedures of the discipline. It was obvious that emergency physicians often faced different problems when performing standard procedures, and that these problems required different solutions than those used by other specialists. Older techniques had to be modified and new ones had to be created to meet the needs of a rapidly expanding specialty. No longer did the otolaryngology text suffice for an emergency physician's approach to epistaxis, nor did the urology text suffice for evaluation of acute genitourinary trauma in the emergency setting by a nonurologist.

A number of experts from a variety of specialties have contributed to this text. The experience and opinions of the contributing authors have been collated by the editors into a textbook that encompasses the majority of procedures performed in clinical emergency medicine. Depending on one's practice, some procedures may be performed frequently, while others may seldom be encountered by even the busiest emergency physician. Some of the procedures are uncommon and may be previously unknown to the reader; others may be extremely well known. In the latter circumstances, one will find objective data upon which to base clinical decisions regarding the technique and often suggestions for modification of familiar techniques that will aid in the future use of the procedure. Each discussion is based on traditional teaching and firm scientific data seasoned with controversy and personal experience.

This book was written to fill the needs of physicians with varied backgrounds and training and can be adapted to a number of practice situations. Specialists in emergency medicine will undoubtedly consider this text an essential ingredient in their practice. Family physicians, pediatricians, general internists, general surgeons, and other specialists will find the text of value for review of infrequently used procedures. Physicians involved in the education of residents and medical students will find the book to be a valuable source of didactic information. Finally, the resident or physician in training will value this text as a ready authoritative source in those lonely hours when a procedure must be performed but on-site consultation is unavailable.

Although the editors had wished that the text could include all procedures that the emergency physician might be called to perform, such a goal is not practical. The text covers such simple procedures as removal of a fish-hook and such complicated procedures as an emergency thoracotomy, but it cannot be exhaustive. Notable exclusions from this text are the basic and advanced life support cardiac resuscitation protocols popularized by the American Heart Association. These protocols have been excluded because of space limitations and the desire to present less commonly available information. In place of the protocols the reader will find extensive discussions on airway, cardiac, and vascular procedures that expand upon the information likely to be garnered from the American Heart Association courses.

Most emergency procedures are gleaned from a "see one, do one, teach one" format, and techniques are handed down from resident to intern to medical student. Often critical detail or basic concepts are lost or distorted in the transmission. The editors have attempted to present a clear and straightforward discussion of each technique. Some points may seem obvious or superfluous to the experienced physician, but they have been provided for thoroughness.

As the field of emergency medicine expands or contracts, some procedures may be added or subtracted from the repertoire. At present, the book provides all the basic information and perspective needed for clinical procedures in emergency medicine.

JAMES R. ROBERTS
JERRIS R. HEDGES

CONTENTS

Section 7 OBSTETRICS AND GYNECOLOGY

Section 8 GASTROENTEROLOGY

1
RESPIRATORY PROCEDURES

1

Emergency Airway Management Procedures

JOSEPH E. CLINTON, M.D.
ERNEST RUIZ, M.D.

Nonsurgical Airway Management Procedures

OVERVIEW

Airway management is generally recognized as the first priority in the management of any seriously ill or injured patient. The principle is so widely acknowledged that it seems almost unnecessary to mention its importance. Any hesitancy to preach airway management is quickly overcome by experience with therapeutic misadventure in emergency care. Despite widespread lip service, a gap exists between intellectual recognition of the need for a patent airway and the reality of application of airway management maneuvers. Whereas appropriate airway management is evident in all smooth resuscitations, inappropriate management often presages a vicious circle of patient deterioration and misplaced therapeutic intervention.

Unfortunately, recognition of the need for airway management is only part of the problem. Once this need has been recognized, maintaining a patent airway may require one of the most difficult maneuvers of the entire resuscitation. The sheer variety of airway obstructions may challenge the most skilled resuscitator. Blood, loose teeth, vomitus, and swollen or distorted landmarks present formidable barriers to successful management. When obstruction is combined with reflex clenching of the jaws and potential cervical spine injury, conventional airway management tools may be rendered useless. Time constraints imposed by cerebral anoxia force difficult decisions concerning the use of potentially complicating therapeutic factors, such as neck motion, paralyzing agents, or invasive procedures. Tools must be at hand, skills must be well practiced, and decision making must be sharp if optimal emergency airway management is to occur.

Solutions to emergency airway management dilemmas will be presented in this chapter. Nonsurgical and minimally invasive approaches to airway establishment and ventilatory control will be described. Description of techniques will be detailed, and a summary of indications, contraindications, and complications of the various procedures will be included. A detailed description of a procedure is not meant to imply that the procedures may be performed in strictly one fashion. Rather, the descriptions are intended to offer an acceptable answer to those "obvious" procedural questions that are nevertheless often left unanswered.

Decision algorithms will be presented to collate the pieces of the airway management puzzle into a logical schema. Study of the algorithms will serve to clarify and facilitate decision making in times of stress. The reader is urged to spend some time with the algorithms and to apply them to hypothetical cases. Coupling of manipulative skills with sound decisions should lead to effective airway management as a prelude to successful resuscitation.

ESTABLISHMENT OF AIRWAY PATENCY

Maneuvers

The first concern in management of the patient in critical condition is adequacy of the airway. Partial or complete airway obstruction must be quickly overcome. The tongue, dentures, swollen or distorted tissues, blood, and vomitus are common obstructing agents that make intubation difficult. Clearing or bypassing these obstructing agents may be complicated by reflex clenching of the patient's teeth. Moreover, neck motion for suction and intubation may be imprudent because of the danger of cervical spine injury in the acutely injured patient.

Partial or complete airway obstruction resulting from lax musculature and tongue occlusion of the posterior pharynx may be overcome by a variety of maneuvers. The relative benefits of various airway opening maneuvers have been examined. In a study of 120 anesthetized patients, Guildner compared the ease of performance of the neck lift–head tilt, jaw thrust, and chin-lift methods. His assessment of the maneuvers led to his conclusion that the chin-lift method was the easiest to perform and produced the greatest airway patency of the three tested.[1] Besides offering greater patency, the chin-lift method has an additional advantage in that neck extension is unnecessary for its success (Fig. 1–1, Tables 1–1 and 1–2). Potential cervical spine injury is a contraindication to the neck lift–head tilt procedure. Some type of jaw thrust or chin-lift maneuver should be performed on every

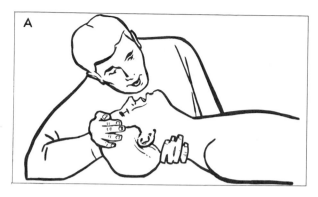
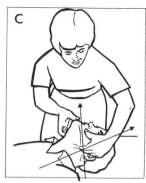
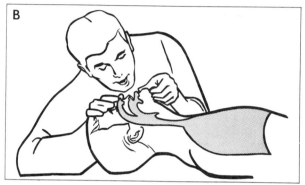

Figure 1–1. Chin-lift maneuver. A, Neck lift; B, Chin lift, and C, Jaw thrust. (From Guildner, C. W.: Resuscitation—opening the airway: A comparative study of techniques for opening an airway obstructed by the tongue. JACEP 5:588, 1976. Used by permission.)

unconscious patient to ensure airway patency. When uncertain about cervical spine status, one must maintain the neck in the neutral position. In the difficult situation in which the patient is found with a flexed or extended neck, the neck is first restored to the neutral position with longitudinal traction. The chin-lift maneuver or the jaw thrust is then performed. A combination of these maneuvers will usually overcome the positional causes of airway obstruction that are often encountered.

The Chin-Lift Maneuver. The tips of the fingers are placed, volar surface superiorly, beneath the patient's chin. The patient's jaw is gently lifted forward. The patient's mouth is opened by drawing down on the lower lip with the thumb of the same hand. Mouth-to-mouth or another means of positive-pressure ventilation is applied if the patient is not spontaneously ventilating.

The Jaw Thrust Maneuver. The jaw thrust maneuver is the second choice of the three, since neck extension is not necessary. One achieves forward traction on the mandible by using two hands to grasp the mandibular rami and to pull them forward. The neck lift–head tilt maneuver as it is described in cardiac life support courses should not be used when cervical spine injury is even a remote possibility, since the extension of the spine produced during the maneuver endangers the spinal cord.[2]

Table 1–1. SUBJECTIVE EVALUATION OF EFFECTIVENESS OF TECHNIQUES ON PATIENTS NOT MAKING ANY RESPIRATORY EFFORT (N = 120)*

Effectiveness	Neck Lift		Chin Lift		Jaw Thrust	
	No.	*%*	*No.*	*%*	*No.*	*%*
Total obstruction Unable to ventilate	7	5.8	–	–	1	0.8
Partial obstruction Inadequate ventilation	8	6.7	2	1.7	2	1.7
Partial obstruction Adequate ventilation but with difficulty	58	48.3	9	7.5	23	19
Good airway Easy ventilation	47	39.2	109	90.8	94	78

*From Guildner, C. W.: Resuscitation—opening the airway: A comparative study of techniques for opening an airway obstructed by the tongue. JACEP 5:588, 1976. Used by permission.

Table 1–2. EFFECTIVENESS OF TECHNIQUES FOR OPENING AIRWAY IN PATIENTS WITH COMPLETE RESPIRATORY OBSTRUCTION BUT MAKING SPONTANEOUS RESPIRATORY EFFORT (N = 30)*

Effectiveness (Tidal Volume)	Neck Lift		Chin Lift		Jaw Thrust	
	No.	*%*	*No.*	*%*	*No.*	*%*
0–50 ml	13	43.3	–	–	1	3.4
50–250 ml	9	30	2	6.7	3	10
250–400 ml	6	20	7	23.3	7	23.3
Over 400 ml	2	6.7	21	70	19	63.3

*From Guildner, C. W.: Resuscitation—opening the airway: A comparative study of techniques for opening an airway obstructed by the tongue. JACEP 5:588, 1976. Used by permission.

Airway Clearing Maneuvers. Clearing the airway of foreign material requires more than a simple jaw thrust. The occasional patient who presents with complete airway obstruction secondary to food aspiration may be treated with the back blows and abdominal thrusts described in the American Heart Association's Basic Cardiac Life Support Course.[3] A more common presentation in the emergency department is that of the patient with a decreased level of consciousness whose airway is partially or completely obstructed as a result of another condition.

Partial or complete airway obstruction is frequently the result of upper airway hemorrhage, accumulation of the patient's own secretions, vomitus, or fractured dentition. Selection of airway clearing maneuvers must take these circumstances into account. Rotation of the head to perform a finger sweep is clearly contraindicated if cervical spine injury is a possibility. Application of the abdominal thrust maneuver should be limited to the supine method described for unconscious victims in cases of trauma. Even then, chest compression may be preferable.[4] Because of the limited applicability of abdominal thrust maneuvers to the trauma patient, we will not discuss them further here. The reader is referred to the American Heart Association's Standards for Cardiopulmonary Resuscitation for a more detailed description.[3] We will focus on patient positioning and suctioning as means of maintaining and clearing the airway of a patient in critical condition.

Positioning of the patient who has sustained multiple trauma injuries can be a dilemma. Spinal injury and airway access priorities dictate that the patient should be kept in the supine position while immobilized on a backboard. Turning the patient on the side will allow upper airway hemorrhage, secretions, and vomitus to drain externally instead of collecting in the patient's mouth to the point of airway obstruction and aspiration.

Guidelines for patient positioning must take into account the status of the patient's spine and the beneficial effects of using gravity to assist in airway maintenance by allowing secretions to drain rather than accumulate in the patient's airway. A judicious approach to the problem in a patient with spontaneous respiration is the following:

1. Initial airway maintenance accomplished by the chin-lift maneuver and application of cervical traction.

2. Immobilization of the patient on a spinal backboard.

3. While the neck is controlled, transportation of the injured patient on the patient's side to facilitate airway drainage.

Suction

Airway opening and clearing maneuvers and patient positioning are often inadequate to achieve the degree of airway patency desired. Ongoing hemorrhage, vomitus, and particulate debris often require suction in order for the respiratory passage to be cleared and maintained. Three basic types of suctioning devices are available, each suited to different types of airway obstruction problems. Figure 1–2 illustrates the three types of suction devices that are of benefit in management of the traumatized patient's airway.

Dental tip suction is most useful for clearing particulate debris from the upper airway. Vomitus is most readily cleared with this tip, since the device is the least likely to become obstructed itself by the particulate matter. The *tonsil* tip suction device is most effectively used to clear upper airway hemorrhage and secretions. Its design is intended to prevent the obstruction of its tip by tissue and clot. The rounded tip is also less traumatic to soft tissues.

Unfortunately, the catheter tip suction device is the most readily available in many hospitals. Often it is the only type of suction available for use in the injured patient presenting to the emergency department. Catheter tip suction is virtually useless during the critical resuscitation of the patient. The catheter tip device is useful only after the patient has been intubated, when it is needed to suction the trachea and the bronchi through the tracheal tube. The dental tip device should be used during the resuscitation period and should be kept ready at the bedside. The dental tip allows rapid clearing of both particulate matter and hemorrhage, thereby expediting airway control.

Optimal suction equipment for stabilization of the multiply injured patient should include all three types of suction tips. The dental suction tip

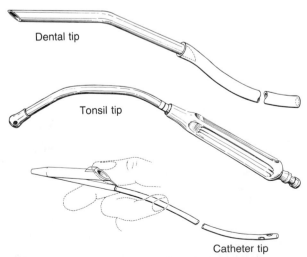

Figure 1–2. Three types of suction tips: dental, tonsil, and catheter tips. (From Clinton, J. E., and Ruiz, E.: Trauma Life Support Manual, 1982.)

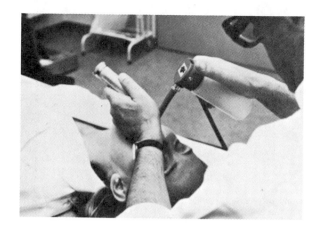

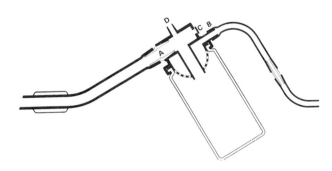

Figure 1–3. Suction booster of Ruben. Ruben's suction booster is designed to allow high-capacity suctioning through the endotracheal tube during intubation. Schematic diagram. *A*, Tracheal tube connection; *B*, Connection to suction; *C*, Introducer opening in the closed position; and *D*, Opening that is kept closed when suction is needed through the tracheal tube. (From Ruben, H., Hansen, E., and Macnaughton, F. I.: High capacity suction technique. Anesthesia 34:349, 1979. Used by permission.)

should be attached to the suction source during the interval between cases, since it is the instrument that most likely will be used at short notice. Both the tonsil tip and the catheter tip should be stored next to the suction source to be readily attached when needed. Latex suction tubing will allow easy interchangeability of the three suction tips. Interposition of a suction trap at the base of the dental tip suction device will prevent clogging of the latex tubing with particulate debris. A trap has been described that fits directly onto a tracheal tube. Use of this device will allow effective suctioning during the act of intubation (Fig. 1–3).[5]

Although no specific contraindications of airway suctioning exist, complications of incorrectly performed suctioning may be significant. Nasal suction is often not required to improve oxygenation (except in infants), since most adult airway obstruction occurs in the mouth and the oropharynx. Induction of epistaxis by vigorous nasal suction may further complicate an already difficult situation. Prolonged suctioning may lead to significant hypoxia. Suctioning should never exceed 15–second intervals without oxygenation.[6] Inadvertent placement of tubes introduced nasally into the brain through basilar skull fractures has been reported (Fig. 1–4).[7, 8] Extreme care should be exercised when a basilar skull or facial fracture is present, since communication between the nasal and intracranial cavities may exist. Generally it is best to perform suctioning *under direct vision* or with the aid of the laryngoscope.[7] Forcing a suction tip blindly into the posterior pharynx may injure tissue or may convert a partial obstructing mass into a complete obstruction.

Figure 1–4. Intracranial intubation. Lateral skull x ray showing nasogastric tube placed into brain through skull fracture. (From Clinton, J. E., and Ruiz, E.: Trauma Life Support Manual, 1982.)

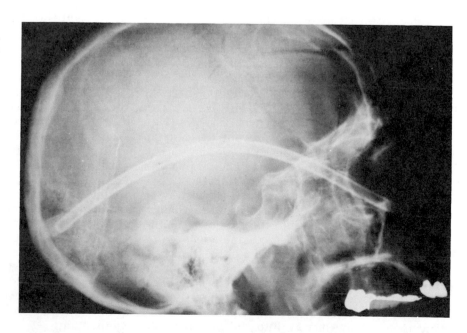

Complications may be avoided by anticipation of problems and appropriate care during performance of the suctioning maneuvers. Epistaxis may be avoided by simple limitation of force during suctioning. Vasoconstrictor drops, such as 1 per cent phenylephrine, will constrict the nasal mucosa and will limit the injury potential in cases in which the need for repeated nasopharyngeal suctioning is anticipated. Holding one's own breath during application of the suctioning will increase awareness of the time and will limit the likelihood of induction of hypoxia. Hyperventilation before and after suctioning has been shown to limit hypoxia. Naigow found that suction induced hypoxia in dogs consistently. Hypoxia was best avoided by hyperventilating the animals before, during, and after suctioning.[6]

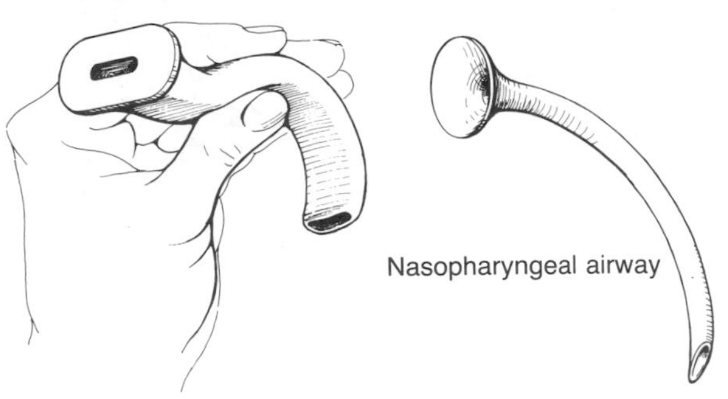

Artificial Airways

Once the airway has been established through these maneuvers and suctioning, the patient may require further temporary support in order for airway patency to be maintained. The semiconscious patient who is breathing at an adequate rate and tidal volume when the chin-lift maneuver is being performed may develop hypoxia caused by recurrent obstruction if the maneuver is discontinued. The use of an artificial airway and oxygen supplementation may be all the support that is necessary. More efficient use of rescuer skills may be achieved and fatigue from the continuous application of the chin-lift or jaw thrust maneuver may be avoided through use of artificial airways.

Positive-pressure ventilation with a bag-valve mask or oxygen-powered breathing device may be necessary to assist the patient's inadequate ventilatory effort or to provide total ventilation in cases of apnea. Artificial airways facilitate this procedure by maintenance of airway patency. A specialized artificial airway, the esophageal obturator airway, is designed for use in the unconscious patient requiring positive-pressure ventilation.

Oropharyngeal and Nasopharyngeal Airways. The simplest forms of artificial airways are the oropharyngeal and nasopharyngeal airways (Fig. 1–5). Both are intended to prevent the tongue from falling back against the posterior pharyngeal wall and obstructing the airway. The oropharyngeal airway may be inserted by either of two procedures. In the first procedure, the airway is inserted in an inverted position along the patient's hard palate. When well into the patient's mouth, the airway is rotated 180 degrees and advanced to its final placement position along the patient's tongue, with the distal end of the airway lying in the hypopharynx. The second procedure involves the performance of a jaw thrust maneuver either manually or with a tongue blade and simple advancement of the airway into the mouth to its

Figure 1–5. Simple artificial airways: oropharyngeal and nasopharyngeal. (From Clinton, J. E., and Ruiz, E.: Trauma Life Support Manual, unpublished, 1982.)

final position. No rotation is performed when the airway is placed in this manner.

The nasopharyngeal airway is placed by gentle advancement of the airway into a nostril. The tip is directed along the floor of the nose toward the nasopharynx. When in final position, the flared external end of the airway should rest at the nasal orifice. Either of these two airways will provide airway patency similar to that achieved by a correctly performed chin-lift maneuver.

Complications of these airways are few but should be considered. The oropharyngeal device may obstruct the patient's own airway if incorrectly placed by pushing the tongue against the posterior pharyngeal wall, contrary to its purpose. Care in placement will prevent this occurrence. Stimulation of the gag reflex may produce retching and emesis in the patient with intact reflexes. A semiconscious patient may not tolerate the oropharyngeal airway. If gagging is a persistent problem, the airway should be removed and tracheal intubation should be considered. If the patient is comatose without a gag reflex, the oropharyngeal airway *should not be used*. Tracheal intubation is the preferred method of airway control in such patients. Occasionally, the oropharyngeal airway is used with tracheal intubation. The oropharyngeal airway will keep the mouth partially open if an orogastric tube is placed for gastric lavage or suction, and it will prevent clenching of the teeth, which may obstruct an orotracheal tube.

One advantage of the nasopharyngeal airway over the oropharyngeal airway is that it is less likely to induce gagging. The same considerations that apply to nasal suctioning apply to placement of the nasopharyngeal airway, i.e., one must exercise care not to induce epistaxis, and extreme caution is indicated in application to patients with a basilar skull fracture or facial injury. All patients with oral or nasopharyngeal airways should be constantly observed, since the devices are temporary measures and do not substitute for tracheal intubation.

Esophageal Obturator Airway. The esophageal obturator airway (EOA), although technically an artificial airway, represents a transitional intervention between airway establishment and true airway control. Tracheal intubation and tracheostomy are true means of airway control. The optimal role of the EOA has yet to be determined. Although it has gained popularity as a prehospital airway device, the EOA has not been widely used in the emergency department. The EOA maintains airway patency similarly to the oral and nasal airways, but it also protects the airway by occluding the esophagus and preventing gastric distention and regurgitation. The face mask permits use of the esophageal airway as a positive-pressure ventilating device. Air insufflated through the airway exits in the hypopharynx and travels down the trachea under pressure (Fig. 1–6). The airway is useful in the apneic patient because it retains much of the simplicity of the artificial airway while adding an important feature of more complicated airways, i.e., some protection against regurgitation and facilitation of ventilation.[9-12]

A significant advantage of the esophageal airway is the speed with which airway control may be achieved. It has been demonstrated that trained individuals may successfully place an esophageal airway in an average of 5 seconds, whereas 20 seconds are required for tracheal intubations by the same individuals.[10] Moreover, neck motion is not necessary with the esophageal airway, as it is with tracheal intubation. For these reasons, the EOA may be an effective adjunct in the management of an unconscious injured patient who requires respiratory assistance. The most difficult aspect of this form of ventilation is securing a tight fit with the mask. Dentures should be left in place to give support to the lips.

There are, however, contraindications to use of the EOA. The EOA cannot be used in the awake patient because of attendant discomfort. Size specifications preclude its use in the pediatric patient. Sixteen years of age is usually quoted as the lower limit of application. The actual limiting factors are esophagus and facial sizes. An adult-sized 14-year-old would certainly tolerate EOA use if needed. On the other hand, a small-sized adult may not receive an appropriate fit. Esophageal injury or conditions predisposing to perforation are considered contraindications. A patient who has ingested a caustic agent or one with a known esophageal stricture should not undergo esophageal intubation. As a precaution against pressure-related complications, it is recommended that the EOA be removed and replaced with tracheal intubation as soon as is feasible. It should be stressed that the EOA is a *temporary* form of airway control. It has been used most frequently in prehospital care.

Placement of the EOA is accomplished with the head in the neutral position. Neck motion is unnecessary. The jaw is grasped by the rescuer and is pulled forward. At this point the assembled airway, with the mask attached, is introduced. The obturator tip is directed into the patient's posterior pharynx with gentle steady pressure. The obturator is advanced down the esophagus until the mask rests flush against the face of the patient. Figure 1–6 illustrates the correct position at placement. The cuff should lie in the esophagus just distal to the carina of the trachea. The balloon is not inflated until proper position is confirmed. The patient is ventilated with a tight mask seal on the face, and the lungs are auscultated. The tight mask seal is mandatory for effective ventilation. Breath sounds should be audible bilaterally. Failure of auscultation or unilateral breath sounds

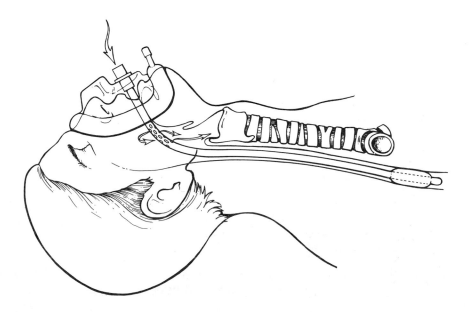

Figure 1–6. Esophageal obturator airway. Correct placement of the esophageal airway with the cuff inflated in the esophagus caudad to the bifurcation of the trachea. (From Clinton, J. E., and Ruiz, E.: Trauma Life Support Manual, unpublished, 1982.)

should lead the rescuer to reassess the airway placement. Pneumothorax or hemothorax may explain unilateral sounds, as may inadvertent main stem bronchus intubation. Tracheal intubation will result in the absence of breath sounds. The possibility of tracheal or bronchial intubation mandates removal and replacement of the airway.[10] Once satisfactorily placed, the esophageal balloon is inflated with 20 ml of air.

A 5 per cent incidence of inadvertent tracheal intubation has been reported by Don Michael in a series of 29,000 placements.[10] Tracheal intubation is obviously a disastrous complication if not quickly rectified, since the patient's airway is occluded in such a situation. Disciplined examination for bilateral breath sounds is critical when this device is used for airway management. Esophageal rupture has been reported in case histories.[13, 14] Since Scholl first reported ruptures at our institution in 1977, we have decreased the balloon inflation volume from 35 to 20 ml. No further ruptures have occurred, and leakage around the 20-ml cuff has not been noted. We therefore recommend that balloon inflation be limited to 20 ml. Factors other than balloon inflation volume that may contribute to rupture include careless removal without balloon deflation and forceful attempts at placement when obstruction is met.

Tracheal intubation must be performed *before* removal of the EOA, since vomiting often occurs following balloon deflation and EOA removal. If the EOA cuff has been overinflated, it may partially occlude the trachea and may make intubation difficult. In such cases, the balloon is partially deflated to facilitate tracheal intubation.

VENTILATORY CONTROL—TRACHEAL INTUBATION

Overview

The critically ill patient must be well oxygenated with a protected airway. In the absence of airway obstruction and the presence of spontaneous adequate respiratory effort, oxygen supplementation and artificial airway placement may suffice. When these qualifications are lacking, as in the patient with a head injury who is hypoventilating or the patient with a flail chest, the airway must be protected and ventilation must be assisted. Breathing is a dynamic function that must be constantly monitored and reassessed. In general, the significantly injured patient with a tidal volume of less than 500 ml and the patient with a respiratory rate of less than 10 or more than 24 breaths per minute are candidates for airway control and assisted ventilation.

All patients who are unconscious from head trauma should be tracheally intubated and hyper-

ventilated. Borderline cases should receive airway control if blood gases indicate hypoxia or acidosis. The presence of a decreased level of consciousness secondary to head injury is considered an indication for hyperventilation to an arterial PCO_2 of 25 mm Hg. Hypovolemic shock that does not rapidly respond to volume replacement oxygen supplementation and will soon manifest clear indications for airway control, such as decreasing level of consciousness, acidosis, hypoxia, or hypoventilation. All unconscious patients without a gag reflex must be intubated to protect against aspiration and to provide ventilation if the condition deteriorates.

Definitive control of the airway by nonsurgical means is, for practical purposes, synonymous with tracheal intubation. Tracheal intubation may be accomplished from a variety of approaches, each with its own advantages and disadvantages. The existence of several differing approaches attests to the difficulty of nonsurgical airway control. Nowhere is the problem more complicated or the variety of approaches more needed than in the multiply injured patient. In this chapter we will describe the various means of passing a tracheal tube either through the mouth or through the nose. The techniques to be described are listed in Table 1–3.

General Cautions

The complication rate of emergency department tracheal intubation is relatively high. In general, the complications of emergency intubation are underestimated and under-recognized by most physicians. Taryle and associates found a total of 38 complications in 24 of 48 consecutive emergency intubations.[63] Common complications included prolonged intubation times, aspiration of gastric contents, and main stem bronchus intubations. Transient vocal cord dysfunction, minor lacerations of lips and mucosa, tooth trauma, and postintubation sore throat are very common following emergency intubation.[63] The specific complications of each intubation procedure will be discussed under each technique. Unless one follows the

Table 1–3. NONSURGICAL AIRWAY MANAGEMENT TECHNIQUES

Direct laryngoscopy
Orotracheal intubation
  With EOA in place
  With jaw spreaders
Pharmacologic adjuncts
  Topical lidocaine
  Succinylcholine
  Pancuronium bromide
Nasotracheal intubation
  Blind
  With laryngoscope and Magill forceps
Retrograde tracheal intubation

postintubation course of emergency patients, one may gain a false sense of security about one's intubation skill and fail to appreciate the incidence of complications.

Special Considerations

Cervical Spine Injury. One must always be cognizant of the potential for cervical spine injury in any patient who has sustained a significant injury. Falls from heights and motor vehicle accidents are common causes of spinal instability. Five to 10 per cent of patients with serious head trauma have been cited as having associated cervical spine injury.[15] Any patient sustaining a fall should be considered as potentially having spinal injury, even if the initial injury was an isolated penetrating injury.

Tracheal intubation involving the use of the laryngoscope is significantly limited by the overriding consideration of potential cervical spine injury in multiply injured patients. Either the patient's ventilation must be maintained by means that do not require neck extension until adequate radiographs of the cervical spine are obtained or some other means of tracheal intubation that does not require neck motion must be achieved.

Methods of positive-pressure ventilation that may be accomplished without neck motion are listed in Table 1–4. Mouth-to-mouth and bag-mask ventilation may be accomplished with minimal neck motion, but these frequently require some degree of neck extension to open the airway. Therefore, they are the least adequate of the methods listed in Table 1–4. The last three methods provide more than temporary control of the airway. Additionally, they protect the airway against aspiration of foreign material. The techniques and limitations will be discussed in detail in the sections to follow.

Teeth Clenching. Hypertonus induced by neurologic dysfunction is a common complicating factor of airway management, especially in the multiply injured patient. Teeth clenching may at times be a lethal complication when it prevents clearing of foreign bodies in the airway. No more difficult airway complications exist than occlusion of the nasal and oral passages by vomitus while the patient's teeth are tightly clenched. Although the hypertonus will gradually give way as the brain

stem becomes progressively hypoxic, respiratory efforts during the interim may lead to severe aspiration. The cerebral hypoxic insult sustained in the process may be irreversible. Similar consequences may result from accumulation of airway hemorrhage or secretions occurring in combination with clenched teeth in various disease states.

Of course, teeth clenching and spine injury may occur together. Fortunately, the nasotracheal routes of intubation may bypass this problem as well as avert further spine injury. At least a small degree of spontaneous air movement should be present for the *blind* nasotracheal approach to be successful. Although a serendipitous success may occur in the apneic patient, it is recommended that time not be wasted on this approach when complete apnea is present. The airway must be nearly free of foreign debris or blood for success of the *bronchoscopic* nasotracheal approach.

A method of opening the mouth is necessary to clear the airway in cases of complete airway obstruction and clenched teeth. Methods of overcoming clenching may be mechanical or pharmacologic. Devices called "jaw spreaders" are available for opening the mouth in spite of resistance, although drug therapy is almost always the preferred method of overcoming clenching. Both neuromuscular depolarizing and nondepolarizing agents may be administered intravenously to the injured patient to induce paralysis that will allow orotracheal intubation. Techniques, precautions, and complications of these techniques will be described.

Time Constraints. Prolonged efforts to intubate may result not only in hypoxia but also in cardiac decompensation. Pharyngeal stimulation can produce profound bradycardia or asystole, and, whenever feasible, an assistant should view the cardiac monitor during intubation of a patient who has not suffered cardiac arrest. Atropine should be available to reverse vagal-induced bradycardia. Prolonged pharyngeal stimulation may also result in laryngospasm, bronchospasm, and apnea.

Selection of the airway management approach must always reflect a consideration of the degree of hypoxic insult imposed prior to and during the maneuver. Thirty seconds is the maximum interval allowable for routine intubation of the apneic patient. Failure to achieve such rapid control demands an interval of positive-pressure ventilation prior to repeated attempts.[16] When ventilation is not achievable, irreversible brain damage may result within minutes.[3] The maximum interval allowable for conservative airway management maneuvers before one should escalate attempts to the level of surgical intervention is approximately 3 minutes. The algorithm at the end of this chapter (see Fig. 1–14) reflects the considerations discussed and collates the many maneuvers into a logical schema for nonsurgical management of the

Table 1–4. AIRWAY MANAGEMENT METHODS NOT REQUIRING SIGNIFICANT NECK MOTION

Mouth-to-mouth ventilation
Bag-valve mask ventilation
Esophageal obturator ventilation
Blind nasotracheal intubation
Bronchoscopic nasotracheal intubation
Retrograde tracheal intubation

airway. The time constraint algorithm in the upper left corner of the figure should be noted.

Priorities in Cardiac Arrest Airway Management. Mouth-to-mouth and bag-mask ventilation may suffice for prehospital care with very short transport times or for the initial few minutes of ventilation in cardiac arrest. Prolonged adequate ventilation with a bag and a mask during cardiopulmonary resuscitation (CPR) in the ambulance is almost impossible. The two methods are adequate and effective for ventilation in the anesthetized or paralyzed patient with an empty stomach in the absence of chest compression, but they are *inadequate* for prolonged ventilation in the cardiac arrest situation. Proper bag-mask ventilation is probably harder to master than is tracheal intubation, and prolonged attempts at bag-mask ventilation during CPR usually only distend the stomach and give the uninitiated a false sense of security. *Patients in cardiac arrest should be tracheally intubated.* The majority of arrests will not be associated with cervical spine injury. Although a high index of suspicion should be maintained, the fear of a cervical spine injury should not preclude tracheal intubation in cardiac arrest in patients who have not sustained trauma or in trauma victims with injuries unlikely to produce cervical spine injuries.

Direct Laryngoscopy

A necessary prerequisite to orotracheal intubation is facility with the use of the direct laryngoscope. Interchangeable blades of various sizes are available to conform to patient size (various adult and pediatric sizes exist). There are two basic blade designs: curved and straight. Slight variation in the technique of laryngoscopy is necessary, depending on whether a curved or a straight blade is used. The choice of blade is often a matter of preference. The straight blade may be more advantageous in children or in patients with a very anterior larynx. The straight blade is more likely to damage teeth in the adult. The wider blades are helpful in keeping the tongue retracted from the field of vision.

Any clinical situation in which visualization of the vocal cords is necessary and neck motion is permissible is an indication for use of the laryngoscope. Direct laryngoscopy is useful in the trauma patient requiring suctioning of the hypopharynx. The most expeditious method of tracheal intubation is the orotracheal route using the laryngoscope. Cervical spine injury or its potential is a contraindication to direct laryngoscopy.

Technique of Direct Laryngoscopy. Figure 1–7 illustrates the use of the curved and the straight laryngoscope blades. Technique is as follows:

1. The laryngoscopist is stationed at the supine patient's head.

2. The patient's head is placed in the "sniffing" position, with the head extended on the neck and the neck slightly flexed in relation to the trunk. Dentures are removed.

3. The laryngoscope is grasped in the rescuer's *left* hand with the blade directed toward the patient from the hypothenar aspect of the rescuer's hand.

4. The patient's lower lip is drawn down by the rescuer's right thumb, and the tip of the laryngoscope is introduced into the *right* side of the patient's mouth.

5. The blade is slid axially along the right side of the patient's tongue, gradually displacing the tongue toward the patient's left as the blade is moved to the center of the patient's mouth. *Failure to move the tongue to the left is a common error in technique that prevents visualization of the cords.*

6. The rescuer exerts force anteriorly along the line of the laryngoscope handle, being careful not to pry the blade on the patient's upper teeth.

7. If needed, suctioning is performed at this point.

8. The epiglottis is visualized. When using a straight blade, one lifts the epiglottis with the tip of the blade. When using a curved blade, one places the tip of the blade anterior to the epiglottis into the vallecula.

9. Continued anterior elevation of the base of the tongue and the epiglottis will expose the vocal cords. Proper neck positioning and pressure on the larynx by an assistant will facilitate visualization and intubation of an anterior larynx.

In a study of 366 patients, McGovern found broken teeth to be the most common complication of laryngoscopy.[17] Laceration of the mucosa of the lips, especially the lower lip, may be easily produced if adequate care is not taken. Failure to visualize the larynx may lead to complications that will be discussed in the section on tracheal intubation.

Tracheal Tubes

Sizing of endotracheal tubes can be a source of confusion because of variations in parameters used to categorize tubes. Three mechanisms of sizing have been used: Magill sizes, French sizes, and internal diameter. Internal diameter is now the most commonly used system. Magill sizes are rarely used but consist of a gradation of diameters ranging from 0 for infants to 10 for adults. French size is roughly equivalent to the external circumference of the tube. Since circumference is given by π times diameter and π equals 3.14, one can calculate the external diameter in millimeters of a

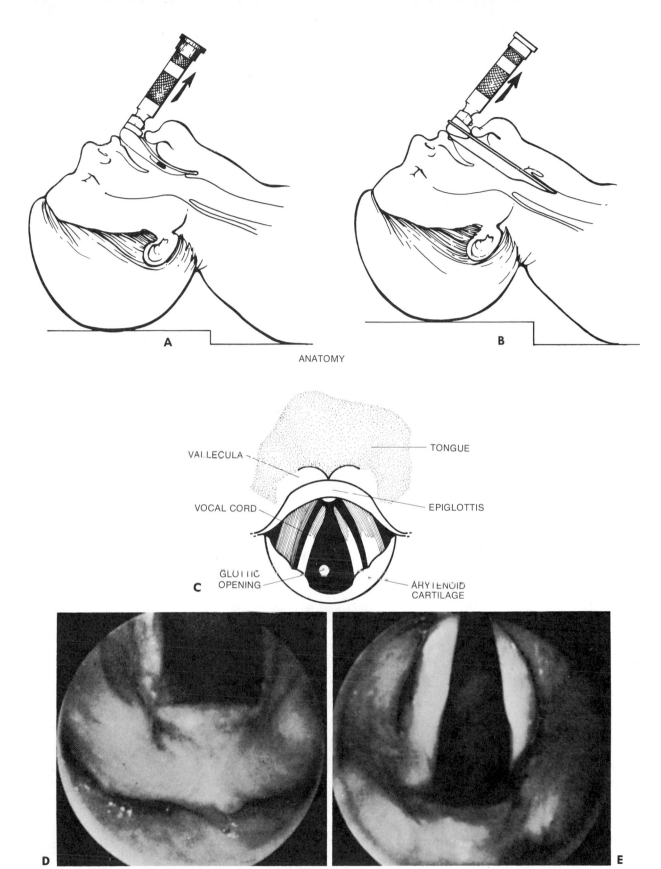

ANATOMY

VALLECULA

TONGUE

VOCAL CORD

EPIGLOTTIS

GLOTTIC OPENING

ARYTENOID CARTILAGE

Figure 1–7. Direct laryngoscopy. *A,* Use of curved laryngoscope blade. *B,* Use of straight laryngoscope blade. (From Clinton, J. E., and Ruiz, E.: Trauma Life Support Manual, 1982.) *C,* Diagram of anatomy of larynx entrance exposed by direct laryngoscopy. (From AHA Advanced Life Support Slide Series, 1976.) *D,* Direct laryngoscopic view during tracheal intubation; exposure of arytenoids. *E,* Direct laryngoscopic view during tracheal intubation; exposure of glottis. The anterior commissure is not fully seen. The posterior commissure is below. (From Holinger, P. H., Anison, G. C., and Johnston, K. C.: Bronchoscopic and esophagoscopic cinematography. J. Thorac. Surg. 17:178, 1948.)

Table 1–5. TRACHEAL TUBE SIZES FOR AVERAGE PATIENTS*†

Age	French Size	Internal Diameter (mm)	Equivalent Tracheotomy Tube Size
Premature			00
newborn	12	2.5	00–0
6 months	16	3.5	0–1
1 year	20	4.5	1–2
2 years	22	5.0	2
4 years	24	5.5	3
6 years	26	6.0	4
8 years	28	6.5	4
10 years	30	7.0	4
12 years	32	7.5	5
14 years	34	8.0	5
Adult			
Female	34–36	7.5–8.5	5
Male	36–40	8.0–9.0	6
Special cases			8–10

*Modified from Applebaum, E. L., and Bruce, D. L.: Tracheal Intubation. Philadelphia, W. B. Saunders Co., 1976.
†A slightly smaller size may be required for nasotracheal intubation.

French tube by dividing the French size by 3. Internal diameter sizing is the most descriptive of parameters and is the preferred method of nomenclature. The diameter in millimeters of the internal lumen is reported in this method of sizing. Internal diameter is 2 to 4 mm less than external diameter, depending on the thickness of the walls of the tube.[18] Internal diameter sizes that are commonly used are listed in Table 1–5.

Most adult females can be intubated with a 7.5- to 8.0-mm tube. Adult males can usually accept a 8.0- to 8.5-mm tube. One can estimate the size for a tube in a child by comparing the diameter of the tube with the diameter of the child's little finger. For nasal intubation a slightly smaller (by 0.5 to 1.0 mm) tube is usually chosen.

All adult tubes will accept a standard adaptor to which the ventilator tubing will fit. Pediatric tubes require a special adaptor with a distal end small enough to accommodate the small tube size. Most tubes with an internal diameter of less than 7 mm do not have inflatable cuffs. They are used in children less than 8 years old. During emergencies, there is a tendency to choose a smaller than adequate tube because it is thought that a smaller tube will pass more easily. In children this is a problem, since a tight seal between the tube and the soft trachea is required to prevent aspiration. Although one can compensate for a small tube by inflating the cuff in an adult, a properly sized tube should be chosen for the first intubation in children.

Orotracheal Intubation

Indications for orotracheal intubation are the same as those that have been described for airway control in general. The only contraindication is potential cervical spine injury.

The most difficult steps in orotracheal intubation technique have been described previously; they are clearing of the airway and visualization of the vocal cords by laryngoscopy. Once the vocal cords have been visualized with the laryngoscope, all that remains is to pass an endotracheal tube of the appropriate size between the vocal cords and (under direct vision) into the trachea. With the laryngoscope in place and the vocal cords visualized, orotracheal intubation is achieved as follows:

Orotracheal Intubation Technique

1. For an adult, the operator selects a tube that is 7.5, 8.0, or 8.5 mm in internal diameter, depending on patient size. (The average adult male takes the largest tube and the average female takes the smallest tube.) For smaller and larger individuals, 7.0- and 9.0-mm tubes are available. Pediatric tube size is chosen as noted in the previous section.

2. The tube is held in the rescuer's right hand while the vocal cords are visualized. The concavity of the tube should be oriented toward the tongue during placement. A wire stylet may be placed in the lumen of the tube to assist in placement by giving the tube some increased stiffness. The stylet should not extend past the tip of the tube.

3. The tube is advanced toward the patient's larynx from an angle rather than along the blade of the laryngoscope. In this way the operator's view of the larynx is not obstructed by the hand or the tube until the last possible moment before the tube enters the larynx.

4. The tube is advanced into the larynx until the proximal aspect of the cuff is observed to pass between the vocal cords out of view. The tube is advanced 2 to 3 cm beyond this point. The tube should be passed during inspiration, when the vocal cords are open.

5. The cuff is inflated with 5 to 10 ml of air to the point of minimal air leak on positive pressure inspiration. In emergency intubation, 10 ml of air is placed in the cuff, and optimal inflation is adjusted after patient stabilization.

6. Both lungs are auscultated under positive-pressure ventilation. Care is taken to auscultate laterally in the lung periphery, since midline auscultation may lead to an erroneus impression of tracheal placement when the tube is actually in the esophagus. Asymmetric breath sounds indicate probable main stem bronchus intubation. The cuff should be deflated and the tube withdrawn until equal breath sounds are present. Persistent asymmetry indicates a probable unilateral pulmonary pathologic condition, e.g., pneumo- or hemothorax. Increased abdominal size or gurgling sounds indicate esophageal misplacement. The patient cannot vocalize when the tube is in the

trachea; the presence of groaning or other sounds should also alert the physician to esophageal misplacement.

7. When satisfied that the tube is correctly placed and the cuff is inflated, the operator secures the tube with umbilical (nonadhesive cloth) tape by tying the tape securely around the tube and around the patient's head.

It should be noted that the vocal cords may close and prevent passage of the tube when they are stimulated. Much of this spasm can be eliminated with the use of local topical anesthetics, but occasionally prolonged spasm presents a problem. One best overcomes spasm by using gentle sustained pressure with the tip of the tracheal tube. At no time should the tube be forced, since permanent damage to the vocal cords may occur. Intense spasm in the face of life-threatening need for intubation may be overcome with diazepam (Valium) or succinylcholine. If vocal cord spasm prevents passage in a child, a chest thrust maneuver may momentarily open the passage.

Tracheal stricture as a result of intubation has been a serious complication of long-term intubation in the past. High-volume, low-pressure cuffs have replaced low-volume, high pressure cuffs on tracheal tubes in recent years. The principle behind this change has been that the high-volume cuffs distribute a lower pressure over a wider area of the trachea. Most feel that this innovation has lessened the degree of tracheal injury associated with long-term intubation.[19-23] Red rubber tubes with high-pressure cuffs are obsolete and should not be used. If these devices are inserted, they should be replaced as soon as possible.

Orotracheal Intubation with EOA in Place. The unconscious patient who requires respiratory assistance may benefit from the temporary use of the esophageal obturator airway, as described earlier. Although this may be an effective manner of airway control, it is a temporary measure. The EOA often does allow rapid effective airway control until cervical spine injury can be ruled out and orotracheal intubation can be accomplished.

Replacement of the EOA with an orotracheal tube requires appropriate care. Removal of the esophageal cuff before placement of the endotracheal tube is fraught with danger. Spontaneous gastric regurgitation often occurs on removal of the EOA. The rescuer must therefore learn to perform endotracheal intubation around the esophageal obturator to protect the patient from aspiration.

The technique for intubation around an EOA should be modified as follows:

1. The patient is hyperventilated with the EOA.
2. The face mask portion of the EOA is removed.
3. The EOA tube is displaced to the left side of the patient's mouth.

4. Laryngoscopy and orotracheal intubation are performed.
5. The esophageal obturator balloon is *completely deflated.*
6. The EOA is gently slid out of the patient's esophagus. If resistance is met, the operator rechecks to be sure the esophageal cuff has been completely deflated.

Complications of the orotracheal intubation procedure include those that have been described for laryngoscopy. The most severe complications are related to tube placement. Placement of the endotracheal tube into the esophagus, if unrecognized, is a disastrous complication for obvious reasons. Esophageal placement is not always immediately apparent. One may hear "normal" breath sounds if only the midline is auscultated. One way to check for tracheal placement is to note if air is felt or heard to exit from the tube following positive-pressure ventilation with cuff inflation. If the lungs are ventilated, the exit of air should be obvious. Inadvertent advancement of the tracheal tube into the main stem bronchus beyond the trachea is one of the most frequent complications seen at our institution. Unilateral atelectasis and hypoxia may result if bronchial intubation goes unrecognized.

Adherence to proper technique will help avoid the complications and will help the clinician to recognize them when they do occur.[24] Routine auscultation of the lungs *and the stomach* after intubation will verify the correct position of the tube. Esophageal intubation is apparent when faint lung sounds and loud gastric sounds are heard together. Asymmetry of lung sounds suggests bronchial intubation. A chest radiograph must be obtained shortly after the intubation to confirm clinical impressions of tube location. Anticipation of complications can help avoid them. The assessment of tube position should also be the first step in the emergency department evaluation of a patient who has been intubated in the field by paramedics.

Mechanical Devices for Overcoming Clenched Jaws. Four devices for opening the mouth and keeping it open are illustrated in Figures 1–8 and 1–9. They are infrequently required and are mentioned for completeness. The Christmas tree jaw spreader is a triangular device with a threaded surface that allows advancement by a twisting motion. Figure 1–9 illustrates two types of mouth gags that are particularly useful in the semiconscious or unconscious patient with clenched teeth. Both the Jennings and Denhard gags operate on a ratchet mechanism. The dental processes of the Jennings gag are placed between the upper and lower incisors, and the jaws are pried open. Operation of the Denhard device is identical, except that the processes are placed between the molars.

Contraindications to the use of the spreaders

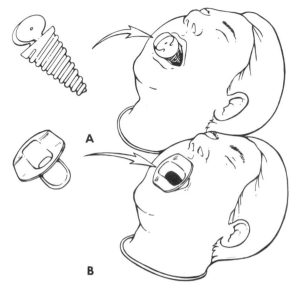

Figure 1–8. *A,* Christmas tree jaw spreader and *B,* Olympus bite block. (From Clinton, J. E., and Ruiz, E.: Trauma Life Support Manual, unpublished, 1982.)

and the gag include maxillary or mandibular fracture, which may be complicated by displacement if the devices are used. Displacement may, of course, have to be accepted if the need for an airway is great enough that use of the jaw spreaders is the only alternative for airway control.

Depending on the situation, any of these devices alone may be sufficient to accomplish the clinical goal of opening the mouth sufficiently to allow orotracheal intubation. More often, however, a combination of the devices is optimal for achievement of this end. An example of the procedure is as follows:

1. The tip of the Christmas tree jaw spreader is placed into a gap in the patient's dentition.

2. The jaw spreader is twisted until maximal separation of the teeth is obtained.

3. The operator inserts the Jennings gag between the upper and lower incisors, spreading the jaws farther as necessary to allow intubation. The Christmas tree spreader is then removed.

4. Orotracheal intubation is performed.

5. The Olympus bite block is placed around the endotracheal tube and between the teeth.

6. The Jennings gag is removed.

The Jennings and Denhard mouth gags are not as effective as the Christmas tree device in obtaining the first few degrees of mouth opening but are more effective for wider opening. The Olympus bite block serves to protect the tube once it is in place.

Complications are limited to local injury to the teeth, the oral mucosa, and the tongue. We have found local injury to be minimal. Damage caused by attempts to intubate without adequate jaw spreading devices may, in fact, be significantly greater than damage caused by a jaw spreader.

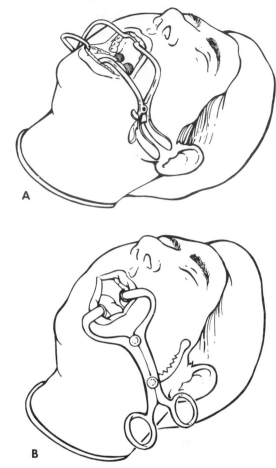

Figure 1–9. Ratchet-type jaw spreaders. *A,* Jennings mouth gag and *B,* Denhard mouth gag. (From Clinton, J. E., and Ruiz, E.: Trauma Life Support Manual, unpublished, 1982.)

Experience with the use of mouth gags and bite blocks quickly impresses one with their limitations. Although effective, they are far from ideal. Significant experience in difficult situations is necessary to develop skill in their use. Reflex tongue motion at times dislodges the jaw spreader, leaving the resuscitator where he started. Continued hypertonus after jaw spreading increases the difficulty of laryngoscopy. Difficult cases are best handled with pharmacologic adjuncts.

Pharmacologic Adjuncts to Intubation

A more aesthetic and efficacious approach to the management of hypertonus is to control it with paralyzing agents. In cases not involving paralysis, topical anesthesia helps to blunt the reflex response of the patient to attempts at intubation with or without the jaw spreader. In this section, we will examine the utility of topical lidocaine, intravenous lidocaine, intravenous succinylcholine, and pancuronium bromide as separate adjuncts of airway control.

Topical Anesthesia. Teeth clenching, gagging,

and tongue motion are often stimulated by attempts at laryngoscopy. These resistive reflexes often may be prevented with topical 4 per cent lidocaine anesthesia.[25-27] One may facilitate intubation by spraying the airway through a laryngotracheal cannula containing multiple side holes, which allow easy coating of the mucosal surfaces. Application of topical anesthesia may be performed under direct vision during laryngoscopy or by cricothyroid puncture. Both methods will be described here.

Direct Vision During Laryngoscopy

1. The lips, the gingival mucosa, and the top of the tongue are sprayed with a topical anesthetic, such as Cetacaine.

2. The operator sprays the proximal one half of the tongue and the pharynx with 4 per cent lidocaine using a laryngeal injection cannula, such as is supplied with the LTA (laryngotracheal anesthesia) kit (Abbott Lab) or the Duo-trach Kit (Astra Pharmaceuticals) (Fig. 1–10).

3. The laryngoscope blade is warmed to decrease reflex gagging and is used to visualize the hypopharynx.

4. The epiglottis and the vocal cords are liberally sprayed with 4 per cent lidocaine.

5. Two ml of 4 per cent lidocaine is injected into the laryngotracheal area with the cannula.

6. Orotracheal intubation is then performed.

Cricothyroid Membrane Puncture

1. The cricothyroid membrane is located between the cricoid and thyroid cartilages in the neck.

2. The membrane is punctured with a 20 gauge needle attached to a syringe containing 2 ml of 4 per cent lidocaine without epinephrine.

3. The operator aspirates during puncture until air is aspirated from the trachea.

4. The operator quickly injects 2 ml of lidocaine into the lumen and withdraws the needle.[26] A cough reflex should distribute the lidocaine adequately.

The total amount of lidocaine used should not exceed 300 mg (7.5 ml of a 4 per cent solution), because there is significant systemic absorption from tracheally instilled lidocaine.[28] The technique is of benefit in patients who have some productive respiratory efforts, in whom 2 to 3 minutes may be expended securing the airway.

Contraindications and complications of this technique both involve time considerations. The technique is contraindicated if immediate intubation is indicated. Hypoxia secondary to prolonged intubation is the most significant complication of the technique. Aspiration through the anesthetized airway is a potential complication should intubation attempts fail in spite of an adequately anesthetized airway.

Systemic Lidocaine. Intubation may cause an undesirable increase in heart rate, blood pressure, and intracranial pressure. The direct administration of lidocaine to the vocal cords decreases the cough reflex but does not prevent deleterious cardiovascular or intracranial pressure changes during intubation. The systemic administration of 1.5 mg per kg of lidocaine intravenously a few minutes prior to intubation has been shown to be superior to topical application in limiting intracranial pressure and blood pressure increases during intubation.[29] This finding, coupled with evidence of decreased cough reflex with systemic administration, indicates that systemic lidocaine may be simpler and more effective than topical lidocaine during intubation.[30] The benefit may be most marked in patients with head trauma.

Succinylcholine. A more potent means of overcoming jaw clenching and hypertonus is to induce complete paralysis by neuromuscular blockade. The rapid induction of the flaccid paralysis may greatly expedite management of the patient with clenched jaws. Succinylcholine is the drug that is most useful. It must be emphasized that paralysis by these agents requires airway control and positive-pressure ventilation until adequate respiratory function returns.

Succinylcholine is a short-acting neuromuscular depolarizing agent that has been used for anesthesia since the 1950s. The drug acts by combining with the neuromuscular end-plate, causing muscle depolarization that is manifested as widespread fasciculation of the body musculature. The onset of paralysis occurs within 1 minute of intravenous administration of a therapeutic dose. The sequence of muscle paralysis is typical. Initially, fascicula-

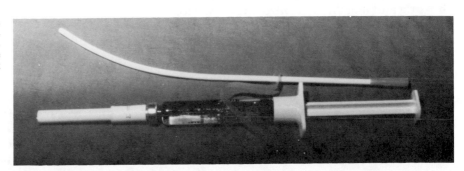

Figure 1–10. Laryngotracheal anesthesia kit. Duo-Trach Kit, Astra Pharmaceuticals. Note the laryngeal applicator—Teflon catheter with multiple side holes for application in larynx during direct laryngoscopy.

tions can be seen across the chest and the abdomen. As paralysis progresses the neck, arm, and leg muscles become paralyzed. Next the facial masticatory, lingual, pharyngeal, and laryngeal muscles are involved. Lastly, the intercostal muscles and the diaphagm become paralyzed. The effect begins to wane at 2 minutes, and muscle tone returns to normal within 8 minutes of injection. The usual dosage is 1 mg per kg intravenously (Anectine 20 mg per ml, Sucostrin 100 mg per ml).[31–33] The dosage per kilogram is increased in children.[34] The dosage of 1.5 mg per kg has been found to be more satisfactory in all multiply injured patients, including adults, in whom rapid immediate effect without the need for redosage is desired.

The use of succinylcholine is indicated in the initial management of the patient in critical condition when the more conservative techniques we have described previously are unsuccessful. As we have gained experience with succinylcholine administration in these situations, we have tended to favor it over the use of jaw spreaders in the management of patients with clenched teeth, such as those with seizures. Failure of orotracheal intubation because of excessive gagging and muscle tension short of teeth clenching is considered an indication for use of succinylcholine.

Two prerequisites must be met before succinylcholine use may be considered. First, the potential of cervical spine injury must have been ruled out or considered so minimal that orotracheal intubation may be safely performed. Secondly, the patient's level of consciousness must be sufficiently depressed so that he will not perceive himself to be paralyzed while conscious. (This has been described as a frightening and painful experience.) One of the indications for premedication with diazepam prior to the use of succinylcholine may be to prevent this occurrence when doubt exists as to the patient's level of perception.[35]

Contraindications to the use of succinylcholine are largely related to the adverse effects of the drug. Since airway management is the first priority in patient management, it must be understood that the contraindications are all relative to the importance of succinylcholine in the attainment of the priority of airway control. Absolute contraindications to succinylcholine are unfamiliarity with the drug and inability to control the airway following paralysis. A list of relative contraindications will be presented in the following section. The narrative following the list explains the circumstances in more detail and attempts to place them in proper perspective.

Relative Contraindications to Succinylcholine
1. Unstable cervical spine injury.
2. Alert patient.
3. Known hypersensitivity to succinylcholine.
4. Long-standing paralysis.
5. Old multiple trauma (greater than 2 weeks).
6. Penetrating ocular injury.
7. Increased intracranial pressure (?).

The first two contraindications have been addressed. True hypersensitivity to succinylcholine is rare.[36] A more common situation is prolonged paralysis following succinylcholine administration because of low levels of plasma cholinesterases which are necessary to metabolize succinylcholine. Low cholinesterase levels may be genetically determined or may be associated with certain disease states, such as cirrhosis, other liver disease, anemia, malnutrition, dehydration, exposure to insecticides or antimalarial drugs, and hypo- or hyperthermia.[37] Prolonged activity can be treated by respiratory support until the paralysis resolves. Severe hyperkalemia has been reported when succinylcholine is given to patients who have had a long-standing pre-existent paralysis. Presumably, this is related to exaggerated response of the denervated musculature to the drug. Similar hyperkalemia has been seen when patients with multiple trauma or burns receive succinylcholine more than 2 weeks after their injury.[38–42] This complication has not been reported when succinylcholine is used during the acute phase of resuscitation of the injured patient and therefore is not a concern in the usual resuscitation following multiple trauma.

Three pressure increases are of concern when succinylcholine is administered: intraocular, intragastric, and intraspinal.[43–45] It is believed that the reason for these pressure increases is muscle fasciculations induced by the drug. Presumably, the pressure changes may be averted by premedication with a small dose of a nondepolarizing paralyzing agent or diazepam.[33, 35] Penetrating injuries to the eye are considered a contraindication to succinylcholine use. Gastric pressures may predispose to regurgitation. Some authors have postulated that the increase in spinal pressure may contraindicate succinylcholine use in the patient with head injuries.

Both intraocular and intraspinal pressures are greatly increased by straining and gagging, which might be induced during any routine airway management maneuver. The management question that must be answered is which is the greater danger—to allow the possibility of increased pressures during routine intubation attempts or to control the situation with succinylcholine, knowing that some degree of pressure increase will occur during the administration of the drug. With penetrating ocular injuries, the prevailing opinion seems to be to avoid succinylcholine. Since penetrating ocular injuries are relatively uncommon in patients requiring intubation, one can easily abide by this requirement. Head injuries are much more common and are often the cause of the hypertonus necessitating intubation. In the face of unquestionable increased intracranial pressures during straining[46] and the questionable evidence of transient rise with the drug,[44] one must conclude that in head injuries succinylcholine is the lesser of the two evils and is of great benefit to the patient because it prevents undue struggling during intubation attempts.

The danger of intragastric pressure increase is compounded by a simultaneous decrease in tone of the gastroesophageal sphincter. The combination of the two produces a high likelihood of regurgitation if the stomach is full at the time of administration of succinylcholine; therefore, great pains should be taken to ensure an empty stomach in preparation for elective surgery of any kind. Again, one must weigh this potential complication against the need for immediate airway control in a patient with clenched teeth who is hypoventilating. Replacement of the problem of clenched teeth with a mouthful of regurgitated stomach contents is not a therapeutic triumph. We believe the procedure that will be outlined for the use of succinylcholine in the critical patient takes this dilemma into account. Cricoid pressure is applied during drug administration and intubation attempts.[47–51] This maneuver has been shown to be capable of withstanding up to 100 cm H_2O esophageal pressure.[49] The rescuers must be prepared to approach the airway surgically if orotracheal intubation fails or if regurgitation is uncontrollable with cricoid pressure. Strict adherence to the protocol that will be described is necessary to avoid complications.

Some additional, but less common, complications of succinylcholine administration that were not mentioned with the contraindications should be discussed. Bradycardia and even asystole of a transient nature have been reported after administration of succinylcholine.[52–54] This seems to be more common in children and may be prevented by premedication with atropine. Malignant hyperthermia has been triggered by succinylcholine. Masseter spasm following administration of a therapeutic dose may occur.[55, 56] The syndrome of malignant hyperthermia may be more common in individuals who develop masseter spasm.[56]

Administration Procedure. In order to minimize the predictable complications of the use of succinylcholine, Thompson devised a protocol requiring a two-person team that is prepared to perform immediate cricothyrotomy in the face of orotracheal intubation failure, regurgitation, or masseter spasm.[57] The procedure is as follows:

1. Preparation includes having a laryngoscope, an endotracheal tube, a cricothyrotomy tube, and instruments all laid out and ready for use. The neck is prepared for a possible surgical approach to the airway.

2. The intubator is stationed at the patient's head. The assistant is at the patient's side and is prepared to perform cricothyrotomy.

3. If the level of consciousness is unclear or if fasciculations are feared, 5 mg of diazepam is administered intravenously. Atropine premedication, 0.01 mg per kg, is given to children. Succinylcholine, 1.5 mg per kg, is administered intravenously while cricoid pressure is exerted and maintained by the assistant.

4. After waiting 30 to 60 seconds for effect of the succinylcholine, the operater attempts orotracheal intubation with a laryngoscope. Preoxygenation with a bag-valve mask is performed prior to intubation when the situation allows.

5. If intubation is unsuccessful, cricothyrotomy is performed.

In a series of 820 emergency endotracheal intubations, Thompson reported the adjunctive use of succinylcholine in 5.9 per cent (48 of 820) of the intubations. Five of the 48 patients ultimately required cricothyrotomy.[57]

Succinylcholine is an important tool in the armamentarium of airway management for the critically ill or injured patient. Its appropriate use renders otherwise unmanageable airway problems manageable without surgery.

The use of succinylcholine outside the operating room is feasible when appropriate precautions are taken. The emergency team must be prepared to resort to surgical airway management if orotracheal intubation fails in the paralyzed patient, especially if gastric regurgitation occurs. Strict adherence to the protocol described here will limit complications and will maximize successful airway control in the critical patient.

Pancuronium Bromide (Pavulon). Longer-acting nondepolarizing agents, such as pancuronium bromide (Pavulon), are also of use in the injured patient. The absence of fasciculation and the longer duration of action are of benefit in certain situations.

Pancuronium bromide is a curariform drug that induces paralysis by blocking the effects of acetylcholine at the myoneural junction. The onset of action is within 45 seconds. The peak effect occurs at approximately 3 minutes. The duration of action is 45 minutes to 1 hour.[58] Pancuronium (Pavulon) is available in 2- and 5-ml ampules in a concentration of 2 mg per ml or in 10-ml vials at a concentration of 1 mg per ml.

The primary use of pancuronium in the injured patient is not usually airway management. Rather, the agent is used to immobilize agitated patients with neurologic injury in order to facilitate their rapid evaluation. The thrashing, agitated patient with multiple injuries may be impossible to evaluate or to treat unless he is effectively immobilized. In such cases, the patient must be intubated and placed on a respirator.

Pancuronium may be used when alternatives to paralysis are less desirable because of more serious side effects. Physical restraint may lead to straining and increased intracranial pressure. Narcotics such as morphine may induce hypotension, which in turn requires reversal. Sedatives such as diazepam have unpredictable effects and dosage requirements.

Occasionally, pancuronium is useful for emergency tracheal intubation when succinylcholine is contraindicated. The patient with penetrating ocular injury and the patient with pre-existent paraplegia are two important examples of individuals in whom succinylcholine may not be used and pancuronium is effective. The time to onset and peak effect is dose dependent. Since the maximum effect is desired in emergency situations, a dosage of 0.1 to 0.15 mg per kg is routinely used.

Contraindications to the use of pancuronium include unfamiliarity with use of the drug or a patient history of adverse reaction to pancuronium. Expertise in both nonsurgical and surgical airway management is a necessary prerequisite to use of the drug.

The protocol of use of pancuronium is identical to that for succinylcholine. It is mandatory to have two rescuers present, with one applying cricoid pressure. As a precaution, preparation should be made for surgical approach, if needed.

Complications are related to duration of action and inadequate support during the period of paralysis. The prolonged effect of the drug is the most common adverse reaction and requires prolonged respiratory support. Certain anesthetics and other drugs may induce this effect.[31] Failure to achieve airway control quickly following administration of the drug can be particularly disastrous because of the prolonged length of action of pancuronium. Pressure rises (intracranial, intraocular, and intragastric) do not pose a problem with pancuronium, as they do with succinylcholine. Any rises in intracranial pressure are caused by carbon dioxide buildup following hypoventilation.[59]

In practice, pancuronium is used in addition to succinylcholine to prolong paralysis. One may use pancuronium to avoid complications associated with succinylcholine by substituting it for succinylcholine entirely or by giving it in small dosages of 0.01 to 0.04 mg per kg as a premedication before succinylcholine administration, thereby avoiding muscle fasciculation when the succinylcholine is given. Whenever pancuronium is used, one must remember that the physical findings of neurologic deterioration have been masked. Therefore, definitive neurologic evaluation in the form of computed tomography, arteriography, or surgery must proceed as rapidly as possible after the administration of the drug.

Nasotracheal Intubation

The technique of nasotracheal intubation can be extremely advantageous in any patient requiring intubation. When in place, the nasotracheal tube traverses the nasal cavity, the nasal hypopharynx, and the larynx, with the tip resting in the trachea. This situation prevents biting of the tube by the patient and manipulation of the tube by the tongue. Oral injuries are cared for without interference by the tube. A nasotracheal tube is more easily stabilized and is generally easier to care for than an orotracheal tube. The nasotracheal tube is better tolerated by the patient and produces less reflex salivation than do the oral tubes. Nasotracheal intubation is the method of intubation preferred by some authors for acute epiglottitis.

The tube may be placed with the aid of the laryngoscope, but placement by blind technique or with the aid of the bronchoscope offers the additional advantage of avoiding the need for neck motion or opening of the mouth. Patients with hypertonus or suspected cervical spine injury may undergo intubation with a minimum of preparation when these techniques are used. Cervical spine films, jaw spreading, or paralyzing agents as prerequisites to airway control may thus be avoided. A specific clinical situation that lends itself to nasotracheal intubation is a decreased level of consciousness in the drug overdose patient. Such patients are often intubated before gastric lavage. They may be awake enough to make orotracheal intubation very difficult but may be breathing sufficiently to facilitate nasotracheal intubation by the blind technique. Blind nasotracheal intubation is possible with the patient in the

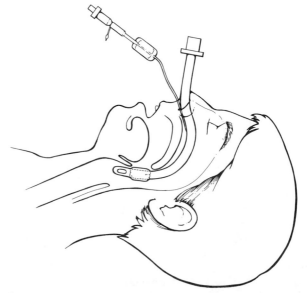

Figure 1–11. Blind nasotracheal intubation. (From Clinton, J. E., and Ruiz, E.: Trauma Life Support Manual, unpublished, 1982.)

sitting position, a distinct advantage in elective intubations of the patient with congestive heart failure or asthma who will not tolerate the supine position.

Placement Under Direct Vision. This technique may be looked on as an equivalent of orotracheal intubation. The indications and precautions are similar to those for orotracheal intubations. It is important to consider cervical spine injury before performance of this technique, and jaw opening by physical or pharmacologic means may be necessary. The primary indication for choice of this route over orotracheal intubation is in the case of an oral injury in which the presence of an orotracheal tube would be a nuisance. The convenience of using a nasotracheal tube rather than an orotracheal tube may lead to operator preference for the former (Fig. 1–11).

Technique is as follows:

1. The nasal mucosa is constricted with 1 per cent phenylephrine or 4 per cent cocaine spray. These agents should be used with caution in hypertensive patients. The most patent nostril is chosen for passage of the tube. The proper nostril is identified by direct vision with a nasal speculum.

2. With adults, a 7.0-, 7.5-, or 8.0-mm internal diameter tracheal tube (nasal or universal nasal/oral type) is lubricated with viscous lidocaine. In addition, some viscous lidocaine is placed in the nostril to be used.

3. The tube is inserted into the nostril directly posteriorly *along the floor of the nasal cavity* until the tip of the tube is in the hypopharynx. This is usually the most traumatic portion of the procedure, and it must be performed gently. Twisting the tube may help bypass soft tissue obstruction.

4. Laryngoscopy is performed as described earlier to visualize the vocal cords and the tip of the endotracheal tube.

5. The physician grasps the tip of the endotracheal tube with the Magill forceps avoiding the cuff and directs the tip toward the larynx.

6. The assistant is instructed to advance the tube gently while the physician directs the tip into the larynx and the trachea. Cricoid pressure may facilitate the passage. If the larynx can be manipulated with the laryngoscope, the physician can advance the tube with the right hand and guide it between the cords without the use of Magill forceps. Occasionally, the natural curve of the tracheal tube guides it through the cords without any manipulation.

7. The cuff is inflated, and both lungs are auscultated to ensure ventilation.

8. When satisfied with placement, the operator secures the tube with cloth tape.

Epistaxis is a common complication of nasotracheal intubation in the emergency situation. This is probably the most common complication. Severe epistaxis was encountered in 5 of 300 cases reported by Danzl.[60] Tintinalli encountered severe bleeding in 1 of 71 cases and less serious bleeding in 12 others.[61] Other complications that have been reported include turbinate fracture, nasal necrosis, intracranial placement through a basilar skull fracture, retropharyngeal laceration or dissection, excessive delay, and failure of successful placement.[8, 59, 62–64]

Many complications may be minimized by selection of a smaller tube and by gentle technique. There is a higher incidence of bacteremia and sinusitis following nasotracheal intubation compared with orotracheal intubation.

The complication of delay deserves some special discussion. Manipulation of the endotracheal tube through the nose and with the Magill forceps involves additional steps, each requiring time. Since time is of the essence in the resuscitation of the critically ill patient, orotracheal intubation may be preferable when time is crucial. *A stylet is never used during nasotracheal* intubation. If the tube is not easily passed through the nose, orotracheal intubation is performed.

Blind Placement. Blind nasotracheal intubation is the most useful airway control maneuver in the multiply injured or critically ill patient who exhibits some degree of spontaneous respiration. The patient's breath sounds are used to guide the tube into the trachea during this maneuver. It is unnecessary for the operator to visualize the larynx. Opening the jaws and extending the neck are unnecessary for success. The technique therefore overcomes two of the most frustrating airway management obstacles—potential cervical spine injury and hypertonus.

Indications for the use of blind nasotracheal intubation in the patient requiring airway control are liberal. Any patient requiring airway control who has some spontaneous ventilation is considered a candidate for this maneuver. Specific indications in which this approach is definitely favored over others are:

1. Inability to open the patient's mouth.
2. Inability to move the patient's neck.
3. Dental injuries.
4. Gagging or resisting the use of the laryngoscope on the part of the patient.
5. Short thick neck or cervical kyphosis making vocal cord visualization difficult.

Apnea is the major contraindication to blind nasotracheal intubation. Attempts to place the tube without respiration as a guide are futile. Relative contraindications include anterior fossa fracture and nasal injury.[7, 8, 65] Significant bleeding may occur if the patient is anticoagulated, making anticoagulation a relative contraindication.

The technique of blind nasotracheal intubation

was first described by Magill in 1930.[66] Little change in technique has occurred since. Modifications have been described to increase the success rate and to limit complications. The description of the technique that follows will incorporate many of the tips for success.

1. The nasal mucosa is constricted with 1 per cent phenylephrine drops. The mucosa is anesthetized with a topical anesthetic, such as 4 per cent cocaine, if the patient is responding to pain.

2. An endotracheal tube (7.0, 7.5, or 8.0 mm in internal diameter for adults) is inserted along the floor of the nasal cavity. The operator listens to breath sounds through the tube as it is advanced. A decrease in resistance indicates passage into the nasopharynx.

3. The tube is advanced into the hypopharynx and is used as a nasopharyngeal airway to ensure ventilation. As long as breath sounds are heard, retropharyngeal placement is unlikely. The neck is maintained in a neutral position, i.e., with the head directed forward. A small towel placed under the patient's occiput helps to align the airway.

4. The tube is advanced during an *inspiratory* effort into the trachea. Often, the patient will cough during this maneuver. Coughing indicates that the tip of the tube is entering the trachea and slow steady pressure is maintained to overcome any vocal cord spasm. One should never use great force in advancing the tube. Continued air passage through the tube indicates that the tube is in the trachea rather than the esophagus. Once the tube is in the trachea, moaning and groaning noises should disappear. Their continuance means esophageal passage.

5. The operator auscultates both lungs while applying positive-pressure ventilation. If only one lung is being ventilated, one should withdraw the tube until both lungs are ventilated.

6. The cuff is inflated with 10 ml of air, and the tube is secured with cloth tape.[66, 67]

Most of the time the endotracheal tube will pass into the trachea when it is advanced gently and swiftly during inspiration. Jacoby has described five possible locations of the misplaced tube:

1. Left piriform sinus.
2. Right piriform sinus.
3. Anterior to epiglottis.
4. In esophagus.
5. Above vocal cords but unable to pass.[67]

Observation of the soft tissues of the neck during attempted passage of the nasotracheal tube will often allow the operator to determine the location of the misplaced tube. Maneuvers to correct the misplacement may be used on the second attempt.[67]

Bulging of the neck laterally and superiorly to the larynx indicates the presence of the tube in the piriform sinus on either side. A midline bulge at the same level suggests positioning anterior to the epiglottis. Esophageal placement is detected by passage of the tube to a greater depth with loss of air movement through the tube. In addition, attempted ventilation while the stomach is auscultated leaves no doubt as to an esophageal placement. If the tube is advanced beyond the larynx level into the esophagus, it is withdrawn back into the hypopharynx. Between attempts at tracheal placement, the tube is not removed from the nose, since this creates additional trauma to the nasal soft tissues. Resistance to passage at the level of the larynx without anterior bulging suggests a location above the vocal cords.

Methods of achieving success when the tube has been misplaced are listed in the following sections.

Piriform Sinus

1. The tube is rotated away from the side of the misplacement, and passage is reattempted.

2. The patient's head is abducted toward the side of the misplacement, and passage is reattempted. For example, a tube placed in the right nostril tends to advance diagonally toward the left piriform sinus. Abducting or cocking the patient's head toward the left tends to straighten the course of the tube toward the larynx, away from the sinus.[67, 68]

Anterior to the Epiglottis

1. Extension of the head on the neck is decreased.

2. A tube with a lesser degree of curvature is used.

Esophageal Placement

1. The tube is withdrawn to the hypopharynx (not out of the nose). Passage is reattempted while cricoid pressure is applied.

2. Extension of the head on the neck is increased during placement.

Placement Above the Cords (as in Laryngospasm)

1. Passage is reattempted with a smaller tube.

2. Laryngeal anesthesia is reassessed. Transcricothyroid anesthesia with 2 ml of 4 per cent lidocaine is administered, and passage is reattempted.[65]

The potential presence of cervical spine injury must be constantly kept in mind when these corrective maneuvers are considered. Any maneuver that significantly moves the neck should not be used when alternatives that do not jeopardize the spinal cord exist.

Complications are similar to those described for nasotracheal intubation with Magill forceps. The dangers of retropharyngeal laceration and esophageal intubation described for nasotracheal intubation with Magill forceps exist. Retropharyngeal laceration and esophageal intubation are more of a threat in blind placement techniques, since they are more likely to go unrecognized.[61] To avoid retropharyngeal laceration, one should advance the tube only while breath sounds are heard. The sudden loss of breath sounds may indicate abutment against soft tissue, and the tube must never be forcibly advanced. Meticulous auscultation of lung fields for bilaterally symmetric sounds must be performed. In addition, auscultation of the epigastrium is a good idea, since it sometimes clarifies esophageal placement more quickly.

Adherence to careful and gentle technique will avoid most of the complications and will allow early recognition of those that do occur. Failure of recognition of complications without corrective action accounts for most of the damage inflicted through complications.

Placement Over Fiberoptic Bronchoscope. Flexible fiberoptic scopes allow placement of endotracheal tubes under direct vision in circumstances in which other techniques are not applicable.[69–71] Two approaches to placement using the fiberoptic scope are available; one is a nasotracheal method, and the other is an orotracheal approach. The nasotracheal method is the most common application, but both will be described here.

Although blind nasotracheal intubation is the technique of choice in the spontaneously breathing patient with potential cervical spine injury, it is occasionally unsuccessful in spite of corrective maneuvers, and it is not feasible in the apneic patient. Failure of blind nasotracheal intubation is a potential indication for use of the fiberoptic bronchoscope. Teeth clenching and potential cervical spine injury remain significant factors in the decision to use this maneuver.

Contraindications to fiberoptic placement of a nasotracheal tube are similar to the contraindications to other forms of nasotracheal intubation. An impediment to this technique is the presence of significant airway hemorrhage, secretions, or foreign material. The degree of obstruction may be significant enough to contraindicate an attempt at fiberoptic placement. Two means of handling mild hemorrhage and secretions exist; the first is to use the suction port of the bronchoscope. This may be effective in mild situations. Another less cumbersome technique is to attach oxygen tubing to the suction port for insufflation of oxygen during intubation. The insufflation serves to keep debris away from the tip of the bronchoscope while providing the patient with at least some oxygen supplementation. Fiberoptic intubation is generally too time-consuming to be used in the apneic patient.

Fiberoptic-Assisted Nasotracheal Intubation Technique

1. The endotracheal tube is inserted without the fiberoptic scope along the floor of the patient's nasal cavity into the nasopharynx or the hypopharynx.

2. The Lubrifax-lubricated bronchoscope is inserted through the endotracheal tube to a premeasured distance corresponding to the point at which the tip of the bronchoscope is at the tip of the endotracheal tube.

3. The operator visualizes the vocal cords through the fiberoptic scope and advances the scope through the endotracheal tube toward the cords without moving the endotracheal tube.

4. The bronchoscope is advanced past the cords into the trachea. The endotracheal tube is then advanced over the bronchoscope into the trachea.

5. The bronchoscope is removed, the cuff is inflated, and the patient is ventilated.

6. Both lungs are auscultated to ensure adequate ventilation. The tube is repositioned if asymmetric ventilation exists.

7. When confident of adequate placement, the operator secures the tube in place with cloth tape.[69]

The complications are identical to those of blind nasotracheal intubation. Excessive delay during attempts is a much greater hazard with the fiberoptic intubation technique. The manipulation is much more complicated, and the operator tends to become intrigued with the procedure and loses awareness of the passage of time. One must be particularly disciplined in timing these attempts to avoid unnecessary hypoxic insult.

Inability to visualize the vocal cords with a laryngoscope because of anatomic variation may necessitate the orotracheal use of the fiberoptic scope as an adjunct for intubation. The patient with a short "bull" neck or patients with spinal deformities may be particularly refractory to direct laryngoscopy. Failure to visualize the vocal cords or anticipation of such a difficulty may lead the operator to choose the fiberoptic scope as an adjunct for *orotracheal* intubation.

Contraindications and complications of this technique are identical to those for orotracheal intubation with a laryngoscope. Again, excessive delay is a greater hazard when the fiberoptic scope is used. Two operators are necessary to perform this technique.

Fiberoptic-Assisted Orotracheal Intubation

1. The fiberoptic scope and the endotracheal tube are assembled by insertion of the scope through the tube lumen until the fiberoptic tip is protruding from the distal end of the tube.

2. The first operator retracts the tongue with

the laryngoscope in a similar manner to that for laryngoscopy.

3. The first operator grasps the assembled fiberoptic scope and the endotracheal tube and slowly advances the combination in the direction of the larynx.

4. The second operator visualizes the vocal cords through the fiberoptic scope as it is advanced toward the larynx. The tip is manipulated with the controls to pass between the vocal cords.

5. The tube is advanced to its final position in the trachea.

6. The fiberoptic scope is removed, and the cuff is inflated.

7. The lungs are auscultated to ensure proper ventilation.

8. When the position is adequate, the tube is secured with cloth tape.

A malleable fiberoptic scope has recently become available.[72] This device is designed for orotracheal intubation in patients whose larynx is difficult to visualize with the laryngoscope. This procedure is also best performed by two rescuers. The first retracts the tongue and advances the tube under the direction of the second rescuer, who visualizes the larynx with the scope.

Retrograde Endotracheal Intubation

The technique for retrograde intubation represents a more invasive procedure than those described thus far. The technique that will be described necessitates puncture of the cricothyroid membrane to place a guide up through the mouth, over which an endotracheal tube may be slid into the trachea. The technique combines elements of both nonsurgical airway control maneuvers already described with cricothyroid membrane puncture.

The technique was originally described in 1960 as a means of intubating patients with a tracheostomy tube in place.[73] Subsequent modifications of the technique have involved its use in conjunction with puncture of the larynx, allowing the technique to be applied in any patient in need of airway control.[74–76]

Since retrograde intubation is a relatively invasive technique, it should be reserved for patients in whom more conservative approaches to management of the airway have failed. It may be particularly useful when too much airway debris prevents fiberoptic scope intubation and neck motion is limited. Retrograde intubation may be the most conservative management procedure short of surgical airway management in some patients. When it can be performed rapidly (after failure of any of the more conservative nonsurgical approaches), it may be a reasonable alternative to emergency surgical management.

Contraindications to this procedure include the ability to secure airway control by less invasive means. Clenched teeth provide the same obstacle to retrograde endotracheal intubation as they do to orotracheal intubation. Cervical spine injury does not pose a problem, since neck motion is unnecessary for retrograde intubation.

Although nasotracheal retrograde intubation has been described, it is too complicated and time-consuming to be of significant benefit to the acutely ill or injured patient.[72] The technique to be described here is the retrograde orotracheal approach.[73, 74]

Retrograde Orotracheal Intubation Technique

Equipment
1. 24-inch intravenous catheter-needle combination
2. Tracheal tube of appropriate size
3. Forceps for grasping the catheter in the posterior pharynx
4. Cloth tape
5. Syringe

Procedure
1. The anatomic landmarks (cricoid cartilage, thyroid cartilage, and hyoid bone) are located.

2. The skin is anesthetized over the cricothyroid membrane.

3. The lower half of the cricothyroid membrane is punctured with the needle directed slightly cephalad. The bevel should also face cephalad.

4. Air is aspirated through the needle to ensure laryngeal lumen location.

5. The catheter is threaded through the needle until the catheter is visible in the patient's mouth.

6. The catheter is grasped with the forceps and is drawn out through the mouth. Sufficient length of the catheter is withdrawn to allow a tracheal tube to be slipped over the catheter with the catheter tip extending from the proximal end of the tracheal tube.

7. The operator slides the tube over the catheter by introducing the catheter through the endotracheal side wall into the lumen and out the proximal end of the tube.

8. The operator applies tension over the catheter by pulling on both its ends.

9. The endotracheal tube is advanced into the larynx over the catheter until resistance is felt at the cricothyroid puncture site.

10. The operator cuts the catheter at the puncture site while simultaneously advancing the endotracheal tube into the trachea.

11. The distal end of the catheter is withdrawn out of the patient's mouth.

12. The cuff is inflated. The operator ventilates the patient and auscultates the patient's lungs.

13. When confident of correct placement, the operator secures the tube with cloth tape.

Complications of the technique are largely related to cricothyroid membrane puncture. They are: failure to achieve intubation, hemorrhage, subcutaneous emphysema, and soft tissue infection.

Authors have stressed two points that are helpful in minimizing failure. The first is that the catheter should be kept taut during passage of the tracheal tube to prevent kinking and obstruction.[73] Secondly, a special technique for threading the catheter up the tracheal tube has been proposed. Figure 1–12 illustrates the recommended method, in which the catheter is threaded up the side hole of the tube rather than the end hole. This allows the maximum length of the tube to be advanced into the larynx before the catheter is cut. There is less chance that the tube will be displaced out of the larynx into the esophagus when the catheter is threaded in this manner.[74] The operator can minimize hemorrhage by taking care to puncture the cricothyroid membrane in its lower half to avoid the cricothyroid artery.[77–79] Subcutaneous

Figure 1–12. Retrograde intubation using a catheter threaded from the larynx by cricothyroid membrane puncture. (From Clinton, J. E., and Ruiz, E.: Trauma Life Support Manual, unpublished, 1982.)

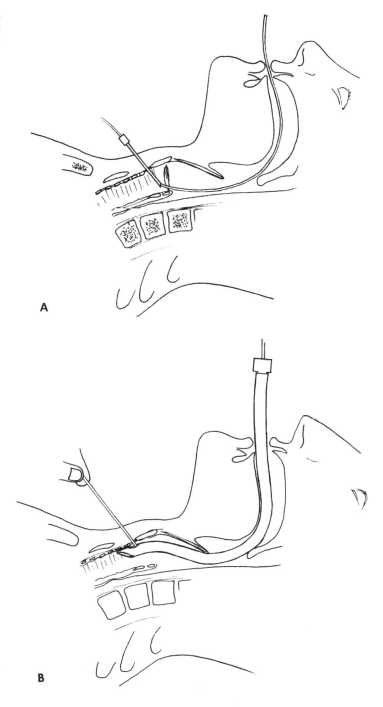

A

B

emphysema may be unavoidable but usually is of little significance, since no air is insufflated during this procedure. A low incidence of soft tissue infection is reported with translaryngeal needle procedures and can be expected to occur with this technique as well.

Retrograde intubation is a useful technique that is available in the armamentarium of airway control procedures for dealing with the critically ill patient. It is a valuable tool under the appropriate circumstances because neck motion and spontaneous respiration are not required and it may be performed quickly.

Surgical Techniques in Emergency Airway Management

Thus far in this chapter we have described several techniques for dealing with many different scenarios of airway compromise in emergency situations. We have discussed the variables of degree of airway obstruction, clenching of teeth, and concomitant cervical spine injury. As yet we have offered no procedure for use in situations in which time is not available to implement some of the more involved techniques that could otherwise be used. Moreover, no procedure has been proposed for use in the patient who presents in cardiac arrest following trauma or the patient who is apneic with airway obstruction and clenched teeth following trauma.

Surgical techniques come into play in situations in which time is not available to accomplish more conservative airway management. Three surgical techniques have been applied in the emergency situation. They are transcricothyroid catheter ventilation, cricothyroidotomy, and tracheotomy. Cricothyroidotomy will be discussed in Chapter 7. Tracheotomy is only rarely applicable as an emergency approach to airway management and will not be described at length in this text. On the next few pages we will describe transcricothyroid ventilation. A discussion of the logic of emergency airway management will be provided, taking into account all the procedures we have discussed as well as cricothyroidotomy and tracheotomy.

TRANSCRICOTHYROID CATHETER VENTILATION

Insufflation of air into the trachea by a catheter introduced through the cricothyroid membrane is a proven method of respiratory support.[80–87] Effective oxygenation of blood with clearing of carbon dioxide may be accomplished through use of this technique. To provide adequate tidal volume, a high pressure oxygen source is necessary. An oxygen source of 50 lbs per square inch easily provides the necessary pressure to deliver adequate tidal volume through a 14 to 16 gauge catheter introduced through the cricothyroid membrane.[82, 88]

Transcricothyroid ventilation may be advantageous when rapid control of ventilation is necessary. When the apparatus is at hand and the technique is properly performed, the speed with which the patient may be ventilated is unmatched by other techniques. This is the only surgical technique that can be viewed as being a reversible temporizing measure. Ventilation in this manner may allow endotracheal intubation by providing time to obtain cervical spine films or to succeed with the technically difficult intubation.

The temporary nature of this airway may be a disadvantage under a different set of circumstances. The flexibility of the catheter requires constant attention to prevent kinking and obstruction during ventilation. A more secure, definitive airway may be chosen as the primary surgical airway when personnel are limited, when a long-term surgical airway is needed, or when attention must be shifted to other critical injuries after airway control is established. The lone physician attempting to resuscitate a multiply injured patient with a severe facial injury or an individual in a state of cardiac arrest may opt to perform cricothyroidotomy primarily rather than transtracheal ventilation.

Transtracheal catheter ventilation is indicated when nonsurgical techniques have failed because of either excessive delay or technical failure. Likewise, judgment by the physician that the risk of failure of more conservative methods is excessive constitutes sufficient indication. A major advantage of the technique is that is can be used in these situations to avoid more radical surgical intervention.

Relative contraindications to the use of the technique include primary laryngeal injury, such as laryngeal fracture. The availability of time, equipment, and skill necessary to achieve airway control by more conservative means should lead to use of a less invasive means of airway control.

Equipment necessary for the application of transcricothyroid ventilation includes:

1. A 14 gauge needle with a Teflon catheter sheath.

2. A three-way stopcock or other manual valve mechanism.

3. Oxygen tubing.

4. An oxygen source of 50 lbs per sq inch (wall or tank O_2).[78–86] If wall oxygen is used, the regulator is opened widely (flush position).

This material must be prepared beforehand if it is to be used in an expeditious manner. The setup should be constantly available in the emergency department for use at short notice.

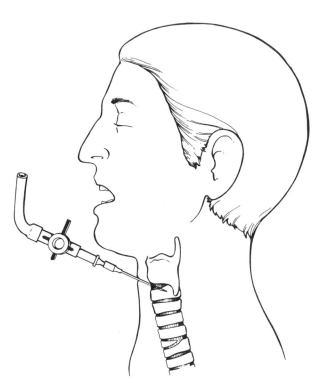

Figure 1–13. Translaryngeal catheter ventilation. (From Clinton J. E., and Ruiz, E.: Trauma Life Support Manual, unpublished, 1982.)

Procedure for Transcricothyroid Catheter Ventilation (Fig. 1–13)

1. A 14 gauge needle and catheter are attached to an empty syringe.

2. The operator palpates the cricoid cartilage, the thyroid cartilage, and the hyoid bone and locates the membrane between the cricoid cartilage and the thyroid cartilage (the cricothyroid membrane.

3. The operator palpates the cricothyroid membrane while grasping the larynx firmly.

4. The grasp is maintained on the larynx during puncture of the cricothyroid membrane.

5. The cricothyroid membrane is punctured at a slight angle from the perpendicular point in a caudad direction.

6. Aspiration is performed during puncture with a syringe until air is obtained, signifying entry into the airway.

7. The catheter is advanced into the trachea, and the needle is removed.

8. The syringe is reattached to the catheter, and air is aspirated again to ensure correct placement.

9. The stopcock is attached to the catheter.

10. The operator alternates lung insufflation with pressurized oxygen and passive exhalation. A 2- to 3-second inspiratory phase has been recommended.[85]

11. The physician prepares a more definitive method of airway control to be performed under more controlled circumstances.

Several complications from transtracheal ventilation have been reported.[78, 79, 88–92] Subcutaneous emphysema, mediastinal emphysema, and hemorrhage are the most significant complications reported. The emphysema is present with most transtracheal techniques and is manageable, provided that it results from a leak around the catheter rather than from direct insufflation into the soft tissues of the neck. Severe subcutaneous emphysema may obscure landmarks and may further complicate attempts at airway access. Hemorrhage is usually minimal and self-limited, but deaths have been reported from laryngeal aspiration techniques related to hemorrhage.[78, 79, 89–92] Puncture in the lower part of the cricothyroid membrane is recommended to avoid the cricothyroid artery, which courses horizontally over the upper part of the membrane.[77]

The complication rate that has been reported in the literature for all transtracheal procedures, including transtracheal aspiration and anesthesia, is 0.03 to 0.8 per cent.[78, 89, 91] Sporadic complications that have been reported with other transtracheal procedures include soft tissue infection, necrosis of the cricoid cartilage, hemoptysis, and arrhythmias. The low complication rate and the minor, self-limited nature of these problems makes this the safest of the surgical approaches.

Transtracheal ventilation is underused in the management of the acutely ill or injured patient in respiratory distress. Prolonged hypoxia during futile intubation attempts should be avoided with this technique. Many emergency cricothyrotomies can be avoided if transcricothyroid ventilation is attempted first.

Decision Making in Airway Management

The physician must have many tools at hand to deal with the emergently compromised airway. Even though the physician may be proficient in the performance of all the previously described procedures, the maneuver to be used is often chosen when no time is available for contemplation. It is critical that the potential scenarios be considered before emergency airway management becomes necessary in the clinical situation. Failure to consider all possibilities will lead to unnecessarily aggressive management in some situations and, worse, irreversible hypoxic injury as a result of delays produced by indecisiveness.

Several parameters must be assessed quickly and judged before an airway management choice can be made. The parameters to be considered are:

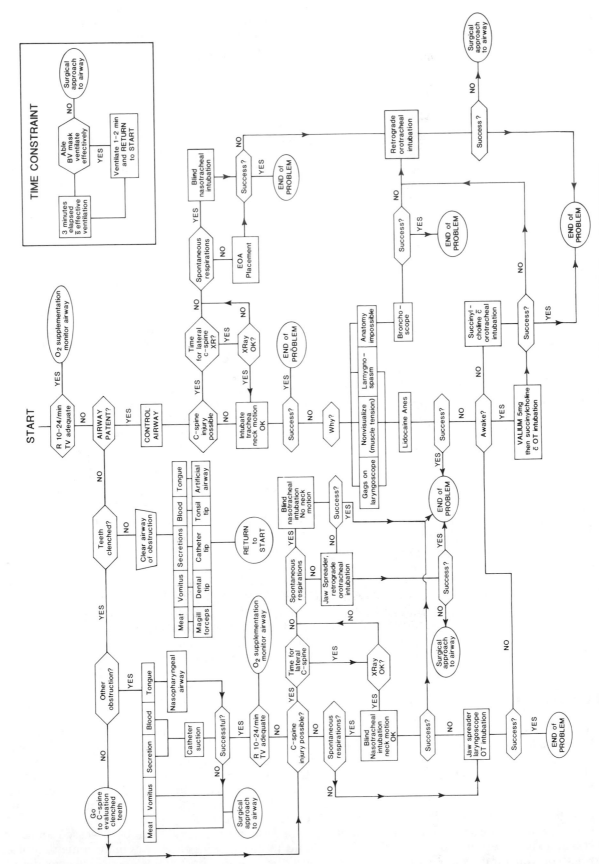

Figure 1-14. Nonsurgical airway management algorithm. (From Clinton, J. E., and Ruiz, E.: Trauma Life Support Manual, unpublished, 1982.)

1. adequacy of current ventilation,
2. time of hypoxia,
3. patency of airway,
4. malleability of jaws (teeth clenching),
5. cervical spine stability, and
6. safety of technique.

Consideration of these factors will allow the physician to choose the optimum procedure from among those we have described. This initial choice is relatively straightforward. The real difficulty is encountered when the initial choice is unsuccessful. Time becomes more of a factor, and the safety of the technique is less important as the borderline of irreversible hypoxic injury is approached. Anxiety increases in such a clinical situation, and the potential for error is compounded. No substitute exists for forethought and practice in making these decisions.

Schemata are offered in Figures 1–14 and 1–15, outlining the logic behind the airway choices. The first diagram is the most complicated. It represents the choices among nonsurgical approaches to the airway we have described. The end point of this diagram is either success or the decision to pursue surgical management. The overriding time-oriented diagram in the upper right corner of the first diagram should be noted. This forces a judgment in favor of surgical airway management when time is running out. The second diagram (Figure 1–15) is much simpler. Once the decision to manage the airway surgically has been made, one needs to choose among three available options. Consideration of patient condition, definitiveness of the airway approach, and degree of invasiveness are contributing factors to the final decision.

Figure 1–15. Surgical airway management algorithm. (From Clinton, J. E., and Ruiz, E.: Trauma Life Support Manual, unpublished, 1982.)

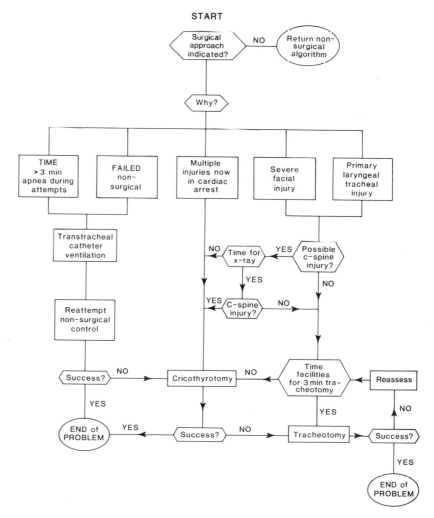

Summary

Airway management in the critically ill or injured patient with acute airway compromise is a most demanding task for the emergency physician. Mastery of several nonsurgical and three surgical techniques of airway control is necessary to meet any emergency situation that might occur. Preparation involving mastery of technique, preparation of equipment, and experience in decision making is essential. Through scenario visualization, one may practice the difficult decision making necessary to provide the patient with the most expeditious and safest means of airway control available under the circumstances. In this chapter we have described the techniques and have offered a logical schema for their use in the patient with an acutely compromised airway.

1. Guildner, C. W.: Resuscitation—opening the airway: A comparative study of techniques for opening an airway obstructed by the tongue. JACEP 5:588, 1976.
2. Kapp, J. P.: Endotracheal intubation in patients with fractures of the cervical spine. J. Neurosurg. 42:731, 1975.
3. American Heart Association: Standards and guidelines for cardiopulmonary resuscitation. JAMA 244:453, 1980.
4. Guildner, C. W., and Williams, D.: Airway obstructed by foreign material: The Heimlich maneuver. JACEP 5:675, 1976.
5. Ruben, H., Hansen, E., and MacNaughton, F. I.: High capacity suction technique. Anaesthesia 34:349, 1979.
6. Naigow, D., and Powasner, M. D.: The effect of different endotracheal suction procedures on arterial blood gases in a controlled experimental model. Heart Lung 6:808, 1977.
7. Bouzarth, W. F.: Intracranial nasogastric tube insertion (editorial). J. Trauma 18:810, 1978.
8. Horellou, M. F., Mathe, D., and Feiss, P.: A hazard of nasotracheal intubation (letter). Anaesthesia 33:73, 1978.
9. Schofferman, J., Oill, P., and Lewis, A. J.: The esophageal obturator airway. A clinical evaluation. Chest 69:67, 1976.
10. Don Michael, T. A.: Esophageal obturator airway. Med. Instrum. 11:231, 1977.
11. Meislin, H. W.: The esophageal obturator airway: A study of respiratory effectiveness. Ann. Emerg. Med. 9:54, 1980.
12. Gordon, A. S.: An improved esophageal obturator airway. In Safar, P. (ed.): Advances in Cardiopulmonary Resuscitation. Berlin, Springer-Verlag, 1977.
13. Johnson, K. R., Genovesi, M. G.,and Lassar, K. H.: Esophageal obturator airway: Use and complications. JACEP 5:36, 1976.
14. Scholl, D. G., and Tsai, S. H.: Esophageal perforation following the use of the esophageal obturator airway. Radiology 122:315, 1977.
15. Bouzarth, W. F.: Trauma to the head. In Schwartz, G. R., et al. (eds.): Principles and Practice of Emergency Medicine. Philadelphia, W. B. Saunders Co., 1978, pp. 608–618.
16. American Heart Association: Advanced Life Support Manual. Dallas, American Heart Association, 1975.
17. McGovern, F. H., Fitz-Hugh, G. S., and Edzeman, L. J.: The hazards of endotracheal intubation. Ann. Otol. Rhinol. Laryngol. 80:556, 1971.
18. Applebaum, E. L., Bruce, D. L.: Tracheal Intubation. Philadelphia, W. B. Saunders Co., 1976, pp. 35–37.
19. Lewis, F. R., Schlobohn, R. M., and Thomas, A. N.: Prevention of complications from prolonged tracheal intubation. Am. J. Surg. 135:452, 1978.
20. Black, A. M. S., and Seegobin, R. D.: Pressures on endotracheal tube cuffs. Anaesthesia 36:498, 1981.
21. Grillo, H. C., Cooper, J. D., Geffin, B., and Pontoppidan, H.: A low pressure cuff for tracheostomy tubes to minimize tracheal injury: A comparative clinical trial. J. Thorac. Cardiovasc. Surg. 62:898, 1971.
22. Vogelhut, M. M., and Downs, J. B.: Prolonged endotracheal intubation. Chest 76:110, 1979.
23. Loeser, E. A., Hodges, M., Gliedman, J., Stanley, T. H., Johansen, R. K., and Yonetani, D.: Tracheal pathology following short-term intubation with low-and high-pressure endotracheal tube cuffs. Anesth. Analg. 57:577, 1979.
24. Salem, M. R., Mathrubhutham, M., and Bennett, E. J.: Difficult intubation. N. Engl. J. Med. 295:879, 1976.
25. Kralemann, H., and Coate, R. A.: Utilizing local spray intubation. J. Am. Assoc. Nurse Anesth. 43(2):150, April 1975.
26. Thomas, J. L.: Awake intubation: Indications, techniques and a review of 25 patients. Anaesthesia 24:28, 1969.
27. D'Hollander, A. A., Monteny, F., Dewacheter, B., Sanders, M., and Dubois-Primo, J.: Intubation under topical supraglottic analgesia in unpremedicated and nonfasting patients: Amnesic effects of subhypnotic doses of diazepam and Innovar. Can. Anaesth. Soc. J. 21:467, 1974.
28. Boster, S. R., Danzl, D. F., Madden, R. J., and Jarboe, C. H.: Translaryngeal absorption of lidocaine. Ann. Emerg. Med. 11:461, 1982.
29. Hamill, J. F., Bedford, R. F., Weaver, D. C., and Colohan, A. R.: Lidocaine before endotracheal intubation: Intravenous or laryngotracheal? Anesthesiology 55:578, 1981.
30. Poulton, T. J., and James, F. M., III: Cough suppression by lidocaine. Anesthesiology 50:470, 1979.
31. Collins, V. J.: Principles of Anesthesia. 2nd ed. Philadelphia, Lea & Febiger, 1976.
32. Burroughs Wellcome Co.: Product information. Triangle Park, N.C., Burroughs Wellcome Co., 1979.
33. Goodman, L. S., and Gilman, A. (eds.): The Pharmacological Basis of Therapeutics. 5th ed. New York, Macmillan Publishing Co., 1975.
34. Nugent, S. K., Laravuso, R., and Roger, M.C.: Pharmacology and use of muscle relaxants in children. J. Pediatr. 94:481, 1979.
35. Fahmey, N. R., Malek, N. S., and Lappas, D. G.: Diazepam prevents some adverse effects of succinylcholine. Clin. Pharmacol. Ther. 26:395, 1979.
36. Royston, D., and Wilkes, R. G.: True anaphylaxis to suxamethonium chloride. Br. J. Anaesth. 50:611, 1978.
37. Whittaker, M.: Genetic aspects of succinylcholine sensitivity. Anesthesiology 32:143, 1970.
38. Brooke, M. M., Donovan, W. H., and Stolov, W. C.: Paraplegia: Succinylcholine induced hyperkalemia and cardiac arrest. Arch. Phys. Med. Rehabil. 59:306, 1978.
39. Gronert, G. A., and Theye, R. A.: Pathophysiology of hyperkalemia induced by succinylcholine. Anesthesiology 43:89, 1975.
40. Schoner, P. J., Brown, R. L., Kirksey, T. D., et al.: Succinylcholine induced hyperkalemia in burn patients. Anesth. Analg. 48:764, 1969.
41. Cooperman, H., Strokel, G. E., and Kennell, E. M.: Massive hyperkalemia after administration of succinylcholine. Anesthesiology 32:161, 1970.
42. Mazze, R. I., Escue, H. M., and Houston, J. B.: Hyperkalemia and cardiovascular collapse following administration of succinylcholine to the traumatized patient. Anesthesiology 31:540, 1969.
43. Andersen, N: Changes in intragastric pressure following the administration of suxamethonium. Br. J. Anaesth. 34:363, 1962.
44. Halldren, M., and Wahlin, A.: Effect of succinylcholine on the intraspinal fluid pressure. Acta Anesth. Scand. 3:155, 1959.
45. Hunter, A. R.: Neurosurgical Anesthesia. Oxford, Blackwell Scientific Publications, 1975, p. 99.

46. Jennett, B., and Teasdale, G.: Management of Head Injuries. Philadelphia, F. A. Davis Co., 1981.
47. Salem, M. R., Sellick, B. A., Elam, J. O.: The historical background of cricoid pressure in anesthesia and resuscitation. Anesth. Analg. 53:230, 1974.
48. Sellick, B. A.: Cricoid pressure to control regurgitation of stomach contents during induction of anesthesia. Lancet 2:404, 1961.
49. Sellick, B. A.: The prevention of regurgitation during induction of anesthesia. Wien. 9:3, 1962.
50. Salem, M. R., Wong, A. Y., Mani, M., et al.: Efficacy of cricoid pressure in preventing gastric inflation during bag-mask ventilation in pediatric patients. Anesthesiology 40:96, 1974.
51. Salem, M. R., Wong, A. Y., and Fizzoth, G. F.: Efficacy of cricoid pressure in preventing aspiration of gastric contents in pediatric patients. Br. J. Anaesth. 44:401, 1972.
52. List, W. F. M.: Succinylcholine induced cardiac arrhythmias. Anesth. Analg. 50:361, 1971.
53. McLeskey, C. H., McLeod, D. S., Hough, T. L., et al.: Prolonged asystole after succinylcholine. Anesth. Analg., 49:208, 1978.
54. Wong, A. L., and Brodsky, J. B.: Asystole in an adult after a single dose of succinylcholine. Anesth. Analg. 57:135, 1978.
55. Barnes, P. K.: Masseter spasm following intravenous suxamethonium. Br. J. Anaesth. 45:759, 1973.
56. Donlon, J. V., Newfield, P., Sreter, F., and Ryan, J. F.: Implications of masseter spasm after succinylcholine. Anesthesiology 49:298, 1978.
57. Thompson, J., Fish, S., and Ruiz, E.: Succinylcholine for endotracheal intubation. Ann. Emerg. Med. 11:526, 1982.
58. Speight, T. M., and Avery, G. S.: Pancuronium bromide: A review of its pharmacologic properties and clinical application. Drugs 4:163, 1972.
59. Gray, T. C., Nunn, J. F., and Utting, J. E.: General Anesthesia, 4th ed. London, Butterworths, 1980.
60. Danzl, D. F., and Thomas, D. M.: Nasotracheal intubation in the emergency department. Crit. Care Med. 8:677, 1980.
61. Tintinalli, J. E., and Claffey, J.: Complications of nasotracheal intubation. Ann. Emerg. Med. 10:142, 1981.
62. Zwillnick, C., and Pierson, D. J.: Nasal necrosis: A common complication of nasotracheal intubation. Chest 64:376, 1973.
63. Taryle, D. A., Chandler, J. G., Good, J. T., Jr., Potts, D. E., and Sahm, S. A.: Emergency room intubations—complications and survival. Chest 75:541, 1979.
64. Blanc, V. F., and Tremblay, N. A.: The complications of tracheal intubation: A new classification with a review of the literature. Anesth. Analg. 53:202, 1974.
65. Iserson, K. V.: Blind nasotracheal intubation. Ann. Emerg. Med. 10:468, 1981.
66. Magill, I. W.: Technique in endotracheal anesthesia. Br. Med. J. 2:817, 1930.
67. Jacoby, J.: Nasal endotracheal intubation by an external visual technique. Anesth. Analg. 49:731, 1970.
68. Collins, V. J.: Principles of Anesthesiology, 2nd ed. Philadelphia, Lea & Febriger, 1976.
69. Taylor, P. A., and Towey, R. M.: The bronchofiberscope as an aid to endotracheal intubation. Br. J. Anesth. 44:611, 1976.
70. Lindholm, C. E., and Grenvik, A.: Flexible fiberoptic bronchoscopy and intubation in intensive care. In Ledingham (ed.): Recent Advances in Intensive Therapy. Edinburgh, Churchill Livingstone, 1977, pp. 47–66.
71. Rucker, R. W., Silva, W. J., and Worcester, C. C.: Fiberoptic bronchoscopic nasotracheal intubation in children. Chest 76:56, 1979.
72. American Optical, Scientific Instrument Division: Fiberoptics. Southbridge, MA, American Optical, 1981.
73. Butler, F. S., and Cirillo, A. A.: Retrograde tracheal intubation. Anesth. Analg. 39:333, 1960.
74. Waters, D. J.: Guided endotracheal intubation for patients with deformities of the upper airway. Anesthesia 18:158, 1963.
75. Powell, W. F., and Ozdel, T.: A translaryngeal guide for tracheal intubation. Anesth. Analg. 46:231, 1967.
76. Bourke, D., and Levesque, P.: Modification of retrograde guide for endotracheal intubation. Anesth. Analg. 53:1013, 1974.
77. Hollingshead, W. H.: Anatomy for Surgeons, vol. I, 2nd ed. New York, Harper & Row, 1968, p. 487.
78. Gold, M. I., and Buechal, D. R.: Translaryngeal anesthesia: A review. Anesthesiology 20:181, 1959.
79. Schillaci, R. F., Iaconani, V. E., and Conte, R. S.: Transtracheal aspiration complicated by fatal endotracheal hemorrhage. N. Engl J. Med. 295:488, 1976.
80. Jacoby, J. J., Hamelberg, W., Reed, J. P., et al.: A simple technique for artificial respiration. Am. J. Physiol. 167:798, 1951.
81. Reed, J. P., Kemph, J. P., Hamelberg, W., Hitchcock, F. A., and Jacoby, J. J.: Studies with transtracheal artificial respiration. Anesthesiology 15:28, 1954.
82. Jacoby, J. J., Hamelberg, W., Ziegler, C. H., Flory, F. A., and Jones, J. R.: Transtracheal resuscitation. JAMA 162:625, 1956.
83. Jacobs, H. B.: Emergency percutaneous transtracheal catheter and ventilator. J. Trauma 12:50, 1972.
84. Attia, R. R., Bettit, G. E., Murphy, J. D.: Transtracheal ventilation. JAMA 234:1152, 1975.
85. Levinson, M. D., Scuderi, P. E., Gibson, R. L., and Comer, P. B.: Emergency percutaneous transtracheal ventilation (PTV). JACEP 8:396, 1979.
86. Dunlap, L. B.: A modified, simple device for the emergency administration of percutaneous transtracheal ventilation. JACEP 7:42, 1978.
87. Smith, R. B., Babinski, M., Klein, M., and Pfaeffle, H.: Percutaneous transtracheal ventilation. JACEP 5:765, 1976.
88. Bangas, T. P., and Cook, C. D.: Pressure-flow characteristics of needles suggested for transtracheal resuscitation. N. Engl. J. Med. 262:511, 1960.
89. Editorial: Transtracheal aspiration. N. Engl. J. Med. 269:703, 1963.
90. Spencer, C. D., and Beatty, H. M.: Complications of transtracheal aspiration. N. Engl. J. Med. 286:304, 1972.
91. Lyons, G. D., Garrett, M. E., and Fourier, D. G.: Complications of percutaneous transtracheal procedures. Ann. Otol. 86:633, 1977.
92. Unger, K. M., and Moser, K. M.: Fatal complications of transtracheal aspiration: A report of 2 cases. Arch. Intern. Med. 132:437, 1973.

2

Inhalation Techniques and Oxygen Delivery

WILLIAM L. MORRISSEY, M.D.
MATTHEW H. SMITH, M.D.

Patient Evaluation

The emergency physician is often the first person to confront the patient with pulmonary disease; thus, he or she must be able to rapidly assess the patient and to institute therapy. Diagnostic decisions and choices of treatment are primarily based on the patient's history and findings on physical examination. Adjunct information can be obtained from the microscopic evaluation of sputum (as discussed in Chapter 72), from chest radiographs, and from blood gas analysis (as discussed in Chapter 26). Spirometry or peak flow measurements can also serve a useful role in guiding therapy.

Spirometry

Patients with reversible bronchospasm frequently present to the emergency department. A spirometer is useful in graphically displaying the pattern of a forced expiration on a volume versus time plot. Spirometry should be performed both in the initial assessment of the patient and in the subsequent evaluation of the patient's response to therapy and to guide further intervention. Spirometry is helpful for all but the most severe cases of bronchospasm. The patient with severe bronchospasm is rarely able to cooperate with this procedure.

EQUIPMENT

Devices that are currently available include the water-sealed spirometer, electronically activated spirometers, and computerized models. The water-sealed spirometer is a simple, reliable instrument and the time-honored standard for lung volume measurement. A spirometer generally measures volume on the vertical (y-axis) and time on the horizontal (x-axis) (Fig. 2–1). Because spirometry measures the changing volume of the lungs with time, it provides a good means of displaying the various lung volumes in addition to the emptying characteristics of the lungs and airways.

TECHNIQUE

Spirometric measurements can be made by two techniques. In both techniques, the patient wears nose clips to ensure that all the gas exchanged is registered by the spirometer.

The first technique is called the *two-stage test*. The patient breathes tidally and is asked to inhale maximally, yet slowly, then to return to tidal breathing, followed by a slow maximal exhalation. This technique determines the unforced (or slow) lung volumes. The test is often performed easily and satisfactorily by the patient and thus can provide a true indication of the vital capacity in the patient with dyspnea.

The second technique is the *forced expiration method*. In this test, the patient is asked to expire forcefully and maximally after maximal inspiration. Because this test is very dependent upon the effort of the patient, a full explanation of the test and the exertional requirements must be given. Spirited coaching by the person administering the test may also help the patient. The patient inspires deeply, retains the volume for 1 to 3 seconds, and then expires as forcefully as possible. Because this test is very dependent upon the efforts of the patient, three separate efforts should be obtained, and the one showing the largest measurable vital capacity or forced expiratory volume should be considered the accepted effort.

INTERPRETATION

Various measurements can be obtained from the two techniques that were just described. The two-stage test will yield all the lung volumes, with the exception of the residual volume (RV), the air remaining in the chest at maximal expiration.

The measurements obtainable from the forced spirogram include the forced vital capacity (FVC), the forced expiratory volume in 1 second (FEV_1), and assessment of the midexpiratory flow. Both airflow obstruction and restrictive lung diseases will decrease the FVC and FEV_1. These two groups of respiratory dysfunction can be distinguished by evaluation of the FEV_1/FVC ratio. The normal range for the FEV_1/FVC ratio is 80 to 90 per cent but may be as low as 70 per cent in older people. Values lower than this generally suggest airflow obstruction, because there has been proportionately less emptying of the lungs.

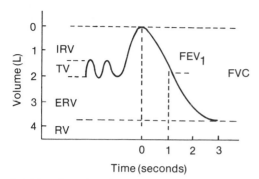

Figure 2–1. Time-forced vital capacity (FVC) is the volume of gas forcibly expelled following a maximal inspiration. Forced expiratory volume in 1 second (FEV$_1$) is the volume of gas expelled during the first second of the forced expiration. The other lung volumes obtainable are the tidal volume (TV), which is the volume of gas moved during quiet respiration; the inspiratory reserve volume (IRV), which is the volume of gas that can be inspired in addition to the tidal gas volume; and the expiratory reserve volume (ERV), which is the volume of gas that can be forcibly expired at the end of a tidal expiration. Some gas cannot be expired and remains in the chest. This is known as the residual volume (RV).

Severity of obstruction is often quantitated by the FEV$_1$/FVC ratio, with a ratio of 70 per cent suggesting mild obstructive disease, 50 per cent suggesting moderate obstructive disease, and less than 35 per cent suggesting severe obstructive disease. An FEV$_1$/FVC of less than 40 per cent is often associated with carbon dioxide retention. Taking serial measurements of FEV$_1$/FVC or FEV$_1$ alone may be a useful method of assessing the need for and the results of therapy in patients with reversible bronchospasm.

Nowak and associates,[1] in an unblinded emergency department study of acute asthmatic patients, determined that an FEV$_1$ of 0.6 L or less prior to treatment or an FEV$_1$ of 1.6 L or less after treatment was associated with an unfavorable course of disease. In this study, 88 per cent of the admitted asthmatic patients met at least one of the criteria. Among all patients with an initial FEV$_1$ of 0.6 L or less, 80 per cent either were admitted or developed subsequent respiratory problems within 24 to 48 hours. Among all patients with a post-treatment FEV$_1$ of 1.6 L or less, 75 per cent either were admitted or developed subsequent respiratory problems.

In restrictive lung diseases, bronchodilators do not help to increase airflow because of a limitation in the volume that the lung can contain. In this family of disorders, the FEV$_1$ will be reduced in proportion to the FVC, and the FEV$_1$/FVC ratio will be normal or slightly increased.

The severity of restrictive lung diseases can also be assessed by an initial spirometric measurement, although this preliminary measurement is often inadequate to quantitate precisely the degree of restriction. The range of severity of restrictive disease parallels that of the obstructive diseases, with FVC and FEV$_1$ reductions to 70 per cent, 50 per cent, and 35 per cent of predicted values representing mild, moderate, and severe restrictive disease, respectively. The assessment of restrictive disease in the presence of significant obstruction is generally not possible using these limited techniques.

When assessing possible decreases in pulmonary function, it is important to remember that the predicted normal value for vital capacity will vary among patients. In Table 2–1, such variability is shown according to age, height, and gender. Furthermore, knowledge of the patient's previous pulmonary function tests (baseline values) often assists in decision-making.

Peak Flow Measurements

As noted previously, the forced spirogram is a test that is dependent upon the effort of the patient, and some patients, including children, may not be able to cooperate adequately for valid test results to be obtained. Because peak airflow is also reduced in obstruction and because peak flow measurements do not depend upon a sustained effort, peak flow measurement is often a preferable test for measuring the degree of bronchospasm, particularly in children.

TECHNIQUE

There are several devices available for recording the peak flow, and all function similarly. The patient is asked to inspire maximally and then to expire forcefully into the flowmeter. A sustained effort is not required. Based upon the peak flow generated during expiration, the peak flowmeter will register a value representing the liters of flow per minute that would occur if the peak flow were sustained.

INTERPRETATION

In children, predicted peak flow rates vary linearly with patient height, from 150 L per min at a height of 42 inches to 550 L per min at a height of 72 inches. In adults, the value varies with both

Table 2–1. MAJOR PARAMETERS DETERMINING PREDICTED FORCED VITAL CAPACITY (FVC) IN ADULTS

Gender	Age (yrs)	Height (in)	FVC (predicted)
Male	20	72	6.0 L
Male	70	64	3.5 L
Female	20	68	4.5 L
Female	70	62	2.5 L

age and height but generally remains between 550 and 650 L per min in males and between 400 and 500 L per min in females.

Nowak and coworkers,[2] in an unblinded prospective clinical study of emergency department patients with acute asthma, found a good correlation of peak expiratory flow rate (PEFR) with FEV_1. Furthermore, they found a good correlation between PEFR and admission to the hospital or a successful outpatient course. Of the patients who had both a pre-treatment PEFR less than 100 L per min and a post-treatment PEFR less than 300 L per min, 92 per cent required admission or had an unsuccessful outpatient course. Of patients who had a pre-treatment PEFR less than 100 L per min and an improvement less than 60 L per min after initial treatment with terbutaline sulfate, 85 per cent were admitted to the hospital or developed respiratory problems after they were discharged.

Martin and colleagues,[3] using slightly different criteria for admission in a blinded prospective study of emergency department asthmatic patients, did not find as clear a distinction between the PEFR values and the decision to admit the patient. Martin and colleagues did note that all patients requiring admission had a PEFR less than 30 per cent predicted prior to treatment and less than 40 per cent predicted after 6 hours of treatment, and a change in PEFR of less than 30 per cent predicted at 20 minutes after a single subcutaneous dose of epinephrine. None of the patients with PEFR measurements greater than these required admission or sustained a relapse within 48 hours.

Martin and associates[4] found the PEFR to be potentially useful for limiting use of arterial blood gases in their population. No patient with a PEFR of 25 per cent or greater predicted had a Pa_{CO_2} greater than 45 mm Hg or a pH less than 7.35. Martin and coworkers estimate that restricting the use of arterial blood gases to patients with a PEFR less than 25 per cent predicted would eliminate the need for blood gases in at least 40 per cent of their emergency department asthmatic population.

The peak flowmeter is also useful in the assessment of upper airway or laryngeal obstruction. In adults with upper airway lesions, a critical obstruction (orifice less than 5 mm) correlates with flows less than 150 L per min and suggests the need for close observation and consideration of elective tracheostomy or intubation.

Oxygen Therapy

After an initial patient assessment has been made, the emergency physician must provide specific therapies aimed toward supporting the im-

paired physiology. For the patient with pulmonary decompensation, such therapy includes techniques to improve the matching of ventilation with perfusion within the lungs, thus decreasing the amount of desaturated blood leaving the lungs. Whereas the later sections of this chapter are mainly concerned with correcting ventilation/perfusion mismatches, in this section we will concentrate on therapy that alleviates the effects of such disturbances. The physician must remember that the actual delivery of oxygen (O_2) to tissues is not determined solely by the arterial oxygen tension (Pa_{O_2}) but also by the cardiac output (CO) and O_2 carrying capability of the blood.

The O_2 carrying capacity of blood is mostly determined by the hemoglobin (Hgb) concentration, with each gram of Hgb being able to carry 1.34 ml O_2 per 100 ml of blood (volume per cent). Other factors include the status of the red blood cell and the quality of hemoglobin within it, but these two factors are usually of minimal concern. Chronic hypoxemia and acidemia may lead to a rightward shift in the oxyhemoglobin dissociation curve (Fig. 2–2). The shift decreases the affinity of hemoglobin for oxygen, resulting in more oxygen being released at the tissue level. Variant hemoglobins with different O_2 affinities can occasionally be of clinical importance.

In the emergency unit, the relative importance of these factors can often be quickly and effectively evaluated with a hematocrit determination and an examination of the bloodsmear or mean corpuscular volume (MCV) determination. When available, direct measurement of oxygen saturation (oximetry) can also be useful. The oxygen saturation routinely reported by the laboratory is generally an ideal value, read from a chart correlating saturation and Pa_{O_2}

Assuming that there is adequate cardiac output and an adequate number of functional red blood cells, restoration of an adequate arterial oxygen tension is the next priority. Although O_2 is ubiquitous in nature, constituting 21 per cent of atmospheric gas at sea level, when given to patients in higher concentrations, it attains the status of a

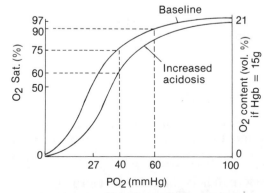

Figure 2–2. O_2-Hgb Dissociation curve.

drug, and it must be used correctly in order to prevent the side effects inherent in the use of any drug. Once the decision has been made that inadequate oxygenation in the presence of respiratory system disease is contributing to tissue hypoxia, an enriched oxygen gas mixture is indicated. Furthermore, because arterial hypoxemia occurs in many patients who are seriously ill, oxygen should be started empirically for any patient with suspected hypoxemia while a baseline arterial blood gas sample is being analyzed. Only in cases of pure neurologic or muscular dysfunction, in which the respiratory system is intact and the hypoxemia is secondary to inadequate function of the bellows mechanism with an elevation of arterial carbon dioxide tension (Pa_{CO_2}), will restoration of ventilation and reduction in Pa_{CO_2} without supplemental O_2 be sufficient to restore an adequate Pa_{O_2} (Table 2–2). This is true because in these situations the lungs retain their normal gas-exchanging function and, if expanded, can adequately participate in normal gas transfer.

Ordinarily, enough supplemental O_2 should be provided to restore the Pa_{O_2} to a level at which the Hgb is at least 90 per cent saturated. Using the oxyhemoglobin dissociation curve, this level is generally assumed to be approximately 60 mm Hg. Because of the shape of the curve, with the plateau segment beginning at approximately a Pa_{O_2} of 60, efforts to increase the Pa_{O_2} further with higher concentrations of supplemental O_2 will yield little further increase in the Hgb saturation but can predispose to O_2 toxicity (see Fig. 2–2).

Although O_2 toxicity is generally not noted in the emergency department setting, inappropriate initiation of high inspired oxygen concentrations may result in continued use of excess oxygen in subsequent patient care. Oxygen toxicity is a clinical syndrome consisting of increasing tracheobronchitis, followed by a picture that is consistent with the adult respiratory distress syndrome. This syndrome consists of decreasing lung compliance, patchy atelectasis, non-cardiogenic pulmonary edema, and eventually, pulmonary fibrosis. The syndrome is caused by exposure of the pulmonary parenchyma to high concentrations of oxygen free radicals that overwhelm the reducing capabilities of the tissues and result in progressive parenchymal destruction.

The area most susceptible to damage by these radicals is the alveolocapillary membrane, possibly because this membrane is in close proximity to increased radical concentrations both in the gas in the alveolus and in the blood in the capillary. Because the concentration of O_2 radicals is directly proportional to the fraction of inspired oxygen (FIO_2), O_2 toxicity can best be avoided by meeting but *not* exceeding the patient's oxygen needs. Oxygen toxicity is generally considered to be a risk only when oxygen concentrations of 60 to 100 per cent are used; however, if the patient has had damage to the pulmonary parenchyma by malnutrition or exposure to irradiation, chemotherapy, or paraquat, toxicity may occur at lower concentrations of 40 to 50 per cent. In addition to causing classic O_2 toxicity, high oxygen concentrations can predispose to other problems, including decreased mucociliary transport, which can impair the clearance of secretions, and atelectasis of poorly ventilated areas secondary to the absorption of O_2 from the alveoli.

It has been shown in patients with pulmonary disease as well as in healthy individuals that the alveolar oxygen tension (PA_{O_2}) rises in a fairly linear manner with the use of increasing concentrations of supplemental O_2. The response of the PA_{O_2} to supplemental oxygen can be calculated quickly and accurately from the alveolar gas equation, whose simplified form is:

$$PA_{O_2} = [(PB - 47) \times FIO_2] - (Pa_{CO_2} \times 1.2)$$

In this equation, PA_{O_2} = alveolar O_2 tension; FIO_2 = fractional inspired O_2 concentration; Pa_{CO_2} = arterial CO_2 tension; PB = barometric pressure; and 47 represents the partial pressure of water vapor in the lungs. The equation can be simplified for calculating PA_{O_2} at sea level ($P_B = 760$) while breathing room air ($F_{IO_2} = 0.21$) as follows:

$$PA_{O_2} = [(760 - 47) \times 0.21] - (Pa_{CO_2} \times 1.2)$$
$$= 150 - 1.2 (Pa_{CO_2})$$

Note that the alveolar air equation used in this chapter represents an approximation of the equa-

Table 2–2. CAUSES OF RESPIRATORY FAILURE*

Neurologic	**Lower Airway**
Drug overdose	Tracheobronchitis
Stroke	Tracheal stenosis
Central hypoventilation	Bronchospasm
Guillain-Barré syndrome	
Head trauma	**Lung Parenchyma**
Poliomyelitis	Adult Respiratory
Botulism	distress syndrome
	Emphysema
Muscles and Chest Wall	Pneumonia
Myopathy	Interstitial pneumonitis
Myasthenia gravis	
Kyphoscoliosis	**Heart**
Flail chest	Pulmonary edema
	Mitral stenosis
Oropharynx	
Foreign body	
Laryngospasm	
Tonsillar hypertrophy	

*Disease at any level of the respiratory system, central or peripheral nervous system, bellows mechanism, or heart may cause respiratory failure.

tion given in Chapter 3. The form used in this chapter is adequate for oxygen therapy decisions.

Because normal people have neither significant ventilation/perfusion (V/Q) mismatch nor diffusion abnormalities, the expected arterial oxygen tension (Pa_{O_2}) depends almost solely upon the alveolar oxygen tension and is generally 5 to 10 mm Hg less than it. At sea level, atmospheric pressure is 760 torr (or mm Hg). The nasopharynx fully humidifies the gas that reaches the lower airway, displacing 47 torr of gas with water vapor. Thus, the sum of partial pressures of the original gases that reach the lower airway is 713 torr. If a patient were breathing 100 per cent oxygen, the partial pressure of inspired oxygen would be 713 torr. The PA_{O_2} in the normal person may be calculated after arterial blood gases (ABG) have been determined. If we assume that the oxygen concentration of room air is 21 per cent and that the ABG values of $Pa_{O_2} = 95$, $Pa_{CO_2} = 40$, then:

$$PA_{O_2} = 0.21 \,(713) - 1.2 \,(40)$$
$$= 150 - 48$$
$$= 102 \text{ torr}$$

Finally, the alveolar-arterial oxygen gradient, or the *difference* between alveolar and arterial oxygen (A–a D_{O_2}), can be determined. If the PA_{O_2} is calculated to be 102 torr and the Pa_{O_2} is measured at 95 torr, the A–a gradient is 7 torr. The calculation of the PA_{O_2} for an individual at sea level breathing a 50 per cent oxygen mixture with a normal Pa_{CO_2} of 38 torr is:

$$PA_{O_2} = 0.5 \,(713) - 1.2 \,(38)$$
$$= 357 - 46$$
$$= 311 \text{ torr}$$

If this individual had normal lungs and a normal alveolar-arterial O_2 *difference* (A–a D_{O_2}) of approximately 10 torr, the Pa_{O_2} would be $311 - 10$, or 301 torr.

In a patient with lung disease, the response to supplemental O_2 is also linear, but the dose-response relationship is different. A more useful formula in some patients with altered pulmonary function is the arterial/alveolar O_2 *ratio* (a/A O_2 ratio). If, as in the aforementioned situation, when breathing 50 per cent O_2, the PA_{O_2} is 311 torr and the patient has a measured Pa_{O_2} of 150 torr, his a/A O_2 *ratio* would equal 150/311 or approximately 0.5. If his oxygen concentration were subsequently decreased to an FIO_2 of 0.28, then:

$$PA_{O_2} = 0.28 \,(713) - 1.2 \,(38)$$
$$= 200 - 46$$
$$= 154 \text{ torr}$$

and with his a/A O_2 ratio of 0.5, we would expect his new Pa_{O_2} to be 0.5×154 torr, or 77 torr.

These concepts are useful in initiating therapy. If, for example, while breathing ambient air, a patient's presenting arterial blood gases were:

$$Pa_{O_2} = 42 \text{ torr; } Pa_{CO_2} = 25 \text{ torr; pH} = 7.55$$

the PA_{O_2}, A–a O_2 difference, and a/A O_2 ratio can be calculated:

$$PA_{O_2} = 0.21 \times (713) - 1.2 \,(25)$$
$$= 150 - 28$$
$$= 122 \text{ torr}$$
$$\text{A–a } D_{O_2} = 122 - 42$$
$$= 80 \text{ torr}$$
$$\text{a/A } O_2 \text{ ratio} = 42/122$$
$$= 0.35$$

To determine the FIO_2 required to achieve a minimally acceptable Pa_{O_2} of 60 torr, assuming that the a/A ratio will remain constant, then:

$$Pa_{O_2}/PA_{O_2} = 0.35$$
$$60/PA_{O_2} = 0.35$$
$$60/0.35 = PA_{O_2}$$
$$176 \text{ torr} = PA_{O_2}$$

Knowing that a PA_{O_2} of 176 torr is needed to get a Pa_{O_2} of 60, the alveolar gas equation is used to determine the requisite FIO_2:

$$PA_{O_2} = FIO_2 \,(713) - 1.2 \,(Pa_{CO2})$$
$$176 = FIO_2 \,(713) - 1.2 \,(25)$$
$$204/713 = FIO_2$$
$$0.29 = FIO_2$$

Thus, a minimum of 29 per cent O_2 should be provided to ensure obtaining a Pa_{O_2} of 60 torr. Because this prediction may not be exact but only a close approximation, a slightly richer O_2 mixture (35 to 40 per cent) should be initiated until repeat arterial blood gases are obtained.

One admonition about the use of oxygen is that it must never be stopped precipitously, particularly in the patient in whom there is the danger of resulting hypoxemia. For example, in a patient with initial blood gases of pH = 7.45, $Pa_{CO_2} = 48$, and $Pa_{O_2} = 52$, if 4 L per min of O_2 by nasal cannula were given, his next ABG could reveal a pH = 7.32, $Pa_{CO_2} = 58$, and $Pa_{O_2} = 95$. In this patient who depended upon the hypoxic ventilatory drive, 4 L O_2 (≈ 37 per cent FIO_2) suppressed this drive and led to CO_2 retention and respiratory acidemia. If the mistake were noted at the time, the immediate tendency would be to remove the oxygen supplementation. The ABG could then revert to a pH = 7.32, Pa_{CO_2} = 58, and Pa_{O_2} = 40, demonstrating worsening hypoxemia when there is persistent CO_2 retention despite an unchanged A–a gradient. Decreasing the supplemental oxygen in such a manner that the patient receives some enrichment, perhaps 2.0 L O_2 flow, would be more appropriate and might result in ABG of pH = 7.36, Pa_{CO_2} = 54, and Pa_{O_2} = 70, thereby avoiding both hypoxemia and further CO_2 retention.

OXYGEN DELIVERY SYSTEMS AND PRIMARY EQUIPMENT

In respiratory therapy, a gas source and the method for delivering the gas to the source outlet are regarded as primary equipment. The equipment that constitutes the remainder of the delivery system, from the source outlet to the patient, is considered secondary equipment. The gas source is generally either a cylinder or a large liquid reservoir system. A cylinder is a hollow container made from high-quality seamless steel capable of withstanding high internal pressures of at least 2200 psi (pounds per square inch). The manufacturer is responsible for re-checking the integrity and pressure testing the cylinder at least once every 5 years. Several gases in addition to oxygen are used in treating patients; thus, cylinders are painted different colors according to the gas that they contain (Table 2–3).

When using cylinders of different sizes (Table 2–4), it is important to know the period of time that the cylinder can provide the desired supply of oxygen. The following equation may be useful in calculating this time period:

$$\text{Time in minutes} = \frac{\text{gauge pressure (psi)} \times \text{cylinder factor}}{\text{flow rate (L per min)}}$$

Example:
A full "E" cylinder of oxygen with a gauge pressure of 2200 psi used at 6 L per min would last:

$$2200 \times 0.28 \div 6 = 103 \text{ min, or about 1.5 hr,}$$

whereas a full "G" cylinder at 2.0 L per min would last:

Table 2–3. COLOR CODES FOR MEDICAL GASES

Oxygen	Green or white
Carbon dioxide	Grey
Helium	Brown
Cyclopropane	Orange
Nitrous oxide	Light blue
Ethylene	Red

Table 2–4. CYLINDERS FOR OXYGEN DELIVERY

Cylinder Size	Height (in.)	Volume (L)	Cylinder Factor
"E"	30	650	0.28
"G"	48	5600	2.41
"H"	54	6900	3.14

$$2200 \times 2.41 \div 2 = 2651 \text{ min, or 44 hours}$$

A cylinder valve is in place when the cylinder is supplied. The gas leaving the cylinder is under high pressure, and a reducing valve must be applied to lower this pressure to the range of 30 to 50 psi, the normal working pressure of the delivery system. This is the same pressure at which gas is provided from wall-mounted outlet stations.

Most hospitals are also equipped with large liquid oxygen reservoir systems. This is understandable from a volume consideration alone, because 1 L of liquid oxygen can expand to form 892 L of gaseous oxygen; therefore, liquid systems conserve storage space. A long series of safety regulations promulgated by the National Fire Protection Association (NFPA) dictates the location of the main reservoir and the characteristics of the piping system. Wall outlets must have either a manual shutoff valve for closing the outlet when it is not in use or a spring-loaded plunger that closes automatically when the striker (or quick connect) is removed from an outlet. The responsibility for ensuring that built-in oxygen systems are functioning appropriately is one that emergency personnel cannot ignore.

Once oxygen is available at a suitable delivery pressure, a flow rate must be chosen. A flowmeter is a device for both indicating and controlling the gas flow. The meter is constructed so that the gas supplied to it is at a standard pressure of 50 psi. Most flowmeters control flow by means of a needle valve that widens and narrows the orifice through which the gas flows. The flow is indicated by the varying level of a marker suspended in a vertical tube of increasing diameter. In a Thorpe tube, the indicator is a ball float; in a kinetic flowmeter, the indicator is a plunger float.

Because most flowmeters are constructed to work in the upright position, laying them on their side or at an angle will affect the accuracy of the reading. Some flowmeters use a dial face to monitor gas flow, and are less dependent upon position. Additionally, because a flowmeter is calibrated to the density characteristics of a single gas, if gases other than the calibration gas are used with the meter, the reading will vary according to the relative densities of the two gases.

Often, a reducing valve and a flowmeter are combined into a single controlling unit known as a *regulator*. Regulators generally contain two dial gauges, one representing cylinder pressure and the other indicating gas flow. Regulators are only used with cylinder systems because no modification of the delivery pressure is needed with wall units. Emergency personnel should be familiar with the technique for providing gas from cylinders.

1. Secure the tank in an upright position so that it will not move or fall while being manipulated.

2. Remove the cylinder seal ("E" tank) or cylinder cap ("G," "H" tank).

3. Turn the cylinder valve on and off quickly to clear ("crack") the valve. On the "E" tank, this is done with a wrench, and on the "G" or "H" tank, it is done with the cylinder handle.

4. Check the yoke to ensure that it is compatible for use with oxygen, and place it on the cylinder, being sure that the fittings are compatible.

5. Tighten the yoke, making certain that any necessary gasket is in place.

6. Close the needle valve.

7. Slowly open the cylinder valve until the pressure maximizes.

8. Observe that the cylinder contains adequate pressure to ensure a reasonable supply of gas.

9. Connect a humidifier or nebulizer unit and the desired form of patient connection (e.g., cannula, mask).

10. Open the needle valve so that the desired oxygen flow registers on the flowmeter.

The outlet of a cylinder valve is indexed according to the gas that it contains. Large ("G," "H") cylinders may be indexed according to thread size and type, right- or left-handed threading, internal or external threading, and the nipple seat design. Indexing of small ("E") cylinders with post-type valves is by means of a Pin-Index Safety System (PISS), whereby two holes are placed in specific locations on the post, corresponding to the locations of two pins in the post valve specific for the gas in question.

SECONDARY OXYGEN DELIVERY SYSTEMS

Gas leaving the flowmeter is dry, and unless a very low flow is used, drying of the upper and lower airways can become annoying to the patient. This effect is amplified in the lower airway if the normal humidification mechanisms of the nasopharynx are bypassed either by high-flow mouth breathing or by direct application of gas through an endotracheal tube.

The capacity of any gas for water vapor increases as a function of its temperature, and a gas that is 100 per cent saturated at room temperature is only slightly more than half saturated at body temperature. Delivery of water to the respiratory tract can be accomplished either by humidification, which provides water in the gas phase, or by nebulization, in which water is aerosolized and presented to the airway as water droplets in a gaseous suspension. Several secondary systems for delivering and humidifying oxygen-enriched gas mixtures are readily available.

Cannula. The simplest and most commonly used oxygen delivery system is the nasal cannula. In this system, the prongs of the cannula extend about 1 cm into the nares and deliver 100 per cent oxygen from the O_2 source at a desired gas flow rate measured in liters per minute. Each liter per minute of flow up to about 6 L per min corresponds to approximately a 3 to 4 per cent increase in O_2 concentration (Table 2–5). The system uses the ambient air in the nasopharynx as its reservoir; therefore, the FIO_2 rarely increases above 45 per cent. Patients who are mouth breathers can still benefit from O_2 enrichment with use of the nasal cannula, because the O_2-enriched gas in the nasopharynx will be entrained as long as the nares are patent.

The advantages of the cannula system include ease in both setup by the therapist and usage by the patient. The system is comfortable and well tolerated by most patients. Because it does not obstruct the mouth, patients can continue to receive oxygen supplementation while eating or talking. Additionally, the cannula system is useful for ambulatory patients, because 50-foot tubing systems are available.

There are a few disadvantages inherent in the use of the nasal cannula. Most important is the unreliability of the final O_2 concentration delivered to the lower airway. The FIO_2 delivered varies with the patient's respiratory pattern. A higher minute ventilation ($\dot{V}_E$) results in proportionately less O_2 enrichment and lower final O_2 concentration than does a low $\dot{V}_E$ that entrains proportionately more O_2. Variability in final O_2 concentration is of importance, particularly in patients with CO_2 retention who depend upon their hypoxic respiratory drive for respiratory stimulation rather than upon the usual, primary hypercapnic drive.

Table 2–5. OXYGEN SUPPLEMENTATION BY NASAL CANNULA

L/Min O_2 Flow	FIO_2 (approx. %)
0	21
1	25
2	29
3	33
4	37
5	41
6	45

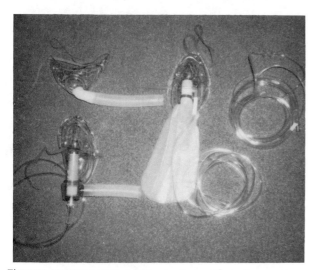

Figure 2–3. Types of O_2 delivery systems. *Clockwise*, Tracheostomy collar, non-rebreathing mask, nasal cannulae, and Venturi mask.

Another disadvantage of the nasal cannula is that the O_2 delivered is often poorly humidified. Clinically, this means that flows greater than about 6 L per min will have a pronounced drying effect on the nasal mucosa and can become uncomfortable and even painful to the patient. Lastly, because of the limited volume of the nasopharyngeal reservoir, flows exceeding 6 L per min usually lead to only small and inconsistent additional increases in the FIO_2. Nevertheless, the nasal cannula is a very useful system in a wide variety of situations in which the amount of O_2 needed does not exceed approximately 40 per cent.

Masks. Several varieties of masks are available (Fig. 2–3). They share several positive and negative features common to their format.

Advantages include higher flow rates than are possible with nasal prongs, permitting both a higher final FIO_2 and better humidification.

Disadvantages are that the masks are of variable fit and are often a cause of patient discomfort. If they are fairly tight, the patient may have facial irritation. In addition, a feeling of suffocation is sometimes present, despite the fact that supplemental O_2 is being provided, because both the nose and mouth are enclosed by the mask. Lastly, the patient must remove the mask to eat, drink, or expectorate. These factors often lead to its being worn either incorrectly or not at all. Facial irritation and anxiety are sometimes reduced with a more open variant of the face mask called the *face tent*.

The adequacy of flow in a system that uses an oxygen reservoir is determined by the patient's minute ventilation. If the $\dot{V}_E$ exceeds the flow in the system, the reservoir will empty and room air will be entrained, decreasing the FIO_2 delivered.

The simple open mask is similar to the nasal cannula in that the final FIO_2 depends, to some degree, upon the patient's respiratory pattern, but since it uses the mask itself as its reservoir, it benefits from less variability. Also, because it is a larger reservoir and covers both the nose and the mouth, it can provide an FIO_2 as high as 50 or 60 per cent at maximum flow rates of 15 L per min.

Venturi masks deliver a well-controlled, final oxygen concentration and are available in FIO_2's of 24, 28, 31, 35, 40, and 50 per cent. The commercially available Venturi systems develop their final oxygen concentration by using the oxygen flow as a jet, entraining a fixed proportion of room air. The characteristics of the most common systems are shown in Table 2–6.

By mixing the gases at a distance from the patient, a stable concentration is delivered to the patient. This limits the maximum oxygen concentration available but also generally fixes the minimum oxygen concentration that the patient receives, because the Venturi systems have such high flow rates. In an individual with normal lungs and a basal minute ventilation ($\dot{V}_E$) of about 5 L, the inspiratory flow rate will average 10 to 15 L per min, varying with the respiratory pattern. In the patient with a higher but sustainable (for short periods) $\dot{V}_E$ of 30 L per min, the average inspiratory flow rate may reach the range of 60 to 100 L per min. Thus with large minute ventilations, even the high flow rates of the Venturi system may be exceeded, resulting in the entrainment of additional room air by the patient and a mild decrease in the final FIO_2.

The obvious benefit of a Venturi system is tighter control of the delivered FIO_2, ensuring that there is an absolute maximum concentration in the system. Moisture in the Venturi system can be provided at the site of gas entrainment (room air), because proportionately more gas enters the system here. This is accomplished by placing a collar around the entrainment orifice into which a nebulizer delivers aerosol. This collar has the added advantage of ensuring that the entrainment ports cannot be inadvertently blocked or occluded. The nebulizer should not be powered by an oxygen source, because this would obviously alter the FIO_2 delivered by the system.

There are two types of masks with reservoir

Table 2–6. CHARACTERISTICS OF COMMON VENTURI SYSTEMS

Delivered FIO_2 (%)	O_2 Flow (L/min)	Entrained Room Air (L/min)	Total Flow (L/min)
24	4	101.0	105.0
28	4	41.1	45.1
31	6	41.4	47.4
35	8	37.1	45.1
40	8	25.2	33.2
50	10	17.2	27.2

bags: partial rebreathing and non-rebreathing. They provide for the highest concentrations of supplemental O_2, approximately 60 per cent in the former and 90 per cent in the latter. Great care must be taken with these masks to ensure a tight fit and good patient compliance so that a high FIO_2 is actually being delivered. The highest concentration of oxygen that can be delivered is obtained by using a non-rebreathing mask with a reservoir. This system may be useful for patients with carbon monoxide poisoning in whom the half-life of carboxyhemoglobin is reduced in proportion to the FIO_2.

Tents. Oxygen and humidity may also be delivered by an oxygen tent. Generally, the use of this system is limited to pediatric patients because of their relatively small size. Tents are cumbersome, and may be fire hazards. Access to the patient for procedures and examinations is limited, and oxygen concentrations are variable.

Disadvantages of oxygen tents are that the maximum oxygen concentration attainable in this type of system is only about 40 per cent, and even this drops precipitously when the tent is opened. There is also little place for the oxygen tent in the emergency department.

CPAP. Another method of oxygen delivery is the tight-fitting mask with continuous positive airway pressure (CPAP). In all the previously described methods, supplemental O_2 is provided without alteration of the normal pressure relationships in the intrathoracic and extrathoracic parts of the respiratory tract. Under normal conditions, gas flow is initiated by movement of the muscles of respiration, and passive filling of the lungs occurs from the negative pressures created. Exhalation is mediated by elastic recoil of the lungs, with airflow resulting from decreasing the negative pressure during recoil. At no time during spontaneous unforced respiration are the airway pressures positive.

There are certain pathologic states, notably pulmonary edema, either cardiogenic or non-cardiogenic, in which the pathophysiology includes instability of alveoli with early closure. This loss of functional alveoli is equivalent to widespread microatelectasis with a loss of gas-exchanging units and a resulting shuntlike effect. Generally, hypoxemia secondary to ventilation/perfusion mismatch responds to oxygen supplementation. In states where hypoxemia is secondary to *shunting* it will *not* improve, because the oxygen-enriched gases still do not have access to the mixed venous blood. Historically, in ventilator-dependent patients with the clinical syndrome of non-cardiogenic pulmonary edema or adult respiratory distress syndrome (ARDS), it has been noted that the maintenance of positive airway pressure at the end of the ventilator cycle (PEEP) permitted some

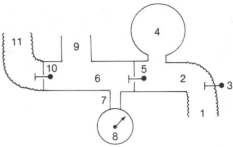

Figure 2–4. CPAP system diagram. *1*, Gas inlet thru large bore flexible tubing; *2*, Inhalation chamber; *3*, One-way safety valve, allows entrainment of room air; *4*, Reservoir (at least 2 L); *5*, One-way valve to patient chamber; *6*, Patient chamber; *7*, Connecting tube for aneroid manometer; *8*, Anaeroid manometer; *9*, Patient connection; *10*, One-way exhalation valve; and *11*, Flexible tube to PEEP valve.

portion of these collapsing alveoli to remain open, thus making them more available for gas exchange. Analogously, in the nonintubated spontaneously breathing patient who otherwise has no need of mechanical ventilation, this same positive airway pressure can be provided by a CPAP system (Fig. 2–4).

In practice, a humidified gas mixture is introduced into an inhalation chamber that is fitted with a reservoir bag. To allow for high patient flows, a one-way safety valve is placed in the chamber, allowing for the entrainment of room air if needed during an emergency. The gas leaves the chamber through another one-way valve and enters the patient chamber. The pressure in this latter chamber is monitored, and the patient is allowed to breathe from the gas in this chamber. Exhaled gas exits from this chamber through a third one-way valve that is connected to a positive-pressure chamber or underwater seal.

CPAP in infants is achieved through different systems than in adults. In one system, a large flow enters one end of a tube. Resistance to flow is achieved by a narrow orifice valve at the opposite end, creating a fixed positive pressure in the tube. The patient then breathes from this chamber and is exposed to the positive pressure within the tube. This system is feasible in infants, because their small tidal volumes do not affect the pressure in the system, but is not practical in adults because of the tremendous flows needed to maintain similar pressures with the much larger adult tidal volumes.

CPAP is most useful in the patient with adult respiratory distress syndrome caused by aspiration, fat embolism secondary to long bone fracture, smoke inhalation, abuse of narcotics or salicylate overdosage, trauma, or neurologic injury.

The obvious advantage of CPAP is its ability to provide positive pressure without the need for intubation. This permits the recovery of the functional residual capacity (FRC) lost by microatelectasis and may reverse life-threatening hypoxemia that has been unresponsive to oxygen. Also, CPAP may permit adequate oxygenation with a lower FIO_2 through the same mechanism and thus avoid oxygen toxicity.

Disadvantages are 1) adverse effects of positive intrathoracic pressure with a possible decrease in venous return and cardiac output, 2) risk of positive airway pressure producing barotrauma such as pneumothorax or pneumomediastinum, 3) patient discomfort or skin damage owing to the tightness of the mask, 4) aerophagia, and 5) mask leaks that may lead to rapid life-threatening hypoxemia.

T-Pieces. The oxygen supply may be connected directly to a tracheal airway already in place using a T-tube arrangement. A T-tube is a system in which high-flow humidified gas in large bore tubing passes by the patient connection. The gas flows by this point into a tail composed of similar tubing. When the patient inhales, gas is entrained from both the main tubing and the tail piece. When the patient exhales, gas fills both limbs of the system. Requirements for the T-piece system are that the tail be long enough so that when the patient inspires, room air is not entrained, and that the gas flow be great enough to allow both limbs of the T-piece to flush during exhalation before the next inhalation is begun.

As in most systems in which true humidification is used, there will be a tendency for water to accumulate in the proximal tubing. Because this tube is directly connected to the trachea via the endotracheal tube, care must be taken to prevent this water from being emptied into the airway. The temperature of the humidified gas must not be allowed to be excessive to the point of causing airway burns. Lastly, the addition of a significant volume of water into the airway decreases the volume of insensible water loss and may lead to positive fluid balance and contribute to volume overload in patients who are otherwise predisposed.

An alternate means of providing supplemental oxygen and humidification to the patient with a tracheostomy is the trach-collar. This device consists of a small plastic dome into which the proximal tubing delivers humidified gas. The collar is similar to the T-piece, but its advantages are that it puts less traction and tension on the tracheostomy tube and thus is more comfortable for both short periods of time and long-term wear, and is less likely to result in water being poured into the airway. The disadvantage of the collar is that it fits looser than a T-piece and can more easily entrain room air from outside the dome and decrease the FIO_2, particularly at greater flow rates.

Aerosols

INTRODUCTION

An aerosol consists of a number of particles of liquid or solid that are suspended in a gas. Natural aerosols include fogs, plant spores, salt spray at the beach, and airborne bacteria. Some manmade aerosols are cigarette smoke, chemical mists, dusts, and combustion products.

Some important properties of an aerosol are the size and shape of its particles, the density of the particles, particle charge, and the nature of the aerosol as a whole. The latter may include the number, concentration, or the number of particles produced per unit volume, and also the uniformity of the particle size and the amount of skew from this size. All these factors can influence lung deposition. An aerosol with particles of widely varying size is called a *polydisperse aerosol,* and most of its mass is contained in relatively few particles. More uniform particle sizes form a *monodisperse aerosol* in which most of the particles have a similar mass.

Because an aerosol is an unstable system, it begins to decay as soon as it is created. The properties of the aerosol as well as the characteristics of the diluent gas determine the relative stability of the system. The suspended particles can interact with one another, with the diluent gases, or with the boundaries of the system.

AEROSOL GENERATORS

Aerosols can be generated in several different ways and most use some combination of the following three methods: 1) atomization of a solution (creation of a polydisperse aerosol), 2) pulverization or the dispersion of dry powder, and 3) condensation of liquid from the gaseous phase.

An *atomizer* is a device that produces polydisperse aerosol. It is appropriate for creating an aerosol intended to impact quickly on a surface and when particle size is relatively unimportant, such as in spraying the throat with a local anesthetic. A *nebulizer* is a device that creates a monodisperse aerosol. It can deliver particles to any desired part of the airway. Examples of common nebulizers include cold steam generators, high-humidity mask systems, and ventilator circuits.

Ultrasonic nebulizers use piezoelectric crystals that vibrate at high frequencies. The vibrations pass through a liquid and produce an aerosol of great uniformity when they contact the air-fluid interface. The particle size is dependent upon frequency. The ultrasonic systems add a great amount of energy to the liquid that they nebulize and raise the temperature of the aerosolized particles. Because higher energies are needed to produce smaller particles, the amount of heat generated is usually the limiting factor in particle size. Cooling is necessary to prevent the fluid from becoming too hot and is provided primarily by gas flow. If there is insufficient gas flow, the aerosol will not cool adequately. At higher flow rates, the density of the aerosol may be reduced, because ultrasonic nebulizers do not use a flow-related mechanism to produce their aerosol.

One benefit of heat produced by the ultrasonic nebulizer is the addition of 100 per cent relative humidity to the high-density aerosol without the need for a separate heating device. Ultrasonic nebulizers are thus useful when a great volume of water needs to be added to the respiratory system. Furthermore, the ultrasonic nebulizer does not need a supplemental oxygen source and therefore can be used when oxygen supplementation is not needed or is contraindicated. Finally, the device is quite efficient at producing a high-density aerosol. Disadvantages of the ultrasonic system are the high initial cost, the relative fragility and higher incidence of system breakdown, and the potential for fluid overload.

Finally, there is the modern hand nebulizer (metered dose inhaler), a pressurized device containing a gas that evaporates at below room temperature. Activating the valve releases a pre-measured jet burst of aerosol. Diluent gas then evaporates as the aerosol particles are inhaled.

HUMIDIFIERS

In contrast to atomizers and nebulizers, which add liquid water to a gas, humidifiers provide only gaseous water, without particulate water, to the system. Often this is accomplished by heating the gas and water or by saturating the gas with water at room temperature, as with a bubble humidifier. The heated units must use high temperatures, because cooling will occur as the gas travels from the humidifier to the patient. With the cooling, condensation will occur, because the gas loses some of its water-carrying capability as its temperature decreases. Care should be taken to direct the conducting tubing downward and away from the patient so that liquid water will not reach the patient.

A popular device for providing heated humidification is the cascade humidifier, which passes the gas through a heated liquid film. Although the cascade humidifier was not primarily designed for patient re-warming, it can be used to increase core temperature via the airways in cases of hypothermia (see Chapter 73).

There are several other classes of humidifiers. Pass-over or blow-by humidifiers direct the gas stream tangentially to the water surface. The low gas-water contact time and small surface area available make this a rather inefficient system. Bubble humidifiers release the gas under water, with the creation of bubbles, which increase the surface area of the gas exposed to water. In jet humidifier/nebulizers, a stream of gas entrains water droplets conducted through a capillary tube. This creates a combination of nebulization and true humidification. When the nebulized particles are removed by a series of baffles, only humidified gas leaves the unit.

Generally, in the emergency setting, the physician is concerned about inducing sputum (ultrasonic nebulizer), providing adequate moisture to patients receiving oxygen therapy (cascade humidifier, bubble humidifier), delivering aerosolized medication (hand nebulizer, side-stream jet nebulizer), or increasing core temperature (heated mainstream nebulizer).

USE OF AEROSOLS: GENERAL CONCEPTS

Aerosols are widely used in the treatment of pulmonary diseases. In the delivery of nebulized particles to various levels of the respiratory system, aerosols of different qualities are required. It is important to understand the constraints of the various aerosol systems.

For the purposes of localizing aerosol deposition, the respiratory tract may be conveniently subdivided into three zones: 1) the nasopharyngeal zone, which is composed of the nares and the larynx; 2) the tracheobronchial zone, which includes the larger airways from the trachea to the terminal bronchioles (greater than 0.7 mm in diameter); and 3) the pulmonary zone, which consists of the respiratory bronchioles, alveoli, and ducts.

In the nasopharynx, the narrow and curving geometry creates a turbulent airflow that favors deposition by impaction. This is further enhanced by interdigitating cilia projecting into the lumen of the nares. Within the tracheobronchial tree, the flow is more laminar; however, turbulence remains at the bifurcations, with impaction being important there. Lastly, in the pulmonary compartment, gas flow is relatively slow owing to the large cross-sectional area. Slow air movement favors diffusion and sedimentation rather than impaction as the methods by which particles deposit.

A functional size gradient exists for particle deposition. Three- to 10-micrometer–sized particles are most subject to inertial forces, particularly at high flow rates, and tend to be removed in the nasopharyngeal zone. Particles between 1 and 3 micrometers in size are usually deposited in the tracheobronchial zone. Functionally, there is a gap in the continuum at this range of particle size. Particles less than 0.1 micrometer in size are retained by diffusion in the pulmonary zone. Those between 1.0 and 0.1 micrometer are not lost by impaction, sedimentation, or diffusion but remain in the flow of air. Approximately 80 per cent of these particles are removed from the lung during exhalation.

Another variable affecting the percentage of aerosol delivered to the lower airways is the pattern of respiration. Maximal deposition in the lower airways is accomplished by having the patient inhale the aerosol through his mouth from functional residual capacity to total lung capacity at low flow rates of 0.5 to 1 L per second. The aerosol inhalation should start at the end of one tidal breath just as the patient initiates the next breath. The inhalation should continue until the patient fully expands his lungs. Retention can also be enhanced by breath-holding, allowing more time for diffusion in the lower airways. The benefits of the breath-holding maneuver are maximized at approximately 10 seconds. Obviously, if the lower airways are not the prime target of therapy, the breathing pattern becomes less important.

Of some concern is the theoretical problem of aerosol distribution when there is airway disease. If the airways are non-uniform, those that need therapy may not receive it. Proximal deposition is enhanced by bronchiectasis, and areas with bronchospasm, excessive secretions, or consolidation may show decreased deposition of aerosol.

On the positive side, obstruction will also decrease aerosol clearance, leading to increased retention at the site of obstruction. This may favor resolution of the obstruction by increasing the concentration of therapeutically active particles at the obstruction site if the blockage is due to bronchospasm. If the blockage is caused by a destructive lung disease, particles may be trapped distally where they are inactive. If a high proportion of particles impact at the sites of reversible obstruction, these areas will experience bronchodilation. The airways distal to these sites may not be exposed to medication during the initial bronchodilator aerosol treatment. Repetition of the treatment at 15-minute intervals can lead to progressive bronchodilation over as many as 6 cycles. When possible, the nebulizer selected should generate particle sizes appropriate for the intended target area.

METHODS OF MEDICATION DELIVERY

Inhaled bronchodilators are the most frequently aerosolized compounds and have proved to be of value. There are several different classes of agents that can promote bronchodilation when inhaled. The most popular and widely used are the $beta_2$-adrenergic agonist agents. In the United States, these include albuterol (Ventolin, Proventil) and metaproterenol (Alupent, Metaprel). The generic name for albuterol in Europe is salbutamol. These agents are available in hand nebulizer (metered dose inhaler) form. Albuterol is currently unavailable in solution for use in a side-stream nebulizer. Another agent frequently used by the inhaled route is isoetharine (Bronkosol). The primary disadvantage of isoetharine is that its duration of action is approximately half that of metaproterenol. The beta agonists promote bronchodilation by accelerating the rate of formation of cyclic adenosine monophosphate (cAMP). The resulting increase in cellular concentration of cAMP decreases smooth muscle tone in the lower bronchial tree where the beta receptors are located. The onset of bronchodilation is rapid after inhalation of bronchodilators, with 75 per cent of the maximum effect seen in 5 minutes, peak effect noted from 30 to 90 minutes, and little decline in effect over 4 hours (as previously noted, the effect of isoetharine may last only 2 to 3 hours). Because these agents are relatively specific for the $beta_2$-adrenergic receptors, they minimize cardiostimulatory activity (mediated by $beta_1$ receptors). Isoproterenol (Isuprel) may result in significant side effects caused by $beta_1$ stimulation and is rarely indicated for inhalation, despite potent $beta_2$ effects.

Inhaled anticholinergics such as atropine are of use in blocking the vagal component of the reflex arc in parasympathetic bronchoconstriction, thereby decreasing levels of cyclic guanosine monophosphate (cGMP) and favoring a reduction in bronchial smooth muscle tone. The onset of action of the anticholinergics is delayed compared with the $beta_2$ agonists, with maximal effects appearing at 3 to 4 hours, but bronchodilation also seems to be more prolonged. Anticholinergics are helpful in bronchospasm secondary to mechanical stimulation of the airways, for example, in patients who are being treated by intubation, in elderly patients, and perhaps in those who have a psychogenic component to their bronchospasm. Despite theoretical concerns that atropine may produce a harmful drying of the airways and predispose to mucous inspiration, no clinically significant drying effect has been noted.

Other inhaled agents sometimes used include the inhaled steroids, cromolyn, antibiotics, and mucolytics. Beclomethasone in doses of 8 to 20 inhalations (400 to 1000 micrograms) per day may be useful in providing topical control of airway inflammation. Inhaled steroids are of limited value when the inflammation is severe or when the disease resides in the parenchyma. Inhaled steroids are *not* indicated in the control of *acute* bronchospasm but are commonly used in long-term control of airway inflammation.

Cromolyn sodium is an aerosol of solid particles. The mode of action is prevention of mediator release, avoiding degranulation of mast cells. Because of the mode of action of cromolyn, it is useful in the *prophylaxis* of bronchospasm, especially if the patient is aware that he is about to encounter a provocative situation. Cromolyn aerosol is *not* useful after an attack has started.

Mucolytic agents such as *N*-acetylcysteine are of little or no proven benefit in therapy. *N*-acetylcysteine theoretically works because its sulfhydryl groups are capable of attacking the disulfide bonds of nucleic acids and glycoproteins in mucus. Mucolytics have been shown to be effective in vitro and after direct tracheal instillation but as yet are not proven to be beneficial when given as an aerosol. Undesirable effects of these agents include bronchospasm, decreased vital capacity, and worsening of arterial blood gases secondary to these effects.

Technique of Administration

Inhaled bronchodilators are easily administered using a side-stream nebulizer. The beta$_2$ agonists (metaproterenol or isoetharine) are diluted (0.2 to 0.5 ml of the bronchodilator solution in 3 ml of normal saline) and placed in the reservoir well of a side-stream nebulizer. The nebulizer should be driven with pressurized oxygen rather than air if the patient is markedly hypoxic. Such patients should have continuous cardiac monitoring and medical observation during and following nebulizer treatments.

The patient is then instructed to inhale through the nebulizer mouthpiece in tidal breaths, with a deep breath once every 3 to 5 respirations. The treatments last 10 to 20 minutes until the solution is depleted. In the emergency situation, treatments may be repeated as often as every 15 to 20 minutes until either the patient obtains relief or a significant increase in the heart rate (20 per cent increase or about 20 beats per minute) or cardiac dysrhythmias signal cardiac stimulation secondary to loss of the beta$_2$ specificity.

Atropine has been used in adults in doses of 2 to 3 mg in 3 to 5 ml of normal saline solution and administered every 4 to 6 hours. Atropine treatments should *not* be immediately repeated, because systemic absorption of the drug may generate tachycardia. Ipratropium bromide (Atrovent), an atropine derivative, has shown less systemic absorption and may soon replace atropine. The recommended dosage of ipratropium is 20 to 40 mg three times daily; however, experience with the drug is limited.

BLAND AEROSOLS

As previously noted, an aerosol vehicle is of proven value for the delivery of bronchodilators and topical glucocorticoids. There are fewer data to support the use of bland aerosols. A bland aerosol is considered to be water or any saline solution. The theoretical benefits of bland aerosols include adding water to the secretions of the lower airways to yield thinner, more easily expectorated sputum. Unfortunately, no more than a small amount (10 per cent) of the water delivered by most available systems is deposited on the lower airways and the viscosity of sputum is not significantly altered.

The main use of bland aerosols is to provide humidity to the upper airways in an effort to counteract drying of the larynx and trachea. Bland aerosol has never been proved to be more effective than 100 per cent humidity generated by humidifiers but may provide a possible alternative to it. On the negative side, the introduction of water particles into the lower airways may produce bronchospasm in some susceptible individuals.

A more controversial use of bland aerosol is in sputum induction. Hypotonic saline solution and water may cause irritation of the upper airway through their osmotic effects. This may lead to an effective cough in patients who are otherwise unable to produce sputum, but it will not produce thinner sputum. In patients who receive frequent aerosol treatments or when aerosol is applied to an endotracheal tube, care must be taken to ensure that no significant volume of water remains in the airway. Cough and suctioning are the primary methods that are recommended for removing secretions in the emergency setting.

Chest Physiotherapy

Chest physiotherapy and postural drainage are often indicated to help clear the lung of secretions, particularly when such secretions are copious or tenacious. Effectively performed, treatments can increase the volume of sputum produced and may transiently increase the Pa$_{O_2}$ and FEV$_1$.

Percussion and postural drainage are most appropriate as part of a long-term home care program in patients with cystic fibrosis, chronic bronchitis, bronchiectasis, and pneumonia in which thick, highly viscous secretions are produced. Dysfunction of the tracheobronchial elevator is often noted in patients who have endotracheal tubes; such patients may also benefit from these procedures. The areas of the chest that will undergo chest physiotherapy and postural drainage should be determined by a combination of physical examination and chest radiography, with attention directed toward areas of atelectasis, rhonchi, bronchial breathing, or consolidation.

INDICATIONS AND CONTRAINDICATIONS

In the emergency situation, chest physiotherapy is indicated as only part of the therapy to help clear secretions. Physiotherapy is not indicated for atelectasis except when collapse is secondary to retained secretions. Chest physiotherapy should be avoided in cases in which secretions do not exist, because the treatment may result in a small reduction in FEV_1 and Pa_{O_2}. Chest physiotherapy is contraindicated if the patient is experiencing any of the following: trauma, flail chest, recent chest surgery, hemoptysis, tuberculosis, and lung abscess. Extra care should be exercised in the osteoporotic patient.

TECHNIQUE

Percussion is performed by placing the cupped hand on the chest wall overlying the desired segment and repetitively striking the chest wall with the cupped hand. The patient should sense the outline of the hand and the air within the cupped portion. The process is continued throughout the respiratory cycle at the rate of 3 to 5 percussions per second. The treatment is generally repeated two to four times daily, and sessions should continue as long as the process is productive but not to the point of operator or patient fatigue. Care should be taken not to percuss the sternum, scapula, or kidney regions.

Vibration is performed by keeping the hand in contact with the chest wall. Repetitive isometric contractions of the shoulder and forearm are carried out. Vibration may be better tolerated than percussion.

Postural drainage is accomplished by aligning the bronchus to be drained in a near vertical position above the trachea. The anatomy of the tracheobronchial tree dictates the most effective position for drainage to proceed under the influence of gravity from the involved lobe into the trachea. Procedures should be carried out in an orderly manner, beginning with the upper lobes and proceeding in a way that minimizes the expenditure of energy by the patient through turning and rolling. After completion of a treatment, suctioning should take place to remove the secretions that have been mobilized, particularly if the patient's own cough mechanisms are weak or suppressed.

A variety of mechanical percussors and vibrators **are** available to assist with these treatments and are of use to patients who must care for themselves; however, they offer no specific advantages over manual therapy.

Intermittent Positive-Pressure Breathing (IPPB) Therapy

Intermittent positive-pressure breathing (IPPB) is the application of a pressure-cycled (or limited) inspiratory phase to a patient's respirations. The patient then exhales spontaneously into the environment. The origins of IPPB date back to the late 1930's. It was first used for pulmonary edema. In the 1950's, IPPB experienced a rapid increase in popularity, unsupported by well-controlled studies but spurred on by the development of practical portable pressure-cycled ventilators (Fig. 2–5).

IPPB is thought of as somewhat of a panacea, being used to treat many varieties of pulmonary disease. Some of the claims for IPPB include optimum delivery of aerosols, improvement in the clearance of secretions, a decrease in the effort required for breathing, improvement in the matching of ventilation/perfusion, and a decrease in airway resistance. Few, if any, of these claims have been proved.

Specifically, IPPB has not been shown to increase the delivery of aerosol over what is obtained by generating the aerosol with a simple nebulizer device. Indeed, delivery to the respiratory tract may be lessened with IPPB, because it can lead to aerophagia and increased deposition in the gastrointestinal tract. Similarly, IPPB has never been documented to improve ventilation/perfusion

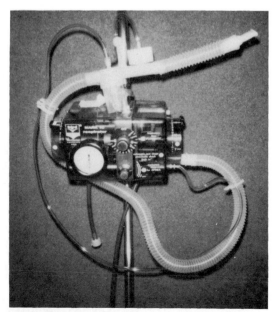

Figure 2–5. Intermittent positive-pressure breathing (IPPB) apparatus.

matching, but it has been shown actually to *increase* the effort required for breathing in some patients. This is especially true in chronic obstructive pulmonary disease. IPPB has been shown to increase expiratory work more than it decreases inspiratory work, resulting in a slight increase in the work of breathing in most patients. There is no proof that it aids in the clearance of secretions.

INDICATIONS AND CONTRAINDICATIONS

In the patient who is weaning from or has just been weaned from mechanical ventilation and who breathes with small tidal volumes, volume-oriented IPPB can be used in a manner similar to that of a frequent sigh mechanism. This may reduce atelectasis and prevent respiratory failure. An IPPB breath may enable a patient to cough more effectively. Aerosol therapy can be delivered as nebulized particles in the IPPB gas stream, although IPPB should not be ordered solely for aerosol delivery, because treatments by mini-nebulizer or other simple nebulizers are equally effective. Another major indication for the use of IPPB is for psychological benefit in those patients who have already come to depend upon it and in whom the sensation of positive pressure assures the adequacy of their therapy. The main benefit of IPPB therapy is in the delivery of increased inspired volume to patients who either cannot or will not take sufficiently deep spontaneous breaths to prevent atelectasis. In the spontaneously breathing patient who is also cooperative, other methods such as incentive spirometry are superior to IPPB in preventing atelectasis.

The usage of IPPB should be restricted to a narrower range of applications than has previously been the case. IPPB is contraindicated in conditions in which positive pressures may cause an exacerbation of the underlying disease. Low cardiac reserve states, severe emphysema with air-trapping (especially with bullous disease), pneumothorax, worsening subcutaneous emphysema, and tracheoesophageal fistula are all contraindications to the use of IPPB. Hemoptysis and active tuberculosis are generally listed as contraindications to IPPB usage, but this belief is anecdotal and not supported by objective data. Obviously, positive pressure usage should be avoided if simpler alternative therapies are available.

TECHNIQUE

IPPB therapy is administered by asking the patient to exert a small negative inspiratory effort, which triggers the pressure-cycled ventilator to deliver a desired oxygen mixture up to a specific pressure limit. The gas most often contains either bland or therapeutic nebulized aerosol. These positive pressure inspiratory and spontaneous expiratory cycles are generally repeated six to eight times per minute for 15 to 20 minutes, three or four times daily. Occasionally, treatments are given more frequently. The therapist should record both the peak airway pressure produced and the corresponding volume delivered by the ventilator cycles (volume-oriented IPPB).

The delivery of volume-oriented IPPB is obtained by measuring the actual expired volume corresponding to a specific pressure on the pressure-cycled ventilator. An arbitrary maximum pressure (less than 40 cm of H_2O) should be preselected. For example, the therapist or nurse may be instructed not to exceed a peak inspiratory pressure of 25 to 30 cm of H_2O pressure while attempting to deliver a 1000 ml tidal volume. Hopefully, the measured volume returned will be 1 L or greater in the averge-sized patient and the peak pressure limit will not be reached. Although a volume of 1 L may seem large, this is not unreasonable when one recalls that most adults have a vital capacity greater than 3 L.

COMPLICATIONS

The use of IPPB carries with it the risks of pneumothorax, decreased cardiac output, and hyperventilation, even to the point of unconsciousness. Although most patients do not experience any of the aforementioned complications, all patients experience the physiologic consequences of applying positive pressure to the airways. Because the positive pressure is transmitted to the pulmonary vasculature with compression of these vessels, blood is initially forced out of the capillaries into the left heart. After this, however, increased pulmonary resistance decreases the transfer of blood from the right to the left heart with subsequent peripheral venous pooling, which may cause a severely decreased cardiac output in the patient with a previously compromised cardiac reserve or hypovolemia. IPPB can also cause bronchospasm by the irritating effects of the bland aerosol and pressure on the airways. Patients may also experience aerophagia or, in patients with air-trapping, hyperinflation.

1. Nowak, R. M., Gordon, K. R., Wroblewski, D. A., et al.: Spirometric evaluation of acute bronchial asthma. JACEP 8:9, 1979.
2. Nowak, R. M., Penslar, M. I., Sarker, D. D., et al.: Comparison of peak expiratory flow and FEV$_1$ admission criteria for acute bronchial asthma. Ann. Emerg. Med. 11:64, 1982.

3. Martin, T. G., Elenbaas, R. M., and Pingleton, S. H.: Failure of peak expiratory flow rate to predict hospital admission in acute asthma. Ann. Emerg. Med. 11:466, 1982.
4. Martin, T. G., Elenbaas, R. M., and Pingleton, S. H.: Use of peak expiratory flow rate to eliminate unnecessary arterial blood gases in acute asthma. Ann. Emerg. Med. 11:70, 1982.

General

1. Burton, G. G., and Gee, Glen N. (eds.): Respiratory Care. Philadelphia, J. B. Lippincott Co., 1977.
2. Schwartz, G. R., et al. (eds.): Principles and Practice of Emergency Medicine. Philadelphia, W. B. Saunders Company, 1978.
3. McPherson, S. P.: Respiratory Therapy Equipment. St. Louis, The C. V. Mosby Co., 1977.
4. National Heart, Lung, and Blood Institute (NHLBI): Proceedings of the 1979 conference on the scientific basis of in-hospital respiratory therapy. Am. Rev. Respir. Dis. 122(2):1, 1980.
5. National Heart and Lung Institute (NHLI): Proceedings of the conference on the scientific basis of respiratory therapy. Am. Rev. Respir. Dis. 110(2):1, 1974.

Aerosols

1. Brain, J. D. and Valberg, P. A.: State of the art review deposition of aerosol in the respiratory tract. Am. Rev. Respir. Dis. 120:1325, 1979.
2. Lourenço, R. V., and Cotromanes, E.: Clinical aerosols. (I) Characterization of aerosols and their diagnostic uses. Arch. Intern. Med. 142:2163, 1982, and (II) Therapeutic aerosols. Arch. Intern. Med. 142:2299, 1982.
3. Rossing, T. H., et al.: Emergency therapy of asthma: comparison of the acute effects of parenteral and inhaled sympathomimetics and infused aminophylline. Am. Rev. Respir. Dis. 122:365, 1980.
4. Ryan, G., et al.: Standardization of inhalation provocation tests: influence of nebulizer output, particle size, and method of inhalation. J. Allergy Clin. Immunol. 67:156, 1981.
5. Dolovitch, M. B., et al.: Optimal delivery of aerosols from metered dose inhalers. Chest 80 (supplement):911, 1981.
6. Newman, S. P., et al.: Simple instructions for using pressurized aerosol bronchodilator. J. Royal Soc. Med. 73:776, 1980.
7. Newhouse, M. T.: Principles of aerosol therapy. Chest 82 (supplement):32, 1982.
8. Newhouse, M. T., and Ruffin, R. E.: Deposition and fate of inhaled aerosols. Chest 73 (supplement):936, 1978.
9. Rossing, T. H., et al.: A controlled trial of the use of single versus combined drug therapy in the treatment of acute episodes of asthma. Am. Rev. Respir. Dis. 123:190, 1981.
10. Nelson, H. S.: Beta adrenergic agonists. Chest 82 (supplement):33, 1982.

11. Pakes, G. E., et al.: Ipratropium bromide: a review of its pharmocologic properties and therapeutic efficacy in asthma and chronic bronchitis. Drugs 20:237, 1980.
12. Rebuck, A. S., et al.: Anticholinergic therapy of asthma. Chest 82 (supplement):55, 1982.
13. Heimer, D., et al.: The effect of sequential inhalation of metaproterenol aerosol in asthma. J. Allergy Clin. Immunol. 66:75, 1980.

Oxygen

1. Altschuler, S. L.: Oxygen therapy in pulmonary disease. Med. Clin. North Am. 57:851, 1973.
2. Mithoefer, J. C., et al.: Response of the arterial PO_2 to oxygen administration in chronic pulmonary disease. Ann. Intern. Med. 74:328, 1971.
3. Mithoefer, J. C., et al.: The $AaDO_2$ and venous admixture at varying inspired oxygen concentrations in COPD. Crit. Care Med. 6:131, 1968.
4. Anthonisen, N. R.: Hypoxemia and O_2 therapy. Am. Rev. Respir. Dis. 126:729, 1982.
5. Covelli, H. D., et al.: Efficacy of continuous positive airway pressure administered by face mask. Chest 81:147, 1982.
6. Greenbaum, D. M., et al.: Continuous positive airway pressure without tracheal intubation in spontaneously breathing patients. Chest 69:615, 1976.
7. Smith, J. P., et al.: Acute respiratory failure in chronic lung disease. Observations on controlled oxygen therapy. Am. Rev. Respir. Dis. 97:791, 1968.
8. Campbell, E. J. M.: Respiratory failure, the relation between oxygen concentrations of inspired air and arterial blood. Lancet 2;10, 1960.
9. Campbell, E. J. M.: A method of controlled oxygen administration which reduces the risk of carbon dioxide retention. Lancet 2;12, 1960.
10. Schiff, M. M., and Massaro, D.: Effect of oxygen administration by a Venturi apparatus on arterial blood gas values in patients with respiratory failure. N. Engl. J. Med. 277:950, 1967.

Other

1. Kelsen, S. G., et al.: Emergency room assessment and treatment of patients with acute asthma. Adequacy of the conventional approach. Am. J. Med. 64:622, 1978.
2. Shim, C. S., and Williams, M. H.: Evaluation of the severity of asthma. Am. J. Med. 68:113, 1980.
3. Williams, M. H., Jr., et al.: Life-threatening asthma. Arch. Intern. Med. 140:1604, 1980.
4. Rebuck, A. S., et al.: Evaluation of the severity of the acute asthmatic attack. Chest 82 (supplement):29, 1982.
5. Godfrey, S., et al.: Spirometry, lung volumes, and airway persistence in normal children aged 5 to 18 years. Br. J. Dis. Chest 64:15, 1970.
6. Schilling, J. P., and Kasik, J. E.: Intermittent positive pressure breathing: a continuing controversy. J. Iowa Med. Soc., March 1980, p. 99.

3

Mechanical Ventilation

WILLIAM DURSTON, M.D.

Mechanical ventilation is a potentially lifesaving mode of therapy with which all physicians involved in emergency or critical care medicine should be thoroughly familiar. Yet the field of ventilator therapy is evolving so rapidly and modern ventilators are so versatile and complex that it is difficult even for those involved in daily care of ventilator patients to maintain mastery of this subject. The purpose of this chapter is to provide a practical yet complete guide to mechanical ventilation. Although the following sections are written primarily with the emergency physician in mind, they are intended to serve as a reference for all practitioners, from medical student to critical care specialist.

Historical Background

The notion that a person who is not breathing on his own can be resuscitated by someone or something breathing for him dates back to at least 850 B.C., when it was recorded in the Bible that the prophet Elisha resuscitated a Shunammite boy: "And he put his mouth on his mouth and the flesh of the child waxed warm."[1] Not until the Industrial Revolution many centuries later was the first mechanical device for artificial ventilation described. In 1864, Alfred E. Jones of Lexington, Kentucky was issued the first patent for a mechanical ventilator, a negative-pressure device that he claimed "cured paralysis, neuralgia, rheumatism, seminal weakness, asthma, bronchitis, and dyspepsia" (Fig. 3–1A).[2] In 1929, Drinker and Shaw patented the first practical iron lung, designed for the treatment of respiratory failure.[3] With this ventilator, the patient lay on a sliding bed with his head outside the apparatus, a rubber collar around his neck, and the remainder of his body inside the metal tank, which was evacuated and recompressed by an electrical pump (Fig. 3–1B). Although it was extremely cumbersome, the Drinker-Shaw iron lung, with few modifications, was used extensively for three decades and contributed to the survival of many polio victims with respiratory insufficiency.[4]

Techniques for positive-pressure ventilation during general anesthesia were developed during the 1920s but were not applied to patients outside of the operating room until the Scandinavian polio epidemic of 1952–53, when the Danish anesthesiologist Bjorn Ibsen showed that survival was improved in patients ventilated through a cuffed endotracheal tube as compared with patients ventilated in iron lungs.[5] The positive pressure for Dr. Ibsen's patients was supplied by teams of nurses, medical students, and interns squeezing rubber anesthesia bags. By 1955, when a polio epidemic struck New England, a positive-pressure ventilator was commercially available, and once again the superiority of positive-pressure ventilation was demonstrated.[6] Respiratory intensive care units soon proliferated, and as the incidence of polio declined, positive-pressure mechanical ventilation came to be used not only in patients with respiratory failure due to neuromuscular disease but also in patients with a variety of other pulmonary and cardiac disorders. The explosive growth in the application of mechanical ventilation is illustrated by the records of Massachusetts General Hospital, where the number of patients treated on ventilators increased from 66 in the year 1958 to approximately 1500 in 1971.[7] In addition to the development of more reliable ventilators, the invention of the clinical blood gas electrode in the early 1960s contributed to the more widespread application of mechanical ventilation.[8]

Almost all patients who require mechanical ventilation today are treated with positive-pressure ventilation by means of an endotracheal tube or a tracheostomy tube. In a few select cases, however, negative-pressure ventilation is the method of choice. Patients with chronic respiratory insufficiency caused by chest wall deformity and patients with intermittent respiratory insufficiency resulting from neurologic diseases, such as "Ondine's curse," have been managed successfully out of the hospital for prolonged periods with cuirass or tank-type negative-pressure ventilators.[9, 10] For the most part, however, negative-pressure ventilators are of historical interest only. In the remainder of this chapter, only positive-pressure ventilation will be discussed. The abbreviations that will be used in this chapter are listed in Table 3–1.

Indications for Mechanical Ventilation

The principal indication for mechanical ventilation is respiratory failure. Respiratory failure can be defined in terms of arterial blood gases, although criteria based upon pulmonary mechanics have also been proposed. The indications for mechanical ventilation are summarized in Table 3–2.

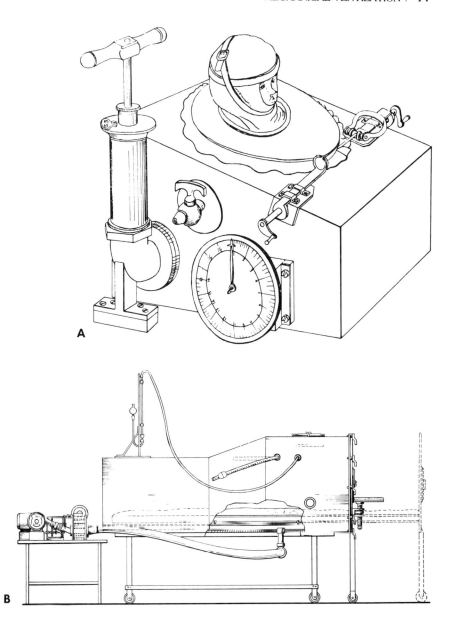

Figure 3–1 A, The first mechanical ventilator, patented by Alfred Jones of Lexington, Kentucky, in 1864. (From Crit. Care Med. 6:310, 1978. Used by permission.) B, The Drinker-Shaw iron lung, patented in 1929, was the standard ventilator for polio victims during the early 1950s. (From Crit. Care Med. 7:226, 1979. Used by permission.)

Respiratory failure in adults is usually defined as a Pa_{O_2} less than 60 mm Hg while the patient is breathing the maximum oxygen concentration achievable by mask or a Pa_{CO_2} greater than 50 mm Hg with a pH less than 7.30. These criteria must sometimes be modified by the clinical situation. For example, a patient with chronic obstructive pulmonary disease (COPD) who is a chronic carbon dioxide retainer but who is no longer maintaining his usual metabolic alkalosis might have blood gases on low-flow oxygen showing a Pa_{O_2} of 55, a Pa_{CO_2} of 50, and a pH of 7.32 and not be considered in respiratory failure, whereas a young asthmatic with the same blood gases might be in need of immediate intubation and mechanical ventilation.[11]

In addition to arterial blood gases, other indices of pulmonary function may be helpful in determining whether or not a patient needs mechanical ventilation. In adults, a respiratory rate of greater than 35 to 40 per minute usually cannot be sustained for prolonged periods, and if this rate is required to maintain a normal pH or Pa_{CO_2}, tachypnea may be an indication for mechanical ventilation. A forced expiratory volume in 1 second (FEV_1) of less than 1000 ml or less than 10 ml per kg indicates severe airway obstruction and, if not readily reversible, predicts that the patient may need ventilatory assistance. A vital capacity less than 15 ml per kg or a maximum inspiratory force (MIF) less than 25 cm H_2O is another indicator that the patient will not be able to maintain ade-

Table 3–1. ABBREVIATIONS USED IN THIS CHAPTER

$A–a\ D_{O_2}$	Alveolar-arterial oxygen difference
C_a	Oxygen content of systemic arterial blood
C_c	Oxygen content of pulmonary capillary blood
C_v	Oxygen content of mixed venous blood
COPD	Chronic obstructive pulmonary disease
CPAP	Continuous positive-airway pressure
EPAP	Expiratory positive-airway pressure (spontaneous breathing with PEEP)
f	Respiratory rate or frequency
FEV_1	Forced expiratory volume in 1 second
$F_{I_{O_2}}$	Per cent oxygen content of inspired gas
IMV	Intermittent mandatory ventilation
MIF	Maximum inspiratory force
MVV	Maximum voluntary minute volume
$P_{A_{CO_2}}$	Alveolar carbon dioxide tension
Pa_{CO_2}	Arterial carbon dioxide tension
$P_{A_{O_2}}$	Alveolar oxygen tension
Pa_{O_2}	Arterial oxygen tension
$P_{E_{CO_2}}$	Tension of carbon dioxide in mixed expired air
PEEP	Positive end-expiratory pressure
Q_s/Q_t	Shunt fraction (ratio of right-to-left shunt to total pulmonary blood flow)
R	Respiratory quotient (ratio of carbon dioxide produced by the body to oxygen consumed)
SIMV	Synchronized intermittent mandatory ventilation
V_A	Alveolar ventilation
$\dot{V}_A$	Alveolar minute ventilation
V_c	Vital capacity
$\dot{V}_{CO_2}$	Carbon dioxide production per minute
V_d	Dead space volume
$\dot{V}_E$	Expired minute volume
V_t	Tidal volume

quate ventilation on his own. Similarly, a dead space to tidal volume ratio (V_d/V_t) of greater than 0.6 implies a high minute volume requirement and a need for ventilatory assistance in most patients.

Table 3–2. INDICATIONS FOR MECHANICAL VENTILATION

Blood gas criteria
  Pa_{O_2} less than 55 to 60 mm Hg on maximum $F_{I_{O_2}}$ by mask
  Pa_{CO_2} greater than 50 mm Hg and pH less than 7.30
Blood gas criteria in neonates
  Patient on CPAP of 5 to 8 cm H_2O and $F_{I_{O_2}}$ up to 0.80
  Pa_{O_2} less than 55 to 60 mm Hg
  Pa_{CO_2} greater than 60 mm Hg
  pH less than 7.25
Criteria based on pulmonary mechanics
  Vital capacity less than 10 ml per kg
  FEV_1 less than 10 ml per kg
  MIF less than 25 cm H_2O
  V_d/V_t greater than 0.6
Indications other than respiratory failure
  Need for hyperventilation
    Increased intracranial pressure
    Tricyclic antidepressant overdose
  Hypothermia
    Mechanical ventilation used as means of core rewarming
  Prophylactic postoperative mechanical ventilation
    In postoperative patients with shock, morbid obesity, COPD, neuromuscular disease, or other debilitating illness or following cardiothoracic surgery

Respiratory failure in adults is usually caused by primary pulmonary disease, cardiac disease, neuromuscular disease, or a combination of factors. In infants, respiratory failure usually results from hyaline membrane disease or meconium aspiration. The blood gas criteria for respiratory failure in infants are somewhat different from those in adults, since more deviation from the physiologic norm is allowed before mechanical ventilation is instituted. Arterial blood gas indications for mechanical ventilation in infants proposed in the literature include a Pa_{O_2} less than 50 to 60 mm Hg or a Pa_{CO_2} greater than 60 to 70 mm Hg with a pH less than 7.25. It is usually stipulated that the patient first be tried on continuous positive-airway pressure (CPAP) of 5 to 8 cm H_2O with an inspired oxygen concentration up to 0.80.[12-14] As with adults, other clinical factors must be weighed in the decision of whether to ventilate mechanically. In infants, these factors include birth weight, gestational age, and the presence or absence of apneic or bradycardic periods.

In the absence of respiratory failure, there are few other indications for mechanical ventilation. Flail chest was formerly considered one of these. The concept of "alkalotic apnea for internal pneumatic stabilization of the critically crushed chest" was proposed in 1956 by Avery, who found that positive-pressure ventilation was more effective and humane in the treatment of flail chest than were the older methods of external stabilization with Hudson traction and towel clips.[15] For two decades following Avery's report, it was largely accepted that most patients with flail chest segments should be treated with mechanical ventilation to minimize chest wall motion caused by spontaneous respiratory effort and to allow the fractured ribs to heal. More recently, it has been recognized that patients who have flail segments but who do not meet usual blood gas criteria for respiratory failure do better if treated only with pain control, including epidural and intercostal blocks, than if treated with mechanical ventilation.[16]

Mechanical ventilation may be instituted in the absence of respiratory failure in patients who require hyperventilation. In patients with increased intracranial pressure, hyperventilation to a Pa_{CO_2} of 25 to 30 mm Hg has been advocated to rapidly reduce cerebral blood flow and brain swelling.[17] Hyperventilation has also been reported to produce a respiratory alkalosis as a means of preventing seizures and ventricular dysrhythmias in patients suffering from tricyclic antidepressant overdose.[18]

In severely hypothermic patients, the administration of warm nebulized air is an effective means of core rewarming.[19] Although such patients usually require mechanical ventilation for other reasons, the need for rewarming might be considered an additional indication. Postoperative mechanical ventilation is also used "prophylactically" in certain surgical patients who are at high risk for the development of respiratory failure, atelectasis, or pneumonia. Conditions that may place a patient in a high risk category include shock, morbid obesity, COPD, neuromuscular disease, or other debilitating illnesses. Patients also are at increased risk for the development of respiratory complications following cardiothoracic surgery.[7]

There are no absolute contraindications to mechanical ventilation. COPD with chronic carbon dioxide retention is considered by some to be a relative contraindication, since patients with this condition are notoriously difficult to wean back to spontaneous breathing. When the COPD patient presents with respiratory failure, however, the condition has usually been precipitated by an acute process, such as a pulmonary infection, which can be reversed while the patient receives ventilatory assistance. The complication rate is unusually high in patients with asthma during mechanical ventilation.[20] The high complication rate merely reflects the severity of their pulmonary disease and should not be considered a contraindication to mechanical ventilation. Finally, in some patients with terminal illness or chronic debilitating disease, a decision not to initiate mechanical ventilation may be made.

Types of Ventilators

Mechanical ventilators manufactured by over a dozen companies are currently available in the United States; most manufacturers offer several different models. Despite the diversity of these machines, they may be grouped and classified according to a few basic characteristics that describe their operation.

INSPIRATORY FLOW

There are basically two types of inspiratory flow patterns built into modern ventilators. The inspiratory flow either is constant during the inspiratory cycle or varies from the start to the end of the cycle. In general, ventilators with constant flow are called "flow generators," whereas ventilators with variable flow are classified as "pressure generators."[21] In a constant-*flow* generator, a high pressure gradient is established between the ventilator and the patient. The machine is built with a high internal resistance so that changes in the resistance and compliance of the patient's airways make relatively little contribution to the total resistance of the system. The result is a constant, or square wave, flow pattern (Fig. 3–2A). In a constant-*pressure* generator, the machine develops a constant pressure that is only slightly above the pressure in the patient's airways. An exponential flow pattern results, with flow approaching zero as the patient's airway pressure approaches the pressure from the ventilator (Fig. 3–2B).

It is apparent that constant-flow generators and constant-pressure generators are not conceptually different but rather are the opposite ends of a spectrum. By reducing internal resistance and machine pressure, one can convert a constant-flow generator into a constant-pressure generator.

In addition to constant-flow and constant-pressure generators, there are also nonconstant-flow generators and nonconstant-pressure generators. In nonconstant-flow generators, the flow varies during the inspiratory period, but the time-dependent flow pattern stays the same from breath to breath despite changes in the patient (Fig. 3–2C). In nonconstant-pressure generators, pressure changes during the inspiratory period, but the time-dependent pressure pattern remains the same from breath to breath (Fig. 3–2D). The flow patterns of ventilators are of more interest to bioengineers than to clinicians, except that some modern ventilators have controls that allow the operator to switch from one flow pattern to another. As discussed in the section on ventilator settings, by changing the flow pattern, one may sometimes effect small but significant improvements in ventilation of the patient.

CYCLING

In addition to being classified according to their inspiratory flow characteristics, ventilators are classified according to the factor that determines when the ventilator cycles from the inspiratory phase to the expiratory phase. Basically, there are three different types: pressure-cycled, volume-cycled, and time-cycled.

Pressure-Cycled. In pressure-cycled ventilators, the inspiratory phase is terminated, and expiration begins when a preset pressure limit is reached. The tidal volume received by the patient is not set directly but depends upon the set pressure limit and the patient's chest and lung compliance and airway resistance. As long as the patient's compliance and resistance do not change, the tidal volume will be the same with each breath. If the patient's compliance falls or resistance increases, the tidal volume will also fall, and hypoventilation may result.

Pressure-cycled ventilators were more popular in the past. Because of the problem of a changing tidal volume caused by changing patient compliance, pressure-cycled ventilators largely have been replaced by volume- or time-cycled ventilators for mechanical ventilation in adults. Another disadvantage of most pressure-cycled machines is that

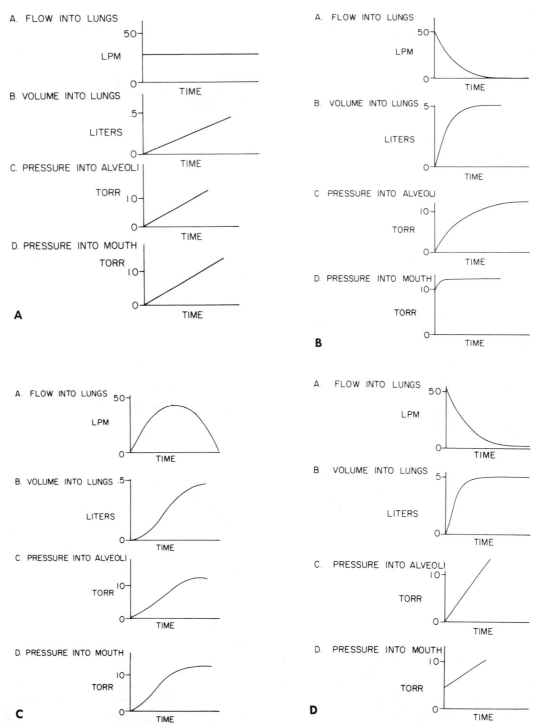

Figure 3–2. *A*, The constant-flow generator delivers constant flow with a linear increase in pressure and volume. *B*, Flow is exponential in a constant-pressure generator, approaching zero as the pressure in the lungs approaches the pressure generated by the ventilator. *C*, The sine wave flow pattern of a nonconstant-flow generator is produced by a piston on an eccentric cam. *D*, In a nonconstant-pressure generator, flow declines exponentially, but pressure increases during the inspiratory cycle. (From Kirby, R. R., Desautels, D. A., Modell, J. H., and Smith, R. A.: Mechanical ventilation. *In* Burton, G. G., Gee, E. N., and Hodgkin, J. E.: Respiratory Care. Philadelphia, J. B. Lippincott Co., 1977. Used by permission.)

the $F_{I_{O_2}}$ cannot be precisely set. Pressure-cycled ventilators still have certain advantages. They are much less expensive than volume- and time-cycled machines. They are more compact and can be run off from a compressed gas source without the need for an electrical source, making them well suited for ambulance transport.

Volume-Cycled. In volume-cycled ventilators, inspiration is terminated and expiration begins when a preset tidal volume is delivered. The gas is usually delivered from a compressible bellows. Since the introduction of the Puritan-Bennett MA-1 volume ventilator in 1968, volume ventilators have become the standard for mechanical ventilation in adults. They have an important advantage over pressure-cycled ventilators: They deliver a relatively constant tidal volume despite changes in the patient's compliance. Even with volume cycled machines, however, the delivered tidal volume will fall slightly if the patient's compliance falls. This is because although a constant volume is delivered from the ventilator bellows, as the patient's lungs become stiffer, more of this gas is lost to expansion of the ventilator tubing. This phenomenon becomes very important in neonates. The compliance of the infant's chest and lungs may be less than the compliance of the ventilator tubing, and more gas will go to expansion of the tubing than to ventilation of the patient.

Most modern volume ventilators have adjustable secondary pressure limits such that when the airway pressure exceeds the set limit, inspiration is terminated. Thus, volume-cycled ventilators may function as pressure-cycled ventilators when the pressure limit is set low enough.

Time Cycled. In time-cycled ventilators, inspiration is terminated and expiration begins after a preset time has elapsed. The tidal volume that is delivered is determined by the product of the inspiratory flow and the inspiratory time. Time-cycled ventilators resemble volume-cycled machines in that they deliver a relatively constant tidal volume despite changes in the patient's compliance. They may also function as pressure-limited ventilators when the secondary pressure limits are adjusted. Time-cycled ventilators are becoming increasingly popular. They allow great flexibility in adjustment of the inspiratory to expiratory ratio, and their internal circuitry is such that they can be manufactured at a lower cost than most volume-cycled machines.

Choosing Ventilator Settings

In order to optimize ventilator therapy, the physician must understand the capabilities of the ventilator at his disposal, the pathophysiology of the patient, and how to match the ventilator settings to the patient's condition to achieve the desired results. In this section, the rational choice of ventilator settings will be discussed. Not all of the settings described in this section are available on every ventilator. To learn the capabilities of a given ventilator, the physician should consult the operating manual supplied with that particular machine. A summary of recommended initial ventilator settings is provided in Table 3–3.

RATE AND TIDAL VOLUME

The two most important settings on a volume-cycled ventilator (and those that are usually set first) are the rate and tidal volume. To provide an understanding of the way in which the rate and tidal volume determine alveolar ventilation and the arterial carbon dioxide tension (Pa_{CO_2}), it is necessary to review briefly some aspects of pulmonary physiology.

Minute Volume and Alveolar Ventilation. The volume of air (or any other gas mixture) that moves in and out of a patient's lungs per minute is termed the minute volume ($\dot{V}_E$). Minute volume is the product of tidal volume (V_t) and respiratory frequency or rate (f):

$$\dot{V}_E = V_t \times f \tag{1}$$

Tidal volume can be further broken down into alveolar ventilation (V_A) and dead space ventilation (V_d):

$$V_t = V_A + V_d \tag{2}$$

In healthy young persons, the anatomic dead space can be accounted for by the trachea and the larger airways and is approximately 1 ml per pound of lean body weight. In disease states, in addition to the anatomic dead space, there is also a variable amount of "pathologic" dead space corresponding to ventilated alveoli and respiratory bronchioles that are not adequately perfused. The sum of the anatomic and pathologic dead spaces is often referred to as the physiologic dead space.

Alveolar minute ventilation ($\dot{V}_A$) is the product of rate times tidal volume minus dead space:

$$\dot{V}_A = (V_t - V_d) \times f. \tag{3}$$

Alveolar minute ventilation and the rate of carbon dioxide production by the body ($\dot{V}_{CO_2}$) determine the partial pressure of carbon dioxide in the alveoli (PA_{CO_2}), which is approximately equal to the systemic arterial carbon dioxide tension (Pa_{CO_2}). This relationship is shown in equation 4:

Table 3–3. RECOMMENDED INITIAL VENTILATOR SETTINGS

Parameter	Recommended Setting	Comment
Tidal volume	10 to 15 ml per kg	8 to 12 ml per kg in infants (see section on rate and tidal volume).
Rate	10 to 14 breaths per minute	Starting rates of 25 to 30 per minute used in infants. Rates of 18 per minute or greater used in adults when hyperventilation is indicated or when V_d/V_t is very high (see section on rate and tidal volume).
FI_{O_2}	0.40	Levels of 0.50 to 1.00 should be ordered initially in patients with known or suspected large A–a D_{O_2} (see section on inspired oxygen concentration).
Ventilator mode	Assist control, IMV, or SIMV	(See section on ventilator mode.)
PEEP	None	Start with PEEP of 5 cm H_2O and increase in 5–cm H_2O increments if Pa_{O_2} less than 60 mm Hg with FI_{O_2} greater than or equal to 0.50 (see section on PEEP and CPAP).
Inspiratory waveform	Square wave	(See section in inspiratory flow.)
Inspiratory flow	50 L per minute	8 to 15 L per minute in infants (see section on inspiratory flow rate).
Inspiratory pause	None	(See section on inspiratory pause.)
I:E ratio	1:2	(See section on inspiratory pause.)
Peak pressure	50 cm H_2O	With pressure-cycled ventilators, starting pressures of 20 to 30 cm H_2O should be used in infants and in adults with normal compliance (see section on peak pressure).
Expiratory retard	None	(See section on expiratory retard.)
Sighs	None	(See section on sighs.)
Humidifier temperature	35°C	Use higher temperature (40°C) for rewarming hypothermic patients, lower temperature for cooling febrile patients.

*See section in text.

$$Pa_{CO_2} \simeq PA_{CO_2} = k \times (\dot{V}_{CO_2}/\dot{V}_A) \qquad (4)$$

Where the value of the constant is 0.863 when the partial pressure of carbon dioxide is measured in mm Hg at 37°C saturated with water vapor, $\dot{V}_{CO_2}$ is measured in milliliters per minute, and $\dot{V}_A$ is measured in liters per minute.

Using equations 3 and 4, one can work through the example of an average 150-lb man with a typical spontaneous tidal volume of 500 ml, respiratory rate of 12 breaths per minute, carbon dioxide production of 200 ml per minute, and dead space of 150 ml, and see that a normal Pa_{CO_2} results:

$$\dot{V}_A = (0.500 - 0.150) \times 12$$
$$= 4.2 \text{ liters/minute}$$

and

$$Pa_{CO_2} = 0.863 \times (200/4.2)$$
$$= 41.0 \text{ mm Hg}$$

If this same 150-lb man were to develop respiratory failure purely on a neurologic basis without any change in his dead space or carbon dioxide production, one might assume that the appropriate ventilator settings would be a tidal volume of 500 ml and a rate of 12 breaths per minute. It has been found empirically, however, that *when patients are ventilated with tidal volumes that are in the normal range for spontaneous breathing, atelectasis and hypoxemia develop*.[7] One can prevent this by ventilating patients at higher tidal volumes, in the range

of 10 to 15 ml per kg. Also, mechanical ventilation alters the normal ventilation/perfusion relationships in the lungs, causing relatively greater ventilation of the less well-perfused upper lung regions, which in turn results in an increase in physiologic dead space.[22] The magnitude of this effect is roughly to double the predicted dead space when a patient converts from spontaneous breathing to mechanical ventilation.[23]

Returning to the case of our 150-lb man, assuming a physiologic dead space on the ventilator of 300 ml, a desired tidal volume of 12 ml per kg (850 ml), and a desired Pa_{CO_2} of 40 mm Hg, one can use equations 3 and 4 to solve for the desired ventilator rate:

$$Pa_{CO_2} = 0.863 \, (\dot{V}_{CO_2}/\dot{V}_A)$$
$$40 = 0.863 \times (200/\dot{V}_A).$$

Solving for $\dot{V}_A$:

$$\dot{V}_A = (0.863 \times 200)/40$$
$$= 4.3 \text{ liters per minute}$$

Putting this value for $\dot{V}_A$ into equation 3 and solving for f:

$$\dot{V}_A = (V_t - V_d) \times f$$
$$4.3 = (0.850 - 0.300) \times f$$
$$f = 4.3 \div (0.850 - 0.300)$$
$$= 7.8 \text{ breaths per minute}$$
$$\simeq 8 \text{ breaths per minute}$$

In practice, such a low rate is rarely prescribed as the initial ventilator setting, because it is usually preferable to risk overventilating a patient slightly rather than to underventilate him. *Starting rates of 10 to 14 breaths per minute are recommended for most patients.*

The well-known Radford nomogram is still referred to in some texts as a means of predicting the minute volume requirements in ventilator patients. First published in 1954,[24] this nomogram was developed and tested using data from polio victims and healthy volunteers and was intended mainly for use in patients under general anesthesia. The Radford nomogram is shown in Figure 3–3. The graph is included mainly for historical interest, since it consistently underestimates the ventilatory requirements of critically ill patients with respiratory failure.[25]

Changes in Pa_{CO_2} as a Result of Changes in Rate and Tidal Volume. Once a patient has been placed on a ventilator at a rate and tidal volume that are deemed appropriate, it is necessary to check arterial blood gases to be sure that the patient is being adequately ventilated and oxygenated. *Arterial blood gases are customarily drawn 15 minutes after the initiation of mechanical ventilation or after changes in ventilator settings.* This interval is supported by indirect evidence suggesting that blood gases reach equilibrium within 15 minutes after ventilator changes in most patients with severe pulmonary disease and much sooner in patients with normal lungs.[26, 27] In most patients, achieving a normal Pa_{CO_2} (36 to 44 mm Hg) is the goal. In some cases, however, a higher or lower Pa_{CO_2} is desired. For example, most experts warn against rapid reduction of Pa_{CO_2} to normal in

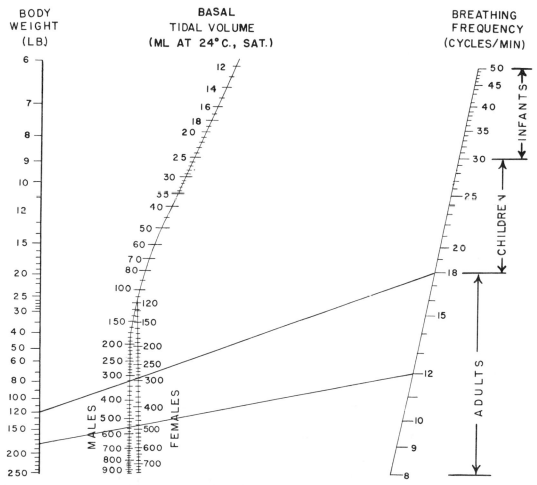

Figure 3–3. The Radford nomogram. Published in 1954 as a guide for prediction of rate and tidal volume in patients undergoing general anesthesia, this nomogram has since been applied to patients on prolonged mechanical ventilation. Note that the nomogram predicts a tidal volume of 550 ml in a 180-lb man breathing at a rate of 12 per minute and a tidal volume of 280 ml in a 120-lb woman breathing at 18 per minute. Although such tidal volumes are in the normal range for spontaneous breathing, much higher tidal volumes, in the range of 10 to 15 ml per kg, are currently recommended for ventilator patients. (See text for further discussion; From Radford, E. P.: Ventilation standard for use in artificial respiration. J. Appl. Physiol. 7:451, 1955. Used by permission.)

patients with chronic carbon dioxide retention. The resultant alkalemia may have many undesirable consequences, including diminished cardiac output, diminished cerebral blood flow, hypokalemia, hypocalcemia with associated seizures, increased airway resistance, and a shift in the hemoglobin-oxygen dissociation curve to the left with impaired release of hemoglobin to the tissues.[22] On the other hand, in patients with increased intracranial pressure due to trauma, infection, or cerebrovascular accident, a lower than normal Pa_{CO_2} may be desired in order to lower intracranial pressure.

Whatever the desired Pa_{CO_2}, if the measured Pa_{CO_2} differs from the desired level, the ventilator rate or tidal volume must be adjusted accordingly. One can easily calculate the amount of change in ventilator settings needed to produce the desired change in Pa_{CO_2} using the relationship

$$\dot{V}_{E_2} = (Pa_{CO_2}^1/Pa_{CO_2}^2) \times \dot{V}_{E_1} \qquad (5)$$

where $\dot{V}_{E_2}$ is the desired minute volume, $\dot{V}_{E_1}$ is the present minute volume, $Pa_{CO_2}^2$ is the desired Pa_{CO_2}, and $Pa_{CO_2}^1$ is the present Pa_{CO_2}. (Strictly speaking, Pa_{CO_2} varies inversely with alveolar minute ventilation and not with total minute ventilation, which includes both alveolar ventilation and wasted, dead-space ventilation. It has been observed empirically, however, that the ratio of V_d/V_t remains relatively constant despite changes in tidal volume.[28] Thus, equation 5 holds whether rate or tidal volume or both are altered.) As an example, suppose that the initial rate is 10, the tidal volume is 900 ml, the observed Pa_{CO_2} is 50 mm Hg, and the desired Pa_{CO_2} is 30 mm Hg. The desired minute volume is calculated as:

$$\dot{V}_{E_2} = (50/30) \times 9.0 \text{ liters per minute}$$
$$= 15 \text{ liters per minute}$$

To obtain a Pa_{CO_2} of 30, the tidal volume could be increased to 1500 ml (although this would be outside of the physiologic range), the rate could be increased to 16 to 17 breaths per minute, or the rate and tidal volume could both be changed so that their product is 15 liters per minute.

Adding Dead Space. Many patients who are placed on ventilators and who are allowed to trigger the machine themselves, as in the assist control mode, will spontaneously hyperventilate. If the Pa_{CO_2} drops as low as 25 to 30 mm Hg in a patient who is used to a normal Pa_{CO_2}, the same complications may develop as described previously for rapidly lowering the carbon dioxide to normal in a chronically hypercapnic patient. An approach that may be useful in dealing with patients who spontaneously hyperventilate is to add dead space to the ventilator tubing so that the patient rebreathes some of his expired air. A

formula has been developed that predicts the amount of dead space that must be added to give a desired increase in Pa_{CO_2}.[29] This formula is somewhat complicated, though, and requires determination of the concentration of carbon dioxide in the expired air. Empirically, it has been found that the addition of 50 ml of dead space will lead to an increase in Pa_{CO_2} of approximately 5 mm Hg in most patients.[29]

Another approach to raising the Pa_{CO_2} in a patient who spontaneously hyperventilates is to add carbon dioxide to the inspired air. A rise of 1 per cent in the inspired carbon dioxide concentration leads to a rise in Pa_{CO_2} of approximately 5 mm Hg.[30] The disadvantage of using this method rather than adding dead space is that it requires an expensive piece of additional equipment, the carbon dioxide mixer. Paradoxically, it has been found that increasing the Pa_{CO_2} by either method leads to a rise, rather than a decline, in Pa_{O_2}.[29, 30] This seems to be a result of the increased cardiac output that occurs with normalization of the Pa_{CO_2}. The problem with adding either dead space or inspired carbon dioxide is that the patient may hyperventilate even more, returning his Pa_{CO_2} to harmfully low levels. If this occurs, the patient should be sedated or changed to a different ventilator mode, as will be discussed subsequently.

The Dead Space to Tidal Volume Ratio (V_d/V_t). As noted earlier, in addition to their anatomic dead space, patients with pulmonary disease have variable amounts of pathologic dead space. The ratio of total dead space to tidal volume (V_d/V_t) is useful to follow as an index of the severity of a patient's pulmonary disease. The normal V_d/V_t ratio is 0.25 to 0.40.[31] Patients with V_d/V_t ratios of 0.6 or greater usually need ventilatory assistance, since they require large minute volumes to maintain adequate alveolar ventilation. The V_d/V_t ratio may be calculated using the Bohr equation:

$$V_d/V_t = (P_{A_{CO_2}} - P_{E_{CO_2}})/P_{A_{CO_2}} \qquad (6)$$

where $P_{E_{CO_2}}$ is the partial pressure of carbon dioxide in mixed expired air and $P_{A_{CO_2}}$ is the partial pressure of carbon dioxide in alveolar air, which is assumed to be the same as Pa_{CO_2}. To use this equation, one must have access to a carbon dioxide analyzer. Although these analyzers are commercially available, they are not standard equipment in most emergency departments or intensive care units. For this reason, a graph has been constructed from which V_d/V_t can be determined if one knows the patient's minute ventilation and Pa_{CO_2} (Fig. 3–4).[32] The graph assumes a normal carbon dioxide production of 200 ml per minute. Although critically ill patients tend to have higher rates of carbon dioxide production, when the V_d/V_t ratio determined from the graph was compared with the V_d/V_t ratio calculated from the Bohr equa-

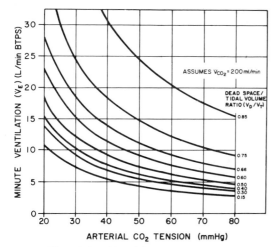

Figure 3–4. The relationship of $\dot{V}_E$ to Pa_{CO_2} is shown graphically for various V_d/V_t ratios. Once $\dot{V}_E$ is deteremined from the ventilator settings and Pa_{CO_2} is determined by blood gas analysis, the V_d/V_t ratio can be read from the graph. Conversely, once the V_d/V_t ratio is known, the change needed in $\dot{V}_E$ to produce a desired change in Pa_{CO_2} can be predicted from the graph. (See text.) Assumptions made in constructing this graph are that $\dot{V}_{CO_2}$ is 200 ml per minute (the basal metabolic rate for a 70-kg man) and that V_d/V_t remains constant whether rate or tidal volume is changed. (From Selecky, P. A., Wasserman, K., Klein, M., and Ziment, I.: A graphic approach to assessing interrelationships among minute ventilation, arterial carbon dioxide tension, and ratio of physiologic dead space to tidal volume in patients on respirators. Am. Rev. Respir. Dis. 117:181, 1978. Used by permission.)

tion on 23 occasions in 9 critically ill patients, a close correlation was found between the graphically determined and measured V_d/V_t ratios.[32] Conversely, when a change in rate or tidal volume was made in a patient with a known V_d/V_t ratio, the graph was accurate in predicting the new Pa_{CO_2}.

Compliance. Measurement of pulmonary compliance is useful in following the progression of a patient's pulmonary disease as well as in determining the optimal tidal volume and level of positive end-expiratory pressure (PEEP—see the following discussion). Compliance is defined as change in volume over change in pressure:

$$\text{Compliance} = \Delta V/\Delta P \qquad (7)$$

Total pulmonary compliance can be subdivided into the compliance of the lung and the compliance of the chest wall. For practical purposes in managing most ventilator patients, only the total compliance need be considered. Total compliance in a ventilator patient may be measured as either static compliance, which is the tidal volume delivered divided by the plateau airway pressure after the patient has been held in full inspiration for 1 second, or as dynamic compliance, which is the tidal volume divided by the peak airway pressure. (When measuring compliance in a patient on PEEP, one considers the change in pressure to be the difference between the peak or plateau inspi-

ratory pressure and the positive end-expiratory pressure level.)

In monitoring ventilator therapy, measurements of static compliance are usually preferred, since dynamic compliance is affected not only by the elastic recoil properties of the patient's chest wall and lungs but also by the patient's airway resistance. Normal static compliance in a healthy young adult undergoing general anesthesia is approximately 50 ml per cm H_2O.[33] It is believed that the tidal volume that leads to the greatest total compliance is that which results in maximal recruitment of alveoli without overdistention. In most patients, the best compliance is found with tidal volumes of 12 to 15 ml per kg.[34] In addition to being affected by tidal volume, compliance is also affected by PEEP and characteristics of inspiratory flow, as will be discussed later.

Set Tidal Volume Versus Delivered Tidal Volume. As was mentioned in the discussion of the different types of ventilators, an advantage of volume- and time-cycled ventilators is that they deliver a relatively constant volume despite changes in the patient's compliance. One must remember that even with volume- and time-cycled ventilators, delivered tidal volume will drop slightly if the patient's compliance goes down. This drop in delivered volume occurs because the ventilator tubing has compliance of its own. Although most of the gas mixture delivered by the ventilator bellows goes to expansion of the patient's lungs, a certain amount is lost to expansion of the ventilator tubing.

The compliance of the tubing varies from ventilator to ventilator. For a typical modern volume ventilator, such as the Bear-2, the compliance of the inflow circuit is 3 ml per cm H_2O.[35] To calculate the difference between the set tidal volume and that actually received by the patient, one can multiply the pressure read from the inspiratory pressure gauge at the end of inspiration times the tubing compliance. For example, if the set tidal volume is 850 ml and the peak inspiratory pressure is 30 cm H_2O, then the volume delivered to the patient is:

$$
\begin{aligned}
\text{delivered volume} &= \text{set volume} - (\text{tubing compliance} \times \text{peak pressure}) \\
&= 850 - (30 \times 3) \\
&= 760 \text{ ml}
\end{aligned}
$$

The lower the patient's compliance, the higher the peak inspiratory pressure will be and the more gas mixture will be captured in the ventilator tubing.

Tidal Volume and Rate in Infants. The recommended tidal volume for neonates is slightly lower than that for adults (in the range of 8 to 12 ml per kg).[12] Starting respiratory rates of 25 to 30 are usually prescribed, although rates up to 60 per minute are sometimes needed in neonates with severe hyaline membrane disease. Most ventilators used for adults and larger children are not capable of delivering the small tidal volumes required in infants and neonates. (An exception is the Siemens-Elema Servo Ventilator.[36]) Therefore, special ventilators have been developed for neonatal intensive care. The compliance and dead space of the ventilator tubing and the valves have special importance in neonates. The total pulmonary compliance of a newborn with hyaline membrane disease may be 1 ml per cm H_2O, which is the same as the compliance of some ventilators designed especially for use in neonates. Thus, with each breath delivered by the machine, one half of the volume goes to expand the patient's lungs and the other half goes to expand the ventilator tubing. This technical problem has to some extent hampered the development of volume ventilators for infants.[37]

INSPIRED OXYGEN CONCENTRATION ($F_{I_{O_2}}$)

After rate and tidal volume have been set, the next variable that the physician usually fixes is the $F_{I_{O_2}}$. The goal should be to deliver the lowest oxygen concentration that provides adequate arterial oxygenation. Adequate arterial oxygenation is difficult to define and may vary from patient to patient. Most experts recommend maintaining a Pa_{O_2} of 60 mm Hg or greater, since a Pa_{O_2} of 60 corresponds to the shoulder on the normal hemoglobin-oxygen dissociation curve at which hemoglobin is 90 per cent saturated with oxygen. Beyond this point, increases in Pa_{O_2} lead to relatively little rise in hemoglobin saturation, whereas below this point, small decrements in Pa_{O_2} cause large drops in hemoglobin saturation. Conditions such as acidemia, fever, hypercarbia, and certain hemoglobinopathies result in a shift in the curve to the right so that at a Pa_{O_2} of 60, the hemoglobin will be less than 90 per cent saturated. Thus, a Pa_{O_2} of 60 mm Hg may not be adequate in such patients.[38]

Oxygen Toxicity. When one is initiating mechanical ventilation, it is better to err on the side of a higher than necessary $F_{I_{O_2}}$ rather than to risk making a patient hypoxemic. $F_{I_{O_2}}$'s in the range of 0.50 to 1.00 are commonly prescribed as initial settings for patients with known cardiopulmonary disease, whereas patients with no known pulmonary pathologic condition are commonly started at an $F_{I_{O_2}}$ of 0.40. With chronic ventilator support, however, a higher than necessary $F_{I_{O_2}}$ may have serious adverse effects. The phenomenon of pulmonary oxygen toxicity has been recognized since the turn of the century, although the pathophysiology is still not completely understood.[39] The syndrome begins with tracheal irritation, cough,

and chest pain, followed by diminished vital capacity and dyspnea. In the later stages, hypoxemia develops with associated alveolar edema and infiltrates on chest radiographs. Finally, as the process becomes irreversible, alveoli become replaced by fibrosis.

Although the exact dose-time relationship of pulmonary oxygen toxicity has not been established, it is known that at atmospheric pressure an $F_{I_{O_2}}$ of 0.40 is well tolerated for 30 days or more, an $F_{I_{O_2}}$ of 0.70 will lead to signs and symptoms of toxicity by 2 days, and an $F_{I_{O_2}}$ of 1.00 leads to toxicity within 30 hours.[39] In general, an $F_{I_{O_2}}$ of 0.50 or greater should be considered potentially toxic if used for more than a few days.

In neonates, two other manifestations of oxygen toxicity may occur: retrolental fibroplasia and bronchopulmonary dysplasia.[40, 41] The dose-time relationship of oxygen administration to the development of these two conditions is even less well established than oxygen toxicity in adults. A recent multicenter cooperative study designed to develop guidelines for the safe administration of oxygen in neonates was unable to yield any firm recommendations.[42]

The Alveolar-Arterial Oxygen Difference. After the patient has been on a given $F_{I_{O_2}}$ for 15 minutes, arterial blood gases should be checked. Besides confirming the adequacy of arterial oxygenation, blood gas results can be used to measure the efficiency of the lungs in oxygenating venous blood. One way to quantitate how well the lungs are doing their job is to compare the oxygen concentration delivered to the alveoli with the oxygen tension in arterial blood. The difference between these two values is known as the alveolar-arterial oxygen difference ($A - a\ D_{O_2}$). The PA_{O_2} is easily obtained by blood gas analysis, and is calculated using the alveolar air equation:

$$PA_{O_2} = [F_{I_{O_2}} \times (P_B - P_{H_2O})] - PA_{CO_2}$$
$$\times \left[F_{I_{O_2}} + \frac{1 - F_{I_{O_2}}}{R} \right] \quad (8)$$

where P_B is barometric pressure (760 mm Hg at sea level), P_{H_2O} is the pressure of water vapor in the patient's lungs (47 mm Hg at 37°C), and R is the respiratory quotient (assumed to be 0.8 unless it has been directly measured). The alveolar carbon dioxide partial pressure, PA_{CO_2}, is assumed to be the same as the arterial carbon dioxide tension, Pa_{CO_2}. When the patient is breathing 100 per cent oxygen, this equation simplifies to

$$PA_{O_2} = 713 - PA_{CO_2} \quad (9)$$

At room air, an approximation that is easy to remember (for sea level calculations) is:

$$PA_{O_2} = 150 - 1.2 \times Pa_{CO_2} \qquad (10)$$

Recall that $A\text{-}a\ D_{O_2} = PA_{O_2} - Pa_{O_2}$. In healthy young adults, the normal $A\text{-}a\ D_{O_2}$ is less than or equal to 10 to 15 mm Hg at room air and 30 to 50 mm Hg at 100 per cent oxygen.[31] Corrected for age, the normal $A\text{-}a\ D_{O_2}$ is approximately 15 plus 1 mm Hg for each decade of life (assuming room air at atmospheric pressure).

The Shunt Fraction (Q_s/Q_t). The width of the alveolar-arterial oxygen gradient reflects the amount of ventilation/perfusion mismatch and right-to-left shunting occurring in the lungs as well as the severity of barriers to diffusion between the alveoli and the pulmonary capillaries. To quantitate further the amount of right-to-left shunting and ventilation/perfusion mismatch, known collectively as venous admixture, the so-called shunt equation can be used. This equation states:

$$Q_s/Q_t = (C_c - C_a)/(C_c - C_v) \qquad (11)$$

where Q_s is the pulmonary blood flow that does not become oxygenated, Q_t is the total pulmonary blood flow, C_c is the oxygen content of pulmonary capillary blood (which is calculated based on the assumption that the oxygen tension in the pulmonary capillaries equals the partial pressure of oxygen in the alveoli), C_a is the oxygen content of systemic arterial blood, and C_v is the oxygen content of mixed venous blood (ideally obtained from the distal port of a pulmonary artery catheter).

With the patient breathing 100 per cent oxygen, the effect of ventilation/perfusion mismatching is eliminated, and calculation of Q_s/Q_t reflects only the true right-to-left shunting. The normal Q_s/Q_t ratio in healthy young adults is 2 to 3 per cent.[31] A Q_s/Q_t ratio of greater than 50 per cent results in severe hypoxemia, even at 100 per cent inspired oxygen. In Figure 3–5, the relationship of Pa_{O_2} to PA_{O_2} is shown for various Q_s/Q_t ratios. It can be seen from this figure that when Q_s/Q_t is small, large increases in PA_{O_2} lead to similarly large increases in Pa_{O_2}. With high Q_s/Q_t ratios, however, large increases in PA_{O_2} lead to only slight increases in Pa_{O_2}. The clinical application of this observation is that diseases characterized mainly by ventilation/perfusion mismatching, such as COPD, respond well to oxygen therapy, whereas in conditions marked by large degrees of right-to-left shunting, such as intracardiac shunts, pneumonia, pulmonary edema, and the adult respiratory distress syndrome, large increases in FI_{O_2} may lead to relatively little improvement in arterial oxygenation.

VENTILATOR MODE

After rate, tidal volume, and FI_{O_2} have been set, the next priority is to set the mode of ventilation. Although not all the modes discussed in this section are available on all ventilators, most modern machines allow the operator to choose more than one mode. The airway pressure and flow characteristics of the different modes are shown diagrammatically in Figure 3–6.

Controlled Ventilation. In this mode, the patient is ventilated at the rate set by the operator. He cannot breathe in between machine breaths. This mode may be used in an unconscious patient with depressed respiratory drive, in a heavily sedated patient, in a patient who has been paralyzed with drugs, or in a patient who is being deliberately hyperventilated. Other patients may attempt to inhale against the closed inspiratory valve, resulting in apprehension, asynchronous chest movement, increased oxygen consumption and carbon dioxide production, and high peak pressures.

Assist Control. In this mode, the operator sets the minimum rate at which he wants the patient to be ventilated. If the patient makes no respiratory effort, he will receive the prescribed number of breaths and no more. If the patient does try to breathe, when he generates a sufficient inspiratory effort, the machine will deliver an extra breath with the same tidal volume as the others. The amount of negative inspiratory pressure that the patient must generate to trigger the machine is controlled by the operator. The sensitivity is set so that it is neither too difficult for the patient to

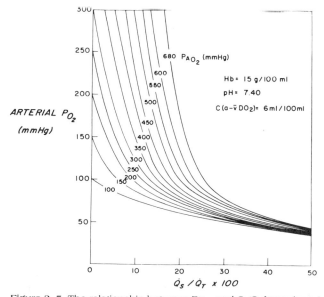

Figure 3–5. The relationship between Pa_{O_2} and Q_s/Q_t for various levels of Pa_{O_2}. This graph is constructed from the shunt equation, assuming normal values for hemoglobin, arterial-mixed venous oxygen difference, and hemoglobin-oxygen dissociation curve. (From Pontoppidan, H., Geffin, B., and Lowenstein, E.: Acute respiratory failure in the adult. N. Engl. J. Med. 287:744, 1982. Used by permission.)

Within the figure:
PA_{O_2} (mmHg)
680, 600, 580, 500, 450, 400, 350, 300, 250, 200, 150, 100
Hb = 15 g/100 ml
pH = 7.40
$C(a-\bar{v}DO_2) = 6\ ml/100ml$

ARTERIAL P_{O_2} (mmHg)

$\dot{Q}_s / \dot{Q}_T \times 100$

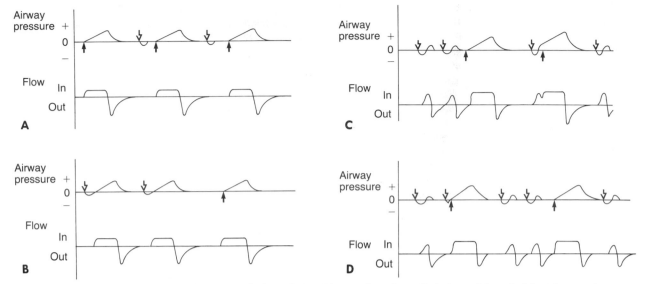

Figure 3–6. Ventilator modes. *A*, Controlled ventilation. The ventilator is cycling at a regular rate *(closed arrows)*. The patient is making inspiratory efforts *(open arrows)* but does not receive any breaths at these times. *B*, Assist control. Each time the patient makes a sufficient inspiratory effort *(open arrows)*, the ventilator delivers a full tidal volume. If the patient's spontaneous rate drops below the set ventilator rate, then the ventilator cycles on its own *(closed arrow)*. *C*, IMV. The patient is breathing at a rate faster than the ventilator is set *(open arrows)*. The ventilator does not assist him but cycles at an independent rate *(closed arrows)*. The second ventilator breath falls coincidentally on top of a spontaneous breath (so-called stacking), leading to a high peak pressure. *D*, SIMV. This mode is the same as IMV, except that the ventilator is programmed to avoid stacking by timing machine breaths either to coincide with the initiation of a spontaneous breath *(first closed arrow)* or to fall in between spontaneous breaths *(second closed arrow)*.

initiate a breath (in which case the ventilator would actually be functioning in the control mode) nor too easy (in which case small movements by the patient might trigger the machine). The advantage of assist control over the control mode is that it allows the patient to regulate his own minute volume in part. This mode is usually preferred in conscious patients. A disadvantage of assist control is that some patients spontaneously hyperventilate to an undesirable degree in this mode.

IMV and SIMV. Intermittent mandatory ventilation (IMV) is a relatively new concept in mechanical ventilation first introduced in the early 1970s.[43, 44] As in the assist control mode, the patient may breathe at a rate faster than the set ventilator frequency. With IMV, however, when the patient initiates a spontaneous breath, the machine does not assist him, and he receives only the tidal volume that he generates on his own. This is usually smaller than the tidal volume delivered by the ventilator. As in the assist control mode, the patient may determine his own minute volume in part. An advantage of IMV is that there is less tendency for the patient to hyperventilate spontaneously. Also, since the patient must work harder to generate a spontaneous breath, it is believed that IMV may help maintain tone of the respiratory muscles. An additional potential advantage of IMV over assist control and controlled ventilation is that mean airway pressures tend to be lower in the IMV mode, resulting in less imped-

ance to return of blood to the right side of the heart.[22] (See the section on complications of mechanical ventilation.) The IMV mode is particularly well suited for weaning a patient from mechanical ventilation. Over a period of hours to days, the IMV rate can be gradually turned down, so that the patient makes a smooth transition from depending mainly on the ventilator to breathing entirely on his own. Some authors have claimed that the use of IMV facilitates weaning in difficult patients,[44] although other authors have questioned the assertion that it speeds the weaning process.[45]

Older ventilators, such as the Puritan-Bennett MA-1, do not have IMV circuits built into them but may be converted to the IMV mode through the use of additional tubing and an independent oxygen source. This system wastes oxygen, since the patient may breathe only a small fraction of the air-oxygen mixture that is continuously flowing through the IMV circuit. Newer ventilators have IMV circuits built into them so that gas flows through the IMV circuit only when the patient initiates a breath. Another problem that occurred with older IMV systems was that the ventilator sometimes delivered a tidal volume just as the patient had completed a spontaneous inspiration. This so-called stacking of a machine breath on top of a spontaneous breath could lead to overdistention of the lungs and dangerously high peak pressures. This problem has been overcome by the development of synchronized IMV (SIMV).

This mode is the same as IMV except that the ventilator times the machine breaths to fall in a pause in the patient's spontaneous respiratory cycle or to coincide with the initiation of a spontaneous breath.

PEEP AND CPAP

Positive end-expiratory pressure (PEEP) and continuous positive-airway pressure (CPAP) were introduced in the late 1960s and early 1970s as means of improving oxygenation in hypoxemic patients. PEEP was originally used in patients with the adult respiratory distress syndrome[46] and CPAP was first used in infants with hyaline membrane disease,[47] but both techniques have since been applied to patients of all ages with hypoxemia from a wide variety of causes.

Some confusion exists in the literature with regard to the usage of the terms PEEP and CPAP. The term PEEP is used most often to denote positive end-expiratory pressure in a patient who is receiving assisted ventilation. In this mode, airway pressure is positive not only at end expiration but also throughout the respiratory cycle. The term CPAP is used most often to denote continuous positive-airway pressure in a patient who is breathing spontaneously. CPAP circuits are designed so that airway pressure drops slightly during inspiration but remains above ambient pressure because of a continuous flow of gas through the inspiratory circuit.

The confusion arises when a patient who has been receiving assisted ventilation with PEEP is weaned to spontaneous breathing while still exhaling against positive pressure. Some authors would say that the patient is now on CPAP. With most ventilators, however, airway pressure must drop below ambient before the patient will receive a breath. Therefore, this mode should not be termed CPAP but rather spontaneous breathing with PEEP, or EPAP (for expiratory positive-airway pressure). The importance in distinguishing between CPAP and EPAP is that mean airway pressure is lower and the work of breathing is greater with EPAP than with CPAP. As will be discussed in the section on complications of mechanical ventilation, the level of mean airway pressure may influence venous return to the heart and cardiac output.

PEEP can be used with the ventilator in the control, assist control, IMV, or SIMV mode. In older ventilators, application of PEEP involved cumbersome extra circuitry. In newer machines, the capability for PEEP is built in, and one sets the level merely by turning a knob. Although CPAP is usually applied by way of an endotracheal **tube** with a ventilator supplying the positive pressure, it can also be applied by means of a tight-fitting mask or a head-enclosing box.[48, 49]

Theoretically, PEEP and CPAP improve oxygenation by keeping alveoli open during expiration. Whether or not they actually work by this mechanism is a moot point.[50] What is known is that they lead to improved oxygenation and narrowing of the A–a D_{O_2} in most patients.

The number of indications for PEEP and CPAP is currently increasing as more experience is being gained with these modes of ventilator therapy. A generally accepted indication for PEEP is failure to achieve adequate oxygenation (e.g, Pa_{O_2} less than 60 mm Hg) with safe levels of inspired oxygen (e.g., Fi_{O_2} less than or equal to 0.50). Other indications are more controversial. There is a prevalent philosophy in the surgical literature that PEEP has prophylactic value in preventing the respiratory distress syndrome or that it hastens its resolution.[51] One basis for this belief is that PEEP alters the appearance of infiltrates on chest films, making them appear less dense. In one study, skilled radiologists interpreted pre- and post-PEEP chest films differently in 25 per cent of cases after patients had been on 10 to 20 cm PEEP for only 15 minutes.[52] Thus, some surgical intensive care units routinely use low levels of PEEP (5 to 8 cm H_2O) in patients who require postoperative ventilation but who are not hypoxemic on safe levels of Fi_{O_2}. The prophylactic and therapeutic value of PEEP has been questioned in the medical literature, however.[53] In one large retrospective study, use of PEEP did not seem to improve survival in critically ill patients.[54] Animal studies designed to assess the influence of PEEP on pulmonary edema have shown either no change or an increase in lung water after institution of PEEP.[55]

Determination of the optimal level of PEEP is also controversial. A conservative approach is to use a level of PEEP that is just enough to provide adequate arterial oxygenation with an inspired oxygen concentration under 50 per cent. In patients requiring higher Fi_{O_2}'s, PEEP may be started at 5 cm H_2O and may be increased in increments of 3 to 5 cm H_2O at 15-minute intervals. At each new level, one should measure and record pulse and blood pressure, static compliance, peak airway pressure, arterial blood gas tension, and cardiac output. The pulmonary artery wedge pressure should probably also be measured, although it may not accurately reflect left ventricular filling pressure in patients on PEEP.[53] The Fi_{O_2} can usually be gradually turned down as PEEP is increased and the A–a D_{O_2} narrows.[56]

Most patients exhibit a fall in cardiac output at levels of PEEP above 12 to 15 cm H_2O. This drop can be at least partially overcome by expansion of intravascular volume.[57] A useful method of determining when a fall in cardiac output negates the effect of a rise in Pa_{O_2} is to calculate the peripheral oxygen delivery at different levels of PEEP.[56, 58] One can calculate the peripheral oxygen delivery by multiplying the cardiac output by the arterial oxygen content:

$$O_2 \text{ delivery to periphery} = \text{cardiac output} \times \text{arterial } O_2 \text{ content} \quad (12)$$

One calculates arterial oxygen content by remembering that 1 gm of hemoglobin, fully saturated, carries 1.34 ml of oxygen and that an additional 0.003 ml of oxygen is dissolved in 100 ml of blood for each mm Hg of oxygen tension.

$$\begin{aligned} &\text{arterial } O_2 \text{ content} \\ &(\text{ml } O_2 \text{ per 100 ml of blood}) \\ &= (\text{Hgb conc} \times \text{Hgb sat} \times 1.34) \\ &\quad + (0.003 \times Pa_{O_2}) \quad (13) \end{aligned}$$

Some authors have recommended that PEEP be increased until the intrapulmonary shunt (Q_s/Q_t) falls below 15 per cent, a level that has been arbitrarily assigned as defining acute respiratory failure.[59] Extremely high levels of PEEP (up to 44 cm H_2O) may be required to reach this goal, however.[60] These levels are associated with a high incidence of barotrauma. Furthermore, as can be seen from Figure 3–5, with Q_s/Q_t ratios of up to 30 per cent, one can usually maintain adequate oxygenation with safe inspired oxygen concentrations.

In patients who do not have pulmonary artery catheters in place, measurement of static compliance has been advocated as a means of determining the optimal level of PEEP. One small study found that the best PEEP from the point of view of oxygen delivery to the periphery coincided with the level at which static compliance was highest, usually in the range of 6 to 12 cm H_2O.[61] Other authors have questioned the reproducibility of this association.

CPAP has been used most extensively in infants with hyaline membrane disease. In this setting, CPAP is usually initiated at levels of 2 to 8 cm H_2O before mechanical ventilation is begun.[12] In some cases, CPAP leads to enough improvement in the A–a D_{O_2} that assisted ventilation can be avoided. Recently, CPAP has also been advocated for adults with a variety of pulmonary diseases who are hypoxemic on high inspired oxygen concentrations but who are able to maintain normal arterial carbon dioxide tensions.[49] CPAP has also been claimed to be of benefit in weaning difficult patients from mechanical ventilation.[62] This indication will be discussed further in the section on weaning.

CHARACTERISTICS OF INSPIRATORY AND EXPIRATORY FLOW

There are many variables of inspiratory and expiratory flow that the operator may alter on modern ventilators. These include inspiratory flow wave form, inspiratory flow rate, inspiratory time, I:E ratio, peak inspiratory pressure, and expiratory resistance. These variables, along with rate and tidal volume, are interrelated, so that a change in one affects the others. Which variable is set by the operator and which variable is secondarily determined depends upon the ventilator design. For example, in a pressure-cycled ventilator, flow and pressure are set and tidal volume is determined, whereas in a volume-cycled ventilator, flow and tidal volume are set and pressure is determined. With a time-cycled ventilator, the I:E ratio is set, whereas with pressure- and volume-cycled ventilators, the I:E ratio is determined. Although changes in the characteristics of inspiratory and expiratory flow tend to result in relatively small changes in the final measures of oxygenation and carbon dioxide elimination, by adjusting these variables appropriately one can fine-tune the ventilator to optimize the therapy of critically ill patients.

Inspiratory Flow. The basic flow pattern built into most ventilators is a constant flow (square wave). In many modern ventilators, this basic pattern can be altered by the operator to produce an accelerating or decelerating (tapered wave) pattern. In most cases, a square wave is chosen as the initial setting, since this leads to lower peak pressures for a given inspiratory time and tidal volume. In some patients with very uneven ventilation of different regions of the lungs, however, use of a tapered inspiratory waveform may result in more even ventilation by allowing more time for the inspired gas to pass through airways with increased resistance to flow.[63]

Inspiratory Flow Rate. In volume- and pressure-cycled ventilators, the inspiratory flow rate is initially set in the range of 40 to 50 liters per minute in adults and 8 to 15 liters per minute in infants. In time-cycled ventilators, one may secondarily determine the inspiratory flow by setting the tidal volume and inspiratory time. An inspiratory flow rate that is too rapid may lead to dangerously high peak pressures or unequal ventilation of lung units with different time constants, whereas an inspiratory flow rate that is too slow may lead to an undesirably long inspiratory time with inadequate time for exhalation.

Inspiratory Pause. Some ventilators allow the operator to add a pause to the end of inspiration, during which time airway pressure is held constant and the patient cannot exhale. Like other maneuvers that prolong the inspiratory phase, an inspiratory pause leads to more even ventilation.[63] The pause may also lead to air trapping. An inspiratory pause is also analogous to PEEP in that by increasing mean airway pressure, it may lead to decreased venous return and decreased cardiac output. An inspiratory pause is usually not initially prescribed but may be added when hypoxemia due to uneven ventilation is a problem.

I:E Ratio. To allow complete exhalation, the expiratory phase of the ventilatory cycle should generally be two to three times the length of the inspiratory phase. Larger I:E ratios (e.g., 1) in adults may lead to air trapping, overdistention, and high peak pressures. In diseases such as asthma and COPD characterized by airway obstruction, even smaller I:E ratios (e.g., 1:4) may be necessary to allow complete exhalation. In infants with hyaline membrane disease, however, it has been found that a so-called inverse I:E ratio of 2:1 may improve oxygenation and thereby decrease the time that the patient must be on PEEP and high FI_{O_2}.[64]

Peak Pressure. With pressure-cycled ventilators, peak pressure is a set variable and determines tidal volume. Starting pressures of 20 to 25 cm H_2O are commonly used in adults with no known pulmonary disease, although pressures of 40 cm H_2O and above are usually required in patients with a pulmonary pathologic condition.

With time- and volume-cycled ventilators, peak pressure is determined mainly by tidal volume. Typical peak pressures for patients with respiratory failure are in the range of 40 to 50 cm H_2O. Peak pressures greater than 60 cm H_2O are not uncommon but are associated with a high incidence of barotrauma. In exceptional cases, peak pressures of 100 cm H_2O and above are required. Modern volume- and time-cycled ventilators have adjustable peak pressure limits such that when the airway pressure exceeds the set limit, inspiration is terminated. The limit is usually set at 10 cm H_2O above the peak pressure that is observed when the patient is initially placed on the ventilator. If the peak pressure alarm sounds later, it is a sign that the patient's compliance has dropped or resistance has increased, and a cause must be sought. (Typical causes of acute increases in peak pressure include attempts by the patient to override, or "buck," the ventilator, development of pneumothorax, migration of the tip of the endotracheal tube into the right main stem bronchus, kinking of the tube, or plugging of the tube or a major airway.)

Expiratory Retard. Many ventilators have an adjustable expiratory resistance, or retard. The development of such a mechanism was inspired by the observation of COPD patients who breathe through pursed lips, apparently in an effort to increase their own expiratory resistance. Theoretically, this resistance to expiration may prevent the premature collapse of small airways and may paradoxically lead to more complete exhalation. Whether this is actually the reason for pursed-lip breathing and whether expiratory retard is a useful setting on a ventilator remain controversial.[21, 65]

Sighs. In the early 1960s, it was shown that patients who were being mechanically ventilated during anesthesia showed a progressive decline in compliance and widening of their A–a D_{O_2}.[66] These changes were thought to be caused by atelectasis and were reversed by intermittent deep breaths. Based on this work, "sigh" functions have been built into mechanical ventilators, allowing the operator to introduce a breath 1 1/2 to 2 times the usual tidal volume at regular intervals. A problem with the original study that demonstrated the benefit of "sighs," however, was that patients were ventilated with low tidal volumes. With tidal volumes in the range of 10 to 15 ml per kg that are used today, it has not been demonstrated that progressive atelectasis occurs. The optimal rate and volume of sighs are unknown, as is whether sighs are beneficial at all. Indeed, it has been argued that incorporation of a sigh function into a ventilator adds only needless extra expense.[67]

HUMIDIFICATION

Normally, inspired air is humidfied and warmed in the oropharynx and the nasopharynx before reaching the lower airway. In an intubated patient, inspired air bypasses the nasopharynx and the oropharynx and is injected directly into the trachea. In order to prevent drying of the mucosa of the lower airways, all modern ventilators are equipped with systems for humidifying and warming inspired air. The setup of these systems varies from ventilator to ventilator and is described in the operating manuals supplied by the manufacturers. A commonly overlooked setting, however, is the temperature of the inspired air. Normally, the air temperature should be 35°C at the point at which the gas enters the endotracheal tube. One should remember that in patients who are hypothermic, heating the inspired air is an effective means of core rewarming.[19] Likewise, cooling the inspired air will lower the body temperature in febrile patients.

MEDICATION NEBULIZERS

Most modern ventilators have in-line medication nebulizers for the administration of bronchodilator drugs. The dosages are the same as those for hand-held medication nebulizers. (See Chapter 2.)

Practical Ventilator Setup

The actual setting up of a ventilator is usually done by a respiratory therapist while the physician specifies the ventilator settings. In some cases, a respiratory therapist may not be readily available. This section on practical ventilator setup is included to aid the physician who finds himself setting up the ventilator alone. Unfortunately, it is not practical to give step-by-step instructions for every ventilator on the market. Rather, I have chosen to describe the setup of three representative machines. The Bear-2 and the Siemens-Elema Servo 900C are presented as representative examples of modern volume- and time-cycled ventilators, respectively. The setup of an adult pressure-cycled ventilator is not included, since pressure-cycled ventilators are used infrequently today. Instead, the setup of the Babybird, which is commonly used for the ventilation of infants, is described. Although this ventilator is actually time-cycled, its design and setup are similar to those of the pressure-cycled ventilators marketed by the Bird Corporation for use in adults.

The descriptions of ventilator setup in this section are not intended to provide "all one needs to know" to use these ventilators safely on a long-term basis. For detailed setup and operating instructions for these and other ventilators, the physician should consult a certified respiratory therapist and the operator manuals supplied by the manufacturers. Copies of the manuals should be filed in all emergency departments or critical care units in which the ventilators are used.

SETUP OF THE BEAR-2 ADULT VOLUME VENTILATOR

The Bear-2 is an extremely versatile modern volume ventilator with built-in features that provide virtually fail-safe ventilation of adults and larger children. Despite its rather formidable control and display panels (Fig. 3–7 and 3–8), the Bear-2 is relatively easy to set up. The appearance of the Bear-2 as it is usually found in the emergency department or critical care unit is shown in Figure 3–9. The ventilator is fully assembled with the humidifier and patient tubing attached. The setup to this point is presented in detail in the manufacturer's instruction manual and will not be discussed further here.

1. The air and oxygen hoses at the back of the ventilator should be connected to house compressed air and oxygen sources. If no compressed air source is available, an internal air compressor is automatically activated. The power supply cord should be plugged into a standard 110-volt AC outlet.

2. The humidifier on the front of the ventilator should be filled with sterile distilled water, and the temperature control should be turned slightly beyond midposition. Up to 30 minutes is required for the water in the humidifier to warm up. The temperature of the inspired air at the patient wye is shown on the display panel (item 4, Fig. 3–8) and should be adjusted to approximately 35°C for normothermic patients.

3. One determines the desired ventilator settings simply by turning the knobs on the ventilator control panel (see Fig. 3–7). The initial critical settings are *ventilator mode, tidal volume,* and *rate,* all located on the top row of the control panel, and *inspired oxygen per cent* and *peak flow,* both located on the bottom row. The *normal pressure limit* (item 6, Fig. 3–7) should also be included as one of the initial settings in order to avoid exposing the patient to excessively high pressures. This setting determines the upper limit of machine pressure beyond which the ventilator will not continue to deliver a tidal volume. Usually, the pressure limit is set at 50 cm H_2O initially and then is adjusted while the patient is on the ventilator to a level 10 to 15 cm H_2O above the machine pressure required to deliver the desired tidal volume. The adjacent *low inspiratory pressure* knob is set 10 to 15 cm H_2O below the observed initial peak pressure. If the machine pressure fails to reach this lower limit, as might occur with a leak in the ventilator tubing, audible and visible alarms are activated.

4. The *multiple sigh* switch (item 7, Fig. 3–7) should be turned off. (See the discussion in the section on sigh.) The *sigh volume* and *sigh pressure limit* knobs should be set the same as the *tidal volume* and *normal pressure limit* controls in case someone later turns on the *multiple sigh* switch.

5. The waveform toggle switch (item 17, Fig. 3–7) may be turned up for square wave inspiratory flow or down for tapered flow. A square wave pattern is usually used initially. (See the discussion in the section on inspiratory flow.) The *proximal airway pressure* toggle switch (item 16, Fig. 3–7) should be left in the neutral position. When one holds the switch to the left, the pressure gauge on the display panel indicates the pressure at the patient circuit outlet of the ventilator. When the switch is released, the pressure gauge indicates the proximal airway pressure. The difference is the pressure drop through the humidifier and patient circuit, which increases with higher flow rates.

6. The amount of effort that the patient must exert to initiate a breath is controlled by the *assist*

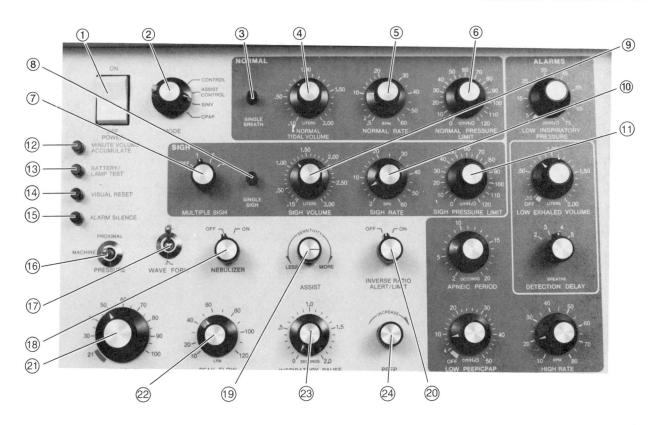

CONTROL PANEL

1. **POWER ON/OFF** — Controls electrical power to the ventilator.

2. **MODE CONTROL** — Selection of mode of operation.

3. **NORMAL SINGLE BREATH** —Manual breath; operable 350 milliseconds after the end of exhalation. Operates in all modes.

4. **TIDAL VOLUME** — 100-2000 ml. When tidal volume is delivered, inspiration ends. (Exhaled tidal volume and minute volume are displayed.)

5. **NORMAL RATE** — 0.5-60 BPM (Rate display indicates the sum of the machine and patient breaths.)

6. **NORMAL PRESSURE LIMIT** —0-120 cmH$_2$O. When the selected pressure is reached, inspiration ends and terminates volume delivery. (Audio-visual alert, PRESSURE LIMIT on display panel shows that pressure limit was reached.)

7. **MULTIPLE SIGH** — Number of sighs to be delivered in succession at preset intervals. (CONTROL and ASSIST-CONTROL modes only.)

8. **SINGLE SIGH** — Manual sigh; operable 350 milliseconds after the end of exhalation when MULTIPLE SIGH is set at 1, 2 or 3 position.

9. **SIGH VOLUME** — 150-3000 ml. When sigh volume is delivered, sigh breath ends.

10. **SIGH RATE** — 2-60 sighs per hour (CONTROL and ASSIST-CONTROL modes only.)

11. **SIGH PRESSURE LIMIT** — 0-120 cmH$_2$O. When the selected sigh pressure is reached, inspiration ends and terminates volume delivery. (Audio-visual alert, PRESSURE LIMIT on display panel shows that pressure limit was reached.)

12. **MINUTE VOLUME ACCUMULATE** — Tidal volume accumulates for one minute, displays for second minute and then automatically returns to tidal volume. (MINUTE VOLUME ACCUMULATE indicator blinks during accumulation and remains lit during the display of minute volume.)

13. **BATTERY/LAMP TEST** —Activates all digital and LED displays, as well as testing the battery powered, power-loss sensing circuit.

14. **VISUAL RESET** — All activated visual alarm/alert indicators remain on, until the VISUAL RESET button is pushed.

15. **ALARM SILENCE** — Allows silencing of all audible alarms except the VENT INOPERATIVE alarm. The alarm system will reset automatically in 60 seconds or can be reset manually by depressing the ALARM SILENCE pushbutton (display panel light shows ALARM SILENCE on).

16. **PROXIMAL PRESSURE SWITCH**—PROXIMAL position: pressure measured at patient wye; MACHINE position: pressure measured upstream of the mainflow bacteria filter. (Read on PROXIMAL AIRWAY PRESSURE gauge.)

17. **WAVE FORM** — Controls flow pattern delivered during positive pressure breaths.

18. **NEBULIZER** — Allows intermittent administration of medication during positive pressure breaths (14 psig at 11 LPM). Does not alter oxygen concentration or tidal volume (display panel light shows NEBULIZER ON).

19. **ASSIST-SENSITIVITY** — Adjustable from LESS (-5cmH$_2$O) to MORE (-1cmH$_2$O). Senses patient effort in ASSIST-CONTROL and SIMV modes to deliver synchronized positive pressure breaths (Display light shows inspiratory source.)

20. **INVERSE RATIO ALERT/LIMIT** — OFF: Allows INVERSE I.E RATIO (visual alert only; display panel light indicates INVERSE RATIO is OFF). ON: Prevents inverse ratio, 1:1 ratio terminates inspiration (Audio-Visual alert).

21. **OXYGEN %** — 21-100% oxygen (±3%). Connect to 30-100 psig oxygen source for concentrations higher than 21%. Audio-Visual alert on display panel shows oxygen source pressure less than 30 psig with OXYGEN % control setting higher than 21%.

22. **PEAK FLOW** — 10-120 LPM. Controls initial flow rate during positive pressure breaths, no effect on spontaneous flow.

23. **INSPIRATORY PAUSE** — 0-2.0 seconds. Delays the beginning of exhalation.

24. **PEEP** — 0-50 cmH$_2$O. Leak compensated in all modes except CONTROL (effective leak compensation is the available flow less the patient demand, as long as PEEP exceeds 1 cmH$_2$O to keep the demand valve open. NOTE: ASSIST sensitivity may be compromised if excessive leak compensation is required.)

CONTROL PANEL

Figure 3–7. Bear-2 control panel. (Reproduced with permission from Bear Medical Systems, Inc., Riverside, California.)

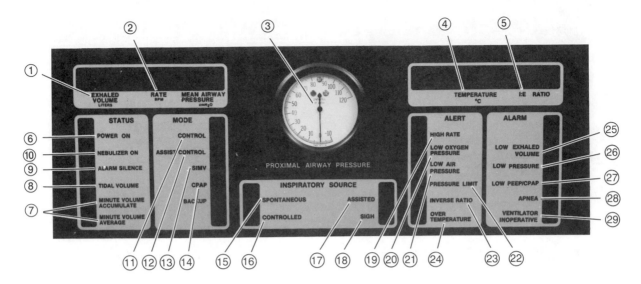

(1) Digital display of **EXHALED VOL-UME** on a breath-to-breath basis or **MINUTE VOLUME.**

(2) Digital display of the number of **BREATHS PER MINUTE.** Shows the average breath rate, based on the total spontaneous and machine breaths in the last twenty seconds and continuously updates every second.

(3) Displays level of pressure at the proximal airway from -10 to 120 cmH_2O. Machine (system) pressure may also be read on the **PROXIMAL AIRWAY PRESSURE GAUGE** by moving the **PROXIMAL PRESSURE** toggle switch to the left or to the right.

(4) Displays the gas temperature at the patient wye.

(5) Digital display of inspiratory time to expiratory time ratio, breath-to-breath in the **CONTROL** and **ASSIST-CONTROL** modes. A flashing display indicates greater than a 1:9.9 machine **I:E RATIO.**

(6) **POWER ON** — The machine is plugged into an operating AC power outlet and the POWER switch is "ON".

(7) **MINUTE VOLUME** — The **EXHALED VOLUME** is being accumulated for one minute (flashing LED indicator) or the minute volume is displayed (continuously illuminated LED indicator).

(8) **TIDAL VOLUME** — The **EXHALED VOLUME** displays the breath-to-breath **TIDAL VOLUME.**

(9) **ALARM SILENCE** — Audible alarm silenced for 60 seconds (except for VENT INOPERATIVE).

(10) **NEBULIZER ON** — Nebulizer is on during mechanical inspiration cycle.

(11) **CONTROL** — Ventilator set in CONTROL mode.

(12) **ASSIST-CONTROL** — Ventilator set in ASSIST-CONTROL mode.

(13) **SIMV** — Ventilator set in SIMV mode.

(14) **CPAP** — Ventilator set in CPAP mode.

(15) **SPONTANEOUS** — Patient breath, unassisted (SIMV, CPAP modes).

(16) **CONTROLLED** — Ventilator initiated positive pressure breath (CONTROL, ASSIST—CONTROL, SIMV modes).

(17) **ASSISTED** — Patient initiated positive pressure breath (ASSIST—CONTROL, SIMV modes).

(18) **SIGH** — Sigh breath delivered (Automatic-CONTROL, ASSIST-CONTROL; Single—all modes).

(19) **HIGH RATE** — The total spontaneous and machine delivered breaths exceeded the HIGH RATE control setting.

(20) **LOW OXYGEN PRESSURE** — Oxygen inlet pressure less than 30 psi and OXYGEN % control set above 21%.

(21) **LOW AIR PRESSURE** — Internal air compressor pressure and external air pressure less than 9.5 psi.

(22) **PRESSURE LIMIT** — Machine pressure has reached preset level and terminated inspiration (exhaled volume may be less than selected tidal volume).

(23) **INVERSE RATIO** — Inspiratory time interval exceeds expiratory time, I:E Ratio less than 1:1. If the INVERSE RATIO ALERT / LIMIT control is ON and the ventilator is in CONTROL mode, the ventilator will terminate inspiration and provide an audible and visual alarm when a 1:1 I:E Ratio is reached.

(24) **OVER TEMPERATURE** — Inspired gas temperature exceeds 41°C, or the electrical connection of the temperature probe inadvertently is disconnected, or the temperature probe is defective.

(25) **LOW EXHALED VOLUME** — Exhaled volume has not exceeded level set on LOW EXHALED VOLUME alarm for the number of consecutive breaths selected with the DETECTION DELAY control. Disconnect of clamshell from flow tube will cause alarm on next breath.

(26) **LOW PRESSURE** — Inspiratory pressure has not exceeded level set on the LOW INSPIRATORY PRESSURE alarm, or the expiratory pressure has not dropped below the level set on the LOW INSPIRATORY PRESSURE alarm.

(27) **LOW PEEP/CPAP** — PEEP / CPAP pressure is less than that set on the PEEP/CPAP control.

(28) **APNEA** — The number of seconds selected on the APNEIC PERIOD control has elapsed since the beginning of the last breath (spontaneous or mechanical).

(29) **VENTILATOR INOPERATIVE** — Indicates total air pressure source or AC power failure, or certain internal electronics failure.

Figure 3–8. Bear-2 display panel. (Reproduced with permission from Bear Medical Systems, Inc., Riverside, California.)

sensitivity knob (item 19, Fig. 3–7). The knob should be set at midposition initially and then should be adjusted with the patient on the ventilator so that he must exert −1 to −3 cm H_2O of pressure to trigger a breath.

7. When PEEP or CPAP is desired, the level of positive pressure is controlled by the *PEEP* knob (item 24, Fig. 3–7). Starting with the knob turned fully counterclockwise, one turns it clockwise until the desired end-expiratory pressure is observed on the *proximal airway pressure* gauge.

8. The *low exhaled volume* knob on the far right side of the control panel should be set approximately 100 ml below the desired tidal volume.

When the exhaled volume falls below this level for the number of consecutive breaths indicated on the *detection delay* knob, audible and visible alarms are activated. In the SIMV or CPAP modes, the *low exhaled volume* alarm must be set below the spontaneous tidal volume.

9. The *low PEEP/CPAP* knob sets a limit below which a fall in expiratory pressure will activate audible and visible alarms. This knob should be set approximately 5 cm H_2O below the desired level of PEEP or CPAP.

10. The *inverse ratio alert/limit* switch (item 20, Fig. 3–7), when turned on, will cause the inspiration to be terminated and audible and visible

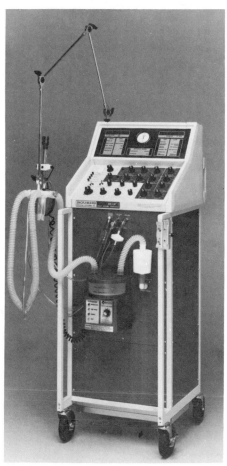

Figure 3–9. The Bear-2 adult volume ventilator. (Reproduced with permission from Bear Medical Systems, Inc., Riverside, California.)

alarms to be activated when the I:E ratio of assisted breaths exceeds 1:1.

11. The *high rate* knob at the bottom right-hand corner of the control panel determines the combined rate of spontaneous and machine breaths allowed before audible and visible alarms are activated. The appropriate setting depends upon the clinical situation, but in most cases the limit should be set in the range of 24 to 26 breaths per minute.

12. The *apneic period* control just above and to the left of the *high rate* knob determines the length of time allowed between breaths (mechanical or spontaneous) before audible and visible alarms are activated. An initial setting of 10 seconds, corresponding to a rate of 6 breaths per minute, is recommended.

13. The *on/off* switch is located at the upper left-hand corner of the control panel (item 1, Fig. 3–7). After the other desired settings have been fixed, the ventilator should be turned on and the patient tubing connected to a test lung. Once it has been established that the prescribed tidal volume is being delivered at the prescribed rate, the ventilator may be connected to the patient.

Displays and Alarms on the Bear-2. The display panel at the top of the ventilator (shown in Fig. 3–8) is for the most part self-explanatory. Of particular note are the *rate* and *exhaled volume* displays. The *rate* display provides a second-by-second update of the total of the spontaneous and mechanical rates based on the average over the preceding 20 seconds. The *exhaled volume* display records the volume of the preceding breath. (As noted in the section on set tidal volume versus delivered tidal volume, the exhaled volume is slightly greater than the tidal volume that the patient receives, because a small fraction of the volume delivered from the ventilator goes to expansion of the ventilator tubing rather than the patient's lungs.) When the *minute volume accumulate* button (item 12, Fig. 3–7) is pushed, the *exhaled volume* display sums the total minute volume over the next 60 seconds, shows that minute volume for 60 seconds, and then returns to displaying breath-to-breath tidal volumes.

The alarms on the right-hand side of the display panel notify the operator of internal malfunctions within the ventilator; critical drops in the pressure of the oxygen or compressed air supplies; and deviations in rate, tidal volume, level of PEEP or CPAP, I:E ratio, and temperature of inspired gas from the set limits. The *alarm silence* button (item 15, Fig. 3–7) turns off the audible alarms for a period of 60 seconds.

Although the Bear-2 may seem extremely complex with its more than 50 knobs, buttons, switches, and displays, in a true emergency it is relatively simple to initiate mechanical ventilation by following the first three aforementioned steps. Attention can be turned to the other controls, alarm limits, and displays once the patient's condition has been stabilized.

SETUP OF THE SIEMENS-ELEMA SERVO VENTILATOR 900C

The Servo 900C is probably the most technologically advanced ventilator currently available. The machine is very compact and operates almost silently. With its many available accessories, it can be used as a ventilator for infants, children, or adults; as an anesthesia machine; or as a diagnostic instrument. Although it is basically a time-cycled ventilator, volume and pressure limits can be set to make it function like either a volume-cycled or a pressure-cycled machine.

The modes available on the Servo 900C deserve special mention, since they are somewhat different from those available on most other ventilators. In the *volume control* mode, the ventilator functions much like a typical volume-cycled ventilator, except that the operator sets the desired minute

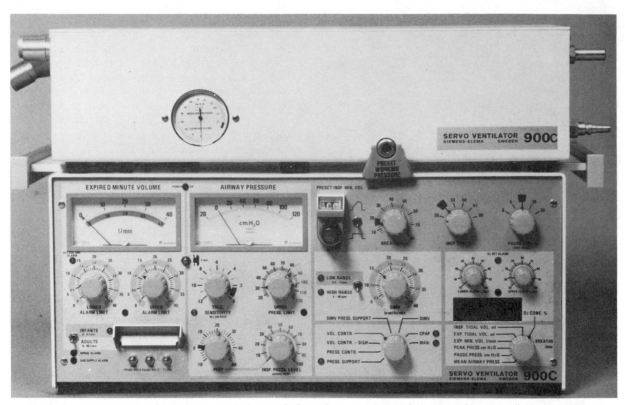

Figure 3–10. Siemens-Elema Servo 900C time-cycled ventilator. (Courtesy of Siemens-Elema Ventilator Systems, Elk Grove Village, Illinois.)

volume rather than the desired tidal volume. He then sets the desired respiratory rate and I:E ratio, and through its internal electronic circuitry, the ventilator determines the inspiratory flow necessary to deliver the set minute volume. A *volume control plus sigh* mode, in which every hundredth breath is delivered with double the basic tidal volume, is also available. By adjusting the *trigger sensitivity* appropriately, the *volume control* mode becomes analogous to *assist control* in a volume-cycled ventilator. In the *pressure control* mode, the ventilator functions as a typical time-cycled, pressure-limited ventilator, with the inspiratory time and inspiratory pressure determining the tidal volume received by the patient. *Pressure support* is a unique mode in which the patient must initiate all breaths on his own but is assisted by positive pressure from the ventilator each time he makes a sufficient inspiratory effort. The tidal volume of each breath depends in part upon the set inspiratory pressure and in part upon the amount of effort made by the patient. This mode is suggested by the manufacturer for weaning patients from anesthesia or from mechanical ventilation.

The *SIMV* mode is the same as that in a volume ventilator, except as for the *volume control* mode, minute volume rather than tidal volume is set. *SIMV plus pressure support* combines these two modes, providing the patient with a set minute

volume at a set rate but allowing him to breathe spontaneously in between machine breaths with the ventilator applying positive pressure during the spontaneous inhalations. The *CPAP* mode is the same as that in a volume ventilator. A *manual* mode is also available for providing manual ventilation during the administration of anesthesia or while a patient is being suctioned.

The external appearance of the Servo 900C is shown in Figure 3–10. The assembly of the ventilator to this point as well as the attachment of the humidifier, the oxygen-air mixer, and the patient tubing are discussed in detail in the manufacturer's instruction manual. The power supply cord, (which must be plugged into a standard 110-volt AC outlet) and the on/off switch are located at the rear of the electronic unit. The further setup of the ventilator is illustrated in Figure 3–11 and will be discussed here. Setup is described for the *assist control* mode, since this is the mode that is most appropriate for initial ventilation of most adult patients in the emergency department or the critical care unit. The setup in other modes varies slightly and is covered in the manufacturer's manual.

1. The *working pressure* adjustment on the pneumatic unit, which is mounted above the electronic unit, determines the maximum pressure that the ventilator will deliver and provides a secondary

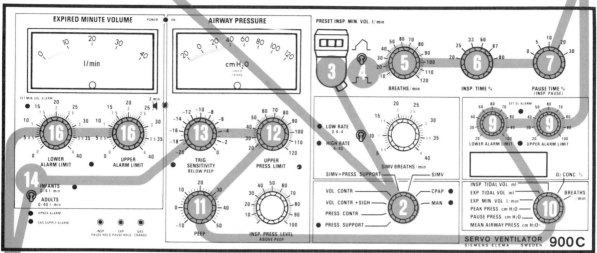

15 Connect the patient.

12 To protect the patient against high pressures, always start from a low value.

1
Set the WORKING PRESSURE.

2
Set the mode selector at VOL. CONTR. or VOL. CONTR.+SIGH.

3
Set the desired minute volume (e.g. by means of a Radford nomogram).

4
Select the curve shape for the inspiration flow.

5
Set the respiratory rate, BREATHS/min.

6
Set the INSP. TIME %.

7
Set the PAUSE TIME %.

8
Set the mixer.

9
Set the LOWER ALARM LIMIT and UPPER ALARM LIMIT for O_2 CONC. %.

10
Set the parameter selector.

11
Set the PEEP-level.

12
Set the UPPER PRESS. LIMIT for AIRWAY PRESSURE to approximately 10 cm H_2O above the patient's airway pressure.

13
Set the TRIG. SENSITIVITY.

14
Set the scale INFANTS/ADULTS.

15
Connect the ventilator to the patient and check:
– that the patient's chest rises and falls in time with the preset respiratory rate.
– the tidal volumes on the digital display and the reading on the EXPIRED MINUTE VOLUME meter.
– that the AIRWAY PRESSURE meter gives a reading during inspiration, and that the reading falls to 0 cm H_2O, or alternatively, to PEEP level, during expiration.

16
Set the LOWER ALARM LIMIT and UPPER ALARM LIMIT for EXPIRED MINUTE VOLUME.

If the VOL. CONTR.+SIGH mode is selected, it may be necessary to increase the UPPER ALARM LIMIT for EXPIRED MINUTE VOLUME, as well as the UPPER PRESS. LIMIT for AIRWAY PRESSURE. This is done in order to avoid activating the alarms when the sigh occurs.

Figure 3–11. Setup of the Servo 900C in the assist control mode. (Courtesy of Siemens-Elema Ventilator Systems, Elk Grove Village, Illinois.)

safeguard against inadvertent exposure of the patient to dangerously high pressures. (The primary safeguard is the *upper pressure limit* setting on the ventilator control panel, described in step 12.) The recommended working pressure for most adult patients is 60 cm H_2O. Higher pressures, up to 120 cm H_2O, may be required in rare cases.

2. The mode selector switch may be turned to either *volume control* or *volume control plus sigh*. As discussed previously, the sigh function is not recommended.

3. The *preset inspiratory minute volume* control determines the minute volume that the ventilator will deliver if the patient initiates no breaths on his own. As discussed in the section on set tidal volume versus delivered tidal volume, not all of the volume delivered by the ventilator actually reaches the patient, since some is lost to compression within the humidifier and the patient tubing. The difference between the *preset inspiratory minute volume* and the minute volume that the patient actually receives is on the order of 400 to 600 ml per minute for a typical adult patient. A method of calculating the exact difference is given in the operating manual.

4. Either a square wave or an accelerating inspiratory flow pattern may be selected. In most cases, a square wave is the appropriate initial setting (see discussion in the section on inspiratory flow).

5. The *breaths/minute* knob determines the minimum number of breaths that the patient will receive. One determines the tidal volume of each breath by dividing the preset inspiratory minute volume by the breaths per minute. The patient may trigger the ventilator at a faster rate than the *breaths/minute* setting, and if he does, he will receive more than the preset inspiratory minute volume. The tidal volume of the ventilator breaths will not change, however.

6 and 7. The *inspiratory time per cent* setting determines the fraction of each respiratory cycle that is spent in inspiration. The *pause time per cent* setting may be used to provide a pause at the end of inspiration that is up to 20 per cent of the respiratory cycle. In combination, the *inspiratory time per cent* and *pause time per cent* settings determine the I:E ratio, which may be set anywhere from 1:4 to 4:1. The recommended initial setting is an inspiratory time of 33 per cent with no pause, resulting in an I:E ratio of 1:2. (See the sections on inspiratory pause and I:E ratio for a discussion of the use of an inspiratory pause and different I:E ratios.)

8. The inspired oxygen concentration is set by a control on the air-oxygen mixer attached to the right side of the ventilator.

9. The *upper* and *lower alarm limit* controls should be set approximately 6 per cent above and below the desired oxygen concentration. When the $F_{I_{O_2}}$ varies outside of the set limits, as detected by the internal oxygen analyzer on the ventilator, visible and audible alarms are activated.

10. The *parameter selector* knob determines which parameter is displayed in the digital readout window on the control panel above the knob. The available parameters include breathing rate (sum of spontaneous and mechanical), actual $F_{I_{O_2}}$, inspiratory tidal volume, expiratory tidal volume, expired minute volume, peak pressure, pause pressure, and mean airway pressure.

11. If PEEP is required, one sets the desired level by turning the *PEEP* knob.

12. The *upper pressure limit* knob allows the operator to set a ceiling for airway pressure above which inspiration is terminated and visible and audible alarms are activated. The limit should be set at approximately 50 cm H_2O initially and should be readjusted with the patient on the ventilator to 10 to 15 cm H_2O above the observed peak pressure. If the upper pressure limit is set above the working pressure (see step 1), inspiration will end when the working pressure is reached, but no alarms will be activated.

13. The *trigger sensitivity* control determines how much inspiratory effort the patient must make to trigger an assisted ventilator breath. The sensitivity is usually set so that an inspiratory effort of -1 to -3 cm H_2O is required.

14. The *expired minute volume* meter at the top left corner of the ventilator control panel has dual scales: from 0 to 40 liters per minute for adults and from 0 to 4 liters per minute for children. The proper scale is selected with the *infants/adults* switch at the lower left corner of the control panel. This switch also sets the scale for the *upper* and *lower alarm limit* controls (see step 16).

15. The ventilator is now connected to the patient. In addition to observing the clinical response of the patient, one should use the *parameter selector* control and *expired minute volume* and *airway pressure* meters to be sure that the rate, tidal volume, minute volume, $F_{I_{O_2}}$, and airway pressures are in the desired range.

16. After the patient has been on the ventilator for a few minutes and it has been determined that he is receiving an appropriate minute volume, the *upper* and *lower alarm limit* controls should be set approximately 20 per cent above and below the desired minute volume. When the expired minute volume deviates from this range, visible and audible alarms are activated.

Alarms on the Servo 900C. The alarms that are included for patient safety are depicted in Figure 3–12. Alarms are given in the form of audible signals as well as flashing red lights. One can switch off most of the audible alarms for 2 minutes by depressing the *alarm silence* button on the control panel.

In addition to the features discussed previously,

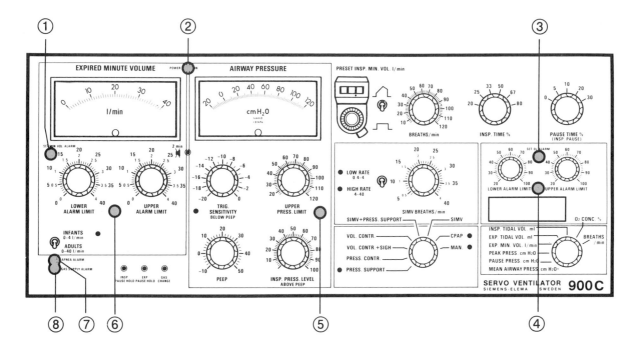

① Set minute volume alarm

Indicates that the alarm limits for expired minute volume have not been set.

② Power supply failure

The green lamp for POWER ON goes out. Slow audible signals which stop after 5–10 minutes.

③ Set O₂ alarm

Indicates that the alarm limits for O₂ concentration have not been set.

④ Alarm limit, O₂ concentration

Upper or lower alarm limit has been passed.

If the O₂ cell is not mounted, neither digital displays nor alarm is given.

A deterioration in the linearity and/or a rapid fall in the values of O₂ concentration, despite adequte O₂ supply, indicates that the O₂ cell is exhausted.

⑤ Upper pressure limit, airway pressure

The airway pressure exceeds the preset upper pressure limit. When the alarm is activated, inspiration and/or pause in progress is immediately terminated and changed to expiration. The alarm is given as a single audible signal and a visual flashing signal.

⑥ Alarm limit, expired minute volume

Upper or lower alarm limit has been passed. There are two alarm limit settings:
UPPER ALARM LIMIT 3–43 l/min (adults)
0–4.3 l/min (infants)
LOWER ALARM LIMIT 0–37 l/min (adults)
0–3.7 l/min (infants)

⑦ Apnea alarm

No attempt to trigger a breath has been made during approx. 15 seconds. Respiratory rates below 4 are not possible in the controlled ventilation modes. The alarm will, therefore, not be activated in these modes. The alarm is disconnected in the MAN mode.

⑧ Gas supply alarm

This alarm is inoperative if the respiratory rate exceeds 80 breaths/min (with inspiration time 20 or 25%).

In the CPAP and PRESS. SUPPORT modes, a patient trig is required to activate the alarm.

Figure 3–12. Alarms on the Servo 900C. (Courtesy of Siemens-Elema Ventilator Systems, Elk Grove Village, Illinois.)

available options on the Servo 900C include a carbon dioxide monitor, which analyzes end tidal carbon dioxide and has alarms for levels of carbon dioxide above or below set limits, a lung mechanics calculator, which calculates airway resistance and compliance, and a paper strip recorder, which can print pressure-flow curves or graphically present the digital displays from the ventilator control panel. With its great versatility and dependability, the Servo 900C is probably the most advanced ventilator on the market. As one would expect, it is also one of the most expensive machines.

SETUP OF THE BABYBIRD INFANT VENTILATOR

The Babybird ventilator is used primarily for the ventilation of the infant weighing 10 kg or less. Although similar in many respects to the pressure-cycled Bird ventilators used for adults, the Babybird is a time-cycled, continuous-flow ventilator with adjustable secondary pressure limits. An optional heater-humidifier requires an electrical power source, but the ventilator itself is entirely pneumatically powered. The Babybird offers only two modes, CPAP and IMV, with IMV rates of from 4 to 100 breaths per minute.

The ventilator is initially set up as shown in Figure 3–13, with the high-flow oxygen blender

mounted above the ventilator and the heater-humidifier mounted below it. The details of setup to this point are covered in the operator's manual supplied by the manufacturer. The remainder of the setup and operation is illustrated in Figure 3–14 and will be discussed here.

1. The oxygen and air supply hoses should be connected to house sources, and the patient tubing should be connected to a test lung.

2. The desired $F_{I_{O_2}}$ is set with the control on the air-oxygen blender.

3. The rotary mode switch at the center of the ventilator panel is turned to the desired mode, either IMV or CPAP (see Fig. 3–14A).

4. The *flow* control knob should be turned so that the adjacent flow gauge records a flow of approximately 15 liters per minute (see Fig. 3–14B). Flows below 10 liters per minute may result in erratic oxygen concentrations. To turn the knob, one must pull out the red locking ring at the base of the knob. After the knob has been adjusted, the locking ring should be pushed back in to prevent accidental changes in flow rate.

5. One determines the rate, tidal volume, and I:E ratio of the mechanical breaths by adjusting the *inspiratory* and *expiratory time* knobs (see Fig. 3–14F). The usual starting point is with both knobs in the 12 o'clock position. From this point, the *inspiratory time* control is used mainly to adjust the tidal volume (shorter inspiratory times lead to

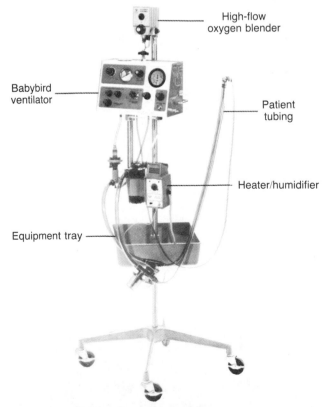

High-flow oxygen blender

Babybird ventilator

Patient tubing

Heater/humidifier

Equipment tray

Figure 3–13. The Babybird infant ventilator. (Courtesy of Bird Products/3M, St. Paul, Minnesota.)

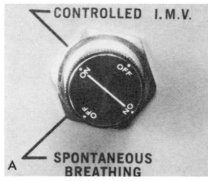

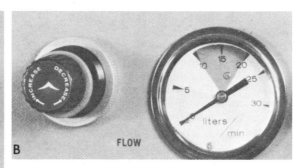

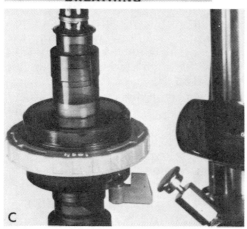

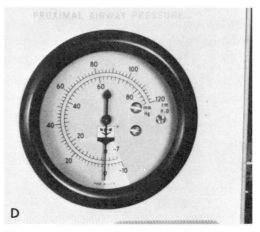

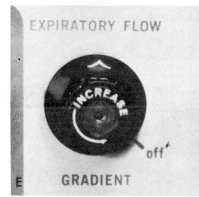

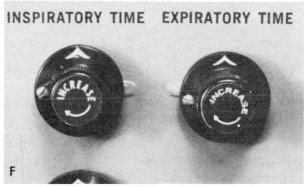

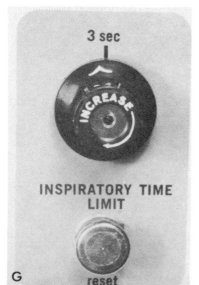

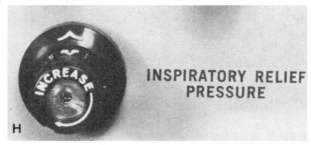

Figure 3–14. Controls on the Babybird. *A,* Mode selector switch. *B,* Flow control and gauge. *C,* Outflow valve and PEEP/CPAP adjustor lever. *D,* Pressure manometer. *E,* Expiratory flow gradient control. *F,* Inspiratory/expiratory time controls. *G,* Inspiratory time limit control. *H,* Inspiratory relief pressure control. (Courtesy of Bird Products/3M, St. Paul, Minnesota.)

lower tidal volumes), and the *expiratory time* control is used mainly to adjust the rate (shorter expiratory times lead to higher rates). It should be noted that there are no monitors on the Babybird to indicate the actual tidal volume, respiratory rate, or I:E ratio. If such quantitative information is desired, one must obtain it by using a separate spirometer for tidal volume and a clock or stopwatch for respiratory rate and I:E ratio.

6. The *inspiratory time limit* control (see Fig. 3–14G) provides a safeguard against locking of the ventilator in inspiration. When turned to the 12 o'clock position, this control causes the ventilator to convert automatically to the spontaneous breathing mode and an audible alarm to be activated if the inspiratory time exceeds 3 seconds.

7. The peak pressure in the inspiratory circuit is limited by the *inspiratory relief pressure* control (see Fig. 3–14H). Because there is no absolute scale printed on this control, one sets it by turning the knob counterclockwise until a plateau is observed on the *proximal airway pressure* manometer at the end of inspiration. This indicates that the airway pressure has exceeded the set limit. The *inspiratory relief pressure* knob should then be turned clockwise a few degrees.

8. After the desired settings have been made using the test lung, the ventilator is connected to the patient. The operator must then recheck to be sure that the desired rate, I:E ratio, and peak airway pressure are maintained.

Alarms on the Babybird. There are four alarms built into the Babybird. Since the ventilator is entirely pneumatically powered, there are no flashing lights to signal malfunctions. Rather, there are audible alarms only, which are generated by the same compressed gases that power the ventilator. The first alarm sounds if there is a 20 psi or greater difference between the inlet pressures of the two source gases, as might occur if either the oxygen or the compressed air supplies have failed. A second alarm sounds if the inlet pressure from the oxygen blender into the main ventilator falls below 43 psi. A third alarm sounds if the length of the inspiratory phase of the ventilator cycle exceeds the limit set on the *inspiratory time limit* control (see step 7). A fourth alarm sounds and pressure is vented to the atmosphere if the circuit pressure exceeds the set value on the pressure relief valve. This valve is adjustable and during assembly of the ventilator should be set at 5 to 10 cm H_2O above the anticipated peak pressure for a given patient. It should be noted that the pressure relief valve is a secondary means of limiting circuit pressure; the *inspiratory pressure relief* control described previously in step 7 is the primary means.

The Babybird does not allow the operator the same degree of precision in controlling and monitoring ventilator settings as does the Servo 900C or the Bear-2. Although the Babybird appears simpler than these other ventilators, it actually requires more expertise on the part of the operator in order to be used safely. Recommending the Babybird, however, are its relatively low cost and the fact that it has been used extensively in neonatal intensive care units across the United States since 1973.

Sedation and Paralysis

Whereas many patients adapt readily to mechanical ventilation and synchronize their own breathing with the ventilator breaths, other patients "fight the machine." By coughing, bucking, and breathing out of phase with the ventilator, they generate high peak airway pressures and increase their oxygen consumption and carbon dioxide production. When their airway pressures exceed the peak pressure limits, they receive less than the prescribed tidal volume, and hypoventilation results. In such cases, *a complication or a mechanical problem must first be ruled out.* One should check the inspired oxygen concentration with an oxygen analyzer to be sure that the set FI_{O_2} is really being delivered. While the patient is being "bagged" by hand, increased resistance to inflow of air, suggesting a plugged or kinked endotracheal tube, can be sensed. Malposition of the endotracheal tube and pneumothorax should be ruled out by auscultation and a chest film. The patient should be suctioned to remove any large airway obstruction due to mucus, blood, and so forth. Other causes for agitation, such as hypotension or pain, should be considered. If the patient is coherent, he should be reassured.

When all of these measures have been taken, no complication or malfunction has been found, and the patient continues to fight the ventilator, sedation should be considered. Diazepam is a very useful drug in this setting. Diazepam acts rapidly and provides excellent relaxation, sedation, and amnesia. The usual starting dose in adults is 2.5 to 5.0 mg intravenously, given at a rate of 2.5 mg per minute. Since the main side effect is respiratory depression, much larger doses, up to 1 mg per kg, can be given in a mechanically ventilated patient, although some cardiac depression occurs at very high doses (greater than 3 mg per kg).[68]

An alternative to diazepam is morphine sulfate. Morphine is usually given in 2- to 4-mg increments intravenously and titrated to effect. As with diazepam, the main side effect of morphine is respiratory depression, which is not a problem in the mechanically ventilated patient with a secure airway. The drug also causes a small drop in blood pressure, probably a result of peripheral vasodilation rather than a direct cardiac depressant effect.[69] Morphine is also known to cause histamine release, which could theoretically lead to increased bronchospasm.[69] Whether this effect is of clinical significance is unknown. Advantages of morphine over diazepam are that it is a potent analgesic and its effect is readily reversible with naloxone (although it has been reported that both the coma[70] and the respiratory depression[71] induced by diazepam are partly reversible with naloxone).

When sedation and analgesia are ineffective in preventing the patient from fighting the ventilator, a paralyzing drug may be used. The use of neuromuscular blockers has recently been reviewed.[72, 73] Pancuronium bromide is the drug of choice for inducing paralysis in ventilator patients. Pancuronium is a nondepolarizing blocker of neuromuscular transmission. The main side effects of the drug are a mild increase in pulse and blood pressure, although it has also been reported to cause severe hypertension, ventricular dysrhythmias, and anaphylactic reactions on rare occasions.

Pancuronium is preferred over d-tubocurarine, which commonly causes hypotension, and the depolarizing agent succinylcholine, which is short-acting and causes fasciculations and cholinergic side effects. The dose of pancuronium is 0.02 to 0.06 mg per kg intravenously. Paralysis occurs within 1 to 3 minutes and lasts 1 to 2 hours, after which time repeat doses may be given. Paralysis induced by pancuronium can be reversed by neostigmine, 0.06 to 0.08 mg per kg intravenously up to a total of 2.5 mg. Physostigmine should *not* be used for reversal, because it crosses the blood brain barrier and may induce seizures. Atropine, 0.01 to 0.02 mg per kg up to a total of 1 mg,

should be given in the same syringe to block the cholinergic side effects of neostigmine. Paralysis with pancuronium has been reported to be particularly effective in asthmatics.[74] This agent is also used frequently in neonates with hyaline membrane disease, in whom it has been shown to increase compliance and Pa_{O_2}.[75]

It is important to remember that although a patient who is paralyzed with pancuronium may appear asleep and calm, the drug has no sedative or analgesic properties. A paralyzed patient must be given liberal doses of sedatives and analgesics at regular intervals. Hospital personnel should treat the patient as if he is fully awake, talking to him in a reassuring manner and avoiding bedside discussion of his case. Finally, the patient must be continually observed and ventilator function and alarms must be checked frequently, since the patient will be entirely unable to breathe on his own should the ventilator fail.

Weaning from Mechanical Ventilation

Deciding when a patient can be safely weaned from mechanical ventilation may be more difficult than deciding when mechanical ventilation should be initiated. The patient who is being considered for weaning is often just recovering from a life-threatening illness, and the physician is usually reluctant to do anything that might further stress him and disturb his precarious equilibrium. On the other hand, the longer the patient remains on a ventilator, the more likely he is to develop a complication. To help the physician in this dilemma, objective criteria have been developed to determine when a patient may be safely weaned.[76-79] These criteria are summarized in Table 3–4. It should be noted that weaning from mechanical ventilation is not necessarily equivalent to extubation. Patients with altered mental status caused by conditions such as stroke, head injury, or drug ingestion may be able to breathe adequately on their own but may not be able to clear their secretions or protect their airways and may therefore require continued intubation after they have been weaned from mechanical ventilation.

The simplest and most reliable predictors of successful weaning are a vital capacity of greater than 10 ml per kg and a maximum inspiratory force of -20 cm H_2O or greater. These parameters are measured easily at the bedside but require cooperation of the patient. In patients with COPD or asthma, either FEV_1 of less than 10 ml per kg or peak flow of less than 25 to 30 per cent of the predicted rate indicates moderately severe airway obstruction and a low likelihood of successful

Table 3–4. WEANING CRITERIA

Measured indices of pulmonary mechanics
  V_c greater than 10 ml per kg
  MIF greater than or equal to -20 cm H_2O
  FEV_1 greater than 10 ml per kg
  Peak flow greater than 25 per cent predicted
  Resting $\dot{V}_E$ less than 10 L per minute
  MVV greater than two times resting $\dot{V}_E$
  Static compliance greater than or equal to 30 ml per cm H_2O

Calculated indices of efficiency of gas exchange
  A–a D_{O_2} on 100 per cent oxygen less than 350 mm Hg
  Q_s/Q_t less than 15 per cent
  V_d/V_t less than 0.6

Clinical indices at the end of 30-minute T piece trial with FI_{O_2} of 0.40
  Pa_{O_2} greater than or equal to 60 mmHg
  Pa_{CO_2} and pH normal (An elevated Pa_{CO_2} may be accepted in a patient with chronic carbon dioxide retention provided that the pH is normal.)
  Blood pressure change (up or down) less than 20 mm Hg
  Pulse less than 110
  Respirations less than 30

weaning. In patients with high carbon dioxide production and oxygen demands, it is useful to measure the resting minute volume. The patient with a resting minute volume of greater than 10 liters per minute is unlikely to be weaned successfully, since he would probably not be able to maintain this minute volume during spontaneous breathing. Also, the patient should have a maximum voluntary ventilation that is at least twice his resting minute volume in order to provide a margin of safety during time of stress. A static compliance of greater than 30 ml per cm H_2O has also been suggested as a useful weaning parameter. The work of breathing may be too great for a patient with a lower compliance.

Calculated indices of the efficiency of gas exchange may be helpful in predicting successful weaning. A patient with an alveolar-arterial oxygen gradient of greater than 300 to 350 mm Hg on 100 per cent O_2 would be hypoxemic on inspired oxygen concentrations that can be readily administered by mask. Likewise, a shunt fraction of greater than 15 per cent is predictive of hypoxemia following extubation. A V_d/V_t ratio of greater than 0.6 corresponds to a high minute volume requirement and predicts the need for continued ventilatory assistance in most patients.

Once the patient has satisfied criteria for weaning, there are several alternative ways to proceed toward spontaneous breathing. Some physicians use a "sink-or-swim" approach, extubating the patient directly from the assist control or control mode. A more cautious approach is to discontinue mechanical ventilation and allow the patient to breathe spontaneously for a period of approximately 30 minutes while still intubated. An oxygen-enriched mixture (usually 40 per cent) is supplied by a T piece from a wall source or from the ventilator. The patient is observed for signs of anxiety or respiratory distress, vital signs are monitored, and at the end of 30 minutes, arterial blood gases are drawn. If the patient appears clinically stable and arterial blood gases are good, he is extubated. If not, mechanical ventilation is reinstituted.

A third approach, and the one most commonly used today, is to wean the patient from the IMV mode. Even before the patient satisfies weaning criteria, he may be placed on an IMV rate that provides adequate ventilation but encourages him to take a few breaths on his own. As the patient's pulmonary status improves, the IMV rate is gradually turned down, until finally the patient is breathing entirely on his own. Although it has not been proved that this approach hastens weaning, it certainly provides a smooth transition from assisted ventilation to spontaneous breathing.

Recently, it has been advocated that patients be weaned to CPAP rather than to breathing at atmospheric pressure.[62] It has been observed that patients breathing spontaneously through an endotracheal tube have a lower Pa_{O_2}, a lower functional residual capacity, and a higher shunt fraction than when they are breathing the same oxygen mixture after extubation. The improvement in Pa_{O_2} after extubation is on the order of 10 mm Hg while the patient is breathing 40 per cent oxygen. If the same patients breathe spontaneously with a CPAP of 5 cm H_2O, their Pa_{O_2}, functional residual capacity, and shunt fraction are the same before and after extubation. Their Pa_{CO_2} is approximately 2 mm Hg higher while they are on CPAP as compared with spontaneous breathing with or without an endotracheal tube. Thus, borderline patients who fail a trial of spontaneous breathing at atmospheric pressure because of hypoxemia may succeed at a CPAP of 5 cm H_2O and go on to be safely extubated.

In addition to the weaning criteria described previously, one should consider other clinical parameters in deciding when a patient may be safely weaned. Weaning should be deferred in patients with unstable, life-threatening cardiac dysrhythmias, since the stress of weaning may exacerbate the dysrhythmias. Also, a cardiac arrest is easier to manage in an intubated patient. Patients with marked anemia may be difficult to wean despite meeting usual weaning criteria, because their oxygen delivery to the periphery is impaired by their low hemoglobin levels. Patients who require heavy doses of sedatives or narcotics may be weanable between doses but lose their respiratory drive when their drugs peak. An example would be a burn patient who receives high doses of narcotics for debridement of his wounds. A patient with a metabolic acidosis may be difficult to wean, since he must hyperventilate to maintain a normal pH. On the other hand, a metabolic alkalosis may be an impediment to weaning in a COPD patient, because it may allow his Pa_{CO_2} to rise to narcotizing levels before the development of acidemia stimulates him to breathe.

In addition, psychological factors play a role. Some patients, particularly elderly individuals with prolonged illnesses, repeatedly fail attempts at weaning despite meeting objective weaning criteria. It seems that their spirits have been broken by the regimentation of their lives and that they have lost the will to do anything for themselves, including breathing. These are the most frustrating patients to wean, but may respond to a combination of reassurance, encouragement, and cajolery.

Complications of Mechanical Ventilation

In a prospective study of 354 episodes of mechanical ventilation at the University of Colorado from 1972 to 1973, there were 400 complications.[80] Although most were minor, some were associated with increased patient mortality. It is probably not surprising that there is a high incidence of complications with mechanical ventilation, since it is an invasive form of therapy using complex equipment in critically ill patients for prolonged periods. To some extent, however, the complications are preventable. Others that are not preventable at present should at least be anticipated so that when they occur, they can be recognized and dealt with promptly.

The potential complications of ventilator therapy are listed in Table 3–5. Complications related to intubation and the presence of an endotracheal tube are dealt with in more detail elsewhere in this text but deserve mention here. Intubation of the right main stem bronchus was one of the most common complications in the University of Colorado study and was associated with other problems, including pneumothorax and atelectasis, as well as with decreased survival. Complications related to pressure from the endotracheal tube cuff have declined since the introduction of high-volume, low-pressure cuffs, which require less than 25 mm Hg to produce a seal. Whereas it was recommended in the older literature that a tracheostomy be performed in patients requiring mechanical ventilation for more than 1 to 2 weeks, more recent studies have reported fewer complications with soft cuff endotracheal tubes in place for up to 3 weeks than with tracheostomies.[81] There has been one report of orotracheal intubation for 2 months without complications.[82] The safety of orotracheal versus nasotracheal intubation has not been studied systematically. In general, nasotracheal intubation is better tolerated by the patient, is more secure, and allows better mouth care. On the other hand, it leads to a higher incidence of sinusitis and necrosis of the nasal mucosa and cartilage.

The incidence of complications related to ventilator malfunction has declined as ventilators have become more reliable, but operator errors remain a significant problem. One of the most common yet potentially serious errors is to turn off a ventilator alarm and forget to turn it back on. This happens most frequently when the patient is disconnected briefly from the ventilator for suctioning. With many older ventilators, such as the Puritan-Bennett MA-1, one can permanently silence the alarm that signals when the patient has failed to receive a full tidal volume by turning off a single switch. If this alarm is not turned back on after the patient has been suctioned, the patient may later turn his head and cause the ventilator tubing to become disconnected from the endotracheal tube. The next indication that something is wrong may be the development of a ventricular dysrhythmia on the cardiac monitor. To prevent this occurrence, many modern ventilators have been designed with alarms that can be turned off by the operator only for 1 to 2 minutes before they reactivate themselves.

Barotrauma remains a relatively common complication of ventilator therapy. Pneumothorax is the most serious form of barotrauma and may be preceded or accompanied by pulmonary interstitial emphysema, pneumomediastinum, subcutaneous emphysema, and pneumoperitoneum. In patients receiving ventilatory assistance, pneumothorax is more often than not of the tension type. The reported incidence of pneumothorax in mechanically ventilated patients varies in the literature from 0.5 to 14 per cent.[60, 83–85] The highest incidence of barotrauma occurs with the use of levels of PEEP greater than 24 cm H_2O,[60] whereas levels of PEEP of 5 cm H_2O and below do not seem to be associated with increased risk.[85] The incidence of pneumothorax is also particularly high in patients with asthma.[20]

It has been reported that the incidence of barotrauma is lower with pressure-cycled than with volume-cycled ventilators.[84] This is not surprising when it is considered that higher pressures are commonly used with volume-cycled ventilators, since it is generally believed that it is safer to risk barotrauma but maintain an adequate tidal volume than to risk hypoventilation by limiting peak pressure. Judicious use of sedation and paralysis may

Table 3–5. POTENTIAL COMPLICATIONS OF MECHANICAL VENTILATION

Complications related to endotracheal or tracheostomy tube
  Tube malfunction (leaking cuff, kinked tube, obstruction caused by herniation of balloon over end of tube)
  Pressure phenomena (nasal and tongue necrosis due to pressure from the tube, laryngeal ulceration and polyps, tracheal stenosis and malacia, fistulae into esophagus and innominate artery)
Complications resulting from machine malfunction and operator error
  Failure of ventilator to deliver set tidal volume, rate, F_{O_2}, and so forth
  Inappropriate settings ordered
  Settings not fixed as ordered (commonly includes wrong rate, tidal volume, and F_{O_2}; assist control sensitivity too high or too low)
  Alarm failure
  Alarm turned off and left off
  Inadequate humidification
  Over- or underheating of inspired air
  Patient accidentally disconnected from ventilator
Direct effects of positive-pressure ventilation
  Barotrauma (pneumothorax, tension pneumothorax, pulmonary interstitial emphysema, subcutaneous emphysema, pneumomediastinum, pneumoperitoneum, air embolism)
  Decreased venous return and cardiac output
Other complications
  Ventilator-associated pneumonia
  Oxygen toxicity and retrolental fibroplasia
  Bronchopulmonary dysplasia

help reduce pressures and thereby lower the risk of pneumothorax. Most importantly, the development of pneumothorax should be anticipated in patients at high risk. A pneumothorax should be suspected whenever there is a sudden deterioration in compliance and blood gases. Pneumothorax should be confirmed by auscultation, palpation of the position of the trachea, and, if time permits, a chest film. In the patient who is deteriorating rapidly, needle thoracostomy is both diagnostic and therapeutic. (See Chapter 5.)

Pneumoperitoneum is a form of barotrauma that deserves special mention. The incidence of pneumoperitoneum and pneumoretroperitoneum has been reported to be as high as 4 per cent in patients on PEEP.[86] Pneumoperitoneum is typically preceded by pulmonary interstitial emphysema, subcutaneous emphysema, and pneumomediastinum and is usually, but not always, accompanied by pneumothorax. Patients with ventilator-induced pneumoperitoneum have been subjected to needless laparotomies in a search for the cause of the free air in their abdomens.[87] Another unusual form of barotrauma is fatal arterial and venous air embolism, which has been reported in association with tension pneumothorax in premature infants receiving mechanical ventilation.[88]

Another potential problem that is a direct effect of positive-pressure ventilation is diminished cardiac output. As discussed in the section on PEEP and CPAP, a clinically significant fall in cardiac output usually occurs at levels of PEEP of 12 to 15 cm H_2O and above. A drop in cardiac output has also been shown to be a result of positive-pressure ventilation without PEEP.[28] The fall in cardiac output seen with mechanical ventilation is thought to be caused by decreased venous return as a result of increased intrathoracic pressure. This effect is greatest when mean airway pressures are highest, as in controlled ventilation with PEEP, and is negligible when low mean airway pressures are used, as in the IMV mode with a low mechanical breathing frequency.[22] It has been shown in the case of PEEP that the fall in cardiac output is at least partly reversible with blood volume expansion.[57] The influence of positive-pressure ventilation on venous return also depends upon the extent to which airway pressure is transmitted to the pleural space. When lung compliance is high and chest wall compliance is low, as in COPD, much of the airway pressure is transmitted to the pleural space, and venous return is impaired more than in conditions such as the adult respiratory distress syndrome, in which lung compliance is low.

It should not be assumed that the effect of positive-pressure ventilation on cardiac function is always detrimental. It has been shown that patients with respiratory distress may generate highly negative intrathoracic pressures during spontaneous breathing and that this negative pressure acts as increased afterload on the heart.[89] Just as venous return into the thorax is enhanced by negative intrathoracic pressure, ejection of blood out of the thorax is impeded, and the more negative the intrathoracic pressure, the harder the left heart must pump to reach a given systemic arterial pressure.[90] Mechanical ventilation substitutes positive for negative intrathoracic pressure, thereby decreasing afterload on the left heart. In most cases, the effect of positive-pressure ventilation in decreasing venous return to the heart outweighs its effect in decreasing afterload, and decreased cardiac output results. In patients breathing spontaneously on PEEP as compared with those breathing spontaneously without PEEP, however, an increased cardiac output has been demonstrated.[91] Positive-pressure ventilation would be expected to be particularly beneficial in the treatment of patients with cardiogenic pulmonary edema, since it would decrease both the increased preload and the increased afterload, which are involved in the pathogenesis of this condition.

Pneumonia is one of the more common complications of intubation and mechanical ventilation. In a review of infections related to medical devices, it was found that ventilator-associated pneumonia was second in frequency only to catheter-related cystitis, and it was estimated that 75,000 ventilator patients a year acquire a nosocomial pneumonia with fatality rate of 40 per cent.[92] In another large-scale retrospective study, the incidence of nosocomial pneumonia was 0.3 per cent in patients not on ventilators, 1.3 per cent in patients ventilated by endotracheal tube, and a surprising 66 per cent in patients ventilated by tracheostomy.[93] No pneumonias developed in patients ventilated less than 24 hours, whereas there was an abrupt rise in risk for patients ventilated more than 5 days.

Most cases of ventilator-associated pneumonia resulted from enteric gram-negative organisms. Ventilator-associated pneumonias may be preventable in part by strict adherence to sterile technique during suctioning and by avoidance of prolonged ventilation or tracheostomy whenever possible. Ventilator humidification systems are a potential source of bacterial contamination, and it is the policy at many hospitals to change the ventilator tubing and humidification system every 24 hours. With the cascade humidifiers used on most modern ventilators, however, there is probably little risk of introducing bacteria into the inspired gas mixture, and it has been shown that the system need not be changed more often than every 48 hours.[94]

Oxygen toxicity was discussed as a potential complication of mechanical ventilation in the section on inspired oxygen concentration. Although the exact dose-time relationship of oxygen toxicity has not been worked out, it should be assumed that an FI_{O_2} of 0.50 or greater is potentially toxic. One can avoid oxygen toxicity in many cases by using measures such as PEEP, which improve the A–a D_{O_2} and allow one to use lower inspired oxygen concentrations.

A final condition that should be included as a potential complication of mechanical ventilation is bronchopulmonary dysplasia. Bronchopulmonary dysplasia is a form of chronic lung disease that occurs in infants who have been mechanically ventilated for severe hyaline membrane disease. It is characterized radiographically by cystic enlargement of the airways with intermingled dense, strand-like infiltrates. The incidence of bronchopulmonary dysplasia is 6 to 11 per cent in survivors of hyaline membrane disease.[41] It is not known whether bronchopulmonary dysplasia results from high inspired oxygen concentrations, high airway pressures, or the evolution of hyaline membrane disease itself. One small study has suggested that intramuscular administration of vitamin E may modify the development of bronchopulmonary dysplasia.[95] Until more is known about the actual cause of this condition, however, it cannot be considered preventable.

Future Developments

The field of mechanical ventilation has changed dramatically over the past 25 years, and it will undoubtedly continue to change. A review of the subject would not be complete without a mention of anticipated future developments.

Probably the most exciting development on the horizon is high-frequency ventilation. This technique differs radically from the traditional approach of using tidal volumes and frequencies in the physiologic range. Instead, volumes of a few milliliters per kilogram are used at rates from 60 to 1200 breaths per minute. One might expect that only the dead space gas would be exchanged and that no alveolar ventilation would occur at all. In fact, however, it has been shown that adequate ventilation does occur with this technique, probably as a result of facilitated diffusion of gases along the vibrating column of air. The advantages of high-frequency ventilation are that very low peak pressures are required and small-diameter, uncuffed endotracheal tubes may be used. Thus, problems related to barotrauma and pressure effects from the endotracheal tube are virtually eliminated. High-frequency ventilation has already found practical application in laryngeal surgery, in which it allows the surgeon a clear view of motionless vocal cords.[96] High-frequency ventila-

tion has also been used for short periods in infants with hyaline membrane disease[97] and in adults with chronic respiratory failure.[98] At present, however, there is no commercially available ventilator designed to provide high-frequency ventilation. Also, it remains to be seen whether patients with severe pulmonary disease can be ventilated by this method for prolonged periods or whether problems such as progressive atelectasis will limit use of this technique.

Another exciting prospect of the future is servocontrol of ventilator parameters. Some manufacturers have already incorporated servomechanisms into the design of their ventilators. For example, in the Siemens-Elema Servo 900C,[99] gas flow to the patient is measured by a transducer, which converts this flow into an electronic signal. This signal is compared with another signal generated by the settings on the ventilator control panel, and if there is a difference, an appropriate change in flow occurs. This concept can be expanded so that the input signals include information from the patient, such as Pa_{O_2}, Pa_{CO_2}, arterial pH, airway pressure, and cardiac output.

It has already been demonstrated in experimental animals that by using indwelling monitors of arterial pH and Pa_{CO_2}, a system can be designed so that the ventilator will adjust its own minute volume to maintain a normal pH despite perturbations in acid-base balance introduced by acid infusion.[100] It is conceivable that a similar system could be designed whereby the ventilator would regulate its own FI_{O_2} and decide the best PEEP, inspiratory waveform, I:E ratio, and so on. In fact, one might imagine that in the critical care unit of the future, the physician will intubate the patient, place the necessary monitors, and type the desired end points into the ventilator-computer, which will then regulate all of its own settings, print out periodic progress reports, and page the physician when the patient has been weaned and is ready for extubation. Unfortunately, the development of such a system depends not only upon the necessary technology, much of which already exists, but also upon a society that has almost unlimited resources to devote to medical care. If present economic trends continue, it seems more likely that the emphasis in the future will be on the development of equally reliable yet simpler and less expensive volume- and time-cycled ventilators than are currently available.

---

1. Brewer, L. A.: Respiration and respiratory treatment. A historical overview. Am. J. Surg. 138:342, 1979.
2. Crit. Care Med. 6:310, 1978.
3. Crit. Care Med. 7:226, 1979.
4. Comroe, J. H.: Man-cans. Am. Rev. Respir. Dis. 116:945, 1977.

5. Shapiro, B. A., Harrison, R. A., and Trout, C. A.: Clinical Application of Respiratory Care, 2nd ed. Chicago, Year Book Medical Publishers, 1979, p. 326.
6. Pontoppidan, H., Wilson, R. S., Rie, M. A., and Schneider, R. C.: Respiratory intensive care. Anesthesiology, 47:96, 1977.
7. Pontoppidan, H., Geffin, B., and Lowenstein, E.: Acute respiratory failure in the adult (3 parts). N. Engl. J. Med. 287:690, 743, 799, 1972.
8. Laver, M. B., and Safen, A.: Measurement of blood oxygen tension in anesthesia. Anesthesiology 26:73, 1965.
9. Downer, D. H., and Hoffman, L. G.: Bedside construction of a custom cuirass for respiratory failure in kyphoscoliosis. Chest 74:469, 1978.
10. Man, G. C. W., Jones, R. L., MacDonald, G. F., and King, E. G.: Primary alveolar hypoventilation managed by negative-pressure ventilators. Chest 76:219, 1979.
11. McFadden, E. R., and Lyons, H. A.: Arterial blood gas tension in asthma. N. Engl. J. Med. 278:1027, 1968.
12. Krauss, A. N.: Assisted ventilation: A critical review. Clin. Perinatol. 7:61, 1980.
13. Spahr, R. C., Klein, A. M., Brown, D. R., MacDonald, H. M., and Holzman, I. R.: Hyaline membrane disease. A controlled study of inspiratory to expiratory ratio and its management by ventilator. Am. J. Dis. Child. 134:373, 1980.
14. Krauss, A. N., and Auld, P. A. M.: Evaluation of methods of assisted ventilation in hyaline membrane disease. Arch. Dis. Child. 53:878, 1978.
15. Avery, E. E., Morch, E. T., and Benson, D. W.: Critically crushed chests. A new method of treatment with continuous mechanical hyperventilation to produce alkalotic apnea and internal pneumatic stabilization. J. Thorac. Cardiovasc. Surg. 32:291, 1956.
16. Shackford, S. R., Virgilia, R. W., and Peters, R. M.: Selective use of ventilator therapy in flail chest injury. J. Thorac. Cardiovasc. Surg. 81:194, 1981.
17. Gordon, G.: Controlled respiration in the management of patients with traumatic brain injury. Acta. Anaesthesiol. Scand. 15:193, 1971.
18. Callaham, M.: Tricyclic antidepressant overdose. JACEP 8:413, 1979.
19. Reuler, J. B.: Hypothermia: Pathophysiology, clinical settings, and management. Ann. Intern. Med. 89:519, 1978.
20. Scoggin, C. H., Sahn, S. A., and Petty, T. L.: Status asthmaticus. A nine-year experience. JAMA 238:1158, 1977.
21. Kirby, R. R., Desautels, D. A., Modell, J. H., and Smith, R. A.: Mechanical ventilation. In Burton, G. G., Gee, E. N., and Hodgkin, J. E. (eds.): Respiratory Care. Philadelphia, J. B. Lippincott Co., 1977, pp. 583–663.
22. Douglas, M. E., and Downs, J. B.: Cardiopulmonary effects of intermittent mandatory ventilation. Int. Anesthesiol. Clin. 18:97, 1980.
23. Downs, J. B., and Mitchell, L. A.: Pulmonary effects of ventilatory pattern following cardiopulmonary bypass. Crit. Care Med. 4:295, 1976.
24. Radford, E. P.: Ventilation standard for use in artificial respiration. J. Appl. Physiol. 7:451, 1955.
25. Pontoppidan, H., Hedley-Whyte, J., Bendixen, H. H., Laver, M. B., and Radford, E. P.: Ventilation and oxygen requirements during prolonged artificial ventilation in patients with respiratory failure. N. Engl. J. Med. 273:401, 1965.
26. Ayres, S. M.: Analysis of ventilation and perfusion abnormalities by washout in alveolar air and arterial blood and continuous measurement of inert gas. Crit. Care Med. 4:261, 1976.
27. Smith, L. L., Walton, D. M., Wilson, D. R., Jackson, C. L., and Hinshaw, D. B.: Continuous blood gas and pH monitoring during cardiovascular surgery. Am. J. Surg. 120:249, 1970.
28. Hedley-Whyte, J., Pontoppidan, H., and Morris, M. J.: The response of patients with respiratory failure and cardiopulmonary disease to different levels of constant volume ventilation. J. Clin. Invest. 45:1543, 1966.
29. Suwa, K., and Bendixen, H. H.: Change in Pa_{CO_2} with mechanical dead space during artificial ventilation. J. Appl. Physiol. 24:556, 1968.
30. Breivik, H., Grenvik, A., Millen, E., and Safar, P.: Normalizing low arterial CO_2 tension during mechanical ventilation. Chest 63:525, 1973.
31. Murray, J. F.: The Normal Lung. Philadelphia, W. B. Saunders Co., 1976, pp. 184–185.
32. Selecky, P. A., Wasserman, K., Klein, M., and Ziment, I.: A graphic approach to assessing interrelationships among minute ventilation, arterial carbon dioxide tension, and ratio of physiologic dead space to tidal volume in patients on respirators. Am. Rev. Respir. Dis. 117:181, 1978.
33. Grimby, G., Hedenstierna, G., and Lofstrom, B.: Chest wall mechanics during artificial ventilation. J. Appl. Physiol. 38:576, 1975.
34. Suter, P. M., Fairley, H. B., and Isenberg, M. D.: Effect of tidal volume and positive end-expiratory pressure on compliance during mechanical ventilation. Chest 73:158, 1978.
35. Bear Medical Systems, Inc.: Bear-2 Adult Volume Ventilator Instruction Manual. Riverside, CA, Bear Medical Systems, Inc.
36. Rawlings, D. J., McComb, R. C., Williams, T. A., and Thompson, T. R.: The Siemens Elema Servo ventilator 900B for the management of newborn infants with severe respiratory distress syndrome. A 22 month trial. Crit. Care Med. 8:307, 1980.
37. Bazaral, M. G.: Volume ventilation systems for infants. Anesthesiology 54:240, 1981.
38. Shapiro, B. A., Harrison, R. A., and Walton, J. R.: Clinical Application of Blood Gases, 2nd ed. Chicago, Year Book Medical Publishers, 1977, pp. 85–86.
39. Menn, S. J., and Tisi, G. M.: Oxygen as a drug. In Burton, G, Gee, G. N., and Hodgkin, J. E. (eds.): Respiratory Care. Philadelphia, J. B. Lippincott Co., 1977, pp. 386–399.
40. Weiter, J. J.: Retrolental fibroplasia: An unsolved problem. N. Engl. J. Med. 305:1404, 1981.
41. Northway, W. H.: Bronchopulmonary dysplasia and vitamin E. N. Engl. J. Med. 299:599, 1978.
42. Kinsey, V. E., et al.: Pa_{O_2} levels and retrolental fibroplasia: A report of the cooperative study. Pediatrics 60:655, 1977.
43. Kirby, R. R., Robison, R. J., Schulz, J., and DeLemos, R.: A new pediatric volume ventilator. Anesth. Analg. 50:533, 1971.
44. Downs, J. B., Klein, E. F., Desautel, S. D., Modell, J. H., and Kirby, R. R.: Intermittent mandatory ventilation: A new approach to weaning patients from mechanical ventilators. Chest 64:331, 1973.
45. Schacter, E. N., Tucked, D., and Beck, G. J.: Does intermittent mandatory ventilation accelerate weaning? JAMA 246:1210, 1981.
46. Ashbaugh, D. G., Bigelow, D. B., Petty, T. L., and Levine, B. E.: Acute respiratory distress in adults. Lancet 2:319, 1967.
47. Gregory, G. A., et al.: Treatment of the idiopathic respiratory distress syndrome with continuous positive airway pressure. N. Engl. J. Med. 284:1333, 1971.
48. Greenbaum, D. M., Milien, J. E., Eross, B., Snyder, J. V., Grenvik, A., and Safar, P.: Continuous positive airway pressure without tracheal intubation in spontaneously breathing patients. Chest 69:615, 1976.
49. Hoff, B. N., Flemming, D. C., and Sasse, F.: Use of positive airway pressure without endotracheal intubation. Crit. Care Med. 7:559, 1979.
50. Dantzker, D. R., Brook, C. J., Dehart, P., Lynch, J. P.,

and Weg, J. G.: Ventilation perfusion distribution in the adult respiratory distress syndrome. Am. Rev. Respir. Dis. 120:1039, 1979.

51. Schmidt, G. B., O'Neill, W. W., Kotb, K., Hwang, K. K., Bennett, E. J., and Bombeck, C. T.: Continuous positive airway pressure in the prophylaxis of the adult respiratory distress syndrome. Surg. Gynecol. Obstet. 143:613, 1976.

52. Zimmerman, J. E., Glodman, L. R., and Shaituari, M. B. G.: Effect of mechanical ventilation and PEEP on chest radiograph. Am. J. Radiol. 133:811, 1979.

53. Weisman, I. M., Rinaldo, J. E., and Rogers, R. M.: Positive end-expiratory pressure in adult respiratory failure. N. Engl. J. Med. 307:1381, 1982.

54. Springer, R. R., and Stevens, P. M.: The influence of PEEP on survival of patients in respiratory failure. A retrospective analysis. Am. J. Med. 66:196, 1979.

55. Rizk, N. W., and Murray, J. F.: PEEP and pulmonary edema. Am. J. Med. 72:381, 1982.

56. Lutch, J. S., and Murray, J. F.: Continuous positive-pressure ventilation: Effects on systemic oxygen transport and tissue oxygenation. Ann. Intern. Med. 76:193, 1972.

57. Jardin, F., Farcot, J., Boisaute, L., Curien, N., Margairaz, A., and Bourdarias, J.: Influence of positive end-expiratory pressure on left ventricular performance. N. Engl. J. Med. 304:387, 1981.

58. Powers, S. R., Mannal, R., Neclerio, M., English, M., Marr, C., Leather, R., Ueda, H., Williams, G., Custead, W., and Dutton, R.: Physiologic consequences of positive end-expiratory pressure ventilation. Ann. Surg. 178:265, 1973.

59. Gallagher, T. J., and Civetta, J. M.: Goal-directed therapy of acute respiratory failure. Anesth. Analg. 59:831, 1980.

60. Kirby, R. R., Downs, J. B., Civetta, J. M., Modell, J. H., Dannermiller, F. J., Klein, E. F., and Hodges, M.: High level positive end-expiratory pressure in acute respiratory insufficiency. Chest 67:156, 1975.

61. Suter, P. M., Fairley, B., and Isenberg, M. D.: Optimum end-expiratory airway pressure in patients with acute pulmonary failure. N. Engl. J. Med. 292:284, 1975.

62. Annest, S. J., Gottlieb, M., Paloski, W. H., Stratton, H., Newell, J. C., Dutton, R., and Powers, S. R.: Detrimental effects of removing end-expiratory pressure prior to endotracheal extubation. Ann. Surg. 191:539, 1980.

63. Dammann, J. F., McAslan, T. C., and Maffeo, C. J.: Optimal flow pattern for mechanical ventilation of the lungs. Crit. Care Med. 6:293, 1978.

64. Spar, R. C., Klein, A. M., Brown, D. R., MacDonald, H. M., and Holzman, I. R.: Hyaline membrane disease. A controlled study of inspiratory to expiratory ratio in its management by ventilator. Am. J. Dis. Child. 134:373, 1980.

65. Shapiro, B. A., Harrison, R. A., and Trout, C. A.: Clinical Application of Respiratory Care, 2nd ed. Chicago, Year Book Medical Publishers, 1979, pp. 349–363.

66. Bendixen, H. H., Hedley-Whyte, J., Chir, B., and Laver, M. B.: Impaired oxygenation in surgical patients during general anesthesia with controlled ventilation. N. Engl. J. Med. 269:991, 1963.

67. Kirby, R. R.: Mechanical ventilation in acute ventilatory failure: Facts, fiction, and fallacies. Curr. Probl. Anesth. Crit. Care Med. 3:5, 1977.

68. Clarke, R. S. J., and Lyons, S. M.: Diazepam and flunitrazepam as induction agents for cardiac surgical operations. Acta. Anaesthesiol. Scand. 21:282, 1977.

69. Jaffe, J. H., and Martin, W. R.: Narcotic analgesics and antagonists. In Goodman, L. S., and Gilman, H. (eds.): The Pharmacological Basis of Therapeutics, 5th ed. New York, Macmillan Inc., 1975, pp. 245–283.

70. Bell, E. F.: The use of naloxone in the treatment of diazepam poisoning. J. Pediatr. 87:803, 1975.

71. Jordan, C., Tech, B., Lehane, J. R., and Jones, G.: Respiratory depression following diazepam. Reversal with high-dose naloxone. Anesthesiology 53:293, 1980.

72. Kravitz, M., and Pace, N. L.: Management of the mechanically ventilated patient receiving pancuronium bromide. Heart Lung 8:81, 1979.

73. DeGarmo, B. H., and Dronen, S.: Pharmacology and clinical use of neuromuscular blocking agents. Ann. Emerg. Med. 12:48, 1983.

74. Levin, N., and Dillow, J. B.: Status asthmaticus and pancuronium bromide. JAMA 222:1265, 1972.

75. Stark, A. R., and Frantz, I. D.: Muscle relaxation in mechanically ventilated infants. J. Pediatr. 94:439, 1979.

76. Freely, T. W., and Hedley-Whyte, J.: Weaning from controlled ventilation and supplemental oxygen. N. Engl. J. Med. 292:903, 1975.

77. Sahn, S. A., Lakshminarayan, S., and Petty, T. L.: Weaning from mechanical ventilation. JAMA 235:2208, 1976.

78. Sahn, S. A., and Lakshminarayan, S.: Bedside criteria for discontinuation of mechanical ventilation. Chest 63:1002, 1973.

79. Bowser, M. A., Hodgkin, J. E., and Burton, G. G.: Techniques of ventilator weaning. In Burton, G., Gee, G. N., and Hodgkin, J. E. (eds.): Respiratory Care. Philadelphia, J. B. Lippincott Co., 1977, pp. 664–671.

80. Zwilich, C. W., Pierson, D. J., Creagh, C. E., Sutton, F. D., Schatz, E., and Petty, T. L.: Complications of assisted ventilation. A prospective study of 354 consecutive episodes. Am. J. Med., 57:161, 1974.

81. Stauffer, J. L., Olson, D. E., and Petty, T. L.: Complications and consequences of endotracheal intubation and tracheostomy. A prospective study of 105 critically ill patients. Am. J. Med. 70:65, 1981.

82. Vogelhut, M. M., and Downs, J. B.: Prolonged endotracheal intubation. Chest 76:110, 1979.

83. Kumar, A., Pontoppidan, H., Falke, K. J., Wilson, R. S., and Laver, M. B.: Pulmonary barotrauma during mechanical ventilation. Crit. Care Med. 1:181, 1973.

84. DeLatorre, F. J., Tomasa, A., Klamburg, J., Leon, C., Soler, M., and Rius, J.: Incidence of pneumothorax and pneumomediastinum in patients with aspiration pneumonia requiring ventilatory support. Chest 72:141, 1977.

85. Cullen, D. J., and Caldera, D. L.: The incidence of ventilator-induced pulmonary barotrauma in critically ill patients. Anesthesiology 50:185, 1979.

86. Altman, A. R., and Johnson, T. H.: Pneumoperitoneum and pneumoretroperitoneum. Consequences of positive end-expiratory pressure therapy. Arch. Surg. 114:208, 1979.

87. Summers, B.: Pneumoperitoneum associated with artificial ventilation. Br. Med. J. 1:1528, 1979.

88. Banagale, R. C.: Massive intracranial air embolism: A complication of mechanical ventilation. Am. J. Dis. Child. 134:799, 1980.

89. Buda, A. J., Pinsky, M. R., Ingels, N. B., Daughters, G. T., Stinson, E. B., and Alderman, E. L.: Effect of intrathoracic pressure on left ventricular performance. N. Engl. J. Med. 301:453, 1979.

90. McGregor, M.: Pulsus paradoxicus. N. Eng. J. Med. 301:480, 1979.

91. Sturgeon, C. L., Douglas, M. E., Downs, J. B., and Dannemiller, F. J.: PEEP and CPAP: Cardiopulmonary effects during spontaneous ventilation. Anesth. Analg. 56:633, 1977.

92. Stamm, W. E.: Infections related to medical devices. Ann. Intern. Med. 89:764, 1978.

93. Cross, A. S., and Roup, B.: Role of respiratory assistance devices in endemic nosocomial pneumonia. Am. J. Med. 70:681, 1981.

94. Craven, D. E., Connolly, M. G., Lichtenberg, D. A.,

Primeau, P. J., and McCabe, W. R.: Contamination of mechanical ventilators with tubing changes every 24 or 48 hours. N. Engl. J. Med. 306:1505, 1982.

95. Ehrenkranz, R. A., Bonta, B. W., Ablow, R. C., and Warshaw, J. B.: Amelioration of bronchopulmonary dysplasia after vitamin E administration. N. Engl. J. Med. 299:564, 1978.

96. Babinski, M., Smith, R. B., and Klain, M.: High frequency jet ventilation for laryngoscopy. Anesthesiology 52:178, 1980.

97. Marchak, B. E., Thompson, W. K., Bryan, A. C., and Froese, A. B.: Treatment of RDS by high-frequency oscil-latory ventilation. A preliminary report. J. Pediatr. 99:287, 1981.

98. Rossing, T. H., Slutsky, A. S., Lehr, J. L., Drinker, P. A., Kamm, R., and Drazen, J. M.: Tidal volume and frequency dependence of carbon dioxide elimination by high-frequency ventilation. N. Engl. J. Med. 305:1375, 1981.

99. Siemens Elema Ventilator Systems: Servo ventilator 900C operating manual. Elk Grove Village, IL, Siemens Elema Ventilator systems.

100. Coon, R. L., Zupericu, E. J., and Kampine, J. B.: Systemic arterial blood pH servocontrol of mechanical ventilation. Anesthesiology 49:201, 1978.

4

Transtracheal Aspiration

STEVEN M. JOYCE, M.D.

Patients presenting to the hospital with signs and symptoms of acute pneumonia require expeditious diagnosis and treatment. Examination and culture of lower respiratory tract secretions is desirable in these patients; sampling is mandatory in those who are critically ill. Although expectorated sputum is always contaminated somewhat with oropharyngeal flora, properly screened expectorated sputum is a sufficient specimen in most cases. Occasionally, results of sputum examination and culture are equivocal, or an adequate specimen simply cannot be obtained. In selected cases, the emergency physician may wish to use the technique of transtracheal aspiration to obtain a specimen of tracheobronchial secretions prior to initiation of antibiotic treatment.

Background

Since the introduction of antibiotics, examination of the Gram stain and culture of expectorated sputum has been a safe and simple method of identifying pathogens in lower respiratory tract infections. In patients who are unable to generate a sputum specimen, bronchoscopic aspiration has been used to collect tracheobronchial secretions. Specimens obtained by the aforementioned methods are subject to contamination by oropharyngeal flora, which can yield inaccurate culture results.

Pecora and Yegian[1] found poor correlation between cultures of expectorated sputum and those of lower respiratory tract secretions obtained by open lung biopsy. Recognizing the need for uncontaminated culture specimens, Pecora[2] introduced transtracheal aspiration, a modification of the technique commonly used for translaryngeal anesthesia.

Cultures of lower respiratory tract secretions obtained by transtracheal aspiration are more predictive of pulmonary infection than are those obtained from expectorated washed sputa[3] or bronchoscopic aspirates.[4, 5] Bartlett[6] found that in a series of 488 patients, cultures of transtracheal aspirates agreed 100 per cent with blood cultures from those patients with bacteremic pneumonias. In that same series, the overall diagnostic accuracy of transtracheal aspirate bacteriologic studies was over 90 per cent, with a 1 per cent false-negative and a 21 per cent false-positive incidence. (False positive results usually reflected an exacerbation of chronic bronchitis.) Transtracheal aspiration specimens have been shown to be especially useful in the diagnosis of unusual pulmonary infections, including those caused by anaerobic bacteria,[7] tuberculosis bacilli[8] *Aspergillus*,[8] and *Pneumocystis carinii*.[9] The technique has also been suggested as an aid to bacteriologic diagnosis in hospital-acquired and partially treated pneumonias.[10]

Indications

Failure to obtain an adequate expectorated sputum is the primary reason for performing transtracheal aspiration. Many patients with pneumonia are obtunded and are unable to produce a coughed sputum specimen. Several authors have suggested that expectorated sputum containing less than 25 squamous epithelial cells per 100× microscopic field and greater than 25 leukocytes per 100× field generally is representative of lower respiratory tract secretions.[3] These criteria can be checked by quick microscopic screening of a coughed sputum sample. Furthermore, when no predominant organism is found or when multiple organisms are seen on the Gram stain of the screened sputum, transtracheal aspiration should be considered (see also Chapter 72).

Patients with complicated or unusual pulmonary infections may benefit from transtracheal aspiration. This is especially true in anaerobic infections. When putrid sputum or necrotizing roentgenographic lesions suggest anaerobic pneumonia or abscess, secretions obtained by transtracheal aspiration are *preferred* over those obtained by expectoration, because contamination of a sputum specimen by oral anaerobic flora may alter the results of anaerobic cultures.

In addition, transtracheal aspiration has been shown to be useful in obtaining specimens of fastidious organisms, such as *Aspergillus, Pneumocystis carinii, Nocardia,* and tubercle bacilli.[11] Patients with hospital-acquired pneumonia or with partially treated but poorly responding infections may also benefit from transtracheal aspiration performed to establish the correct pathogen.

Contraindications

Absolute contraindications involve patient safety. Uncooperative patients are most likely to suffer tracheal damage and bleeding. Patients with bleeding diatheses should not be considered for the procedure.

A bleeding diathesis may be suspected by documentation of a prothrombin time greater than twice normal, a platelet count less than 100,000, or a prolonged bleeding time.[12] Hypoxia may predispose patients to potentially dangerous cardiac dysrhythmias. Supplemental oxygen should be administered, and an arterial PO_2 of greater than 70 mm Hg should be documented prior to the procedure.[12] In addition, the inability to identify the proper anatomic landmarks for cricothyroid puncture should preclude use of this technique.

A relative contraindication to the use of transtracheal aspiration is chronic respiratory disease. The transtracheal aspirate from the patient with chronic bronchitis may yield false positive culture results. A severe paroxysmal cough increases the likelihood of subsequent subcutaneous emphysema and hence is also a relative contraindication.

Finally, transtracheal aspiration should never be used when an adequate expectorated sputum specimen can be obtained and is suitable for proper diagnosis.

Equipment

The equipment needed for transtracheal aspiration is minimal and is usually readily available.

Material for sterile preparation of the neck includes gloves, drapes, and a povidone-iodine or isopropyl alcohol solution. One per cent or 2 per cent lidocaine (with or without epinephrine) and a syringe for administration of local anesthetic should be available. Commercially available intravenous catheter sets consisting of either a 14 or a 16 gauge needle with a 6- to 8-inch through-the-needle polyethylene catheter are commonly used. A large (10 to 50 ml) syringe should be used to collect the sample. Two to 5 ml of *nonbacteriostatic* normal saline in a syringe should be available. Cardiac monitoring is desirable, and resuscitative drugs should be available.

Procedure

Transtracheal aspiration can be performed safely when precautions are taken. The patient or family should be counseled regarding the procedure, and informed consent should be obtained. The patient's ability to suppress a cough on command should be assessed, since coughing while the needle is being inserted may result in tracheal laceration. Supplemental oxygen should be applied well in advance of the procedure.

When time permits, results of clotting studies and arterial blood gas evaluation should be obtained and confirmed to be within the acceptable limits discussed previously. A functioning intravenous line and a prefilled syringe with atropine are desirable for the immediate treatment of any clinically significant bradycardia. Premedication

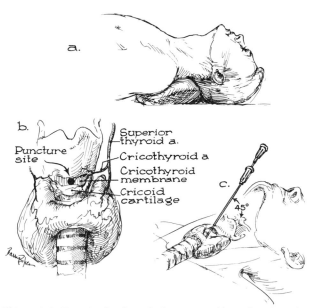

Figure 4–1. Transtracheal aspiration: *a*, position of patient; *b*, anatomic landmarks; *c*, technique of puncture. The Intracath needle is inserted just above the cricoid cartilage through the cricothyroid membrane with its bevel up at a 45-degree angle to the skin. (From Eknoyen: Medical Procedures Manual. Chicago, Year Book Medical Publishers, 1981. Used by permission.)

with atropine, 0.4 mg intramuscularly, 20 to 30 minutes prior to the procedure may minimize the incidence of bradycardia. The procedure should be performed with cardiographic monitoring.

The patient is positioned as shown in Figure 4–1A, with a pillow or rolled towel between the shoulder blades to allow full extension of the neck. The neck is sterilized and draped. The operator then palpates the cricothyroid membrane, and a small intradermal wheal is raised with local anesthetic directly over the membrane (Fig. 4–1B).

Next, the 14 or 16 gauge needle is introduced in the midline through the lower portion of the cricothyroid membrane while the larynx is stabilized (with the application of bilateral support) by the operator or an assistant. The tip of the needle should be angulated approximately 45 degrees caudad to avoid injury to laryngeal structures. A "pop" or a sudden give will be felt as the needle enters the tracheal lumen, and air will be easily aspirated into a syringe attached to the needle. As soon as tracheal entry is confirmed, the needle should be advanced *only a few millimeters* to ensure that the entire needle tip is within the lumen. The needle should then be stabilized and advanced *no further* (to avoid injury to the posterior tracheal wall or adjacent structures).

The polyethylene catheter is then inserted quickly through the needle to its full length, and the needle tip is immediately withdrawn through the skin surface. A vigorous cough will almost always be produced when the catheter is introduced, so the needle should be withdrawn as soon as possible to minimize the chance of laryngeal injury. Once inserted, *the catheter must never be withdrawn through the needle*—catheter fragments are easily sheared off by the needle bevel and may become lodged in the trachea.

As soon as the catheter is in place, a 10- to 50-ml syringe is attached to the catheter hub and suction is applied. Usually, a specimen of secretions is easily obtained. Enough fluid to fill the catheter hub is sufficient for analysis.

If a specimen is not forthcoming, 2 to 5 ml of sterile, nonbacteriostatic saline may be rapidly injected through the catheter; suction should be reapplied immediately. Saline will dilute the sample, however, and may decrease the yield of positive cultures. In addition, small volumes of saline may temporarily depress arterial oxygen tension.

As soon as a suitable amount of sample is obtained, the catheter is withdrawn and direct pressure is applied to the puncture site. The patient is instructed to avoid coughing as much as possible in the next 24 hours and should not receive intermittent positive-pressure breathing (IPPB) treatments or other forms of therapy that stimulate coughing during this period.

Proper handling and screening of the aspirate is essential. The catheter and syringe assembly should be transported promptly to the bacteriology laboratory for processing. A smear for Gram stain is made, and cultures are plated as soon as possible, including anaerobic cultures. One may inspect the Gram stain under $100\times$ dry magnification to ascertain that the specimen meets criteria for lower respiratory tract secretions (less than 25 squamous epithelial cells; greater than 25 leukocytes per field). Oil immersion magnification should reveal a predominant organism in bacterial infections, and antibiotic therapy may be started immediately based on organism morphology, epidemiology, and roentgenographic appearance of the infiltrate(s). Subsequent culture results should confirm the diagnosis and, as mentioned, are highly accurate when specimens are obtained by transtracheal aspiration.

Complications

When proper precautions are taken and patients are selected appropriately the complication rate of transtracheal aspiration is very low. The overall mortality in over 1500 cases reviewed in the literature is less than 0.1 per cent. Complications will be discussed from most to least common, and treatment will be outlined.

Subcutaneous emphysema may be observed in up to 20 per cent of patients. It is usually confined to the anterior neck and is self-limiting without specific treatment. One may minimize the incidence of subcutaneous emphysema following transtracheal aspiration by instructing the patient to avoid strenuous coughing, by forgoing (for 24 hours) IPPB and other treatments that stimulate coughing, and by avoiding positive-pressure ventilation when possible. Mediastinal emphysema is very rare and is likewise self-limited.

Some minimal hemoptysis may occur for 1 to 2 minutes following the procedure, but sustained hemoptysis is rare (1 to 2 per cent of cases). Careful assessment of the patient's clotting studies and caution in needle placement (with prompt needle withdrawal) will minimize the risk of injury to the cricothyroid arteries. Digital pressure over the cricothyroid puncture site for 5 minutes will prevent prolonged intratracheal or paratracheal hemorrhage in most instances. Persistent intratracheal hemorrhage has caused death from asphyxia in at least one case.[13] Prompt recognition of intratracheal hemorrhage, placement of a cuffed endotracheal tube, and correction of any coagulopathies will prevent aspiration and serious complications.

Cardiac dysrhythmias are probably secondary to vagal stimulation during tracheal suctioning and occur with an unknown frequency. Cardiac monitoring is recommended. Hypoxia most certainly potentiates dysrhythmias and is easily prevented by administration of supplemental oxygen and monitoring of the arterial P_{O_2}. Premedication with atropine as described should offer some protection against vagally mediated bradycardia. Atropine as well as other cardioresuscitative drugs and equipment should be immediately available during the procedure.[14]

Anterior cervical infections following transtracheal aspiration have been reported (0.4 to 0.8 per cent of cases).[11] The pathogen is usually the same as that isolated from the transtracheal aspirate. Treatment consists of appropriate antibiotic therapy and incision and drainage of abscesses. Mediastinitis from inadvertent esophageal puncture has not been reported.

Catheter fragments may be sheared free when the catheter is withdrawn without concurrent needle removal. Fragments can be located radiographically and removed by bronchoscopy. Other rare complications, such as pneumothorax, are treated by observation or tube thoracostomy as indicated.

Interpretation

When properly obtained, screened, and processed, cultures of transtracheal aspirate secretion are highly predictive of the pathogen responsible for pulmonary infection. Careful screening by Gram stain minimizes the likelihood of oral contaminants and gives preliminary information as to the identity of the pathogen.

Gram-stained slides of aspirated material that contain fewer than 25 squamous epithelial cells and greater than 25 leukocytes per $100 \times$ field may be considered to represent lower respiratory tract specimens (approximately 66 per cent accuracy).[3] Antibiotic treatment may be instituted immediately, based upon the morphology of stained organisms and the patient's history, clinical presentation, and roentgenographic and laboratory tests. Special staining, as for acid-fast bacilli, should be done when clinically indicated.

Specimens containing more than 25 squamous epithelial cells per $100 \times$ field should be considered to be contaminated by oral secretions. In these instances, repeat transtracheal aspiration may be attempted, or the physician may proceed with treatment with the understanding that the culture of such material is likely to contain oral flora, which may obscure or suppress growth of the actual pathogen.[3]

The accuracy of culture results from properly handled specimens is very high in most studies. Bartlett[6] found an incidence of 1 per cent false-negative and 21 per cent false-positive cultures in 488 samples obtained by transtracheal aspiration. A negative culture was found to indicate an alternative diagnosis in 60 per cent of cases and suppression of growth by prior antibiotic treat-

ment in 37 per cent of cases. Of the false-positive cultures, 25 per cent were considered to reflect exacerbated chronic bronchitis, whereas 75 per cent of the false-positive cultures were presumed to be caused by oral flora contamination. When correctly processed, materials from transtracheal aspiration are highly predictive even of fastidious pathogens or unusual infections, including anaerobic pulmonary infections.[7, 8]

Conclusion

In the infrequent instances in which tracheobronchial secretions are not obtainable from expectorated sputum and accurate bacteriologic diagnosis is essential to care of the patient with suspected pulmonary infection, transtracheal aspiration is a safe, practical method for obtaining such a sample. When one adheres to the precautions and guidelines presented herein, the procedure has low morbidity, high yield, and high diagnostic accuracy.

1. Pecora, D. V., and Yegian, D.: Bacteriology of the lower respiratory tract in health and chronic diseases. N. Engl. J. Med. 258:71, 1958.
2. Pecora, D. V.: A method of securing uncontaminated tracheal secretions for bacterial examination. J. Thorac. Surg. 37:653, 1959.
3. Geckler, R. W., Gremillion, D. H., AcAllister, C. K., and Ellenbogen, C.: Microscopic and bacteriologic comparison of paired sputa and transtracheal aspirates. J. Clin. Microbiol. 6:396, 1977.
4. Jordan, G. W., Wong, G. A., and Hoeprich, P. D.: Bacteriology of the lower respiratory tract as determined by fiberoptic bronchoscopy and transtracheal aspiration. J. Infect. Dis. 134:428, 1976.
5. Pecora, D. V.: A comparison of transtracheal aspiration with other methods of determining the bacterial flora of the lower respiratory tract. N. Engl. J. Med. 269:664, 1963.
6. Bartlett, J. G.: Diagnostic accuracy of transtracheal aspiration bacteriologic studies. Am. Rev. Respir. Dis. 115:777, 1977.
7. Bartlett, J. G., Rosenblatt, J. E., and Finegold, S. M.: Percutaneous transtracheal aspiration in the diagnosis of anaerobic pulmonary infection. Ann. Intern. Med. 79:535, 1973.
8. Schouteus, E., Dekoster, J. P., Vereerstraeten, J., et al.: Use of transtracheal aspiration in the bacteriological diagnosis of bronchopulmonary infection. Biomedicine 19:160, 1973.
9. Lau, W. K., Young, L. S., and Remington, J. S.: Pneumocystis carinii pneumonia: Diagnosis by examination of pulmonary secretions. JAMA 236:2399, 1976.
10. Jay, S. J., and Stonehill, R. D. (eds.): Manual of Pulmonary Procedures. Philadelphia, W. B. Saunders Co., 1980, pp. 170–179.
11. Eknoyan, G.: Medical Procedures Manual. Chicago, Year Book Medical Publishers, 1981.
12. Pratter, M. R., and Irwin, R. S.: Transtracheal aspiration, guidelines for safety. Chest 76:518, 1979.
13. Schillaci, R. F., Iacovoni, V. E., and Conte, R. S.: Transtracheal aspiration complicated by fatal endotracheal hemorrhage. N. Engl. J. Med. 295:488, 1976.
14. Shim, C., Fine, N., Fernandez, R., et al.: Cardiac arrhythmias resulting from tracheal suctioning. Ann. Intern. Med. 71:1149, 1969.

5

Thoracentesis

DAVID S. ROSS, M.D.

Introduction

The term thoracentesis is derived from the Greek "thorakos" (chest) and "kentesis" (to pierce). Although a broad definition could include the introduction of any object into the chest, including thoracostomy tubes, common usage is confined to the temporary insertion of a needle or small catheter into the pleural space. Traditionally, we think of thoracentesis as the method of removing a pleural effusion for diagnostic or therapeutic purposes. In the emergency situation, the removal of air from the pleural space (e.g., from a tension pneumothorax) may also be referred to as thoracentesis. In this chapter, both aspects are discussed. (Tube thoracostomy is discussed in Chapter 6.)

Thoracentesis may be performed whenever the appropriate indications are evident and suitable equipment is available. Because a tension pneumothorax may quickly cause death, all physicians should be familiar with the method of its presentation and the appropriate indications and techniques for relief of this life-threatening situation. In many communities, paramedical and nursing personnel are trained in needle thoracentesis for treatment of tension pneumothorax.

The pleural space is a potential space between the visceral and parietal pleura and contains a thin physiologic layer of pleural fluid. With normal inspiration, a negative pressure is developed within the thorax and is transmitted through the pleural space to the pulmonary parenchyma, allowing normal influx of air. During expiration, the elasticity of the pulmonary parenchyma allows exhalation.

If there is an accumulation of fluid, blood, or air in the pleural space, normal ventilatory mechanisms may be affected. If the volume of fluid or air is large, respiratory compromise may be the result. If the accumulation is rapid and progressive (e.g., tension pneumothorax), there may also be cardiovascular compromise. The underlying etiology of an effusion may also play a part in the severity of symptoms.

Historical Background

Thoracentesis (paracentesis thoracis) was first described by Hippocrates and later was recommended by Cicero for relief of empyema. Various operative approaches using trochars or open drainage were advocated during the ensuing centuries. In the late eighteenth century, both Alexander Monro (Secundus) of Edinburgh and William Hewson of Northumberland reported the use of thoracentesis for treatment of pneumothorax.[1] Glinz credits the French internist, René Laënnec (1781–1826) with the use of thoracentesis for the relief of an apparent tension pneumothorax with associated pneumomediastinum.[2]

In the nineteenth century, more interest developed in thoracentesis. John Snow of York developed a trochar in 1841. Other early pioneers in the use of thoracentesis for pleural effusion and empyema were Armand Trousseau in Paris (1843) and Henry Bowditch in Boston (1851).[1] The use of thoracentesis was followed by the development of continuous pleural drainage for empyema.[3] In World War II, thoracentesis and chest drainage replaced routine thoracotomy for most chest injuries, and during the Korean conflict, repeated thoracentesis was advocated for penetrating chest wounds.[2, 4] At the time of the war in Vietnam, the improvement in thoracostomy tubes made them more effective and tube thoracostomy came to be preferred to simple or repeated thoracentesis.[5]

Indications

At the present time, thoracentesis remains as a useful diagnostic and therapeutic tool in the treatment of pleural effusions. This technique is also frequently used as a temporary lifesaving intervention for the alleviation of tension pneumothorax. A list of current indications is summarized in Table 5–1.

TENSION PNEUMOTHORAX

Mechanism

A tension pneumothorax is a type of pneumothorax that is marked by the progressive collection of air in the pleural space, with subsequent shift of the mediastinum away from the side of the

Table 5–1. INDICATIONS FOR THORACENTESIS

Emergency diagnosis and treatment of suspected tension pneumothorax (prior to tube thoracostomy).
Diagnostic analysis of pleural effusion.
Acute treatment for symptomatic pleural effusions.
Evacuation of simple stable pneumothorax. (This is a controversial issue.)

pneumothorax. During inspiration, negative intrapleural pressure facilitates inward flow by relative bronchiolar and alveolar dilatation. During expiration in the patient with a tension pneumothorax, air is less able to exit the pleural space owing to collapse of the rent in the airway and there is a relative compression of the bronchioli and alveoli owing to positive intrathoracic pressure. This creates a ball-valve mechanism, which favors collection and trapping of additional air in the pleural space.

As the volume of intrapleural air continues to expand, the intrapleural pressure rises. This pressure is transmitted against the lungs, causing a continued decrease in functioning lung volume. First the ipsilateral and then the contralateral lung become compressed. This collapse leads to respiratory compromise as ventilation/perfusion mismatching develops and hypoxia and acidosis ensue. In addition, the increase in the volume of the intrapleural air causes a shift of the mediastinum away from the side of the tension pneumothorax. There is a subsequent drop in the systemic venous return due to a combination of increased intrathoracic pressure and mechanical collapse of the venae cavae. The compromised venous return results in diminished cardiac output and may lead to cardiovascular collapse. The rapidity with which these events occur is variable. They can proceed quickly and lead to death in a matter of minutes. Therapeutic intervention may often be necessary before full diagnostic evaluation can be carried out.

Etiology

A tension pneumothorax may develop as a result of any of the usual causes of pneumothorax or pneumohemothorax (see Chapter 6). The tension pneumothorax may develop either primarily as a complication of a previously stable pneumothorax or pneumohemothorax or as a result of changes in the ventilatory mechanisms. Certain factors may predispose to the development of a tension pneumothorax in a patient with an otherwise stable pneumothorax. A primary predisposing factor is the use of positive-pressure ventilation, either by bag-valve devices or by mechanical ventilators.[5a] The addition of positive end–expiratory pressure (PEEP) may further increase the risk of developing a tension pneumothorax.[5b] Finally, an open pneumothorax can occasionally be converted to a tension pneumothorax following application of an airtight seal at the site of the thoracic wound.

Diagnosis

Tension pneumothorax should always be suspected in any patient when there is sudden respiratory or cardiopulmonary deterioration. The clinical presentation in the patient who is awake includes the sudden development of dyspnea, agitation, or diminished consciousness. Tachypnea, tachycardia, and hypotension may be present and may progress to cardiac or respiratory arrest. The classic but inconsistent constellation of findings are hyperresonance to percussion, decreased breath sounds over the involved hemithorax, tracheal deviation toward the contralateral side, and the presence of an overinflated, immobile, ipsilateral hemithorax.[6] Other signs of chest trauma or respiratory distress should prompt one to consider the possibility of an underlying pneumothorax with potential tension.

In the patient who suddenly deteriorates, other diagnostic considerations should include massive pulmonary embolus, pericardial tamponade, pneumomediastinum, respiratory failure, and myocardial infarction. Traumatic diaphragmatic hernia has also been reported to simulate a tension pneumothorax.[6a] The patient with a tension pneumothorax who is being mechanically ventilated will show signs of increased airway resistance, evidenced by increased ventilatory pressures, prolonged inspiratory times, and elevated central venous pressure.

Diagnosis by a portable chest radiograph is warranted only in the patient who is relatively stable or who has moderate respiratory compromise but no physical evidence of a tension pneumothorax. A pneumothorax with a partially or completely collapsed lung and a shift of the mediastinum is diagnostic of a tension pneumothorax.[7] If a patient has even the most remote possibility of a tension pneumothorax, he should never be sent to the radiology suite unless accompanied by a physician who is prepared to perform immediate thoracentesis or tube thoracostomy. Despite an increased awareness of the possibility of a tension pneumothorax on clinical grounds, the diagnosis is often not recognized until a chest film has been taken.[7a]

When the patient is in extremis, the diagnosis should be made by needle or catheter thoracentesis. The successful relief of a tension pneumothorax is marked by the rapid efflux of air through the thoracentesis needle during both inspiration and expiration. If a syringe is attached to the thoracentesis needle, the plunger may be driven outward if sufficient pressure has developed. In a similar manner, a flutter-valve apparatus attached to the needle may continue to show evidence of massive air efflux. In addition, the patient will show clinical improvement following needle thoracentesis. If the patient is intubated and is being ventilated, *diagnostic tube thoracostomy is preferred to thoracentesis* when time permits. There is a theoretical risk of creating a tension pneumothorax by indiscriminate thoracentesis in the patient who is receiving positive-pressure ventilation.

Treatment

Treatment of a tension pneumothorax depends upon the clinical setting. It should be emphasized that *the preferred and definitive treatment is immediate tube thoracostomy* (see Chapter 6); however, this may not be possible in many clinical settings. If a patient develops acute deterioration and rapid tube thoracostomy is not immediately possible, thoracentesis is an appropriate treatment and may be lifesaving. Thoracentesis is most commonly performed by simple needle or catheter aspiration in the mid-clavicular line, 2nd intercostal space.

In the pre-hospital care setting, when a patient in extremis is suspected to have a tension pneumothorax, thoracentesis is indicated.[7b] To facilitate the continued drainage of the pneumothorax, an expedient flutter-valve may be made or a one-way valve may be attached.[8] A McSwain Dart (Medical Dynamics, Inc.) with a flutter-valve attachment has been suggested as an alternative to thoracentesis in the pre-hospital care setting or in a hospital setting where tube thoracostomy may be delayed (see Chapter 6).[9]

PLEURAL EFFUSION

Mechanism

Normal pleural fluid is created as a result of several physiologic mechanisms, including hydrostatic pressure, colloid osmotic pressure, lymphatic absorption, and intrapleural pressure. With normal pleura, the hydrostatic pressure of the systemic capillaries in the *parietal* pleura is 30 cm H_2O. Likewise, the hydrostatic pressure of the pulmonary capillaries in the *visceral* pleura is approximately 11 cm H_2O. This creates a gradient that allows for the formation of normal fluid at the parietal pleura and absorption by the visceral pleura. A summary of the homeostatic forces involved is shown in Figure 5–1.

The integrity of this system can be disrupted by changes in hydrostatic pressure, colloid osmotic pressure, lymphatic flow, intrapleural pressure, capillary permeability, and perhaps pleural fluid surfactant composition.[10] Increased pleural fluid can be produced secondary to the following general mechanisms. Congestive heart failure can increase pulmonary and systemic vascular hydrostatic pressure. Colloid osmotic pressure is diminished secondary to hypoalbuminemic states, as seen with the nephrotic syndrome and cirrhosis. Trauma to the lymphatic duct or other disease within the lymphatic system may alter thoracic lymphatic flow. Intrapleural pressure may be ab-

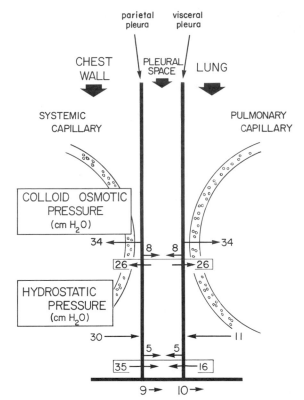

Figure 5–1. Diagrammatic representation of the pressures involved in the formation and absorption of pleural fluid. (From Fraser, R. G., and Paré, J. A. P.: Diagnosis of Diseases of the Chest. Philadelphia, W. B. Saunders Company, 1970, p. 416. Used by permission.)

normally decreased in the presence of atelectasis. Inflammation, infection, pulmonary infarction, and neoplasm can alter capillary permeability.

Etiology

Numerous etiologies may account for the formation of abnormal pleural fluid. Rapid or relatively acute accumulations may be seen with hemothorax, thoracic duct injury, esophageal rupture, pulmonary infarction, infection, empyema, obstructive uropathy, or iatrogenic causes (such as intrapleural placement of a subclavian vein catheter). More chronic effusions may also be seen and are commonly classified as transudates or exudates. Transudates typically have a low specific gravity and low protein concentration. Exudates usually have an increased specific gravity and high protein concentration. Common causes of both are listed in Table 5–2.

Physical Diagnosis

A pleural effusion may be asymptomatic or may produce varying degrees of dyspnea or pleuritic pain. Other symptoms may be present and related to the underlying cause of the effusion.

Table 5–2. CAUSES OF PLEURAL EFFUSION

Common Causes of Transudates
Congestive heart failure
Cirrhosis with ascites
Nephrotic syndrome
Hypoproteinemia
Acute atelectasis
Acute glomerulonephritis
Myxedema
Peritoneal dialysis
Superior vena caval obstruction

Common Causes of Exudates
Pulmonary infarction
Lung abscess
Bacterial pneumonia (parapneumonic effusion)
Neoplasm
Viral illness
Tuberculosis
Fungal illness
Rickettsia
Certain parasites
Collagen vascular disease (especially lupus erythematosus or rheumatoid pleuritis)
Pancreatitis
Drug reactions (nitrofurantoin, methysergide, practolol)
Asbestosis
Meigs' syndrome
Dressler's syndrome
Lymphatic disease
Trapped lung
Subphrenic and hepatic abscess
Sarcoidosis
Chronic atelectasis
Uremia
Chylothorax

The physical signs of pleural effusion vary according to its size. Less than 300 ml of fluid accumulation will not usually produce physical findings. Effusions of greater than 300 to 500 ml can produce physical findings over the area of the effusion. Breath sounds may be diminished, there may be dullness to percussion, and tactile fremitus may be decreased. When the patient is in an upright position, a decrease in movement of the lower chest may be noted. Fluid collections of greater than 1000 ml generally produce all the aforementioned findings. In addition, breath sounds may change from vesicular to bronchovesicular as compression of the underlying lung occurs. Egophony may be heard, and as additional fluid collects, breath sounds may be absent. Large accumulations of fluid may produce mediastinal shift, with accompanying tracheal deviation and displacement of the cardiac impulse. In such cases, bulging of the intercostal spaces may be noted.

Radiographic Diagnosis

Radiographic findings with pleural effusions also correlate with the amount of fluid present. Displacement of the costophrenic angle away from the ribs may occur prior to obvious costophrenic angle blunting.[11] Up to 500 ml of fluid may be needed in order for blunting of the costophrenic angle to be seen on an upright chest film.[12] A fluid level with an upwardly concave meniscus indicates a considerably larger effusion. A fluid level without a meniscus is indicative of a coexisting pneumothorax.

From the upright chest film, the upper level of the effusion can be determined. Smaller amounts of fluid may be seen on a lateral decubitus chest film. Slight elevation of the hemidiaphragm or lateral displacement of the diaphragmatic dome on the posteroanterior (PA) chest film suggests a small subpulmonic effusion. Thickening of the pleural fissures may also be seen.

On a supine anteroposterior (AP) film, a generalized haziness, particularly of the lower lung fields, may be suggestive of a pleural effusion. A lateral decubitus or upright chest film will help confirm this diagnosis. Loculated effusions along the pleural border may occasionally be seen following previous hemothorax or empyema. Elliptical thickening of the fissures is suggestive of loculated effusions. Computed tomography (CT) or ultrasonic examination of the chest may help differentiate loculated effusions from solid tumors.

Pleural Fluid Analysis

The most frequent indication for thoracentesis in the patient with a pleural effusion is for determining the cause of the effusion. An exception to the need for diagnostic thoracentesis is an obvious case of congestive heart failure. Determining whether an effusion is hemorrhagic, purulent, or chylous may be done quickly by visual examination of aspirated pleural fluid. A bloody effusion is usually the result of trauma. A blood-tinged effusion may result from several mechanisms that can be clarified by the red blood cell (RBC) count as described later. White or milky fluid suggests a chylothorax or a chyliform effusion. Grossly purulent effusions may be thick and opaque. Turbid effusions may occur either with an elevated white blood cell (WBC) count or in the presence of chylothorax.

Further diagnostic differentiation can be made by separating effusions into transudates or exudates. The traditional approach had been to define an exudate as an effusion with a protein level greater than 3 gm per 100 ml and a specific gravity greater than 1.016. Light and associates have suggested alternative diagnostic criteria that appear to be more accurate. They define an exudate by the presence of any of the following criteria: 1) a ratio of pleural fluid protein to serum protein of greater than 0.5, 2) a lactate dehydrogenase (LDH) level in the pleural fluid of greater than 200 IU per ml, or 3) a ratio of pleural fluid LDH to serum LDH of greater than 0.6.[13]

Other laboratory determinations may also be helpful. A WBC count greater than 1000 per mm³ suggests an exudate. A WBC count greater than 25,000 per mm³ is suggestive of empyema. The differential cell count of the fluid may be helpful. Polymorphic neutrophils are seen in greater numbers in pneumonia, pulmonary infarction, empyema, and pancreatitis. Monocytes follow the appearance of neutrophils and are found in more chronic forms of these processes. Monocytes may also be seen in transudates or exudates found with tuberculosis (TB), lymphoma, carcinoma, uremia, and rheumatic disease. Lymphocytes are seen in greater numbers in cases of TB or malignancy. Often, pleural macrophages may precede the appearance of the lymphocytes.[14, 15] An eosinophil count of greater than 10 per cent of the differential may be seen secondary to a recent pneumothorax or hemothorax. Eosinophilia may also be seen with pulmonary embolus, asthma, and polyarteritis, and in parasitic or fungal diseases.

An RBC count greater than 5000 to 10,000 per mm³ may be seen with TB, pulmonary infarction, congestive heart failure, or malignancy. An RBC count greater than 100,000 per mm³ suggests trauma, pulmonary infarction, or malignancy. A hematocrit level of the pleural fluid that equals the serum hematocrit suggests a hemothorax or a traumatic thoracentesis. Other abnormal cells, such as mesothelial cells in mesothelioma, may also be seen. Cytology may reveal malignant cells in a large percentage of patients with malignancies within the lung and pleura.[16]

Chemical analysis may be helpful in establishing the diagnosis. A pleural glucose is considered to be normal if it is greater than 60 mg per dl or has a ratio to the serum glucose of greater than 0.5. Lower levels are seen in rheumatoid disease, empyema, carcinoma, TB, esophageal rupture (anaerobic empyema), and lupus erythematosus.[17, 18] The pleural fluid amylase is considered to be elevated when its levels are above 160 Somogyi units per dl or when it has a ratio to the serum amylase of greater than 2.0. Causes include pancreatitis, pancreatic pseudocyst, esophageal rupture, and lung carcinoma.[18, 19] A pleural fluid pH of less than 7.30 is seen in exudates secondary to empyema, parapneumonic effusions, malignancy, rheumatoid disease, lupus erythematosus, TB, and esophageal rupture.[20, 21] A pleural fluid creatinine greater than the serum creatinine may suggest obstructive uropathy and retroperitoneal urine collection as a cause of the pleural effusion.[21a]

There are two types of milky pleural effusions, chylous and chyliform. Both contain increased lipids. Chylothorax results from chyle draining directly into the pleura from trauma to the thoracic duct or from damage to the lymphatic system owing to lymphoma. These effusions contain chylomicrons and triglycerides. Chylomicrons and triglycerides can be seen in chylous effusions stained with Sudan III.[22, 23] Chyliform effusions are characterized by high cholesterol, which does not stain with Sudan III. Chyliform effusions are seen in TB, rheumatoid disease, and trapped lung. A laboratory determination of the levels of triglycerides and cholesterol may also be made.

Wright's stain will allow identification of LE cells as seen in lupus erythematosus. A Gram stain may be positive for bacteria in the presence of empyema or a parapneumonic effusion. A stain for acid-fast bacillus (AFB) may be positive with TB pleural effusion.[24] Appropriate cultures for aerobic and anaerobic bacteria, TB, and fungal disease should also be taken.

A comprehensive review of pleural fluid analysis, which covers these features in more detail, has been prepared by Sahn[25] (see Table 5–3).

Treatment

The management of a pleural effusion is directed toward treating the underlying etiology. Therefore, thoracentesis is primarily indicated for diagnosis. In the case of congestive heart failure, the etiology is usually obvious clinically and the effusion generally responds well to medical therapy without thoracentesis. Occasionally, with very large or rapidly accumulating effusions, the presence of the effusion itself may impair normal respiratory mechanics, causing significant pulmonary symptoms and respiratory compromise. If this is the case, pleural fluid may be removed for symptomatic reasons.

In certain cases, removal of pleural fluid by thoracentesis should be followed by tube thoracostomy. The presence of an empyema is best managed by continuous drainage through a thoracostomy tube. The finding of hemopneumothorax will require tube thoracostomy. A ruptured esophagus, discovered by thoracentesis, requires operative thoracotomy and surgical repair. Repeated thoracentesis may be required for large symptomatic pleural effusions. Chylothorax due to thoracic trauma can often be managed by repeated thoracentesis or by tube thoracostomy; parenteral alimentation and bed rest are recommended.[26]

STABLE PNEUMOTHORAX

Stable pneumothorax is usually managed by observation or tube thoracostomy as discussed in Chapter 6. The use of thoracentesis to treat small pneumothoraces has been suggested.[27, 28] In such cases, the pneumothorax is considered stable and thoracentesis is advocated to decrease the time

Table 5-3. PLEURAL FLUID CHARACTERISTICS IN COMMON DISEASES*

Diagnosis	Appearance	Total Leukocytes (per mm³)	Predominant Leukocytes	RBC (per mm³)	Protein	Glucose	LDH	Amylase	pH	Comment
Transudates										
Congestive heart failure	Clear, straw-colored	<1,000	M	0–1,000	PF/S<0.5	PF=S	PF/S<0.6 <200 IU/L	≤S	>7.40	Usually presence of biventricular failure
Cirrhosis	Clear, straw-colored	<500	M	<1,000	PF/S<0.5	PF=S	PF/S<0.6 <200 IU/L	≤S	>7.40	Incidence 5% of cirrhotic patients with ascites
Exudates										
Parapneumonic (uncomplicated)	Turbid	5,000–25,000	P	<5,000	PF/S>0.5	PF=S	PF/S>0.6	≤S	< or >7.30	Resolves with antibiotics only
Empyema	Turbid to purulent	25,000–100,000	P	<5,000	PF/S>0.5	0–60 mg/dl PF/S<0.5	PF/S>0.6 some >1,000 IU/L	≤S	<7.30	Requires tube drainage
Pulmonary infarction	Straw-colored to bloody	5,000–15,000	P	1,000–100,000	PF/S>0.5	PF=S	PF/S>0.6	≤S	>7.30	Small effusion with basal alveolar infiltrate and elevated diaphragm
Tuberculosis	Straw-colored to serosanguineous	5,000–10,000	M	<10,000	PF/S>0.5	PF=S or <60 mg/dl	PF/S>0.6	≤S	< or >7.30	Positive PPD, AFB stain and culture of pleural tissue often diagnostic
Rheumatoid disease	Turbid, green to yellow	1,000–20,000	M or P	<1,000	PF/S>0.5	<30 mg/dl	Often >1,000 IU/L	≤S	<7.30	Men, rheumatoid nodules, low pleural fluid complement
Carcinoma	Turbid to bloody	<10,000	M	1,000 to several 100,000	PF/S>0.5	PF=S or <60 mg/dl	PF/S>0.6	≤S	< or >7.30	Cytology and pleural biopsy enable diagnosis in 80% of cases
Pancreatitis	Turbid	5,000–20,000	P	1,000–10,000	PF/S>0.5	PF=S	PF/S>0.6	PF/S>2	>7.30	Occurs in 6% of cases of pancreatitis: left-sided in 70% of cases

RBC = red blood cells; LDH = lactate dehydrogenase; M = mononuclear; PF = pleural fluid; S = serum; P = polymorphonuclear; PPD = tuberculin skin test with purified protein derivative; AFB = acid-fast bacilli.

*Reproduced with permission from Sahn, S. A.: Pulmonary disease. In Reller, L. B., et al. (eds.): Clinical Internal Medicine. Boston, Little, Brown and Co., 1979, pp. 106–107.

needed for the spontaneous resorption of the intrapleural air. Such a compromise between conservative observation and more invasive tube thoracostomy may be reasonable in selected cases.

HEMOTHORAX

Historically, repeated thoracentesis has been used to evacuate hemothoraces. With the advent of effective tube thoracostomy, however, this method has become nearly obsolete. There are three major reasons for the discontinuation of this practice. First, repeated violation of the pleura may increase the risk of infection. Second, the effectiveness of evacuation is inferior to that of tube thoracostomy with continuous suction. Failure of complete resorption of a hemothorax creates a fibrous "peel," which can lead to "trapped lung" and may subsequently require open thoracotomy. Finally, tamponade of the bleeding source is theoretically enhanced by complete expansion of the lung. (Traumatic hemothorax is discussed in depth in Chapter 6.)

Contraindications

In clinical situations in which there is a suspected tension pneumothorax, there are several relative contraindications to the use of thoracentesis. If tube thoracostomy is readily available, it may be the preferred procedure and thoracentesis may only serve to delay the more definitive treatment. In patients who are being ventilated manually or by respirator, extreme caution should be exercised when performing thoracentesis. If the presumptive diagnosis of a tension pneumothorax is incorrect, the insertion of a thoracentesis needle may actually create a pneumothorax, which may be converted into a tension pneumothorax by the positive ventilation pressure.

The removal of pleural fluid by thoracentesis should be avoided in patients with bleeding dyscrasias prior to correction of the clotting deficits. Thoracentesis is also contraindicated if the patient has a ruptured diaphragm. Extreme caution should be used when a thoracentesis is being performed in a patient who has pleural adhesions, such as from previous TB, hemopneumothorax, or empyema, because of the danger of piercing the closely approximated visceral pleura and lung.

Equipment

The equipment needed to perform rapid thoracentesis for tension pneumothorax or aspiration of a spontaneous pneumothorax is listed in Table

Table 5–4. EQUIPMENT NEEDED FOR THORACENTESIS EVACUATION OF TENSION PNEUMOTHORAX

Antiseptic solution and sterile gauze sponges
14 to 16 gauge needles (1½–2 inches) or 14 gauge intravenous catheter
Optional equipment for one-way needle drainage
5–10 ml pre-moistened syringe or flutter-valve fashioned from a sterile glove fingertip or finger cot or sterile IV tubing with water-filled basin

5–4. Because several techniques will be described, equipment for all techniques is included in this list. Evacuation of a tension pneumothorax can be accomplished by insertion of a needle only, a through-the-needle catheter, or an over-the-needle catheter. Although the needle insertion technique is the technique that can be most rapidly performed, the catheter insertion techniques may theoretically be safer, allowing continued drainage of the relieved tension pneumothorax without the presence of a rigid needle in the thorax. The drawbacks to the use of a catheter are the possibility of the catheter crimping and increased resistance to drainage owing to the catheter's length. The catheter technique is preferred in relief of tension pneumothorax in the pre-hospital setting.[7b]

For removal of fluids, more equipment is necessary. The additional equipment permits more thorough patient preparation, more adequate anesthesia, controlled evacuation of fluid, and careful collection of specimens. In Table 5–5, the basic and alternative equipment is listed. The simple needle method has the potential risk of perforating the visceral pleura as the fluid is withdrawn, whereas a catheter of narrow diameter and long length may limit the removal of thick, tenacious fluids.

Table 5–5. EQUIPMENT NEEDED FOR STANDARD THORACENTESIS

Basin for preparation solution
Antiseptic solution (providone-iodine)
Sterile gauze sponges
Sterile towels
5- to 10-ml syringes (non-Luerlock) with 22 and 25 gauge needles for anesthetic infiltration
Local anesthetic (e.g., 1% lidocaine)—10 ml
50-ml syringe (non-Luerlock) for aspiration
15 to 18 gauge needle—2 inch for aspiration or 14 gauge intravenous catheter
Two curved hemostats
Three-way stopcock
Sterile IV extension tubing
Specimen bowl (may be calibrated for volume measurement) or sterile vacuum bottle with IV tubing
Sterile dressing and adhesive tape

Procedure

There are two approaches to performing thoracentesis. The first is the anterior approach, which is used primarily for diagnosis and relief of tension pneumothorax. Because treatment is urgently required, the procedure chosen should be performed in an appropriately expedient manner. Likewise, the amount of preparation and equipment needed will be dictated by each particular clinical situation. Informed consent will probably be impossible to obtain in such cases.

The second approach to thoracentesis is the posterior (or lateral) approach, which is used primarily for diagnosis or relief of symptomatic pleural effusions. This is generally an elective procedure and should be performed after adequate diagnostic radiographic studies have been obtained. The procedure should be carried out with adequate preparation, after all available equipment has been tested, and under properly controlled circumstances. Informed consent should usually be obtained and documented.

INSERTION SITE AND PATIENT POSITION

Tension Pneumothorax

The conventional approach has been to evacuate tension pneumothoraces by using the anterior approach, with the patient in a supine position, with the head of the stretcher elevated 30 degrees. The recommended insertion site is the 2nd intercostal space in the mid-clavicular line (Fig. 5–2). This intercostal space can be readily found by palpating the sternal angle of Louis, which attaches to the 2nd rib, directly above the 2nd intercostal space. The rationale for this approach is that free pleural air will rise to the anterior upper chest. With tension pneumothorax, however, the collapsed lung is moved away from the entire ipsilateral chest wall, making a lateral approach also possible. If the patient is in a supine position and if the anterior chest is obscured (subclavian vein catheter bandage, chest monitoring leads, subcutaneous emphysema), a lateral approach may be more practical. A lateral approach is accomplished by inserting the needle into the 4th or 5th intercostal space in the mid-axillary line. This location can be quickly identified in males by extending the horizontal nipple line laterally into the axilla. In females who have large breasts, reliable approximation can be made by extending an imaginary horizontal line between the inferior tips of the scapulae laterally into the axilla.

There are two major problems when the lateral

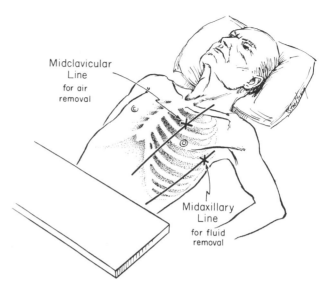

Figure 5–2. For relief of a tension pneumothorax, the 2nd intercostal space in the mid-clavicular line is preferred. The head of the stretcher is elevated 30 degrees. The mid-axillary line, 4th or 5th intercostal space site, has been used for thoracentesis of pleural fluid (see text). (From Fishman, N. H.: Thoracic Damage: A Manual of Procedures. Chicago, Year Book Medical Publishers, Inc., 1983, p. 26. Used by permission.)

approach is chosen. The first is a greater risk of parenchymal injury when either no tension pneumothorax or only a small pneumothorax is present. The second problem is the danger of adhesions. Previous empyema, hemothorax, and other inflammatory processes may cause pleural adhesions, which frequently occur in dependent portions of the thorax. Therefore, the anterior approach is theoretically safer and is recommended for most cases in which relief of tension pneumothorax is required.

Pleural Fluid

The choice of insertion site for removal of pleural fluid depends upon many clinical factors. If the fluid collection is large and if the patient is able to sit upright for a prolonged period of time, the following approach is recommended. The patient is seated, leaning forward *slightly*, supported by the back of a chair or a table (Fig. 5–3). The site chosen for aspiration is the mid-scapular line or the posterior axillary line at a level below the top of the fluid. This level may be determined clinically by the height of dullness to percussion and the decrease of tactile fremitus or from a chest film of the patient in an upright position. Radiographic determination of fluid levels may occasionally be misleading, because the position of the fluid changes with respiration and patient position. In addition, Fishman contends that the fluid level seen on a chest film of a patient in an upright position represents only the bottom of the fluid

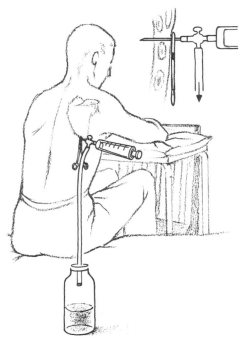

Figure 5–3. Upright positioning of patient for drainage of pleural fluid. Note the use of the hemostat to limit the depth of penetration of the thoracentesis needle. (From Nealon, T. F., Jr.: Fundamental Skills in Surgery, 3rd ed. Philadelphia, W. B. Saunders Company, 1979, p. 291. Used by permission.)

meniscus.[29] Because the lung exerts pressure that varies according to distance from the hilum, the actual fluid level at the chest wall may be higher, forming the raised edge of the meniscus. An exception to this distribution of pleural fluid may occur with combined pneumothorax and pleural effusion, producing a flat air-fluid level. In all cases, the lowest level recommended for thoracentesis is the 8th intercostal space. The highest level clinically indicated is generally chosen in order to minimize inadvertent abdominal insertion of the needle. If a plastic catheter has been inserted, the patient can subsequently be repositioned to make the insertion site more dependent.

The following two alternative approaches have been described. If the patient is unable to remain seated, Fishman suggests that a plastic catheter (either through-the-needle or over-the-needle) can be inserted into the mid-axillary line in the 4th intercostal space while the patient is in a supine position[29] (see Fig. 5–2). It may be prudent to evaluate the height of the fluid both clinically and radiographically in this position prior to attempting this approach. If there is only a small amount of fluid and there is a great need for diagnostic analysis, fluid can be aspirated from the mid-axillary line with the patient in the lateral decubitus position.[30] This technique requires that the patient be placed across an open space in such a way that the physician can aspirate from below.

NEEDLE/CATHETER INSERTION FOR TENSION PNEUMOTHORAX

Patient Preparation

The patient is positioned as previously discussed. An explanation of the procedure is appropriate if the patient is awake, but it should not delay the procedure. Because the patient is usually in extremis, sedation is contraindicated. Restraining the patient may be necessary if the patient is hypoxic and confused. The insertion site is rapidly swabbed with povidone-iodine or another suitable antiseptic, when time permits.

Anesthesia

Local anesthesia is usually inappropriate in the case of relieving a tension pneumothorax and will only delay the procedure. If the patient has a slowly progressive tension pneumothorax and is not in extremis, local anesthesia with 0.5 to 1 per cent lidocaine may be used. It is administered through a 5- to 10-ml syringe with a 25 to 27 gauge needle. An intradermal wheal is raised over the upper edge of the 3rd rib. Anesthetic is infiltrated down to the periosteum. The needle is then removed.

Insertion Techniques

A 14 to 16 gauge needle is selected and attached to a 5- to 10-ml syringe, if time allows. The 2nd intercostal space is identified by palpation. The needle is inserted perpendicularly in the mid-clavicular line over the upper edge of the 3rd rib. As the rib is encountered, the needle is walked over the rib and into the lower portion of the 2nd intercostal space to avoid the intercostal vessels positioned near the lower border of each rib, as indicated in Figure 5–4. The syringe is gently aspirated as the needle is advanced. A "pop" may be felt as the pleural space is entered and air is encountered. A pneumothorax under tension should create enough pressure to drive the plunger of a pre-moistened syringe the length of the barrel without manually withdrawing it. If the needle has been inserted without a syringe attached, a rush of air exiting the chest may be heard in inspiration as well as during expiration. Either of these findings will confirm the presence of a tension pneumothorax. Inserting a needle without an attached syringe or other drainage device invites the possibility of creating a pneumothorax. If a tension pneumothorax is confirmed, a one-way drainage device should be attached as soon as possible.

Alternate methods of relief of a tension pneumothorax include the use of standard intravenous needle and catheter insertion sets (Fig. 5–5). This

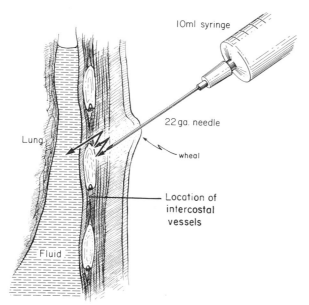

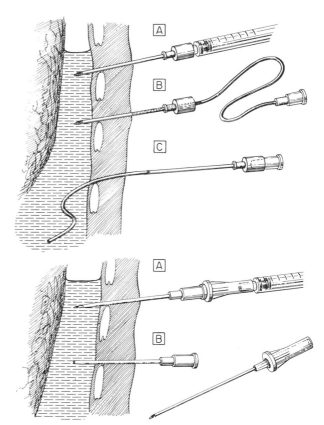

Figure 5–4. Walking the anesthetic needle over the superior aspect of the rib. (From Fishman, N. H.: Thoracic Damage: A Manual of Procedures. Chicago, Year Book Medical Publishers, Inc., 1983, p. 28. Used by permission.)

Figure 5–5. Insertion technique for through-the-needle and over-the-needle catheters. Separate intercostal spaces depict the steps (A, B, C) that occur at a single intercostal space. (From Fishman, N. H.: Thoracic Damage: A Manual of Procedures. Chicago, Year Book Medical Publishers, Inc., 1983, p. 30. Used by permission.)

can be accomplished by attaching the syringe to the hub of an over-the-needle catheter (with a 14 to 16 gauge needle). The 2nd intercostal space is entered as previously described, and the catheter is advanced over the needle into the pleural space. The needle is then removed, and the syringe or another drainage device is attached to the hub of the catheter. A tension pneumothorax is confirmed by the same findings as those previously discussed. The catheter should be secured with adhesive tape or sutures.

A through-the-needle catheter (14 gauge) of the shortest available length may also be used. Once the needle has entered the pleural space, the catheter is advanced fully into the thorax through the needle. The needle is then withdrawn, and a drainage device is attached to the catheter hub. The "needle guard" should be attached to prevent a laceration of the catheter by the surrounding needle. The catheter is then secured with tape or by suturing it to the chest wall.

Drainage

After the diagnosis of a tension pneumothorax has been made, drainage should be continued until a thoracostomy tube can be placed. Continuous drainage can be accomplished by attaching the distal end of an intravenous tubing set to the needle or catheter hub. The proximal end of the intravenous tubing is placed 2 to 5 cm under water in a basin in order to create an underwater seal. This prevents air from entering the pleural space. Continuous bubbling from the intravenous tubing during inspiration and expiration is also diagnostic

of a tension pneumothorax. A commercial flutter valve may be attached or an alternative device may be made using a finger that has been cut from a sterile examination glove (see Fig. 5–6). As the needle is inserted into the chest and a tension pneumothorax is encountered, the cut edge of the glove finger will act as a one-way flutter-valve.

If a tension pneumothorax is found and confirmed by any of the aforementioned methods, a thoracostomy tube should be placed as soon as possible. A chest film is also indicated following any of the previously discussed procedures to confirm the position of the catheters (or thoracostomy tube), the successful relief of the tension pneumothorax, and the lack of a persistent pneumothorax. This is best accomplished with an upright expiratory chest film or a lateral decubitus film.

NEEDLE/CATHETER INSERTION FOR PLEURAL FLUID

Patient Preparation

The patient should be placed in the appropriate position, as described previously. Proper expla-

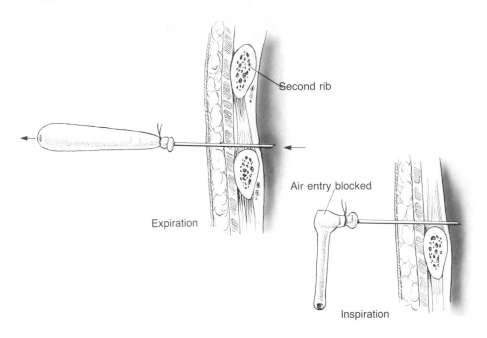

Second rib

Expiration

Air entry blocked

Inspiration

Figure 5–6. Use of a needle and a sterile finger cot or a finger from a sterile glove to fashion a one-way (flutter) valve for emergency evacuation of a tension pneumothorax. (Redrawn from Cosgniff, J. H.: An Atlas of Diagnostic and Therapeutic Procedures for Emergency Personnel. Philadelphia, J. B. Lippincott Co., 1978, p. 243.)

nation of the procedure is essential when there is adequate time. If the patient is comfortable and cooperative, sedation is not needed. When the patient is uncooperative and in extremis, it may be necessary to restrain the patient. If the patient is restrained, there must be clear access to the insertion site and the ability to manage the patient must not be compromised. Sedation is generally not recommended and is contraindicated in patients in extremis. Supplementary oxygen by nasal prongs or mask should be used if clinically indicated and may minimize postevacuation hypoxia (see Complications of Thoracentesis). A wide area about the thoracentesis site should be prepared, using povidone-iodine or another suitable antiseptic, to allow selection of several intercostal spaces or the rapid placement of tube thoracostomy when thoracostomy follows the procedure. When the patient is recumbent, sterile towels should be draped around the site.

Anesthesia

Local anesthesia should be used prior to removal of pleural fluid. A 0.5 to 1 per cent solution of lidocaine is frequently used. The lidocaine (5 to 10 ml) is drawn into a syringe, and a 25 or 27 gauge needle is attached. The previously selected insertion site is relocated by palpation. A skin wheal is raised at the upper edge of the rib, directly inferior to the selected intercostal space. The syringe is withdrawn, and a 22 gauge needle is inserted through the wheal toward the upper border of the rib. The subcutaneous tissue and muscle are infiltrated down to the periosteum of the rib. At this point, the needle is "walked" above the upper

edge of the rib and infiltration is continued through the intercostal space until the pleura is entered (see Fig. 5–4). A "pop" may be felt, and fluid or air should be aspirated to ensure that the pleural space has been reached. If no fluid is encountered, the chosen intercostal space may be too low and a higher site may be indicated. If air is encountered, the chosen intercostal space may be too high and a lower site may be indicated. Once fluid or air is aspirated, a curved hemostat may be applied to the needle at the skin surface to indicate the proper depth of penetration. The needle and hemostat should be removed together.

Needle Insertion Technique

The following technique has traditionally been recommended. A large 15 to 18 gauge needle and a 50-ml syringe are attached to a three-way stopcock. A drainage tube is also attached to the stopcock, as shown in Figure 5–3. The lever of the stopcock is set to allow passage of fluid between the needle and the syringe. The depth of the pleural space as determined from the anesthetic needle and hemostat is now marked on the larger aspiration needle with a second hemostat or by transferring the first hemostat. The pleural space is again entered through the previous anesthetic site. The attached hemostat guide will prevent inserting the needle farther than necessary, decreasing the chance of lacerating the underlying lung. Fluid is first aspirated with the syringe. The stopcock lever is then turned, and the fluid is expelled through the drainage tube into a sterile basin, sterile vacuum bottle, or into open specimen tubes. An assistant will be needed to handle the specimen tubes. The process of aspirating and ejecting the fluid through the drainage tubing is repeated until an adequate amount of fluid to accommodate all needed specimens has been drained. If thoracentesis was performed for diagnostic purposes, removal of 50 to 100 ml should be adequate. The specimens obtained are listed in Table 5–6. It is suggested that individual laboratories be contacted to ensure the optimal collection technique for a specific analysis. It may, for example, be best to collect fluid for cytology in the morning to ensure fresh cells. If the purpose of the thoracentesis is therapeutic drainage, the fluid is removed in 50-ml aliquots until the respiratory distress appears to be relieved. It is usually recommended that no more than 1000 ml of pleural fluid be removed because of the potential for excessive loss of serum protein as the pleural fluid gradually re-accumulates. Once the desired amount of fluid has been removed, the equipment is withdrawn. A sterile dressing is applied over the insertion site. An upright expiratory chest film is taken to ensure that an iatrogenic pneumothorax was not created.

Catheter Insertion Techniques
(see Fig. 5–5)

An alternative method of removing the pleural fluid can be accomplished by either of the following techniques. A large-bore over-the-needle catheter (14 to 16 gauge needle) is attached to the 50-ml syringe. The proper depth of the pleural space is indicated on the catheter by grasping it between a gloved index finger and thumb. The needle and catheter are inserted into the pleural space as previously described. As fluid is encountered, the needle and the catheter are angled slightly caudally. The catheter is advanced into the pleural space, and the needle is withdrawn. The exposed lumen of the catheter hub is covered with a gloved finger to prevent the entry of air. A three-way stopcock with an attached 50-ml syringe and a drainage tube are again attached to the catheter hub. Fluid is removed following the same process for the needle insertion technique. Aftercare is also the same.

A final alternative method involves the use of a through-the-needle catheter (14 gauge needle). The catheter is withdrawn from the needle prior to the procedure. A three-way stopcock is attached to the catheter hub and adjusted to close the catheter to the passage of air or fluid. The catheter and stopcock are temporarily set aside. The empty outer needle is attached to a 50-ml syringe. A curved hemostat is attached to the needle, as previously described, to mark the depth of the pleural fluid as measured from the anesthetic needle. The needle is inserted into the pleural space through the anesthetized area. Once fluid is encountered, the needle is angled caudally and held securely as the syringe is removed. Again, it is essential to cover the needle hub with a gloved finger. The catheter is inserted through the needle into the pleural space and advanced its full distance. The needle is withdrawn from the chest wall, and the "needle guard" is attached to the needle tip to prevent shearing off of the catheter. The catheter must not be drawn back through the needle, because this may lacerate the catheter and allow its free entry into the pleural space. Once the catheter has been placed securely within the pleural space, the syringe is reattached to the stopcock and the stopcock lever is turned to allow passage of fluid into the syringe. Fluid is withdrawn and ejected through the drainage tube, as with the previously described needle technique. After an adequate amount of fluid has been withdrawn, the catheter is removed and the entry site is covered with a sterile bandage. A follow-up chest film is again indicated.

THORACENTESIS IN PEDIATRIC PATIENTS

Etiology

Children may develop a pneumothorax or tension pneumothorax due to most of the same causes as adults. In addition, the neonatal period appears to be associated with an increased incidence of

---

Table 5–6. DIAGNOSTIC PLEURAL FLUID SPECIMENS

5 ml plain specimen tube (red top)
  Amylase
  Cholesterol
  LDH
  Glucose
  Protein
  Triglycerides

5 ml EDTA specimen tube (lavender top)
  Appearance
  Color
  pH
  Specific gravity
  Cell counts
  Differential counts

10 ml sterile container
  Gram stain
  Aerobic and anaerobic cultures
  AFB culture and stain
  Fungal culture and stain

10–50 ml plain specimen tube (red top)
  Cytology

5 ml heparinized specimen tube (green top)
  LE cells

pneumothorax.[31-33] Pneumothorax may be associated with fetal distress, difficult delivery, meconium aspiration, resuscitation, hyaline membrane disease, or the use of mechanical ventilation, particularly PEEP. Occasionally, a simple pneumothorax may progress and become a tension pneumothorax.

In the older child, trauma, asthma, bronchiolitis, cystic fibrosis, staphylococcal pneumonia, metastatic carcinoma, and, rarely, dermatomyositis are potential causes of pneumothoraces. On occasion, these may advance to a tension pneumothorax. Cystic fibrosis seems to have a high incidence of tension pneumothorax that is occasionally bilateral.[34]

Pleural effusions may be encountered in the pediatric age group. These effusions have been found to be due to most of the same processes that cause effusions in adults. Juvenile rheumatoid arthritis and systemic lupus erythematosus are also common etiologic causes.[35]

Diagnosis

The newborn child with a tension pneumothorax presents with increasing respiratory difficulty marked by grunting, tachypnea, intercostal retractions, and nasal flaring. Cyanosis and cardiovascular collapse may occur. The classic physical findings of a tracheal shift, displacement of cardiac impulse, and ipsilateral hyperresonance to percussion may be found but are not consistent findings. A hyperinflated, relatively immobile hemithorax and decreased breath sounds may occasionally be seen but are frequently absent. This is in part owing to the fact that the small chest in a neonate easily transmits breath sounds from the uninvolved side to the side of the tension pneumothorax.

In the older child, the presentation of tension pneumothorax may be more obvious, with progressive dyspnea and respiratory distress. Chest pain may be present and is usually pleuritic. Tachycardia, tachypnea, agitation, use of accessory muscles, nasal flaring, and cyanosis are nonspecific signs of respiratory compromise that may be seen. Cardiovascular collapse is a sign of progression of a tension pneumothorax.

In the pediatric population, pleural effusions may be asymptomatic or may present with respiratory compromise, pleuritic chest pain, or signs and symptoms of underlying systemic illness. A moderate to large pleural effusion may be recognized on physical examination by the presence of decreased breath sounds, dullness to percussion, pleural friction rub, and decreased excursions of the ipsilateral hemithorax.

In evaluating a possible tension pneumothorax, an upright posteroanterior chest film will confirm the diagnosis. It is appropriate to relieve the tension pneumothorax by needle or catheter aspiration when it is recognized clinically. Radiographic diagnosis is only indicated in a relatively stable patient when the diagnosis of tension pneumothorax is in doubt. A bilateral tension pneumothorax may be difficult to diagnose clinically and may present without a mediastinal shift. On a chest film, microcardia and the bilateral absence of lung markings is seen. In such a case, bilateral chest decompression will confirm the diagnosis.

Large pleural effusions may be seen on a standard chest film. For small effusions, lateral decubitus films may be necessary.

Treatment

The indications for thoracentesis in children are the same as in adults. Immobilization of the child may be a significant problem because of the child's small size as well as the inability of the frightened child to comprehend the explanation for the procedure. Gentle and simple explanations are appropriate for older children.

A neonate may be held securely by an assistant. If a small child requires restraint, a standard "papoose" restraining board may be helpful. It is important to position the small child in the same position as described for adults in order to provide the proper access to the insertion site. To relieve a tension pneumothorax, a larger child may be positioned supinely on a stretcher, with the head elevated 30 degrees. For removal of pleural fluid, the child should be seated, leaning against the back of a chair or table in the same manner as indicated for adults.

The insertion sites for relieving tension pneumothorax and removing pleural effusion are essentially the same as those recommended for adults. The use of a standard needle, a butterfly "scalp vein" needle, or an intravenous catheter/needle set have all been recommended. In the smaller child, a slightly smaller gauge needle than would be used for an adult is recommended.

Complications

The most frequent complication caused by inserting a thoracentesis needle or catheter into the thorax from any approach is the creation of a pneumothorax. Although many patients may already have a small pneumothorax, it may become larger or even become a tension pneumothorax during the procedure. In the case of removal of pleural fluid by thoracentesis, it is well documented that pneumothorax is a frequent complication. The mechanism for this complication seems to be a laceration of the underlying lung, inadequately covering of the hub of the needle or catheter after the pleural space is entered, an inadequate drainage system, or the presence of an air leak in the drainage system or thoracentesis apparatus.[36-38] The risk of pneumothorax secondary to lung puncture may be increased with patients who are intubated and being positive pressure ventilated. If a pneumothorax is found on a follow-up chest film, tube thoracostomy may also be indicated, according to the criteria in Chapter 6.

Unilateral pulmonary edema may occur following thoracentesis. This phenomenon was initially noted as a complication of draining pleural effusions[39] but has also been seen following relief of a pneumothorax or tension pneumothorax.[40, 41] The pulmonary dysfunction may result from local hypoxia in the atelectatic lung, with resultant changes in the basement membrane or loss of surfactant, as well as from excessive pleural negative suction pressure. When performing thoracentesis, one can minimize these changes by first applying a passive underwater seal, followed by gradually increasing the negative suction pressure, as needed. Once pulmonary edema develops, administering oxygen may relieve the hypoxia. Rarely, PEEP may be needed to correct this complication.[41a]

Hypoxia has been noted as a consistent finding after thoracentesis. Hypoxia appears predictably and seems to be self-limited according to Brandstetter and Cohen.[42] There appears to be a ventilation/perfusion mismatch with perfusion of atelectatic lung or areas of localized pulmonary edema. Although the hypoxia rarely attains clinically significant proportions, oxygen administration may be indicated, particularly in the patient with minimal respiratory reserve.

Hemothorax and hemoperitoneum are potential complications of thoracentesis. Hemothorax may be due to laceration of the lung or diaphragm, intercostal vessels, or internal mammary vessels. Careful attention to technique, such as avoiding the superior portion of the intercostal space, never puncturing medial to the mid-clavicular line to avoid the internal mammary vessels, and not penetrating too deeply into the thorax during needle insertion, is an excellent preventative measure. Hemoperitoneum may result from puncture of the spleen or liver through the diaphragm. This may occur with a low posterior approach during expiration. If a hemothorax is noted on a post-thoracentesis upright chest film, evacuation with a thoracostomy tube may be indicated, according to the criteria in Chapter 6. If laceration of intraabdominal contents has occurred, close observation is essential and an exploratory laparotomy may be indicated.

As with all surgical procedures, there is the potential of infection. The risk of infection is lessened with proper attention to patient preparation and sterile technique. In the case of rapid relief of a tension pneumothorax, preparation will be minimal, although simple needle thoracentesis is rarely associated with infection.

Inadvertent shearing of the plastic catheter may occur when a catheter through-the-needle technique is used. This complication is prevented by securing the needle with a needle guard after it has been withdrawn from the chest. In addition, it is essential to avoid withdrawing the catheter back through the needle at any time. Air embolus could occur if the thoracentesis device is left open to air and if the needle or catheter is inadvertently inserted into a pulmonary or intrathoracic blood vessel. Hypoproteinemia may occur after removal of a large pleural effusion. A thick pleural "peel" may accumulate secondary to inadequate drainage of a hemothorax or an empyema. This complication is avoided by the use of tube thoracostomy to completely drain blood or empyema rather than using thoracentesis.

1. Garrison, F. H.: An Introduction to the History of Medicine, 4th ed. Philadelphia, W. B. Saunders Company, 1929.
2. Glinz, W.: Chest Trauma. New York, Springer-Verlag, 1981.
3. Hewett, F. C.: Thoracentesis: the plan of continuous aspiration. Br. Med. J. 1:317, 1876.
4. Valle, A. R.: An analysis of 2811 chest casualties of the Korean conflict. Dis. Chest 26:623, 1964.
5. McNamara, J. J., Messersmith, J. K., Dunn, R. A., et al.: Thoracic injuries in combat casualties in Vietnam. Ann. Thorac. Surg. 10:389, 1970.
5a. Zwillich, C. W., Pierson, D. J., Creogh, C. E., et al.: Complications of assisted ventilation. Am. J. Med. 57:161, 1974.
5b. Steirer, M., Ching, N., Roberts, E. B., et al.: Pneumothorax complicating ventilatory support. J. Thorac. Cardiovasc. Surg. 67:17, 1974.
6. Vukich, D. J., and Markovich, V. J.: Pneumothorax. In Rosen, P., et al. (eds.): Emergency Medicine Concepts and Clinical Practice. The C. V. Mosby Co., St. Louis, 1983.
6a. Lernau, O., Bar-Maor, J. A., and Nissan, S.: Traumatic diaphragmatic hernia simulating acute tension pneumothorax. J. Trauma 14:880, 1974.
7. Wiot, J. F.: The radiologic manifestations of blunt chest trauma. JAMA 231:500, 1975.
7a. Blair, E., Topuzlu, C., and Davis, J. H.: Missed diagnosis in blunt chest trauma. J. Trauma 11:129, 1971.
7b. American Academy of Orthopedic Surgeons: Emergency Care and Transportation of the Sick and Injured, 3rd ed. American Academy of Orthopedic Surgeons, 1981, pp. 50–51.
8. Heimlich, J. H.: Valve drainage of the pleural cavity. Dis. Chest 52:282, 1968.
9. McSwain, N. E.: A thoracostomy tube for field and emergency department use. JACEP 6:324, 1977.
10. Hills, B. S., and Bryan-Brown, C. W.: Role of surfactant in the lung and other organs. Crit. Care Med. 11:951, 1983.
11. Rudikoff, J. C.: Early detection of pleural fluid. Chest 77:109, 1980.

12. Harris, J. H., and Harris, W. H.: The Radiology of Emergency Medicine, 2nd ed. Baltimore, Williams & Wilkins, 1981, p. 293.
13. Light, R. W., MacGregor, I., Luchsinger, P. C., et al.: The diagnostic separation of transudates and exudates. Ann. Intern. Med. 77:507, 1972.
14. Light, R. W., Erozan, Y. S., Ball, W. C., et al.: Cells in pleural fluid: their value in differential diagnosis. Arch. Intern. Med. 132:854, 1973.
15. Dines, D. E., Pierre, R. V., and Franzen, S. J.: The value of cells in the pleural fluid in the differential diagnosis. Mayo Clin. Proc. 50:571, 1975.
16. Jarvi, O. H., Kunnas, R. J., Laito, M. T., et al.: The accuracy and significance of cytologic cancer diagnosis of pleural effusion: a follow-up study of 338 patients. Acta Cytol. 16:152, 1972.
17. Calnan, W. L., Winfield, B. J. O., Crowley, M. F., et al.: Diagnostic value of the glucose content of serous pleural effusions. Br. Med. J. 1:1239, 1951.
18. Light, R. W., and Ball, W. C.: Glucose and amylase in pleural effusions. JAMA 225:257, 1973.
19. Kaye, M. D.: Pleuropulmonary complications of pancreatitis. Thorax 23:297, 1968.
20. Potts, D. E., Levin, D. C., and Sahn, S. A.: Pleural fluid pH in parapneumonic effusions. Chest 70:328, 1976.
21. Light, R. W., MacGregor, M. I., Ball, W. C., Jr., et al.: Diagnostic significance of pleural fluid pH and PCO_2. Chest 64:591, 1973.
21a. Stark, D. D., Shanes, J. G., Baron, R. L., et al.: Biochemical features of urinothorax. Arch. Intern. Med. 142:1509, 1982.
22. Roy, P. H., Carr, D. T., and Payne, W. S.: The problem of chylothorax. Mayo Clin. Proc. 42:457, 1967.
23. Ferguson, G.: Cholesterol pleural effusion in rheumatoid lung disease. Thorax 21:577, 1966.
24. Sibley, J. C.: A study of 200 cases of tuberculous pleurisy with effusion. Am. Rev. Tuberculosis 62:314, 1950.
25. Sahn, S. A.: The differential diagnosis of pleural effusions. West. J. Med. 137:99, 1982.
26. Selle, J. G., Snyder, W. H., and Schreiber, J. T.: Chylothorax: indications for surgery. Ann. Surg. 177:245, 1973.
27. Brooks, J. W.: Thoracotomy in the management of spontaneous pneumothorax. Ann. Surg. 177:1973.
28. Raja, O. G., and Lalor, A. J.: Simple aspiration of spontaneous pneumothorax. Br. J. Dis. Chest 75:207, 1981.
29. Fishman, N. H.: Thoracic Drainage: A Manual of Procedures. Chicago, Year Book Medical Publshers, Inc., 1983, pp. 21–25.
30. Stackhouse, C.: How to perform safe thoracocentesis. Hospital Physician, October:46, 1982.
31. Chernick, V., and Reed, M. H.: Pneumothorax and chylothorax in the neonatal period. J. Pediatr. 76:624, 1970.
32. Monin, J., and Vert, P.: Pneumothorax. Clin. Perinatol. 5:335, 1978.
33. Yu, V. Y., Liew, S. W., and Robertson, N. R.: Pneumothorax in the newborn. Changing pattern. Arch. Dis. Child 50:449, 1975.
34. Scanlin, T. F.: Cystic fibrosis. In Fleisher, G. R., and Ludwig, S. (eds.): Textbook of Pediatric Emergency Medicine. Baltimore, Williams & Wilkins, 1983.
35. Athreya, B. H., and Yancey, C. L.: Rheumatologic emergencies. In Fleisher, G. R., and Ludwig, S. (eds.): Textbook of Pediatric Emergency Medicine. Baltimore, Williams & Wilkins, 1983.
36. Cameron, G. R.: Pulmonary edema. Br. Med. J. 1:965, 1948.
37. Luisada, A. A., and Cardi, L.: Acute pulmonary edema: pathology, physiology, and clinical management. Circulation 13:113, 1956.
38. Van Heerden, J. A., and Laufenberg, H. J.: Simplified thoracentesis. Mayo Clin. Proc. 43:311, 1965.
39. Trapnell, D. H., and Thurston, J. G. B.: Unilateral pulmonary edema after pleural aspiration. Lancet 1:1367, 1970.
40. Steckel, R. J.: Unilateral pulmonary edema after pneumothorax. N. Engl. J. Med. 289:621, 1973.
41. Ziskind, M. M., Weil, H., and George, R. A.: Acute pulmonary edema following the treatment of spontaneous pneumothorax with excessive negative intrapleural pressure. Am. Rev. Respir. Dis. 92:632, 1965.
41a. Murphy, K., and Tomlanovich, M. C.: Unilateral pulmonary edema after drainage of spontaneous pneumothorax: case report and review of the world literature. J. Emerg. Med. 1:29, 1983.
42. Brandstetter, R. D., and Cohen, R. P.: Hypoxemia after thoracentesis: a predictable and treatable condition. JAMA 242:1060, 1979.

Introduction

Tube thoracostomy is a commonly performed procedure. The purpose is to evacuate an abnormal collection of air or fluid from the pleural space. Normally, the visceral and parietal pleurae are closely approximated. The potential space between them is occupied by only a thin film of fluid. The addition of air, blood or other fluid, or (rarely) tissue to this space disrupts the normal ventilatory mechanism, producing subjective dyspnea and interference with normal gas exchange. The amount of pulmonary and cardiovascular dysfunction is generally proportional to the amount of the abnormal collection and the rate at which it accumulates. Respiratory and cardiovascular embarrassment result from multiple mechanisms, including intrapulmonary shunting; mechanical compression of the mediastinum, the heart, and the great vessels; increased intrathoracic pressure; and altered diaphragmatic motion.[1]

Continuous intercostal tube drainage was first introduced for the treatment of empyema by Buelaw, a German internist, in 1875[2] and was described in the English literature 1 year later.[3] It is believed that the increased use of such tubes as both initial and definitive treatment of wartime thoracic trauma led to much of the decrease in mortality from such injuries in battles following World War II.[4, 5] Today, the procedure is used in individuals who have sustained penetrating chest trauma during violent crimes or blunt trauma in highway accidents. Tube thoracostomy is also used frequently in cases of spontaneous pneumothorax. Other indications are listed in Table 6–1.

Indications

TRAUMATIC PNEUMOTHORAX, HEMOTHORAX, OR HEMOPNEUMOTHORAX

Mechanism

Pneumothorax and hemopneumothorax are common after blunt or penetrating thoracic trauma. Pneumothorax alone occurs in 15 to 50 per cent of significant injuries resulting from blunt chest trauma and is usually attributed to lung puncture from a rib fracture. Following trauma, a definite rib fracture may not always be evident on radiographs. In the absence of fractures, pneumothorax is believed to result from rupture of an alveolus secondary to abrupt increases in intrathoracic and intra-alveolar pressures against a

6

Tube Thoracostomy*

KENNETH FRUMKIN, M.D., Ph.D.

closed glottis. The air leak may be self-limited, or a ball-valve mechanism may lead to a tension pneumothorax (see later). Esophageal rupture or injuries to the tracheobronchial tree may also be responsible for pneumothorax and are often manifested by persistent air leaks or food particles in the intercostal tube drainage.[6] Penetrating injuries result in simple pneumothorax by allowing air to enter the chest, either through a persistent chest wall defect or by direct injury to underlying lung.

Hemothorax may result from bleeding from the heart, the lungs, the great vessels or their branches, the intercostal arteries or veins, the mediastinal veins, the diaphragm, the chest wall vessels, fractured ribs, or torn pulmonary adhesions. Bleeding from the lung parenchyma is usually self-limited because of the relatively low-pressure vascular supply of the lung and the high concentration of tissue thromboplastins. In addition, re-expansion of the collapsed lung generally tamponades low-pressure bleeding sites. Partially severed intercostal arteries bleed particularly briskly, since all but the first two come directly

---

*The opinions or assertions contained herein are the private views of the author and are not to be construed as official or reflecting the views of the Department of Defense or the Department of the Army.

Table 6–1. INDICATIONS FOR TUBE THORACOSTOMY

Traumatic conditions
  Pneumothorax
  Hemothorax
  Hemopneumothorax
  Conditions requiring "prophylactic" surgical management
  Open pneumothorax
  Iatrogenic indications—post-CVP hemopneumothorax

Spontaneous pneumothorax

Tension pneumothorax

Drainage of recurrent pleural effusion

Empyema

Chylothorax

Following thoracotomy

from the aorta. In addition, the partially lacerated internal mammary artery will rarely cease bleeding without surgical intervention.

Diagnosis

Physical Examination. Alert patients with a pneumo-, hemo-, or hemopneumothorax may complain of chest pain and shortness of breath. Pneumothorax alone may be manifested by increased resonance to percussion, decreased tactile fremitus, decreased or absent breath sounds, or subcutaneous emphysema. With isolated hemothorax breath sounds will be decreased as well, but the percussion note is dull. A succussion splash has been described when air *and* fluid are both present. It is important to note that physical examination is often misleading, and many pneumothoraces may go undetected by physical examination alone.

Hemothorax alone may also be difficult to detect. Patients can rapidly lose 30 to 40 per cent of their blood volume into the pleural space with little resistance from the compliant lung. They may then present primarily with signs of shock.[7] The presence of shock in a patient with a chest injury should also raise the question of pericardial tamponade, which may not be manifested by distended neck veins in the hypovolemic patient (see Chapter 14). Evidence of mediastinal shift or compression (distended neck veins, shifted trachea) may represent massive blood or fluid accumulation or, more likely, tension pneumothorax. In contrast, a small hemothorax (less than 400 ml) may produce few clinical findings.

Radiographic Diagnosis. A standard, 6-foot posteroanterior (PA) upright chest radiograph is the diagnostic procedure of choice for hemo- or pneumothorax. One can often obtain a sitting (portable) 6-foot PA film in patients (who may require some assistance) by having them sit up and "hug" the x-ray plate to their chest. The machine is placed at the standard distance behind the patient. This view more closely approximates standard technique and allows a better evaluation of mediastinal size. Otherwise, anteroposterior (AP) films should be taken with the patient sitting in as erect a position as possible. When one is interpreting a supine chest film, it is important to compare the relative densities of both lung fields. On a supine chest radiograph, even as much as 1000 ml of blood may be manifested only as a slight homogeneous increase in the density of one hemithorax. Up to 500 ml of blood may be required to produce blunting of the costophrenic angle on an upright film. Subpulmonic collections can resemble an elevated hemidiaphragm. Lateral decubitus films may be required to demonstrate either of these findings. If an air-fluid level, as opposed to a fluid meniscus, is seen, a pneumothorax must also be present (Fig. 6–1).

Treatment

In a patient in extremis with evidence of major thoracic trauma (subcutaneous emphysema, palpable rib fractures, flail chest), no further diagnostic studies need be undertaken. Needle aspiration (if tension is suspected) or immediate tube thoracostomy is indicated on the suspected side of injury. Tube thoracostomy allows egress of the fluid or air and provides a means of continuous drainage and monitoring of the pleural space. Further drainage can be quantified, and the need for other intervention can thus be assessed. Observation of the drainage and collection devices allows for the diagnosis of persistent air leak or other problems that may require additional treatment.

Small pneumothoraces and hemothoraces (less than 400 ml) have been treated with observation alone if the patient is relatively asymptomatic, otherwise healthy, and not likely to require positive-pressure ventilation. Resolution occurs in 10 to 14 days.[6] Patients with larger or more symptomatic traumatic hemo-, pneumo-, or hemopneumothoraces should have a large-bore intercostal tube placed.

A tube should be placed "prophylactically" in a patient with evidence of a penetrating injury to the chest even without demonstrable intrathoracic injury if anesthesia and positive-pressure ventilation are required or if the patient will be transported a long distance for definitive care of other injuries. Such patients are at high risk for developing a tension pneumothorax when subjected to positive airway pressures. They may also develop a simple or tension pneumothorax during transport when definitive treatment may be difficult or impossible.

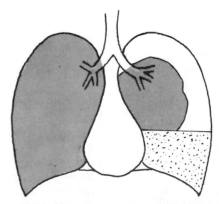

Figure 6–1. Hemopneumothorax. Note that the fluid level produces a straight line as opposed to a meniscus when a pneumothorax is present with the pleural fluid.

Table 6–2. INDICATIONS FOR SURGERY AFTER TUBE THORACOSTOMY*

Massive hemothorax (over 1000 ml)

Bleeding
    Rapid (over 300 to 500 ml in first hour)
    Continued (over 200 ml per hour for first 3 or more hours)
    Increasing size of hemothorax on chest film

Persistent hemothorax
    After two functioning tubes placed
    Clotted hemothorax

Large air leak preventing effective ventilation

Persistent air leak after placement of second tube or inability to expand lung fully

Documented bronchial injury

Ruptured esophagus

Ruptured diaphragm

Upper mediastinal entrance wound

Pericardial tamponade

Cardiac arrest; secondary to penetrating trauma

Great vessel injury

Cardiac injury

Open pneumothorax

Gross intrapleural contamination from a foreign body

*Data from references 5, 6, 7, 10, 25, 45, 50, 51, 52, 53, and 55.

Early institution of blood replacement is recommended in patients with massive hemothorax (over 2000 ml) before evacuation is begun. The blood in the chest may be functioning to tamponade a briskly bleeding vessel, and marked hypo-tension potentially could result from precipitous evacuation without prior fluid resuscitation.[7, 8] A number of commercial devices are available for the collection, filtration, anticoagulation, and autotransfusion of blood obtained by tube thoracostomy (see Chapter 29). Autotransfusion is indicated in instances of massive hemothorax when such facilities are available.

Seventy-two to 82 per cent of patients with traumatic hemothorax can have their injury managed successfully by tube thoracostomy and volume replacement alone.[5, 9, 10] In the remaining patients, immediate or delayed elective thoracotomy may be required. There is disagreement among different authors concerning the indications for surgery. Table 6–2 provides a summary of surgical indications.

OPEN PNEUMOTHORAX (Fig. 6–2)

Open pneumothorax ("sucking chest wound") most commonly results from shotgun or combat injuries with a loss of chest wall integrity. Such wounds can produce markedly deficient gas exchange and cardiovascular function when the negative intrapleural pressure is replaced with atmospheric pressure. If the chest wall defect is larger in cross-sectional area than the trachea, air will move preferentially through the chest wall with diaphragmatic excursions, and no ventilation will occur. With smaller defects, a tension pneumothorax (see below) may develop. Clinically, a chest

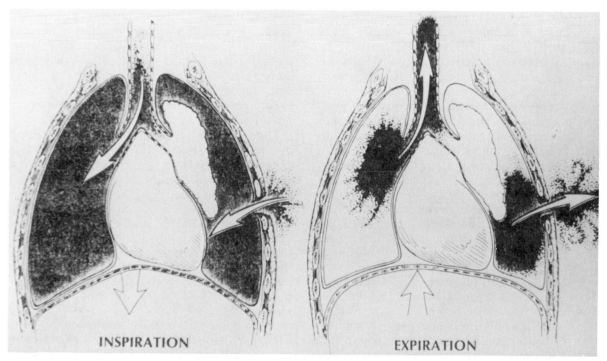

INSPIRATION   EXPIRATION

Figure 6–2. Simple open pneumothorax without tension.

wall defect and subcutaneous emphysema are seen in a patient with marked respiratory distress. Emergency (prehospital) treatment involves the application of a (preferably sterile) dressing to act as a one-way (flap) valve, allowing air to exit the pleural space while blocking re-entry. In the field, anything (palm, plastic wrap, gauze) can be used. The patient is instructed to perform a Valsalva maneuver after deep inspiration or to cough just as the dressing is placed. Ideally, a sterile dressing of petrolatum-impregnated gauze extending 3 to 5 inches beyond the wound in all directions is used. This underlying dressing should be covered by gauze dressings and secured on *three* sides only. An airtight dressing could predispose to tension pneumothorax in the presence of a continued intrapleural air leak. This dressing may be sealed after tube thoracostomy through a separate site is performed to allow continued evacuation of air or fluid. The presence of the open wound is an indication for operative debridement and closure of the chest wall defect with continued tube drainage of the pleural space.[6, 7, 11]

SPONTANEOUS PNEUMOTHORAX

Pathophysiology

Spontaneous pneumothorax is the cause of one in every 1000 general hospital admissions and usually occurs in males less than 40 years of age.[12] Although as many as 40 per cent of affected patients do not have *known* underlying lung disease, the most common predisposing factor is emphysema.[13, 14] Other associated potential etiologic factors are chronic bronchitis, asthma, tuberculosis, pneumonia, bronchiectasis, atelectasis, pulmonary fibrosis, trauma (exertion, cough, injuries), and various connective tissue diseases, such as scleroderma or eosinophilic granuloma. Tuberous sclerosis, rupture of a hydatid cyst, pulmonary infarct, empyema, pleurisy, subphrenic abscess, a foreign body, and alpha$_1$- antitrypsin deficiency have all been implicated. Neoplasm is a consideration in older patients. Recurrent pneumothoraces attributed to pleural/diaphragmatic endometriosis occur in some women at the time of menstruation.[12, 13, 15]

The rupture of an emphysematous bleb, an alveolar septum, or the bronchial wall causes air to flow freely into the pleural space. Seventy to 80 per cent of cases occur when the patients are at rest; and 70 per cent of affected individuals seek medical attention within 24 hours of onset. Five to 7 per cent of cases are bilateral. The symptoms correlate with the amount of collapse, the mobility of the mediastinum, the amount of respiratory reserve, the presence of underlying disease, and the degree of compression of the rest of the lung.

Diagnosis

Almost all patients with a spontaneous pneumothorax (95 per cent) complain of chest or shoulder (or, rarely, back or abdominal) pain that is usually sudden in onset, sharp, pleuritic, and cutting. Tightness may be described. Sixty per cent have dyspnea in addition to these symptoms, and a mild cough occurs in 12 per cent.[15] Breathlessness and anxiety are more common in older patients, and the morbidity and mortality are increased in patients with underlying disease.[16] Half may attribute the onset of pain to a sudden mild exertion (cough, sneeze) or trauma. Varying degrees of respiratory distress may be manifested. Subcutaneous emphysema rarely occurs. Decreased breath sounds, decreased tactile fremitus, and hyper-resonance to percussion may be noted in an uncomplicated spontaneous pneumothorax, although the physical examination may reveal no abnormalities if the pneumothorax is small.

The diagnosis is made on a standard upright PA chest film. Small pneumothoraces are best seen by radiography with the patient in full expiration. During expiration, the volume of air in the pleural space remains the same, but the expiratory decrease in the volume of the collapsed lung on the affected side increases the apparent relative size of the pneumothorax. A lateral film helps rule out complications (see later) and may help define the etiology when the pneumothorax is secondary to some other intrathoracic pathology. In pediatric patients or in those who are uncooperative for other reasons, radiographs in both decubitus positions may successfully demonstrate a small pneumothorax. If the patient is placed in the lateral decubitus position with the affected side up, air will collect in the uppermost portion of the pleural space, and the pneumothorax may be more perceptible. Also when the *affected* side is *dependent*, the dependent lung will be partially deflated as on an expiratory film accentuating a small pneumothorax.

The size of the pneumothorax can be estimated by the method outlined in Figure 6–3.[17] The area of the collapsed lung is subtracted from the area of the involved hemithorax. One calculates the area of the collapsed lung in the figure using the area of a rectangle drawn to include the extreme superior (*a*), lateral (*b*), and inferior (*c*) margins of the collapsed lung and the center of the mediastinum (*d*). One then subtracts this number from the area of a rectangle encompassing the entire affected hemithorax, measured from the inferior border of the first rib (*A*), the inner border of the mid–lateral chest wall (*B*), the tip of the costophrenic angle (*C*), and the center of the mediastinum (*D*). One divides the difference between the area of the hemithorax and the area of the collapsed lung by the area of the hemithorax to yield

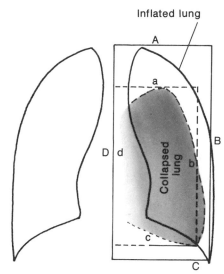

Inflated lung

A

a

D d

Collapsed lung

B

b

c

C

Figure 6–3. Method of calculating the area of a pneumothorax. [Area of hemithorax (A × B) − Area of collapsed lung (a × b)] ÷ Area of hemithorax (A × B).[29] The shaded area is the collapsed lung.

the percentage of pneumothorax. A simpler way of monitoring the size of the pneumothorax involves measuring from the lateral lung margin to the lateral chest wall on full inspiration. It is important to have some easily reproducible means of repeatedly recording the size of a pneumothorax, particularly if the patient is to be examined by different physicians.

In the patient with chest pain, pneumothorax must be differentiated from myocardial infarction, dissecting aneurysm, pericarditis, spontaneous esophageal rupture, perforated peptic ulcer, and biliary or renal colic. Radiographically, giant bullae or lung cysts may mimic a pneumothorax and these must be carefully differentiated, occasionally with tomography.

Treatment

The treatment varies with the age of the patient, the symptoms, the degree of respiratory compromise, the bilaterality, the need for general anesthesia, the size of the pneumothorax, and whether or not the current episode represents a recurrence. Otherwise healthy and asymptomatic patients with small (less than 10 per cent or less than 1 cm collapse laterally) pneumothoraces may be treated by observation alone. A period of hospital observation (with the length depending on the amount of time the pneumothorax has been present) is recommended to ensure that the pneumothorax is not expanding. Re-expansion is estimated to occur at 1.25 per cent of lung volume daily.[17] Affected patients must be instructed to return immediately if symptoms increase, to minimize their activities, and to have follow-up chest x-rays to document

resolution. Needle aspiration (see Chapter 5) of small pneumothoraces has been recommended by some and has been successful in 50 to 70 per cent of the patients in whom it has been attempted.[13, 18] Needle aspiration does carry a slight chance of increasing the size of the pneumothorax if the lung is punctured. Traditional therapy of a spontaneous pneumothorax is tube thoracostomy and water seal drainage with or without the addition of suction. The tube evacuates the intrapleural air, prevents further accumulation, and allows monitoring for persistent air leaks. The local irritation of the tube is believed to aid in scar formation and in preventing recurrence. The tube is left for 24 hours after all evidence of continued air leak has disappeared.

A number of authors have reported successful outpatient management of chest tubes in 74 to 88 per cent of their patients with spontaneous pneumothorax.[19-21] Stable patients are selected; these individuals should be free of significant underlying disease or persistent air leaks and should have satisfactory lung re-expansion after 1 to 12 hours of observation in the emergency department. They are sent home with a flutter (Heimlich) valve attached and are seen 3 to 4 days later for tube removal if complete re-expansion is maintained.

Surgical treatment (usually thoracotomy with abrasion of pleural surfaces) is advocated at the time of the first or second recurrence.[12] Patients who have had one pneumothorax have a 30 to 50 per cent chance of ipsilateral recurrence within 1 to 2 years. After a second spontaneous pneumothorax, the probability of a third rises to 50 to 80 per cent.[13, 15, 22] Surgery may be recommended on the occasion of a patient's first pneumothorax in a number of situations: life-threatening tension pneumothorax, massive air leaks with incomplete re-expansion, an air leak persisting 4 to 5 days after a second intercostal tube has been placed, associated hemothorax with complications (see later), cases of identifiable bullous disease, and failure of easy re-expansion in patients with cystic fibrosis.[13, 23]

TENSION PNEUMOTHORAX (Fig. 6–4)

Etiology

Tension pneumothorax may be a complication of both spontaneous pneumothorax and traumatic hemopneumothorax. Fractures of the trachea or the bronchi, the presence of an occlusive dressing over an open pneumothorax, or a ruptured esophagus may also result in tension pneumothorax. The risk is markedly increased in patients with chest trauma undergoing positive-pressure ventilation. Because of this, a patient with penetrating thoracic injury (even without immediate evidence

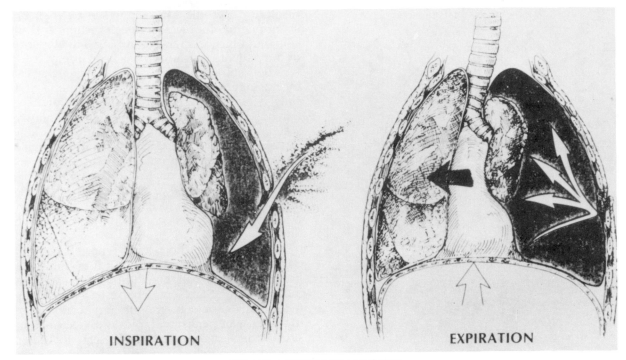

INSPIRATION   EXPIRATION

Figure 6–4. Tension pneumothorax.

of intrathoracic bleeding or air) should still have a "prophylactic" chest tube placed prior to surgery. A "tension *hemo*thorax" does not occur in the absence of massive fluid replacement, because the volume of blood required to produce a shift of mediastinal structures requires nearly total exsanguination into the chest.

Pathophysiology

Classically, a pulmonary parenchymal or bronchial tear creates a ball-valve mechanism. The increased endobronchial diameter and intrathoracic negative pressure during inspiration allow air to pass into the pleural space. The decrease in bronchial diameter and the relatively elevated intrathoracic pressure during expiration cause the leak to close. This mechanism traps increasing amounts of air in the pleural space with each respiratory cycle. As intrapleural pressure rises, venous return to the right heart declines and cardiac output drops. The mediastinum shifts toward the uninvolved side, mechanically interfering with right atrial filling. Ventilation of both the involved lung and the opposite lung is compromised, and hypoxemia or acidosis, or both, result from ventilation/perfusion inequalities. Tension pneumothorax may develop at any time after injury, during resuscitation, or with cardiopulmonary resuscitation (CPR). It should be considered as a possible cause for deterioration in any susceptible patient, particularly if positive-pressure ventilation is being used.

Diagnosis

Clinically, patients with tension pneumothorax may present with or rapidly develop restlessness, dyspnea, agitation, or cyanosis. Hypotension, tachypnea, tachycardia, nasal flaring, and retractions may occur. Pulsus paradoxus may be evident. There is hyperresonance to percussion and decreased breath sounds on the affected side. Obvious chest trauma, rib fractures, or subcutaneous emphysema should alert one to the possibility of tension pneumothorax. The trachea and the cardiac apex are displaced toward the uninvolved side. Neck veins may be distended but can be flat in the hypovolemic patient. The prominent, fixed, and overinflated hemithorax may be obvious when the semi-sitting patient is inspected from the head or the foot of the bed.[21] Increased airway resistance in an intubated patient (one of the first signs of a tension pneumothorax) may be manifested by increased difficulty in manual ventilation or increased ventilatory pressures when a volume-cycled respirator is used. A quick check is to compare the patient's airway resistance with one's own by a brief trial of mouth-to-tube ventilation. Increased resistance is readily apparent, and tension pneumothorax is one of the most likely causes. If there is time, a chest radiograph that shows a depressed hemidiaphragm and lung collapse on the affected side with a shift of the mediastinum to the opposite side is confirmatory.

Pericardial tamponade figures strongly in the differential diagnosis and should be considered in the trauma patient when mediastinal shift, hyperresonance, and decreased breath sounds are not prominent clinical features or when needle aspiration of the hemithorax fails to bring prompt relief.

Treatment

If the patient is *in extremis* and the diagnosis is suspected clinically, needle aspiration of the involved side should be undertaken without further delay (see Chapter 5). Even if no facilities are available for chest tube placement, a large needle inserted into the chest to convert a tension pneumothorax to an open pneumothorax can be lifesaving. A 14 gauge needle is commonly placed in the second anterior intercostal space but is effective anywhere in the pleural space. A field-expedient flutter valve may be fashioned from the fingers of a rubber surgical glove until definitive treatment is available. The definitive treatment of a tension pneumothorax is tube thoracostomy.

OTHER INDICATIONS

Drainage of Recurrent Pleural Effusions

Initially, most pleural effusions can be managed by thoracentesis (see Chapter 5), but recurrent effusions may require tube thoracostomy.

Empyema

Empyema was one of the first recorded indications for continuous intercostal drainage in adults[3] and children[24] and remains a prominent one today.

Chylothorax

Chylothorax can be a rare complication of thoracic trauma. It may result directly from penetrating injury or from a fall from a height. Chyle will collect extrapleurally and 2 to 10 days may elapse before it enters the pleural cavity. Initially, the few clinical manifestations may be masked by other injuries. As fluid accumulates in large amounts, dyspnea and the physical findings of a pleural effusion become prominent. Thoracentesis reveals a milky, white liquid with a high lymphocyte count, 4 to 5 g per dl of protein, and a high fat content. Repeated thoracentesis or tube thoracostomy is combined with bed rest and parenteral alimentation until the volume of chyle declines.[6]

Postoperative Thoracotomy

Chest tubes are nearly always placed under direct vision when open thoracotomy is performed.

Contraindications

A list of contraindications may be found in Table 6–3. There are probably no absolute contraindications in the case of a patient in distress who requires the procedure, although some relative contraindications exist. Multiple pleural adhesions, emphysematous blebs, and scarring should mandate caution in a stable patient. *It is important to note that a giant emphysematous bleb or bulla in adults and congenital lobar emphysema in infants may be extremely difficult to differentiate from a pneumothorax on chest films.* A second or third spontaneous pneumothorax in a stable patient may be an indication to proceed directly to surgery instead of attempting another tube thoracostomy. A patient requiring immediate open thoracotomy (i.e., in the case of cardiac arrest after penetrating trauma) may not benefit from chest tube placement. The presence of a massive hemothorax usually requires rapid blood or crystalloid replacement with or without immediate surgery. Tube thoracostomy before fluid replacement is believed by some to promote further bleeding.[7, 25] Treatment of respiratory distress because of a massive hemothorax, however, must take precedence over the theoretical risk of aggravating bleeding by immediate institution of chest tube drainage. Bleeding dyscrasias prior to clotting factor replacement may be a relative contraindication.

Procedure

The ideal procedure performed under ideal circumstances will be described. The degree of urgency as determined by the patient's condition and the available resources will dictate how closely to the ideal any one chest tube insertion will come. Under the best circumstances, the diagnosis should be established prior to the procedure and the appropriate radiographs should be taken. The preferred films are upright PA and lateral chest radiographs and should be approximated whenever feasible. The nature and necessity of the procedure should be explained to the patient as completely as possible, and (preferably) informed consent should be obtained and documented.

Table 6–3. RELATIVE CONTRAINDICATIONS TO TUBE THORACOSTOMY

Multiple adhesions, blebs
Recurrent pneumothorax mandating surgical treatment
Need for immediate open thoracotomy
Massive hemothorax without adequate volume replacement
Bleeding dyscrasia

Table 6–4. INSTRUMENT TRAY FOR TUBE THORACOSTOMY

Prep razor
Sterile towels—4
Basin for prep solution
Gauze pads
Towel clips (optional)—4
10- to 20-ml syringe and assorted needles for infiltration of local anesthetic
Medicine cup for local anesthetic
Large, straight (suture) scissors
Large, curved (Mayo) scissors
Large clamps (Kelly)—2
Medium clamps (Kelly)—2 to 4
Needle holder
Number 0 or 1–0 silk on large cutting needles—several
Knife handle #4—1
#10 scalpel blades
Forceps

EQUIPMENT

Instruments

The instruments required for performing tube thoracostomy by the method detailed here are listed in Table 6–4. Prepared "trays" are available in hospitals and often contain many more instruments than required or described here. In addition to the instruments, a number of other materials are needed; these are listed in Table 6–5. All the necessary items should be assembled and tested prior to the start of the procedure. If the tape is torn as desired, the solutions are poured, the packages are opened, and a check list (mental or written) is followed prior to beginning, the procedure will go much more smoothly.

Chest Tubes

The size, shape, and characteristics of tubes used for thoracostomy vary considerably. The

Table 6–5. OTHER MATERIALS REQUIRED FOR TUBE THORACOSTOMY

Local anesthetic
Antiseptic solution
Arm restraints (padded)
Vaseline-impregnated gauze
Tincture of benzoin
Adhesive tape—cloth-backed
Chest tubes
    28 to 36 French for adults
    16, 20, 24 French for children
    Right-angled tubes (36 French)
Plastic tubing—clear, sterile in 6-foot lengths; 1/2-inch diameter
Hard plastic serrated connectors
Drainage apparatus with sterile water for water seal
High-flow, high-volume regulated suction pump (Emerson)
Y connectors

most commonly used devices are clear plastic straight tubes (Argyle) with a series of holes at one end. They have a radiopaque strip that is commonly interrupted by the last fenestration. Angled (90 degrees) tubes are also available. A wide variety of soft rubber tubes (including Malecot, de Pezzer, and Foley catheters) have been used, most commonly for simple pneumothoraces. They are particularly useful for second anterior intercostal space placement, in which the fenestrated segment of the standard tubes may be too long and may project outside the skin. Sizes used for adults have varied from 12 to 42 French. Most authorities believe that 22 to 32 French is adequate for pneumothorax alone, whereas the larger tubes (a minimum of 36 French) are best when blood or pus is to be drained. It is a mistake to attempt to drain a hemothorax with a small chest tube. For pediatric patients, 16, 20, and 24 French tubes are adequate.[26] The right-angled tubes are used in various ways—most often to fit in the posterior costophrenic sulcus when a single straight tube fails to drain a dependent fluid accumulation adequately.

TUBE LOCATION (Fig. 6–5)

The classic approach has always been to place tubes anteriorly in the second intercostal space, mid–clavicular line (usually 2 inches from the lateral border of the sternum) for pneumothorax alone, and dependently in the mid– or posterior axillary line and directed posteriorly for fluid removal. *In an emergency, a tube placed anywhere in the pleural space should be adequate.* The second intercostal space is nearly always mentioned as a location for tube placement but in practice is less

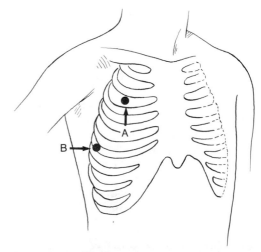

Figure 6–5. Standard sites for tube thoracostomy. A. Second intercostal space, mid–clavicular line, for air. B. Fifth intercostal space, mid–axillary line, for fluid.

often used. Disadvantages include the need to dissect through several inches of muscle mass and the resulting unsightly and highly visible scar, which is particularly undesirable in women. Some sources have advocated using the lateral insertion for women but retaining the anterior site for men.[20]

Authors of recent articles have suggested avoiding the second intercostal space entirely and recommend a mid–axillary line placement for all indications. It is cosmetically preferred and better tolerated and is believed to result in increased pleural involvement and scarring.[13, 23] If the tube is placed slightly anteriorly, the patients may lie on their backs more comfortably. Gill and Long have stated, however, that the "practice of attempting to drain both air and fluid through a single tube inserted in the mid–axillary line has been unsatisfactory and often leads to multiple tube insertions and reinsertions."[27] Hegarty randomly placed tubes in either the second intercostal space, mid–clavicular line or the fifth intercostal space, mid–axillary line in 131 cases of pneumo- or combined hemopneumothorax. He found that the time of removal of the tube was not influenced by location, regardless of whether air, blood, or both were being drained.[28] Duponselle studied 156 randomly placed chest tubes and found no unsatisfactory results with pneumothorax regardless of tube position.[29] Logically, as the collapsed lung expands and the parietal and visceral pleurae become more tightly opposed, either air or fluid will follow the path of least resistance and will enter a functioning drainage tube, regardless of its location. Although some clots may remain in the pleural space because of brisk bleeding and rapid clotting, Broadie and coworkers[30] demonstrated that blood that is drained from the chest cavity has no demonstratable fibrinogen and is thus *incoagulable*. Therefore, a tube anywhere in the pleural space should adequately drain a hemothorax of unclotted blood, as long as there are no adhesions.

Specific recommendations for lateral placement have varied from anterior to posterior axillary lines and from the fourth to the eighth intercostal space. If time permits and the physician who will subsequently be caring for the patient can be consulted, his or her preference should be followed. For all indications for "routine" placement in the emergency department, the fourth or fifth intercostal space in the mid–axillary line to the slightly anterior axillary line is suggested for chest tubes. This is roughly at the level of the nipple or the inferior scapular border in most patients. The tube is directed posteriorly and toward the apex of the lung. This has proved satisfactory for drainage of either fluid or air. If fluid continues to accumulate, a second tube may be placed in the posterior axillary line at the same interspace or one inter-

space lower. Obviously, the location of the diaphragm varies with the position of the patient and can rise quite high when the patient is supine. The phase of respiration and other associated injuries (diaphragmatic hernia, abdominal distention) can also alter its position. The most reliable means of preventing inadvertent damage to lung or the abdominal viscera is a thorough digital exploration of the pleura before tube insertion. If the patient breathes during this procedure, the location of the diaphragm can often be verified and intrapleural placement can be assured.

TUBE INSERTION

Patient Preparation

For axillary line insertions, the patient is ideally placed with the head of the bed elevated 30 to 60 degrees (Fig. 6–6). Inserting a chest tube while the patient is lying flat increases the chances of injury to the diaphragm, the spleen, or the liver. When the patient is lying down, the diaphragm may rise as high as the third intercostal space. The arm on the affected side is placed over the patient's head and restrained in that position with wide strips of adhesive tape or by other means. The other arm can be restrained comfortably at the patient's side. (Even in the conscious and seemingly cooperative

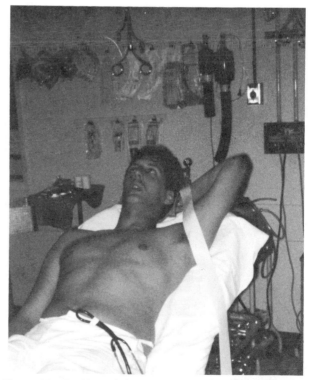

Figure 6–6. Position of the patient for axillary line chest tube insertions. Whenever possible, the patient should be semi-erect at a 30- to 60-degree angle.

patient, judicious use of comfortable restraints prior to painful or frightening procedures often allows more rapid and efficient completion.) When no contraindications exist, sedation or parenteral analgesia should be considered. For anterior mid–clavicular line placements, the patient's arms may be placed at his side. Nasal oxygen should be used, since it helps to decrease subjective dyspnea. Monitoring of arterial blood gases should be considered, since significant pulmonary shunting can occur even with small pneumothoraces. The area where the tube is to be placed should be identified, and the surrounding skin should be shaved if necessary. The area should be sterilized with a povidone-iodine solution or another suitable antiseptic and draped with sterile towels.

Anesthesia

A local anesthetic should be used generously; careful anesthesia can render the procedure nearly painless (Fig. 6–7). One half to 1 per cent lidocaine (Xylocaine) with epinephrine (1:100,000) is most commonly used. The maximum dose of 5 mg per kg should not be exceeded.[31] A skin wheal should be raised with a 25 to 26 gauge short (1/2- to 5/8-inch) needle in the area of the skin incision. Many authors advocate locating the skin wound one intercostal space below the one through which the tube will pass. The "tunneling" up and over the next rib that is required if this is to be done is believed to provide a better seal against air leaks both while the tube is in place and during and after its removal (see Fig. 6–10). A larger (23 gauge, 1 1/2-inch) needle is used to infiltrate the subcutaneous tissues, the muscle, the periosteum, and the parietal pleura in the areas through which the tube will pass (Fig. 6–8). The syringe should be kept readily available because further anesthesia is often required. *A common error is inadequate local anesthesia.* Intercostal nerve (rib) blocks above and

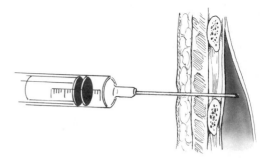

Figure 6–8. Use of a needle to puncture the pleura and establish the presence of blood or air in the pleural space. This not only is diagnostic but also may be a *temporary* therapeutic maneuver in a tension pneumothorax. (Redrawn from Richards, V.: Tube thoracostomy. J. Fam. Pract. 6:631, 1978.)

below the incision and insertion rib spaces are also helpful but add the risk of intercostal vessel injury. The anesthetic needle and syringe should be used to aspirate the pleural cavity in the area of insertion. If air or fluid is not obtained and the patient's condition is stable, the diagnostic evaluation may need to be repeated or the insertion site changed. This simple and extremely useful technique to verify the location and the character of the intrapleural accumulation is often forgotten.

Insertion

One measures the length of the tube to be inserted by holding it near the chest wall. The distance from the incision site to the apex of the lung is estimated, and a clamp is placed on the tube at the point at which it should enter the chest

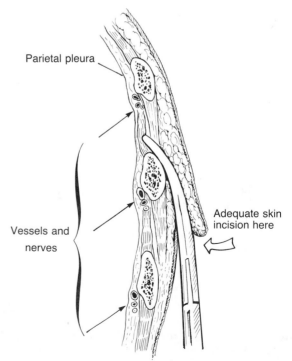

Figure 6–9. Location of the intercostal neurovascular bundle. (From Millikan, J. S. et al.: Complications of tube thoracostomy for acute trauma. Am. J. Surg. 140:739, 1980.)

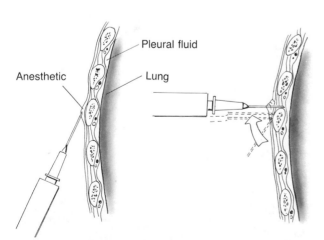

Figure 6–7. Infiltration of skin and pleura with local anesthetic. (Redrawn from Hughes, W. T., and Buescher, E. S.: Pediatric Procedures, 2nd ed. Philadelphia, W. B. Saunders Co., 1980, p. 234.)

wall. The beveled end of the tube is often cut squarely at this time so that it fits the commonly available connectors better.

A *generous* 2- to 4-cm transverse skin incision is made through the skin and the subcutaneous tissues directly over the rib one interspace beneath the rib the tube will pass over. *It is a common error to attempt to place a chest tube through an inadequately sized incision.* This incision is extended by *blunt* dissection to the fascia overlying the intercostal muscles. A scalpel is needed *only* to make the skin incision. Care must be taken to avoid the intercostal vessels and the nerve located on the inferior margin of each rib (Fig. 6–9). One uses a large Kelly clamp to tunnel superiorly through the subcutaneous tissues over the rib above, pushing forward with the closed points and then spreading and pulling back with the points spread (Fig. 6–10). Some physicians used a curved Mayo scissors

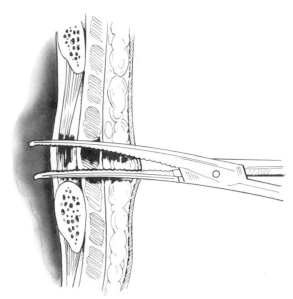

Figure 6–11. One accomplishes blunt dissection by forcing the closed points of the clamp forward and then spreading the tips and pulling back with the points spread. One must be certain to make an adequate opening in the pleura. (From Bricker, D. L.: Safe, effective tube thoracostomy. E. R. Reports 2:49–52, 1981.)

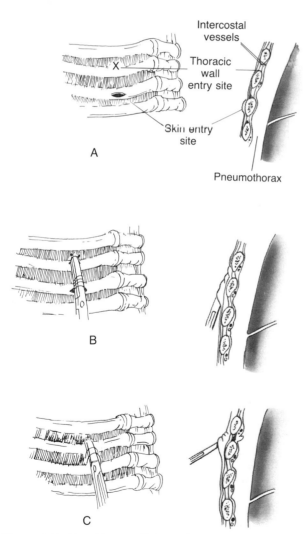

Figure 6–10. The skin wound is made one intercostal space below the space through which the tube will pass (A). Blunt dissection is carried subcutaneously (B) and into the pleural space (C). A common error in technique is to attempt to insert a large chest tube through a skin incision that is too small. (Redrawn from Hughes, W. T., and Buescher, E. S.: Pediatric Procedures, Philadelphia, W. B. Saunders Co., 1980, p. 237.)

in the same manner as a Kelly clamp as a blunt dissecting instrument. The closed points of the heavy clamp are then pushed with some force through the muscles, and the parietal pleura immediately overlying the rib and the pleural cavity is entered. A twisting or drilling motion will enhance pleural penetration. A rush of air or fluid should occur at this point. The tips of the clamp, still within the pleural cavity are spread widely and withdrawn (Fig. 6–11). One must be certain to make an adequate incision in the pleura.

Next is one of the most important parts of the procedure: *the insertion of a gloved finger into the chest to verify that the pleura has been entered and that pleural adhesions are absent.* The finger should sweep completely around the hole in the chest wall. Dense adhesions may mandate an alternative site for tube placement. The finger is left in the pleural space. The tube is then grasped with the curved clamp, with the tube tip protruding from the jaws (Fig. 6–12). (Another technique is to pass one jaw of the clamp inside the tube through a distal fenestration.) *With the finger in the chest cavity as a guide,* the tip is placed into the pleural space (Fig. 6–13). The finger is used to verify intrapleural placement of the chest tube. The curve in the clamp is used to guide the tip superiorly and posteriorly. The clamp is released, and the tube is pushed superiorly, medially, and posteriorly until the marker clamp that was previously attached to measure the insertion distance touches the chest wall. All the holes in the chest tube *must* be within the pleural space.

Alternatively, the tube may be advanced until pain is felt or until resistance is met and then

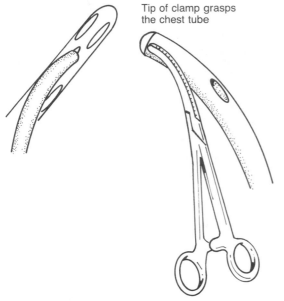

Figure 6–12. The tube is grasped with the curved clamp, with the tip protruding from the jaws.

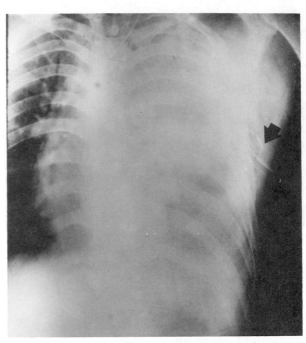

Figure 6–14. Subcutaneous placement of a chest tube *(arrow)*. The incorrect placement was not appreciated until the radiograph was taken.

pulled back 2 to 3 cm. *Subcutaneous placement is a frequent complication that can simulate entry into the chest cavity* (Fig. 6–14). Therefore, a finger should again be inserted to verify that the tube enters the pleural space. Entry into the thoracic cavity is suggested by condensation on the inside of the tube coincident with respiratory movements, audible movement of air through the tube during respiration, free flow of blood or fluid, and the

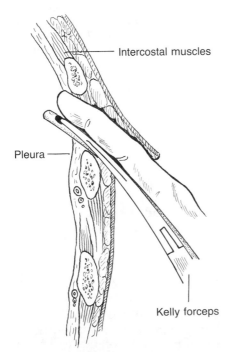

Figure 6–13. Using the finger as a guide, one places the tip into the pleural cavity. (From Millikan, J. S., et al.: Complications of tube thoracostomy for acute trauma. Am. J. Surg. 140:739, 1980.)

ability of the operator to rotate the tube freely after insertion. The tube is attached to the previously assembled water seal or suction set-up by means of a sterile serrated connector before the clamp is released. Asking the patient to cough and observing bubbles in the water seal device is a good way to check system patency.

Securing the Tube

There are as many ways of fastening a chest tube in place as there are physicians who place the device. More important than the individual technique chosen is the need to communicate the method used effectively to the person who will be caring for the patient, particularly the one who will be removing the tube. A reasonable approach is as follows: A number 0 or 1-0 silk suture on a cutting needle is used. The first suture is placed next to the tube to close the lateral margin of the skin incision and is tied firmly (Fig. 6–15). The ends of this suture are left long, and these are then tied repeatedly around the chest tube and knotted securely to hold it in place. The sutures must be tied tightly enough to indent the chest tube slightly in order to avoid slippage (Fig. 6–16). A horizontal mattress suture is then placed around the tube approximately 1 cm across the incision on either side of the tube (Fig. 6–17). This will be used to close the incision after the tube is removed. No knots are tied initially, but the skin should be pulled snugly together and held with a

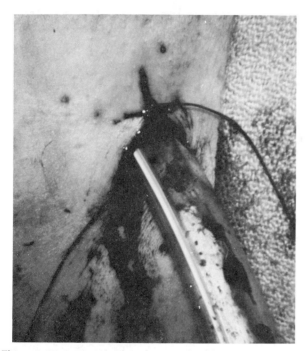

Figure 6–15. A suture is placed next to the tube to close the skin incision. The ends are left long.

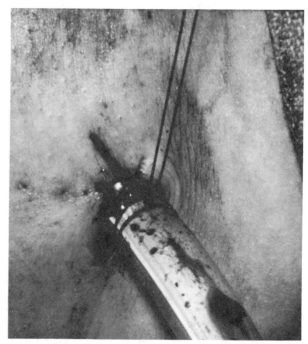

Figure 6–16. The ends of the suture are wound twice about the tube tightly enough to indent the tube slightly and are tied securely.

surgeon's knot (double throw). The loose ends are repeatedly wound tightly around the chest tube as it enters the skin with occasional repeated surgeon's knots tied tightly enough to indent the

tube gently. The final knot is a bow, which should clearly identify the suture as one not to be cut.

An occlusive dressing of Vaseline-impregnated gauze should be placed where the tube enters the

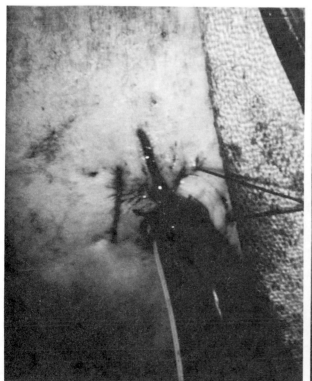

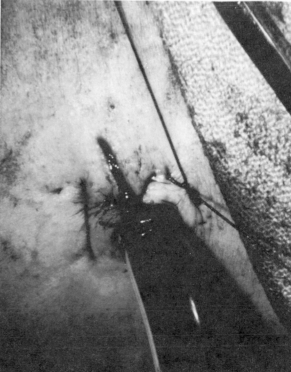

Figure 6–17. A horizontal mattress suture is placed around the tube and is held only with a surgeon's knot.

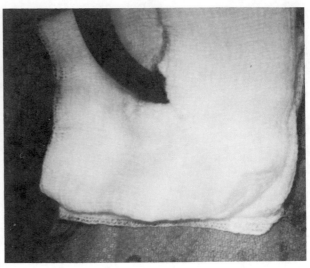

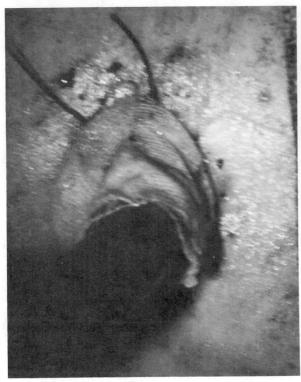

Figure 6–18. A dressing consisting of Vaseline-impregnated gauze and gauze sponges is applied to the entry site.

skin. Overlying this should be two or more gauze pads with a Y-shaped cut from the middle of one side to the center. These are oriented at 90 degrees to each other (Fig. 6–18). The shaved skin and the tube may be coated with tincture of benzoin and wide (3-inch) cloth adhesive tape used to hold the tube more securely in place. Two strips of tape applied with an "elephant-ear" technique at 90 degrees to each other provide an excellent method of securing the tube in place (Fig. 6–19). The tape is torn so that one end is split into three pieces extending halfway to the center. The two outside pieces are placed on the skin on either side of the tube site, and the center piece is wrapped tightly around the tube. This is repeated with a second piece of tape, which is torn similarly and placed

at 90 degrees to the first. A third simple piece of tape may be used elsewhere on the chest to prevent the tube from accidentally being pulled loose. The connections are then securely taped.

Repeat PA and lateral chest radiographs must be taken to confirm tube placement and to document the degree of resolution. In a stable patient, it is often better to obtain the post-procedure films with a less elaborate temporary dressing in place, in case tube repositioning is required. It is important to note that a simple pneumothorax should be completely re-expanded within a few minutes of continual suction. If the film taken following chest tube insertion shows that the lung is still collapsed, one should consider three possibilities: (1) The tube may be in the wrong place. (This is the most easily corrected problem.) (2) A persistent air leak, usually from a large bronchus or the trachea, may be delaying expansion. (3) Plugging of a main bronchus with blood, mucus, or aspirated material may be delaying resolution of the pneumothorax.

Gauze pad

Figure 6–19. The tube is secured with two strips of wide adhesive tape. (Redrawn from Suratt, P. M., and Gibson, R. S.: Manual of Medical Procedures. St. Louis, C.V. Mosby, 1982.)

DRAINAGE SYSTEM

Physicians who place chest tubes infrequently or who do not participate in the ongoing care of patients who have undergone this procedure may have little familiarity with the physiology and mechanics of chest tube drainage systems. Life-

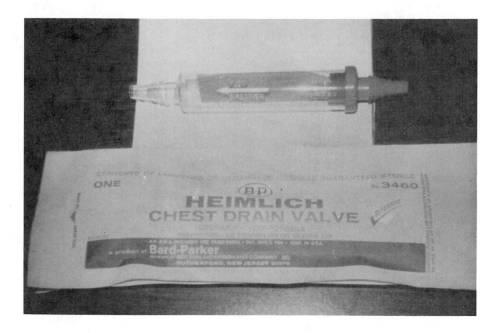

Figure 6–20. Heimlich valve.

threatening complications may arise from improper use of these devices, however, and the physician must be knowledgeable about the salient features of the system.

With the availability of modern closed drainage systems, the classic glass bottle collection system is rather cumbersome and largely antiquated. Nevertheless, the principles of the various drainage systems will be discussed here. The simplest drainage device is a flutter (Heimlich) valve (commonly used only for pneumothorax) attached to the end of the chest tube itself (Fig. 6–20). Such valves allow one way flow of air from the chest but collapse to prevent air from passing back into the chest. Normal respiration (assisted by coughing) gradually removes the excess air from the pleural space, and the lung re-expands to fill the thoracic cage.

The simplest device that may be used to remove small amounts of either fluid or air is the underwater seal (single-bottle) device (Fig. 6–21). The chest tube is connected to a second plastic tube, which runs into a closed glass or plastic container. The tube extends 2 to 4 cm below the surface of the (sterile) water placed in the drainage bottle. The water provides a "seal" against the entering of further air into the chest. The water also acts as a one-way valve. The intrathoracic pressure need only be greater than the depth of immersion of the tip of the drainage tube in the collection bottle to cause the intrathoracic air or fluid to exit into the bottle. This is easily accomplished with simple coughing.

In order for air to enter back into the pleural space through the chest tube, the patient must generate enough negative intrathoracic pressure to pull the water in the collection bottle up to the

height of the chest. Normal inspiration is not forceful enough to do this *if the bottle is kept on the floor*. The normal fluctuation in the height of the fluid level in the long tube during respiration provides proof that free communication exists with the pleural space and that the tube is functioning normally. An absence of respiratory fluctuation or a decrease in the drainage implies blockage or, if the tube has been in for a long enough period, full expansion of the lung and obliteration of the pleural space. The two situations (blockage and full expansion) should be distinguishable by clinical and radiographic means.

On the other hand, an *increase* in respiratory fluctuation may imply an increased inspiratory effort due to airway obstruction or atelectasis. If blocked, the tube may be changed or "milked" or "stripped" to dislodge clots.[21] "Milking" refers to

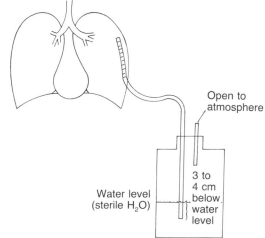

Open to atmosphere

3 to 4 cm below water level

Water level (sterile H₂O)

Figure 6–21. Single-bottle (water seal) collection device. (From Bricker, D. L.: Safe, effective tube thoracostomy. E. R. Reports 2:49–52, 1981.)

forcing air or fluid back into the chest by pinching or clamping the tube distally and, with the other hand, compressing the tube and forcing the contents proximally. This can dislodge a blocking intrathoracic clot and can obviate the need for tube replacement when radiographic or clinical examination suggests incomplete expansion or drainage. "Stripping" involves proximal pinching or clamping and progressive distal compression followed by release of the proximal aspect. This allows the tube to spring open. The sudden increase in negative pressure may extract clots and fluid from a more proximal location. These procedures are more effective with soft latex tubing than with clear plastic tubes. Persistent bubbling in the tube in both expiration and inspiration implies an air leak, the most common source of which is the drainage system connections. These should be taped thoroughly and rechecked frequently.

Another source of leakage may be failure to get the last opening of the chest tube inside the chest wall. One may best manage leaking at the skin incision side by initially tunneling up one interspace and by using effective suture technique and a Vaseline-impregnated gauze dressing. Of course, the bottle must always remain dependent, since gravity contributes a great deal to the proper drainage of the pleural space. Elevating the bottle above the chest can cause fluid to re-enter the chest and can increase the probability of infection. If a bronchopleural fistula exists, drowning can also occur.[16] The length of the tubing must be carefully controlled so that dependent loops of fluid do not form. Such loops of accumulated liquid must be displaced before more air or fluid can pass. The amount of positive intrapleural pressure required for air to pass to dependent loop of fluid is greater than the vertical elevation of the fluid in the loop (Fig. 6–22). If the fluid loop becomes high enough (15 to 25 cm of water), egress of air may be blocked to a degree sufficient to cause a tension pneumothorax.[32] Similarly, as

fluid accumulates in the water seal, the immersed tip of the tube must be raised so that it stays 2 to 4 cm below the water surface. Otherwise, a similarly progressive increase in intrathoracic pressure will be required to continue emptying the pleural space.

Sometimes a second "trap," or collecting bottle, is placed proximally to the water seal (Fig. 6–23). This has the advantage of keeping the level of fluid in the water seal bottle constant and allows for better measurement of collected drainage. A disadvantage is that air can enter the chest tube from the first bottle with accidental disconnection of any of the tubes or with a significant increase in negative intrapleural pressure. The dead space provided by the dry trap can produce an air-lock effect and can lead to to-and-fro pressure changes with ventilation without effective drainage.[21] More commonly, when a two-bottle system is used, it is connected to suction. The amount of suction in tube 1 is regulated not by the pressure reading on the wall suction valve but by the depth of water in the second bottle above tube 3 and by the depth of tube 1 (Fig. 6–24). When suction exceeds the depth of the water in bottle 2, air enters from the top of the third tube to prevent further increases. The internal diameter of the various tubes (especially 3) also contributes to the amount of suction that can be created.

The more complex the system, the more problems that can occur. Evaporation occurs quickly, and fluid levels must be maintained to keep pressures from steadily decreasing. Vigorous bubbling in the first bottle may cause foam to rise and to be suctioned into the second, either breaking the water seal or changing the pressure regulation. A few drops of a chemical agent (caprylic alcohol)

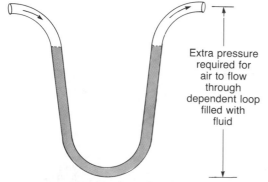

Extra pressure required for air to flow through dependent loop filled with fluid

Figure 6–22. Dependent loops of fluid-filled tubing require positive intrapleural pressure greater than the vertical height of the fluid-filled loop for drainage to occur. (From Batchelder, T. L., et al.: Critical factors in determining adequate pleural drainage in both the operated and non-operated chest. Am. Surg. 28:298, 1962.)

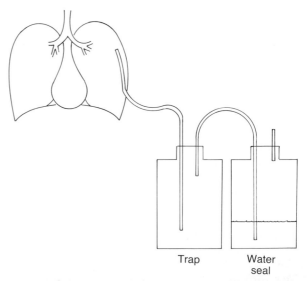

Trap   Water seal

Figure 6–23. A "trap" proximal to the water seal is sometimes used. (From Bricker, D. L.: Safe, effective tube thoracostomy. E. R. Reports 2:49–52, 1981.)

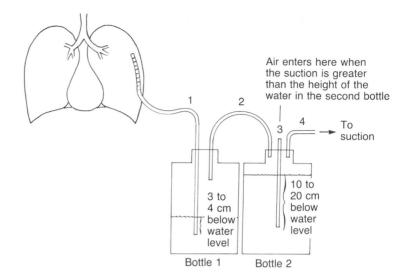

Figure 6–24. A two-bottle system for applying regulated suction to the pleural space. The height of the column of water in bottle 2 regulates the amount of suction applied, independent of the pressure on the suction valve. (From Bricker, D. L.: Safe, effective tube thoracostomy. E. R. Reports 2:49–52, 1981.)

can be used in bottle 1 to prevent this. As the first bottle fills with fluid, the effective suction decreases because of an increase in hydrostatic pressure at the bottom of tube 1. Although a two-bottle system (water seal plus suction regulator) is adequate for nearly all emergency department applications,[26] a number of self-contained setups that avoid the bulky bottle system are commercially available.

Some add a dry trap (third bottle) to collect fluids. The commercially available Pleur-Evac system mimics this setup with one piece of molded plastic and two tubes (Fig. 6–25). Because glass bottles are cumbersome and time-consuming to assemble, the editors strongly urge emergency departments to use the convenient, disposable devices, such as the Pleur-Evac.

Occlusive clamping of chest tubes should be performed only with great trepidation and physician supervision, particularly in the first 24 hours after the tubes are placed. Clamping with a persistent intrathoracic air leak or fluid accumulation may rapidly lead to a tension pneumo- or hemothorax. Clamping is appropriate only to change the underwater seal bottle rapidly. Patients with chest tubes in place are best transported without clamping—on water seal only, with the bottle placed well below chest level.

ROLE OF SUCTION

Most sources recommend suction at least initially in all patients with chest tubes placed for either pneumo- or hemothorax.[6, 12, 13, 33] Ideally, a suction machine must have high flow (up to 20 L per minute) and a regulated constant suction (0 to 60 cm of water). Gill and Long recommend suction only if the air leak is massive, if the lung fails to re-expand, or if bleeding continues.[27] The continuous bubbling and the lack of respiratory variation with suction can mask the presence of air leak. With extensive bleeding, excessive suction may actually increase the rate of blood loss, particularly when the bleeding is from a relatively low-pressure pulmonary vessel. Intermittent clamping or water seal may be preferred. With a massive air leak, excess suction may cause respiratory distress by removing inspired air before alveolar gas exchange can occur.[1] Suction may be useful for rapid initial expansion and drainage. Because of the added complexity and complications, suction should be replaced by simple underwater seal drainage as long as expansion and drainage are satisfactory and no persistent air leak exists. When suction is applied, 20 cm of water is normally used.

TUBE REMOVAL

Recommendations vary, but chest tubes should generally be removed when there has been no drainage of fluid or air for a minimum of 24 hours, when respiratory variations in the water seal have ceased, and when high-quality radiographs reveal satisfactory resolution. Because of pleural irritation, small amounts of serous fluid (less than 200 ml per day) may continue to drain without contraindicating removal. The patient should be placed in a semi-erect position, and the dressings should be removed. Sedation or restraints may be helpful. The area should be sterilized and draped, and sterile technique should be followed. The only instruments required are sterile basins, heavy scissors to cut the suture, dressing materials, and instruments to tie the previously placed purse-string suture or to place a new one. Facilities and

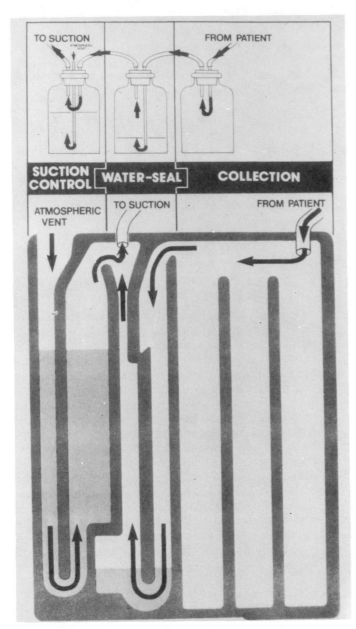

Water seal chamber: If one notices air bubbles going through this section, there is a continual air leak in the patient or in the collection system.

Figure 6–25. Three-bottle suction system: the "classic" three-bottle system versus the commercially available Pleur-Evac device.

equipment should be available to reinsert a new chest tube properly if it should become necessary. The suture holding the tube to the skin should be removed from the tube, and the purse-string suture that was placed previously should be loosened and readied for tying. A second (gloved) assistant is helpful. The tube should be clamped, and the connecting tubing should be removed. A Vaseline- or antibiotic-impregnated gauze dressing should be prepared. The patient should exhale fully and should perform a mild Valsalva maneuver. The tube is removed in one swift motion while the patient holds his breath. Two fingers hold the skin edges shut, and the purse-string suture is tied. The occlusive dressing is placed and taped securely. A period of observation (minimum 2 to 6 hours) is recommended if the patient is to be sent home, with a chest film at the end of that time. Any increase in symptoms should call for prompt re-evaluation. After 48 hours, the dressing may be removed and the wound managed as any sutured skin wound would be.

PNEUMOTHORAX IN PEDIATRIC PATIENTS

Incidence

Pneumothorax occurs more commonly during the neonatal period than at any other time of life. When chest radiographs are taken of all newborns in large series, the incidence of pneumothorax is high (1 to 2 per cent). The incidence does not seem to change when normal (term) vaginal deliveries are compared with premature births or with delivery by cesarean section. The incidence of *symptomatic* pneumothorax in newborn infants, however, is consistently only 0.05 to 0.07 per cent. Of newborns with pneumothorax, several studies report twice as many males as females. Some studies report more instances of right-sided collapse. Ten to 20 per cent of cases are bilateral.[34-37]

It should be noted that lobar emphysema in a newborn may cause severe respiratory symptoms shortly after birth (Fig. 6–26). The physical examination may detect decreased breath sounds in a hemithorax and even evidence of mediastinal shift. Lobar emphysema often looks like a tension pneumothorax radiographically, and the unwary physician may rush to insert a chest tube. The treatment in this case is surgical removal of the diseased lobe, and a chest tube may worsen the clinical condition.

Pathophysiology

There seem to be two groups of newborns who develop pneumothorax. The first are term or post-term neonates with a history of fetal distress; difficult delivery; need for resuscitation; or aspiration of meconium, amniotic fluid, or blood. These infants tend to become symptomatic within the first 2 hours of life and generally fare quite well. The mechanism in this group is believed to be an excess intra-alveolar pressure generated at birth. With the first breath, the transpulmonary pressure rises from 40 to as much as 100 cm of water. Compression of the chest during vaginal delivery places the diaphragm and the muscles of respiration at a marked mechanical advantage. With mechanical obstruction of some alveoli or bronchioles, as can occur with aspiration, the intense transpulmonary pressure is transmitted to the normally aerated alveoli, which can overdistend and rupture. Mechanical ventilation, end-expiratory pressure, and resuscitative efforts can also precipitate alveolar rupture.

The second group of newborns with pneumothorax are those who have underlying pulmonary disease (most notably hyaline membrane disease [respiratory distress syndrome]) or congenital abnormalities. These infants commonly develop their pneumothoraces in the second day of life, often while being treated with positive airway pressures. The prognosis in these cases is much worse.[35, 37]

Clinical Findings

The physical examination of the newborn with pneumothorax can yield findings ranging from no abnormalities whatsoever to complete cardiovascular collapse. Grunting respirations and tachypnea (to a respiratory rate as high as 120) are often seen. Retractions or nasal flaring can be seen. Cyanosis may be present or may occur only with crying or feeding. Irritability, restlessness, apneic periods, bradycardia, or tachycardia may be the only manifestation. Distention and tympany of the affected side may be found. A decrease in breath sounds is difficult to appreciate in the newborn. With tension pneumothorax, the cardiac impulse and the trachea may be shifted away from the affected side.

Diagnosis

The definitive diagnosis is made with high-quality radiographs taken in both the anteroposterior and the horizontal beam (cross-table) lateral projections. Small pneumothoraces may be seen only on the lateral view, as the air collects at the top of the thoracic cavity. Bilateral tension pneumothorax can appear as microcardia, without any mediastinal shift. Further radiologic studies may be needed to differentiate this condition from lung cysts, lobar emphysema, and skin folds.

Transillumination of the chest with a high-intensity fiberoptic light source has been used with great success to detect and follow pneumothorax and pneumomediastinum in newborns.[38]

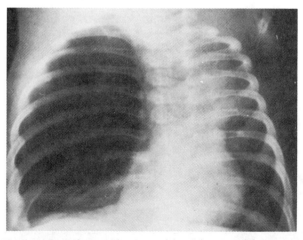

Figure 6–26. Lobar emphysema of the right upper lobe simulating a tension pneumothorax.

Monin and Vert have noted that abrupt changes in transthoracic impedance in infants on respiratory monitors have been related to the appearance of pneumothorax.[35] Such changes should initiate prompt re-evaluation of the patient's respiratory status.

Treatment

In general, tube thoracostomy is the treatment of choice. When signs of tension pneumothorax are present, aspiration with a plastic catheter-over-the-needle device is recommended. Small pneumothoraces (less than 20 per cent of the hemithorax) in relatively asymptomatic infants (who are without other problems and who do not require positive airway pressures) can be merely monitored by close observation.

Repeated films or transillumination and frequent monitoring of vital signs and arterial blood gases are indicated. Breathing 100 per cent oxygen is believed to hasten reabsorption by as much as six-fold.[34, 39] The risks of retrolental fibroplasia and pulmonary oxygen toxicity must be carefully assessed, however.

When evacuation of the pleural space is elected, needle aspiration using a 50-ml syringe, an 18 gauge catheter-over-the-needle device, and a three-way stopcock may be attempted once (see Chapter 5).[40] This may suffice in patients without a continued air leak, although the risk of lung puncture is considerable.

Technique

The technique of tube thoracostomy in pediatric patients varies little from that already described. Small, commercially available thoracostomy tubes (Argyle) or standard "red rubber" catheters with extra holes cut in the tip can be used. No. 8 to 10 French catheters are used in premature infants, and 10 to 12 French catheters are used in larger newborns. Blunt dissection minimizes the complications of lung puncture, hemorrhage, and traumatic fistula formation, which are seen more often with trocar insertion.[41, 42]

Various tube locations have been proposed. In their controlled trial, Allen and associates compared the effectiveness of lateral (fourth to fifth intercostal space, anterior axillary line) and superior (first to third intercostal space, mid–clavicular line) placements of 149 chest tubes for their effectiveness in evacuating pneumothorax.[43] The most important factor was the eventual location of the tube rather than the site of insertion. Anterior tubes were effective 96 per cent of the time, whereas only 42 per cent of the tubes directed posteriorly functioned satisfactorily.

Placement in the third intercostal space, mid–axillary line with the tip directed under the sterum appears to be a good compromise.[35] Care must be taken to avoid the nipple, which can be difficult to identify in the premature infant. Water seal with 10 to 20 cm of water for suction is usually recommended until re-expansion occurs and the absence of continued air leakage is verified.

Smaller collecting bottles are recommended to measure drainage more accurately. Hughes and Beuscher have described a miniature water seal apparatus using a 50-ml multiple-use saline bottle, standard intravenous tubing, and one long and one short needle (Fig. 6–27).[44]

OTHER DEVICES

Trocar Insertion

The blunt dissection technique described previously is the one that is commonly advocated by authorities on chest tube placement. Many practitioners have become proficient in using a trocar for the percutaneous introduction of chest tubes. The trocar device that is currently commercially available consists of a siliconized plastic catheter that is generally smaller than 34 French and has fewer fenestrations than do the other (Argyle) tubes. It fits over a central pointed steel or aluminum rod with a plastic ball handle at one end and

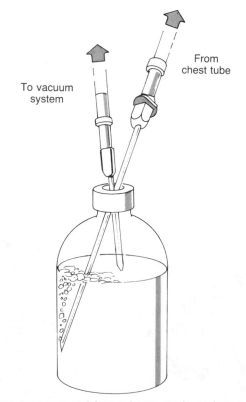

To vacuum system

From chest tube

Figure 6–27. Water seal for newborns. (Redrawn from Hughes, W. T., and Beuscher, E. S.: Pediatric Procedures, 2nd ed. Philadelphia, W. B. Saunders Co., 1980, p. 239.)

a small portion of the sharpened tip protruding through the fenestrated end. The positioning, preparation, and local anesthesia that were described previously are used. A skin incision as before is made with a number 11 blade. With the tip of the catheter held firmly in one hand for control and the ball held in the other hand, one forces the trocar point through the intercostal muscles and the parietal pleura. As the pleural space is entered, the catheter is pushed from the stylet into the pleural space and is secured in the usual fashion.[45] Other trocars contain a sharp obturator and a hollow metal tube through which a rubber catheter may be passed and secured.[6] Millikan and coworkers reviewed 1249 patients undergoing tube thoracostomy for acute trauma from 1967 to 1978. The authors abandoned the trocar in 1974 in favor of a blunt technique because of "major technical complications," such as damage to lung and solid organs, and concluded that "the trocar should never be used."[33] Bricker in his recent review also noted that "most authorities

condemn" such devices.[1] The editors of this text do *not* recommend the use of the trocar technique to puncture the pleura, although the trocar may be used instead of a Kelly clamp to introduce or guide the chest tube *after the pleura has been opened* (Fig. 6–28).

McSwain Dart (Fig. 6–29)

McSwain has developed an ingenious percutaneous catheter suitable for rapid treatment of pneumothorax and tension pneumothorax. It is a 15-cm, 16 French polyethylene catheter that fits over a metal stylet. It has a retractable winged flange at its tip to secure it in the thoracic cavity. Plastic tubing leads to a one-way (Heimlich) valve and can be connected to suction. The device is placed through a stab skin wound over a rib and has been advocated for both prehospital and in-hospital use by physicians and paramedic personnel. Complications in one series of 40 patients were minor.[46] Bayne has recently documented the

Figure 6–28. Sequence of steps in the use of a hollow metal trocar to insert a catheter into the pleural space. Before starting, one must determine that the entire length of the catheter can pass through the trocar. *Note:* Although the trocar apparatus may be used to introduce the chest tube *after the pleura has been opened,* the editors do *not* recommend the use of the trocar method to puncture the pleura. (Redrawn from Cosgniff, J. H.: An Atlas of Diagnostic and Therapeutic Procedures for Emergency Personnel. Philadelphia, J. B. Lippincott Co., 1978, pp. 257–258.)

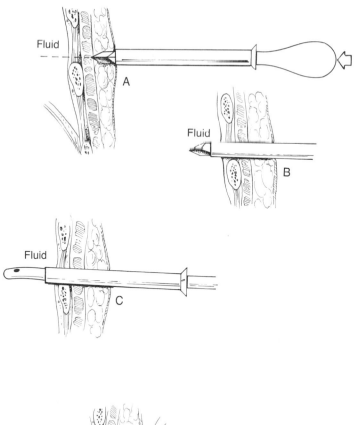

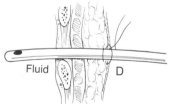

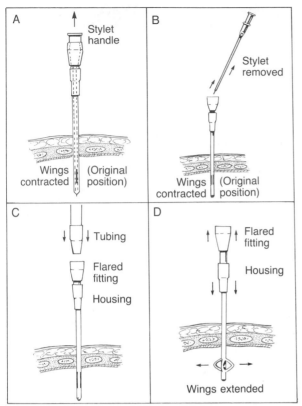

Figure 6–29. Operation of the McSwain Dart. (From Medical Dynamics, Inc.)

need for accurate diagnosis prior to insertion, however, noting consistent parenchymal lung damage when fully expanded lungs were encountered.[8] The editors recommend that this device be used only when the standard method of blunt dissection tube thoracostomy is not available.

COMPLICATIONS

As with any surgical procedure, complications can and will occur (Table 6–6).[33, 47] Millikan and colleagues noted a 1 per cent incidence of technical complications (visceral perforation) in their series of 447 patients undergoing tube thoracostomy for trauma.[33] Pneumonia and atelectasis are attributed to a decrease in coughing and failure to clear secretions because of pain. As for any postoperative patient, early ambulation and vigorous pulmonary toilet are indicated. Empyema is uncommon,[33] since tube thoracostomy remains a useful treatment for this problem. Empyema tends to occur with loculated effusions or those that are inadequately drained.

Local infection at the site of insertion is common and may reflect the often hurried performance of this procedure in the emergency setting. Meticulous technique provides the most effective prev-

Table 6–6. COMPLICATIONS OF TUBE THORACOSTOMY

Infection
    Pneumonia
    Empyema
    Local incision infection
    Osteomyelitis

Bleeding
    Local incision hematoma
    Intercostal artery or vein laceration
    Internal mammary artery laceration (with mid–clavicular line placement)
    Pulmonary vein or artery injury
    Great vessel injury (rarely)

Laceration or puncture of solid organs
    Lung
    Liver
    Spleen
    Diaphragm
    Stomach
    Colon
    Long thoracic nerve
    Intercostal nerve (may result in intercostal neuritis/neuralgia)
    Intercostal muscles (intercostal myalgia)

Mechanical problems
    Chest tube dislodgement from chest wall
    Incorrect tube position
        Subcutaneous placement
        Intra-abdominal placement

Air leaks
    Leaks from tubing or drainage bottles
    Last tube fenestration not entirely within pleural space
    Leaks from skin site

Flow of drainage bottle contents into chest from inadvertently elevating drainage bottles

Blocked drainage
    Kinked chest tube or drainage tubes
    Clots

Miscellaneous
    Allergic reactions to surgical preparation or anesthesia
    Pulmonary atelectasis
    Persistent pneumothorax
    Retained hemothorax
    Clotted hemothorax or fibrothorax
    Subcutaneous or mediastinal emphysema
    Re-expansion pulmonary edema
    Recurrence of pneumothorax after chest tube removal

entative. Osteomyelitis has been reported in settings in which tubes have been kept in place for a long time. Careful dissection may prevent a local hematoma. Intercostal arteries or veins may be lacerated at the time of tube insertions. Such lacerations can be minimized if sharp dissection is carried only to the fascia and the tube is carefully placed just above the rib. The tube may adequately tamponade such bleeding, but if tamponade is insufficient, the incision may need to be extended in order to expose or ligate the bleeding vessel. If a lacerated intercostal artery does not stop bleeding, one may attempt to insert a Foley catheter into the incision, inflate the balloon, and withdraw the catheter to tamponade the vessel. Anterior chest wall placement carried to the midline may result in internal mammary artery laceration. This is notoriously difficult to control and may require thoracotomy. Damage to the lung parenchyma or the intrapulmonary vessels can readily occur. This is more common with trocar insertion and is minimized by blunt dissection and the use of manual exploration of the pleura to exclude or free adhesions. Use of the anesthetizing needle to document air or fluid in the area in which the tube is to be placed can minimize this problem.

Careful attention to the anatomy, with recognition of exactly how high the diaphragm may rise (especially if the abdomen is filled with blood), can minimize injuries to the diaphragm or the intra-abdominal organs. Blunt dissection and manual exploration prior to tube insertion also work well in this instance. Careful preinsertion measurement of the distance a tube is to be placed may minimize the chance that it will impinge upon or injure the large nerves and vessels at the lung apex. Persistent pain may result from pressure on the intercostal nerves and muscles and may respond to intercostal nerve blocks or infiltration with a long-acting local anesthetic.

Mechanical problems commonly result in air leaks with failed re-expansion or inadequate drainage. Tension pneumothorax can occur if a blockage in the drainage system at any point is associated with an air leak. Failure of re-expansion or incomplete re-expansion of a pneumothorax may be due to a mechanical air leak, but it may also indicate a bronchopleural fistula, a continued parenchymal lung leak, or a bronchial injury. Retained hemothorax may result from clotting or poor tube function. The largest possible tube should be used for drainage of a hemothorax. Reinsertion or placement of a second tube may be indicated if the first tube is not functioning properly. Often, an angled tube in the posterior diaphragmatic sulcus will promote drainage of a dependent fluid colleciton. Clotted hemothorax or fibrothorax is an indication for elective decortication and pleurodesis. Subcutaneous emphysema can occur if the chest tube is partially extruded or plugged.

Re-expansion pulmonary edema is a sometimes fatal consequence of thoracentesis or tube thoracostomy for pleural effusion or pneumothorax.[48, 49] Pulmonary edema, typically ipisilateral, can appear as soon as 1 to 2 hours after lung re-expansion. Edema commonly occurs when collapse has been present for longer than 72 hours and when 1000 ml or more is removed. Suction seems to worsen the edema. This complication is believed to be secondary to anoxic injury to large areas of the lung caused by altered pulmonary circulation in areas of atelectasis and resultant increased capillary permeability. Rapid removal of fluid or air may result in abrupt return of circulation and transudation of protein and fluid into the alveolar space. Treatment has included steroids, colloids, diuretics, continuous positive airway pressure, and positive-pressure ventilation. The best course would be to attempt to prevent this complication by slow, staged removal of large effusions or collections of air (especially if they have been present for several days), avoiding suction if possible.

If a chest tube is not functioning properly or has not reversed the pathologic condition as expected, one must carefully re-evaluate the position of the chest tube. In an emergency situation, the tube may have been placed subcutaneously, and the incorrect placement may not be obvious to the physician. If the tube dissects in a fascial plane posteriorly along a rib, even the postinsertion film may appear to confirm proper placement. Such a condition may be lethal. As a general rule, if a chest tube is not functioning properly and the patient is deteriorating, the tube should be removed and inserted again, or another tube should be inserted.

1. Bricker, D. L.: Safe effective tube thoracostomy. Part I: Pathophysiology, diagnosis, indications. Part II: Insertion, collection, transport, complications. E. R. Reports 2:45, 1981.
2. Nissen, R., and Wilson, R. H. L.: Pages in the history of chest surgery. Springfield, IL, Charles C Thomas, 1960.
3. Hewett, F. C.: Thoracentesis: The plan of continuous aspiration. Br. Med J. 1:317, 1876.
4. Brewer, L. A.: Wounds of the chest in war and peace, 1943–1968. Ann. Thorac. Surg. 7:387, 1969.
5. McNamara, J. J., Messersmith, J. K., Dunn, R. A., et al.: Thoracic injuries in combat casualties in Vietnam. Ann. Thorac. Surg. 10:389, 1970.
6. Kirsh, M. M., and Sloan, H.: Blunt Chest Trauma. Boston, Little, Brown & Co., 1977, pp. 49–79.
7. Jones, K. W.: Thoracic trauma. Surg. Clin. North Am. 60:957, 1980.
8. Bayne, C. G.: Pulmonary complications of the McSwain Dart. Ann. Emerg. Med. 11:136, 1982.
9. Beall, A. C., Crawford, H. W., and DeBakey, M. E.: Considerations in the management of acute traumatic hemothorax. J. Thorac. Cardiovasc. Surg. 52:351, 1966.
10. Siemons, R., Polk, H. C., Gray, L. A., Jr., et al: Indications for thoracotomy following penetrating thoracic injury. J. Trauma 17:493, 1977.
11. Shefts, L M.: The Initial Management of Thoracic and Thoraco-abdominal Trauma. Springfield, IL, Charles C Thomas, 1956.
12. DeVries, W. C., and Wolfe, W. G.: The management of spontaneous pneumothorax and bullous emphysema. Surg. Clin. North. Am. 60:851, 1980.
13. Brooks, J. W.: Thoracotomy in the management of spontaneous pneumothorax. Ann. Surg. 177:798, 1973.
14. Ruckley, C. V., and McCormack, R. J.: The management of spontaneous pneumothorax. Thorax 21:139, 1966.

15. Clark, T. A., Hutchison, D. E., Deaner, R. M., et al: Spontaneous pneumothorax. Am. J. Surg. 124:728, 1972.

16. Borrie, J.: Management of Thoracic Emergencies, 3rd ed. New York, Appleton-Century-Crofts, 1980.

17. Kircher, L. T., Jr., and Swartzel, R. L.: Spontaneous pneumothorax and its treatment. JAMA 155:24, 1954.

18. Raja, O. G., and Lalor, A. J.: Simple aspiration of spontaneous pneumothorax. Br. J. Dis. Chest 75:207, 1981.

19. Cannon, W. B., Mark, J. B. D., and Jamplis, R. W.: Pneumothorax: A therapeutic update. Am. J. Surg. 142:26, 1981.

20. Mercier, C., Page, A., Verdant, A., et al.: Outpatient management of intercostal tube drainage in spontaneous pneumothorax. Ann. Thorac. Surg. 22:163, 1976.

21. Von Hippel, A.: A Manual of Thoracic Surgery. Springfield, IL, Charles C Thomas, 1978.

22. Seremetis, M. G.: The management of spontaneous pneumothorax. Chest 57:65, 1970.

23. Gazzaniga, A. B.: Surgical considerations in pulmonary disease. In Burton, G. G., Gee, G. N., and Hodgkin, J. E. (eds.): Respiratory Care. Philadelphia, J. B. Lippincott Co., 1977.

24. Kenyan, J. H.: A preliminary report of a method of treatment of empyema in young children. Med. Rec. 80:816, 1911.

25. American College of Surgeons Committee on Trauma: Advanced Trauma Life Support Course, 1981.

26. Munnell, E. R., and Thomas, E. K.: Current concepts in thoracic drainage systems. Ann. Thorac. Surg. 19:261, 1975.

27. Gill, W., and Long, W. B. (eds.): Shock Trauma Manual. Baltimore, Williams & Wilkins, 1979.

28. Hegarty, M. M.: A conservative approach to penetrating injuries of the chest. Injury 8:53, 1976.

29. Duponselle, E. F. C.: The level of the intercostal drain and other determinant factors in the conservative approach to penetrating chest injuries. Cent. Afr. J. Med. 26:52, 1980.

30. Broadie, T. A., Glover, J. L., and Bang, N.: Clotting competence of intracavitary blood in trauma victims. Ann. Emerg. Med. 10:127, 1981.

31. Gilman, A. G., Goodman, L. S., and Gilman, A. (eds.): Goodman and Gilman's The Pharamacological Basis of Therapeutics, 6th ed. New York, Macmillan Publishing Co., Inc., 1980.

32. Batchelder, T. L., and Morris, K. A.: Critical factors in determining adequate pleural drainage in both the operated and non-operated chest. Am. Surg. 28:296, 1962.

33. Millikan, J. S., Moore, E. E., Steiner, E., et al.: Complications of tube thoracostomy for acute trauma. Am. J. Surg. 140:738, 1980.

34. Chernick, V., and Reed, M. H.: Pneumothorax and chylothorax in the neonatal period. J. Pediatr. 76:624, 1970.

35. Monin, P., and Vert, P.: Pneumothorax. Clin. Perinatol. 5:335, 1978.

36. Steele, R. W., Metz, J. R., Bass, J. W., et al.: Pneumothorax and pneumomediastinum in the newborn. Radiology 98:629, 1971.

37. Yu, V. Y. H., Liew, S. W., and Robertson, N. R. C.: Pneumothorax in the newborn: Changing pattern. Arch. Dis. Child. 50:449, 1975.

38. Kuhns, L. R., Bednarek, F. J., Wyman, M. L., et al.: Diagnosis of pneumothorax or pneumomediastinum in the neonate by transilluminaiton. Pediatrics 56:355, 1975.

39. Chernick, V., and Avery, M. E.: Spontaneous alveolar rupture at birth. Pediatrics 32:816, 1963.

40. Moore, G. C., Mills, L. J., and Mast, C. P.: Thoracentesis and chest tube insertion. In Levin, D. L., Moriss, F. C., and Moore, G. C. (eds.): A Practical Guide to Pediatric Intensive Care. St. Louis, C. V. Mosby, 1979, pp. 415–422.

41. Banagale, R. C., Outerbridge, E. W., and Aranda, J. V.: Lung perforation: A complication of chest tube insertion in neonatal pneumothorax. J. Pediatr. 94:973, 1979.

42. Moessinger, A. C., Driscoll, J. M., Jr.,and Wigger, H. J.: High incidence of lung perforation by chest tube in neonatal pneumothorax. J. Pediatr. 92:635, 1978.

43. Allen, R. W., Jr., Jung, A. L., and Lester, P. D.: Effectiveness of chest tube evacuation of pneumothorax in neonates. J. Pediatr. 99:629, 1981.

44. Hughes, W. T., and Buescher, E. S.: Pediatric Procedures, 2nd ed. Philadelphia, W. B. Saunders Co., 1980.

45. Richardson, J. D.: Management of noncardiac thoracic trauma. Heart Lung 7:286, 1978.

46. Wayne, M. A., and McSwain, N. E.: Clinical evaluation of a new device for the treatment of tension pneumothorax. Ann. Surg. 191:760, 1980.

47. Artz, C. P., and Hardy, J. D.: Management of Surgical Complications, 3rd ed. Philadelphia, W. B. Saunders Co., 1975.

48. Johnstone, W.: Reexpansion pulmonary edema. Va. Med. 107:790, 1980.

49. Sewell, R. W., Fewel, J. C., Grover, F. T., et al.: Experimental evaluation of reexpansion pulmonary edema. Ann. Thorac. Surg. 26:126, 1978.

50. American College of Surgeons Committee on Trauma: Early Care of the Injured Patient, 2nd ed. Philadelphia, W. B. Saunders Co., 1976, pp. 161–173.

51. Hood, R. M., and Spencer, F. C. (eds.): Management of Thoracic Injuries. Springfield, IL, Charles C Thomas, 1969.

52. Kish, G., Kozloff, L., Joseph, W. L., et al.: Indications for early thoracotomy in the management of chest trauma. Ann. Thorac. Surg. 22:23, 1976.

53. Mulder, D. S.: Chest trauma: Current concepts. Can. J. Surg. 23:340, 1980.

54. Richards, V.: Tube thoracostomy. J. Fam. Pract. 6:629, 1978.

55. Thomas, A. W.: Penetrating thoracic trauma (Trauma rounds). West. J. Med. 121:510, 1974.

7

Emergency Cricothyroidotomy

CHARLES O. BRANTIGAN, M.D.

The importance of access to and control of the airway in an emergency has been recognized since antiquity. The critical nature of acute airway obstruction has also been recognized. Lack of physician intervention is rapidly fatal. The wrong action by a physician or the right action carried out slowly or inexpertly is also a cause of death.

Intubation of the airway using an orotracheal tube, a nasotracheal tube, or a rigid bronchoscope constitutes emergency airway management in most hospital situations. Other approaches are used only when it is impossible or inadvisable to intubate the patient. Three such approaches have been considered: needle tracheotomy, standard tracheotomy, and cricothyroidotomy. Insertion of a large-bore needle into the trachea to allow the patient to breathe has been proposed, and occasional case reports that advocate temporary airway support by needle tracheostomy in *partial* airway obstruction have appeared; however, needle tracheostomy is, for the most part, unrealistic. The largest commonly available needle in the hospital setting is 14 gauge. Although a study of the physics of breathing through such a needle led Bouga and Cook[1] to reject the concept in 1960, the use of a needle with high-pressure ventilatory equipment (not available in most hospitals), however, may be practical in some situations.

Standard emergency tracheotomy as described by Jackson is still advocated by some.

In regard to the execution of the operation in the urgent cases, two incisions are better than one. The first should penetrate to the trachea, which is then felt like a wash-board under the left forefinger. This finger acts as a guide for the second incision, which should follow the first in a second's time. With the wound a well of blood, there is little need for a light until the vessels are to be caught up, which should not be attempted until the respiration has been started. . . .[2]

This bloody technique has largely been abandoned by physicians who are called to perform such operations on the front lines of our emergency facilities. Cricothyroidotomy has replaced this brutal procedure.

The purpose of this chapter is to outline the development of cricothyroidotomy and to summarize the pertinent current literature. The relevant anatomy and the technical aspects of the operation will be described, with particular attention paid to the complications of the procedure and how they might be avoided.

Historical Background

Although little was known about proper techniques and even less about asepsis and wound healing, tracheotomy was practiced before 1900 by some brave surgeons. The results of such surgery were described in 1886 by Colles.[3] The mortality of the procedure itself was approximately 50 per cent, the incidence of airway stenosis in survivors was high, and such stenosis was generally fatal. The first reported case of cricothyroidotomy, performed by a patient on herself in a suicide attempt, terminated in fatal airway stenosis.[4] Although good results in survivors caused physicians to maintain interest in the procedure, they limited its use to the terminally ill because of the mortality and the rate of complications. Conservative physicians would not allow the procedure to be used at all. Dr. E. C. Dick, in caring for George Washington during his final illness, reported, "I proposed to perforate the trachea as a means of prolonging life and of affording time for the removal of the obstruction to respiration in the larynx, which manifestly threatened immediate dissolution."[5] Dick was overruled by his colleagues, and the patient died. Attempts at tracheotomy, if made at all, were often made on patients who were too hypoxic to be resuscitated, and this further increased operative mortality. As Hupp described the situation in 1914, "Certainly the delay due to this great dread of tracheotomy was itself largely accountable for the fatality attending its performance."[6] It appears that during this period, patients with airway obstruction died as a result of either physician action or physician inaction.

Against this background, Chevalier Jackson in 1909 described the basic principles that made the procedure safe.[7] These principles are critically important today. The best possible airway control must be achieved before surgery is attempted. Jackson recommended the use of local anesthesia and condemned sedation and general anesthesia, because such measures often cause airway collapse and respiratory arrest in patients with a compromised airway. Only if the patient is intubated is general anesthesia or sedation safe. All equipment and supplies must be present and organized before the procedure is undertaken. The operation must be carried out precisely and in a controlled fashion with the best possible exposure, even if the situation is emergent. Correctly shaped tubes of inert material must be used. Careful postoperative care is critical. Using the aforementioned principles, Jackson was able to report a surgical mortality of 3 per cent, which compares favorably with current series. These principles apply equally well to cricothyroidotomy.

Jackson's landmark work with tracheotomy and his monumental contributions to bronchoscopy and endoscopic surgery made him internationally famous. Patients with decannulation problems and other tracheotomy complications were referred to him from all over the world. In 1921, when the devastating nature of chronic subglottic stenosis became apparent, he published another landmark paper, "High Tracheotomy and Other Errors, the Chief Causes of Chronic Laryngeal Stenosis."[2]

This paper was a study of stenosis rather than of tracheotomy. Two hundred tracheotomy patients were referred to him because the referring physician had been unable to perform decannulation. In 30 patients, stenosis was caused by the condition necessitating the tracheotomy. Of the remaining 170 patients, 93 per cent had stenosis resulting from "high tracheostomy." Included in this category were patients who had worn cannulas placed through the cricothyroid membrane, the thyroid cartilage, the cricoid cartilage, or even the lateral walls of the larynx. Many of the operations were for conditions that are unusual today, such as aspirated foreign bodies, epiglottitis, Ludwig's angina, angioneurotic edema, diphtherial pharyngitis, syphilis or tuberculosis of the larynx, or even perichondritis or typhoid of the larynx. Most of the indications for the procedure were local inflammatory conditions of the larynx, and the introduction of a foreign body into a diseased larynx encouraged development of airway stenosis.

The medical profession accepted Jackson's condemnation of cricothyroidotomy with the same enthusiasm with which Galen's teachings had been embraced 18 centuries before. Just as Jackson lamented that "unfortunately, the literature of tracheotomy, one of the oldest operations in surgery, is full of obsolete ideas handed down from textbook to textbook, generation to generation,"[8] so his teachings were passed on anecdotally to succeeding generations of physicians. With the exception of Nelson's limited animal study on cricothyroidotomy[9] and Caparosa and Zavatsky's[10] classic anatomic description, little research was done in this area. There were few advocates of cricothyroidotomy, even as a lifesaving procedure. Those who recommended its use in emergency situations all advocated rapid conversion to a standard tracheotomy.[11]

In the early days of cardiac surgery, John B. Grow, Sr., a student of Chevalier Jackson, began to question Jackson's teachings. Needing a rapid and safe method of tracheotomy isolated from the median sternotomy wound, he began (cautiously at first) to perform cricothyroidotomy under emergency circumstances. The dreaded subglottic stenosis proved not to be a problem; in fact, the incidence of all complications proved less than that associated with the method taught by his former teacher. Cricothyroidotomy gradually became Grow's operation of choice for all patients requiring tracheotomy in the absence of an acute laryngeal pathologic condition.

In 1976, Brantigan and Grow[12] reported the results of 655 patients undergoing cricothyroidotomy for respiratory support. Most of the patients had multisystemic disease, including various combinations of shock, respiratory failure, sepsis, liver failure, renal and liver failure, and altered consciousness. Cricothyroidotomy was not converted to standard tracheotomy, and the duration of intubation averaged 7 days.

Neither the use of the operating room nor the urgency of the procedure correlated with the results or complications, which occurred in 6.1 per cent of patients. These complications (Table 7–1) included many of those associated with standard tracheotomy. Operative misadventures and major vessel hemorrhage were notably absent. Of the eight patients who developed airway stenotic problems, none had chronic subglottic stenosis. Brantigan and Grow concluded that although Jackson's condemnation of high tracheotomy was valid at the time, there were four important differences

Table 7–1. COMPLICATIONS OF ELECTIVE CRICOTHYROIDOTOMY IN 655 PATIENTS*

Complication	Number of Patients
Postoperative bleeding (one with coagulopathy)	10
Late bleeding (two anticoagulated)	4
Abscess behind packing	1
Cellulitis of neck	2
Subcutaneous emphysema	1
Voice change	7
Feeling of lump in thorat	6
Persistent stoma (suture sinus)	1
Obstructive problems	
Cuff site granuloma	2
Cuff site stricture	5
Subglottic granulations†	1

*Data from Brantigan, C. O., and Grow, J. B., Sr.: Cricothyroidotomy: Elective use in respiratory problems requiring tracheotomy. J. Thorac. Cardiovasc. Surg. 71:72, 1976.

†One additional patient had sublottic granulations before cricothyroidotomy. These were endoscopically resected postoperatively.

between the patients in the two series. Jackson's patients underwent crude operations by a variety of surgeons, not precise operations of the type generally advocated by Jackson and carried out by the small number of thoracic surgeons who performed the operations in the 1976 series. Antibiotics were not available in 1921. Jackson's patients were intubated with a variety of devices, not necessarily Jackson's physiologically shaped inert tubes. Most importantly, the pathologic conditions leading to the tracheotomy in the two groups were entirely different. In Jackson's series, all the patients had acute stenosis of the larynx that required tracheotomy. Inserting a foreign body into the area of an acute stenosis would be expected to lead to an even more severe stenosis, and it did. The 1976 series included only patients who required tracheotomy for respiratory support.

Since the publication of the 1976 article, confirmatory studies have been carried out by a number of investigators. Romita, Colvin, and Boyd, using a variety of techniques, performed cricothyroidotomies on 32 dogs without producing subglottic stenosis.[13] They then evaluated cricothyroidotomy in 147 patients at the New York University Medical Center and Booth Memorial Medical Center.[14, 15] Healing of the stoma was observed by means of the flexible bronchoscope in 35 patients 5 to 7 days after removal of the cricothyroidotomy tube.

In 1977, Habel, an otolaryngologist, reported a series of 30 patients in whom cricothyroidotomy was carried out for respiratory management.[16] In the initial series, not only were there no cases of chronic subglottic stenosis, but also there were no significant complications. Habel subsequently observed one patient who developed subglottic stenosis. Details concerning the magnitude of the problem and the circumstances surrounding the complication are not available. In 1979, Koopman and coworkers[17, 18] investigated the effects of trauma, the denudation of the mucous membrane of the anterior half of the cricoid cartilage, and the prophylactic administration of antibiotics on airway narrowing in 40 dogs that had undergone cricothyroidotomy. None of the dogs developed clinically significant airway narrowing. In 1980, Morain described 16 patients who underwent cricothyroidotomy as an airway management technique in conjunction with reconstructive surgery of the head and the neck.[19] There were no complications in his series, even though one patient was intubated for 14 months. In 1982, Greisz and coworkers[20] reported the results of 61 elective cricothyroidotomies carried out at the bedside in an intensive care unit setting. Complications occurred in 8 per cent of patients, and no patient developed laryngeal stenosis. Other favorable reports have been published as well, but for the most part these contain no objective data.[21-23]

Not all material published since the 1976 report has been favorable. In 1980, Kennedy[24] denounced the procedure; his condemnation was based on the cases of two patients who developed stenosis of the larynx. In these two patients, however, the procedures were carried out in the presence of acute laryngeal pathology, which is a specific contraindication to cricothyroidotomy.[24, 25] In the series of letters to the editor that followed Morain's article, Montagano and Passy stated that they had seen many patients who developed subglottic stenosis following the procedure, but they have not published these bad results.[26] The most articulate condemnation of cricothyroidotomy was published by Mitchell in 1979.[27] In his article he reviewed the objections raised by Jackson but, unfortunately, added no new data. At present, all objective data that have been published support the finding that when cricothyroidotomy is used as described in the 1976 article, the procedure is generally safe.

In reviewing the controversy surrounding this procedure, the editors of *Selected Readings in General Surgery* concluded that

Routine use of cricothyroidotomy is a controversial issue. Brantigan and Grow's series is admirable because of its low complication rate, which is probably at least partially due to the authors' expertise. Whether or not cricothyroidotomy should be routinely performed for upper airway management is uncertain. . . . In the opinion of the Editors of *Selected Readings*, the best information about cricothyroidotomy is that from Brantigan and Grow. It would seem that if the procedure is done "carefully," as outlined by these authors, that a low complication rate should be expected. However, if the cricothyroidotomy is performed under emergency conditions and damage to the cartilaginous structures is suspected, then it would seem prudent to convert that cricothyroidotomy to a standard tracheostomy. The key issue is the avoidance of injury to the cricoid or thyroid cartilages.[28]

Anatomy

Except in cases of tumor, inflammation, or trauma, the airway is generally located in the midline of the neck. Before a tracheotomy of any type is performed, the location of the airway must be determined with certainty. The larynx is a series of cartilages adapted for phonation that cap the trachea and the esophagus. The laryngeal framework is made up of the thyroid cartilage and the cricoid cartilage. The shield-like thyroid cartilage is the prominent "Adam's apple" that is often seen in men. At the superior aspect of the shield is a prominent notch that is easily palpable through the skin. *This notch is the only reliable landmark in the neck.* Attempting to find the thyroid cartilage in women or in people with short, fat

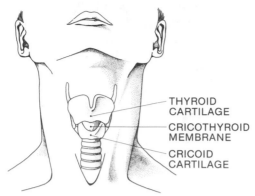

THYROID
CARTILAGE

CRICOTHYROID
MEMBRANE

CRICOID
CARTILAGE

Figure 7–1. Basic anatomy. Note that the notch of the thyroid cartilage is the most consistently identifiable structure in the neck.

necks is difficult if this notch is not sought, because the hyoid bone or the cricoid cartilage may easily be misidentified as the thyroid cartilage with disastrous surgical results. Once the thyroid cartilage is identified, the airway is followed caudally by palpation until the first complete ring is found. This is the cricoid ring, the only circumferential ring in the airway. This cartilage is shaped like a high school class ring with the shield located posteriorly. The membrane connecting the cartilages is the cricothyroid membrane (Fig. 7–1).

The cricothyroid membrane covers a space that is roughly trapezoidal in shape. This membrane is larger than is commonly believed. In a study of 51 adult larynges, Caparosa and Zavatsky[10] found that the distance between the lower border of the thyroid cartilage and the upper border of the cricoid cartilage ranged from 0.5 cm to 1.2 cm, with the average being 0.9 cm. The usable width of the cricothyroid space varied from 2.7 to 3.2 cm with the mean being 3 cm. The distance between the true cords and the midhorizontal plane of the cricothyroid space averaged 1.3 cm. Safar and Penninckx confirmed these measurements in a study of an additional 20 cadaver larynges.[29] The lumen of the airway through the cricoid ring is the narrowest portion of the airway in an adult, but it must be remembered that endotracheal tubes pass through this narrow area nicely. The membrane and the lumen of the airway at this point are clearly large enough to accommodate a standard tracheotomy tube without interference with the vocal cords. In fact, there is generally enough clearance to enable patients to speak around cricothyroidotomy tubes if they are given the opportunity.

The space between the skin and the cricothyroid membrane is remarkably devoid of other structures. There are no major nerves or vessels in the area. The thyroid gland is generally lower, and even the vascular anomalies that occasionally cause a major artery to cross the midline of the neck are almost invariably located lower in the

neck. Superficial veins are sometimes seen in this area and should be looked for. The cricothyroid artery, a branch of the superior thyroid artery, passes across the cricothyroid membrane to anastomose with its fellow on the other side. This artery has not proved clinically significant in the performance of cricothyroidotomy.

Indications

Cricothyroidotomy is seldom indicated as an emergency procedure in the hospital setting. Endotracheal intubation using nasotracheal or orotracheal technique is always preferable. Once control of the airway has been obtained by intubation, the emergency is over, and cricothyroidotomy can be carried out electively as needed. Emergency cricothyroidotomy should be reserved for patients in whom such intubation cannot be safely accomplished. Patients falling into this category include those thought to have unstable neck fractures and patients with massive facial trauma or acute laryngeal obstruction by cancer, Ludwig's angina, acute epiglottitis, peritonsillar abscess, or laryngeal trauma. Patients developing airway obstruction outside the hospital where endotracheal tubes are not available may be candidates for the procedure as well. Although acute inflammatory conditions of the larynx are relative contraindications to cricothyroidotomy, it is better to have a live patient with a complication than a patient who died from lack of an airway.

The use of cricothyroidotomy in children has never been adequately investigated. Since the major studies of the technique have included few children, the long-term effects of such procedures on the developing airway are unknown. Tracheotomy or cricothyrodotomy in the small child is clearly more formidable than in the adult, since the important structures in the neck are more easily confused. Because of the technical difficulties in performing cricothyroidotomy in an infant or a child, the procedure should be attempted only under clearly life-threatening circumstances. The immediate risk of emergency cricothyroidotomy is still substantially less than that of emergency tracheotomy, and for this reason alone, cricothyroidotomy should be elected when control of the airway cannot be achieved by endotracheal intubation. Decisions concerning converting to standard tracheotomy or leaving the cricothyroidotomy tube in place can then be made electively after due consideration of the patient's clinical situation.

Equipment

The equipment used in the performance of cricothyroidotomy varies with the circumstances under which the procedure is undertaken. In an emergency situation outside the hospital, the physician must use whatever is available. Some sort of sharp instrument is necessary (even a kitchen knife will do), as is any sort of hollow tube to keep the new airway open. In a pinch, the kitchen knife can be wedged sideways into the cricothyroidostomy incision, spreading the cartilages and thus keeping the orifice open.

If the physician is more fortunate, a tracheotome may be available. Many tracheotomes have been manufactured to allow such operations under adverse circumstances, but the devices are seldom available when needed. The physician who is not familiar with the tracheotome at hand, however, will probably do better with a kitchen knife.

In the emergency department, a set of instruments should be immediately available at all times for performance of this operation. The basic equipment that should be included in such a set of instruments is listed in Table 7–2. The use of a tracheotome in the emergency department is a matter of individual preference. To many physicians, the tracheotome represents an attempt to substitute a clever device for knowledge of a procedure and clinical judgment. It should be remembered that a tracheotome, no matter how foolproof its design, can be an instrument of disaster if used improperly. As Jackson pointed out, some of the incisions made in the course of tracheotomy carry the same mortality as similar incisions made with homicidal intent.[7]

Technique

Before undertaking cricothyroidotomy, the physician should review Jackson's principles. *The best possible airway control must be obtained before starting.* The time taken to ensure an airway is time well spent. Simple expedients, such as having an assistant maintain an open airway using the manuevers described in Chapter 1, may improve the situation considerably. In an emergency situation, sedation and general anesthesia are contraindicated, and there may not be enough time even for local anesthesia. Endotracheal intubation is ideal, but if such intubation could be accomplished, emer-

Table 7–2. REQUIRED INSTRUMENTS FOR CRICOTHYROIDOTOMY

Tracheotomy tube
Two-blade Trousseau dilator
Curved Mayo scissors
Two curved hemostats
Scalpel with number 11 blade
Two 10-ml syringes
22 gauge needle
25 gauge needle
Suction apparatus
Gauze pads

gency tracheotomy would not be necessary. *All equipment must be present and organized.* Even though this equipment may be just a knife and the barrel of a pen, the operator must have a clear idea of how the operation will be accomplished with the equipment available. *The operation must be precise.* Even if the operation is performed under battlefield conditions, it must be undertaken with deliberation and precision to ensure success and to minimize permanent laryngeal damage.

Attentive postoperative care is critical. The operator should know what will be done with the patient after the operation is accomplished. In the prehospital setting, one of the spectators should be arranging transport; in the hospital, a ventilator should be on the way. Significant morbidity will be avoided if the operator thinks through these principles before starting.

CRICOTHYROIDOTOMY USING THE TOYE TRACHEOTOME

The main problem with the tracheotome is that it can be easily introduced into the wrong structure. On occasion, the aorta has been cannulated with a tracheotome, and the results have been undesirable. The Toye tracheotome is but one of many such devices available for the performance of emergency tracheotomy (Fig. 7–2).[30] The tracheotome consists of five pieces: a 16 gauge needle, which fits inside a winged, slotted 13 gauge needle; thin polyethylene tubing reinforced with a guide wire, which in turn is fixed to a handled introducer; and a 5 mm metal tracheotomy tube or a 5-mm cuffed plastic tracheotomy tube, which fits onto the introducer. The device is available as a disposable or a reusable kit.*

The patient is positioned with the neck extended as much as possible without further compromise of the airway. The skin is prepared with an antiseptic solution and draped as the circumstances allow. If anesthesia is practical, the skin is anesthesized. The landmarks in the neck are identified. One hand is used to stabilize the thyroid cartilage; the other hand is used to insert the needle through the cricothyroid membrane at a 45-degree angle so that the needle passes cleanly down the trachea. If the patient is breathing, there should be an egress of air at this point. The thin polyethylene tube attached to the introducer is then passed through the needle and into the airway. The tubing must advance freely before one proceeds to the next step. One then removes the needle, allowing the tubing that passed through the slot in the needle to remain in the airway. The tubing, with its enclosed guide wire, is passed into the

---

*A video tape demonstrating this device is available from Pertrach Company, Long Beach, California.

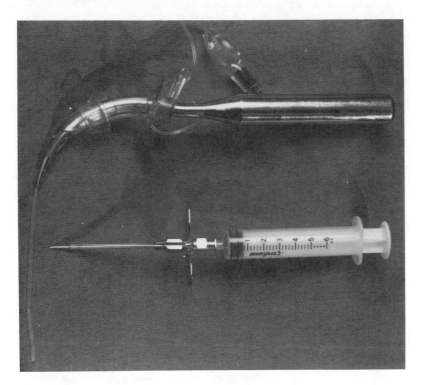

Figure 7–2. Emergency percutaneous Toye tracheotome. (Courtesy of Pertrach Company, Long Beach, California.)

airway, and the introducer is advanced following the guide wire. The introducer dilates the opening to allow passage of the tracheotomy tube that rides on its shaft. A small recessed knife blade cuts tissue under tension but is sufficiently recessed to prevent unnecessary tissue damage. After the whole assembly has been introduced, the tracheotomy tube is left in place while the introducer is withdrawn. The tube is firmly held in place until secured with tapes.

CRICOTHYROIDOTOMY USING SURGICAL INSTRUMENTS

A standard low-pressure, cuffed tracheotomy tube is selected (Lanz, Shiley, American). The tube should be the same size as the endotracheal tube that would be selected for the same patient. If the operator is in doubt, a tube with a 7-mm internal diameter, although small, should be large enough for most adults and will pass with ease. The cuff should be tested and then completely deflated to allow easy passage. Tapes should be attached so that they will be ready to secure the tube as soon as the procedure is completed. If a standard tracheostomy tube is not available, an endotracheal tube will temporarily suffice.

The patient is positioned with the neck extended as much as possible without causing further airway compromise. It is important to maintain extension throughout the procedure. The skin is prepared with an antiseptic solution and is draped with surgical drapes as circumstances allow. If there is time, the skin is injected with local anesthetic. The thyroid cartilage should first be identified by its notch (see Fig. 7–1). The thyroid cartilage is then stabilized with one hand. The other hand is used to introduce the scalpel with a number 11 blade *transversely* through the cricothyroid membrane (Fig. 7–3). One should be sure that the scalpel blade is *transverse* to the longitudinal axis of the neck and that only a stab incision perpendicular to the skin is made. No further skin incision is required or desirable.* The knife is

---

Editor's note: A recent study[41] has suggested that in an emergency when landmarks may be difficult to identify, a *2- to 3-cm longitudinal* **skin** incision may help identify the cricothyroid space and may facilitate the subsequent *transverse* **stab** incision of the membrane. Under no circumstances should a horizontal skin incision be made in the neck!

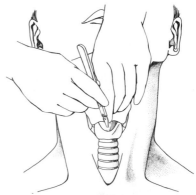

Figure 7–3. A transverse stab incision is made into the cricothyroid membrane.

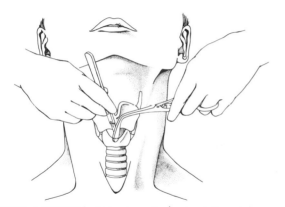

Figure 7–4. With the knife in place, the tracheal dilator is inserted.

inserted transversely to avoid possible damage to the laryngeal cartilages. It is essential that no attempt be made to enlarge the hole with the knife, since this will just cause bleeding. If an endotracheal tube is in place, the operator will be heartened by the feel of the knife blade impacting on the tube. If there is no tube in place, the blade will meet no resistance. The blade should not be removed at this point. Care should be taken to avoid injuring the posterior trachea during the stab incision, although the wide posterior cricoid cartilage offers some degree of safety.

With the knife blade in place, one introduces a two-bladed Trousseau tracheal dilator into the airway by sliding it down the blade (Fig. 7–4). The blades of the dilator are kept parallel to the transversely held knife. Although a standard spreader will work well, the procedure is facilitated if the blades have been flattened before use. The knife blade is then removed, and the spreader is gently but forcefully spread to enlarge the hole in a vertical direction. The goal here is to separate the cartilages rather than to fracture them. A pair of Mayo scissors is then used to enlarge the hole in

the transverse plane (Fig. 7–5). The opening is dilated in both directions until it is large enough to accept the tracheotomy tube. At this point the surgeon should be able to see the tracheal mucosa and air movement if the patient is breathing. Suction may be helpful in removing secretions at this point. After the mucosa is visualized, the dilator is rotated so that the blades point toward the lungs (blades parallel to the trachea). A gentle lifting force is applied to straighten out the airway, and the tracheotomy tube, with the obturator in place, is inserted between the blades (Fig. 7–6). The obturator is quickly removed when the tube is in place. The presence of a free airway is ascertained either by the observation of air motion through the tube or by the free passage of a suction catheter into the bronchial tree. The tracheotomy tube is then held firmly until it is securely tied in place.

Attempts at hemostasis using clamps or cautery are seldom necessary when this procedure is undertaken. Since tissue is stretched more than cut, its elastic nature tends to tamponade bleeders against the tube. It goes without saying that it is the responsibility of the surgeon to remain in constant attendance until the patient's airway is clear of secretions and blood and until the airway has stabilized.

Complications

Cricothyroidotomy is associated with many of the same complications that occur with standard tracheotomy. Although complication rates with cricothyroidotomy, as with any surgical procedure, are largely a function of the experience and skill of the surgeon, it appears that the overall complication rate is lower for cricothyroidotomy than for other techniques. Table 7–3 lists the complication rates for some of the larger series in which tracheotomy and cricothyroidotomy were performed. It should be noted that this table includes complications of cricothyroidotomy per-

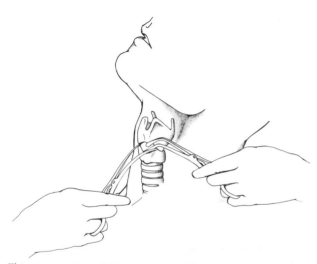

Figure 7–5. Mayo scissors are used to enlarge the hole in a transverse plane.

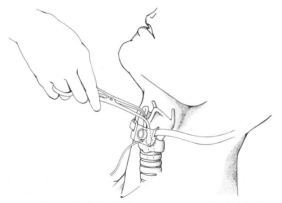

Figure 7–6. When the tube is in place, the dilator is withdrawn.

Table 7–3. RATE OF COMPLICATIONS

Study	Number of Patients	Complica-tion Rate
Skaggs and Cogbill, 1969[31] Tracheotomy	389	66%
Head, 1961[32] Tracheotomy	462	41%
Arola, 1981[33] Tracheotomy	794	71%
Brantigan and Grow, 1976[12] Cricothyroidotomy	655	6.1%
Greisz et al., 1982[20] Cricothyroidotomy	61	8%
Boyd et al., 1979[15] Cricrothyroidotomy	147	8.6%

formed under both elective and emergent conditions and may not reflect the complication rate of the procedure when it is performed in a true emergency, such as in cardiac arrest.

Complications shared by tracheotomy and cricothyroidotomy include acute airway obstruction, infection, and tracheoesophageal fistula. Acute airway obstruction is most commonly produced by a mucous plug. Since the plug may cause a one-way valve effect, when it occurs the entire tube may have to be changed. Acute airway obstruction may be produced by overinflation of the balloon in such a way that it herniates over the tip of the tube. The tracheotomy tube may be passed into a subcutaneous plane instead of into the trachea either during insertion or, more commonly, during a tube change. This form of acute airway obstruction occurs more frequently after standard tracheotomy, particularly if the tube becomes dislodged in the immediate postoperative period before a clear tract becomes established. In the standard tracheotomy, the hole is comparatively deep and is difficult to cannulate.

Essentially all indwelling endotracheal tubes and tracheotomy tubes become colonized by bacteria regardless of the precautions that are taken. Such colonization can lead to frank infection either of the tracheobronchial tree or of the tissues of the neck itself. The pressure of the tracheotomy cuff against the walls of the trachea, and particularly against a nasogastric tube, can lead to the formation of a tracheoesophageal fistula. Bacterial colonization compounds the risk. The consequences may be devastating.

Some of the more uncommon complications of standard tracheotomy are not found with cricothyroidotomy, primarily for anatomic reasons. Pneumothorax has never been reported with cricothyroidotomy, because the higher and more superficial position of the incision avoids the cupulas of the lungs. Major vessel hemorrhage has never been reported, since the incision and the eventual location of the cuff and the tip of the cannula are safely away from the innominate artery, the most common vessel of origin of such a hemorrhage. Acute tracheoesophageal fistula occurring during performance of the operation is prevented in cricothyroidotomy, because the esophagus is protected by the posterior flaring of the cricoid ring. Cardiac arrest during performance of tracheotomy is generally a result of hypoxia rather than of vagal reaction. Hypoxia is caused by the time required to perform the procedure. Since cricothyroidotomy is one of the fastest and most reliable ways of gaining airway control, hypoxic arrest should be much less common with this procedure.

Some complications, although shared by both procedures, merit individual consideration. These include operative bleeding and airway stenosis.

Since there are no major vessels (either arteries or veins) overlying the cricothyroid membrane, the incidence of significant operative hemorrhage is lower with cricothyroidotomy than with standard tracheotomy. Superficial veins are often seen in the area of skin puncture, however. The incision should be made in such a way as to avoid the superficial veins, or, if necessary, they can be secured above and below the planned incision by suture ligature before the stab incision is made. Much has been made in individual case reports of the possibility of inadvertent puncture of the cricothyroid artery, because its branches course across the membrane to anastomose with those of its fellow.[34] Although bleeding from this vessel can be bothersome, it caused no problems in the 655 elective patients described in the 1976 article and has been encountered by the author on only one occasion. It should be remembered that in all cases of post-tracheotomy hemorrhage, if the tracheotomy tube is in place and the cuff is inflated, the airway is protected. With the airway protected, the bleeding vessel can be sought in a leisurely fashion, or the bleeding can be controlled by pressure until more help arrives. The deaths attributed to tracheotomy bleeding, even from a major artery, have occurred not from blood loss but from obstruction of the airway by blood.[35]

Airway stenosis is the occasional consequence of any form of intubation of the airway. By choosing the form of intubation, the physician selects the location of possible development of stenosis. Orotracheal and nasotracheal intubation uniformly produce laryngeal damage at the site of the balloon cuff. Although the significance of the injury produced has been hotly debated, several facts have emerged from the discussions. Endotracheal intubation is currently the most common cause of chronic subglottic stenosis.[36] In addition, the mucosal injuries produced by these tubes are consistently infected. Airway stenosis produced by standard tracheotomy and cricothyroidotomy is usually a tracheal stenosis located at the cuff site.

This lesion following standard tracheotomy is located fairly distally in the trachea and may be difficult to reach for repair. The mucosal injury produced by the balloon cuff and the point of entrance of the tube into the trachea are both uniformly colonized by bacteria. When the space between mucosal injuries caused by an endotracheal tube and the subsequent tracheotomy becomes infected as well, the resulting stenosis is even more difficult.[37] Prolonged endotracheal intubation followed by tracheotomy of any type carries a higher rate of airway stenosis than does either procedure alone.[38]

Chronic subglottic stenosis is a dreaded complication with no entirely satisfactory solutions. Since the time of Jackson, the concern that this problem will develop has prevented wider use of cricothyroidotomy. Yet this complication has not occurred in any of the reported series involving cricothyroidotomy. The four differences between Jackson's series and more current series have been discussed previously. Although all four factors are important, the most important has to do with the disease leading to tracheotomy. In all of Jackson's patients, acute inflammatory conditions of the larynx produced stenosis. Brantigan and Grow[39] studied ten patients who developed chronic subglottic stenosis after cricothyroidotomy, and in all cases the procedures were performed in the face of an acute laryngeal pathologic condition. Except in a dire emergency, an acute infectious laryngeal condition must be considered a contraindication to cricothyroidotomy. Cricothyroidotomy under these circumstances should probably be converted to standard tracheotomy as soon as practical so that the incision has a chance to heal before becoming colonized.

Although gunshot wounds to the pharynx and fractures of the larynx are obvious sources of laryngeal damage, a more subtle and important source of such damage is the endotracheal tube. Laryngoscopy should be carried out in patients who have been intubated more than 48 to 72 hours before cricothyroidotomy. If laryngeal damage is found, standard tracheotomy is preferred. I have seen one patient develop chronic subglottic stenosis under these circumstances following standard tracheotomy.

The subglottic space or the area of a standard tracheotomy can become acutely obstructed, most commonly by granulation tissue. The proper management of such granulation tissue has not been defined. Tracheotomy stomas and cuff injuries heal by formation of granulation tissue followed by re-epithelialization. Only when the granulations significantly narrow the airway do they become a problem. It appears, however, that when extensive granulation occurs, a vigorous surgical approach will minimize the incidence of chronic airway stenosis.

The importance of intraluminal granulation tissue as a prodrome to the development of chronic airway stenosis was recognized as early as 1886, when C. J. Colles[3] recommended that such tissue, when encountered, be removed. Since that time, his opinion has been confirmed by Hawkins and associates,[40] who successfully maintained an airway in 16 of 20 patients who experienced subglottic stenosis after endotracheal intubation. Their protocol included antibiotics, steroids, and dilations of obstructions. Endoscopic resection of granulations using the laser is a particularly promising approach to this problem. In reviewing their experience, Hawkins and coworkers reported, "The earlier we started endoscopic treatment and the more persistent we were, the earlier we were able to remove the tracheostomy." Although acute obstruction of the airway by granulation tissue is an uncommon complication of cricothyroidotomy, Brantigan and Grow's[39] review of seven such cases confirmed the value of aggressive management.

The Emergency Medicine Experience

Although it would be highly desirable to perform cricothyroidotomy under an elective or semiurgent controlled situation in the operating suite and under the guidance of an experienced surgeon, the definition of emergency care implies that the procedure will be performed, on occasion, under adverse circumstances and by less experienced physicians. Although it has been stated that the procedure can be easily performed in less than 2 minutes, even the easiest surgical procedure can quickly become complicated. Equipment may become difficult to locate and well-known anatomy may become difficult to identify in the excitement of the moment.

The majority of cases reported in the surgical literature consist of elective or semi-urgent situations. Many of the patients in these studies had a controlled airway prior to cricothyroidotomy. At present there is a shortage of hard data to evaluate the procedure in a clinical setting that is less than ideal and involves patients with a number of concurrent life-threatening insults. McGill and coworkers[41] reported the results of 38 truly emergent cricothyroidotomy procedures that were performed by house staff in the emergency department. Twenty-six of the 38 patients were trauma victims requiring airway support, and 13 patients were in cardiac arrest. Only 12 of 38 patients lived to be discharged, underscoring the seriousness of the clinical condition. McGill and coworkers' complication rate for cricothyroidotomy was almost 40 per cent. The tracheostomy tube was incorrectly placed in five patients, with the tube being misplaced superior to the thyroid cartilage in four of the five cases. Other complications included prolonged procedure, unsuccessful tracheal cannulation, and hemorrhage.

Conclusions

The ultimate role of cricothyroidotomy in the surgical repertoire is yet to be clearly defined. Although all of the reported series to date have documented that the procedure is safe and comparatively free of complications, many physicians still fear the possibility of subglottic stenosis to such a degree that they would never use the procedure electively. It is clear, however, that the elective use of this procedure in the presence of an acute laryngeal pathologic condition is, as one would expect, associated with an unacceptable incidence of subglottic stenosis.

In contradistinction to the elective use of this operation, the value of its use in the emergency situation is well established. Cricothyroidotomy should be reserved for patients who cannot or should not be intubated with an endotracheal tube. Even though a misdirected surgical approach to the airway can instantly turn a would-be lifesaver into an assassin by producing an irretrievable complication, cricothyroidotomy can be safely used by physicians with little training to gain control of a patient's airway rapidly and safely. If the procedure is performed carefully and in a controlled fashion, there is no need to convert it to a standard tracheotomy.

1. Bouga, T. P., and Cook, C. B.: Pressure flow characteristics of needles suggested for transtracheal resuscitation. N. Engl. J. Med. 262:511, 1960.
2. Jackson, C.: High tracheotomy and other errors the chief causes of chronic laryngeal stenosis. Surg. Gynecol. Obstet. 32:392, 1921.
3. Colles, C. J.: On stenosis of the trachea after tracheotomy for croup and diphtheria. Ann. Surg. 3:499, 1886.
4. Upham, J. B.: Report of a case of incised wound of the throat resulting in closure of the larynx by cicatrix. New Hampshire J. Med. 2:206, 1852.
5. Marx, R.: A medical profile of George Washington. American Heritage, Aug: 43, 1955.
6. Hupp, F. L.: Tracheotomy: A new retractor and tube pilot for the emergency operation. Surg. Gynecol. Obstet. 19:671, 1914.
7. Jackson, C.: Tracheotomy. Laryngoscope 18:285, 1909.
8. Jackson, C., and Jackson C. L.: Surgery of the larynx, trachea, and endoscopic surgery of the bronchi. In Southwick, H. W. (ed.): Lewis Practice of Surgery, Vol. 4. New York, Harper & Row, 1974.
9. Nelson, T. G.: Tracheotomy: Clinical and experimental study. Am. Surg. 23:660, 1957.
10. Caparosa, R. J., and Zavatsky, A. R.: Practical aspects of the cricothyroid space. Laryngoscope 47:577, 1957.
11. Nicholas, T. H., and Rumer, G. F.: Emergency airway—a plan of action. JAMA 174:1930, 1960.

12. Brantigan, C. O., and Grow, J. B., Sr.: Cricothyroidotomy: Elective use in respiratory problems requiring tracheotomy. J. Thorac. Cardiovasc. Surg. 71:72, 1976.
13. Romita, M. C., et al.: Cricothyroidotomy—its healing and complications. Surg. Forum 28:175, 1977.
14. Boyd, A. D., and Conlan, A. A.: Emergency cricothyroidotomy: Is its use justified? Surg. Rounds 12:19, 1979.
15. Boyd, A. D., et al.: A clinical evaluation of cricothyroidotomy. Surg. Gynecol. Obstet. 149:365, 1979.
16. Habel, D. W.: Cricothyroidotomy as a site for elective tracheotomy. Trans. Pac. Coast Otoophthalmol. Soc. Annu. Meet. 58:181, 1977.
17. Koopman, C. F., et al.: Effects of antibiotics and injury of cricoid cartilage in cricothyreotomy. Surg. Forum 30:507, 1979.
18. Koopman, C. F., et al.: The effect of cricoid cartilage injury and antibiotics in cricothyroidotomy. Am. J. Otol. 2:123, 1981.
19. Morain, W. D.: Cricothyroidostomy in head and neck surgery. Plast. Reconstr. Surg. 65:425, 1980.
20. Greisz, H., et al.: Elective cricothyroidotomy: A clinical and histopathologic study. Crit. Care Med. 10:387, 1982.
21. Schechter, W. P., and Wilson, R. S.: Management of upper airway obstruction in the intensive care unit. Crit. Care Med. 9:577, 1981.
22. Kress, T. K., and Balasubramaniam, S.: Cricothyroidotomy. Ann. Emerg. Med. 11:197, 1982.
23. Orringer, M. B.: Endotrachial intubation and tracheostomy indications, techniques, and complications. Surg. Clin. North Am. 60:1447, 1980.
24. Kennedy, T. L.: Epiglottic reconstruction of laryngeal stenosis secondary to cricothyroidostomy. Laryngoscope 90:1130, 1980.
25. Brantigan, C. O.: Cricothyroidotomy—letter to the editor. Laryngoscope 90:1898, 1980.
26. Montagano, J., and Passy, V.: Letter to the editor. Plast. Reconstr. Surg. 67:98, 1981.
27. Mitchell, S. A.: Cricothyroidostomy revisited. Ear Nose Throat J. 58:54, 1979.
28. Selected Readings in General Surgery 9:34, 1982.
29. Safar, P., and Penninckx, J.: Cricothyroid membrane puncture with a special cannula. Anesthesiology 28:943, 1967.
30. Toye, F. J., and Weinstein, J. D.: A percutaneous tracheostomy device. Surgery 65:384, 1969.
31. Skaggs, J. A., and Cogbill, C. L.: Tracheostomy: Management, mortality, complications. Am. Surg. 35:293, 1969.
32. Head, J. M.: Tracheostomy in the management of respiratory problems. N. Engl. J. Med. 264:587, 1961.
33. Arola, M. K.: Tracheostomy and its complications—a retrospective study of 794 tracheostomized patients. Ann. Chir. Gynaecol. 70:96, 1981.
34. Schillaci, R. F., et al.: Transtracheal aspiration complicated by fatal endotracheal hemorrhage. N. Engl. J. Med. 95:488, 1976.
35. Brantigan, C. O.: Delayed major vessel hemorrhage following tracheostomy. J. Trauma 13:235, 1973.
36. Wong, M. L., et al.: Vascularized hyoid interposition for subglottic and upper tracheal stenosis. Ann. Otol. 87:491, 1978.
37. Sasaki, C. T., et al.: Tracheotomy related subglottic stenosis: Bacteriologic pathogenesis. Laryngoscope 89:857, 1979.
38. McGovern, F. H., et al.: The hazards of endotracheal intubation. Ann. Surg. 80:556, 1971.
39. Brantigan, C. O., and Grow, J. B., Sr.: Subglottic stenosis after cricothyroidotomy. Surgery 91:217, 1982.
40. Hawkins, D. B.: Glottic and subglottic stenosis from endotracheal intubation. Laryngoscope 87:339, 1977.
41. McGill, J., Clinton, J. W., and Ruiz, E.: Cricothyrotomy in the emergency department. Ann. Emerg. Med. 11:361, 1982.

Introduction

Historically, tracheotomies have been performed since ancient times. The exact origin, though often attributed to Hippocrates, is uncertain. Throughout modern medicine, tracheotomy has proved to be a lifesaving operation. It is primarily indicated to relieve upper airway obstruction, to provide mechanical access to the trachea and lower airway for respiratory assistance, and to assist with lower respiratory toilet. Appelbaum has categorized the conditions that may require tracheotomy into skeletal, neuromuscular, central nervous system, upper respiratory tract, pulmonary, and cardiovascular.[1]

Care of the tracheotomy begins prior to the surgical procedure. Judgments made by the operative surgeon prior to surgery significantly contribute to the ease or difficulty of tracheotomy care. The position and size of the incision, the amount of deep dissection, and the method of entering the trachea itself may either increase or decrease the extent of direct wound care required. The size and type of tracheotomy tube used, as well as the method of its attachment to the neck, are also significant factors.

Tracheotomy tubes are made of many materials, including metal, Silastic, Teflon, polyethylene, and rubber. They may be cuffed or uncuffed (Fig. 8–1). They may have a single lumen or an inner cannula (Fig. 8–2). It is important that the emergency physician recognize these factors; however, the basic care of the tracheotomy itself is relatively independent of the type of tube used.

The key to optimal care is cleanliness.

Immediate Postoperative Care

In the immediate postoperative period, high humidity must be provided. Humidity may be provided through a neck collar attached to a nebulizer or vaporizer or through a controlled environment, such as in a tent or steam room. *High humidity* is critical in maintaining liquefaction of the patient's mucus for adequate suctioning.

Suctioning of the tracheotomy tube should be done routinely, approximately every 1 to 2 hours in the immediate postoperative period, but is gradually reduced according to each patient's needs. When suctioning, relatively sterile techniques should be used. The suction catheter should be introduced into the tracheotomy lumen by a gloved hand.

The size of the catheter used is dictated by the size of the tracheotomy tube; the largest size that can be passed without difficulty is best. When the catheter has been introduced into the trachea itself (it need not be introduced further), suction is

8

Tracheotomy Care

ROBERT L. KATZ, M.D.

applied and the catheter is slowly removed, aspirating the produced mucus (Fig. 8–3). When the catheter touches the tracheal mucosa, coughing may result. Unless excessive, coughing is desirable, because it not only brings mucus into the trachea for aspiration but also expands the distal alveoli, which may collapse in the absence of laryngeal resistance. Excessive stimulation, however, may abuse the tracheal mucosa as the catheter rubs against the tracheal wall during the coughing effort. Coughing can be suppressed by the instillation of a topical mucosal anesthetic. The suctioning should be repeated until the trachea has been cleared of secretions and as often as necessary to keep the airway clear. Prolonged suctioning may produce significant hypoxia, and short periods of suctioning (5 to 8 seconds) with oxygen supplementation in between are preferred.

In the infant with limited respiratory reserve, active support of respiration by Ambu bag or mechanical ventilator with supplemental oxygen is encouraged, particularly prior to and between suctioning efforts. Mucus plugs can often be softened for aspiration by the instillation of saline or acetylcysteine (Mucomyst) drops instilled prior to suctioning.

The neck wound should be kept clean with hydrogen peroxide as needed. Antibiotic ointments can also be used.

During the first 24 to 48 hours following tracheotomy, careful and constant observation is required. It is during this period of time that the tracheotomy tube can most easily become dislodged, or malpositioned. Early recognition of these abnormalities may be lifesaving to the patient. Cardiac and respiratory monitors should be used, and constant, attentive nursing care is mandatory.

Changing a Tracheotomy Tube

When long-term tracheotomy care is required, the previously discussed philosophies hold true but are modified according to need. The degree of humidity required gradually lessens. Suctioning,

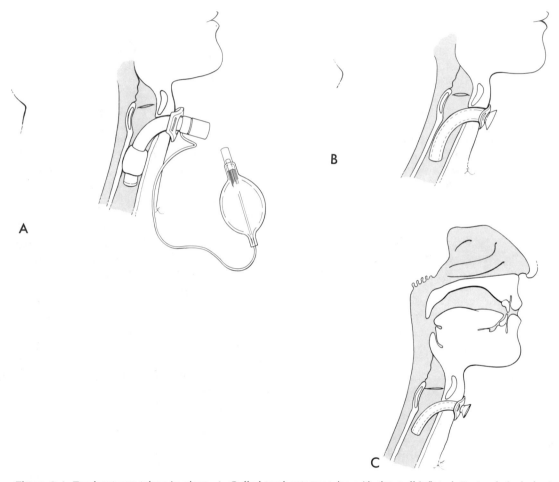

Figure 8–1. Tracheotomy tubes in place. *A*, Cuffed tracheotomy tube with the cuff inflated. *B*, A relatively large uncuffed tube. *C*, This smaller uncuffed tracheotomy tube permits the passage of air up through the vocal cords. If, during expiration, the patient's finger is placed over the tube, all expired air will pass through the vocal cords, permitting vocalization. (From Alperin, K., Levine, H., and Grover, M.: Tracheostomy Care Manual. New York, Thieme-Stratton Inc., 1982. Used by permission.)

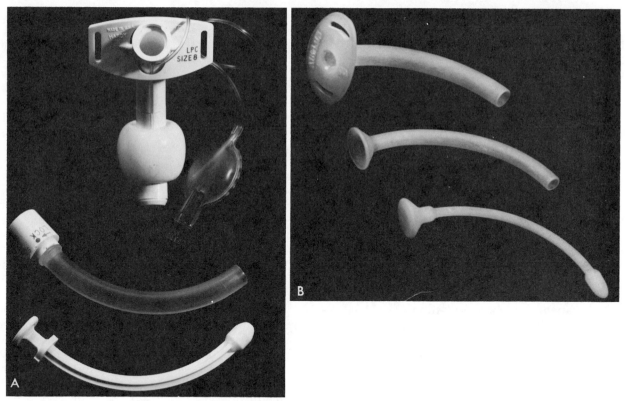

Figure 8–2. Cuffed tracheotomy tube with the cuff inflated. The tube has a translucent plastic inner cannula that can be removed for cleaning. An obturator, which is used only during insertion of the tracheotomy tube, is also illustrated. *B*, A plastic uncuffed tracheotomy tube with inner cannula and obturator. Some uncuffed tracheotomy tubes such as those designed by Jackson are made of metal. (From Alperin, K., Levine, H., and Grover, M.: Tracheostomy Care Manual. New York, Thieme-Stratton Inc., 1982. Used by permission.)

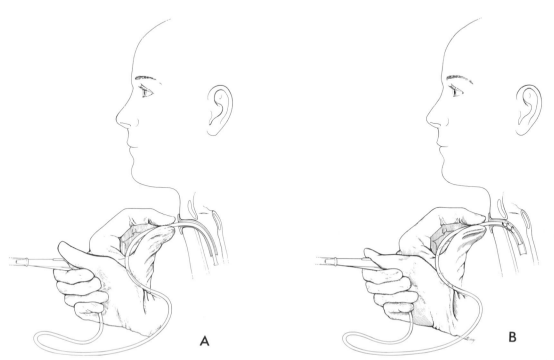

Figure 8–3. Suctioning of a tracheotomy tube is carried out as an aid to removal of secretions or is done in an emergency setting to evaluate the patency of a tracheotomy tube. *A*, The suction catheter is inserted only a short distance past the end of the tracheotomy tube. The thumb is kept off the hole in the suction catheter during placement. Suction is applied only during withdrawal. *B*, The suction catheter can be twisted during removal. (From Alperin, K., Levine, M., and Grover, M.: Tracheostomy Care Manual. New York, Thieme-Stratton Inc., 1982. Used by permission.) Short periods of suctioning (5 to 8 seconds) with respiratory support and supplemental oxygen are necessary in infants and hypoxic adults.

135

though needed periodically, is often replaced by an effective cough, and long-term monitoring is rarely required except in children.

Once the tracheotomy wound has matured, generally at about 5 days, routine changing of the tracheotomy tubes (see Figure 8–4) can be carried out safely and *must* be done in order to clean them satisfactorily. Prior to changing the tracheotomy tube, the new tube should be carefully checked. One must be certain that all component parts fit together comfortably and that if a cuffed tube is being used, the integrity of the cuff under pressure is checked. Once this has been accomplished, the patient is placed in a controlled, comfortable position with his *neck hyperextended,* when possible. Adults may sit or lie down; however, children should be lying down and held firmly in the controlled position.

The patient's tracheotomy tube should be removed in a single sweeping motion, and the new tube, which has been readied with the obturator in position, should be gently and immediately inserted into the stoma with the same sweeping circular motion. This is most easily accomplished by wetting or slightly lubricating the tube and inserting it during inspiration. There should be no force exerted, because creating false passages may prove to be disastrous.

Once the tracheotomy tube is in position, the obturator is removed and the inner cannula (if needed) is placed. The tracheotomy tube should be tied snugly around the patient's neck while his head is held in flexion. The physician should be certain that the tape is in direct approximation to the skin all around the neck and that nothing is intervening that when removed would result in a loose tape and possible extubation. The tape should be tied with a square knot and double checked when it is in place. If an inner cannula is being used, it should be removed and cleaned, usually with hydrogen peroxide, pipe cleaners, and small wire brushes, as often as necessary to keep it mucus-free.

The entire tube should be changed approximately once a week, and the inner cannula should be cleaned twice daily. If the tubes need to be changed and cleaned more often, this should be done in order to keep them mucus-free and functioning optimally.

Obstructed Tracheotomy Tube

A tracheotomy patient who presents to the emergency physician with respiratory distress should be *assumed to have a plugged tracheotomy tube.* Such patients should immediately be placed on high-flow humidified oxygen, with the flow directed either at the tracheotomy tube or over the mouth, if appropriate. *The usual cause of obstruction is inspissated mucus,* which commonly occurs in the winter because of the low humidity of inspired air.

Immediate suctioning is appropriate in an attempt to clear the tracheotomy tube (see Fig. 8–3). If an inner cannula is present, it should be cleaned and obstructing plugs should be removed. If suctioning and removal of the inner cannula do not immediately clear the airway obstruction, the entire tracheotomy tube should be removed and replaced with a new tube. Hesitancy at total removal and changing of tubes may be a fatal mistake. In an emergency, *one should not hesitate to remove a tracheotomy tube,* because most patients are able to breathe easier through a stoma than through a partially blocked tube.

A tracheotomy patient may present with the tracheotomy tube in hand, stating that the tube came out, either during cleaning or coughing, and that he has been unable to replace the tube because the stoma was closing. It is appropriate to accept the patient's judgment that the tube will not fit. Forceful attempts to insert the tube may create false passages and traumatic edema, making reintubation almost impossible. The patient's tube should be inspected to identify its size, which can usually be found on the flange of the outer cannula. The sizes of tubes are designated by numbers progressing sequentially from 00 to 10, from smallest to largest. When the size of the patient's tube has been determined, a new tracheotomy tube one or two sizes smaller can generally be inserted with relative ease. *Care should be taken to avoid false passages.* The tube should be inserted with ease, not forced. Once the smaller tube has been inserted to maintain the trachea stoma, it may gradually be enlarged on a daily basis until the appropriate-sized maintenance tube can again be worn.

A stressful situation can develop when a blocked tracheotomy tube has been removed and the proper passage for easy insertion of a new tube cannot be found. Often, simple extension of the neck will line up tissue planes and facilitate passage. If time permits, it is safer and certainly less stressful for the inexperienced physician to insert a small red rubber catheter into the tracheotomy tube for a short distance down the trachea before the old tracheotomy tube is removed (Fig. 8–4). When the old tracheotomy tube is withdrawn, the catheter remains in the passage to serve as a guide for atraumatic insertion of a new tube. Once the new tube is in place, the catheter can be easily removed.

A flexible pediatric laryngoscope can, on occasion, be used to identify the lumen and the entrance into the trachea. In difficult situations, a tracheotomy tube can be introduced over the flex-

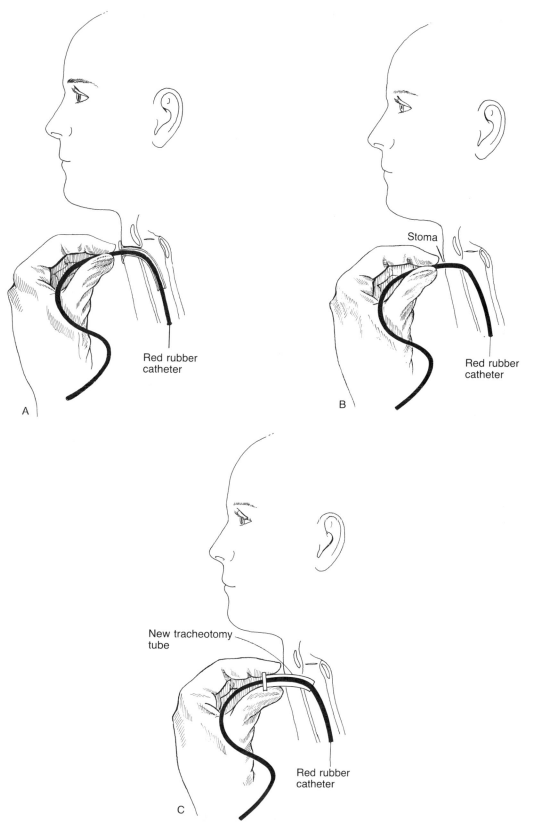

Red rubber
catheter

A

Stoma

Red rubber
catheter

B

New tracheotomy
tube

Red rubber
catheter

C

Figure 8–4. Changing a tracheotomy tube. *A,* Before the old tube is removed, a small red rubber catheter is passed into the proximal trachea. *B,* The tracheotomy tube has been removed, and only the rubber catheter remains in the trachea. The catheter serves as a guide for easy and atraumatic insertion of a new tube. Note that the neck should be slightly hyperextended. *C,* A new tracheotomy tube is threaded over the guide catheter; once the tube is in place, the catheter is removed.

ible laryngoscope. The appropriate-sized tracheotomy tube should be threaded over the laryngoscope prior to its insertion. The stenosed stoma should be carefully suctioned free of mucus. The laryngoscope can then be introduced into the stoma, and under direct observation, the tracheal lumen can be identified. Once the laryngoscope is comfortably in place within the trachea, the tracheotomy tube can be advanced over the laryngoscope, which functions as a lumen guide.

1. Applebaum, E. L., and Bruce, D. L.: Tracheal Intubation. Philadelphia, W. B. Saunders Company, 1976.
2. Alperin, K., Levine, H., and Grover, M.: Tracheostomy Care Manual. New York, Thieme-Stratton, Inc., 1982.

2

CARDIOLOGY

9

Carotid Sinus Massage

STEVEN GAZAK, M.D.

In 1961, Bernard Lown stated that "in recent years, insufficient attention has been given to the carotid sinus test."[1] This statement continues to apply to practice today. Generally speaking, carotid sinus massage (CSM) is either glossed over hastily or neglected entirely during the training of medical students and house officers alike.

The human cardiovascular system is richly supplied with specialized sensory nerve endings, known as baroreceptors, which autoregulate heart rate and blood pressure. The carotid sinus is part of this autoregulatory system, along with additional baroreceptors located at the level of the aortic arch, the atria, the ventricles, and the pulmonary veins. The carotid sinus, however, maintains a privileged position by virtue of its unique accessibility to external manipulation.

The word *carotid* is derived from the Greek *karos*, meaning deep sleep.[2] The soporific properties of carotid sinus stimulation have been exploited by warriors and physicians alike since antiquity. Carotid sinus massage (CSM) remains an important diagnostic and therapeutic maneuver in modern-day medicine because of its profound effects on the cardiovascular system. With practice and continual refinement of technique, it is a safe and potentially useful tool for any physician summoned regularly to evaluate patients with cardiac dysrhythmias.

Anatomy and Physiology

The bifurcation of the common carotid artery possesses an abundant supply of sensory nerve endings located within the adventitia of the vessel wall (Fig. 9–1). These nerves have a characteristic spiral configuration, continually intertwining along their course and eventually uniting to form the sinus nerve of Hering. This small nerve travels but a short distance before joining the glossopharyngeal nerve, which then terminates in the cardiac and vasomotor centers of the medulla.[3] This pathway constitutes the afferent loop of the carotid sinus circuit. The efferent loop, in turn, has two parts. The vagus nerve exits the dorsal motor nucleus of cranial nerves IX and X in the medulla to supply the sinus node and the atrioventricular (AV) node. In addition, there are sympathetic inhibitory fibers that leave the medullary vasoconstrictor center and travel, by way of the sympathetic chain, to supply the heart and the peripheral vasculature. Hering initially delineated these anatomic pathways in the 1920s.[1]

The afferent nerve endings located within the carotid sinus are sensitive to mean arterial pressure as well as the rate of change of pressure.[4] Generally speaking, pulsatile stimuli are more effective than sustained pressure in evoking a response.[1] Increasing stretch on the baroreceptors, which occurs in the presence of relative hypertension, leads to increased firing of the afferent nerve endings. The reverse occurs when pressures are low.[5] There is greater sensitivity in response to hypotensive states, a phenomenon that seems teleologically sound.[6]

Both the parasympathetic and the sympathetic nervous systems play a role in the carotid sinus reflex. Increased firing of the carotid sinus results in reflex stimulation of vagal activity, while simultaneously there is a reflex reduction in sympathetic output. From a clinical standpoint, the vagal effect has the most significance. The parasympathetic effect is almost immediate, occurring within the first second. The sympathetic effect, however, becomes manifest only after several seconds and may not take effect until 1 minute has elapsed.[7]

Carotid sinus stimulation has a variety of effects. The two of greatest clinical importance are the cardioinhibitory and vasodepressor effects. These are independent phenomena. The fall in heart rate is blocked by the administration of atropine, whereas epinephrine blocks the reduction in blood pressure. A third effect of carotid sinus stimulation is a cerebral response, manifested by varying degrees of alteration of consciousness; the cerebral response is independent of the reduction in heart rate and blood pressure.[8] The cerebral effect is not blocked by the administration of atropine or epinephrine.[9] The etiology of this response remains controversial, although many feel that it is a reflection of carotid occlusive disease that is exacerbated by application of carotid sinus pressure too vigorously.[2, 10] The respiratory effects of carotid sinus stimulation include bronchoconstriction (CSM may induce wheezing), a decrease in respiratory rate, and pulmonary hypotension.

The parasympathetic branch of the carotid sinus reflex supplies the sinus node and the AV node. The sinoatrial pacemaker is more likely to be affected than is the AV node, except when digitalis has been administered. In order of decreasing frequency, the changes seen clinically with CSM include (1) sinoatrial slowing, occurring in approximately 75 per cent of cases and leading to sinus arrest approximately 3 per cent of the time; (2)

AFFERENT   EFFERENT

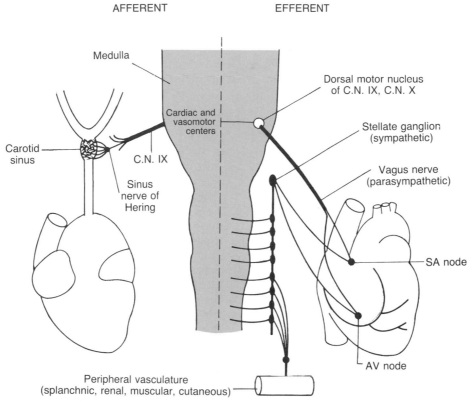

Figure 9–1. Anatomy of the carotid sinus reflex. Carotid receptors send impulses to the medulla by way of the sinus nerve of Hering and cranial nerve IX. Efferent nerves are shown on the right. (Adapted from Scher, A.M.: Control of arterial blood pressure. *In* Ruch, T.C., and Patton, H.D.: Physiology and Biophysics, 20th ed., vol. 2. Philadelphia, W.B. Saunders Company, 1974.)

atrial conduction defects, manifested by an increase in width of the P wave on the electrocardiogram; (3) prolongation of the PR interval and higher degrees of AV block, seen in approximately 10 per cent of cases; (4) nodal escape rhythms; (5) complete asystole, defined as sinus arrest without ventricular escape lasting greater than 3 seconds, occurring in 4 per cent of cases; and (6) premature ventricular contractions.[1, 11] CSM does not exert an effect on the configuration of the QRS complex, since the ventricle is not directly influenced by the vagus nerve.

The sympathetic branch of the reflex during stimulation is less important from a clinical standpoint. It exerts its effect through the stellate ganglion by sending inhibitory fibers to the sinus node and the AV node and thus further decreases heart rate. Efferents to heart muscle fibers cause a generalized decrease in cardiac contractility. Nerve endings supplying the peripheral vasculature cause a generalized vasodilation of the splanchnic, renal, muscular, and cutaneous arterial circulation.[4]

Although the carotid sinus mechanism has been described as "one of the oldest and best known of the cardiovascular reflexes,"[1] there is still much controversy and uncertainty regarding its total function. Early literature, for example, implicated

the carotid sinus reflex in the development of essential hypertension, speculating that chronic elevation of blood pressure might simply reflect a basic defect in the autoregulatory capacity of the cardiovascular system. This theory was never substantiated, and it is now apparent that the carotid sinus pressor reflex acts as a "shock absorber" within the cardiovascular tree, reducing the minute-to-minute fluctuations in blood pressure to approximately 50 per cent of what they would be if the system were not operative.[4] It plays a minimal role in the long-term control of hypertension. Current topics of interest include the role of the carotid sinus in the regulation of body fluids[12] and its effect on renin secretion.[13]

Clinical Use of Carotid Sinus Massage

The most valuable application of CSM is in the diagnosis and treatment of tachydysrhythmias, particularly when the QRS complex is wide and the differentiation between supraventricular and ventricular tachycardia must be made quickly.[14] It should be emphasized, however, that CSM is potentially useful when one is confronted with a dysrhythmia at any rate, including bradycardias.[1]

Lown summarizes the indications for CSM with the statement that "when a patient shows a rhythm disorder that is not readily deciphered, complete investigation requires determination of the response of the heart to vagal stimulation. Carotid sinus massage is usually the simplest and safest way of achieving this."[1] Although CSM is primarily used in the management of dysrhythmias, at one time the indications for it were broader, and the technique was used in the management of angina pectoris and pulmonary edema.[1, 15] It may also be helpful in the evaluation of the patient with palpitations and a normal electrocardiogram (EKG) as well as during auscultation of the heart in the patient with tachycardia and in the investigation of syncope.

BRADYCARDIA

At rates between 30 and 60 beats per minute when the rhythm is regular, CSM may differentiate between sinus bradycardia and various degrees of partial or complete heart block. If smooth, gradual slowing of the ventricular rate is achieved, then the mechanism is sinus. Under these circumstances, cessation of CSM is accompanied by a gradual return to the original heart rate. A jerky or irregular decrease in heart rate suggests the presence of second-degree heart block. The irregular slowing is a consequence of increasing AV block, and nonconducted P waves may be demonstrated. An additional clue to the presence of second-degree heart block is the precipitation of paradoxic acceleration of the ventricular rate during CSM. As was discussed earlier, the carotid sinus reflex is more likely to affect the sinoatrial pacemaker rather than the AV node. In the presence of AV block, the initial response to CSM is

likely to be slowing of the atrial rate by slowing of the sinoatrial node. The previously blocked impulse now reaches the AV node when it is no longer refractory to conduction. Theoretically, this could convert 2:1 conduction to 1:1 conduction and could actually increase the heart rate (Fig. 9–2).

The ventricular rate in complete heart block is unaffected by CSM, and complete heart block is ruled out if some effect on ventricular rate is achieved with the procedure. If the procedure has no effect, an independent ventricular source for the dysrhythmia is suggested. The lack of a response to carotid sinus massage is essentially nondiagnostic, however, since the failure of response may be a result of other factors as well, including an insensitive carotid sinus reflex or faulty technique on the part of the examiner. CSM may be helpful in the diagnosis of complete heart block if the procedure affects the atrial, but not the ventricular, rate. If the atrial rate is slowed but the ventricular rate is unaffected, previously hidden P waves may now be demonstrated. A decreased atrial rate is easily measured on a rhythm strip. This is useful both in slow ventricular rates and in the investigation of ventricular tachycardia (Fig. 9–3).

NORMAL HEART RATE

At normal rates, carotid sinus massage is also helpful diagnostically. Smooth, gradual alterations in the heart rate suggest a sinus mechanism. An abrupt slowing or an exact halving of the heart rate may occur in the presence of either paroxysmal atrial tachycardia (PAT) with block or atrial flutter. Atrial flutter with a 2:1 conduction may be indistinguishable on the EKG from a sinus tachycardia. If the rate is 150 to 160 beats per minute with a sinus mechanism, the P wave will be

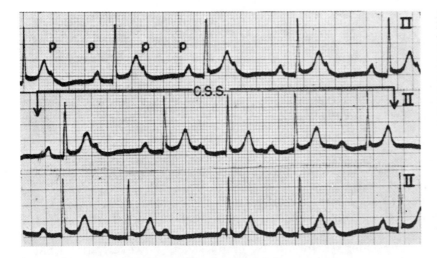

Figure 9–2. Acceleration of ventricular rate by carotid sinus stimulation (CSS). Continuous tracing. Upper strip shows 2:1 atrioventricular block: atrial rate = 102; ventricular rate = 51. The second and third strips were recorded during and after CSS, when the atrial rate was reduced to 68; a 1:1 response occurs. (From Lown, B., and Levine, S.A.: Carotid sinus—clinical value of its stimulation. Circulation 23:766, 1961. Used by permission.)

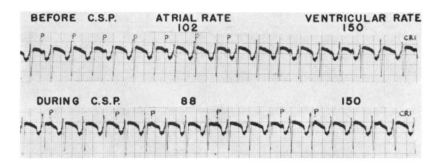

Figure 9–3. Carotid sinus pressure (C.S.P.) slows atria but not ventricles, thus establishing the presence of atrioventricular dissociation, supporting the diagnosis of ventricular tachycardia. The QRS measures 0.16 second. Note atrial slowing from 102 to 88 while the ventricular rate is unaffected. (From Lown, B., and Levine, S. A.: Carotid sinus—clinical value of its stimulation. Circulation 23:766, 1961. Used by permission.)

hidden in the QRS complex but will be demonstrated if CSM slows the ventricular rate. PAT with block is often an elusive and misleading rhythm that is commonly a result of digitalis toxicity. PAT owing to digitalis toxicity is suggested by the emergence of nonconducted P waves when CSM increases AV block (Fig. 9–4). The *atrial* rate in PAT with block is characteristically less than 200 beats per minute, whereas the *atrial* rate in atrial flutter is characteristically 300 beats per minute and in a sawtooth pattern. It is important to note that the underlying cause for atrial tachycardia is almost always digitalis toxicity if CSM changes AV block to a higher degree without affecting the atrial mechanism.[16]

TACHYCARDIA

At rapid heart rates, CSM has its greatest clinical application, since it is useful from both a diagnostic and a therapeutic standpoint (Table 9–1). If ventricular slowing is achieved with CSM, then ventricular tachycardia is most probably ruled out. The procedure may be helpful in diagnosis of ventricular tachycardia if the atrial rate is slowed while the ventricular rate remains constant or if P waves can be demonstrated to indicate AV dissociation (see Fig. 9–3). Ventricular tachycardia will not be terminated by CSM in the vast majority of cases. It is generally believed that autonomic tone has little effect on ventricular dysrhythmias, but

Hess and associates[17] recently reported two cases of ventricular tachycardia that were terminated by CSM. Other sporadic cases[18] have been reported, and the consensus that CSM will not terminate ventricular tachycardia is not an absolute rule. In the Hess cases the termination of ventricular tachycardia was thought to be secondary to CSM-induced AV nodal echo beats in one patient and direct vagal effects on the ventricular muscle or the ventricular conduction system in the other. The vast majority of cases of ventricular tachycardia, however, will not be terminated by CSM.

Smooth slowing of a rapid ventricular rate with gradual resumption of the original rate following termination of CSM indicates a sinus mechanism. Slowing may unmask P waves that were hidden in the QRS complex of a rapid sinus tachycardia (Fig. 9–5). Occasionally, varying degrees of heart block may be precipitated during CSM with an underlying sinus rhythm (Fig. 9–6). If the tachycardia stops abruptly and sinus rhythm is maintained, either paroxysmal atrial or nodal tachycardia was present (Fig. 9–7). If paroxysmal atrial tachycardia (PAT) or paroxysmal nodal tachycardia is known to be present and the response to CSM is a decrease in AV conduction without conversion, the dysrhythmia is usually secondary to digitalis excess.[14] CSM has no effect on nonparoxysmal junctional tachycardia and should not be attempted if this rhythm is known to exist, since more serious dysrhythmias may be precipitated. Nonparoxysmal junctional tachycardia is often seen with digitalis toxicity. If slowing of the heart

Figure 9–4. Carotid sinus pressure uncovers P waves hidden in the ventricular complex. Upper strip resembles atrial flutter or atrial fibrillation with ventricular ectopic beats. Lower strip shows PAT with variable block at an atrial rate of 166. (From Lown, B., and Levine, S.A.: Carotid sinus—clinical value of its stimulation. Circulation 23:766, 1961. Used by permission.)

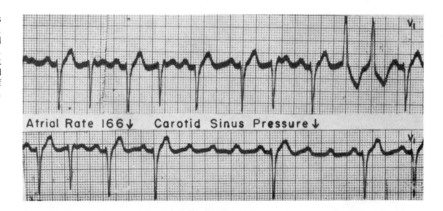

Table 9–1.   EFFECTS OF CAROTID SINUS MASSAGE ON VARIOUS CARDIAC RHYTHMS

Cardiac Rhythm	Usual Response to Carotid Sinus Massage (CSM)
Sinus rhythm	1. Smooth and gradual slowing of ventricular rate with return to original rate with termination of CSM. (The procedure may bring out diagnostic P waves.) 2. Occasionally produces varying degrees of heart block. 3. *Caution:* Possible prolonged asystole with hypersensitive carotid sinus syndrome.
Atrial flutter or atrial fibrillation	1. Irregular slowing of ventricular rate by increasing AV block. 2. An effect is rarely absent. 3. CSM does not terminate the rhythm but may bring out diagnostic flutter or fibrillation waves. 4. *Caution:* Ventricular standstill may occur if CSM is prolonged.
Paroxysmal atrial tachycardia (PAT)	No effect or abrupt termination of dysrhythmia.
Paroxysmal atrial tachycardia (Wolff-Parkinson-White syndrome)	1. Varying results (slowing, no effect, termination). 2. CSM may unmask W-P-W syndrome by increasing anomalous AV conduction.
Paroxysmal AV junctional tachycardia	No effect or termination of dysrhythmia.
Nonparoxysmal junctional tachycardia	1. No response. 2. *Caution:* CSM may be dangerous if rhythm results from digitalis toxicity.
Ventricular tachycardia	1. No response in ventricular rate. 2. CSM may uncover AV dissociation by demonstrating P waves or a decrease in atrial rate. 3. If rhythm is ventricular parasystole, response may be variable.
Digitalis-toxic rhythms	CSM should not be attempted.

rate is abrupt but temporary with a jerky, irregular return, then atrial flutter, atrial fibrillation, or PAT with block is present. The ventricular rate of PAT with block is rarely over 100 beats per minute and hence PAT with block is unlikely to be confused with the more common tachydysrhythmias.

In the presence of fast but *irregular* rhythms, the major conditions to be ruled out are atrial fibrillation, atrial flutter with varying block, sinus tachycardia with premature atrial contractions (PACs), and PAT with variable block. Atrial fibrillation, atrial flutter, and PAT with block respond to CSM

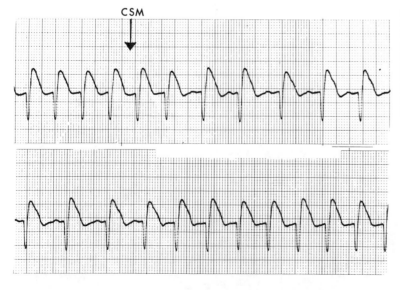

Figure 9–5. Sinus tachycardia. The sinus P wave is obscured within the descending limb of the T wave. Carotid sinus massage (CSM) transiently slows the sinus rate and exposes the P wave. The rate then increases. The strips are continuous. (From Silverman, M.E.: Recognition and treatment of arrhythmias. *In* Schwartz, G.R., et al.: Principles and Practice of Emergency Medicine, vol. 2. Philadelphia, W.B. Saunders Company, 1978. Used by permission.)

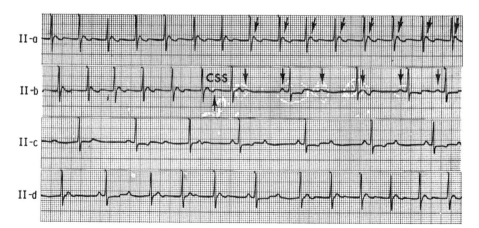

Figure 9–6. Arrows indicate sinus P waves. Strips II-a to -d are continuous. The basic rhythm is sinus, but marked first-degree atrioventricular block is present. High-degree (advanced) atrioventricular block associated with transient slowing of sinus rate is produced by carotid sinus stimulation (CSS). (From Chung, E.K.: Electrocardiography, 2nd ed. New York, Harper & Row, 1980. Used by permission.)

in a similar fashion, with an increase in AV block. The diagnosis of atrial flutter is confirmed if CSM slows the ventricular rate and demonstrates typical flutter waves. The atrial rate in atrial flutter is characteristic—300 beats per minute (Fig. 9–8). A regular rhythm of 150 to 160 beats per minute with a narrow QRS complex should always raise the suspicion of atrial flutter with 2:1 conduction. Atrial flutter may closely resemble sinus tachycardia on the EKG and may be differentiated only with CSM. In atrial fibrillation, CSM transiently slows the ventricular rate and reveals a fibrillating baseline (Fig. 9–9). Long periods of ventricular standstill may occur following CSM in both atrial flutter and atrial fibrillation. As a rule, neither atrial flutter nor atrial fibrillation converts to a sinus rhythm with CSM. Sinus tachycardia with PACs responds in the usual fashion, with gradual slowing of the ventricular rate.

The following six "rules of massage" essentially summarize the clinical features of carotid sinus massage at any heart rate:

1. A positive effect on the ventricular rate essentially rules out a ventricular dysrhythmia,[17] except in the rare instances in which ventricular tachycardia occurs secondary to a parasystolic mechanism. (CSM may slow the heart rate in this circumstance.[14]) CSM may slow the atrial rate in ventricular tachycardia or complete heart block and may demonstrate P waves or obvious AV dissociation.

2. Abrupt changes in the heart rate without conversion are a result of increasing AV block.

3. Gradual slowing of the ventricular rate suggests the presence of a sinus rhythm. Only rarely will CSM decrease AV conduction in the presence of a sinus mechanism.

4. The dysrhythmias most likely to convert to sinus rhythm are paroxysmal atrial tachycardia and paroxysmal nodal tachycardia.

5. Dysrhythmias that are associated with AV conduction defects (PAT with block, atrial flutter, atrial fibrillation) infrequently convert to a sinus rhythm,[14] but the ventricular rate invariably slows.

6. A negative response to CSM is nondiagnostic.

OTHER CLINICAL CONSIDERATIONS

The success rates for conversion of PAT and paroxysmal nodal tachycardia to sinus rhythm vary considerably in the literature. White reported only a 10 per cent rate of conversion,[36] whereas others noted success in 80 per cent of cases. Success rates are even higher when parasympa-

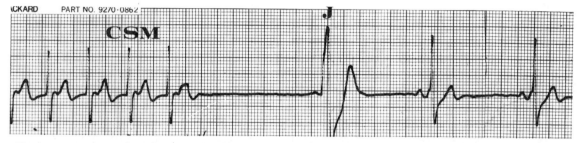

Figure 9–7. Paroxysmal atrial tachycardia. Carotid sinus massage (CSM) abolishes the dysrhythmia and results in a period of sinus suppression with a junctional (J) escape beat. Prolonged periods of asystole may produce anxiety in the physician who is waiting for the resumption of a sinus pacemaker. (From Silverman, M.E.: Recognition and treatment of arrhythmias. In Schwartz, G.R., et al.: Principles and Practice of Emergency Medicine, vol. 2. Philadelphia, W.B. Saunders Company, 1978, Used by permission.)

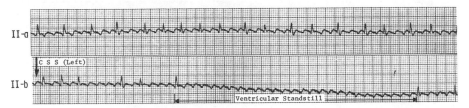

Figure 9–8. Carotid sinus stimulation (CSS, *downward arrow*) produces marked slowing of the ventricular rate in atrial flutter. Note the obvious flutter waves with an atrial rate of 300 and a long period of ventricular standstill. Strips are continuous. (From Chung, E.K.: Electrocardiography, 2nd ed. New York, Harper & Row, 1980. Used by permission.)

thomimetic agents, such as edrophonium (Tensilon), are used in conjunction with CSM.[4] Young patients with recurrent attacks of PAT can be taught CSM to abolish attacks without fear of producing serious side effects.[19]

CSM may also be helpful in those patients who present with palpitations, or "fluttering in the chest," and a normal EKG.[1] The differentiation between an organic and a functional etiology is difficult at times, and the temptation often is to diagnose the disorder as functional in origin. CSM may supply useful information in these cases. Because the sinus rate is slowed, an ectopic focus may emerge, or AV conduction defects may be unmasked (Fig. 9–10). In patients with Wolff-Parkinson-White (W-P-W) syndrome, reflex vagal stimulation impairs conduction down the normal AV bundle, thus favoring conduction through the accessory pathway. Actual (antegrade) tachycardia associated with the W-P-W syndrome can frequently be terminated by CSM, according to Chung,[20] but the effects of CSM in W-P-W syndrome are variable. Since CSM impairs conduction in the normal AV pathways in W-P-W syndrome, the favoring of conduction through the anomalous bundles may facilitate the diagnosis of W-P-W syndrome.

CSM can be a diagnostic aid during auscultation of the heart in the presence of tachycardia. If the rate is fast, it may be impossible to distinguish between the first and second heart sounds. By slowing the heart rate and lengthening diastole, CSM facilitates the differentiation. Likewise, CSM has been useful in eliciting the diastolic rumble of mitral stenosis, a murmur that is often difficult to appreciate.

In his extensive review of CSM, Lown pointed out an interesting, but little appreciated, phenomenon; namely, that this maneuver is helpful diagnostically and therapeutically in the evaluation of the patient with suspected angina pectoris.[1] CSM has recently been supplanted by newer pharmacologic agents and more sophisticated studies, such as cardiac catheterization and myocardial scanning. Nevertheless, from a physiologic and historical standpoint, the relationship between CSM and "chest pain of uncertain etiology" deserves brief discussion.

According to Wasserman, "carotid sinus massage may provide relief unobtainable by other means" in the presence of angina pectoris and may be followed by complete disappearance of the pain after only a few seconds.[37] According to Lown, relief of pain is a function of cardiac slowing.[1] More recent work has shown that relief is not accompanied by slowing of the heart rate in all cases. Bronk further suggested that relief may be secondary to inhibition of sympathetic discharge from the stellate ganglion.[21] Certainly, the speed with which relief is obtained favors a reflex neurogenic mechanism. Lown states that if chest pain is relieved by CSM, then it is anginal in origin. Pain from gastrointestinal disorder is not affected by CSM, and functional chest pain may be worsened by this procedure.[1] If there is no relief with CSM, then the test is inconclusive. These considerations suggest that CSM could have a role in the emergency department evaluation of the patient with chest pain of uncertain etiology. One should be aware that patients with coronary artery disease, especially during an acute anginal attack, may be exquisitely sensitive to CSM and are at risk for the development of dangerous cardiac dysrhythmias.[3, 22]

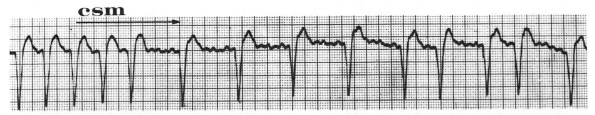

Figure 9–9. Atrial fibrillation. Carotid sinus massage (CSM) transiently slows the ventricular response, revealing the fibrillating baseline. The ventricular rate will subsequently accelerate. (From Silverman, M.E.: Recognition and treatment of arrhythmias. In Schwartz, G.R., et al.: Principles and Practice of Emergency Medicine, vol. 2. Philadelphia, W.B. Saunders Company, 1978. Used by permission.)

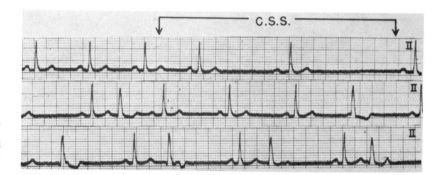

Figure 9–10. Carotid sinus stimulation (CSS), reveals ventricular extrasystoles, thereby explaining the cause of palpitation in this case. (From Lown, B., and Levine, S.A.: Carotid sinus—clinical value of its stimulation. Circulation 23:766, 1961. Used by permission.)

According to Alzamora-Castro, relief can be obtained in 80 per cent of patients with pulmonary edema through the use of CSM.[15] The proposed mechanism is peripheral vasodilation secondary to reflex sympathetic inhibition as well as relative bradycardia leading to more efficient diastolic filling. The following quotation from Lown reflects the enthusiasm that earlier clinicians had for this procedure in the presence of acute pulmonary edema:

> The patient is promptly able to lie flat. Pain, dyspnea, and chest oppression disappear, perspiration lessens, and pallor vanishes. Pulmonary rales decrease or clear entirely, respirations become less labored, heart sounds diminish in intensity, and the apex impulse becomes less forceful. The episode is frequently completely reversed.[1]

Despite this, CSM is not generally advocated as a first-line treatment of pulmonary edema. CSM must be maintained for extended periods in this setting, thus increasing the risk of side effects. Furthermore, the disorder can usually be handled adequately by more conventional means.

An uncommon cause of dizziness and actual syncope may be the hypersensitive carotid sinus syndrome (Fig. 9–11). Most affected patients are older and have associated diabetes or vascular disease. Some clinicians advocate the controlled use of CSM in the work-up of syncope to investigate this syndrome as a cause for clinical symptoms. Specific cautions for the diagnostic use of CSM under these circumstances are listed later.

Contraindications

CSM is essentially contraindicated in two groups of patients: (1) those at significant risk for the development of a cerebrovascular accident during the procedure as a consequence of atherosclerosis of the carotid arteries, and (2) those at risk for the development of life-threatening dysrhythmias as a manifestation of a hypersensitive carotid sinus reflex.[23, 24] Patients in this latter category may develop a syncopal episode simply by coughing, sneezing, or quickly turning the head.[9] A hypersensitive carotid sinus reflex is defined as (1) asystole lasting greater than 3 seconds and unaccompanied by the emergence of a ventricular escape rhythm, (2) a fall in the systolic blood pressure by 50 mm Hg, and (3) reproducible results following CSM. Slowing of the heart rate by 30 to 50 per cent of the original value or a decrease in the systolic blood pressure by 30 mm Hg is considered a borderline response.[23] Patients lacking a history of carotid sinus hypersensitivity should nevertheless be carefully evaluated before the procedure is attempted if the history and physical examination uncover any of the factors known to enhance the sensitivity of the carotid sinus reflex, particularly the presence of coronary artery disease or a history of digitalis use.

A basic list of contraindications to CSM include (1) the presence of carotid bruits on physical examination; (2) age above 75; (3) a history or suspicion of sick sinus syndrome (since a hypersen-

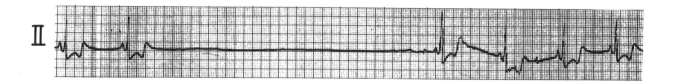

Figure 9–11. Hyper-reactive carotid sinus reflex. Gentle pressure was applied to the carotid sinus for 3 seconds (indicated by the black bar over the electrocardiographic tracing), resulting in a pause in sinus rhythm of approximately 7 seconds. This syndrome may be the cause of syncope. (From Bigger, J.T., Jr.: Mechanisms and diagnosis of arrhythmias. In Braunwald, E.: Heart Disease, vol. 1. Philadelphia, W.B. Saunders Company, 1980. Used by permission.)

sitive carotid sinus may be the presenting feature of previously undiagnosed sick sinus syndrome); (4) possible digitalis toxicity; and (5) the presence of nonparoxysmal junctional tachycardia (since this rhythm is unresponsive to carotid sinus massage, and, more importantly, because it is frequently a manifestation of digitalis toxicity[14]). CSM should be used cautiously in patients with a history or suspicion of a hypersensitive carotid sinus. The presence of coronary artery disease or ingestion of drugs known to heighten the sensitivity of the carotid sinus may render the carotid sinus hypersensitive. The use of CSM under controlled circumstances may be the only definitive test to diagnose a hypersensitive carotid sinus and may be required when a patient with debilitating symptoms is evaluated. Cardiac pacing may be indicated in such patients.

Technique of Carotid Sinus Massage

Given an examiner who knows how and when to massage the carotid sinus, the procedure is effective and carries minimal risk to the patient. It works best in patients with long, narrow necks.[19] In any situation, however, it is essential to have a relaxed patient. A tense platysma muscle makes palpation of the carotid sinus difficult. Furthermore, an anxious patient will be less sensitive to carotid sinus massage as a result of heightened sympathetic tone. Mild sedation of selected patients has been recommended by some authors.[19]

Before attempting CSM, the clinician should start an intravenous line; normal saline is preferred as a precaution against hypotension. Atropine should be readily available at the bedside as well as resuscitative equipment, including a transvenous pacemaker, in the event that a life-threatening bradycardia occurs.

One should always auscultate for carotid bruits on both sides of the neck before attempting CSM, *since the detection of bruits is a contraindication to massage*. The patient requires continuous electrocardiographic monitoring. One should monitor a lead that is most likely to demonstrate a P wave. This is usually lead II or lead V_1 or V_2. One may use the Lewis lead modification, in which the right and left arm leads are placed at the second and fourth intercostal spaces, respectively, just to the right of the sternum. With the Lewis leads in place, the EKG machine should record on the lead I setting. It is preferable to have a nurse or other assistant available at the bedside; this person can document on the monitor strip the times of initiation and termination of massage. The examiner should begin on the right side[25] and should stand slightly behind the patient, with the cardiac monitor always in full view. It is conventional to begin

massage on the right side for two reasons. First, the success rate is higher with right-sided massage,[9] and second, there is a greater incidence of escape rhythms associated with right-sided carotid sinus massage.[26] Escape rhythms are a desirable safety mechanism should CSM produce prolonged asystole. The explanation for these clinical observations remains a mystery but may reflect a subtle asymmetry of neural input from side to side.[4] Simultaneous bilateral CSM is absolutely contraindicated, since there are no data indicating that it is more effective than unilateral CSM, and cerebral circulation may be severely compromised.

The examiner should observe the monitor, not the patient, during CSM. An assistant may watch the patient, or the examiner may have the patient count aloud to ten during the procedure.[19] This serves several purposes: First, it places an upper limit on the duration of massage; second, it continually monitors the patient's level of consciousness during CSM (as long as the patient is counting, the examiner knows that he is awake); and third, it may distract the patient from the occasional discomfort associated with the procedure.

The patient should assume the recumbent position as a precaution against syncope.[1] The head is tilted backward and slightly to the opposite side,[27] until the expansile body is readily palpated in the neck. This is usually accomplished just below the angle of the mandible at the upper level of the thyroid cartilage and anterior to the sternocleidomastoid muscle.[1] Once the expansile body is identified, one should use the thumb[9] or the tips of the fingers to administer CSM in a posteromedial direction, aiming toward the vertebral column.[25] At this point, it must be re-emphasized that the procedure is truly *massage*.[8] Simple compression of the vessel is contraindicated, since it is more dangerous and less effective. Furthermore, pulsatile stimuli are more likely to evoke a response than is sustained pressure.

CSM should be firm, yet not so vigorous as to occlude the pulse of the carotid artery. One can check this tendency by simultaneously palpating the superficial temporal artery with the opposite hand.[2, 8] As long as this vessel can be felt, patency of the carotid artery is assured. CSM should be administered up and down the length of the vessel—a distance of approximately 3 cm.[19] The massage should be continued until the desired effect is achieved, asystole develops, or 5 to 10 seconds elapse. If unsuccessful, CSM may be repeated after 30 seconds. If the procedure is still unsuccessful, the opposite carotid sinus may be massaged in a similar fashion. A simultaneous Valsalva maneuver may enhance carotid sinus sensitivity. If the CSM is used therapeutically but is unsuccessful initially, it can be repeated after the administration of digitalis, edrophonium (Tensilon), or propranolol. CSM may be more effective following the administration of these medications and may result in termination of the dysrhythmia on a second attempt after the medication renders the carotid sinus more sensitive.

The literature reflects a lack of full standardization of the technique of CSM. Massage is advocated for anywhere from 5 to 30 seconds, and occasionally even longer.[25] In this discussion, the lower limits of time are recommended, simply because CSM should be effective within the first few seconds if done properly. In any event, the greatest obstacle to successful CSM is faulty technique, not duration of massage. Many observers believe that high failure rates reflect carotid *artery* massage, rather than massage of the sinus.[4] As Greenwood stated, "the drama of effective carotid sinus pressure by the fingers of a skilled physician is impressive."[28] This skill is certainly within the reach of any physician willing to practice and refine the technique.

Side Effects

There are two major deleterious side effects of CSM: further deterioration in the cardiac rhythm and decreased level of consciousness, which can occasionally precipitate a transient ischemic attack or a cerebrovascular accident as a result of interference with cerebral circulation. Lown stated that "permanent cessation of the heartbeat or serious ventricular arrhythmias are almost unheard of."[1] Since that statement was made, however, it has become apparent that in rare cases prolonged asystole or ventricular fibrillation may result from CSM. It is common, for instance, to have 3 to 5 seconds of asystole, a few escape PVCs, or a short run of ventricular beats following conversion of PAT with carotid sinus massage; the straight line on the EKG will invariably disappear but can produce a few anxious moments.

Dysrhythmias are largely preventable by proper patient selection. Avoidance of CSM in patients with a history or suspicion of a hypersensitive carotid sinus reflex should eliminate cases of prolonged asystole. Furthermore, *all* cases of ventricular fibrillation following CSM have occurred in patients taking digitalis glycosides. Ventricular fibrillation should not occur if massage is withheld in patients who have digitalis toxicity. No clear danger of CSM has been demonstrated in patients with *therapeutic* levels of digitalis, but the procedure is definitely contraindicated in the presence of digitalis *toxicity*.

From time to time, authors have commented on the risk of precipitating permanent neurologic sequelae by CSM.[29] In 1945, Askey conducted an extensive review of this issue, presenting case reports of seven patients who became hemiplegic following CSM.[30] All patients in his series were elderly and had a history of advanced atherosclerosis. Again, proper patient selection should virtually eliminate this potential complication.

Factors Affecting Sensitivity of the Carotid Sinus

The presence of diffuse, advanced atherosclerosis is associated with increased sensitivity of the carotid sinus reflex, particularly when the coronary or cerebral arteries are involved. The association between coronary artery disease and carotid sinus hypersensitivity is profound.[3, 31] The exaggerated response of affected patients reflects the increased vagal tone that is invariably present. The hypersensitivity is further augmented during an anginal attack or an acute myocardial infarction. An article by Brown and coworkers showed that the degree of carotid sinus hypersensitivity was directly proportional to the severity of coronary artery disease documented by cardiac catheterization in a study of 66 patients.[32] Increased sensitivity of the carotid sinus reflex is likewise associated with hypertension and the sick sinus syndrome.

The response of the cardiovascular system to CSM is markedly age-related. A positive effect is seen in about 80 per cent of patients over 40 years of age, as opposed to approximately 20 per cent of patients under 40 years old.[1] Whether this is strictly a function of age or whether it is caused by some other factor (such as atherosclerosis, which is associated with the process of aging) remains open to discussion. Males are somewhat more sensitive than females at any given age. Organic diseases that enhance vagal tone, such as cholecystitis, are associated with increased carotid sinus sensitivity.[33] Other miscellaneous conditions cited in the literature that enhance the sensitivity of the carotid sinus include fatigue, inflamed cervical lymph nodes, and the presence of acidosis.

There are a wide variety of pharmacologic agents that may render the carotid sinus hypersensitive. Digitalis must be mentioned first, because in addition to sensitizing the carotid sinus to the effects of CSM, it is a precipitating factor in the development of dysrhythmias and is frequently "on board" in those patients under consideration for therapeutic carotid sinus massage. Carotid sinus massage should not be used in patients with possible digitalis toxicity, although it may be used cautiously in patients with therapeutic digitalis levels. Other agents that may render the carotid sinus hypersensitive to massage include cholinergic agents, such as edrophonium (Tensilon), methyldopa (Aldomet),[34] propranolol,[20] morphine sulfate, nitrites, calcium, salicylates, and insulin.[35]

Conditions predisposing to sinus tachycardia or creating a state of heightened sympathetic tone are associated with a decreased sensitivity of the carotid sinus reflex. Such conditions include fever, anemia, thyrotoxicosis, pneumonia, chronic obstructive pulmonary disease, anxiety states, and hyperventilation.[9] Several drugs, including the sympathomimetics, alcohol, quinidine, and vagolytic agents, have been implicated in the production of an insensitive carotid sinus reflex. Other miscellaneous factors include hypocalcemia, hypoxia, and high spinal anesthesia.

Summary

CSM, the "oldest and best known cardiovascular reflex," can be useful diagnostically and therapeutically when the physician is confronted with a cardiac dysrhythmia. The major limitation to its usefulness seems to be improper technique. If the procedure is to be helpful and simultaneously is to do no harm, it must be performed properly and in the correct clinical setting. CSM is often included early in the protocol for management of cardiac dysrhythmias. CSM is to be avoided in patients with carotid bruits or a suspicion of digitalis toxicity. The procedure must be used cautiously in the elderly and in those with a history of coronary artery disease.

1. Lown, B., and Levine, S. A.: Carotid sinus—clinical value of its stimulation. Circulation 23:766, 1961.
2. Silverstein, A., et al.: Manual compression of the carotid vessels, carotid sinus hypersensitivity and carotid artery occlusions. Ann. Intern. Med. 52:172, 1960.
3. Sigler, L. H.: Hyperactive cardioinhibitory carotid sinus reflex as an aid in the diagnosis of coronary disease—its value compared with that of the electrocardiogram. N. Engl. J. Med. 226:46, 1942.
4. Scher, A.: Carotid and aortic regulation of arterial blood pressure. Circulation 56:521, 1977.
5. Bjurstedt, H., Rosenhamer, G., and Tyden, G.: Cardiovascular responses to changes in carotid sinus transmural pressure in man. Acta Physiol. Scand. 94:497, 1975.
6. Mancia, G., et al.: Controls of blood pressure by carotid sinus baroreceptors in human beings. Am. J. Cardiol. 44:895, 1979.
7. Wang, S. C., and Borison, H. L.: An analysis of the carotid sinus mechanism. Am. J. Physiol. 150:712, 1947.
8. Toole, J. F.: Stimulation of the carotid sinus in man. 1. The cerebral response. 2. The significance of head positioning. Am. J. Med. 17:952, 1959.
9. Evans, E.: The carotid sinus: Its clinical importance. JAMA 149:46, 1952.
10. Gurdjian, E. J., Webster, J. E., and Linder, D. W.: On the nonexistence of the cerebral form of "irritable carotid sinus." Trans. Am. Neurol. Assoc. 49, 1958.
11. Purks, W. K.: Electrocardiographic findings following carotid sinus stimulation. Ann. Intern. Med. 13:270, 1939.
12. Lindblad, L., et al.: Circulatory effects of carotid sinus stimulation and changes in blood volume distribution in hypertensive man. Acta Physiol. Scand. 111:299, 1981.
13. Cunningham, S. G., et al.: Carotid sinus reflex influence on plasma renin activity. Am. J. Physiol. 234:H670, 1978.
14. Read, E. A., and Scott, J. C.: Factors influencing the carotid sinus cardioinhibitory reflex. Am. J. Physiol. 181:21, 1955.
15. Alzamora-Castro, V., Battiliana, G., et al.: Acute left ventricular failure and carotid sinus stimulation. JAMA 157:226, 1955.
16. Chung, E. K. (ed.): Electrocardiography: Practical Applications with Vectorial Principles, 2nd ed. New York, Harper & Row, 1980.
17. Hess, D. S., Hanlon, T., Scheinman, M., et al.: Termination of ventricular tachycardia by carotid sinus massage. Circulation 65:627, 1982.
18. Waxman, M. B., and Wald, R. W.: Termination of ventricular tachycardia by an increase in cardiac vagal drive. Circulation 56:385, 1977.
19. Prinzmetal, M.: The Auricular Arrhythmias. Springfield, IL, Charles C Thomas, 1952.
20. Chung, E.: Cardiac Emergency Care, 2nd ed. Philadelphia, Lea & Febiger, 1980.
21. Bronk, D. W., et al.: Inhibition of cardiac accelerator impulses by the carotid sinus. Proc. Soc. Exp. Biol. Med. 31:579, 1933–34.
22. Sigler, L. H.: The hyperactive cardioinhibitory carotid sinus reflex: A possible aid in the diagnosis of coronary artery disease. Arch. Intern. Med. 67:177, 1941.
23. Trout, H. H., III, Brown, L. L., and Thompson, J. E.: Carotid sinus syndrome—treatment by carotid sinus denervation. Ann. Surg. 189:575, 1979.
24. Chughtai, A., et al.: Carotid sinus syncope. Report of two cases. JAMA 237:2320, 1977.
25. Gould, L., et al.: Usefulness of carotid sinus pressure in detecting the sick sinus syndrome. J. Electrocardiography 11:261, 1978.
26. Rizzon, P., and DiBiase, M.: Effect of carotid sinus reflex on cardiac impulse formation and conduction: Electrophysiologic study. In Schwartz, P. J., Brown, A. M., Malliani, A., and Zanchetti, A. (eds.): Neural Mechanisms in Cardiac Arrhythmias. New York, Raven Press, 1978.
27. Sigler, L. H.: The cardioinhibitory carotid sinus reflex—its importance as a vagocardiosensitivity test. Am. J. Cardiol. 12:175, 1963.
28. Greenwood, R. J., and Dupler, D. A.: Death following carotid sinus pressure. JAMA 181:605, 1962.
29. Brannon, E. S.: Hemiplegia following carotid sinus stimulation. Am. Heart J. 36:299, 1948.
30. Askey, J. M.: Hemiplegia following carotid sinus stimulation. Am. Heart J. 31:131, 1946.
31. Reed, E. A., and Scott, J. C.: Factors influencing the carotid sinus cardioinhibitory reflex. Am. J. Physiol. 181:21, 1955.
32. Brown, K., et al.: Carotid sinus reflex in patients undergoing coronary angiography: Relationship of degree and location of coronary artery disease to response to carotid sinus massage. Circulation 62:697, 1980.
33. Engel, G. L., and Engel, F. L.: Significance of the carotid sinus reflex and biliary tract disease. N. Engl. J. Med. 227:470, 1942.
34. Bauernfeind, R., et al.: Carotid sinus hypersensitivity with alpha methyldopa. Ann. Intern. Med. 88:214, 1978.
35. Rudnikoff, I.: Insulin and the carotid sinus. Arch. Intern. Med. 34:1382, 1951.
36. White, P. D.: Alternation of the pulse—still a common and important clinical condition. Concepts of Cardiovasc. Dis. 22:174, 1953.
37. Wasserman, S.: Acute Cardiac Pulmonary Edema. Springfield, Illinois, Charles C Thomas, Publisher, 1959.

Introduction

Cardioversion is the use of direct current electricity to convert a cardiac dysrhythmia to a sinus mechanism. The use of electrical current to terminate ventricular fibrillation is termed defibrillation. Cardioversion is performed with the aid of a synchronizer, which assures a timed discharge of electrical current during a specific phase of the cardiac cycle. In defibrillation, electrical current is immediately discharged asynchronously, that is, regardless of the underlying chaotic cardiac activity.

In many cases, direct current cardioversion has specific advantages over drug therapy. The speed and simplicity of electrical cardioversion enhance its usefulness in the emergency department setting. Cardioversion is effective almost immediately, has few side effects, and is often more successful than drug therapy in terminating dysrhythmias. In addition, the effective dose of many antidysrhythmic medications has not been standardized, and there is often a small margin between therapeutic and toxic dosages. Although they suppress an undesired rhythm, drugs may also suppress a normal sinus mechanism or may create toxic manifestations that are more severe than the dysrhythmia being treated. In the clinical setting of hypotension or acute cardiopulmonary collapse, cardioversion may be lifesaving.

The earliest recorded experimentation in "therapeutic" electroshock was performed by Abildgaard in 1775, when he demonstrated that dead fowl could be revived by means of an electrical shock of a certain amplitude.[1] In 1899, Provost and Batelli observed that a relatively small current of electricity induced ventricular fibrillation, whereas a stronger current discharged over a short interval terminated ventricular fibrillation.[2]

In 1947, Beck was the first to defibrillate the human heart successfully, and in the early 1960s, electrical energy was used to treat dysrhythmias other than ventricular fibrillation for the first time. Alternating current remained in vogue until 1962, when Lown advocated direct current countershock as the method of choice for terminating atrial fibrillation.[3] This advance culminated years of investigation that had suggested that direct current was safer and more effective than alternating current in the treatment of dysrhythmias. Ventricular fibrillation follows alternating current countershock in an alarming number of cases. The switch to direct current immediately led to a ten-fold decrease in the incidence of ventricular fibrillation following countershock.

Theoretical Considerations

In 1934, King noted that discharge of a low-intensity current would precipitate ventricular fib-

10

Direct Current Electrical Cardioversion

STEVEN GAZAK, M.D.

rillation only when current was applied during a specific phase of the cardiac cycle. This 30-millisecond interval immediately preceding the apex of the T wave on the electrocardiogram was termed the "vulnerable period."[4] The vulnerable period represents the phase of early repolarization in the cardiac cycle. During this phase, a variably excitable field results from asynchronous recovery of individual myocardial cells. An electrical impulse interspersed during this period may precipitate a re-entrant dysrhythmia, which can degenerate into ventricular fibrillation. The synchronizer on the cardioverter is programmed to discharge a direct current shock, which is timed to avoid the vulnerable period of the T wave. At delivered currents exceeding 1 ampere (greater than 100 joules), the entire ventricle is depolarized, and the risk of ventricular fibrillation by stimulation in the vulnerable period is thus eliminated.

The relative safety of direct current countershock is easily explained. The duration of direct current discharge is exceedingly brief (1.5 to 4 milliseconds) and thus can be programmed to avoid the vulnerable period. In contrast, the standard 60-Hz sinusoidal waveform of alternating current has a duration of 0.2 second. Because of the relatively lengthy duration of this waveform, it is difficult to guarantee discharge of alternating current shock outside the vulnerable period during cardioversion (Fig. 10–1).

The basic concept of cardioversion is that electrical shock momentarily causes depolarization of the majority of cardiac cells and allows the sinus node to resume normal pacemaker function. In re-entrant dysrhythmias, such as paroxysmal supraventricular tachycardia and ventricular tachycardia, cardioversion restores sinus rhythm by interrupting a self-perpetuating re-entrant circuit. Re-entry is similar to an advancing wavefront that "chases its tail" in a cyclic journey around the conducting tissue of the heart. This advancing wavefront is separated from its tail by a stretch of nonrefractory tissue, the so-called excitable gap (Fig. 10–2). Cardioversion succeeds by depolariz-

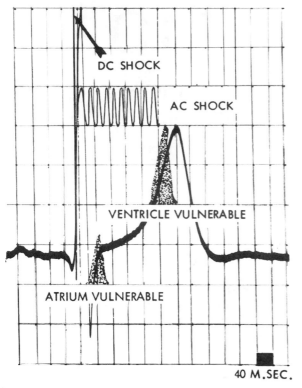

Figure 10–1. Phases of vulnerability for atrium and ventricle. Note that an alternating current shock of 1/5 second may end at the T wave even when synchronized with the R wave of the electrocardiogram. (From Resnekov, L.: Theory and practice of electroversion in cardiac dysrhythmias. Med. Clin. North Am. 60:325, 1976. Used by permission.)

ing a segment of the excitable gap, which is then refractory when the wave of depolarization arrives.[2] The self-perpetrating cardiac dysrhythmia is thus abolished, and the sinus node resumes its function as a pacemaker. Cardioversion is much less effective in terminating tachycardias resulting from augmented normal automaticity, such as digitalis-induced dysrhythmias.

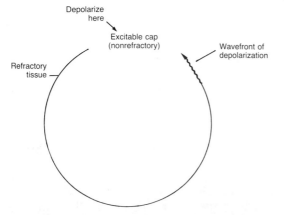

Figure 10–2. Schematic representation of the mechanism of termination of a cardiac dysrhythmia by cardioversion. See text.

Equipment and Preparation for Cardioversion

The cardioverter device consists of five components (Fig. 10–3): (1) a direct current depolarizer, which provides varying amounts of electrical current; (2) an oscilloscope screen for monitoring heart rate and rhythm; (3) access to a continuous electrocardiogram (EKG) readout to document the patient's course and response to treatment; (4) two removable electrode paddles, which can be applied easily to the patient's chest wall; and (5) a synchronizer, permitting discharge of energy outside the vulnerable period of the cardiac cycle. The synchronizer permits triggering of the electrical discharge by the R or S wave of the EKG.

The actual size of the electrode paddle is of no great significance, but paddles must be large enough to depolarize the majority of heart fibers simultaneously. In addition, since current is discharged over a greater surface area, larger paddles limit the risk of myocardial injury by decreasing the current density passing through each unit of myocardium. Most conventional paddles have an electrode diameter of at least 4 inches.

The ideal placement of the paddle on the chest wall has been debated ever since the inception of cardioversion. Two systems have been used traditionally in clinical practice: (1) the anterolateral position, with one paddle placed in the left fourth to fifth intercostal space, mid–axillary line and the other just to the right of the sternal margin in the second to third intercostal space (Fig. 10–4); and (2) the anteroposterior position, with one paddle placed anteriorly over the sternum and the other on the back between the scapulae (Fig. 10–5). Many of the newer cardioverter-defibrillators are specifically designed for anterolateral paddle placement. Anteroposterior paddle placement may be more convenient in elective cases, since the operator manipulates only one paddle during the procedure of cardioversion, but this position of paddle placement may be inconvenient in an emergency. Either method of paddle placement is acceptable in clinical practice. Kerber and associates demonstrated that transthoracic resistance, paddle size, or paddle position has no relationship to the energy required or the incidence of successful elective cardioversion in patients with atrial flutter or atrial fibrillation.[5]

Generous use of EKG paste or defibrillator gel pads on the underside and, especially, along the edges of the electrode paddles is essential, both to reduce transthoracic impedance and to prevent skin burns. Paste should be applied liberally but must never run between paddles if the anterolateral approach is used, since the paste may cause current (which always seeks the path of least resistance) to be diverted over the skin surface

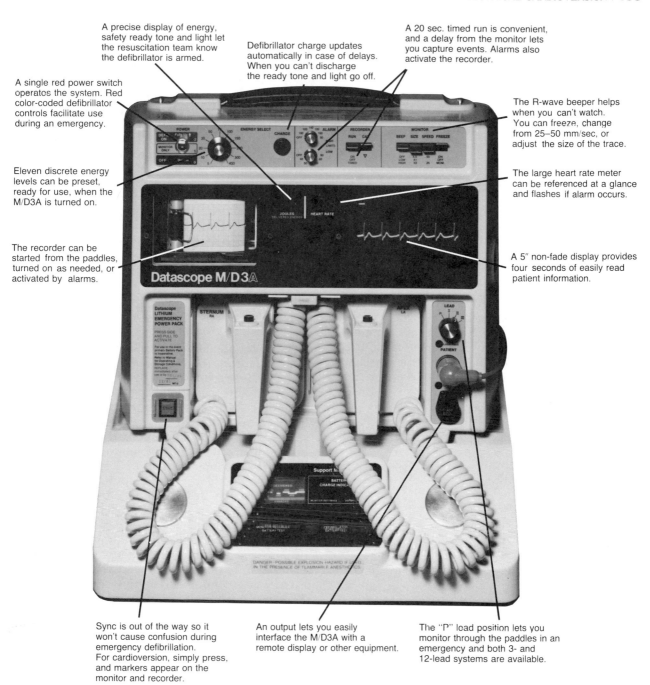

A precise display of energy, safety ready tone and light let the resuscitation team know the defibrillator is armed.

A single red power switch operates the system. Red color-coded defibrillator controls facilitate use during an emergency.

Defibrillator charge updates automatically in case of delays. When you can't discharge the ready tone and light go off.

A 20 sec. timed run is convenient, and a delay from the monitor lets you capture events. Alarms also activate the recorder.

The R-wave beeper helps when you can't watch. You can freeze, change from 25–50 mm/sec, or adjust the size of the trace.

Eleven discrete energy levels can be preset, ready for use, when the M/D3A is turned on.

The large heart rate meter can be referenced at a glance and flashes if alarm occurs.

The recorder can be started from the paddles, turned on as needed, or activated by alarms.

A 5″ non-fade display provides four seconds of easily read patient information.

Sync is out of the way so it won't cause confusion during emergency defibrillation. For cardioversion, simply press, and markers appear on the monitor and recorder.

An output lets you easily interface the M/D3A with a remote display or other equipment.

The "P" load position lets you monitor through the paddles in an emergency and both 3- and 12-lead systems are available.

Figure 10–3. Typical converter–defibrillator monitor with display screen and readout. (Courtesy of Datascope Corporation, Paramus, New Jersey.)

and away from the heart. This is a crucial consideration, since (even under ideal circumstances) only 10 to 30 per cent of the total current passes through the heart. Saline-soaked pads are generally not practical or safe for the aforementioned reasons.

Before cardioversion, the patient should assume the prone position and should be as relaxed as possible, with an intravenous line and supplemental oxygen in place. The cardiac rhythm is under constant surveillance by the oscilloscope on the cardioverter. In order to ensure discharge of the current at the appropriate time, one should choose the lead that displays the highest R wave amplitude. When it is activated in the synchronized mode, the cardioverter will automatically discharge when it "reads" a regular recurrent R wave. It is preferred to have the monitor sense the electrical activity through standard electrode leads rather than through the paddles.

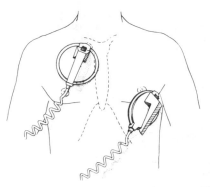

Figure 10–4. Anteroapical paddle electrode position. (From Suratt, P. M., and Gibson, R. S.: Manual of Medical Procedures. St. Louis, C. V. Mosby, 1982. Used by permission.)

Anesthesia is required in the conscious patient.[6] Intravenous diazepam (Valium) is an excellent amnestic, and it is preferred by most physicians for this purpose.[7] The dosage is 5 mg initially, followed by increments of 2.5 mg every 3 minutes until adequate sedation is achieved. Slurred speech or nystagmus on lateral gaze correlates well with effective sedation. The average dose required for sedation is 15 mg, but there is consid-

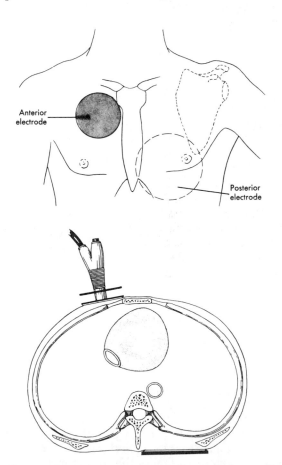

Figure 10–5. Anteroposterior paddle electrode position. (From Suratt, P. M., and Gibson, R. S.: Manual of Medical Procedures. St. Louis, C.V. Mosby, 1982. Used by permission.)

erable patient-to-patient variability. Because of its negative inotropic effect, however, diazepam must be used cautiously in the patient with congestive heart failure. In addition, apparatus for endotracheal intubation must be available in the event that respiratory depression becomes profound. Some clinicians prefer a short-acting barbiturate,[8] such as methohexital sodium (Brevital), for anesthesia, since this agent is more effective than diazepam as an amnestic and has a shorter duration of action. The dosage is 5 to 12 ml of a 1 per cent solution.

Ampules of lidocaine, atropine, and other antidysrhythmics must be immediately available at the bedside should life-threatening ventricular ectopy or bradycardia ensue following attempts at cardioversion.

Technique of Cardioversion

The technique of cardioversion is essentially the same regardless of the dysrhythmia.[9] One proceeds to the cardioverter, turning the power on and setting the unit on the synchronized mode. A common error in an emergency is to neglect to set the machine in the synchronized mode, since most equipment is routinely stored in the nonsynchronized mode in anticipation of ventricular fibrillation. Two to 10 seconds are required for the capacitor to warm up and the charge button to light up. One selects the desired energy by choosing the corresponding number on the dial labeled "energy select." One should begin at the lowest practical energy for the specific dysrhythmia and should increase the power gradually if cardioversion is unsuccessful and the clinical situation permits. A useful role of thumb in elective cases is to begin at 25 joules in adults, increasing to 50, 100, 150, 200, 250, 300, 350, and 400 joules in succession as needed. If the patient is taking digitalis, one should begin at 5 to 10 joules and should proceed in increments of 5 to 10 joules.[4] In the clinical setting of acute coronary or cerebral ischemia, myocardial infarction, pulmonary edema, or cardiovascular collapse aggravated or caused by the patient's dysrhythmia, one should select an energy that is most likely to produce immediate cardioversion. In the adult, a 150- to 200-joule initial shock is acceptable. In a child, the initial energy setting of 2 joules per kg is satisfactory. *Note: One should always be prepared for the development of ventricular fibrillation or asystole following cardioversion.*

Irregular rhythms, such as atrial fibrillation or atrial flutter with variable block, may not be converted with the synchronized mode and may require unsynchronized shock. The chance occurrence of ventricular fibrillation following unsynchronized cardioversion is approximately 2 per cent,[4] although some authors will routinely use no synchronizer during the procedure.[10] If no synchronizer is used, it is important to use a higher energy level to ensure depolarization of all myocardial fibers and to lessen the chance for ventricular fibrillation.

Prior to cardioversion with the monitor sensing the rhythm through standard leads, the operator should check the accuracy of discharge within the cardiac cycle by placing the paddles against each other and discharging the current.[3] One should observe where the blip discharge artifact occurs on the monitor. The blip must coincide with the peak of the R wave. One must be absolutely certain that the monitor screen is free of artifact before proceeding to the patient. The capacitor may inadvertently interpret artifact as R waves, with potentially disastrous results. Likewise, improper synchronization may occur in the patient with tall T waves or in the presence of right bundle branch block. The lead that best shows the R wave should always be chosen for monitoring, since the cardioverter only "senses" the QRS complex that appears on the screen.

The patient's skin must never be in contact with metal on the stretcher, and all bystanders must remove themselves from the stretcher prior to cardioversion. The operator should place the well-lubricated paddles firmly against the chest wall in the appropriate positions. Firm paddle contact is essential in order to minimize transthoracic impedance and to ensure proper contact. Approximately 20 lb of contact pressure is desired. *The operator should not be in contact with the stretcher or the patient at the time of cardioversion in order to avoid the potential of self-injury.* One should warn ancillary staff that countershock is imminent by shouting "all clear." The operator should press the buttons on the paddles to discharge current during exhalation when the thoracic impedance is minimized. There will be a delay of a few moments before the current is discharged, so one must maintain constant contact with the chest wall. The patient's response is heralded by a twitch of the thoracic muscles, a jerk of the arms, and an audible sigh. If cardioversion is successful, the monitor will usually reveal sinus bradycardia initially. This will be followed by a gradually accelerating rate as the sinus node warms up.[11] If normal sinus rhythm is obtained, the operator should stop. If the dysrhythmia persists, patient clinical status permitting, one should wait at least 3 minutes before proceeding to the next energy level. If ventricular fibrillation occurs, one should *switch off the synchronizer* and defibrillate *immediately*. Following successful cardioversion, the patient should be monitored in a critical care setting for at least 24 hours; proper antidysrhythmic medication should be given to prevent recurrence.

Drug Therapy and Cardioversion

All efforts should be made to ensure that there is a proper electrolyte and acid-base balance and adequate oxygenation before cardioversion is attempted.

There is no convincing evidence that quinidine or any other antidysrhythmic drug given *routinely* immediately before cardioversion reduces the energy requirements, increases the chance for success, or helps maintain sinus rhythm afterward. Medication may, however, prevent premature beats following cardioversion. In elective cases, some physicians prefer to have patients receive maintenance quinidine therapy before cardioversion of atrial fibrillation and to withhold digitalis for 48 hours prior to cardioversion. Such protocols are impossible in the unstable patient requiring emergency cardioversion.

As a routine approach to patients requiring emergency cardioversion of *non–digitalis-toxic* rhythms, no prophylactic medications are given. If premature ventricular beats occur following unsuccessful cardioversion, they should be suppressed with intravenous lidocaine in 50- to 75-mg bolus injections (or equivalent doses of procainamide) before one proceeds to the next higher energy level. It should be remembered that such drugs may depress pacemaker function as well as suppress ectopic beats. If persistent after successful cardioversion, premature ventricular contractions (PVCs) may indicate digitalis toxicity or electrolyte disturbance and should be treated accordingly. Lidocaine, procainamide, or phenytoin may be helpful. A few transient PVCs frequently occur following cardioversion and need not be treated. Persistent bradycardia or asystole following cardioversion should be treated with intravenous atropine (1.0 to 2.0 mg).

Patients with *digitalis-toxic* rhythms present a particularly difficult problem. Fortunately, most digitalis-toxic rhythms need not be treated with cardioversion. Digitalis significantly lowers the direct current threshold for ventricular tachycardia and ventricular fibrillation in dogs, but direct current cardioversion appears safe in converting supraventricular dysrhythmias in patients receiving maintenance digitalis therapy who have no evidence of digitalis toxicity, acute myocardial ischemia, or electrolyte disturbance.[12] The potential for malignant ventricular rhythms or ventricular fibrillation following cardioversion in the presence of digitalis toxicity has long been recognized (Fig. 10–6). When emergency cardioversion is required in patients with digitalis toxicity, it appears prudent to pretreat with prophylactic intravenous lidocaine (75 to 100 mg), phenytoin (100 to 200 mg), or procainamide (75 to 100 mg) *before* cardioversion and to check serum potassium levels on a

AFTER 200 WATT SECS COUNTERSHOCK

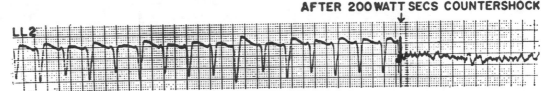

Figure 10–6. Ventricular fibrillation following countershock in the presence of digitalis toxicity (lead 2). Control shows junctional paroxysmal tachycardia (rate, 150 beats per minute), probably the result of digitalis toxicity. Note the occurrence of ventricular fibrillation following countershock at arrow. (From Bellet, S.: Clinical Disorders of the Heart Beat, 3rd ed. Philadelphia, Lea & Febiger, 1971. Used by permission.)

stat basis. Propranolol has been advocated, but it should be administered with the concomitant use of atropine to prevent asystole or bradycardia following cardioversion. In addition to administering prophylactic medication, one should reduce the energy used in this situation by 10 to 15 joules.[13-15]

Indications and Contraindications

Cardioversion is indicated on an emergency basis when cardiac dysrhythmias are complicated by the presence of significant hypotension, congestive heart failure, chest pain suggesting myocardial ischemia, or evidence of cerebral ischemia. Rapid cardioversion is also advocated when the ventricular rate exceeds 180, especially in the elderly patient, because of the risk of imminent hemodynamic compromise.[11] Cardioversion is useful on a less urgent basis in the patient with a cardiac dysrhythmia refractory to conventional drug therapy. It is a common tendency and a common error to delay cardioversion in a compromised patient in the hope that drug therapy will prove successful. Such a timid approach should be avoided, since the outcome of procrastination may be cardiac arrest.

A history or suspicion of digitalis toxicity is a relative contraindication to the use of emergency cardioversion; alternatives to cardioversion are preferable in this case. A therapeutic digitalis level, however, is not a contraindication to cardioversion. Slow atrial fibrillation, usually secondary to ischemic heart disease if not digitalis-related, is also a relative contraindication. Restoration of sinus rhythm in this setting may result in an even slower ventricular rate, which may worsen the patient's condition. Likewise, patients known to be in the tachycardiac phase of sick sinus syndrome may develop asystole following cardioversion, and thus the procedure is also contraindicated in this instance. Intravenous overdrive pacing is preferable in these settings. The presence of myocardial infarction is *not* a contraindication to cardioversion.

Specific Dysrhythmias Treatable by Cardioversion

Cardioversion is effective in terminating a variety of cardiac dysrhythmias. In an emergency situation, any dysrhythmia associated with a rapid ventricular rate may be treated with cardioversion. Specific indications are discussed in the following paragraphs.

VENTRICULAR TACHYCARDIA

Cardioversion is successful in converting ventricular tachycardia in over 95 per cent of cases.[4] In the stable patient, drug therapy is advocated as the first-line treatment. The energy required for effective termination of ventricular tachycardia is almost always less than 100 joules, and 10 joules will convert approximately 80 per cent of cases. An initial setting of 25 to 50 joules is suggested.

If ventricular tachycardia occurs at rapid rates with bizarre and widened QRS intervals, a broad, prominent T wave may not be distinguished from the QRS complex. This has been termed "ventricular tachycardia of the vulnerable period," or ventricular flutter.[2] In such a setting, the cardioverter apparatus may not be able to separate the T wave from the QRS complex. Synchronized cardioversion under these circumstances may be dangerous, since there is a 50 per cent chance that current will be discharged during the peak of the T wave or the vulnerable period of the cardiac cycle. Nonsynchronized cardioversion of at least 100 joules is preferable in these instances. The chance occurrence of ventricular fibrillation in association with asynchronized cardioversion is 2 per cent, and one may minimize this small risk further by delivering a shock of sufficient energy to depolarize all myocardial fibers instantaneously. This requires an electrical current of at least 1 ampere. In clinical practice, a shock of 100 joules or greater will accomplish this. Immediately following conversion of ventricular tachycardia, antidysrhythmic medication should be given to prevent recurrence.

ATRIAL FLUTTER

Atrial flutter is ideally suited to cardioversion. Atrial flutter is difficult to convert with drug therapy, which must often be given to the point of toxicity, but sinus rhythm is easily achieved through cardioversion. Success has been reported in 72 to 100 per cent of cases,[2, 4, 16, 17] with most investigators reporting success in over 90 per cent of patients. Cardioversion is now considered the treatment of choice for atrial flutter, even in stable patients. Low energies generally will suffice, and a shock of 25 to 50 joules is usually successful on the first attempt.[2] Some cases that do not immediately change to sinus rhythm may instead convert to atrial fibrillation,[18] especially after an initial countershock of low intensity (10 to 20 joules). These cases will usually convert to sinus rhythm with the use of higher energies.

ATRIAL FIBRILLATION

Cardioversion is effective in the majority of cases of atrial fibrillation, the most common disorder of the heart beat, although there is a smaller immediate and long-term success rate than in cases of atrial flutter.[2-4, 19-22] If atrial fibrillation in the absence of demonstrable heart disease (idiopathic, or "lone," atrial fibrillation) is excluded, success rates approach 90 per cent. Atrial fibrillation seldom requires cardioversion on an emergency basis, and chronic or recurrent cases are best managed with drug therapy.

Duration of the rhythm is the single most important factor affecting successful cardioversion of atrial fibrillation. An average of 100 joules is required when atrial fibrillation has been present for less than 3 months, in contrast to an average of 150 joules when the rhythm has persisted for more than 6 months.[2] The chance of successful conversion or the maintenance of sinus rhythm is decreased in the presence of an enlarged left atrium, atrial fibrillation of longer than 1 year's duration, chronic mitral valve disease, and atrial fibrillation in the setting of left ventricular failure. If slow atrial fibrillation is encountered in the absence of cardiac medication, the use of cardioversion is dangerous and the procedure should not be attempted, since serious bradycardia may result.

The size of the fibrillatory, or F, wave in the V_1 lead is a reliable predictor of the energy requirements for conversion of atrial fibrillation to sinus rhythm.[2] The energy is inversely proportional to the size of the F wave. On the average, 140 joules is needed when the F wave is 1 mm in height, whereas approximately 90 joules is required when the F wave measures 2 mm.

SUPRAVENTRICULAR TACHYCARDIA

Most cases of supraventricular tachycardia can be treated with carotid sinus massage (see Chapter 9) or drug therapy, but in a series studied by Vassaux and Lown, cardioversion was successful in terminating 70 per cent of cases of supraventricular tachycardia (paroxysmal atrial tachycardia [PAT] with block, paroxysmal atrial tachycardia, and junctional tachycardias).[23] Most failures occurred in the presence of PAT with block, a rhythm that is often a manifestation of digitalis toxicity. When PAT with block is successfully converted to sinus rhythm, it often occurs at low energies. Patients who fail to convert generally respond as though they are overdigitalized, with further deterioration of the rhythm.

The most important factor complicating the approach in the case of the patient with supraventricular tachycardia is the presence of digitalis. Cardioversion is dangerous in the patient who is taking digitalis, and low energies must always be used in this setting.[13-15]

Cardioversion may actually be helpful diagnostically in determining whether a dysrhythmia is digitalis-related.[24] If attempts at cardioversion are met with increasing degrees of atrioventricular block or PVCs, then digitalis toxicity should be suspected. If the atrial rate increases following unsuccessful cardioversion, then digitalis toxicity is invariably present.

Paroxysmal atrial tachycardia is a common dysrhythmia during pregnancy, especially in the third trimester. Schroeder and Harrison used cardioversion successfully during all three trimesters of pregnancy without serious side effects to mother or fetus.[25] Fetal rhythm should be monitored when cardioversion is attempted during the third trimester of pregnancy, although the risk of inducing fetal dysrhythmias is small, since the effective energy reaching the fetus is exceedingly low.[2]

Complications

In 1970, Resnekov reported a 14.5 per cent overall incidence of complications following cardioversion, excluding minor complications, such as superficial skin burns, slight muscle discomfort, and transient bradycardia immediately after shock. The complication rate is profoundly dose-related (Fig. 10–7). At 150 joules, the incidence of complications is only 6 per cent, whereas at 400 joules, the incidence rises to greater than 30 per cent.[4]

Dysrhythmias are a frequent complication following cardioversion.[26] Usually, they are benign and transient. The establishment of a temporary nodal rhythm before the sinus node takes over is

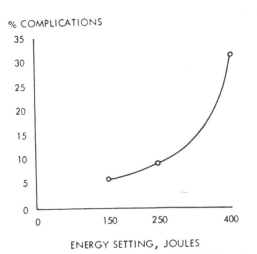

% COMPLICATIONS

ENERGY SETTING, JOULES

Figure 10–7. Percentage of complications in 220 patients treated by countershock related to the maximum energy setting used. ≦150 joules, 108 patients; ≦250 joules, 55 patients; ≦400 joules 37 patients. (From Resnekov, L.: Theory and practice of electroversion in cardiac dysrhythmias. Med. Clin. North Am. 60:325, 1976. Used by permission.)

quite common, as are PVCs and bigeminy. These transient dysrhythmias need not be treated if they follow conversion of a supraventricular rhythm. Frequent or multifocal PVCs are a warning of impending ventricular dysrhythmias and should be abolished with intravenous medication. Antidysrhythmic medication should always be given following cardioversion of ventricular tachycardia.

The incidence of serious ventricular dysrhythmias following cardioversion is proportional to the energy requirement.[26] Lown observed that the risk of ventricular tachycardia in dogs was 3 per cent at 100 joules, rose to 25 per cent at 200 joules, and was 65 per cent at 400 joules. He likewise reemphasized the danger of cardioversion in the presence of digitalis by demonstrating an 8000-fold increase in sensitivity to electrical shock in dog models following administration of toxic doses of ouabain.[2] Patients with enlarged hearts are also at increased risk of developing ventricular dysrhythmias following cardioversion.

The incidence of ventricular fibrillation has been reported to be 0.8 per cent following synchronized cardioversion and is essentially of two types. The first (more benign) variety occurs immediately after countershock and is easily reversed by a second, nonsynchronized shock. This type of ventricular fibrillation results from improper synchronization, with discharge of current occurring during the vulnerable period. The second variety, which is more ominous, occurs approximately 30 seconds to a few minutes following attempted cardioversion. This dysrhythmia is characteristically preceded by the development of PAT with block or a junctional rhythm. In affected patients, it may be very difficult to convert the dysrhythmia to a sinus rhythm. This phenomenon occurs in

patients who have been taking digitalis glycosides and is presumably a manifestation of digitalis toxicity.[27, 28]

An increase in serum enzyme levels (CPK, LDH, SGOT) may also occur following cardioversion, and the incidence has been reported to be between 10 and 70 per cent.[2, 4, 27] The enzyme rise is usually a consequence of skeletal muscle injury rather than myocardial damage. Transient ST segment elevation occurs in 3 per cent of cases but does not necessarily indicate myocardial injury, as subsequent cardiac scanning of these patients has shown.[29] Cardioversion does not alter the enzyme profile of patients with myocardial infarction.[30]

Myocardial damage may occur as a consequence of countershock and is usually subepicardial in location.[2] The risk is a function of many variables, including the strength and number of shocks; impedance of the heart, the ribs, and the skin; the size of the electrodes; the use of EKG paste versus saline pads and creams; and the interval between successive shocks.[31] In general, smaller and fewer shocks, lower impedance, large electrodes, use of EKG paste or gel pads, and intervals of at least 3 minutes between shocks will minimize the risk of myocardial injury.

Pulmonary and systemic embolization occurs in approximately 1.5 per cent of patients following cardioversion.[2, 4, 22] This risk, however, is negligible in patients who have previously undergone anticoagulation therapy. Lown reported that the incidence of embolism following cardioversion of atrial fibrillation was 1.2 per cent in a series of 450 patients, with a zero incidence in the 100 patients who received anticoagulation therapy before countershock. Such observations raise the issue of the value of prophylactic anticoagulation before cardioversion. Although this measure may be impractical in the emergency situation, the use of intravenous heparin has been advocated when there is an increased risk of embolism, such as in patients with myocardial infarction, coronary artery disease, mitral valve disease, cardiomyopathy, prosthetic heart valves, or history of a previous embolic event.[2]

A puzzling complication of cardioversion that has been reported periodically is the development of pulmonary edema approximately 1 to 3 hours following successful cardioversion.[32-35] With the exception of one case, it has occurred exclusively following conversion to normal sinus rhythm, thus developing paradoxically in cases in which improved cardiac output would be expected. Myocardial damage secondary to countershock was originally implicated in these cases of pulmonary edema, but it has since been shown that this complication occurs regardless of the strength or the number of shocks, factors that are known to increase the risk of myocardial injury. One of the more popular current theories is that the development of pulmonary edema represents a defect in contractile capacity of the left atrium relative to the right atrium.

Other miscellaneous complications that have been reported in the literature include pericarditis,[36] pneumonitis, hypotension, ocular damage,[37] transient left recurrent laryngeal nerve paralysis, and compression fractures of the thoracic vertebrae.[38]

Summary

The overall success rate of direct current cardioversion in the presence of cardiac dysrhythmias approaches 90 per cent. Countershock is a relatively recent therapeutic modality that combines safety, ease of operation, and efficacy when used properly. It is an invaluable tool in the emergency department setting when cardiac dysrhythmias are complicated by the presence or threat of hemodynamic compromise. Extreme caution must be exercised in patients who are taking digitalis as well as those with sick sinus syndrome, and electrical cardioversion is relatively contraindicated in these groups. Cardioversion is most effective in the presence of ventricular tachycardia and atrial flutter, although it is also frequently successful in cases of atrial fibrillation and a variety of supraventricular tachycardias. The lowest practical energy setting should be used initially, since complications are directly proportional to shock strength.

1. Driscol, T., Ratnoff, O., and Nygaard, O. F.: The remarkable Dr. Abildgaard and countershock. Ann. Intern. Med. 83:878, 1972.
2. DeSilva, R. A., et al.: Cardioversion and defibrillation. Am. Heart J. 100:881, 1980.
3. Lown, B., et al.: "Cardioversion" of atrial fibrillation. N. Engl. J. Med. 269:325, 1963.
4. Resnekov, L.: Theory and practice of electroversion in cardiac dysrhythmias. Med. Clin. North Am. 60:325, 1976.
5. Kerber, R. E., et al.: Elective cardioversion: Influence of paddle-electrode location and size on success rates and energy requirements. N. Engl. J. Med. 305:658, 1981.
6. Orko, R.: Anesthesia for cardioversion: A comparison of diazepam, thiopentone, and propanidid. Br. J. Anaesth. 48:257, 1976.
7. Kahler, R. I., Burrow, G. H., and Felig, P.: Diazepam-induced amnesia for cardioversion. JAMA 200:997, 1967.
8. Coe, E.: Anesthesia for elective cardioversion. (letter) N. Engl. J. Med. 299:262, 1978.
9. Lown, B., Klieger, R., and Wolff, G.: The technique of cardioversion. Am. Heart J. 67:282, 1964.
10. Kreus, K. E., Salokannel, S. J., and Waris, E. K.: Non-synchronized and synchronized direct-current countershock in cardiac arrhythmias. Lancet 2:405, 1966.
11. Isselbacher, K. J., et al. (eds.): Harrison's Principles and Practice of Internal Medicine, 9th ed. New York, McGraw-Hill, 1980, pp. 1072–1073.
12. Ditchey, R. V., and Karlinger, J. S.: Safety of electrical cardioversion without digitalis toxicity. Ann. Intern. Med. 95:676, 1981.
13. Hagemeijer, F., and Van Houwe, E.: Titrated energy cardioversion of patients on digitalis. Br. Heart J. 37:1303, 1975.
14. Szekely, P., Wynne, N. A., Pearson, D. T., Barson, G. A., and Sideris, D. A.: Direct current shock and digitalis. Br. Heart J. 31:91, 1969.
15. Klieger, R., and Lown, B.: Cardioversion and digitalis II: Clinical studies. Circulation 33:878, 1966.
16. Morris, J. J., et al.: Experience with cardioversion of atrial fibrillation and flutter. Am. J. Cardiol. 14:94, 1964.
17. Frithz, G., and Aberg, H.: Direct current cardioversion of atrial flutter. Acta Med. Scand. 187:271, 1970.
18. Guiney, T. E., and Lown, B.: Electrical conversion of atrial flutter to atrial fibrillation-flutter mechanism in man. Br. Heart J. 34:1215, 1972.
19. Morris, J. J., Peter, R. H., and MacIntosh, H. D.: Electrical conversion of atrial fibrillation—immediate and long term results and selection of patients. Ann. Intern. Med. 65:216, 1966.
20. Szekely, P., Batson, G., and Stark, D. C.: Direct current shock treatment of cardiac arrhythmias. Br. Heart J. 28:366, 1966.
21. Bjerkelund, C., and Ornig, O. M.: Evaluation of direct current shock therapy of atrial arrhythmias. Acta Med. Scand. 184:481, 1968.
22. Razavi, M., Duarte, E., and Tahmooressi, P.: Cardioversion: Ten year Cleveland clinic experience. Cleve. Clin. Q. 43:175, 1976.
23. Vassaux, C., and Lown, B.: Cardioversion of supraventricular tachycardia. Circulation 39:791, 1969.
24. Gilbert, R., and Cuddy, R. P.: Digitalis intoxication following cardioversion to sinus rhythm. Circulation 32:58, 1965.
25. Schroeder, J. S., and Harrison, D. C.: Repeated cardioversion during pregnancy. Am. J. Cardiol. 27:445, 1971.
26. Donoso, E., et al.: Ventricular arrhythmias after precordial shock. Am. Heart J. 73:595, 1967.
27. Aberg, H., and Cullhed, I.: Direct current countershock complications. Acta Med. Scand. 183:415, 1968.
28. Ross, E. M.: Cardioversion causing ventricular fibrillation. Arch. Intern. Med. 114:811, 1964.
29. Chun, P., Davia, J., and Donohue, D.: ST-segment elevation with elective DC cardioversion. Circulation 63:220, 1981.
30. Reiffel, J., McCarthy, D. M., and Leahey, E. B.: Does DC cardioversion affect isoenzyme recognition of myocardial infarction? Am. Heart J. 97:6, 1979.
31. Dahl, C. F., Ewy, G. A., Warner, E. D., and Thomas, E. D.: Myocardial necrosis from direct current discharge. Effect of paddle electrode size and time interval between discharges. Circulation 50:956, 1974.
32. Sutton, R. B., and Tsagaris, T. O.: Pulmonary edema following direct current cardioversion. Chest 57:191, 1970.
33. Resnekov, L., and McDonald, L.: Pulmonary edema following treatment of arrhythmias by direct current shock. Lancet 1:506, 1965.
34. Budow, J., Natarajan, P., and Kroop, I. G.: Pulmonary edema following direct current cardioversion for atrial arrhythmias. JAMA 218:1803, 1971.
35. Lindsey, J., Jr.: Pulmonary edema following cardioversion. Am. Heart J. 74:434, 1967.
36. Strom, S.: Pericarditis following cardioversion. A case report. Acta Med. Scand. 195:431, 1974.
37. Berger, R. O.: Ocular complications of cardioversion. Ann. Ophthalmol. 10:161, 1978.
38. Okel, B. B.: Vertebral fracture from cardioversion shock (letter). JAMA 203:369, 1968.

11

Defibrillation

MICHAEL I. GREENBERG, M.D.
JERRIS R. HEDGES, M.D.

Introduction

Defibrillation is the conversion of ventricular fibrillation to an alternative (preferably supraventricular) rhythm. Ventricular fibrillation (VF) is incompatible with life. VF is often associated with myocardial ischemia or infarction, marked electrolyte disturbances, electrical injuries, pronounced hypothermia, or drug toxicity (e.g., that caused by tricyclic antidepressants, quinidine, and digitalis). Although brief periods of VF with spontaneous reversion to a sinus rhythm have been recorded, VF is usually irreversible without electrical countershock.[1]

VF is the primary cause of sudden cardiac death.[2] The majority of victims of sudden death have *not* suffered a myocardial infarction, although most have advanced coronary disease and often have poor ventricular function.[2-4] Furthermore, survivors of sudden death attributable to VF are at increased risk of suffering a recurrence.[2, 4, 5]

With the advent of portable defibrillation units and prehospital cardiac resuscitation teams, the challenge of early defibrillation of the sudden death patient in VF is being aggressively addressed. More than 40 per cent of prehospital VF cardiac arrest victims can be saved if cardiac massage and ventilation are provided promptly (in less than 4 minutes) and followed by advanced cardiac resuscitation (within 8 minutes).[6-8] Prompt, effective defibrillation is equally important for in-hospital VF cardiac arrests; physicians and nurses alike must be thoroughly familiar with this procedure.

Background

The concept of electrical shock therapy in resuscitation can be traced to the experiments of Abildgaard in the eighteenth century. Abildgaard described chickens as "lifeless" following electrical shocks and noted successful resuscitation after the use of additional shocks. Subsequent animal stud-

ies were reported by Preust and Batell.[9] In 1947 the first successful human defibrillation using the direct application of electrical current to the heart was reported by Beck and coworkers.[10] Nine years later, Zoll and associates reported the first successful cardiac defibrillation using an alternating current (AC) electrical shock applied externally to the thorax.[11]

Portable direct current (DC) defibrillators were introduced by Lown and colleagues[12] and Edmark and coworkers[94] during the 1960s. DC defibrillators opened the way for prehospital defibrillation.[2, 4, 6, 13] Although the basic design of modern defibrillators has changed little since the 1960s, modifications in paddle size, energy delivered, energy waveform, conducting materials, and pharmacologic enhancement of defibrillation have been recent areas of research. These topics will be discussed later in this chapter.

Indications and Contraindications

Electrical defibrillation of the heart in VF is indicated whenever immediate spontaneous conversion to a perfusing rhythm does not occur. The need to ensure that the sudden death patient is in VF prior to defibrillation is no longer an issue with the advent of "quick-look" paddles, which permit immediate monitoring of the patient's rhythm prior to electrical defibrillation. Unresponsive patients with regular tachydysrhythmias are best treated with synchronized cardioversion (see Chapter 10), although if monitoring capabilities are not immediately available, an initial unsynchronized countershock may be lifesaving.

Although the timing of defibrillation has been debated, an initial electrical shock applied to the sudden death patient prior to drug administration is currently recommended.[14, 15] In most resuscitations, cardiac massage and ventilations are initiated while the defibrillator is being readied. If the patient is unconscious, apneic, and pulseless, it is reasonable to assume that an episode of VF is taking place if cardiac monitoring is not available. In such instances, an immediate attempt at defibrillation is warranted. Although asystole and, more rarely, ventricular tachycardia may occur in a similar fashion, an immediate countershock is unlikely to affect either clinical situation adversely. Defibrillation countershock is otherwise contraindicated in the patient with a rhythm other than VF, or perhaps ventricular flutter. Since VF can occasionally masquerade as ventricular standstill or asystole, monitoring paddle electrodes should be rotated 90 degrees from their original position before the decision *not* to defibrillate the sudden death patient is made (Fig. 11–1).[16] Low-voltage VF likewise is *not* a contraindication to defibrillation, since this may reflect low monitor gain or

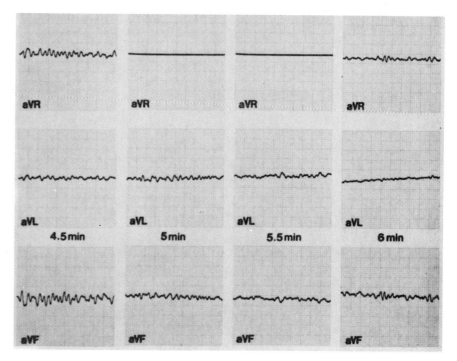

Figure 11–1. Leads aVR, aVL, and aVF from an animal with electrically induced VF. From onset to 4½ minutes, VF waves were obvious in all six frontal plane leads. At 5 minutes and 5½ minutes, lead aVR was a straight line. Note that aVR is the electrical sum of leads aVL and aVF. By 6 minutes, the null vector had changed and VF was again evident in all six frontal plane leads. (From Ewy, G. A., et al.: Ventricular fibrillation masquerading as ventricular standstill. Crit. Care Med. 9:841, 1981. Used by permission.)

monitor lead/paddle placement. *Repeated* countershocks are contraindicated before optimal oxygenation, acid/base status, and body temperature have been reached, since these derangements may make the heart refractory to countershock. In addition, repeated countershocks may produce tissue damage.

Characteristics of Ventricular Fibrillation

Electrocardiographically, VF is characterized by the presence of low-amplitude baseline undulations that are variable in both amplitude and periodicity. Although often considered to represent an electrically random process, electrical directionality to depolarization (i.e., wavefronts) may exist.[16] Mechanically, VF represents an uncoordinated, disorderly contractile process. The absence of effective contractile function abolishes tissue perfusion and leads to death.

At the tissue level, VF represents a disorganization of the orderly depolarization sequence that usually occurs in the ventricles. Normally, the refractory period of depolarized muscle prevents the development of re-entrant ventricular rhythms. When ischemia, electrolyte disorders, cardiac drug toxicities, rapid ventricular rates, hypothermia, and certain other disorders exist, refractory periods may shorten or conduction velocities may increase in certain areas of the ventricle.

Wandering depolarization wavefronts that become self-perpetuating can develop. A combination of disorders of impulse formation (automaticity) and impulse conduction (re-entry) generally contribute to the development of VF.[17, 18] The tendency for VF is enhanced by, but is not dependent upon, premature ventricular impulses occurring during the "vulnerable" period of the cardiac cycle represented by early ventricular repolarization (T wave).[95]

Asynchronous ventricular depolarization may be confined to a small area of the ventricle if the remaining ventricle is refractory to further stimulation. Several studies have shown that a critical muscle mass is required for VF to be self-sustaining.[19, 20] A large mass of muscle involved in asynchronous depolarization having a brief refractory period and a slow conduction velocity will increase the tendency for the ventricles to fibrillate.

BASIS FOR DEFIBRILLATION

Electrical defibrillation represents the simultaneous depolarization of sufficient ventricular tissue to render the tissue ahead of the VF wavefronts refractory to further electrical conduction. Following generalized depolarization, the sinus node or other pacemaker region of the heart with the highest degree of automaticity can then acquire dominance of a well-ordered depolarization-repolarization sequence.

Defibrillator Characteristics

General standards[21] and product evaluations[22] for cardiac defibrillation devices are beyond the scope of this chapter. This section will discuss the major components and design configurations of a defibrillator and how they relate to effective defibrillation.

WAVEFORMS

Although the first successful human defibrillation was performed using alternating current,[10] Lown and coworkers were able to demonstrate that direct current is more effective than alternating current in defibrillation and produces a much lower incidence of postcardioversion arrhythmias.[12] Only DC defibrillators are in clinical use today. Most of the modern defibrillators use a damped half-sinusoidal waveform or a trapezoidal (truncated exponential decay) waveform. The trapezoidal waveform can be modified to resemble a square waveform. The more square the waveform, the more effective it is for experimental defibrillation.[23, 24] Furthermore, in a comparison of square waveforms and damped half-sinusoidal waveforms for animal defibrillation, it was found that less peak current per kilogram was needed with the square waveforms, although the average current levels were equivalent.[25] Furthermore, the delivered waveform is dependent upon thoracic resistance.[24] In clinical practice, however, there is little difference in the effectiveness of the currently available waveforms.

STORED ENERGY

Since the ability to defibrillate is dependent upon current delivered to the myocardium, the stored energy is one factor that, coupled with transthoracic impedance and internal defibrillator energy loss, contributes to successful defibrillation. Each defibrillator is calibrated by measuring the current delivered as a function of time across a 50-ohm impedance. Defibrillators do not always deliver the energy indicated on the device. With a "stored" energy of 400 watt-sec (400 J), anywhere from 155 to 410 watt-sec may be delivered.[26-28] Obviously, any increase in transthoracic impedance will further reduce delivered energy.

DEVICE SWITCHES

Many portable (capable of battery operation) defibrillators have separate power switches for the accompanying monitor and recorder and for the defibrillator. Before attempting defibrillation, the physician must be familiar with the location and operation of the controls lest he attempt to defibrillate a patient when the defibrillator portion has yet to be turned on. One defibrillator in common usage is shown in Figure 10–3.

Defibrillators also have a control permitting synchronous cardioversion. The physician must be sure that the control is set to the asynchronous mode to permit defibrillation; otherwise, the device in the synchronous mode would wait indefinitely for a nonexistent repetitive series of R waves prior to discharging.

Energy settings may be determined by a switch or a dial setting or may be read off a meter permitting a continuous range of settings. In each case the physician must be aware of the need for initially charging the device and recharging after each discharge. The mechanism of charging the device may be intrinsic to the setting of the dial or meter but more commonly requires the use of a separate charge button on the device control panel or paddle handle. Full charge accumulation usually takes 2 to 5 seconds following activation of the charging mechanism.

Discharge controls are generally present on the paddle handles, allowing the operator to place the paddles and to deliver the charge as desired. Alternatively, there may be a separate control on the panel. Usually the simultaneous activation of the control on both paddles is required for energy discharge.

Monitor controls permit alteration of lead-monitored image size, and often allow the selection of chest lead electrode versus paddle electrode monitoring. The latter is desirable when an initial "quick-look" rhythm evaluation is desired prior to placement of the chest lead electrodes. A hard copy paper recorder for documenting rhythms seen on the monitor may operate in a real-time, delay, or standby mode.

PADDLES

Most commercial defibrillator devices have adult paddle electrodes with diameters between 8 and 9 cm. Canine studies have shown that slightly larger (12.8 cm diameter) paddles are more effective for defibrillation[29] and produce less myocardial injury.[30] Paddles that are slightly smaller (4.5 cm diameter) produce greater damage at the same energies. The larger paddles may permit a greater amount of muscle to be depolarized while minimizing the potentially damaging current density. If the paddles are too large with respect to the heart (e.g., if adult paddles are used during infant resuscitation), the current density is less and the defibrillator is less effective.[31] The recommended minimum diameter for pediatric transthoracic paddles is 2.2 cm.[21]

Some defibrillators have a flat posterior ground shield rather than a second paddle for lateral chest wall placement. With the two-paddle system, charge and discharge controls are generally present on the paddles.

The metal composition of the paddle electrode will affect transthoracic impedance to the defibrillation discharge. Most modern defibrillators use stainless steel because of its durability, although copper alloys and several other metals provide a lower transthoracic impedance.[32]

CONDUCTIVE MATERIALS

Transthoracic impedance varies with the type of conductive material applied between the paddles and the chest wall.[33, 34] For paddles that are 8.0 cm in diameter, the transthoracic impedance is 91 ± 20 ohms for bare contact, 71 ± 11 ohms for saline-soaked gauze, and 64 ± 15 ohms for Redux Paste.[35] Ewy recommends that Corgel, Redux Paste, American Writer, GE Gel, Electrode Jelly, or Trucon Electrode Paste be used to minimize impedance.[34] Saline-soaked gauze pads may be used, although one must be careful not to allow the saline to bridge the skin between the electrodes.

Procedure

Sudden death victims suspected to be in VF should be defibrillated as soon as possible. When adequate personnel are available, cardiopulmonary resuscitation should be initiated while the defibrillator device is being readied.

Following the application of conductive material to the entirety of the paddle conductive surface, the paddles are firmly applied to the chest. One paddle should be positioned to the right of the upper sternum below the clavicle; the second paddle is placed just to the left of the nipple in the anterior axillary line and is centered in the fifth intercostal space (see Fig. 10–4). In some paddle sets, each paddle is labeled "sternum" or "apex" so that any rhythm detected on the monitor can be properly aligned. This is irrelevant for defibrillation but is important for cardioversion. The anteroposterior paddle positioning is also acceptable and may deliver more current to the heart.[36, 37] The anterior paddle is placed to the left of the sternum over the precordium and the posterior electrode just to the left of the spine directly posterior to the heart (see Fig. 10–5).

With the monitor turned on and set to display the "paddle" electrodes, the rhythm is evaluated. If a flatline rhythm is detected, the monitor gain is increased fully to rule out a "fine VF" tracing. Should the tracing remain flat during a pause in closed-chest cardiac massage, the paddles are rotated 90 degrees from the original position and the rhythm is reassessed. Should a bradycardiac or asystolic rhythm be detected, standard resuscitation measures, including basic cardiopulmonary resuscitation, correction of hypoxia and acidosis, administration of catecholamines, correction of volume or cardiac filling deficiencies, and emergency cardiac pacing (see Chapters 12 and 13), should be initiated.

In cases of "fine" VF when a patient is wearing an implanted (subcutaneous) pacemaker, the pacer spikes may initially appear to be a paced but nonconducted rhythm; attention to the baseline and lack of ST changes characteristic of capture should reveal the true nature of the dysrhythmia. Since injury to the pacemaker pulse generator[38] and to the myocardium can occur by transmission of current down the pacing electrode,[39] the physician must be careful to situate the defibrillator paddle at least 5 inches away from the pulse generator.

In the presence of VF, the paddles should be immediately charged to a stored energy of 2 watt-sec per kg for children and 200 watt-sec for adults. Separate power switches may be needed to turn on the defibrillator and to store the charge. The amount of charge is usually set by a button or a dial on the control panel. In most devices, the preset level of charge (energy) can be stored if a button on the "apex" paddle is pressed. The physician must check to be certain that the defibrillator is *not* in the synchronous mode.

Once the paddles are charged, the physician should instruct all personnel to stand back from the patient and the stretcher to avoid stray discharge. The operator in particular must be sure that the only contact he makes is with dry paddle handles. The patient is allowed to exhale passively to minimize transthoracic impedance[40] while firm (25 lb) pressure is applied through the paddles to the thorax.[41, 42] The energy in the paddles is discharged through the chest as soon as possible following charging to minimize energy decay inside the device. Simultaneous depression of both paddle discharge buttons is essential for discharge. Anticipation of patient extremity motion subsequent to discharge of the paddles will minimize operator injury.

Should no skeletal muscle contraction occur following simultaneous depression of the discharge buttons, the physician should ensure that firm chest wall contact is made (some devices will not discharge without adequate contact), that the device is in the asynchronous mode, that a charge has been stored and the defibrillator (not just the monitor) is turned on, and that the battery is not low (when operating off the storage battery). If there is no muscle contraction even though these factors have been ruled out, a back-up defibrillator should be brought into use.

After the first countershock, the paddles should remain in place for 5 to 10 seconds to enable the physician to check for an organized rhythm while ventilation is continued. Should VF persist, another countershock should be administered immediately. When the second countershock is unsuccessful, closed-chest cardiac massage should be continued, hypoxia and acidosis corrected, and α-*agonist catecholamines administered to elevate the diastolic pressure and to improve coronary perfusion.*[43-46] A third countershock should follow these measures after adequate time for circulation of the catecholamines has passed. This countershock should be at 360 to 400 watt-sec for adults. Repeated countershocks in children should be at 4 watt-sec per kg. Infants who develop VF are often taking digitalis preparations. Since excessive defibrillation energy may produce irreversible VF in the digitalis-toxic patient, the lowest available energy level should be used for the initial defibrillation.[14] If the initial energy dose is unsuccessful, the energy can be cautiously increased for successive countershocks.

Additional therapy can be undertaken to enhance defibrillation; this will be discussed in the following section. Adequate ventilation, cardiac massage, and correction of electrolyte and acid/base disorders are intrinsic to every resuscitation and will not be discussed further. In addition, evaluation of the patient for hypothermia and rapid core rewarming when indicated (see Chapter 73) should not be overlooked.

When practical, electronic monitoring devices and transvenous pacemakers should be turned off or, preferably, disconnected from the patient to avoid equipment damage. Recently manufactured patient monitoring devices, however, have built-in protective filter circuitry, which makes equipment damage an unlikely occurrence.

Enhancing Defibrillation Success

EARLY DEFIBRILLATION

Energy requirements for conversion of VF may increase dramatically shortly after the onset of VF.[47, 48] Yakaitis and coworkers observed immediate defibrillation success when dogs were placed in VF for only 1 minute prior to defibrillation.[43] Animals in VF for longer than 3 minutes required cardiopulmonary resuscitation and an epinephrine infusion prior to defibrillation. The rationale for early defibrillation is that in the absence of adequate coronary perfusion, cellular metabolism continues with the depletion of energy substrates and the accumulation of toxic metabolites. Electro-physiologic changes secondary to cellular ischemia develop and contribute to continued asynchronous transmission of VF wavefronts.

Once these electrophysiologic changes develop, coronary perfusion for the reversal of advanced tissue ischemia may be needed prior to successful countershock. Yakaitis and associates have shown that in the *non*ischemic canine heart fibrillated for a short period (75 seconds), pure hypoxia or acidosis (respiratory and metabolic situations studied individually) for 10 to 20 minutes prior to VF did not significantly alter the ability to convert VF.[49] Animals with hypoxia or metabolic acidosis, however, were rarely able to resume circulation spontaneously following defibrillation. This condition could clinically lead to redevelopment of VF.

TRANSTHORACIC IMPEDANCE

Delivery of energy to the heart is dependent upon energy supplied to the paddles and the impedance to transmission of that energy. Reported values for human transthoracic impedance using electrodes 8.0 cm in diameter range from 50 to 100 ohms with a mean of 75 ohms.[99] We have previously discussed the importance of paddle electrode composition[32] and size,[29] conductive materials,[33-35] applied paddle-to-chest-wall pressure,[41, 42] state of ventilation,[40] and location of the paddle on the chest wall.[36, 37]

The transthoracic impedance of direct current discharge also decreases with higher energy shocks,[50] increasing number of previous countershocks delivered,[42, 51, 52] and decreasing interval between the discharges.[52] Unfortunately, each of the aforementioned maneuvers is also associated with an increased potential for myocardial injury. Nonetheless, one may be faced with the need to defibrillate a very obese patient who is unresponsive to standard paddle placement and maximum device energies. Should such a situation exist, the patient can be rolled on his side and anteroposterior defibrillation attempted. Should this prove unsuccessful, a second defibrillating device can be simultaneously charged and used to administer countershock *immediately* following discharge of the first defibrillator.

ENERGY CHOICE

Defibrillation is dependent upon the simultaneous depolarization of a sizable mass of the myocardium by the passage of current through the heart. For a given thorax, defibrillation device, and defibrillation technique, more current will be passed through the heart and, hence, more tissue will be depolarized with larger energies. Once sufficient tissue has been depolarized, however, additional current is not desirable and may in fact produce additional tissue injury.

Several studies have supported the concept that a weight-adjusted dosage of energy is preferred for converting VF.[53, 54] Indeed, a dose based on weight concept has been found clinically useful for treating children in VF.[55] More recent prospective human adult studies have questioned the importance of dose strength to conversion of VF.[56–59] Weaver and coworkers alternated treatment protocols to determine prospectively the merits of 175 watt-sec (200 J stored energy) versus 320 watt-sec (400 J stored) countershocks for defibrillation.[60] On test days, VF patients were initially shocked with one or two 175 watt-sec discharges, and all subsequent shocks needed were 320 watt-sec. On alternate days, only 320 watt-sec shocks were given. The investigators found that 73 per cent (n = 76) of the patients were defibrillated following the first two shocks in the low-energy group, whereas 81 per cent (n = 77) of the patients were initially defibrillated in the high-energy group (difference not statistically significant). Asystole occurred in 19 per cent of patients shocked with high energy and in 12 per cent receiving low energy. Transient or persistent heart block occurred in 25 per cent of patients shocked with high energy versus 11 per cent of patients receiving low energy. Survival to hospital discharge was inversely related to the number of shocks required; no patients requiring more than eight shocks survived.

Weaver and associates concluded that low-energy (175 watt-sec delivered) countershocks were safe, effective, and less cardiotoxic. Obviously, many factors besides discharged energy play a role in successful defibrillation. Most authorities now believe that although high-energy shocks may be needed in some patients, most patients will respond to a delivered energy of 175 watt-sec and rarely is a delivered energy of greater than 320 watt-sec indicated.

DRUG THERAPY

The role of correcting hypoxia, acidosis, and electrolyte disorders in the treatment of VF has previously been discussed. The benefit of α-agonist catecholamines used to enhance aortic diastolic pressure and to improve coronary perfusion has also been outlined in the section on early therapy.

Bretylium Tosylate. Bretylium tosylate has been used to facilitate ventricular defibrillation.[61–63] Bretylium (Bretylol) has been shown to decrease the threshold shock strength required for defibrillation.[64] The drug increases the effective refractory period in normal ventricular muscle and Purkinje fibers[65] and enhances electrical uniformity throughout the myocardium, thus tending to terminate conditions supportive of re-entrant rhythms.[66] Spontaneous chemical defibrillation has been reported in myocardial infarction patients given bretylium by intravenous drip rather than by bolus perfusion during cardiopulmonary resuscitation.[67]

For VF, 5 to 10 mg per kg of bretylium is given by rapid intravenous push and cardiac massage is performed for 1 to 2 minutes to permit circulation of the drug prior to defibrillation attempts. If after 2 minutes the initial therapy is unsuccessful, a repeat dose of 10 mg per kg is given, and defibrillatory efforts are continued. Successful defibrillation may be followed by hypotension; the physician must be prepared to administer volume or pressor agents to support the blood pressure. A recent retrospective study suggests that the early use of bretylium tosylate during VF sudden death may enhance survival.[68]

Lidocaine. Lidocaine has long been used to facilitate defibrillation.[69, 70] The rationale for use of lidocaine in VF is primarily based upon anecdotal experience. Recently, a nonischemic canine model has demonstrated that lidocaine *increases* the energy required for electrical defibrillation.[71] Lidocaine has complex effects on membrane responsiveness—little change in conduction velocity occurs in normal myocardium, whereas conduction in ischemic tissue is decreased.[72] Lidocaine increases uniformity of the action-potential duration and refractory period throughout the ventricles[73] and can terminate ventricular re-entrant rhythms.[74]

Lidocaine is initially given as a bolus of 1 mg per kg to the VF sudden death patient who is refractory to conventional defibrillatory efforts. A second 1 mg per kg bolus can be given in 10 to 15 minutes. Alternatively, an infusion of 1 to 2 mg per minute following the initial bolus can be used to maintain blood levels during drug redistribution.

One retrospective study of prehospital VF arrests documented a small but statistically *insignificant* improvement in both defibrillation rate and survival when patients refractory to conventional therapy for VF were given lidocaine during the course of their resuscitation.[75] Unfortunately, strict drug and therapy protocols were not followed, and variations in treatment may have masked a beneficial effect of lidocaine administration. A comparison study of prehospital lidocaine and bretylium use for refractory VF showed similar conversion and survival rates in the two drug treatment groups.[76] Although the role of lidocaine and bretylium in the facilitation of defibrillation remains to be more clearly defined, clinical experience suggests that both drugs have value in aiding defibrillation. Although one drug may be more beneficial than the other in a given patient, broader generalizations cannot be made. Certainly both drugs are useful for preventing degeneration of a supraventricular rhythm once effective defibrillation occurs.

Complications

The major complications of direct current defibrillation are (1) injury to skin and other soft tissue, (2) myocardial injury, and (3) cardiac dysrhythmias.

SOFT TISSUE INJURY

When firm skin contact along with a conductive material between the paddles and the chest wall is applied, contact burns are minimal. Nonetheless, repeated countershocks can produce erythema resembling superficial skin burns. The presence of liquids (blood, intravenous solutions, vomitus, urine, excessive sweat, and so forth) may permit the passage of current across the trunk. This electrical arcing will produce thermal burns (third-degree at times) and ineffective defibrillation. Intrathoracic injuries (extrinsic to the heart) are likely to occur but are difficult to document during the postresuscitative period and to separate from cardiac injury (e.g., pulmonary edema).[77-79]

MYOCARDIAL INJURY

The direct application of electrical countershock to the heart has long been known to produce epicardial and myocardial injury.[80] Lown and coworkers demonstrated that closed-chest defibrillation could produce cardiac injury. This suggested that electrical current rather than direct thermal injury produced injury.[12] Multiple countershocks have been shown in animals to produce ST segment elevation and gradual cell necrosis (over days) with subsequent fibrosis.[81, 82] The lesions are primarily subepicardial at the points of current entrance and exit wounds. Animals receiving less than twice the defibrillation threshold value do not develop significant necrosis.[83] The degree of cardiac injury correlates with increasing energy exposure.

The ability to document anatomic injury to the human heart is limited by the natural reparative process, concurrent ischemic processes producing similar microscopic changes, and the fact that several days are needed for the injuries to manifest themselves. Cardiac isoenzyme (CK MB) levels were shown to rise in patients undergoing elective cardioversion only if the cumulative *delivered* energy was greater than 475 watt-sec.[84] Therefore *standard* defibrillation does not invalidate enzymatic diagnosis of myocardial infarction given that defibrillations were not excessive and that isoenzymes are measured. Although myocardial scintigraphy with technetium 99m pyrophosphate is a sensitive means of demonstrating canine myocardial injury due to transthoracic countershocks,[85] Werner and associates were unable to detect injury in defibrillated sudden death patients who received standard delivered energies.[86] Nonetheless, it is likely that cardiac injury from defibrillation is possible, and data from animal injury studies are expected to be valid for patients.

Animal studies have shown that ST segment elevation and pathologic changes are increased with more rapidly delivered discharges (1 or 3 seconds versus 15 seconds between discharges).[81] Furthermore, the cumulative energy correlates with myocardial injury for a given dosing schedule.[81-83, 97]

CARDIAC DYSRHYTHMIAS

The rhythm that one obtains following defibrillation may be ventricular, supraventricular, or flatline (asystole). Laboratory studies have suggested a correlation between the severity of postdefibrillation dysrhythmias and the degree of myocardial damage produced.[96, 98] Reducing the peak current delivered to the heart by changing the waveform of the discharge was associated with fewer dysrhythmias.[87] Weaver and coworkers noted that asystole occurred in 19 per cent of prehospital VF patients receiving high energy and in 12 per cent of patients shocked with low energy.[60] Furthermore, transient heart block occurred significantly more frequently (25 per cent versus 11 per cent) in the patients shocked with high energy.

INJURIES TO HEALTH CARE PROVIDERS

All electrical devices, including defibrillators when improperly grounded or insulated, can cause injury to the device operator.[88, 89] Other participants in a resuscitation who touch the patient or the stretcher can also serve as a ground for the defibrillator charge and can sustain electrical injury. Improper use of the device for cranial countershock can also produce short-term memory loss.[90]

Special Topics in Defibrillation

THUMP DEFIBRILLATION

The precordial thump is a firm, rapid blow applied to the midsternum with a closed fist from a height of 12 to 15 inches above the pulseless patient. The precordial thump is of no proven value in VF. Miller and associates noted no VF conversion in 15 prehospital arrest patients.[91] They did note that rhythm was improved in two of the ten ventricular tachycardia patients after a precordial thump, although the rhythm deteriorated in six of the ten and did not change in the other two.

AUTOMATIC IMPLANTED DEFIBRILLATORS

Automatic implanted defibrillators are in limited clinical use, although they hold great promise for patients with recurrent VF who are unresponsive to drug therapy. The current models (manufactured by Medrad, Inc., Pittsburgh, Pennsylvania) physically resemble early pacemakers. The defibrillator is surgically placed with one electrode passed transvenously in the superior vena cava and the other (cuplike in shape) placed over the cardiac apex extrapericardially.[92] Although the device discharges internally at a potential of 700 volts, the surface voltage at the time of discharge would be on the order of tens of volts.[93] A discharge during cardiopulmonary resuscitation is likely to startle the rescuer, although injury is unlikely. Standard monitoring units should also be well protected electrically in the event that the device discharges.[93]

Refractory Ventricular Fibrillation

A number of clinical conditions may result in the inability to convert VF initially or the recurrence of VF following the first successful defibrillation. Patients with severe hypothermia are often refractory to initial defibrillation and require rapid core rewarming to be treated effectively. Severe bradycardia will predispose to lethal escape rhythms, and emergency cardiac pacing may be required. Severe electrolyte disturbances, such as hypokalemia, hypomagnesemia, and hypocalcemia may precipitate refractory VF and be amenable only to the rapid infusion of the deficient electrolyte. Such cases may be seen in fad dieters or abusers of diuretics. Uncorrected acidosis or hypoxia, such as seen with drowning, may be the cause of persistent VF. In addition, excessive adrenergic stimulation, such as seen with cocaine or amphetamine overdose, may require the use of propranolol infusion prior to successful defibrillation. As a final note, following defibrillation all patients should be treated with prophylactic lidocaine (or other appropriate antidysrhythmic therapy) to minimize the chance of recurrent VF.

Conclusions

Electrical defibrillation is the preferred treatment for VF sudden death. Treatment should be initiated early with attention to proper energy selection and minimization of transthoracic impedance. Although repetitive high-energy shocks may be associated with myocardial injury, this feature has not been clinically found to be common at the currently recommended energy levels.

1. Bigger, J. T.: Mechanism and diagnosis of arrhythmias. *In* Braunwald, E. (ed.): Heart Disease: A Textbook of Cardiovascular Medicine. Philadelphia, W. B. Saunders Co., 1980, pp. 609–670.
2. Cobb, L. A., Baum, T. L. S., Alvarez, H., III, et al.: Resuscitation from out-of-hospital ventricular filbrillation: 4 years follow-up. Circulation 52(Suppl III):223, 1975.
3. Liberthson, R. R., Nagle, E. L., Hirschman, J. C., et al.: Prehospital ventricular defibrillation; prognosis and follow-up course. N. Engl. J. Med. 291:317, 1974.
4. Schaffer, W. A., and Cobb, L. A.: Recurrent ventricular fibrillation and modes of death in survivors of out-of-hospital ventricular fibrillation. N. Engl. J. Med. 293:259, 1975.
5. Myerburg, R. J., Kessler, K. M., Zaman, L., et al.: Survivors of prehospital cardiac arrest. JAMA 247:1485, 1982.
6. Eisenberg, M. S., Bergner, L., and Hallstrom, A.: Cardiac resuscitation in the community. Importance of rapid provision and implications for program planning. JAMA 241:1905, 1979.
7. Thompson, R. G., Hallstrom, A. P., and Cobb, L. A.: Bystander initiated cardiopulmonary resuscitation in the management of ventricular fibrillation. Ann. Intern. Med. 90:737, 1979.
8. Lund, I., and Skulberg, A.: Cardiopulmonary resuscitation by lay people. Lancet 2:702, 1976.
9. Preuot, J. I , and Batelli, F.: Sur quelques effets des décharges électriques sur le coeur des mammiferes. C. R. Acad. Sci. (Paris) 129:1267, 1899.
10. Beck, C. S., Pritchard, W. H., and Feil, H.: Ventricular fibrillation of long duration abolished by electrical shock. JAMA 135:985, 1947.
11. Zoll, P. M., Linenthal, A. J., Gibson, W., et al.: Termination of ventricular fibrillation in man by an externally applied electric countershock. N. Engl. J. Med. 254:727, 1956.
12. Lown, B., Neuman, J., Amarasingham, R., et al.: Comparison of alternating current with direct current countershock across the closed chest. Am. J. Cardiol. 10:223, 1962.
13. Eisenberg, M. S., Copass, M. K., Hallstrom, A. P., et al.: Treatment of out-of-hospital cardiac arrests with rapid defibrillation by emergency medical technicians. N. Engl. J. Med. 302:1379, 1980.
14. Creed, J. D., Packard, J. M., Lambren, C. T., et al.: Defibrillation synchronized cardioversion. *In* American Heart Association: Textbook of Advanced Cardiac Life Support. Dallas, American Heart Association, 1981.
15. Parmley, W. H., Hatcher, C. R., Ewy, G. A., et al.: Thirteenth Bethesda Conference: Emergency cardiac care, task force V.: Physical interventions and adjunctive therapy. Am. J. Cardiol. 50:409, 1982.
16. Ewy, G. A., Dahl, D. F., Zimmerman, M., et al.: Ventricular fibrillation masquerading as ventricular standstill. Crit. Care Med. 9:841, 1981.
17. Zipes, D. P.: Electrophysiological mechanisms involved in ventricular fibrillation. Circulation 52(Suppl. III):120, 1975.

18. Cranefield, P. F.: Ventricular fibrillation. N. Engl. J. Med. 289:732, 1973.

19. Garrey, W. E.: The nature of fibrillatory contraction of the heart—its relation to tissue mass and form. Am. J. Physiol. 35:397, 1979.

20. Zipes, D. P., Fisher, J., King, R. M., et al.: Termination of ventricular fibrillation in dogs by depolarizing a critical amount of myocardium. Am. J. Cardiol. 36:37, 1975.

21. American National Standard for Cardiac Defibrillator Devices. Arlington, VA, Association for the Advancement of Medical Instrumentation, 1981.

22. Battery-powered defibrillator monitors. Health Devices, April 1980, pp. 135–163.

23. Schuder, J. C., Rahmoeller, G. A., and Stueckle, H.: Transthoracic ventricular defibrillation in the triangular and trapezoidal waveforms. Circ. Res. 19:689, 1966.

24. Tacker, W. A., Geddes, L. A., Bourland, J. D., et al.: The effect of tilt on the strength duration curve for trans-chest ventricular defibrillation. In Proceedings of the 12th Annual Meeting, Association for the Advancement of Medical Instrumentation. 1977, p. 403.

25. Geddes, L. A., Tacker, W. A., Bourland, M. D., et al.: Comparative efficacy of square and damped sine wave current for ventricular defibrillation. In Proceedings of the 12th Annual Meeting, Association for the Advancement of Medical Instrumentation. 1977, p. 404.

26. Ewy, G. A., Fletcher, R. D., and Ewy, M. D.: Comparative analysis of direct current defibrillators. J. Electrocardiol. 5:349, 1972.

27. Ewy, G. A.: Defibrillation output. In Proceedings of the Cardiac Defibrillation Conference. West Lafayette, Indiana, Purdue University, 1975, p. 33.

28. Sloman, G., Storckey, J., Kowadlow, E., et al.: Direct current defibrillator testing. Med. J. Aust. 1:597, 1983.

29. Thomas, E. D., Ewy, G. A., Dahl, C. F., et al.: Effectiveness of direct current defibrillation: Role of paddle electrode size. Am. Heart J. 93:436, 1977.

30. Dahl, C. F., Ewy, G. A., Warner, E. D., et al.: Myocardial necrosis from direct current countershock. Circulation 50:956, 1974.

31. Ewy, G. A., and Horan, W. J.: Effectiveness of direct current defibrillation: Role of paddle electrode size II. Am. Heart J. 93:674, 1977.

32. Ewy, G. A., Eerman, S. G., Alferness, C., et al.: Effect of electrode metal on the transthoracic impedance to defibrillator discharge. In Proceedings of the 15th Annual Meeting, Association for the Advancement of Medical Instrumentation. San Francisco, April 13–17, 1980, p. 43.

33. Ewy, G. A., and Taren, D.: Impedance to transthoracic direct current discharge: A model for testing interface material. Med. Instrum. 12:47, 1978.

34. Ewy, G. A., and Taren, D.: Relative impedance of gels to defibrillation discharge. Med. Instrum. 13:295, 1979.

35. Connell, P. N., Ewy, G. A., Dahl, C. F., et al.: Transthoracic impedance to defibrillation discharge; effect of electrode size and electrode-chest wall interface. J. Electorcardiol. 6:313, 1973.

36. Nachlas, M., et al.: Observations on defibrillation and synchronized countershock. Progr. Cardiovasc. Dis. 9:64, 1966.

37. Dolan, A. M., Horucek, B. M., and Rantaharju, P. M.: Evaluation of cardiac defibrillation using a computer model of the thorax (abstr.). Med. Instrum. 12:54, 1978.

38. Lan, F. Y. K., Bilitch, M., and Wintrab, A. J.: Protection of implanted pacemakers from excessive electrical energy of DC shock. Am. J. Cardiol. 23:244, 1969.

39. Aylward, P., Blood, R., and Tonkin, A.: Complications of defibrillation with permanent pacemaker in situ. Pace 2:462, 1979.

40. Ewy, G. A., Hellman, D. A., McClung, S., et al.: Influence of ventilation place on transthoracic impedance and defibrillation effectiveness. Crit. Care Med. 8:164, 1980.

41. Kerber, R. E., Grayzel, J., Hoyt, R., et al.: Transthoracic resistance in human defibrillation: Effects of body weight, chest size, serial same energy shocks, paddle size, and paddle contact pressure (abstr.). Med. Instrum. 14:156, 1980.

42. Kerber, P., Hoyt, R., Grayzel, J., et al.: Transthoracic resistance in defibrillation: Effects of repeated same energy shocks and paddle contact pressure. Circulation 59 and 60(Suppl. II):127, 1979.

43. Yakaitis, R. W., Ewy, G. A., Otto, W., et al.: Influence of time and therapy on ventricular defibrillation in dogs. Crit. Care Med. 8:147, 1980.

44. Chandra, N., Tsitlik, J., and Weisfeldt, M. L.: Coronary flow during cardiopulmonary resuscitation in the dog (abstr.). Crit. Care Med. 9:165, 1981.

45. Yakaitis, R. W., Otto, E. W., and Blitt, C. B.: Relative importance of α^3 and β adrenergic receptors during resuscitation. Crit. Care Med. 7:293, 1979.

46. Redding, J. G., and Pearson, J. W.: Evaluation of drugs for cardiac resuscitation. Anesthesiology 24:203, 1963.

47. Wolff, G. A., Veith, F., et al.: Vulnerable period for ventricular tachycardia following myocardial infarction. Cardiovasc. Res. 2:111, 1968.

48. Kerber, R. E., and Sarnat, W.: Factors influencing the success of ventricular defibrillation in man. Circulation 60:226, 1979.

49. Yakaitis, R. W., Thomas, J. D., and Mahaffey, J. E.: Influence of pH and hypoxia on the success of defibrillation. Crit. Care Med. 3:139, 1975.

50. Ewy, G. A., Ewy, M. D., Nuttall, A. J., et al.: Canine transthoracic resistance. J. Appl. Physiol. 32:91, 1972.

51. Geddes, L. A., Tacker, W. A., Cabler, P., et al.: The decrease in transthoracic impedance during successive ventricular defibrillation trials. Med. Instrum. 9:139, 1975.

52. Dahl, C. F., Ewy, G. A., Ewy, M. D., et al.: Transthoracic impedance to direct current discharge: Effect of repeated countershocks. Med. Instrum. 10:151, 1976.

53. Geddes, L. A., Tacker, W. A., Rosborough, J. P., et al.: Electrical dose for ventricular defibrillation of large and small animals using precordial electrodes. J. Clin. Invest. 53:310, 1974.

54. Tacker, W. A., Galiato, F. M., Giuliani, E., et al.: Energy dosage for human trans-chest electrical ventricular defibrillation. N. Engl. J. Med. 290:214, 1974.

55. Gutzesell, H. P., Tacker, W. A., Geddes, L. A., et al.: Energy dose for defibrillation in children. Pediatrics 58:898, 1976.

56. Partridge, J. R., Adgey, A. A. J., Webb, S. W., et al.: Electric requirements for ventricular defibrillation. Br. Med. J. 2:313, 1975.

57. Adgey, A. A.: Electrical energy requirements for ventricular defibrillation. Br. Heart J. 40:1197, 1978.

58. Gasche, J. A., Crampton, R. S., Cherwek, M. L., et al.: Determinants of ventricular defibrillation in adults. Circulation 60:231, 1979.

59. Crampton, J. A., Crampton, R. S., Sipes, J. N., et al.: Energy levels and patient weight in ventricular defibrillation. JAMA 242:1380, 1979.

60. Weaver, W. D., Thurman, C., Copass, M. K., et al.: Ventricular defibrillation: A prospective comparative trial of 175 joule and 320 joule energies. In Proceedings of the 16th Annual Meeting, Association for the Advancement of Medical Instrumentation. Washington, D.C., May 1981, p. 68.

61. Heissenbuttel, T. L. H., and Bigger, J. R.: Bretylium tosylate: A newly available antiarrhythmic drug for ventricular arrhythmias. Ann. Intern. Med. 91:229, 1979.

62. Bernstein, J. G., and Koch-Weser, J.: Effectiveness of bretylium tosylate against refractory ventricular arrhythmias. Circulation 45:1024, 1972.

63. Holder, D. A., Sniderman, A. D., Fraser, G., et al.: Experience with bretylium tosylate by a hospital cardiac arrest team. Circulation 55:541, 1977.

64. Tacker, W. A., et al.: The effect of newer antiarrhythmic

drugs on defibrillation threshold. Crit. Care Med. 8:177, 1980.

65. Bigger, J. T., Jr., and Jaffee, C. C.: The effects of bretylium tosylate on the electrophysiologic properties of ventricular muscle and Purkinje fibers. Am. J. Cardiol. 27:82, 1971.

66. Cardinal, R., and Sasyniuk, B. J.: Electrophysiological effects of bretylium tosylate on subendocardial Purkinje fibers from infarcted canine hearts. J. Pharmacol. Exp. Ther. 204:159, 1978.

67. Sanna, G., and Arcidiacono, R.: Chemical ventricular defibrillation of the human heart with bretylium tosylate. Am. J. Cardiol. 32:982, 1973.

68. Harrison, E. E., and Amey, B. D.: The use of bretylium in prehospital ventricular fibrillation. Am. J. Emerg. Med. 1:1, 1983.

69. Standards and guidelines for cardiopulmonary resuscitation (CPR) and emergency cardiac care (ECC). JAMA 244:453, 1980.

70. Goldberg, A. H.: Cardiopulmonary arrest. N. Engl. J. Med. 290:1974.

71. Babbs, C. F., Yim, G. K. W., Whistler, S. T., et al.: Elevation of ventricular defibrillation threshold in dogs by antiarrhythmic drugs. Am. Heart J. 98:345, 1979.

72. Kupersmith, J., Antman, E. M., and Hoffman, B. F.: In vivo electrophysiological effects of lidocaine in canine acute myocardial infarction. Circ. Res. 36:84, 1975.

73. Wittig, J., Harrison, L. A., and Wallace, A. G.: Electrophysiological effects of lidocaine on distal Purkinje fibers of canine heart. Am. Heart J. 86:69, 1978.

74. El-Sherif, N., et al.: Reentrant ventricular arrhythmias in the late myocardial infarction period. IV. Mechanism of action of lidocaine. Circulation 56:395, 1977.

75. Harrison, E. E.: Lidocaine in prehospital countershock refractory ventricular fibrillation. Ann. Emerg. Med. 10:420, 1981.

76. Hayes, R. E., Chinn, T. L., Copass, M. R., et al.: Comparison of bretylium tosylate and lidocaine in the management of out-of-hospital ventricular fibrillation: A randomized clinical trial. Am. J. Cardiol. 48:353, 1981.

77. Resnekov, L., and McDonald, L.: Pulmonary oedema following treatment of arhythmias by direct current therapy. Lancet 1:506, 1965.

78. Honey, M., Nicholls, T. T., and Towers, M. K.: Pulmonary oedema following direct current defibrillation. Lancet 1:765, 1965.

79. Palcheimo, J. A.: Pulmonary oedema after defibrillation. Lancet 2:439, 1965.

80. Tedeschi, C. G., and White, C. W., Jr.: Morphologic study of canine hearts subjected to fibrillation, electrical defibrillation and manual compression. Circulation 9:916, 1954.

81. Dahl, C. F., Ewy, G. A., Warner, E. D., et al.: Myocardial necrosis from direct current countershock. Circulation 50:956, 1974.

82. Warner, E. D., Dahl, C., and Ewy, G. A.: Myocardial injury from transthoracic defibrillation countershock. Arch. Pathol. 99:55, 1975.

83. Davis, J. S., Lie, J. T., et al.: Cardiac damage due to electric current and energy. In Proceedings of the Cardiac Defibrillation Conference. West Lafayette, Indiana, Purdue University, 1975, p. 27.

84. Ehsani, A., Ewy, G. A., Sobel, B. E.: Effects of electrical countershock on serum creatinine phosphokinase (CPK) isoenzyme activity. Am. J. Cardiol. 87:12, 1976.

85. DiCala, U. C., Freedman, G. S., Downing, S. E., et al.: Myocardial uptake of technetium-99m stannous pyrophosphate following direct current transthoracic countershock. Circulation 54:980, 1976.

86. Werner, J. A., Potkin, R. T., Botvinick, E. H., et al.: Scintigraphic and enzymatic findings in survivors of sudden cardiac death. Clin. Res. 1:73A, 1977.

87. Peleska, B.: Cardiac arrhythmias following condenser discharge led through an inductance; comparison with effects of pure condenser discharges. Circ. Res. 16:11, 1965.

88. Hopps, J. A.: The electric shock hazard in hospitals. Can. Med. Assoc. J. 21:1002, 1968.

89. Edmark, K. W., Proctor, R. L., Thomas, G. I., et al.: DC defibrillator failure. J. Thorac. Cardiovasc. Surg. 5:741, 1968.

90. Iserson, E. V., Barsan, W. G.: Accidental "cranial" defibrillation. JACEP 7:24, 1979.

91. Miller, J., Tresch, D., Horwitz, L., et al.: The precordial thump—useful or detrimental? (abstr.). Ann. Emerg. Med. 12:246, 1983.

92. Mirowski, M., Mower, M. M., Bhagavan, B. S., et al.: The implantable automatic defibrillator. Cardiovasc. Med. 4:851, 1979.

93. Tacker, W. A.: Problems of clinical significance—current clinical trends in cardiac defibrillation: Monitors and defibrillators. In Cardiac Monitoring in a Complex Patient Care Environment. AAMI Technology Assessment Report. Arlington, VA, Association for the Advancement of Medical Instrumentation, 1982, pp. 13–14.

94. Edmark, K. W., Thomas, G. I., and Jones, T. W.: DC pulse defibrillation. J. Thorac. Cardiovasc. Surg. 51:326, 1966.

95. Wiggers, C. J., and Wegria, R.: Ventricular fibrillation due to a single, localized induction and condenser shocks applied during the vulnerable phase of ventricular systole. Am. J. Physiol. 128:500, 1940.

96. Peleska, B.: Cardiac arrhythmias following condenser discharges and their dependence upon strength of current and phase of cardiac cycle. Circ. Res. 13:21, 1963.

97. Ewy, G. A., et al.: Comparison of myocardial damage from defibrillator discharge at various dosages. Med. Instrum. 14:10, 1980.

98. Jones, J. L., and Jones, R. E.: Postshock arrhythmias: A possible cause of unsuccessful defibrillation. Crit. Care Med. 8:167, 1980.

99. Ewy, G. A.: Defibrillation. In Harwood, A. L. (ed.): Cardiopulmonary Resuscitation. Baltimore, Williams & Wilkins, 1982, pp. 89–126.

12

Emergency Transvenous Cardiac Pacing*

GEORGES C. BENJAMIN, M.D.

Introduction

The purpose of transvenous cardiac pacing is to restore or ensure effective cardiac depolarization. Several approaches to pacing exist, including transcutaneous, transthoracic, epicardial, endocardial, and, most recently, esophageal (see also Chapter 13). The transvenous method of endocardial pacing is used most frequently and is both safe and effective. In skilled hands, the semi-floating transvenous catheter is successfully placed under electrocardiographic guidance in 80 per cent of patients.[1] The technique can be performed in less than 20 minutes in 72 per cent of patients and in less than 5 minutes in 30 per cent of patients. As with other medical procedures, it should not be performed without a thorough understanding of both its indications and contraindications.

Background

The ability of muscle to be artificially depolarized was recognized as early as the 18th century. Over the succeeding years, several scattered experiments were reported, and in 1951, Callaghan and Bigelow first used the transvenous approach to stimulate the asystolic heart in hypothermic dogs.[2] Zoll demonstrated the first clinical use of cardiac pacing in humans in 1952.[3] He reported the successful use of an external transcutaneous electrical stimulator in two patients with ventricular standstill.

Furmkn and Schwedel demonstrated the transvenous endocardial approach in humans in 1959.[4] They treated two patients with complete heart block and Stokes-Adams seizures, reconfirming

that low-voltage pacing could completely control myocardial depolarization. The catheter remained in their second patient for 96 days without complication. Other clinical studies by Muller and Bellet,[5] Siddons and Davies,[6] and DeSanctis[7] have proved that transvenous pacing is a valuable procedure in medicine. Fluoroscopic guidance was used for placement of the pacing catheter in all these studies.

In 1964, Vogel and colleagues demonstrated the use of a flexible catheter passed without fluoroscopic guidance for intracardiac electrocardiography.[8] One year later, this technique was used by Kimball and Killip to insert an endocardial pacemaker at the bedside.[9] They noted technical difficulties, including intermittent capture, difficulty passing the catheter, and catheter knotting, in 20 per cent of their patients. During the same year, Harris and associates confirmed the ease and speed with which this procedure could be accomplished.[10]

Prior to 1965, all intracardiac pacing was done asynchronously, which meant that the pacing catheter could cause electrical stimulation during any phase of the cardiac cycle. Asynchronous pacing frequently resulted in the pacemaker firing during the vulnerable period of an intrinsic depolarization; this occasionally caused ventricular tachycardia or fibrillation. In 1966, Goetz and coworkers demonstrated a pacing generator that sensed intrinsic depolarizations and inhibited the pacemaker for a predetermined period of time.[11] In 1967, this form of *demand* pacemaker was used successfully by Zuckerman and associates in six patients.[12]

A further improvement in the pacing catheter was made by Rosenberg and colleagues when they introduced the Elecath semi-floating pacing wire.[1] The Elecath was stiffer than the Flexon steel wire electrode. Rosenberg and coworkers achieved pacing in 72 per cent of patients, with an average procedure time of 18 minutes. They also noted that 30 per cent of their patients were paced in 5 minutes or less. Bedside insertion resulted in successful pacing for an average of 4 days. Six of 111 patients developed minor complications, including pneumothorax, local infection, and arterial bleeding, resulting in a complication rate of 7 per cent. Inconsistent pacing occurred in 14 per cent of patients and required simple bedside repositioning.[1]

The technique of heart catheterization using a flow-directed balloon-tipped catheter was introduced by Swan and associates in 1970.[13] This concept was used successfully by Schnitzler and coworkers for the placement of a right ventricular pacemaker in 15 of 17 patients.[14]

In 1981, Lang and colleagues compared the bedside use of the flow-directed balloon-tipped catheter with insertion of a semi-rigid electrode

*The opinions or assertions contained herein are the private views of the author and are not to be construed as official or reflecting the views of the Department of Defense or the Department of the Army.

Table 12–1. HISTORY OF TRANSVENOUS PACING

Date	Investigator	Event
1700	Early investigators	First restimulation studies
1951	Callaghan and Bigelow	First transvenous approach in dogs
1952	Zoll	Transcutaneous cardiac stimulator
1958	Falkmann and Walkins	Implanted pacing wires post surgery
1959	Furman and Robinson	First transvenous pacer in man
1964	Vogel and associates	Flexible electrocardiographic catheter without fluoroscopy
1965	Kimball and Killip	First bedside transvenous pacing
1966	Goetz and associates	Demand pacemaker developed
1967	Zuckerman and associates	Use of demand pacemaker clinically
1969	Rosenberg and associates	Semi-floating pacing catheter
1973	Schnitzler and associates	Balloon-tipped pacers

Table 12–2. INDICATIONS FOR CARDIAC PACING

Bradycardias
  Without myocardial infarction
    Symptomatic sinus node dysfunction (sinus arrest, tachy-brady (sick sinus) syndrome, sinus bradycardia)
    Second and third degree heart block
    Atrial fibrillation with slow ventricular response
  With myocardial infarction
    Symptomatic sinus node dysfunction
    Mobitz II second degree and third degree heart block
    Left bundle branch block (LBBB), right bundle branch block (RBBB), bifascicular block, and alternating bundle branch block
  Trauma patient with hypotension and unresponsive bradycardia
  Prophylaxis — cardiac catheterization, post open heart surgery, threatened bradycardia during drug trials for tachydysrhythmias
  Malfunction of implanted pacemaker
  Asystolic arrest patient—not clear

Tachycardias
  Supraventricular dysrhythmias
  Ventricular dysrhythmias
  Prophylaxis — cardiac catheterization, post open heart surgery

catheter in 111 patients.[15] These researchers found a significantly shorter insertion time (6 minutes 45 seconds compared with 13 minutes 30 seconds), a lower incidence of serious arrhythmias (1.5 per cent compared with 20.4 per cent), and a lower incidence of catheter displacement (13.4 per cent compared with 32 per cent) with the balloon-tipped catheter. The concluded that the balloon-tipped catheter was the method of choice for temporary transvenous pacing (Table 12–1).

Indications

The purpose of cardiac pacing is to resume effective cardiac depolarization. In most cases, the specific indications for cardiac pacing are clear; however, some controversial areas remain. The decision to pace on an emergent basis requires knowledge of the presence or absence of hemodynamic compromise, the etiology of the rhythm disturbance, the status of the atrioventricular (AV) conduction system, and the type of dysrhythmia. In general, the indications can be grouped into those that cause either tachycardias or bradycardias (Table 12–2).

BRADYCARDIAS

Sinus Node Dysfunction. In a review of 200 initial pacemaker implants at Montefiore Hospital during 1975, 36.5 per cent were used for sinus node dysfunction, 11.3 per cent were used for sinus arrest, 20.2 per cent were used for tachy-brady (sick sinus) syndrome, and 5 per cent were used for sinus bradycardia.[16] Patients without myocardial infarction who present with symptomatic sinus node dysfunction should be promptly paced if medical therapy fails. Escher and Furman note that pacing is indicated until the etiology of

the dysrhythmia is clarified and stability is ensured.[17]

In the asymptomatic patient, a more intensive cardiac evaluation is required to decide whether pacing will be beneficial. This evaluation frequently includes 24-hour Holter monitoring, noting sinus node recovery times, and coronary care unit monitoring.

Sinus bradycardia occurs in an average of 17 per cent of patients with acute myocardial infarction.[18–21] Sinus bradycardia occurs more frequently in inferior than in anterior infarction and has a relatively good prognosis when accompanied by a hemodynamically tolerable escape rhythm. Sinus bradycardia is not a benign rhythm in this situation; it has a mortality rate of 2 per cent with inferior infarction and 9 per cent with anterior infarction.[22] Several mechanisms have been suggested to explain sinus node dysfunction with infarction. Among these, ischemia of the node[20] or its neurologic controls[21–24] and reflex slowing secondary to pain play dominant roles.[25] Sinus node dysfunction will frequently respond to medical therapy but requires prompt pacing if this fails.

Asystolic Arrest. The role of transvenous pacing in the asystolic patient is unclear. In one recent study of 13 patients with cardiac arrest, capture of the myocardium was noted in four patients but there were no survivors.[26] Hazard speculated that the absence of forward blood flow and the dislodging effect of closed chest massage played important roles in his lack of success.[26] Frequently, cardiac pacing is used as a "last ditch" effort in asystolic patients; therefore, any benefits from its early use are as yet unknown. A more complete discussion of pacing in brady-asystolic cardiac arrest appears in Chapter 13.

Atrioventricular Block. Atrioventricular block is the classic indication for pacemaker therapy. In symptomatic patients without myocardial infarction and in the asymptomatic patient with a ventricular rate below 40, pacemaker therapy is indicated.[27]

In patients with acute myocardial infarction, 15 to 19 per cent progress to heartblock: approximately 8 per cent develop first degree block, 5 per cent develop second degree block, and 6 per cent develop third degree block.[28, 29] First degree block progresses to second or third degree block 33 per cent of the time, and second degree block progresses to third degree block about one third of the time.[30]

Atrioventricular block occurring during anterior infarction is believed to occur because of diffuse ischemia to the septum and conduction tissue infranodally. Patients with atrioventricular block tend to progress to high degree block without warning and should be prophylactically paced temporarily if conduction abnormalities develop, even without hemodynamic compromise.

During inferior infarction, early septal ischemia is the exception and block develops serially from first degree to Mobitz type I second degree then to third degree. These conduction abnormalities frequently result in hemodynamically tolerable escape rhythms because of sparing of the bundle branches. The hemodynamically unstable patient who is unresponsive to medical therapy should be paced promptly. When the stable patient should be paced has not been determined.

One study in which the indications for temporary and permanent pacemaker insertion were reviewed in 432 patients with myocardial infarction concluded that patients with second or third degree atrioventricular block should be paced, because a higher incidence of sudden death or recurrent high degree block over the following year was found in patients who were not continuously paced.[31]

Bundle Branch Block. Bundle branch block, occurring in acute myocardial infarction, is associated with a higher mortality rate and a greater incidence of third degree heart block than uncomplicated infarction. Atkins and associates noted that 18 per cent of patients had bundle branch block with myocardial infarction.[32] Of these patients, complete heart block developed in 43 per cent who had right bundle branch block and left axis deviation, 17 per cent who had left bundle branch block, 19 per cent who had left anterior hemiblock, and 6 per cent who had no conduction block. The authors concluded that right bundle branch block with left axis deviation should be prophylactically paced.

A later study by Hindman and colleagues confirmed the natural history of bundle branch block during myocardial infarction.[33] In their study, the presence or absence of first degree atrioventricular block, the type of bundle branch block, and the age (new vs. old) of the block were used to determine the relative risk of progression to type II second degree or third degree block (Table 12–3).

Because of the increased risk, most physicians would pace new onset left bundle branch block, right bundle branch block with left axis deviation or other bifascicular block, and alternating bundle branch block.[31–34] One authority recommends prophylactic pacing for all new bundle branch blocks when myocardial infarction is evident.[35]

Trauma. In the patient with nonpenetrating chest trauma, several rhythm and conduction disturbances have been documented.[36–38] In these patients, traumatic injury to the specialized conduction system may predispose the patient to life-threatening dysrhythmias and blocks that can be treated by cardiac pacing.[39]

Hypovolemia and hypotension can cause ischemia of conduction tissue and cardiac dysfunction.[40, 41] Continued marked bradydysrhythmias

Table 12–3. THE INFLUENCE OF DIFFERENT VARIABLES ON RISK OF HIGH DEGREE ATRIOVENTRICULAR BLOCK IN PATIENTS WITH BUNDLE BRANCH BLOCK DURING MYOCARDIAL INFARCTION

	Patients	Hi° AV Block (%)
Infarct location		
Anterior	272	25
Indeterminant	77	12
Inferior or posterior	83	20
PR Interval		
> 0.20 sec	169	25
≤ 0.20 sec	263	19
Type BBB		
LBBB	163	13
RBBB	48	14
RBBB + LAFB	149	27
RBBB + LPFB	45	29
ABBB	27	44
Onset BBB		
Definitely old	91	13
Possibly new	95	25
Probably new	65	26
Definitely new	181	23

Abbreviations: Hi° ABV = high degree AV block; BBB = bundle branch block; LBBB = left bundle branch block; RBBB = right bundle branch block; LAFB = left anterior fascicular hemiblock; LPFB = left posterior fascicular hemiblock; ABBB = alternating bundle branch block. (Reprinted by permission of the American Heart Association from Hindman, M. C., et al.: The clinical significance of bundle branch block complicating acute myocardial infarction. 2. Indications of temporary and permanent pacemaker insertion. Circulation, 58:690, 1978.)

after vigorous volume replacement may respond to cardiac pacing in patients with such trauma.[42]

Tachycardias

Hemodynamically compromising tachycardias are usually treated by medical means or cardioversion (see Chapters 9 and 10). Over the last 15 years, there has been an increasing interest in pacing therapy for symptomatic tachycardias. In 1960, two groups reported that asynchronous pacing prevented ventricular tachycardia and fibrillation in patients with bradycardia and heart block.[43, 44] Over the next four to five years, several investigators noted that supraventricular dysrhythmias could be suppressed, even in the absence of heart block.[45-47] It was also learned that pharmacologic and pacing therapies could augment each other when used concurrently.

Supraventricular dysrhythmias, with the exception of atrial fibrillation, respond well to atrial pacing. By pacing the atria at rates 10 to 20 beats per minute faster than the underlying rhythm, the atria become intrained, and when the rate is slowed, the rhythm frequently returns to normal sinus. A similar procedure is done for ventricular dysrhythmias.[45, 48-50]

Transvenous pacing is especially useful in patients with digitalis-induced dysrhythmias in whom direct current (DC) cardioversion may be dangerous or in patients in whom there is further concern about myocardial depression with drugs.[49]

Equipment

Several items are required in order to adequately insert a transvenous pacemaker. Like most special procedures, a prearranged tray is convenient. The usual components required to insert a transvenous cardiac pacemaker are listed in Table 12–4.

Many different pacing generators are available, but in general, they all have the same basic features. The on/off switch frequently will have a locking feature to prevent the generator from inadvertently being switched off. An amperage knob allows the operator to control the amount of electrical current delivered to the myocardium and usually ranges from 0.1 to 20 milliamperes (ma). The pacing control mode is the gain control for the sensing function of the generator. By moving this knob, one can convert the unit from a fixed rate (asynchronous mode) to a demand (synchronous mode) pacemaker. In the fixed rate mode, the unit will fire despite the underlying intrinsic rhythm; the unit does not sense any intrinsic electrical activity. In the full demand mode, how-

Table 12–4. EQUIPMENT

Pacemaker Tray
10 ml syringe
1% lidocaine
Alcohol wipes
Betadine
Several gauze pads
4 sterile drapes
No. 11 scalpel blade
0.9 normal saline—2 ampules
Sterile gloves
Needle holder
2—22 gauge needles
Scissors (suture)
2—4-0 silk sutures on needles
Sterile basin

Electrical Hardware
Spare 9 volt battery
Medtronic pacing unit No. 5375
3F Balectrode Pacing Kit (catalog No. 11—KBE1)
12 lead EKG (well grounded)

ever, the pacemaker will sense the underlying ventricular depolarizations and the unit will not fire as long as the patient's ventricular rate is equal to or faster than the set rate of the pacing generator. A sensing indicator meter and rate control knob are also present. An example of a pacing generator is shown in Figure 13–2.

Several sizes and brands of pacing catheters are available. In general, most range from 3 French to 5 French in size and are approximately 100 cm in length. Along the catheter surface, there are lines that are marked at approximately 10 cm intervals, which can be used to estimate catheter position during insertion. Two basic types of pacing catheters are currently in use: the flexible semi-floating or floating catheter and the rigid fixed-position catheter.[51]

The flexible catheters are more advantageous than the rigid catheter in their ability to be inserted in low flow states as well as in their decreased tendency to perforate the ventricle. For emergency pacing, the 4 French semifloating bipolar electrode with or without the balloon tip is used most frequently (Fig. 12–1). The balloon holds approximately 1.5 ml of air or carbon dioxide, and some of them have a locking lever to secure balloon expansion. Prior to insertion, the balloon is checked for air leakage by inflating it and immersing it in sterile water (Fig. 12–2). The presence of an air leak is noted by a stream of bubbles arising at the surface of the water. An inflated balloon helps the catheter "float" into the heart in low flow states but is obviously not advantageous in the cardiac arrest situation.

For all practical purposes, temporary transvenous pacing is accomplished with a bipolar pacing catheter. The terms *unipolar* and *bipolar* refer to the

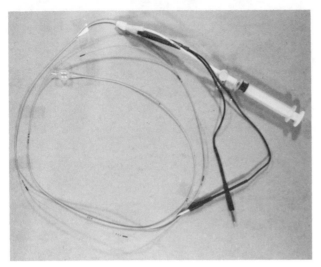

Figure 12–1. Pacing balloon-tipped catheter.

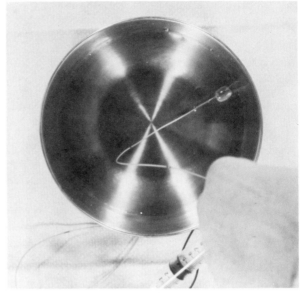

Figure 12–2. Testing balloon for leakage.

number of electrodes in contact with that portion of the heart that is to be stimulated. All pacemaker systems must have both a positive (anode) and a negative (cathode) electrode, and all stimulation is *bipolar*. The typical bipolar catheter that is used for temporary transvenous pacing has the cathode (stimulating electrode) at the tip of the pacing catheter. The anode is located 1 to 2 cm proximal to the tip, and the two electrodes may be separated by a balloon or an insulated wire. The electrodes are usually platinum rings that encircle the pacing catheter. When properly positioned, both electrodes will be within the right ventricle so that a field of electrical excitation is set up between the electrodes. With the bipolar catheter, the cathode does not need to be in direct contact with the endocardium in order for pacing to occur, although it is preferable to have direct contact.

A unipolar system is also effective but is infrequently used for temporary transvenous pacing. In a unipolar system, the cathode is at the tip of the pacing catheter and the anode is located either in the pacing generator itself, more proximal on the catheter (outside the ventricle), or underneath the skin on the patient's chest. The bipolar system may be converted to a unipolar system by simply disconnecting the positive proximal connection of the bipolar catheter from the pacing generator and running a new wire from the positive terminal to the patient's chest wall. Such a conversion may be required in the unlikely event of failure of one lead of the bipolar system.

Theoretically, the field of electrical stimulation of a pacing catheter is equal to the distance between the electrodes. If the field of excitation is not close enough to the myocardium, depolariza-

tion will not occur. When a catheter is passed blindly in an emergency, it seems advantageous to ensure the best chance of capture by separating the electrodes more than the standard 1 to 2 cm. A pacing catheter that uses this configuration (Davison pacing lead, Electro-Catheter Corp.) is a hybrid of the standard bipolar and unipolar catheters. This catheter has the cathode at the tip, but the anode is situated 19 cm proximal to the tip. This configuration allows pacing with a very wide field of excitation. Pacing has been reported to occur with this catheter when the catheter is placed anywhere within the thoracic venous system.[52] The catheter is a hybrid because both electrodes are present on the same catheter (bipolar), but both electrodes will not be positioned in the same cardiac chamber (unipolar).

An electrocardiograph can be used to record the heart's inherent electrical activity during pacer insertion and to aid in localization of the catheter tip without fluoroscopy. The electrocardiograph machine must be well grounded to prevent leakage of alternating current, which can cause ventricular fibrillation. Such leakage should be suspected if 50 to 60 cycle per second (Hz) interference is noted on the electrocardiograph.

The electrocardiograph machine should be placed in such a manner to allow easy visibility of the rhythm during insertion. One method is to place the machine on the same side of the patient as the operator at the level of the midthorax (Fig. 12–3). Note that the operator stands at the head of the patient during internal jugular or subclavian vein passage of the catheter and at the midabdomen for femoral or brachiocephalic vein insertion.

An introducer set or sheath is required for venous access (see Chapter 19). Some pacing catheters are pre-packaged with the appropriate equipment, whereas others require a separate set. The introducer set is used to enhance passage of the pacing catheter through the skin, subcutaneous tissue, and vessel wall. To allow passage of the pacing catheter, the sheath must be one size larger than the pacing catheter. A makeshift sheath can be made with an appropriate sized intravenous catheter. For the 3F balloon-tipped catheter, a 14 gauge, 1.5 to 2 inch intravenous catheter is suitable.

Overall, the key to success with this procedure is preparation. It is imperative that one examines all the components of the tray before starting the procedure and ensures that all wires, sheaths, dilators, and syringes fit as expected.

Procedure

PATIENT PREPARATION

Patient instruction is an extremely important aspect of any procedure. Frequently, there is not enough time to give the patient a detailed explanation. Nonetheless, sufficient information should be provided so that the patient feels at ease. The patient should be assured that he will feel no discomfort after the venipuncture site has been anesthetized and that he will feel better when the catheter is in place and is functional. Continued reassurance is required during the procedure, because the patient is usually facing away from the operator and often has his face covered and is therefore unsure of what is occurring.

SITE SELECTION

The four venous channels that provide an easy access to the right ventricle are the brachial, subclavian, femoral, and internal jugular veins (Table 12–5). The route selected is often one of personal

Table 12–5. ADVANTAGES AND DISADVANTAGES OF PACEMAKER PLACEMENT SITES

Venous Channels	Advantages	Disadvantages
Brachial	Very safe route Vessel easily accessible — either by cutdown or percutaneous approach	Often requires cutdown Easily displaced and poor patient mobility Not reusable if cutdown technique is performed Catheter is more difficult to advance than with central or larger vessels
Subclavian	Direct access to right heart (especially via left subclavian) Rapid insertion time Reusable Good patient mobility	Pneumothorax and other intrathoracic trauma is possible
Femoral	Direct access to right heart Rapid insertion time Reusable	Increased incidence of thrombophlebitis Can be dislodged by leg movement and poor patient mobility Infection
Internal jugular	Direct access to right heart (especially via right internal jugular) Rapid insertion time Reusable	Possible carotid artery puncture Dislodgement with movement of the head Thrombophlebitis

Figure 12–3. Position of EKG device during femoral vein insertion of pacemaker catheter.

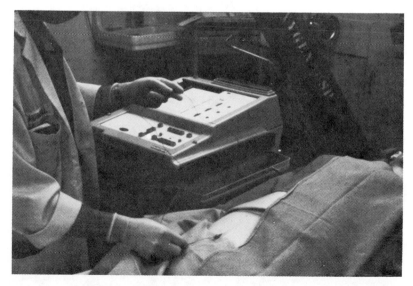

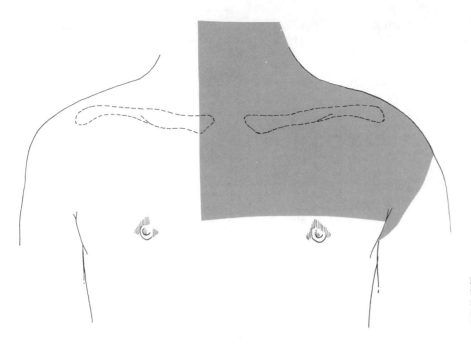

Figure 12–4. Cleaned skin for left infraclavicular approach—a preferred route. Note that the prepped infraclavicular area extends up the neck and to the opposite sternal border.

Figure 12–5. Cleaned skin for supraclavicular or right internal jugular approach.

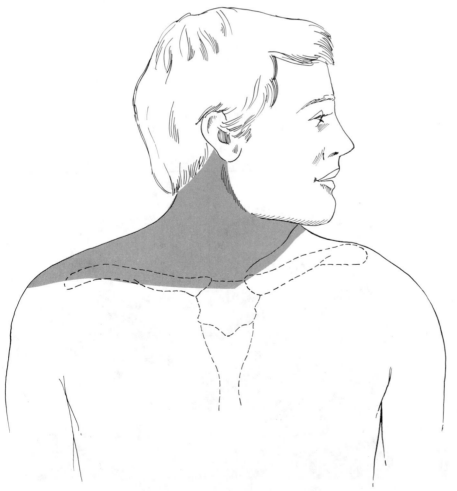

or institutional preference. The right internal jugular and the left subclavian veins have the straightest anatomic pathway to the right ventricle and are generally preferred for temporary transvenous pacing. In some centers, a particular site is preferred for *permanent* transvenous pacemaker placement and, if possible, this site should be avoided for temporary placement.

The subclavian vein can be accessed by both an infraclavicular and a supraclavicular approach; the infraclavicular approach is most commonly reported for all temporary transvenous pacemaker insertions. This route is preferred because of its easy accessibility, close proximity to the heart, and ease in catheter maintenance and stability. The supraclavicular approach, although described in the literature for several years, has only recently gained popularity among some authors.[53] The left subclavian vein is preferred because of the less acute angle traversed when compared with the right-sided approach.

Some physicians believe the internal jugular approach to be as easy and safer than subclavian catheterization.[54] The right internal jugular vein is preferred due to the direct line to the superior vena cava. Problems with this approach include dislodgment of the pacemaker with movement of the head, carotid artery puncture, and thrombophlebitis (see Chapter 22).

Femoral veins, like the neck veins, are reusable and easily catheterized. Problems include easy dislodgment, infection, and increased risk of thrombophlebitis.[55-57]

Brachial vein catheterization is easy to perform but results in a high incidence of infection and vessel thrombosis.[58] In addition, the catheter is easily dislodged with arm motion. This approach is seldom used in the emergency setting.

SKIN PREPARATION

The skin over the venipuncture site is cleaned twice with an antiseptic solution such as povidone-iodine and isopropyl alcohol. A wide area is prepared because of the tendency for guidewires and catheters to spring from the hands of the unsuspecting operator. For the infraclavicular approach to the subclavian, the skin between the opposite sternal border, the nipple line, the anterior axillary line, and the posterior aspect of the clavicle must be cleaned (Fig. 12–4). For the supraclavicular and internal jugular approach, an area enclosing the sternal notch, clavicle, midshoulder, and lateral neck from the midline to the ramus of the mandible (Fig. 12–5) should be prepared. For the femoral approach, skin preparation includes an area 2 inches above and 6 inches below the in-guinal ligament, from the mid inner thigh to its lateral border (Fig. 12–6).

Similarly, wide draping is carried out in the standard manner to maintain a sterile field and to allow clear visibility of the venipuncture site.

OBTAINING VENOUS ACCESS

The infraclavicular approach is used in this chapter to illustrate venous access, although the mechanics are generally the same for other vascular approaches. The reader is referred to Chapters 21 and 22 for the specific techniques of venous access. The subclavian approach is outlined in Figure 12–7, A–C.

Occasionally, a patient who already has a central venous line in place will require the emergent placement of a pacing catheter. An existing central venous pressure (CVP) line can be used to place the pacing catheter if the catheter lumen is large enough to accept a guide wire. The CVP line should be withdrawn 1 to 2 inches to expose an area of sterile tubing. The tubing is transected through a sterile area while being held firmly at the skin level (see Fig. 12–8). A guide wire can then be passed through the tubing, and the tubing can be withdrawn, leaving only the wire in the vein (see Fig. 12–9). The guide wire and the tubing should never be released, because embolization

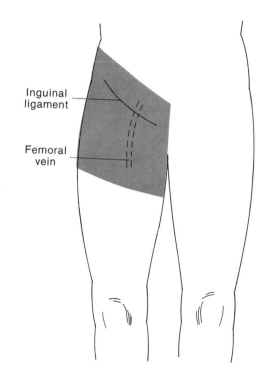

Figure 12–6. Area of skin preparation for femoral approach.

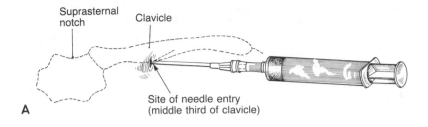

Suprasternal notch

Clavicle

Site of needle entry (middle third of clavicle)

A

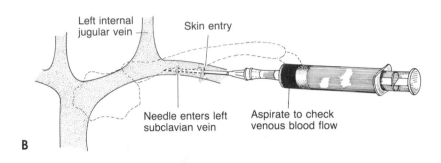

Left internal jugular vein

Skin entry

Needle enters left subclavian vein

Aspirate to check venous blood flow

B

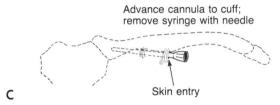

Advance cannula to cuff; remove syringe with needle

C

Skin entry

Figure 12–7. Infraclavicular approach to the subclavian vein. A, Skin entry. B, Cannulation of the vessel. C, Insertion of the introducer sheath. Note that the exposed catheter hub must be covered with a gloved thumb to avoid air embolization.

may result. An introducer unit can then be passed over the guide wire, as is done in the Seldinger technique (see Chapter 18), and the pacing catheter can be placed (Fig. 12–10).

PACEMAKER PLACEMENT (ELECTROCARDIOGRAPHIC GUIDANCE)

The patient should be connected to the limb leads of an electrocardiographic (EKG) machine, and the indicator should be turned to record the chest (V) lead. The pacing wire should be inserted about 10 to 12 cm into the selected vein. The *distal* terminal of the pacing catheter must be connected to the V lead of the EKG machine by a male-to-male connector (Fig. 12–11) or by an insulated wire with an alligator clip on each end (Fig. 12–12). The pacing catheter is thus an exploring electrode that creates a unipolar electrode for intracardiac electrocardiographic recording. The EKG recorded from the electrode tip localizes the position of the tip of the pacing electrode. If a balloon-tipped catheter is used, the balloon is inflated with air or carbon dioxide *after* the catheter enters the superior vena cava. Carbon dioxide is preferred because of its rapid absorption if balloon rupture occurs, although carbon dioxide is not usually available.

The pacing catheter should be advanced both quickly and smoothly. The V lead should be monitored, and the P wave and QRS complex should be observed to ascertain the location of the pacing catheter tip. The use of an EKG to guide the placement of a pacing catheter is based on two concepts: First, the complex will vary in size depending upon which chamber is entered. For example, when the tip of the pacing catheter is in the atrium, one will see large P waves, often larger than the corresponding QRS complex. Second, the sum of the electrical forces will be negative if the depolarization is moving away from the catheter tip and will be positive if the depolarization is moving toward the catheter tip. Therefore, if the catheter tip is *above* the atrium, both the P wave and the QRS complex will be negative. As the tip progresses inferiorly in the atrium, the P wave will become isoelectric (biphasic) and will eventually become positive as the wave of atrial depolarization advances toward the catheter tip. The elec-

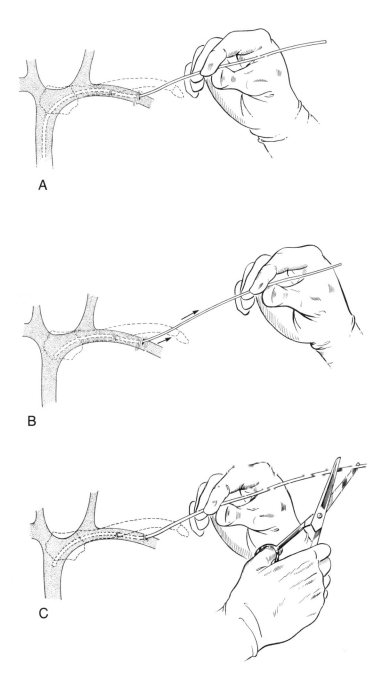

Figure 12–8. Preparing the central line for guide wire insertion. The existing CVP line is grasped (A), withdrawn a few inches (B), and transected (C). Note that the remaining CVP line must be considerably shorter than the guide wire to permit continuous control of the guide wire.

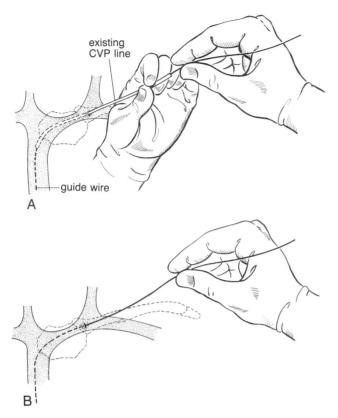

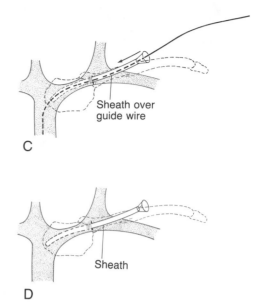

Figure 12–9. Using the central line to insert the guide wire. The guide is passed through the transected CVP line into the central circulation (A), and the existing CVP line is then withdrawn, leaving only the guide wire in the vein (B). C. The passage of an introducer sheath over the guide wire. The guide wire is then removed (D), and the pacemaker is subsequently inserted through the sheath (see Fig. 12–10).

trocardiogram resembles an aVR lead initially when in the left subclavian vein (Fig. 12–13A) or midsuperior vena cava (Fig. 12–13B). At the high right atrium, both the P wave and QRS complex are negative; the P wave is larger than the QRS complex and is deeply inverted (Fig. 12–13C and D). As the center of the atrium is approached, the P wave becomes large and biphasic (Fig. 12–13E). As the catheter approaches the lower atrium (Fig. 12–13F), the P wave becomes smaller and upright. The QRS complex is fairly normal. When striking the right atrial wall, an injury pattern with a P–Ta segment is seen (Fig. 12–13G). As the electrode passes through the triscupid valve, the P wave becomes smaller and the QRS complex becomes larger (Fig. 12–13H). Placement in the inferior vena cava may be recognized by a change in the morphology of the P wave and a decrease in the

amplitude of both the P wave and the QRS complex (Fig. 12–13I).

Once the pacing catheter is in the desired position, the balloon is deflated by unlocking it and allowing the air to passively fill the syringe. One should avoid drawing back on the syringe, because this may cause balloon rupture. If the plunger does not move back spontaneously, assume that the balloon ruptured and do not subsequently place more air into the port. The pacing catheter should be withdrawn, and the balloon

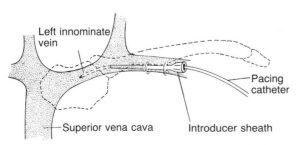

Figure 12–10. Insertion of pacing catheter through introducer sheath.

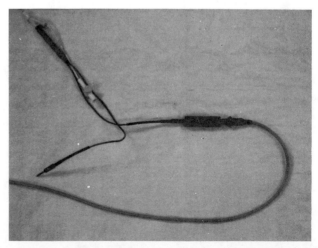

Figure 12–11. Connecting the temporary pacemaker to the V lead of an EKG machine with a male–to–male connecter.

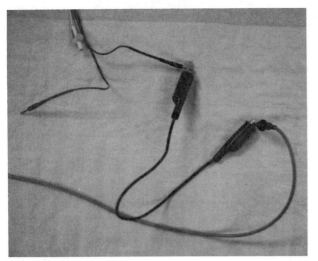

Figure 12–12. Using alligator clips to connect the pacemaker to the V lead of an EKG machine.

should be checked for leaks. If a leak is found, the pacing catheter should be replaced.

After successful placement of the catheter within the right ventricle, the tip should be advanced until contact is made with the endocardial wall. When this occurs, the QRS segment will show ST segment elevation (Fig. 12–13*J*). Ideally, the tip of the catheter should be lodged in the trabeculae at the apex of the right ventricle; however, pacing may be successful if the catheter is in various other positions within the ventricle or outflow tract.

If the pacer enters the pulmonary artery outflow tract, the P wave again becomes negative and the QRS amplitude diminishes (Fig. 12–13*K*). If the catheter is in the pulmonary artery, the pacing catheter should be withdrawn into the right ventricle and readvanced. Sometimes, a clockwise or counterclockwise twist of the catheter will redirect its path in a more favorable direction. If catheter-

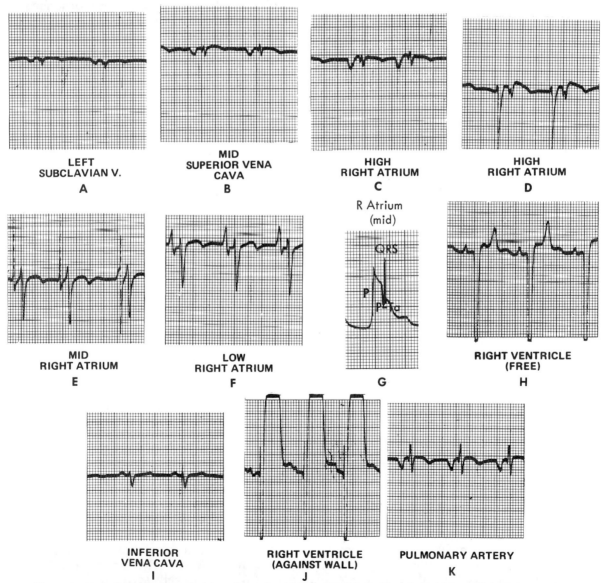

Figure 12–13. *A–K,* Intracardiac electrocardiography. (*A–F* and *H–K,* from Bing, O. H., McDowell, J. W., Hantman, J., et al.: Pacemaker placement by electrocardiographic monitoring. N. Engl. J. Med. 287:651, 1972. *G,* from Goldberger, E.: Treatment of Cardiac Emergencies, 3rd ed. St. Louis, The C. V. Mosby Co., 1982, p. 252.)

induced ectopy develops, the catheter should be slightly withdrawn until the ectopy stops; then it should be readvanced. Occasionally, an antidys-rhythmic drug such as lidocaine may need to be given to desensitize the myocardium. Once ventricular endocardial contact is made, the catheter is disconnected from the EKG machine. The proximal positive and negative leads are connected to their respective terminals on the pacing generator. The pacing generator is then set to a rate of 80 beats per minute or 10 beats per minute faster than the underlying ventricular rhythm, whichever is higher. The full demand mode is selected with an output of about 5 ma. The pacing generator is then turned on. If complete capture does not occur or if it is intermittent, the pacer will need to be repositioned. When proper capture occurs, the pacer is tested for optimal positioning. This is done by testing the thresholds for sensing and pacing, by chest radiographs, by physical examination, and by electrocardiograph.

CATHETER PLACEMENT (WITHOUT AN ELECTROCARDIOGRAPH)

Occasionally, it is necessary to use a transvenous pacemaker in an emergency setting when a well-grounded electrocardiograph machine is not available.

Emergency Blind Placement

Blind insertion of the transvenous pacing catheter is a safe and effective alternative to electrocardiographic guidance. In this technique, the pacing catheter is placed 10 to 12 cm into the venous port and is connected to the pacing generator as noted previously. The pacing rate is selected at *twice* the intrinsic heart rate, and the output is set at an amperage that is too low to capture the ventricle, usually less than 0.2 ma. The unit is then turned on, and the pacing is begun in order to *sense* but *not* to pace. Upon entering the ventricle, the pacer will sense on every other beat. The balloon can then be deflated, the amperage can be increased to 4 to 5 ma, and the pacemaker can be advanced to capture the ventricle. If this does not occur within an additional 10 cm, the pacing catheter should be withdrawn to its original position and then advanced again. As with electrocardiographic placement, proper positioning must be ensured.

Fluoroscopy is a valuable tool in the placement of transvenous pacemakers. Its use depends upon the operator's preference, the patient's condition, and its availability. Pacemakers should not be inserted under fluoroscopy without electrocardiographic monitoring because of the high incidence of ventricular dysrhythmias.[51]

If the cardiac output is too low to "float" a pacing catheter or if the patient is in extremis, there often is not enough time to advance a pacing catheter under EKG guidance. Such a situation would be asystole or complete heart block with malignant ventricular escape rhythms (although one can make a case for transthoracic or transcutaneous pacing in such conditions). In the emergency blind placement technique, the pacing catheper is connected to the energy source, the output is turned to the maximum amperage, and the asynchronous mode is selected. The catheter is then blindly advanced, in hopes that it will enter the right ventricle and that pacing will be accomplished. The pacing catheter is rotated, advanced, withdrawn, or otherwise manipulated according to the clinical response. The left subclavian approach is the most practical access route in this situation. In such instances, there is the theoretical advantage of using the previously described Davison catheter, because one is only interested in rapid capture until the patient is stabilized.

TESTING THRESHOLD

The threshold is the minimum current necessary to obtain capture. Ideally, this is less than 1.0 ma, and usually it is between 0.3 and 0.7 ma. If the threshold is in this ideal range, good contact with the endocardium can be presumed.

To determine the threshold, the pacing generator should be placed in the full demand mode at 5 ma with a rate of approximately 80 beats per minute. The amperage (output) should then be reduced slowly until capture is lost. This current is the threshold. This maneuver should be carried out two or three times to ensure that this value is consistent; the amperage should then be increased to two and one half times the threshold to ensure consistency of capture (usually between 2 and 3 ma).

If one reduces the output to below the threshold and then slowly increases it, there may be a difference in the point at which capture returns. This difference is called hysteresis and represents the time interval between sensing and pacemaker firing. If the difference in capture current is greater than 20 per cent, the pacing catheter should be repositioned, because serious dysrhythmias may result if the pacemaker fires during the vulnerable period of repolarization.[51, 59]

TESTING SENSING

The sensing function should be tested in patients who have underlying rhythms. The pacemaker system is again set in full demand mode with complete capture, and the rate is decreased

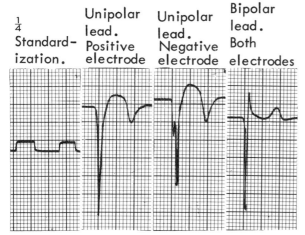

Figure 12–14. Testing unipolar sensing with a bipolar system. (From Goldberger, E.: Treatment of Cardiac Emergencies, 3rd ed. St. Louis, The C. V. Mosby Co., 1982.)

until it is suppressed by the patient's intrinsic rhythm. This is done several times to ensure accuracy of the sensing function.

In bipolar systems, another method of evaluating the sensing mode is to take a unipolar electrocardiogram from each end of the bipolar lead on a chest lead at one-fourth standardization to permit observation of the entire complex.[51] The voltage of the QRS complex is multiplied by four and, if adequate, should be greater than the sensing threshold by more than 1 mv (Fig. 12–14). Another method is to set the electrocardiograph machine on lead 1 and to connect the wires from the proximal electrode to the right arm lead and the left arm lead to the distal electrode (Fig. 12–15). A lead 1 is created, which, when the QRS voltage is multiplied by four, should also be at least 1 mv greater than the sensing threshold.

SECURING AND FINAL ASSESSMENT

After the pacemaker's position has been tested for electrical accuracy, the introducer sheath should be withdrawn (Fig. 12–16) and the catheter should be secured to the skin with 4–0 silk suture. A fastening suture should be sewn to the skin, and the catheter should be tied securely in place. The excess pacing catheter should be coiled and secured in a sterile manner along with the introducer (Fig. 12–17). A large sterile dressing should be applied. Pacemaker function should again be assessed and a chest film should be taken to ensure proper positioning. Ideal positioning of the

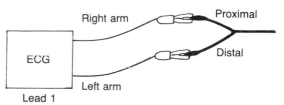

Figure 12–15. Pacemaker lead attachment to EKG machine for lead 1 monitoring of sensing function.

Figure 12–16. Pulling back the introducer sheath (cannula).

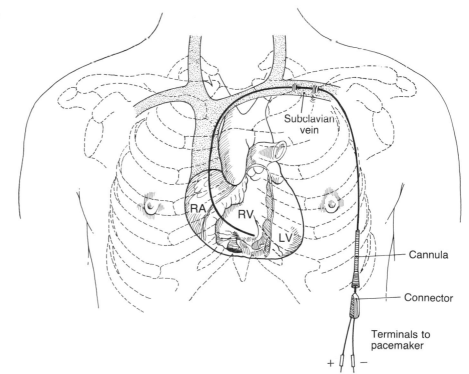

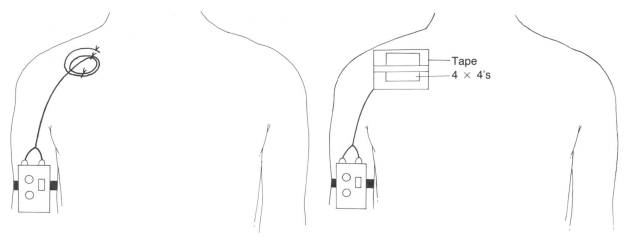

Figure 12–17. Securing the pacemaker.

pacing catheter is at the apex of the right ventricle (Fig. 12–18).

A 12 lead electrocardiogram should be obtained after placement. If the catheter is within the right ventricle, a left bundle branch pattern with left axis deviation should be evident in paced beats (Fig. 12–19). If a right bundle branch block pattern is noted, coronary sinus placement or left ventricular pacing due to septal penetration should be suspected.

With a properly functioning ventricular pacemaker, large cannon waves will be noted on inspection of the venous pulsations at the neck. This is caused by the atria contracting against a closed triscupid valve. On auscultation of the heart, a slight murmur secondary to tricuspid insufficiency from the catheter interfering with the tricuspid valve apparatus may be evident.[60] A clicking sound heard best during expiration following each pacemaker impulse may also be noted here and is believed to represent either intercostal or dia-

phragmatic muscular contractions caused by the pacemaker.[61-63] Note that this can also be a sign of cardiac perforation.[64] On auscultation of the second heart sound, paradoxical splitting may be noted. This represents a delay in closure of the aortic valve because of delayed left ventricular depolarization.

As in any procedure, the patient should then be assessed for improvement and clinical status. An evaluation of vital signs, mentation, improvement in congestive symptoms, and urinary output must be noted. In addition, complications secondary to the procedure should be sought and treated as needed.

Complications

The complications of emergency transvenous cardiac pacing are numerous and represent a compendium of those related to central venous cath-

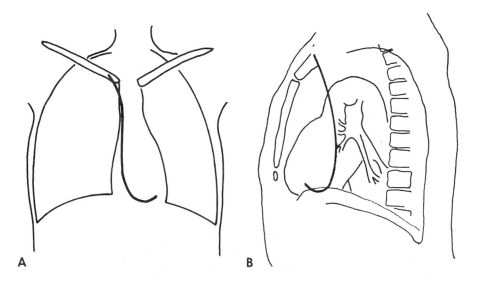

Figure 12–18. Normal pacemaker position on posteroanterior (A) and lateral (B) chest films. (From Goldberger, E.: Treatment of Cardiac Emergencies, 3rd ed. St. Louis, The C. V. Mosby Co., 1982.)

A   B

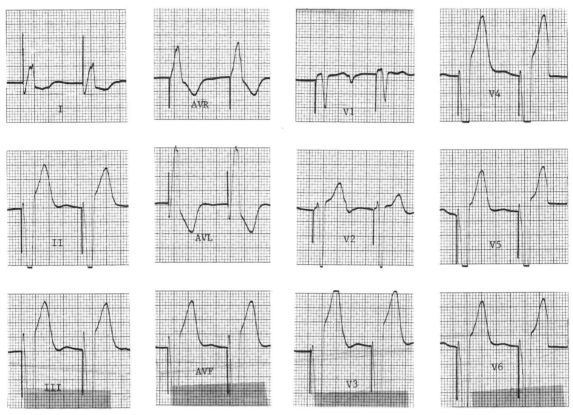

Figure 12–19. EKG pattern of right ventricular pacemaker.

eterization, right heart catheterization, and those unique to the pacing catheter itself.

PROBLEMS RELATED TO CENTRAL VENOUS CATHETERIZATION

Inadvertent arterial puncture is a well-known complication of the percutaneous approach to the venous system.[65] This problem is usually quickly recognized by the rapid return of arterial blood. Firm compression over the puncture site will almost always result in hemostasis in 5 minutes or less.

Venous thrombosis and thrombophlebitis are also potential problems with central venous catheterization. Thrombophlebitis, which occurs early after insertion, is said to be a rare complication. Some experts believe that it can be managed without removal of the catheter or anticoagulation.[58] When thrombophlebitis occurs in chronically implanted pacemakers, removal and anticoagulation may be required. In one series, only 0.1 per cent of permanent pacemakers were in this category and, in a small percentage of these, occult malignancies were found.[58] Complete thrombosis of the innominate vein is also a rare problem, with pul-

monary embolism an even more uncommon event.[66] Femoral vein thrombosis, on the other hand, appears to be a much more common event associated with femoral vein catheterization.[55-57] Recent studies using noninvasive techniques have shown a 37 per cent incidence of femoral vein thrombosis, with 55 per cent of these having ventilation-perfusion scan evidence of pulmonary embolism.[56]

Pneumothorax is consistently a problem with the various approaches to the veins at the base of the neck. Various techniques have been introduced to lessen the chance of pneumothorax, but in general, this complication probably relates to the lack of skill and patience of the operator and to the presence of anatomic variation, such as the apex of the lung being located higher than expected. The decision to place a chest tube in patients with this complication depends upon the extent of the air leak and the clinical status of the patient (see Chapter 6). In addition, laceration of the subclavian with hemothorax, thoracic duct laceration with chylothorax, air embolism, wound infections, pneumomediastinum and hemomediastinum, phrenic nerve injury, fracture of the guide wire with embolization, and catheter or guide wire knotting are all potential complications.[51, 67-75]

COMPLICATIONS OF RIGHT HEART CATHETERIZATION

A very common complication of the pacing catheter is dysrhythmia, with premature ventricular contractions being a common occurence in this author's experience. One study noted a 1.5 per cent incidence of serious dysrhythmias with a balloon-tipped catheter using electrocardiographic guidance compared with a 32 per cent incidence rate with the semi-rigid catheter and fluoroscopic guidance, suggesting that the balloon catheter was the preferred type of catheter.[15] Another study noted a 6 per cent incidence of ventricular tachycardia during insertion.[55] It is well known that the ischemic heart is more prone to dysrhythmias than the non-ischemic heart.[76, 77] The therapy for catheter-induced ectopy involves withdrawing the catheter from the ventricle. This usually stops the ectopy; however, if after repeated attempts it is found that the catheter cannot be passed without ectopy, myocardial suppressant therapy may be used to desensitize the myocardium.

Misplacement of the pacing catheter has been well studied. Passage of the catheter into the pulmonary artery can be diagnosed cardiographically by observing return of an inverted P wave and a decrease in the voltage of the QRS complex.

Misplacement in the coronary sinus may occur and should be suspected in the patient in whom a paced right bundle branch pattern on the electrocardiogram is seen with right ventricular pacing (Fig. 12–20). Rarely, a right bundle branch pattern can be seen with a normal right ventricular position; therefore, all right bundle branch patterns do not represent coronary sinus pacing.[81] Further evidence for coronary sinus location can be obtained by viewing the lateral chest film. Normally, the catheter tip should point anteriorly toward the apex of the heart; however, with coronary sinus placement, the catheter tip is displaced posteriorly and several centimeters away from the sternum (Fig. 12–21). Other potential forms of misplacement include left ventricular pacing through an atrial septal defect or ventricular septal defect, septal puncture, extraluminal insertion, and arterial insertions.[82]

Perforation of the ventricle is also a well-described complication that can result in loss of capture, hemopericardium, and tamponade.[83–85] Reported symptoms and signs of this problem include chest pain, pericardial friction rub, and diaphragmatic or chest wall muscular pacing.[86] At least one case of a post–pericardiotomy-like syndrome and two cases of endocardial friction rub have been reported without perforation.[87, 88] Un-

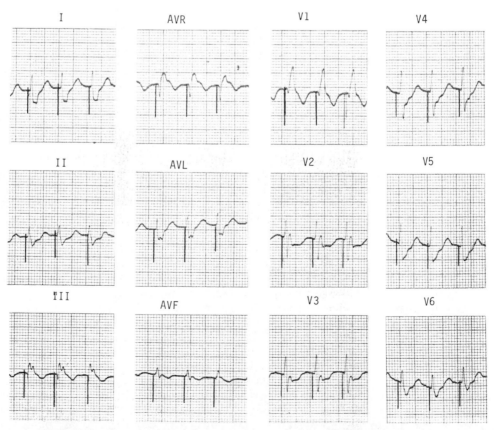

Figure 12–20. Coronary sinus pacing. Note the paced right bundle branch block pattern.

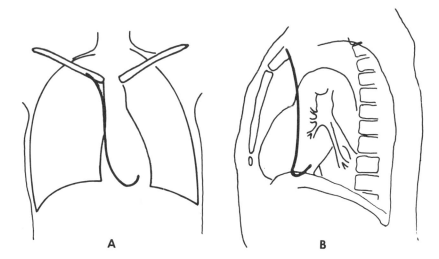

Figure 12–21. Coronary sinus position. *A*, Posteroanterior view. *B*, Lateral view. (From Goldberger, E.: Treatment of Cardiac Emergencies, 3rd ed. St. Louis, The C. V. Mosby Co., 1982.)

complicated perforation can usually be treated by simply pulling back the catheter and repositioning it in the right ventricle.

During the insertion of a permanent pacing catheter when a temporary catheter is in place, there is a small risk of entanglement or knotting. This potential also exists with other central lines and Swan-Ganz catheters. Frequently, these lines can be untangled under fluoroscopy using specialized catheters.

Although local infection does not always require removal of a permanent pacing catheter, systemic infection always does. The most common organism responsible for this infection is *Staphylococcus aureus* followed by *Staphylococcus epidermidis*.[58] One should be certain of the diagnosis of bacteremia before removing the pacing catheter. Therapy for bacteremia usually requires removal of the catheter, placement of a temporary transvenous pacemaker, and 6 weeks of intravenous antibiotics.[89, 90] Sometimes it is difficult to remove a permanent catheter due to entrapment from endothelialization and scar formation. A technique for removing these pacing catheters using a constant traction device has been described.[91] This method may be useful before considering open thoracotomy.

Balloon rupture, pulmonary infarction, phrenic nerve pacing, and rupture of the chorda tendineae are also potential complications.[92–94]

COMPLICATIONS OF THE PACING ELECTRODE

The complications related to the pacing electrode can be separated into three groups: mechanical, organic, and electrical.

Mechanical failures include displacement, fracture of the catheter, and loose leads. Displacement can result in intermittent or complete loss of capture or improper sensing, malignant dysrhyth

mias, diaphragmatic pacing, or perforation. Displacement should be suspected with changes in amplitude or vector changes greater than 90 degrees or with a change in threshold.[95] Fracture of the catheter or loose leads have been reported after chest trauma or even after physical exertion.[96, 97] Frequently, catheter fractures may be detected by careful review of the chest film (Fig. 12–22) or may be suspected because of a change in the sensing threshold. As with displacement, intermittent or complete loss of capture may result. This problem usually does not occur until 30 or more days after placement of permanent pace-

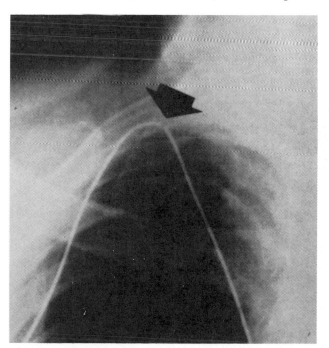

Figure 12–22. Posteroanterior roentgenogram shows transvenous pacemaker electrode in supraclavicular area. Lead is fractured at exit of lead from jugular vein (*arrow*). (From Tegtmeyer, C. J., Bezirdjian, D. R., Irani, F. A., and Landis, J. D.: Cardiac pacemaker failure: a complication of trauma. South. Med. J. 74:378, 1981. Used by permission.)

makers; however, it may occur sooner in temporary units.

Organic causes of pacemaker failure result in changes in the threshold or sensing function. Progressive inflammation, fibrosis, and thrombosis may result in more than doubling of the original threshold. This may occur in 3 to 4 weeks and should be expected in prolonged temporary or permanent pacemakers. Physiologic and pharmacologic factors that affect threshold have been studied. Sleeping, eating a heavy meal, lowered aldosterone concentration, potassium infusions, and myxedema all increase threshold by raising the resting membrane potential. The threshold to cardiac pacing tends to decrease with exercise, sympathetic amines, glucocorticoids, and toxic levels of procainamide.[98–102]

In some patients, the atrial contribution to ventricular filling is extremely important. Transvenous ventricular pacing results in the loss of the atrial kick and ultimately a decrease in left ventricular stroke volume. This phenomenon is called post-pacer syndrome and occasionally is severe enough to preclude the use of a pacemaker.[103] A sequential pacemaker that stimulates the atria and ventricles in sequential fashion is a viable alternative for patients unable to tolerate the loss of the atrial kick. This device is currently only used for permanent pacing.

Electrical problems with pacing include battery failure, dysrhythmias, and outside interference. Battery failure is usually detected by a slowing of the heart rate.[98] With the old mercury battery system, sensing capability was usually lost first, followed by a relatively rapid loss in capture. With the new lithium and nuclear units, a slow, progressive rate decrease occurs naturally. These units found in permanent pacemaker systems are usually replaced electively after the rate decreases approximately 10 per cent. When they do fail, however, the underlying intrinsic rhythm may require emergency pacing. Occasionally, runaway pacemaking with rates greater than 200 may be a manifestation of battery failure. In an emergency situation, the skin pocket that contains the pacemaker generator can be opened under sterile technique. The wires may be cut close to the generator and connected to a temporary unit. The pacemaker generator can then be replaced electively.

In the first type of units available, outside interference, caused by television transmitters, electric tooth brushes, electric razors, magnetic fields, microwave ovens, and airport surveillance equipment, frequently resulted in pacemaker inhibition because of inappropriate sensing.[104–109] Although current models are designed to prevent this type of complication, problems still occur, usually converting the unit to a fixed mode.

Table 12–6. COMPLICATIONS OF TRANSVENOUS CARDIAC PACING

Year	Author	Patients	Catheter	Route	Result
1969	Rosenberg, A. S., et al.[1]	111	Flexon steelwire vs. unipolar semi-floating (EKG)	96 subclavian 5 basilic 1 external jugular	12 inconsistent pacing, 3 local infection, 2 pneumothorax, 1 subclavian artery puncture; 16% complication rate
1973	Schnitzler, R. N., et al.[14]	17	3F bipolar semi-floating balloon (EKG)	Antecubital vein	2 PVCs, stable pacing, no thrombophlebitis
1973	Weinstein, J., et al.[16]	100	6F bipolar (U.S.C.I.) (fluoroscopy)	Femoral	2 ventricular tachycardia, 2 perforations, 2 required repositionings, 1 questionable thrombophlebitis and pulmonary embolism, 1 local infection
1973	Lumia, F. J., and Rios, J. C.[112]	142 insertions in 113 patients	Bipolar (fluoroscopy)	61 brachial 81 femoral	12 ventricular tachycardia and fibrillation in 9 patients, 3 perforations in 2 patients; local hematoma, abscess, and bleeding in 30%; 16.9% complication rate
1980	Pandian, N. G., et al.[57]	20	5F bipolar (fluoroscopy)	Femoral	25% deep venous thrombosis
1980	Nolewajka, A. T., et al.[56]	29	6F cordis (fluoroscopy)	Femoral	34% venous thrombosis by venogram with 60% of these with pulmonary embolism by VQ scan
1981	Lang, R., et al.[15]	111	Balloon, semi-floating vs. semi-rigid	Subclavian	Serious dysrhythmia: 1.5% balloon-tipped, 20.4% semi-rigid; Catheter displacement: 13.6% ± 4.4 days balloon-tipped; 32% ± 1.9 day semi-rigid
1982	Austin, J. L., et al.[55]	113 insertions in 100 patients	4–7F bipolar (fluoroscopy)	Brachial Femoral	Failure to sense or pace in 37%; repositioning in 37% of brachial insertions; repositioning in 9% of femoral insertions; fever, sepsis, local infection only in femoral insertions; 20% complication rate

Although ventricular tachycardia and ventricular fibrillation have been reported to result from pacemakers, these dysrhythmias are rare. Because of this, patients who present with such dysrhythmias should be evaluated for a non-pacemaker etiology.[110]

DC cardioversion and electroshock therapy are safe procedures to carry out in patients who have pacemakers as long as the current does not directly go over the generator pack.[98, 111]

Table 12–6 summarizes the complications found in several studies on cardiac pacing.

Conclusion

Temporary transvenous pacing is a rapid, safe, and reliable method for achieving effective electrical stimulation of the heart. It can and should be mastered by any physician who is responsible for the care of the critically ill or injured patients. Symptomatic bradycardias unresponsive to pharmacologic means and some tachycardias are indications for its use. In acute myocardial infarction, it serves both a therapeutic and prophylactic function. Transvenous pacing in the trauma patient may be advocated more frequently in the future.

1. Rosenberg, A. S., et al.: Bedside transvenous cardiac pacing. Am. Heart J. 77:697, 1969.
2. Callaghan, J. C., and Bigelow, W. G.: Electrical artificial pacemaker for standstill of heart. Ann. Surg. 134:8, 1951.
3. Zoll, P. M.: Resuscitation of the heart in ventricular standstill by external electrical stimulation. N. Engl. J. Med. 247:768, 1952.
4. Furman, S., and Schwedel, J. B.: Intracardiac pacemaker for Stokes-Adams seizures. N. Engl. J. Med. 261:943, 1959.
5. Muller, O. F., and Bellet, S.: Treatment of intractable heart failure in the presence of complete atrioventricular heart block by the use of internal cardiac packemaker. Report of two cases. N. Engl. J. Med. 265:768, 1961.
6. Siddons, H. and Davies, J. G.: A new technique for internal cardiac pacing. Lancet 12:1204, 1963.
7. DeSanctis, R. W.: Short-term use of intravenous electrode in heart block. JAMA 184:130, 1963.
8. Vogel, J. H. K., et al.: A simple technique for identifying P waves in complex arrhythmias. Am. Heart J. 67:158, 1964.
9. Kimball, J. T., and Killip, T.: A simple bedside method for transvenous intracardiac pacing. Am. Heart J. 70:35, 1965.
10. Harris, C. W., et al.: Percutaneous technique for cardiac pacing with a platinum-tipped electrode catheter. Am. J. Cardiol. 15:48, 1965.
11. Goetz, R. H., et al.: Pacing on demand in the treatment of atrioventricular conduction disturbances of the heart. Lancet 7464:599, 1966.
12. Zuckerman, W., et al.: Clinical experience with a new implantable demand pacemaker. Am. J. Cardiol. 20:232, 1967.
13. Swan, H. J., et al.: Catheterization of the heart in man with use of a flow-directed balloon-tipped catheter. N. Engl. J. Med. 283:447, 1970.
14. Schnitzler, R. N., et al.: "Floating" catheter for temporary transvenous ventricular pacing. Am. J. Cardiol. 31:351, 1973.
15. Snag, R., et al.: The use of the balloon-tipped floating catheter in temporary transvenous cardiac pacing. PACE 4:491, 1981.
16. Furman, S.: Cardiac pacing and pacemaker. I. Indications for pacing bradyarrhythmias. Am. Heart J. 93:523, 1977.
17. Escher, D. J., and Furman, S.: Emergency treatment of cardiac arrhythmias. Emphasis on use of electrical pacing. JAMA 214:2028, 1970.
18. Julian, D. G., et al.: Disturbances of rate, rhythm, and conduction in acute myocardial infarction: a prospective study of 100 consecutive unselected patients with the aid of electrocardiographic monitoring. Am. J. Med. 37:915, 1965.
19. Adgey, A. A. J., et al.: Incidence, significance, and management of early bradyarrhthmias complicating acute myocardial infarction. Lancet 2:1097, 1968.
20. Haden, R. F., et al.: The significance of sinus bradycardia in acute myocardial infarction. Dis. Chest 44:168, 1963.
21. Rotman, M.: Bradyarrhythmias in acute myocardial infarction. Circulation 45:703, 1972.
22. Baba, N.: Experimental cardiac ischemia, observation of the sinoatrial and atrioventricular node. Lab. Invest. 23:168, 1970.
23. James, T. N.: Cardiac innervation: anatomic and pharmacologic relations. Bull. N.Y. Acad. Med. 43:1041, 1967.
24. Constantin, L.: Extracardiac factors contributing to hypotension during coronary occlusion. Am. J. Cardiol. 11:205, 1963.
25. Wolf, S.: Bradycardia of the dive reflex: a possible mechanism of sudden death. Trans. Am. Clin. Climatol. Assoc. 76:142, 1964.
26. Hazard, P. B.: Transvenous cardiac pacing in cardiopulmonary resuscitation. Crit. Care Med. 9:666, 1981.
27. Conklin, E. F., et al.: Four hundred consecutive patients with permanent transvenous pacemakers. J. Thorac. Cardiovasc. Surg. 69:1, 1975.
28. Escher, D. J.: The use of artificial pacemakers in acute myocardial infarction. In Chung, E. K. (ed.): Controversy in Cardiology: A Practical Clinical Approach. New York, Springer Verlag, 1976, p. 51
29. Simon, A. B., et al.: Atrioventricular block in acute myocardial infarction. Chest 62:156, 1972.
30. Resuekov, L., and Lipp, H.: Pacemaking in acute myocardial infarction. Prog. Cardiovasc. Dis. 14:475, 1972.
31. Hindman, M. C., et al.: The clinical significance of bundle branch block complicating acute myocardial infarction. 2. Indications of temporary and permanent pacemaker insertion. Circulation 58:689, 1978.
32. Atkins, J. M., et al.: Ventricular conduction blocks and sudden death in acute myocardial infarction. N. Engl. J. Med. 288:281, 1978.
33. Hindman, M. C., et al.: The clinical significance of bundle branch block complicating acute myocardial infarction. 1. Clinical characteristics, hospital mortality, and one year follow-up. Circulation 58:679, 1978.
34. Jocobson, C. B., et al.: Management of acute bundle branch block and bradyarrhythmias. Med. Clin. North Am. 63:93, 1979.
35. Escher, D. J.: The use of cardiac pacemakers. In Braunwald, E. (ed.): Heart Disease: A Textbook of Cardiovascular Medicine. Philadelphia, W. B. Saunders Company, 1980, p. 749.
36. Bharati, S., et al.: Atrial arrhythmias related to trauma to sinoatrial node. Chest 61:331, 1972.
37. Dreifus, L. S.: Dysrhythmias related to cardiac trauma. Chest 61:310, 1972.
38. Miller, M. S., and Scott, S. F.: Cardiac contusion and right bundle branch block. JACEP 6:504, 1977.
39. Bognolo, D. A., et al.: Traumatic sinus node dysfunction. Ann. Emerg. Med. 11:319, 1982.

40. Mazor, A., and Roger, S.: Cardiac aspects of shock. Ann. Surg. 178:128, 1973.

41. White, B. C., et al.: HIS electrocardiographic characterization of terminal arrhythmias of hemorrhagic shock in dogs. JACEP 8:298, 1979.

42. Millikan, J. S., et al.: Temporary cardiac pacing in traumatic arrest victims. Ann. Emerg. Med. 9:591, 1980.

43. Schwedel, J. B., et al.: Use of intracardiac pacemaker in treatment of Stokes-Adams seizures. Prog. Cardiovasc. Dis. 3:170, 1960.

44. Zoll, P. M., et al.: Ventricular fibrillation: treatment and prevention by external electric currents. N. Engl. J. Med. 262:105, 1960.

45. Haft, J. L.: Treatment of arrhythmias by intracardiac electrical stimulation. Prog. Cardiovasc. Dis. 16:539, 1974.

46. Cheng, T. O.: Transvenous ventricular pacing in the treatment of paroxysmal atrial tachyarrhythmias alternating with sinus bradycardia and standstill. Am. J. Cardiol. 22:874, 1968.

47. Kastor, J. A.: Transvenous atrial pacing in the treatment of refractory ventricular irritability. Ann. Intern. Med. 66:439, 1967.

48. Barold, S. S., and Linhart, J. W.: Recent advances in the treatment of ectopic tachycardias by electrical pacing. Am. J. Cardiol. 25:698, 1970.

49. Weiner, I.: Pacing techniques in the treatment of tachycardias. Ann. Intern. Med. 93:326, 1980.

50. DeSanctis, R. W., and Kastor, J. A.: Rapid intracardiac pacing for treatment of recurrent ventricular arrhythmias in the absence of heart block. Am. Heart J. 76:168, 1968.

51. Goldberger, E.: Temporary cardiac pacing. In Goldberger, E., and Wheet, M. W., Jr. (eds.): Treatment of Cardiac Emergencies, 3rd ed. St. Louis, The C. V. Mosby Co., 1982, p. 233.

52. Personal communication with Electro-Catheter Corp.

53. Dronen, S., et al.: Subclavian vein catheterization during cardiopulmonary resucitation. JAMA 247:3227, 1982.

54. Mostert, M. D., et al.: Safe placement of central venous catheter into the internal jugular veins. Arch. Surg. 101:431, 1970.

55. Austin, J. L., et al.: Analysis of pacemaker malfunction and complications of temporary pacing in the coronary care unit. Am. J. Cardiol. 44:301, 1982.

56. Nolewajka, A. T., et al.: Temporary transvenous pacing and femoral vein thrombosis. Am. J. Cardiol. 45:459, 1980.

57. Pandian, N. G., et al.: Transfemoral temporary pacing and deep vein thrombosis. Am. Heart J. 100:847, 1980.

58. Furman, S.: Pacemaker emergencies. Med. Clin. North Am. 63:113, 1979.

59. Thompson, M. E., and Shaver, J. A.: Undesirable cardiac arrhythmias associated with rate hysteresis pacemakers. Am. J. Cardiol. 38:685, 1976.

60. Nachnani, G. H., et al.: Systolic murmurs induced by pacemaker catheters. Arch. Intern. Med. 24:202, 1969.

61. Kluge, W. F.: Pacemaker sound and its origin. Am. J. Cardiol. 25:362, 1970.

62. Korn, M., et al.: The pacemaker sound. Am. J. Med. 49:451, 1970.

63. Pupillo, G. A., et al.: "Pacemaker heart sound" caused by diaphragmatic contractions. Am. Heart J. 82:711, 1971.

64. Kramer, D. H., et al.: Mechanisms and significance of pacemaker-induced extracardiac sound. Am. J. Cardiol. 25:367, 1970.

65. Herbst, C. A.: Indications, management, and complications of percutaneous subclavian catheters. Arch. Surg. 113:1421, 1978.

66. Sethi, G. K., et al.: Innominate venous thrombosis: a rare complication of transvenous pacemaker electrodes. Am. Heart J. 87:770, 1974.

67. Johnson, C. L., et al.: Subclavian venipuncture, preventable complications. Mayo Clin. Proc. 45:719, 1970.

68. Woods, R. R.: Technic of subclavian vein cannulization to eliminate danger of pneumothorax. South. Med. J. 70:1111, 1977.

69. Arbitman, M., and Kart, B. H.: Hydromediastinum after aberrant central venous catheter placement. Crit. Care Med. 7:27, 1979.

70. Drachler, D. H., et al.: Phrenic nerve injury from subclavian vein catheterization. JAMA 236:2880, 1976.

71. Cope, C.: Intravascular breakage of seldinger spring guide wires. JAMA 180:1061, 1962.

72. Schwartz, A. J., et al.: Guide wires—a caution. Crit. Care Med. 9:347, 1981.

73. Johansson, L., et al.: Intracardiac knotting of the catheter in heart catheterization. J. Thorac. Surg. 27:605, 1954.

74. Boal, B. H., et al.: Complication of intracardiac electrical pacing—knotting together of temporary and permanent electrodes. N. Engl. J. Med. 280:650, 1969.

75. Lipp, H., et al.: Knotting of a flow-directed balloon catheter. N. Engl. J. Med. 284:220, 1971.

76. Mehra, R., et al.: Vulnerability of the mildly ischemic ventricle to cathodal, anodal, and bipolar stimulation. Circ. Res. 41:159, 1977.

77. Chatterjee, K., et al.: The risk of pacing after infarction and current recommendations. Lancet 2:1061, 1969.

78. Maytin, O., et al.: Unusual QRS complexes produced by pacemaker stimuli. Am. Heart J. 77:732, 1969.

79. Nower, M. M.: Unusual patterns of conduction produced by pacemaker stimuli. Am. Heart J. 74:24, 1967.

80. Spitzberg, J.: An unusual site of ventricular pacing occurring during the use of transvenous catheter pacemaker. Am. Heart J. 77:529, 1979.

81. Abernathy, W. S., and Crevey, B. J.: Right bundle branch block during transvenous ventricular pacing. Am. Heart J. 90:774, 1975.

82. Campo, I., et al.: Complications of pacing by pervenous subclavian semifloating electrodes including extraluminal insertions. Am. J. Cardiol. 26:627, 1970.

83. Goswani, M., et al.: Perforation of the heart by flexible transvenous pacemaker. JAMA 216:2013, 1971.

84. Danielson, G. K., et al.: Failure of endocardial pacemaker due to myocardial perforation. J. Thorac. Cardiovasc. Surg. 54:42, 1967.

85. Kalloor, G. J.: Cardiac tamponade. Report of a case after insertion of transvenous endocardial electrode. Am. Heart J. 88:88, 1974.

86. Jorgensen, E. O., et al.: Unusual sign of perforation of a pacemaker catheter. Am. Heart J. 74:732, 1967.

87. Kaye, D., et al.: Probable postcardiotomy syndrome following implantation of a transvenous pacemaker: report of the first case. Am. Heart J. 90:627, 1975.

88. Glassman, R. D., et al.: Pacemaker-induced endocardial friction rub. Am. J. Cardiol. 40:811, 1977.

89. Furman, R. W., et al.: Infected permanent cardiac pacemaker. Management with removal. Ann. Thorac. Surg. 14:54, 1972.

90. Kennelly, B. M., and Diller, L. W.: Management of infected transvenous permanent pacemakers. Br. Heart J. 36:1133, 1974.

91. Bilgulay, A. M., et al.: Incarceration of transvenous pacemaker electrode. Removal by traction. Am. Heart J. 77:377, 1969.

92. Foote, G. A., et al.: Pulmonary complications of the flow-directed balloon-tipped catheter. N. Engl. J. Med. 290:927, 1974.

93. Sprinkle, J. D., et al.: Phrenic nerve stimulation as a complication of implantable cardiac pacemaker. Circulation 28:114, 1963.

94. Escher, D. J., et al.: Transvenous pacing of the phrenic nerve. Am. Heart J. 72:283, 1977.

95. Preston, T. A.: Electrocardiographic diagnosis of pacemaker catheter displacement. Am. Heart J. 854:445, 1973.

96. Kronzon, I., and Mehta, S. S.: Broken wire in multiple trauma: a case report. J. Trauma 14:82, 1974.
97. Ohm, O.: Displacement and fracture of pacemaker electrode during physical exertion: report of three cases. Acta Med. Scand. 192:33, 1972.
98. Smith, N. D.: Pacemaker dysfunction. In Greenberg, M. I., and Roberts, J. R. (eds.): Emergency Medicine: A Clinical Approach to Challenging Problems. Philadelphia, F. A. Davis Co., 1982, p. 355.
99. Preston, T. A., et al.: Changes in myocardial threshold, physiologic, and pharmacologic factors in patients with implanted pacemakers. Am. Heart J. 74:235, 1967.
100. Gay, R. J., and Brown, D. F.: Pacemaker failure due to procainamide toxicity. Am. J. Cardiol. 34:728, 1974.
101. Walker, W. J., et al.: Effect of potassium in restoring myocardial response to a subthreshold cardiac pacemaker. N. Engl. J. Med. 271:12, 1964.
102. Basu, D., and Chatterjee, K.: Unusually high pacemaker threshold in severe myxedema. Decrease with thyroid hormone therapy. Chest 70:677, 1976.
103. Haas, J. M., and Strait, G. B.: Pacemaker-induced cardiovascular failure. Am. J. Cardiol. 33:295, 1974.
104. D'Cunha, G. F., et al.: Syncopal attacks arising from erratic demand pacemaker function in the vicinity of a television transmitter. Am. J. Cardiol. 31:789, 1973.
105. Escher, D. J., et al.: Pacemaker triggering (inhibition) by electric toothbrush. Am. J. Cardiol. 38:126, 1976.
106. Furman, S.: Electric razor interference with cardiac pacemakers. JAMA 222:1658, 1972.
107. Escher, D. J., et al.: Influence of alternating magnetic fields on triggered pacemakers. Circulation 44:162, 1971.
108. Editorial: Microwaves and pacemakers: just how well do they go together? JAMA 221:957, 1972.
109. Mitchell, J. C., et al.: Empirical studies of cardiac pacemaker interference. Aerospace Med. 45:189, 1974.
110. Leung, F. W., and Oill, P. A.: Ticket of admission unexplained syncopal attacks in patients with cardiac pacemaker. Ann. Emerg. Med. 9:527, 1980.
111. Youmans, R. C., et al.: Electroshock therapy and cardiac pacemakers. Am. J. Surg. 118:931, 1969.
112. Lumia, F. J., and Rios, J. C.: Temporary transvenous pacemaker therapy: an analysis of complications. Chest 64:604, 1973.

13

Transthoracic Transcutaneous Cardiac Pacing

EMERGENCY TRANSTHORACIC PACEMAKER*

JAMES R. ROBERTS, M.D.

Introduction

The history of electrical stimulation of the heart began in the mid-18th century when crude attempts were made to revive dead animals and humans with electrical current from a Leyden jar.[1] The first successful clinical application of external cardiac pacing was accomplished by Zoll (1952) using a method of externally applied closed chest pacing for Stokes-Adams disease.[2] In the 1960's, a popular technique involved the use of percutaneous wires implanted directly into the myocardium through the chest wall.[3] The apparatus most commonly used today for transthoracic pacing is the transmyocardial pacemaker, a bipolar pacing wire that is placed into the ventricular cavity using an intracardiac stick with a needle introducer.

With the development of sophisticated transvenous pacemaker electrodes, the technique of transthoracic wire implantation for emergency pacing became less prevalent. Recent advancements in technology and the development of the specialty of emergency medicine have sparked a new interest in the concept of emergency transthoracic pacing.

Although in most textbooks the use of the transthoracic route is mentioned only briefly or not at all,[4-7] approximately 40,000 units are used annually in the United States. The device is supplied to more than 1000 hospitals.[8] Considering such wide usage, it is surprising to find such a paucity of recent literature on this subject.

It is the purpose of this chapter to review the development, concepts, and technique of transthoracic pacemaker insertion and to offer a rational approach to current application of the procedure in the emergency department. All references to transthoracic pacing that follow apply to percutaneous pacing wires introduced through a transthoracic needle and do not apply to electrodes inserted into the myocardium by a thoracotomy or under direct vision. Some of the conclusions and recommendations are the opinions of the author based on a review of the literature and personal clinical experience.

*Reproduced from Roberts, J.R. Greenberg, M. I.: Emergency transthoracic pacemaker. Ann. Emerg. Med. 10:600–612, 1981. Used with permission.

Historical Development

In reviewing the medical literature, the author found many articles concerning the clinical use of emergency transthoracic pacing.[2, 7, 9–18]

Before the development of reliable transvenous electrodes, initial attempts at transthoracic pacing consisted of two external needle electrodes placed subcutaneously on the chest wall with the wires attached to an external energy source.[2, 16, 17] Pacing of the heart through the chest wall by this minimally invasive method was generally successful, although extremely high voltages were sometimes required and capture was intermittent. With this technique, the entire thorax and the diaphragm were also stimulated, resulting in painful muscle contractions. Skin burns occasionally occurred, and the unsedated patient had difficulty tolerating the discomfort. Although clinically successful, this impractical technique was short lived. Recent advances in technology have made transcutaneous pacing more feasible; thus, over the next few years, there may be a revival in *transcutaneous* pacing.

Thevenet and associates[3] published the first description of a *transthoracic* technique incorporating the percutaneous implantation of a unipolar wire electrode (cathode) into the myocardial wall of the right ventricle. The uninsulated wire was inserted through a spinal needle using a left parasternal approach. The indifferent electrode (anode) was a wire placed subcutaneously in the chest wall near the cardiac apex. The experimental animals in this study had surgical interruption of the AV node and bundle of His and were in complete heart block. Transthoracic pacing was successful in controlling the heart rate in all experimental animals, and no harmful effects to the myocardium or pericardium were noted at autopsy. One dog was paced for 10 days. In addition, a percutaneous wire was successfully placed in the ventricles of seven human cadavers, thus demonstrating the clinical feasibility of the technique. Thevenet and coworkers concluded that the procedure was safe, easy, and effective and that it had no significant associated morbidity. Other authors reported success with percutaneous pacing in experimental animals and in humans when a wire was implanted into the ventricular wall, although the procedure and equipment varied slightly with each report.[9–13]

A review of the relatively sparse medical literature substantiates the fact that the transthoracic pacer can be easily introduced, is relatively safe, and is effective in treating selected pathology. Of the 44 human cases reported in the older literature to have been successfully treated with the transthoracic pacemaker, two patients had non-lethal pericardial bleeding. There are no reported cases of pneumothorax, coronary artery lacerations, major organ or vessel injury, or a fatality directly attributed to the technique. The majority of pacemakers were not introduced during cardiopulmonary resuscitation (CPR), a situation that would most likely increase the complication rate. Most older studies involve complete heart block, and all are retrospective in nature. There are no prospective studies in the literature that address the efficacy of the transthoracic pacemaker in treating cardiac arrest.

Tintinalli and White[18] reported a retrospective series of 21 unsuccessful resuscitations in which the transthoracic pacer was used in bradyasystolic arrest. The study used an older model of the transthoracic pacer, and the device was used for some conditions for which a pacer could not have been expected to be of benefit. In addition, the device was used as a last resort, approximately 30 to 45 minutes into the resuscitation and only after extensive drug therapy had failed. Despite the late use of the pacer in the study, capture occurred in 8 of 21 cases and a transient blood pressure was recorded in two patients. A cardiac tamponade occurred in one patient, and this complication may have contributed to an unsuccessful outcome. The authors concluded that the transthoracic pacer did not alter outcome in bradyasystolic arrest when standard advanced cardiac life support (ACLS) therapy was unsuccessful.

Roberts and colleagues[19] reported the successful use of the transthoracic pacemaker in six patients with bradyasystolic cardiac arrest. Pathology included asystole, AV dissociation, and supraventricular bradycardia. The severity of the underlying disease did not allow for long-term survival in three patients, but the initial resuscitation of all patients was attributed to the technique of transthoracic pacing.

Ornato and coworkers reported the results of patients in bradyasystolic cardiac arrest who after failing standard pharmacologic therapy were treated with transthoracic cardiac pacing.[61] Electrical capture was noted in 30 of 48 patients (63 per cent); 2 of the patients developed a pulse; and 1 of the patients survived to admission but died in the hospital. Although there was a trend for electrical capture to be more likely if the patient was paced shortly after cardiac arrest, the authors were unable to show statistical significance to this trend. White and Brown recently reported a prospective trial of transthoracic pacing used as an initial method of emergency department therapy for 48 asystolic arrest patients.[62] Their patients had failed pharmacologic resuscitation in the prehospital phase and they did not report the duration of cardiac arrest prior to transthoracic pacing. White and Brown demonstrated electrical capture in 23 per cent of the patients and a palpable pulse in 17 per cent. With subsequent intracardiac sodium bicarbonate and epinephrine therapy, the capture rate rose to 46 per cent with a transient pulse or blood pressure in 33 per cent. One of their patients survived to be admitted but there were no long-term survivors. They concluded that *immediate* transthoracic pacing is temporarily effective in restoring electrical activity in a substantial number of asystolic patients.

Indications for Emergency Transthoracic Pacing

Although the absolute indications for emergency transthoracic pacing are not described, most authors express a vague consensus about contraindications. General guidelines suggest that when the time and clinical situation permits, cardiac pacing should be done using the transvenous route with fluoroscopy or flow-directed pacemaker catheters (see Chapter 12). The transthoracic route is contraindicated in the stable or awake patient or in situations in which the cardiac emergency can quickly and easily be managed by drug therapy.[4] Obviously, these are imprecise criteria that are subject to various interpretations. For the sake of discussion concerning the use of emergency transthoracic pacing, patients can be divided into two general categories: those who are "unstable," including critically ill patients in heart block, recurrent ventricular tachycardia, or profound bradycardia; and all patients in cardiac arrest.

UNSTABLE PATIENTS

The specific use of transthoracic pacing in unstable patients is poorly addressed in the modern literature. Early studies demonstrated the efficacy of the procedure in animals and in a few patients with complete heart block. With the availability of current pharmacology and with the development of sophisticated transvenous pacing methods, it is questionable whether the transthoracic route is currently indicated for most unstable patients with third degree AV block or with other forms of symptomatic bradycardia. Because the procedure has been shown to be relatively safe, rapid, and effective in complete heart block, I believe that it is reasonable to consider emergency transthoracic pacing in patients with severe *drug-resistant* ventricular bradycardias producing pulmonary edema, seizures, recurrent ventricular fibrillation, or ventricular tachycardia. These are patients in whom a transvenous pacemaker cannot be rapidly inserted.

Transthoracic pacing is technically a relatively simple procedure when compared to transvenous pacemaker placement. Transthoracic pacing can be accomplished rapidly when one considers the time required for a cutdown or securing of a large-bore central cannula. Therefore, the transthoracic route may be advantageous in selected situations that produce an unstable clinical picture. A special advantage is that no blood flow is required to float the transthoracic pacemaker into proper position.

It is my opinion that a *rapidly deteriorating patient* with complete AV dissociation or other type of ventricular bradycardia should be considered a candidate for emergency transthoracic pacing if transvenous pacing cannot be immediately instituted. The frequency of instituting such therapy would naturally depend upon the availability of consultation and the expertise of the emergency physician.

CARDIAC ARREST

The use of transthoracic pacing during cardiac arrest is a controversial subject. Cardiology texts usually dismiss the procedure with brevity. One text on pacing is illustrative and states that the procedure is "dangerous and should be used only in an emergency."[20] Because cardiac arrest is an emergency, one would assume that the technique would be supported in such cases. A more recent text takes a firm stand and advocates the use of a transthoracic pacemaker in bradyasystolic cardiac arrest.[21]

Many physicians report poor results with transthoracic pacing in cardiac arrest, whereas others have reasonable (although largely anecdotal) success. Preston[22] estimates a 40 per cent success rate in achieving pacing by the transthoracic route and attributes this expectation to the moribund condition of most patients in whom the procedure is used. Iseri and associates[23] suggest that because bradyasystolic cardiac arrest is associated with an almost certain fatal outcome, transthoracic pacing may be one of the techniques that can be explored to alter this rather dismal prognosis. Accurate statistics are not available concerning the efficacy of emergency transthoracic pacing. Because resuscitation from cardiac arrest is successful in only approximately 15 per cent of the cases[24] (range 8.5 to 28.6 per cent[25–27]), any technique or drug therapy will be associated with a poor result. The issue of transthoracic pacing during cardiac arrest becomes even more controversial when one considers two additional points: at what point during the resuscitation is pacing attempted, and what constitutes the underlying cause of the cardiac arrest.

Rationale for Use in Cardiac Arrest

I do not believe that the routine use of any form of emergency cardiac pacing will drastically alter the survival rate in cases of bradyasystolic cardiac arrest, and transthoracic pacing should in no way be considered a panacea for cardiac arrest. Emergency pacing, however, will certainly be lifesaving in selected clinical situations. Emergency pacing, by definition, does not include those patients who are able to tolerate delays in treatment or various diagnostic techniques; rather, the term *emergency* is used to refer to patients in cardiac arrest or in other truly life-threatening conditions.

Because no clear-cut indications or guidelines exist for use of transthoracic cardiac pacing during cardiac arrest and because there are, as yet, few controlled, prospective studies addressing its success rate, it is impossible to comment on changes in survival rate, percentage of capture, or frequency of complication if the procedure were used routinely.

Nonetheless, some logical deductions can be made from the sparse information that does exist. One would expect that emergency transthoracic pacing would be most effective following cardiac arrest from primary cardiac disease. This would account for approximately 80 per cent of cardiac arrests.[2] One would expect that cardiac collapse secondary to hypovolemia (such as that which may occur secondary to trauma) or severe electrolyte or acid-base abnormalities, sepsis, or drug intoxication would be less likely to respond to cardiac pacing. These severe metabolic derangements would certainly make resuscitation difficult, and perhaps no form of therapy can be expected to be successful in such a hostile milieu. In early animal studies, Bellet[10] demonstrated that pacing was not effective in cases of severe hyperkalemia or cardiac arrest secondary to poisoning with procainamide, whereas pacing was effective in cases of primary cardiac pathology, such as AV dissociation.

Although cardiac arrest may initially be caused by rhythms that would not benefit from pacing, one might raise the academic question of using a pacemaker in all cases of bradyasystolic cardiac arrest. Such logic would be predicated on the expected development of a treatable rhythm during the course of the resuscitation. For example, although ventricular fibrillation would not be affected by pacing, asystole (straight line) frequently follows defibrillation, and asystole may be treatable by pacing. In such a circumstance, the presence of a functioning pacer, prophylactically inserted, may be of value.

Any discussion concerning the use of pacing in cardiac arrest must consider the time during the arrest at which pacing should be instituted. Bellet[10] demonstrated that a pacemaker was ineffective in patients with prolonged cardiac arrest. Patients with cardiac arrest for more than 5 to 10 minutes could not be resuscitated with the use of pacing but patients who had a pacemaker placed within 2 to 7 minutes after cardiac standstill were suc-

cessfully resuscitated. It is logical to assume that a severely acidotic, anoxic heart would benefit little from pacing. If pacing is expected to be of any value, it should be instituted as soon as possible, rather than after exhaustive medical therapy has failed. The standard argument against the use of transthoracic pacing is that anecdotal clinical experience indicates lack of appreciable success with the procedure, even after all other methods and multiple drug therapy have failed.[18] This "last ditch" or "final effort" approach may have led to much of the negativism associated with the procedure.

All rhythms encountered during cardiac arrest are not amenable to pacing. One would not expect pacing by any route to be effective in the treatment of electromechanical dissociation. Electromechanical dissociation, which can result from primary cardiac disease or from hypovolemia or cardiac tamponade from trauma, can be defined as electrical activity at an appropriate rate (occasionally a relatively normal-looking QRS complex on EKG is seen) with the absence of a pulse, blood pressure, or audible heart sounds. Because electrical stimulation is believed to be intact in this primarily mechanical derangement, the addition of another electrical stimulation would not be beneficial,[4, 26] unless the electrical activity occurred at an unacceptably slow rate.[4, 28] Pacing would be without value in the treatment of ventricular fibrillation. With the onset of ventricular fibrillation, the heart becomes insensitive to pacemaker activity and a pacemaker spike may be observed to "march" through an EKG. The probable ineffectiveness of pacing in both electromechanical dissociation and ventricular fibrillation is supported by various reviews of therapy that fail to recommend pacing in the presence of these disorders.[6, 7, 20, 28]

Although trauma frequently results in death from electromechanical dissociation secondary to anoxia, acidosis, or hypovolemia, cardiac collapse from trauma occasionally is manifested as severe drug-resistant bradycardia.[29, 30] Millikan and colleagues[31] recently reported lifesaving benefit from emergency pacing (epicardial pacemaker used during surgery) in two patients with penetrating thoracic injuries with bradycardia unresponsive to cardioactive medication and volume replacement. It is unlikely that most trauma-related cardiac arrests would be responsive to pacing, especially those associated with severe acidosis, hypovolemia, or pericardial tamponade. When bradycardia or asystole persists despite correction of the underlying pathology, the use of temporary emergency pacing to correct conduction abnormalities secondary to prolonged ischemia during hypovolemic shock may be lifesaving.

Certain clinical situations that arise during cardiac arrest may benefit from emergency transthoracic cardiac pacing. These are asystole (or more appropriately, straight line on the EKG) and slow idioventricular rhythm. Both asystole and the wide, slow, bizarre QRS complex rhythm without pulses (termed pulseless idioventricular rhythm) are associated with mortality rates of almost 100 per cent.[23] Both rhythms are an indication for emergency pacing,[21, 32, 33] and both lend themselves to the rapid transthoracic approach. The severely hypoxic or acidotic heart has little chance for resuscitation by any method; thus, it is reasonable to institute pacing efforts in the early stages of therapy, when the heart is most likely to respond to pacemaker stimulation. Simultaneous measures to correct acidosis and anoxia should be started. If all other methods of therapy for asystole have failed, it is reasonable to expect that a pacemaker placed as a terminal gesture is also doomed to failure. A summary of clinical recommendations for transthoracic pacing is shown in Table 13–1.

Complications

The type and incidence of complications from emergency transthoracic pacing cannot be accurately assessed. Although animal studies have not demonstrated serious complications from the procedure and a limited number of clinical trials in humans have failed to register a single fatality directly related to transthoracic pacing, the procedure must not be used indiscriminately. One might expect complications similar to those associated with other conditions requiring intracardiac injections of drugs, such as pericardial tamponade, pneumothorax, myocardial laceration, or coronary artery or other major vessel laceration. Although intracardiac injections are much maligned and the technique is usually not recommended,[34–36] data in the literature do not support this hard-line approach.

Zoll[2] reported a 600-ml pericardial effusion and a myocardial wall hematoma at autopsy in a patient who had 34 intracardiac injections within a 4-hour period, but neither coronary artery laceration nor pneumothorax was noted.

Amey[37] demonstrated that intracardiac injections by paramedics in the pre-hospital care of cardiac arrest patients are accomplished with ease and with only a slight increase in complications over control groups. In this small series of 47 intracardiac injections, there were no cases of endocarditis, air embolism, or pericardial effusion. There were four cases of pneumothorax, but these were associated with vigorous CPR and rib fractures.

In a series of 147 intracardiac injections during CPR for the purpose of transthoracic pacemaker insertion or drug therapy, Davidson and coworkers[38] demonstrated that percutaneous puncture of the heart using the subxyphoid approach seldom results in complications of any serious consequence. In this study, small pericardial effusions secondary to bleeding were relatively common (about 30 per cent of the cases), but there were no cases of pericardial tamponade or myocardial or coronary artery laceration. In addition, only 1 of the 40 patients in whom circulation had been restored had a pneumothorax, even though most patients (62 per cent) continued to receive positive pressure ventilation after CPR.

Tintinalli and White[18] and Roberts and Greenberg[19] have each reported a case of pericardial tamponade that probably was a direct result of a transthoracic pacer and may have contributed to the death of the patient.

Considering the dismal outcome of cardiac arrest, an intracardiac needle stick for the purpose of pacemaker insertion is justified if the procedure itself is assumed to be of potential value. If the pacer were inserted during CPR, the complication rate would be expected to be greater. Especially worrisome would be the development of a tension pneumothorax if the lung were punctured during positive-pressure ventilation or pericardial tamponade if the patient were anticoagulated or had another bleeding diathesis. It has been my experience (in a small series of six patients) that some pericardial bleeding occurs in all patients who undergo transthoracic pacing combined with CPR. There were no cases of tamponade in my series, and the amount of pericardial bleeding ranged from a few milliliters to 120 ml of blood found at autopsy.[19] Pericardial tamponade, however, is a complication that must be recognized following transthoracic pacing.

Table 13–1. RECOMMENDATIONS FOR EMERGENCY TRANSTHORACIC PACING WHEN TRANSVENOUS PACING NOT IMMEDIATELY AVAILABLE

Indications*	Contraindications
Asystole	Stable patient
Any severe bradycardia	Pathology quickly and easily corrected by medication
Pulseless idioventricular rhythm	
A-V dissociation with inadequate ventricular response or recurrent V-fibrillation or V-tachycardia	Presence of functioning transvenous pacemaker
	Cannot Be Expected to Benefit
Unstable sinus bradycardia/junctional bradycardia/atrial fibrillation with high-degree AV block	Electromechanical dissociation
	Ventricular fibrillation

*Consider the use of pacing in trauma arrest if the patient is unresponsive to other forms of therapy. (From Roberts, J. R., and Greenberg, M. I.: Emergency transthoracic pacemaker. Ann. Emerg. Med. 10:603, 1981.)

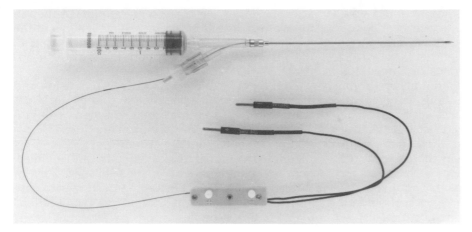

Figure 13–1. Elecath Pacejector transthoracic pacemaker. A bipolar pacing wire is preloaded through a side port and threaded to the tip of the needle. The pacing wire, as shown, is attached to the connector, which will be hooked up to the pacing energy source. (Courtesy of Electrocatheter Corporation, Rahway, NJ.)

Instrumentation

The most widely used instrumentation for transthoracic pacing is a sterile, one-time use, prepackaged kit. A representative device is the Elecath Pacejector (Fig. 13–1). The Pacejector consists of a 13-cm 17 gauge needle, a 10-ml syringe, and a 30-cm bipolar pacing wire that is preloaded via a side port in the needle hub. The syringe is used to confirm intracavitary placement of the needle tip and to inject intracardiac medications, if so desired. Because the pacing wire is already threaded to the tip of the needle, once the cardiac chamber has been entered one simply advances the wire a few centimeters. The entire introducing assembly is then removed, leaving the pacing wire in the right ventricle. A variety of external pacemaker energy sources are available (Fig. 13–2). In the standard bipolar pacing wire, the negative electrode (cathode), situated at the tip of the pacing wire, and the positive electrode (anode), situated 10 cm proximal to the tip, are separated by an insulating sleeve. The separation of the electrodes in this configuration theoretically develops a wider field of electrical excitation than did the older models that placed the electrodes adjacent at the tip of the pacing stylet.

One model has the trademark "transmyocardial" as opposed to "transthoracic" pacer (Electro-Catheter Corp). When the transmyocardial pacing wire is properly positioned, the cathode lies within the ventricle and the anode lies within the myocardium or on the outer surface of the heart. Although the tip of the pacing wire is situated within the ventricular cavity, direct contact with the endocardium is not necessary for successful pacemaker function, and the tip often floats freely within the ventricle.

Technique

The transmyocardial pacing wire can be properly positioned by an experienced physician in approximately 30 to 45 seconds. CPR can be continued during most of the procedure but should be stopped while the intracardiac needle is being placed to avoid possible myocardial or lung damage. Theoretically, the procedure is applicable for field use by paramedics.

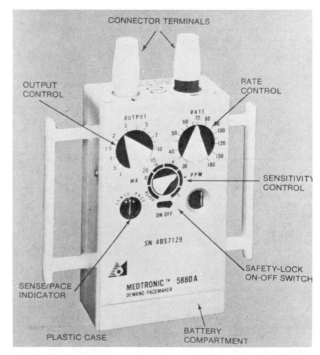

Figure 13–2. Medtronic pacemaker energy source. Unit has (+) and (−) connector terminals, rate control, output control, and sensitivity control.

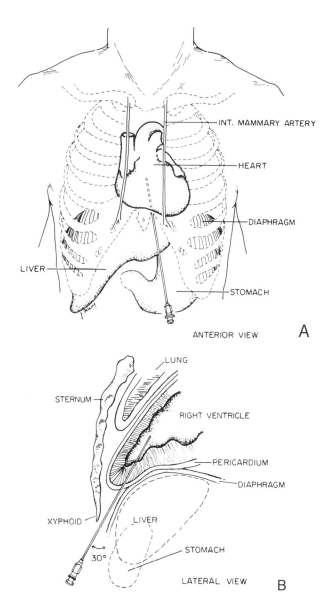

Figure 13–3. Subxyphoid approach to the right ventricle. A, Frontal view. B, Lateral view. Note proximity of stomach and liver to entrance point.

The ideal position for the wire is within the right ventricular cavity. Atrial pacing or left ventricular pacing may be successful, but I recommend right ventricular pacing. Atrial pacing would be of no value in heart block. The left ventricle is not easily accessible through the transthoracic route, and its thick wall may be an obstacle to easy positioning of the electrode. Although some physicians prefer the left parasternal approach, most authors recommend that the subxyphoid approach be used. There is less chance of pneumothorax or coronary artery or other major vessel injury with the subxyphoid approach, and the right ventricle is easily accessible.

After CPR has been briefly stopped, the trans-

thoracic needle is inserted subxyphoidally at a 30 to 45 degree angle to the skin (Fig. 13–3). The right ventricle is easily entered if the left xyphocostal notch is utilized and if the needle is directed toward the sternal notch. Some physicians prefer aiming toward the right or left shoulder, but I have had most success by aiming toward the sternal notch (Fig. 13–4). Certain conditions, such as dextrocardia, severe emphysema, or scoliosis, make successful placement more difficult. It is imperative that the angle between the skin and the needle not exceed 45 degrees. A greater angle may direct the needle too far posteriorly and miss the heart or risk injury to the left lobe of the liver or the stomach, both of which are dangerously close to the xyphoid. The needle is advanced approximately three fourths of its length.

Aspiration of blood with the syringe confirms proper positioning. (As an aside, an intracardiac injection of cardioactive drugs may be given through the intracardiac needle at this time if a central intravenous line has not already been obtained.) If no blood is aspirated, the needle is withdrawn and re-inserted. When the intracavitary placement of the needle tip is confirmed by the aspiration of blood, the pacing wire is advanced a few centimeters via the side port. The introducing needle is now withdrawn and CPR is again instituted. Some physicians prefer to insert an introducing needle with an inner trocar as a unit directly into the ventricle. Removal of the trocar reveals free flowing blood when the transthoracic needle is correctly located in the ventricle. A pacing wire is then passed, and the introducing needle is withdrawn as before. If one grasps the pacing wire, the pacing stylet will not be acciden-

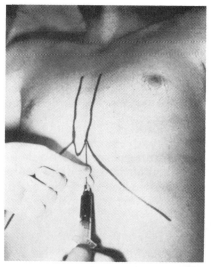

Figure 13–4. Using the left xiphoid-costal notch and aiming toward the sternal notch will usually allow one to enter the right ventricle at 3 to 6 cm depth.

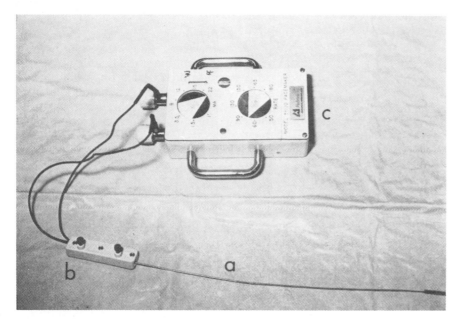

Figure 13–5. Proper connection of pacing wire (A), plastic connector (B), and pacemaker box (C).

tally pulled out as the needle is withdrawn. Now only the pacing stylet exits from the chest.

The proximal end of the pacing wire is inserted into the plastic connector and secured by the screws in the body of the connector. The pacing wire must be inserted all the way into the connector to ensure proper contact. The positive and negative wire from the plastic connector is then secured to the respective terminals on the external energy source, and electrical stimulation is initiated (Fig. 13–5).

The external energy source should initially be used as a fixed rate (asynchronous) pacemaker, with pacing being initiated without regard for the intrinsic rate of the patient. The rate is set at 70 to 90 beats per minitue. The current output control is turned to the maximum milliamperes possible to facilitate capture. The sensitivity control (which senses the patient's R wave) is turned to the "off" or "asynchronous" position.

There is no real danger of injuring the heart from too strong a stimulating current or production of ventricular dysrhythmias if a paced beat falls on an intrinsic QRS-T complex. If spontaneous cardiac activity becomes apparent, the fixed-rate pacemaker can easily become a demand pacemaker by activating the sensitivity control, which senses the patient's electrical complex and inhibits the pacemaker's own output. The pacemaker should be disconnected during the defibrillation whenever possible. A summary of the operation of the pacemaker energy source is given in Table 13–2.

If pacing is not successful, the pacing wire should be manipulated to change its position and the connections should be checked. Regardless of the clinical situation, a pacing spike should be noted on the EKG, although the spike may fail to capture. One must be careful not to interpret artifact on the EKG as a paced beat (Fig. 13–6). It has been my experience that failure to observe a pacing spike on the EKG results either from poor contact between the pacing wire and the electrical connector or from rundown batteries in the pacemaker energy source.

The position of the pacing wire should be verified with both AP and lateral chest films (Fig. 13–7). It is imperative to examine the chest film for evidence of a pneumothorax. A 12 lead EKG

Table 13–2. OPERATION OF AN EXTERNAL PACEMAKER (MEDTRONIC MODEL 5880-A)

To operate the External Pacemaker in the *asynchronous* or fixed rate mode:

1. Set rate between 70 and 90, or at a rate to exceed intrinsic rate of the patient.
2. Turn current output control clockwise to maximum.
3. Turn sensitivity control to "off" or to the "async" mode.
4. Turn pacemaker to "on" position.
5. Check for activation of the pacing indicator needle, which should deflect to the "PACE" indication.

To convert to a *demand* mode:

1. Turn *sensitivity* control to maximum clockwise position. This will then sense the R wave if there is intrinsic electrical activity.
2. Turn *rate* control to 10 beats lower than patient's intrinsic rate. This should stop the pacemaker, and the needle indicator should deflect to the "SENSE" indication or "PACE" if the patient's rate drops below the reading set on the rate control.

Note: The pacemaker should be disconnected during defibrillation whenever possible.

(From Roberts, J. R., and Greenberg, M. I.: Emergency transthoracic pacemaker. Ann. Emerg. Med. 10:607, 1981.)

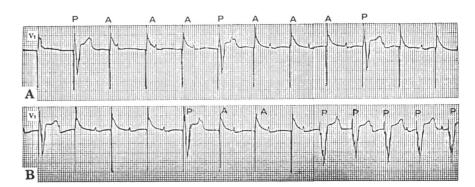

Figure 13–6. Pacemaker spike with failure to pace. Only beats marked "P" are paced beats. During decay of a pacer spike of high voltage, an artifact may be produced which can simulate a QRS complex (A).

should be obtained to document capture. The position of the pacing wire can be confirmed by the QRS configuration in the EKG. If the stylet is pacing from the right ventricle, there should be a positive QRS complex in leads I and V_6 and a negative QRS in lead V_1 (Fig. 13–8). This occurs because depolarization is from right to left ventricle and simulates a left bundle branch block pattern. If the stylet is pacing from the left ventricle, a right bundle branch block pattern is observed, and because depolarization is from left to right, the QRS complex is positive in V_1 and negative in I and V_6.

When the pacemaker is functioning properly, the entire apparatus should be securely taped to the patient (Fig. 13–9). Should the pacing box fall from the patient, the pliable pacing wire will be accidentally pulled out. The entire apparatus should remain in place until a transvenous pacing stylet is in place and functioning.

Occasionally during cardiac arrest from trauma, an emergency thoracotomy is performed in the emergency department or in the operating room. If pacing is required in such a situation on a truly stat basis, the author prefers using a sew-in epicardial pacing wire as pictured in Figure 13–10, as

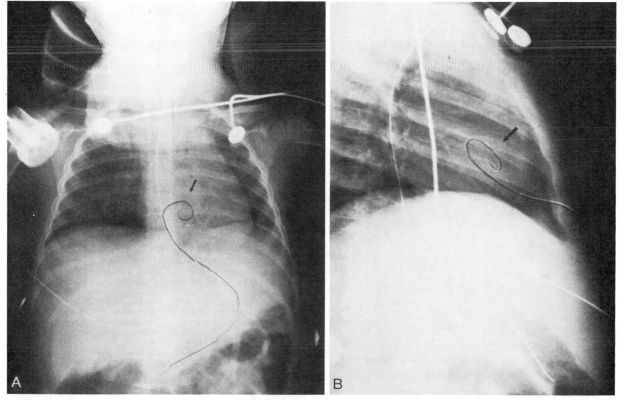

Figure 13–7. Chest films demonstrating transthoracic pacing wire (arrow) in right ventricle. A, AP view. B, Lateral view.

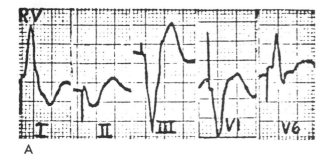

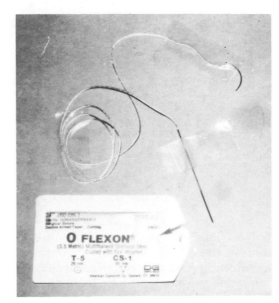

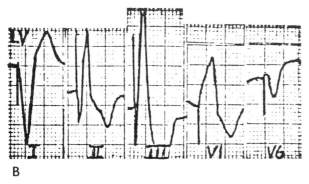

Figure 13–10. Sew-in epicardial pacing wires. This material is Flexon from Davis and Geck Company. The curved needle is used to sew in the wire. The straight wire was designed to guide the wire through the chest wall for easy pull-out of the wire. Once the curved needle is used to penetrate the myocardium, the needle is cut off so that only the wire remains attached. During an emergency thoracotomy the straight needle can be inserted into the pacemaker box to give contact.

Figure 13–8. QRS configuration seen with pacing wire in right *(A)* and left *(B)* ventricles.

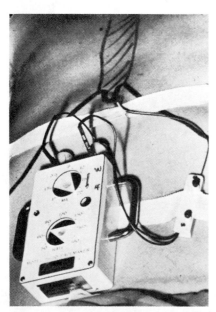

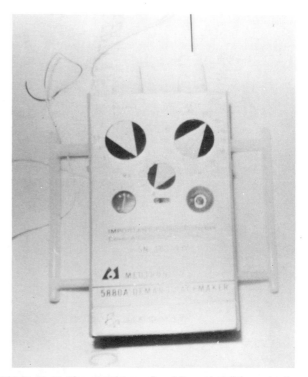

Figure 13–11. The straight needle of the epicardial sew-in electrode is inserted into the negative terminal of the pacing box. Another wire will be added to the positive terminal to complete the circuit.

Figure 13–9. Secured pacemaker and wire.

opposed to placing a transthoracic pacer under direct vision. The material pictured in Figure 13–11 is a steel wire with a curved needle on one end and a straight needle on the other end. The needles are separated by an insulating material along the length of the suture material. One sews two wires into the epicardium approximately 2 cm apart, using the curved needles. The straight needles are then inserted into the terminals on the pacing power source (see Fig. 13–11). These electrodes are often used prophylactically after cardiac surgery.

Conclusion and Recommendations

The technique of transthoracic cardiac pacing has been clinically feasible for the past 20 years, yet the procedure remains somewhat controversial. The procedure is not dealt with adequately in the current literature, in terms of either technique or specific indications. In addition, the effect of pacing on the outcome of cardiac arrest is unknown. Although the transthoracic pacemaker is associated with potentially serious complications and the procedure should not be used indiscriminately, transthoracic placement of pacing wires is accomplished rapidly and easily and is effective in selected clinical situations.

There is no debate that cardiac pacing itself is a valuable clinical procedure, although most non-arrest situations can probably be best handled with transvenous pacing. The exception to this is the unstable patient with drug-resistant bradycardia producing cardiovascular collapse or lethal escape rhythms whose clinical condition does not warrant delay in therapy. In the case of cardiac arrest, delay of specific therapy for even a few minutes may mean the difference between a successful resuscitation and a dead patient. Also, the lack of circulation during cardiac arrest hinders the proper placement of flow-directed pacemakers, and fluoroscopy is impossible during cardiac arrest.

Obviously cardiac arrest secondary to a rhythm that is amenable to pacing affords the best chance for success. Asystole is a rhythm for which pacing is indicated. Based on current evidence, asystole is an indication for emergency transthoracic pacing. Pacing is also recommended in cardiac collapse exhibiting a slow pulseless idioventricular rhythm. Pacing in these rhythms should be a first-line treatment, not a therapy used as a last resort after extensive drug therapy has been unsuccessful. It is unlikely that a pacemaker is of benefit in electromechanical dissociation. In trauma-related cardiac arrest when severe bradycardia persists despite correction of hypovolemia, acidosis, or hypoxia, pacing should be instituted by the transthoracic method or under direct vision if a thoracotomy has been performed. Pacing would most likely be effective in cases of primary cardiac disease and less effective in cases in which there is severe metabolic disturbance. A severely hypoxic or acidotic heart cannot reasonably be expected to respond to electrical stimulation, and pacemaker therapy must be complemented by vigorous correction of ventilation defects and acid-base abnormalities.

Although it is an intriguing concept, the possibility of prophylactic use of transthoracic pacing in all cases of cardiac arrest is difficult to assess. Certainly, many cases of ventricular fibrillation can be treated with defibrillation and drug therapy with a successful outcome and without the development of a rhythm for which pacing would have been beneficial. Because asystole and pulseless idioventricular rhythm are almost universally fatal, a prospective, controlled study on the early use of transthoracic pacing in cardiac arrest would more clearly define the role of this procedure. It is hoped that the dismal outcome of these conditions can be favorably altered as more aggressive methods of resuscitation are investigated.

Introduction

Transcutaneous cardiac pacing is a rapid, minimally invasive method of treating severe bradycardias and asystole. An electrode is applied to the anterior and posterior chest walls, and pacing is initiated with a portable pulse generator. In an emergency setting, this pacing technique is faster and easier to use than transvenous or transthoracic pacing. Pulse generators are sufficiently portable to be used in emergency departments, hospital wards, intensive care units, and mobile paramedic vehicles. Clinical trials are in progress to define the role of emergency transcutaneous pacing.

TRANSCUTANEOUS CARDIAC PACING

SCOTT A. SYVERUD, M.D.

Historical Development

In 1872, Duchenne reported a successful resuscitation of a child by attaching one electrode to a limb while a second electrode was rhythmically touched to the precordium of the thorax.[39] Successful overdrive pacing of the human heart, using a precordial electrode, was reported by Von-Ziemssen in 1882.[40]

In 1952, Zoll introduced the first practical means of transcutaneous cardiac pacing. Using a ground electrode attached to the skin and a subcutaneous needle electrode over the precordium, he reported the successful resuscitation of two patients in ventricular standstill.[2] One patient was paced for 5 days and subsequently discharged from the hospital. Zoll later introduced a machine that delivered impulses lasting 2 msec through 3-cm diameter paddles pressed firmly against the anterior chest wall. This device was the first commercial transcutaneous cardiac pacemaker. During the 1950's, Zoll and Leatham demonstrated the effectiveness of transcutaneous pacing in patients with bradycardia and asystole.[42–45] Leatham used larger electrodes (4 × 6 cm) and a longer pulse duration (20 msec) to successfully pace two patients with bradydysrhythmias.[45]

Until the late 1950's, transcutaneous pacing was the only clinically accepted method of cardiac pacing. The technique, however, had adverse effects, including local tissue burns, muscle contraction, and severe pain.[41, 45] With the development of the first implantable pacemakers from 1958 through 1960 and the improvement of transvenous electrodes during the early 1960's, transcutaneous pacing was rapidly discarded.[46]

Transvenous pacing requires access to the central venous circulation and is difficult and time consuming when trying to resuscitate patients with severe bradycardia or asystole. Flow-directed catheters are difficult to advance in patients with hypotensive states, and the catheter tip frequently does not seat in the right ventricle. Successful capture and ultimate survival using transvenous or transthoracic pacing for cardiac arrest remain poor under current management.[47, 48] Conventional pharmacologic therapy for asystolic or bradycardic arrests is rarely successful. In one series of patients who arrested while paramedics were on the scene and in whom conventional Advanced Cardiac Life Support (ACLS) guidelines were followed, there was not a single survivor whose initial rhythm was asystole or pulseless bradycardia.[49] The limitations of invasive emergency pacing techniques, the poor efficacy of pharmacologic therapy, and an interest in prehospital pacing led contemporary investigators to re-examine transcutaneous pacing as an emergency procedure.[50, 51]

Three recent clinical studies have demonstrated the safety and efficacy of transcutaneous pacing in pre-hospital, emergency department, and hospital settings.[63–65] In a pre-hospital study of patients with asystole or life-threatening bradycardia, Falk reported a 37 per cent electrical capturerate (7 of 19 patients) using a 20-msec pulse duration transcutaneous pacer.[63] One of the 19 patients had a pulseless bradycardia and was successfully paced transcutaneously until a transvenous pacing wire could be passed. The patient was a long-term survivor. In an emergency department study, Dalsey and coworkers reported a 50 per cent electrical capture rate (26 of 52 patients) when transcutaneous pacing was used late in the course of cardiac arrests.[64] They found no significant difference in electrical capture rates between asystolic and pulseless bradycardic groups. Four of the 52 patients developed detectable blood pressures and were short-term survivors. There were no long-term survivors. In 25 of the 52 patients, transvenous pacing was also attempted. The electrical capture rate was 20 per cent (5 of 25 patients). It was noted that all patients who had electrical capture with transvenous pacing also had capture with transcutaneous pacing. Conversely, transvenous pacing failed to produce capture in 5 patients in whom transcutaneous pacing successfully produced electrical capture.

Both studies just discussed used transcutaneous pacing after conventional pharmacologic management failed. In perhaps the most promising series to date, Falk and coworkers used a 40-msec pulse duration transcutaneous pacemaker as first-line therapy in 4 hospitalized patients who suddenly developed asystole.[65] Pacing produced pulses and blood pressures in 3 of the 4 patients. Pulses and blood pressures were also noted in 9 of 11 hospitalized patients in whom transcutaneous pacing was used for bradycardias or conduction defects. Falk and coworkers also successfully paced normal volunteers transcutaneously at a mean capture threshold of 54 ma. They noted that the mean transcutaneous pacing capture threshold in the 4 patients who developed asystole was 78 ma. These results raise the possibility that early transcutaneous pacing might improve the dismal survival rate now associated with bradyasystolic cardiac arrest.

Some of the disadvantages of earlier transcutaneous pacing techniques have been overcome in newer pacing unit designs. The original transcutaneous pacemakers used short duration electrical impulses of relatively large amplitude. These impulses closely resemble the electrical characteristics of muscle action potential. In comparison, cardiac action potentials are of much longer duration. Increasing the pulse duration of the transcutaneous impulse decreases both muscle stimulation and the current required for cardiac capture. Combining increased pulse duration with larger surface area electrodes has resulted in effective transcutaneous pacing with minimal muscle contraction or soft-tissue damage. A cardiac pacemaker incorporating these characteristics is now commercially available (Pace*Aid Model 50, Car-

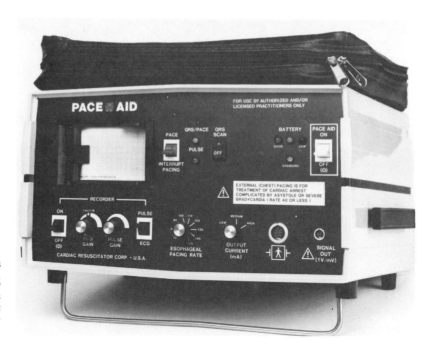

Figure 13–12. Commercial transcutaneous pacing device. Note location of ON/OFF, PACE/INTERRUPT PACING, and recorder ON/OFF switches. Discussion of control settings is provided in the text. (Provided by Cardiac Resuscitator Corporation, Wilsonville, Oregon.)

diac Resuscitator Corp., Wilsonville, Oregon) and has been approved by the Food and Drug Administration (FDA) for use in humans. Other commercial units may be available soon.

Equipment

Transcutaneous pacing is not in wide clinical use but prototype equipment have been developed. The Pace*Aid device (Cardiac Resuscitator Corp., Wilsonville, Oregon, Fig. 13–12) weighs approximately 7 kg and may be run from wall current or by a self-contained rechargeable battery. Pulse duration is fixed at 20 msec; rate is fixed at 80 beats per minute; and current settings available include 50, 100, and 200 ma. At the 100-ma setting, assuming human chest wall resistance is 50 ohms, a single pacing impulse delivers approximately 0.01 watt-sec.[52] The 8-cm diameter conducting surface of the electrodes is surrounded by an adhesive rim. One electrode is placed over the mid dorsal spine, and the other is placed over the left anterior chest (Fig. 13–13). The posterior electrode serves as the ground. Chest compressions can be administered directly over the anterior electrode. Personnel who carry out procedures are not in danger of sustaining electrical injury during pacing.

Indications for Transcutaneous Cardiac Pacing

The FDA has approved transcutaneous cardiac pacing for use in unconscious patients with a heart rate of 40 or less and for patients in asystole. Use of the device in conscious patients with bradycardias is currently under investigation. Potential applications include overdrive pacing of tachycardias and treatment of transient heart block associated with myocardial infarction. The latter application may be especially critical if the patient has received streptokinase therapy. In that situation, central venous access for passage of a transvenous catheter can lead to disastrous hemorrhagic complications. Overdrive pacing would require a variable-rate pacing device. Absolute contraindications to transcutaneous pacing have not been identified, although electrodes available at the present time can produce pain in the conscious patient, especially at the highest current setting.

Technique

The pacing electrodes are applied as shown in Figure 13–13 and are attached to the instrument cable as labeled. Electrocardiogram sensing electrodes are placed on the chest wall and connected to the instrument cable (Fig. 13–14). The pacing unit monitor (recorder) is then activated. Because the rate and pulse duration are fixed, only the milliamperage setting needs to be selected. When the operator is ready to initiate pacing, the unit power switch should be in the "on" position. The monitor should be turned to the EKG mode. The QRS scanner should be turned off. The activator switch should then be turned to the "pace" position. Pacing impulses will commence after a 5-sec delay.

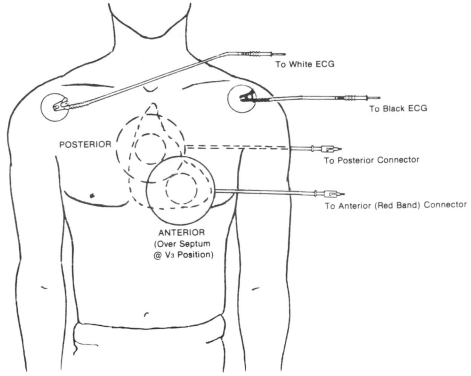

Figure 13–13. Placement of external electrode pads. Note that monitor leads are also shown in place on upper thorax. (Provided by Cardiac Resuscitator Corporation, Wilsonville, Oregon.)

Commonly, the operator begins at the 100-ma setting, increasing to 200 ma or decreasing to 50 ma, depending upon the response of the patient. Once pacing has begun, capture can be determined by the electrocardiographic complex displayed on the stripchart (Fig. 13–15). Identification of successful pacing may be difficult due to the large amplitude of the pacer spike and frequent monitor artifact. Therefore, determining the presence or absence of pulses during pacing is an important monitoring parameter. Because of minor muscle contractions generated by the device, pulses may be difficult to assess by palpation. Assessment of peripheral pulses using a Doppler device or intra-arterial pressure monitoring is more reliable. The finger pulse sensor that accompanies

this device is not reliable in low-flow states. Anterior sternal and left lateral placement of the electrodes may be required in the massively obese patient to reduce tissue resistance. Reversing electrode cables (i.e., connecting anterior electrode to cable marked *posterior*) may also enhance capture.

If electrical capture or pulses cannot be obtained with transcutaneous pacing, the clinical situation may warrant an attempt at passage of a transvenous or transthoracic pacer. If transcutaneous pacing is successful, insertion of a transvenous pacemaker is generally recommended to limit the potential hazards of prolonged transcutaneous pacing. Passage of the transvenous electrode will be facilitated by the forward flow generated by the transcutaneous pacer. With a functioning pa-

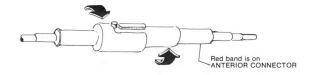

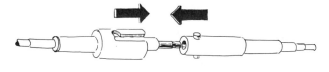

PUSH TOGETHER AND ROTATE CLOCKWISE

Red band is on
ANTERIOR CONNECTOR

Figure 13–14. Connecting external pacing electrodes to pacing cable. (Provided by Cardiac Resuscitator Corporation, Wilsonville, Oregon.)

Figure 13–15. Monitoring of EKG during pacing. Upper tracing shows pacing without capture, whereas lower tracing shows pacing with capture. The device pacing stimulus is so strong compared to the underlying EKG signal that standard EKG monitors or recorders are usually overloaded, and their EKG display may not be interpretative. The PACE∗AID incorporates special circuitry within its EKG detection system to enable EKG monitoring of the heart's response to the pacing stimulus and any spontaneous cardiac activity between stimuli. The chest lead I position is generally used, since it minimizes interference with other therapy, although lead II may be required for adequate QRS signal strength for sensing. (Provided by Cardiac Resuscitator Corporation, Wilsonville, Oregon.)

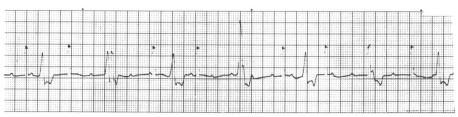

PACING WITHOUT CAPTURE

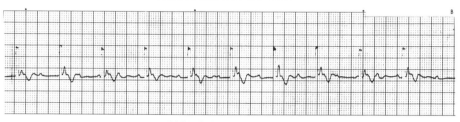

PACING WITH CAPTURE

cer in place, the operator will have time to perform a controlled transvenous procedure without the impediment of simultaneous chest compressions.

COMPLICATIONS

Potential complications of transcutaneous pacing include induction of dysrhythmias, pain from stimulation, and tissue damage. With epicardial electrodes, the threshold current required to induce ventricular fibrillation decreases as impulse duration increases. At a 10-msec impulse duration, ventricular fibrillation can be induced with currents as low as 25 ma delivered through epicardial electrodes.[53] Because transcutaneous pacing impulses are of even longer duration (20 msec) and of higher current (50 to 200 ma), there has been concern about possible induction of ventricular fibrillation during transcutaneous pacing. Recent studies of fibrillation thresholds using large *precordial* electrodes have shown the relationship of threshold to impulse duration to be opposite to that seen with *epicardial* electrodes. With *cutaneous* electrodes, the current required to induce fibrillation *increases* as pulse duration *increases*.[54] The apparent paradox may be explained by the differing nature of the electrodes. Epicardial electrodes are localized on one small area of the myocardium, whereas transcutaneous electrodes deliver a broad electrical charge to the myocardium as a whole. The implication is that longer impulse durations, although more dangerous with internal pacing, seem to decrease the chance of inducing ventricular fibrillation with transcutaneous pacing. In the author's clinical experience, patients uncommonly develop ventricular fibrillation during transcutaneous pacing; it is not possible to establish whether the fibrillation is induced by pacing or

whether pacing is coincidental to it. Further experience with the technique in humans should delineate the incidence and importance of this potential complication.

Pain from electrical skin and muscle stimulation was a significant complication of earlier transcutaneous pacemakers and was one factor that led the FDA to recommend the use of the device only for unconscious patients. In the study of Falk and coworkers, only 2 of 30 subjects (patients and volunteers) who were transcutaneously paced while conscious required discontinuation of pacing owing to discomfort.[65] Most reported the discomfort as "mild or moderate and easily tolerable." Sedation would presumably improve a conscious patient's ability to tolerate transcutaneous pacing.

Previous experience with transcutaneous pacing in humans has not been extensive. Zoll reported 25 humans paced for up to 108 hours with transcutaneous impulses of a 2-msec duration.[44] Pacer-induced dysrhythmias did not occur. Leatham paced one patient for 68 hours with impulses of a 20-msec duration.[45] The patient died two days after pacing was discontinued. Pathologic examination revealed no evidence of pacer-induced myocardial damage. Studies of repetitive DC countershocks in dogs have shown that energy levels required to induce tissue damage are 1000 times greater than those required to transcutaneously pace the heart. In a canine study, ten animals that were stimulated over their intrinsic rhythms for 30 minutes (20-msec duration at 80 beats per minute with 8-cm diameter cutaneous electrodes) did not develop pacer-related dysrhythmias. Serial cardiograms and cardiac enzymes revealed no evidence of ischemia or infarction. Pathologic examination of the canine hearts after sacrifice 72 hours post pacing did not reveal clinically significant myocardial damage.[51] A single primate paced for one hour with 20-msec impulses of 400 ma had no evidence of tissue damage at autopsy and at microscopic examination after sacrifice 24 hours later.[55] Based on these studies, transcutaneous pacing appears to be safe for short-term use in humans.

Conclusions

Devices that transcutaneously pace the heart have been available for clinical use since 1952. Recent technological improvements have minimized the complications associated with earlier use of the transcutaneous route and have enabled the reapplication of this relatively old pacing technique to a selected subset of cardiac emergencies. The need for a rapid, noninvasive method to pace the heart during periods of severe bradycardia and asystole is apparent to physicians who render emergency care. The recent development of commercially available transcutaneous pacemakers may fulfill this need. Instituting pacing earlier in the course of bradycardic or asystolic arrests, including the pre-hospital phase of care, may increase the poor survival rate now associated with these conditions.

TRANSESOPHAGEAL PACING

SCOTT A. SYVERUD, M.D.

Introduction

Another method of rapid, minimally invasive cardiac pacing involves passing a pacing electrode down the esophagus to the area just behind the right atrium. Transesophageal resistance is high (approximately 600 ohms) requiring high voltages (up to 30 v) for cardiac capture.[53, 54] The close proximity of the esophagus to heart keeps current requirements for capture relatively low (5 to 20 ma). An emergency transesophageal pacing system is commercially available in Europe, but at present, none has been approved for use in humans in the United States. Several case reports of successful resuscitation using transesophageal pacing have appeared in the recent medical literature.[56–59]

Procedure

Transesophageal pacing requires passage of an electrode-bearing nasogastric tube and correct positioning of the tube so that the electrode lies directly behind the right atrium. This technique may be more difficult to use during a cardiac arrest than transcutaneous pacing. Even when properly placed in the esophagus behind the heart, the electrode could be displaced by chest compressions or patient movement during transport. This technique offers advantages over transvenous and transthoracic pacing in terms of the ease and rapidity with which pacing can be established.

The nasogastric pacing catheter can be passed by paramedics at the scene of cardiac arrests. Lower current is required for transesophageal pacing than for transcutaneous pacing. Prophylactic insertion of the nasogastric pacing catheter during surgical procedures in which bradycardia might be encounted seems to be the most immediate practical application of transesophageal emergency pacing.[60] Investigations of its use during cardiac arrest have not as yet been carried out. Further development and investigation of transesophageal pacing await commercial availability of pulse generators and catheters as well as FDA approval of the technique.

Emergency Transthoracic Pacemaker

1. Registers of the Royal Humane Society of London. Nichols & Sons, 1774–1784.
2. Zoll, P. M.: Resuscitation of the heart in ventricular standstill by external electric stimulation. N. Engl. J. Med. 247:768, 1952.
3. Thevenet, A., Hodges, P. C., and Lillehei, C. W.: The use of myocardial electrode inserted percutaneously for control of complete atrioventricular block by an artificial pacemaker. Dis. Chest 34:621, 1958.
4. Braunwald, E. (ed.): Heart Disease. Philadelphia, W. B. Saunders Company, 1980.
5. Schwartz, G., Safar, P., Stone, D., et al. (eds.): Principles and Practice of Emergency Medicine. Philadelphia, W. B. Saunders Company, 1978.
6. Gottlieb, R., and Chung, E. K.: Techniques of temporary pacing. *In* Chung, E. K. (eds.): Artificial Cardiac Pacing—A Practical Approach. Baltimore, Williams & Wilkins, 1978, pp. 150–160.
7. Daicoff, G. R., and Miscia, V. E.: Shock, pacemakers, and surgical therapy. *In* Eliot, R. S. (ed.): The Acute Cardiac Emergency. Mount Kisco, New York, Futura Publishing Co., Inc., 1972, p. 253.
8. Personal communication with Electro-Catheter Corp.
9. Ross, S. M., and Hoffman, B. E.: A bipolar pacemaker for immediate treatment of cardiac arrest. J. Appl. Physiol. 15:974, 1960.
10. Bellet, S., Muller, O. F. DeLeon, A. C., et al.: The use of an internal pacemaker in the treatment of cardiac arrest and slow heart rates. Arch. Intern. Med. 105:361, 1960.

11. Lillehei, C. W., Levy, M. J., Bonnabeau, R. C., et al.: Direct wire electrical stimulation for acute postsurgical and postinfarction complete heart block. Ann. N.Y. Acad. Sci. 111:938, 1964.

12. Roe, B. B.: Intractable Stokes-Adams disease: a method of emergency management. Am. Heart J. 69:470, 1965.

13. Roe, B. B., and Katz, H. J.: Complete heart block with intractable asystole and recurrent ventricular fibrillation with survival. Am. J. Cardiol. 15:401, 1965.

14. Kodjababian, G. H., Gray, R. E., Keenan, R. L., et al.: Percutaneous implantation of cardiac pacemaker electrodes. Am. J. Cardiol. 19:372, 1967.

15. Morris, J. H., Gillette, P. C., and Barrett, F. F.: Atrioventricular block complicating meningitis: treatment with emergency cardiac pacing. Pediatrics 58:866, 1976.

16. Zoll, P. M., Linenthal, A. J., and Norman, L. R.: Treatment of Stokes-Adams disease by external electric stimulation of the heart. Circulation 9:482, 1954.

17. Zoll, P. M., Linenthal, A. J., Norman, L. R., et al.: Use of the external electric pacemaker in cardiac arrest. JAMA 159:1428, 1955.

18. Tintinalli, J. E., and White, B. C.: Transthoracic pacing during CPR. Ann. Emerg. Med. 10:113, 1981.

19. Roberts, J. R., and Greenberg, M. I.: Emergency transthoracic pacemaker. Ann. Emerg. Med., 10:600, 1981.

20. Dreifus, L. S., Chaudry, K. R., and Otawa, S.: Temporary and emergency cardiac pacing. In Varriate, P., and Naclerio, E. (eds.): Cardiac Pacing. Philadelphia, Lea and Febiger, 1979, pp. 133–143.

21. Johnson, R. A., Haber, E., and Austen, W. G. (eds.): The Practice of Cardiology. Boston, Little, Brown, and Co., 1981, p. 28.

22. Preston, T. A.: The use of pacemaking for the treatment of acute arrhythmias. Heart Lung 6:249, 1977.

23. Iseri, L. T., Humphrey, S. B., and Siner, E. J.: Prehospital brady-asystolic cardiac arrest. Ann. Intern. Med. 88:741, 1978.

24. Shriver, J. A.: Results of cardipulmonary resuscitation: a review. Top. Emerg. Med. 1:103, 1979.

25. Lund, I., and Skulberg, A.: Resuscitation of cardiac arrest outside hospitals: experience with a mobile intensive care unit in Oslo. Acta Anaesthesiol. Scand. 53:13, 1973.

26. Hollingsworth, J. H.: The result of cardiopulmonary resuscitation: a three-year university hospital experience. Ann. Intern. Med. 71:459, 1969.

27. Lemire, J. G., and Johnson, A. L.: Is cardiac resuscitation worthwhile? A decade of experience. N. Engl. J. Med. 286:970, 1972.

28. Raizes, G., Wagner, G., and Hackel, D.: Instantaneous non-arrhythmic cardiac death in acute myocardial infarction. Am. J. Cardiol. 39:1, 1977.

29. Mazor, A., and Rogel, S.: Cardiac aspects of shock. Ann. Surg. 178:128, 1973.

30. White, B., Hoehner, P. J., Petinga, T. J., et al.: His electrocardiographic characterization of terminal arrhythmias of hemorrhagic shock in dogs. JACEP 8:298, 1979.

31. Millikan, J. S., Moore, E. E., Dunn, E. L., et al.: Temporary cardiac pacing in trauma arrest victims. Ann. Emerg. Med. 9:591, 1980.

32. Meltzer, L. E., and Cohen, H. E.: The incidence of arrhythmias associated with acute myocardial infarction. In Meltzer, L. E., and Dunning, A. J. (eds.): Textbook of Coronary Care. Philadelphia, Charles Press, 1972.

33. Escher, D. J., and Furman, S.: Emergency treatment of cardiac arrhythmias. Emphasis on use of electrical pacing. JAMA 214:228, 1970.

34. Schechter, D. C.: Transthoracic epinephrine injection in heart resuscitation is dangerous. JAMA 234:1184, 1975.

35. Goldberg, A. H.: Cardiopulmonary arrest. N. Engl. J. Med. 290:381, 1974.

36. Vijay, N. K., and Schoonaker, F. W.: Cardiopulmonary arrest and resuscitation. Am. Fam. Phys. 26:85, 1975.

37. Amey, B. D., Harrison, E. E., Staub, E. J., et al.: Paramedic use of intracardiac medications in pre-hospital sudden cardiac death. JACEP 7:130, 1978.

38. Davidson, R., Barresi, V., Parker M., et al.: Intracardiac injections during cardiopulmonary resuscitation—a low risk procedure. JAMA 244:111, 1980.

Transcutaneous Cardiac Pacing

39. Duchenne de Boulogne. De l'électrisation localise et son application a la pathologique et a la therapeutique. Paris, Bailliere, 1872.

40. VonZiemssen, H.: Studien ueber die Bewegungsvorgaenge am menschlichen Herzen, slwie ueber die mechanische und elektrische Erregbarkeit des Herzens und des Nervus phrenicus, angelstellt an dem freiliegenden Herzen der Catherina Serafin. Arch. Klin. Med. 30:20, 1882.

41. Zoll, P. M.: Resuscitation of the heart in ventricular standstill by external electrical stimulation. N. Engl. J. Med. 24:68, 1952.

42. Zoll, P. M., Linenthal, A. J., Norman, L. R., et al.: Treatment of unexpected cardiac arrest by external electric stimulation of heart. N. Engl. J. Med. 254:541, 1956.

43. Zoll, P. M., Linenthal, A. J., and Norman, L. R.: Treatment of Stokes-Adams disease by external stimulation of the heart. Circulation 9:482, 1954.

44. Zoll, P. M., Linenthal, A. J., Norman, L. R., et al.: External electric stimulation of the heart in cardiac arrest. Arch. Intern. Med. 96:639, 1955.

45. Leatham, A., Cook, P., and Davis, J. G.: External electric stimulator for treatment of ventricular standstill. Lancet Dec 8, 1956, p. 1185.

46. Chardack, W. M., Gage, A. A., and Greatbatch, W.: A transistorized self-contained, implantable pacemaker for the long-term correction of complete heartblock. Surgery 48:643, 1960.

47. Hazard, P. B., Benton, C., and Milnor, P.: Transvenous cardiac pacing in cardiopulmonary resuscitation. Crit. Care Med. 9:666, 1981.

48. Tintinalli, J. E., and White, B. C.: Transthoracic pacing during CPR. Ann. Emerg. Med. 10:113, 1981.

49. Iseri, L. T., Siner, E. J., Humphrey, S. B., et al.: Prehospital cardiac arrest after arrival of the paramedic unit. JACEP 6:530, 1977.

50. Zoll, P. M.: External noninvasive electric stimulation of the heart. Crit. Care Med. 9:393, 1981.

51. Syverud, S. A., Dalsey, W. C., Hedges, J. R., et al.: Transcutaneous cardiac pacing: determination of myocardial injury in a canine model. Ann. Emerg. Med. 12:261, 1983.

52. Dalsey, W. C., Syverud, S. A., and Trott, Z.: Transcutaneous cardiac pacing. J. Emerg. Med. 1:201, 1984.

53. Jones, M., and Geddes, L. A.: Strength duration curves for cardiac pacemaking and ventricular fibrillation. Cardiovasc. Res. Bull. 15:101, 1977.

54. Varghese, P. J., Bren, G., and Ross, A.: Electrophysiology of external pacing: a comparative study with endocardial pacing. Circulation 66:349, 1982.

55. Varghese, J., Bren, G., and Ross, A.: Absence of Tissue Injury After Prolonged Transcutaneous Pacing. The Scientific and Technical Basis of External Cardiac Pacing. Cardiac Resuscitator Corporation, Wilsonville, OR, 1982.

Transesophageal Pacing

56. Burack, B., and Furman, S.: Transesophageal cardiac pacing. Am. J. Cardiol. 23:469, 1969.

57. Rowe, G. C., Ward, T., and Neblett, I.: Cardiac pacing with an esophageal electrode. Am. J. Cardiol. 24:549, 1969.

58. Shaw, R. J., Berman, L. H., and Hinton, J. M.: Successful emergency transesophageal cardiac pacing with subsequent endoscopy. Br. Med. J. 284:309, 1982.

59. Colquhoun, M.: Emergency transesophageal cardiac pacing. Br. Med. J. 284:1263, 1982.

60. Hartley, J. M.: Transesophageal cardiac pacing. Anaesthesia 37:192, 1982.
61. Oranto, J. P., Carveth, W. L., Windle, J. R., et al.: Pacemaker insertion for prehospital bradyasystolic cardiac arrest. Ann. Emerg. Med. 13:101, 1984.
62. White, J. D., and Brown, C.: Immediate transthoracic pacing for asystole. (submitted for publication).
63. Falk, R. H., Jacobs, L., Sinclair, A., et al.: External noninvasive cardiac pacing in out-of-hospital cardiac arrest. Crit. Care Med. 11:779, 1983.
64. Dalsey, W. C., Syverud, S. A., and Hedges, J. R.: Emergency department use of transcutaneous pacing for cardiac arrests. (abstract) Crit. Care Med. (March), 1984.
65. Falk, R. H., Zoll, P. M., and Zoll, R. H.: Safety and efficacy of non-invasive cardiac pacing. N. Engl. J. Med. 309:1166, 1983.

14

Pericardiocentesis

MICHAEL CALLAHAM, M.D.

Introduction

The mechanics of cardiac tamponade from accumulation of intrapericardial fluid were first demonstrated in 1889.[1] Pericardiotomy under direct vision was first done in 1815. In 1840, the first blind approach for drainage using a trocar was carried out successfully on a patient with tamponade from malignancy.[2] By the end of the nineteenth century, the trocar and cannula method of pericardiocentesis was commonly used. The subxiphoid approach was described in 1911. In the past three decades, there has been renewed interest in the best direct surgical approach for the treatment of cardiac tamponade; however, at present there is considerable controversy as to which surgical technique is most useful.[3]

Pericardiocentesis is a commonly performed procedure that is occasionally lifesaving. The details of the procedure should be thoroughly understood by all physicians. The medical literature concerning pericardiocentesis tends to fall into two very distinct categories: studies of traumatic hemopericardium, and studies of pericardial effusion from other causes. This separation is not entirely artificial, because these two clinical entities are quite different in their time course, etiology, and treatment. In the following section, these two categories, traumatic and nontraumatic, respectively, will be discussed, with the understanding that the former involves acute hemopericardium, and the latter involves nontraumatic pericardial effusion.

Etiology of Effusion and Tamponade

There are many disease processes that can cause pericardial effusion and eventually produce cardiac tamponade, ranging from the common to the very rare (Table 14–1). The etiology and clinical course of pericardial effusion vary widely, and the potential for an effusion to develop into tamponade must be considered when contemplating therapy.

TRAUMATIC

In trauma, a discrete event (such as a knife wound to the heart or a misdirected cardiac catheter) causes bleeding into the pericardial sac. Intracavitary blood as from a penetrating wound or blood from a bleeding myocardium generally accumulates in the pericardial space much faster than exudate or transudate. Tamponade from hemorrhage occurs frequently because often such bleeding does not stop spontaneously and the pericardial sac cannot acutely change size to accomodate the extra volume. If tamponade develops following penetrating chest trauma, the patient or the physician is usually immediately aware of an abnormal state. The exceptions to the "self-declaring" nature of traumatic tamponade include the more subtle tamponade as a complication of closed chest cardiopulmonary resuscitation (CPR), cardiac catheterizations, bleeding diathesis, and dissecting aortic aneurysm.

Closed chest CPR is a rare cause of tamponade. Theoretically, this may occur secondary to the blunt trauma of overenthusiastic CPR, broken ribs, or intracardiac injections. In one recent study, however, only 12 per cent of 26 CPR patients studied by echocardiography had a pericardial effusion, despite the fact that 31 per cent had received an intracardiac injection. None of these effusions were clinically significant; tamponade did not ensue.[4]

A bleeding diathesis may cause spontaneous bleeding into the pericardial sac. The incidence of spontaneous pericardial tamponade in patients

Table 14–1. CAUSES OF PERICARDIAL EFFUSION

Neoplasm	Mesothelioma
	Lung
	Breast
	Melanoma
	Lymphoma
Pericarditis	Radiation (especially after Hodgkin's disease)
	Viral
	Bacterial
	Fungal
	Tuberculosis
	Amebiasis
	Toxoplasmosis
	Idiopathic
	Staphylococcus
	Pneumococcus
	Haemophilus
Connective Tissue Disease	Systemic lupus erythematosus
	Scleroderma
	Rheumatoid arthritis
	Acute rheumatic fever
Metabolic Disorders	Myxedema
	Uremia
	Cholesterol pericarditis
	Bleeding diatheses
Cardiac Disease	Acute myocardial infarction
	Dissecting aortic aneurysm
	Congestive heart failure
	Coronary aneurysm
Drugs	Hydralazine
	Phenytoin
	Anticoagulants
	Procaine amide
Trauma	Blunt
	Major trauma
	Closed chest CPR
	Penetrating
	Major penetrating trauma
	Intracardiac injections
	Transthoracic and transvenous pacing wires
	Pericardiocentesis
	Cardiac catheterization
	CVP catheter
Miscellaneous	Serum sickness
	Chylous effusion
	Löffler's syndrome
	Reiter's syndrome
	Behçet's syndrome
	Pancreatitis
	Postpericardiotomy
	Amyloidosis

Data from Guberman, B. A., Fowler, N. O., Engel, P. J., et al.: Cardiac tamponade in medical patients. Circulation 64:633, 1981; and Pories, W. J., and Gaudiani, V. A.: Cardiac tamponade. Surg. Clin. North Am. 55:573, 1975.

experiencing anticoagulation has been reported to range from 2.5 to 11 per cent.[5, 6] If patients are anticoagulated, pericardial blood will not clot and can be easily aspirated, unlike the situation in traumatic tamponade where clots are frequent, making diagnosis more difficult and pericardiocentesis less beneficial.

An aneurysm of the ascending aorta may dissect around the base of the aorta into the pericardial sac, causing dramatic, rapid, and often fatal tamponade. Such aneurysms may be caused by syphilis, Marfan's syndrome, atherosclerosis, or deceleration injuries in motor vehicle accidents. Diagnosis of this mechanism of tamponade depends upon maintaining a high index of suspicion.

Traumatic tamponade is the most acutely life-threatening form of tamponade, because it may occur very rapidly. Most commonly, tamponade is the result of a stab wound to the heart,[7] presumably because the pericardium seals itself, preventing automatic decompression into the pleural space.[7, 8] About 80 to 90 per cent of stab wounds to the heart demonstrate tamponade,[7, 9] compared with 20 per cent of gunshot wounds. Larger pericardial wounds from gunshots generally drain into the pleural space and produce a hemothorax.[10] Cardiac tamponade is often suspected with anterior chest wounds, but it is imperative that one remember that any penetrating wound of the lateral chest, back, or upper abdomen may involve the heart.

Iatrogenic causes of cardiac tamponade are uncommon, but tamponade may result from invasive or diagnostic procedures. Pacemaker insertion (either transthoracic or transvenous) and cardiac catheterization are two of the main causes, resulting in tamponade when cardiac chambers or coronary vessels are inadvertently penetrated.[10, 11] Tamponade is also seen as a complication after cardiac surgery, although it is usually anticipated, and mediastinal or pericardial drainage helps to control and prevent it.[11, 12] Pericardiocentesis itself can cause tamponade by lacerating myocardium or coronary vessels.[13, 14] Cardiac tamponade may result from perforation of the right atrium or, less commonly, from the right ventricle or superior vena cava, by a central venous pressure catheter. Perforation may occur during placement or secondary to pressure erosion of an indwelling catheter. Tamponade from medical intervention such as transvenous pacing or CVP line placement is not often seen in the emergency department but may be the cause of sudden decompensation after a diagnostic or therapeutic procedure.

Blunt trauma may cause hemopericardium. Significant trauma (such as in a motor vehicle accident) is usually required. Major chest injury with associated bruises or rib and sternal fractures is often obvious. Cases have been reported, however, in which tamponade occurred in major blunt trauma with no immediate obvious signs of injury to the thorax.[15] This may be more common than is clinically recognized, judging by the reports of constrictive pericarditis and pericardial defects

Table 14–2. ETIOLOGY OF PERICARDIAL EFFUSION IN TWO STUDIES

	Krikorian[6] (120 patients) (%)	Guberman[5] (56 patients) (%)
Neoplastic disease	—	32
Pericardial invasion	16	—
Radiation pericarditis	7.5	4
Etiology uncertain	18	—
Traumatic hemopericardium	9	—
Hemopericardium, nontraumatic	2.5	—
Rheumatic disease	12	2
Uremia/dialysis	5	9
Bacterial infection	2.5	12.5
Congestive heart failure (CHF)	1.5	—
Uncertain etiology	12.5	—
Idiopathic pericarditis	13.5	14
Cardiac infarction	—	—
Iatrogenic diagnostic procedures	—	7.5
Myxedema	—	4
Aneurysm	—	4
Anticoagulation and cardiac disease	—	11
Post-pericardiotomy	—	2

months to years later in trauma patients who were not originally noted to have effusion.

Severe deceleration injury may cause aortic dissection and tamponade. However, fewer than 14 per cent of people with severe aortic injury reach the hospital alive.[16] In one series, only 1 of 28 patients with concomitant aortic injury developed tamponade. Interestingly, in the same series, 5 of 72 blunt trauma victims without aortic injuries developed tamponade. In another series, only 1 of 43 patients with aortic injury had hemopericardium; thus, tamponade is a relatively uncommon development of aortic deceleration injury.[17]

An interesting but very rare cause of cardiac tamponade is pneumopericardium. Pneumopericardium is most commonly seen with pneumothorax and pneumomediastinum as a complication of respiratory therapy in infants. However, it has also been reported as a spontaneous development in asthma[18] and following blunt chest injury.[19] Pneumopericardium rarely causes tamponade, although life-threatening tamponade from this cause has been reported as a complication of pericardiectomy.[20]

NONTRAUMATIC

There are many causes of nontraumatic pericardial effusion and cardiac tamponade (see Tables 14–1 and 14–2). Nontraumatic effusions can be of tremendous size, because their gradual development over weeks or months usually allows time for the pericardium to stretch to accommodate the fluid, a process that the pericardium cannot do acutely.[21] This stretching prevents rapid rises in intrapericardial pressure, and as a result, tamponade is much less frequent than in the rapidly

accumulating traumatic effusion. Infrequently, the patient with a nontraumatic tamponade may be severely ill when first seen and may require immediate therapy. Alternatively, the patient is often stable long enough so that pericardiocentesis (or another therapeutic procedure) can be performed under orderly and controlled conditions. The differentiation between nontraumatic and traumatic tamponade is usually obvious but is a distinction that must be made, because the etiology determines the aggressiveness, type, and speed of treatment.

The etiology of nontraumatic tamponade may not be obvious upon examination in the emergency department, and tamponade is frequently misdiagnosed as congestive heart failure or other pulmonary pathology. Cancer is a prominent cause; the pericardium is involved in 20 per cent of patients with disseminated tumors.[1]

There is primary pericardial involvement in 69 per cent of acute leukemias, in 64 per cent of malignant melanomas, and in 24 per cent of lymphomas; however, the incidence of actual tamponade in these malignancies is not known. Of metastases to the pericardium, 35 per cent originate in the lung, 35 per cent in breast, 15 per cent in lymphomas, and 10 per cent in melanomas. Thus, any patient who is known to have one of these malignancies should be considered at risk for tamponade. Metastasis to the heart is usually a late finding in cancer, and other foci located elsewhere are usually evident.[22] Radiation pericarditis, particularly after treatment for Hodgkin's disease, is a common cause of effusion.[23] Effusion occurs in approximately 5 per cent of those patients who receive 4000 rads to the heart. Cardiac tamponade was the presenting manifestation of pericarditis in 81 per cent of Guberman's patients with that diagnosis; however, most of those patients also had chest pain. Thirty per cent of myxedema patients may have pericardial effusions, but few have tamponade.[5] Large pericardial effusion (up to 1500 cc or more) is common in uremia and occurs in 7 per cent of chronic dialysis patients.[24] Tamponade occurs in 34 per cent of uremic patients who have effusions, but the effusion may be managed with dialysis alone in most cases. In many cases of nontraumatic effusion, tamponade does not occur and the effusion may resolve with treatment of the underlying disease or may be managed successfully by pericardiocentesis.

Most of the other etiologies listed in Table 14–1 are isolated case reports, and their incidences in large series have not been determined.

Pathophysiology of Tamponade

The pericardium is a tough, leathery sac that encloses the heart. The pericardial sac cannot expand quickly, although it is quite distensible under prolonged pressure. Its compliance varies considerably in different individuals and disease states. This compliance helps to determine the pressure/volume response curves shown in Figures 14–1 and 14–2.[23]

The pericardial sac normally contains about 25 to 35 ml of serous fluid.[25] As more fluid accumulates, the first 80 to 120 ml are easily accommodated in the pericardial recesses without significantly affecting pericardial pressure (see Fig. 14–1).[26] Beyond this amount, however, the intrapericardial pressure rises substantially, and an

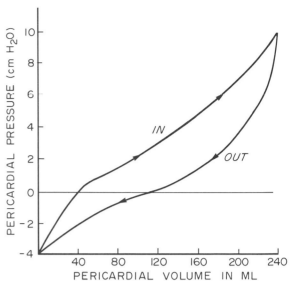

Figure 14–2. Relationship of intrapericardial pressure to volume of pericardial fluid. Note that pressure drops more rapidly when fluid is removed than when it accumulates. (From Pories, W., and Gaudiani, V.: Cardiac tamponade. Surg. Clin. North Am. 55:573, 1975. Used by permission.)

additional 20 to 40 ml almost doubles the intrapericardial pressure, often leading to sudden decompensation. This pressure/volume relationship demonstrates hysteresis; the withdrawal of a quantity of fluid drops the pressure more than its addition raised it (see Fig. 14–2).[21] For example, adding 160 ml of fluid would raise pressure about 9 cm of H_2O, but only 80 ml would have to be removed to return the pressure to the original value.[1]

As fluid accumulates, the increased intrapericardial pressure is transmitted through the ventricular wall and causes increased ventricular diastolic pressure. This decreases the pressure gradient across the mitral and tricuspid valves, thereby decreasing ventricular filling. The net result is a decrease of ventricular filling in diastole, with a resultant decreased stroke volume, contractile force, and cardiac output. The increased intraventricular pressure is reflected in increased atrial and central venous pressures (CVP). Pulse pressure narrows as left ventricular end-diastolic pressure rises and reflex sympathetic stimulation increases. Coronary perfusion is diminished due to lower aortic pressure and increased diastolic pressure.

Because stroke volume is decreased, heart rate increases to maintain cardiac output. Sympathetic discharge causes both arterial and venous vasoconstriction.[27] Vasoconstriction increases venous pressure, which helps to restore the normal venous-atrial and atrioventricular filling gradients. These mechanisms are often very effective and may permit establishment of a new homeostasis with normal cardiac output.

If, however, intrapericardial pressure continues

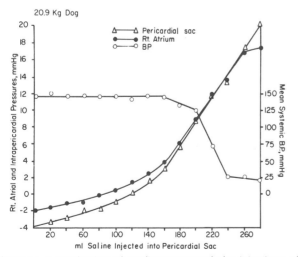

Figure 14–1. Production of cardiac tamponade by injections of saline into the pericardial sac. Note steep increases in pressure and drop in blood pressure at about 200 ml of saline. (From Fowler, N. O.: Physiology of cardiac tamponade and pulsus paradoxus. II: physiological, circulatory, and pharmacological responses in cardiac tamponade. Mod. Concepts Cardiovasc. Dis. 47:116, 1978. Used by permission of the American Heart Association, Inc.)

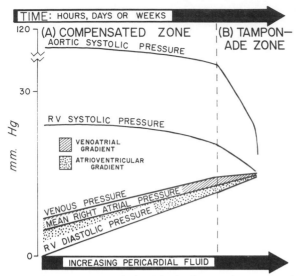

Figure 14–3. Summary of physiologic changes in tamponade. (From Shoemaker, W. C., Carey, S. J., Yao, S. T., et al.: Hemodynamic monitoring for physiological evaluation, diagnosis, and therapy of acute hemopericardial tamponade from penetrating wounds and Spodick, D.: Acute cardiac tamponade: Pathologic physiology, diagnosis, and management. Prog. Cardiovasc. Dis. 10:65, 1967. Used by permission.)

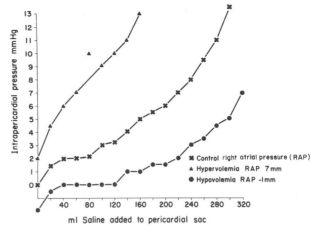

Figure 14–4. Experimental pericardial pressure-volume curve in three states: control, hypovolemia, and hypervolemia. (From Fowler, N. O.: Physiology of cardiac tamponade and pulsus paradoxus. II: physiological, circulatory, and pharmacological responses in cardiac tamponade. Mod. Concepts Cardiovasc. Dis. 47:117, 1978. Used by permission of the American Heart Association, Inc.)

to rise, these compensatory mechanisms will fail. Lactic acidosis may result from poor tissue perfusion and be the triggering event that lowers myocardial contractility and disrupts the uneasy equilibrium.[28] Atrial pressure rises rapidly (see Figs. 14–1 and 14–3). Right ventricular end-diastolic pressure rises. The pulmonary circulation, being at much lower pressure than the systemic arterial pressure, is more vulnerable to the rising atrial pressure. A "pressure plateau" occurs in which right atrial pressure, right ventricular diastolic pressure, pulmonary artery diastolic pressure, and pulmonary capillary wedge pressure are virtually identical. With a continued rise in intrapericardial pressure, pulmonary blood flow ceases and cardiac arrest shortly follows.[28]

Total blood volume intimately affects cardiac compensation, and it is possible to encounter a "low pressure" cardiac tamponade. The hypovolemic patient with tamponade will have a decreased venous pressure, which not only decreases cardiac output but also may obscure the diagnosis, because distended neck veins or an elevated CVP will not be present (Fig. 14–4). Conversely, increasing blood volume in hypovolemia will increase CVP enough to provide a higher filling pressure, thus, at least temporarily, offsetting increased intrapericardial and ventricular pressure. In a patient with a chronic pericardial effusion, the onset of hypovolemia can lower filling pressure enough to precipitate tamponade. The result is tamponade in the presence of low right atrial and central venous pressure, despite

the fact that tamponade is usually associated with an *elevated* CVP.[29]

Diagnosis of Cardiac Tamponade

The diagnosis of pericardial effusion may be difficult in the emergency department and may require extensive evaluation, but pericardial tamponade is usually diagnosed on clinical grounds alone.

The classical physical findings of tamponade were first characterized by Beck in 1935. He described two triads, one for acute and one for chronic compression.[30] The triad in acute compression consists of elevated venous pressure, decreased arterial pressure, and muffled heart sounds. Unfortunately, in most major trauma series, only about one third of the patients demonstrate the complete triad,[28, 31] although almost 90 per cent have one or more signs.[7] It should be noted that the simultaneous occurrence of all three physical signs is a very late manifestation of tamponade and is usually only seen shortly before cardiac arrest (Fig. 14–3). Careful hemodynamic monitoring reveals much earlier changes that indicate the progression of tamponade (Table 14–3).[32] In Grade I tamponade, cardiac output and arterial pressure are normal, but central venous pressure (CVP) and heart rate are increased. In Grade II tamponade, blood pressure is normal or slightly decreased, CVP is increased, and tachycardia persists. In Grade III tamponade, the classic findings of Beck's triad occur. Although this sequence represents the natural history of acute

Table 14–3. SHOEMAKER SYSTEM OF GRADING CARDIAC TAMPONADE

Grade	Pericardial Volume (ml)	Cardiac Index	Stroke Index	Mean Arterial Pressure	CVP	Heart Rate	Beck's Triad
I	< 200	normal or ↑	normal or ↓	normal	↑	↑	Venous distension, hypotension, muffled heart sounds usually not present
II	≥ 200	↓	↓	normal or ↓	↑ (≥12 cm H₂O)	↑	May or may not be present
III	> 200	↓↓	↓↓	↓↓	↑↑ (up to 30–40 cm H₂O)	↓	Usually present

From Shoemaker, W. C., Carey, S. J., Yao, S. T., et al.: Hemodynamic monitoring for physiologic evaluation, diagnosis, and therapy of acute hemopericardial tamponade from penetrating wounds. J. Trauma 13:36, 1973.

tamponade, the time course varies. Some patients are stable at a given stage or hours; others proceed to cardiac arrest within minutes.[28, 32]

Beck also described a triad of high CVP, ascites, and a small, quiet heart in chronic compression. The diagnosis of tamponade is made by careful evaluation and correlation of the following parameters.

PULSUS PARADOXUS

Pulsus paradoxus is essentially a normal phenomen that occurs to a slight degree during normal respiration, and an exaggerated respiration will often produce a clinically detectable change in blood pressure during inspiration.

Paradoxical pulse is one of the classical physical signs of tamponade, although it is not pathognomic, because it is also caused by pulmonary emphysema, asthma, obesity, cardiac failure, constrictive pericarditis, pulmonary embolism, and cardiogenic shock.[7, 21, 28] Paradoxical pulse is defined as an exaggeration of the normal inspiratory fall in blood pressure.[27, 31] To demonstrate paradoxical pulse, the patient should be lying comfortably, at a 30 to 45 degree angle, breathing normally and in an unlabored fashion, because any abnormal respiration may accentuate pulsus paradoxus.[27] The blood pressure cuff is inflated well above systolic pressure and slowly deflated until one first hears the systolic sounds that are synchronous with expiration (Fig. 14–5). Initially, one will hear the arterial pulse only during expiration, and it will disappear during inspiration. The cuff is then further deflated until arterial sounds are heard throughout the respiratory cycle. If the difference between these two pressures is greater than 10 mm Hg, the paradoxical pulse is considered abnormal. Most patients with proven tamponade will have a difference of 20 to 30 mm Hg or more during the respiratory cycle,[7, 21, 28] but

this absolute figure is not reliable. Patients with very narrow pulse pressures (typical of Grade III tamponade) will have a deceptively "small" paradoxical pulse of 5 to 15 mmHg, because paradoxical pulse is a function of actual pulse pressure. The inspiratory systolic pressure may be below the level at which diastolic sounds disappear.[27] For this reason, the ratio of paradoxical pulse to the size of the pulse pressure is a more reliable measure. Paradoxic pulse greater than 50 per cent of the pulse pressure is abnormal.[27] The exact cause of pulsus paradoxus is unknown, but two physiologic principles have traditionally been thought to be contributory factors. During inspiration, blood is preferentially drawn into the right ventricle. This increase in right ventricular volume shifts the intraventricular septum to the left, and, by this shift in the septum, the compression of the left ventricle may decrease left ventricular filling enough to decrease left ventricular outflow via the Frank-Starling effect. Secondly, with inspiration, blood pools in the pulmonary veins, thereby reducing left ventricular filling enough to have an effect on left ventricular output. Pressure in the pericardial space secondary to pericardial fluid may accentuate these normal physiologic events enough to be clinically significant.

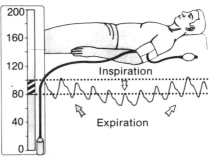

Figure 14–5. Measurement of pulsus paradoxus. (From Stein, L., Shubin, H., and Weil, M.: Recognition and management of pericardial tamponade. JAMA 225:504, 1973. Used by permission.)

Measuring paradoxical pulse is difficult and time consuming, and any frightened, hypotensive patient with labored breathing can have it. Although the mean paradoxical pulse was 49 mm Hg in one series of nontraumatic tamponade,[5] 23 per cent of the patients had a paradox of less than 20 mm Hg and one had no paradox. One half of the uremic patients with tamponade had no pulsus paradoxus.[24]

Pulsus paradoxus has been reported to be *absent* in tamponade when there is an atrial septal defect, aortic insufficiency, localized collections of pericardial blood, extreme tamponade with hypotension, or when left ventricular diastolic pressure is intrinsically elevated.[29] In traumatic tamponade, it is deemed unreliable;[7, 34, 35] in one study, only 35 per cent of the patients had paradoxical pulse when elevated CVP and decreased heart sounds were present.[35] In another study of 197 traumatic cases, only 8.6 per cent of the diagnoses of tamponade were arrived at by finding pulsus paradoxus.[36]

It seems clear that when a large paradoxical pulse is present, it is useful, particularly in a nontrauma patient in whom tamponade might not be suspected initially. Paradoxical pulse can be palpated if it is very large; during palpation, the pulse may completely disappear during inspiration. Palpation for this purpose is best done at peripheral arteries such as the radial or femoral. Similarly, when arterial pressure monitors are already in place, paradoxical pulse can be measured rapidly and accurately. Its presence is significant, because it appears in *late* tamponade, when left ventricular end-diastolic volume has already fallen to 48 per cent of normal and coronary blood flow has been cut in half.[37] Whether or not time is taken to actually *measure* the paradoxical pulse depends upon the patient's status. If the patient is moribund or rapidly deteriorating, this would obviously be a poor choice of priorities.

VENOUS DISTENTION

Venous distention, reflecting increased CVP, is also a late sign in cardiac tamponade (see Fig. 14–3). It may be masked by venoconstriction due to vasopressors (such as dopamine) or intrinsic sympathetic discharge or by hypovolemia,[8, 21, 28, 32, 34] a common finding in the trauma patient. Neck vein distention may be obvious clinically, but the measured CVP is more reliable than the state of venous distention. A CVP line may be placed immediately in all patients who have penetrating chest trauma, and the position should be verified by radiologic examination. The CVP reading should take into account positive-pressure ventilation and the effects of a Valsalva maneuver. Most patients with significant tamponade will have a CVP of 12 to 14 cm H_2O or greater.[34] Hypovolemia changes the intrapericardial pressure/volume curve in tamponade and will lower the CVP reading at any given stage in the tamponade process, as opposed to normovolemic values.

Animal studies have documented that right atrial pressure can be normal in hypovolemia with tamponade. One case of low-pressure cardiac tamponade was reported in a patient with no jugular venous distention, no paradoxical pulse, and a right atrial pressure of 8 mm Hg.[29] Thus, although the initial CVP reading is useful and diagnostic if grossly elevated, for example, 20 to 30 cm H_2O,[20, 34] it is actually the *trend* of CVP readings that is the most sensitive diagnostic tool.[34] A rising CVP, especially when there is persistent hypotension, is extremely suggestive of tamponade in the trauma patient. In the rare case of the hypovolemic patient who is suspected of tamponade but who demonstrates a low CVP, a fluid challenge will help clarify the situation and also improve the cardiac output.[29]

CHEST RADIOGRAPHS

Chest radiographs are not useful in the diagnosis of acute traumatic tamponade, because the cardiac size and shape does not change acutely. They may, however, reveal hemothorax, bullet location, or even pneumopericardium. In the unstable trauma patient with clinical tamponade, time should not be wasted in obtaining films. In the nontrauma patient with chronic effusion, a chest film will often reveal an enlarged sac-like "water bottle" cardiac shadow. Unfortunately, radiographic findings cannot accurately differentiate pericardial from myocardial enlargement, nor can they distinguish between simple pericardial effusion and tamponade.

The value of a chest film is that it may suggest the diagnosis and indicate further investigation. Another useful finding on the plain chest film is the epicardial fat pad sign, seen in 41 per cent of lateral and 23 per cent of frontal chest films in proven pericardial effusion.[38] The water-density space between the radiolucent epicardial fat and the mediastinal fat represents the pericardial tissues and is normally less than 2 mm. An increase in this width suggests pericardial fluid or thickening (Fig. 14–6).

ELECTROCARDIOGRAM

The electrocardiogram (ECG) is seldom of diagnostic value, because most changes of tamponade, such as altered ST segments, low-voltage QRS complexes, and T inversions are nonspecific.[21]

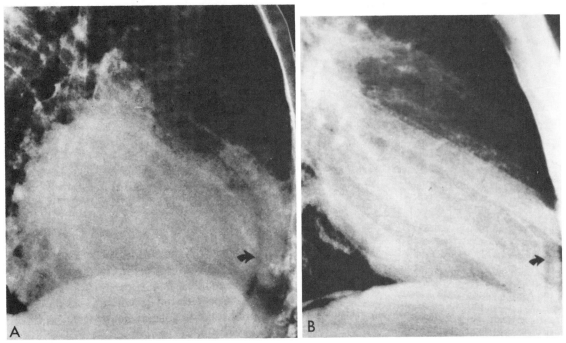

Figure 14–6. Epicardial fat pad sign. The water-density space between the radiolucent epicardial fat and mediastinal fat represents the pericardium, and its contents and should be 2 mm or less. An increase suggests pericardial fluid or thickening. A, Posteroanterior chest film. B, Lateral chest film.

Electrical alternans of both the P wave and the QRS complex (total electrical alternans) is a rare finding but, when seen, is thought to be pathognomic of tamponade (Fig. 14–7).[21, 39] Electrical alternans is caused by pendular motion of the heart within the pericardial sac.[40] Alternans does not always appear in the standard ECG leads; a bipolar chest lead (Lewis lead) may be needed to detect it. Electromechanical dissociation and profound bradycardia are terminal events.[41]

ECHOCARDIOGRAPHY

Echocardiography is the most accurate technique for diagnosing pericardial effusion,[8] but it may take too much time for its use to be justified in patients who are deteriorating rapidly. Both M-mode and two-dimensional echo are used.

In the relatively stable patient in whom CVP and peripheral IV lines are in place and in whom a fluid challenge is being administered, echocardiography can be a useful technique. This is particularly true in the patient with nontraumatic tamponade. The availability of echocardiography and skilled interpretation of it vary from institution to institution; however, when it is available, echocardiography is a benign, noninvasive procedure that can definitely determine the presence of an effusion and tamponade with considerable accuracy.[42] In a stable situation, it can save the patient an unnecessary pericardiocentesis.

Fluoroscopy, x-ray contrast techniques, and radioisotope techniques have been used but are too slow and difficult to arrange for emergency department purposes.

PATIENT PROFILE

Small and slowly developing pericardial effusion may produce few or no symptoms. Respiratory symptoms, such as dyspnea on exertion, may suggest pulmonary pathology, and pericardial ef-

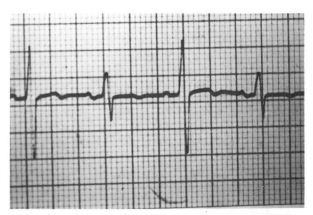

Figure 14–7. Lewis lead EKG showing total electrical alternans of both amplitude and configuration of P and QRS complexes. This is pathognomonic of tamponade. (From Sotolongo, R. P., and Horton, J. D.: Total electrical alternans in pericardial tamponade. Am. Heart J. 101:854, 1981. Used by permission.)

fusion is often mistaken for congestive heart failure. It is said that CHF produces orthopnea more consistently than pericardial effusions, but such a distinction is not always evident.

Acutely, pericardial tamponade may resemble tension pneumothorax, acute hemothorax, hypovolemia, pulmonary edema, or pulmonary embolism. The patient is often agitated or panic-stricken, confused, uncooperative, restless, cyanotic, diaphoretic, and acutely short of breath. In the late stages, the patient is moribund. Hypotension in the presence of severe cyanosis and distended neck veins is a helpful finding, but diagnosis of tamponade on purely clinical grounds may be difficult to ascertain.

Indications

DIAGNOSTIC PERICARDIOCENTESIS

Two indications for pericardiocentesis have been stated: to diagnose the cause or presence of a pericardial effusion and or to relieve tamponade. Detailed discussion of these indications and associated concerns is provided in the following sections.

The use of pericardiocentesis for diagnosis of the *etiology* of effusions is widespread and frequently recommended.[23, 43] Neoplastic cells, blood, bacteria, and chyle can be sought. The results of a recent, large series of pericardiocentesis for non-traumatic effusions cast some doubt on diagnostic accuracy, however, because although fluid was obtained in 90 per cent of the taps, specific etiologic diagnoses were obtained from only 24 per cent of the fluid specimens.[6] In the Krikorian series, in patients with normal venous pressure, only 14 per cent of the taps provided a diagnosis.[6] Fluid was falsely negative for cytology in several cases of lymphoma and mesothelioma. Overall it was concluded that although 68 per cent of the patients with elevated venous pressure benefited in some hemodynamic manner from the procedure, only 11 per cent of those with normal venous pressure received any benefit. There were several complications, including death, delays of surgery, purulent pericarditis, hemopericardium secondary to the procedure, and ventricular tachycardia. The risks were thought to exceed those of other methods of diagnosis.

On the other hand, several recent studies have indicated that subxiphoid pericardiotomy is a much safer technique than pericardiocentesis and involves few major complications. In addition, pericardial biopsy provides a definite diagnosis in virtually all cases.[3, 44] It has been stated that diagnostic pericardiocentesis is inappropriate and that pericardiocentesis is indicated only for the emergency relief of tamponade.[45]

Because cardiac tamponade is a clinical diagnosis, the use of pericardiocentesis to diagnose traumatic tamponade is unequivocally inappropriate. As a diagnostic measure to determine the presence of pericardial bleeding in trauma, the procedure has a false-negative rate of between 20 and 40 per cent.[9, 34, 35, 46–48] An "inconclusive" tap is one in which no fluid is obtained, although many authors have equated a dry tap with a negative tap. A true negative tap would recover a few milliliters of clear serous fluid, but such fluid is almost never obtained because of the very small amount of fluid that is normally present in the pericardial sac. The reason for the high false-negative rate (defined as no blood aspirated) is well demonstrated by a typical study of stab wounds of the heart.[9] Ninety-six per cent of the patients had blood in the pericardium; however, it was clotted in 41 per cent of the patients and partially clotted in another 24 per cent. In only 19 per cent was the blood completely fluid. Obviously, pericardiocentesis will be negative in the presence of clotted blood, and importantly, it will fail to fully relieve tamponade when secondary to clotted blood.

THERAPEUTIC PERICARDIOCENTESIS

Use in Nontraumatic Effusion/Tamponade

The clinical relevance to emergency treatment is that pericardiocentesis is often therapeutic in cardiac tamponade. Most nontraumatic effusions are liquids that can be easily drained through a small needle. Removal of even a small amount of fluid can dramatically improve blood pressure, cardiac output, and perfusion in a patient with tamponade (Fig. 14–8). Pericardiocentesis has relieved tamponade due to nontraumatic effusions in 60 to 90 per cent of the cases.[5, 6] Those patients in whom it failed often had purulent pericarditis or malignant invasion of the pericardium. The procedure is less useful for long-term management; 26 per cent of the patients in Guberman's series eventually required pericardial resection.[5] In Krikorian's series, 24 per cent of the patients were managed successfully with one pericardiocentesis, and 37 per cent had multiple taps or an indwelling catheter, and 39 per cent required surgical drainage. Fifty-five per cent of the latter group had traumatic hemopericardium. The risk of performing pericardiocentesis without echocardiographic determination of pericardial fluid is shown in the Krikorian series.[6] Of the patients with a clinical picture of tamponade, 17 per cent had constrictive pericarditis, 16 per cent had CHF–fluid overload, and 5 per cent had obstruction of the superior vena cava. None of these patients could be expected to benefit from pericardiocentesis and all would be at much higher risk of complications.

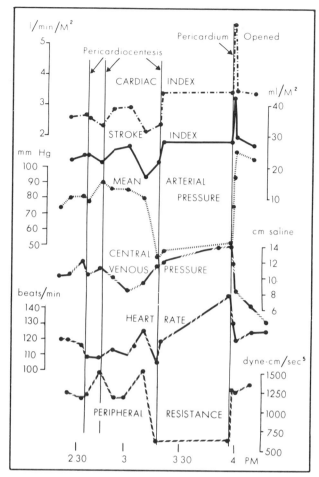

Figure 14–8. Effect of pericardiocentesis in a patient with tamponade. On two of the three occasions, pericardiocentesis was productive of 30 ml of non-clotting blood, with favorable effects on hemodynamic parameters. (From Shoemaker, W. C.: Algorithm for early recognition and management of cardiac tamponade. Crit. Care Med. 3:62, 1975. Used by permission of Williams & Wilkins Co., Baltimore.)

It is clear that with properly confirmed evidence of effusion and a clinical picture of tamponade, pericardiocentesis is therapeutic in a significant number of cases. Certain subgroups, however, may be better managed by alternative methods. Approximately 7 per cent of all dialysis patients will develop a large pericardial effusion. In one series, 63 per cent of these patients were sucessfully managed with dialysis alone, and only 6 per cent needed surgical treatment over the long term.[6] An alogrithm for the emergency management of *nontraumatic* cardiac tamponade is shown in Figure 14–9.

In summary, pericardiocentesis is therapeutic in many patients with nontraumatic tamponade. These patients tend to accumulate effusions slowly, allowing the pericardium to stretch to accommodate up to 2000 ml of fluid.[23] This slower accumulation of fluid (compared with the rapid accumulation of blood in traumatic tamponade) means that even in a moderately hypotensive

patient more time may be available for work-up. If possible, an echocardiogram should be obtained, and the procedure is best carried out under controlled situations, such as in a catheterization lab. Uremic patients may be more safely managed by dialysis.

Use in Traumatic Tamponade

In distinct contrast to its significant role in the therapy of medical tamponade, pericardiocentesis may be misleading or perhaps even dangerous in traumatic effusion. The high incidence of pericardial clots has already been discussed under diagnostic pericardiocentesis; thus, failure to obtain fluid does not rule out pericardial bleeding.

Even if the pericardiocentesis confirms the suspicion of pericardial bleeding, it is seldom used as definitive treatment in traumatic tamponade.[49, 50] Although aspiration of a small quantity of fluid may cause dramatic improvement, blood often reaccumulates.[21, 39] Repeated taps will be necessary, increasing the risk of complications. A plastic catheter may be left in place, but it cannot prevent or remove intrapericardial clots. Such a catheter may give a false sense of security. A positive tap does not provide information regarding the size or nature of the cardiac injury. Thus, ultimately, patients with pericardial hemorrhage require thoracotomy to explore and repair the cardiac wound.

One of the greatest potential drawbacks of pericardiocentesis in traumatic tamponade is that significant time may be spent with nondefinitive therapy, either delaying thoracotomy or creating a false sense of security. In one study of 25 trauma patients with cardiac injury,[49] all those who were operated on within 2 hr of injury survived, regardless of age or type of wound. With greater delay, none survived. Sugg and colleagues,[47] in a study of 459 similar patients, found a mortality rate of 43 per cent when pericardiocentesis was the sole treatment but a mortality rate of only 16 per cent when surgery was performed. Most authors agree that with early thoracotomy and little or no reliance on pericardiocentesis the number of deaths due to stab wounds has decreased.[9, 11, 34, 46, 48, 50, 51] Mortality rates dropped from 26 to 5 per cent in one series.[47]

With a similar change in approach, Symbas reported a drop in the mortality rate, from 17.6 per cent when relying heavily on pericardiocentesis to 5 per cent with surgery, using pericardiocentesis only to gain time. By comparison, Sugg and associates report that 10 of 18 patients with traumatic tamponade who were managed by repeated pericardiocentesis alone died within 1 to 2 hr.[47] At autopsy, all patients had completely repairable wounds.

Thoracotomy has a low complication rate and essentially no mortality.[8, 41] Emergency thoracot-

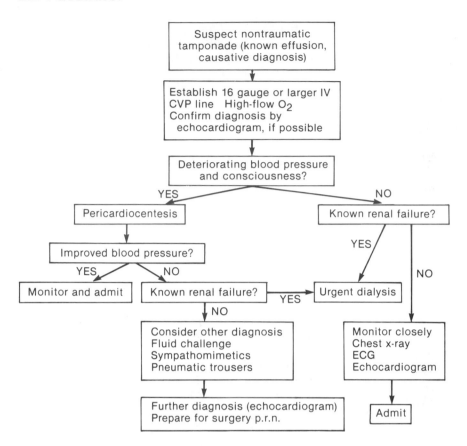

Figure 14–9. Management of *nontraumatic* cardiac tamponade.

omy is reported to result in an infection rate of 6.8 per cent or less,[51] with most studies reporting no infection,[7, 47, 50] even when a completely unsterile thoracotomy was carried out with the physician in street clothes using bare hands.[49] Thus, it is clear that pericardiocentesis is not acceptable as definitive treatment for traumatic tamponade, and rapid surgical treatment is the standard method of care.

Pericardiocentesis is, however, mandated treatment when the emergency physician is faced with a deteriorating patient, when other treatments have been unsuccessful (see Fig. 14–10) and surgical consultation has already been initiated. If a patient with clinical signs of tamponade is deteriorating to the stage of unconsciousness as a result of hypotension, cardiac arrest is not far off. In that case, the emergency physician who is not experienced in emergency thoracotomy or subxiphoid pericardiotomy must attempt therapeutic pericardiocentesis, because it is the only option available and it may be lifesaving.

Some experimental evidence supports the usefulness of pericardiocentesis as a temporizing measure while preparing for definitive surgical treatment. In a study of 174 patients with tamponade from penetrating trauma, 96 had operating room (OR) thoracotomy, 44 had emergency department (ED) thoracotomy, and 34 received only pericardiocentesis and were observed.[36] Of those

with OR thoracotomy, 68 per cent were hemodynamically unstable and preoperative pericardiocentesis decreased the mortality rate from 25 to 11 per cent. Ninety-one per cent of those with ED thoracotomy were unstable, and prethoracotomy pericardiocentesis decreased the mortality rate from 94 to 63 per cent. Of those observed after pericardiocentesis, 50 per cent were unstable and the mortality rate was 15 per cent. Thirty-five per cent of the latter group had recurrent tamponade, which was treated with repeat pericardiocentesis. Recent experimental work shows that the early stages of tamponade produce endocardial followed by epicardial ischemia and that this ischemia causes myocardial decompensation, which contributes to the tamponade process.[37] Intrapericardial pressure rapidly exceeds diastolic and even right ventricular systolic pressure. Combined with decreased aortic pressure and tachycardia, this results in reduced coronary flow and ventricular work (see Fig. 14–8).[27] Enzyme changes and myocardial necrosis have been found in experimental animals.[53]

In summary, pericardiocentesis has no role as the *definitive* treatment of traumantic tamponade. Nonetheless, while other treatments (such as fluid challenge, vasopressors, and pneumatic antishock garment) are instituted and while arrangements for definitive surgical treatment are being made, pericardiocentesis may help reduce myocardial is-

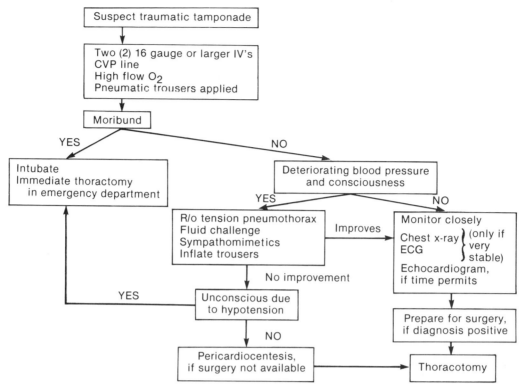

Figure 14–10. Management of *traumatic* cardiac tamponade.

chemia and improve the outcome. Pericardiocentesis should be used only to temporize and only in patients in extremis. For the unconscious, hypotensive, or agonal patient, emergency thoracotomy is an accepted alternative treatment (see Chapter 17). *No trauma patient should die of presumed hypovolemic shock without cardiac tamponade first being ruled out.*

Contraindications

The contraindications to pericardiocentesis are relative, not absolute. They include lack of familiarity with the procedure and its complications, absence of proper equipment (especially monitors, defibrillators, and resuscitation equipment), and the immediate availability of a better treatment modality (e.g., dialysis for uremic patients and immediate surgery for trauma patients). For diagnostic or non-emergency pericardiocentesis, absence of a confirmed diagnosis of effusion (e.g., echocardiographic proof) is a contraindication, because the complication rate increases dramatically under such circumstances.

Equipment

Although the procedure can be performed with only a syringe and a spinal needle, monitoring is desirable. An alligator clamp is useful for connecting the needle to the V lead of an electrocardiograph (ECG) device (Fig. 14–11). A 3- to 5-inch 18 gauge needle is used, preferably of the spinal type, with an obturator. A short bevel is preferred in order to reduce the chance of myocardial lacerations.

A similar gauge over-the-needle catheter may be used. This device allows the plastic catheter, which is less likely to cause myocardial damage, to be left in place for continuous drainage. Alternatively, a Seldinger technique, using a catheter over J wire method, may be used. With this technique, a much smaller gauge needle may be used.[54] A three-way stopcock can be attached to the needle or catheter to allow removal of more than one syringeful without much movement of the needle. The continuous motion of the heart may require the need for minor changes in needle position during the procedure.

Procedure

It is critical that all necessary equipment be functional and laid out in advance. In addition, full resuscitation equipment must be on hand, including a defibrillator. The patient must have an intravenous line in place and be attached to a cardiac monitor. The non-emergency patient may require sedation, but on a emergency basis, peri-

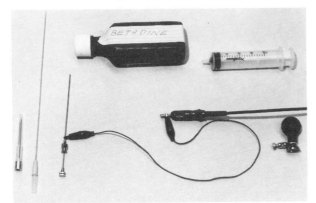

Figure 14–11. Equipment for pericardiocentesis: bactericidal solution (povidone-iodine); long, 18 gauge spinal needle; wire with alligator clips for connection to the ECG machine; and syringe (three-way stopcock optional). A local anesthetic is also required.

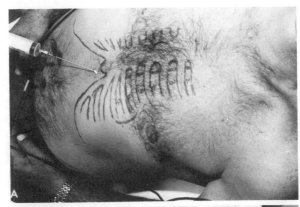

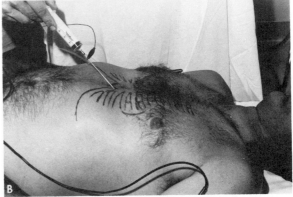

Figure 14–12. Xiphosternal approach for pericardiocentesis. The needle is aimed for the sternal notch or left shoulder. Note ECG monitoring. Although the patient is shown in the supine position, he should preferably be sitting at a 45-degree angle, if his clinical condition permits.

cardiocentesis is usually performed on patients who are already obtunded or unresponsive as a result of low cardiac output. Premedication of the patient with atropine may help to prevent vasovagal reactions. If possible, the presence of pericardial effusion should have already been determined by echocardiography. If surgery *may* be needed, preparations should be under way.

The patient should be sitting at a 45-degree angle to bring the heart closer to the anterior chest wall. If the abdomen is distended because of gastric contents or previous CPR, a nasogastric tube should be used to decompress the stomach. The entire lower xiphoid and epigastric area should be carefully prepped with povidone-iodine 10 per cent solution and sterilely draped, if time permits.

If the patient is awake, the skin and the proposed route of the pericardial needle should be anesthesized by infiltration with 1 per cent plain lidocaine. The pericardium is very sensitive and should be anesthesized in patients who are awake.[54]

The xiphosternal approach is preferred. The needle is inserted between the xiphoid process and the left costal margin at a 30 to 45 degree angle to the skin (Fig. 14–12). Because the heart is an anterior structure, an angle greater than 45 degrees may injure the liver or stomach. In this approach, the needle enters the pericardium at the angle at which it becomes the diaphragmatic pericardium. Recommendations as to where to aim the needle vary from the right shoulder to the left shoulder and all points in between. Aiming toward the sternal notch is a reasonable first choice.[45, 54]

After the skin has been punctured but before the pericardial needle is advanced, ECG monitoring is begun by attaching a sterile cord with alligator clips (see Fig. 14–11) from the pericardial needle to the precordial lead (V lead) of the ECG

machine. The V lead is then recorded, as the needle becomes an "exploring electrode." The machine must be properly tested and internally grounded; small current leaks can induce dysrhythmias.[21] The purpose of the ECG monitoring is to prevent ventricular puncture. When the needle touches the epicardium, a current of injury pattern is noted on the ECG. This current of injury may be local and could be missed if a lead other than the V lead is monitored. Usually one notes ST segment elevation upon contact with the heart or pericardium in the absence of an effusion, but a premature contraction or other ventricular dysrhythmia may also be induced by the direct mechanical stimulation of the ventricular epicardium by the needle. Contact with the atrium will cause atrial dysrhythmias, marked elevation of the PR segment, or atrioventricular dissociation.[13] If there is abnormal myocardial scarring secondary to infarction or other diseases or if there is malignant infiltration of myocardium, there may be no current of injury generated.[14] Thus, ECG monitoring is not infallible in preventing myocardial penetration.

With constant ECG monitoring, the operator slowly advances the needle and syringe, aspirating constantly. The needle will penetrate the pericar-

Withdraw

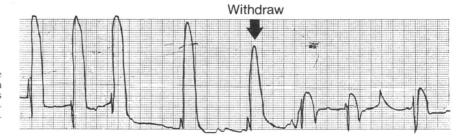

Figure 14–13. Current of injury: There is an obvious change in the EKG when the pericardiocentesis needle touches the epicardium. Following slight withdrawal (arrow) the ST elevation diminishes.

dium (a barrier whose penetration usually cannot be palpated) at about 6 to 8 cm below the skin in adults and 5 cm or less below the skin in children.[25] The patient who is awake may complain of sharp chest pain as the sensitive pericardium is entered. When a current of injury is noted (Fig. 14–13), the needle is touching epicardium and can easily lacerate myocardium or coronary vessels. The needle should be withdrawn a few millimeters until the current of injury disappears. At this point, the needle should be safely positioned in the pericardial space.

An attempt is then made to drain pericardial fluid or blood. If blood is obtained, a hematocrit can be done on both the presumed pericardial sample and venous blood; pericardial blood has a lower hematocrit than vascular blood, and substantially different values rule out the possibility that the needle was in a cardiac chamber. Bloody pericardial fluid may clot, particularly in traumatic situations when bleeding is brisk, so clotting of the aspirated blood does not eliminate the possibility of a pericardial source in favor of an intracardiac source. Nonclotting blood is indicative of pericardial blood.

Interpreting the results of pericardiocentesis has been previously discussed. In the non-emergent situation, if the pericardial needle is thought to be in a cardiac chamber, this possibility may be diagnosed by injecting Decholin or sodium fluorescein into the needle and asking the patient to describe the taste or by observing a flush of the skin under ultraviolet light;[27] however, this procedure is rarely performed.

Most ventricular punctures occur in the lower aspect of the right ventricle. Because the pressure is lower here than in the left ventricle,[25] there should be less bleeding; however, the ventricular wall is also thinner and more vulnerable to laceration.

As much fluid as possible should be aspirated from the pericardium. The removal of even 30 to 50 ml may result in a marked clinical improvement in patients with tamponade. If diagnosis is a consideration, fluid should be taken for cell counts, Gram stain, cytology, culture, and other routine tests. If desired, air can be injected into the pericardium to allow delineation of the pericardial space on a chest film. Repeat films will allow monitoring of the re-accumulation of fluid.[24] This should be done only if the fluid obtained contained no blood; injection of air into the heart can cause fatal air embolism. An indwelling plastic catheter may be left in place if continued drainage is desired. A chest film should be obtained after the procedure to rule out iatrogenic pneumothorax, and patients should be monitored closely for 24 hours for signs of re-accumulating fluid or iatrogenic complications from the procedure.

Alternatively, but less, desirable, pericardiocentesis may be performed in the left 5th intercostal space medial to the border of cardiac dullness, with the needle perpendicular to the skin (Fig. 14–14). The puncture site should be at least 3 to 4 cm lateral to the sternal border to avoid the internal thoracic artery. Pneumothorax is more common by this route, and the left coronary artery or its branches may be lacerated.[21] This route is not usually recommended. Another approach is the apical one; the needle is inserted 1 cm outside the apex beat in the intercostal space below it, within the area of cardiac dullness, and aimed toward the right shoulder.[34] If the apex cannot be palpated, the needle is inserted just inside the area of cardiac dullness. This area is very close to the lingula and left pleural space, and pneumothorax is more frequent; a concomitant pleural effusion

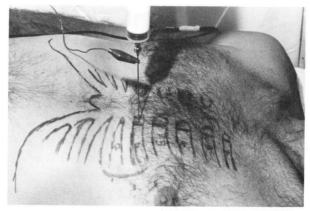

Figure 14–14. Parasternal approach for pericardiocentesis. This route should only be used if the subxiphoid route is unsuccessful. Note proximity to the internal mammary thoracic artery, coronary vessels, and lingula. The patient is depicted in a supine position, although preferably he should be sitting at an angle of 45 degrees, if his clinical condition permits.

may be inadvertently tapped. Supporting this technique are the facts that the coronary vessels are small at the apex, and if the ventricle is entered, it is the thick-walled left ventricle. There are insufficient data to state whether these theoretical advantages are real in practice.

Complications

One of the most common "complications" of pericardiocentesis is the high false-negative rate, which was discussed previously. The pericardial needle can injure any organ within its reach, causing pneumothorax or myocardial or coronary vessel laceration, thus causing hemopericardium.[51] Venous air embolism may be caused by air entering the heart.[55] The pericardial needle can also induce dysrhythmias from direct irritation of the epicardium or from small currents leaking from the connected ECG machine.[2]

Although many complications of pericardiocentesis have been reported anecdotally in the literature since 1896,[2] only recently have their incidence been reported in large series of patients. The first series reporting incidence of complications was that of Kotte and McGuire,[56] who reported that 18 of 21 physicians polled had seen at least one

fatality due to pericardiocentesis. Bishop and associates[57] reported six ventricular punctures in 40 procedures. Kilpatrick and Chapman[2] reported seven ventricular punctures in 20 procedures, with three patients developing hypotension and one death. Frederiksen and colleagues[58] reported three cardiac chamber punctures in 21 procedures; Pradham and Ikins[59] reported one iatrogenic tamponade in five procedures; and Silverberg and coworkers[60] reported one cardiac arrest in 21 procedures. Many of these smaller studies were not detailed. It is important to separate the problems inherent in a potentially fatal process such as tamponade from those caused by the procedure itself. Four large, recent studies are summarized in Table 14–4, which indicates that early, ominous reports of the risks of pericardiocentesis were not overstated. The major complications will be discussed individually.

CARDIAC ARREST AND DEATH

This combination of complications occurred in approximately 2 per cent of the patients in the three largest series in Table 14–4. An exact causal relationship between pericardiocentesis and sudden death, however, is difficult to substantiate. In

Table 14–4. INCIDENCE OF COMPLICATIONS OF PERICARDIOCENTESIS

	Wong (1979)	Guberman[5] (1981)	Krikorian[6] (1978)	Kwasnik[24] (1978)
Number of cases	52	56	123	34
Environment	Cath lab with echo, fluoroscopy, no trauma	Cardiology service with echo, fluoroscopy, etc., no trauma	University hospital, most in cath lab, 9% trauma	All uremic patients
Success in obtaining fluid (%)	69	87	86	—
Diagnosis from taps (%)	50	60 (malignancy only)	18	—
Cardiac arrest (% resuscitated)	2	2	—	—
Death (%)	2	2	1.6(3.2)*	—
Ventricular puncture or laceration (%)	9	6.5	—	—
False-negative taps (%)	7.6	—	—	—
Surgery needed for tamponade (%)	—	26	39	—
New hemopericardium (%)	—	—	10.5	—
Major dysrhythmias (%)	—	—	0.08	—
Hypotensive episode (% vasovagal)	—	—	2	—
Pneumothorax (%)	—	—	—	3
Pneumoperitoneum (%)	—	—	—	3

*1.6% indicates directly attributable deaths; 3.2% also includes contributory deaths.

Wong's series of 52 patients, the one death occurred in a patient in cardiogenic shock who had a nonproductive pericardiocentesis and who, on post mortem, had severe arteriosclerotic heart disease, not tamponade. There was an additional case of cardiac arrest that was successfully resuscitated, also in a patient with a nonproductive pericardiocentesis; the exact cause of the arrest was not discussed.

In Guberman's series of 56 patients, there was also one death during pericardiocentesis; details are not given. Another patient with tamponade had right ventricular laceration by the pericardial needle, causing cardiac arrest; she was resuscitated and had emergency pericardiotomy but suffered hypoxic brain damage and died 2 weeks later.

In Krikorian's series of 123 patients, there were two deaths reported, both in seriously ill patients who had other medical problems. One suffered right ventricular laceration and iatrogenic tamponade. Effusion had not been present prior to pericardiocentesis, which was done with echocardiogram. Another patient with large effusion but no tamponade died shortly after periocardiocentesis was performed; the exact cause of death was not known. A third patient, in whom an indwelling catheter was left in place for 5 days to drain pericardial effusion, developed purulent pericarditis and died. Two additional patients in Krikorian's series died after pericardiocentesis; the time spent performing the procedure delayed definitive surgery and was believed to contribute substantially to death. If these patients are included, the mortality rate in this series rises to 3.2 per cent.

Most deaths associated with pericardiocentesis occur in patients who were already seriously ill. It should be noted that Wong found the most complications in patients who retrospectively had no effusion. With increased use of echocardiography, the rate of complications from pericardiocentesis decreased.

CARDIAC CHAMBER OR LUNG LACERATION

This complication occurs in 6 to 9 per cent of patients, even in the hands of experienced physicians under controlled situations. Nonfatal cardiac puncture, pneumothorax, and pneumoperitoneum have been reported,[24] as well as suppurative costochondritis that requires resection of cartilage. In the Krikorian series, 13 of 123 patients developed hemopericardium as a result of pericardiocentesis, one as a result of a lacerated coronary artery. One patient died from a punctured ventricle. Surgical control was necessary for four patients who developed tamponade, whereas eight patients did not develop tamponade and were managed conservatively. Several cases of induced tamponade occurred in patients with platelet counts greater than 50,000.

Guberman reported three right ventricular lacerations in 46 patients; one was fatal. Wong found five right ventricular punctures, four in patients with nonproductive pericardiocentesis, but none causing "any adverse sequelae."

A review of the literature reveals 22 ventricular punctures and 6 iatrogenic tamponades caused by 230 pericardiocenteses, for an overall ventricular puncture rate of 10 per cent. Authors differ in their opinions as to the adverse effects of ventricular puncture. Atrial puncture has also been reported.[13]

DYSRHYTHMIAS

Serious dysrhythmias induced by pericardiocentesis are rare, although premature ventricular contractions (PVCs) occur commonly during the procedure and are benign in most cases. Wong, Guberman, and Kwasnik reported no dysrhythmias. Krikorian reported only one episode of ventricular tachycardia and "several" hypotensive vasovagal reactions, which were associated with bradycardia and responded to atropine and fluid loading.

Conclusions

In *nontraumatic patients*, tamponade should always be considered in the differential diagnosis of shock, especially in patients who are on anticoagulants, with recent myocardial infarction or with pericardial disease. Tamponade should also be considered in the differential diagnosis when hypotension persists following closed-chest CPR, CVP line placement, or attempts at cardiac pacing.

In any patient with blunt or penetrating chest or upper abdominal trauma, the possibility of *traumatic tamponade* must be considered. If clinical deterioration occurs in the ED pending operative care, pericardiocentesis should be considered if other therapy fails. When such a trauma patient arrives with no obtainable blood pressure or in profound shock and unconscious, immediate thoracotomy and pericardiotomy is indicated after intubation.[50, 61, 62] Pericardiocentesis would entail a dangerous delay in this situation.

In summary, management of either traumatic or nontraumatic tamponade requires a sound understanding of pathophysiology, an ever-vigilant attitude, and the willingness, if it is necessary, to perform relatively high-risk procedures such as pericardiocentesis on critically ill or injured patients.

1. Stein, L., Shubin, H., and Weil, M.: Recognition and management of pericardial tamponade. JAMA 225:503, 1973.
2. Kilpatrick, Z. M., and Chapman, C. B.: On pericardiocentesis. Am. J. Cardiol. 16:722, 1965.
3. Prager, R. L., Wilson, C. H., and Bender, H. W.: The subxiphoid approach to pericardial disease. Ann. Thorac. Surg. 34:6, 1981.
4. Glasser, S. P., Harrison, E. E., Amey, B. D., et al.: Echocardiographic incidence of pericardial effusion in patients resuscitated by emergency medical technicians. JACEP 8:6, 1979.
5. Guberman, B. A., Fowler, N. O., Engel, P. J., et al.: Cardiac tamponade in medical patients. Circulation 64:633, 1981.
6. Krikorian, J. G., Hancock, E. W.: Pericardiocentesis. Am. J. Med. 65:808, 1978.
7. Symbas, P. N., Harlafhs, N., and Waldo, W. J.: Penetrating cardiac wounds: a comparison of different therapeutic methods. Ann. Surg. 183:377, 1976.
8. Schwartz, S. I.: Principles of Surgery. New York, McGraw-Hill, Inc., 1974, pp. 787–790.
9. Borja, A. R., Lansing, A., and Randell, H.: Immediate operative treatment for stab wounds of the heart. J. Thorac. Cardiovasc. Surg. 59:662, 1970.
10. Blair, E., Tapuzla, C., and Dean, R.: Chest trauma. In Hardy, J. D. (ed.): Critical Surgical Illness. Philadelphia, W. B. Saunders Company, 1971, pp. 175–185.
11. Thomas, T.: Emergency evacuation of acute pericardial tamponade. Ann. Thorac. Surg. 10:566, 1970.
12. Frater, R. W.: Intrapericardial pressure and pericardial tamponade in cardiac surgery. Ann. Thorac. Surg. 10:563, 1970.
13. Kerber, R. E., Ridges, J. D., and Harrison, D. C.: Electrocardiographic indications of atrial puncture during pericardiocentesis. N. Engl. J. Med. 282:1142, 1979.
14. Sobol, S. M., Thomas, H. M., and Evans, R. W.: Myocardial laceration not demonstrated by continuous electrocardiographic monitoring occurring during pericardiocentesis. N. Engl. J. Med. 292:1222, 1979.
15. Ramp, J., Harkins, J., and Mason, G.: Cardiac tamponade secondary to blunt trauma. J. Trauma 14:767, 1974.
16. Roe, B.: Cardiac trauma including injury of great vessels. Surg. Clin. North Am. 52:573, 1972.
17. Kirsh, M. M., Behrendt, D. M., Orringer, M. B., et al.: The treatment of acute traumatic rupture of the aorta. Ann. Surg. 184:308, 1976.
18. Toledo, T. M., Moore, W. L., Nash, D. A., et al.: Spontaneous pneumopericardium in acute asthma: case report and review of the literature. Chest 16:118, 1972.
19. Hacker, P. K., and Dorsey, D. J.: Pneumopericardium and pneumomediastinum following closed chest injury. JACEP 8:409, 1979.
20. Khan, R. M. A.: Air tamponade and tension pneumopericardium. J. Thorac. Cardiovasc. Surg. 68:328, 1974.
21. Pories, W., and Gaudiani, A.: Cardiac tamponade. Surg. Clin. North Am. 55:573, 1975.
22. Hanfling, S. M.: Metastatic cancer in the heart. Circulation 22:474, 1960.
23. Hancock, E. W.: Management of pericardial disease. Mod. Concepts Cardiovasc. Dis. 48:1, 1979.
24. Kwasnick, E. M., Kostes, J. K., Lazarus, J. M., et al.: Conservative management of uremic pericardial effusions. J. Thorac. Cardiovasc. Surg. 76:629, 1978.
25. Baue, A. E., and Blakemore, W. S.: The pericardium. Ann. Thorac. Surg. 14:81, 1972.
26. Shabetai, R., Fowler, N., and Guntheroth, W.: The hemodynamics of cardiac tamponade and constrictive pericarditis. Am. J. Cardiol. 26:480, 1970.
27. Spodick, D. H.: Acute cardiac tamponade. Pathologic physiology, diagnosis and management. Prog. Cardiovasc. Dis. 10:64, 1967.
28. Shoemaker, W. C., Carey, S. J., Yao, S. T., et al.: Hemodynamic monitoring for physiologic evaluation, diagnosis, and therapy of acute hemopericardial tamponade from penetrating wounds. J. Trauma 13:36, 1973.
29. Antman, E. M., Cargill, V., and Grossman, W.: Low-pressure cardiac tamponade. Ann. Intern. Med. 91:403, 1979.
30. Beck, C. A.: Two cardiac compression triads. JAMA 104:715, 1935.
31. Dipasquale, J. A., and Pluth, J. R.: Penetrating wounds of the heart and cardiac tamponade. Postgrad. Med. 49:114, 1971.
32. Shoemaker, W. C., Carey, J. S., Jao, S. T., et al.: Hemodynamic alterations in acute cardiac tamponade after penetrating injuries of the heart. Surgery 67:754, 1970.
33. Fowler, N. O.: Physiology of cardiac tamponade and pulsus paradoxus. II: physiological, circulatory, and pharmacological responses in cardiac tamponade. Mod. Concepts Cardiovasc. Dis. 47:115, 1978.
34. Shoemaker, W. C.: Algorithm for early recognition and management of cardiac tamponade. Crit. Care Med. 3:59, 1975.
35. Trinkle, J. K., Marcas, J., Grover, F., et al.: Management of the wounded heart. Ann. Thorac. Surg. 17:230, 1974.
36. Breaux, E. P., Dupont, J. B., Jr. Albert, H. M., et al.: Cardiac tamponade following penetrating mediastinal injuries: improved survival with early pericardiocentesis. J. Trauma 19:461, 1979.
37. Friedman, H. S., Sakura, H., Choe, S., et al.: Pulsus paradoxus: a manifestation of a marked reduction of left ventricular end-diastolic volume in cardiac tamponade. J. Thorac. Cardiovasc. Surg. 79:74, 1980.
38. Carsky, E. W., Azimi, F. A., and Maucer, R.: Epicardial fat sign in the diagnosis of pericardial effusion. JAMA 244:2762, 1980.
39. Spodick, D. H.: Electrical alternative of the heart. Its relation to the kinetics and physiology of the heart during cardiac tamponade. Am. J. Cardiol. 10:155, 1962.
40. Sotolongo, R. P., and Horton, J. D.: Total electrical alternans in pericardial tamponade. Am. Heart J. 101:853, 1981.
41. Friedman, H., Gomer, J., Tardio, A., et al.: The electrocardiographic feature of acute cardiac tamponade. Circulation 50:260, 1974.
42. Asinger, R. W., Rourke, T., Hodges, M., et al.: Role of echocardiography in emergencies. Minn. Med. 63:855, 1980.
43. Memon, A., and Zawadzki, Z. A.: Malignant effusions: diagnostic evaluation and therapeutic strategy. Curr. Probl. Cancer 5:1, 1981.
44. Alcan, K. E., Zabetakis, P. M., Marino, N. D., et al.: Management of acute cardiac tamponade by subxiphoid pericardiotomy. JAMA 247:1143, 1982.
45. Fowler, N. O.: Recognition and management of pericardial disease and its complications. In Hurst, J. W. (ed.): The Heart, 4th ed. New York, McGraw-Hill, Inc., 1978.
46. Bolanowski, P., Swaminathan, A. P., and Neville, W.: Aggressive surgical management of penetrating cardiac injuries. J. Thorac. Cardiovasc. Surg. 66:52, 1973.
47. Sugg, W. L., Rea, W. J., Ecker, R. R., et al.: Penetrating wounds of the heart. An analysis of 459 cases. J. Thorac. Cardiovasc. Surg. 56:531, 1968.
48. Arom, K., Richardson, J. D., Webb, G., et al.: Subxiphoid pericardial window in patients with suspected traumatic pericardial tamponade. Ann. Thorac. Sug. 23:545, 1977.
49. Boyd, T., and Strieder, J.: Immediate surgery for traumatic heart disease. J. Thorac. Cardiovasc. Surg. 50:305, 1965.
50. Siemens, R., Polk, H., Gray, L., et al.: Indications for thoracotomy following penetrating thoracic injury. J. Trauma 17:493, 1977.
51. Beall, A., Gasior, R., and Bricker, D.: Gunshot wounds of the heart: changing patterns of surgical management. Ann. Thorac. Surg. 11:523, 1972.
52. Wechsler, A. S., Auerbach, B. J., and Graham, T. C.:

Distribution of intramyocardial blood flow during pericardial tamponade correlated with microscopic anatomy and intrinsic myocardial contractility. J. Thorac. Cardiovasc. Surg. 68:847, 1974.

53. Wertheimer, W. I., Bloom, S., and Hughes, R. K.: Myocardial effects of pericardial tamponade. Ann. Thorac. Surg. 14:494, 1972.

54. Treasure, T., and Cotter, L.: Practical procedures: how to aspirate the pericardium. Br. J. Hosp. Med. 24:488, 1980.

55. Kizer, K. W., and Goodman, P. C.: Radiologic manifestations of venous air embolism. Diag. Radiol. 144:35, 1982.

56. Kotte, J. H., and McGuire, J.: Pericardial paracentesis. Mod. Concepts Cardiovasc. Dis. 20:102, 1951.

57. Bishop, L. H., Estes, E. H., and McIntosh, H. D.: The electrocardiogram as a safeguard in pericardiocentesis. JAMA 62:264, 1956.

58. Frederiksen, R. T., Cohen, L. S., and Mullins, C. B.: Pericardial windows or pericardiocentesis for pericardial effusion. Am. Heart J. 82:158, 1971.

59. Pradham, D. J., and Ikins, P. M.: The role of pericardiectomy in the treatment of pericarditis with effusion. Am. Surg. 42:257, 1976.

60. Silverberg, S., Oreopoulos, D. G., Wise, D. G., et al.: Pericarditis in patients undergoing long-term hemodialysis and peritoneal dialysis. Am. J. Med. 63:874, 1977.

61. Mattox, K., Beall, A., Jordan, G., et al.: Cardiography in the emergency center. J. Thorac. Cardiovasc. Surg. 68:886, 1974.

62. Fulton, R.: Penetrating wounds of the heart. Heart Lung 7:262, 1978.

15

Intracardiac Injections

RICHARD DAVISON, M.D.
THOMAS G. FROHLICH, M.D.

Introduction

Successful resuscitation from cardiac arrest has been shown to depend upon the speed with which spontaneous, effective circulation is restored.[1] The prompt administration of certain drugs is an important part of advanced cardiac life support (ACLS) and seems to play a crucial role in the termination of circulatory arrest.[2, 3] It is estimated that in 1981 over 300,000 deaths from cardiac arrests occurred outside the hospital, and surely many others involved hospitalized patients without an intravenous line at the time of the arrest.[4] It follows that rapid intravascular access is crucial in the setting of cardiac arrest.

Throughout the 1960s, intracardiac injection (ICI) was recommended as the most expeditious route of drug administration during cardiac arrest.[3, 5] In the years that followed, the technique fell into disfavor for several reasons. (1) Several authors emphasized the potential for serious complications resulting from ICI.[6–8] (2) Safe and simple percutaneous techniques were developed that allowed entry into the central venous circulation (i.e., subclavian, internal jugular, or femoral vein puncture). (3) Concern was expressed about the cessation of cardiopulmonary resuscitation (CPR) maneuvers during the performance of ICI.[6] (4) Experimental evidence suggested that the administration of drugs through ICI offered no advantage over injection into peripheral veins.[9] (5) The endotracheal route of drug administration was validated.[10, 11]

We believe that although ICI is not the preferred route for drug administration during CPR, intracardiac injection can still be useful in those cases in which prompt intravenous (IV) access is unattainable or when drug administration by other routes has proved ineffective. The technique of ICI is easily taught and requires little equipment.

Studies have shown that there is a low incidence of complications during its use.[12, 13]

Most likely, the frequency with which intracardiac injection is performed will depend on the skill of the operator in the initiation of intravenous lines. ICI may be necessary only in exceptional circumstances; nonetheless, it behooves those individuals involved in the delivery of ACLS to become familiar with this technique.

Historical Development

The technique of intracardiac injection appears to have originated in the latter part of the nineteenth century. Fantus attributed its first use to a German physiologist, Schiff, around 1880.[14] Over the next 40 years, scattered case reports appeared of successful resuscitation from cardiac arrest with the use of various intracardiac medications.[15, 16] In a 1923 case report, Bodon[17] reviewed the literature and found 90 cases of intracardiac administration of medication, with 24 successful resuscitations. The technique of the injection varied widely, and so did the substances injected, including camphor, caffeine, strophanthin, Pituitrin, strychnine, and epinephrine, the last of which Bodon recommended as the most effective.

By 1930, over 250 case reports had appeared in the literature, with approximately a 25 per cent success rate in terms of prolonged survival. Many of these cases were instances of cardiac arrest secondary to chloroform anesthesia. Yet use of intracardiac injections remained controversial. A *JAMA* editorial in 1930 proclaimed that "reports of resuscitation by intracardiac injection belong with the miracles."[18] In that same year, the Special Committee on Intracardiac Therapy of the Witkin Foundation published its report.[19] Hyman, the author of this detailed paper, concluded that the beneficial effect of intracardiac injection was not from the medication itself but from the irritant effect of the needle upon the myocardium. He recommended that right atrial puncture (without injection of medication) be used in the treatment of all cases of cardiac arrest. Hyman's point of view was still popular 17 years later, when Beecher and Linton reported a case of intraoperative cardiac arrest that failed to respond to repeated right atrial punctures until two injections of epinephrine into the right atrium restored a normal sinus rhythm.[20] They concluded that the epinephrine, and not the needle stick itself, was responsible for the successful resuscitation.

In 1951, Kay published one of the first modern experimental studies of the treatment of cardiac arrest.[21] Following the induction of asystole and ventricular fibrillation in dogs, he performed open chest cardiac massage and injected different substances into the cardiac chambers. He concluded that ventricular standstill was effectively treated by cardiac massage plus intracardiac injection of epinephrine, but he did not recommend epinephrine for the treatment of ventricular fibrillation. By the mid-1950s, intracardiac epinephrine had become part of the standard treatment for cardiac arrest,[5, 22] and with the advent of closed chest cardiac massage in the 1960s, the intracardiac route of drug administration remained popular.[8, 23, 24] By the mid-1970s, the popularity of ICI had declined. Goldberg warned of the numerous potential complications and advised against the use of ICI, except when it was "absolutely necessary" or during open chest cardiac massage.[6] Schechter, in a letter to *JAMA* in 1975, harshly condemned the intracardiac injection of epinephrine and stated that "the technique has been obsolete for about 20 years."[25]

Indications and Contraindications

The circulation time during CPR has been measured in a few instances and has been shown to be quite prolonged,[26] suggesting that the beneficial effect of a drug could be considerably delayed when the agent is administered into a peripheral site. Kuhn and associates[27] have demonstrated that medication injected in a peripheral intravenous site is delayed in reaching the arterial circulation during CPR in cardiac arrest patients. Although they did not study intracardiac injections, the data from their study indicate a distinct advantage in delivery time to the systemic arteries, when medication is injected into a central versus a peripheral intravenous site. In dogs with experimentally induced asystole, Pearson and coworkers found epinephrine given by the intravenous, intracardiac, and intratracheal routes to be equally effective in restoring circulation.[36] Furthermore, recent reports have confirmed the rapid attainment of blood levels and have documented the clinical success of epinephrine when administered intratracheally.[10, 11]

To date, there are no experimental or clinical data to suggest an advantage of the intracardiac route for drug delivery during cardiac resuscitation. Thus, the primary indication for the intracardiac injection of medications during cardiopulmonary resuscitation is restricted to the circumstance in which the administration of an essential drug by other routes would result in an intolerable delay.

Based exclusively on anecdotal information, several authors have suggested that the intracardiac administration of epinephrine may be more effective than the intravenous route in treatment of asystole or electromechanical dissociation.[28-31] As a secondary indication, then, if intravenous epinephrine fails to reverse asystole or electromechanical dissociation, it would seem appropriate to readminister it by intracardiac puncture.

In either of the aforementioned two circumstances, there are no true contraindications to this technique. Certain associated conditions, such as the presence of a pre-existent pneumothorax or the hyperinflated chest of chronic lung disease, will make the procedure more difficult. Anticoagulation has been shown to be associated with a greater incidence of hemopericardium, but this rarely results in hemodynamic embarrassment.[24]

Equipment and Drugs

A 3½-inch-long 18 gauge needle is most often used for the performance of ICI. Syringes prefilled with a standard dose of epinephrine (1 mg in 10 ml) and calcium chloride (1 gm in 10 ml = 14 mEq of calcium) are provided by the manufacturer with an "intracardiac needle" (Abboject or Bristoject). If these are not available, an 18 gauge spinal needle can be fitted to the end of a regular medication syringe (Fig. 15–1). Spinal needles of narrower gauge may be used but are more prone to bending

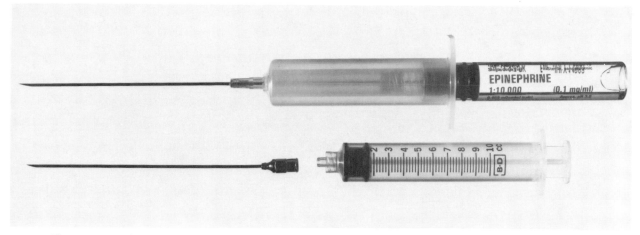

Figure 15–1. Equipment for intracardiac injections. "Intracardiac" needles are available in prefilled syringes *(top).* A 3½-inch, 18 gauge spinal needle can be fitted onto a regular syringe *(bottom).*

and occlusion by tissue plugs—we discourage their use.

Sodium bicarbonate given by the intracardiac route is well described in the pediatric literature.[32-34] In the adult,[13] the relatively large volume of solution that is required imposes a lengthy injection time and a dangerous prolongation of the period during which CPR maneuvers are withheld. Furthermore, the usual commercial syringes containing bicarbonate are prefitted with short needles. If one believes that the intracardiac administration of bicarbonate in an adult is desirable, one can break off the needle by grasping it with the needle guard and bending the short needle close to the hub from side to side. Once the short needle is broken off, the spinal needle can be fitted onto the hub of the syringe.

Procedure

For many years, the "correct" technique for ICI was in dispute. In fact, there was even disagreement concerning the appropriate cardiac chamber to enter. Hyman's contention[19] that right atrial injection would be as effective as a ventricular injection and would be less likely to cause ventricular fibrillation has never been confirmed and retains only historical interest. In the 1950s and 1960s, many authors recommended that the injections be made into the left ventricle.[2, 8, 21, 35] Theoretically, this approach would have the advantage of a more direct delivery of the drugs into the coronary arteries. In addition, the thick left ventricular wall is more likely to seal off a puncture hole and is less susceptible to being torn than the thinner right ventricular wall. In spite of these considerations, no clear difference in effectiveness between right and left ventricular injections has been demonstrated.[36] In fact, based on observa-

tions accumulated during the performance of transthoracic cardiac ventriculography, it is at times difficult to predict which chamber will be entered during the insertion of the transthoracic needle into the heart.[37]

THE SUBXIPHOID APPROACH

A needle entering the heart through its diaphragmatic surface is unlikely to encounter a large epicardial coronary artery or interposed lung tissue. Two studies that relied mainly on the subxiphoid technique showed it to be associated with a low incidence of complications.[12, 13] It is therefore the preferred approach for the performance of ICI. This route of injection usually involves the right ventricle.

Technique. Without interrupting CPR, the left costoxiphoid area is prepared with an antiseptic solution. The syringe with the drug to be injected is freed of all air bubbles. At this point, the lungs are allowed to deflate, and CPR maneuvers are stopped. With the bevel up, the tip of the needle is inserted in the xiphocostal notch (approximately 1 cm to the left of the tip of the xiphoid process). The needle is directed cephalad toward the middle of the left clavicle at a 30- to 45-degree angle with the skin of the abdominal wall (Fig. 15–2). As soon as the skin is punctured, constant negative pressure is applied to the syringe, and the needle is advanced rapidly. When blood spurts into the syringe, the needle advancement is stopped, and the medication is injected as quickly as possible. The needle is withdrawn immediately, and CPR is resumed. *An intracardiac injection should not interrupt CPR for more than 5 to 10 seconds.* If after full insertion of the needle there is no blood return, the needle must be withdrawn immediately, and CPR must be resumed before another attempt is

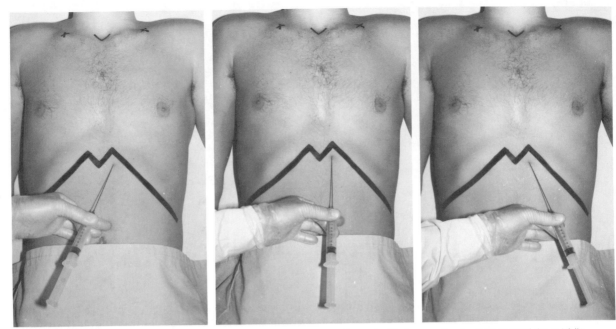

Figure 15–2. The subxiphoid approach. The initial attempt is performed with the needle directed toward the middle of the left clavicle *(left)*. If this attempt is unsuccessful, the needle should be redirected straight up *(middle)*. One can make a third attempt by aiming toward the mid–right clavicle *(right)*.

made. One may then attempt penetration again, this time with the needle directed straight up toward the suprasternal notch. If this fails, a third attempt with the needle directed toward the mid–right clavicle is recommended. If this is also unsuccessful, the left parasternal approach should be tried.

THE LEFT PARASTERNAL APPROACH

Although with this technique the chance of entering the cardiac chambers may be greater, the potential for complications may also be greater. Specific risks include laceration of the internal mammary artery, damage to the left anterior descending coronary, and pneumothorax secondary to puncture of the lingula.

Technique. For this approach, an area surrounding the left fourth intercostal space along the sternal border is prepared with antiseptic solution. After the lungs are allowed to deflate passively, the needle is inserted just over the fifth rib, two fingerbreadths from the left sternal border. The needle is perpendicular to the frontal plane or angled slightly medially (Fig. 15–3). While exerting suction on the syringe, one rapidly advances the needle until an abrupt blood return is observed. At this time, the medication is injected as rapidly as possible, the needle is withdrawn, and CPR is resumed immediately. One author suggests using the same interspace but entering

directly adjacent to the sternum of the adult to minimize the risk of pneumothorax or coronary artery laceration.[38]

ICI IN INFANTS AND CHILDREN

The injection technique for infants and children is essentially the same as that for adults. Both the left parasternal and the subxiphoid routes may be used, but the latter is preferred. The chest wall in children is thinner and more pliable than in adults, and injection with a 20 or 22 gauge spinal needle has been recommended.[33, 34] Prepackaged pediatric doses of cardiac drugs are also available with an "intracardiac needle." For the subxiphoid approach, the point of insertion and the angulation of the needle are identical to those used in adult patients.[34] If the left parasternal approach is used, the needle is inserted in the fourth or fifth intercostal space, 2 to 5 cm from the left sternal border; the younger the child, the closer to the sternum.[33] The needle may be angled slightly medially and cephalad. Because of the relative difficulty in obtaining intravenous access in infants and children, ICI is used more frequently in these age groups.

Complications

A reviewer of the literature on ICI will probably be baffled by the disparity between the anticipated

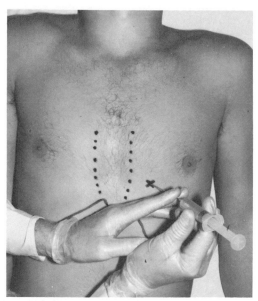

Figure 15–3. The left parasternal approach. The needle is inserted at a point perpendicular to the frontal plane, just over the fifth rib, two fingerbreadths from the left sternal border.

high frequency of complications and the paucity of instances in which they have actually been documented (Table 15–1).

Coronary artery laceration is one of the most feared and frequently mentioned potential complications of ICI. Bodon, in his 1923 review of 90 cases,[17] found no instance of coronary artery laceration and quoted Brunning's calculation that the area occupied by the coronaries is less than 1/1000 of the area of the free walls of the heart. In 1954 Smith, reporting on percutaneous ventriculography experiments in dogs, found one instance of left anterior descending artery (LAD) laceration following 15 left parasternal injections.[39] Subsequently, 60 subxiphoid injections were accomplished without laceration. In over 300 human ventriculographies involving subxiphoid injection, Lehman found no evidence of coronary artery laceration.[43] At a symposium on resuscitation in 1968, Holmdahl mentioned two instances of coronary artery laceration in his group's experience

with human CPR, but the technique of injection was not specified. At that same symposium, Jude reported never having seen this complication.[40] Amey studied 29 survivors of cardiac arrests who had received a total of 47 intracardiac injections. He compared this group with 67 patients who had survived cardiac arrest without the use of intracardiac medication. There were no significant differences between these two groups in the incidence of acute myocardial infarctions.[13] Davison studied 53 patients who had received a total of 147 intracardiac injections during cardiac arrest.[12] In the 24 nonsurvivors in whom an autopsy was performed, no evidence of coronary artery laceration was found. In the 29 survivors there was no clinical evidence to suggest coronary artery puncture or laceration. Saphir found no coronary artery lacerations at autopsy in 62 patients who had received a total of 155 intracardiac injections during unsuccessful resuscitation.[24] Thus, although coronary artery laceration is frequently mentioned as a hazard of ICI,[6–9, 39, 41] only two poorly documented instances could be found in the literature.

Hemopericardium, on the other hand, appears to be relatively common following intracardiac injection. In a series of left ventriculographies using the intercostal approach, Bjork found four instances of hemopericardium among 27 patients who underwent surgery following cardiac puncture.[42] In the same series, there were six instances of cardiac tamponade among 138 patients. Lehman found three instances of tamponade in over 300 patients receiving transthoracic ventriculography by the subxiphoid approach.[43] Saphir reported nine cases of hemopericardium at autopsy in 62 patients following unsuccessful CPR and noted that this complication is associated with intracardiac injection.[24] Another study found evidence of hemopericardium in 12 of 39 patients by echocardiography or post mortem but no clinical evidence of tamponade in 29 survivors.[12]

Intuitively, one would expect *pneumothorax* to be a common occurrence following intracardiac injection. Bjork reported pneumothorax in 8 of 138 patients in whom contrast was injected into the

Table 15–1. COMPLICATIONS OF INTRACARDIAC INJECTIONS

Study	Technique	Coronary Laceration*	Hemopericardium	Tamponade	Pneumothorax	Intramyocardial Injection
Pondsmenech, 1951[45]	subxiphoid	0(30)	0(30)	0(30)	0(30)	0(30)
Lehman, 1957[37]	subxiphoid	0(60)	11(35)	0(60)	0(60)	0(60)
McCaughan, 1957[44]	subxiphoid	0(29)	—	0(29)	2(29)	2(29)
Lehman, 1959[43]	subxiphoid	0(300)	—	3(300)	—	2(300)
Bjork, 1961[42]	parasternal	1(137)	4(27)	6(137)	8(137)	—
Amey, 1978[13]	parasternal and subxiphoid	0(33)	1(8)	0(8)	3(33)	—
Davison, 1980[12]	subxiphoid	0(53)	12(39)	0(29)	1(29)	—
Chen, 1981[38]	parasternal	—	—	—	5(16)	—
Total		1(642)	28(139)	9(593)	19(334)	4(419)

*Numbers in parentheses indicate number of patients examined for evidence of each complication.

heart by the left parasternal approach.[42] Mc-Caughan found two instances of this complication in 134 patients studied by the subxiphoid approach.[44] Chen identified a pneumothorax in 5 of 16 patients receiving left parasternal injections during CPR.[38] In Amey's study, 3 of 29 patients receiving ICI developed a pneumothorax, compared with only 1 of 64 who did not receive intracardiac injections during CPR.[13] Davison found only one instance of pneumothorax in 40 patients receiving ICI.[12] Thus, the incidence of pneumothorax appears to be relatively low, especially if the subxiphoid approach is used.

The *intramyocardial injection* of contrast material has been associated with intractable ventricular fibrillation and death.[43] The combined results of two ventriculography series involving the subxiphoid approach showed that 4 of 434 patients underwent intramyocardial injections with subsequent ventricular fibrillation.[43, 44] This situation is probably not comparable with intracardiac injections during CPR when the heart is not beating and injection must be made without the benefit of fluoroscopic guidance. It is unlikely that the true incidence of this dire complication, which may result in the same rhythm as was originally being treated, will ever be known.

Other potential complications include infection, laceration of other organs, and air embolism. Although Bodon in 1923 reported a case of fulminant pericarditis following intracardiac injection,[17] no subsequent reports of pericarditis or endocarditis could be found. The subxiphoid approach brings the injecting needle close to the left lobe of the liver and the stomach, and Smith reported hepatic laceration during subxiphoid injection in dog experiments.[39] No instance of internal organ laceration following intracardiac injections in humans appears in the literature, however. Similarly, air embolism has never been reported.

Careful attention to technique will minimize the risk of some of these complications. During subxiphoid injection, the needle should form an angle of 30 to 45 degrees with the skin of the abdominal wall. A more vertical position may cause the needle to pass posterior to the heart and cause damage to the liver or the stomach. Applying constant suction on the syringe during insertion of the needle is necessary to ensure proper intracavitary positioning and thus to prevent intramyocardial injection. One may lessen the risk of pneumothorax by using the subxiphoid approach and by allowing passive deflation of the lungs before injection. Following a successful resuscitation, a chest film should be examined for evidence of pneumothorax.

By far the most common error in technique that we have observed is the repeated attempt at ICI after an initial failure *without the reinstitution of CPR.*

Conclusions

For almost 100 years, the intracardiac route has been used to deliver medication during cardiac arrest. Although the technique has been shown to be effective, its popularity has declined because of the fear of potential complications. A review of the literature suggests that these fears are overstated. Although intracardiac puncture is not recommended as the initial route of injection, it should be retained as a valid technique for the administration of emergency drugs during cardiopulmonary resuscitation when other routes are not readily available.

1. Eisenberg, M. S., et al.: Cardiac resuscitation in the community. JAMA 241:1905, 1979.
2. Redding, J. S., and Pearson, J. W.: Evaluation of drugs for cardiac resuscitation. Anesthesiology 24:203, 1963.
3. Pearson, J. W., and Redding, J. S.: Epinephrine in cardiac resuscitation. Am. Heart J. 66:210, 1963.
4. McIntyre, K. M., and Lewis, A. J. (eds.): Textbook of Advanced Cardiac Life Supports. Dallas, American Heart Association, 1981.
5. Massey, F. C. (ed.): Clinical cardiology. Baltimore, William & Wilkins, 1953, p. 872.
6. Goldberg, A. H.: Cardiopulmonary arrest. N. Engl. J. Med. 290:381, 1974.
7. Enarson, D. A., and Gracey, D. R.: Complications of cardiopulmonary resuscitation. Heart Lung 5:805, 1976.
8. Philips, J. H., and Burch, G. E.: Management of cardiac arrest. Am. Heart J. 67:265, 1964.
9. Redding, J. S., et al.: Effective routes of drug administration during cardiac arrest. Anesth. Analg. 46:253, 1967.
10. Roberts, J. R., et al.: Endotracheal epinephrine in cardiorespiratory collapse. JACEP 8:515, 1979.
11. Roberts, J. R., et al.: Blood levels following intravenous and endotracheal epinephrine administration. JACEP 8:53, 1979.
12. Davison, R., et al.: Intracardiac injections during cardiopulmonary resuscitation. JAMA 244:1110, 1980.
13. Amey, B. D., et al.: Paramedic use of intracardiac medication in prehospital sudden cardiac death. JACEP 7:130, 1978.
14. Fantus, B.: The technic of medication. JAMA 87:563, 1926.
15. Zuntz, H.: Wiederbelebung durch intracardiale. Injektion. Munch. Med. Wschr. 21:562, 1919.
16. Rüdiger, G.: Die intracardiale Injektion. Wien. Med. Wochenschr. 1916, #4.
17. Bodon, C.: The intracardiac injection of adrenalin. Lancet 1:586, 1923.
18. Editorial: Resuscitations and intracardiac injections. JAMA 94:107, 1930.
19. Hyman, A. S.: Resuscitation of the stopped heart by intracardiac therapy. Arch. Intern. Med. 46:553, 1930.
20. Beecher, H. K., and Linton, R. R.: Epinephrine in cardiac resuscitation. JAMA 135(2):1947.
21. Kay, J. H.: The treatment of cardiac arrest. Surg. Gynecol. Obstet. 93:682, 1951.
22. Gerbode, F.: The cardiac emergency. Ann. Surg. 135(3):1952.
23. Lillehei, C. W., et al.: Four years' experience with external cardiac resuscitation. JAMA 193:85, 1965.
24. Saphir, R.: External cardiac massage. Medicine 47:73, 1968.
25. Schechter, D. C.: Transthoracic epinephrine injection in heart resuscitation is dangerous. JAMA 234:1184, 1975.

26. Del Guercio, L. R. M., et al.: Cardiac output and other hemodynamic variables during external cardiac massage in man. N. Engl. J. Med. 269:1398, 1963.

27. Kuhn, G. J., et al.: Peripheral versus central circulation times during CPR: A pilot study. Ann. Emerg. Med. 10:417, 1981.

28. Iseri, L. T., et al.: Prehospital brady-asystolic cardiac arrest. Ann. Intern. Med. 88:741, 1978.

29. Hurst, J. W.: Cardiopulmonary resuscitation. *In* Hurst, J. W. (ed): New York, McGraw-Hill, 1978, pp. 734–744.

30. American Heart Association: Standards and guidelines for cardiopulmonary resuscitation (CPR) and emergency cardiac care (ECC). JAMA 244:453, 1980.

31. McIntyre, K. M., and Lewis, A. J. (eds): Textbook of Advanced Cardiac Life Support. Dallas, American Heart Association, 1981.

32. Riker, W. L.: Cardiac arrest in infants and children. Pediatr. Clin. North Am. 16:661, 1969.

33. Anthony, C. L., Jr., et al.: Management of cardiac and respiratory arrest in children. Clin. Pediatr. 8:647, 1969.

34. Scarpelli, E. M., Auld, P. A. M., and Goldman, H. S.: Airway management, mechanical ventilation and cardiopulmonary resuscitation. *In* Scarpelli, E. M., et al. (eds.): Pulmonary Disease of the Fetus, Newborn and Child. Philadelphia, Lea & Febiger, 1978, p. 123.

35. Huszar, R. J.: Emergency Cardiac Care. Bowie, Maryland, Robert J. Brady, 1974, p. 200.

36. Pearson, J. W.: Historical and experimental approaches to modern resuscitation. Springfield, IL, Charles C Thomas, 1965, p. 70.

37. Lehman, J. S., et al.: Cardiac ventriculography. Am. J. Roentgenol. Rad. Ther. Nuclear Med. 77:207, 1957.

38. Chen, H. H.: Closed-chest intracardiac injection. Resuscitation 9:103, 1981.

39. Smith, P. W., et al.: Cardioangiography. J. Thorac. Surg. 28:273, 1954.

40. Jude, J. R., et al.: Vasopressor-cardiotonic drugs in cardiac resuscitation. Acta Anesth. Scand. (Suppl.) 9:147, 1968.

41. Enarson, D. A., and Gracey, D. R.: Complications of cardiopulmonary resuscitation. Heart Lung 5:805, 1976.

42. Bjork, V. O., et al.: Sequelae of left ventricular puncture with angiocardiography. Circulation 24:204, 1961.

43. Lehman, J. S.: Cardiac ventriculography: Practical considerations. Prog. Cardiovasc. Dis. 2:52, 1959.

44. McCaughan, J. J. Jr., and Pate, J. W.: Aortography utilizing percutaneous left ventricular puncture. Arch. Surg. 75:746, 1957.

45. Pondsmenech, E. R.: Heart puncture in man for diodrast visualization of the ventricular chambers and great arteries. Am. Heart J. 41:643, 1951.

16

Mechanical Adjuncts for CPR

NISHA CHANDRA, M.D.

Introduction

The history of resuscitation is replete with descriptions of mechanical devices and maneuvers that were designed to improve both ventilation and circulation. In the eighteenth century, it was common practice to throw a person in respiratory arrest over a trotting horse to facilitate ventilation and, it was hoped, to resuscitate the patient. A more ingenious technique (and one that was more probably effective) was to use air bellows to inflate the lungs.[1] The current technique of using chest compression at the sternum and oral ventilation during cardiopulmonary resuscitation (CPR) is a recent development.

Closed-chest cardiac massage was shown in 1960[2, 3] to be an effective technique for maintaining vital organ perfusion during periods of circulatory arrest. In 1961, the necessity of ensuring adequate ventilation during resuscitation was demonstrated.[4] These two initial observations heralded an era of universal implementation of these CPR techniques. Recent studies have led to a better understanding of the hemodynamics of cardiac and pulmonary function during cardiac arrest. Based on this knowledge, techniques and mechanical devices have been developed in an effort to improve the quality of resuscitation. It is imperative to have a basic understanding of the mechanism of movement of blood during CPR if the role and applicability of various mechanical adjuncts in current use are to be fully understood.

Mechanisms of Blood Flow During CPR

BACKGROUND

The classical view of blood flow during CPR as proposed by Jude, Kouvenhowen, and Knickerbocker was that blood flow during external chest compression resulted from the heart being mechanically squeezed between the sternum and the vertebral column.[3] Closure of the atrioventricular valves during chest compression was postulated to prevent regurgitant blood flow, thus generating antegrade arterial blood flow. During the release phase of chest compression, blood returned to the heart by a suction effect. Numerous recent studies,[5, 6] however, question this hypothesis of cardiac compression during CPR.

One of the most important observations was that coughing enabled a patient in ventricular fibrillation to maintain consciousness for 45 seconds.[7] The most important physiologic effect of a cough is not cardiac compression but rather a significant rise in intrathoracic pressure. The importance of intrathoracic pressure during CPR was further suggested by the observation that patients with chronic obstructive pulmonary disease, in whom cardiac compression during external chest compression is least likely to occur (because of their increased anteroposterior chest diameter), could often be successfully resuscitated. Also noted was the inability to generate adequate arterial pressures in an arrested patient with a flail sternum (in whom cardiac compression would be most easily achieved because of increased sternal mobility) until paradoxical chest movement was prevented and intrathoracic pressure was thereby raised.

ANIMAL STUDIES

In order for flow to occur in any fluid-filled system, there must be a pressure gradient. If a pump is responsible for generating this gradient, then there must be a pressure gradient across the pump. Hence, to prove that the heart is the "pump" during CPR, one would need to demonstrate a pressure gradient across the heart. Studies in dogs, pigs, and baboons during cardiac arrest showed that external chest compression resulted in a rise in intrathoracic pressure.[6, 8, 9] The lack of a pressure gradient across the heart during chest compression, together with the similarity of all intrathoracic vascular pressures to the pleural pressure, suggests that the heart is not the pump responsible for generating blood flow during CPR (Fig. 16–1).

During chest compression, pressure from the thick-walled intrathoracic aorta is transmitted relatively unchanged to the thick-walled extrathoracic carotid artery.[10] Venous valves at the thoracic inlet,[8] however, prevent the transmission of intrathoracic venous pressure to the extrathoracic venous system. Venous valves in humans have been shown to be competent in preventing venous flow cephalad during cough at transvalvular pressure gradients of greater than 100 mm Hg.[11] In addition, it is likely that at the thoracic inlet (where veins exit from an intrathoracic high-pressure zone to an extrathoracic low-pressure zone), venous collapse aids in the generation of the intra- to extrathoracic venous pressure gradient. Thus, during chest compression intrathoracic vascular pressures rise; the differential transmission of this pressure to peripheral vessels generates an extrathoracic arteriovenous pressure gradient. This gradient, in turn, results in the forward flow of blood.

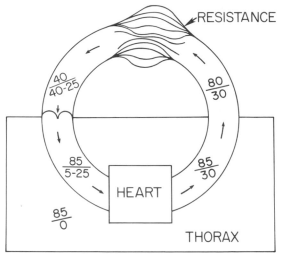

ALL PRESSURES IN mmHg

Figure 16–1. Representative pressures as recorded during cardiopulmonary resuscitation with forward carotid flow. Veins are depicted on the left side of the heart, with arteries on the right. The numerator for each pressure displayed refers to pressures recorded during chest compression. Intrathoracic pressures were indexed from esophageal pressure. During chest compression there is no significant pressure gradient across the heart, and all intrathoracic vascular pressures are equal. The extrathoracic arterial pressure is similar to the intrathoracic arterial pressure. The extrathoracic venous pressure is markedly lower than the intrathoracic venous (right atrial) pressure because of a competent venous valve at the thoracic inlet. There is an extrathoracic arteriovenous pressure gradient, which results in forward flow. The denominator for each pressure displayed refers to pressures recorded during the release of chest compression. The gradient between the intrathoracic aorta and the right atrium during release of chest compression results in coronary flow.

During CPR, when chest compression is released, intrathoracic and extrathoracic vascular pressures fall toward zero; the higher extrathoracic venous pressure results in the inflow of blood from extrathoracic to intrathoracic structures. Cineangiographic studies[8] and radionuclide angiography[12] have both confirmed that during the release phase of chest compression blood moves rapidly from extrathoracic veins through the right heart and an open tricuspid valve into the lungs. With the onset of chest compression the pulmonic valve probably closes (since there is little regurgitant flow into the right ventricle), and blood can be demonstrated to move as a column from the lungs through the left heart and open mitral and aortic valves into the aorta and the carotid bed. Thus, during CPR the heart functions as a passive conduit and blood moves largely because of changes in intrathoracic pressure. Also, during the release phase of chest compression an aortic to right atrial pressure gradient is present. Blood flow into the coronary bed during CPR occurs during this phase and is determined by the magnitude of the aortic to right atrial pressure gradient.[13]

Based on the observation that maneuvers that increased intrathoracic pressure during external chest compression resulted in higher carotid flows,[6] simultaneous compression ventilation CPR (SCV CPR) was developed as a technique to provide safe, cyclic incremental rises in intrathoracic pressure. This technique was shown to improve not only carotid flow but also brain and myocardial blood flow as compared with conventional CPR.[9, 14]

Other animal studies identified simpler and less sophisticated techniques for increasing intrathoracic pressure and improving blood flow during CPR. Redding and coworkers showed that abdominal binding during CPR increased survival following defibrillation.[15] Rudikoff and associates demonstrated that abdominal binding during conventional CPR increased intrathoracic pressure, mobilized blood volume, and probably redistributed flow toward thoracic and cranial vascular beds.[6] Conventional CPR plus abdominal binding resulted in higher carotid flow than did conventional CPR alone.[6]

Subsequent studies using the concept of changing intrathoracic pressure during CPR to produce blood flow showed that adequate blood flow could be generated during CPR without the use of sternal compression.[16, 17] Luce and colleagues produced cyclic changes in intrathoracic pressure during CPR by using a pneumatic vest around the thorax and again demonstrated that carotid, myocardial, and brain flow are significantly improved by this technique as compared with conventional CPR.[16]

It is important to realize that changing intrathoracic pressure is not the sole mechanism of blood flow during CPR. It has been shown that in some large animals, occasionally in humans, and often in small flat-chested animals, vascular or cardiac compression does occur during CPR. Cardiac compression during CPR is suggested by a rise in intrathoracic vascular pressures that exceeds the measured rise in intrapleural pressure.[18]

HUMAN STUDIES

Data in humans with regard to the primary mechanism of blood movement are still inconclusive. Taylor and coworkers[19] showed that during conventional CPR, the mean arterial blood pressure and the Doppler carotid flow index were significantly improved by an increase in chest compression duration. This would be the expected result when manipulation of intrathoracic pressure generated blood flow, since the longer period of chest compression would enable the arteriovenous pressure gradient to be maintained for a longer time and would thereby generate increased forward blood flow. Our recent studies in which intra- and extrathoracic venous and arterial pressures were monitored demonstrated similar intrathoracic venous and peripheral arterial pressures,

the presence of an intra- to extrathoracic venous gradient, and a definite peripheral arterial and venous pressure gradient during chest compression. This hemodynamic pattern (similar to that seen in Fig. 16–1) would favor movement of blood by manipulation of intrathoracic pressure. Studies in a few patients have also shown that maneuvers that increase intrathoracic pressure improve the arterial pressure and the Doppler flow index.[20, 21]

Two-dimensional echocardiographic studies in humans during CPR have been interpreted as showing little cardiac or vascular compression, since they have failed to demonstrate distortion of left ventricular or aortic cavity size during chest compression.[22, 23] These studies showed that the mitral valve remains open during chest compression. This is contrary to the classical cardiac compression hypothesis[2] but is in keeping with animal data showing movement of blood by changing intrathoracic pressure.

Nonetheless, in a few patients with thin chests and cardiomyopathy, we have clearly demonstrated arterial pressures that are significantly higher than intrathoracic venous pressures. This pattern would indicate probable vascular or cardiac compression during CPR. It is important to realize that although two mechanisms exist for generating blood flow during CPR, these mechanisms are not mutually exclusive but can coexist and can be additive.

During chest compression when significant vascular compression occurs, a higher cerebral flow should result, since the increase in arterial pressure is greater than the associated increase in intrathoracic and intracranial pressure; higher cerebral perfusion pressures are thus achieved.[14, 24] Also as a result of cardiac compression, aortic volume is likely to be increased. This greater aortic volume would facilitate sustained and augmented peripheral arterial pressure and flow during movement of blood by manipulation of intrathoracic pressure.[10]

Building on this basic understanding of the mechanism of blood flow during CPR, mechanical adjuncts have been developed to improve resuscitation. Some of these aid chest compression during CPR, and others facilitate both ventilation and chest compression. Many helpful adjuncts are in current use and other devices, which use the principle of improving blood flow by manipulation of intrathoracic pressure, are being developed and are undergoing initial clinical testing.

Devices for Chest Compression

In 1960, following the observations of Jude, Kouvenhowen, and Knickerbocker that external chest compression could maintain adequate circulation during CPR,[3] attempts at mechanizing the process of external chest compression were initiated. Currently used devices can be divided into three categories:

1. Manually operated chest compressors,
2. Gas-powered chest compressors, and
3. Devices designed to improve or control manually performed chest compression.

In an exhaustive review, the Emergency Care Research Institute (ECRI) outlined design criteria for gas-powered and manual chest compressors.[25] They recommend that such equipment be:

1. Lightweight, portable, and able to withstand rough handling.
2. Easy to deploy, simple to operate with a conforming piston pack of appropriate size, and with non-slip characteristics.
3. Able to allow access to the patient's thorax and not inhibiting of procedures such as central venous catheter placement or application of defibrillation paddles.

Additional recommendations for gas-powered chest compressors were:

1. The device should be fitted for variable sternal compression force with a gauge to indicate sternal deflection.
2. A compression rate of 60 per minute with systolic:diastolic time ratios of 1:1 should be a feature.
3. The design should facilitate airway control and should not limit expansion of the thorax during ventilation. Inspiratory oxygen content should be greater than 50 per cent and flow rate greater than 120 L per minute. Limiting inspiratory pressures should be continuously adjustable over the range of 20 to 60 cm of water to accommodate variable lung compliances.
4. A non-rebreathing valve should be situated close to the patient to minimize dead space. Inspiratory pressures and flow characteristics should not permit pressures within the oropharynx to exceed 30 cm H_2O for the nonintubated patient, since excessive pressure would divert inspiratory gas to the stomach and would result in gastric distention and regurgitation.

Indications and Contraindications

Mechanical devices have certain significant advantages over manual CPR in some settings:

1. By providing both ventilation and compression, the devices will free personnel to attend to other matters during an arrest. This is of significant benefit in situations in which few skilled personnel are available and support services are limited. Because of this feature, many paramedic units are using these devices during out-of-hospital cardiac arrests.
2. The devices overcome operator fatigue and provide constant, adequate, sustained, and con-

trolled chest compression. This becomes especially important during prolonged resuscitations (e.g., in patients with hypothermia or drug overdose). Also, the quality of chest compression is far superior to that usually performed by most lay people. The Thumper (see Fig. 16–2) is capable of running for 15 to 20 minutes on two ''D'' tanks of portable oxygen.

3. Chest compression during transportation of patients can be easily continued with these devices, and an acceptable electrocardiogram can be recorded with the compressor in operation. Hence, for situations in which patients suffering cardiac arrest are being transported, mechanical devices are ideal, because they also maintain uniformity of chest compression.

4. When mechanical devices are used, chest compression does not have to be interrupted during defibrillation. During attempted defibrillation, 10 to 30 seconds often elapse when chest compression is interrupted. It is important to remember that this is a period of total anoxia for the patient; it can only be detrimental to have many such periods. Furthermore, the initial chest wall incision for an emergency thoracotomy can be made with the Thumper device in place.

5. In situations in which a standardized form of resuscitation is desirable, e.g., in therapeutic trials, mechanical devices are preferred.

Drawbacks of these devices are that they are somewhat cumbersome and expensive and the more popular devices need to be powered from oxygen tanks or constant oxygen delivery sources. Time is spent in setting up the devices. In addition, mechanical assist devices are contraindicated when the rescuer is unfamiliar with the equipment, since excessive or inadequate force or misplaced compressions can easily occur. Adequacy of blood flow should be carefully assessed in large patients when such devices are used since low chest wall compliance may necessitate the use of a compression force that is higher than usual. Finally, most mechanical devices (with the exception of the Thumper) are not indicated for use with children.

Gas-Powered Chest Compressors

Two gas-powered devices are currently in fairly broad use: the Michigan Institute Life Aid ''Thumper'' and Brunswick Manufacturing Company's HLR ''Quick Fit.''

THUMPER

The Thumper (Fig. 16–2) is a pneumatically powered chest compressor with an accompanying base plate that contains controls, gauges, and

compression at a rate of 40 per minute in patients with endotracheal intubation. Airway pressure during ventilation is adjustable from 0 to 120 cm of water. The device is also capable of delivering conventional CPR and can change from this to SCV-CPR by alteration of a switch position. This device delivers five low-pressure, 1-second "sigh" breaths every 1 minute when in the SCV mode to ensure adequacy of gas exchange. Safety features in the device prevent high airway pressure ventilation from occurring if chest compression is inadequate. Thus, the chance of lung trauma is minimized. This device is not commercially available; it is the only device that is capable of providing SCV-CPR.

COMPARISON OF THE GAS-POWERED DEVICES

The major advantage of the HLR over the Thumper is its size and the possibility of providing 100 per cent oxygen for ventilation. Studies from the ECRI, however, showed that application and assembly time and chances of sternal pack migration were less with the Thumper than with the HLR device. The maximal sternal deflection capability of the Thumper is higher than that of the HLR, making the Thumper a better device to use on larger patients. The rise and dwell times of chest compression are also quicker and longer, respectively, with the Thumper, thus likely ensuring higher mean arterial pressures.[26]

In terms of ventilation, the Thumper provides higher volumes at lower face mask pressures without dead space as compared with the HLR device. The Thumper can be used (although cautiously) on pediatric patients. The manufacturers of the HLR device state in their instruction manual that children less than 27 kg (60 lbs) do not "lend themselves to resuscitation with the HLR unit."

Studies using the Thumper have shown it to be as effective as manual CPR in terms of survival and with no greater incidence of side effects or complications.[27] McDonald and coworkers demonstrated higher mean arterial pressures but lower peak pressure during CPR with the Thumper as compared with manual CPR.[26]

Manually Operated and Hand-Held Chest Compressors

The Bowen pulsator and the Rentsch cardiac press are essentially *hand-powered pistons* for use during external chest compression. The Rentsch press consists of a base plate, which is positioned under the patient. An inverted U-shaped frame is connected to a hand-held lever; the lever thus provides a mechanical advantage in applying compression and reduces operator fatigue (Fig. 16–4).[28] The Bowen pulsator consists of a base plate (positioned behind the patient) and a vertical arm (mounted on an adjustable vertical column) fitted with a piston. The piston is similarly operated from a lever. Both the units have mechanical stops to maintain uniform, constant sternal displacement.

The Harrigan resuscitator is one of the most commonly used *hand-held pressure sensors*. These instruments are suggested for immediate use in an arrest to ensure better chest compression. The Harrigan device consists of a compression pad equipped with a gauge to indicate when the force of chest compression is adequate. Other devices similar to this are additionally equipped with timer signals to "pace" the operator at a rate of 60 chest compressions per minute. They undoubtedly encourage and facilitate uniformity of chest compression. It is my opinion that since these devices are precalibrated for *force*, they may well allow *excessive* force to be used in situations in which chest compliance is increased and therefore chest displacement cannot be gauged. Also, most of these devices have no ability to monitor the duration of chest compression. If the goal of these instruments is to "hit a certain point" on a gauge, the operator may well be encouraged to jab quickly and hard at the chest, producing chest compressions that are short in duration and, probably, produce lower mean arterial pressures.

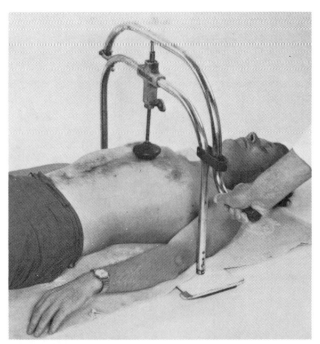

Figure 16–4. One hand-operated mechanical press device for performing chest compression. (From Vaagenes, P., Lund, I., Skulberg, A., and Osterud, A.: On the technique of external cardiac compression. Crit. Care Med. 6:176, 1978. Used by permission.)

Other Mechanical Augmentation Devices

ANTI-SHOCK GARMENTS AND PNEUMATIC ABDOMINAL BINDERS

The usefulness of anti-shock garments in the setting of hypovolemic shock has been well documented.[29] These devices have been shown to increase peripheral vascular resistance, to increase circulating volume, and thereby to maintain vital organ perfusion and function. Their usefulness in terms of vital organ perfusion and survival during CPR in humans without obvious hypovolemia has not been demonstrated.

Some animal studies of anti-shock garments used during CPR have shown no improvement in survival and a high incidence of abdominal visceral injury.[30] Other studies using pneumatic abdominal binders have shown improved carotid flow, higher carotid arterial and cerebral perfusion pressures during conventional CPR, no abdominal visceral injury, and improved survival.[6, 14, 15] Chandra and coworkers[21] examined the effect of abdominal binding on 11 patients with cardiac arrest undergoing conventional CPR. Abdominal binding was produced by the use of a pneumatic cuff positioned around the abdomen and inflated to 110 cm H_2O pressure. With abdominal binding, the mean arterial pressure increased from 53.9 ± 7.1 to 67.2 ± 8.4 mm Hg and could be sustained for 5 minutes. Although this study demonstrated a significant increase in arterial pressure during the release phase of chest compression (i.e., diastole), it did not assess the effect of abdominal binding on the aortic to right atrial pressure gradient in diastole. It is possible that because of lower circulating blood volumes and high venous compliance during conventional CPR, the rise in right atrial pressure produced by abdominal binding is minimal. If so, the aortic to right atrial pressure gradient during diastole would be increased during CPR with abdominal binding. On the other hand, if right atrial and arterial pressure rise equally, there would be no net change or, possibly, a decrease in this gradient. Therefore, although abdominal binding can significantly improve carotid perfusion, its effect on coronary perfusion during conventional CPR in humans is unclear.

Mahoney and associates[31] studied the efficacy of anti-shock garments during CPR in patients undergoing out-of-hospital resuscitation who had failed to respond to three defibrillation attempts and appropriate drug therapy. The investigators demonstrated that in a small subset of patients (16.6 per cent) with pulseless idioventricular rhythm, the application of anti-shock garments resulted in a significant improvement in resuscitation and discharge rates as compared with conventional techniques of resuscitation. In the overall analysis of the treatment group versus the control group, although there was improved survival, the difference was not statistically significant. Nonetheless, it is encouraging to note that in the 66 patients on whom pneumatic anti-shock garments were used, no complications attributable to the use of the pneumatic trousers (specifically, abdominal visceral tears) could be found and ventilation was considered adequate.[31] The current practice in most prehospital situations is that if arrest occurs in a patient in hypovolemic shock, CPR is initiated with the anti-shock garment inflated.

Harris and associates evaluated abdominal binding during CPR in dogs.[30] Abdominal binding was produced by the application of manual pressure over the abdomen. These investigators found a high incidence of liver rupture with this technique and hence concluded that its usefulness during CPR was nil. Redding and colleagues and Rudikoff and coworkers, however, used a pneumatic binder to produce abdominal compression during CPR and demonstrated higher arterial pressures and no abdominal visceral injury with this technique.[6, 15] Patient studies similarly showed that there was no evidence of abdominal visceral injury during CPR with pneumatic suits or binders.[24, 31] These differences can likely be explained by the fact that abdominal binding with a pneumatic cuff ensures a more uniform rise in abdominal pressure and prevents localized increases in abdominal pressure and, hence, visceral injury. The potential for abdominal visceral injury and serious side effects, however, does exist when anti-shock garments and binders are used. Therefore, the routine use of these devices during arrest should be discouraged unless specific indications exist.

Interposed Abdominal Compressions

Recently, Babbs and coworkers[32] reported that abdominal compressions of 100 to 150 mm Hg applied alternately with standard closed-chest compressions improved diastolic blood pressure, cardiac output, and oxygen consumption in experimental animals in cardiac arrest when compared with conventional CPR. Abdominal compressions were applied manually to the mid-abdomen over a standard blood pressure cuff 12 cm in width folded to 12×15 cm and inflated with air to a thickness of approximately 3 cm. The bladder of the cuff was attached to an aneroid manometer to regulate the pressure applied to the abdomen. Using an electrical analog model, Babbs and Geddes[33] found that the elevation of aortic diastolic pressure and concurrent retrograde volume flow produced by interposed abdominal compression are beneficial during CPR regardless of the actual mechanism of blood flow during chest compression. Berryman and Phillips recently reported six subjects in whom IAC-CPR was noted to raise mean arterial pressure.[37] Clinical efficacy of this technique for improving organ perfusion and ultimate survival has yet to be demonstrated.

Pneumatic Vests

Pneumatic vests have also been used in animal studies during CPR. Rabson and associates showed that rhythmic inflation and deflation of a pneumatic vest resulted in a cyclic rise in thoracic pressure and significant carotid blood flow during arrest.[34] Other investigators have shown that flow generated during arrest with chest compression is comparable with flow generated by using only a pneumatic vest to cycle intrathoracic pressure.[35] Unfortunately, no comparable human data are available. It is possible that in cases of diffuse severe chest trauma, a pneumatic vest may be preferable to conventional chest compression when efforts are made to minimize chest wall excursion and visceral injury. Nonetheless, when one considers human resuscitation, it is likely that in some instances chest compression results in vascular compression. Because direct cardiac compression is a potent mechanism for blood flow during CPR, it is currently preferable that any technique of resuscitation designed for routine field use consist of chest compression, thus allowing for the possibility of vascular compression.

Caution

It is important to realize that although these mechanical augmentation devices appear to be potentially beneficial during cardiac arrest, their routine use is not recommended by the American Heart Association. The potential for abdominal visceral injury and serious side effects exists, particularly when anti-shock garments and binders are used. Many investigators are currently studying the role of these techniques in large field trials. Until the results of these studies become available and the effect on survival and cerebral function is known, these techniques should be used only as research tools.

INTRA-AORTIC BALLOON PUMPS

Intra-aortic balloon counterpulsation devices have been used during resuscitation. They have been shown to be beneficial in rare instances.[36] Although the technique is capable of providing some circulation, the drawbacks are extensive, making its use limited. Intra-aortic balloon counterpulsation is an invasive and expensive method of support that is available only in highly specialized centers and requires skilled personnel for its implementation.

Complications of Mechanical Adjuncts to CPR

Although sternal fractures and rib and visceral injuries have been reported with these devices, the incidence of complications is no greater than that with manual CPR alone.[27] As in manual CPR, these complications are more common when excessive or misplaced force is applied. Skillful operation is also important; this will ensure that adequate compressions are performed to provide clinically acceptable blood flow. As mentioned previously, the newer experimental devices may have their own specific complications. Large field trials will be needed to determine the incidence of these potential complications.

Conclusion

Numerous devices exist and many more are being developed, as the physiology of CPR becomes clearer, in an effort to improve cardiopulmonary resuscitation. The weight of responsibility rests on the shoulders of physicians to evaluate these various adjuncts critically and to use only those that have been clinically validated and proven useful. Some of the adjuncts discussed in this chapter should be considered only exciting developmental techniques until they have been shown to be safe and efficacious in an arrest. In choosing devices to aid in resuscitation, the clinician must also keep in mind the environment in which they will be used and the training of personnel who handle the equipment.

Before we succumb to the mechanization of the twentieth century, it behooves each physician to realize that the best immediate resource during an arrest is an individual well trained in manual CPR!

1. Debard, M. L.: The history of cardiopulmonary resuscitation. Ann. Emerg. Med. 9:273, 1980.
2. Kouvenhowen, W. B., Jude, J. R., and Knickerbocker, G. G.: Closed chest cardiac massage. JAMA 173:1064, 1960.
3. Jude, J. R., Kouvenhowen, W. B., and Knickerbocker, G. G.: Cardiac arrest: Report of application of external cardiac massage on 118 patients. JAMA 178:1063, 1961.
4. Safar, P., Brown, T. C., Holtey, W. J., and Wilder, R. J.: Ventilation and circulation with closed-chest cardiac massage in man. JAMA 176:564, 1961.
5. Thomsen, J. E., Stenlund, R. R., and Rowe, G. G.: Intracardiac pressures during closed chest massage. JAMA 205:46, 1968.
6. Rudikoff, M. T., Maughan, W. L., Effron, M., Freund, P., and Weisfeldt, M. L.: Mechanisms of flow during cardiopulmonary resuscitation. Circulation 61:345, 1980.

7. Criley, J. M., Blaufuss, A. N., and Kissel, G. L.: Cough-induced cardiac compression. JAMA 236:1246, 1976.

8. Niemann, J. T., Rosborough, J. P., Hausknecht, M., Garner, D., and Criley, J. M.: Pressure synchronized cineangiography during experimental cardiopulmonary resuscitation. Circulation 64:985, 1981.

9. Chandra, N., Weisfeldt, M. L., Tsitlik, J., Vaghaiwalla, F., Snyder, L., Hoffecker, M., and Rudikoff, M.: Augmentation of carotid flow during CPR in dogs by ventilation at high airway pressures simultaneous with chest compression. Am. J. Cardiol. 48:1053, 1981.

10. Yin, F. C. P., Cohen, J. M., Tsitlik, J., Zola, B., and Weisfeldt, M. L.: Role of carotid artery resistance to collapse during high-intrathoracic-pressure CPR. Am. J. Physiol. 243:H259, 1982.

11. Fisher, J., Vaghaiwalla, F., Tsitlik, J., Levin, H., Brinker, J., Weisfeldt, M. L., and Yin, F.: Determinants and clinical significance of jugular venous valve competence. Circulation 65:188, 1982.

12. Cohen, J. M., Chandra, N., Alderson, P. O., VanAswegen, A., Tsitlik, J., and Weisfeldt, M. L.: Timing of pulmonary and systemic blood flow during intermittent high intrathoracic pressure cardiopulmonary resuscitation in the dog. Am. J. Cardiol. 49:1883, 1982.

13. Niemann, J., Rosborough, J., Ung, S., and Criley, J. M.: Coronary perfusion pressure during experimental cardiopulmonary resuscitation. Ann. Emerg. Med. 11:127, 1982.

14. Koehler, R. C., Chandra, N., Guerci, A. D., Tsitlik, J., Traystman, R. J., Rogers, M. C., and Weisfeldt, M. L.: Augmentation of cerebral perfusion by simultaneous chest compression and lung inflation with abdominal binding following cardiac arrest in dogs. Circulation 67:266, 1983.

15. Redding, J. S.: Abdominal compression in cardiopulmonary resuscitation. Anesth. Analg. 50:668, 1971.

16. Luce, J. M., Ross, B. K. O'Quinn, R. J., Culver, B. H., Sivarajan, M., Amory, D. W., Niskanen, R. A., Alferness, C. A., Kirk, W. L., Pierson, L. B., and Butler, J.: Regional blood flow during cardiopulmonary resuscitation in dogs using simultaneous and nonsimultaneous compression and ventilation. Circulation 67:258, 1983.

17. Rosborough, J. P., Niemann, J. T., Criley, J. M., O'Bannon, W., and Rouse, D.: Lower abdominal compression with synchronized ventilation: A CPR modality. Circulation 64:IV-303, 1981.

18. Chandra, N., Guerci, A., and Weisfeldt, M. L.: Contrasts between intrathoracic pressures during external chest compression and cardiac massage. Crit. Care Med. 9:789, 1981.

19. Taylor, G. J., Rubin, R., Tucker, M., Greene, H. L., Rudikoff, M., and Weisfeldt, M. L.: External cardiac compression: A randomized comparison of mechanical and manual techniques. JAMA 240:644, 1978.

20. Chandra, N., Rudikoff, M., and Weisfeldt, M. L.: Simultaneous chest compression and ventilation at high airway pressure during cardiopulmonary resuscitation. Lancet 1:175, 1980.

21. Chandra, N., Snyder, L. D., and Weisfeldt, M. L.: Abdominal binding during CPR in man. JAMA 246:351, 1981.

22. Werner, J. A., Greene, H. L., Janko, C. L., and Cobb, L. A.: Visualization of cardiac valve motion in man during external chest compression using two-dimensional echocardiography. Implications regarding the mechanism of blood flow. Circulation 63:1417, 1981.

23. Rich, S., Wix, H. L., and Shapiro, E. P.: Clinical assessment of heart chamber size and valve motion during cardiopulmonary resuscitation by two-dimensional echocardiography. Am. Heart J. 102:368, 1981.

24. Guerci, A., Chandra, N., Levin, H., Koehler, R. C., Tsitlik, J. E., Traystman, R. J., Rogers, M. C., and Weisfeldt, M. L.: Hemodynamic determinants of intracranial pressure during resuscitation. Circulation 64:IV-304, 1981.

25. ERCI report. Health Devices 2:6, 1973.

26. McDonald, J. L.: Systolic and mean arterial pressure during manual mechanical CPR in humans. Crit. Care Med. 9:382, 1981.

27. Taylor, G. J., Rubin, R., Tucker, M., Greene, H. L., Rudikoff, M., and Weisfeldt, M. L.: External cardiac compression: A randomized comparison of mechanical and manual techniques. JAMA 240:644, 1978.

28. Vaagenes, P., Lund, I., Skulberg, A., et al.: On the technique of external cardiac compression. Crit. Care Med. 6:176, 1978.

29. Wayne, M. A.: The MAST suit in the treatment of cardiogenic shock. JACEP 7:107, 1978.

30. Harris, L. C., Kirimli, B., and Safar, P.: Augmentation of artificial circulation during cardiopulmonary resuscitation. Anesthesiology 28:730, 1967.

31. Mahoney, B. D., and Mirick, M. J.: Efficacy of pneumatic trousers in refractory prehospital cardiopulmonary arrest. Ann. Emerg. Med. 12:27, 1983.

32. Babbs, C. F., Ralston, S. H., and Voorhees, W. D., III: Improved cardiac output during CPR with interposed abdominal compressions. Ann. Emerg. Med. 12:246, 1983.

33. Babbs, C. F., and Geddes, L. A.: Effects of abdominal counterpulsation in CPR as demonstrated in a simple electrical model of the circulation. Ann. Emerg. Med. 12:247, 1983.

34. Rabson, J., Goldberg, H., Bromberger-Barnea, B., and Permutt, S.: The use of a pneumatic vest to generate carotid flow in a canine model of circulatory arrest. Circulation 59 and 60:II-196, 1979.

35. Chandra, N., Tsitlik, J., and Weisfeldt, M. L.: Optimization of carotid flow during CPR in arrested dogs. Crit. Care Med. 9:379, 1981.

36. Kennedy, J. H.: The role of assisted circulation in cardiac resuscitation. JAMA 197:615, 1966.

37. Berryman, C. R., and Phillips, G. M.: Interposed abdominal compression-CPR in human subjects. Ann. Emerg. Med. 13:226, 1983.

17

Resuscitative Thoracotomy

ROBERT L. BARTLETT, M.D.

Introduction

As a multidisciplinary specialist, the emergency physician will at times find it necessary to use procedures previously considered to be the province of one of the surgical specialities. The emergency thoracotomy is the most invasive and controversial of these procedures.[1-7] "The days when an individual specialty could restrict the use of a technical skill are long gone. Pertinent to technical skills are appropriate training, skills maintainence, and judgment as to when to apply them or when to withhold them."[8]

In the past two decades, the development of sophisticated emergency medical systems using well-trained paramedics, advanced life support, and rapid transport has increased the number of patients arriving at the emergency department in various stages of shock.[9-11] With increasing frequency, emergency physicians are being given the opportunity to resuscitate patients who previously would have expired at the scene. For some, survival is possible if an aggressive approach using emergency thoracotomy is taken. Therefore, with such a broad spectrum of patients, knowing who may respond to thoracotomy becomes an important issue.

This chapter will discuss the factors that influence the outcome of an emergency thoracotomy and the pathophysiology, diagnosis, and treatment of those injuries that require such an invasive procedure. The heart, the lungs, and the great vessels are the three vital structures in which injuries may require the use of a resuscitative thoracotomy. The mechanism of injury, prehospital vital signs, and the systolic blood pressure following thoracotomy form the basic structure of a resuscitative algorithm.

Indications and Contraindications

The current trend toward more aggressive management of trauma was pioneered in the mid-1960s and early 1970s by Sugg,[12] Mattox,[13, 14] and others. Most simply, the indication for thoracotomy in the emergency care unit has been the absence of vital signs on admission or the loss of pulse and blood pressure during the resuscitation of a trauma victim. Initially, thoracotomy with cross-clamping of the aorta was applied to all moribund patients, regardless of the mechanism of injury. The high success rates for the initial resuscitation (75 per cent) and the long-term survival rates (8 to 31 per cent) were cited as support for such indiscriminate use of emergency thoracotomies. A closer review of these early reports reveals the mechanism of injury and prehospital vital signs as major determinants of a successful outcome.[14-16] Blunt and penetrating trauma are the

two categories of injury that subsequently will be considered. The importance of making this distinction becomes apparent when published survival rates are reviewed.

RESUSCITATIVE THORACOTOMY IN *BLUNT* TRAUMA

When other methods of resuscitation fail, *blunt* trauma victims may respond following thoracotomy. Unfortunately, the *survival* rate for these cases is negligible. In the past 10 years there have been seven published reports evaluating the role of emergency thoracotomy in blunt trauma.[7, 13, 15-19] The overall survival rate was only 2.9 per cent. Patients rarely survived when their vital signs were lost prior to admission, and there were no survivors when the electrocardiogram (EKG) demonstrated asystole.[15, 17]

To date, Bodai has published the most detailed study of blunt trauma resuscitation with emergency thoracotomy.[18] Only those patients who exhibited a pulse or respiratory efforts at the scene were studied. Half of the patients arrived in the emergency department within 30 minutes of injury, yet more than 85 per cent of patients had no obtainable vital signs or were *agonal* upon arrival. "Agonal" was defined as having irregular respiration or thready pulse without measurable blood pressure. From this group of 38 patients, 56 per cent were resuscitated following thoracotomy and transferred to the operating room. This initial resuscitation rate is impressive; however, only 10 per cent (4 of 38) survived the surgical procedures, and each of these individuals expired shortly thereafter. Two died from brain injuries, one from multiple organ failure, and one from disseminated intravascular coagulation. Thus, there were no long-term survivors in this series.

Hemodynamic Response to Emergency Thoracotomy

A report of emergency department thoracotomies for blunt and penetrating trauma from Denver General Hospital related the hemodynamic response to thoracotomy to patient outcome.[15] Of the 146 cases reviewed, 45 patients (31 per cent) were transferred to the operating room following initial resuscitation and aortic cross-clamping when necessary. For those patients surviving with full neurologic recovery, the average systolic blood pressure after the first 30 minutes of resuscitation was 110 mm Hg. In those who were long-term survivors but had developed significant brain damage, the average systolic blood pressure was 85 mm Hg. There were no survivors when the mean systolic blood pressure was less than 70 mm Hg. Thus, the blood pressure response to emergency thoracotomy becomes predictive of survival. For those patients who remain lifeless with systolic blood pressures below 70 mm Hg despite control of hemorrhage, volume replacement, and cross-clamping for 30 minutes, the authors recommended that "heroic measures should be discontinued." Transfer of these patients to the operating suite for definitive repair would be nonproductive.

In summary, emergency thoracotomy for *blunt* trauma is limited in its ability to resuscitate patients who develop cardiac arrest or who arrive with agonal signs. Until more encouraging results are advanced, this resuscitative procedure should be reserved for those patients who arrive in the emergency care unit with pulse, respiratory efforts, and reactive pupils.[15, 18, 21]

EMERGENCY THORACOTOMY FOR *PENETRATING* TRAUMA

Following the unsuccessful attempt of Cappelen[22] and Farina[23] to repair a wound of the heart in 1896, Paget[24] stated that "the surgery of the heart has probably reached the limits set by nature to all surgery. No new method or discovery can overcome the natural difficulties that attend a wound of the heart." Yet that same year Rehm[25] successfully relieved a pericardial tamponade and repaired an actively bleeding wound of the right ventricle. Over the next 50 years, the effectiveness of cardiorrhaphy for penetrating wounds of the heart and the great vessels was firmly established, with survival figures ranging from 50 per cent to 65 per cent.[26-34] These reports, however, involved patients who were transported directly to the operating theater and tolerated their wounds in the absence of prehospital emergency care.

The prehospital mortality for penetrating chest wounds depends on the structures involved. For heart wounds in particular, the prehospital mortality is approximately 80 per cent. Nonetheless, if any signs of life are present during the prehospital phase, these patients may be salvaged. Recently, the vital importance of speed and the use of the emergency department as the site of thora-

cotomy has been emphasized. Mattox, in describing 37 emergency thoracotomies in emergency center patients in cardiac arrest shortly before or after arrival, stated that there was "no question that these patients could not have survived the short trip to the operating room. This group represents patients who, in former years, probably would have died at the scene or en route to the hospital."[14] MacDonald, commenting on his series of 28 emergency thoracotomies in a community hospital, observed that "resuscitation can be hampered by significant delays in assembling the necessary operating room staff. These delays sometimes mean that a trauma patient will be detained for a significant amount of time in the emergency department before a definitive procedure can be performed in the operating room."[7]

When the patient's vital signs suggest that cardiac arrest is imminent despite airway control and the initiation of volume replacement, a thoracotomy should be performed immediately. A tragic death may result if the physician should allow a cardiac arrest to occur while waiting for a possible response to ancillary therapy or while transporting the patient to the operating table. Beal[35] compared the mortality figures for emergency thoracotomies performed for penetrating cardiac injuries in patients with and without cardiac arrest. Only those patients whose arrest had occurred in the hospital were studied. For the group receiving thoracotomy prior to cardiopulmonary arrest the mortality was 15 per cent. If the thoracotomy was performed after cardiopulmonary arrest, the mortality increased to 60 per cent. Reul[36] compared the mortality figures for emergency thoracotomies performed on patients with mixed trauma (blunt and penetrating) to the thoracic great vessels. Again, only those patients whose arrest had occurred in the hospital were studied. When the thoracotomy was performed prior to arrest, the mortality was 18 per cent. If arrest occurred prior to thoracotomy, the mortality was 73 per cent.

Unfortunately, the preceding data do not permit a more detailed analysis, and it must be acknowledged that patients who suffer cardiac arrest may have more severe injuries. Nonetheless, it should be clear that every effort, including thoracotomy, should be made to avert a cardiac arrest. As stated by Siemens and coworkers, "delay and observation in the shocked, bleeding, or tamponading injury can only lead to prolongation of hypotension, acidosis, excessive requirement of blood and crystalloids, and on occasion sudden ventricular fibrillation or standstill."[38] If the etiology of the patient's deterioration is hemorrhage, Beall and coworkers believe that "surgery should not await resuscitation but is an integral part of resuscitation, as only when bleeding is controlled can the circulating blood volume be restored adequately."[37]

With penetrating thoracic trauma, the frequency of organ injury corresponds to the relative exposure of each organ. The lung is the most commonly injured organ, followed by the heart, the great vessels, the tracheobronchial tree, and the esophagus. Approximately 80 per cent of penetrating chest injuries can be managed conservatively with tube thoracostomy if the only significant injury is a pneumothorax[38–41] (see Chapter 6).

When heart wounds in particular are considered, the distribution of injuries reflects the relative exposure of each chamber and the intracardiac vessels. A review of the distribution of 1802 cardiac wounds showed an incidence of 43 per cent for right ventricular injuries, 33 per cent for left ventricular injuries, 14 per cent for right atrial injuries, and 5 per cent for injuries to the intrapericardial vessels.[42] The percentage of anterior chest wall exposure of these structures is 55 per cent for the right ventricle, 20 per cent for the left ventricle, 10 per cent for the right atrium, 10 per cent for the great vessels, and 5 per cent for the vena cava.[43]

The combined survival rate in nine recent reports of penetrating chest injuries requiring emergency department thoracotomy was 34 per cent for gunshot wounds and 45 per cent for stab wounds.[42] Gunshot wounds are the most common form of penetrating injury. When they involve the heart, the associated blast effect usually results in exsanguination rather than tamponade.[44] In contrast, 80 to 90 per cent of stab wounds to the heart will result in tamponade. The development of tamponade may be temporizing during the prehospital phase. If tamponade does not occur, most patients with myocardial stab wounds will exsanguinate.[45, 46]

Two additional factors that influence the development of tamponade are wound size and chamber involvement. Wounds of the myocardium less than 1 cm may spontaneously seal, depending on the location. Wounds larger than 1 cm will usually continue to bleed regardless of the chamber involved.[46, 47] The low-pressured atria will usually clot off before tamponade develops.[43] On the other hand, a wound of the right ventricle is often associated with tamponade. This is the result of a thin wall (3 mm) with little occlusive potential and a higher systolic pressure than the atria. In contrast, the thicker-walled left ventricle (120 mm Hg average) may spontaneously seal stab wounds up to 1 cm in length. Thus, tamponade may be absent even though the left ventricle has been lacerated.[46]

Improved survival figures support the use of emergency department thoracotomy. *This procedure is most effective when it is used to prevent a cardiac arrest rather than to treat it.* Four factors are closely associated with patient outcome following resuscitative thoracotomy: (1) mechanism of injury; (2) presence or absence of pulse, pupil reactivity, and respiratory effort at the scene and on admission; (3) EKG activity; and (4) systolic blood pressure after cross-clamping. The following guidelines should be considered:

1. Blunt trauma victims who lose their vital signs while en route to the emergency department rarely survive, despite thoracotomy.

2. Penetrating trauma victims who lose their vital signs while en route to the emergency department may still survive and should receive an immediate thoracotomy.

3. Thoracotomy should be considered when the systolic blood pressure cannot be maintained above 70 mm Hg with aggressive management and the use of the pneumatic anti-shock garment.

4. Further efforts should be discontinued following thoracotomy when patients do not exhibit cardiac activity and were not suffering from tamponade.

5. Further efforts should be discontinued following thoracotomy if the systolic pressure cannot be raised above 70 mm Hg.

CARDIAC TAMPONADE*

Diagnosis and Pathophysiology

Cardiac tamponade is defined as the *decompensated* phase of cardiac function resulting from increased intrapericardial pressure.[48] The clinical diagnosis of pericardial tamponade in the unstable trauma patient is difficult because of the combined effect of hemorrhagic and cardiogenic shock. The classical signs of Beck's triad (distended neck veins, hypotension, and decreased heart sounds) have limited diagnostic value for acute penetrating cardiac trauma. In most series, the complete triad was found in only 35 per cent of patients.[52–55] Additional signs of tamponade include tachycardia, pulsus paradoxicus, elevated central venous pressure, agitation and confusion (reflecting decreased cerebral perfusion), air hunger, and cold, clammy skin.[49–51]

The pericardial sac has a potential space of 80 to 120 ml.[48] After the normal pericardial recesses have been filled, intrapericardial pressure rises quickly with continued bleeding. Rapid accumulation of as little as 150 ml can produce fatal tamponade. Only in the chronic situation does the pericardium distend to accommodate the large volumes that produce the "water bottle heart" on the chest radiograph.

The physiologic changes seen with tamponade are the result of the limited diastolic expansion of the ventricles. This limitation produces an early rise in ventricular diastolic pressure and a corresponding reduction of the atrioventricular filling

*See also Chapter 14.

gradient. With poor ventricular filling, stroke volume and cardiac output are decreased.

Secondary pathophysiologic mechanisms further compromise cardiac output by decreasing coronary blood flow. The coronary perfusion gradient is adversely affected by the elevated ventricular diastolic pressure and the reduced arterial pressure. With a lowered stroke volume, heart rate will increase. As the rate increases, the proportion of the cardiac cycle occupied by diastole decreases. Because coronary perfusion occurs primarily during diastole, the effective perfusion period is shortened. Additional limitation of coronary flow may occur through compression of coronary arteries and veins.[48, 56] This may result from pressure alone or from a localized mechanical effect of blood clots within the pericardium.[56] The combined effect of a decreased coronary perfusion pressure, a shortened perfusion period, and compression of coronary vessels is decreased ventricular function.[57]

Reactive tachycardia during the hypotensive phase of tamponade is the usual finding, but for some patients a bradycardia may be present. Several studies involving rapid induction of cardiac tamponade failed to find significant changes in heart rate.[59] These findings may reflect vagally mediated cardiac depressor reflexes. Receptors for these reflexes have been identified in the left and right atria, the left coronary artery, the myocardium, and the epicardium.[59–62] Using a dog model for rapid induction of tamponade, Friedman[58] observed the appearance of cardiac dysrhythmias, including sinus bradycardia, sinoatrial block, junctional or idioventricular escape rhythm with the onset of marked hypotension (undefined by authors), and electromechanical dissociation. Severing both vagus nerves immediately reversed these dysrhythmias. Rapid evacuation of fluid from the pericardial sac was followed by a slower recovery. Even in the absence of tamponade, a significant vagal response to cardiac wounds may occur. In such cases, administration of atropine will produce dramatic improvement.[63]

Reactive tachycardia is one of three major compensatory mechanisms. An elevation of the central venous pressure is another. Although this secondarily reflects poor atrioventricular filling, it is primarily the result of increased venomotor tone, which improves the effective filling pressure of the ventricles. The third compensatory mechanism is an increased peripheral vascular resistance that preserves arterial pressure in the face of falling cardiac output. When hypotension does appear, it is an ominous sign.

An elevated central venous pressure has been used as an indicator of tamponade. In the acute situation with persistent hypotension one cannot rely on the central venous pressure. Many affected patients have marked volume depletion and are incapable of elevating their central venous pressure despite advanced tamponade. This is further compounded by the metabolic acidosis of shock, which lowers vasomotor tone by decreasing the action of catecholamines. These patients should be rapidly transfused with crystalloid and blood. Their acid/base status should also be assessed and treated accordingly. If hypotension persists and the central venous pressure (CVP) rises, the patient should be presumed to have cardiac tamponade. One should be aware that in some cases there may be a poor correlation between the CVP and the extent of tamponade even when the blood volume has been corrected.[68, 69]

When the central venous pressure is elevated, other factors should also be considered. These include rapid administration or over-administration of fluids; vasopressors; increased intrathoracic pressure from pneumothorax, hemothorax, airway obstruction, positive end-expiratory pressure (PEEP); a nonfunctioning clotted CVP line; kinking or malposition of the catheter; pneumatic anti-shock garment inflation; shivering; straining or muscular guarding.[70] The position of the CVP catheter should always be checked by a chest film. An attempt should be made to relax the abdomen to avoid falsely elevated values. It has been suggested that trends in CVP are more useful and would allow for earlier recognition and management of cardiac tamponade.[70]

Pericardiocentesis as a Diagnostic Test

Pericardiocentesis was once felt to be a reliable method of diagnosing and treating acute hemorrhagic tamponade. Observations from several large series now suggest that this is no longer the case. The diagnostic ability of pericardiocentesis is limited by a high rate of false positive and false negative results in proven cardiac trauma. There is a false negative rate of 20 to 40 per cent.[63, 71] The use of predictive value theory illustrates the diagnostic limitations of pericardiocentesis.[72–75] Using data from Trinkle,[71] the sensitivity of pericardiocentesis as a test for tamponade in penetrating chest wounds was 53 per cent and the specificity was 50 per cent. The predictive value of a positive test was 72 per cent, and that of a negative test was 33 per cent. The test efficiency, which indicates the percentage of patients correctly classified, was only 52 per cent.

Clotted blood that cannot be aspirated is the most common cause of a false negative tap. The presence of clots depends on the rate of bleeding and the elapsed time. Classical "nonclotting blood" implies that there has been sufficient time for a given volume of blood to undergo fibrinolysis and fibrinogenolysis. Thus, blood obtained by pericardiocentesis from patients with an acute hemopericardium has been observed to clot.[12, 49, 76]

In summarizing pericardiocentesis as a diagnostic test for acute hemorrhagic tamponade, one may draw the following conclusions:

1. The efficiency of pericardiocentesis as single test for acute tamponade is just marginally better than a 50:50 chance prediction.

2. The predictive value of a positive aspirate is greater than that of a negative aspirate.

3. A negative aspirate does not rule out pericardial tamponade. If there are signs of deterioration or persistence of hypotension, emergency thoracotomy is indicated.

4. If the withdrawn blood remains unclotted, one can be confident of the diagnosis of tamponade. If the blood clots, no conclusions can be made.

Pericardiocentesis as a Therapeutic Technique

Use of pericardiocentesis as a therapeutic technique for suspected tamponade depends on the clinical state of the patient. Pericardiocentesis has been advocated as a nonoperative treatment of heart wounds with associated tamponade and no active bleeding.[77]

Because of improved survival figures for patients undergoing emergency thoracotomy, pericardiocentesis is now considered a preoperative, temporizing procedure.[14–16, 78, 79] As mentioned, pericardiocentesis can be negative in 15 per cent to 37 per cent of surgically proven cases of tamponade. When pericardiocentesis is positive it may fail to relieve tamponade completely.[32, 49]

Recently, there has been a concern that physicians may be abandoning this procedure in an attempt to rush patients to the operating suite. In an effort to minimize early subendocardial ischemia, Breaux[80] investigated the use of immediate decompressive pericardiocentesis, for any degree of tamponade, as soon as the diagnosis was suspected. Even patients who were to have an immediate thoracotomy received pericardiocentesis. Overall mortality dropped from 55 per cent in patients who did not undergo pericardiocentesis to 19 per cent in those treated with pericardiocentesis prior to either emergency department or operating suite thoracotomy. It was the investigators' conclusion that the improved operative and overall survival rates justified the slight delay for pericardial decompression.

Pericardiocentesis appears to improve survival by providing a more rapid (but less complete) relief of tamponade. Decompression of the pericardium prior to thoracotomy may also improve survival by preventing "anesthetic arrests." Several authors have commented on the common occurrence of cardiac arrest during the induction of anesthesia.[47, 49, 81] Such "anesthetic arrests" result from the loss of the compensatory increase in vascular resistence. Evans[49] reported that pericardiocentesis did not completely relieve tamponade in any of nine patients but did produce a transient rise in blood pressure, allowing safer anesthesia.

Pericardiocentesis is not without significant hazards. Pories[65] has reported fatalities and complications resulting from right ventricular tears, transient asystole, laceration of coronary arteries, ventricular fibrillation, and vasovagal arrest. Because of these complications and the high incidence of false positives and negatives, several authors now advocate the use of a subxiphoid pericardial window whenever possible.[42, 49, 81] In experienced hands this procedure can be completed in less than 5 minutes (Fig. 17–1). As a diagnostic test it is 100 per cent efficient (having no false positives or negatives). As a therapeutic maneuver it is more effective in removing clots that cannot be aspirated. Finally, it has a much lower complication rate than standard pericardiocentesis. Arome[81] reported no deaths or complications in 50 patients in whom a subxiphoid pericardial window was used for suspected traumatic cardiac tamponade.

Treatment of Cardiac Tamponade

The definitive therapy for acute tamponade is surgical decompression and repair. The adjunctive therapies include rapid volume expansion, atropine, isoproterenol, pericardiocentesis or a subxiphoid window, and the use of a vasopressor with alpha activity during the induction of anesthesia.

Because of the steep slope of the curve relating blood pressure to intrapericardial pressure, cardiac tamponade may behave in a very labile manner, depending upon the treatment used.[52, 70] Rapid volume expansion with blood or colloids should be the first form of therapy. In spite of severe tamponade, volume expansion alone, which further increases the venous pressure, may temporarily normalize cardiac output and arterial pressure.[56] A high CVP is not necessarily a sign of fluid overload but rather is a sign of poor ventricular filling and increased venous tone. Improved circulatory dynamics may occur with only minimal increases (5 to 6 cm H_2O) in CVP.[70]

At present, isoproterenol is the catecholamine of choice for short-term cardiovascular support. The use of catecholamines with alpha activity may further depress cardiac output by increasing an already elevated systemic vascular resistance. Shoemaker[52] studied the hemodynamic response to isoproterenol and found that stroke volume and cardiac index were increased significantly. There was a decline in the systemic vascular resistance and a modest increase in CVP. The algebraic effect of these changes is an increased cardiac output with the same or slightly increased mean arterial pressure.

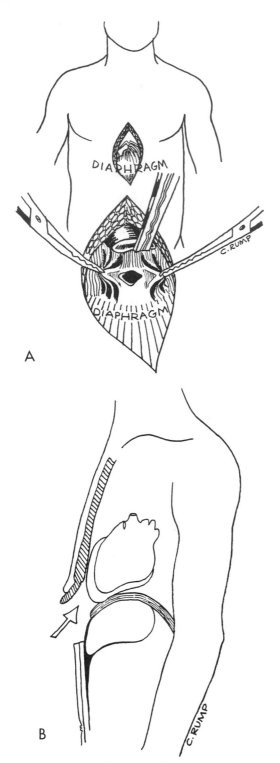

A

B

Figure 17–1. *A* and *B*, Placement of a pericardial window. An extrapleural window is created in the pericardium for diagnosis and decompression of cardiac tamponade. The xiphoid may be removed for better access to the pericardium.

To prevent the loss of vascular tone during the induction of anesthesia, a vasopressor with alpha receptor activity should be administered immediately prior to induction. Even if the patient is being supported with isoproterenol, a pressor with alpha activity should be added. Since the use of catecholamines with alpha activity prior to the induction of anesthesia may have a deleterious effect on the cardiac output, the vasopressor should be used only to maintain an adequate level of vascular resistance while the cardiovascular reflexes are depressed by anesthesia.[49]

TREATMENT SUMMARY OF PERICARDIAL TAMPONADE

Agonal patients should receive an immediate thoracotomy.

Unstable patients with suspected tamponade and a systolic pressure less than 90 mm Hg[38] or a pulsus that is 50 per cent of the pulse pressure should receive an immediate pericardiocentesis while preparations for a thoracotomy are being made.[48]

If pericardiocentesis is used and the aspirate is negative or the patient fails to improve immediately, one should proceed directly to thoracotomy.

Use of a vasopressor is mandatory for maintenance of the compensatory increase in peripheral vascular resistance during the induction of anesthesia.

Ideally, patients should receive pericardial decompression by means of a subxiphoid pericardial window with local anesthesia.[81, 49]

Anesthesia should not be induced until all personnel are ready to begin the thoracotomy.

PULMONARY INJURIES AND EMERGENCY THORACOTOMY

Pulmonary injuries can be divided into three types: parenchymal, tracheobronchial, and large vessel. Parenchymal and tracheobronchial injuries rarely create a situation requiring thoracotomy in the emergency department. The vast majority of these injuries can be adequately treated by tube thoracostomy during initial resuscitation (see Chapter 6).

Tracheobronchial injuries may be incurred from penetrating trauma; however, blunt trauma is the more usual etiology. Many affected patients expire at the scene. A comprehensive study of 1178 motor vehicle fatalities revealed the presence of this injury in 33 cases.[82] Unfortunately, because this injury is not always associated with severe thoracic trauma, it may be overlooked. In 12 of 80 bronchial tears reported by Hood and Sloan,[83] the tracheobronchial injury was the only major intrathoracic wound.

With this injury, the airway is usually maintained, even in the face of a complete transection. The stiff tracheobronchial cartilage tends to hold the lumen open while the peritracheal and peribronchial fasciae preserve the relationship of proximal to distal bronchi.[84] Ninety per cent of tracheobronchial tears occur within 1 inch of the carina.

These tears most commonly involve the main stem bronchi. Less frequently, vertical tears may occur along the membranous cartilage line of the trachea. Complete division of the trachea is extremely rare. Depending on the size and the location of the injury, patients may present with one or more of the following: massive hemoptysis when bronchial vessels are involved, airway obstruction, and pneumomediastinum or pneumothorax with or without tension.

Fatalities are the result of associated injuries or a tension pneumothorax. The build-up of pleural air under pressure impairs venous return directly by partially or fully collapsing the vena cava and indirectly by mediastinal shifts that distort the caval-atrial junction.[85] A large chest tube is usually sufficient treatment. If the leak is large, a point is reached at which the rate of removal of pleural air prevents adequate intake of air into the lungs. In this event, the emergency physician must settle for a pneumothorax without tension and must discontinue further attempts to expand the lung fully. Affected patients require urgent thoracotomy in the operating suite. Relief of the tension pneumothorax should allow sufficient time for safe transfer. In the presence of profuse hemorrhage or if the site of injury can be determined, the use of a bifid endotracheal tube or unilateral intubation of a main stem bronchus will secure the airway.

Lacerations of the parenchyma unaccompanied by major vessel injuries also respond well to a tube thoracostomy. Although the associated hemothorax may be significant, the pulmonary vascular system is of sufficiently low pressure that re-expansion of the lung will often halt or reduce bleeding. Reduction of parenchymal bleeding by negative pressure coaptation of the pleural surfaces is successful in 72 to 98 per cent of cases.[38, 86] If the initial chest tube drainage is more than 800 ml with continued drainage at a rate of 50 ml every 10 minutes or there is persistent hypotension, immediate thoracotomy should be considered.[38, 87] Such patients rarely have simple parenchymal injuries; major vascular structures are usually involved. A complication of parenchymal injuries that will require immediate thoracotomy is the development of air embolism.

AIR EMBOLISM

Suspicion of air embolism following trauma is considered to be an indication for emergency thoracotomy. Until recently, the occurrence of air embolism following penetrating injuries of the lung has not been widely recognized, although it may be a significant cause of morbidity and mortality.[88, 89]

The preoperative and postmortem diagnosis of air embolism is difficult. Air embolism is comfirmed at thoracotomy by needle aspiration of a foamy air-blood admixture from the left or right heart or by visualization of air within the coronary arteries. Preoperative demonstration of air by aspiration from a central venous catheter or the femoral artery is rare but has been reported.[89, 90]

Air embolism may appear in either the right or the left side of the circulatory system. Involvement of the right side of the circulation is referred to as "venous" or "pulmonary" air embolism. Generally, venous air is well tolerated, but death may occur when the volume of air reaches 5 to 8 ml per kg. The rate at which air moves into the circulation and the body position are important determinants of the volume that can be tolerated. Death usually results from obstruction of the right ventricle or the pulmonary circulation. If the mean pulmonary arterial pressure exceeds 22 mm Hg, air may pass into the systemic circulation. Paradoxical air embolism may also occur in the 15 to 25 per cent of patients who have a potentially patent foramen ovale.

The most common cause of venous air embolism is management error with intravenous therapy.[89, 91, 92] Air embolism fatalities have been reported with subclavian venipuncture.[91] A pressure difference of 5 cm H_2O across a 14 gauge needle will allow the introduction of 100 ml of air per second. Injuries of the vena cava or the right heart would also create obvious portals of entry into the right circulatory system.

Air embolism involving the left side of the circulatory system is referred to as "arterial" or "systemic" air embolism. The lethal volume depends upon the organs to which it is distributed. As little as 0.5 ml of air in the left anterior descending coronary artery has led to ventricular fibrillation. Arterial air will traverse systemic capillaries more readily than those in the pulmonary system. The pressure threshold for the passage of air through these capillaries is usually less than the normal systemic arterial pressure.[93] Air can pass from the femoral artery to the femoral vein with pressures as low as 20 mm Hg. The required pressure for visceral capillaries is higher and has a much larger range. Experimental pressures as high as 180 mm Hg have occasionally been required. Unfortunately, not all of the air will traverse the capillaries, and some will remain and obstruct blood flow. Air that passes through to the right side of the circulation is referred to as "secondary venous embolism." Clinical manifestations of arterial air embolism are related to the involvement of the coronary or cerebral circulation. The distribution of arterial air is partly a function of body position.

Systemic air embolism following injury of the lung has only recently been described.[93, 94] The formation of traumatic bronchovenous fistulae creates the potential entry points for air to move into the left side of the circulatory system. The only requirement is the formation of an air-blood gradient conducive to the inward movement of air. Although a lowered intravascular pressure from hemorrhage is a risk factor, the most important element in all reports of air embolism has been the use of positive-pressure ventilation.[90] Clinically, measurements of peak airway pressures during manual ventilation are often found to exceed 90 mm Hg. Dogs with penetrating lung injuries that are ventilated using peak pressures of 90 mm Hg have uniformly developed fatal systemic air embolism within 5 minutes of ventilation.[90]

Air embolization has even been shown to occur in the absence of penetrating lung injuries. In the canine model, the threshold airway pressure for systemic air embolism is 65 mm Hg with or without a penetrating injury. For intratracheal pressures less than 65 mm Hg, air embolism does not occur. In the canine model, the presence of a penetrating lung injury does not appear to alter the threshold for embolization. It does, however, significantly increase the volume of air embolized for any given pressure beyond the threshold pressure.[95, 96]

In a review of 447 cases of major thoracic trauma, Yee found adequate chart data to diagnose air embolism in 61 patients.[88] This incidence of 14 per cent is remarkable in light of the small number of reported cases prior to 1973.[93] A mechanism of blunt injury should not preclude a consideration of this diagnosis, since 25 per cent of patients with air embolism reported by Yee had blunt trauma with associated lung injury secondary to multiple rib fractures of hilar disruption.[88] The overall mortality was 56 per cent (34 of 61 patients). Refractory cardiac arrest accounted for 63 per cent of the operative deaths, with exsanguination as the cause in the remaining 27 per cent.

The diagnosis of air embolism is easily overlooked because of the similarity of the signs and symptoms of this condition to those of hypovolemic shock. Two valuble signs that were present in 36 per cent of patients are hemoptysis and the occurrence of cardiac arrest after intubation and ventilation. The diagnosis of air embolism should also be considered when there is sudden development of unconsciousness followed by convulsions in a lung injury patient on positive-pressure ventilation.[97]

Treatment of Air Embolism

A high index of suspicion with rapid control of the source of air embolism is vital. The patient should immediately be placed in the Trendelenburg (head-down) position so as to minimize cerebral involvement by directing the air emboli to less critical organs. This is followed by a left anterolateral thoracotomy. Peripheral bronchovenous fistulae can be identified by the bloody froth created during positive-pressure ventilation.

A quick search for hilar injuries should be carried out in the patient with blunt trauma. If the source of air embolism is not readily apparent, a contralateral thoracotomy is performed. Once the bronchovenous communication is controlled, needle aspiration of the residual air that commonly remains in the left heart and the aorta should be performed. If the patient is hypotensive, the aorta may now be cross-clamped. "Reflex" cross-clamping of the aorta prior to control of bronchovenous fistulae and removal of residual air will result in further dissemination of air to the heart and the brain.

Adjunctive Therapy. As mentioned earlier, air emboli will traverse capillary beds if the blood pressure is high enough.[93] A brief period of proximal aortic hypertension can be produced by cross-clamping of the decending aorta. Systemic arterial pressure should be maintained with adequate fluid resuscitation. If vasopressors are required, metaraminol (Aramine) appears to be the drug of choice. Goldstone and coworkers,[94] using a rat model, investigated the effect of metaraminol, dopamine, and phenylephrine on the time required to clear air emboli. In their model, the use of metaraminol cleared emboli within 1 minute of administration. When dopamine was used, 5 to 7 minutes were required. The use of phenylephrine produced such intense vasoconstriction of the larger arterioles (75 to 100 microns) that no movement of air bubbles occurred.

Left atrial pressure should be maintained at a high level. The ventilator inspiratory pressures should be kept as low as possible, and 100 per cent oxygen should be used to facilitate diffusion of nitrogen from emboli. Pharmacotherapy may include steroids, mannitol, aspirin, and barbiturates in conjunction with hypothermia.[97-102] The most important therapy will be the use of a hyperbaric chamber.[97-100]

Hyperbaric oxygen therapy is beneficial because it (1) compresses air bubbles, (2) establishes a high diffusion gradient that greatly speeds the dissolution of the bubbles, and (3) improves the oxygenation of ischemic tissues and lowers intracranial pressure. Hyperbaric oxygen therapy should be sought even though it may be many hours before it can be initiated. The effectiveness of hyperbaric oxygen therapy is illustrated by cases of success and improvement even when as many as 36 hours elapsed before pressurization.

MAJOR VASCULAR INJURIES

Major vascular injury resulting in rapid deterioration following blunt or penetrating trauma will require the use of an emergency thoracotomy for diagnosis, resuscitation, and control of hemorrhage. Even with immediate intervention, survival rates are low (14 to 29 per cent). Mavroudis reviewed 76 patients with thoracic vascular injury from mixed trauma who received emergency department thoracotomy because they were moribund or an immediate thoracotomy in the operating suite for hemodynamic instability.[103] The three most common sites of vascular injuries were pulmonary artery (28 per cent of cases), intercostal artery (23 per cent of cases), and pulmonary vein (20 per cent of cases). Aortic injuries accounted for only 12.5 per cent of the injuries requiring immediate surgical intervention. No attempt was made to perform arteriography in unstable patients. Air embolism was the cause of death in 18 per cent of cases.

The clinical approach to patients with suspected vascular injury will depend upon their hemodynamic status, the mechanism of injury, and the presence of associated injuries. If the patient is sufficiently stable, angiography is a valuable diagnostic measure, although the risk of sudden deterioration necessitates constant monitoring. If the patient is deteriorating rapidly and vascular injury is suspected, emergency thoracotomy will play a dual role as a diagnostic and a resuscitative procedure. It must be emphasized that patients with seemingly trivial penetrating wounds may appear stable and yet may precipitously exsanguinate and suffer an arrest from 5 minutes to 2 hours after admission.[40, 103]

Thoracotomy with cross-clamping of the thoracic aorta to control hemorrhage from penetrating abdominal injuries has been advocated, but survival rates have been poor for those undergoing this procedure. The collective survival rate in 194 cases described in the literature is only 5 per cent.[7, 14–17, 19] Three factors contribute to this low figure. First, aortic occlusion will not substantially affect the rate and volume of bleeding from major venous injuries. Second, most patients had lost all vital signs by the time of thoracotomy. Third, multiple collateral pathways around the cross-clamped aorta may diminish the effectiveness of this procedure.[104]

Aortic cross-clamping for massive hemoperitoneum was originally conceived as a preoperative "prophylactic" procedure to prevent sudden hypotension following abdominal decompression.[105–106] In this role, it has clearly been beneficial when systolic pressure cannot be raised above 80 mm Hg prior to laparotomy.[106]

As discussed earlier, emergency thoracotomy following blunt trauma should be selectively applied according to vital signs. The diagnosis of a ruptured aorta should be considered in anyone sustaining severe blunt chest trauma. Isolated traumatic rupture of the descending thoracic aorta has been described in approximately 10 per cent of fatal motor vehicle accident victims. One third

of these individuals died from their aortic rupture and not from associated injuries.[107] Of those who do reach a hospital, 40 per cent will be expected to expire within 24 hours if they do not receive prompt diagnosis and treatment.[107–109]

Aortic tears may occur near the root of the aorta and may present as cardiac tamponade. Much more commonly, the site of injury is just distal to the origin of the subclavian artery and the ligamentum arteriosum. The mechanism of injury is a multifactorial result of (1) direct displacement of the aorta by distorted ribs and sternum, producing a shearing effect at the relatively fixed ligamentum arteriosum, (2) indirect displacement of the aorta during deceleration as a result of mass/inertia effect, and (3) sudden elevation of aortic pressure, which may exceed 1000 mm Hg.[110, 111]

Unfortunately, few symptoms are present with aortic tears. A complaint of retrosternal or interscapular pain and, more rarely, hoarseness, dyspnea, or dysphagia should immediately raise one's index of suspicion. Physical findings that would allow diagnosis are present in fewer than 30 per cent of cases. Such findings include pseudocoarctation with upper extremity hypertension and lower extremity hypotension, pulse difference, interscapular systolic murmur, paraplegia, and deviation of the trachea.[112]

The primary radiographic sign of aortic rupture is widening of the mediastinum. A mediastinum greater than 7.5 cm to 8.0 cm at the level of the aortic knob seen on a 100-cm supine film is considered significant.[113, 114] Although direct measurement is helpful, a recent study found that measurement of mediastinal width was not as reliable as the subjective interpretation of mediastinal widening because of the wide variation in measurements among observers and the fact that a significant fraction of patients with traumatic rupture and widened mediastinum do not have direct measurements greater than the statistical cutoff of 7.5 to 8 cm.[113] Other radiographic signs are often secondary to mediastinal widening and include shift of the trachea to the right, obscuring of the aortic knob, loss of the aortic pulmonary window, depression of the left main stem bronchus, displacement of the right paraspinous line, deviation of a nasogastric tube to the right, and loss of the sharp medial apical contour of the left upper lobe.[115–119] One sign that is occasionally described in the absence of a widened mediastinum and may be one of the earliest signs of this injury is a left apical cap.[112]

For blunt trauma victims with deteriorating vital signs, a presumptive diagnosis of ruptured thoracic aorta should be made. "In few situations is it as axiomatic as with an aortic injury that operation does not await resuscitation but is an integral part therefore."[37]

OPEN CHEST RESUSCITATION FOR NONTRAUMATIC ARREST

Failure to resuscitate patients from cardiac arrest is a result of (1) a delay in the onset of cardiopulmonary resuscitation (CPR), (2) the use of less than optimal resuscitative techniques, or (3) the intractability of the underlying disease process.[120] The development of closed chest resuscitation, which is quickly and easily applied, coupled with the development of more advanced prehospital care has dramatically reduced the number of failures caused by a delay in the onset of CPR.[121] The new frontier is now in the area of improving resuscitative techniques. Recent evidence suggests that standard closed chest resuscitation does not meet coronary and cerebral needs for a sufficient period to allow successful resuscitation.[122–127] Consequently, some investigators are calling for a critical re-evaluation of current CPR techniques—a first step, they hope, toward something better.

Current studies have focused attention on the changes in intrathoracic pressure during closed chest resuscitation.[128–134] It is now generally accepted that blood flow during CPR is primarily the result of intrathoracic pressure changes rather than direct cardiac compression, as was previously thought (see Chapter 14). During CPR the heart is essentially a conduit. Such a concept has important implications for coronary blood flow because it suggests that closed chest resuscitation may not provide an effective perfusion gradient for coronary circulation. The work of Ditchey and Niemann supports this hypothesis.[122, 123] In canine models using standard CPR, the coronary blood flow is less than 1 per cent of prearrest values. For practical purposes there is no coronary blood flow when standard closed chest resuscitation is used.

Disappointing results were also found when investigators evaluated common carotid blood flows using standard CPR methods. In animal models, carotid blood flows vary from 7 to 17 per cent of the prearrest value.[124–127] Irreversible brain damage occurs quickly when carotid blood flow cannot be maintained at more than 10 per cent of normal.[126, 135] It is important to recall that the common carotid artery contributes to both the external and the internal carotid. Thus, changes in common carotid blood flows do not necessarily correlate with changes in cerebral blood flow. Measurements of regional cerebral cortical blood flow during CPR by White and associates suggest that adequate cortical perfusion is *not* achieved.[136] White and coworkers found cortical blood flows to be less than 10 per cent of normal. This value is in agreement with previous microsphere studies that found cerebral blood flows to be only 5 per cent of normal when conventional CPR was used.[124]

There is no question that closed chest resuscitation has saved countless lives. The length of time that closed chest resuscitation can maintain life, however, appears to be more limited than was previously suspected. Observations by Eliastam, Jeresaty, and others suggest that there are rarely any long-term survivors after 30 minutes of *continuous* advanced cardiac life support.[137–142] The two exceptions to this rule are those patients with hypothermia and those suffering from drug overdose.

In view of the preceding studies, open chest methods of resuscitation are being reconsidered.[143, 144] Direct compression of the heart produces higher arterial pressures and greater blood flows than do current closed chest techniques.[125–127, 145–150] Del Guercio measured the comparative hemodynamics of open and closed methods during cardiac resuscitation of patients.[147–149] The cardiac index was more than doubled by open chest massage. The cardiac index produced by the closed chest method was 0.6 L per minute per m². With an open chest method the cardiac index increased to 1.3 L per minute per m². Equally important is the return of coronary blood flow with open chest resuscitation.[122, 127]

In a comparative study of closed and open resuscitation using a canine model, Bartlett demonstrated improved survival and neurologic outcome with open chest cardiac compression method. Only 10 per cent of control animals could be resuscitated after 50 minutes of closed chest resuscitation, and all had fixed and dilated pupils. An experimental group received 10 minutes of closed chest resuscitation followed by 40 minutes of open chest resuscitation for a total arrest time of 50 minutes. *All* of these dogs were resuscitated; equally important was the preservation of the pupillary light reflex in 90 per cent of these animals.[151, 152]

At present the precise role of open chest resuscitation for nontraumatic arrests is poorly defined. Although several indications have been suggested, only two can be readily accepted. The first indication is for resuscitation of patients with hypothermic arrest (see Chapter 73). When cardiopulmonary bypass is not readily available, asystole unresponsive to pacing or ventricular fibrillation unresponsive to cardioversion may be treated with internal massage and direct rewarming of the heart.[153–156] The second indication is for use in medical arrests unresponsive to external resuscitation. Unfortunately, there is no clear method for determining the point at which unresponsiveness occurs, nor is it easy to determine when signs of tissue perfusion exist.[144, 157–159] A palpable pulse does not ensure flow. A pulse with CPR indicates only that a continuous fluid column capable of transmitting shock waves is present.[157]

There have been several reports of successful

open chest resuscitation occurring after closed chest resuscitation had failed.[148, 149, 157, 158] Cohn and Del Guercio reported long-term survival in 11 patients who were resuscitated after closed chest resuscitation was abandoned in favor of the direct internal approach.[148, 149] Sykes reported 4 survivors out of 36 patients resuscitated with internal massage after external massage failed.[158] The renewal of coronary perfusion with internal massage may supply sufficient oxygen and substrate to restore effective electrical or mechanical activity.[157] Based on the previously mentioned observations of Eliastam, Jeresaty, and Szczygiel and case reports of successful open chest resuscitation following attempted closed chest resuscitation, the following guidelines may be helpful.

Duration of Advanced Cardiac Life Support (ACLS). There are rarely any long-term survivors when the duration of ACLS is *continuous* for more than 30 minutes without cardiac response. The probability of long-term survival is approximately 86 per cent during the first 10 minutes of ACLS.[137] This is reduced to 30 per cent by 16 minutes[139] and becomes less than 1 per cent after 30 minutes.[140–142] (This analysis assumes that basic life support begins within 4 minutes and that advanced life support is initiated within 8 minutes.)

Onset of Asystole. When asystole occurs, regardless of the ACLS duration, there will rarely be any survivors if standard methods are used. In most large series, the fatality rate for asystole is 100 per cent.[160, 161] Shocket observed that some affected patients actually are in fine ventricular fibrillation.[157] The return of coronary blood flow with internal massage may restore coordinated electrical and mechanical activity[157] or may convert the fine ventricular fibrillation into the more responsive coarse fibrillation.

Onset of Electromechanical Dissociation (EMD) or Pulseless Idioventricular Rhythm. Possible causes of EMD, such as tension pneumothorax, volume depletion, and pericardial tamponade, should be rapidly excluded. If the patient does not respond immediately to conventional therapy, the outcome is generally fatal.[161] Therefore, open chest methods should be considered.

Onset of Nonreactive Pupils. The pupillary light reflex should be noted as soon as possible and should be observed continually. Loss of this reflex during resuscitation indicates inadequate cerebral and brain stem perfusion. During resuscitation, this is the only clinical sign of perfusion that can be assessed. Although complete neurologic recovery is possible, the loss of this reflex is an ominous sign[152] and should not be tolerated for more than a few minutes. Unfortunately, the administration of pharmacologic agents during resuscitation may alter the value of this parameter.

Presence of Hypoxia. Arterial blood gases should be determined prior to attempting open resuscitation. If significant hypoxia has developed, internal massage may be of little benefit. The relationship of hypoxia to arteriovenous shunting and its reversibility with increased blood flow is unknown.

Although closed chest resuscitation will continue to be the first-line method of handling medical cardiac arrests, there is sufficient experimental and clinical evidence to support the use of open chest resuscitation if standard closed chest methods fail. At present, the criteria for and the timing of open chest resuscitation must rest with the individual physician.

Equipment for Resuscitative Thoracotomy

The physician must carefully consider the instruments to be included in a resuscitation thoracotomy tray. The inclusion of too many instruments will make the tray cumbersome and will delay the procedure. Nonessential instruments are best kept available in the resuscitation room in case they are needed for specific repair (e.g., Foley catheter for stellate wound tamponade).

The following items are essential for a thoracotomy tray:

Scalpel with attached number 20 blade,
Mayo scissors,
Rib spreaders,
Tissue forceps (10-inch),
Vascular clamps (two needed, Satinsky),
Needle holder (10-inch, Hegar),
2-0 or larger silk on large curve needle, and
Suture scissors.

The following items are optional for the tray and can be supplied as needed by an assistant:

Towel clips (six),
Hemostats (four to six, curved and straight),
Metzenbaum scissors,
Right-angled clamp,
Liebsche knife,
Foley catheter (20 French, 30-ml balloon),
Chest tube (number 30, Argyle),
Lap sponges (12) or gauze pads
Towels (six),
Cloth tape, and
Teflon patches.

In addition, functioning suction and sterile suction tips, antiseptic solution, sterile gloves, a defibrillator with internal paddles, and overhead surgical lights are needed in the resuscitation room. In the unlikely event that the patient awakens during the procedure, diazepam or narcotics can be administered for sedation, amnesia, and pain control.

Procedure

If a potential survivor is to benefit from a resuscitative thoracotomy, the emergency physician must act swiftly and skillfully. A thoracotomy per se does not save lives; it is the repairs and adjunctive therapies used that determine the outcome.

PRELIMINARY CONSIDERATIONS

For all trauma victims presenting to the emergency department with hypotension, the initial working diagnosis must be one of volume depletion. Other possibilities should be rapidly excluded, e.g., tension pneumothorax, cardiac tamponade, air embolism, and neurogenic or cardiogenic shock.

The importance of rapidly reversing shock was emphasized in a review of 1136 patients seen in the emergency department of North Detroit General Hospital with chest trauma and shock on arrival.[162] The authors defined shock as a systolic blood pressure less than 90 mm Hg. In the subgroup of patients with a systolic pressure less than 70 mm Hg, the mortality was 18 per cent. For those patients presenting with a systolic pressure greater than 70 mm Hg, the mortality was only 3 per cent. In moribund patients, the time required for volume replacement will be a critical determinant of success.

There is no single site for rapid volume delivery that can be universally used for trauma resuscitation (see Chapter 20). With thoracic injuries, consideration should be given to the use of the proximal saphenous or femoral vein.[49, 163–165] A recent study evaluated the relationship of catheter choice to flow rate.[166] The USCI 9 French introducer (C.R. Bard Inc., Ellerica, Massachusetts) was found to have the fastest flow rate. With a pressure infusion cuff at 200 mm Hg, the USCI introducer had a flow rate of 556 ml per minute with water and 343 ml per minute with diluted packed red blood cells (PRBCs) (Hct 45 per cent). In contrast, intravenous extension tubing, which requires a delay for cutdown, had flow rates of 500 ml per minute and 312 ml per minute for water and diluted PRBCs, respectively. The commonly used 14 gauge Deseret subclavian jugular catheter has unacceptable flow rates for patients with shock and severe volume depletion: 341 ml per minute with water and only 171 ml per minute with diluted PRBCs using a pressure infusion cuff. In addition to catheter choice, Mateer and coworkers reported the effect of diluting PRBCs to a 45 per cent Hct.[166] Diluting a unit of PRBCs with 200 ml of normal saline tripled the flow rate and caused a twofold increase in the red cell mass delivery rate.

Use of the preceding techniques will allow for more rapid blood transfusions. When massive transfusion is indicated, concern for the possible adverse side effects of a large and rapid transfusion should not slow the rate of administration. The increased morbidity and mortality associated with massive transfusions appear to be related more to the duration and severity of shock than to the rate or volume of blood used. From a study of 402 patients requiring massive transfusions,[167] the following observations were made: (1) Patients with adequate tissue perfusion will tolerate the acid pH, electrolyte concentrations, and low temperature of stored blood. When prolonged shock was prevented by immediate transfusion, the mortality was 62 per cent. (2) The theoretic possibility of hyperkalemia has been overemphasized; most patients remain normokalemic. The incidence of hypokalemia (10 per cent) was as common as that of hyperkalemia (12 per cent). (3) In transfusions with only group O blood, the reaction rate was only 0.16 per cent. (Wilson and associates continued with only group O blood if three or more units had been transfused.)[167]

Because a large amount of blood may be lost into the chest, an autotransfusion system should be available (see Chapter 29). The use of autotransfusion has several benefits.[169, 170] The most important advantages are: (1) immediate availability of "compatible," warm blood, (2) significantly higher levels of 2,3-DPG than in stored blood, and (3) less risk of exhausting the banked supply of the patient's blood type. This third point can be crucial when there are blood bank shortages or when there are cross-match problems.

Another factor to be considered is ensuring adequate ventilation and oxygenation of the hypotensive patient. Intubation with controlled ventilation is desirable for all agonal patients and crucial in the management of the thoracotomy patient. Antiseptic preparation of the chest wall by necessity is abbreviated during resuscitative thoracotomy and is best performed by an assistant while the physician is putting on surgical gloves.

SUBXIPHOID PERICARDIAL WINDOW

Most patients with suspected cardiac injury should receive a subxiphoid pericardial window for diagnosis and decompression.[81, 171–173] Preferably, this procedure is performed in the operating suite. If the patient is unstable, the pericardial window operation is performed in the emergency department. At the same time there should be a thoracotomy tray open and ready. This precaution is important in the event of sudden patient deterioration or profuse and uncontrollable hemorrhage when the pericardium is decompressed.

With the patient under local anesthesia, a 10-cm midline incision is placed over the xiphoid process (see Fig. 17–1). The tip of the xiphoid is elevated and separated from the rectus sheath on either side. A plane is developed behind the xiphoid, and the sternal attachment of the diaphragm is separated. If needed, the xiphoid can be removed at the xiphisternal joint to facilitate exposure. Using a sponge for traction, an assistant depresses the diaphragm and elevates the sternum with a small retractor. Fat must be dissected away before the pericardium can be visualized. The anterior inferior "shelf" of the pericardium is then grasped with a fine-toothed forceps and is incised.

ANTEROLATERAL THORACOTOMY INCISION

When the site of injury is unknown and the patient's status requires immediate intervention for possible intrathoracic injuries, a left anterolateral incision in the fourth intercostal space will provide the best access to the heart and the great vessels. In the setting of cardiac arrest, time should not be taken to count the rib spaces. An incision just beneath the nipple in the male or along the inframammary fold in the female will approximate the fourth intercostal space. Closed chest compressions are continued during the initial incision. The first sweep of the scalpel (number 20 blade) should separate skin, subcutaneous fat, and the superficial portions of the pectoralis and serratus muscles. When dividing the intercostal muscles with a scalpel or Mayo scissors, one should be careful not to lacerate the lung. With the first opening of the pleura, ventilations should be stopped momentarily. This will allow the lung to collapse away from the chest wall. The intercostal incision just over the top of the fifth rib can then be carried quickly and safely to completion. Some surgeons prefer to begin the thoracotomy incision over the sternum, whereas others begin 2 cm lateral to the edge of the sternum, hoping to avoid the internal mammary artery. Should the internal mammary artery be transected during the procedure, hemorrhage is generally minimal until after perfusion is re-established. At that time the patient can exsanguinate from a lacerated internal mammary artery. Therefore, all internal mammary artery lacerations should be ligated once perfusion is established.

The intercostal space is spread and a chest wall retractor (rib spreader) is placed with the handle and ratchet bar down (Fig. 17–2). If the retractor is placed with the handle up, the ratchet bar will prevent extension of the incision into the right chest. When the site of injury is to the right of the heart and cannot be reached, a trans-sternal extension into the right chest is performed with a Liebsche knife.

It is important to establish wide exposure from the outset by extending the skin incision past the posterior axillary line. One can facilitate this by quickly wedging towels or sheets under the left posterior chest and by placing the patient's left arm above his head. Inadequate exposure, rib fractures, and additional delays occur when the skin incision is too limited. In patients with suspected left subclavian vessel injuries or aortic arch injuries, better exposure and control will be obtained when the third intercostal space is used. If access is still difficult, the ribs may be separated at the costochondral junction.

Figure 17–2. Left anterolateral thoracotomy. An incision is made between the fourth and fifth interspaces. It is important to stay as close to the top of the fifth rib as possible to avoid the intercostal artery. The rib spreader should be placed with the handle down. Pericardiotomy is started near the diaphragm and anterior to the phrenic nerve.

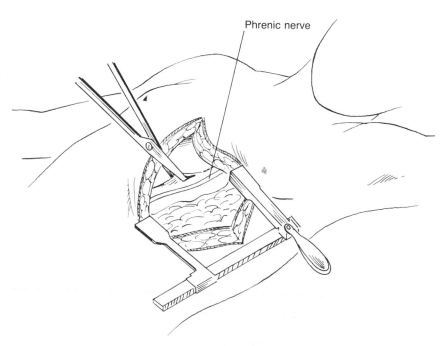

Phrenic nerve

PERICARDIOTOMY

If cardiac arrest has occurred, the question of whether to open the pericardial sac arises. If the myocardium cannot be visualized, the pericardium should be opened, but in the majority of cases the myocardium can be evaluated through the intact pericardium. If a tamponade is not present it is usually best to leave the pericardial sac closed. From a physiologic standpoint, compression of the heart is more efficient when it is performed with the pericardium open because pressure is transmitted only to the ventricles. Opening the pericardium, however, will only increase the risk of added complications. The delay in beginning cardiac compressions will add to the risk of cerebral damage. The myocardium or a coronary vessel may be injured. The left phrenic nerve may be cut by mistake and if there has been previous pericardial disease, adhesions may be present. If attempts are made to separate these adhesions rapidly, tears of the atrial or right ventricular wall can occur. The incidence of traumatic rupture of the atria or the right ventricle during massage is greater when the pericardium is open. With an intact pericardium, pressure is distributed over a larger area and the pericardial fluid seldom allows the compression fingers to remain in one spot for a prolonged period.

Patients with tamponade will require pericardiotomy. This is performed in a location anterior and parallel to the left phrenic nerve. The incision should start near the diaphragm to avoid possible injury of the coronary arteries. When the pericardium is under tension, it may be very difficult to grasp the pericardium with forceps. In that case, sharp, straight Mayo scissors are used to divide the pericardium by layers. If the heart is in arrest, speed is important, and sharp scissors should be used to "catch" the pericardium and to start the pericardiotomy. To do this, the point of the scissors is held almost parallel to the surface of the heart with enough pressure to create a wrinkle in the pericardium that can be punctured as the scissors are moved forward. Moderate pressure must be used to puncture the fibrous pericardium. The sudden give that occurs when the pericardium opens may result in a laceration of the myocardium if the point of the scissors is unnecessarily angled toward the heart. Clots of blood are removed from the pericardial sac by the sweeping motion of a gloved hand or with sterile lap sponges or gauze pads.

DIRECT CARDIAC COMPRESSIONS

Three techniques for cardiac compression have been advocated: one-handed compression, one-handed with sternal compression, and two-handed, or bimanual, compression. Of these three, single-handed compression of the heart against the anterior chest wall is considerably less effective and is not recommended. This method can produce only 50 per cent of the blood flow that is obtained by the other two methods.[174] The effectiveness of the other two methods seems to vary more with the individual than with the method used. Compression is performed using the *entire palmar surface* of the fingers. Fingertip pressure should be avoided at all times. The fingers should be positioned so that the coronary arteries will not be occluded. It is also important to maintain a relatively anatomic position of the heart to prevent kinking of the great vessels. Venous inflow is especially sensitive to changes in position. Rapid establishment of intra-arterial pressure monitoring is of tremendous value for assessing the consistency and effectiveness of compressions.

A difference of opinion exists regarding the optimal rate at which the heart should be compressed. Most of the literature has recommended a rate of 50 to 60 compressions per minute; however, there are few data to support such a recommendation. Johnson and Kirby studied the relationship of compression rate to cardiac output and blood pressure and found these parameters to be directly related.[174] Although their work has been disputed,[175] a more recent study has confirmed these findings.[176] Using an animal model, compression rates of 60 and 90 were compared. The cardiac index and mean arterial pressure were increased by almost 20 per cent and 25 per cent, respectively, when the compression rate was increased to 90 per minute.

CONTROL OF HEMORRHAGIC CARDIAC WOUNDS

One may partially control active bleeding from ventricular wounds by placing the finger of one hand over the wound while using the other hand to stabilize the beating heart. The wound is repaired by placement of several horizontal mattress sutures under the tamponading finger (Fig. 17–3). Nonabsorbable 2-0 silk sutures are customarily used. Smaller sutures should *not* be used, and nylon sutures should be avoided. Some physicians prefer to use even larger silk sutures, such as Number 1 or 2 [(note that this is *not* 0 (1–0) or 0–0 (2–0).] When multiple sutures are needed, they should all be in place before they are tied. This allows for a rapid and equal distribution of wound tension, which prevents tearing of the myocardium.[46, 78] Passing the suture through Teflon pledgets also prevents the suture from cutting through the myocardium. It is especially important to use Teflon pledgets for reinforcement when the myocardium has been weakened by the blast effect of a bullet.[49, 50] With large wounds that cannot be

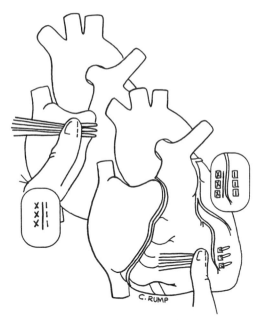

Figure 17–3. Technique of repair. Multiple horizontal mattress sutures are placed 6 mm from the wound edge before tying. The wound is closed just enough to stop bleeding. Teflon pledgets are used for reinforcement. For repairs near a coronary artery, care is taken to pass the suture under the artery.

palpably controlled, an incomplete horizontal mattress suture should be placed on either side of the wound (Fig. 17–4). The free ends are then crossed to stop the bleeding. The actual reparative sutures can then be accurately placed. It must be stressed that suturing the myocardium requires good technique. Excessive tension may tear the myocardium and aggravate the situation. Keys to success include the use of appropriate sized suture, a generous "bite" with the needle, and application of only enough tension as needed to control bleeding.

If exsanguinating hemorrhage is not controlled by the aforementioned methods, temporary inflow occlusion can be used. Inflow occlusion may be applied intermittently for 60 to 90 seconds. During occlusion the heart shrinks, hemorrhage is con-

trolled, and sutures can be placed in a decompressed injury. Three techniques have been described: (1) vascular clamping of the superior and inferior vena cava for partial inflow occlusion,[76] (2) use of the Sauerbruch grip (Fig. 17–5) for occlusion of the vena cava between the ring and the middle finger of the left hand for partial inflow occlusion,[34] and (3) use of a venous mesocardial snare for total inflow occlusion.[177] The mesocardial snare for total inflow occlusion is formed with heavy cloth tape (Fig. 17–6). The tape is passed through the transverse sinus and encircles the inferior surface of the heart. The oblique sinus is then packed with gauze pads. Constriction of the umbilical tape will now compress the horseshoe-shaped venous mesocardium against the gauze tampon. This particular method has several advantages: (1) Preliminary placement of a venous mesocardial snare prior to opening the pericardium allows the physician to "shut off" the entire circulation instantly in the event of uncontrollable hemorrhage; (2) one can perform the procedure intermittently by simply tightening and relaxing the snare; (3) with total inflow occlusion venous return from the lungs will not be lost through left heart wounds; and (4) it does not interfere with the operative field.

Insertion of a Foley catheter (20 French with a 30-ml balloon) through a wound is another technique for controlling hemorrhage.[44, 46, 178–180] Following insertion of the catheter, the balloon is inflated, the catheter is clamped, and gentle traction is applied (Fig. 17–7). Enough traction is applied to slow the bleeding to an acceptable level for visualization and repair. Attempts to achieve complete hemostasis with excessive traction may pull the catheter out and potentially enlarge the wound. The balloon will effectively occlude the wound internally. When repairing the wound, the

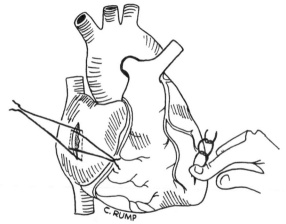

Figure 17–4. Control of bleeding using digital pressure and by crossing two widely placed incomplete mattress sutures.

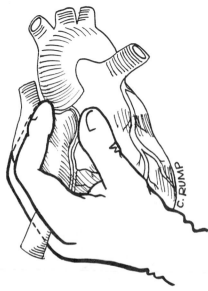

Figure 17–5. Sauerbruch's maneuver: Venous inflow occlusion is achieved by using the first and second or second and third fingers as a clamp.

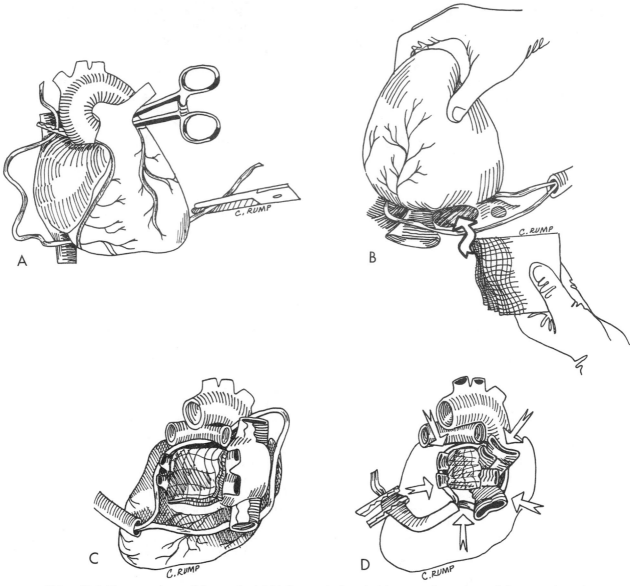

Figure 17–6. Venous mesocardial snare for total inflow occlusion. *A,* A hemostat is used to pull the snare through the transverse sinus. *B,* Inferior view. Arrow indicates the shallow oblique sinus, which is packed with gauze. The heart has been elevated for illustration. Clinically, excessive lifting of the heart can produce cardiac arrest. *C,* Posterior view, with snare and tampon in place. *D,* Posterior view during venous occlusion.

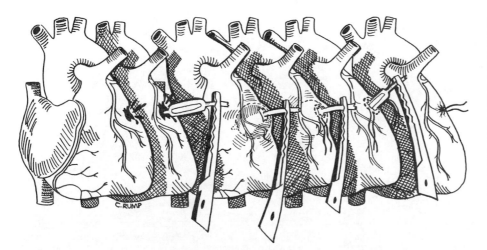

Figure 17–7. Serial illustration. Gentle traction on an inflated Foley catheter will control hemorrhage and allow easy repair. The balloon is inflated with saline, and care is taken to avoid rupturing the balloon with the suture needle. This technique is particularly useful with injuries of the inferior caval-atrial junction, with posterior wounds, and during cardiac massage. Volume loading can be obtained by infusion of blood or crystalloid solutions through the lumen of the catheter. Care should be taken to avoid an air embolus through the lumen of the catheter during placement.

operator must be careful with the suture needle to prevent rupturing the balloon. Temporarily pushing the balloon into the ventricular lumen during needle passage is helpful. It is important to use normal saline when inflating the balloon. Use of air will result in air embolism if the balloon is ruptured by the suture needle.

Foley catheters have several advantages over other methods of controlling cardiac wounds. With the digital method, the fingertip will often slip if there is a strong heartbeat, the wound cannot be visualized during repair, and digital pressure significantly interferes with cardiac massage. Total venous inflow occlusion is an effective method of controlling bleeding and decompressing the heart, but such control will be at the expense of a poor cardiac output. Comparatively, the Foley catheter causes very little cardiovascular interference, although inflation near the base of the ventricle may obstruct blood flow. Attempts to elevate the heart for control and repair of posterior cardiac wounds will often result in cardiac arrest by reduction of both venous and arterial flows. With posterior injuries, one cannot continuously view the wound for digital control of bleeding. Use of a catheter does not require continued viewing after the initial placement. If bleeding can be controlled, repairs in this location should await full volume expansion or cardiopulmonary bypass.[16, 50, 181] Regardless of location, the most valuable feature of using a Foley catheter, is its ability to control hemorrhage without interfering with cardiac compression.

Deliberate fibrillation should be considered as a last resort for repair of difficult wounds of the ventricle or the proximal aorta. Elective cardiac arrest is best tolerated if there is adequate blood volume and oxygenation prior to fibrillation.[14] For fibrillation, the internal cardiac paddles are placed perpendicular to the surface of the heart and discharged at 20 watt-sec (Fig. 17–8).[76] The heart should be massaged intermittently during repair, and the duration of fibrillation should not exceed 3 to 4 minutes.

Defibrillation is accomplished while the internal paddles are firmly pressed over the right and left ventricles. Following repair, the epicardium is often dry and should be moistened with saline to improve electrical conduction. An energy level of 20 watt-sec is used. If the initial attempt is unsuccessful, repeated shocks at the same setting should be used. Higher energy levels can cause myocardial necrosis.[186] Defibrillation through an intact pericardium should begin with 20 watt-sec. If unsuccessful, the shock should be repeated once and then increased to 40 to 60 watt-sec.

Management of the wounded heart that has spontaneously arrested is controversial. Some authors have recommended a rapid repair of ventricular wounds while the heart is arrested. Others

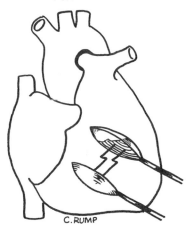

Figure 17–8. Technique for elective fibrillation. Twenty joules (watt-sec) are delivered through internal defibrillating paddles placed perpendicular to the epicardium. Coronary vessels should be avoided during paddle placement.

consider immediate cardiac massage and reversal of cardiac arrest to be more important. Immediate cardiac massage to maintain blood flow is probably the best approach. When cardiac arrest occurs, physiologic reserves have been depleted, and a delay for repair during arrest would only diminish the chance of a successful resuscitation.

Wounds of the atria are managed with partial occlusion clamps (Fig. 17–9). Because of the thin structure and instability of the atrial wall, digital pressure will not effectively stop bleeding. Injuries near the caval-atrial junction are not amenable to clamping. In this location a Foley catheter should be used to tamponade the wound (Fig. 17–10).[179–182] Care must be exerted to avoid obstruction of atrial filling with the inflated balloon. During wound closure, the catheter should be pushed away from the ventricular wall to avoid rupture of the balloon.

Wounds of the septae, the valves, and the coronary arteries require definitive repair in the operating suite. Hemorrhage from a coronary artery can generally be controlled with digital pressure. Ligation of a coronary artery should be avoided when possible.

CONTROL OF HEMORRHAGIC GREAT VESSEL WOUNDS

Wounds of the great vessels can be controlled with digital pressure or partial occlusion clamps.[181] Exsanguinating hemorrhage from the left subclavian artery can be prevented by cross-clamping of the intrathoracic portion of the artery. Cross-clamping of the right subclavian artery is very difficult. For injuries of this vessel, compression with laparotomy pads in the apex of the pleura from below and the supraclavicular fossa from

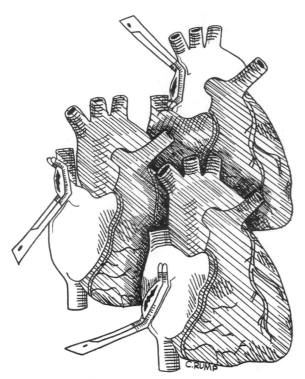

Figure 17–9. Use of a partial occluding clamp in different locations for control of bleeding and repair.

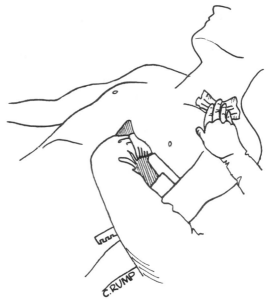

Figure 17–11. Cross-clamping for control of subclavian bleeding is difficult and time-consuming. Compression with laparotomy pads in the apical pleura from below and the supraclavicular fossa from above will control hemorrhage while the patient is stabilized.

above (Fig. 17–11) will prevent further bleeding as the patient is stabilized and moved to the operating suite.[183]

Large or difficult vena caval injuries should be controlled with a temporary intravascular shunt to maintain venous return while providing vascular

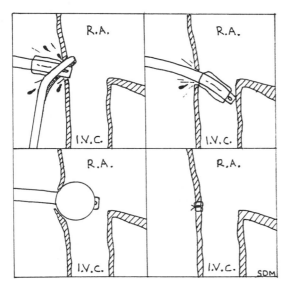

Figure 17–10. Wounds of the inferior caval–atrial junction are difficult to manage with simple vascular clamping. Use of a Foley catheter will provide satisfactory control.

isolation of the injured segment.[163, 179] Ideally, heparin-bonded tubing should be used.[16] If this is not available, a number 30 Argyle plastic chest tube will be a satisfactory alternative.[179] The tube is placed through a pursestring suture in the right atrium, and the tip is advanced beyond the site of the injury (Fig. 17–12). Flow is established by creation of several large ports in the proximal portion of the tube, which is then advanced into the atrium. Next, a clamp is placed across the tube just outside the atrium. Finally, vascular isolation of the injury is completed by placement of tourniquets above and below the site of injury (Fig. 17–13).

When the systolic pressure cannot be raised above 70 mm Hg, temporary occlusion of the descending thoracic aorta will maintain myocardial and cerebral perfusion (Fig. 17–14). Selective clamping will be necessary when the aorta has been injured with blunt trauma (Fig. 17–15). Aortic occlusion has a limited role in controlling hemorrhage below the diaphragm.[21, 104] When there is a tense abdomen with massive hemoperitoneum, aortic cross-clamping is clearly beneficial when applied just before laparotomy. This has been referred to as "prophylactic cross-clamping" to prevent a sudden drop in blood pressure when the abdomen is decompressed.[105–106] As a preoperative procedure, cross-clamping should be applied when the systolic pressure is less than 80 mm Hg in the setting of a tense abdomen.[106]

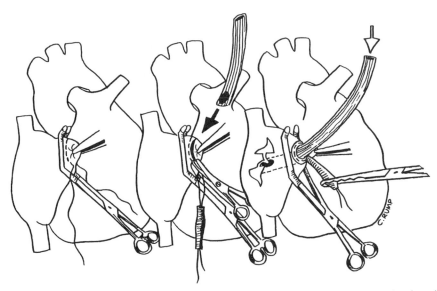

Figure 17–12. Technique for placing an atrial line or vascular shunt. A purse-string suture is placed, the atrial appendage is clamped, and an incision is made. A catheter or intravascular shunt is inserted, and the purse string is tightened.

To expose the descending aorta, the left lung is retracted in a superior-medial direction by an assistant. To achieve adequate exposure, it is sometimes necessary to divide the inferior pulmonary ligament (Fig. 17–16). The aorta can be quickly identified by advancement of the fingers of the left hand along the thoracic cage toward the vertebral column. On some occasions, the operator may choose to have an assistant simply occlude the aorta with digital pressure. To locate the aorta, one uses a DeBakey aortic clamp or a curved Kelly clamp for blunt dissection and spreads open the pleura above and below the aorta (Fig. 17–17). The esophagus, which lies medially and slightly anteriorly, is separated from the vessel. When the aorta is completely isolated, the index finger of the left hand is flexed around the vessel and a vascular clamp is applied with the right hand. The brachial blood pressure should be checked immediately after the occlusion. If the systolic pressure is more than 120 mm Hg, the clamp should be slowly released and adjusted to maintain a systolic pressure of 120 mm Hg.[106]

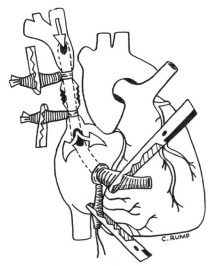

Figure 17–13. Temporary intravascular shunt. With complicated injuries, this technique controls bleeding and provides continued blood flow. A proximal port must be cut in the tube, which is inserted through the atrial appendage as shown in Figure 17–12.

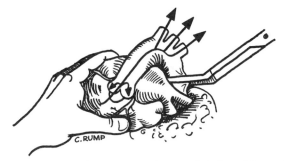

Figure 17–14. Manual massage and cross-clamping of the aorta to increase coronary and cerebral perfusion selectively.

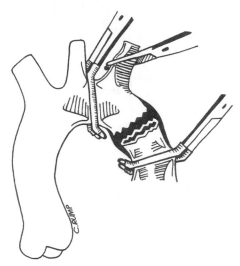

Figure 17–15. Traumatic rupture of the aorta. Three clamps are required for control. Back-bleeding will occur if fewer than three clamps are used.

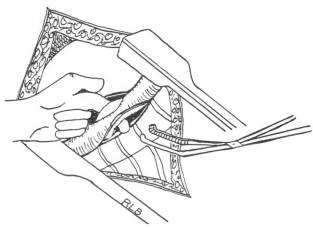

Figure 17–17. Aortic cross-clamping: Using blunt dissection, one spreads the pleura above and below the aorta. The vessel should be fully mobilized and clearly separated from the esophagus prior to clamping.

The issue of whether aortic cross-clamping is beneficial in hypovolemia because it increases coronary perfusion or whether it is detrimental because it increases afterload to an ischemic heart has recently been addressed. Dunn,[184] using a canine shock model, measured ventricular contractility before and after aortic occlusion. Contractility was impaired during the period of hypotension prior to cross-clamping. Following aortic occlusion, contractility returned to normal.

Potential complications of aortic cross-clamping are multiple: Ischemia of the spinal cord, liver, bowel, and kidneys as well as iatrogenic injury of the aorta and the esophagus may occur.[106] Failure to monitor blood pressure every 60 seconds during aortic occlusion may result in cerebral hemorrhage or left ventricular failure if there is excessive elevation of pressure. Fortunately, these complications are infrequent. In a report of 12 patients surviving emergency department thoracotomy with cross-clamping for as long as 60 minutes, there were no lasting impairments of renal, myocardial, or neurologic function.[185] Whenever possible, the aorta was unclamped for 30 to 60 seconds every 10 minutes to increase renal perfusion. Final release of the aorta is always performed gradually.

Treatment of Hypothermia

Prolonged resuscitation and the administration of cold crystalloid solutions or blood can lead to hypothermia in the traumatic and nontraumatic arrest situation. Under such conditions, core rewarming may be required prior to re-establishment of cardiac function.[155–157] Tap water at a temperature of 40°C can be infused directly about the heart and thorax during open chest cardiac compression to enhance rewarming. Sterile saline heated in a microwave oven to the same temperature is equally effective and somewhat more hygienic.

Complications

There are a variety of postoperative complications that may occur in patients surviving emer-

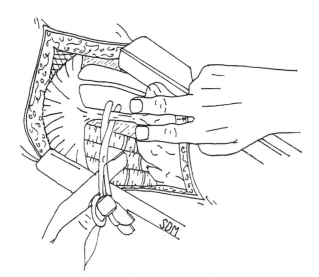

Figure 17–16. Adequate exposure of the descending aorta may require division of the inferior pulmonary ligament.

gency thoracotomy.[12, 16, 187, 188] Most of these complications stem from the particular injuries of each patient and must be considered on an individual basis. The complications of open chest resuscitation are relatively insignificant when compared with a fatal outcome. There are two post-thoracotomy complications that are frequently discussed. One is thoracic sepsis. This is a rare complication, and excessive concern with preparation may unnecessarily delay a thoracotomy. In a combined series of 142 emergency department thoracotomies there were no reports of wound infections.[38, 78, 170] It should be noted that most patients received antibiotics just before or during the procedure. Thus, the concern for infection as a complication of a thoracotomy performed with less than sterile technique is unwarranted, although a short course of antibiotics should be administered as soon as possible.

A second complication that is frequently feared and may actually deter a lifesaving thoracotomy is the threat that the patient will survive but will be in a vegetative neurologic state. This complication is also rare and such apprehension appears unjustified. Likewise, the concern of "tying up intensive care unit beds" with patients who have "fatal" injuries has been overemphasized. The first 24 hours following injury will rapidly separate those patients who will become long-term survivors; most patients with fatal injuries expire within 24 hours. The San Francisco experience with 168 emergency thoracotomies for mixed trauma illustrates this point.[189] Of those patients surviving the first 24 hours, 80 per cent (33 of 41) recovered and left the hospital. Full neurologic recovery occurred for 90 per cent of these survivors. Overall, only 2.4 per cent (4 of 168) remained severely disabled or in a persistent vegetative state. Of these four patients, only one (0.6 per cent) lived beyond 2 months; he eventually expired at 14 months from sepsis.

The report by Moore[15] in Denver describing 146 emergency thoracotomies for mixed trauma was comparable with the report from San Francisco. Moore reported 15 patients who survived the surgical repairs in the operating suite. Eighty per cent (12 of 15) of these patients went on to become long-term survivors; 75 per cent had full neurologic recovery. In the Denver study, two valuable observations were made regarding the presence or absence of various signs. First, all survivors with full neurologic recovery had respiratory efforts at the scene; in 75 per cent of these patients respiratory efforts were still present on arrival in the emergency care unit. Second, the presence or absence of a palpable pulse is not a reliable prognostic indicator. Sixty-six per cent of long-term survivors (11 penetrating cases and 1 blunt case) had no detectable pulse on arrival in the emergency care unit.

Conclusions

The recent advances in prehospital care have increased the number of patients requiring advanced resuscitation. For selected patients, an emergency thoracotomy will substantially reduce morbidity and mortality. The effectiveness of using this procedure for resuscitation has been well documented. The mechanism of injury and the status of vital signs "at the scene" and on arrival to the hospital should be considered before an emergency thoracotomy is performed. Victims of penetrating trauma who had any vital signs present at the scene are candidates for resuscitative thoracotomy and have a very good chance of survival. In contrast, the survival rates for victims of blunt trauma are negligible. With blunt trauma, resuscitative thoracotomy should be considered only when vital signs are still present on arrival to the emergency care unit. Following emergency thoracotomy, the systolic blood pressure after the first 30 minutes of resuscitation may be used as a decision point for further treatment. This response of blood pressure to thoracotomy applies to both blunt and penetrating trauma. With injuries of the heart, the lungs, and the great vessels, successful resuscitation will depend on rapid restoration of an effective blood volume and surgical intervention through a thoracotomy. The pathophysiology and treatment of those injuries that require resuscitative thoracotomy have been discussed. Pericardial tamponade, hemorrhagic shock, air embolism, and cardiac arrest may all require this procedure.

Debate over who should perform an emergency thoracotomy is not necessary. It stands to reason that whoever uses this resuscitative procedure must be prepared to manage the patient. Emergency physicians must possess the knowledge and skills necessary to enable the optimal survival of as many patients as possible. Whenever possible, a pre-established plan of chest wound management and post-thoracotomy care should be established with the emergency physician's surgical backup. With such a plan, a team approach to resuscitation and, hence, optimal patient care will be possible.

1. Mattox, K. L.: Emergency department thoracotomy (editorial). JACEP 7:455, 1978.
2. Denny, M. K.: Emergency department thoracotomy question raises larger issues. JACEP 8:385, 1979.
3. MacDonald, J. R.: Emergency department thoracotomy (correspondence). JACEP 8:441, 1979.
4. Page, J. R.: Emergency department thoracotomy (correspondence). JACEP 8:441, 1979.
5. Johnson, L. A.: Emergency department thoracotomy (correspondence). JACEP 8:441, 1979.
6. Mattox, K. L.: Emergency department thoracotomy (correspondence). JACEP 8:443, 1979.
7. MacDonald, F. R., and McDowell, R. M.: Emergency

department thoracotomies in a community hospital. JA-CEP 7:423, 1978.

8. Rosen, P., Baker, F. J., Braen, R. G., Daily, R. H., and Levy, R. C.: Emergency Medicine: Concepts and Clinical Practice. St. Louis, C. V. Mosby Co., 1983, p. 3.

9. Hirshman, J. C., Nussenfeld, S. R., and Nagel, E. L.: Mobile physician command: A new dimension in civilian telemetry-rescue systems. JAMA 230:255, 1974.

10. Cobb, L. A., Conn, R. D., and Samson, W. E.: Prehospital coronary care: The role of a rapid mobile intensive care system. Circulation 43 and 44 (Suppl. II):45, 1971.

11. American Medical Association: Recommendations of the Conferences on the Guidelines for the Categorization of Hospital Emergency Capabilities, Chicago, American Medical Association, 1971.

12. Sugg, W. L., Rea, W. J, Ecker, R. R., et al.: Penetrating wounds of the heart: An analysis of 459 cases. J. Thorac. Cardiovasc. Surg. 56:531, 1968.

13. Mattox, K. L., Espanda, R., Beall, A. C., et al.: Performing thoracotomy in the emergency center. JACEP 3:13, 1974.

14. Mattox, K. L., Beall, A. C., Jordan, G. L., et al.: Cardiorrhaphy in the emergency center. J. Thorac. Cardiovasc. Surg. 68:886, 1974.

15. Moore, E. E., Moore, J. B., Gallaway, A. C., et al.: Post injury thoracotomy in the emergency department—a critical evaluation. Surgery 86:590, 1979.

16. Baker, C. C., Thomas, A. N., and Trunkey, D. D.: The role of emergency room thoracotomy in trauma. J. Trauma 20:848, 1980.

17. Harnar, T. J., Oreskovich, M. R., Copass, M. K., et al.: Role of emergency thoracotomy in the resuscitation of moribund trauma victims. Am. J. Surg. 142:96, 1981.

18. Bodai, B. I., Mith, J. P., and Blaisdell, F. W. The role of emergency thoracotomy in blunt trauma. J. Trauma 22:487, 1982.

19. Flynn, T. C., Ward, R. E., and Miller, P. W.: Emergency department thoracotomy. Ann. Emerg. Med. 11:413, 1982.

20. Willimas, J. W., Beutler, E., Ersley, A. J., and Rundles, R. W.: Hematology, 2nd ed. New York, McGraw-Hill Book Co. 1977, p. 392.

21. Bodai, B. I., Smith, P. J., Ward, R. E., et al.: Emergency thoracotomy in the management of trauma. JAMA 249:1891, 1983.

22. Capplelen, A.: Vulnus cordis sutur of hjertet. Nord. Mag. f Laegenvid 11:285, 1896.

23. Farina, G.: Discussion (cited by Durante). Zentralbl. Chir. 23:1224, 1896.

24. Peek, C. H.: Operative treatment of heart wounds. Ann. Surg. 50:101, 1909.

25. Rehn, L.: Veber Penetriren den Herzwunden und Hertnacht. Arch. Chn. Chir. 55:315, 1897.

26. Bigger, I. A.: Heart wounds. J. Thorac. Surg. 8:239, 1939.

27. Bigger, I. A.: Diagnosis and treatment of heart wounds with summary of 34 cases. Med. Ann. Distr. Columbia 9:390, 1940.

28. Elkin, D. C.: Diagnosis and treatment of cardiac trauma. Ann. Surg. 114:169, 1941.

29. Elkin, D. C.: Wounds of the heart. Ann. Surg. 120:817, 1944.

30. Griswald, R. A., and Maguire, C. H.: Penetrating wounds of the heart and pericardium. Surg. Gynecol. Obstet. 74:406, 1946.

31. Nelson, H.: Penetrating wounds of the heart. Arch. Surg. 47:517, 1943.

32. Linder, H., and Hodo, H.: Stab wounds of the heart and pericardium. South. Med. J. 37:261, 1944.

33. Blau, M. H.: Wounds of the heart. Am. J. Med. Sci. 210:252, 1945.

34. Maynard, A. D. I., Cordice, J. W., and Naclerio, E. A.: Penetrating wounds of the heart. A report of 81 cases. Surg. Gynecol. Obstet. 94:605, 1952.

35. Beall, A. C., Diethrich, E. B., Crawford, H. W., et al.: Surgical management of penetrating cardiac injuries. Am. J. Surg. 112:686, 1966.

36. Reul, G. J. Beall, A. C., Jordan, G. L., and Mattox, K. L.: The early operative management of injuries to the great vessels. Surgery 74:862, 1973.

37. Beall, A. C., Diethrich, E. B., Cooley, D. A., and DeBakey, M. E.: Surgical management of penetrating cardiovascular trauma. South. Med. J. 60:698, 1967.

38. Siemens, R., Polk, M. C., Jr., et al.: Indications for thoracotomy following penetrating thoracic injury. J. Trauma 17:493, 1977.

39. Beall, A. C., Bricker, D. L., Crawford, H. W., Noon, G. P., and DeBakey, M. E.: Considerations in the management of penetrating thoracic trauma. J. Trauma 8:408, 1968.

40. Oparah, S. S., and Mandal, A. K.: Operative management of penetrating wounds of the chest in civilian practice. Review of indications in 125 cases. J. Thorac. Carciovasc. Surg. 77:162, 1979.

41. Oparah, S. S., and Mandall, A. K.: Penetrating wounds of the chest—experience with 200 consecutive cases. J. Trauma 16:868, 1976.

42. Karrel, R., Shaffer, M. A., and Franasek, J. B.: Emergency diagnosis, resuscitation and treatment of acute penetrating cardiac trauma. Ann. Emerg. Med. 11:504, 1982.

43. Symbas, P. N.: Trauma to the Heart and the Great Vessels. New York, Grune and Stratton, 1976, p. 17.

44. Tassi, A., and Davies, A. L.: Pericardial tamponade due to penetrating fragment wounds of the heart. Am. J. Surg. 118:535, 1969.

45. Carrasguilla, C., Wilson, R. F., Wait, A. F., et al.: Gunshot wounds of the heart. Ann. Thorac. Surg. 13:208, 1972.

46. Asfaw, I., and Austin, A.: Penetrating wounds of the pericardium and heart. Surg. Clin. North Am. 57:37, 1977.

47. Beach, P. M., Bognolo, E., and Hutchison, J. E.: Penetrating cardiac trauma—experience with 34 patients in hospital without cardiopulmonary bypass capability. Am. J. Surg. 131:411, 1976.

48. Spodick, D.: Acute cardiac tamponade: Pathophysiology, diagnosis, and management. Prog. Cardiovasc. Dis. 10:64, 1967.

49. Evans, J., Gray, L. A., Rayner, A., et al.: Principles for the management of penetrating cardiac wounds. Ann. Surg. 189:777, 1979.

50. Symbas, P. N., Harlaffis, N., and Waldo, W. J.: Penetrating cardiac wounds. A comparison of different therapeutic methods. Ann. Surg. 183–377, 1976.

51. Broja, A. R., and Ransell, H. T.: Treatment of penetrating gunshot wounds of the chest: Experience with 145 cases. Am. J. Surg. 122:81, 1971.

52. Shoemaker, W. C., Carey, J. S., Yao, S. T., et al.: Hemodynamic alterations in acute cardiac tamponade after penetrating injuries of the heart. Surgery 67:754, 1970.

53. Beall, A. C., Ochsner J. L., Morris G. C., et al: Penetrating wounds of the heart. J. Trauma 1:195, 1961.

54. Naclerio, E. A.: Penetrating wounds of the heart—experience with 249 patients. Dis. Chest 46:1, 1964.

55. Wilson, R. F., and Basset, J. S.: Penetrating wounds of the pericardium and its contents. JAMA 195:513, 1966.

56. Carey, J. S., Yao, S. T., Kho, L. K., et al.: Cardiovascular responses to hemopericardium, compression by balloon tamponade and acute coronary occlusion. J. Thorac. Cardiovasc. Surg. 54:65, 1967.

57. Isaacs, J. P., Bergulund, E., and Sarnoff, S. J.: Ventricular function III. Pathologic physiology of acute cardiac tamponade studied by means of ventricular function curves. Am. Heart J. 28:66, 1954.

58. Friedman, H. S., Gomers, J. A., Tardio, A. R., et al.: The electrocardiographic features of acute cardiac tamponade. Circulation 50:260, 1974.

59. Jarisch, A., and Zotterman, Y.: Depressor reflexes from the heart. Acta Physiol. Scand. 16:31, 1948.

60. Coleridge, H. M., Coleridge, J. C. G., and Kidd, C.: Cardiac receptors of the dog with particular reference to two types of afferent endings in the ventricular wall. J. Physiol. 174:323, 1964.

61. Brown, A. M.: The depressor reflex arising from the left coronary artery of the cat. J. Physiol. 184:825, 1966.

62. Sleight, P., and Widdicomb, J. G.: Action potentials in fibers from receptors in the epicardium and myocardium of the dog's left ventricle. J. Physiol. 181:235, 1965.

63. Bolanowski, P. J. D., Swaminathan, A. D., and Neville, W. E.: Aggressive surgical management of penetrating cardiac injuries. J. Thorac. Cardiovasc. Surg. 66:1, 1973.

64. DeGowin, E. L., and Degowin, R. L.: Bedside Diagnostic Examination, 3rd ed. New York, Macmillan Publishing Co., Inc., 1976, p. 396.

65. Pories, W., and Guadiani, V.: Cardiac tamponade. Surg. Clin. North Am. 55:573, 1975.

66. Kussmaul, A.: Uber Schwielige mediastino-pericarditis und den paradoxen. Puls. Klin. Wochenschr. 10:433, 1873.

67. Dornhorst, A. C., Howard, P., and Leathart, A. I.: Pulsus paradoxus. Lancet 1:476, 1952.

68. Roe, B. B.: Cardiac trauma including injury of the great vessels. Surg. Clin. North Am. 52:573, 1972.

69. Beall, A. C., and Wilson, R. F.: Penetrating wounds of the heart: Changing patterns of surgical management (correspondence). J. Trauma 12:6, 1972.

70. Shoemaker, W. C.: Algorithm for early recognition and management of cardiac tamponade. Crit. Care Med. 3:59, 1975.

71. Trinkle, J. K., Marcos, J., Grover, F. L., et al.: Management of the wounded heart. Ann. Thorac. Surg. 17:230, 1974.

72. Galen, R. S.: Predictive value of laboratory testing. Pediatr. Clin. North Am. 27:861, 1980.

73. Galen, R. S., and Gambino, S. R.: Beyond Normality: The Predictive Value and Efficiency of Medical Diagnoses. New York, John Wiley & Sons, 1975.

74. Griner, P. F., Mayewski, R. J., Mushlin, A. I., and Greenland, P.: Test selection and use. Ann. Intern. Med. 94(Part 2):599, 1981.

75. Griner, P. F., Mayewski, R. J. Mushlin, A. I., and Greenland, P.. Principles of test interpretation. Ann. Intern. Med. 94 (part 2):565, 1981.

76. Trinkle, J. K., Toon, R. S., Franz, J. L., et al.. Affairs of the wounded heart: Penetrating cardiac wounds. J. Trauma 19:467, 1979.

77. Blalock, A., and Ravitch, M. M.: A consideration of the nonoperative treatment of cardiac tamponade resulting from wounds of the heart. Surgery 14:157, 1943.

78. Mattox, K. L., Von Kock, L., Beall, A. C., Jr., et al.: Logistic and technical considerations in the treatment of the wounded heart. Circulation 51,52:210, 1975.

79. DeGennaro, V. A., Bonfils-Roberts, E. A., Ching, N., et al.: Aggressive management of potential penetrating cardiac injuries. J. Thorac. Cardiovasc. Surg. 79:833, 1980.

80. Breaux, E. P., Dupont, J. B., Albert, H. M., et al.: Cardiac tamponade following penetrating mediastinal injuries: Improved survival with early pericardiocentesis. J. Trauma 19:461, 1979.

81. Arom, K. V., Richardson, J. D., Webb, G., et al.: Subxiphoid pericardial window in patients with suspected traumatic pericardial tamponade. Ann. Thorac. Surg. 23:545, 1977.

82. Bertelsen, S., and Howitz, P.: Injuries of the trachea and bronchi. Thorax 27:188, 1972.

83. Hood, R. M., and Sloan, H. E.: Injuries of the trachea and major bronchi. J. Thorac. Cardiovasc. Surg. 38:458, 1959.

84. Guest, J. L., and Anderson, J. N.: Major airway injury in closed chest trauma. Chest 72:63, 1977.

85. Rutherford, R. B., Hurt, H. H., Brickman, R. D., and Tubb, J. M.: The pathophysiology and treatment of progressive tension pneumothorax. J. Trauma 8:212, 1968.

86. Schwartz, G. R., and Wagner, D. J.: Emergency therapy: Penetrating trauma to the chest, heart, and great vessels. JACEP 2:196, 1973.

87. Borja, A. R., and Ransdell, H.: Treatment of thoracoabdominal gunshot wounds in civilian practice: Experience with 44 cases. Am. J. Surg. 121:580, 1971.

88. Yee, E. S., Verrie, E. D., and Thomas, A. N.: Management of air embolism in blunt, and penetrating thoracic trauma. J. Thorac. Cardiovasc. Surg. 85:661, 1983.

89. Thomas, N. A., and Stephens, G. B.: Air embolism: A cause of morbidity and death after penetrating chest trauma. J. Trauma 14:633, 1974.

90. Graham, M. J., Beall, C. A., Mattox, K. L., et al.: Systemic air embolism following penetrating trauma to the lung. Chest 72:449, 1977.

91. Flanagan, J. P., Frandisaria, I. A., Gross, R. J., et al.: Air embolism—a lethal complication of subclavian venipuncture. N Engl. J. Med. 281:488, 1969.

92. Doblar, D. D., Hinkel, J. C., Fay, M. L., et al.: Air embolism associated with pulmonary artery catheter introducer kit. Anesthesiology 53:307, 1982.

93. Thomas, A. N., and Roe, B. B.: Air embolism following penetrating lung injuries. J. Thorac. Cardiovasc. Surg. 66:553, 1973.

94. Goldstone, J., Towan, H. J., and Ellis, R. J.: Rationale for use of vasopressors in treatment of coronary air embolism. Surg. Forum 29:237, 1978.

95. Meier, G. H., and Symbas, P. N.: Systemic air embolization; factors involved in its production following penetrating lung injury. Am. J. Surg. 12:765, 1978.

96. Meier, G. H. Wood, W. J., and Symbas, P. N.: Systemic air embolization from penetrating lung injury. Ann. Thorac. Surg. 27:161, 1978.

97. Halpern, P., Greenstein, A., Malamed, Y., et al.: Arterial air embolism after penetrating lung injury. Crit. Care Med. 11:392, 1983.

98. Peirce, E. C.: Specific therapy for arterial air embolism. Ann. Thorac. Surg. 29:300, 1980.

99. Tomatis, L., Nemiroff, M., Riahi, M., et al.: Massive arterial air embolism due to rupture of pulsatile assist device: Successful treatment in the hyperbaric chamber. Ann. Thorac. Surg. 32:604, 1981.

100. Warren, P. A., Phillips, R. B., and Inwood, M. J. The ultrastructural morphology of air embolism platelet adhesion to the interface and endothelial damage. Br. J. Exp. Pathol. 54:163, 1973.

101. Dicthrich, E. B., Koopot, R., Maze, A., and Dyess, N.: Successful reversal of brain damage from iatrogenic air embolism. Surg. Gynecol. Obstet. 154:572, 1982.

102. Mills, N. L., and Ochsner, J. L.: Massive air embolism during cardiopulmonary bypass. J. Thorac. Cardiovasc. Surg. 80:708, 1980.

103. Marvoudis, C., Roon, A. J., Baker, C., et al.: Management of acute cervicothoracic vascular injuries. J. Thorac. Cardiovasc. Surg. 80:342, 1980.

104. Brotmans, S., Oster-Granite, M., and Cox, E. F.: Failure of cross clamping the thoracic aorta to control intra-abdominal bleeding. Ann. Emerg. Med. 11:147, 1982.

105. Sankaran, S., Lucas, C., and Walt, A. J.: Thoracic aortic clamping for prophylaxis against sudden cardiac arrest during laparotomy for acute massive hemoperitoneum. J. Trauma 15:290, 1975.

106. Ledgerwood, A. M., Krazmers, M., and Lucas, E. C.: The role of thoracic aortic occlusion for massive hemoperitoneum. J. Trauma 16:610, 1976.

107. Parmley, L. F., Marion, W. C., and Mattingly, T. W.: Nonpenetrating traumatic injury of the heart. Circulation 18:371, 1958.

108. Bodily, K., Perry, J. F., Strat, R. G., et al.: The salvageability of patients with post-traumatic rupture of the descending thoracic aorta in a primary trauma center. J. Trauma 17:754, 1977.

109. Greedyke, R. M.: Traumatic rupture of the aorta. JAMA 195:119, 1966.

110. Commack, K., Rapport, R. L., Paul, J., and Baird, W. C.:

Deceleration injuries of the thoracic aorta. Arch. Surg. 79:244, 1959.

111. Pickard, L. R., Mattox, K. L., Espanada, R., et al.: Transection of the descending thoracic aorta secondary to blunt trauma. J. Trauma 17:749, 1977.

112. Simeone, J. F., Deren, M. M., and Cagle, F.: The value of the left apical cap in the diagnosis of aortic rupture. Diag. Radiol. 139:35, 1981.

113. Gundry, S. R., Burnery, R. E., Mackenzie, J. R., et al.: Assessment of mediastinal widening associated with traumatic rupture of the aorta. J. Trauma 23:293, 1983.

114. Marsh, D. G., and Sturm, J. T.: Traumatic aortic rupture: Roentgenographic indications for angiography. Ann. Thorac. Surg. 21:337, 1976.

115. Cole, D. C., Knopp, R., Wales, L. R., et al.: Nasogastric tube displacement to the right as a sign of acute traumatic rupture of the thoracic aorta. Ann. Emerg. Med. 10:623, 1981.

116. Symbas, P. N., Tyras, D. H., Ware, R. E., et al.: Traumatic rupture of the aorta. Ann. Surg. 178:6, 1973.

117. Kirsh, M. M., Crane, J. D., Kahn, D. R., et al.: Roentgenographic evaluation of traumatic rupture of the aorta. Surg. Gynecol. Obstet. 131:900, 1970.

118. Peters, D. R., and Gansu, G.: Displacement of the right paraspinous interface: A radiographic sign of acute traumatic rupture of the aorta. Radiology 134:599, 1980.

119. Ayella, R. J., Hankins, J. R., Turney, S. Z., et al.: Ruptured thoracic aorta due to blunt trauma. J. Trauma 17:199, 1977.

120. Babbs, C. F.: A renaissance of CPR research. Crit. Care Med. 8:119, 1980.

121. Kouwenhoven, W. B., Jude, J. R., and Knickerbocker, G. G.: Closed-chest cardiac massage. JAMA 173:94, 1960.

122. Ditchey, R. V., Winkler, J. V., and Rhodes, C. A.: Relative lack of coronary blood flow during closed-chest resuscitation in dogs. Circulation 66:297, 1982.

123. Niemann, J. T., Rosborough, J. P., Ung, S., et al.: Coronary perfusion pressure during experimental cardiopulmonary resuscitation. Ann. Emerg. Med. 11:127, 1982.

124. Luce, J. M., Ross, B. K., O'Quinn, R. J., et al.: Regional blood flow during cardiopulmonary resuscitation in dogs using simultaneous and nonsimultaneous compression and ventilation. Circulation 67:258, 1983.

125. Bircher, N., Safar, P., and Stewart, R.: A comparison of standard, "MAST"-augmented, and open-chest CPR in dogs. Crit. Care Med. 8:147, 1980.

126. Bircher, N., and Safar, P.: Comparison of standard and "new" closed-chest CPR and open-chest CPR in dogs. Crit. Care Med. 9:384, 1981.

127. Byrne, D., Pass, H. I., Neely, W. A., et al.: External versus internal cardiac massage in normal and chronically ischemic dogs. Am. Surg. 46:657, 1980.

128. Babbs, C. F.: Knowledge gaps in CPR. Crit. Care Med. 8:181, 1980.

129. Criley, J. M., Niemann, J. T., Rosborough, J. P., et al.: The heart is a conduit in CPR. Crit. Care Med. 9:373, 1981.

130. Weisfeldt, M. L., Chandra, N., and Tsitlik, J.: Increased intrathoracic pressure—not direct heart compression—causes the rise in intrathoracic vascular pressures during CPR in dogs and pigs. Crit. Care Med. 9:377, 1981.

131. Babbs, C. F.: New versus old theories of blood flow during CPR. Crit. Care Med. 8:191, 1980.

132. Chandra, N., Guerci, A., Weisfeldt, M. L., et al.: Contrasts between intrathoracic pressures during external chest compression and cardiac massage. Crit. Care Med. 9:789, 1981.

133. Rudikoff, M. T., Maughan, W. L., Effron, M., et al.: Mechanisms of blood flow during cardiopulmonary resuscitation. Circulation 61:345, 1980.

134. Niemann, J. T., Rosborough, J. P., Hausknecht, M., et al.: Pressure-synchronized cineangiography during experimental cardiopulmonary resuscitation. Circulation 64:985, 1981.

135. Kovach, A. G. B., and Sandor, P.: Cerebral blood flow and brain function during hypotension and shock. Annu. Rev. Physiol. 38:571, 1976.

136. Jackson, R. E., Joyce, K., White, B., et al.: Blood flow in the cerebral cortex during cardiac resuscitation in dogs. Ann. Emerg. Med. 12:257, 1983.

137. Szczygiel, M., Wright, R., Wagner, E., et al.: Prognostic indicators of ultimate long-term survival following advanced life support. Ann. Emerg. Med. 10:566, 1981.

138. DeBard, M.: Cardiopulmonary resuscitation: Analysis of six years' experience and review of the literature. Ann. Emerg. Med. 10:408, 1981.

139. Eisenberg, M., Bergner, L., and Hallstrom, A.: Cardiac resuscitation in the community. JAMA 241:1905, 1979.

140. Eliastam, M., Duralde, T., Martinez, F., et al.: Cardiac arrest in the emergency medical service system: Guidelines for resuscitation. JACEP 6:525, 1977.

141. Eliastam, M.: When to stop cardiopulmonary resuscitation. In Bander, J. J., et al. (eds.): Cardiac Arrest and CPR. Rockville, MD, Aspen Systems Corp., 1980, p. 161.

142. Jeresaty, R. M., Godar, T. J., and Liss, J. P.: External cardiac resuscitation in a community hospital. Arch. Intern. Med. 124:588, 1969.

143. Bartlett, R. L., Raymond, J. I., Anstadt, G. L., et al.: Clinical research: Use of direct mechanical ventricular assistance in cardiopulmonary resuscitation. Richland Memorial Hospital Investigational Review Board, Columbia, S.C., 1982.

144. Stephenson, H. E.: An increasing role for surgeons in cardiac resuscitation. Surg. Gynecol. Obstet. 152:822, 1981.

145. Barsan, W. G., and Levy, R. C.: Experimental design for study of cardiopulmonary resuscitation in dogs. Ann. Emerg. Med. 10:135, 1981.

146. Weiser, F. M., Adler, L. N., and Kuhn, L. A.: Hemodynamic effects of closed and open chest cardiac resuscitation in normal dogs and those with acute myocardial infarction. Am. J. Cardiol. 10:555, 1962.

147. Del Guercio, L. R. M., Coomarswamy, R. P., and State, D.: Cardiac output and other hemodynamic variables during external cardiac massage in man. New Engl. J. Med. 269:1398, 1963.

148. Del Guercio, L. R. M., Feins, N. R., Cohn, J. D., et al.: Comparison of blood flow during external and internal cardiac massage in man. Circulation 31 (Suppl. 1):171, 1965.

149. Cohn, J. D., and Del Guercio, L. R. M.: Cardiorespiratory analysis of cardiac arrest and resuscitation. Surg. Gynecol. Obstet. 23:1066, 1966.

150. Redding, J. S., and Cozine, R. A.: A comparison of open-chest and closed-chest cardiac massage in dogs. Anesthesiology 22:280, 1961.

151. Bartlett, R. L., Stewart, N. J., Raymond, J. I., and Martin, S. D.: A comparative study of closed and open resuscitation: effects on survival and neurologic damage. (Submitted for publication).

152. Longstreth, W. T., Diehr, P., and Inui, T. S.: Prediction of awakening after out-of-hospital cardiac arrest. N. Engl. J. Med. 308:1378, 1983.

153. Miller, J. W., Danzl, D. F., and Thomas, D. M.: Urban accidental hypothermia: 135 cases. Ann. Emerg. Med. 9:456, 1980.

154. Wickstrom, P., Ruix, E., Lija, G. P., et al.: Accidental hypothermia. Am. J. Surg. 131:622, 1976.

155. Truscott, D. G., Firor, W. B., and Clein, L. J.: Accidental profound hypothermia. Arch. Surg. 106:216, 1973.

156. Althaus, U., Aeberhard, P., Schupbach, P., et al.: Management of profound accidental hypothermia with cardiorespiratory arrest. Ann. Surg. 195:492, 1982.

157. Shocket, E., and Rosenblum, R.: Successful open cardiac

massage after 75 minutes of closed massage. JAMA 200:157, 1967.

158. Sykes, M. K., and Ahmed, N.: Emergency treatment of cardiac arrest. Lancet 2:347, 1963.

159. Bayer, M. J.: Emergency thoracotomy and internal cardiac massage. Topics Emerg. Med., 1979, p. 95.

160. Castagna, J., Weil, M. H., and Shubin, H.: Factors determining survival in patients with cardiac arrest. Chest 65:527, 1974.

161. Iseri, L. T., Siner, E. J., Humphrey, S. B., and Mann, S.: Prehospital cardiac arrest after arrival of the paramedic unit. JACEP 6:530, 1977.

162. Wilson, R. F., Gibson, D. B., and Antonenko, D.: Shock and acute respiratory failure after chest trauma. J. Trauma 17:697, 1971.

163. Bricker, D. L., Morton, J. R., Okies, J. E., et al.: Surgical management of injuries to vena cava—changing patterns of injury and newer techniques of repair. J. Trauma 11:725, 1971.

164. Dronen, S. C., Yee, A. S., and Tomlanovich, M. C.: Proximal saphenous vein cutdown. Ann. Emerg. Med. 10:328, 1981.

165. Knopp, R.: Venous cutdowns in the emergency department. JACEP 7:439, 1978.

166. Mateer, J. R., Thompson, B. M., Aprahamion, C., et al.: Rapid fluid resuscitation with central venous catheters. Ann. Emerg. Med. 12:149, 1983.

167. Wilson, R. F., Mammen, B., and Walt, A. J.: Eight years of experience with massive blood transfusion. J. Trauma 11:275, 1971.

168. Harrigan, C., Lucas, C., and Ledgerwood, A.: Significance of hypocalcemia following hypovolemic shock. J. Trauma 23:488, 1983.

169. Young, G. P.: Emergency autotransfusion. Ann. Emerg. Med. 12:180, 1983.

170. Reul, G. J., Mattox, K. L., Beall, A. C., et al.: Recent advances in the operative management of massive chest trauma. Ann. Thorac. Surg. 16:52, 1973.

171. Snow, N., Lucas, A. E.: Subxiphoid pericardiotomy. Am. Surg. 49:249, 1983.

172. Santos, G. H., and Frater, R. W. M.: The subxiphoid in the treatment of pericardial effusion. Ann. Thorac. Surg. 23:467, 1977.

173. Alcan, K. E., Zabetakis, P. M., Marino, N. D., et al.: Management of acute cardiac tamponade by subxiphoid pericardiotomy. JAMA 247:1143, 1982.

174. Johnson, J., and Kirby, C. K.: An experimental study of cardiac massage. Surgery 26:472, 1949.

175. Stephenson, H. E.: Cardiac Arrest and Resuscitation, 4th ed. St. Louis, C. V. Mosby, 1974.

176. Barlett, R. L., Stewart, N. J., Raymond, J. I., and Martin, S. D.: Open chest resuscitation: The relationship of compression rate to cardiac output and blood pressure (submitted for publication).

177. Cooper, P.: The Craft of Surgery, 2nd ed., vol. 1. Boston, Little, Brown & Co., 1971, pp. 29–31.

178. McQuillan, R. F., McCormack, T., and Heligan, M. C.: Penetrating left ventricular stab wound: A method of control during resuscitation and prior to repair. Injury 12:63, 1980.

179. Levitsky, S.: New insights in cardiac trauma. Surg. Clin. North Am. 55:43, 1975.

180. Pearce, C. W., McCool, E., and Schimdt, F. E.: Control of bleeding from cardiovascular wounds. Ann. Surg. 163:257, 1966.

181. Reul, G. J., Beall, A. C., Jordan, G. L., and Mattox, K. L.: The early operative management of injuries to the great vessels. Surgery 74:862, 1973.

182. Hoffman, J. R.: Emergency department thoracotomy. Ann. Emerg. Med. 10:275, 1981.

183. Feliciano, D. V., and Mattox, K. L.: Indications, technique, and pitfalls of emergency center thoracotomy. Surg. Rounds, Dec. 1981, p. 32.

184. Dunn, E. L., Moore, E. E., and Moore, J. B.: Hemodynamic effects of aortic occlusion during hemorrhagic shock. Ann. Emerg. Med. 11:238, 1982.

185. Garcia-Rinaldi, R., Defore, W. W., Mattox, K. L., and Beall, A. C.: Unimpaired renal, myocardial and neurologic function after cross clamping of the thoracic aorta. Surg. Gynecol. Obstet. 143:249, 1976.

186. Kerber, R. E., Carter, J., Klein, S., et al.: Open chest defibrillation during cardiac surgery. Am. J. Cardiol. 46:393, 1980.

187. Symbas, P. N., Diorio, D. A., Tyras, D. H., et al.: Penetrating cardiac wounds—significant residual and delayed sequelae. J. Thorac. Cardiovasc. Surg. 66:526, 1973.

188. Heller, R. F., Rahimtolla, S. H., Ehsani, A., et al.: Cardiac complications—results of penetrating chest wounds including the heart. Arch. Intern. Med. 134:491, 1974.

189. Baker, C. C., Caronna, J. J., and Trunkey, D. D.: Neurologic outcome after emergency room thoracotomy for trauma. Am. J. Surg. 139:677, 1980.

190. Molokhia, F. A., Ponn, B. A., and Robinson, W. J.: A method of augmenting coronary perfusion during internal massage. Chest 62:610, 1972.

3

VASCULAR ACCESS AND ADMINISTRATION OF FLUIDS

18

Vascular Access and Blood Sampling Techniques in Infants and Children

RICHARD L. SCHREINER, M.D.
JAMES A. LEMONS, M.D.
THOMAS R. WEBER, M.D.

Capillary Blood Sampling

Many clinicians are not experienced in the technique of venous or arterial puncture in infants. There is a limit to the number of times that small arteries and veins can be successfully entered; there also are fewer such vessels available in small infants compared with older children and adults. Because of these limitations, heel punctures are frequently performed in small infants. This section will discuss the proper technique of heel stick puncture for routine blood sampling and how it relates specifically to the procurement of "arterialized" blood for blood gas analysis. The technique described also applies to capillary blood sampling from finger, toe, and ear lobe sites in older children.

Capillary blood can also be used to produce a blood smear for obtaining a white blood count and differential as well as for red cell and platelet analysis. The blood collected in a capillary tube may also be spun to obtain a hematocrit. The use of blood chemistry devices analyzing small sample sizes permits determination of most routine blood chemistries from capillary blood.

INDICATIONS AND CONTRAINDICATIONS

Capillary blood sampling is indicated whenever an adequate sample of blood can be obtained for analysis by the puncture technique and when an alternative technique (e.g., indwelling arterial line) is not more readily available. The technique is most appropriate for patients requiring repeated venous or arterial sampling. Judicious use of the technique minimizes vascular trauma from repeated vessel puncture.

Sampling from an area of inflammation should be avoided. Repetitive sampling from the same site may induce inflammation and subsequent scarring and hence should be avoided. In general, heel stick sampling is *not* ideal for blood gas analysis in the following situations: (1) when the infant is hypotensive; (2) when the heel is markedly bruised; or (3) when there is evidence of peripheral vasoconstriction. In addition, when the capillary P_{O_2} is greater than 60 mm Hg, the arterial P_{O_2} may be considerably higher, with possibly dangerous consequences to infants receiving supplemental oxygen. In this situation, either an arterial P_{O_2} should be obtained or the $F_{I_{O_2}}$ should be decreased and another capillary sample obtained for P_{O_2} determination.

PROCEDURE

A 3-mm lancet should be used to perform this procedure; a scalpel blade should never be used. After the heel is cleansed with alcohol and allowed to dry, the skin is punctured with the lancet on the lateral or medial portion[1] of the plantar surface of the heel (anterior to the posterior margin of the heel) (Fig. 18–1). The use of a 3-mm lancet will prevent the puncture from penetrating more than the maximum safe distance. The full 3 mm of the lancet should be used; a more superficial incision will not bleed adequately. Prewarming the foot in a hot towel will produce hyperemia and will enhance blood flow. Squeezing of the foot should be avoided, since this may inhibit capillary filling and may actually decrease blood flow. Furthermore, squeezing may dilute the sample with serum or tissue fluid and may make analysis less accurate. If blood does not flow freely, another puncture may be required.

The first small drop of blood is wiped away with gauze, and another drop is allowed to form.

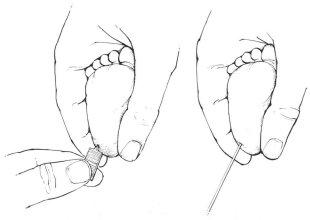

Figure 18–1. The heel stick is performed on the lateral or medial aspect of the heel. Blood is allowed to flow into the capillary tube, thereby avoiding air bubbles.

A heparinized capillary tube is placed in the drop of blood, and the tube is allowed to fill by capillary action. The tube (or tubes, if several tests will be needed) is sealed at one end before being sent to the laboratory. A dry dressing is applied to the puncture site.

When a heel stick is performed for arterialized blood samples, the technique used is similar to that discussed previously for routine blood sampling, with the following differences: The infant's foot *must* be wrapped with a warm cloth for a few minutes. The first drop of blood *must* be discarded and the remaining blood allowed to flow freely into a heparinized capillary tube. The tip of the tube should be placed as near the puncture site as possible to minimize exposure of the blood to environmental oxygen. Collection of air in the tube as well as excessive squeezing of the foot should be avoided, because this may artificially lower the PO_2. Approximately 0.2 to 0.3 ml of blood should be collected in the heparinized capillary tube.

COMPLICATIONS

When properly performed, heel sticks are associated with a low incidence of complications. Lacerations should not occur when the procedure is performed with a lancet rather than a scalpel blade. Heel sticks may cause infection (local infection, bacteremia,[2] or osteomyelitis[3]), scarring, and calcified nodules.[4] When the heel stick technique is used for the procurement of "arterialized" blood for pH, PCO_2, and PO_2 analysis, the most important potential error is that false information (inaccurate PO_2) may result in the exposure of the infant to improper amounts of supplemental oxygen.

INTERPRETATION

Numerous studies have compared the reliability of the capillary blood with that of arterial blood for determination of pH, PCO_2, and PO_2. Although the results have been quite variable,[5-10] most investigations have documented a close correlation between the arterial and capillary samples for pH and PCO_2 determinations (except when the patient is in shock or has an extremely high PCO_2). Unfortunately, the PO_2 determination has not been found to be as reliable when performed on blood obtained by capillary or "arterialized" sampling. Most studies indicate that the capillary (heel stick) PO_2 correlates poorly with the arterial PO_2, especially if the arterial PO_2 is greater than 60 mm Hg. For example, a capillary PO_2 of 70 mm Hg may reflect an arterial PO_2 of 70 to 200 mm Hg. In nearly all situations, the capillary PO_2 is equal to or less than the arterial PO_2, but in any individual case, one does not know how closely the capillary value approximates the arterial level. Therefore reliance on a capillary sample of blood for PO_2 measurement in an acutely sick infant may be fraught with potential risks. "Arterialized" blood samples obtained from finger and toe sticks might be more reliable for PO_2 determination than those obtained from heel sticks, but the data are controversial.[11-14]

Venous Sampling and Catheterization

VENIPUNCTURE

Although many laboratory tests for the small infant may be performed on blood obtained by heel sticks, a larger volume of blood than is obtainable by heel stick may be necessary. Venipuncture is the usual method used for obtaining large quantities of blood as well as samples for blood culture. In an emergency, blood for laboratory analysis may alternatively be obtained from an arterial puncture.

Procedure

Sites that are reasonably accessible for obtaining venous blood include the antecubital veins (Fig. 18–2), the external jugular veins, or any easily visible peripheral vein (e.g., on the scalp, the hands, or the feet). If an extremity vein is to be used, a tourniquet should be applied proximal to the selected vein; in small infants, a rubber band will serve as an adequate tourniquet, but one must be certain to remove the rubber band following venipuncture. The tourniquet should not be so tight that arterial filling is obstructed. The area surrounding the planned site of penetration of the skin is cleaned with alcohol. An appropriately sized syringe (approximately 3 ml) is attached to

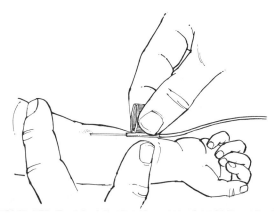

Figure 18–2. Technique for obtaining blood by antecubital venipuncture with a butterfly needle and a syringe. Once blood is obtained, the butterfly needle may serve as an infusion site.

a butterfly scalp vein needle (usually 21 to 25 gauge). A small gauge butterfly needle is usually preferred over a needle and syringe for obtaining blood in infants. It is difficult to manipulate standard needles and syringes in tiny veins, and better control is obtained with the butterfly needle. Suction is also more controlled with the butterfly needle and syringe. The butterfly needle may also serve as an infusion line once adequate amounts of blood are obtained. If a straight needle and syringe are used, the technique is similar to that described later for percutaneous arterial puncture, except that a peripheral vein is punctured.

Once the needle penetrates the skin, one must apply suction by gently and slowly withdrawing the plunger of the syringe. If the suction is excessive, the vein will collapse and blood flow will stop. If a butterfly or scalp vein needle technique is used, the procedure is similar to that described later for placement of a peripheral intravenous line. An assistant can help attach the syringe to the catheter of the butterfly needle apparatus and can withdraw the blood while the physician concentrates on keeping the needle within the vein and immobilizing the arm. After the required amount of blood is withdrawn, the needle is removed, and a sterile dressing is applied to the skin.

It should be emphasized that immobilization of the extremity is mandatory. Prior stabilization of the extremity on a board is especially important if the butterfly scalp vein needle is to be used for subsequent infusion.

The external jugular vein also may be used in infants for the performance of a venipuncture. The vein lies in a line from the angle of the jaw to the middle of the clavicle and is usually visible on the surface of the skin. The vein is more prominent when the baby is crying. An assistant is needed to restrain the infant in a supine position with the head and neck extended over the edge of the bed. The head is turned approximately 40 to 70 degrees from the midline (Fig. 18–3), and the skin surrounding the area to be punctured is cleaned with alcohol. A finger may be placed just above the clavicle to distend the jugular vein. Using a 21 to 25 gauge straight needle with a syringe, a 21 to 25 gauge butterfly scalp vein needle attached to a syringe, or a 19 to 23 gauge plastic catheter (Angiocath, Medicut, or another similar catheter), the clinician punctures the skin and advances the needle slowly until the jugular vein is entered. The syringe is connected to the needle or the catheter at all times to maintain a constant negative pressure in order to avoid air embolism. After the appropriate amount of blood is obtained, the needle is withdrawn and slight pressure is applied to the vessel. The infant should be placed in an upright position after the needle is removed, and

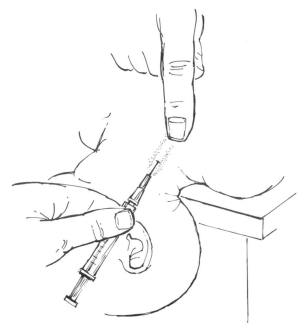

Figure 18–3. External jugular venipuncture. Either a syringe or a butterfly needle may be used. This vein becomes distended when the infant cries.

slight pressure should be continued for 3 to 5 minutes. Close observation of the puncture site should follow.

Complications

Complications of venipuncture include hematoma formation, local infection, injury to structures adjacent to vessels, and phlebitis. All of these complications are uncommon. Special care should be used when puncture of the external jugular vein is attempted. Inadvertent deep puncture in the neck can produce injury to the carotid artery, the vagus or phrenic nerve, or the apex of the lung. Such structures are unlikely to be injured if proper technique is practiced, however.

BLOOD CULTURES

Although the heel stick procedure has been used in some centers for the procurement of blood from infants for cultures,[15, 16] there is a significant incidence of false positive results with the technique, and therefore it is not generally recommended if venous blood is available. Venipunctures continue to be the main source of blood for culture in small infants. In the newborn infant, blood may be obtained for culture from an umbilical arterial or venous catheter, if it is obtained immediately after sterile insertion; even then, there is considerable controversy concerning the incidence of false positive cultures.

Procedure

The technique of venipuncture for a blood culture is similar to that described previously for general blood sampling, with the following differences: The puncture site should be doubly prepared, first with a povidine-iodine solution and then with alcohol. (Following completion of the procedure, all of the iodine solution should be removed from the infant's skin to prevent irritation.) The volume of blood required for a blood culture depends upon the size of the infant. In the neonate with bacteremia there is a greater number of organisms per milliliter of blood;[17] a sample size of 0.5 to 1 ml is probably sufficient. In older infants, 2 to 3 ml of blood is ideal. After the appropriate volume of blood is withdrawn, the needle that was used to penetrate the skin is removed, and a sterile needle is attached to the syringe. Half of the specimen should be placed in an anaerobic culture bottle and half in an aerobic bottle.

PERIPHERAL INTRAVENOUS (IV) PLACEMENT: PERCUTANEOUS

Indications

Peripheral IV lines are used for maintenance of fluid balance, administration of medication, nutrition, and prevention of hypoglycemia. In general, peripheral IV lines are indicated when the patient is unable to attain medical and nutritional goals with enteral therapy.

Equipment

Materials needed for placement of a peripheral IV line in an infant include: (1) a 21 to 27 gauge butterfly scalp vein infusion set or a 21 to 23 gauge plastic catheter, such as Angiocath, Medicut, or Quikcath; (2) 1/2-inch tape; (3) a plastic medicine cup; (4) a bottle of intravenous fluid; (5) an intravenous fluid chamber with microdrip; and (6) a continuous infusion pump. One must carefully monitor fluid administration in an infant. Macrodrip tubing and liter bottles should *not* be used; inadvertent infusion of large amounts of fluids to an infant may be disastrous. An infusion pump is an ideal way of limiting fluid infusion while keeping the vein open.

Procedure

A number of IV sites are available for the placement of a peripheral intravenous needle or catheter in the infant.[18, 19] The scalp veins are probably the easiest to cannulate, but many clinicians prefer the veins on the dorsa of the hands and feet. The antecubital veins are often easily cannulated in the older infant. If one is using a peripheral vein on the hands, the feet, or the antecubital fossa, one should first immobilize the extremity by taping it to an armboard, a splint, or a sandbag. The particular site is a matter of preference, and the physician should choose the vein that appears to be the easiest to cannulate.

If the scalp veins are used, the area surrounding the planned site of insertion should be shaved and cleaned with an iodine solution. Arteries and veins can usually be differentiated on the scalp by the fact that arteries are more tortuous than veins. In addition, the arteries fill from below, whereas the veins fill from above. If an artery is entered during placement of the needle and fluid is infused, blanching will occur in the area. If this happens, the catheter or needle should be removed, light pressure should be maintained for several minutes, and the procedure should be repeated in another site. A rubber band may be used as a tourniquet around the head to produce venous dilation. One should always check that the rubber band is removed after venous cannulation. If a peripheral extremity is used, a tourniquet may be placed proximal to the planned site of entry.

The tubing of the scalp vein butterfly infusion set or the catheter should be flushed before venipuncture with a sterile intravenous solution, such as D_5W or normal saline, to prevent air embolism. If a plastic catheter is used,[20] the catheter with stylet in place is directed through the skin at a 10- to 20-degree angle. The catheter with stylet is slowly advanced until blood return is noted. One then advances the catheter over the stylet into the vein using the forefinger of the guiding hand.

If a scalp vein butterfly infusion set is used, the wings of the butterfly are grasped between the thumb and forefinger and are introduced beneath the skin approximately 0.5 cm distal to the anticipated site of vein entrance (Fig. 18–4). The needle is advanced slowly toward the vessel until blood appears in the tubing, indicating that the vessel has been entered. The tourniquet should then be removed. The needle should be flushed with 0.5 to 2 ml of intravenous fluid such as D_5W or normal saline, to ensure that the needle is properly in place within the vein. If infiltration occurs, as noted by a subcutaneous bump, the IV line should be removed, and the process should be repeated at another site.

The needle assembly may be taped, as shown in Figure 18–5. After the wings are secured with tape, the tubing of the butterfly set should be taped in a loop on the scalp so that it is not accidentally pulled. A wisp of cotton may be placed under the wings of the butterfly if the infusion is positional. A small plastic medicine cup or half of a paper cup may be taped over the

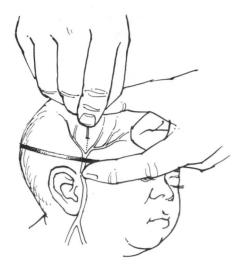

Figure 18–4. The needle is introduced approximately 0.5 cm distal to the anticipated site of vessel puncture in a scalp vein.

Figure 18–5. Technique for taping the intravenous line. A wisp of cotton may be placed under the wings of the butterfly needle if the infusion is positional.

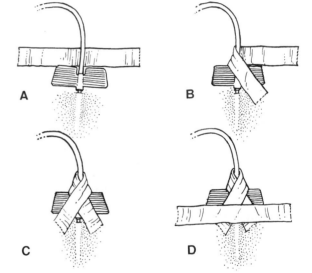

Figure 18–6. Protecting the intravenous line with a plastic medicine cup.

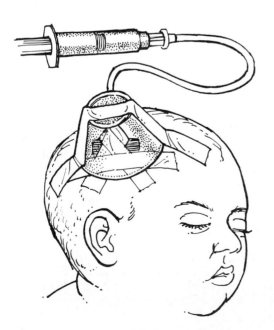

wings and the needle to protect the intravenous line (Fig. 18–6). The catheter of the butterfly set should then be connected to the tubing from the intravenous system, and the IV pump should be started.

If a catheter is used for placement of the intravenous line, the stylet is removed and the intravenous line is connected to the hub of the catheter by means of a T piece connector. The catheter is fixed to the skin with a piece of 1/2-inch tape placed adhesive side uppermost under the catheter hub and crossed over the catheter in a V shape. A second piece of tape is passed around and over the catheter hub and is fixed to the skin.

Complications

Complications of intravenous fluid therapy include infection,[21] injection of sclerosing agents into the subcutaneous space with resultant necrosis and sloughing of the skin[22] (especially in small infants), air embolism,[23] and administration of inappropriate volumes of fluid. The incidence of infection secondary to peripheral intravenous therapy may be decreased by routine periodic replacement of the needles. Because the life span of an intravenous needle or catheter is usually fairly short (less than 72 hours) in the small infant, the decision concerning elective removal and replacement of the intravenous system is not usually a problem. Of course, it is important to pay meticulous attention to sterility during insertion and maintenance of the intravenous system in order to decrease the risk of infection.

A simulator (Medical Plastics Laboratory, Gatesville, Texas) is available to demonstrate and practice the proper technique of placement of peripheral intravenous needles in infants.[24]

VENOUS CUTDOWN CATHETERIZATION

With the development of small intravenous catheters and "scalp vein" needles, peripheral venous cutdown is rarely used in infants. Nonetheless, when rapid venous access is needed in an infant (particularly for the infant in shock, in whom few veins are visible), venous cutdown can be lifesaving. For the purpose of illustration, the exposure and cannulation of the saphenous vein will be discussed (Fig. 18–7). The same principles apply when a cutdown is performed on an arm vein (see also Chapter 20).

Equipment

Successful venous catheterization in the small infant requires sterile instruments, an assistant, good lighting, and a selection of catheters. Cer-

tainly, previous clinical experience is helpful. The use of self-retaining retractors is a personal preference. Because of temperature instability, a warming light or an overhead radiant warmer is frequently useful. Silastic catheters, which can be obtained in 2, 3, and 4 French sizes (Dow-Corning Co.), seem to remain patent longer and can be sterilized with the instruments to make a "cutdown tray." Polyethylene catheters can also be used but tend to infiltrate more readily due to the rigid catheter perforating the vein wall.

Procedure

The clinician should begin with complete immobilization of the thigh, the leg, the ankle, and the foot by taping them to a padded armboard, which in turn is attached to the table or bed where the procedure is being performed (see Fig. 18–7A). The area around the medial malleolus is prepared with a povidone-iodine solution and draped with sterile towels. Local anesthesia is accomplished by a superficial infiltration with 0.25 to 1 per cent lidocaine (Xylocaine) in an area proximal and anterior to the superior portion of the medial malleolus. Fortunately, there are no major nerves or tendons that accompany the vein in this location.

A tourniquet is placed in the mid-leg, and a transverse skin incision is made; a small mosquito hemostat is inserted into the wound, with the concavity of the clamp upward. The tip of the hemostat is advanced to the bone in one corner of the wound, and all tissues lying against the bone and in the subcutaneous region are "scooped up" with the hemostat (see Fig. 18–7B). This will invariably lift the vein out of the wound with surrounding tissues. Fine forceps or a mosquito hemostat is used to separate and remove all nonvenous structures, leaving only the saphenous vein tented over the hemostat (see Fig. 18–7C). To avoid injury to the vein during dissection, one spreads the ends of the hemostat parallel to the direction of the vein—never transversely.

Two 4–0 silk sutures are passed under the vein; one silk suture is pulled distal to stabilize the vein, and the other suture is pulled proximal to the site of venipuncture. The distal suture is commonly tied. Some clinicians will not tie the distal suture, however, using it only for stabilization. Removal of the untied distal suture following vein cannulation may allow for subsequent vein recannulation following eventual catheter removal. If the distal suture is left untied, longitudinal traction on it permits hemostasis and continued exposure of the vein above the wound. Fine scissors or a scalpel blade may be used to make an oblique or V-shaped incision in the upper vein wall between the sutures (see Fig. 18–7D). The catheter (beveled at its tip) is then filled with saline.

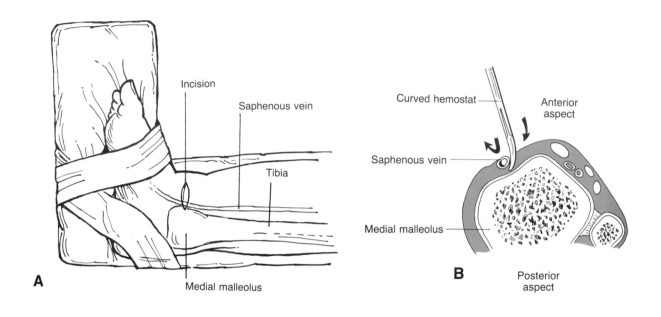

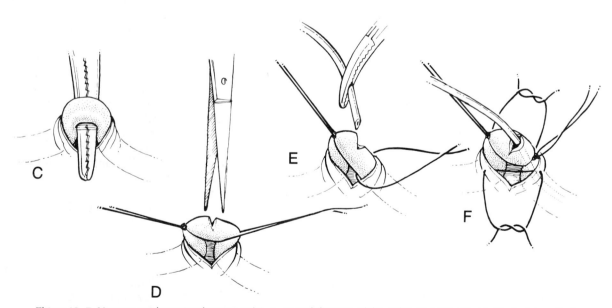

Figure 18–7. Venous cutdown (saphenous vein). *A*, Immobilization of the ankle and the site of skin incision. *B*, A curved hemostat scoops up the vein. The point of the hemostat should be kept against the bone. *C*, The vein is dissected free. (From Surah and Gibson: Manual of Medical Procedures. St. Louis, C. V. Mosby Co., 1900. Used by permission.) *D*, With a proximal and distal tie to stabilize the vein and to control bleeding, a V-shaped incision is made in the upper one third of the vein. *E* and *F*, The infusion catheter is threaded into the vein lumen and advanced.

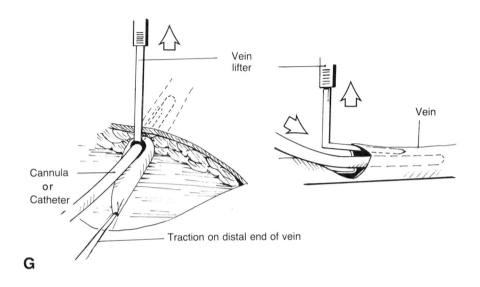

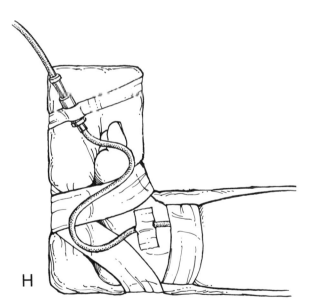

Figure 18– 7 *(Continued). G,* A vein lifter/dilator facilitates the placement of the catheter into the vein lumen. *H,* The incision is sutured, and the catheter is secured.

The catheter is grasped with a forcep and is advanced into the vein for a distance of 2 to 3 cm (see Fig. 18–7E and F). This is usually the most difficult and time-consuming portion of the procedure. A vein dilator or forceps may be used to hold open the incision in the vein (see Fig. 18–7G). Downward pull on the distal tie will give countertraction and will stabilize the vein during catheter advancement. The tourniquet is then removed. One ties the proximal suture around the vein with the catheter inside, taking care not to occlude the catheter by tying the suture too tight. If it was not tied, the distal suture is now removed. When the distal suture is left untied, the proximal suture is still tied to secure the catheter, but the ends are left long so that the suture can be pulled out of the incision and removed to allow recannulation once the infusion catheter is removed. Continued infusion of saline through the catheter from an attached syringe will ensure patency. The catheter is oriented into either corner of the incision, and the incision is closed with interrupted 4–0 nylon sutures. The skin suture nearest the catheter is wrapped around the catheter and tied to hold the catheter in place. Bleeding can be controlled with direct pressure. Antibiotic ointment is placed over the wound, and a sterile, occlusive dressing is applied. The intravenous tubing is connected and taped securely to the footboard to prevent inadvertent removal of the catheter (see Fig. 18–7H).

One should change the dressing carefully every day, using sterile technique with reapplication of antibiotic ointment. When cared for properly, the catheters can remain in place for as long as 7 to 10 days. Obviously, at the first sign of infiltration or infection the catheter must be removed. Unfortunately, once the vein has been used for a cutdown, it is usually rendered useless for future venous cannulation.

Mini-cutdown. The cannulation of a small vein with a catheter or tube may be difficult and very time-consuming if one is not experienced in the technique. As an alternative, the mini-cutdown procedure may be used. Once the vein is exposed through a skin incision and subcutaneous dissection, it is cannulated directly with a standard intravenous catheter (Medicut, Angiocath) rather than nicked with a scalpel (Fig. 18–8). A silk suture or hemostat may be placed under the vein to immobilize it during puncture, but with the mini-cutdown technique the vein is not tied off after being cannulated. The catheter will not be as secure with this modification, but the technique is useful when time is critical. The vein is not destroyed with this technique. In essence, the mini-cutdown uses the percutaneous technique of cannulation, except that venipuncture is performed through a skin incision under direct visualization (see also Chapter 20).

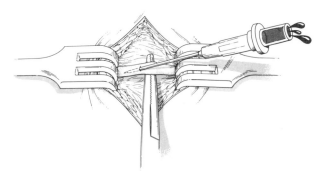

Figure 18–8. The mini-cutdown procedure is technically easier than a full cutdown and may be preferred in an emergency. (From Vander Salm, T. J.: Atlas of Bedside Procedures. Boston, Little, Brown & Co., 1979. Used by permission.)

Suggestions

In an emergency, a saphenous cutdown in infants may not be an easy procedure. The technique requires practice and may consume 5 to 15 minutes of resuscitation time. One common error is making an improper skin incision. The incision must be through all layers of the skin without severing the vein. Subcutaneous fat should be visible through the incision. The subcutaneous incision should be carried to the end of the skin incision in order for the clinician to take full advantage of the skin incision. A 2-cm incision is usually required, and one should not try to work through a skin incision that is too small.

One should perform dissection only with a blunt technique, spreading the hemostat parallel to the course of the vein. Inadvertent severance of the vein may occur during dissection, and one can best control bleeding by pulling the silk ties taut. The incision in the vessel may be a source of frustration. One must incise completely into the lumen of the vessel; a superficial nick, although it will bleed, will not allow for catheter passage. If the vein is severed completely, it will retract from view and will be difficult to find. Generally, an incision should include one third of the vessel diameter. Placing the catheter into the vessel lumen is usually the most difficult part of the procedure, and it is easy to create a false lumen. Small plastic vein dilators are available to facilitate entering into the lumen. If a valve is encountered during passage, one should turn the IV up full force and rotate the catheter.

Complications

In addition to the problems discussed previously, venous cutdowns can result in wound infections and phlebitis. Adjacent structures may be injured during the incision and subsequent blunt dissection. When the mini-cutdown technique without ligatures is used, extravasation of infusate may result. Light pressure on the closed wound will generally prevent continued extravasation.

Arterial Blood Sampling

The arterial blood gas is an important laboratory test for evaluation of an infant or child with respiratory distress (see also Chapter 26). Arterial blood may also be used for routine laboratory analysis if venous blood cannot be obtained. Possible sites of arterial blood sampling include (1) radial, brachial, temporal, dorsalis pedis, and posterior tibial arteries; (2) umbilical arteries in the newborn infant; and (3) capillaries ("arterialized"). Femoral arteries should not be used for obtaining blood samples from the infant or child.[25] Transcutaneous electrodes for P_{O_2} and P_{CO_2} analysis may provide a useful adjunct to arterial sampling in many patients. Nonetheless, they do not replace intermittent arterial sampling, which remains necessary for the stabilization of infants and for verification of the accuracy of transcutaneous methods.

PERIPHERAL ARTERY PUNCTURE

Peripheral artery punctures may be performed in the radial, brachial, temporal, dorsalis pedis, and posterior tibial arteries. There is no vein or nerve immediately adjacent to the radial artery; this minimizes the risk of obtaining venous blood or damaging a nerve. This is not the case with the brachial artery, and the risk of both complications appears to be greater when this artery is used.[26] The temporal artery is also adjacent to a vein, and if the patient's head is in an oxygen hood it is nearly impossible to obtain a sample in a steady state.

The radial artery (Fig. 18–9) is most frequently used to obtain intermittent arterial samples from infants and children. We prefer not to use the ulnar artery for arterial puncture in order to preserve the collateral circulation to the hand, although some clinicians advocate performing punctures and catheterization of the ulnar artery. The median nerve is in the midline and the ulnar nerve is near the ulnar artery; these areas should therefore be avoided.

Procedure

In preparation for a radial artery puncture, one should first heparinize a tuberculin syringe. All heparin should be ejected from the syringe; a 25 or 26 gauge needle should then be attached to the syringe. The amount of heparin coating the barrel of the syringe is adequate to anticoagulate the sample; excess heparin may result in inaccurate P_{CO_2} determinations because of dilution of the blood sample.[27-30]

The clinician should hold the infant's wrist and

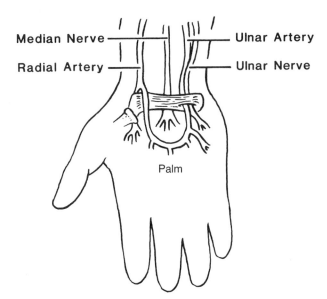

Figure 18–9. Anatomy of the volar surface of the wrist and the palm.

hand in the left hand (if the clinician is right-handed) and should palpate the pulsations of the radial artery just proximal to the transverse wrist creases. Some clinicians prefer to immobilize the wrist by taping it to a sandbag or another restraint.[31] The area is cleansed with alcohol. Some practitioners advocate the use of subcutaneous lidocaine. The skin is penetrated at a 30- to 45-degree angle (Fig. 18–10), and while the plunger of the syringe is withdrawn, the needle is advanced slowly until the radial artery is punctured or until resistance is met (Fig. 18–11). In contrast with adults, with infants it is necessary to provide continuous suction on the plunger of the syringe. One can be sure that the radial artery is punctured when blood appears in the hub of the needle. Some clinicians prefer to use a 25 gauge scalp vein butterfly needle connected to a syringe. This allows better control of the needle while an assistant aspirates the syringe and may also permit a larger volume of blood to be withdrawn. One may place a transilluminator on the underside (dorsum) of the wrist to visualize the radial artery.

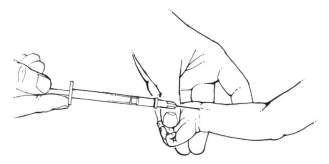

Figure 18–10. For arterial blood gas analysis, needle should be inserted under the skin at a 30-to 45-degree angle. A butterfly needle and syringe are used if larger volumes of blood are required.

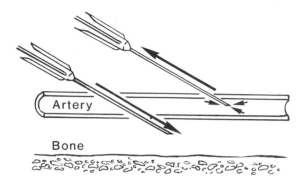

Figure 18–11. If resistance is met, this usually indicates contact with the bone. The needle should be withdrawn slowly; if the needle has traversed both walls of the artery, blood will be obtained as the needle is slowly withdrawn into the arterial lumen.

If one meets resistance while pushing the needle deeper, one slowly withdraws the needle to the point at which only the distal needle tip remains beneath the skin and then repeats the procedure. After 0.3 ml of blood is obtained, the needle is removed, and light pressure is applied for 5 minutes or longer to prevent any bleeding.[32]

A simulator (Medical Plastics Laboratory, Gatesville, Texas) may be used to teach and practice the technique of radial artery puncture in infants.[32]

Complications

The complications of radial artery puncture include infection, hematoma formation, and nerve damage.[33] With the use of proper technique, however, the complication rate is extremely low. The most common concern with puncture of a radial artery (or any peripheral artery) in infants is that the baby may start to cry before blood is obtained, thus changing the P_{O_2} and P_{CO_2} from the values of the quiet state.[34, 35]

Another potential problem is the dilutional effect of heparin on the P_{CO_2}. The heparin in the dead space of the tuberculin syringe may decrease the P_{CO_2} by 15 to 25 per cent when 0.2 ml of blood is obtained and by approximately 10 per cent with 0.4 ml of blood. This emphasizes the need for all heparin to be ejected from the dead space of the syringe before the needle is applied. The use of a syringe (e.g., Becton-Dickinson 1-ml U-100 insulin syringe) with minimal dead space or the use of lyophilized heparin eliminates this problem[36] (see also Chapter 26).

UMBILICAL ARTERY CATHETERIZATION

Umbilical artery catheterization is a useful procedure in the care of newborn infants who require frequent arterial blood gas and blood pressure assessment, although it is imperative for the clinician to remain aware of potential complica-

tions.[37-39] One of the two umbilical arteries may be cannulated for resuscitation purposes, but an umbilical vein is generally technically easier to cannulate and may be preferred in an emergency.

Procedure

The supplies and equipment for catheterization are listed in Table 18–1. The infant is placed beneath a radiant warmer, and the extremities are restrained. The skin temperature is maintained at 35.8°C (96.5°F). Oxygen is administered as needed, and the audible beep on the cardiac monitor is turned on. The operator should wear a surgical cap and mask and a sterile gown and gloves.

The umbilicus is scrubbed with a bactericidal solution. Pooling of liquid at the infant's side should be avoided, because this may be associated with blistering of the skin under a radiant warmer. The umbilical area is draped in a sterile fashion with the infant's head left exposed for observation.

To provide hemostasis and to anchor the line after placement, a pursestring suture is placed at the junction of the skin and the cord (Fig. 18–12). Alternatively, a constricting loop of umbilical tape in the same position may be used. The cord is cut 3 to 5 mm from the skin, and the vessels are identified. The vein is usually located at 12 o'clock and has a thin wall and large lumen, whereas the two arteries have thicker walls and smaller lumina.

The cord is grasped with a curved hemostat near the selected artery, providing clear visualization and stabilization of the vessel. Using the curved iris forceps without teeth, one gently dilates the artery. Umbilical artery spasm may make the procedure difficult. A 3.5 to 5 French catheter is attached to a three-way stopcock and is flushed with the sterile heparinized solution. The catheter may then be introduced into the dilated artery. A 3.5 to 4 French catheter is recommended for infants weighing less than 2 kg and a 5 French catheter for those weighing more than 2 kg.

When the catheter is being inserted, tension should be placed cephalad on the cord, and the

Table 18–1. UMBILICAL ARTERY CATHETERIZATION EQUIPMENT

Line fluid usually consists of $D_{5-10}W$ with electrolytes. Some physicians also add 1 unit heparin per ml fluid (to "prevent" clotting in the catheter).
Fluid chamber, intravenous tubing, infusion pump, filter (0.22 μ), short length of intravenous tubing, three-way stopcock.
Umbilical artery catheter (3.5 to 5 French).
3–0 silk suture on a curved needle.
Curved iris forceps without teeth.
Small clamps, forceps, scissors, needle holder.
Sterile drapes.
Light source.
10 ml of heparinized solution for flush (1 to 2 units Na^+ heparin per ml fluid).
Surgical cap, mask, gown, and gloves.

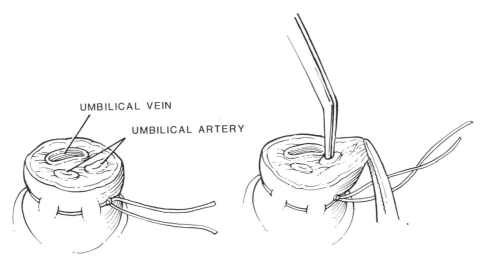

Figure 18–12. A purse-string suture or umbilical tape is placed around the base of the cord to provide hemostasis. The umbilical artery is dilated with curved iris forceps.

catheter should be advanced with slow, constant pressure toward the feet (Fig. 18–13). Resistance is occasionally felt at 1 to 2 cm. Resistance should be overcome by gentle, sustained pressure. If the catheter passes 4 to 5 cm and meets resistance, this generally indicates that a "false passage" through the vessel wall has occurred. Occasionally, one may bypass the perforation by attempting catheterization with the larger 5 French catheter.

If a low (L-3 to L-4) position is desired, the catheter may be advanced 7 to 8 cm in a 1-kg premature infant or 12 to 13 cm in a full-term infant. Graphs are available to estimate the proper length of insertion for a high or low catheter location.[40, 41] Once sterile technique is broken, the line may not be advanced. It is therefore preferable to position the catheter too high and to withdraw as necessary according to the location on a radiograph. After it has been positioned appropriately, the catheter should be tied with the previously placed suture (see Fig. 18–13) and taped to the

abdominal wall (Fig. 18–14). A radiograph should be obtained, and the catheter should be repositioned, if necessary, with the tip at the lower border of the L-3 vertebra. Some clinicians prefer to place the catheter high (above the diaphragm). There are no unequivocal data to support either preference.[42, 43]

Radiographs of an arterial catheter (Fig. 18–15) will show the catheter proceeding from the umbilicus down toward the pelvis, making an acute turn into the internal iliac artery, continuing toward the head into the bifurcation of the aorta, and then moving up the aorta slightly to the left of the vertebral column.[44]

Most unsuccessful umbilical artery catheterization attempts fail because the catheter perforates the arterial wall approximately 1 cm below the umbilical stump where the umbilical artery begins curving toward the feet.[45] In this instance, the catheter is advanced in the extraluminal space, and resistance is met at 4 to 6 cm. The following

Figure 18–13. The catheter is introduced into the dilated artery and advanced toward the feet. The suture placed around the base of the cord is tied to the catheter.

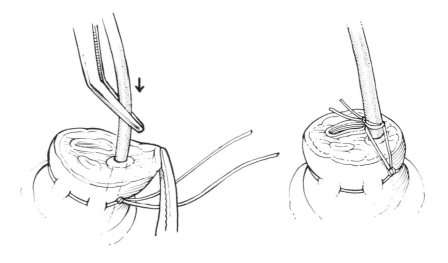

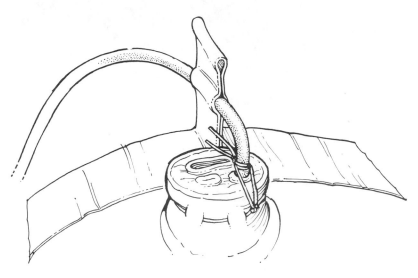

Figure 18–14. The tape is pleated above and below the catheter.

maneuvers make it possible to avoid perforating the umbilical arterial wall in most cases:

1. The catheter should be advanced slowly. When slight resistance is met at approximately 1 cm, the catheter should be advanced very gently with steady pressure. The catheter should never be forced, because it will likely perforate the wall. A catheter or feeding tube with a molded tip should be used. A catheter tip that has been cut with scissors is more difficult to insert and advance.

2. Because the artery curves toward the feet, the umbilical stump should be held with a curved clamp and should be pulled toward the head so that the catheter is inserted toward the feet in as straight a direction as possible.

The use of a placenta[46] or a commercially available simulator[47] (Medical Plastics Laboratory, Gatesville, Texas) makes it relatively easy to demonstrate and practice the proper technique of umbilical artery catheterization.

Complications

If the catheter becomes plugged or fails to function properly or if there is blanching or discoloration of the buttocks, the heels, or the toes, the catheter should be removed at once. Umbilical arteries are most easily cannulated in the first few hours of life but may be a viable vascular route as late as 5 to 7 days of age.

Complications include hemorrhage,[48, 49] infection,[50–53] thromboembolic phenomena (especially to the kidneys, the gastrointestinal tract, and the lower extremities),[54–59] vasospasm, air embolism, vessel perforation, electrical hazards, peritoneal perforation, hypertension,[60–62] and possible effects of plasticizers.[63]

UMBILICAL VEIN CATHETERIZATION

The major indication for umbilical vein catheterization is access to the vascular system for

Figure 18–15. The umbilical artery catheter makes a loop downward before heading cephalad (schematic drawing of an x-ray interpretation).

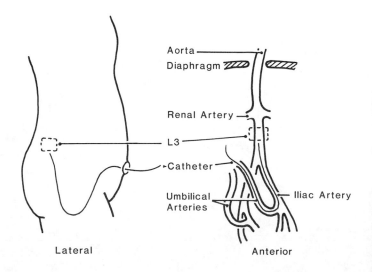

emergency resuscitation and stabilization of the newborn. The umbilical vein may also be used for exchange transfusions in newborns. The umbilical vein may be cannulated up to the age of 5 to 7 days, but after 1 week of life the technique is not generally used. The procedure is technically easier than umbilical artery cannulation. Umbilical vein catheterization is not an acceptable alternative after the baby leaves the hospital (for example, the procedure would not be used should a 2- to 4-week-old infant present to the emergency department).

Procedure

The technique of umbilical vein catheterization is similar to that described for umbilical arterial catheterization in the preceding section. Occasionally, a persistent urachus may be mistaken for the umbilical vein, but the return of urine should identify the mistake.

The catheter (3.5 to 8.0 French), which has been flushed with heparinized saline, is placed in the lumen of the umbilical vein and is advanced gently. The catheter is inserted only 4 to 5 cm in a term-sized infant, and the suitable length should be marked before the catheter is advanced. If the catheter is pushed farther than 4 to 5 cm, it will do one of two things: (1) It may enter the ductus venosus and then move into the inferior vena cava. (The catheter must be inserted approximately 10 to 12 cm in a term-sized infant in order to reach the inferior vena cava.) (2) It may enter a branch of the portal vein within the liver (evidenced by obstruction at 5 to 10 cm). Ideally, radiographs should be obtained to document the placement of the catheter; an umbilical venous catheter will proceed directly cephalad (without making a downward loop) until it passes through the ductus venosus (Fig. 18–16). Of course, in a resuscitation radiographic documentation is not possible. Therefore, it is generally recommended that the catheter be inserted approximately 4 to 5 cm to minimize the risk of injecting sclerosing solutions into the liver.

Air embolism may occur at the time of catheter removal if the infant generates sufficient negative intrathoracic pressure (as during crying) to cause air to be drawn into the patent umbilical vein. Therefore, caution must be used during catheter removal to ensure that the vein is promptly occluded (by tightening a purse-string suture or applying pressure on or just cephalad to the umbilicus).

Complications

Complications of umbilical venous catheters include hemorrhage, infection, injection of sclerosing substances into the liver (resulting in hepatic necrosis), air embolism, and vessel perforation. It is most important that one follow careful technique in insertion and maintenance of catheters in order to minimize such complications.

PERCUTANEOUS ARTERIAL CATHETERIZATION

A percutaneous peripheral arterial catheter may be indicated when there is a need for frequent blood gas sampling or continuous arterial pressure monitoring, or both. Arteries used for peripheral catheters in infants include the radial,[64–67] ulnar,[66] temporal,[68, 69] and posterior tibial arteries.

Only the procedure for radial artery cannulation will be described here, but cannulation of other vessels is similar. The procedure should be performed with good lighting and an adequate work area while the infant's heart and respiratory rates are monitored closely.

Contraindications

The following are contraindications to peripheral arterial catheterization: (1) situations in which

Figure 18–16. An umbilical vein catheter is directed toward the head and remains anterior until it passes through the ductus venosus into the inferior vena cava.

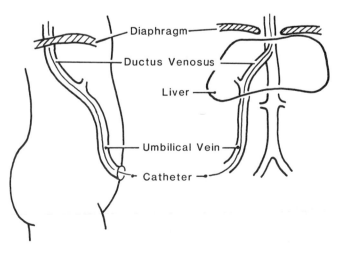

adequate peripheral arterial samples can be obtained by percutaneous punctures, (2) situations in which circulation of the extremity to be catheterized is compromised, and (3) situations in which occlusion of the vessel to be catheterized results in compromised perfusion of that extremity.

Procedure

The radial artery may be palpated proximally to the transverse wrist crease on the palmar surface of the wrist, medial to the styloid process of the radius. The artery is then compressed, and the hand and fingers are observed for color change. If blanching or cyanosis is noted (indicating poor collateral circulation), catheterization is not performed.

A fiber optic transilluminator may be used to localize the artery. With the overhead lights off, the transilluminator head (with a rubber shield or filter to prevent overheating the skin[70, 71]) is positioned beneath the wrist, and the artery is visualized as a dark, pulsatile shadow.

The equipment includes a 22 gauge catheter with hollow metal stylet, T piece connector, and stopcock. One should connect the T piece and the stopcock, and then fill them with an isotonic solution.

The area over the radial artery is prepared with a povidone-iodine solution and washed with alcohol. With the infant's hand and forearm held firmly between the thumb and forefingers of one of the clinician's hands, the catheter with stylet is inserted through the skin just proximal to the transverse wrist crease at a 10- to 20-degree angle (Fig. 18–17). It should be noted that this is less of an angle than is used for arterial puncture. The catheter with stylet is advanced slowly until blood return is noted from the hollow metal stylet. One then pushes the catheter over the stylet using the forefinger of the guiding hand (Fig. 18–18). The

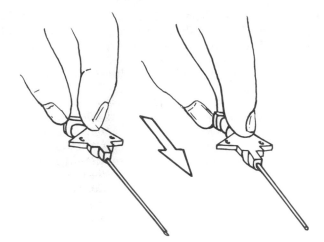

Figure 18–18. The forefinger advances the catheter over the needle.

stylet is removed, and the stopcock and T piece connector are attached to the catheter hub. The stopcock is opened to the syringe to confirm pulsatile blood return. It is then flushed with 0.5 ml heparinized flush solution very gently to clear the catheter while the fingers and the hand are observed for evidence of blanching or cyanosis.

The catheter is fixed to the skin by a thin piece of tape placed adhesive side uppermost under the catheter hub and crossed over the catheter in a V shape. A second piece of tape is passed around and over the catheter hub and is fixed to the wrist. The hand and wrist are stabilized on a tongue depressor splint with the hand slightly dorsiflexed and the palmar surface uppermost and with a gauze pad or a cotton ball underneath the wrist (Fig. 18–19). A small piece of tape is used to attach the T piece connector to the wrist area or to the splint. The fingers should be easily visible.

An isotonic solution of either glucose or electrolytes is used for infusion. Some clinicians prefer to add 1 to 2 units of heparin per milliliter of infusion solution infused at 1 to 2 ml per hour.

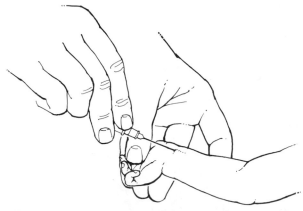

Figure 18–17. The catheter assembly is introduced into the radial artery through skin at a 10- to 20-degree angle. This is less of an angle than is used for arterial puncture.

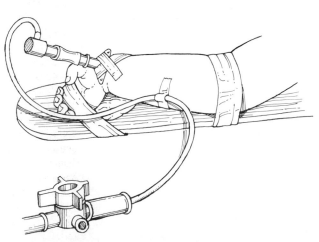

Figure 18–19. Technique of taping the arterial catheter.

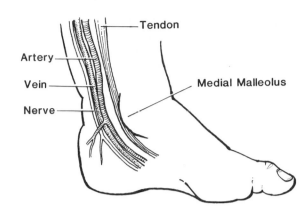

Figure 18–20. Anatomy of the posterior tibial artery and surrounding structures.

Medications, blood or blood products, amino acid solutions, intravenous fat solutions, or hypertonic solutions are not infused through the catheter.

The catheter must be removed when there is evidence of blanching or cyanosis or when it is impossible to withdraw blood from the catheter or difficult to flush the catheter.

Complications

Complications, which have been reported with every type of arterial catheter,[72–74] include hemorrhage, thrombosis, spasm, infection, scars, and nerve damage. Thrombosis or spasm may result in blanching or cyanosis of the extremity or skin. There is potential for loss of digits, an entire extremity, or large areas of skin, as well as cerebral infarction with temporal artery catheters.

ARTERIAL CUTDOWN CATHETERIZATION

Indications and Contraindications

Arterial catheterization by cutdown on the posterior tibial artery,[75] radial artery, and temporal artery[76–78] may be indicated when the need exists for frequent monitoring of arterial blood gases or blood pressure and when percutaneous access is not possible. Arterial cutdowns are contraindicated when (1) adequate peripheral blood gas samples can be obtained by percutaneous punctures or catheterization, (2) circulation of the extremity to be catheterized is compromised, and (3) occlusion of the vessel to be catheterized results in compromised perfusion of that extremity.

Procedure

The anatomy and technique for posterior tibial arterial cutdown will be described in detail (Fig. 18–20). The same technique is applicable for the radial artery. The clinician stabilizes the foot in a neutral position by taping the externally rotated lower leg to a splint. The posterior tibial artery is then localized by Doppler ultrasound just *posterior to the medial malleolus.* The operator prepares for the procedure by scrubbing and donning a gown and gloves; the foot is prepared with a povidone-iodine solution. The following materials may be used: T connector, stopcock, and syringe filled

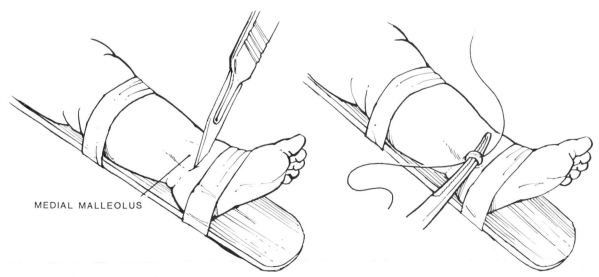

MEDIAL MALLEOLUS

Figure 18–21. With the foot prepared and immobilized, a 5- to 7-mm incision is made in the skin posterior to and at the midline of the medial malleolus. Curved forceps and a silk suture are inserted beneath the posterior tibial artery, which courses just posterior to the medial malleolus.

with flush solution (D$_5$W with 1 to 2 units of heparin per ml); silk suture ties; and a 22 gauge Quikcath (Vicar Division of Travenol Laboratories, Inc., Dallas, Texas) or equivalent catheter.

Following subcutaneous injection of 1 per cent lidocaine, a 5- to 7-mm transverse incision is made in the skin over the artery posterior to and at the midlevel of the medial malleolus (Fig. 18–21). With blunt dissection in a vertical direction (parallel to the vessels) the tissue is separated with a small, curved forceps, and the artery is identified. The artery courses with the vein just anterior and superficial to the nerve and is usually pulsatile. One isolates the artery by sliding a small, curved forceps beneath it and gently elevating the vessel (see Fig. 18–21). Excessive manipulation of the artery can cause spasm; if this occurs, a few drops of 1 per cent lidocaine applied locally may result in dilation. A silk tie (without a needle) is then placed beneath the artery to stabilize it during cannulation.

At a 10-degree angle, a 22 gauge Quikcath with the catheter bevel down is inserted into the artery over the surface of the forceps. When blood return is seen, the catheter is advanced over the stylet to its full length (Fig. 18–22). The needle stylet is then removed, the catheter is connected to the T connector, and the three-way stopcock is prefilled with heparinized flush solution. Patency is checked by observation of blood return with pulsations; the catheter is then flushed slowly and gently. The silk suture is removed, and the skin incision is sutured. The Quikcath wings are sutured to the skin over the heel. Collodion is applied over the incision and at the stopcock

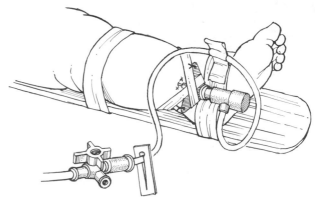

Figure 18–23. The skin incision is closed, the catheter wings are sutured to the skin, and the catheter is taped in place.

connection, and the catheter is further secured (Fig. 18–23). The stopcock is then connected to the infusion line.

Complications

The complications of arterial cutdown are similar to those of percutaneous arterial catheterization. They include hemorrhage, thrombosis, or spasm resulting in loss of tissue; infections; permanent scars; and nerve damage. Complications have been reported with all types of arterial cutdown. Follow-up data and computed tomography data suggest an association between temporal artery catheterization by the cutdown technique and cerebral infarct that may result in hemiparesis.[79] Therefore, we advocate that temporal artery catheterization be the last choice for arterial catheterization.

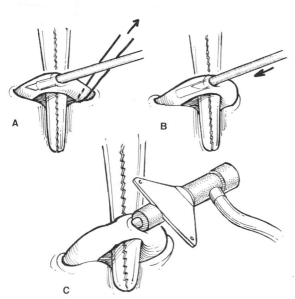

Figure 18–22. Technique of inserting the arterial catheter. A silk tie is used to stabilize the artery during cannulation. One inserts the catheter under direct vision without making an incision in the vessel.

1. Blumenfeld, T. A., Turi, G. K., and Blanc, W. A.: Recommended site and depth of newborn heel skin punctures based on anatomical measurements and histopathology. Lancet 1:230, 1979.
2. Lauer, B. A., and Altenburger, K. M.: Outbreak of staphylococcal infections following heel puncture for blood sampling. Am. J. Dis. Child, 135:277, 1981.
3. Lilien, L. D., Harris, V. J., Ramamurthy, R. S., and Pildes, R. S.: Neonatal osteomyelitis of the calcaneus: Complication of heel puncture. J. Pediatr. 88:478, 1976.
4. Sell, E. J., Hansen, R. C., and Struck-Pierce, S.: Calcified nodules on the heel: A complication of neonatal intensive care. J. Pediatr. 96:473, 1980.
5. Folger, G. M., Kouri, P., and Sabbah, H. N.: Arterialized capillary blood sampling in the neonate: A reappraisal. Heart Lung 9:521, 1980.
6. Hunt, C. E.: Capillary blood sampling in the infant: Usefulness and limitations of two methods of sampling, compared with arterial blood. Pediatrics 51:501, 1973.
7. Desai, S. D., Holloway, R., Thambiran, A. K., and Wesley, A. G.: A comparison between arterial and arterialized capillary blood in infants. S. Afr. Med. J. 41:13, 1967.
8. Glasgow, J. F. T., Flynn, D. M., and Swyer, P. R.: A comparison of descending aortic and "arterialized" capillary blood in the sick newborn. Can. Med. Assoc. J. 106:660, 1972.

9. Banister, A.: Comparison of arterial and arterialized capillary blood in infants with respiratory distress. Arch. Dis. Child., 44:726, 1969.
10. Koch, G., and Wendel, H.: Comparison of pH, carbon dioxide tension, standard bicarbonate and oxygen tension in capillary blood and in arterial blood during the neonatal period. Acta Paediatr. Scand. 56:10, 1967.
11. Corbet, A. J. S., and Burnard, E. D.: Oxygen tension measurements on digital blood in the newborn. Pediatrics 46:780, 1970.
12. Duc, G. V., and Cumarasamy, N.: Digital arteriolar oxygen tension as a guide to oxygen therapy of the newborn. Biol. Neonate 24:134, 1974.
13. Karna, P., and Poland, R. L.: Monitoring critically ill newborn infants with digital capillary blood samples: An alternative. J. Pediatr. 92:270, 1978.
14. Power, W. F.: Digital capillary sampling. J. Pediatr. 93:729, 1978.
15. Knudson, R. P., and Alden, E. R.: Neonatal heelstick blood culture. Pediatrics 65:505, 1980.
16. Holt, R. J., Frankcombe, C. H., and Newman, R. L.: Capillary blood cultures. Arch. Dis. Child. 49:318, 1974.
17. Fischer, G. W., Crumrine, M. H., and Jennings, P. B.: Experimental *Escherichia coli* sepsis in rabbits. J. Pediatr. 85:117, 1974.
18. Clarke, T. A., and Reddy, P. G.: Intravenous infusion technique in the newborn. Clin. Pediatr. 18:550, 1979.
19. Hanid, T. K.: Intravenous injections and infusions in infants. Pediatrics 56:1080, 1975.
20. Filston, H. C., and Johnson, D. G.: Percutaneous venous cannulation in neonates and infants: A method for catheter insertion without "cut-down." Pediatrics 48:896, 1971.
21. Stamm, W. E., Kolff, C. A., Dones, E. M., Javariz, R., Anderson, R. L., Farmer, J. J., III, and de Quinones, H. R.: A nursery outbreak caused by *Serratia marcescens*— scalp-vein needles as a portal of entry. J. Pediatr. 89:96, 1976.
22. Gaze, N. R.: Tissue necrosis caused by commonly used intravenous infusions. Lancet 2:417, 1978.
23. Willis, J., Duncan, C., and Gottschalk, S.: Paraplegia due to peripheral venous air embolus in a neonate: A case report. Pediatrics 67:472, 1981.
24. Hildebrand, W. L., Schreiner, R. L., Yacko, M. S., Gosling, C., and Sternecker, C.: Placing a needle in an infant's scalp vein. Am. Fam. Physician 21:139, 1980.
25. Feldman, S., Goodgold, J., Levy, H., and Zaleznak, B. D.: Acute thrombosis of the femoral artery in an infant. J. Pediatr. 38:498, 1951.
26. Pape, K. E., Armstrong, D. L., and Fitzhardinge, P. M.: Peripheral median nerve damage secondary to brachial arterial blood gas sampling. J. Pediatr. 93:852, 1978.
27. Gast, L. R., Scacci, R., and Miller, W. F.: The effect of heparin dilution on hemoglobin measurement from arterial blood samples. Resp. Care 23:149, 1978.
28. Fan, L. L., Dellinger, K. T., Mills, A. L., and Howard, R. E.: Potential errors in neonatal blood gas measurements. J. Pediatr. 97:650, 1980.
29. Bageant, R. A.: Variations in arterial blood gas measurements due to sampling techniques. Resp. Care 20:565, 1975.
30. Accurso, F. J., Bailey, D. L., and Cotton, E. K.: Effect of syringe heparinization technique on arterial blood gas determination. Pediatr. Res. 14:588, 1980.
31. Curran, J. S., and Ruge, W.: A restraint and transillumination device for neonatal arterial/venipuncture: Efficacy and thermal safety. Pediatrics 66:128, 1980.
32. Schreiner, R. L., Gresham, E. L., Gosling, C. G., and Escobedo, M. B.: Neonatal radial artery puncture: A teaching simulator. Pediatrics (Suppl. 6) 59:1054, 1977.
33. Koenigsberger, M. R., and Moessinger, A. C.: Iatrogenic carpal tunnel syndrome in the newborn infant. J. Pediatr. 91:443, 1977.
34. Speidel, B. D.: Adverse effects of routine procedures on preterm infants. Lancet 1:864, 1978.
35. Long, J. G., Philip, A. G. S., and Lucey, J. F.: Excessive handling as a cause of hypoxemia. Pediatrics 65:203, 1980.
36. Crockett, A. J., McIntyre, E., Ruffin, R., and Alpers, J. H.: Evaluation of lyophilized heparin syringes for the collection of arterial blood for acid base analysis. Anaesth. Intens. Care 9:40, 1981.
37. Lemons, J. A., and Honeyfield, P. R.: Umbilical artery catheterization. Perinatal Care 2:17, 1978.
38. Dorand, R. D., Cook, L. N., and Andrews, B. F.: Umbilical vessel catheterization—the low incidence of complications in a series of 200 newborn infants. Clin. Pediatr. 16:569, 1977.
39. Tooley, W. H., and Myerberg, D. Z.: Should we put catheters in the umbilical artery? Pediatrics 62:853, 1978.
40. Weaver, R. L., and Ahlgren, E. W.: Umbilical artery catheterization in neonates. Am. J. Dis. Child 122:499, 1971.
41. Rosenfeld, W., Biagtan, J., Schaeffer, H., Evans, H., Flicker, S., Salazar, D., and Jhaveri, R.: A new graph for insertion of umbilical artery catheters. J. Pediatr. 96:735, 1980.
42. Mokrohisky, S. T., Levine, R. L., Blumhagen, J. D., Wesenberg, R. L., and Simmons, M. A.: Low positioning of umbilical-artery catheters increases associated complications in newborn infants. N. Engl. J. Med. 299:561, 1978.
43. Harris, M. S., and Little, G. A.: Umbilical artery catheters: High, low, or no. Perinatal Med. 6:15, 1978.
44. Paster, S. B., and Middleton, P.: Roentgenographic evaluation of umbilical artery and vein catheters. JAMA 231:742, 1975.
45. Clark, J. M., and Jung, A. L.: Umbilical artery catheterization by a cutdown procedure. Pediatrics (Suppl. 6) 59:1036, 1977.
46. Clarke, T. A., Levy, L., and Mannino, F.: Use of the placenta as a teaching model. Pediatrics 62:234, 1978.
47. Schreiner, R. L., Gresham, E. L., Escobedo, M. B., and Gosling, C. G.: Umbilical vessel catheterization—a teaching simulator. Clin. Pediatr. 17:506, 1978.
48. Hilliard, J., Schreiner, R. L., and Priest, J.: Hemoperitoneum associated with exchange transfusion through an umbilical arterial catheter. Am. J. Dis. Child 133:216, 1979.
49. Miller, D., Kirkpatrick, B. V., Kodroff, M., Ehrlich, F. E., and Salzberg, A. M.: Pelvic exsanguination following umbilical artery catheterization in neonates. J. Pediatr. Surg. 14:264, 1979.
50. Krauss, A. N., Albert, R. F., and Kannan, M. M.: Contamination of umbilical catheters in the newborn infant. J. Pediatr. 77:965, 1970.
51. Bard, H., Albert, G., Teasdale, F., Doray, B., and Martineau, B.: Prophylactic antibiotics in chronic umbilical artery catheterization in respiratory distress syndrome. Arch. Dis. Child. 48:630, 1973.
52. Cowett, R. M., Peter, G., Hakanson, D. O., Stern, L., and Oh, W.: Prophylactic antibiotics in neonates with umbilical artery catheter placement—a prospective study of 137 patients. Yale J. Biol. Med. 50:457, 1977.
53. Lim, M. O., Gresham, E. L., Franken, E. A., Jr., and Leake, R. D.: Osteomyelitis as a complication of umbilical artery catheterization. Am. J. Dis. Child 131:142, 1977.
54. Goetzman, B. W., Stadalnik, R. C., Bogren, H. G., Blankenship, W. J., Ikeda, R. M., and Thayer, J.: Thrombotic complications of umbilical artery catheters: A clinical and radiographic study. Pediatrics 56:374, 1975.
55. Neal, W. A., Reynolds, J. W., Jarvis, C. W., and Williams, H. J.: Umbilical artery catheterization: Demonstration of arterial thrombosis by aortography. Pediatrics 50:6, 1972.
56. Purohit, D. M., Levkoff, A. H., and deVito, P. C.: Gluteal necrosis with foot-drop—complications associated with umbilical artery catheterization. Am. J. Dis. Child 132:897, 1978.

57. Rudolph, N., Wang, H., and Dragutsky, D.: Gangrene of the buttock: A complication of umbilical artery catheterization. Pediatrics 53:106, 1974.

58. Aziz, E. M., and Robertson, A. F.: Paraplegia: A complication of umbilical artery catheterization. J. Pediatr. 82:1051, 1973.

59. Krishnamoorthy, K. S., Fernandez, R. J., Todres, I. D., and DeLong, G. R.: Paraplegia associated with umbilical artery catheterization in the newborn. Pediatrics 58:443, 1976.

60. Bauer, S. B., Feldman, S. M., Gellis, S. S., and Retik, A. B.: Neonatal hypertension—a complication of umbilical-artery catheterization. N. Engl. J. Med. 293:1032, 1975.

61. Merten, D. F., Vogel, J. M., Adelman, R. D., Goetzman, B. W., and Bogren, H. G.: Renovascular hypertension as a complication of umbilical arterial catheterization. Radiology 126:751, 1978.

62. Plumer, L. B., Kaplan, G. W., and Mendoza, S. A.: Hypertension in infants—a complication of umbilical arterial catheterization. J. Pediatr. 89:802, 1976.

63. Hillman, L. S., Goodwin, S. L., and Sherman, W. R.: Identification and measurement of plasticizer in neonatal tissues after umbilical catheters and blood products. N. Engl. J. Med. 292:381, 1975.

64. Adams, J. M., and Rudolph, A. J.: The use of indwelling radial artery catheters in neonates. Pediatrics 55:261, 1975.

65. Amato, J. J., Solod, E., and Cleveland, R. J.: A "second" radial artery for monitoring the perioperative pediatric cardiac patient. J. Pediatr. Surg. 12:715, 1977.

66. Barr, P. A., Sumners, J., Wirtschafter, D., Porter, R. C., and Cassady, G.: Percutaneous peripheral arterial cannulation in the neonate. Pediatrics (Suppl. 6) 59:1058, 1977.

67. Todres, I. D., Rogers, M. C., Shannon, D. C., Moylan, F. M. B., and Ryan, J. F.: Percutaneous catheterization of the radial artery in the critically ill neonate. J. Pediatr. 87:273, 1975.

68. Schlueter, M. A., Johnson, B. B., Sudman, D. A., Wang, L. Y., Namkung, P., Heasley, S. V., Haddock, S. A., and Tooley, W. H.: Blood sampling from scalp arteries in infants. Pediatrics 51:120, 1973.

69. Au-Yeung, Y. B., Sugg, V. M., Kantor, N. M., Chiu, T. T. W., and Garrison, R. D.: Percutaneous catheterization of scalp arteries in sick infants. J. Pediatr. 91:106, 1977.

70. McArtor, R. D., and Saunders, B. S.: Iatrogenic second-degree burn caused by a transilluminator. Pediatrics 63:422, 1979.

71. Pearse, R. G.: Percutaneous catheterization of the radial artery in newborn babies using transillumination. Arch. Dis. Child. 53:549, 1978.

72. Adams, J. M., Speer, M. E., and Rudolph, A. J.: Bacterial colonization of radial artery catheters. Pediatrics 65:94, 1980.

73. Cartwright, G. W., and Schreiner, R. L.: Major complication secondary to percutaneous radial artery catheterization in the neonate. Pediatrics 65:139, 1980.

74. Mayer, T., Matlak, M. E., and Thompson, J. A.: Necrosis of the forearm following radial artery catheterization in a patient with Reye's syndrome. Pediatrics 65:141, 1980.

75. Spahr, R. C., MacDonald, H. M., and Holzman, I. R.: Catheterization of the posterior tibial artery in the neonate. Am. J. Dis. Child 133:945, 1979.

76. Prian, G. W.: Temporal artery catheterization for arterial access to the high risk newborn. Surgery 82:734, 1977.

77. Prian, G. W.: Complications and sequelae of temporal artery catheterization in the high-risk newborn. J. Pediatr. Surg. 12:829, 1977.

78. McGovern, G., and Baker, A. R.: Temporal artery catheterization for the monitoring of blood gases in infants. Surg. Gynecol. Obstet. 127:601, 1968.

79. Bull, M. J., Schreiner, R. L., Garg, B. P., Hutton, N. M., Lemons, J. A., and Gresham, E. L.: Neurologic complications following temporal artery catheterization. J. Pediatr. 96:1071, 1980.

19

Large–Bore Infusion Catheters (Seldinger Technique of Vascular Access)

ALFRED SACCHETTI, M.D.

Introduction

The expeditious placement of large-bore or central intravenous catheters can be a frustrating task, especially in the hypovolemic or critically ill patient. Not infrequently, the physician is faced with the problem of being unable to locate a suitable vein or, even more frustrating, finding a vein but not being able to cannulate it. The Seldinger technique of catheter introduction may be the optimal solution to difficult vascular access in an emergency department.

There are four basic intravenous access systems: the metal needle technique, the catheter-over-the-needle technique, the catheter-through-the-needle technique, and the Seldinger wire guide technique, each with its own advantages and disadvantages (Fig. 19–1).

Metal needles, or butterfly systems, are unsuitable for most large-bore fluid infusions and are inadequate for central venous catheterization. They are valuable for peripheral intravenous (IV) use in pediatric, septic, or immunosuppressed patients, although even in these cases they are unstable and prone to easy dislodgement.

Catheter-over-the-needle devices are usually the first choice for fluid resuscitation because of their ease of placement, their stability, and their potential for relatively rapid volume infusions. These systems can be used for central lines but have two

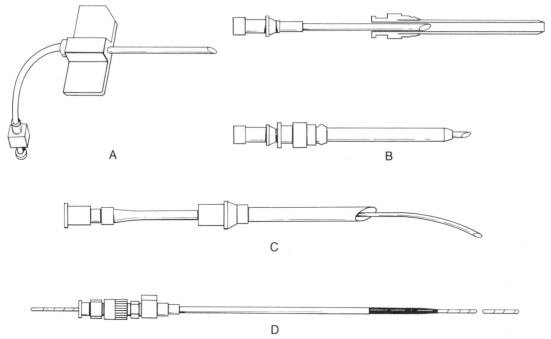

Figure 19–1. Intravenous access systems. *A*, Butterfly. *B*, Catheter over the needle. *C*, Catheter through the needle. *D*, Seldinger-type catheter and guide wire.

disadvantages. The first is that because of the design of the system, the needle will enter the vessel lumen, and a blood return will be observed while the catheter is still outside the vessel wall (Fig. 19–2). If the needle is removed at this point, the catheter will remain outside the vein or artery. The proper technique is to advance the catheter off the needle when a blood return is observed. Even with this approach, however, the catheter may push the vein ahead of it and may still not enter the lumen. The second disadvantage is that the size of the needle is directly related to the size of the catheter. A 14 gauge catheter requires approximately a 14 gauge needle. This is of little concern in peripheral veins but is a major consideration when one is searching for hidden vessels in the chest or the neck.

The catheter-through-the-needle set-ups are designed mainly for central venous cannulations.

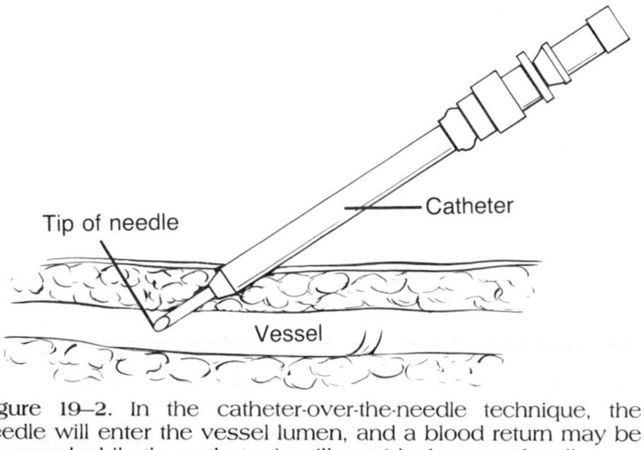

There is a much greater probability of successfully advancing the catheter into the lumen with this system, since the catheter is threaded through the needle. There is the very real risk of catheter embolism, however, because the catheter may be sheared off if it is withdrawn through the needle. In a tense, rushed environment this can happen quite easily. In addition, the needle size is determined by the gauge of the catheter, as in catheter-over the needle devices, and since the catheter must be small enough to fit through the introducing needle, the catheter must be smaller than the needle. As a result the puncture site in the vessel wall is larger than the final indwelling device, which may result in leakage around the insertion site. These devices have little place in current vascular access systems.

The Seldinger technique offers the advantages of rapid intravenous access with none of the aforementioned hazards. The technique is also excellent for the placement of temporary transvenous pacemakers or Swan-Ganz catheters.

The guide-wire-through-the-needle technique was originally described in 1953 by S. I. Seldinger as a method for catheter placement in percutaneous arteriography.[1] The basic approach is extremely simple and has been adapted for placement of any catheter in any hollow-lumened structure or body cavity. A needle much smaller than the infusion catheter is used to enter a vessel, and a wire is threaded through the needle. The needle is removed, the wire is left in the vessel, and the catheter is advanced over the wire using the wire as a guide into the lumen. The major advantage of this system is the rapid placement

Figure 19–2. In the catheter-over-the-needle technique, the needle will enter the vessel lumen, and a blood return may be observed while the catheter is still outside the vessel wall.

Table 19–1. RELATIVE FLOW RATES FOR VARIOUSLY SIZED CATHETERS*

Catheter Size	Flow (ml/min)
8.5 French × 12 cm†	108
8.0 French × 13 cm†	96
14 gauge × 5.7 cm	94
14 gauge × 13.3 cm	83
16 gauge × 5.7 cm	83
16 gauge × 13.3 cm	57
16 gauge × 20 cm	25
18 gauge × 4.3 cm	55

*These flow rates are only comparative and represent the rate of emptying of 1-L bottles of normal saline solution over a gradient of 3 m. The absolute rate of flow of these catheters is variable and is determined by the clinical situation.
†Cook Corp. High-Flo Desilets-Hoffman sheaths.

of variously sized catheters in the peripheral or central circulation using small-gauge needles to initially puncture the vessel.

Indications

In situations requiring volume expansion, the rate of fluid resuscitation is determined directly by the size and length of the intravenous catheter. Poiseuille and Hagen's law states that the flow of fluid through a catheter is proportional to the fourth power of the diameter of the device and the inverse of its length.[2] Table 19–1 shows the relative flow rates of various IV catheters. It should be noted that the flow rate through a 5.7-cm, 16 gauge catheter is more than three times faster than that through a catheter of identical diameter with a 20-cm length. As is often the case, patients in most need of large vascular infusions may be the ones in whom access is the most difficult. With the use of a needle much smaller than the final catheter size, the probability of finding and entering a collapsed or hidden vessel is greatly increased. In addition, the smaller needle reduces the damage caused by inadvertent entering of the wrong vessel or adjacent structures. These advantages are magnified even more in the pediatric patient, in whom finding any vascular access can be difficult. Table 19–2 lists catheters of various sizes and their introducer needle sizes. It should be noted that one may introduce a 3 French catheter using a rather small 21 gauge needle.

Table 19–2. CATHETER AND NEEDLE SIZES

Patient	Catheter Size	Needle Gauge
Less than 10 kg	3 French*	21
Less than 10 kg	4.0–4.5 French	20
10 kg to 40 kg	5.0–6.0 French	20–19
Over 40 kg	6.0–8.5 French	19–18

*This size supplied only as simple catheter. All others are available as Desilets-Hoffman sheath introducers.

Because it involves the percutaneous cannulation of vessels, the Seldinger technique is faster and more versatile than any cutdown approach. Seldinger-technique catheters may be placed in any vessel but are particularly valuable in central venous locations. External jugular, internal jugular, subclavian, basilic, cephalic, saphenous, and femoral veins as well as any peripheral or central artery can be cannulated using the Seldinger technique.

One can readily appreciate the way in which the ability to introduce an 8.5 French catheter quickly through an 18 gauge needle can alter the course of fluid resuscitation in a patient with vascular collapse. This technique can rapidly convert an 18 gauge peripheral IV catheter placed in the field by paramedics into a large-bore access route for blood fluids within seconds of the arrival of the patient at the emergency department.

Although large-bore fluid resuscitation has been stressed, other devices may be introduced with this technique. The wire acts as an ideal guide for the subsequent placement of Swan-Ganz catheters, pacemakers, and arteriography tools. Although the Seldinger technique may not always be required initially, one should be certain that all central venous pressure (CVP) lines placed are large enough to accommodate the guide wire. Should a patient with a standard CVP line deteriorate, one simply passes the guide wire through the already existing CVP line. With the aid of the dilator-introducer, one now has a ready access for a transvenous pacemaker or Swan-Ganz catheter without needing to cannulate another central vein.

Equipment

The equipment needed for the Seldinger wire guide technique of vascular access is listed in Table 19–3. All of the equipment, with the exception of the needle, the wire, and the catheter, is standard emergency department stock. It is preferable not to use a Luer-Lok syringe in this situation, because the added twisting needed to remove the syringe from the needle may dislodge a needle that is tenuously located in a vein.

Table 19–3. NECESSARY EQUIPMENT FOR SELDINGER TECHNIQUE

Introducing needle	Lidocaine
Guide wire	3-ml syringe
Catheter or sheath introducer	(for anesthetizing)
Prep solution (iodine)	3- to 5-ml syringe
Sterile gloves	Suture (00–000)
Small anesthetizing needle	Drapes
(25 gauge)	Antibiotic ointment
Gauze pads	Completed radiograph
Prep razor	request
Number 11 scalpel	

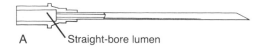

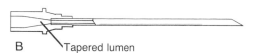

Figure 19–3. Introducing needles. *A*, Ordinary needle with straight-bore lumen. *B*, Seldinger needle with tapered lumen.

Many of the companies that produce this equipment market it within kits containing the three main items: the needle, the wire, and the catheter. Although any of these items can be purchased separately, it should be mentioned that in the midst of a hectic resuscitation asking a nurse for one item (the kit) rather than three is more than a mere convenience.

NEEDLE

Virtually any needle or catheter can be used to introduce a guide wire into a vessel; however, two factors must be kept in mind. First, the needle must be large enough to accommodate the desired wire. The needles contained in prepared sets are usually thin-walled, and therefore a smaller gauge can accommodate a larger wire. If a needle that is not thin-walled is used, a size one gauge larger than that listed in Table 19–2 should be used. Most standard peripheral IV catheters of 18 gauge or larger will accept the guide wire, and in an emergency one should first attempt to convert the

peripheral IV rather than search for another accessible vein. Another factor in the selection of the introducing needle is the taper of the lumen at the proximal end. Seldinger needles have a funnel-shaped taper that guides the wire directly into the needle (Fig. 19–3). Ordinary needles may have a straight-bore lumen leading squarely into the needle. These needles can present a problem when the wire abuts against the flat end-plate surface.

GUIDE WIRE

The guide wires used are of two basic types; straight or J-shaped. The straight wires are for use in vessels with a linear configuration, and the J wires are for use in tortuous vessels. Both wires have essentially the same internal design (Fig. 19–4A). The flexibility of the wire is a result of a stainless steel coil or helix that forms the bulk of the guide wire. Within the central lumen of the helix is a straight central core wire, called a mandrel. The mandrel is fixed at one end of the helix and terminates 0.5 to 3 cm from the other end. The mandrel adds rigidity to the portion of the wire that contains it, whereas the rest of the wire without the mandrel is floppy and flexible. Many guide wires also contain a straight safety wire that runs parallel to the mandrel to keep the wire from kinking or shearing.

The floppy end of the straight wire allows atraumatic passage of the guide wire through a relatively straight vessel. The J wire is useful in areas where vessels turn at sharp angles or are tortuous and in vessels with valves. The internal structure of the J wire is similar to that of the straight wire, except that the flexible tip remains a J shape. This gives the leading edge of the wire a rounded surface that may be turned, twisted, or otherwise manipulated around corners or valves in an atrau-

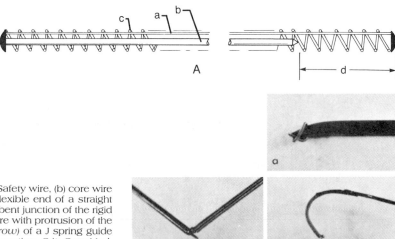

Figure 19–4. *A*, Guide wire internal structure. (a) Safety wire, (b) core wire (mandrel), (c) coiled wire, (d) flexible tip. *B*, (a) Flexible end of a straight spring guide wire knotted on a vessel dilator, (b) bent junction of the rigid and flexible portions of a straight spring guide wire with protrusion of the central core *(arrow)*, (c) partially fractured tip *(arrow)* of a J spring guide wire. (From Schwartz, A., et al.: Guide wires—a caution. Crit. Care Med. 9:348, 1981. Used by permission.)

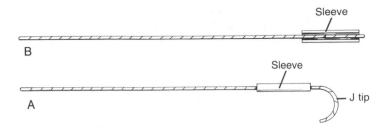

Figure 19–5. J wire. *A*, Plastic sleeve in retracted position demonstrating J tip, *B*, Plastic sleeve advanced to straighten curve.

matic fashion. The J wire is most commonly used for external jugular vein catheterization to help negotiate the junction of the external jugular vein with the subclavian vein and to bypass the valves in the external jugular vein.

One easily introduces the straight wire by threading the flexible end of the wire into the proximal hub of the indwelling needle. To introduce the J wire, a plastic sleeve contained in the kit is advanced to the floppy end of the wire to straighten out the J shape. This end is now introduced into the proximal hub of the indwelling needle. Once the J wire has been advanced, the sleeve is removed and discarded (Fig. 19–5).

It is important to emphasize that the guide wires are delicate and may bend, kink, break, or unwind. A force of 4 to 6 lbs will result in rupture of the wire. Repeated or excessive manipulation of the wires will predispose them to fracture or will promote separation of the coiled portion. Embolization of portions of the guide wire is possible, and sharp defects in the wire may perforate vessel walls (Fig. 19–4*B*). One should carefully inspect wires before use for defects, such as kinks, sharp ends or spurs, and weak points. Wires should be threaded easily and smoothly and should never be forced.

CATHETERS

Once a guide wire is in place and the needle is removed, any of a number of devices may be introduced. Simple catheters for central venous pressure monitoring or arterial lines are threaded directly over the wire into the appropriate vessels. These catheters are exactly identical to non–Seldinger-type catheters and function well for low-flow infusions, drug administrations, and monitoring. This technique will not work for large-bore catheters and nonlumened devices, such as pacemakers. To place these devices, a Desilets-Hoffman–type sheath introducer unit is used. This introducer unit was designed by D. T. Desilets and R. Hoffman in 1965 to aid in arteriography procedures requiring multiple catheter changes.[3] The sheath introducer unit consists basically of two catheters, one inside another (Fig. 19–6). The first catheter, termed the *dilator*, is hard, with an inner lumen to fit over the guide wire. This catheter is longer and thinner than its sheath and has a tapered end; it serves as a *dilator* when the unit is passed through subcutaneous tissue and into the vessel. The second catheter, termed the *sheath*, has a blunt end and is simply a catheter with a large diameter. This sheath may be used as an

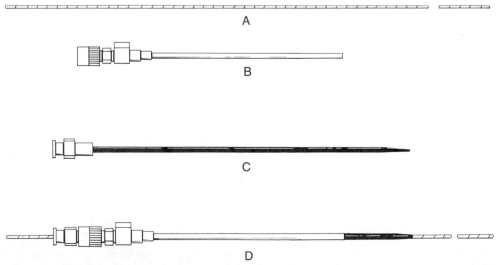

Figure 19–6. Desilets-Hoffman sheath introducer. *A*, Guide wire. *B*, Sheath. *C*, Dilator. *D*, Assembled device.

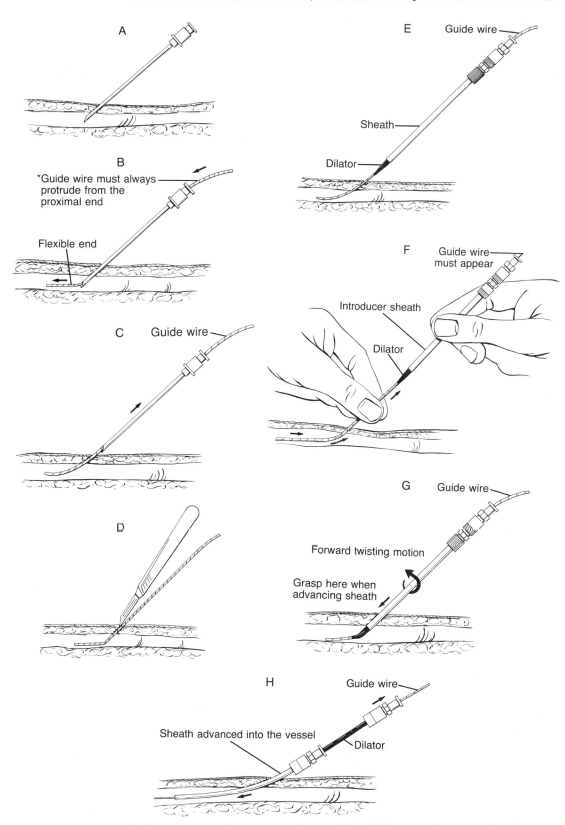

Figure 19–7. Procedure for placement of Seldinger-type guide wire catheter. *A,* The selected vessel is cannulated. *B,* The guide wire is threaded through the vessel with the flexible end first into the lumen of the vessel. *C,* The needle is removed so that only the wire now exits from the vessel. *D,* The skin entry site is enlarged with a number 11 scalpel. *E,* The catheter sheath and the dilator are threaded over the wire and advanced to the skin. The wire must be visible through the back of the device. *F,* If the proximal wire is *not* visible, it is pulled from the skin through the catheter until it appears at the back of the catheter. *G,* The sheath and the dilator are advanced as a unit into the skin with a twisting motion. It is best to grasp the unit at the junction of the sheath and the dilator to prevent bunching up of the sheath. *H,* Once the sheath and the dilator are well within the vessel, the wire guide and the dilator are removed.

infusion catheter or may serve as a guide for passage of a pacemaker or a Swan-Ganz catheter.

Many modifications of the sheath exist, with side arms and diaphragms to aid in placement of Swan-Ganz catheters and pacemakers. Care must be taken in the use of side arm sets for rapid fluid administration, since some catheters may be 8.5 French but may have only a 5 French side arm. If faced with this problem, one can introduce an 8 French feeding tube through the diaphragm at the catheter hub for rapid fluid administration.

Procedure

The actual procedure for placement of Seldinger-type guide wire catheters is quite simple:

Sterile technique is maintained. The area of vascular access is prepared and cleaned as described in the section on central venous access. The first step is to place the guide wire into the desired vessel. An introducing needle or a standard over-the-needle catheter that is large enough to accommodate the guide wire is selected. The needle is attached to a small syringe (Fig. 19–7). The needle and syringe are introduced together, and the selected vessel is cannulated. Once a free return of blood is obtained, the syringe is removed, and the flexible end of the guide wire is threaded through the needle. If an IV catheter is already in place, the wire is passed through it before the catheter is removed from the vein.

When working with large central veins, one must take care to avoid aspiration of air through the exposed needle. A finger should thus be placed over the hub after the syringe is removed until passage of the wire. The wire should thread smoothly. If resistance is met, the wire should not be forced but should be removed from the needle, and the syringe should be reattached to confirm intravascular placement. Occasionally, the wire must be teased into the vessel; rotating the needle or the wire itself can often help in difficult placements. The guide wire should be threaded until at least one quarter of the wire is within the patient's blood vessel. Once this is accomplished, the needle or IV catheter is removed. Now only the guide wire remains in the vessel. At this point a small incision is made in the skin at the site of the wire. The incision should be approximately the size of the catheter to be introduced. Alternatively, some physicians prefer to make the skin nick first and to introduce the needle through this incision. The disadvantage of this approach is that if the vessel is displaced, the physician is forced to attempt a difficult entry through the existing incision or to make a second incision.

Once the incision is made, the sheath with dilator is threaded over the wire to a point 1 cm from the surface of the skin. *At this point, the wire should be protruding from the back end of the introducer unit.* This is a critically important procedural point. If the wire is not protruding from the proximal end of the introducer unit, it may be lost in the vessel and may migrate to the central circulation. If the wire is not visible, it is carefully withdrawn from the vein until it exits from the proximal end of the introducer unit. *The wire must always be visible and graspable from the back end of the catheter throughout the remainder of the procedure.* Guide wires are always longer than the catheters. The guide wire needs to be advanced only a few inches into the vessel for the procedure to be performed correctly; advancing the wire more than a few inches may result in losing the wire completely. With experience it becomes easy to judge the optimal distance to thread the wire in order to ensure good introducer placement as well as to leave enough wire protruding from the proximal end of the catheter.

Once the wire is visible, it is grasped and held. The introducer unit is threaded into the skin with a twisting motion until it is well within the vessel. When one uses the sheath and dilator, it is best to grasp the unit at the junction of the sheath and the dilator. This prevents the thinner sheath from kinking or bending at the tip or from bunching up at the coupler end. The dilator need only be advanced a few centimeters into the vessel, because it only serves to dilate the vessel so that it will accept the sheath. Once the vessel has been dilated, the sheath is advanced over the dilator to its full length within the vessel. The wire and the dilator are then removed, leaving the sheath in the selected vessel. The device is usually affixed with one or two sutures, and infusion or monitoring is begun.

The Seldinger technique can be used for the placement of catheters in any body cavity (for example, for passing a guide for peritoneal lavage). The approach is identical to that described for vascular access, except that blood will not be aspirated through the introducing needle. Other situations in which this technique is used include intra-abdominal abscess drainage, percutaneous nephrostomy and cystostomy, cricothyrotomy, and pericardiocentesis.

Complications

Vascular access using the Seldinger technique holds the promise of fewer injuries to vessels and adjacent structures by virtue of the use of a small locator needle rather than direct large-bore needle cannulation of a vessel. Nonetheless, injuries similar to those reported for conventional vessel cannulation (see Chapters 21, 22, and 26) may occur.

Complications unique to the Seldinger technique include guide wire migration and trauma from defective guidewire tips (see Fig. 19–4B).[4]

1. Seldinger, S. I.: Catheter replacement of needle in percutaneous arteriography. Acta Radiol. 39:368, 1953.
2. Macintosh, R., Mushin, W. W., and Epstein, H. G.: Physics for the Anaesthetist, 2nd ed. Springfield, IL, Charles C Thomas, 1958.
3. Desilets, D. T., and Hoffman, R.: A new method of percutaneous catheterization. Radiology 85:145, 1965.
4. Schwartz, A., Horrow, J., Jobes, D., and Ellison, N.: Guide wires—a caution. Crit. Care Med. 9:4, 1981.
5. McIntyre, K., and Lewis, A. J.: Textbook of Advanced Cardiac Life Support. Dallas, American Heart Association, 1981.

20

Venous Cutdown

STEVEN C. DRONEN, M.D.

Introduction

"The standard cutdown is well known to all surgeons and needs no description."[1] Were this a true statement, the remainder of this chapter would be superfluous; however, physician training in the technique of venous cutdown has been largely informal. For four decades, the mechanics of venous cutdown have been handed down from house officer to house officer as one of the rites of internship. There are, in fact, few detailed descriptions of the procedure in the medical literature, and the scientific data documenting its usefulness or complication rate are sparse.

The frequency with which the venous cutdown is performed is impossible to estimate. The growing popularity of central venous cannulation by the internal jugular and subclavian routes has most probably decreased the frequency of venisection. Nevertheless, the cutdown remains an excellent method of obtaining venous access in several emergent clinical situations.

Although a cutdown is mechanically simple to perform, ease of performance does not guarantee that the procedure will be performed efficiently and without complications. This can be achieved only by a thorough knowledge of the procedure and by attention to its many details.

Historical Background

An early description of the technique of venous cutdown was provided by Keeley in 1940. He offered the procedure as an alternative to venipuncture in patients in shock or in individuals with small, thin veins.[2] In 1945, Kirkham gave the first detailed description of the saphenous vein cutdown at the ankle.[3] Although the article is now somewhat dated, most of the steps remain unchanged today.

The most significant changes over the past four decades have involved not the technique itself but the cannulas that are used. Keeley and Kirkham used metal needles. With the advent of plastic cannulas in the mid-1940s, the cutdown became more popular as a means of providing long-term intravenous (IV) infusion. In recent years, physicians have used IV tubing, feeding tubes, and even nasogastric tubes as cannulas in the management of hypovolemic patients.

Indications

There are no absolute indications for venous cutdown, simply because several options for venous access usually exist. The indications for use of the procedure are relative, depending to a great extent upon physician experience and preference. There are several clinical situations in which the venous cutdown may be used.

Venous Access in Infants. Small children present a unique challenge to the clinician who does not perform pediatric venipuncture regularly. The challenge is greater still if the procedure must be performed rapidly in a critically ill child. The distal saphenous vein is large enough to cannulate in most children and has a predictable anatomic location. Consequently, venous cutdown at the ankle is commonly used for both emergent and long-term venous access.[4, 5]

A venous cutdown may be performed when all accessible peripheral sites have been exhausted. Alternatively many physicians would cannulate the subclavian or internal jugular veins under these circumstances.

The rapid percutaneous insertion of large-bore (14 gauge) catheters is appropriate in most cases of hypovolemic shock. Unfortunately, peripheral vessels frequently collapse in hypovolemia or have been rendered useless by intravenous drug abuse or previous venous catheterization. The venous cutdown is an acceptable alternative in these instances. When the procedure is efficiently performed, time is not wasted searching for a vein, and under direct control it is easy to insert catheters of large diameter. The use of the cutdown as a vehicle for the insertion of intravenous extension tubing and rapid transfusion was popularized during the Vietnam war.[6] The technique has also been found useful in civilian practice for the resuscitation of patients with profound hypovolemia.[7] The superiority of large-bore lines is determined by physical laws, which state that flow is proportional to the fourth power of cannula radius and inversely proportional to cannula length and fluid viscosity. The flow rate for saline through a standard IV extension set (3 mm inside diameter) cut to a length of 12 inches and inserted directly into the vein is 15 to 30 per cent greater than that through a 2-inch, 14 gauge catheter. The difference is greater if pressure is applied to the system; blood products also flow much faster through large-bore lines because of viscosity factors, which slow the passage of blood through small gauge tubing.[7, 8] One can transfuse a unit of blood in 3 minutes using IV extension tubing inserted intravenously. Consequently, large-bore lines placed by venous cutdown are an excellent mechanism for the treatment of severe hypovolemia.

Contraindications

Venous cutdown is contraindicated when less invasive alternatives exist or when excessive delay would be required for the procedure to be performed.[9] Percutaneous insertion of large-bore catheters is the preferred method of fluid resuscitation unless very high flow rates are required or peripheral vessels are collapsed. Another method of rapid fluid infusion that is technically easier than venisection is the percutaneous insertion of large-bore introducer devices into the subclavian, internal jugular, or large peripheral veins (see Chapter 19). The use of these vessels is also preferable to the cutdown for long-term applications.

Other contraindications are relative. In the presence of coagulation disorders, impaired healing, or compromised host defense mechanisms, the need to perform a cutdown should be weighed carefully against the potential complications.

Anatomy

Detailed knowledge of anatomy is critically important to the success of this procedure. Veins in both the upper and the lower extremities may be used. The choice of a particular vein should be governed by its accessibility and size and by the physician's experience and training. The anatomy of individual vessels and their relative merits as cutdown sites are described in the following paragraphs.

The Greater Saphenous Vein. The greater saphenous vein is the longest vein and runs subcutaneously throughout much of its course (Fig. 20–1). It is most easily accessible at the ankle but may also be cannulated above the knee and below the femoral triangle. The greater saphenous vein begins at the ankle where it is the continuation of the medial marginal vein of the foot. The vein crosses 1 cm anterior to the medial malleolus and continues up the anteromedial aspect of the leg.[10] At the level of the malleolus, the vein lies adjacent to the periosteum and is accompanied by the relatively insignificant saphenous nerve, which if

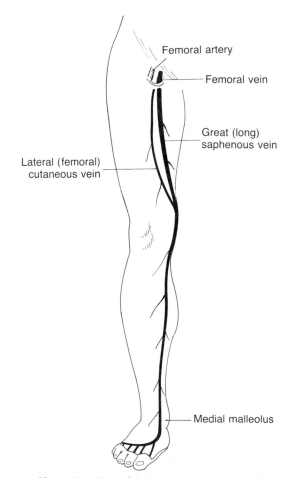

Femoral artery

Femoral vein

Great (long) saphenous vein

Lateral (femoral) cutaneous vein

Medial malleolus

Figure 20–1. Superficial veins of the lower limb.

transected causes little or no sensory loss along the medial aspect of the foot. At the ankle, the vessel can be exposed with minimal blunt dissection. The vein's superficial, predictable, and isolated location has made the distal saphenous vein the classical pediatric cutdown site.[11]

The saphenous vein lies superficially on the medial aspect of the knee. A cutdown performed 1 to 4 cm below the knee and immediately posterior to the tibia is described in the pediatric literature.[4] This site is distal enough to avoid interference with the performance of other resuscitative procedures, yet proximal enough to allow the passage of a long line into the central circulation.[12] This site of venous cutdown is seldom used, however. Disadvantages of this technique include kinking of the line as the leg is flexed and the risk of injury to associated structures. Improper placement of the incision may injure the saphenous branch of the genicular artery and the saphenous nerve.[13]

In the thigh, the saphenous vein begins on the medial aspect of the knee and crosses anterolaterally as it ascends toward the femoral triangle. Proximally, it enters the fossa ovalis and joins the femoral vein. Three to 4 cm distal to the inguinal ligament the saphenous vein is of large caliber (4 to 5 mm outside diameter) and is easily isolated from the surrounding fat. Also lying anteromedially in the thigh is the lateral femoral cutaneous vein, which has a smaller diameter (2 to 3 mm) and lies lateral to the greater saphenous vein.[14, 15]

The accessibility and large diameter of the greater saphenous vein in the thigh make it an excellent choice in the treatment of profound hypovolemia.[7]

The Basilic Vein. The basilic vein is the preferred site for venous cutdown in the upper extremity. Veins of the dorsal venous network of the hand unite to form the cephalic and basilic veins, traveling along the radial and ulnar sides of the forearm, respectively (Fig. 20–2). At the level of the mid-forearm, the basilic vein crosses anterolaterally and is consistently found 1 to 2 cm lateral to the medial epicondyle on the anterior surface of the upper arm. The median cubital vein crosses over from the radial side of the arm to join the basilic vein just above the medial epicondyle. The basilic vein then continues proximally, occupying a superficial position between the biceps and pronator teres muscles. In this segment it lies in close association with the medial cutaneous nerve, which supplies sensation to the ulnar side of the forearm. The vein penetrates the brachial fascia in the distal third of the upper arm and then occupies a deeper position.[16]

The basilic vein is generally cannulated at the antecubital fossa a few centimeters proximal to the flexor skin crease. It is exposed through a transverse incision on the medial aspect of the proximal antecubital fossa. This vein is of sufficient size to be easily located even in the hypotensive or hypovolemic patient. Large catheters, such as intravenous extension tubing and pediatric feeding tubes, can generally be passed without difficulty.

Figure 20–2. The veins of the upper limb.

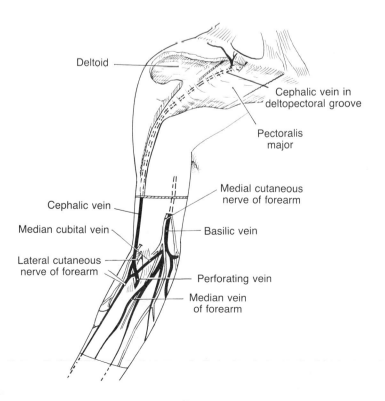

Deltoid

Cephalic vein in deltopectoral groove

Pectoralis major

Medial cutaneous nerve of forearm

Cephalic vein

Median cubital vein

Basilic vein

Lateral cutaneous nerve of forearm

Perforating vein

Median vein of forearm

The median cubital vein is accessible through the same incision. Superficially at this level there are no important associated structures, but the brachial artery and the median nerve are found deep to the basilic vein. In the distal third of the upper arm there is risk of injury to the medial cutaneous nerve, which can result in sensory loss on the ulnar side of the forearm.

The Cephalic Vein. This vessel begins on the radial aspect of the wrist and crosses anteromedially, ascending toward the antecubital fossa (see Fig. 20–2). In the forearm it lies in close association with the lateral cutaneous nerve, which supplies sensory innervation to the radial aspect of the forearm. In the antecubital fossa it lies subcutaneously, just lateral to the midline, and then ascends in the upper arm, overlying the lateral aspect of the biceps muscle. At the shoulder the cephalic vein lies in the deltopectoral groove. Just below the clavicle, it passes deep to end in the axillary vein.[16]

Venisection is easily performed on the cephalic vein because of its large diameter and superficial location. In the forearm it is important to avoid the lateral cutaneous nerve. The best location is in the antecubital fossa at the distal flexor crease. The cephalic vein may also be entered in the deltopectoral groove. The slightly deeper position and physical interference with the performance of other procedures make this approach more difficult.

The Brachial Veins. The brachial veins are small, paired vessels lying on either side of the brachial artery. In contrast with the vessels described earlier, these are not superficial and will not accommodate large cannulas. Their most superficial location is 1 to 2 cm above the antecubital fossa just medial to the biceps muscle. Palpation of the brachial pulse serves as a useful landmark, but the artery may be inadvertently cannulated in the pulseless patient. Additionally, there is the risk of injury to the closely associated median nerve. Time-consuming blunt dissection is generally required. Consequently, the brachial vein cutdown is not recommended as an emergency venous access route[9] and should be used only in the absence of a suitable alternative. This site may be acceptable when time and vessel size are not critical factors, but it is difficult to justify the deep dissection that is required.

The External Jugular Vein. The external jugular vein begins below the angle of the mandible formed by confluence of the posterior auricular and retromandibular veins. It descends posterolaterally across the surface of the sternocleidomastoid muscle and then pierces the fascia to join the subclavian vein deep to the clavicular head of this muscle. The greater auricular nerve, which supplies sensation to the external ear, travels parallel to the external jugular vein.[10]

A venous cutdown may be performed on the external jugular vein at its superficial location on the sternocleidomastoid muscle. This is not recommended as a first-line means of venous access for the following reasons: (1) There is risk of injury to the greater auricular nerve; (2) performance of a cutdown may cause physical interference with airway management and central venous cannulation; (3) it is difficult to immobilize the area adequately; and (4) it is a hazardous procedure in the uncooperative patient.[9] As a general rule, cutdown on the external jugular vein should be performed only when other means of venous access are exhausted. The external jugular vein is an acceptable site for emergency percutaneous venous cannulation, however, especially in children.

Equipment

The materials required are listed in Table 20–1. All necessary instruments should be available on a sterile tray before the procedure is begun. The standard cutdown tray is shown in Figure 20–3. A time-consuming search for the proper instrument can be avoided if only necessary instruments are included. The appropriate catheter should also be placed on this tray. Catheter choice depends upon the function of the venous line. When a central position is required, the catheter chosen must be long enough to reach the superior vena cava (SVC). The average distance from the antecubital fossa to the SVC is 54 cm in the adult male. One can approximate this distance by aligning the catheter over the chest with the tip at the level of the manubrial-sternal junction. Lumen size is relatively unimportant when the line is intended to measure central venous pressure (CVP) or to infuse drugs, but it is a critical factor in the treatment of hypovolemia. Short, large-bore catheters are preferred when fluids must be rapidly delivered. Silastic catheters are preferred by some over plastic tubing. A pediatric 5 or 8 French feeding tube may

Table 20–1. MATERIALS REQUIRED FOR VENOUS CUTDOWN*

Curved Kelly hemostat
Scalpel with number 11 blade
Small mosquito hemostat
Tissue spreader
Iris scissors
Plastic venous dilator or lifter
4–0 silk suture ties
4–0 nylon suture on cutting needle
Antibiotic ointment
Gauze sponges
1-inch tape
Armboard
Intravenous catheter
Rolled gauze bandage

*See Figure 20–3.

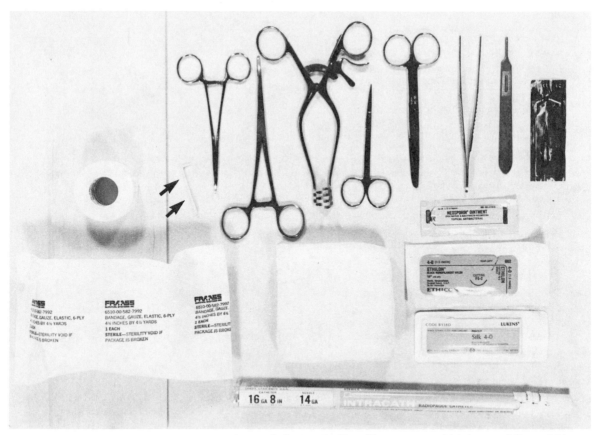

Figure 20–3. Venous cutdown tray. Note the small plastic vein dilator/lifter *(arrows)*, which is especially useful in children.

also be used as an infusion catheter. Tables 20–2, 20–3, and 20–4 list the flow rate of fluids through some of the commonly used devices. Knowledge of relative flow rates is essential if maximal benefit is to be obtained from the time spent performing the cutdown. One can achieve optimal flow rates by threading intravenous tubing (sterile tubing may be cut to the appropriate length) directly into the vein or by using a 2-inch, 14 gauge catheter.[17] It is particularly important to note the low rate of infusion using long 16 gauge catheters. These are commonly, but inappropriately, used in the treatment of hypovolemic patients. Their flow rate is less than half that provided by 3-mm internal diameter IV extension tubing.[7] These differences are accentuated when blood is infused.[8]

Technique

The technique of venous cutdown is essentially the same regardless of the vessel cannulated (Figs. 20–4 through 20–13). Detailed knowledge of the local anatomy is important if the procedure is to be performed rapidly without injury to associated structures. Even in emergent situations, reasonable precautions should be taken to avoid infec-

tion. The area of the skin incision should be widely prepared with an antiseptic solution and then draped. A tourniquet placed proximal to the cutdown site will help in the visualization of the vein.

In the conscious patient, the site is infiltrated with 1 per cent lidocaine (Xylocaine). A skin incision is made transverse to the course of the vessel (see Fig. 20–4). A longitudinal incision may decrease the risk of transecting neurovascular structures but does not provide sufficient exposure. A transverse incision involving all layers of the skin is the best approach. Subcutaneous fat should bulge from the incision. One bluntly dissects subcutaneous tissue by spreading the tissue gently with a curved hemostat. The tissue is spread in a direction parallel to the course of the vein. Bleeding is usually minimal, unless the vein is nicked. A tissue spreader or a self-retaining retractor may be used to provide a wider field. The vein is then isolated from the adjacent tissue and mobilized for 1 to 3 cm (see Fig. 20–5).

After the vein is mobilized, proximal and distal silk ties are passed under it. The distal ligature may or may not be tied at this point, but if it is tied it should not be cut, because it is useful in controlling the vein (see Fig. 20–6). Some prefer not to tie off the vein so that the vein may be used

Table 20–2. COMPARATIVE AVERAGE FLOW RATES (ml/min) FOR TAP WATER*

Catheter	Pressure 200 mm Hg (95% CI)†	Gravity (95% CI)
Central Venous Catheters		
USCI 9 French Introducer Internal diameter 0.117 in., length 5½ in.	566 (±16)	247 (±2)
USCI 8 French Introducer Internal diameter 0.104 in., length 5½ in.	540‡	243 (±5)
Deseret Angiocath Gauge 14, length 5¼ in.	341 (±6)	157 (±6)
Deseret Angiocath Gauge 16, length 5¼ in.	195 (±4)	91 (±2)
Deseret Subclavian Jugular Catheter Gauge 16, length 12 in.	142 (±4)	54 (±3)
Peripheral Venous Catheters		
IV Extension Tubing Internal diameter 0.12 in., length 12 in.	500 (±21)	222 (±4)
Argyle Medicut Gauge 14, length 2 in.	484 (±8)	194 (±5)
Deseret Angiocath Gauge 14, length 2 in.	405 (±2)	173 (±4)
Vicra Quick-Cath Gauge 14, length 2¼ in.	—	167 (±1)
Argyle Medicut Gauge 16, length 2 in.	353 (±4)	151 (±3)
Deseret Angiocath Gauge 16, length 2 in.	231 (±1)	108 (±1)
Vicra Quick-Cath Gauge 16, length 2 in.	—	108 (±1)

*Mean of three trials with hydrostatic pressure head of 1 m.
†CI = confidence interval.
‡95% confidence interval not calculated because all three trials resulted in 11.1 sec for 100-ml flow.
(From Mateer, J. R., et al.: Rapid fluid resuscitation with central venous catheters. Ann. Emerg. Med. 12:150, 1983. Used by permission.)

Table 20–3. COMPARATIVE AVERAGE FLOW RATES (ml/min, 200 mm Hg Pressure) FOR RED BLOOD CELLS

Catheter	Diluted PRBCs Hct 45% (95% CI)	Diluted PRBCs Hct 45% Through Blood Warmer (95% CI)	PRBCs Hct 65% (95% CI)
Central Venous Catheters			
USCI 9 French Introducer Internal diameter 0.117 in., length 5½ in.	343 (±21)	218 (±26)	124 (±2)
USCI 8 French Introducer Internal diameter 0.104 in., length 5½ in.	324 (±23)	—	—
Deseret Angiocath Gauge 14, length 5¼ in.	210 (±7)	171 (±9)	63 (±6)
Deseret Angiocath Gauge 16, length 5¼ in.	125 (±4)	—	—
Peripheral Venous Catheters			
IV Extension Tubing Internal diameter 0.12 in., length 12 in.	312 (±1)	—	—
Argyle Medicut Gauge 14, length 2 in.	287 (±21)	192 (±15)	96 (±6)
Deseret Angiocath Gauge 14, length 2 in.	257 (±11)	—	—
Argyle Medicut Gauge 16, length 2 in.	220 (±5)	—	—
Deseret Angiocath Gauge 16, length 2 in.	158 (±14)	—	—

(From Mateer, J. R., et al.: Rapid fluid resuscitation with central venous catheters. Ann. Emerg. Med. 12:151, 1983. Used by permission.)

Table 20–4. COMPARATIVE AVERAGE FLOW RATES IN (ml/min)

Catheter	Tap Water at 200 mm Hg	Diluted PRBCs at 200 mm Hg	Tap Water Gravity	Diluted PRBCs Blood Warmer at 200 mm Hg	PRBCs at 200 mm Hg
Central Venous Catheters					
USCI 9 French Introducer Internal diameter 0.117 in., length 5½ in.	566 (±16)	343 (±21)	247 (±2)	218 (±26)	124 (±2)
USCI 8 French Introducer Internal diameter 0.104 in., length 5½ in.	540*	324 (±23)	243 (±5)	—	—
Deseret Angiocath Gauge 14, length 5¼ in.	341 (±6)	210 (±7)	157 (±6)	171 (±9)	63 (±6)
Peripheral Venous Catheters					
IV Extension Tubing Internal diameter 0.12 in., length 12 in.	500 (±21)	312 (±1)	222 (±4)	—	—
Argyle Medicut Gauge 14, length 2 in.	484 (±8)	287 (±21)	194 (±5)	192 (±15)	96 (±6)
Argyle Medicut Gauge 16, length 2 in.	353 (±4)	220 (±5)	151 (±3)	—	—

*95% confidence interval not calculated because all three trials resulted in 11.1 sec for 100-ml flow.
(From Mateer, J. R., et al.: Rapid fluid resuscitation with central venous catheters. Ann. Emerg. Med. 12:151, 1983. Used by permission.)

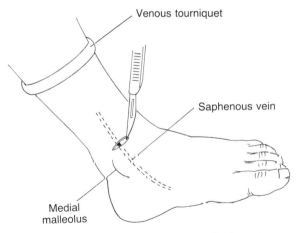

Figure 20–4. A skin incision is made perpendicular to the course of the vein.

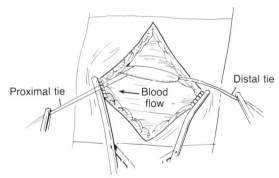

Figure 20–6. Proximal and distal ties are passed under the vein. If the vein is to be sacrificed, the distal suture is tied to prevent bleeding, and the ends are left long to help stabilize the vein during cannulation. The proximal tie is not tied at this point, but traction on it will control back bleeding. (From Vander Salm, T. J., et al.: Atlas of Bedside Procedures. Boston, Little Brown & Co., 1979. Used by permission.)

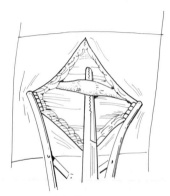

Figure 20–5. Skin retracted and vein exposed. (From Vander Salm, T. J., et al.: Atlas of Bedside Procedures. Boston, Little, Brown & Co., 1979. Used by permission.)

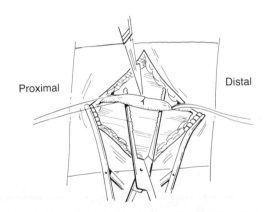

Figure 20–7. The vein is stretched flat and incised at a 45-degree angle. Approximately one third of the lumen must be exposed. Traction on the proximal tie will control back bleeding.

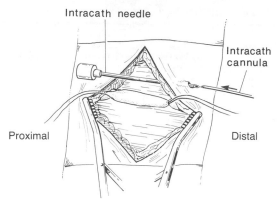

Figure 20–8. Use of the Intracath needle to produce a separate stab incision. The cannula is introduced into the wound by retrograde passage through the introducing needle. (From Van der Salm, T. J., et al.: Atlas on Bedside Procedures. Boston, Little, Brown & Co., 1979. Used by permission.)

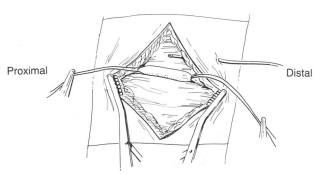

Figure 20–9. Cannula threaded through the stab incision. Intracath needle has been withdrawn following introduction of the cannula into the wound. (From Vander Salm, T. J., et al.: Atlas of Bedside Procedures. Boston, Little, Brown & Co., 1979. Used by permission.)

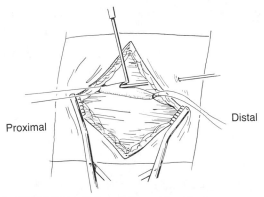

Figure 20–10. Threading catheter with aid of venous dilator (lifter). This is technically the most difficult part of the procedure. The lifter is especially helpful in small veins.

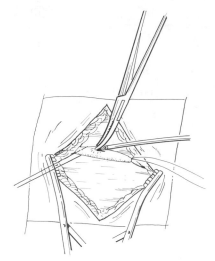

Figure 20–11. In larger veins, a mosquito hemostat can facilitate the placement of the cannula by opening the lumen and providing countertraction.

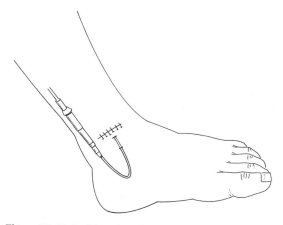

Figure 20–12. Incision closed and catheter sutured in place.

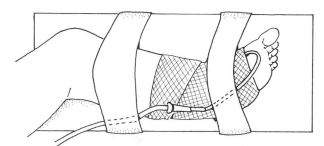

Figure 20–13. Cutdown site securely dressed and splinted.

again once the cannula is removed. Using a hemostat, one then elevates the vessel and stretches it flat. This provides good visualization and control of the vessel and limits bleeding when the vessel is incised. Alternatively, placing gentle traction on the proximal tie will control oozing around the puncture site. The vessel is incised at a 45-degree angle, through one third to one half of its diameter (see Fig. 20–7). A number 11 blade (as illustrated) or iris scissors may be used to incise the vessel. Too small an incision may cause threading of the catheter into a false channel in the adventitia; conversely, the vessel may be torn completely and may retract from the field if the incision is too large.[18] A longitudinal incision is sometimes used to avoid transecting the vessel, but the lumen is more difficult to identify with this technique. The incision must enter the actual lumen of the vein, although some bleeding will occur after the vein has merely been nicked. Incision of the vessel is unnecessary when an IV catheter with an introducing needle is used. The vessel is simply punctured, as in percutaneous venous cannulation. (See the section on the mini-cutdown procedure.)

Prior to its introduction into the vessel, the cannula is beveled at a 45-degree angle. A short bevel is preferred, and a sharply pointed tip is to be avoided, because it may pierce the posterior wall or otherwise damage the vein. The rounded tip of a feeding tube may be more difficult to introduce, but it may be advanced less traumatically. The cannula may be introduced directly through the skin incision or through a separate stab wound. The latter method is illustrated in Figures 20–8 and 20–9. Theoretically, the percutaneous approach reduces the risk of infection.[19] The beveled catheter is then threaded into the vessel lumen. Threading the catheter into the vein is usually the most difficult portion of the procedure and is often time-consuming.

Difficulty in threading may be encountered for several reasons. The lumen may have been incorrectly identified, or a false passage may have been created. This frequently occurs and may be difficult to recognize, because the catheter can easily advance between layers of the vessel wall. Other causes of difficult threading are penetration of the posterior vessel wall or use of a catheter that is too large for the vessel being cannulated. Identification of the vessel lumen may be facilitated through use of a plastic venous dilator or lifter (Becton-Dickinson #X10152). The small, pointed tip of the device is threaded into the vessel to expose the lumen in advance of the catheter (see Fig. 20–10). This device is useful in pediatric cutdowns but is generally unnecessary in adults. One can facilitate the threading of very large catheters in adults by grasping the proximal surgical edge of the vessel with small forceps or a mosquito hemostat. Countertraction is applied as the catheter is advanced (see Fig. 20–11). At no time should one force a catheter that will not advance.

Once the catheter is advanced into the lumen, air is back-bled from the cannula, which is then connected to IV tubing. The proximal ligature is tied around the vessel wall and the intraluminal cannula. The tie may be removed instead of tied, but oozing at the puncture site often occurs. The tourniquet is now removed, the catheter is affixed to the skin, and the incision is closed (see Fig. 20–12). An antibiotic ointment is applied at the point at which the catheter passes through the skin, and the wound is dressed. Adequate immobilization must be provided to prevent displacement of the line. This is especially important in children (see Fig. 20–13).

MINI-CUTDOWN

An alternative method that is designed to preserve the vein[20] and to bypass the time-consuming step of placing a catheter into the vessel has been described. A skin incision and blunt dissection are used to locate the vessel. Once identified, the vein is punctured under direct vision with a standard percutaneous venous catheter. The needle may be introduced through a separate stab incision or through the skin incision. If a separate incision is used, the cannula is threaded through the needle into the vein, and the needle is withdrawn to the skin surface (Fig. 20–14). A guard is placed on the needle tip, the catheter device is fixed to the skin, and the incision is closed. An over-the-needle device (Angiocath, Medicut) may also be used, in which case the needle would be withdrawn and discarded. This method eliminates the need for tying or cutting the vein, thereby permitting repeated catheterization. Venipuncture is easier, and the technique uses the same equipment as for percutaneous venous cannulation. The mini-cutdown is therefore used in treatment of chronically ill patients requiring long-term intravenous therapy or in children having limited accessible veins. A simple skin incision may also permit direct visualization of veins in the obese patient and may facilitate standard percutaneous venipuncture.

Removal of catheters inserted by cutdown requires only cutting of skin stitches holding the catheter in place, followed by withdrawal of the catheter. Back-bleeding from the proximal venous end is controlled by a simple pressure dressing and is generally not a significant problem.

Hansbrough and coworkers[20a] recently described the mini-cutdown procedure with a new 10 gauge intravenous catheter (Deseret 10 gauge Angiocath). The flow rates of blood and saline with this catheter are equal to the rates obtained when intravenous extension tubing is placed in a vein using the more time-consuming standard venous cutdown technique. This catheter allows one to infuse a unit of whole blood in 2 to 3 minutes if pressure and oversized intravenous tubing (urology irrigating tubing) are used.

Complications

The complications of venous cutdown include local hematoma and infection, sepsis, phlebitis, embolization, wound dehiscence, and injury to associated structures. An indirect, but significant, complication is deterioration of an unstable patient during a time-consuming cutdown attempt. Doc-

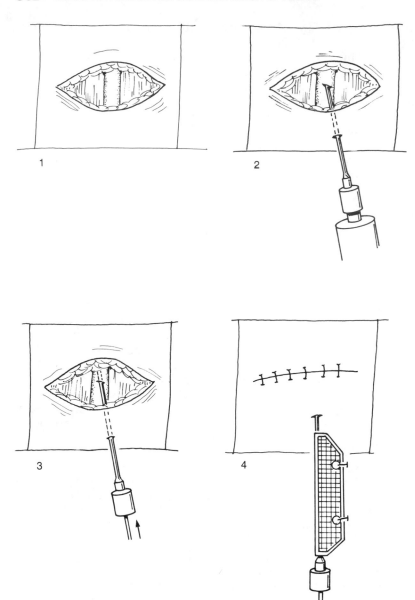

Figure 20–14. The mini-cutdown technique is an alternative to the venous cutdown method. The vein is cannulated under direct vision using standard percutaneous catheters. A separate entry site (shown) may be used, or the vein can be cannulated through the skin incision. Note that the vein is not tied off with this technique.

umentation of complications and their frequency has been sparse. Bogen reported a 15 per cent complication rate in 234 cases.[21] Infection and phlebitis each occurred at a rate of 4 per cent. Infectious complications may result from introduction of pathogens during line placement, transcutaneous invasion along the course of the cannula, or deposition of blood-borne organisms on the catheter tip.[22] A clear correlation exists between the incidence of infectious complications and the length of time that a catheter is left in place. Moran and associates found that the infection rate rose from 50 per cent to 78 per cent when a catheter was left in place for more than 48 hours.[23] Druskin and Siegel, studying a mixed population of patients who had undergone cutdowns and those who had had catheters percutaneously inserted,

found that the incidence of culture-positive catheter tips rose from 0 to 52 per cent after 48 hours.[22] In Moran's study, *Staphylococcus albus* was the predominant organism that was isolated, but organisms more commonly thought of as pathogenic (*S. aureus*, enterococcus, and *Proteus*) were isolated with greater frequency from cutdowns that had been in place for long periods.[23]

There is some evidence that the rate of infectious complications decreases when a broad-spectrum antibiotic ointment is applied to the cutdown site. Moran and coworkers found a rate of infectious complications of 18 per cent when topical Neosporin was used, compared with a 78 per cent rate in a placebo-treated group.[23] In this study, it was also shown that topical antibiotic use results in only a moderate decrease in the incidence of phlebitis (from 53 to 37 per cent) but a significant decrease in the incidence of phlebitis associated with positive cultures (from 86 to 14 per cent). This suggests that phlebitis is primarily a chemical or an irritative process rather than an infective process.[23] Whatever the cause, the incidence of phlebitis is clearly related to the duration of catheterization.[6, 21, 24] Early removal is a key factor in the prevention of both phlebitis and the infectious complications of venous cutdown. This is especially true of lines inserted during emergency resuscitative treatment. Such lines should be removed as soon as the patient's condition stabilizes and alternative routes exist.[7,9]

Proper attention to the details of surgical technique will limit the occurrence of minor complications, such as local hematoma, abscess, and wound dehiscence. One can avoid injury to associated structures by selecting a site in which the vein is isolated and, specifically, avoiding brachial vein cutdown.

Conclusion

The venous cutdown is a time-honored, simple surgical technique that is useful in the management of seriously ill patients. It is an excellent means of venous access in children and in markedly hypovolemic patients. Complications are potentially serious but can be controlled by good surgical technique and prompt removal of the line following clinical improvement.

1. Craig, R. G., Jones, R. A., and Sproul, G. L.: The alternate methods of central venous system catheterization. Am. Surg. 3:131, 1968.
2. Keeley, J. L.: Intravenous injections and infusions. Am. J. Surg. 50:485, 1940.
3. Kirkham, J. H.: Infusion into the internal saphenous vein at the ankle. Lancet 2:815, 1945.
4. Aldeman, S.: An emergency intravenous route for the pediatric population. JACEP 5:596, 1976.
5. Alexander, E., Small, W., and Campbell, J. B.: A dependable method for constant intravenous therapy in infants using polyethylene tubing. Ann. Surg. 127:1212, 1948.
6. Dudley, H. A. F. (ed.): Hamilton Bailey's Emergency Surgery, 10th ed. Bristol, John Wright & Sons, 1977, p. 28.
7. Dronen, S. C., Yee, A. S., and Tomlanovich, M. C.: Proximal saphenous vein cutdown. Ann. Emerg. Med. 10:328, 1981.
8. Westaby, S.: Ryle's tube for rapid intravenous transfusion. Lancet 1:360, 1979.
9. Knopp, R.: Venous cutdowns in the emergency department. JACEP 7:429, 1978.
10. Hollinshead, W. H. (ed.): Textbook of Anatomy, 2nd ed. New York, Harper & Row, 1967, p. 442.
11. Randolph, J.: Technique for insertion of plastic catheters into the saphenous vein. Pediatrics 24:631, 1959.
12. Preston, G.: Emergency venous access and cannulation. JACEP 11:642, 1982.
13. Anderson, J. E. (ed.): Grant's Atlas of Anatomy, 7th ed. Baltimore, Williams & Wilkins, 1978, pp. 4.6, 4.11.
14. Ficcara, B. J.: Saphenous vein alimentation. Angiology 21:563, 1970.
15. Gray, H.: The veins. In Goss, C. M. (ed.): Anatomy of the Human Body, 29th ed. Philadelphia, Lea & Febiger, 1973, p. 717.
16. Warwick, R., and Williams, P.: Gray's Anatomy, 35th ed. Philadelphia, W. B. Saunders Co., 1973, p. 669.
17. Graber, D.: Catheter flow rates updated. JACEP 6:518, 1977.
18. Stanley-Brown, E. G.: The venous cutdown. Arch. Pediatr. 75:480, 1958.
19. Priouleau, W. H.: Technique of venesection in infants. Surg. Gynecol. Obstet. 122:838, 1966.
20. Shiu, M. H.: A method for conservation of veins in the surgical cutdown. Surg. Gynecol. Obstet. 134:315, 1972.
20a. Hansbrough, J. F., Cain, T. L., and Millikan, J. S.: Placement of 10 gauge catheter by cutdown for rapid fluid replacement. J. Trauma 23:231, 1983.
21. Bogen, J. E.: Local complications in 167 patients with indwelling venous catheters. Surg. Gynecol. Obstet. 110:112, 1960.
22. Druskin, M. S., and Siegel, P. D.: Bacterial contamination of indwelling intravenous polyethylene catheters. JAMA 185:966, 1963.
23. Moran, J. M., Atwood, R. P., and Rowe, M.: A clinical and bacteriologic study of infections associated with venous cutdown. N. Engl. J. Med. 272:554, 1963.
24. Collins, R. N., Braun, P. A., Zinner, S. H., et al.: Risk of local and systemic infection with polyethylene intravenous catheters. N. Engl. J. Med. 279:340, 1968.

21

Subclavian Venipuncture

STEVEN C. DRONEN, M.D.

Introduction

The popularity of subclavian venipuncture has paralleled the medical advances of the past 20 years. The development of sophisticated monitoring techniques, transvenous pacemaker devices, total parenteral nutrition, and emergency resuscitative protocols has created a need for rapid and reliable methods of central venous access. Peripheral venous sites can be used for some of these procedures but necessitate the use of long catheters that must be accurately threaded into the superior vena cava. Peripheral veins may be collapsed, thrombosed, buried in subcutaneous fat, or otherwise difficult to locate. The subclavian vein has a predictable relationship to easily identified anatomic landmarks and can be cannulated within minutes. Consequently, subclavian venipuncture has become a common practice in a variety of clinical settings. Supraclavicular (SC) and infraclavicular (IC) approaches have been described.

Historical Development

The technique of subclavian venipuncture was first described in the French literature in 1952, and numerous articles soon appeared to support the use of the technique.[1-8] Wilson, who described the role of central venous pressure (CVP) monitoring in the maintenance of optimal blood volume, is credited with popularizing the procedure in the United States. He used the subclavian vein for the introduction of CVP catheters, arguing that this approach is easier, safer, and more accurate than other methods.[9]

Multiple reports of clinical experience with the IC technique followed Wilson's article. These stressed the clinical usefulness of the procedure, the ease with which it is performed, and the low complication rate. Subclavian venipuncture was described as useful in the management of hypovolemia, burns, cardiac arrest, chronic intravenous (IV) therapy, and septic shock.[10-14]

Early enthusiasm for IC subclavian venipuncture was countered by a growing awareness of serious and occasionally fatal complications. Yarom was the first to warn of the potential dangers in 1964.[15] A year later, Matz called for the abandonment of the technique, labeling it a "disease of medical progress." He encountered six complications, including two fatalities, in 1 week.[16] Smith and coworkers reported eight complications over a 2-year period and concluded that the subclavian vein should be cannulated only when other means have been exhausted.[17]

The reported complications of the IC subclavian approach suggested the need for a safer method. In 1965, Yoffa described the SC approach. Anatomic dissections had shown that the route to the subclavian vein is more direct when approached from above the clavicle. In a series of 130 patients, he reported no fatalities or serious complications when the SC approach was used.[18] Other studies have substantiated the utility of this approach.[19-25] Dronen and associates compared the two approaches during the performance of cardiopulmonary resuscitation (CPR) and found a significant decrease in catheter tip malposition and CPR interruption when the SC approach was used.[26]

Irrespective of the approach that is used, subclavian vein cannulation has increased dramatically over the past 20 years. It would be difficult to estimate the frequency with which this procedure is performed today, but it is a commonplace practice in hospitals throughout the world. Other methods of central venous cannulation have been developed simultaneously. These include the passage of long lines through the basilic vein and cannulation of the internal jugular vein (see Chapter 22). Each has its relative merits (Table 21–1). Any physician involved in the care of critically ill patients should master several of these techniques.

Indications

INFRACLAVICULAR APPROACH

There are no absolute indications for IC subclavian venipuncture. Since this technique is one of several venous access routes, its use depends to a great extent upon physician experience. There are several clinical situations in which its use is applicable.

CVP Monitoring. Wilson described the placement of a catheter into the superior vena cava as a means of assessing blood volume.[9] Although supplanted to some extent by more sophisticated methods, this remains an excellent tool in the treatment of hypovolemic patients (see Chapter 23).

Volume Loading. Subclavian venipuncture has been widely used as a vehicle for rapid volume resuscitation. Unfortunately, it is often misused in this regard. The flow rate of saline through a

Table 21–1. ADVANTAGES AND DISADVANTAGES OF TECHNIQUES*

Technique	Advantages	Disadvantages
Basilic (peripheral) puncture	Low incidence of major complications Performed under direct visualization of vein Allows large quantities of fluid to be given rapidly	Greater incidence of minor complications of infection, phlebitis, and thrombosis Hinders free movement of arms More difficult to place catheter in correct position for central venous pressure monitoring
Internal jugular puncture	Good external landmarks Lesser risk of pneumothorax than with subclavian puncture Bleeding can be recognized and controlled Malposition of catheter is rare Almost a straight course to the superior vena cava on the right side Carotid artery easily identified Useful alternative approach to cutdown in children under the age of 2 years	"Blind" procedure Has a slightly higher incidence of failures than subclavian More difficult and inconvenient to secure
Infraclavicular subclavian puncture	Good external landmarks	Higher incidence of complications, especially in hypovolemic shock "Blind" procedure Should not be attempted in children under 2 years of age
Supraclavicular (subclavian) puncuture	Good landmarks Less risk of pneumothorax than with infraclavicular puncture Most practical method of inserting a central line in cardiorespiratory arrest Malposition of catheter is uncommon	"Blind" procedure

*Modified from Knopp, R., and Dailey, R. H.: Central venous cannulation and pressure monitoring. JACEP 6:358, 1977.

peripheral 2-inch, 14 gauge catheter is roughly twice the rate of that through an 8-inch, 16 gauge central venous catheter, with equivalent pressure heads.[27, 28] The difference in flow is even greater for blood products because of viscosity factors, which slow the passage of red cells through small gauge catheters.[28, 29] Consequently, *the placement of peripheral large-bore catheters is the preferred method of rapid volume loading, unless time would be lost searching for venipuncture sites.* An excellent alternative to the use of standard small-bore, low-flow subclavian catheters for fluid resuscitation is the passage of an introducer device into the subclavian vein with the Seldinger technique. This is technically more complicated than routine subclavian venipuncture but uses a catheter that even exceeds the flow capabilities of commonly used IV tubing.[30] In trained hands this is an ideal method of rapid fluid resuscitation (see Chapter 19).

Emergency Venous Access. The predictable anatomic location of the subclavian vein and the speed with which it can be cannulated (15 to 30 seconds) have prompted its use in cardiac arrest and other emergency situations. Although subclavian venipuncture by the infraclavicular route is an ideal means of rapid venous access, it may not be the best technique to use during CPR. Chest wall motion and physical interference with the performance of effective CPR make IC venipunc-

ture more difficult and perhaps more dangerous in this setting.[26] The need for a central line during CPR is controversial, although many clinicians advocate use of a central line routinely. It has been suggested that therapeutic drug levels are reached more rapidly if given centrally. This was verified with the use of lidocaine in an animal study, but the differences were not thought to be clinically significant.[31] A cadaver study demonstrated significant delay in the arrival of peripherally injected dye in the arterial circulation.[32] Further study is needed to clarify this issue. In my opinion, central venous cannulation is preferred over peripheral venous access because it provides a rapid and reliable route for the administration of drugs to the patient in cardiac arrest.

Routine Venous Cannulation. Drug abusers, burn victims, and obese or chronically hospitalized patients may have inadequate peripheral IV sites. Subclavian vein cannulation may be indicated under these circumstances.

Routine Blood Drawing. Despite the claim of Kalcev that subclavian venipuncture is a "safe and easy method" of obtaining blood specimens,[8] the potential complications of this procedure do not justify its use in routine blood sampling. Lines already in place may be used for this purpose if properly cleared of IV fluid. An 8-inch, 16 gauge catheter contains 0.3 ml of fluid, so at least this much must be withdrawn to avoid dilution of blood samples. Because of the increased risk of infectious complications, air embolus, and venous back-bleeding, the IV tubing should not be repeatedly disconnected from the catheter hub. Interposition of a three-way stopcock in the IV tubing simplifies access and is an acceptable method of blood sampling in the intensive care unit setting.

Hyperalimentation. In 1969, Dudrick described beneficial results of long-term parenteral nutrition in patients with various gastrointestinal disorders. Intravenous hyperalimentation by way of the subclavian vein was found to be safe and reliable.[33] Use of the infraclavicular technique frees the patient's extremities and neck; this procedure is therefore well suited to long-term applications.[34] Strict aseptic technique is necessary to minimize infectious complications.[35]

Infusion of Concentrated Solutions. Hyperosmolar or irritating solutions, potentially causing thrombophlebitis if given through small peripheral vessels, are frequently infused by way of the subclavian vein. Examples are potassium chloride (greater than 40 mEq per ml), hyperosmolar saline, and acidifying solutions, such as ammonium chloride.

Other indications for central venous access include the placement of a Swan-Ganz catheter or a temporary transvenous pacemaker, the performance of cardiac catheterization and pulmonary angiography, and hemodialysis. Dialysis catheters, such as Vas-Cath, have been developed. These make the subclavian vein a useful site for hemodialysis.

SUPRACLAVICULAR APPROACH

The indications for SC venipuncture are essentially the same as those for the IC procedure. During CPR the SC route is often preferred, however, because it minimizes physical interference with the functions of chest compression and airway management. The IC technique requires deep penetration of a moving chest wall and frequently demands an interruption of chest compression. SC subclavian venipuncture can be performed without cessation of CPR and involves superficial penetration of the relatively motionless neck.[26] This technique also avoids interference with airway management, which commonly occurs when the internal jugular vein is cannulated.[36] When a true central location is required, the SC approach is superior to the IC and long peripheral line insertion techniques because of the low incidence of catheter tip malposition with the SC approach.[22, 26] Additionally, the SC technique has been performed in the sitting position in patients with severe orthopnea. Placement of a central line

with a patient in the sitting position would be virtually impossible with other central venous access routes.[19, 37] Finally, the low complication rate reported for SC subclavian venipuncture makes it a more attractive alternative, especially in the seriously ill patient.[18-23]

Contraindications

The contraindications to subclavian venipuncture have been described in several reviews.[36, 38, 39] They are listed in Table 21–2. Subclavian venipuncture is generally contraindicated in patients with distortion of the local anatomy or landmarks. These include patients who have undergone previous surgery or trauma involving the clavicle, the first rib, or the subclavian vessels; patients who have undergone previous radiation therapy to the clavicular area; patients with significant chest wall deformities; and those with marked cachexia or obesity. Physicians in many burn centers will routinely place a central catheter through a burned area, however. Patients with unilateral deformities not associated with pneumothorax (e.g., fractured clavicle) should be catheterized on the opposite side.

Subclavian venipuncture is not contraindicated in patients who have penetrating thoracic wounds unless the injuries involve the superior vena cava. Generally, the vein on the *same side* as the chest wound should be cannulated to avoid the possibility of bilateral pneumothoraces, unless one suspects that the subclavian vessels have been injured. In such instances, the opposite side is cannulated.[40] In penetrating wounds that may involve the superior vena cava, neither subclavian vessel should be cannulated and venous access below the diaphragm should be sought. Use of the subclavian approach in patients with coagulation disorders or in those receiving heparin

Table 21–2. CONTRAINDICATIONS TO SUBCLAVIAN VENIPUNCTURE

Distorted local anatomy*
Chest wall deformities
Extremes of weight
Vasculitis
Prior long-term subclavian cannulation
Prior injection of sclerosing agents
Suspected superior vena cava injury
Suspected subclavian vessel injury*
Previous radiation surgery*
Pneumothorax†
Bleeding disorders
Anticoagulant therapy
Combative patients
Inexperienced, unsupervised physician

*May cannulate contralateral side.
†May cannulate ipsilateral side.

therapy is contraindicated. A more visible and accessible site should be chosen (preferably percutaneous cannulation of a peripheral vein), because it is impossible to apply direct pressure to an oozing subclavian vein. The procedure should not be performed in combative patients because of the greater possibility of pneumothorax, vessel laceration, air embolism, and septic complications. Subclavian venipuncture is also contraindicated in children less than 2 years of age because of the high risk of complications. Internal jugular cannulation is an acceptable alternative in young children. Relative contraindications include those conditions predisposing to sclerosis or thrombosis of the central veins, such as vasculitis, long-term subclavian cannulation, or intravenous drug abuse via the jugular system. Finally, the procedure

should not be performed by unsupervised physicians who are inexperienced in the technique.

Anatomy

The subclavian vein begins as a continuation of the axillary vein at the outer edge of the first rib (Figs. 21–1 and 21–2). It joins the internal jugular vein to become the innominate vein 3 to 4 cm proximally. It has a diameter of 10 to 20 mm and is valveless. After crossing the first rib, the vein lies posteriorly to the medial third of the clavicle. It is only in this area that there is an intimate association between the clavicle and the subclavian vein. The costoclavicular ligament lies anterior and inferior to the subclavian vein, and the fascia

Figure 21–1. A and B, Subclavian vein and local anatomy. (Part A from Linos, D., Mucha, P., and von Heerden, J.: The subclavian vein: A golden route. Mayo Clin. Proc. 55:316, 1980. Part B from Davidson, J. J., Ben-Hur, N., and Nathan, H.: Subclavian venepuncture. Lancet 2:1140, 1963. Used by permission.)

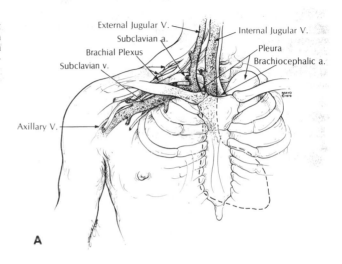

A

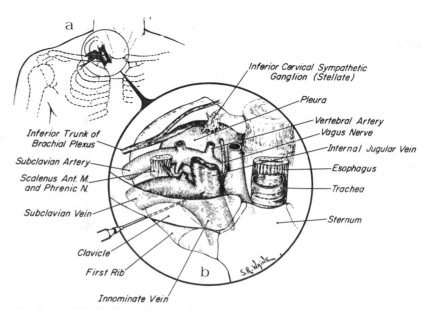

B

a, Point of insertion and direction of needle.
b, Oblique anterosuperior view of root of neck.

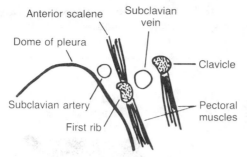

Figure 21–2. Subclavian area, sagittal section. (From Bramos, G.: Central venous catheterization, SC approach. J. Trauma 17:873, 1977. Used by permission.)

contiguous to this ligament invests the vessel. Posterior to the vein, separating it from the subclavian artery, lies the anterior scalene muscle, which has a thickness of 10 to 15 mm. The phrenic nerve passes over the anterior surface of the scalene muscle and runs immediately behind the junction of the subclavian and internal jugular veins. The thoracic duct (on the left) and the lymphatic duct (on the right) pass over the anterior scalene muscle and enter the subclavian vein near its junction with the internal jugular vein. Superior and posterior to the subclavian artery lies the brachial plexus. The dome of the *left* lung may extend above the first rib, but the right lung rarely extends this high.

Materials

The materials required for subclavian venipuncture are listed in Table 21–3. The catheter may be of the "over-the-needle" or the "through-the-needle" variety (Fig. 21–3). Over-the-needle devices (such as the Angiocath) use a tapered plastic catheter that passes through the vessel wall into

Table 21–3. MATERIALS FOR SUBCLAVIAN VENIPUNCTURE

1 per cent lidocaine (Xylocaine)
26 gauge needle
2-ml Luer-Lok syringe
10-ml non–Luer-Lok syringe
Swabs
Prep solution
Gloves
Drapes
Catheter device
IV tubing
IV solution
Needle holder
4–0 silk sutures
Suture scissors
Antibiotic ointment
Gauze pads
Tincture of benzoin
Cloth tape

the lumen using the needle tip as a guide. There are several advantages of this system. The catheter does not pass through a sharp needle, and the risk of shearing with resultant catheter embolization is thus decreased. The needle is removed following cannulation, making a guard unnecessary. The hole made by the needle in the vessel wall is smaller than the catheter, producing a tighter seal. The main disadvantage is the length of the catheter, which is generally limited to 2 to 3 inches. Also, catheter threading is made more difficult by the longer length of the needle relative to the catheter. With over-the-needle catheters, the needle extends a few millimeters past the tip of the catheter. A blood return will be obtained when the tip of the needle is in the vein, but the catheter may actually be outside the lumen. If the needle is withdrawn before the catheter is advanced, the catheter tip will remain outside the vein. One must be certain to keep the needle steady and to advance the catheter forward over the needle to ensure intravascular placement.

Through-the-needle devices (such as the Intracath) use a catheter of smaller gauge than the puncturing needle. Generally, the needle is 14 gauge and the catheter is 16 gauge. This catheter is threaded through the lumen of the needle after the vessel is entered by the needle tip. After the threading, the needle is withdrawn and is left on the skin surface with a plastic guard protecting the patient and the catheter. A modification of this system uses a detachable hub on the catheter so that the needle can be removed. The main advantage of through-the-needle systems is that catheters of any length may be used. Also, the rate of successful entry of the catheter into the vessel lumen is generally higher. The main disadvantage of this system is the potential for catheter shearing during or after insertion. Systems using a detachable catheter hub (Deseret 755) allow the needle to be completely removed following insertion but require assembly of small plastic parts. This is undesirable in an emergency. Another disadvantage of through-the-needle devices is that the caliber of the catheter must be smaller than that of the needle. Standard catheters are 16 gauge, a size not optimal for rapid infusion of blood.

At least one device takes advantage of both over-the-needle and through-the-needle technology. The Argyle Intramedicut catheter has a short over-the-needle catheter that serves as an introducer for a longer (30 cm) infusion catheter. Following successful cannulation of the vein with the introducing catheter, the needle is withdrawn and the infusion catheter is advanced through the introducing catheter.

Catheter length and size are also important considerations. The superior vena cava begins at the level of the manubrial-sternal junction and terminates in the right atrium, approximately 2

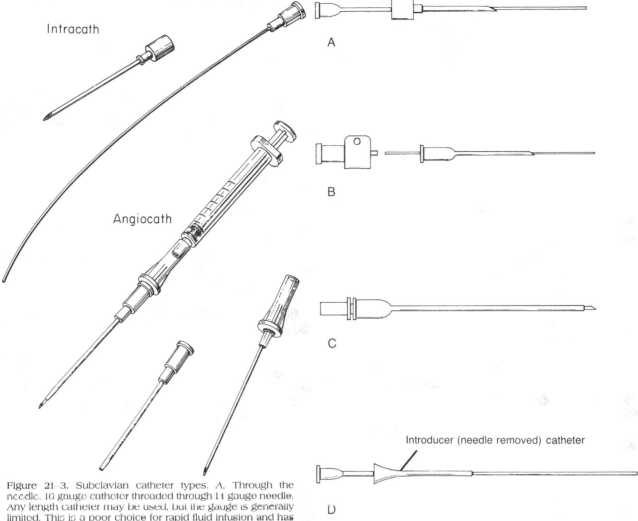

Intracath

Angiocath

A

B

C

Introducer (needle removed) catheter

D

E

Figure 21-3. Subclavian catheter types. A, Through the needle. 16 gauge catheter threaded through 14 gauge needle. Any length catheter may be used, but the gauge is generally limited. This is a poor choice for rapid fluid infusion and has the potential for catheter embolization. Examples: Intracath, upper left. B, Deseret 3162. Through the needle, detachable hub. Modification of A in which needle is withdrawn over catheter before hub is attached. Eliminates the need for a needle guard, but assembly of small parts is required. Example: C, Deseret 755. Over the needle. 14 gauge catheter advanced over 16 gauge needle. This permits use of a larger bore catheter than A, B, or D, but the catheter length is limited. Threading is more difficult than with through-the-needle devices. Example: Angiocath, lower left. D, Intramedicut. Long 16 gauge catheter is threaded through a short 14 gauge catheter previously advanced over a 16 gauge needle. This eliminates the risk of catheter shearing and the need for a needle guard. Has the same low flow rate as do through-the-needle devices. Example: Argyle Intramedicut. E, Introducer set. Large-bore catheter advanced over a venous dilator. This permits very rapid fluid infusion, but insertion is more complicated than with other devices.

inches lower.[41] *The proper position of the catheter is in the superior vena cava, not the right atrium or ventricle.* Therefore, the catheter should be threaded approximately 1 inch below the manubrial-sternal junction. One can estimate this distance by placing the catheter parallel to the chest wall prior to insertion. The standard catheters marketed for subclavian venipuncture are 8 inches long. This is a good size for the average adult

male, but it may be necessary to cut off 1 to 4 inches in smaller adult patients. Proper placement is best assessed by a chest film, not by predetermined measurements.

Subclavian veins are often cannulated in seriously ill patients who will require subsequent Swan-Ganz monitoring or transvenous pacemakers. Any CVP catheter that is initially inserted should have a lumen that is large enough to accept the guide wire for an introducer sheath (Seldinger technique) that can be used to insert the afore-mentioned devices. Not all of the commercially available CVP catheters will accept a guide wire through the lumen. As long as one is cannulating the vein, it is reasonable to use a catheter that can later be converted via the Seldinger technique for other purposes.

A number of different subclavian catheters are currently manufactured. It is *not* advisable to stock several different catheter types. This practice adds unnecessary confusion to the duties of supply clerks and nurses, not to mention the physician who might be handed an unfamiliar brand during a cardiac arrest. It is better to use one brand routinely and to see that all medical personnel are thoroughly schooled in its use.

Technique

The technique of subclavian venipuncture has been described in several reports.[14, 36, 42-49] Undue attention has been given to descriptions of angles and landmarks and to myths concerning the effects of patient positioning. The important factors governing success or failure are knowledge of the anatomy and meticulous attention to the details of the procedure.[50]

Strict adherence to the principles of sterile technique is important if septic complications are to be avoided. Violation of these principles for the sake of speed is seldom justified. The few extra seconds required to put on gloves and to swab and drape the chest will rarely make a critical difference in patient survival. It is recognized that the optimum practice of aseptic technique often cannot take place during a resuscitation. For this reason, all central lines placed in this setting should be replaced at the earliest possible opportunity.

The area of the needle puncture should be widely prepared with an iodophor solution. In iodine-allergic patients, pHisoHex is an acceptable alternative. The area that is prepared should include puncture sites for the IC and SC subclavian and internal jugular approaches. This permits the physician to change the site following an unsuccessful attempt without repeating the preparation. A standard preparation should include the ipsilateral anterior neck, the supraclavicular fossa, and the anterior chest 1 to 2 inches past the midline and the same distance above the nipple line.

The need to perform an operating suite–style preparation (gowns, surgical scrub, and so forth) in patients receiving hyperalimentation is unproven. In a study of 63 patients with long-term subclavian catheterization for hyperalimentation, Merk reported only one infection using a simple iodophor spray preparation. He emphasized the role of experienced personnel as having prime importance in the prevention of infection.[35]

INFRACLAVICULAR APPROACH

The patient is placed in the supine position with the arm adducted. Placing the patient in the Trendelenburg position (10 to 15 degrees) decreases the risk of air embolism. The claim that this position distends the vein[47] is unsubstantiated. Land has demonstrated by venographic studies that there is no change in the diameter of the subclavian vein associated with the Trendelenburg position.[51] Because his patients were normovolemic, this finding cannot necessarily be extrapolated to hypovolemic patients. Nonetheless, the vessel is hemmed by the semi-rigid costoclavicular ligament on its anterior-inferior aspect and therefore will not distend in a direction facilitating IC venipuncture.[18]

Abduction of the arm has been recommended to flatten the deltoid bulge.[52] This is sometimes a helpful maneuver in muscular individuals but is not generally necessary. Land has demonstrated that abduction moves medially the point at which the subclavian vein passes beneath the clavicle.[51]

Turning the head to the opposite side, as advocated by Borja,[42] has no effect on the vessel size or on the relative positions of the vessel and the clavicle.[51] Turning the head away may help to prevent contamination of the venipuncture site and prevents the patient from observing a frightening procedure. Placing a pillow under the back will make the clavicle more prominent but is seldom necessary.[42] Moreover, as the shoulder falls backward, the space between the clavicle and first rib narrows, making the subclavian vein less accessible.[52]

The right subclavian vein is usually cannulated because of the lower pleural dome on the right and because of the need to avoid the left-sided thoracic duct. The anatomically more direct route between the left subclavian vein and the superior vena cava is a theoretic advantage of left-sided subclavian venipuncture over the right-sided approach. It is as yet unproved if there is a higher incidence of catheter malposition when the right IC approach is used.

In the conscious patient, the point of needle entry is anesthetized with 1 per cent lidocaine (Xylocaine). Subcutaneous infiltration to the periosteum of the clavicle will make the procedure painless but is not always necessary. When using a through-the-needle device, one attaches the 14 gauge needle to a 10-ml non–Luer-Lok syringe. It is advised that the needle not be left attached to the catheter as it is packaged (Deseret 3162), because this gives less control over the needle tip. It also makes threading more difficult, since the catheter slides back and forth in the plastic envelope (Fig. 21–4).

Opinions vary as to the best point of needle entry. The junction of the middle and medial thirds of the clavicle is the standard site.[41] There the vein lies just posteriorly to the clavicle and just above the first rib, which acts as a barrier to penetration of the pleura. This protective effect is lost when a more lateral location is chosen. Westreich advocates entry just laterally and inferiorly to the junction of the clavicle and the first rib, with the needle aiming at this junction.[39] Simon advocates entry at the site of a small tubercle in the medial aspect of the deltopectoral groove.[49] In my opinion, the point of entry is less important than the direction taken by the needle after entry. Points lateral to the mid-clavicle should be avoided, because this location requires a deeper puncture and potentially increases the risk of pneumothorax. Orientation of the needle bevel is important. It should be oriented inferomedially to direct the catheter toward the innominate vein rather than toward the opposite vessel wall or up the internal jugular vein (Fig. 21–5). Alignment of the needle bevel with markings on the barrel of the syringe permits awareness of bevel orientation after skin puncture. Some authors advise puncturing the skin with a number 11 scalpel blade to avoid skin plugs in the needle. Others suggest filling the syringe with a few milliliters of local anesthetic both to anesthetize the subcutaneous tissue and to flush the needle.

The mechanics of IC subclavian venipuncture using a through-the-needle device are illustrated in Figures 21–6 through 21–9. Prior to insertion, the left index finger is placed in the suprasternal notch and the thumb is positioned at the costoclavicular junction.[39] These serve as reference points for the direction of needle travel. The needle is aimed immediately above and posteriorly to the index finger. Vessel entry, signaled by a flashback of dark venous blood, usually occurs at a depth of 3 to 4 cm. If the needle tip is truly intraluminal, there will be a free flow of blood. The return of a pulsatile flow signifies arterial puncture. A single arterial puncture without laceration rarely causes serious harm. Use of this technique eliminates the need to measure angles, to "walk" the clavicle, or to concentrate excessively on maintaining the needle parallel to the chest wall. All of these techniques are based upon fear of complications rather than knowledge of anatomy.[53] Mogil has advocated changing the direction of the needle after it passes posteriorly to the lower edge of the clavicle.[14] In my opinion, this adds a step that is not only unnecessary but also dangerous. One should avoid any sweeping motions of the needle tip to prevent unseen injuries. In patients who are being ventilated with positive pressure, it is advisable to halt ventilations momentarily as the needle penetrates the chest wall. Interruptions should be kept to a minimum and should not exceed the 30-second standard.[54]

After a venous flashback is obtained, the syringe is detached from the needle. Removing the syringe is a step that causes frustration for many physicians. Removal of the syringe may displace the needle tip from the vein lumen, necessitating repuncture. If the syringe is tightly attached to the needle, a hemostat can be used to grasp and secure the needle during detachment of the syringe. Needle tip displacement may also occur if blood specimens are drawn at this stage in the procedure. Blood drawing should be delayed until the catheter is threaded well into the vessel lumen. *The needle hub should be covered with the thumb at this time to prevent air embolus.* Additionally, the patient may be asked to exhale, hum, or perform a Valsalva maneuver in order to raise intrathoracic pressure. The catheter is then threaded through the needle.

When an over-the-needle system is used, the

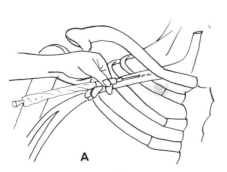 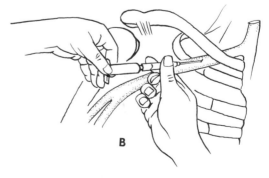

Figure 21–4. *A,* Insertion of "through-the-needle" device, as packaged. *B,* It is advisable to remove the packaged catheter and to puncture the vein with a syringe attached to the needle. (Redrawn from Gallitano, A. L., Kundi, E. S., et al.: A safe approach to the subclavian vein. Surg. Gynecol. Obstet. 135:97, 1972. By permission of Surgery, Gynecology & Obstetrics.)

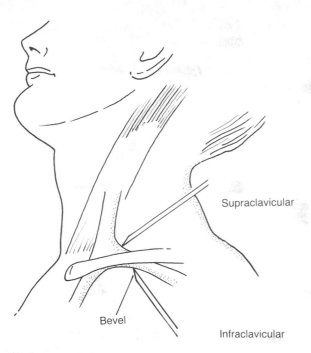

Figure 21–5. Needle bevel orientation using supraclavicular and infraclavicular venipuncture. The orientation of the needle bevel may help in proper positioning of the catheter by guiding the direction of the catheter during advancement.

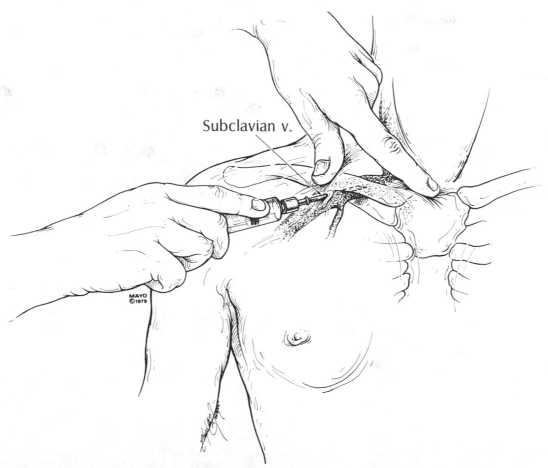

Figure 21–6. Hand position during subclavian venipuncture. (From Linos, D., Mucha, P., and von Heerden, J.: Subclavian vein: a golden route. Mayo Clin. Proc. 55:318, 1980. Used by permission.)

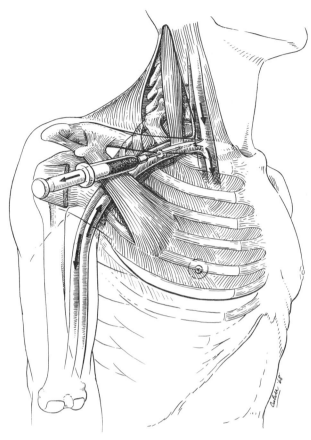

Figure 21–7. Subclavian venipuncture, venous backflow. After venipuncture, the syringe is carefully removed to avoid inadvertent motion of the needle tip, which may dislodge the needle from the vein lumen. A hemostat may help hold the needle hub to prevent motion during withdrawal of the syringe. (From Phillips, S. J.: Technique of percutaneous subclavian vein catheterization. Surg. Gynecol. Obstet. 127:1080, 1968. By permission of Surgery, Gynecology & Obstetrics.)

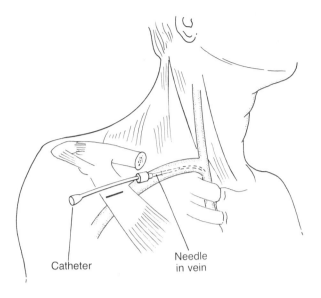

After removal of syringe,
thread catheter fully into needle

Figure 21–8. Catheter threading.

hub (through-the-needle system) is used, the catheter is threaded through the needle to 2 inches from its proximal end. The needle is then withdrawn over the catheter, and the catheter hub is attached (Fig. 21–10).

Prior to infusion of fluids, the intravenous bottle is lowered below the patient, and the line is

needle is advanced into the vein until there is free venous backflow. At this point the needle tip, but not necessarily the catheter, is in the vessel lumen. The needle is not withdrawn; rather, the catheter is advanced over the needle into the vessel lumen. Once threaded, the needle and the syringe are removed, with the thumb kept over the open catheter hub, until the IV tubing is attached.

A properly placed catheter should thread easily. Difficulty in catheter threading may be caused by passage out of the vessel lumen, trapping against the opposite vessel wall, kinking, or angulation up the internal jugular vein. Rotating the needle bevel may alleviate catheter trapping. At no time should the catheter be withdrawn through the needle or forced when it will not thread. Should it thread smoothly into the vessel, it is advanced fully into the needle hub, and the needle is withdrawn from the skin. The guard should be placed immediately. The wire stylet is then removed, and the IV tubing is connected. When a detachable

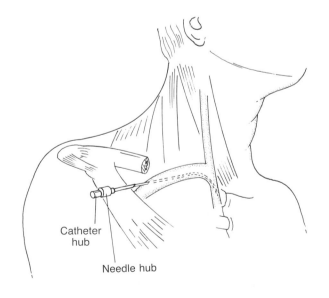

Withdraw needle tip from skin,
leaving catheter in vein

Figure 21–9. Withdrawal of needle leaves only the infusion catheter exiting from the skin. (From James, P., and Myers, R.: Central venous pressure monitoring. Ann. Surg. 175:695, 1972. Used by permission.)

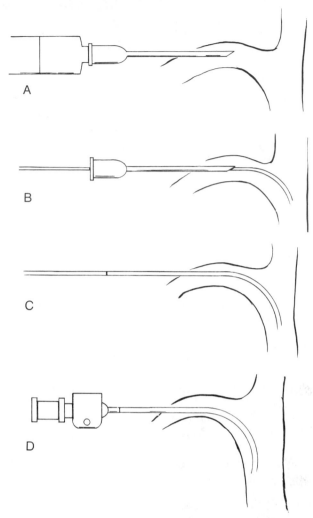

Figure 21–10. Detachable hub catheter system. *A,* Puncture vein, aspirate blood. *B,* Detach syringe, thread catheter. *C,* Withdraw needle over catheter end. *D,* Attach Luer-Lok adapter to catheter.

An antibacterial ointment is applied to the skin puncture site. Antibiotic ointment has been shown to reduce the rate of infectious complications following venous cutdown[57] and may have a beneficial effect in percutaneous venous cannulation.[55, 58] The guard must be firmly secured to prevent dislodgement, disconnection of the catheter–intravenous tubing junction, or skin maceration. A small gauze pad is placed between the plastic guard and the skin, and a large gauze pad folded in half is placed parallel over the guard. Tincture

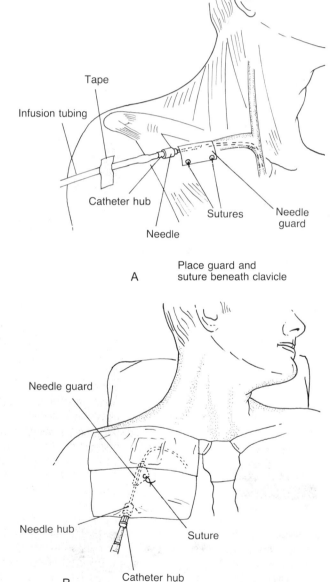

Figure 21–11. *A,* Suture guard to skin. *Note:* Be sure that the catheter fits into the specially designed groove in the plastic needle guard to avoid crushing the catheter when the guard is closed. *B,* Alternative method of securing the subclavian catheter to allow free use of the arm. Note the slight bend in the catheter as it exits from the skin. Also note that the needle guard is sutured to the skin with a single suture. A second suture for fixation should be placed near the needle hub. (From Vander Salm, T. J., et al.: Atlas of Bedside Procedures. Boston, Little, Brown & Co., 1979. Used by permission.)

checked for backflow of blood. *The free backflow of blood is suggestive, but not diagnostic, of intravascular placement.* Backflow may occur with a hematoma or a hemothorax if the catheter is free in the pleural space. One may attach a syringe directly to the catheter hub to check for the free aspiration of blood, which also *suggests* intraluminal catheter tip placement. The guard is sutured to the chest wall parallel to and just below the clavicle (Fig. 21–11). A silk suture (4–0) is used to fix the guard at two points. This prevents excessive motion, which would kink the catheter at the point at which it exits the guard. Fixation also limits to-and-fro catheter motion, which is postulated to traumatize the vessel and to increase the risk of thrombophlebitis, infection, and vascular perforation.[55, 56] It is important to be certain that the catheter fits into the groove in the needle guard. Occasionally, the catheter is misplaced, and when the guard is clamped it occludes the catheter lumen.

of benzoin is applied 2 inches in all directions around the large gauze pad and the gauze is secured with cloth adhesive tape. The catheter hub is included within the tape; this prevents accidental disconnection and allows future use of this site for routine blood drawing.

Following the procedure, the lungs should be auscultated to detect inequality of lung sounds suggesting a pneumo- or hemothorax. One should obtain a chest film as soon as possible, checking for hemothorax, pneumothorax, and catheter tip position. Because small amounts of fluid or air may layer out parallel to the x-ray plate with the patient in the supine position, the film should be taken in the upright or semi-upright position whenever possible. Proper catheter tip position is shown in Figure 21–12. *Misplaced catheters should be repositioned.*

SUPRACLAVICULAR APPROACH

The goal of the supraclavicular technique is to puncture the subclavian vein in its superior aspect just as it joins the internal jugular vein. The needle is inserted above and behind the clavicle, lateral to the sternocleidomastoid muscle. It advances in an avascular plane, away from the subclavian artery and the dome of the pleura. The right side is preferred because of the lower pleural dome, because it is the direct route to the superior vena cava, and because the thoracic duct is on the left side. The Trendelenburg position may be helpful in distending the vein, because the vein is not

bound by fasciae on its superior aspect.[22] The patient's head is turned to the opposite side to help identify the landmarks.

The technique has been well described by Brahos.[22] After the area of the supraclavicular fossa has been prepared and draped, a point is identified 1 cm lateral to the clavicular head of the sternocleidomastoid and 1 cm posterior to the clavicle (Fig. 21–13). The area is anesthetized with 1 per cent lidocaine. If a 1¼-inch needle is used for anesthesia, it may also be used to locate the

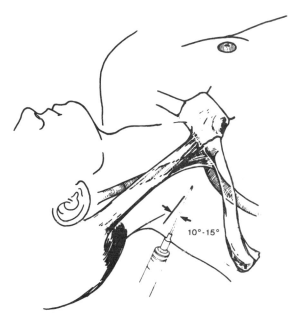

1. Insert needle at a point 1 cm lateral to the sternocleidomastoid muscle and 1 cm cephalad to the clavicle.
2. Direct needle at a 45° angle from the transverse and sagittal planes, angling slightly upward (10°-15°) from the horizontal plane toward the contralateral nipple (in the male).
3. If vein is not entered, withdraw the needle and redirect it in a slightly more cephalad direction.
4. Ensure blood flow and thread catheter.

A

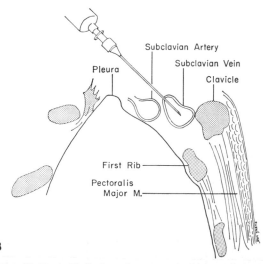

B

Figure 21–13. *A,* Technique for supraclavicular subclavian approach. (From Dronen, S., Thompson, B., Nowak, R. M., and Tomlanovich, M.: Subclavian vein catheterization during cardiopulmonary resuscitation. JAMA 247:3228, 1982. Used by permission.) *B,* Sagittal section.

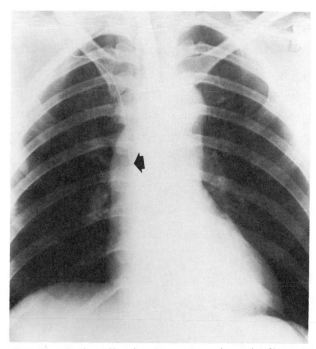

Figure 21–12. Chest film showing proper catheter tip placement in the superior vena cava *(arrow).* The tip should *not* lie within the right atrium or the right ventricle.

vessel in a relatively atraumatic manner. The subclavian vein can almost always be located with this needle because of its superficial location and the absence of bony structures in the path of the needle. A 14 gauge needle is then advanced with gentle negative pressure applied to an attached syringe. The needle is aimed so as to bisect the clavicosternomastoid angle, with the tip pointing just caudad to the contralateral nipple. The bevel is oriented medially to prevent catheter trapping against the inferior vessel wall. The axis of the syringe is pointed 10 degrees above the horizontal. Successful vessel puncture generally occurs at a depth of 2 to 3 cm. The mechanics of catheter insertion are the same as for the IC technique. Generally, a shorter length of catheter is needed for superior vena caval placement with the SC approach. The guard is best secured to the skin in the supraclavicular fossa parallel to the clavicle. As in the IC technique, a chest film must always be obtained following this procedure. *Misplaced catheters should be repositioned.*

Multiple or Unsuccessful Attempts

Cannulation of the subclavian vein may not be successful on the first attempt. It is reasonable to try again, but after three or four unsuccessful attempts it is best to try another approach or to allow a colleague to attempt the procedure. One must use a new setup each time blood is obtained, because clots and tissue will clog the needle and will mislead the physician even if subsequent procedures are performed correctly. If multiple attempts are made, the admitting physician or anesthesiologist must be informed so that proper precautions are taken to identify subsequent complications. It is advisable to obtain radiographs of the chest even after unsuccessful attempts if multiple needle sticks were performed. For aesthetic reasons, one should use the same needle hole for subsequent attempts to avoid an embarrassing pincushion appearance of the upper chest. If the subclavian route is unsuccessful on one side, it is best to attempt an internal jugular catheterization on the *same side* rather than attempt a subclavian catheterization on the opposite side. In this manner, bilateral complications are avoided.

Redirection of Misplaced Catheters

One common complication of central venous line placement is misdirection of the catheter into an inappropriate vein. Although infusions can still be made, CVP readings are inaccurate, and irritating solutions may produce phlebitis. Most commonly, the catheter is misdirected into the internal jugular vein. A number of options are available to remedy this problem. Schaefer[59] has described a novel technique in which a 2 French Fogarty

catheter is inserted through the lumen of the central line and advanced 3 cm beyond the tip. The entire assembly is withdrawn until only the Fogarty catheter is in the subclavian vein. One milliliter of air is injected into the balloon, and the Fogarty catheter is advanced. It is hoped that the blood flow will direct the assembly into the superior vena cava. The balloon is deflated and the central line is advanced over the Fogarty catheter, which is then withdrawn. Other manipulations with guide wires have been suggested, but often reinsertion with another puncture is required in order for the misplaced catheter to be correctly positioned.

Complications

INFRACLAVICULAR APPROACH

The medical literature is replete with reports of the complications of subclavian venipuncture. Initial descriptions of the procedure stressed its clinical usefulness rather than its potential complications.[1-3, 9-13, 46] Shortly after it became popular as a route for CVP monitoring, reports of serious and occasionally fatal complications began to appear.[15-17] Large series have reported complication rates ranging from 0.4 per cent to 11.1 per cent.[60]

Table 21–4. COMPLICATIONS OF SUBCLAVIAN VENIPUNCTURE

Pulmonary
Pneumothorax
Hemothorax
Hydrothorax
Hemomediastinum
Hydromediastinum
Tracheal perforation
Endotracheal cuff perforation
Intrathoracic catheter fragmentation
Vascular
Air embolus
Subclavian artery puncture
Pericardial tamponade
Thrombophlebitis
Catheter embolus
Volume depletion
Arteriovenous fistula
Superior vena cava obstruction
Thoracic duct laceration
Local hematoma
Infectious
Generalized sepsis
Local cellulitis
Osteomyelitis
Septic arthritis
Neurologic
Phrenic nerve injury
Brachial plexus injury
Miscellaneous
Dysrythmias
Ascites
Catheter knotting
Catheter malposition

The average complication rate reported is 4.8 per cent.[61] To date, at least 27 different complications of the IC technique have been described.[52, 60, 62] These are listed in Table 21–4. One can anticipate potential problems by reviewing the anatomic structures associated with the subclavian vein (Table 21–5). These can be categorized according to the major organ system involved.

Pulmonary. Pulmonary complications of subclavian venipuncture include pneumothorax, hemothorax, hydrothorax, hemomediastinum, hydromediastinum, tracheal perforation, and endotracheal tube cuff perforation. Pneumothorax is the most frequently reported complication, occurring in up to 6 per cent of subclavian venipunctures.[62] Initially the importance of this complication was minimized, but reports of fatalities caused by tension pneumothorax, bilateral pneumothorax, and combined hemopneumothorax followed.[16, 63, 64] One would expect a higher incidence of pneumothorax if the procedure were performed during CPR or positive-pressure ventilation. A small pneumothorax can quickly become a life-threatening tension pneumothorax under positive-pressure ventilation. Hemothorax may occur following subclavian vein or artery laceration,[17, 65] pulmonary artery puncture,[66] or intrathoracic infusion of blood.[15, 17, 67] Hydrothorax occurs as a result of infusion of IV fluid into the pleural space.[16, 60] Hydromediastinum is an uncommonly reported complication that is potentially fatal.[68] I have observed this complication on two occasions in patients receiving IV fluids through introducer devices in the subclavian vein. Both patients recovered without significant sequelae.

Vascular. Air embolism is a potentially fatal complication of subclavian venipuncture.[60, 69-72]

There were 5 fatalities in 13 reported cases.[62] The first case was reported by Flanagan, who determined that a 14 gauge needle can transmit 100 ml of air per second with a 5-cm H_2O pressure difference across the needle.[69] This is a potential complication of several invasive procedures about the head and the neck and is not specifically a result of subclavian venipuncture. Air embolism may occur if the line is left open to air during catheterization or if it subsequently becomes disconnected. The recommended treatment is to place the patient in the left lateral decubitus position to relieve the air bubble occlusion of the right ventricular outflow tract.[73] If this is unsuccessful, aspiration with a catheter advanced into the right ventricle has been advocated.[74, 75]

Catheter embolization resulting from shearing of the catheter by the needle tip is a serious complication. This occurs when the catheter is withdrawn through the needle or if the guard is not properly secured. Transvenous retrieval techniques are usually attempted and are followed by surgery if they are unsuccessful.[60]

Perforation or laceration of vascular structures may cause hemothorax, hemomediastinum, and volume depletion. These are rarely serious complications, but fatalities have been reported.[65] Surgical repair is occasionally required.[76] Arteriovenous fistula formation has also been reported.[77]

Perforation of the myocardium is a very rare but generally fatal complication of central venous cannulation by any route.[78-82] The presumed mechanism is prolonged contact of the rigid catheter tip with the beating myocardium.[53] The catheter perforates the myocardial wall and causes a tamponade by either bleeding from the involved chamber or infusion of IV fluid into the pericardium. The

Table 21–5. ANATOMIC STRUCTURES THAT CAN BE INJURED BY SUBCLAVIAN CANNULATION*

Structure	Anatomic Relation to Subclavian Vein (SV)	Error in Procedure	Injury
Subclavian artery	Posterior and slightly superior, separated by scalenus anterior—10 to 15 mm in the adult, 5 to 8 mm in children	Insertion too deep or lateral	Hemorrhage, hematoma, and possible hemothorax
Brachial plexus	Posterior to and separated from SV by the scalenus anterior and the subclavian artery (20 mm)	Same as with subclavian artery	Possible motor or sensory deficits of hand, arm, or shoulder
Parietal pleura	Contact with posterior inferior side of the SV, medial to the attachment of the anterior scalenus muscle to the first rib	Needle penetrates beneath or through both walls of the SV	Pneumothorax
Phrenic nerve	Same as with parietal pleura	Placement of needle above or behind the vein or by penetration of both its walls	Paralysis of the ipsilateral hemidiaphragm
Thoracic duct	Cross the scalenus anterior and enter the superior margin of the SV near the internal jugular junction	Same as with phrenic nerve	Soft tissue lymphedema or chylothorax on left

*From Knopp, R., and Dailey, R. H.: Central venous cannulation and pressure monitoring. JACEP 6:358, 1977. Used by permission.

right atrium is involved more commonly than the right ventricle.[83] This complication can be prevented by repositioning improperly placed catheters. Premature atrial or ventricular beats may be observed if the catheter tip is in contact with the endocardium. Serious dysrhythmias do not occur, and the ectopic beats may be abolished if the catheter is repositioned.

Catheter knotting or kinking may occur if the catheter is forced or repositioned or if an excessively long catheter is used.[84] The most common result of kinking is poor flow of intravenous fluids. Johnson and associates reported a case of superior vena caval obstruction caused by a kinked catheter.[85]

Thrombosis and thrombophlebitis occur rarely because of the large caliber and high flow rates of the vessels involved.[53] It is important to determine that the catheter tip rests in the superior vena cava, especially during the infusion of irritating or hypertonic fluids.[85]

Thoracic duct laceration is a frequently discussed complication of left-sided subclavian venipuncture; however, it is extremely uncommon. McGoon cites this as a complication of internal jugular cannulation, but not subclavian cannulation.[62]

Infectious. Infectious complications include local cellulitis, thrombophlebitis, generalized septicemia, osteomyelitis, and septic arthritis.[62] The incidence of septic complications varies from 0 to 25 per cent.[86, 87] In a retrospective audit, Herbst documented only one culture-proven infectious complication in a series of 117 patients.[61] The frequency with which infectious complications are seen is directly related to the attention given to aseptic technique in insertion and aftercare of the catheter.

Neurologic. Neurologic complications are extremely rare and are presumably caused by direct trauma from the needle during venipuncture. Brachial plexus palsy[17] and phrenic nerve injury with paralysis of the hemidiaphragm[88, 89] have been reported.

Miscellaneous. Improper catheter tip position occurs commonly and has been associated with myocardial perforation,[82] hydrothorax,[60] hemothorax,[17] ascites,[90] chest wall abscesses,[91] and embolization to the pleural space.[92] More commonly, improper location yields inaccurate measurements of the central venous pressure[93] or is associated with poor flow caused by kinking.

SUPRACLAVICULAR APPROACH

The claim by Moosman[52] that the SC approach is more likely to be accompanied by complications is not substantiated by the medical literature. In all reported series the complication rate has been low, ranging from 0 to 6 per cent.[18-23, 25] A compilation of the data from these series yields an overall complication rate of 1.3 per cent. The most significant complications have been pneumothorax and subclavian artery puncture; the highest incidence of pneumothorax is 2.4 per cent.[19] Adherence to Yoffa's technique[18] decreases the risk of these complications, because the needle is directed away from the pleural dome and the subclavian artery. The relatively superficial location of the vein when approached from above (1.5 to 3.5 cm) lessens the risk of puncture or laceration of deep structures.

Catheter tip malposition is also quite low because of the more direct path to the superior vena cava. For those series in which malposition has been reported, the overall rate is 1.1 per cent.[19, 22, 26] Fischer noted a malposition rate of 27.6 per cent using the IC technique,[94] and Herbst has reported a range of 1.7 to 24 per cent.[61] The highest incidence of malposition using the SC technique is 7 per cent and occurred during the performance of CPR.[26] In the same series, a 26 per cent malposition rate was reported for the IC technique.

The incidence of failure to establish a functioning intravenous line ranges from 0 to 5 per cent,[18-26] with an overall rate of 4 per cent. The failure rate reported for the IC technique ranges from 2.5 to 8 per cent.[53] One death has been reported as a result of air embolism, a complication not specifically related to the SC technique.[20]

Prevention of Complications

The reference to subclavian venipuncture as "a favorite clinical whipping boy" made over a decade ago[95] remains appropriate today. It is unfortunate that a procedure that is clinically useful, easy to perform, and relatively safe has been criticized to such a great extent. It is clear that many of the reported complications are avoidable when proper technique is used. Attention to specific details of patient selection, anatomy, surgical technique, and equipment must be stressed, since this *will* prevent complications. Adherence to the following guidelines is particularly important:

1. Patients should be selected properly. Obese, cachectic, emphysematous, and combative patients are poor candidates.

2. The physician should know the anatomy in detail. A poor understanding of the relationship of the subclavian vessels to the clavicle and the first rib is a major cause of complications, especially pneumothorax.[39]

3. Inexperienced personnel should not be allowed to perform the procedure unsupervised. The complication rate is inversely proportional to the level of physician experience.[61] The many small steps designed to prevent complications are often forgotten or ignored by the novice.

4. The procedure should be performed frequently or not at all. In Herbst's retrospective audit, 46 per cent of the procedures during which complications occurred were performed by physicians who attempted an average of only one subclavian venipuncture in a year.[61] Complications were also higher among gynecologists, who started an average of only 8 subclavian lines during the year.

5. Aseptic technique should be practiced throughout, and lines placed during resuscitations should be removed as soon as possible. Antibiotic ointments placed at the skin puncture site may have a role in limiting septic complications.[55, 57, 58]

6. All measures designed to prevent air embolus should be practiced. These include use of the Trendelenburg position, active exhalation, occlusion of the open needle hub, and adequate measures to prevent air entry into IV tubing.

7. One should never pull the catheter through the needle or use through-the-needle devices without the needle guard.

8. One should always lower the IV bag and check for venous backflow or withdraw blood directly from the catheter before infusing fluids. It should be noted that a blood return is only suggestive of intravascular placement.

9. The procedure should always be followed by a chest film. The physician should personally check the film for the presence of hemo- or pneumothorax and for catheter position.

10. Kinked or malpositioned lines should always be replaced or repositioned.

11. During CPR, the supraclavicular technique should be used when a subclavian line is indicated.[26]

12. Excessive punctures should not be made if initial attempts are unsuccessful. An alternative route should be used. If multiple punctures are required, the admitting physician should be alerted for possible complications.

Conclusion

Subclavian venipuncture is a widely used clinical tool despite reports of potentially fatal complications. Its usefulness has been demonstrated in a variety of clinical settings. It is a relatively safe and simple procedure that should be associated with few significant problems. The keys to successful application of this technique are in-depth knowledge of the anatomy and meticulous attention to the details of the procedure.

1. Aubaniac, R.: L'injection intraveineuse sous-claviculaire. Avantages et techniques. Press. Med. 60:1456, 1952.
2. Aubaniac, R.: Une nouvelle voie d'injection ou de ponction veineuse: La voie sous-claviculaire. Sem. Hop. Paris 28:3445, 1952.
3. Aubaniac, R.: L'intraveineuse sous-claviculaire: Avantages et technique. Afr. Fr. Chir. 3–4:131, 1952.
4. Lepp, H.: Uber eine neue intravenose Injektions und Punktions-methode; die infraklavikulare Punktion der vena subclavia. Dtsch. Kahnaerztl. Z.8:511, 1953.
5. Lepp, H.: Die infraklavikulare Punktion der vena subclavia nach Aubaniac. Munch. Med. Wochenschr. 96:1392, 1954.
6. Villafane, P. E.: Technica de la transfusion por via subclavicular. Prensa Med. Argent. 40:2379, 1953.
7. Keeri-Szanto, M.: The subclavian vein, a constant and convenient intravenous injection site. Arch. Surg. 72:179, 1956.
8. Kalcev, B.: Subclavian venepuncture, letter to the editor. Lancet 1:45, 1964.
9. Wilson, J. W., Grow, J. B., and Demong, C. V.: Central venous pressure in optimal blood volume maintenance. Arch. Surg. 85:563, 1962.
10. Ashbaugh, D., and Thompson, J. W. W.: Subclavian-vein infusion. Lancet 2:1138, 1963.
11. Davidson, J. T., Ben-Hur, N., and Nathen, H.: Subclavian venepuncture. Lancet 2:1139, 1963.
12. Malinak, L. R., Gulde, R. E., and Faris, A. M.: Percutaneous subclavian catheterization for central venous pressure monitoring. Applications in obstetrical and gynecological problems. Am. J. Obstet. Gynecol. 92:477, 1965.
13. Giles, H. V.: The subclavian vein: Its usefulness in burn cases. Plast. Reconstr. Surg. 38:519, 1966.
14. Mogil, R. A., DeLaurentis, D. A., and Rosemond, G. P.: The infraclavicular venepuncture: Value in various clinical situations including central venous pressure monitoring. Arch. Surg. 95:320, 1967.
15. Yarom, R.: Subclavian venepuncture, letter to the editor. Lancet 1:45, 1964.
16. Matz, R.: Complications of determining the central venous pressure. N. Engl. J. Med. 273:703, 1965.
17. Smith, B. E., Modell, J. H., and Gaub, M. L.: Complications of subclavian vein catheterization. Arch. Surg. 90:228, 1965.
18. Yoffa, D.: Supraclavicular subclavian venepuncture and catheterisation. Lancet 2:614, 1965.
19. Garcia, J. M., Mispireta, L. A., and Pinho, R. V.: Percutaneous supraclavicular superior vena caval cannulation. Surg. Gynecol. Obstet. 134:839, 1972.
20. James, P. M., and Myers, R. T.: Central venous pressure monitoring: Misinterpretation, abuses, indications and a new technique. Ann. Surg. 175:693, 1972.
21. Nugent, R. P.: Supraclavicular catheterization of the subclavian vein. Aust. N. Z. J. Surg. 43:41, 1973.
22. Brahos, G. H.: Central venous catheterization via the supraclavicular approach. J. Trauma 17:872, 1977.
23. Craig, R. G., Jones, R. A., and Sproul, G. L.: The alternate method of central venous system catheterization. Am. Surg. 34:131, 1968.
24. Defalque, R. J.: Subclavian venepuncture: A review. Anesth. Analg. 47:677, 1968.
25. Brahos, G. H., and Cohen, M. J.: Supraclavicular central venous catheterization: Technique and experience in 250 cases. Wis. Med. J. 80:36, 1981.
26. Dronen, S. C., Thompson, B., and Nowak, R.: Subclavian vein catheterization during cardiopulmonary resuscitation. JAMA 247:3227, 1982.
27. Graber, D., and Dailey, R. H.: Catheter flow rates updated, letter to the editor. JACEP 6:518, 1977.
28. Dronen, S. C., Yee, A. S., and Tomlanovich, M. C.: Proximal saphenous vein cutdown. Ann. Emerg. Med. 10:328, 1981.
29. Westaby, S.: Ryles tube for rapid intravenous transfusion. Lancet 1:360, 1979.
30. Haynes, B. E.: Catheter introducers for hypovolemic patients, letter to the editor. Ann. Emerg. Med. 11:642, 1982.
31. Barsan, W. G., Levy, R. C., and Weir, H.: Lidocaine levels during CPR: Differences after peripheral venous, central venous, and intracardiac injections. Ann. Emerg. Med. 10:73, 1981.

32. Kuhn, G. J., White, B. C., Swetnam, R. E., et al.: Peripheral vs. central circulation times during CPR: A pilot study. Ann. Emerg. Med. 10:417, 1981.

33. Dudrick, S. J., Wilmore, D. W., and Vars, H. M.: Can intravenous feeding as the sole means of nutrition support growth in the child and restore weight loss in an adult? Ann. Surg. 169:974, 1969.

34. Dudrick, S. J., and Wilmore, D. W.: Long term parenteral feeding. Hosp. Pract. 3:65, 1968.

35. Merk, E. A., and Rush, B. F.: Emergency subclavian vein catheterization and intravenous hyperalimentation. Am. J. Surg. 129:266, 1975.

36. Knopp, R., and Dailey, R. H.: Central venous cannulation and pressure monitoring. JACEP 6:358, 1977.

37. Nowak, R. M.: Personal communication, Detroit, Michigan. April, 1981.

38. Mitty, W. F., and Nealon, T. F.: Complications of subclavian sticks. JACEP 4:24, 1975.

39. Westreich, M.: Preventing complications of subclavian vein catheterization. JACEP 7:368, 1978.

40. Simpson, E. T., and Aitchison, J. M.: Percutaneous infraclavicular subclavian vein catheterization in shocked patients: A prospective study in 172 patients. J. Trauma 22:781, 1982.

41. McIntyre, K. M., and Lewis, A. J. (eds.): Textbook of Advanced Cardiac Life Support. Dallas, American Heart Association, 1981.

42. Borja, A. R., and Hinshaw, J. R.: A safe way to perform infraclavicular subclavian vein catheterization. Surg. Gynecol. Obstet. 130:673, 1970.

43. Tofield, J. J.: A safer technique of percutaneous catheterization of the subclavian vein. Surg. Gynecol. Obstet. 128:1069, 1969.

44. Sullivan, R., and Pomerantz, M.: Central venous pressure monitoring: The subclavian approach. Surg. Clin. North Am. 49:1489, 1969.

45. Gallitano, A. L., Kondi, E. S., and Deckers, P. J.: A safe approach to the subclavian vein. Surg. Gynecol. Obstet. 135:96, 1972.

46. Longerbeam, J. K., Vannix, R., Wagner, W., et al.: Central venous pressure monitoring. Am. J. Surg. 110:220, 1965.

47. Phillips, S. J.: Technique of percutaneous subclavian vein catheterization. Surg. Gynecol. Obstet. 127:1079, 1968.

48. Buchman, R. J.: Subclavian venipuncture. Milit. Med. 134:451, 1969.

49. Simon, R. R.: A new technique for subclavian puncture. JACEP 7:409, 1978.

50. Feiler, E. M., and de Alva, W. E.: Infraclavicular percutaneous subclavian vein puncture. Am. J. Surg. 118:906, 1969.

51. Land, R. E.: Anatomic relationships of the right subclavian vein. Arch. Surg. 102:178, 1971.

52. Moosman, D. A.: The anatomy of infraclavicular subclavian vein catheterization and its complications. Surg. Gynecol. Obstet. 136:71, 1973.

53. Borja, A. R.: Current status of infraclavicular subclavian vein catheterization. Ann. Thorac. Surg. 13:615, 1972.

54. American Heart Association: Standards and guidelines for cardiopulmonary resuscitation and emergency cardiac care. JAMA 244:453, 1980.

55. Collins, R. N., Braun, P. A., Zinner, S. H., et al.: Risk of local and systemic infection with polyethylene intravenous catheters. N. Engl. J. Med. 279:340, 1968.

56. Feliciano, D.: Complications of percutaneous subclavian vein catheters. Curr. Concepts Trauma Care, 9, Fall 1980.

57. Moran, J. M., Atwood, R. P., and Rowe, M. I.: A clinical and bacteriologic study of infections associated with venous cutdowns. N. Engl. J. Med. 272:554, 1963.

58. Henzel, J. H., and DeWeese, M. S.: Morbid and mortal complications associated with prolonged central venous cannulation. Am. J. Surg. 121:600, 1971.

59. Schaefer, C. J.: Redirection of misplaced central venous catheters. Arch. Surg. 115:789, 1980.

60. Feliciano, D., Mattox, K., Graham, J., et al.: Major complications of percutaneous subclavian vein catheters. Am. J. Surg. 138:869, 1979.

61. Herbst, C.: Indications, management and complications of percutaneous subclavian catheters. Arch. Surg. 113:1421, 1978.

62. McGoon, M., Benedetto, P., and Greene, B.: Complications of percutaneous central venous catheterization: A report of 2 cases and a review of the literature. Johns Hopkins Med. J. 145:1, 1979.

63. Schapira, M., and Stern, W.: Hazards of subclavian vein cannulation for CVP monitoring. JAMA 201:111, 1967.

64. Maggs, P. R., and Schwaber, J. R.: Fatal bilateral pneumothoraces complicating subclavian vein catheterization. Chest 71:552, 1977.

65. Goldman, L. I.: Another complication of subclavian puncture: Arterial laceration. JAMA 217:78, 1971.

66. Holt, S., Kirkham, N., and Myerscough, E.: Hemothorax after subclavian vein cannulation. Thorax 32:101, 1977.

67. Fontanelle, L. J., Dooley, B. N., and Cuello, L.: Subclavian venipuncture and its complications. Ann. Thorac. Surg. 11:331, 1971.

68. Adar, R., and Mozes, M.: Hydromediastinum. JAMA 214:372, 1970.

69. Flanagan, J., Gradisar, I., and Gross, R.: Air embolus—a lethal complication of subclavian venipuncture. N. Engl. J. Med. 281:488, 1969.

70. Lucas, C., and Irani, F.: Air embolus via subclavian catheter. N. Engl. J. Med. 281:966, 1969.

71. Levinsky, W.: Fatal air embolism during insertion of CVP monitoring apparatus. JAMA 209:1721, 1969.

72. Peters, J. L., and Armstrong, R.: Air embolism as a complication of central venous catheterization. Ann. Surg. 187:375, 1978.

73. Durant, T. M., Long, J. W., and Oppenheimer, M. J.: Pulmonary (venous) air embolism. Am. Heart J. 33:269, 1947.

74. Michenfelder, J. D., Terry, H. R., and Daw, E. F.: Air embolism during neurosurgery. A new method of treatment. Anesth. Analg. 45:390, 1966.

75. Sink, J. D., Comer, P. B., James, P. M., et al.: Evaluation of catheter placement in the treatment of venous air embolism. Ann. Surg. 183:58, 1976.

76. Lefrak, E., and Noon, G.: Management of arterial injury secondary to attempted subclavian vein catheterization. Ann. Thorac. Surg. 14:294, 1972.

77. Farhat, K., Nakhjavan, K., Cope, C., et al.: Iatrogenic arteriovenous fistula. A complication of percutaneous subclavian vein puncture. Chest 67:480, 1975.

78. Thomas, C. S., Carter, J. W., and Lowden, S. C.: Pericardial tamponade from central venous catheters. Arch. Surg. 98:217, 1969.

79. Fitts, C. T., Barnett, L. T., Webb, C. M., et al.: Perforating wounds of the heart caused by central venous catheters. J. Trauma 10:764, 1970.

80. Bone, D. K., Maddrey, W. C., Eagen, J., et al.: Cardiac tamponade: A fatal complication of central venous catheterization. Arch. Surg. 106:868, 1973.

81. Brandt, R. L., Foley, W. J., Fink, G. H., et al.: Mechanism of perforation of the heart with production of a hydropericardium by a venous catheter and its prevention. Am. J. Surg. 119:311, 1970.

82. Friedman, B. A., and Jurgeleit, H. C.: Perforation of the atrium by polyethylene central venous catheters. JAMA 203:1141, 1968.

83. Sheep, R. E., and Guiney, W. B.: Fatal cardiac tamponade. JAMA 248:1632, 1982.

84. Nicolas, F.: Knotting of subclavian central venous catheters. JAMA 214:373, 1970.

85. Johnson, C. L., and Lazarchick, J.: Subclavian venipuncture: Preventable complications, report of two cases. Mayo Clin. Proc. 45:712, 1970.
86. Wilmore, D. W., and Dudrick, S. J.: Safe long term venous catheterization. Arch. Surg. 98:256, 1967.
87. Wilmore, D. W., and Dudrick, S. J.: Guarding against complications in subclavian vein catheterization. Hosp. Phys. 6:82, 1970.
88. Drachler, D., Koepke, G., and Weg, J.: Phrenic nerve injury from subclavian vein catheterization: diagnosis by electromyography. JAMA 236:2880, 1976.
89. Obel, I. W.: Transient phrenic nerve paralysis following subclavian venipuncture. Anesthesiology 33:369, 1970.
90. Allsop, J. R., and Askew, A. R.: Subclavian vein cannulation: A new complication. Br. Med. J. 4:262, 1975.

91. Oakes, D. D., and Wilson, R. E.: Malposition of subclavian lines. JAMA 233:532, 1975.
92. Hegarty, M. M.: The hazards of subclavian vein catheterization: Practical considerations and an unusual case report. S. Afr. Med. J. 52:240, 1977.
93. Thomas, T.: Location of catheter tip and its importance on central venous pressure. Chest 61:668, 1972.
94. Fischer, J., Lundstrom, J., Ohand, H. G.: Central venous cannulation: A radiological determination of catheter positions and immediate intrathoracic complications. Acta Anaesthesiol. Scand. 21:45, 1977.
95. Russo, J.: The subclavian catheter, letter to the editor. N. Engl. J. Med. 281:1425, 1969.

22

Central Venous Catheterization: Internal Jugular Approach and Alternatives

STEVEN R. WYTE, M.D.
WILLIAM J. BARKER, M.D.

Introduction and Background

There are several alternatives to subclavian vein cannulation when access to the central venous circulation is needed. The venae cavae may be readily reached from the internal and external jugular, femoral, basilic, and cephalic veins. The internal jugular (IJ) route is the most useful for the emergency physician, although all of these alternative methods have their merit.

The internal jugular approach was first mentioned in the United States in a pediatric handbook by Silver and coworkers in 1963.[1] Although puncture of the superior jugular bulb at the base of the skull had been used by neurologists for quite some time, the approach was too dangerous for use in routine catheterization.[2] Internal jugular vein catheterization in the adult was first described by Hemosura in 1966.[3] He discussed a variation of what is now commonly termed the central approach. Over the next several years, other methods were proposed by Civetta, Daily, English, Jernigan, and others.[4-10] Defalque reviewed 17 methods in 1974 and grouped them into three major approaches: central, anterior, and posterior.[2] These methods will be discussed in detail later in the chapter.

The femoral, basilic, and cephalic approaches have developed primarily as routes for passage of transvenous pacemakers and Swan-Ganz pressure catheters. The development of commercial flexible wire introducer sets (Seldinger technique) has also permitted central venous cannulation by way of the external jugular vein.[11, 12]

All of these techniques have a place in the practice of emergency medicine, and often the choice of a certain method is determined solely by the confidence of the individual physician in his or her ability to perform them. The internal jugular and subclavian (supra- and infraclavicular) approaches discussed in the preceding chapter are favorites of the emergency physician because of the rapid manner in which access can be obtained.

Indications and Contraindications

The indications and contraindications for the alternative routes of central venous cannulation are generally the same as for subclavian central access, as stated in the preceding chapter, and therefore will be discussed only when important differences exist between the techniques. Before the following techniques are attempted, a thorough understanding of the principles of central venous catheterization is required. The reader is referred to Chapter 21 for a comprehensive discussion of these principles.

INTERNAL JUGULAR APPROACH

As is true of the supraclavicular subclavian approach, the IJ technique is useful for securing routine central venous access and for emergency venous access during cardiopulmonary resuscitation (CPR). The approach is desirable during CPR because the site is removed from the area of chest compressions. Only one prospective comparison trial of IJ cannulation and subclavian cannulation has been performed. In that randomized study, Kaiser and associates[13] found a significantly greater incidence of proper venipuncture and catheter passage with the infraclavicular subclavian approach as compared with the posterior IJ method (98 per cent versus 84 per cent). A 20 per cent rate of catheter malposition was noted with each method. Eisenhauer and colleagues[14] in a retrospective study found that only 0.4 per cent of 248 IJ cannulations resulted in clinically significant morbidity compared with 4.2 per cent of 298 subclavian insertions, even though the overall complication rate was similar. Although there may be a slight difference in complications between the two routes, in the absence of specific contraindications, the physician should use the technique of central venous cannulation with which he or she is most familiar. The IJ route is slightly more difficult technically than the subclavian route, but it is faster and easier than a venous cutdown.

Cervical trauma with swelling or anatomic distortion at the intended site of IJ venipuncture is a specific contraindication to the IJ approach. Neck motion is limited when the IJ central line is in place and represents a relative contraindication in the conscious patient. Furthermore, a short, thick neck may preclude the necessary needle manipulation for IJ catheterization. Although bleeding disorders are relative contraindications to central venous cannulation, the IJ approach is preferred in patients with coagulopathies, since the area may be directly compressed should bleeding occur; compression of the subclavian vein is not possible. Carotid artery disease (plaque or obstruction) is a relative contraindication to IJ cannulation. Inadvertent puncture of the artery may dislodge a plaque, and prolonged compression of the artery to control bleeding may impair cerebral circulation if collateral blood flow is compromised. If a preceding subclavian catheterization has been unsuccessful, the ipsilateral IJ route is generally preferred for a subsequent attempt. In this manner, *bilateral* iatrogenic complications are avoided.

EXTERNAL JUGULAR APPROACH

In instances in which alternative methods of central venous catheterization are not possible, one may obtain access to the central venous system by way of the external jugular vein.[11, 12] Although the external jugular vein is a ready emergency intravenous access route when standard peripheral intravenous catheters are used, the valves and tortuosity of the external jugular system often preclude placement of standard central venous catheters. Successful central vein cannulation is generally possible only with the use of guide wires. The external jugular vein must be readily visible for percutaneous cannulation to be successful. The technique is valuable because it avoids the complications of pneumothorax, carotid artery puncture, and hidden hemorrhage.

The procedure can be used in both children and adults, but success is more common in adults.[15, 16] Central venous catheterization by the external jugular route is technically more difficult than internal jugular cannulation, but it is successful 76 to 100 per cent of the time in adults.[11, 12, 16, 17] Both the straight guide wires and the J-tipped wires have been used. Use of the J-tipped wires is more reliable and is the preferred technique.[12, 16] The J wires are more easily advanced because the rounded tip bounces off vessel walls and more easily navigates sharp angulations in the vessel course.

Despite the increased success of central cannulation via the external jugular route with J wires, the technique is extremely time-consuming.[12] Hence, this approach is contraindicated when *immediate* central access is desired (e.g., cardiac arrest, shock). Nonetheless, simple external jugular cannulation *without* attempts to pass a catheter may itself serve as a useful alternative for the *rapid* administration of fluid and drugs.

FEMORAL APPROACH

Although femoral cannulation is a useful method of central venous access, the femoral vein technique is seldom indicated for central venous line placement when other more proximal sites are available. Nonetheless, the femoral vein is easily cannulated in low-flow states and can serve as a stable site for passage of a transvenous pacemaker or a pressure catheter in the critically ill patient. Fluid resuscitation through a long femoral central venous line is restricted by the large resistance of the tubing. Furthermore, passage of a femoral line is contraindicated in abdominal trauma when intra-abdominal vascular injury is suspected.

BASILIC-CEPHALIC APPROACH

When rapidity of access to the central venous circulation is not important, this approach should be considered, since it has the lowest incidence of major complications. The location of the basilic and cephalic veins away from vital organs and major arteries accounts for this low incidence of major problems. When the patient is upright, the basilic vein is preferred over the cephalic vein because of a higher incidence of successful catheter passage into the subclavian vein, although the overall success rate of superior vena cava cannulation is similar for both techniques in the supine patient.[18-20] Nonetheless, both veins have valves, which may impede catheter advancement.[21-24]

In a cardiac arrest situation in which access for drug or fluid delivery is of primary concern, cannulation of these veins with a standard intravenous (short) large-bore catheter (14 to 18 gauge, 1¼ inches) is preferred over cannulation with longer central catheters. Drug delivery to the heart is almost as expeditious with the shorter catheters, and fluid volume delivery is more rapid.[25, 26] The presence of previous phlebitis and shoulder or proximal extremity trauma is a contraindication to placement of a basilic or a cephalic line. Furthermore, the prolonged use of the catheter may induce phlebitis and hence render the vessel useless for future cannulation. Therefore, the intended future use of the basilic and cephalic vessels for other purposes (e.g., transvenous pacemaker placement or venipuncture) is a relative contraindication to basilic and cephalic catheterization. The arm should also be immobilized following catheter placement to minimize catheter motion or kinking caused by extremity motion. The technique is therefore undesirable in the combative patient.

Procedure

The equipment for internal jugular, femoral, and basilic-cephalic cannulation is the same as that used for the subclavian route (see Table 21–3), with the addition of a 22 gauge locator needle and a 36-inch catheter for the femoral and basilic-cephalic approaches. As stated earlier, central venous cannulation via the external jugular approach should be undertaken with the guide wire (Seldinger) technique, using a curved wire (J wire).

INTERNAL JUGULAR CANNULATION

Anatomy of the Internal Jugular Vein. The anatomy of the IJ vein is relatively constant, regardless of body habitus. The vein drains the cranium, beginning as the superior jugular bulb, which is separated from the floor of the middle ear by a delicate bony plate. The IJ vein emerges deep to the posterior belly of the digastric muscle. At its origin the IJ vein courses adjacent to the spinal accessory, vagus, and hypoglossal nerves

as well as the internal carotid artery. Several tributary veins enter the IJ vein at the level of the hyoid bone. The IJ vein, the internal (and, later, the common) carotid artery, and the vagus nerve course together in the carotid sheath. The IJ vein occupies the anterior lateral position in the carotid sheath.[27] The only structure that maintains a fixed anatomic relationship with the IJ vein is the carotid artery. The vein invariably lies lateral and slightly anterior to the carotid artery, and the course of the artery serves as a guide to venous cannulation. At the level of the thyroid cartilage, the IJ vein can be found just deep to the sternocleidomastoid muscle (SCM) (Fig. 22–1).

The IJ vein emerges from under the apex of the triangle of the two heads of the sternocleidomastoid muscle and joins the subclavian vein behind the clavicle. As the vein approaches its supraclavicular junction with the subclavian vein, it assumes a more medial position in the triangle formed by the sternocleidomastoid muscles, following the anterior border of the lateral head. In this lower cervical region the common carotid artery assumes a deep paratracheal location. The brachial plexus is separated from the IJ vein by the scalenus anterior muscle. The phrenic nerve is anterior to the scalenus anterior muscle. Although quite deep, the stellate ganglion lies anterior to the lower brachial plexus.

Unlike the subclavian vein, the IJ vein is quite distensible. The vessel diameter is increased with the Valsalva maneuver and the head-down (Trendelenburg) tilt position. The diameter of the vein should theoretically increase with the application of the pneumatic anti-shock garment (PASG), although this has not been studied. The PASG minimally increases venous return but can significantly increase intrathoracic pressure and hence decrease emptying of the IJ vein. Prolonged palpation of the carotid pulse will decrease the diameter of the IJ vein.[27] Rotation of the head 90 degrees toward the opposite side or extending the neck will not significantly change the size of the IJ vessel. Severe rotation of the head, however, will bring the SCM anterior or medial to the IJ vein. Severe rotation may make it impossible to cannulate the IJ vein without first traversing the carotid artery when the anterior approach is used. The diameter of the IJ vessel is largest below the cricoid ring,[27] where it may reach 2 to 2.5 cm.

Technique. Defalque[2] reviewed methods of IJ cannulation and organized the approaches into three groups defined by the anatomy of the SCM. In preparation for all three methods, the patient is tilted 15 to 30 degrees in the Trendelenburg position and the head turned away from the side of venipuncture. The internal jugular vein is distensible, and tilting the patient increases the diameter of the vessel. If the patient is awake, he or she should be instructed to perform a Valsalva

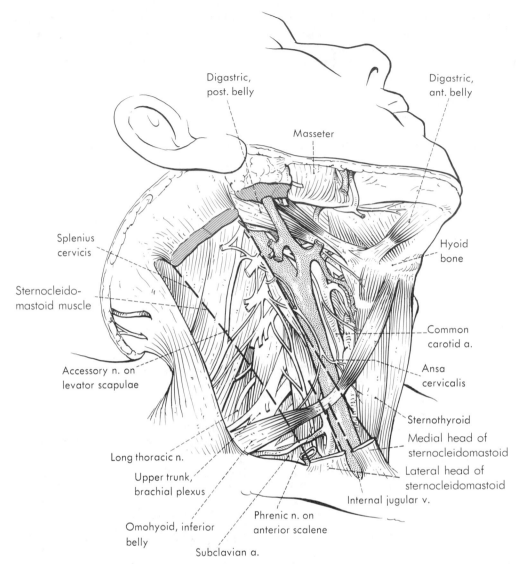

Digastric, post. belly

Digastric, ant. belly

Masseter

Splenius cervicis

Hyoid bone

Sternocleido-mastoid muscle

Common carotid a.

Ansa cervicalis

Accessory n. on levator scapulae

Sternothyroid

Medial head of sternocleidomastoid

Lateral head of sternocleidomastoid

Long thoracic n.

Internal jugular v.

Upper trunk, brachial plexus

Phrenic n. on anterior scalene

Omohyoid, inferior belly

Subclavian a.

Figure 22–1. Structures in a dissection of the neck. The superficial veins and the sternocleidomastoid muscle have been removed, as have the submandibular gland and a segment of the facial vein. The cutaneous nerves have been cut down to short stumps arising from the second, third, and fourth cervical nerves. The internal jugular vein is drawn somewhat more medial in this illustration than is commonly found. (From Hollinshead, W. H.: Textbook of Anatomy, 3rd ed. New York, Harper & Row, 1974, p. 765. Used by permission.)

maneuver during vessel cannulation. In the unconscious patient, abdominal compression by an assistant can be used to help distend the vein.

Familiarity with the anatomy of the neck is important both to increase the probability of successful cannulation and to avoid complications. Most authors favor cannulation of the right side of the neck, which provides a more direct route to the superior vena cava (SVC) and avoids the thoracic duct. Although it is probably clinically insignificant, the cupola of the pleura is also slightly lower on the right side. The left internal jugular approach is more circuitous and, when used with a stiff Teflon catheter, may produce major venous puncture leading to hydrothorax, hydromediastinum, and even pericardial tampon-

ade.[28] When time permits, the skin is prepared with povidone-iodine solution and is draped with sterile towels. Preparation should include the subclavian area in case of failure of the IJ approach. The procedure should be briefly described to the conscious patient, and each step should be restated as it is about to be performed. The area to be punctured should be anesthetized with local anesthetic using a 25 gauge needle. As noted previously, it is advisable to attempt a subclavian approach on the same side if the internal jugular approach is unsuccessful rather than to attempt an IJ route on the opposite side. A bilateral iatrogenic pathologic condition may thus be prevented.

Central Route. This approach is favored by Daily[5] and Kaplan,[29] who believe that the incidence of cannulation of the carotid artery is decreased and the cupola of the lung is avoided with this method. The triangle formed by the clavicle and the sternal and clavicular heads of the SCM is first palpated and identified. The carotid pulse is palpated, and the artery is retracted medially. Alternatively, the lateral border of the carotid pulse can be marked by a local anesthetic skin wheal or a marking pen and all subsequent needle puncture performed laterally to that point.

Some practitioners prefer to attempt cannulation with the catheter apparatus initially. Other clinicians use a small gauge "locator" needle to locate the vein. The smaller needle allows one to ascertain the location of the vein and minimizes injury to the deep structures, which can occur with a larger needle. Use of a "locator" needle can be time-consuming in a cardiac arrest situation. With the exploring technique a 22 gauge, 1½-inch needle attached to a 5- to 10-ml syringe is introduced near the rostral apex of the triangle and is directed caudally at an angle 30 to 40 degrees to the skin. The needle should initially be directed parallel and slightly laterally to the course of the carotid artery (Fig. 22–2). If three fingers are placed over the course of the carotid artery, the parallel course of the IJ vein can be estimated. The vein consistently lies just lateral to the carotid artery. Prolonged deep palpation of the carotid artery may decrease the size of the vein, and the three-finger technique should be used only long enough to identify the course of the artery.

Negative pressure should be maintained on the syringe at all times as the needle is advanced or retracted. The vein is more superficial than might be expected, and deep probing with the needle should be avoided; the vein is usually encountered at a depth of 1 to 1.5 cm. If the internal jugular vein is not entered at a depth of 3 to 5 cm, the needle should be withdrawn to just below the skin surface and directed toward the ipsilateral nipple underneath the medial border of the lateral (clavicular) head of the SCM. The vein should be entered at 1 to 3 cm, and dark blood should be easily aspirated. (Bright red blood indicates carotid artery penetration.) The "locator" needle is withdrawn and is replaced with a 14 gauge, 2-inch needle attached to a syringe.[4] A drop of the aspirated blood from the "locator" needle can be placed at the edge of the sterile field in line with the point of vessel entry, thus serving as a guide to recannulation.

The larger needle is advanced through the skin along the tract determined by the smaller needle until blood is aspirated. Care must be taken to cover the needle hub with a gloved thumb whenever the needle lumen is exposed to air. This will prevent an air embolus when the patient inspires.[30] A catheter and stylet are then passed through the needle into the SVC. Alternatively, an over-the-needle catheter may be used. The over-the-needle catheter is less desirable, since it may not reach the intrathoracic central venous circulation.

One secures the catheter in place by placing a suture through the skin, tying three square knots, and then tying the suture around the catheter. The catheter will be both secure and functional if the knot is tied tightly enough to indent the catheter; the stylet is left in place while the knot is tied to prevent catheter occlusion. Two other skin sutures should be placed on either side (or through standard openings) of the needle guard. To avoid crimping of the catheter, one usually loops the catheter around the ipsilateral ear (Fig 22–3). Antibiotic ointment is then applied to the

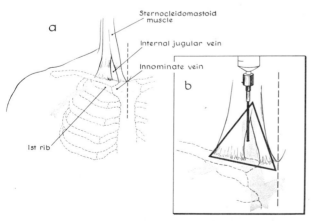

Figure 22–2. Central approach to internal jugular vein. *a.* Relationship of sternocleidomastoid muscle to chest. *b.* Course of internal jugular vein; note its sagittal course. (From Daily, P. O., Griepp, R. B., and Shumway, N. E.: Percutaneous internal jugular vein cannulation. Arch. Surg. 101:534, 1970. Used by permission.)

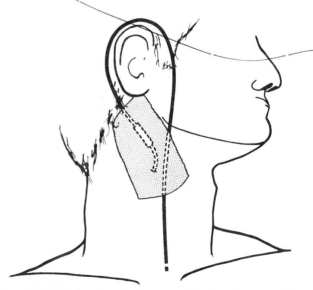

Figure 22–3. Internal jugular line secured by looping around the ear. (From Boulanger, M., et al.: Une nouvelle voie d'abord de la veine jugulaire interne. Can. Anaesth. Soc. J. 23:609, 1976. Used by permission.)

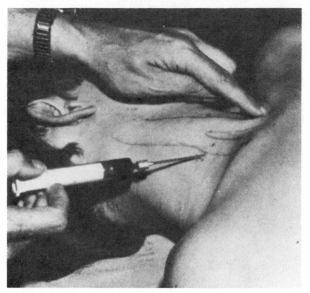

Figure 22–4. Posterior approach to the internal jugular vein. (From Delfaque, R. J.: Percutaneous catheterization of the internal jugular vein. Anesth. Analg. 53:116, 1974. Used by permission.)

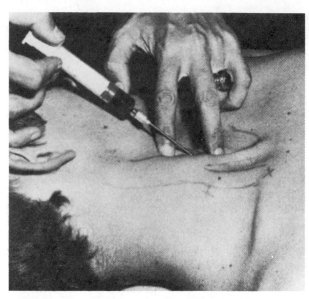

Figure 22–5. Anterior approach to the internal jugular vein. (From Delfaque, R. J.: Percutaneous catheterization of the internal jugular vein. Anesth. Analg. 53:116, 1974. Used by permission.)

puncture site, and a sterile dressing is placed. The intravenous tubing should be securely fastened to the catheter with tape to prevent air embolism or blood loss.

Posterior and Anterior Routes. The techniques of manipulating needles, syringes, and catheters for these approaches are identical to those for the central route; only the landmarks and needle directions vary. For the posterior approach, the skin is entered at the lateral edge of the SCM one third of the way from the clavicle to the mastoid process (Fig. 22–4). The locator needle is directed caudally and medially under the lateral border of the SCM toward the sternal notch until blood is aspirated.

To perform the anterior approach described by Mostert and coworkers,[7] one often retracts the carotid artery medially with the left hand (Fig. 22–5). The three-finger technique to identify the course of the carotid artery may alternatively be used. The small needle should then enter the skin at the midpoint of the medial aspect of the SCM. The needle is directed at an angle of 30 to 45 degrees to the coronal plane caudad toward the ipsilateral nipple. Kaplan alters this approach by starting at the level of the thyroid notch.[29] The proximity of the carotid artery in the alternative anterior approach, with the needle directed cephalad, may prohibit venous cannulation without carotid puncture.[27]

Internal Jugular Vein Catheterization in Infants and Children. Prince and coworkers[31] reported a high success rate (40 of 54 cases) in patients from the ages of 6 weeks to 14 years. Success was dependent on infant size (better above 10 kg) and central venous pressure (better over 10 cm H_2O). Using Daily's[5] central approach with needle punc-

ture at the apex of the triangle bordered by the two heads of the SCM and the clavicle, one passes a 22 gauge needle attached to a 2- to 5-ml Luer syringe into the skin at a 45-degree angle and directs it caudally and laterally toward the ipsilateral nipple. The vessel is usually entered at a depth of 1 to 2 cm. The "locator" needle is then withdrawn, and a 17 to 19 gauge Intracath needle is inserted into the skin and passed along the track of the 22 gauge needle until the IJ vein is penetrated. A catheter is inserted through the needle and is secured in place.

EXTERNAL JUGULAR VEIN CATHETERIZATION

With the patient prepared and in the Trendelenburg position, the external jugular vein is entered with a 16 or 18 gauge needle or a standard over-the-needle peripheral intravenous catheter. Local anesthesia is essential in the conscious patient. The needle or catheter must be able to accept a guide wire through its lumen. When the vein has been cannulated with a needle or a catheter, a J wire is passed through the lumen and into the central venous circulation. If an introducing needle is used, it is now withdrawn to avoid shearing off the guide wire during manipulation. A Teflon over-the-needle catheter is preferred over a needle, since it may stay in the vein during guide wire passage or may serve as a temporary peripheral venous line if the central circulation cannot be cannulated. One advances the guide wire into the thorax by rotating, teasing, or otherwise manipulating the tip until the wire is within the

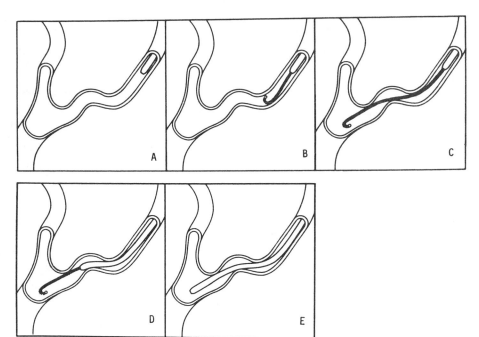

Figure 22–6. Insertion of a catheter over a wire via the external jugular vein. (From Blitt, C. D., Wright, W. A., and Petty, W. C.: Central venous catheterization via the external jugular vein, a technique employing the J-wire. JAMA 229:817, 1974. Used by permission.)

central venous circulation (Fig. 22–6). Guide wire advancement is the most difficult and time-consuming portion of the procedure, and this time constraint limits the usefulness of the technique in an emergency. Once the wire is in the correct position, a standard central venous catheter may be threaded over the wire, or a sheath introducer may be passed (with the aid of a vein dilator, as described in Chapter 19) to facilitate the introduction of a transvenous pacemaker or a pulmonary artery catheter. Even with central placement of the guide wire, the catheter may not pass centrally. After catheter placement, the guide wire is removed and the intravenous line is attached.

Central venous cannulation via the external jugular vein is time-consuming and often difficult. For these reasons, it is not recommended in an emergency. Nonetheless, the external jugular approach may provide central venous access in selected stable patients. Furthermore, simple cannulation with a short catheter may be useful for fluid and drug administration during an emergency.

FEMORAL VEIN CATHETERIZATION

The femoral vein is most easily cannulated percutaneously in patients with a palpable femoral pulse. The femoral vein lies just medially to the artery in the femoral canal below the inguinal ligament. Beneath the femoral vessels lie the psoas muscle and the hip.

After skin preparation, the pulse should be briefly palpated, and the femoral vein should be approached medial to the pulse. During cardi-

opulmonary resuscitation, palpable pulsations may represent venous pressure waves.[32] Hence, if initial attempts are unsuccessful in a cardiac arrest, a more lateral approach over the pulsation is recommended. When the femoral artery pulsation is not palpable, the femoral artery bisects a line that can be drawn from the anterior superior iliac crest to the pubic symphysis.

After local anesthesia is used in the conscious patient, a 14 gauge, 2-inch needle attached to a saline-filled syringe is inserted 1 cm medial to the artery. Negative pressure is maintained with the syringe at all times while the needle is under the skin. The needle is directed posteriorly and is advanced until the vein is entered, as identified by a flash of dark, nonpulsating blood. If the vessel is penetrated when the syringe is not being aspirated, the blood flash may be seen only as the needle is being withdrawn.

Once in the vein, the needle is stabilized; often a hemostat is helpful for holding the needle during removal of the syringe. A premeasured section of a 36-inch catheter may then be inserted through the needle. One determines the appropriate length by holding the catheter over the patient's body and estimating the distance from the skin puncture site to the right atrium. Contamination of the catheter must be avoided while this maneuver is performed. Once the catheter is placed, it is secured with sutures and is dressed in the same manner as other central lines. A "locator" needle with or without a guide wire may minimize vessel injury during location and cannulation of the femoral vein.

In situations requiring rapid volume infusion, in the absence of intra-abdominal trauma, the

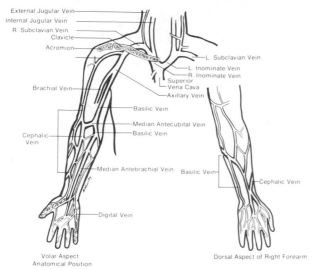

Figure 22–7. Major veins of the upper half of the body. (From Hedges, J. R.: Vascular access. Curr. Top. Emerg. Med. 2:1, 1981. Used by permission.)

femoral vein may be cannulated with the Seldinger technique, as described in Chapter 19. The sheath introducer will allow the rapid transfusion of large volumes of blood or crystalloid for fluid resuscitation.

BASILIC AND CEPHALIC CANNULATION

Anatomy of the Basilic and Cephalic Veins. Considerable variation is present in the venous vasculature of the upper extremities. Nonetheless, the cephalic and basilic veins can usually be located in the volar antecubital region (Fig. 22–7). The interconnecting median antecubital vein is often the most prominent, thus making it a popular site for venipuncture during blood sampling. The basilic vein merges proximally with the bra-

chial vein to form the axillary vein, which subsequently meets the cephalic vein to form the subclavian vein near the distal clavicle. The internal and external jugular veins join the subclavian vein to form the innominate vein bilaterally. Many venous valves exist in the peripheral vessels. Vascular anastomoses may permit aberrant advancement of a long line from the upper extremity. In particular, lines threaded up the cephalic vein may dead-end in a venous plexus or may enter the external jugular vein (Fig. 22–8). Furthermore, lines passed through the basilic vein may easily enter the internal jugular vein.

Technique. Basilic and cephalic venous systems are entered through the large veins in the antecubital fossa (see Fig. 22–7). Tourniquet placement aids venous distention and initial venous puncture. Cannulation can often be performed percutaneously with a 14 gauge needle under direct visualization. When veins are not visible, they may be reached with a cutdown procedure, as described in Chapter 20. The basilic vein, located on the medial aspect of the antecubital fossa, is generally larger than the radially located cephalic vein. Furthermore, the basilic vein generally provides a more direct route for passage into the axillary subclavian vein and superior vena cava. Once a vein has been entered, a premeasured length of a 36-inch catheter is threaded aseptically into the superior vena cava. Catheter length is estimated using the combined distance from the puncture site to the axilla and from the axilla to the middle of the manubrium.

Inability to pass the catheter is common. The cephalic vein may terminate inches above the antecubital fossa or may bifurcate before entering the axillary vein, sending a branch to the external jugular vein. The cephalic vein may also enter the axillary vein at right angles, defeating any attempt to pass the catheter centrally. Furthermore, both

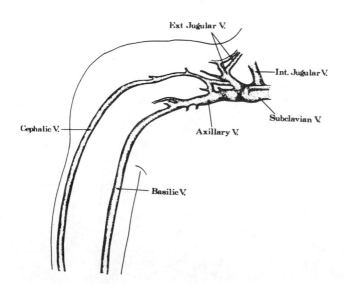

Figure 22–8. Proximal anatomy of the basilic-cephalic venous system. (From Webre, D. R., and Arens, J. F.: Use of the cephalic and basilic veins for introduction of central venous catheters. Anesthesiology 33:389, 1973. Used by permission.)

the basilic system and the cephalic system contain valves that may impede catheterization. Abduction of the shoulder may help to advance the catheter if resistance near the axillary vein occurs. The incidence of failure to place the catheter in the superior vena cava ranges from a high of 40 per cent to a low of 2 per cent.[20, 21, 23] Holt[21] believes that there is a higher incidence of success if crystalloid solution is continuously infused during the passage of the catheter. This contention is not supported by Bridges and coworkers,[20] who found an 80 to 84 per cent success rate with slow catheter advancement without infusion versus a 44 per cent success rate with crystalloid infusion in the supine patient.

The greatest success rate (98 per cent) that has been reported was obtained with slow catheter advancement with the patient in a 45- to 90-degree upright position.[20] Flexible Bard (C. R. Bard, Inc., Murray Hill, N.J.) (16 gauge) catheters were introduced into the basilic vein until the tip was judged to be proximal to the junction of the cephalic and basilic veins and distal to the junction of the internal jugular vein with the innominate vein (see Fig. 22–8). The wire stylet was withdrawn 6 inches and the catheters were advanced slowly ½ inch at a time, with 2 seconds allowed between each ½-inch insertion. The natural flexibility of the Bard catheters contributed to negotiation into the superior vena cava when the patient was upright. Obviously, this time-consuming technique is contraindicated when the patient cannot tolerate an upright position.

FURTHER COMMENTS

All of the percutaneous methods of central venous cannulation can also be performed with the Seldinger guide wire technique described in Chapter 19. Furthermore, when puncturing the skin with a large-bore needle, one should start with 1 to 2 ml of normal saline in the attached syringe. After the skin has been entered, a small amount of this fluid should be expelled in order to remove any plug of skin that might be present and that could interfere with aspiration of blood. The needle bevel should routinely be aligned with the numeric markings on the syringe to aid in bevel location once the skin is entered.

Immediately after any central line has been placed, blood should be aspirated from the catheter. Alternatively, one should place the intravenous bag at a level below the patient to check for blood return in the intravenous tubing. It should be noted that blood return is *presumptive* evidence of intravascular placement and does not substitute for radiographic confirmation. When this gravity flow method is used, it is important to check the intravenous tubing for the presence of a one-way flow valve. A one-way valve will prevent a flash-back of blood. The flashback of blood should also be observed for pulsations that may indicate line placement in an artery, tricuspid regurgitation, atrial fibrillation, or ventricular tachycardia. A chest film should also be obtained after central line placement to confirm catheter placement and to rule out hemo- or pneumothorax.

Complications

The complications of subclavian venipuncture have been extensively discussed in the preceding chapter. Many of these same complications have been reported with the alternative techniques. The following discussion is supplemental to the complication section of Chapter 21.

INTERNAL JUGULAR APPROACH

The complications of IJ cannulation are similar to those that have been discussed in the preceding chapter for the supraclavicular (SC) approach to the subclavian vein. One fairly common complication unique to the IJ approach is a hematoma in the neck. With the IJ approach, pressure can be maintained easily on the area of swelling, and most hematomas will resolve spontaneously. If arterial puncture is recognized and treated with compression, carotid artery puncture rarely causes significant morbidity unless there is marked atherosclerotic carotid artery disease. If the carotid artery is punctured, one may again attempt IJ cannulation on the same side following appropriate compression. Alternatively, the subclavian vein on the same side may be cannulated. A rapidly expanding hematoma from puncture of the internal carotid artery may rarely produce tracheal compression and deviation. Prolonged (15 to 20 *minutes*) firm pressure over the puncture site should be applied after a known or suspected arterial puncture.

Arterial puncture is a contraindication to attempting the IJ route on the opposite side, since bilateral hemorrhage may occur. The physician should also be prepared to rapidly intubate the patient should airway compromise occur. Even in the face of coagulopathies, the IJ approach has been found successful (99.3 per cent of cases) and safe (less than 1 per cent complication rate).[33] Neurologic injury (brachial plexus, phrenic and recurrent laryngeal nerves), although rare, is more common with the IJ technique than with other central venous approaches.[34, 35]

FEMORAL APPROACH

Femoral lines are associated with less severe complications than are IJ or subclavian approaches because of the avoidance of thoracic trauma. The peritoneum can, however, be violated with possible resulting perforation of the bowel. Bowel penetration is especially likely if the patient has a femoral hernia.[36] Injury to the bowel is likely to be minimal and is unlikely to require specific treatment. Nonetheless, the potential bacterial contamination of the femoral puncture site may pose a significant problem. The aspiration of air upon placement of a femoral line necessitates removal of the catheter and reinsertion at another site. A psoas abscess may result from penetration of the underlying psoas fascia.[36] The bladder, when distended, can also be punctured during femoral cannulation, although bladder puncture is unlikely to require therapy beyond removal of the aberrantly placed catheter. Strict aseptic technique should be maintained to prevent septic arthritis in the unlikely event that the hip capsule is punctured. This complication has been reported in infants.[37]

The most common complications of femoral venipuncture are accidental arterial and venous perforation. Prolonged (greater than 15 minutes) pressure should stop any hemorrhage in a patient with normal clotting mechanisms. The femoral nerve can also be injured by an errant needle puncture.[36, 37] One report[38] of 5306 femoral vein cannulations using the Seldinger technique reported five severe complications (three episodes of severe retroperitoneal bleeding after external iliac puncture, one case of fatal femoral artery hemorrhage, and one reversible femoral nerve injury). Complications will be minimized if the patient has a pulse and the femoral vein is approached medial to the femoral pulsations. A helpful mnemonic is NAVEL, which describes the anatomy of the region from *lateral to medial:* nerve, artery, vein, empty space, and inguinal ligament.

Thrombophlebitic complications occur more frequently with femoral lines than with IJ and SC methods.[36] Thrombophlebitis is usually seen only with prolonged cannulation. There have even been reports (2 of 24 patients) of pulmonary emboli thought to result from the thrombosis caused by prolonged (3 to 14 days) femoral cannulation.[39]

BASILIC-CEPHALIC APPROACH

Cannulation of the central venous system through the arm veins has the lowest major complication rate of all. Superficial local infections are common (10 to 20 per cent incidence) and rarely may lead to more serious problems, including sepsis. Catheter malposition is common, and studies have shown this to happen in 10 to 40 per cent of placements.[21-23] One nuisance with this type of catheter is the need to immobilize an entire extremity and the shoulder to prevent catheter movement and kinking.

COMMENTS

The methods of preventing complications that were discussed in the preceding chapter should be heeded when the approaches to central venous access mentioned in this chapter are used. Several cautions in particular need to be re-emphasized. When performing any of these procedures, an individual should have a thorough knowledge of the anatomy or should be supervised by someone who does. One must also remember to replace as soon as possible all lines that were placed during an arrest or in other less than optimally sterile situations. Furthermore, all central lines should be discontinued at the earliest clinical opportunity. Finally, it is incumbent upon the physician who placed the line to check the chest film personally for proper catheter position and possible complications.

Conclusions

There is no "ideal" location for cannulation of the central venous circulation. Factors such as urgency, availability of access site, duration of catheterization, and skill of the physician are the most important determinants of cannulation route.

The major advantage of IJ cannulation compared with subclavian cannulation is the decreased incidence of pleural puncture. If a hematoma occurs as a result of inadvertent puncture of the carotid artery, compression is easily maintained with the IJ approach. In addition, the right IJ route provides a straight anatomic course to the right atrium, thus ensuring successful placement of the catheter tip. This is an obvious advantage if a pacemaker or a Swan-Ganz catheter will be passed.

The major disadvantages of the IJ route are that the vessel is more variable in size, more easily displaced, and more difficult to locate than the subclavian vein. In patients with short, thick necks, the IJ route can be virtually impossible, since the needle and the syringe cannot be manipulated in the small area between the head and the clavicle.

Peripheral insertion of a catheter through the basilic-cephalic vein systems is generally free from major complications but is time-consuming. In addition, the tip location is variable. External jugular insertion using a guide wire avoids the hazards of carotid puncture, brachial plexus injury, and pneumothorax. Frequent cannulation of the superior vena cava from the external jugular vein indicates that this technique can minimize risk and maximizes central location of the catheter tip.[11, 12, 15] Unfortunately, the external jugular approach using guide wires can be prohibitively time-consuming, especially if one is unfamiliar with the method. Schwartz and coworkers found that central cannulation through the external jugular vein with the guide wire technique took 5 to 25 minutes.[12] The same group had a significantly better success rate with curved J wires rather than straight guide wires (86 per cent versus 61 per cent).

Insertion of a central line during cardiac arrest and resuscitation should be secondary in importance to peripheral venous cannulation. Central venous cannulation is indicated when venous collapse or vasoconstriction makes peripheral cannulation impossible, when the need for a rapid central access for drug administration is imperative, or when central venous cannulation can be accomplished more quickly than peripheral venous cannulation in an emergency. In a cardiac arrest situation, a cutdown on a peripheral vein may be too time-consuming. Furthermore, both external and internal jugular cannulation may be difficult, since access to the head is limited by the need to maintain an airway and to ventilate the patient. Cardiac massage may interfere with the placement of a subclavian catheter and increases the risk of a pneumothorax or subclavian vein or artery laceration. Femoral cannulation may be a safe alternative, but cannulation can be difficult in the absence of an easily palpable pulse. Each technique of central cannulation has its drawback during a cardiac arrest. Thus, every physician who may be faced with venous cannulation of the cardiac arrest patient should be familiar with at least one of these techniques for placement of an appropriate line within a short period. Ideally, emergency physicians and others who deal with these extremely urgent situations should familiarize themselves fully with as many alternatives as possible.

1. Silver, J. H., Kemp, C. H., and Bruyn, H. B: Handbook of Pediatrics, 5th Edition. Los Altos, CA, Lange Medical Publications, 1963, pp. 37–38.
2. Defalque, R. H.: Percutaneous catheterization of the internal jugular vein. Anesth. Analg. 53:116, 1974.
3. Hemosura, B.: Measurement of pressure during intravenous therapy. JAMA 195:181, 1966.
4. Civetta, J. M., Gabel, J. C., and Gemer, M.: Internal jugular vein puncture with a margin of safety. Anesthesiology 36:622, 1972.
5. Daily, P. A., Griepp, R. B., and Shumway, N. E.: Percutaneous internal jugular vein cannulation. Arch. Surg. 101:534, 1970.
6. Jernigan, W. R., Gardener, W. C., Mahr, M. M., and Milburn, I. L.: Use of the internal jugular vein for placement of central venous catheter. Surg. Gynecol. Obstet. 130:520, 1970.
7. Mostert, J. W., Kenny, G. M., and Murphy, G. P.: Safe placement of cardiovascular catheters into the jugular vein. Arch. Surg. 101:431, 1970.
8. English, I. C. W., Frew, R. M., Pigott, J. E. G., and Zaki, M.: Percutaneous cannulation of the internal jugular vein. Thorax 24:496, 1969.
9. English, I. C. W., Frew, R. M., Pigott, J. F., and Zaki, M.: Percutaneous catheterization of the internal jugular vein. Anaesthesia 24:521, 1969.
10. Craig, R. G., Jones, R. A., Sproul, G. J., and Kinyon, G. E.: The alternate methods of central venous system catheterization. Am. Surg. 34:131, 1968.
11. Blitt, C. D., Wright, W. A., and Petty, W. C.: Central venous catheterization via the external jugular vein: A technique employing the J-wire. JAMA 229:817, 1974.
12. Schwartz, A. J., Jobes, D. R., Levy, W. J., et al.: Intrathoracic vascular catheterization via the external jugular vein. Anesthesiology 56:400, 1982.
13. Kaiser, C. W., Koornick, A. R., Smith, N., and Soroff, H. S.: Choice of route for central venous cannulation: Subclavian or internal jugular vein? A prospective randomized study. J. Surg. Oncol. 17:345, 1981.
14. Eisenhauer, E. D., Derveloy, R. J., and Hastings, P. R.: Prospective evaluation of central venous (CVP) catheters in a large city-county hospital. Ann. Surg. 196:560, 1982.
15. Humphrey, M. J., and Blitt, C. D.: Central venous access in children via the external jugular vein. Anesthesiology 57:50, 1982.
16. Blitt, C. D., Carlson, G. L., Wright, W. A., et al.: J-wire versus straight wire for central venous system cannulation via the external jugular vein. Anesth. Analg. 61:536, 1982.
17. Belani, K. G., Buckley, J. J., Gordon, J. R., et al.: Percutaneous cervical central venous line placement: A comparison of the internal and external jugular vein routes. Anesth. Analg. 59:40, 1980.
18. Woods, D. G., Lumley, J., Russell, W. J., et al.: The position of central venous catheters inserted through the arm veins: A primary report. Anaesth. Intensive Care 2:43, 1947.
19. Lumley, J., and Russell, W. J.: Insertion of central venous catheters through arm veins. Anaesth. Intensive Care 3:101, 1975.
20. Bridges, B. B., Carden, E., and Takacs, F. A.: Introduction of central venous pressure catheters through arm veins with a high success rate. Can. Anaesth. Soc. J. 26:128, 1979.
21. Holt, M. H.: Central venous pressures via peripheral veins. Anaesthesiology 25:1093, 1967.
22. Johnston, A. O., and Clark, R. G.: Malpositioning of central venous catheters. Lancet 2:1395, 1972.
23. Longston, L. S.: The aberrant central venous catheter and its complications. Radiology 100:55, 1971.
24. Webre, D. R., and Arens, J. F.: Use of the cephalic and basilic veins for introduction of central venous catheters. Anesthesiology 38:389, 1973.
25. Barsan, W. G., Levy, R. C., and Weir, H.: Lidocaine levels during CPR: Differences after peripheral venous, central venous, and intracardiac injections. Ann. Emerg. Med. 10:73, 1981.
26. Graber, D., and Daily, R. H.: Catheter flow rates updated (letter to the editor). JACEP 6:518, 1977.
27. Bazaral, M., and Harlan, S.: Ultrasonographic anatomy of the internal jugular vein relevant to percutaneous cannulation. Crit. Care Med. 9:307, 1981.
28. Sheep, R. E., and Guiney, W. B.: Fatal cardiac tamponade: Occurrence after left internal jugular vein catheterization. JAMA 248:1632, 1982.
29. Kaplan, J. A., and Miller, E. D.: Internal jugular vein catheterization. Anesth. Rev. 21, 1976.
30. O'Quin, R. J., and Lakschminaraan, S.: Venous air embolism. Arch. Intern. Med. 142:2173, 1982.
31. Prince, S. R., Sullivan, R. L., and Hackel, A.: Percutaneous

catheterization of the internal jugular vein in infants and children. Anesthesiology 44:170, 1976.

32. Coletti, R. H., Hartjen, B., Gozdziewskis, S. et al.: Origin of canine femoral pulses during standard CPR (abstract). Crit. Care Med. 11:218, 1983.

33. Goldfarb, G., and Lebrec, D.: Percutaneous cannulation of the internal jugular vein in patients with coagulopathies: An experience based on 1000 attempts. Anesthesiology 56:321, 1982.

34. Frasquet, F. J., and Belda, F. J.: Permanent paralysis of C-5 after cannulation of the internal jugular vein. Anesthesiology 54:528, 1981.

35. Briscoe, C. E., Bushman, J. A., and McDonald, W. I.:

36. Bosch, D. T., Kengeter, J. P., and Beling, C. A.: Femoral venipuncture. Am. J. Surg. 79:722, 1950.

37. Agnes, R. S., and Arendar, G. M.: Septic arthritis of the hip: A complication of femoral venipuncture. Pediatrics 38:837, 1966.

38. Fuchs, J. H., et al.: Percutaneous puncture of the femoral vein for hemodialysis: Report of 5000 punctures. Dtsch. Med. Wochenschr. 102:1280, 1977.

39. Walters, M. B., Stanger, H. A. D., and Rotem, C. E.: Complications with percutaneous central venous catheters. JAMA 220:1455, 1972.

Extensive neurological damage after cannulation of internal jugular vein. Br. Med. J. 1:314, 1974.

23

Central Venous Pressure Measurement

ALICE M. DONAHUE, R.N., M.S.N.

Introduction

For the past two decades, central venous pressure (CVP) monitoring has been used to assess cardiac performance and to guide fluid therapy for critically ill patients. Although the concept was first demonstrated by Forssman in 1931, it was not until the early 1960s that cannulation of the central veins and measurement of the central venous pressure became commonplace.[1, 2]

Simply stated, CVP is the pressure exerted by the blood against the walls of the right atrium. Since the pressure in the great veins of the thorax is generally within 1 mm Hg of the right atrial pressure, the CVP reflects the pressure under which blood is returned to the superior vena cava and the right atrium.[3, 4] The pressure in the central veins has two significant hemodynamic effects. First, the pressure promotes filling of the heart during diastole, a factor that helps determine cardiac output. Second, the CVP is also the back pressure of the systemic circulation, opposing the return of blood from the peripheral blood vessels into the heart.[4] CVP therefore affects both the ability of the heart to pump blood and the tendency for blood to flow from the peripheral

veins.[3, 5] The CVP reading is determined by a complex interaction of intravascular volume, right ventricular function, venomotor tone, and intrathoracic pressure.[2]

One can measure CVP accurately by placing the tip of a pressure-monitoring catheter into any of the great systemic veins of the thorax or into the right atrium.[4] The right atrium is theoretically the ideal site for measurement of CVP but since the risks of catheter placement in the atrium include atrial perforation and cardiac dysrhythmias, any large vein within the thorax is an acceptable alternative. The preferred site for the tip of the CVP catheter is the superior vena cava.[6] The catheter is connected to a water manometer, and pressure is expressed in relation to the height, in centimeters, of a column of water above the level of the tricuspid valve. The level of the tricuspid valve is chosen as the standard reference point for measurement, since at this point the hydrostatic pressure does not affect the measurement significantly.[3]

Clinically, CVP measurements are most frequently used as a guide for determination of a patient's volume status and fluid requirements and for investigation of the possibility of cardiac tamponade.[7-10] Critical commentaries have been written by many authors who regard CVP monitoring as ineffective, outmoded, and unreliable.[11-14] The astute clinician, however, can maximize the usefulness of this diagnostic tool by careful consideration of its indications and limitations. The CVP is one of many variables that must be correlated in the development of an overall management plan for the care of critically ill patients.

Indications for CVP Monitoring

The major indications for CVP monitoring include the following clinical situations:

1. acute circulatory failure,

2. anticipated massive blood or fluid replacement therapy,

3. cautious fluid replacement in patients with compromised cardiovascular status, and

4. suspected cardiac tamponade.

Limitations of CVP Monitoring

The greatest misconception regarding CVP measurement is the incorrect assumption that right atrial pressure consistently reflects pressures found in the left side of the heart.[13] The measurement that best reflects left ventricular pressure changes and reserve is the left atrial pressure, or pulmonary capillary wedge pressure (PCWP). The development of the flow-directed pulmonary artery catheter has allowed repeated measurements of PCWP, thus permitting accurate assessment of left atrial pressure.

The central venous pressure is most helpful in patients without significant pre-existing cardiopulmonary disease. No consistent correlation between isolated right atrial and left atrial pressure measurements has been demonstrated in patients with prior cardiopulmonary diseases. Forrester and coworkers, in a study of 50 patients with myocardial infarction, demonstrated that CVP measurements had no consistent relationship to PCWP.[14] DiLaurentis and associates, in their study of 32 surgical patients without myocardial infarction, found that CVP and pulmonary arterial pressure correlated in only 50 per cent of their patients.[13] James and colleagues[15] studied three parameters—CVP, pulmonary arterial pressure, and PCWP—in 116 patients who either were in shock or had undergone major surgery. In 76 of 116 instances, the PCWP differed significantly from the CVP. An early rise in the PCWP was noted before the rise in the CVP. Samii and coworkers[12] studied 13 relatively elderly patients (mean age of 62) without obvious cardiac or respiratory disease and found a disparity between the right and left ventricular filling pressures. They concluded that CVP may be a misleading index for predicting PCWP in elderly patients.

Toussaint and associates[16] reported a significant *correlation* between CVP and PCWP in 14 patients with no prior history of cardiopulmonary disease. Yet in the same study, a poor correlation between CVP and PCWP was shown in 13 patients with a history of cardiopulmonary disease. These findings suggest that *CVP provides a reliable assessment of cardiac function only in the absence of cardiopulmonary disease.*[16]

Fluid Challenge

CVP monitoring is helpful as a practical guide for fluid therapy.[8, 10] Serial CVP measurement provides a fairly reliable indication of the capability of the right heart to accept an additional volume load. Although the PCWP is a more sensitive index of left heart fluid needs (and in some clinical situations PCWP measurement is absolutely essential), the serial measurement of CVP can provide significant information.

A fluid challenge can help assess both volume deficits and pump failure. Although a fluid challenge can be used with either PCWP monitoring or CVP monitoring, only the fluid challenge for CVP monitoring will be discussed here. Slight variations in the methodology of fluid challenge are reported in the literature. Generally, aliquots of 50 to 200 ml of crystalloid fluid (isotonic saline or lactated Ringer's solution) or smaller aliquots of colloid (5 per cent albumin solution) are sequentially administered, and measurements of CVP levels are obtained after a 10-minute observation period.[9, 10, 15, 17]

The fluid challenge as described by Weil[10] is generally carried out in the following manner: Fluid is administered by a route other than that used for monitoring. An initial CVP reading is taken, and fluid is infused at a rate of 20 ml per minute over a 10-minute period. The infused volume is allowed to equilibrate for 10 minutes, and a reading is again taken. If the CVP is greater than 5 cm of H_2O over the initial measurement, the fluid challenge is discontinued and one assumes that the right ventricle is unable to handle an additional fluid load. Increases of between 3 and 5 cm H_2O over the initial CVP reading are equivocal, and additional measurements are taken over the next 30 minutes if this reading is obtained. Increases of less than 2 cm H_2O over the original reading or a return of higher readings to this level within 30 minutes is indicative of volume depletion. The fluid challenge is repeated until measurements indicate that adequate volume expansion has been obtained. Fluid challenge is discontinued as soon as hemodynamic signs of shock are reversed or signs of cardiac incompetence are evident.

Cardiac Tamponade

In cardiac tamponade, *pericardial* pressure rises to equal right ventricular end-diastolic pressure. The *pericardial* pressure encountered in pericardial tamponade characteristically produces an elevated central venous pressure. The degree of CVP elevation is variable, and one must interpret measurements cautiously. CVP readings in the range of 16 to 18 cm H_2O are typically seen in acute tamponade,[18] but elevations of up to 30 cm H_2O may be encountered. The exact CVP reading is often lower than one might intuitively expect, and it is not uncommon to encounter tamponade with a CVP of 10 to 12 cm H_2O. A normal, or even a low, CVP reading may be seen if the tamponade is associated with significant hypovolemia.

An excessive rise in CVP following a fluid challenge may be more important than a single reading in the diagnosis of pericardial tamponade. It is interesting to note that Shoemaker and associates[18] report a decrease in CVP just prior to cardiovascular collapse in patients with pericardial tamponade.

Excessive straining, agitation, pneumatic antishock garment inflation, positive-pressure ventilation, or tension pneumothorax may raise intrathoracic pressure, producing a high CVP reading, and may erroneously suggest the diagnosis of pericardial tamponade. Increases in vascular tone as seen with the use of dopamine or other vasopressors may also elevate the CVP, mimicking tamponade and complicating volume estimation.

Methods of Measuring CVP

CVP is usually expressed as centimeters of water, indicating the height of a column of water above the zero point on the manometer. Although CVP measurements can be obtained electronically from the level of the right atrium through the proximal port of a pulmonary artery catheter, manometric measurements are more frequently used in the emergency situation and will be the focus of this discussion.[19] The reading on a properly placed CVP catheter will fluctuate 1 to 3 cm of H_2O during normal respiration. The reading decreases with inspiration and increases with expiration, straining, or coughing. Readings should be taken at the end of expiration of a normal breath. If the patient is on a respirator, the CVP changes during the respiratory cycle are reversed, rising with positive-pressure inspiration and decreasing with expiration.

A prepackaged disposable plastic or glass manometer with a three-way stopcock and standard infusion tubing is most commonly used for measuring CVP (see Fig. 23–1). The equipment is connected to a standard intravenous solution bottle. One primes the tubing by turning the stopcock to the position that directs flow of the intravenous solution through the distal end of the catheter, bypassing the manometer. One then primes the manometer with fluid by turning the stopcock to direct the fluid flow from the intravenous solution bottle to the manometer (Fig. 23–2). The distal end of the primed set is now connected to the central catheter, and the stopcock (closed to the manometer) directs fluid from the intravenous bottle to the patient (Fig. 23–3). To obtain a reading the stopcock (closed to the bottle) is directed to open the system from the patient to the manometer. The patient's CVP is reflected by the height of the water in the manometer. The fluid level is allowed to fall spontaneously until it stabilizes before a reading is taken (Fig. 23–4). Between readings, the fluid is turned off to the manometer, and the CVP catheter serves as a standard intravenous infusion site. The rate of infusion should be capable of maintaining catheter patency and meeting fluid needs of the patient. A small amount of heparin (1000 units per liter) may be added to the intravenous solution bottle to minimize catheter tip clotting without altering systemic coagulation.[2]

When preparing the CVP manometer system, one must be certain to remove all air bubbles from the manometer. Bubbles in the manometer fluid column will decrease the accuracy of the reading.

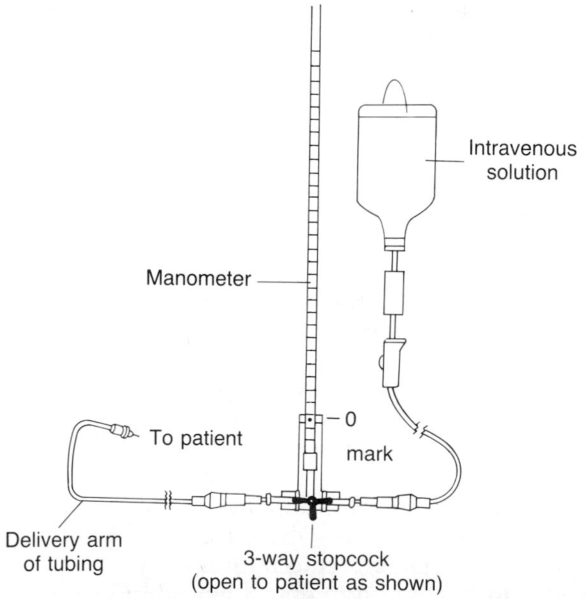

Manometer — | Intravenous solution
To patient | 0 mark
Delivery arm of tubing | 3-way stopcock (open to patient as shown)

Figure 23–1. Standard CVP equipment.

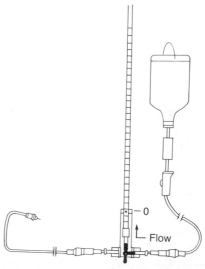

Figure 23–2. The stopcock is turned to fill the manometer to 25 cm H_2O.

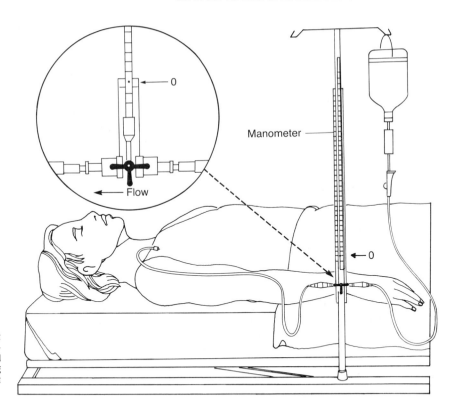

Figure 23–3. Stopcock turned to direct flow to patient, bypassing the manometer. This is the position that is maintained to keep the catheter patent. The tubing is always flushed prior to connecting it to the patient's CVP catheter.

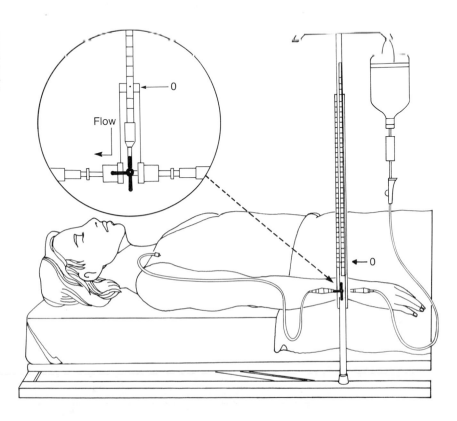

Figure 23–4. The stopcock is opened to the patient, and the column of water in the manometer is allowed to fall and stabilize before a reading is taken. Note that the zero mark is horizontally aligned with the tricuspid valve (midaxillary line in supine patient).

The manometer column is initially raised to approximately 20 to 25 cm. Care must be taken so the water column does not reach the top. Water at the manometer top dampens the cotton and impedes air movement into and out of the chamber. The wet cotton is also a potential source of contamination. If the water column reaches the manometer top, a new setup should be prepared. The addition of multiple vitamins (such as Berocca-C) has been suggested to color the fluid and to enhance the visibility of the fluid column in the manometer. The manometer is preferably secured to an IV pole, which is attached to the patient's bed. A floor model IV pole is less desirable because of its instability.[20]

A reading may be taken after proper assembly of the equipment and after accurate placement of the tip of the catheter has been established. Proper placement is best checked by chest film. The presence of respiratory fluctuations does not ensure superior vena caval placement. Fluctuations with movement of the head suggest improper placement of the catheter in the internal jugular system.

To ensure optimal measurement, the patient should be in a supine position. Two points have been identified in CVP measurements:[21, 22]

1. The patient reference point: This is the point on the patient's lateral chest wall that indicates the position of the tip of the CVP catheter.

2. The zero mark on the manometer: This is the zero line on the manometer, which is aligned with the reference point of the patient's chest.

One determines the patient reference point by locating an external landmark on the thorax at the approximate level of the right atrium.[23] Although a number of anatomic sites have been described[4, 5, 21, 22] and recommended, the most frequently used site is the mid-axillary line in the fourth intercostal space. One should clearly mark the reference point with a marking pen, placing a line or an X on the patient's thorax.

Since the absolute zero level is less important than maintaining consistency in serial measurements, all readings should be taken at the same location and in the same manner. Readings are taken with the zero point on the manometer matched with the horizontal level of the patient reference point (Fig. 23–5). All readings are ideally taken while the patient is supine.[26] If the patient cannot tolerate this position, however, the two reference points are matched in the mid-axillary line at the estimated base of the heart. The position of the patient is noted, and measurements are recorded. Serial measurements must reflect the identical position of the patient for meaningful interpretation of CVP variation with therapy.

Factors Affecting Accuracy of Reading

A number of extrinsic factors may alter the accuracy of the CVP reading (Table 23–1).[2, 5, 24, 25] In addition to the position of the patient, changes

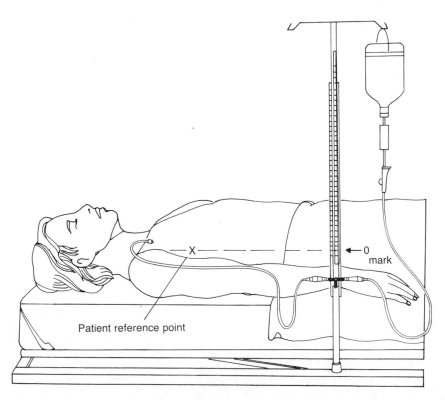

Figure 23–5. The zero mark (not the bottom of the manometer) is aligned with the patient's estimated reference point (see text).

X

0 mark

Patient reference point

Table 23–1. FAULTY CENTRAL VENOUS PRESSURE READINGS

Increased intrathoracic pressure (ventilator, straining, coughing)
Reference points in error
Malposition of catheter tip
Blocking or ball valve obstruction of catheter
Fluids run into manometer during CVP measurement
Air bubbles in the manometer
Vasopressors (presumed)

in intrathoracic pressure affect the CVP reading.[26] A patient on a respirator has an elevated intrathoracic pressure, which reflects a falsely elevated CVP reading. Usually, positive-pressure ventilation raises the CVP reading by only a few centimeters of water. If disconnection can be tolerated, the patient should be temporarily disconnected from the respirator to provide a more reliable measurement. Activities that increase intrathoracic pressure, such as coughing and straining, may also cause spuriously high measurements. The patient should be relaxed at the time of measurement and should be breathing normally. The position of the manometer must also be consistent. The zero point on the manometer must be opposite the patient reference point at the level of the right atrium. Use of varied reference points may result in inaccurate measurements that may be interpreted as a change in the patient's status when none has actually occurred.[2, 21, 22, 24]

Another reason for faulty readings is malposition of the catheter tip. If the catheter tip is not passed far enough into the central venous system, peripheral venous spasm and venous valves may yield pressure readings that are inconsistent with the true CVP.[5, 24]

If the catheter tip is passed into the right ventricle, a falsely high CVP is obtained. This situation should be suspected when excessive fluctuations (6 to 10 cm H_2O) of the manometer fluid column are observed. Such fluctuations may be seen in correctly placed CVP lines when tricuspid regurgitation or atrioventricular dissociation is present.

Inaccurate low venous pressure readings are seen when a valve-like obstruction at the catheter tip occurs either by clot formation or by contact against the vein wall. The negative intrathoracic pressures seen during inspiration will drop the manometer water level, but when the catheter is occluded during expiration, the manometer is unable to sense the true CVP.[19, 24] Air bubbles in the manometer or tubing will also yield faulty readings.

Another reason for faulty readings is unrecognized infusion of fluid running into the manometer system during the time of measurement. Some authors mention a falsely elevated CVP in patients who are receiving vasopressors, but controlled data on this aberration are lacking.

Interpretation of CVP Measurement

Since determination of CVP aids the clinician in assessment of the critically ill patient, it is paramount that the clinician know the normal values and the variables that may alter these values and recognize the pathologic conditions that correlate with abnormal values.

Although early articles reported varying normal ranges for CVP measurements, recent cardiac catheterization studies have demonstrated that the normal range extends from -2 to $+7$ cm H_2O.

Gowen reports from his clinical experience that a reading of 7 cm H_2O is the upper limit of normal and a reading of 8 to 10 cm H_2O is a borderline elevation, whereas levels greater than 12 cm H_2O are consistent with impending heart failure.[17] Weil and coworkers, however, describe the normal CVP as ranging from 2 to 10 cm H_2O and consider a high CVP to be greater than 15 cm H_2O.[9] Other authors describe similar variations. A rough guideline that reflects a consensus in the literature[5, 9, 10, 17] and informal opinions of colleagues follows:

Low	Less than 5 cm H_2O
Normal	5 to 12 cm H_2O
High	Greater than 12 cm H_2O

In the late stages of pregnancy (30 to 42 weeks), the CVP is physiologically elevated, and normal readings are 5 to 8 cm H_2O higher than in nonpregnant women.

A CVP reading of less than 5 cm H_2O is consistent with low right atrial pressure and reflects a decrease in the return of blood volume to the right heart. This may indicate that the patient requires additional fluid or blood. A low CVP reading is also obtained when vasomotor tone is decreased, as in sepsis, an anaphylactic reaction, or another form of sympathetic interruption.[9, 10, 17]

A CVP reading falling within a normal range is viewed in relationship to the clinical situation. A reading of greater than 12 cm H_2O indicates that the heart is not effectively circulating the volume presented to it. This situation may occur in the case of either a normovolemic patient with cardiac decompensation or a patient with a normal heart who is overhydrated or overtransfused. A high CVP is also related to variables other than pump failure, which include pericardial tamponade, restrictive pericarditis, pulmonary stenosis, and pulmonary embolus.[17]

Changes in blood volume, vessel tone, and cardiac function may occur alone or in combination with one another; therefore, it is possible to have a normal or a high CVP in the presence of normovolemia, hypovolemia, and hypervolemia. One must interpret the specific CVP values with respect to the entire clinical picture; *the response of the CVP to an infusion is more important than the initial reading.*

Conclusion

With the introduction of the pulmonary artery catheter and the ability to measure pulmonary capillary wedge pressure, some clinicians have discouraged the use of CVP monitoring. Nonetheless, CVP monitoring continues to be an important adjunct in the care of the critically ill patient in the acute phase of volume resuscitation.

CVP measurements performed in the appropriate clinical situation can be useful when the patient's cardiac function in relation to blood volume is assessed. Initial readings, serial measurements, and trends following fluid infusion provide a guide to therapy in acutely ill or injured patients. Proper interpretation of specific readings requires knowledge of the cardiovascular dynamics as well as an appreciation for extrinsic factors that may alter CVP readings. The clinician is reminded to evaluate the data in relation to the entire clinical situation.

1. Huberty, J., Schwartz, R., and Emich, J.: Central venous pressure monitoring. Obstet. Gynecol. 30:842, 1967.
2. Wilson, J. N., et al.: Central venous pressure in optimal blood volume maintenance. Arch. Surg. 85:563, 1962.
3. Guyton, A. C.: Textbook of Medical Physiology, 4th ed. Philadelphia, W. B. Saunders Co., 1971, p. 227.
4. Guyton, A., and Jones, C.: Central venous pressure: Physiological significance and clinical implications. Am. Heart J. 86:431, 1973.
5. Knopp, R., and Dailey, R. H.: Central venous cannulation and pressure monitoring. JACEP 6:358, 1977.
6. Dunbar, R. D., et al.: Aberrant locations of central venous catheters. Lancet 1:71, 1981.
7. Cohn, J. N.: Central venous pressure as a guide to volume expansion. Ann. Intern. Med. 66:1283, 1967.
8. MacLean, L. D., and Duff, J. H.: The use of central venous pressure as a guide to volume replacement in shock. Dis. Chest 48:199, 1965.
9. Weil, M. H., Shubin, H., and Rosoff, L.: Fluid repletion in circulatory shock. Central venous pressure and other practical guides. JAMA 192:668, 1965.
10. Greenall, M. J., Blewitt, R. W., and McMahon, M. J.: Cardiac tamponade and central venous catheters. Brit. Med. J. 2:595, 1975.
11. Swan, H. J. C.: Central venous pressure monitoring is an outmoded procedure of limited practical value. In Ingelfinger, F. J., et al. (eds.): Controversy in Internal Medicine II. Philadelphia, W. B. Saunders Co., 1974, pp. 185–193.
12. Samii, K., Conseiller, C., and Viars, P.: Central venous pressure and pulmonary wedge pressure. A comparative study in anesthetized patients. Arch. Surg. 111:1122, 1976.
13. DeLaurentis, D., Hayes, M., and Matsumoto, T.: Does central venous pressure accurately reflect hemodynamic and fluid volume patterns in the critical surgical patient? Am. J. Surg. 126:415, 1973.
14. Forrester, J. S., et al.: Filling pressures in the right and left sides of the heart in acute myocardial infarction. N. Engl. J. Med. 285:190, 1971.
15. James, P., and Myers, R.: Central venous pressure monitoring. Ann. Surg. 175:693, 1972.
16. Toussaint, G. P. M., Burgess, J. H., and Hampson, L. G.: Central venous pressure and pulmonary wedge pressure in critical illness. A comparison. Arch. Surg. 109:265, 1974.
17. Gowen, F.: Interpretation of central venous pressure. Surg. Clin. North Am. 86:432, 1973.
18. Shoemaker, W. C., Carey, J. S., and Yao, S. T.: Hemodynamic monitoring for physiologic evaluation, diagnosis, and therapy of acute hemopericardial tamponade from penetrating wounds. J. Trauma 13:36, 1973.
19. Mann, R. L., Carlon, G. C., and Turnbull, A. D.: Comparison of electronic and manometric central venous pressures. Influence of access route. Crit. Care Med. 9:98, 1981.
20. Fisher, R. E.: Measuring central venous pressure: How to do it accurately and safely. Nursing 79:74, 1979.
21. Pennington, L. A., and Smith, C.: Leveling when monitoring central blood pressures: An alternative method. Heart Lung 9:1053, 1980.
22. Debrunner, F., and Bühler, F.: "Normal central venous pressure," significance of reference point and normal range. Br. Med. J. 3:148, 1969.
23. Winsor, T., and Bruch, G. E.: Phlebostatic axis and phlebostatic level, reference levels for venous pressure measurements in man. Proc. Soc. Exp. Biol. Med. 58:165, 1945.
24. Wilson J., and Owens, J.: Pitfalls in monitoring central venous pressure. Hosp. Med. 6:86, 1970.
25. Haughey, B.: CVP lines: Monitoring and maintaining. Am. J. Nurs. 78:635, 1978.
26. Woods, S. L., and Mansfield, L. W.: Effect of body position upon pulmonary artery and pulmonary capillary wedge pressures in noncritically ill patients. Heart Lung 5:87, 1976.

Introduction

The treatment of life-threatening emergencies with lifesaving drugs and fluids requires rapid access to the venous circulation. Establishing venous access in patients who are near death by directly cannulating a vein often requires a considerable amount of skill, and even in the best hands the procedure can sometimes be frustratingly difficult and time-consuming. Alternative methods of administering vital fluids or drugs have been suggested and include subcutaneous, intramuscular, intraperitoneal, intracardiac, endotracheal and intraosseous injections. The subcutaneous, intramuscular, and intraperitoneal routes cause unacceptable delay in uptake by the venous circulation, and intracardiac injections involve additional risk. The intraosseous route of injection can be quickly, safely, and reliably established and permits rapid venous uptake of drugs and fluids; consequently, it is a viable alternative to direct intravenous cannulation and is quite suitable when used in emergency resuscitation.

Background

Tocantins first described the administration of fluids into the general circulation by way of the bone marrow in the early 1940s.[1] At the time, parenteral therapy in general was relatively new, and intravenous techniques in particular were still in their infancy. Tocantins' animal and human studies suggested that the uptake kinetics of fluids or drugs injected into the marrow cavity were very similar to the uptake kinetics of intravenously injected materials.[1-4] Very shortly thereafter, Papper and Rovenstine used intramedullary infusions of fluids and drugs (such as thiopental sodium) and found that the method worked "as rapidly and as easily as by intravenous injection."[5, 6] The intramedullary technique quickly became popular for use in pediatric patients, in whom it could be especially troublesome to establish and maintain intravenous cannulae; numerous case studies attested to the safety and utility of the procedure.[7-12] Some authors even advocated that the intramedullary route be used routinely in place of intravenous therapy.[11] A much more recent report describes the successful use of intraosseous infusion under emergency circumstances in 15 patients without complications.[13]

Physiology and Functional Anatomy

The ability of the bone marrow to accept an infusion with subsequent effects like those of an intravenous injection has been well documented.

24

Intraosseous Infusions*

STEPHEN N. ROGERS, M.D.
JONATHAN L. BENUMOF, M.D.

A review of the literature reveals that a number of fluids, including blood, plasma, saline, and dextrose solutions, have been infused into the bone marrow of adults, children, and even premature infants.[1-12] Infusions have been carried out for various lengths of time and at various flow rates, sometimes resulting in a very large volume of infused fluid (greater than 42 L).[13] Intraosseously infused tracer substances produce effects identical to those of intravenous injection. Schoor and associates have shown that in sheep the hemodynamic response to intramedullary epinephrine and ephedrine is as rapid as after intravenous injection.[14] They also found that normal saline could be infused at an average rate of 2.4 L per hour through a 13 gauge intramedullary needle under an infusion pressure of 300 mm Hg. Average flow rates of 600 ml per hour were achieved with gravity infusion. Indocyanine green dye injected into the medullary cavity of a fibrillating dog's hind limb can reach the left atrium in less than 15 seconds during internal cardiac massage (Rogers and Benumof, unpublished data).

An explanation for the apparent "intravenous injection" is found in anatomic and radiographic studies that demonstrate a rich venous drainage from the bone marrow.[15, 16, 17] The marrow of long bones contains spacious venous sinusoids that drain into large central medullary venous channels and then, by way of nutrient or emissary veins, into the systemic venous system (Fig. 24–1).[15] Radiopaque dye, even when injected forcefully into the marrow, rarely spreads more than a few centimeters before rapidly entering the venous circulation.[16]

Indications

Intraosseous infusion is indicated in emergency situations when lifesaving fluids or drugs need to be rapidly introduced into the circulation and

*This work was supported by the University of California Medical Center, San Diego, Department of Anesthesia.

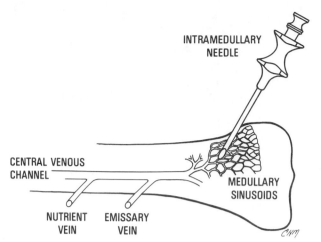

Figure 24–1. A schematic diagram illustrating the venous drainage from the marrow of a long bone with an intramedullary needle in place.

intravenous cannulation is either too difficult or too time-consuming to perform. Today, because intravenous cannulation techniques have become so sophisticated and widely practiced, intraosseous infusion is rarely used. Still, intraosseous infusion should be considered as a potentially lifesaving option under the conditions outlined. Patients in whom this procedure might be most useful include those suffering from cardiac arrest, shock, widespread burns, and massive trauma. Other patients in whom intravenous cannulation might be exceedingly difficult and who are therefore candidates for this procedure include severely obese individuals and patients with peripheral edema, a history of intravenous drug abuse, or prolonged intravenous therapy. This technique is also useful in pediatric patients. We wish to stress that we consider intramedullary infusion an emergency resuscitative procedure that should be replaced by more conventional intravenous therapy when the clinical situation becomes less urgent.

This route of access can be used to obtain blood samples for type and cross matching, although one would not wish to rely upon marrow aspirate when measuring the patient's white or red blood cell count. Blood chemistries measured from marrow aspirate samples, such as electrolyte, glucose, and blood urea nitrogen levels, should be representative of levels obtainable from serum samples, although this is not addressed in the literature. With the possible exception of drugs that are considered marrow-toxic (e.g., certain antibiotics), most drugs compatible with intravenous infusion may be given by intramedullary infusion. Drug administration by this route, however, has not been studied systematically.

Contraindications to this procedure are few, especially in urgent situations, when the alternative may be death. The only absolute contraindication is gross infection at the intended site of puncture. Generalized sepsis is a relative contraindication in view of the possibility of seeding infection into bone, but again this must be weighed against the need for lifesaving therapy.

Equipment

A minimum of equipment is required for this technique. A large-bore (approximately 16 gauge) metal needle with a stylet that is sturdy enough for passage through bony cortex will work. Needles used routinely by hematologists for bone marrow aspiration or biopsy are ideal. They include the short Rosenthal or Osgood needles (16 gauge × 1⁵/₁₆ inches) (left panel, Fig. 24–2) and the larger Silverman-type biopsy needle used without the split inner cannula (10 gauge × 3 inches), all of which are available from Becton-Dickinson. A special sternal bone marrow infusion needle with a trephine-type inner cannula is also available from Becton-Dickinson (right panel, Fig.

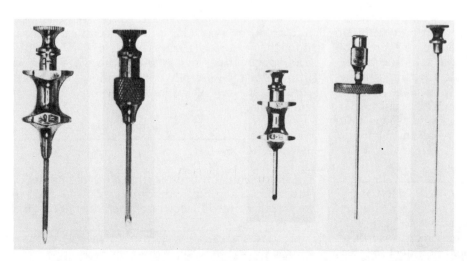

Figure 24–2. Needles used for bone marrow infusion. *Left,* The Rosenthal and Osgood bone marrow aspiration needles with stylets. *Right,* The special sternal bone marrow infusion needle with its trephine-type inner cannula and stylet. The short needle is placed into the periosteum, and the trephine inner cannula is used to drill through the cortex. The short needle is then pushed through the hole into the marrow cavity.

12–2), but its use may be time-consuming and is not necessary for this procedure. In desperate situations, the sturdiest needle that is immediately available should be used.

The authors have found standard phlebotomy and intravenous needles unsatisfactory. These needles tend to bend upon penetration of the adult bony cortex. Although we have had no experience with the use of these needles for intraosseous infusion in children, the softer cortex of the bones of children may be more penetrable with standard phlebotomy needles (16 gauge or larger diameter). We recommend that the emergency physician intent upon using this technique obtain several marrow needles and have them kept in sterile set-ups in the resuscitation room. A 5- or 10-ml syringe to confirm placement by aspiration and to flush the needle should also be available, plus a smaller syringe and needle for administering local anesthesia, if necessary.

Site Preference

Any marrow-containing cavity is a potential site for infusion. Many locations have been used successfully, including the sternum, the greater trochanter, the distal femur, the tibial tuberosity, the medial and lateral malleoli, and the os calcis.[6, 12, 16] The sternum has been the most popular site in adults, because it is easily accessible. In addition, its thin cortex and abundant marrow make insertion easy. Sternal puncture may also produce a number of serious complications. The proximity of the underlying pleura and great vessels is a potential cause of disaster (tension pneumothorax and vascular rupture). Additionally, a sternal needle may interfere with effective chest compression during cardiopulmonary resuscitation. A less dangerous and usually more easily accessible site is the tibial (medial) malleolus. Used frequently

for intraosseous venography,[16, 17] it is the site of choice in adults. In children and infants the locations of choice are the proximal tibia and, less commonly, the distal femur. In children, care should be taken to avoid the epiphyseal plates.

Procedure

Under most circumstances, this procedure should be performed simply and expeditiously. The skin at the site of puncture is wiped with alcohol. The skin and the periosteum may be anesthetized with lidocaine, although in obtunded or moribund patients this may not be necessary. In adults, a site approximately 2 cm proximal to the tip of the medial malleolus is selected, with the needle directed slightly cephalad (Fig. 24–3). Firm pressure and a rotary motion are used to push the needle through the skin and the bony cortex. Entrance into the marrow cavity is indicated by a loss of resistance. The needle will feel firmly fixed by the bone at this point, and removal of the stylet will usually allow free flow of blood from the needle. One obtains confirmation of position by freely aspirating blood or marrow contents into the syringe. Aspiration may be uncomfortable for the patient. The syringe should be flushed with fluid, and a continuous infusion should be begun or the stylet replaced before clotting can occur. The needle should be fixed by the bone firmly enough to remain secure with only a sterile dressing. In infants and children, a point 2 cm below the cartilaginous tibial tubercle on the anteromedial surface is used, with the needle directed distally, away from the epiphyseal line (Fig. 24–4).

Occasionally, one may encounter difficulty in penetrating the cortex or aspirating marrow. If penetration is difficult, another site such as the lateral malleolus or the more proximal tibia should

Figure 24–3. A diagrammatic representation of intramedullary needle placement in the tibial malleolus of an adult. The needle is placed 2 to 3 cm proximal to the medial malleolus and is directed slightly cephalad. Confirmation of intramedullary placement is obtained by aspiration of blood or marrow with a syringe.

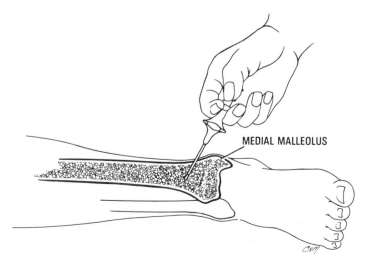

MEDIAL MALLEOLUS

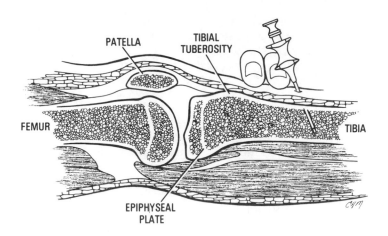

Figure 24–4. A diagrammatic representation of intramedullary needle placement in infants and children. A point two fingerbreadths below the tibial tuberosity is selected. The needle is directed distally to avoid the epiphyseal growth plate.

be chosen. Rarely, if the needle does not fit snugly into the cortex or if a previous cortical puncture site is nearby, fluid may escape out of the medullary cavity and infiltrate surrounding tissue (Fig. 24–5). This is remedied by firm external pressure over the bone at the leak site or by replacement of the needle at another site. Standard intravenous tubing is used to connect the marrow needle to the intravenous bag or bottle. Although gravity drainage may suffice for many infusions, pressurized infusions (by use of a blood pump or syringe and stopcock system) may be needed during resuscitation to increase the flow rate.

Complications

The reported complication rate is low and consists mainly of minor incidents. Specifically, the much-feared complication of fat embolization has not been reported, even with pressurized high-volume infusions.[18, 19] Papper reported the postoperative death of a patient who received a sternal bone marrow infusion intraoperatively.[5] Postmortem examination revealed 2 L of 5 per cent dextrose in the pleural spaces (an example of the dangers of sternal puncture). A few cases of osteomyelitis secondary to intraosseous infusions have been reported.[18] In most of these cases, sepsis combined with difficulty in needle placement or prolonged infusion probably contributed to the complications.

Conclusions

Even though it is rarely used today because of our proficiency in intravenous cannulation, the technique of intraosseous infusion is a valuable addition to a physician's armamentarium of emergency procedures. The technique is easily and rapidly performed, and few associated complications have been reported. In life-threatening situations when venous access is required but not immediately obtainable, intraosseous infusion may be lifesaving. The technique can be used for volume resuscitation or drug administration until more conventional intravenous access can be established.

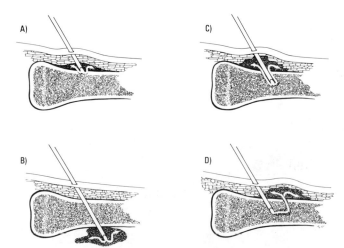

Figure 24–5. A schematic diagram of possible problems encountered with intraosseous infusions. A, Incomplete penetration of the bony cortex. B, Penetration of the posterior cortex. C, Fluid escaping around the needle through the puncture site. D, Fluid leaking through a nearby previous cortical puncture site.

1. Tocantins, L. M.: Rapid absorption of substances injected into the bone marrow. Proc. Soc. Exp. Biol. Med. 45:292, 1940.
2. Tocantins, L. M., and O'Neill, J. F.: Infusion of blood and other fluids into the circulation via the bone marrow. Proc. Soc. Exp. Biol. Med. 45:782, 1940.
3. Tocantins, L. M., and O'Neill, J. F.: Infusions of blood and other fluids into the general circulation via the bone marrow. Surg. Gynecol. Obstet. 73:281, 1941.
4. Tocantins, L. M., O'Neill, J. F., and Jones, H. W.: Infusions of blood and other fluids via the bone marrow. JAMA 117:1229, 1941.
5. Papper, E. M.: The bone marrow route for injecting fluid and drugs into the general circulation. Anesthesiology 3:307, 1942.
6. Papper, E. M., and Rovenstine, E. A.: Utility of marrow cavity of sternum for parenteral fluid therapy. War Med. 2:177, 1942.
7. Arbeiter, H. I., and Greengard, J.: Tibial bone marrow infusions in infancy. J. Pediatr. 25:1, 1944.
8. Behr, G.: Bone-marrow infusions for infants. Lancet 2:472, 1944.
9. Dowd, E. A., and Pysell, J. E.: Massive intramedullary infusions. JAMA 120:1212, 1942.
10. Reisman, H. A., and Tansky, I. A.: Bone marrow as alternate route of transfusion in pediatrics. Am. J. Dis. Child 68:253, 1944.
11. Meola, F.: Bone marrow infusions as routine procedures in children. J. Pediatr. 25:13, 1944.
12. Elston, J. T., Jaynes, R. V., Kaump, D. H., and Irwin, W. A.: Intraosseous infusion in infants. Am. J. Clin. Pathol. 17:143, 1947.
13. Valdes, M. M.: Intraosseous fluid administration in emergencies. Lancet 1:1235, 1977.
14. Shoor, P. M., Berryhill, R. E., and Benumof, J. L.: Intraosseous infusion: Pressure-flow relationship in pharmacokinetics. J. Trauma 19:772, 1979.
15. Root, W. S.: The flow of blood through bones and joints. In Hamilton, W. F. (ed.): Handbook of Physiology. Vol. 2. Baltimore, Williams & Wilkins, 1966, pp. 1651–1655.
16. Begg, A. C.: Intraosseous venography of the lower limb and pelvis. Br. J. Radiol. 27:218, 1954.
17. Kwaan, J. H. M., Jones, R. N., and Connolly, J. E.: Simplified technique for the management of refractory varicose ulcers. Surgery 80:743, 1976.
18. O'Neill, J. F.: Complications of intraosseous therapy. Ann. Surg. 2:266, 1945.
19. Bisgard, J. D., and Baker, C.: Experimental fat embolism. Am. J. Surg. 47:466, 1940.

25

Endotracheal Drug Administration

J. THOMAS WARD, JR., M.D.

Introduction

Endotracheal drug administration is a simple and effective alternative for the systemic administration of selected medications. The technique is reserved for use in those settings in which a patient's condition warrants immediate pharmacologic intervention and no intravenous access is readily available. Such settings occur infrequently; however, when they do occur, knowledge of the appropriate drugs and dosages that can be effectively delivered by this route may prove to be lifesaving. Thus, it is mandatory that physicians be familiar with the concept and method of endotracheal drug delivery.

Background

The history of endotracheal drug administration dates back to the mid-1800's, when the ability of the lung to rapidly absorb solutions was first demonstrated. In the year 1857, Bernard performed an experiment in which he instilled a solution of curare into the upper respiratory tract of dogs by way of a tracheostomy.[1] After the dogs were tilted to an upright position, they died within 7 to 8 minutes, and Bernard concluded that the alveoli were permeable to curare. Over the next several decades, other investigators demonstrated that solutions of substances such as salicylates, atropine, potassium iodide, strychnine, and chloral hydrate were also rapidly absorbed from the lung and excreted in the urine after injection of their aqueous solutions into the tracheas of experimental animals.[2]

In 1915, Kline and Winternitz made several important observations. They noted that in the later stages of pneumonia in rabbits, the circulation to the lungs appeared to be impaired. By contrast, intrabronchial injection of 10 ml of a 1 per cent solution of trypan blue resulted in a uniform and intensely stained section of the lung. Because of these findings, they suggested that "direct medication" of the lung might be an efficient therapeutic route.[3, 4] This philosophy of treating pulmonary diseases gained further acceptance in 1935 when Graeser and Rowe demonstrated that the inhalation of epinephrine mist dramatically relieved symptoms of acute asthma.[5] This mode of treatment for asthma soon became the first widely accepted method of therapy that involved the direct medication of the lung with a therapeutic substance.

In the late 1930's and early 1940's certain chronic suppurative disorders of the lung failed to respond to the conventional use of penicillin and sulfa, and the philosophy of "direct medication" of the lung was once again instituted. Intitially, the antibiotics were delivered by inhaled mist[6-18] (as with epinephrine); later, they were injected in solution endotracheally.[16-22] Several observations were soon made. It was noted that penicillin was absorbed into the bloodstream from the lung and then excreted into the urine. Absorption from the lung occurred in a manner that differed from that of intramuscular (IM) injection: the endotracheal delivery of the drug resulted in a therapeutic blood level of penicillin that lasted twice as long as that after IM injection, a "depot effect."[16] Also, it was found that various diluents mixed with penicillin solution could affect both the rate and the degree of absorption of the drug from the lungs.[17] Both observations have important implications concerning the use of endotracheally delivered drugs and still await further investigation as to their potential applications.

In order for solutions of antibiotics to be injected endotracheally, patients' cough reflexes had to be abolished with local anesthetics and sedatives. This procedure was soon realized to be detrimental in patients with advanced pulmonary disease, and the endotracheal administration of antibiotics soon fell into disuse by physicians, thus ending an important era in endotracheal therapy.

In the 1950's, other important research concerning the endotracheal administration of drugs was carried out by investigators who were attempting to elucidate the mechanism responsible for "anesthetic reactions."[23-26] Results from this research demonstrated several points. First, the rate of absorption of drugs from the mucous membranes varied with the location of their application: drugs that were delivered endotracheally were absorbed much more rapidly than those applied to the posterior pharynx.[26, 27] Second, the rapid absorption of drugs applied locally to the larynx and trachea resulted in blood levels significant enough to be considered a cause for some of the "anesthetic reactions."[26, 27]

In 1967, Redding, Asuncion, and Pearson considered the possibility of using the endotracheal route of drug delivery as a primary means of rapid systemic drug administration.[28] They administered epinephrine by the intravenous, intracardiac, and intratracheal routes, and then evaluated its effectiveness in the resuscitation of dogs that had undergone both respiratory and circulatory arrests secondary to hypoxia. Redding and coworkers found that the intravenous, intracardiac, and intratracheal (diluted) routes of drug administration were equally effective in restoring the circulation of dogs in cardiac arrest. They concluded that "whichever of these routes is most immediately available should be used."[28] Thus, it was demonstrated that the endotracheal route of drug delivery served as an effective window to the systemic circulation.

A decade passed before further research was published concerning the use of the endotracheal route of drug delivery as an alternate means of systemic drug administration. Roberts and associates revived the study of endotracheal drugs with a series of papers concerning both the experimental and clinical administration of endotracheal epinephrine.[29-33] This renewed interest in endotracheal drug therapy was further evidenced by other papers that dealt with endotracheal administration of atropine,[34] lidocaine,[35] naloxone,[36, 37] and diazepam.[38]

Indications

The basic indication for endotracheal drug therapy in a given patient is the need for rapid pharmacologic intervention in a setting in which no intravenous access to the circulation is readily available. Unfortunately, not *all* drugs that can be given safely by the intravenous route can be given safely and effectively by the endotracheal route. The classic example of this is sodium bicarbonate, which appears to inactivate pulmonary surfactant when given endotracheally. At present, only a limited number of drugs have been shown to be effective when delivered by the endotracheal route, and only three of these have been used in clinical settings for the purpose of cardiopulmonary resuscitation (Table 25–1). Indications for the use of a specific drug in endotracheal drug administration are the same as those for intravenous administration. At present, the most appropriate dose for the endotracheal delivery of a given drug in a setting of cardiopulmonary resuscitation is not known. The drug dosages that have been investigated (largely in non-shock non-CPR settings) are included in Table 25–1. At present, *it appears that the endotracheal dose of a drug should at least equal the intravenous dose and should be delivered in a volume of 5 to 10 ml.*

Contraindications

At present, the only definite contraindication to the endotracheal delivery of an *appropriate* drug is

Table 25–1. DRUGS DELIVERED BY THE ENDOTRACHEAL ROUTE AND FOUND TO BE EFFECTIVE IN CLINICAL OR EXPERIMENTAL SETTINGS

Drug	Method of Investigation	Doses Used	Time Until Therapeutic Level or Physiologic Effect	Duration of Therapeutic Level or Physiologic Effect	Comments
Epinephrine	Animal models	0.005–0.27 mg/kg	Within 60 sec	At least 25–30 min	Non-CPR model[29, 30]
	Clinical case reports	10.01 mg—infant 1 mg—adult	Within 60 sec	Not reported	Patients were pulseless and apneic[32, 33]
Lidocaine	Clinical studies	2.4–7.7 mg/kg	5 min	30–60 min	Data obtained from human subjects in a non-shock/ non-CPR setting[35, 47, 48]
Atropine	Animal model	2 mg	11–21 sec	4 times longer than IV dose	Drug delivered intrabronchially[39]
	Clinical case report	1 mg	Within 30 sec	Not reported	Patient was pulseless and apneic[34]
Naloxone	Animal model	0.4 mg	Within 5 min	Not reported	No controls in study[36]
	Clinical case report	0.8 mg × 2	Within 60 sec	Not known	Detectable serum levels after 2 hr[37]
Diazepam	Animal model only	0.5 mg/kg	Within 60 sec	15–20 min	95% ethanol used as a diluent[38]

the presence of another access to the systemic circulation through which the needed drug can be delivered rapidly and effectively. The pharmacokinetics and effectiveness of endotracheally delivered drugs given in various states of cardiovascular or pulmonary compromise are to a large extent unknown, and for that reason, more conventional routes of rapid and effective drug administration should be used when available.

A complete list of drugs that are "contraindicated" relative to their delivery by the endotracheal method is not available. Thus far, those drugs that have been been shown to be *detrimental* or *ineffective* when delivered by the endotracheal route (in animals) include sodium bicarbonate,[39] calcium chloride,[32] and bretylium tosylate.[40] No drug should be delivered by the endotracheal route without experimental or clinical evidence to support its effectiveness and safety.

It should be noted that the endotracheal delivery of some drugs in solution may result in transient decreases in the arterial partial pressure of oxygen (Po₂).[38]

Equipment

Patients in need of endotracheal drug therapy first require management of their airway, usually in the form of tracheal intubation. Once this procedure has been performed (see Chapter 1), little other equipment is needed for the endotracheal delivery of a drug.

In the following section, several different techniques for endotracheal drug administration are described. The equipment necessary for each of the various techniques is minimal and is listed for each of the following techniques.

Technique 1

1. A pre-filled syringe of the required drug solution (Abboject, Bristoject). If a pre-filled syringe is not available or if the concentration of a solution is inappropriate, a Luer-Lok syringe (10 to 20 ml) with a No. 18 or No. 19 gauge needle should be used along with the required drug solution. If necessary, a sterile diluent of either normal saline or distilled water can be used so that the total volume of drug solution to be administered will be 5 to 10 ml for adults and 1 ml for infants.

2. A mechanical ventilation device capable of delivering a fraction of inspired oxygen (FI$_{O_2}$) of at least 50 per cent.

Technique 2

1. A No. 18 or No. 19 gauge needle.

2. A 10 to 20 ml Luer-Lok syringe filled with the appropriate drug solution. Again, the concentration of the solution should be such that the dose to be delivered results in a total volume of 5 to 10 ml for adults and 1 ml for infants.

3. A mechanical ventilation device capable of delivering an FI$_{O_2}$ of at least 50 per cent.

Technique 3

1. An n-doMED device (Fig. 25–1) or a 12-inch central venous (CVP) catheter of approximately 16 gauge size. The n-doMED device can be obtained from Ackrad Laboratories, 70 Jackson Drive, Cranford, NJ 07016.

2. A pre-filled syringe or regular syringe of the drug solution to be administered. Again, the total volume of solution to be delivered should be 5 to 10 ml for adults and approximately 1 ml for infants.

3. A mechanical ventilation device capable of delivering an FI$_{O_2}$ of at least 50 per cent.

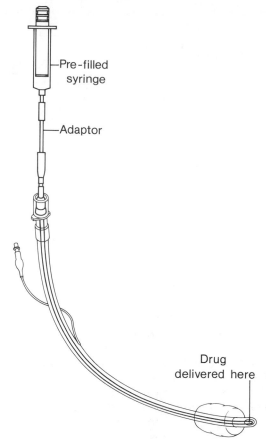

- Pre-filled syringe

- Adaptor

Drug delivered here

Figure 25–1. Line drawing of an n-doMED device. (Courtesy of AKrad Labs.)

Technique 4

1. A No. 22 or No. 23 gauge needle.

2. A Luer-Lok syringe of the specific drug solution, with a total volume of 5 to 10 ml for adults.

3. An alcohol sponge.

4. A mechanical ventilation device capable of delivering an FI_{O_2} of at least 50 per cent.

Procedure

Several techniques for the endotracheal administration of drugs have been described.[32–34, 41] Each technique is quite simple and requires very little skill or experience to perform. The most effective technique has yet to be determined, and for that reason, each will be discussed. There is no special significance to the order in which the techniques are discussed.

Techniques 1, 2, and 3 require that the patient be intubated prior to drug delivery. Each of these methods basically involves the delivery of a drug through the endotracheal tube and into the trachea and bronchi. The differences among the techniques are due to the *manner* by which the drug is delivered through the tube. Technique 1 simply involves squirting the drug into the endotracheal tube and following it by insufflations of a mechanical ventilation device. Technique 2 is somewhat similar but delivers the drug at the same time that the patient is being ventilated. Technique 3 involves delivering the drug to the distal trachea and bronchi *through* the endotracheal tube by means of a catheter.

A fourth technique of drug delivery into the laryngotracheobronchial tree is also discussed. This technique is not a method of endotracheal drug delivery in a strict sense but is instead a method of translaryngeal drug delivery used primarily for anesthesia of the larynx *prior to intubation*.[35, 42, 43] Because this method of drug delivery may result in therapeutic levels of lidocaine by absorption of the drug from the larynx and the trachea, it is included here.[35]

TECHNIQUE 1

This technique can be performed only if management of the patient's airway during initial resusciation required tracheal intubation. After intubation (see Chapter 1), the endotracheal tube should be adequately secured by tape or string so that the tube is not likely to be expelled during a forceful cough. In addition, the cuff of the tube should obviously be inflated.

The patient should be ventilated with a mechanical ventilation device, using supplemental oxygen. The required drug should be drawn up in either a 10 or 20-ml syringe (preferably of the Luer-Lok type to avoid needle dislodgement during injection) and, if necessary, diluted with either sterile normal saline or distilled water to a total volume of 5 to 10 ml. The plunger of the syringe should be drawn back further to enable an equal volume of air to be present with the drug solution in the barrel of the syringe. A No. 18 or No. 19 gauge needle is then *firmly* affixed to the end of the syringe. The connection between the tip of the endotracheal tube and the ventilation device should be interrupted. The syringe is inverted, and the needle is placed within the lumen of the endotracheal tube. The solution is forcefully and rapidly injected into the lumen of the tube, followed by the 5 to 10 ml of air that helps in the emptying of the contents of the syringe. If the patient makes an effort to cough, place your thumb (preferably gloved) over the opening of the tube to prevent expulsion of the solution. If the endotracheal tube has not been properly secured by this time, the tube itself can also be expelled during reflex coughing. Also if external cardiac massage is being performed, it should be interrupted for a few seconds during drug delivery, because chest compression may expel the drug.

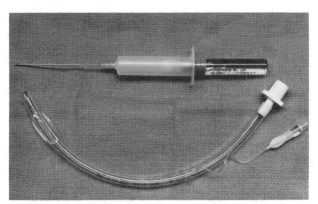

Figure 25–2. Example of pre-filled syringe frequently used in endotracheal therapy.

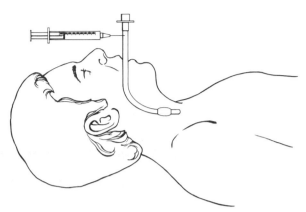

Figure 25–3. Method for drug injection as described in Technique 2.

As soon as possible after injection of the solution, the ventilation device should be re-attached to the endotracheal tube and five rapid insufflations should be done in an effort to promote more distal delivery of the drug solution. Again, one should be sure to use a mechanical ventilation device with supplemental oxygen capable of delivering an FI_{O_2} of at least 50 per cent, because endotracheal drug delivery may cause a transient decrease in arterial P_{O_2}.[38]

Pre-filled syringes of the Abboject type (Fig. 25–2) can be used (and are often preferred) instead of "drawing up" the required drug solution into a regular syringe. These syringes may save time as well as prevent the inadvertent loss of a needle down the endotracheal tube. Most drug solutions used for endotracheal therapy are available in this form; these unit dose syringes usually contain a total volume of 5 to 10 ml.

TECHNIQUE 2

This technique is performed in a method similar to that of Technique 1. Rather than injecting the solution into the open proximal lumen of the tube, however, in Technique 2 the No. 18 or No. 19 gauge needle is inserted through the side of the endotracheal tube into the tube lumen (Fig. 25–3). The syringe is attached, and the solution is injected into the tube *during* the inspiratory phase of ventilation. This method does not require interruption of the connection between the endotracheal tube and the ventilation device, and it also offers the theoretical advantage of "forcing the drug into the lungs" with ventilation as it is being injected. Note that with this method of drug delivery one has also removed the forceful longitudinal injection of the drug solution down the tube lumen. To what degree these factors affect both delivery and absorption of the administered drug is unknown.

TECHNIQUE 3

Recent animal data suggest that this technique may be advantageous in the setting of cardiac arrest.[49] For this reason, the author recommends this technique as a preferred method of endotracheal drug delivery.

With this technique, a catheter is used to inject the drug solution through the endotracheal tube into the distal trachea and bronchi. After the endotracheal tube has been adequately secured with tape or string, the patient should be ventilated while the necessary drug solution is drawn up. A 10- to 20-ml syringe should be used to draw up the drug solution (and equal volume of air) as described in Technique 1. This syringe is then securely attached to the CVP catheter or n-doMED device (Fig. 25–4 A–C) and placed within the lumen of the tube. Once again, the solution should be forcefully and rapidly injected into the trachea and bronchi, followed by air to empty the catheter. If the patient is undergoing CPR, chest compressions should be interrupted for a few seconds. The catheter is then removed, the proximal lumen of the endotracheal tube is momentarily covered by the thumb, the patient is re-attached to the ventilation device, and five rapid insufflations are delivered to promote distal drug delivery.

The n-doMED device is designed to direct the drug solution into the two main stem bronchi by way of the two pairs of small holes located in the rounded tip of the catheter. The CVP catheter performs a similar function but delivers the drug in a single stream of solution. Both methods deliver the drug solution *through* the endotracheal tube directly into the distal trachea and bronchi, thus preventing loss of drug on the walls of the endotracheal tube and promoting a more distal delivery of the drug. Whether or not these methods actually result in more effective drug delivery and absorption is not known, but contrast material delivered in this manner is clearly dispersed more

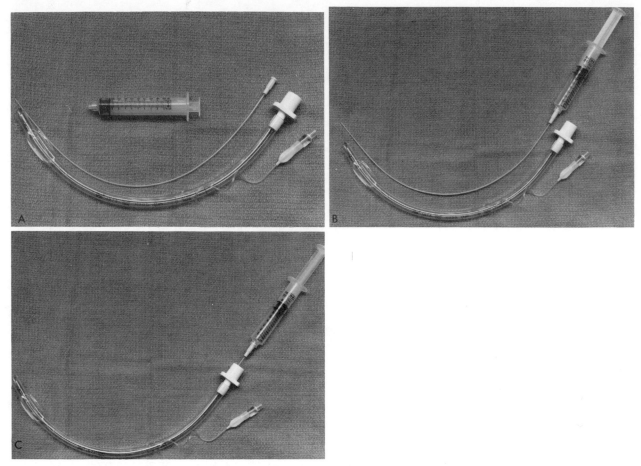

Figure 25–4. Use of a central venous catheter for endotracheal drug delivery.

efficiently and reaches the distal alveoli more rapidly than by other methods.[44] Recent physiologic data also support distal drug delivery during CPR.[49]

Pre-filled syringes can also be used with the n-doMED device. An adapter of the proper length (two are included in the kit) is first placed over the needle, then the assembly is connected to the n-doMED tube and placed within the lumen of the endotracheal tube. These unit dose syringes can also be used with routine CVP catheters, but first the needle must be broken off just distal to the tip of the plastic nipple.

TECHNIQUE 4

As mentioned previously, this technique is more accurately termed *translaryngeal drug administration* than endotracheal drug administration. As with the endotracheal method of drug delivery, drug administration using Technique 4 has been reported to deliver therapeutic blood levels of at least one drug (lidocaine) within approximately 5 minutes. The primary purpose of the technique has been to supply local anesthesia to the larynx and proximal trachea prior to intubation. Because experience with this form of drug delivery is limited to local anesthetics, it is not recommended at present for the delivery of other endotracheal drugs.

The technique of translaryngeal drug delivery is quite simple and has been used for the purpose of providing local anesthesia to the larynx and proximal trachea since the early 1900's. The cricothyroid space is first identified (Fig. 25–5) as described in Chapters 4 (Transtracheal Aspiration) and 7 (Emergency Cricothyroidotomy). This area is then cleansed with an alcohol sponge, and the index finger is used to palpate the superior border of the cricoid cartilage. The cricothyroid membrane is then punctured with a 1-inch No. 21 or No. 22 gauge needle on a 3- to 5-ml syringe (Fig. 25–6). The needle must be in the midline and perpendicular to the membrane. The needle will puncture only four structures as it moves from without inward: skin, subcutaneous tissue, cricothyroid membrane, and endolaryngeal mucosa. When no

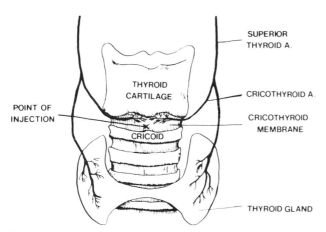

Figure 25–5. Anatomic relationships in translaryngeal anesthesia, anterior view. (From Danzl, D. F., and Thomas, D. M.: Nasotracheal intubations in the emergency department. Crit. Care Med. 8:677, 1980. Used by permission.)

further resistance is felt, air is aspirated to confirm the presence of the needle tip within the lumen of the larynx. The drug solution is then swiftly injected, and the needle is rapidly withdrawn. Drug injection may precipitate a cough in patients who are semiconscious or conscious. After removal of the needle, the site is pressed firmly with a finger to prevent development of a hematoma or subcutaneous emphysema.

The volume of solution required for translaryngeal drug delivery seems to be less than that required for endotracheal drug delivery. Frequently, 1.5 to 3.5 ml of a 4 per cent solution of lidocaine is used for the purpose of translaryngeal anesthesia; however, as much as 9 ml of anesthetic has been delivered by this method.[35, 42, 43]

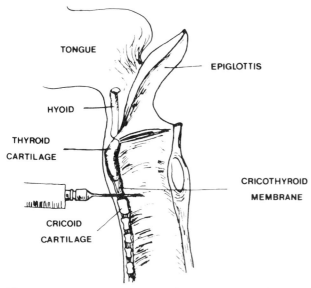

Figure 25–6. Anatomic relationships in translaryngeal anesthesia, cross-sectional view. (From Danzl, D. F., and Thomas, D. M.: Nasotracheal intubations in the emergency department. Crit. Care Med. 8:677, 1980. Used by permission.)

Complications

It is difficult to obtain accurate information concerning the complications of endotracheal drug therapy. This is due in part to the infrequent use of this method of drug therapy. In addition, most patients who receive this form of therapy are either critically ill or have sustained cardiopulmonary arrest. In such a setting, it becomes difficult to determine whether the endotracheal delivery of a drug has any adverse effects on the patient's status because of the large number of variables involved.

Concerning the *techniques* of endotracheal drug administration, no complications have been reported. The only theoretical complication would be loss of a needle or catheter during forceful administration of the drug. If one were to include translaryngeal anesthesia as a method of endotracheal drug delivery, other complications would arise, although their frequency would be extremely low. Gold and Buechel reviewed 17,500 cricothyroid punctures for translaryngeal anesthesia and noted eight complications with no fatalities.[42] There were two cases of severe laryngospasm, four soft-tissue infections of the neck, and two broken needles that were retrieved. Thus, the *techniques* of endotracheal drug administration seem to provide a safe method of drug delivery.

As for the *adverse effects* of endotracheally delivered drugs, two potential undesirable effects are realized. The first of these concerns a transient drop in the arterial oxygen content. Greenberg and associates reported that when 2 ml per kg of normal saline was instilled endotracheally in dogs, the arterial PO_2 decreased to a level of approximately 80 per cent of baseline values for about 20 minutes.[45] Likewise, it was reported that 2 ml per kg of distilled water that was instilled endotracheally produced a drop in arterial PO_2 to a level of approximately 60 per cent of baseline values and persisted for at least 20 minutes. Although the volume of fluid in these experiments represents a dose of fluid much greater than what is usually delivered endotracheally to human subjects (in a single dose), the findings show that if large volumes of fluid are delivered endotracheally, a resultant decrease in arterial PO_2 will develop.

In an experiment reported by Barsan and colleagues, 0.5 mg per kg of diazepam diluted to a total volume of 5 ml with 95 per cent ethanol was administered endotracheally to dogs.[38] Using this much smaller volume of solution, compared with the study of Greenberg and associates, and 95 per cent ethanol as the diluent, these investigators reported the largest change in mean arterial PO_2 to be 12.2 mm Hg from the mean control value. This change occurred at 60 minutes post drug delivery and returned toward control values at 90 minutes. Thus, Barsan and colleagues also reported a transient drop in arterial P_{O_2} after drug delivery, although not as large a drop as that reported by Greenberg and associates.

Obviously, any decrease in arterial P_{O_2} in a critically ill patient, regardless of how small or how transient, may have deleterious effects. This possibility should always be considered when administering drugs by the endotracheal route. Supplemental oxygen should always be administered in an effort to improve oxygenation and to possibly decrease the significance of the transient decrease in arterial oxygen content.

The second potential ill effect from endotracheal drug administration is that of drug toxicity. The kinetics of endotracheally delivered drugs have been partially elucidated in non-shock, non-CPR settings, but the degree to which the kinetics vary in the setting of cardiac or pulmonary dysfunction is not known. Thus, the potential for drug toxicity must always be considered when drugs are delivered endotracheally during cardiopulmonary resuscitation. Drug toxicity would most likely become apparent during the post-resuscitative state, when the improved hemodynamic status of the patient might enhance the absorption of the drug previously delivered to the lungs. Additional research in this area is necessary.

Conclusion

Several questions concerning the endotracheal method of drug delivery have yet to be answered.[46] Most important of these is how the settings of CPR and "near arrest" states affect both the absorption and pharmacokinetics of the drugs administered. In addition, the most effective technique of endotracheal administration has yet to be delineated. The question of just how far into the pulmonary tree a drug should be delivered remains unanswered. One of the most exciting areas yet to be fully investigated is that of drug diluents for the drugs to be administered. Finally, those properties of drugs that either allow or prevent them from being absorbed require investigation.[46]

Endotracheal drug administration during resuscitation is a technique that is still in the very early stages of investigation, and for that reason, it should be reserved for use in those settings in which another rapid and effective alternative means of drug delivery is not available. Knowledge of this method of drug delivery may prove to be of benefit in the resuscitation of certain patients.

1. Bernard, C.: Leçons sur les effets des substances toxiques et méditcamenteuses. Paris, 286, 1857.
2. Mutch, N.: Inhalation of chemotherapeutic substances. Lancet 2:775, 1944.
3. Kline, B. S., and Winternitz, M. D.: Studies upon experimental pneumonia in rabbits. VIII. Intra vitam staining in experimental pneumonia, and the circulation in the pneumonic lung. J. Exp. Med. 21:311, 1915.
4. Winternitz, M. C., and Smith, G. H.: Preliminary Studies in Intratracheal Therapy: Collected Studies on the Pathology of War Gas Poisoning. New Haven, Connecticut, Yale University Press, 1920.
5. Graeser, J. B., and Rowe, A. H.: Inhalation of epinephrine for the relief of asthmatic symptoms. J. Allergy 6:415, 1935.
6. Barach, A. L. Molomut, N., and Soroka, M.: Inhalation of nebulized Promin in experimental tuberculosis. Am. Rev. Tuberc. 46:268, 1942.
7. Stacey, J. W.: The inhalation of nebulized solution of sulfonamides in the treatment of bronchiectasis. Dis. Chest 9:302, 1943.
8. Harris, T. N., Sommer, H. E., and Chapple, C. C.: The administration of sulfonamide micro-crystals by inhalation. Am. J. Med. Sci. 205:1, 1943.
9. Chapple, C. C., and Lynch, H. M.: A study of sulfonamide aerosol inhalation: a supplemental note. Am. J. Med. Sci. 205:488, 1943.
10. Applebaum, I. L.: The treatment of bronchial lesions by the inhalation of nebulized solution of sodium sulfathiazole. Dis. Chest 10:415, 1944.
11. Edlin, J. S., Bobrowitz, I. D., et al.: Promin inhalation therapy in pulmonary tuberculosis. Am. Rev. Tuberc. 50:543, 1944.
12. Bryson, V., Sansome, E., and Laskin, S.: Aerosolization of penicillin solutions. Science 100:33, 1944.
13. Barach, A. L., Silberstein, F. H. et al.: Inhalation of penicillin aerosol in patients with bronchial asthma, chronic bronchitis, bronchiectasis, and lung abscess. A preliminary report. Ann. Intern. Med. 22:485, 1944.
14. Segal, M. S., and Ryder, C. M.: Penicillin aerosolization in the treatment of serious respiratory infections. N. Engl. J. Med. 233:747, 1945.
15. Segal, M. S., Levinson, L., and Miller, D.: Penicillin inhalation therapy in respiratory infections. JAMA 134:762, 1947.
16. Gaensler, E. A., Beakey, J. F., and Segal, M. S.: Pharmacodynamics of pulmonary absorption in man. I. Aerosol and intratracheal penicillin. Ann. Int. Med. 31:582, 1949.
17. Beakey, J. F., Gaensler, E. A., and Segal, M. S.: Pharmacodynamics of pulmonary absorption in man. II. The influence of various diluents on aerosol and intratracheal penicillin. Ann Int. Med. 31:805, 1949.
18. Gaensler, E. A., Beakey, J. F., and Segal, M. S.: Relative effectiveness of parenteral, intratracheal, and aerosol penicillin in chronic suppurative diseases of lung. J. Thorac. Surg. 18:546, 1949.
19. May, H. B., and Floyer, M. A.: Infected bronchiectasis treated with intratracheal penicillin. Br. Med. J. 1:907, 1945.
20. Norris, C. M.: Sulfonamides in bronchial secretion. JAMA 123:667, 1943.
21. Vinson, P. P.: Treatment of chronic non-tuberculous pulmonary infection by bronchoscopy and insufflation of sulfonamide compounds. Ann. Otol. Rhinol. Laryngol. 53:787, 1944.
22. Kay, E. B., and Meade, R. H.: Penicillin in the treatment of chronic infections of the lungs and bronchi. JAMA 129:200, 1945.
23. Derbes, V. J., and Englehardt, H. T.: Deaths following the use of local anesthetics in transcricoid therapy: a critical review. J. Lab. Clin. Med. 29:478, 1944.

24. Rubin, H. J., and Kully, B. M.: Speed of administration as related to the toxicity of certain topical anesthetics. Ann. Otol. Rhinol. Laryngol. 69:627, 1951.

25. Steinhaus, J. E.: A comparative study of the experimental toxicity of local anesthetic agents. Anesthesiology 13:577, 1952.

26. Adriani, J., and Campbell, D.: Deaths following topical application of local anesthetics to mucous membranes. JAMA 162:1527, 1956.

27. Campbell, D., and Adriani, J.: Absorption of local anesthetics. JAMA 168:873, 1958.

28. Redding, J. S., Asuncion, F. S., and Pearson, J. W.: Effective routes of drug administration during cardiac arrest. Anesth. Analg. 46:253, 1967.

29. Roberts, J. R., Greenberg, M. I., et al.: Comparison of the pharmacological effects of epinephrine administered by the intravenous and endotracheal routes. JACEP 7:260, 1978.

30. Roberts, J. R., Greenberg, M. I., et al.: Blood levels following intravenous and endotracheal epinephrine administration. JACEP 8:53, 1979.

31. Greenberg, M. I., Roberts, J. R., et al.: Endotracheal epinephrine in a canine anaphylactic shock model. JACEP 8:500, 1979.

32. Roberts, J. R., Greenberg, M. I., and Baskin, S. I.: Endotracheal epinephrine in cardiorespiratory collapse. JACEP 8:515, 1979.

33. Greenberg, M. I., Roberts, F. R., and Baskin, S. I.: Use of endotracheally administered epinephrine in a pediatric patient. Am. J. Dis. Child 135:767, 1981.

34. Greenberg, M. E., Mayeda, D. V., et al.: Endotracheal administration of atropine sulfate. Ann. Emerg. Med. 11:546, 1982.

35. Boster, S. R., Danzl, D. F., et al.: Translaryngeal absorption of lidocaine. Ann. Emerg. Med. 11:461, 1982.

36. Greenberg, M. I., Roberts, J. R., and Baskin, S. I.: Endotracheal naloxone reversal of morphine-induced respiratory depression in rabbits. Ann. Emerg. Med. 9:289, 1980.

37. Tandberg, D., and Abercrombie, D.: Treatment of heroin overdose with endotracheal naloxone. Ann. Emerg. Med. 11:443, 1982.

38. Barsan, W. G., Ward, J. T., and Otten, E. T.: Blood levels of diazepam after endotracheal administration in dogs. Ann. Emerg. Med. 11:242, 1982.

39. Elam, J. O.: The intrapulmonary route for CPR drugs. In Safar, P. (ed.): Advances in Cardiopulmonary Resuscitation. New York, Springer-Verlag New York, Inc., 1977, p. 132.

40. Murphy, K., Caplen, S., et al.: Endotracheal bretylium tosylate in the canine model. Ann. Emerg. Med. 12:260, 1983.

41. Feferman, I., and Leblanc, L.: A simple method for administering endotracheal medication. Ann. Emerg. Med. 12:196, 1983.

42. Gold, M. I., and Buechel, D. R.: Translaryngeal anesthesia: a review. Anesthesiology 20:181, 1959.

43. Danzl, D. F., and Thomas, D. M.: Nasotracheal intubations in the emergency department. Crit. Care Med. 8:677, 1980.

44. Greenberg, M. I., and Spivey, W.: Comparison of deep vs shallow endotracheal medication administration in dogs (abstract). Ann. Emerg. Med. 12:242, 1983.

45. Greenberg, M. I., Baskin, S. I., et al.: Effects of endotracheally administered distilled water and normal saline on the arterial blood gases of dogs. Ann. Emerg. Med. 11:600, 1982.

46. Ward, J. T.: Endotracheal drug therapy. Am. J. Emerg. Med. 1:71, 1983.

47. Telivuo, L.: An experimental study on the absorption of some local anaesthetics through the lower respiratory tract. Acta Anaesth. Scand. Suppl 16:121, 1965.

48. Chu, S. S., Rah, K. H., et al.: Plasma concentration of lidocaine after endotracheal spray. Anesth. Analg. 54:438, 1975.

49. Ralston, S. H., Voorhees, W. D., and Babbs, C. F.: Intrapulmonary epinephrine during prolonged cardiopulmonary resuscitation: improved regional blood flow and resuscitation in dogs. Ann. Emerg. Med. 13:79, 1984.

26

Arterial Puncture and Cannulation

WILLIAM J. BARKER, M.D.
STEPHEN R. WYTE, M.D.

Introduction

Arterial blood gas evaluation provides useful information that is essentially unavailable by other means. The respiratory status and acid/base equilibrium of individuals with pulmonary disorders, drug overdoses, and metabolic diseases may be evaluated through this procedure. The current sophistication of critical care medicine would be impossible without arterial access, permitting continuous arterial pressure monitoring and frequent blood sampling for metabolic and hematologic indices.

Originally, pressure monitoring was done with mercury or water columns. These devices are accurate only for the mean arterial pressure. Today's transducers convert a fluid pressure wave into an electronic signal. The increased frequency response of modern electromechanical transducers permits the clinician to follow pressure waveforms as well as systolic and diastolic pressures.

Background

Access to the arterial system may now be obtained easily in most patients. Many improvements in arterial access methodology and equipment have occurred since Hale, in 1733, first used a technique similar to today's cutdown technique to attach a fluid column for measurement of the blood pressure of a horse.[1] J. L. M. Poiseville first introduced the use of a mercury manometer for the measurement of blood pressure in 1828. In 1847, Carl Ludwig graphically recorded blood pressure fluctuations by placing a float with a pointer on the mercury column, permitting the pointer to scratch a smoked drum rotating adjacent to the column. Today's manometers, transducers, and recorders are quite different from these early devices but are direct descendants of them. Furthermore, the information one may obtain about

the clinical status of a patient from arterial puncture is more extensive with modern technology.

Indications and Contraindications

Many patients who are seen in the emergency department benefit from arterial puncture or cannulation (see Table 26–1). Most commonly, arterial blood gases are used to evaluate individuals who have significant respiratory pathology. Although most patients with respiratory illness may be managed without arterial puncture, arterial blood gas determination is imperative when they are severely ill. Critically ill patients with nonrespiratory disease may need frequent metabolic and electrolyte monitoring. For instance, the patient with severe diabetic ketoacidosis cannot be properly managed without frequent pH, electrolyte, and glucose measurements. Although arterial blood gas analysis is the most frequent indication for arterial puncture, all blood chemistries can be performed from an arterial sample. When frequent blood sampling is required, it is easier and certainly more humane to insert an indwelling arterial cannula. The nurse who is caring for the patient may then sample the blood as needed.

The most common indication for long-term arterial cannulation is continuous monitoring of arterial blood pressure. An electromechanical pressure transducer attached to an oscilloscope screen allows continuous observation of arterial systolic and diastolic pressures. This capability is most useful in a critical care unit but is also helpful when available in an emergency department. Many situations, such as during the use of vasoactive drugs (e.g., nitroprusside and dopamine), require continuous arterial pressure monitoring. The response of trauma and cardiac patients to resuscitative efforts also may be easily followed in this manner.

Another common use of arterial puncture is radiologic diagnostic imaging of the arterial system. Obviously, this is an uncommon indication

Table 26–1. ARTERIAL PUNCTURE AND CANNULATION

Indications	Contraindications
Blood gas sampling	Relative
Continuous pressure monitoring	Previous surgery in the area, especially cutdown
Frequent blood sampling for any purpose	Anticoagulation
Diagnostic angiography	Coagulopathy
Therapeutic embolization	Skin infection at site
	Atherosclerosis
	Decreased collateral flow
	Absolute
	None

in the emergency department but may be considered for suspected cases of peripheral arterial embolism. Although this procedure is fairly simple to perform, arterial access for diagnostic imaging will most often be performed by a radiologist. Arterial puncture is also used by cardiologists and radiologists for coronary, cerebral, renal, and other central arterial angiography. Aortography can be very important for chest trauma and suspected cases of dissecting or leaking aneurysms.

Few contraindications to arterial puncture exist; none are absolute. Arterial puncture performed in patients who are anticoagulated or who have other coagulopathies should be undertaken with extreme care. Luce and associates[2] reported seven patients with compression neuropathies secondary to hematoma after arterial puncture, all of whom were anticoagulated at the time of puncture. Repeated arterial sampling in these patients may necessitate insertion of an indwelling cannula to minimize the number of puncture sites in the arterial wall.

The presence of severe atherosclerosis, with or without diminution of flow, is a relative contraindication to arterial puncture, especially when followed by cannulation. The existence of a bruit or a palpable decrease in the pulse should warn the physician of the presence of intravascular disease. If either is noted and if the arterial puncture is imperative, an alternative site should be selected.

Evidence of decreased or absent collateral flow in areas in which flow normally exists should also lead one to choose an alternative site. A positive Allen's test (discussed in the technique section) should eliminate the radial and ulnar arteries as possible sites of cannulation. One should also avoid puncture of an artery where infection, burn, or other damage to cutaneous defenses exists in the overlying skin.

Equipment

The equipment used for arterial cannulation has a great influence on the accuracy of pressure measurements. Frequency responses of tubing, transducers, and other components of the monitoring system influence the measurement accuracy of systolic and diastolic pressures.

The dynamic response characteristics of the monitoring system are of minimal importance if the clinician is interested primarily in the mean arterial pressure (MAP).[3] In the emergency department, trends in the MAP are more useful than absolute values for systolic and diastolic pressures.

The various catheter types have been shown to have similar frequency response characteristics, but studies have shown more variable effects on complication rates. Teflon catheters have been implicated in increased complications due to

thrombosis in one study,[4] whereas other studies deny any such effect.[5-7] The diameter of the indwelling cannula seems to have a more consistent effect; the incidence of thrombosis is inversely related to the ratio of vessel lumen to catheter diameter.[8] Thus for a given vessel size, the incidence of thrombosis will increase as the catheter diameter decreases. Catheter choice should be influenced by availability and convenience of use of a particular brand. A short catheter is ideal for peripheral artery cannulation, whereas a longer over-the-needle catheter is preferable for the femoral artery (Fig. 26–1). Downs and associates suggest that thrombosis is less likely with a nontapered catheter.[9] An 18 to 20 gauge catheter should be used in adults. Small children and infants require a 22 to 24 gauge catheter, which may need to be inserted through a cutdown technique.

The tubing that connects the catheter to the pressure transducer has a more significant effect on monitoring systems. The higher the frequency response of the whole system, the more accurate will be the determination of systolic and diastolic pressure.[3, 10] A stiff, low-capacitance plastic tubing should be used, and the manometer should be placed as close as possible to the patient, because the frequency response of a tube is inversely related to its length.[10-12]

After the pressure wave is transmitted from the artery through the catheter and connecting tubing, a measuring device is required to obtain a numerical value for the arterial pressure. Most commonly used today is an electromechanical pressure transducer that changes a mechanical pressure pulse, the fluid wave, into an electrical signal, which is then fed into an oscilloscope. Additional circuitry can be added to display the systolic and diastolic pressure as numerical values. Various mini-computer systems that allow computation of mean

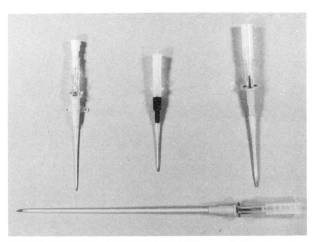

Figure 26–1. Catheters that may be used for arterial line insertion. Short, small gauge over-the-needle catheters are ideal for peripheral artery cannulation (top). The long over-the-needle catheter is used for femoral arterial lines (bottom).

arterial pressure, trend monitoring, and other capabilities in addition to displaying the systolic and diastolic pressures are available. So many transducer and oscilloscope combinations exist that a discussion of their relative merits is beyond the scope of this chapter.

Intravascular transducers are also available but have many potential disadvantages and are used infrequently. They are fragile, temperature sensitive, of variable quality, and much more difficult to place into a vessel than is a catheter. Fibrin deposition on the device is also a common finding. The greatest, and possibly only, advantage of these intravascular transducers is the elimination of potential error induced by catheters, stopcocks, and connecting tubing.

Less expensive means of deriving a number representative of the arterial pressure are available, especially if one is interested in determining only the MAP. Zorab describes the use of an

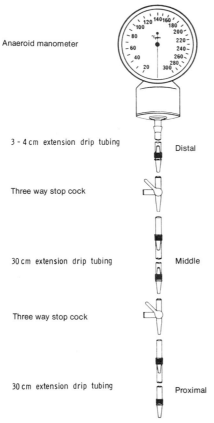

Figure 26–2. Assembly technique for anaeroid manometer system. The middle and proximal extension tubings contain heparinized saline. The middle extension tubing is arranged to form a fluid meniscus at the same level as the heart when the proximal stopcock is closed to the middle tubing (i.e., no pressure input). The distal extension tubing is air-filled and held vertically so that there is no saline contamination of the manometer at maximal pressures. Approximately 10 to 12 cm of air in the distal and middle tubings is optimal. The same system can be used with a mercury manometer in place of the anaeroid manometer. Sterility of the extension tubing and stopcocks is essential. (From Zorab, J.S.M.: Continuous display of the arterial pressure: a simple manometric technique. Anaesthesia 24:433, 1969. Copyright © 1969 by the Association of Anaesthetists of Great Britain and Ireland. Used by permission.)

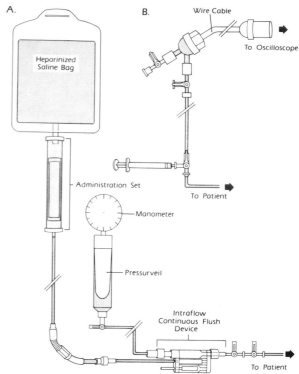

Figure 26–3. Arterial pressure monitoring systems. A, System for continuous flush. Heparin (2 ml of 1:1000 unit solution) is added to a 1 L bag of normal saline, and the bag is pressurized to 300 mm Hg using a metered blood pump (not shown). The continuous flush device is set to deliver 3 ml of the heparinized saline per hour. A mechanical pressure transducer (Pressurveil, Concept Co.) is depicted. The transducer device is a sterile, inexpensive, fully assembled monitor that can be used during patient transfer. Alternatively, the electronic transducer depicted in B may be used. B, System for manual flush. A heparinized saline flush solution can be manually injected through a syringe at the proximal or distal port. The transducer dome should be maintained at the level of the patient's heart. (From Beal, J.M. (ed.): Critical Care for Surgical Patients. New York, Macmillan Publishing Co., Inc., 1982. Used by permission.)

anaeroid manometer connected to the arterial system by a catheter filled with heparinized saline.[13] The catheter is arranged to have a fluid meniscus at the same level as the heart when there is no pressure input. The meniscus is below an air column in a vertical tube that is long enough to avoid saline contamination of the manometer at maximal pressures (Fig. 26–2). A mercury manometer, especially a J tube, may also be used in place of an anaeroid manometer in the previously described system for measurement of MAP.

For continuous arterial pressure monitoring, some method of flushing the system is necessary to maintain patency of the catheter lumen. This may be as simple as a three-way stopcock through which the tubing is intermittently flushed with heparinized saline. There are continuous flush devices that are designed to push a set amount of fluid (usually 2 to 3 ml per hr) through the line. A typical monitoring system that includes this device is shown in Figure 26–3. The pressure transducer is usually mounted at the level of the patient's heart on a bedside pole.

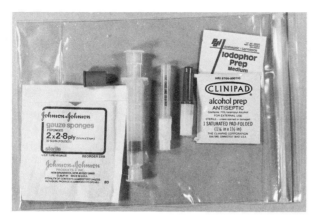

Figure 26–4. Arterial blood gas kit. Contents include: skin prep pads, pre-filled heparinized syringe, stopper for syringe, needles, gauze sponges, and plastic bag for crushed ice.

The equipment needed to percutaneously obtain a single sample for arterial blood gas analysis is simple and readily available in any hospital, often in the form of a pre-packaged kit (Fig. 26–4). The necessary items for arterial line placement are listed in Table 26–2 and referred to in the section describing procedures. Obtaining a sample from an indwelling arterial line requires only two syringes, one of which has been heparinized.

Site Selection

Selection of an arterial site is the first step in placing an indwelling cannula or in obtaining a sample of arterial blood for a blood gas analysis. Successful cannulation of the radial, ulnar, brachial, axillary, dorsalis pedis, and femoral arteries in children and adults is possible. The temporal

Table 26–2. EQUIPMENT FOR INSERTION AND MAINTENANCE OF AN INDWELLING ARTERIAL CANNULA

Percutaneous Insertion
  Alcohol or iodophor solution
  1% lidocaine or other local anesthetic solution
  3–0 nylon or silk suture on skin needle
  4 × 4 dressing sponges
  Adhesive tape
  Iodophor ointment
  Arm board for brachial, radial, or ulnar cannulations
  Syringes
  Pressure tubing
  Two three-way stopcocks
  Pressure transducer
  Connecting wire
  Oscilloscope, thermal graph or other output display
  Heparinized saline
  Pressure blood infusor, set up with continuous flush device

Additional Equipment Required for Cutdown Insertion
    Technique
  Scalpel blade (No. 10)
  0-silk sutures (2 or more)
  Small hemostat
  Forceps

and umbilical arteries are often cannulated in infants and neonates. The radial, brachial, and femoral arteries are usually punctured for blood gas sampling in adults.

The potential consequence of total loss of blood flow through a vessel owing to intraluminal thrombosis is one of several variables that must be considered when choosing a site for arterial puncture. Arteries known to have good collateral blood flow, such as the radial and dorsalis pedis, are thus favored. Determining the effect of the site chosen on the ease of patient care will be appreciated by those who will subsequently be providing direct care. An arterial line in the lower extremities may be preferred during a procedure on the upper body, and a femoral or axillary line may be poorly tolerated by the patient who is capable of positioning himself. Characteristics of the common arterial sites are discussed following general descriptions of the techniques of arterial puncture and cannulation.

Techniques

PERCUTANEOUS TECHNIQUE FOR SINGLE ARTERIAL PUNCTURE

To obtain a single sample of arterial blood by the percutaneous method, a small (5-ml) syringe is attached to a 20 to 22 gauge needle. A smaller needle may be required for young children or individuals who have had many previous punctures. To prevent clotting of the sample, 1 or 2 ml of a heparinized saline solution (1000 IU per ml) are drawn into the syringe to coat the barrel and needle and are then ejected through the needle shortly before puncture. All the visible heparin is ejected, so that all that remains is only enough anticoagulant to fill the dead space of the syringe and needle, minimizing heparin related errors. Because of the air-fluid boundary in the heparin storage bottle, heparin has a higher PO_2 and a lower PCO_2 than blood, and changes in these parameters reflect a dilutional effect. The addition of 0.4 ml of heparin to a 2-ml sample of blood (dilution of 20 per cent) will lower the PCO_2 by 16 per cent and a falsely low PCO_2 is the most clinically significant change caused by excess heparin.[14] PO_2 levels are not significantly altered by the addition of heparin in most instances, although a slight increase in PO_2 has been reported. The pH is affected (lowered) only if high concentrations of heparin are used (25,000 IU per ml), but generally the tremendous buffering capacity of blood maintains a normal pH. The dead space of a 5-ml Luer-Lok glass syringe and a 22 gauge, 1 1/2-inch needle is 0.2 ml. Therefore, to minimize heparin related error, *at least 3 ml of blood should be collected*, even though blood gas analysis equipment requires only a 0.5-ml sample.

The arterial pulse is palpated to ascertain the

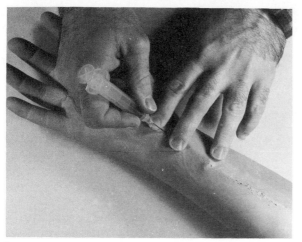

Figure 26–5. Arterial puncture at the wrist. The index and middle fingers are used to isolate the pulsating artery before insertion of the needle.

location of the vessel, and the overlying skin is sterilely prepared with an iodophor or other antiseptic solution. The patient's skin should then be anesthetized with a wheal of local anesthetic placed through a small (25 or 27) gauge needle. If the patient is unresponsive to pain in the area, this step may be omitted. Care must be taken to use a small amount of local anesthetic, because a large wheal may obscure the pulse.

The arterial pulsation is then isolated between the index and middle fingers of the nondominant hand (Fig. 26–5). The skin should be punctured through the anesthetic wheal, and the needle should be advanced toward the pulsating vessel. The needle should form an angle of about 15 to 20 degrees with the skin. A larger angle is required

for femoral artery puncture. Once the needle has entered the arterial lumen, the syringe plunger should be allowed to rise with the arterial pressure to minimize the chance of venous sampling. If no blood flow is obtained, the needle should be withdrawn slowly, because both walls of the vessel may have been punctured. A sample may be obtained during withdrawal. Redirection of the needle should occur only when the needle has been retracted to a location just deep to the dermis.

After a sample of at least 3 ml of blood has been obtained, the needle is removed from the artery and firm pressure is applied at the puncture site for a minimum of 5 minutes. Ten to 15 minutes of pressure is required if the patient is on anticoagulant therapy or has another coagulopathy.

Proper handling of the sample is very important. When the needle is withdrawn, it is imperative to expel any air bubbles that are present in the syringe to avoid false elevation of the PO_2.[15] Air in the sample will significantly increase the PO_2 (mean increase of 11 mmHg) after 20 minutes of storage, even if kept at 4°C. The pH and PCO_2 are not significantly altered by air bubbles if the blood is stored at 4°C for 20 minutes.

Removal of air is neatly and easily accomplished by placing an alcohol wipe or gauze sponge on the needle and tapping the inverted syringe to force any air to the top. Air is then pushed out of the needle, and any blood that is spilled will be caught by the sponge (Fig. 26–6). The needle is then plugged or removed, and the syringe is capped to ensure anaerobic conditions. Blood gas analysis is ideally performed immediately, but if this is not feasible, the sample may be stored in

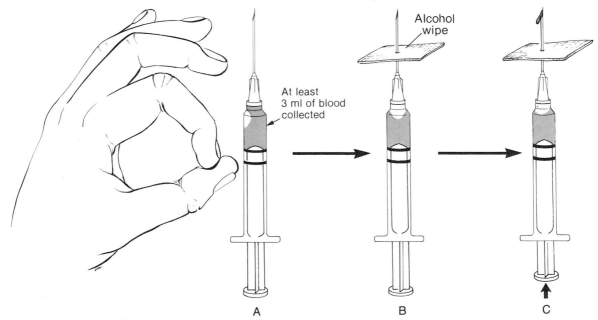

Figure 26–6. Removal of air bubbles from the syringe. A, Air bubbles are finger-tapped to the top of the syringe. B, Alcohol swab is placed over the top of the needle. C, Plunger is advanced to expel air while drops of blood are collected on the alcohol swab. After removal of the bubbles, the syringe is capped and sent to the laboratory.

ice water for 1 hour with limited deterioration.[15, 16] If the sample is stored anaerobically, regardless of the temperature, the PO_2, PCO_2, and pH are relatively stable for up to 20 minutes. If blood is stored at room temperature for longer than 20 minutes, the PCO_2 will increase and the pH will decrease, probably as a result of leukocyte metabolism. In a stored sample, the PO_2 varies to such an extent that the change is unpredictable for chemical interpretation at 30 minutes, regardless of storage method. High leukocyte counts, such as those seen in leukemic patients, may shorten acceptable storage intervals. Local anesthesia will make the procedures of arterial puncture easier for both the patient and the physician; however, one study found no significant alteration of PCO_2 or pH from the pain or anxiety of an unanesthetized arterial puncture (Table 26–3).[17]

PERCUTANEOUS TECHNIQUE FOR ARTERIAL CANNULATION

Percutaneous puncture is the preferred method for arterial cannulation. It is also the method of choice for obtaining an isolated blood gas sample (see the preceding section) when an indwelling cannula has not been placed.

The artery is entered as described in the preceding section, using a 20 gauge catheter-over-the-needle apparatus. Once the artery has been entered, bright red blood should be visible in the flash chamber of the cannula. Advance the needle about 1 mm into the vessel lumen (Fig. 26–7), then fix the needle while threading the catheter further into the lumen. When the needle is withdrawn, blood will pulsate from the catheter hub. Inadvertent puncture of the back wall of the artery can occur, and indeed, a variation of the percutaneous

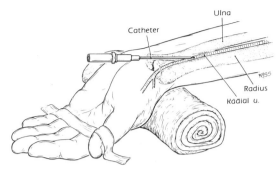

Figure 26–7. Percutaneous arterial cannulation at the wrist. The catheter unit is advanced 1 to 2 mm into the vessel lumen after blood first appears in the flash chamber. While the needle is fixed, the catheter is threaded over the needle. (From Beal, J.M. (ed.): Critical Care for Surgical Patients. New York, Macmillan Publishing Co., Inc., 1982. Used by permission.)

technique is to puncture both walls of the vessel with a single pass. If the back wall is punctured, the needle is withdrawn from the catheter and the catheter is slowly pulled back until a steady stream of blood flows from its hub. The catheter is then carefully advanced further into the lumen. The double puncture method is especially useful for cannulating small vessels.

Once the vessel has been entered, occasionally one will encounter difficulty advancing the catheter into the lumen. The "liquid stylet" method may aid further passage of the catheter.[18] A 10-ml syringe should be filled with about 5 ml of sterile normal saline. The syringe is then attached to the catheter hub, and 1 to 2 ml of blood should be easily aspirated to confirm intraluminal position. The fluid from the syringe is then slowly injected, and the catheter is advanced behind the fluid wave. One catheter set contains a wire stylet which permits a modified Seldinger technique for catheter placement; the over-the-needle catheter follows the self-contained guide wire during cannulation.

Once the catheter has been successfully placed, it should be advanced until the hub is in contact with the skin. The catheter is then secured by fastening it to the skin with suture material. To accomplish this, a moderate bite of skin is taken with the needle and a knot is tied in the suture. Care should be taken to avoid pinching the skin too tightly. The loose ends of the suture are then tied around the catheter without occluding the lumen by constriction.

After tying the catheter in place, a drop of antibiotic ointment is applied to the puncture site, and a self-adhesive dressing is applied over the area. The catheter and its connecting tubing are further secured with sterile sponges and adhesive tape. All tubing connections must be tight and secure. If the tubing inadvertently becomes disconnected, the patient may rapidly exsanguinate.

When successful arterial cannulation has been performed, the catheter should be attached to a

Table 26–3. PARAMETERS THAT AFFECT INTERPRETATION OF ABG

Parameter	Heparin*	Air Bubble in Sample	Delayed Analysis§
PO_2	No significant change**	Elevated	Variable‖
PCO_2	Lowered†	No significant change‡	Elevated¶
pH	Unchanged†	No significant change‡	Lowered¶

*Use only 1000 IU per ml concentration; fill dead space of needle and syringe only, and collect 3 ml of blood.
**There are reports of slight increases in PO_2 with excessive heparin.
†The falsely lowered PCO_2 that occurs with added heparin is the most clinically significant change noted.
‡If stored at 4°C for 20 minutes.
§Anaerobic storage at room temperature for 20 minutes results in no significant change.
‖Changes unpredictable at 30 minutes, regardless of storage method.
¶Minimal changes up to 2 hours, if stored at 4°C.

pressurized fluid-filled system. If the catheter has been placed for monitoring arterial blood pressure, it should be connected to a mechanical or electrical transducer by a short length of rigid plastic tubing filled with saline. A three-way stopcock is interposed between the patient and the transducer for blood gas sampling and to allow flushing of the system with heparinized saline (2 ml 1:1000 heparin per liter of saline). Flushing can be periodic or continuous at a rate of 3 to 4 ml per hour through a continuous flow device (see Fig. 26–3). Procurement of a blood sample from this system is easily performed. A syringe is attached to the three-way stopcock, and 4 to 5 ml of blood are aspirated and discarded to clear the line. A second syringe, which has been heparinized, is then attached, and 3 ml of blood are aspirated and sent for blood gas analysis. If the blood is to be used for other tests, the second syringe does not need to be heparinized. The stopcock and line should be flushed after sampling to avoid clotting.

SELDINGER TECHNIQUE FOR ARTERIAL CANNULATION

An alternative method of placing an indwelling cannula is by the Seldinger technique,[19] which is described in detail for venipuncture in Chapter 19. A needle is percutaneously placed into the arterial lumen, as described previously. A guide wire is then placed through the needle into the vessel lumen, and the needle is removed. A catheter is then threaded over the wire, and the wire is pulled out. As just mentioned, one commercial catheter permits the Seldinger technique to be performed without separate guidewire manipulation.

CUTDOWN TECHNIQUE FOR ARTERIAL CANNULATION

The cutdown technique is another common method of obtaining arterial access. Cannulation is performed after direct visualization of the vessel. A cutdown can be performed on any artery but is most commonly reserved for the brachial and other distal limb arteries. After a site has been selected, the overlying skin should be surgically prepared with an iodophor solution. The physician then puts on sterile gloves and drapes the extremity. Local anesthetic solution is injected subcutaneously in a horizontal line 2 to 3 cm long and perpendicular to the artery. Local anesthesia is not necessary if the patient is unconscious or is otherwise anesthetic at the cutdown site.

Using a scalpel with a No. 10 or 15 blade, the skin is incised along the anesthetic wheal. Underlying tissues are spread parallel to the artery with

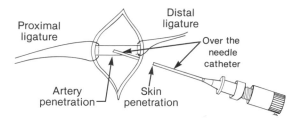

Figure 26–8. Placement of arterial line using cutdown technique. Note that the catheter enters the surgical wound percutaneously to minimize bacterial entry into the healing wound and to permit better stabilization of the catheter. Catheter entry of the vessel is more parallel to the vessel than illustrated.

a mosquito clamp. The pulse is palpated repeatedly throughout the procedure to ensure proper positioning. Once the surrounding soft tissue has been removed, exposing the artery for a distance of approximately 1 cm, the artery should be isolated by passing two silk sutures underneath it. Strip away only enough perivascular tissue to expose the artery. If it is cleaned totally, excessive bleeding may occur after catheter removal. Perivascular tissue will help to limit bleeding. A catheter-over-the-needle device, such as that used in the percutaneous method, is now introduced through the skin just distal to the incision and advanced into the surgical site (Fig. 26–8).[20] The arterial wall is punctured with the needle tip, and the catheter is threaded into the vessel lumen. When this has been accomplished, the two silk sutures, which have been used only to control the vessel, are removed and the skin incision is closed. The artery is not tied off as the vessel would be during a venous cutdown. Firm pressure, as used following arterial puncture, should be applied over the cutdown site. The separation of the soft tissue during the procedure may allow considerable hemorrhage into the tissue if pressure is not applied. The catheter is secured to the skin in the same manner as with the percutaneous method.

Arteries

RADIAL AND ULNAR

The radial artery is the artery that has most frequently been used for prolonged cannulation. A widespread collateral flow exists in the wrist. There are two major palmar anastomoses, known as *arches* (Fig. 26–9). The superficial palmar arch lies between the aponeurosis palmaris and the tendons of the flexor digitorum sublimis. The arch is formed mainly by the terminal ulnar artery and the superficial palmar branch of the radial artery. The other major communication of these two vessels, the deep palmar arch, is formed by connections of the terminal radial artery with the deep palmar branches of the ulnar artery.[21] Some collateral flow is almost always present at the wrist,

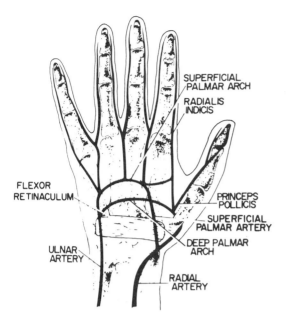

Figure 26–9. Arterial anatomy of the hand and wrist. (From Ramanathan, S., Chalon, J., and Turndorf, H.: Determining patency of palmar arches by retrograde radial pulsation. Anesthesiology 42:758, 1975. Used by permission.)

with the deep arch alone being complete in 97 per cent of 650 hand dissections.[22] In spite of Coleman's findings at autopsy, Friedman noted the absence of palpable ulnar pulses in 10 of 290 (3.4 per cent) healthy children and young adults.[23] Interestingly, this was always a bilateral finding. The radial pulses were present in 100 per cent of the subjects.

Fortunately, there is a simple test to determine the presence of collateral flow in the hand. This procedure has seen many modifications[24, 25] since being described by Allen in 1929.[26] In a cooperative patient, the basic Allen's test is performed as follows: The examiner occludes the radial and ulnar arteries with his hand, and the patient is asked to tightly clench his fist repetitively in order to exsanguinate his hand. The hand is then opened, and the examiner releases the occlusion of the ulnar artery (Fig. 26–10). After several minutes, the test is repeated with release of the radial artery. Rubor should rapidly return to the hand with release of either vessel.

A positive Allen's test, indicative of inadequate collateralization, is defined as the continued presence of pallor 5 to 15 seconds after release of the artery.[8, 21, 27, 28] If the return of color takes longer than 5 to 10 seconds, radial artery puncture should not be performed. One must be careful to avoid overextension of the hand with wide separation of the digits, because this may compress the palmar arches between fascial planes and give a false-positive result.[27] Barber and associates[24] report a modified Allen's test that is useful in unconscious or anesthetized patients who cannot clench their fists. An Esmarch bandage is used to exsanguinate

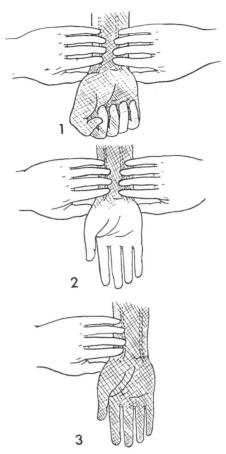

Figure 26–10. Allen's test. Before instrumenting the radial artery it is important to be sure that a competent ulnar artery is present. This can be done as follows:
1. The examiner compresses both arteries and the patient repeatedly makes a tight fist to squeeze all the blood out of the hand.
2. The patient then extends the fingers, and the examiner observes the blanched hand.
3. Compression of the ulnar artery is released, and the examiner observes the hand fill with blood. If filling does not occur within 5 to 10 seconds, radial artery puncture should not be done. If brisk filling occurs, the test is then repeated with release of the radial artery to assess radial artery patency. If both radial and ulnar arteries demonstrate patency, the wrist may be used for arterial puncture. (From Schwartz, G. R. (ed.): Principles and Practice of Emergency Medicine. Philadelphia, W. B. Saunders Company, 1978, p. 354. Used by permission.)

the hand, and the test is performed as previously described. Some variation of the Allen's test is indicated for every patient before ulnar or radial puncture for cannulation or blood gas sampling.

Once adequate collateral flow has been ascertained, arterial puncture may be performed. At the wrist, the radial artery rests on the flexor digitorium superficialis, flexor pollicus longus, the pronator quadratus, and against the radius.[22] Just distal to the styloid process of the radius, the artery winds around the lateral aspect of the wrist to the dorsum of the hand. The pulsation of the artery should be isolated on the palmar surface of the wrist where it is superficial. Dorsiflexing the wrist at about a 60 degree angle over a towel or sandbag, with or without fixing the wrist to an armboard, will help isolate and fix the artery (see Fig. 26-7).[8, 29, 30]

The ulnar artery may occasionally be used but is technically more difficult to puncture than the radial artery because of its smaller size. At the wrist, the ulnar artery runs along the palmar margin of the flexor carpi ulnaris in the space between it and the flexor digitorum sublimis.[22] In this area, it is in intimate contact with the ulnar nerve. The ulnar nerve and artery pass into the hand just radial to the pisiform bone. The ulnar artery can often be made more accessible with dorsiflexion of the wrist.

BRACHIAL

Barnes and colleagues[6] monitored 54 patients with an 18 or 20 gauge Teflon catheter percutaneously placed in the left brachial artery at the antecubital fossa. None of these patients developed Doppler evidence of brachial artery obstruction; however, partial to complete obstruction of the radial artery was noted in two patients and of the ulnar artery in one patient. None of these three patients exhibited ischemic symptoms. These authors also noted no clinical evidence of ischemia in 1000 brachial catheterizations over a period of 3 years. Thus, the brachial artery appears to be a safe site for arterial puncture, although collateral circulation in this area is not as great as in the hand.

The brachial artery begins as the continuation of the axillary artery and ends at the head of the radius, where it splits into the ulnar and radial arteries. The preferred site of puncture of the brachial artery is in or just proximal to the antecubital fossa. In this region, the vessel lies on top of the brachialis muscle and enters the fossa underneath the bicipital aponeurosis (Fig. 26-11). The median nerve runs along the medial side of the artery. Owing to reduced collateral circulation and the necessity of managing the arm in extension for puncture or prolonged cannulation, more distal vessels are preferred when the upper extremity is chosen for cannulation.

AXILLARY

Axillary artery cannulation as described by Adler and coworkers[31] is also a safe means of monitoring arterial blood pressure for a long period of time. The left axillary artery is preferred in order to decrease the possibility of cerebral embolization of flush solution or thrombus. The path from the left subclavian to the left carotid artery is less direct than on the right side, whereas the vertebrals are equally vulnerable.

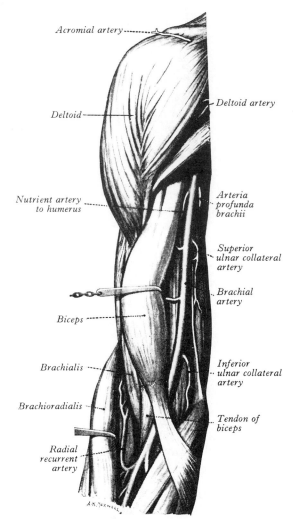

Figure 26-11. The right brachial artery and its branches. (From Warwick, R., and Williams, P. L. (eds.): Gray's Anatomy, 35th ed. Edinburgh, Churchill Livingstone, 1973, p. 650. Used by permission.)

To cannulate the axillary artery, the arm is held in 90 degree abduction. The axillary pulse is then palpated high in the axilla between the insertion of the pectoralis major and the deltoid muscles. The artery may then be cannulated percutaneously with or without a Seldinger guide wire. This site is technically more difficult and time consuming and probably should be avoided in the emergency department. No studies have been reported regarding large numbers of axillary punctures; therefore, the relative safety of this location cannot be determined.

DORSALIS PEDIS

The dorsalis pedis artery is a continuation of the anterior tibial artery. Anterior to the ankle joint, the dorsalis pedis runs from approximately half the way between the malleoli to the posterior end

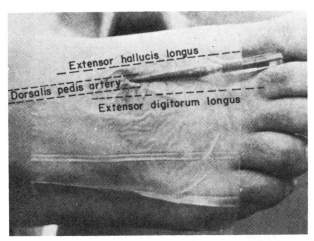

Figure 26–12. A No. 20 gauge catheter in the dorsalis pedis artery, illustrating the relationship to surrounding tendons. The catheter is secured with Steri-drape. Splinting is not needed. (From Johnstone, R. E., and Greenhow, D. E.: Catheterization of the dorsalis pedis artery. Anesthesiology 39:655, 1973. Used by permission.)

of the 1st metatarsal space, where it forms the dorsal metatarsal and deep plantar arteries. The lateral plantar artery, which is a branch of the posterior tibial, passes obliquely across the foot to the base of the 5th metatarsal. The plantar arch is completed where the lateral plantar artery joins the deep plantar artery between the 1st and 2nd metatarsals. On the dorsum of the foot, the dorsalis pedis artery lies in the subcutaneous tissue parallel to the extensor hallucis longus tendon, between it and the extensor digitorum longus (Fig. 26–12).[3] The artery should be cannulated in the midfoot region. Although this vessel is amenable to cutdown, the vascular anatomy of the foot is quite variable. This is of no consequence if a pulse can be palpated, but, Huber, in his dissection of 200 feet, noted the dorsalis pedis artery to be absent in 12 per cent.[32] In 16 per cent of patients, the dorsalis pedis artery provides the main blood supply to the toes.[33] Collateral flow can be determined with a modified Allen's test using the posterior tibial and dorsalis pedis arteries, but this is not as easily performed in the foot as in the hand. The pressure wave obtained with an electronic transducer attached to the dorsalis pedis artery will be 5 to 20 torr higher than that of the radial artery, and in addition, it will be delayed by about one tenth of a second.[34]

FEMORAL

Currently, the femoral artery is the second most commonly used vessel for prolonged arterial cannulation. Several studies have demonstrated the efficacy and safety of using this vessel, and indeed, several authors suggest that it should prob-

ably be the vessel of choice.[35–38] The femoral artery is the direct continuation of the iliac artery. The femoral artery enters the thigh after passing behind the inguinal ligament, where, in most patients, it may be easily palpated at a point midway between the pubic symphysis and the anterior superior iliac spine. When puncturing this vessel, care must be taken to avoid the femoral nerve and vein, which are in close proximity to the artery on the lateral and medial sides, respectively (Fig. 26–13).

A longer cannula is required for the femoral artery owing to the relatively greater depth at which it lies. The Seldinger technique is especially useful for this site, enabling the placement of a 6- to 8-inch plastic catheter for prolonged monitoring. Catheter-over-the-needle devices may also be used but should be at least 4 inches long. Use of catheter-through-the-needle devices has been reported[38] but should be avoided because of the possibility of leakage around the catheter, which may occur with high arterial pressures owing to the loose fit of the cannula in the hole in the vessel wall. Regardless of the device used, the needle should enter the skin at an angle of about 45 degrees instead of the usual 15 to 20 degree angle.

The large ratio of arterial diameter to that of the catheter is felt to beneficially reduce the incidence of thrombus, particularly total occlusion. In fact, no occlusions have been reported with femoral puncture for monitoring purposes.

A commonly postulated disadvantage of this site is the possibility of increased bacterial contamination because of its proximity to the warm, moist groin and perineum; however, no studies confirm this hypothesis. The femoral area is inconvenient for the patient who is awake and mobile, especially if he is capable of sitting in a chair. In spite of these theoretical difficulties, some large hospitals use femoral arterial lines almost exclusively, and the intensive care nursing staff is often more comfortable caring for these lines than those at other sites.

UMBILICAL AND TEMPORAL

In the neonate, arterial access can be accomplished through the umbilical artery for a short period of time. After this artery closes, the temporal artery provides a safe alternative. Prian describes the use of the temporal artery, noting its accessibility and the lack of clinical sequelae if it undergoes thrombosis.[39] The cutdown method should be used with a 22 gauge catheter after the artery's course has been traced with an ultrasonic flow detector. Because of the increasing accuracy of ear oximeters and the use of capillary blood gases for pH determination, prolonged arterial

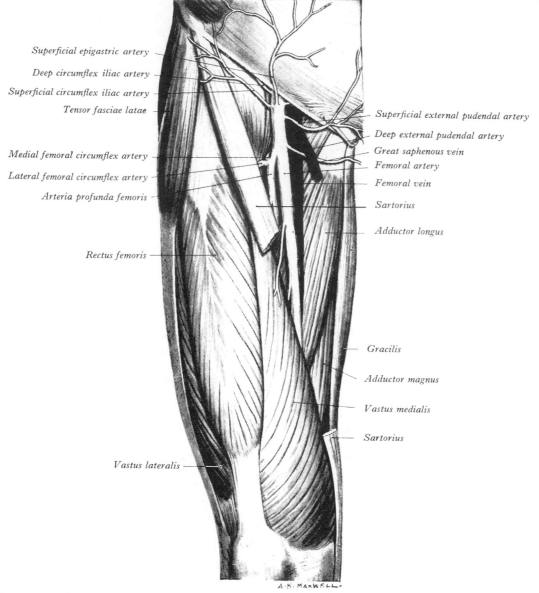

Figure 26–13. The right femoral vessels and some of their branches. The femoral nerve (not shown) lies lateral to the artery and may be deep to the artery. (From Warwick, R., and Williams, P. L. (eds.): Gray's Anatomy, 35th ed. Edinburgh, Churchill Livingstone, 1973, p. 676. Used by permission.)

cannulation will become less frequent during infant care. Further discussion of infant arterial cannulation is provided in Chapter 18.

Complications

Long-term arterial cannulation is safe if care is taken to avoid complications. Almost all the difficulties one may encounter can be avoided or their incidence markedly decreased if one adheres to a few simple principles. Reported clinical sequelae of arterial puncture and cannulation range from simple hematomas to life-threatening infections and exsanguination. The incidence of complica-

tions varies with the site and method of cannulation and with the skill and concern of the patient's physicians and nurses. It is difficult to compare complication rates at various sites, because most published studies have primarily used the radial artery. Many studies also report complications of puncture for arteriography and other procedures unrelated to long-term cannulation.

A commonly encountered problem is hematoma formation at the puncture site. Zorab[13] reported this complication in 50 per cent of catheterizations. The bruising was of minimal clinical significance in Zorab's study, but leakage, when it occurs, around the catheter or from the puncture site after its removal can be of danger to the patient.

Compression neuropathy secondary to bleeding has been reported after brachial artery puncture in anticoagulated patients; in some cases, surgical decompression was necessary.[2] The large amount of soft tissue surrounding the femoral artery makes bleeding in this area difficult to control.[40] Large hematomas are not uncommon after femoral artery catheterization; indeed, Soderstrom and associates[35] report two cases of bleeding that required transfusion after femoral puncture. Another patient suffered a large hematoma that became infected and required incision and drainage.

Prevention of bleeding complications may be accomplished with frequent careful inspection of the puncture site and with the use of prolonged compression after removal of the catheter or needle. Firm pressure should be maintained for at least 10 minutes after removal of a peripheral artery catheter and for a longer period of time after femoral cannulation or if the patient is anticoagulated. Five minutes of pressure is sufficient after puncture for a blood gas sample in an individual with normal coagulation. Exsanguination, a related complication, may occur if the arterial line apparatus becomes disconnected. This is more common in the obtunded or combative patient, and restraints are often required for patients with indwelling arterial cannulas. Exsanguination should not occur if tight connections are maintained throughout the system and if frequent, careful inspections of both the circuit and the patient are made.

Infection may be a complication of prolonged cannulation. Most catheter related infections begin as local infections at the puncture site and remain localized, although systemic sepsis has been reported.[40] Arterial cannulas are more prone to infectious complications than other vascular catheters. Many mechanisms have been proposed for this.[41–43] The arterial pressure monitoring system usually consists of a long column of fairly stagnant fluid and is subject to frequent manipulation. Stamm and colleagues[42] found that patients were at greater risk for systemic infection if they had an arterial line and required frequent blood gas determinations than if they had the cannula alone.[42] The sampling stopcock is a site of frequent bacterial contamination.

The risk of infection also increases as the duration of cannulation is prolonged. Catheters should be changed after 4 days if continued monitoring is necessary.[44] In addition, Makai and associates[43] recommend changing the entire fluid-filled system, including transducer chamber-domes and continuous flow devices, every 48 hours. Shinozaki and coworkers[45] demonstrated a marked reduction in equipment contamination when the continuous flush device was located just distal to the transducer, as opposed to the device being

positioned closer to the three-way stopcock used for sampling. This setup reduces the length of the static column of fluid between the sampling stopcock and the transducer. As mentioned previously, a drop of iodophor or antibiotic ointment applied to the puncture site will decrease the incidence of local wound infection.[44]

Thrombosis of the vessel in which the cannula is placed is another frequently encountered problem. The incidence with which this occurs varies with the method used to determine the presence of the clot. Bedford and Wollman[5] found a greater than 40 per cent occlusion rate when radial artery catheters were left in place for more than 20 hours. All these occluded vessels eventually recanalized. Angiographic studies show deposition of fibrin on 100 per cent of the catheters left in place for more than 1 day, although clinical evidence of ischemia secondary to occlusion with thrombus is present in less than 1 per cent in most studies.[4] Most reports of nonangiographic catheterizations that mention thrombosis study the radial artery. Therefore, it is difficult to compare the incidence of thrombosis at other sites, although during the 176 femoral catheterizations of Soderstrom and Ersoz[35, 38] dorsalis pedis pulses were decreased in only two patients and no clinical signs of ischemia were noted. Larger catheter sizes, trauma during cannulation, and the presence of atherosclerosis have all been postulated to increase the incidence of thrombosis; however, conflicting studies abound. Downs and colleagues associated tapered catheters with an increased incidence of thrombosis.[9]

Arterial spasm after puncture can predispose to thrombus formation and can even lead to ischemic changes without fibrin deposition. Successful reversal of spasm after intra-arterial lidocaine, reserpine, and phentolamine, has been reported, but no reliable studies of efficacy in this situation have been published.[46] Thrombosis can be minimized by decreasing the duration of catheterization, by proper flushing, and by using larger arteries. Surgical embolectomy or thrombectomy is rarely required, because the smaller vessels that are most likely to occlude usually have good collateral circulation. The performance of an Allen's test or a similar test before cannulating peripheral arteries is obviously important to ensure collateral flow. The larger femoral artery, which has poor collateralization, rarely if ever occludes with catheterization for monitoring purposes.

Another complication of thrombosis that must be mentioned is occlusion of the catheter. Times until occlusion of radial and femoral artery catheters were compared, and it was noted that radial cannulas became occluded at an average of 3.8 days, whereas femoral cannulas occluded after 7.3 days.[35] The importance of this comparison is minimal if the clinician follows infection prophylaxis guidelines and changes arterial catheters after 4 days.

A few less common complications are easily prevented. One such complication, which occurs only with the percutaneous catheter-through-the-needle method, is catheter embolization. Once the catheter has been placed through the needle, it should never be pulled back, because the end of the catheter may be sheared off by the sharp needle bevel. If this occurs, surgical removal of the catheter tip is necessary.

Skin necrosis is a complication of radial artery cannulation, involving an area of the volar forearm proximal to the cannula.[47, 48] Wyatt and colleagues[47] believe this is secondary to the poor blood supply of this area and state that the precautionary steps described previously will prevent or decrease the incidence of necrosis. One feared complication of indwelling radial and brachial arterial catheters is the occurrence of a cerebrovascular accident secondary to embolization from flushing of the catheters.[9, 49] As little as 3 to 12 ml of flush solution has been shown to reflux to the junction of subclavian and vertebral arteries.[49] This type of cerebral embolization can be prevented with the use of continuous flush systems (3 ml per hr) or with very small volumes (2 ml) of intermittent flush solution.

Complication rates also vary according to the method of arterial cannulation. Mortensen[50] studied the three main techniques, discussed in the section entitled Techniques, but unfortunately, most of these arterial cannulations were for angiographic purposes. The complications associated with prolonged cannulation time are therefore under-represented. For Mortenson's series, cutdown arteriotomy exhibited the lowest incidence of complications (7.7 per cent), whereas the Seldinger technique had a complications incidence of 17.7 per cent. Complications of percutaneous cannulation were 11.3 per cent. Apparently, false passage of the guide wire and/or the catheter were associated with increased intimal damage and complications. *It is imperative to advance the wire or catheter only if no resistance is met!*

In actuality, arterial puncture and cannulation are very safe procedures when care is taken and when a few basic principles are kept in mind. The operator should be skilled and concerned, thereby providing for an atraumatic insertion. Once the monitoring system has been set up, it should be manipulated as little as possible. Any handling should be performed with a flawless aseptic technique. The tubing and other fluid-filled devices should be changed every 48 hours, and catheters should be inserted into a vessel that provides a vessel-to-catheter ratio that is as great as possible without compromising other needs. If these principles are followed and if the patient and system

are carefully inspected at frequent intervals, complications of arterial puncture and cannulation will be greatly minimized.

Interpretation

An indwelling arterial cannula can provide valuable information about the hemodynamic status of a patient (continuous pressure monitoring) and about his respiratory and metabolic status (through intermittent sampling for blood gas analysis and other blood tests). The partial pressure of carbon dioxide and pH of the blood can be used to define four major groups of metabolic derangement: respiratory acidosis or alkalosis, and metabolic acidosis or alkalosis. Rarely will a disorder be strictly classified into one of these groups; however, a simple chart such as that shown in Figure 26–14 will assist one in determining the relative effects of metabolic and respiratory influence on the blood pH. A rough estimate of the contribution of respiratory factors may be made by assuming that for every 10 torr that the P_{CO_2} varies from 40, the pH will inversely vary 0.08 pH unit from 7.4. Adequacy of oxygenation of the blood can be determined from the measured P_{O_2} of the arterial blood and from the known concentration of oxygen that the patient is inspiring. To avoid iatrogenic complications of intensive care, one must be absolutely certain that the data are

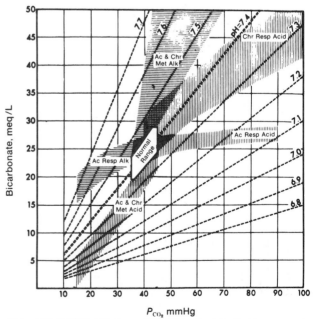

Figure 26–14. In vivo nomogram showing bands for uncomplicated respiratory or metabolic acid-base disturbances. Each "confidence" band represents the mean ± 2 S. D. for the compensatory response of normal subjects or patients to a given primary disorder. (Ac = acute, Chr = chronic, Resp = respiratory, Met = metabolic, Alk = alkalosis, Acid = acidosis) (From Thorn, G. W., Adams R. D., Braunwald, E., et al. (eds.): Harrison's Principles of Internal Medicine, 8th ed. New York, McGraw-Hill, Inc., 1977, p. 377. Used by permission.)

from an arterial sample that has been properly analyzed before basing one's treatment decisions on the numbers obtained. Not uncommonly, one may accidentally puncture a vein when attempting to obtain an arterial blood sample. Furthermore, false readings may result if the sample is not free of air bubbles, not promptly chilled, not analyzed within 20 to 30 minutes, or not corrected for body temperature.

An indwelling arterial catheter also provides continuous blood pressure monitoring. The trend of a patient's pressure helps one assess the effect of various therapeutic interventions. The absolute systolic and diastolic pressures measured will vary at different catheter sites, with higher peak systolic pressures measured at the periphery; the pressures will also be higher when measured in the distal lower limb.[10, 34] A wide variance between direct arterial pressure and that measured with a standard pneumatic cuff will always exist in some patients. Data averaged over a population group, however, compare fairly well.[10] For this reason, the cuff pressure and that displayed on the monitor should be compared regularly. A change in their relationship may be the first indication of difficulties with the direct measuring system. Auscultatory methods usually give a slightly lower value than direct measuring systems.

Waveform analysis may also provide an early indication of thrombosis in the arterial catheter. Many variables affect the waveform, including cardiac valvular disease, arteriosclerosis, and other peculiarities of an individual's cardiovascular system. Waveforms may vary tremendously between patients, but after an adequate monitoring system has been established, a change in an individual's pressure wave is usually indicative of thrombosis or other malfunction in the monitoring system. A change in waveform may also indicate a change in the patient's cardiovascular status, such as a papillary muscle rupture. Once again, before making a therapeutic decision based on an electronically generated number, the patient should be rechecked with a pneumatic cuff; this device is less fallible than the electromechanical system.

Conclusion

As intensive care knowledge and technology grow and develop, cannulation of the arterial system may become a more routine procedure. Nonetheless, devices are currently being developed, which, in some cases, may decrease the frequency with which this procedure is performed. Oximeters can determine the quality of oxygenation of the blood percutaneously and are becoming more accurate and sophisticated. Electronic sphygmomanometers are being refined for continuous indirect blood pressure monitoring. However, these devices will not soon replace the indwelling arterial cannula, because of the need for frequent blood sampling for chemical and hematologic analysis.

Arterial puncture and cannulation are invaluable aids to the emergency and critical care physician. Long-term catheterization is a safe procedure when care is taken from the time of insertion until after removal of the catheter. The radial artery is currently the most favored location for puncture, but as more experience is gained and reported with femoral artery catheterization, the latter may become a more frequently used site. Selection of either site is associated with a low complication rate and should be determined by the skill of the physician and his nursing team and the relative convenience and comfort of the patient.

1. Geddes, L. A.: The Direct and Indirect Measurement of Blood Pressure. Chicago, Year Book Medical Publishers, Inc., 1970.
2. Luce, E. A., Futrell, J. W., Wilgis, E. F., et al.: Compression neuropathy following brachial arterial puncture in anticoagulated patients. J. Trauma 16:717, 1976.
3. Gardner, R. M.: Direct blood pressure measurement. Dynamic response requirements. Anesthesiology 54:227, 1981.
4. Formanek, G., Frech, R. S., and Amplatz, K.: Arterial thrombus formation during clinical percutaneous catheterization. Circulation 41:833, 1970.
5. Bedford, R. F., and Wollman, H.: Complications of percutaneous radial-artery cannulation: an objective prospective study in man. Anesthesiology 38:228, 1973.
6. Barnes, R. W., Foster, E. J., Janssen, G. A., et al.: Safety of brachial arterial catheters as monitors in the intensive care unit prospective evaluation with the Doppler ultrasonic velocity detector. Anesthesiology 44:260, 1976.
7. Brown, A. E., Sweeney, D. B. Lumley, J.: Percutaneous radial artery cannulation. Anaesthesia 24:532, 1969.
8. Bedford, R. F.: Radial arterial function following percutaneous cannulation with 18 and 20 gauge catheters. Anesthesiology 47:37, 1977.
9. Downs, J. B., Rackstein, A. D., Klein, E. F., et al.: Hazards of radial-artery catheterization. Anesthesiology 38:283, 1973.
10. Bruner, J. M., Krenis, L. J., Kunsman, J. M., et al.: Comparison of direct and indirect methods of measuring arterial blood pressure (Parts I, II, III). Med. Instrum. 15:11–21, 97–101, 182–188, 1981.
11. McCutcheon, E. P., Evans, J. M., and Stanifer, R. R.: Direct blood pressure measurement: Gadgets vs progress. Anesth. Analg. 51:746, 1972.
12. Rothe, C. F., and Kim, K. C.: Measuring systolic arterial blood pressure. Possible errors from extension tubes or disposable transducer domes. Crit. Care Med. 18:683, 1980.
13. Zorab, J. S. M.: Continuous display of the arterial pressure: a simple manometric technique. Anaesthesia 24:431, 1969.
14. Goodwin, N. M., and Schreiber, M. T.: Effects of anticoagulants on acid-base and blood gas estimations. Crit. Care Med. 7:473, 1979.
15. Madiedo, G., Sciacca, R., and Hause, L.: Air bubbles and temperatures affect on blood gas analysis. J. Clin. Pathol. 33:864, 1980.
16. Beetham, R.: A review of blood pH and blood gas analysis. Ann. Clin. Biochem. 19:198, 1982.
17. Morgan, E. J.: The effects of unanesthetized arterial puncture on P_{CO_2} and pH. Am. Rev. Respir. Dis. 120:795, 1979.

18. Stirt, J. A.: "Liquid Stylet" for percutaneous radial artery cannulation. Can. Anaesth. Soc. J. 29:492, 1982.

19. Seldinger, S. I.: Catheter replacement of the needle in percutaneous angiography: a new technique. Acta Radiol. 39:368, 1953.

20. Bradley, M. N.: A technique for prolonged intra-arterial catheterization. Surg. Gynecol. Obstet. 119:117, 1964.

21. Ramanathan, S., Chalon, J., and Trundorf, H.: Determining patency of palmar arches by retrograde radial pulsation. Anesthesiology 42:756, 1975.

22. Coleman, S. S., and Anson, J. J.: Arterial patterns in the hand based upon a study of 650 specimens. Surg. Gynecol. Obstet. 113:409, 1961.

23. Friedman, S. A.: Prevalence of palpable wrist pulses. Br. Heart J. 32:316, 1970.

24. Barber, J. D., Wright, D. J., and Ellis, R. H.: Radial artery puncture: a simple screening test of the ulnar anastomotic circulation. Anaesthesia 2:291, 1973.

25. Ryan, J. F., Raines, J., Dalton, B. C., et al.: Arterial dynamics of radial artery cannulation. Anesth. Analg. 52:1017, 1973.

26. Allen, E. V.: Thromboangitis obliterans; methods of diagnosis of chronic occlusive arterial lesions distal to the wrist with illustrative cases. Am. J. Med. Sci. 178:237, 1929.

27. Palm, T.: Evaluation of peripheral arterial pressure on the thumb following radial artery cannulation. Br. J. Anaesth. 49:819, 1977.

28. Greenhow, D. E.: Incorrect performance of Allen's test—ulnar artery flow erroneously presumed inadequate. Anesthesiology 37:356, 1972.

29. Llamas, R., Gupta, S. K., and Baum, G. L.: A simple technique for prolonged arterial cannulation. Anesthesiology 31:289, 1969.

30. Brown, A. E., Sweeney, D. B., and Lumley, J.: Percutaneous radial artery cannualtion. Anaesthesia 24:532, 1969.

31. Adler, D. C., and Bryan-Brown, C. W.: Use of the axillary artery for intravascular monitoring. Crit. Care Med. 1:148, 1973.

32. Huber, J. F.: The arterial network supplying the dorsum of the foot. Anat. Rec. 80:373, 1941.

33. Spoerel, W. E., Deimling, P., and Aitkin, R.: Direct arterial pressure monitoring from the dorsalis pedis artery. Can. Anaesth. Soc. J. 22:91, 1975.

34. Johnstone, R. E., and Greenhow, D. E.: Catheterization of the dorsalis pedis artery. Anesthesiology 39:654, 1973.

35. Soderstrom, C. A., Wasserman, D. H., Dunham, C. M., et al.: Superiority of the femoral artery for monitoring: a prospective study. Am. J. Surg. 144:309, 1982.

36. Russell, J. A., Joel, M., Hudson, R. J., et al.: A prospective evaluation of radial and femoral artery catheterization sites in critically ill patients (abstr). Crit. Care Med. 9:144, 1981.

37. Gurman, G., and Schachar, J.: Femoral artery cannulation in critically ill patients (abstr). Crit. Care Med. 9:202, 1981.

38. Ersoz, C., J., Hedden, M., and Lain, L.: Prolonged femoral arterial catheterization for intensive care. Anesth. Analg. 49:160, 1970.

39. Prian, G. W.: Temporal artery catheterization for arterial access in the high risk newborn. Surgery, 82:734, 1977.

40. Berneus, B., Carlsten, A., Holmgren, A., et al.: Percutaneous catheterization of peripheral arteries as a method for blood sampling. Scand. J. Clin. Lab. Invest. 6:217, 1954.

41. Makai, D. G.: Nosocomial bacteremia: an epidemiologic overview. Am. J. Med. 70:719, 1981.

42. Stamm, W. E., Colella, J. J., Anderson, R. L., et al.: Indwelling arterial catheters as a source of nosocomial bacteremia: an outbreak caused by flavobacterium species. N. Engl. J. Med. 292:1099, 1975.

43. Makai, D. G., and Hassemer, C. A.: Endemic rate of fluid contamination and related septicemia in arterial pressure monitoring. Am. J. Med. 70:733, 1981.

44. Makai, D. G., and Bank, J. D.: A comparative study of polyantibiotic and iodophor ointments in prevention of vascular catheter-related infection. Am. J. Med. 70:739, 1981.

45. Shinozaki, T., Deane, R. S., Mazuzan, J. E., et al.: Bacterial contamination of arterial lines. A prospective study. JAMA 249:223, 1983.

46. Dalton, B., and Laver, M.: Vasospasm with an indwelling radial artery cannula. Anesthesiology 34:194, 1971.

47. Wyatt, R., Glaves, I., and Cooper, D. J.: Proximal skin necrosis after radial-artery cannulation. Lancet 1:1135, 1974.

48. Johnson, R. W.: A complication of radial-artery cannulation. Anesthesiology 40:598, 1974.

49. Lowenstein, E., Little, J. W., and Lo, H. H.: Prevention of cerebral embolization from flushing radial-artery cannulas. N. Engl. J. Med. 285:414, 1971.

50. Mortensen, J. D.: Clinical sequelae from arterial needle puncture, cannulation, and incision. Circulation 35:1118, 1967.

27

The Clinical Use of Orthostatic Vital Signs

TERRY M. WILLIAMS, M.D.
ROBERT KNOPP, M.D.

Introduction

The clinician is frequently faced with the need for determining the amount of blood loss or volume depletion in a patient in the emergency department. When the clinical syndrome of shock exists, assessment of blood volume deficit poses little difficulty. It is preferable, however, that volume loss be detected before physiologic compensation is overcome and clinical shock occurs.

Many techniques have been advocated to assess volume status. Unfortunately, most of these procedures lack a data base on which to judge their reliability. Methods that have been recommended include evaluation of the following parameters: skin color; skin turgor; skin temperature; supine, serial, and orthostatic vital signs; neck vein status; transcutaneous oxymetry; and hemodynamic monitoring techniques, such as monitoring of central venous and pulmonary artery pressure. Serial vital signs have been used but do not reliably detect small degrees of blood loss.[1–5] *Up to 15 per cent of the total blood volume can be lost with minimal hemodynamic changes or alteration of the supine vital signs.*[1, 6–8] A decrease in the pulse pressure occurs with acute blood loss,[5, 6, 9] but often the patient's baseline blood pressure values are unknown. Clinical examination of neck veins adds useful information but is less precise than measurement of central venous pressure. Most clinicians use skin color, temperature, and moisture as a reflection of skin perfusion and sympathetic tone but not as an accurate guide to circulatory volume, since the vasomotor tone of the skin is affected by numerous diseases as well as emotional and enviromental factors. Measurement of the urinary output provides an excellent means of monitoring the patient but is not useful in the rapid bedside assessment of acute blood loss or volume depletion.

Central venous pressure and pulmonary artery pressure measurements add useful information in determining volume status but require invasive techniques and are not without complications.[10] The central venous pressure is dependent on four independent variables: intravascular volume, venomotor tone, right ventricular function, and intrathoracic pressure. The complex interaction of these variables can make interpretation of central venous pressure readings difficult. For example, a healthy patient may be able to accept a large intravascular volume overload with little change in the central venous pressure. A patient with isolated left heart failure, however, may have relative volume overload with no elevation in the central venous pressure. Pulmonary artery pressure provides more accurate assessment of left heart function but is usually not practical in the emergency department.[10]

Radionuclide blood volume determinations are accurate but not feasible in the acute setting of the emergency department. Transcutaneous oxymetry is noninvasive, but further study is required to determine its limitations during clinical assessment of volume depletion.[11]

The ideal test for determining volume status would rapidly and accurately detect volume depletion of 5 per cent or more using a noninvasive technique. At present, no such test exists. Orthostatic vital signs meet the criteria of being noninvasive and easily used at the bedside, although, in patients with acute blood loss of less than 20 per cent of their total blood volume, orthostatic vital signs lack both sensitivity and specificity.[12]

Orthostatic vital signs tend to be misused in clinical practice, largely because of confusion regarding what constitutes a positive or negative test. Bates[13] and others [14–16] have stated that postural hypotension or postural tachycardia will occur with varying degrees of hypovolemia but do not define specific criteria for a positive test. Other sources (without documentation) have perpetuated the notion that relatively small changes in the orthostatic blood pressure or the pulse are reliable in detecting hypovolemia.[17–19] Hayes and Briggs[17] state that a "decrease of 10 mm Hg or more on assuming the sitting position indicates significant hypovolemia." Jacobson[18] notes that "especially upon standing . . . a drop in systolic blood pressure of 10 mm Hg or an increased pulse of 10 beats per minute is consistent with hypovolemia." Watkins[19] states that with a 15-degree tilt "a pulse increase of more than 10 beats per minute, or a drop in blood pressure of more than 10 mm Hg, indicates hypovolemia."

In this chapter we will discuss the physiologic compensatory mechanisms that are activated by hypovolemia and postural tilting and the clinical use of orthostatic vital signs.

Physiologic Response to Hypovolemia

Acute blood loss decreases the pressure gradient between the venules and the right atrium. A fall in this pressure gradient decreases venous return.[20] As a result, cardiac output falls and the clinical manifestations of shock ensue.[7] Several homeostatic mechanisms are initiated by blood loss (Table 27–1). At first, the dominant compensatory mechanism in shock is a reduction in carotid sinus baroreceptor inhibition of sympathetic outflow to the cardiovascular system.[21] This increased sympathetic outflow results in several effects: (1) arteriolar vasoconstriction, which greatly increases total peripheral vascular resistance; (2) constriction of venous capacitance vessels, thereby increasing venous return to the heart; and (3) an increase of heart rate and force of contraction, which helps to maintain cardiac output in spite of significant volume loss.[7] These sympathetic reflexes are geared more for the maintenance of arterial pressure than for the maintenance of cardiac output (Fig. 27–1), because the increase in peripheral vascular resistance has no direct beneficial effect on cardiac output.[7] The value of sympathetic reflex compensation is illustrated by the fact that 30 to 40 per cent of the blood volume can be lost before death will occur, while these reflexes are intact.[7] When the sympathetic reflexes are absent, loss of only 15 to 20 per cent of the blood volume may cause death.[7, 8]

Several other reflexes serve to maintain cardiac output in the presence of volume loss. The central nervous system ischemic response elicits a powerful sympathetic stimulation after the arterial pressure falls below 50 mm Hg and is responsible for the second plateau on the arterial pressure curve (see Fig. 27–1).[7] Other compensatory mechanisms that tend to restore the blood volume to normal include the formation of angiotensin and

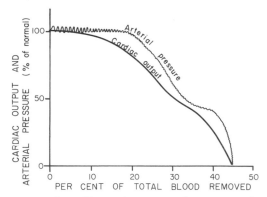

Figure 27–1. Effect of hemorrhage on cardiac output and arterial pressure. (From Guyton, A. C.: Textbook of Medical Physiology, 6th ed. Philadelphia, W. B. Saunders Company, 1981. Used by permission.)

antidiuretic hormone, which cause arteriolar vasoconstriction and conservation of salt and water by the kidneys.[7, 22] There is also a fluid shift from the interstitium to the intravascular space that works to restore blood volume over a longer period (1 to 40 hours).[7, 23, 24]

When blood loss results in anemia, part of the loss in oxygen-carrying capacity is countered by an increase in tissue oxygen extraction.[25] Finally, the lost red cell mass is slowly replaced by erythropoiesis.

Several investigators examined the changes in blood pressure and pulse that occur with blood loss. Ebert and coworkers[2] acutely removed 15.5 to 19.7 per cent of the total blood volume from six volunteers. Five of the six developed a pulse increase of 14 to 30 beats per minute followed by a fall in arterial pressure and bradycardia (36 to 40 beats per minute). Skillman and associates[3] found that after a loss of 15 per cent of the blood volume there is a modest increase in the pulse (9 beats per minute) and a transient fall in the blood pressure followed by a return of the blood pressure to normal. Others[1, 4, 5] have noted a variable response to blood loss of up to 1 L. The inability to detect volume loss with supine vital signs and the observation that patients with acute volume loss frequently develop syncope on arising has led to the use of orthostatic vital signs. Ironically, few data exist regarding this simple bedside test in our present era of advanced technology and invasive monitoring.

Table 27–1. HOMEOSTATIC MECHANISMS IN HEMORRHAGIC SHOCK

Sympathetic reflex compensation
   Arteriolar vasoconstriction
   Venous capacitance vasoconstriction
   Increased inotropic and chronotropic cardiac activity
   Central nervous system ischemic response

Selective increase in cerebral and coronary perfusion by
   means of local autoregulation

Increased oxygen unloading in tissues

Restoration of blood volume
   Renin-angiotensin-aldosterone axis activation
   Antidiuretic hormone secretion
   Transcapillary refill
   Increased thirst resulting in increased fluid intake
   Increased erythropoiesis

Physiologic Response to Tilting

When an individual assumes the upright posture, complex homeostatic mechanisms compensate for the effects of gravity on the circulation in order to maintain cerebral perfusion. These responses include (1) baroreceptor-mediated arteriolar vasoconstriction, (2) venous constriction and increased muscle tone in the legs and the abdomen to augment venous return, (3) sympathetic-mediated inotropic and chronotropic effects on the heart, and (4) activation of the renin-angiotensin-aldosterone system.[26]

These compensatory mechanisms preserve cerebral perfusion in the upright position with minimal changes in vital signs. Currens[27] found that when *normal* subjects stand, there is an average pulse increase of 13 beats per minute, no change or a small drop in systolic blood pressure, and either no change or a small rise in diastolic blood pressure. These changes have been confirmed by others.[12, 28, 29]

The Trendelenburg position (head-down tilt) has long been assumed to have beneficial effects on venous return, cardiac output, and cerebral perfusion in hypotensive patients. These effects can be considered the converse of the circulatory changes that occur in the erect position. Unfortunately, few data substantiating a beneficial hemodynamic effect of the Trendelenburg position exist, and the use and actual clinical value of the position have been questioned by some authors. Sibbald and coworkers[30] failed to detect any consistent or beneficial effect of the Trendelenburg position in hypotensive patients. The authors argue against the use of the head-down tilt in critically ill patients because of detrimental effects on pulmonary physiology.[30]

Many conditions affect the compensatory mechanisms that allow us to assume the upright posture (Table 27–2).[26] Because of decreased vasomotor tone, limited chronotropic response, and other factors, the elderly have a higher incidence of orthostatic hypotension, which can lead to syncope and fall-related injury.[31] One should note that drugs (such as beta-blocking agents and vasodilating drugs) that pharmacologically antagonize the normal autonomic compensatory mechanisms can also produce orthostatic changes. The changes are often enough to produce frank syncope, espcially in the elderly. Even in normal subjects, passive tilting will generate a high incidence of orthostatic syncope.[32] Patients with chronic anemia (and a compensated blood volume) seem to have the same postural response as normal subjects.[33, 34] Most of the conditions that affect postural blood pressure regulation have a sympathetic nervous system pathologic condition as a common denominator.

Few data exist on the effect of acute blood loss on postural vital signs. Shenkin and associates[5] studied 23 young adult volunteers bled from 500 to 1200 ml. They found no reliable change in the postural blood pressure but a postural increase in the pulse of 35 to 40 per cent after a 500-ml blood loss. In the six subjects who were bled approximately 1 L, only two were able to tolerate standing; each of them had postural increases in pulse of more than 30 beats per minute. The other four

Table 27–2. CLASSIFICATION OF DISORDERS OF POSTURAL BLOOD PRESSURE REGULATION*

I. Poor postural adjustment
    Tall, asthenic habitus
    Advanced age
    Physical exhaustion
    Prolonged recumbency
    Pregnancy
    Gastrectomy
II. Orthostatic hypotension
  A. Secondary orthostatic hypotension
    1. Endocrinologic-metabolic disorders
        Diabetes mellitus
        Primary amyloidosis
        Primary and secondary adrenal insufficiency
        Pheochromocytoma
        Primary aldosteronism with marked hypokalemia
        Porphyria
    2. Central and peripheral nervous system disorders
        Intracranial tumors (parasellar and posterior fossa)
        Idiopathic paralysis agitans
        Wernicke's encephalopathy
        Multiple cerebral infarcts
        Brain stem lesions
        Tabes dorsalis
        Syringomyelia
        Traumatic and inflammatory myelopathies
        Guillain-Barré syndrome
        Chronic inflammatory polyradiculoneuropathy
        Peripheral neuropathies
        Familial dysautonomia (Riley-Day syndrome)
    3. Miscellaneous disorders
        Hypovolemia
        Hypochromic anemia
        Electrolyte disturbance
        Psychotropic and antihypertensive drugs
        Extensive surgical sympathectomy
        Chronic hemodialysis
        Anorexia nervosa
        Hyperbradykininism
  B. Primary or idiopathic orthostatic hypotension
    Idiopathic orthostatic hypotension
    Idiopathic orthostatic hypotension with somatic neurologic deficit (Shy-Drager syndrome)

*From Thomas, J. E., Schirger, A., Fealey, R. D., et al.: Orthostatic hypotension. Mayo Clin. Proc. 56:117, 1981. Used by permission.

subjects experienced severe symptoms on standing followed by a marked bradycardia and syncope if they were not allowed to lie down.

Green and Metheny[34] studied the effect of passive tilting to 75 degrees in normal subjects and volunteers bled 500 to 1500 ml. Before phlebotomy, the pulse increase on tilting never exceeded 25 beats per minute. After a blood loss of 1000 ml, the pulse increase on tilting always exceeded 25 beats per minute. The investigators were unable to detect blood loss of 500 ml using these criteria and did not find reliable postural blood pressure changes after phlebotomy. These results have limited direct bedside application, because a tilt table was used.

Knopp and colleagues[12] phlebotomized 100 subjects from 450 to 1000 ml. By using the criteria of a pulse increase of 30 beats per minute or the presence of severe symptoms (syncope or near syncope) during a supine-to-standing test, they were able to distinguish accurately between a 1000-ml blood loss and no blood loss. It should be noted that some patients may become syncopal with a transiently normal blood pressure if vaso-constriction on standing preserves blood pressure at the expense of cerebral blood flow. Changes in blood pressure and pulse were not evaluated in the symptomatic subjects. Most likely, these patients would have had more pronounced blood pressure changes than asymptomatic patients had they not been permitted to lie down immediately. In the study population of normal healthy volunteers with acute blood loss, the sensitivity and specificity using the aforementioned criteria for detecting a 1000-ml blood loss were both 98 per cent, giving an accuracy of 96 per cent (2 per cent false-negatives and 2 per cent false-positives). The investigators were unable to detect blood loss of 500 ml consistently by using these criteria.

Another complicating factor in interpreting orthostatic vital signs is the development of paradoxic bradycardia in the presence of blood loss. Shenkin,[5] Ebert,[2] and Green[34] noted that when orthostatic syncope occurred, it was accompanied by hypotension and bradycardia. Stair[35] and Cobb[36] recently described women with hemoperitoneum secondary to ruptured ectopic pregnancy who were hypotensive but not tachycardic. The absence of tachycardia persisted with standing, but orthostatic symptoms occurred.[37] Knopp and associates[12] included orthostatic symptoms (syncope or near syncope requiring the patient to lie down) as one of the criteria for a positive tilt test. Jansen[38] reviewed other cases of this "relative bradycardia" that occurred in hypotensive patients with acute intraperitoneal bleeding and postulated a parasympathetic mechanism triggered by the presence of free blood in the peritoneal cavity. This bradycardia is reversed with atropine. Several central nervous system factors can contribute to vagal-mediated syncope in emergency department patients with acute traumatic blood loss. These factors include pain, the sight of blood, stress, and nausea. The incidence of paradoxic bradycardia in patients with profound intravascular volume loss or shock from other causes is unknown. *When the patient's clinical presentation is consistent with volume loss or shock, the clinician should not allow the absence of tachycardia to change his assessment.*

Clinical Use of Orthostatic Vital Signs

INDICATIONS AND CONTRAINDICATIONS

When the volume status of a patient is assessed by use of orthostatic vital signs, several points

should be remembered. Many factors influence orthostatic blood pressure, including age, pre-existing medical conditions, the use of medication, and idiopathic orthostatic hypotension (see Table 27–2). Data relating the effect of blood loss to orthostatic vital signs are limited to phlebotomized healthy volunteers. *These results should be extrapolated with great care to patients with anemia, dehydration, or painful trauma, and the limitations of these studies should be recognized.* The clinician must consider the clinical condition of the patient as well as orthostatic vital signs in evaluating a patient for volume depletion.

Orthostatic vital signs are indicated as part of the evaluation of any patient with known or suspected volume loss or a history of syncope, except in the case of the following contraindications: The use of orthostatic vital signs is unnecessary and dangerous in a patient who manifests the clinical syndrome of shock. Orthostatic vital sign evaluation is also contraindicated in patients with a severely altered mental status, in the setting of possible spinal injuries, and in patients with lower extremity or pelvic fractures.

TECHNIQUE

Once the decision to obtain orthostatic vital signs has been made, the blood pressure and pulse are recorded after the patient has been in the supine position for 2 to 3 minutes (Table 27–3). The patient should be resting quietly. No painful or invasive procedures should be performed during the test. Anxiety, fever, and other causes of resting tachycardia may make the test uninterpretable.[39] The use of antihypertensive medications may also invalidate the test.

The patient is then asked to *stand*, and the examiner should be prepared to assist the patient if he develops severe symptoms or syncope. The supine-to-standing test is more accurate than a

Table 27–3. SUMMARY OF ORTHOSTATIC TILT TESTING

Procedure
1. Blood pressure and pulse are recorded after patient has been supine for 2 to 3 minutes.
2. Blood pressure, pulse, and symptoms are recorded *after patient has been standing for 1 minute.* The patient should be permitted to resume a supine position immediately should syncope or near syncope develop.

Positive Test
1. Increase in pulse of 30 beats per minute or more.
2. Presence of symptoms of hypovolemia (dizziness, syncope).
3. Drop in systolic blood pressure of greater than 30 mm Hg.*

*Arbitrary number based on editors' clinical experience. (See text for explanation.)

supine-to-sitting evaluation. Knopp and coworkers[12] found that the supine-to-sitting test was not reliable for detecting 1000 ml of blood loss (55 per cent false-negatives). If the patient develops severe symptoms (defined as syncope or extreme dizziness requiring him to lie down) on standing, the test is positive and should be terminated. If the patient is not symptomatic, the blood pressure and pulse should be recorded after the patient has been standing for one minute. This interval resulted in the greatest difference between the control and 1000-ml phlebotomy groups in Knopp's study.[12]

In the setting of possible blood loss, if the patient has a pulse rise of 30 beats per minute or severe symptoms and if other complicating factors have been excluded, then blood loss is highly likely (2 per cent false-positive rate).[12] The presence of a negative test indicates only that an acute blood loss of 1000 ml is unlikely (2 per cent false-negative rate); a blood loss of 500 ml cannot be excluded (43 per cent false-negative rate).[12]

Criteria for significant blood pressure changes cannot be emphasized because of the lack of correlation between blood pressure in the phlebotomy and control groups in Knopp's study,[12] but certainly a drop of systolic blood pressure of more than 30 mm Hg should be viewed as suggestive of significant hypovolemia.

COMPLICATIONS

The possible complications of orthostatic vital sign assessment can be avoided if the aforementioned contraindications and precautions are remembered. Complications include syncope with a resulting fall and injury and the possibility of exacerbating an existing fracture or spinal cord injury.

Conclusions

Orthostatic vital signs can provide valuable information in the overall assessment of patients suffering from blood loss or volume depletion. Unfortunately, few studies provide us with an adequate data base on which to interpret the results of this test. Orthostatic vital signs are generally overinterpreted in clinical medicine. In the setting of acute blood loss in otherwise healthy patients, a pulse increase of 30 beats per minute or severe symptoms on standing indicates that blood loss has occurred (96 per cent accuracy). The proper interpretation of orthostatic vital signs should enable the clinician to detect volume loss before the clinical syndrome of shock develops.

1. Burri, C., Henkemeyer, H., Passler, H. H., et al.: Evaluation of acute blood loss by means of simple hemodynamic parameters. Prog. Surg. 11:109, 1973.
2. Ebert, R. V., Stead, E. A., and Gibson, J. G.: Response of normal subjects to acute blood loss. Arch. Intern. Med. 68:578, 1941.
3. Skillman, J. J., Olson, J. E., Lyons, J. H., and Moore, F. D.: The hemodynamic effect of acute blood loss in normal man, with observations on the effect of the Valsalva maneuver and breath holding. Am. Surg. 166:713, 1967.
4. Shenkin, H. A., Cheney, R. H., Govons, S. R., et al.: Effects of acute hemorrhage of known amount on the circulation of essentially normal persons (abstract). Am. J. Med. Sci. 206:806, 1943.
5. Shenkin, H. A., Cheney, R. H., Govons, S. R., et al.: On the diagnosis of hemorrhage in man, a study of volunteers bled large amounts. Am. J. Med. Sci. 208:421, 1944.
6. Walt, A. J. (ed.): Early Care of the Injured Patient. Philadelphia, W. B. Saunders Co., 1982.
7. Guyton, A. C.: Textbook of Medical Physiology, 6th ed. Philadelphia, W. B. Saunders Co., 1981.
8. Zuidema, G. D. (ed.): The Management of Trauma, 3rd ed. Philadelphia, W. B. Saunders Co., 1979.
9. American College of Surgeons Committee on Trauma: Advanced Trauma Life Support Course Student Manual. American College of Surgeons, Chicago, Illinois, 1981.
10. Hartong, J. M., and Dixon, R. S.: Monitoring resuscitation of the injured patient. JAMA 237:242, 1977.
11. Podolsky, S., Baraff, L. J., Geehr, E., et al.: Transcutaneous oxymetry measurements during acute blood loss. Ann. Emerg. Med. 11:523, 1982.
12. Knopp, R., Claypool, R., and Leonardi, D.: Use of the tilt test in measuring acute blood loss. Ann. Emerg. Med. 9:29, 1980.
13. Bates, B.: A guide to physical examination. Philadelphia, J. B. Lippincott Co., 1979.
14. Delp, M. H., and Manning, R. T.: Major's Physical Diagnosis: An Introduction to the Clinical Process, 9th ed. Philadelphia, W. B. Saunders Co., 1981.
15. Prior, J. A., Silberstein, J. S., and Stang, J. M.: Physical Diagnosis: The History and Examination of the Patient, 6th ed. St. Louis, C. V. Mosby, 1981.
16. Weil, M. H., and Shubin, H.: Diagnosis and Treatment of Shock. Baltimore, Williams & Wilkins, 1967.
17. Hayes, H. R., and Briggs, B. A.: MGH Textbook of Emergency Medicine. Baltimore, Williams & Wilkins, 1978.
18. Jacobson, S.: Errors in emergency practice. Emerg. Med. 10:124, 1978.
19. Watkins, G. M.: Diagnosing multiple trauma, insights into the art of recognizing automobile injuries. Curr. Concepts Trauma Care, June, 1978, p. 3.
20. Holcroft, J. W.: Impairment of venous return in hemorrhagic shock. Surg. Clin. North Am. 62:17, 1982.
21. Berne, R. M. (ed.): Handbook of Physiology, vol. 1. Bethesda, American Physiological Society, 1979, p. 645.
22. Gann, D. S.: Endocrine control of plasma protein and volume. Surg. Clin. North Am. 56:1135, 1976.
23. Drucker, W. R., Chadwick, C. D. J., and Gann, D. S.: Transcapillary refill in hemorrhage and shock. Arch. Surg. 116:1344, 1981.
24. Moore, F. D.: The effects of hemorrhage on body composition. N. Engl. J. Med. 273:567, 1965.
25. Watkins, G. M., Rabelo, A., Bevilacqua, R. G., et al.: Bodily changes in repeated hemorrhage. Surg. Gynecol. Obstet. 139:161, 1974.
26. Thomas, J. E., Schirger, A., Fealey, R. D., et al.: Orthostatic hypotension. Mayo Clin. Proc. 56:117, 1981.
27. Currens, J. H.: A comparison of the blood pressure in the lying and standing positions: A study of five hundred men and five hundred women. Am. Heart J. 35:646, 1948.
28. Hull, D. H., Wolthius, R. A., Cortese, T., et al.: Borderline

hypertension versus normotension. Differential response to orthostatic stress. Am. Heart J. 94:414, 1977.

29. Stair, I.: Clinical studies in incoordination of the circulation as determined by the response to arising. J. Clin. Invest. 22:813, 1943.

30. Sibbald, W. J., Paterson, N. A. M., Holliday, R. L., et al.: The Trendelenburg position: Hemodynamic effects in hypotensive and normotensive patients. Crit. Care Med. 7:218, 1979.

31. Caird, F. I., Andrews, G.R., and Kennedy, R. D.: Effect of posture on blood pressure in the elderly. Br. Heart J. 35:527, 1973.

32. Stevens, P. M.: Cardiovascular dynamics during orthostatism and the influence of intravascular instrumentation. Am. J. Cardiol. 17:211, 1966.

33. Duke, M., and Abelmann, W. H.: The hemodynamic response to chronic anemia. Circulation 39:503, 1969.

34. Green, D. M., and Metheny, D.: The estimation of acute blood loss by the tilt test. Surg. Gynecol. Obstet. 84:1045, 1947.

35. Stair, T.: Orthostatic tachycardia and ectopic pregnancy (letter). Ann. Emerg. Med. 11:284, 1982.

36. Cobb, T. L.: Orthostatic tachycardia and ectopic pregnancy. Normal pulse rate in the presence of massive hemorrhage (letter). Ann. Emerg. Med. 11:589, 1982.

37. Stair, T.: Orthostatic tachycardia and ectopic pregnancy (reply). Ann. Emerg. Med. 11:590, 1982.

38. Jansen, R. P. S.: Relative bradycardia: A sign of acute intraperitoneal bleeding. Aust. N.Z. J. Obstet. Gynaecol. 18:206, 1978.

39. Bergman, G. E., Reisner, F. F., and Anwar, R. A. H.: Orthostatic changes in normovolemic children: an analysis of the "tilt test." J. Emerg. Med. 1:137, 1983.

28

Transfusion Therapy: Blood and Blood Products

GARRETT E. BERGMAN, M.D.

Introduction

Transfusion of whole blood or its components (red cells, white cells, platelets, whole plasma or plasma fractions) is indicated to replace certain deficiencies manifested by patients. The indications for the transfusion of *whole* blood have diminished as recent technical advances have made specific component replacement more feasible. Appropriate administration of blood products may be a lifesaving procedure in some emergency circumstances but may also be indicated as a prophylactic measure in less urgent situations. By law, transfusions can be given only by a physician; potential life-threatening complications can result, as is true of any intravenous infusion. Almost all physicians have participated in (or independently performed) a blood transfusion *without necessarily knowing* the indications, benefits, proper procedures, risks, or potential complications.

In this chapter, techniques related to transfusion of blood and its components will be presented to provide a comprehensive overview of a very common procedure. Equipment will be discussed, but commercially available equipment systems will *not* be described at length. Representative devices or material will be arbitrarily chosen and described as prototypes; some comparable items produced by other manufacturers will be mentioned, and significant differences or advantages will be highlighted. The reader should bear in mind that several manufacturers may produce similar products of similar utility.

Background and Historical Perspective

Blood Groups. In the seventeenth century, radically daring physicians were experimenting with the transfusion of blood from animals into humans to treat a variety of ills.[1, 2] Around the beginning of the century it became obvious that only human blood was fit for humans. Landsteiner found that most human serum contained naturally occurring substances that would react with the red cells of some, but not all, other humans, thereby discovering the ABO red cell antigen-antibody system.

Red Cell Antigens and Antibodies. An integral part of the red cell membrane is a series of glycoprotein moieties, or antigens, which give the cell an individual identity. Two different genetically determined antigens, type A and type B, occur on the surface of red blood cells (RBCs). The RBCs of any individual may have one, both, or neither of these antigens. Because the type A and type B antigens on the cell surface make the RBC susceptible to agglutination, these antigens are termed agglutinogens. The presence or absence of the agglutinogens makes up the ABO blood group classification. If neither the A nor the B agglutinogen is present, the blood group is O. When only type A agglutinogen is present, the blood is group A, and when only type B agglutinogen is present, the blood is group B. When both A and B agglutinogens are present, the blood is group AB. The relative frequencies of the different blood groups are listed in Table 28–1.

Genes on adjacent chromosomes determine the ABO blood group. These allelomorphic genes can be only one of the three different types—that is, A, B, or O—allowing for six possible combinations of genes (OO, OA, OB, AA, BB, and AB). There is no dominance among the three different allelomorphs; however, the type O is basically functionless, in that it causes such weak agglutination that it is normally insignificant. The different combinations of genes signify the individual's genotype, and each person is one of six different genotypes. The resultant blood groups for the various genotypes are listed in Table 28–2.

When type A agglutinogen is *absent* on a person's RBC, antibodies known as anti-A will spontaneously develop in the plasma. Likewise, when type B agglutinogen is *absent*, anti-B antibodies develop in the plasma, and when the blood is group O, both anti-A and anti-B antibodies will develop. These antibodies are termed agglutinins. It follows, then, that group AB blood, which contains the agglutinogens A and B, contains no agglutinins at all in the plasma. Immediately after birth, the quantity of agglutinins in the plasma is near zero, but titers begin to develop in the first year of life and reach their maximum titer when the individual is between 8 and 10 years of age. This titer gradually declines throughout the remaining years of life.

The agglutinins are gamma globulins of the IgM and IgG type and are probably produced by exposure to agglutinogens in food, bacteria, or exogenous substances other than blood transfusions. The antibodies (agglutinins) in the plasma of one blood type react with the antigens (agglutinogens) on the RBC of another blood type. This initiates the agglutination and hemolysis that are encountered in a transfusion reaction.

Table 28–1. FREQUENCY OF BLOOD GROUPS IN THE GENERAL POPULATION

Type	Per Cent
O	47
A	41
B	9
AB	3
Rh −	15
Rh +	85

From Guyton, A. C.: Textbook of Medical Physiology, 6th ed. Philadelphia, W. B. Saunders Company, 1981.

Table 28–2. THE BLOOD GROUPS WITH THEIR GENOTYPES AND THEIR CONSTITUENT AGGLUTINOGENS AND AGGLUTININS

Genotypes	Blood Groups	Agglutinogens	Agglutinins
OO	O	−	Anti-A and anti-B
OA or AA	A	A	Anti-B
OB or BB	B	B	Anti-A
AB	AB	A and B	−

From Guyton, A. C.: Textbook of Medical Physiology, 6th ed. Philadelphia, W. B. Saunders Company, 1981.

Many other antigenic proteins (as many as 300 of different potency) are present in the red cells of different persons. Some are of academic or legal importance, whereas others are important for their ability to produce transfusion reactions.

Clinically, the importance of antibodies directed against red cell antigens is determined by their frequency and whether they can cause red cell destruction in the circulation. The ABO system is the most important. With the first transfusion of ABO-*incompatible* blood, severe, potentially fatal reactions can occur. The Rh system is likewise very important, because there is a high likelihood (30 to 50 per cent) that an Rh(D)-negative person will form antibodies after exposure to Rh-positive red cells; these antibodies would then be capable of causing severe hemolysis when red cells containing the antigen are transfused a second time. Of the 40 antigens in the Rh system, D is the most antigenic, but others can also stimulate the production of antibodies in recipients lacking the antigen (e.g., E), thus complicating future transfusions. Other antigen systems in which antibodies could potentially cause hemolytic reactions are the Kell (K and k alleles), Duffy (Fy^a and Fy^b), Kidd (Jk^a and Jk^b), and MNS (M and N; closely linked S and s) systems. Other antigen systems are very rarely important in transfusion therapy.

Cross-Matching. Compatibility testing, or *cross-matching*, is the procedure by which the red cells and serum of the donor unit of blood are mixed, respectively, with the serum and red cells of the recipient to identify the presence of any antibodies and, hence, the potential for a transfusion reaction. These antibodies, after attaching to the appropriate red cell surface antigen, have the potential to cause agglutination and hemolysis of either donor or recipient red cells. This hemolysis may be immediate or delayed. "Major" and "minor" cross-match procedures are outlined in Table 28–3. The end point of all cross-matches is the presence of red cell agglutination (either gross or microscopic) or hemolysis. Testing is performed immediately after mixing, after incubation at 37°C for varying times, and with and without an antiglobulin reagent to identify surface immunoglob-

Table 28–3. CROSS-MATCH PROCEDURES

	Major Cross-Match	Minor Cross-Match
Donor	Red cells	Serum
Recipient	Serum	Red cells
End point	Agglutination or hemolysis at 37°C	

ulin or complement. Each unit of blood product, when properly cross-matched, can be administered with the expectation of safety.

Transfusion Reactions. When incompatible blood is given, the result to the patient may range from no effect to a fatality. If the recipient does *not* have antibodies (naturally occurring or acquired) directed against the foreign red cell antigen he receives, he will have no immediate reaction but may within weeks develop antibodies to the infused blood, which will limit the safety of subsequent transfusions from the same donor or same antigenic type. If the recipient *has* preformed antibodies in his serum directed against the donor red cells (incompatibility in the *major* cross-match), he will within seconds or minutes begin to hemolyze the transfused (donor) cells.

In most cases of major cross-match reactions, red cells of the *donor* blood are agglutinated and hemolyzed. It is very rare that the transfused blood ever produces agglutination of the recipient's cells. Donor blood is affected because the plasma portion of the donor blood immediately becomes diluted by the plasma of the recipient, thereby diluting the titer of the infused agglutinins to a level too low to cause agglutination. Because the recipient's plasma is not diluted to any significant degree, the recipient's agglutinins can still agglutinate the donor cells. Mismatched blood groups eventually cause hemolysis of the RBCs. Occasionally, antibodies are potent enough to cause immediate hemolysis. More often, the cells first agglutinate, then are trapped in peripheral vessels and, over a period of hours to days, become phagocytized, releasing hemoglobin into the circulatory system.

Clinical manifestations of acute hemolysis are chills, fever, tachycardia, abdominal pain, back pain, hypotension, fainting, and an anxious "feeling of impending doom." From the liberation of intracellular material associated with hemolysis, vasoactive substances may aggravate a pre-existing hypotension causing shock; other substances may precipitate disseminated intravascular coagulation, and high-output cardiac failure or anoxic acute renal failure may result. *Fatalities can occur!*

An incompatibility in the *minor* cross-match usually causes no serious reaction, although the recipient's (patient's) red cells could be hemolyzed if the titer of the antibody were great. Even when

major and minor cross-match compatibility indicates the safety of a transfusion, a delayed hemolytic transfusion reaction can occur days to weeks later. Usually seen in multiply transfused patients (or in multigravidas), these reactions may be unavoidable without complete red cell antigen typing, a procedure occasionally indicated for recipients of numerous repeated transfusions. Fortunately, 90 per cent of transfusions are now given as packed red cells that contain a small volume of plasma, minimizing the chance for a transfusion reaction due to donor sensitization.

Additional antibodies *not* caused by sensitization from transfused red cells include autoantibodies (both cold- and warm-reacting) and various agglutinins. Autoantibodies can be "cold," reacting with red cells *more strongly at 4°C* than at 37°C. These antibodies are common and are usually harmless; however, they may be associated with disease states in higher titers (e.g., anti-I in mycoplasma infections). If active at higher temperatures (up to 28 to 32°C), pathologic cold antibodies may cause hemolysis or may even lead to enough red cell agglutination to cause obstruction of blood flow through the small vessels of the hands and the feet upon cold exposure. These would also be present and identifiable at 37°C. The primary significance of cold antibodies stems from their ability to complicate cross-matching procedures in the blood bank.

Warm antibodies, reacting *more strongly at 37°C* than at lower temperatures, can be harmless or can be responsible for a hemolytic anemia of variable severity. Characteristics of the IgG antibody itself determine its significance to the patient. Usually harmless warm autoantibodies that can occasionally cause hemolysis are seen in patients taking α-methyldopa. Harmful warm autoantibodies are encountered in approximately 80 per cent of patients with autoimmune hemolytic anemia.

Additional problems in pretransfusion testing may occur with antibodies directed against various substances that can attach themselves to the red cell surfaces and can cause agglutination of the "innocent bystanders." Examples are the fatty acid–dependent agglutinins; penicillin and cephalosporin antibodies; bacterial polysaccharides; and nonspecific agglutination associated with a high erythrocyte sedimentation rate, caused by high levels of the acute phase reactants: fibrinogen, α-2-macroglobulin, and IgM. A delay in pretransfusion testing may occur when the blood bank has to undertake procedures to identify various proteins on red cell surfaces in order to ascertain their clinical significance.

Miscellaneous Transfusion Problems. Pyogenic transfusion reactions, such as fever and chills, are rather common and result from the presence in the donor plasma of proteins to which the recipient is allergic. Occasional full-blown anaphylactic reactions can result.

Theoretically, citrate salts, which are the usual anticoagulants in donor blood, may combine with ionized calcium in the plasma, producing hypocalcemia. In clinical practice, the hemodynamic consequences of citrate-induced hypocalcemia are minimal, although the QT interval may be prolonged on the electrocardiogram (EKG) with citrate infusion. Supplemental calcium administration is usually not necessary even during massive blood replacement as long as circulating volume is maintained, since the liver is able to remove citrate from the blood within a few minutes. Alterations in this recommendation may be necessary in the presence of severe liver disease.

Hypothermia of varying degree may occur following the transfusion of cold blood or packed cells. All blood should be warmed with a standard blood warmer before infusion to limit the degree to which cold blood aggravates the hypothermia that accompanies shock.

Use of Blood Products

Blood products are divided into components and fractions.[3] Blood components, such as fresh frozen plasma, packed red blood cells, granulocytes, cryoprecipitate, and platelets, are prepared from a single donor and are separated by physical means and transfused as single units. The risk of hepatitis is lower when the blood components are obtained from volunteer donors rather than paid donors. Autotransfusion is the safest method of blood transfusion, reducing both the risk of infectious diseases and the risk of transfusion reactions.

Albumin, plasma protein fraction, and factor IX complex are termed blood fractions (as opposed to components) and are commercially prepared from a plasma pool of multiple donors. Some fractions may be heat-treated to reduce the risk of hepatitis, but since the source of such fractions is largely paid donors, the risk of hepatitis is high with transfusion of blood fractions. Table 28–4

Table 28–4. CHARACTERISTICS OF BLOOD AND ITS COMPONENTS

Component	Volume	Shelf Life	Requirements for Transfusion

Whole blood*
  ACD
  CPD
  CPD-A
	450 ml blood
	63 ml anticoagulant
	  preservative
	35 to 40% hematocrit
		21 days at 4°C
		
		35 days at 4°C
			Cross-matched

Packed red cells
  concentrate
  washed
	280 ml
	70% hematocrit
	250 ml
	70% hematocrit
		Same as for whole blood
		
		1 day at 4°C
			Cross-matched
			
			Cross-matched

Frozen-thawed—red cells†	250 ml 70% hematocrit	? years when frozen, 1 day after thawing	Cross-matched

Platelet concentrate	30 ml
	10^{10} platelets
		5 days at 22°C	Type-specific
			  if possible, but
			  not essential,
			  not cross-
			  matched

Fresh frozen plasma	200 to 250 ml	1 year at 18°C,
		  24 hours after
		  thawing‡
			ABO-compatible;
			  random donor,
			  not cross-
			  matched

Cryoprecipitate	10 to 25 ml per bag
	60 to 120 units
	  of factor VIII
		1 year at −18°C,
		  6 hours after
		  thawing
			ABO-compatible;
			  random donor,
			  not cross-
			  matched

Factor IX
  or Prothrombin
  concentrate
	25 ml per vial	Check label	None required

Granulocyte†
  concentrate
	400 ml
	10^{10} leukocytes
		Transfuse within
		  24 hours at 22°C
			Specific donors
			  for each patient,
			  cross-matched

*ACD = Acid-citrate-dextrose; CPD = Citrate-phosphate-dextrose; CPD-A = Citrate-phosphate-dextrose-adenine.
†Special order—few hospitals have facility in-house.
‡Use immediately to correct deficiency of coagulation factors.

lists some characteristics of blood and its components.

Whole Blood. Individuals normally have 70 to 80 ml per kg of whole blood. Whole blood provides a source of red cells for oxygenation, proteins for coagulation factors and oncotic pressure, and volume for rapid restoration of hypovolemia. Whole blood is indicated only for massive transfusion or exchange transfusion and usually is appropriately used only in treatment of patients with a decreased red cell oxygen-delivering ability and hypovolemic shock, e.g., after multiple trauma. Whole blood is *not* the indicated treatment for hypovolemic shock that can be treated effectively with crystalloid (lactated Ringer's, 0.9 per cent sodium chloride) or colloid (plasma protein, albumin); it is *not* indicated for correction of thrombocytopenia, replacement of coagulation factors, or treatment of anemia that can be treated with replacement iron, vitamin B_{12}, or folic acid. Most blood banks currently do *not* stock significant quantities of whole blood.

Whole blood is collected from donors into plastic bags containing 63 ml of citrate-phosphate-dextrose (CPD) anticoagulant and preservative in a total volume of 515 ± 50 ml and resultant hematocrit of 35 to 40 per cent. All red blood cells stored for over 24 hours develop a metabolic defect in oxygen-carrying capacity (lower 2,3 diphosphoglyceric acid [2,3-DPG] levels and higher P_{50} levels) that is partially corrected within 24 to 48 hours after transfusion into a patient. Most patients compensate imperceptibly for this defect by increasing their cardiac output slightly. Some blood banks now also add adenine (in the form of CDPA) to whole blood to preserve levels of ATP, thus extending the survival of transfused RBC's. This increases shelf life from 21 to 35 days.

Whole blood donors are screened for the presence of infectious disease and anemia, although non-A, non-B hepatitis currently cannot be detected. The risk of hepatitis is 0.1 to 1 per cent when whole blood is transfused, and the incidence rises with multiple transfusions. If more than 24 hours old, whole blood is essentially devoid of normally functioning platelets and other clotting factors, especially the labile clotting factors V and VIII. After storage for 21 days, the pH of blood is approximately 6.6, and the plasma potassium and the ammonia levels are quite elevated (Table 28–5). Whole blood contains antigenic leukocytes and serum proteins, which may produce allergic reactions (a risk of 1 per cent).

The incidence of transfusion reactions following transfusion with whole blood is approximately two and one half times greater than the incidence of reactions following transfusion with packed red cells.[4] Although it is certainly true that patients bleed whole blood, not packed cells, it is often recommended that even acute blood loss be

Table 28–5. COMPARISON OF COMPONENTS OF WHOLE BLOOD AND PACKED CELLS (21-DAY STORAGE)*

	Whole Blood	Packed Red Blood Cells
Volume	450–500 ml	300 ml
Red blood cell mass	200 ml	200 ml
Citrate	63 ml	22 ml
Plasma	250 ml	78 ml
Albumin	12.50 g	4 g
Globulin	6.25 g	2 g
Total protein	48.75 g	36 g
Hemoglobin	30 g	30 g
Hematocrit	39%	70%
Plasma sodium	45 mEq	15 mEq
Plasma potassium	15 mEq	4 mEq
Plasma acid (citric-lactic) pH 6.6	80 nanoEq	25 nanoEq
Plasma ammonia	2159 µg	680 µg
Protein antigens	Maximal	Minimal
Protein antibodies	Maximal	Minimal

*From Nathan, D. G., and Oski, F. A.: Hematology of Infancy and Childhood, vol. 2. Philadelphia, W. B. Saunders Co., 1981. Used by permission.

treated with packed cells as opposed to whole blood; many authorities, however, will defend the continued use of whole blood.[5] One unit of whole blood will raise the hematocrit approximately 3 per cent. The plasma of whole blood is no more effective than 5 per cent albumin as a volume expander.

Packed Red Blood Cells. Packed red cells provide oxygen-carrying capacity and volume expansion. Packed red cells (PRBC's) are prepared by centrifugation and removal of most of the plasma from citrated whole blood. PRBC's that have been grouped and that have had the Rh factor determined should be the most common blood component used to treat anemia not amenable to nutritional correction. Hazards of metabolic derangements, donor antibodies, volume overload and (possibly) hepatitis are lessened with packed red cells as compared with whole blood. Patients with severe or chronic anemia or heart disease or those who otherwise require fluid restriction can receive packed cells more safely than whole blood. Furthermore, to prevent circulatory overload in susceptible patients, a rapid-acting diuretic, such as furosemide or ethacrynic acid, can be administered intravenously at the beginning of the transfusion. One unit of packed cells contains the same red cell mass as one unit of whole blood at approximately one half the volume and twice the hematocrit (70 to 80 per cent). One unit of packed cells will raise the hematocrit approximately 3 per cent in an adult. In children, there is an approximate rise in hematocrit of 1 per cent for each ml per kg of packed cells. For example, if 5 ml per kg of packed cells is transfused, the hematocrit will rise by approximately 5 per cent. Actual changes are dependent upon the state of hydration and the rate of bleeding.

When washed to remove leukocytes, platelets, microaggregates, and plasma proteins, red cells cause fewer transfusion reactions than does whole blood. Red cells are not routinely washed before transfusion, but washing reduces the titer of anti-A and anti-B, permitting safer transfusion of type O packed red cells in non-O recipients. Washing does not totally eliminate the risk of hepatitis. Washed red cells are prepared in the blood bank by centrifugation, filtration, or use of sedimenting agents or by washing the unit of whole blood or packed red cells.

Frozen deglycerolized red cells likewise are free of platelets, plasma, and white cells, having been washed after an indefinite period of frozen storage in glycerol. Frozen red cells and fresh red cells function similarly; frozen red cells provide normal levels of 2,3-DPG. Washed or frozen preparations should be given to patients who have had febrile (nonhemolytic) reactions to previous transfusions as a result of leukocyte antibodies or IgA sensitization. Blood bank procedures require that these be prepared to order, with routine cross-matching. Considerable delay (6 hours) may occur if the transfusion service does not have the capability of washing red cells.

Packed red cells contain less sodium, potassium, ammonia, citrate, and antigenic protein and fewer hydrogen ions than does whole blood. This may offer an advantage in patients with reduced cardiovascular, renal, or hepatic function. The rate of urticaria is still relatively high, at 1 to 3 per cent of transfusions, but the incidence of adverse reactions to packed cells is approximately one third that seen with whole blood.

Many physicians use packed cells during surgery and for replacement treatment of acute blood loss of any cause. As is true of whole blood, packed cells can be stored up to 21 days by law, although newer preservatives may allow 35-day storage. Red cell viability decreases approximately 1 per cent per day.

Fresh Frozen Plasma. Fresh frozen plasma should be given to patients with a hereditary or acquired deficiency of coagulation factors, provided that a preparation of the specific deficient factor is not available. Each unit has a volume of approximately 200 to 250 ml and is prepared by freezing the plasma separated from single-donor whole blood within 4 to 6 hours of collection. Plasma should be compatible in terms of the recipient's ABO group, since anti-A and anti-B is present in the plasma of individuals lacking the corresponding antigen. Rh compatibility is not considered essential.

Fresh frozen plasma contains all soluble coagulation factors of the intrinsic and extrinsic clotting systems, including the labile factors V and VIII. Fresh frozen plasma also contains fibrinogen, although not as much as does cryoprecipitate. Fresh frozen plasma has a shelf life of up to 1 year, and plasma stored for 3 months will retain approximately 60 per cent of the normal factor VIII activity. Fresh frozen plasma contains no platelets.

Fresh frozen plasma is indicated for the clotting factor deficiencies resulting from the diluting effect of massive blood replacement. One unit of fresh frozen plasma per 5 units of packed cells or whole blood is a reasonable replacement formula if specific clotting tests are not rapidly available, but plasma replacement is best dictated by evaluation of prothrombin time and partial thromboplastin time. Fresh frozen plasma is indicated for rapid reversal of serious bleeding from warfarin (Coumadin) anticoagulants. In an emergency situation, 5 to 10 ml per kg of fresh frozen plasma will effect a rapid reversal of the vitamin K–dependent factors II, VII, IX, and X. In *life-threatening* hemorrhage from coumadin excess, factor IX concentrate (Konyne, Proplex) may be used but such therapy should not be routine because of the high incidence of hepatitis with these products. Fresh frozen plasma may be valuable in patients with other clotting abnormalities, such as von Willebrand's syndrome, hemophilia A and hemophilia B, or hypofibrinogenemia; however, the effectiveness is limited in severe clotting abnormalities because of the large volume that is generally required. For example, fresh frozen plasma may be successful in the treatment of hemarthrosis or other minor bleeding tendencies in hemophilia, but specific factor replacement is preferred.

Because of the high risk of hepatitis, packed plasma is no longer available. Reactions to fresh frozen plasma include fever, chills, allergic responses, and a risk of hepatitis that is similar to the risk with whole blood.

Fresh frozen plasma should be infused rapidly and given immediately after thawing because of the rapid loss of labile clotting factors.

Cryoprecipitate. Cryoprecipitate is used specifically to correct a deficiency of coagulation factor VIII (in hemophilia A and in von Willebrand's syndrome), factor XIII, or fibrinogen. The precipitate is prepared from single-donor plasma by gradual thawing of rapidly frozen plasma, which results in an undissolved protein that is collected and stored at very low temperatures. Cryoprecipitate is a plasma product and as such requires ABO and Rh compatibility, but cross-matching is not necessary.

Cryoprecipitate contains approximately 30 to 50 per cent of the original plasma content of factors VIII and XIII and fibrinogen. Each 15- to 25-ml bag of cryoprecipitate contains 60 to 120 units of factor VIII, 125 to 250 mg of fibrinogen, and an unknown amount of von Willebrand's factor. Cryoprecipitate is of no value in the treatment of factor IX deficiency (hemophilia B).

Once spontaneous bleeding has occurred in hemophilia or von Willebrand's syndrome, it will usually *not stop until the deficient factor is replaced*. It is best to treat early to prevent minor bleeding from developing into a significant hemorrhage. The goal of therapy is to achieve at least 50 per cent of normal factor VIII activity. In spontaneous intracranial hemorrhage, one should seek 100 per cent activity. The amount of cryoprecipitate required to correct coagulation defects ranges from 10 to 20 units per kg for minor bleeding, such as hemarthrosis, to 50 units per kg for bleeding control in surgery or trauma, but specific replacement should be guided by laboratory assay of factor VIII activity. One bag of cryoprecipitate per 5 kg of body weight will raise the recipient's factor VIII level to approximately 50 per cent of normal. The half-life of factor VIII in plasma is 8 to 12 hours. Mild deficiencies of factor VIII are considered to exist at 10 to 30 per cent of normal, and severe deficiencies exist at less than 3 per cent of normal activity. Many patients know their level of factor VIII and such levels remain relatively constant.

Rarely, cryoprecipitate may be required to correct significant hypofibrinogenemia (less than 100 mg per dl). Fresh frozen plasma may also be used to treat mild degrees of hypofibrinogenemia.

Factor IX Concentrate (Prothrombin Complex)

Prothrombin complex concentrate, or factor IX concentrate (Konyne or Proplex), is prepared from pooled human plasma and is available as a lyophilized powder. Factor IX concentrate contains the liver-synthesized, vitamin K–dependent factors: II (prothrombin), VII, IX, and X. The actual factor IX activity of each vial is stated on the label. Each vial is reconstituted to a volume of 25 ml and contains approximately 500 units of factor IX, 300 units of factors VII and X, and 200 units of factor II. The use of this product carries a very high risk of hepatitis transmission (almost 100 per cent), and, because of this, it is rarely used. Post treatment hyperthrombosis may also occur.

Factor IX concentrate is used almost exclusively in the treatment of hemophilia B, because cryoprecipitate is effective only for the treatment of hemophilia A (factor VIII deficiency). Patients with hemophilia should always be asked about which deficiency they manifest, because the treatment of each type is different. Although factor VIII deficiency is much more common, the routine treatment of all patients with "hemophilia" with cryoprecipitate is not warranted. Factor IX

concentrate may theoretically be used instead of fresh frozen plasma in the rare instance where volume must be kept at a minimum. The use of prothrombin complex is also warranted when there is the possibility of *life-threatening* hemorrhage, such as intracranial bleeding, in patients with *coumadin-induced* hemorrhage. Vitamin K and fresh frozen plasma, however, are definitely preferred in the noncritical patient with coumadin-induced bleeding.

In hemophilia B, the aim of therapy is to achieve 20 to 30 per cent of normal values of factor IX. Higher levels are desired in intracranial bleeding. Most patients know the level of their deficiency, and the deficiency remains relatively constant. Treatment of factor IX deficient patients with 25 to 50 units of factor IX concentrate per kg body weight, once or twice a day, usually results in normal hemostasis, but individual responses to therapy may vary. Minor bleeding (soft tissue, joints) may be controlled with 10 to 20 units per kg body weight. It is a common error to assume that a minor spontaneous bleeding episode will be self-limited in patients with either form of hemophilia. Once spontaneous bleeding occurs, however, it rarely will stop spontaneously and treatment with replacement factors will be necessary.

Platelet Concentrates. Platelet concentrates are prepared by rapid centrifugation of platelet-rich plasma, which is obtained by slow centrifugation of freshly collected whole blood to separate the red cells. Platelet concentrates contain most of the platelets from 1 unit of blood in 30 to 50 ml of plasma; they are given to raise a patient's platelet count and to correct bleeding from thrombocytopenia. One unit (pack) of platelets per 7 kg of body weight will raise the platelet count by 50,000 per mm^3 in the absence of antibodies; therefore, 1 unit of platelet concentrate raises the platelet count by 5 to 10,000 per mm^3. The usual adult dose given is 6 to 10 units of platelet concentrate, depending upon the clinical condition. Some hospital blood banks prepare platelet concentrates regularly; in some cities a central blood bank service, such as the American Red Cross, prepares platelet concentrates regularly and delivers units on an "as-needed" basis within 1 to 2 hours of the request. Platelet concentrates are viable for 5 days when kept at *room temperature* and gently agitated at intermittent periods or when kept in motion. They should not be refrigerated.

Spontaneous bleeding rarely occurs if the platelet count is above 30,000 per mm^3. It is generally recommended that active hemorrhage be treated with platelet transfusion if the platelet count is below 50,000 per mm^3.

Cross-matching is unnecessary for platelet transfusion, but the donor and the recipient should be ABO- and Rh-compatible. Note that platelet concentrates contain enough red cells to sensitize an Rh-negative individual. There may be a diluting effect to the platelet count resulting in thrombocytopenia with massive blood transfusions. When more than 8 to 10 units of blood are transfused, the platelet count must be routinely evaluated, and platelets must be replaced accordingly. Clinically significant platelet depletion rarely occurs if less than 15 units of blood (or 1.5 to 2 times blood volume) have been transfused.

Granulocyte Transfusions. Granulocyte transfusions are given in those unique instances in which a severely neutropenic patient has a suspected or proven bacterial infection not responding to appropriate treatment. They are rarely given in an emergency unit. White cell transfusions require prior arrangements with a large blood bank service that has the capabilities of collecting granulocytes from a suitable donor; the collection procedure takes 4 to 6 hours on a continuous flow cell separator. Transfusions need to be repeated frequently (every 12 hours) to provide a sufficient number of white cells to help the patient.

Blood Products for Jehovah's Witnesses. There are more than one and one half million Jehovah's Witnesses in America. Members of this religion do not accept transfusions of whole blood, packed cells, white cells, platelets, or plasma or autotransfusion of predeposited blood. Some may permit infusion of albumin, hemophiliac preparations, or dextran or other plasma expanders and intraoperative autotransfusion.[6] Jehovah's Witnesses will sign standard release forms to relieve physicians and hospitals from liability. Legal opinion should be sought whenever possible in the case of minors or unconscious patients who may die without the infusion of blood products. State laws have varied on the issue of forced treatment. The editors suggest that in *life-threatening* circumstances, transfusion therapy be performed using standard clinical criteria, since legal precedents against physicians are lacking.

Administration of Blood Components

When it has been decided that a patient needs a transfusion, the physician should question the patient or his relatives concerning any previous transfusion reactions and whether the patient abides by any religious prohibitions to transfusions. A tube of blood (approximately 2 ml for every unit of blood product to be cross-matched) should be drawn from the patient and put into a red-topped, nonanticoagulated tube. The tube must *not* contain a serum separator gel. The label should be signed by the physician. This identifying signature will be used in the blood bank's cross-matching procedures.

Emergency Transfusion. In an emergency or life-threatening situation, three alternatives to fully cross-matched blood exist. The preferred substitute is type-specific blood with an abbreviated cross-match. The abbreviated cross-match includes ABO and Rh compatibility. In addition, the recipient's serum is screened for unexpected antibodies, and an "immediate spin" cross-match is performed at room temperature. This abbreviated cross-match requires approximately 30 minutes, and many institutions are now using this procedure as their standard cross-match for most patients. The safety and utility of the type-specific abbreviated cross-match has been demonstrated repeatedly, and transfusion reactions should occur only rarely.[4, 7]

The second preference for an alternative to fully cross-matched blood is type-specific blood that is only ABO- and Rh-compatible, without screen or immediate spin cross-match. The patient's ABO group and Rh factor can be determined within 2 minutes, and, in an emergency, typing of the blood group and the Rh factor is all that is necessary before transfusion. Type-specific blood that is not cross-matched has been given in numerous military and civilian series without serious consequences.[3] While the type-specific blood is being transfused, the antibody screen and the cross-match are carried out in the laboratory; the transfusion should be stopped if an incompatibility is found to exist.

Ideally, type-specific blood should be similar in Rh factor as well as in ABO group; however, blood with the opposite Rh factor may be used in an extreme emergency or in times of disaster or blood shortage. The patient may develop sensitization to the Rh factor. This may affect a subsequent pregnancy if an Rh-negative woman is given Rh-positive type-specific blood. A male patient may likewise be sensitized to subsequent Rh-incompatible transfusions.

The third preference for an alternative to fully cross-matched blood for an emergency transfusion is group O blood. In general, type-specific blood is preferable to group O blood. There is rarely a situation in which a few minutes cannot safely be expended to allow the blood bank to release type-specific blood. Nevertheless, exceptions may occur, in which case type O blood may be required. Such exceptions would be a trauma victim or a patient with a ruptured aneurysm who has not responded to crystalloid resuscitation in the field.

When type and Rh determination creates an unacceptable delay in transfusion, group O blood (either as whole blood or as packed cells) is transfused. Packed cells are preferred over whole blood. Group O negative *whole* blood was in the past designated the "universal donor" blood, because a recipient's naturally occurring antibodies (anti-A and anti-B) will not react with donor group O red cells. Nonetheless, some donor serum may have a high-titer of naturally occurring anti-A and anti-B antibodies capable of hemolyzing the recipient's (patient's) red cells if large quantities of blood are transfused. True universal donor blood is low in anti-A and anti-B titer. Because group O donors are not regularly screened for unsafe levels of anti-A and anti-B titers, the use of even small amounts of group O whole blood that is not cross-matched is potentially dangerous. The significance of varying titers of anti-A and anti-B antibodies in the donor whole blood may be essentially eliminated if *packed cells* are used instead of whole blood. Other red cell antigens on type O red cells may sensitize the patient or may cause antibody production, complicating future cross-matching or possibly causing future hemolytic transfusion reactions.

Approximately 25 per cent of patients receiving a transfusion of 5 or more units of type O whole blood will develop hyperbilirubinemia suggestive of a minor hemolytic reaction. Large amounts of group O whole blood may cause the patient to acquire significant amounts of anti-A and anti-B that have been passively transfused; hemolysis of red cells may then occur when the recipient's original blood group is subsequently transfused. In a resuscitation, one should continue to use group O blood if large amounts (over two units) of whole blood have already been given.

One may transfuse both Rh-positive and Rh-negative group O packed cells in patients who are in critical condition. In most patients, there is no particular advantage in the Rh factor determination. Many advise the routine use of O Rh-positive packed cells in all patients for whom the Rh factor has not been determined, except in females of childbearing years, for whom future Rh sensitization may be an important consideration. Since individuals with O Rh-negative blood represent only 15 per cent of the population and the blood may be in short supply, it is reasonable to save O Rh-negative blood for Rh-negative females of childbearing potential and to use group O Rh-positive packed cells routinely as the first choice for *emergency* transfusions.[8–10]

Transfusion Coagulopathy. Within the past 10 years it has been appreciated that pathologic hemostasis occurs following massive blood transfusions.[11–13] The exact cause of the transfusion coagulopathy is poorly defined and poorly understood. Although such abnormalities will rarely develop within the time frame of the initial resuscitation in the emergency department, an understanding of the problem will lead to a more intelligent approach to transfusion practices and the anticipation of potential problems. The term "massive transfusion" is loosely defined but is usually considered to be the transfusion of more than 10 units of blood within 24 hours. In patients who are given a transfusion that is equal to two blood volumes, only approximately 10 per cent of the original elements will remain. Considering the significant alteration in blood and blood products that occurs during storage, one can readily appreciate the underlying problem associated with such massive transfusions. The development of transfusion coagulopathy is multifactorial but can be related to two specific areas: platelets and plasma clotting factors.

Platelets. Transfusion coagulopathy is related partly, but not wholly, to a diluting effect of the transfusion of blood deficient in platelets. A dilutional coagulopathy is the most common cause of bleeding associated with massive transfusions. Disseminated intravascular coagulopathy plays a second role in post-transfusion bleeding.

Banked whole blood and packed cells are devoid of functioning platelets. Dilutional thrombocytopenia is a well-recognized complication of massive transfusion, and a platelet count should be obtained routinely if more than 5 units of blood are transfused. As a general guideline, platelet therapy should be considered after the first 10 units of blood have been given, although the most useful parameter for estimating the need for platelet transfusions is the platelet count.

Plasma Clotting Factors. Factors V and VIII are labile in stored blood and absent in packed cells. Fibrinogen is relatively stable in stored blood but is absent in packed cells. A deficiency of most clotting factors, especially factors V and VIII and fibrinogen, occurs with massive transfusions. This deficiency probably occurs on a "wash-out," or dilutional, basis, although the dynamics are poorly understood. The replacement of these factors may be required. Specific assays for the individual factors are available, but it is more practical to measure activated partial thromboplastin time and prothrombin time. Fibrinogen is readily measured in most hospitals. Fresh frozen plasma has been used to correct clotting factor abnormalities secondary to dilution from massive transfusions, but its effectiveness has not been firmly established. Cryoprecipitate has also been used to replace factor VIII and fibrinogen, but it is rarely required, since fresh frozen plasma contains some fibrinogen. Fresh frozen plasma should be infused to correct the coagulopathy as indicated by clotting studies, but as a general guide, 1 to 2 units of fresh frozen plasma may be given empirically for each 5 to 6 units of blood in the massively traumatized or bleeding patient. Cryoprecipitate may be required if fibrinogen levels fall below 100 mg per dl and are not adequately supplemented with fresh frozen plasma.

Ordering of Blood

Ordering a type and cross-match procedure on a blood product implies that the decision has already been made to administer a transfusion. A "type and hold" (no cross-match) request alerts the blood bank to the *possibility* that a blood product will be required for the patient, so appropriate units can be acquired and kept on hand. A type and cross-match procedure takes 45 minutes and restricts a unit of blood to a specific patient. This limits a valuable resource and should not be requested lightly. In the emergency unit, a cross-match procedure should be requested for a blood product only if the adult patient (1) manifests shock, (2) has *symptomatic* anemia (usually associated with a hemoglobin less than 10 gm per dl) in the emergency unit, (3) has a documented loss of 1000 ml of blood, or (4) will require a blood-losing operation immediately (e.g., thoracotomy).[14] A type and hold can safely be requested for all other situations in which a blood transfusion is considered possible during the patient's care; a desirable ratio of units cross-matched to units transfused can thus be achieved.

The number of units to be requested for a cross-match procedure will be determined by the size of the patient, the response of the patient to his injury and subsequent emergency treatment, and whether the patient has ongoing losses (e.g., arterial or massive gastrointestinal bleeding). In the majority of fatalities from massive hemorrhage, the patients die from hypovolemia rather than from lack of oxygen-carrying capacity. Specific guidelines for the administration of blood components are given in Table 28–6.

Red blood cell preparations for transfusion are not routinely tested for the presence of sickle hemoglobin. Donors with sickle trait are not excluded, and blood with sickle trait can safely be given to almost every patient, because occlusion of blood flow, caused by intravascular sickling would occur only in extreme conditions of acidity, hypoxia, or hypothermia that are unlikely to be compatible with life. Nonetheless, when transfusion is being performed in infants and patients with known sickle cell anemia, the blood bank should be alerted, and a "sickle prep" should be requested for donor blood to avoid the infusion of sickle-trait blood into such patients. There have been rare instances in which blood from a donor with a mild variant, such as S-C disease, caused massive intravascular sickling and death in a sick, hypoxic, acidotic infant.[15]

Blood Request Forms. The most important part of ordering blood components for a patient is proper identification of the patient and the intended unit of blood. Transfusion of an incorrect unit is a potentially fatal error. Most transfusion mistakes are clerical errors. Several identification systems have been established to minimize the risk of improper transfusions: a prototype is the

Table 28–6. TRANSFUSION OF BLOOD PRODUCTS

Blood Product	Waiting Time to Receive in Emergency Department	Initial Amount to Transfuse	Expected Response in 70-kg Adult
Uncross-matched O Rh-negative red cells	5 minutes		Stabilize patient in shock
Uncross-matched type-specific whole blood	15 minutes		Change in hemoglobin/hematocrit depends on hydration and rate of bleeding
Typed and screened whole blood	25 minutes	2 to 10 units, 10 to 20 ml per kg per hour or as needed based on clinical condition	
Cross-matched whole blood	1¼ hours		Approximate rise of 1 to 1.5 gm per 100 ml hemoglobin per unit
Packed red cells	1½ hours		Each unit raises hematocrit 2 to 3 per cent
Frozen red cells	4 to 6 hours (if not prepared in-house)		In children, each ml per kg of packed cells raises hematocrit by 1 per cent
Platelet concentrate	5 minutes if available	1 unit per 10 kg, usually 10 units per transfusion in an adult	Rise of 5000 to 10,000 platelets per mm³ per unit
Cryoprecipitate	20 minutes	1 to 2 bags per 10 kg (7 to 15 bags) 10-minute push or 20–50 units/kg	Rise of 3 per cent in factor VIII level per bag (40 to 100 per cent activity desired)
Factor IX or prothrombin concentrate	Immediately available (reconstituted powder)	10–50 units/kg	30–100 per cent rise in factor IX activity
Fresh frozen plasma	40 minutes	1 bag per 7 kg (4 to 10 bags for adult) 10-minute push* 3 to 10 ml per kg, depending on clinical condition	Correction in coagulation status

*Administer 1 bag per 4 to 6 units of blood transfused to replace diluted and inactivated coagulation factors.

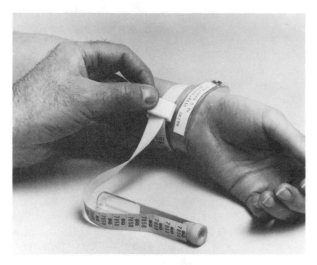

Figure 28–1. The Typenex blood recipient identification system. The identity of the patient and the blood sample are insured by numbered labels on the tube and on the bracelet. (Courtesy of Fenwal Laboratories, Deerfield, Illinois.)

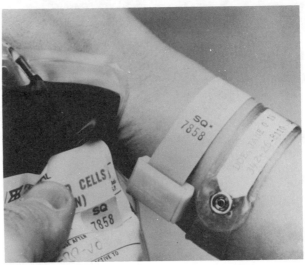

Figure 28–3. Prior to administration of the blood unit, the numbered labels on the patient's bracelet and on the unit of blood are checked for identity. (Courtesy of Fenwal Laboratories, Deerfield, Illinois.)

Typenex Blood Recipient Identification System (Fenwal Laboratories, Inc., Deerfield, Illinois—Fig. 28–1). A strip of adhesive-backed identically numbered labels is attached to a *second* identically numbered patient identification bracelet. The tube containing a blood sample for cross-match is sent to the blood bank with several adhesive-backed numbered labels attached. These can be removed and affixed to the units of blood prepared for the patient. Just prior to administering the blood, the nurse or physician checks the identity of the numbered labels. In addition, the blood bank labora-

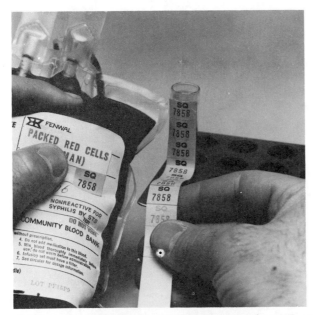

Figure 28–2. In the blood bank, cross-matched units of blood are identified with numbered labels from the patient's blood sample. (Courtesy of Fenwal Laboratories, Deerfield, Illinois.)

tory slip should identify the patient by name and number and should also contain the identification number of the unit of blood. One cannot be overcautious in these identification procedures (Fig. 28–2).

Usual procedures require a separate *blood bank request form* for each unit of red blood cells or whole blood that is ordered. Multiple units of fresh frozen plasma, cryoprecipitate, and platelet concentrates may be ordered on one form with proper identification (depending on individual blood bank procedures). When the blood bank indicates that the units ordered are ready, the person picking up the blood, along with the blood bank technician, checks the notation on the *blood release form* (transfusion form) to verify the identity of the patient (name, hospital number) and to ensure that the blood unit has been prepared for him (blood group and type, unit number). Immediately prior to administering the blood to the patient, the nurse or physician hanging the unit should check the release form, blood unit, and patient tag for identity as well as the expiration date of the unit (Fig. 28–3).

Intravenous Administration

One should not open the unit of blood until and unless a free-flowing intravenous (IV) access line has been established in a large-bore vein. A 14 gauge intravenous catheter is preferred, both to minimize hemolysis and for rapid infusion of fluid for the treatment of hypovolemia or hypotension. When large amounts of blood must be given rapidly, administration by means of a 5 to 8 French introducer sheath is preferred (see Chapter 19).

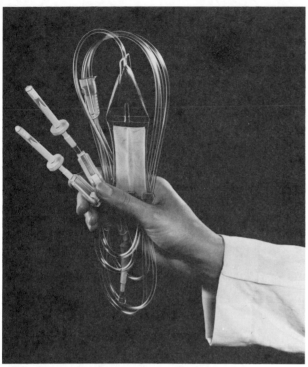

Figure 28–4. An example of a blood administration Y set with two adapters for insertion into a unit of blood or saline; note the in-line filter. (Courtesy of Fenwal Laboratories, Deerfield, Illinois.)

Standard central venous pressure (CVP) lines are generally too small for adequate volume resuscitation in patients in critical condition. Likewise, the purpose of a large-bore infusion line is defeated if blood is piggy-backed with an 18 to 20 gauge needle through a side port in the infusion tubing. For an elective transfusion, however, blood may be given through a smaller needle. No significant hemolysis occurs when small gauge (21, 23, 25, and 27 gauge) short needles are used for transfusion of fresh blood or packed cells in infants and children and when the maximum rate of infusion is less than 100 ml per hour.[16] For rapid infusion, however, the blood administration tubing is connected directly to the infusion catheter. The infusion site should be monitored for infiltration, infection, or local reactions. Antiseptic technique is essential.

Each institution has its own preference for cleansing agents, such as a povidone-iodine solution followed by alcohol. One could follow the same procedures that are used for cleansing the skin prior to drawing a blood culture. Care should be taken to avoid touching the injection site until the needle is under the skin. The area should be kept clean and dry thereafter. Some practitioners routinely cover the site with topical antibiotic and gauze after securing the needle to the skin.

If the patient already has a suitable intravenous line in place, a solution of 0.9 per cent normal saline only should be used to flush the system prior to administering the blood. Other intravenous fluids are *not* to be used because of the risks of hemolysis or aggregation (with 5 per cent dextrose in water) or clotting (with lactated Ringer's solution). No medications can be placed into the unit of blood or added to the infusion line for the same reasons.

ADMINISTRATION TUBING SETS

Both straight and Y-type tubing sets are commercially available to attach the unit of blood to the needle in the patient. Multi-lead (Y) sets (Figs. 28–4 through 28–8) bearing two hard plastic spikes for entering a blood unit or bottle of IV solution are preferred. These provide the option of infusing normal saline while switching blood units or waiting for additional units to be obtained. One should use the sequence in Table 28–7 for flushing the tubing of the blood administration set with normal saline before attaching and administering the unit of blood.

FILTERS

All blood and blood products should be infused only through an appropriate filter, such as those

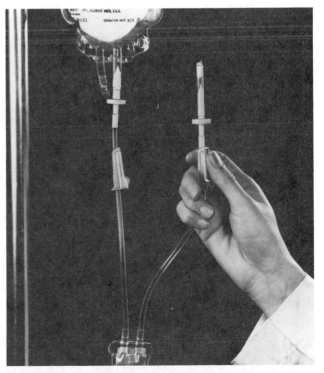

Figure 28–5. One upper adapter has been inserted into a bag containing normal (0.9 per cent) saline. (Courtesy of Fenwal Laboratories, Deerfield, Illinois.)

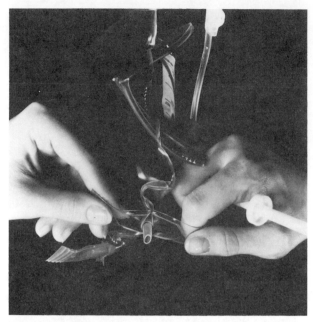

Figure 28–6. The entry site of the unit of blood, into which the other upper adapter of the Y set should be inserted. (Courtesy of Fenwal Laboratories, Deerfield, Illinois.)

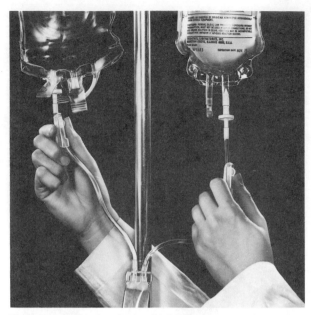

Figure 28–8. After the plastic tubing has been primed with saline, the blood flows through into the patient. (Courtesy of Fenwal Laboratories, Deerfield, Illinois.)

supplied in-line in the blood administration tubing sets. In the past, filtration was required merely to keep the intravenous line from becoming blocked by clots but the adverse consequences to the patient that result from infusing unfiltered blood products have now been recognized. Debris consisting of clots and aggregates of fibrin, white cells, platelets, and intertwined red cells (ranging in size from 15 to 200 microns) will accumulate progressively during storage of the blood unit from the first day of collection. The usual filter,

made of a single layer of plastic with multiple 170-micron pores, will trap larger particles and yet will allow for the rapid infusion of blood for 2 to 3 units before flow is greatly obstructed.

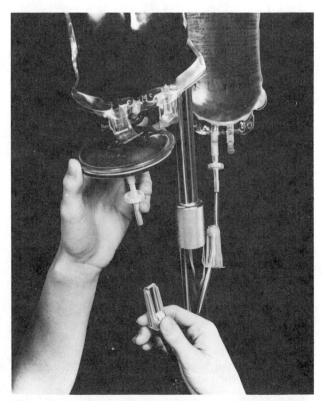

Figure 28–9. Administration of blood through a microaggregate filter attached between the unit of blood and the hard plastic spike of the administration set. (Courtesy of Fenwal Laboratories, Deerfield, Illinois.)

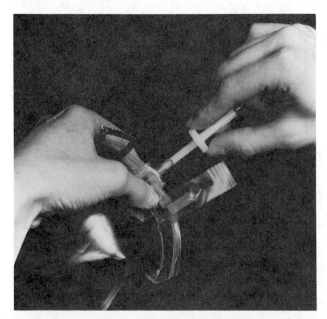

Figure 28–7. Inserting the hard plastic spike of the upper adapter. (Courtesy of Fenwal Laboratories, Deerfield, Illinois.)

Table 28–7. SEQUENCE FOR INFUSING BLOOD

1. Close the two upper and one lower Flo-trol plastic clamps.
2. Insert one of the upper plastic spikes into a bottle of normal saline (250 ml or more) using standard aseptic technique (see Fig. 28–5).
3. Open both plastic clamps on the upper arms of the Y and allow saline to fill the filter. Saline will also flow back up the second arm (blood port) to the end. Close the clamp on the free, unattached upper tube when this occurs.
4. Open the plastic clamp on the lower, longer tube and allow saline to flow to the end of the infusion line. Close the clamp.
5. Attach the infusion tube to the patient's intravenous site and establish a free flow of saline through the IV site.
6. Connect the unit of blood (properly indentified) to the short, unattached tubing leading to the filter by finding the portal of entry to the unit. Grasp one plastic tab in each hand and separate them to expose the entry site. With a twisting back-and-forth motion, push the pointed plastic spike of the tubing into the entry site, puncturing it. Use absolute sterile technique (see Figs. 28–6 and 28–7).
7. When ready to transfuse the blood, close off the upper tube leading directly from the saline bottle and open the clamp on the upper tube from the blood. Blood should now be flowing through the upper tubing, the filter, and the lower tubing to the patient (see Fig. 28–8).

It has been suggested that microaggregates of debris, which could pass through a 170-micron filter, may in part contribute to the syndrome of "shock lung" seen after transfusions of multiple units of blood in patients suffering from severe trauma and hemorrhage. Some practitioners therefore recommend the use of a microaggregate blood infusion filter with a mesh pore size of 40 microns (Fig. 28–9) when multiple units of blood are administered to a trauma victim, to a patient with compromised pulmonary function, or to a neonate. Filters as small as 20 microns have been suggested.[17] Microaggregate filters tend to become blocked, impeding the rate of infusion more quickly, and are not commonly required in the emergency setting. In addition, whether the infusion of microaggregates (between 40 and 170 microns in size) is in fact harmful is still a moot point. Standard filters should be replaced after 2 to 3 units of blood product have been administered; most microaggregate filters should be changed after each unit. It is generally agreed that a significant number of platelets are removed by microaggregate filters, and some advise against using these filters when platelet packs are infused. Others believe that, although platelets are removed with the microaggregate filters, the trapped platelets can be removed with saline flush without any significant loss.[18] Table 28–8 lists some available microaggregate filters.

RATE OF INFUSION

One unit of whole blood can safely be administered to a patient *in shock* at a rate of 20 ml per kg per hour or at an even greater rate in the presence of continued hemorrhage. In the stable

Table 28–8. IN-LINE FILTERS FOR BLOOD TRANSFUSION

Filter	Pore Size	Use and Contraindications
Standard		
Fenwal STD Blood Filter	170 μ	All blood components
McGaw STD Blood Filter	170 μ	All blood components
Special Use		
Fenwal 4C2100	170 μ	Platelets, cryoprecipitate, antihemophilic factor concentrates, fresh whole blood
Microaggregate Filters		
Fenwal Microaggregate Blood Filter 4C2423 or 4C2131	20 μ	
Fenwal PDF-10 4C2428		
Intersept Blood Filter (Johnson & Johnson Co., New Brunswick, NJ)	20 μ	
Alpha Micron-40 (Alpha Therapeutics Corp., Los Angeles, CA)	40 μ	Can be used for all blood products in all patients. Will remove most platelets and leukocytes from blood being transfused. Do not use with fresh whole blood or concentrates of platelets or white cells. Primarily indicated for use with patients receiving *multiple transfusions* of stored blood and patients with *compromised pulmonary function* and for use in patients undergoing cardiopulmonary bypass. Recommended for use in most newborns.
Bentley Disposable Blood Filter PF 127 (Bentley Labs., Inc., Irvine, CA)	27 μ	
Hemonate (Gesco Labs., San Antonio, TX)	40 μ	
Swank In-Line Blood Filter IL-700 (Pioneer Filters, Inc., Beaverton, OR)	20 μ	
Pall Ultipor SQ405 (Pall Biomedical Products Corp., Glen Cove, NY 11542)	40 μ	

patient, 1 unit of whole blood (500 ml) should be administered over approximately a 2-hour period (3 to 4 ml per kg per hour). After this time, red cells begin to lose metabolic activity in addition to the "storage defect"; the unit of blood, which is an excellent culture medium, is likely to become contaminated if bacteria and fungi are allowed to grow at room temperature. Packed cells should be given at approximately the same rate; plasma products may be given more rapidly. In a patient with a healthy cardiovascular system, one should administer fresh frozen plasma more rapidly (about 15 to 20 minutes per unit) to correct coagulation deficits, because the coagulant activity begins to deteriorate rapidly after 20 to 30 minutes of thawing. In patients with severe anemia or congestive heart failure, a rapidly acting diuretic, such as furosemide, can be given (0.5 mg per kg IV) at the onset of transfusion to obviate circulatory overload.

If a transfusion of blood must be interrupted or delayed for some reason, the remainder of the blood unit should be returned to the blood bank. More convenient refrigerators in the emergency unit or on the floor are *not* temperature-controlled or continuously monitored and *should not* be used to store blood products.

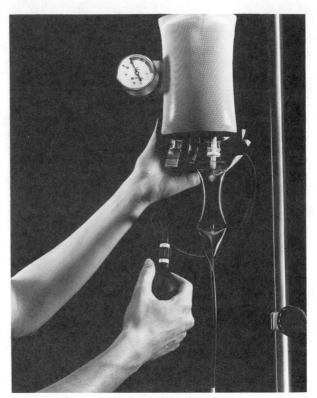

Figure 28–11. A rubber bladder is pumped up, and the blood unit is squeezed uniformly against a reinforced mesh. (Courtesy of Fenwal Laboratories, Deerfield, Illinois.)

Patients who are in hemorrhagic shock can receive blood through two large-bore catheters at different sites. At least one company provides a pressure-augmented device through which the blood unit can be hung to create increased infusion pressure. Usually, gravity provides a sufficient pressure gradient if the unit is raised higher above the patient to increase the rate of infusion when the clamps are wide open. If a pressure pump is used (e.g., a device made by the Sorenson Research Corporation, Salt Lake City, Utah), the infusion can be more rapid (Figs. 28–10 and 28–11).[19] A standard sphygmomanometer cuff should never be wrapped around a unit of blood to create increased infusion pressure, because the nonuniform application of pressure could burst the plastic bag containing the blood component.

One can dilute packed red cells with normal saline (0.9 per cent) before infusion simply by opening the clamps on the upper tubes of the Y infusion set with the lower (recipient end) closed. Dilution will allow for more rapid infusion by decreasing the blood viscosity, which is dependent on hematocrit, at the risk of increased volume. Alternatively, the direct addition of approximately 200 ml of normal saline to the bag of packed red cells has been recommended to bring the hematocrit in the blood bag to approximately 45 per cent.

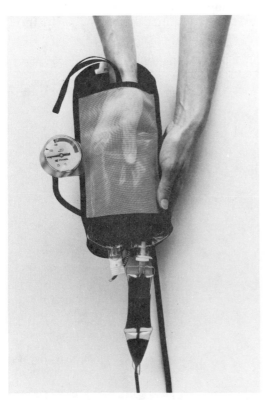

Figure 28–10. A controlled-pressure administration device for rapid infusion of blood products. (Courtesy of Fenwal Laboratories, Deerfield, Illinois.)

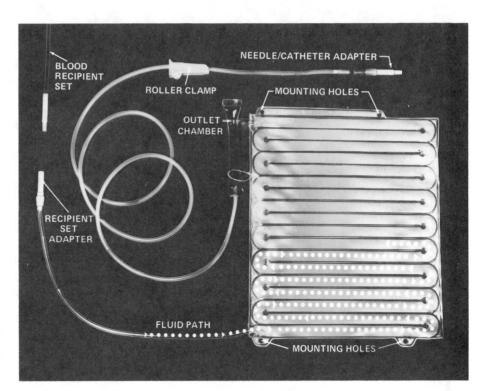

Figure 28–12. Schematic representation of a blood-warming administration set showing the path of blood flow from bottom to top of the set. (Courtesy of Fenwal Laboratories, Deerfield, Illinois.)

REWARMING

The administration of large volumes of blood that have been stored in the blood bank refrigerator and have not been rewarmed can be hazardous to any patient, particularly to the young or to those who are in shock. In addition, cold blood flows very slowly through the infusion tubing. To prevent overheating of the blood and resultant hemolysis, one should warm the blood "in-line" just prior to infusion. One should use a commercially available blood warmer (Fenwal Laboratories' dry heat blood warmer no. 4R4305) that uses electric heating plates to warm a formed coil of plastic tubing "in-line" to the recipient in a continuously monitored and controlled manner. Patients with cold agglutinin diseases should receive only warmed blood products. (Figs. 28–12 through 28–14).

The rapid infusion of large amounts of cold blood may result in significant hypothermia in the recipient. This may aggravate the hypothermia that is invariably present in shock states. At present, there is no satisfactory method of quickly warming large amounts of blood for rapid infusion. Some centers use warmed saline; others simply put the cold blood packs in a bath of hot water, but there is little standardization of techniques. Standard blood warmers should be used routinely, but they lead to unacceptable flow resistance for the patient in shock, who must receive blood rapidly.

MONITORING

During the first 5 to 10 minutes and then every 15 minutes during a transfusion of any blood product, the patient must be carefully monitored

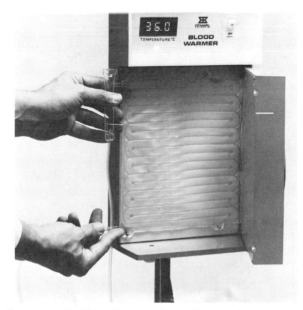

Figure 28–13. The blood-warming administration set being placed inside the dry-heat warmer. The bag should be placed into the warmer and the unit door closed before the tubing is primed with normal saline. Note the temperature display. The entire unit can be mounted on a vertical pole. (Courtesy of Fenwal Laboratories, Deerfield, Illinois.)

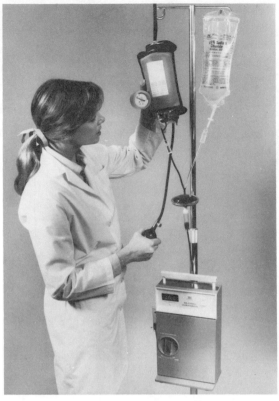

Figure 28–14. Physician administering blood under pressure through a blood warmer. Note that the increased resistance of the blood warmer tubing requires increased pressurization to maintain good flow rates. (Courtesy of Fenwal Laboratories, Deerfield, Illinois.)

for evidence of a transfusion reaction. Signs and symptoms that one may encounter are hives, chills, diarrhea, fever, pruritus, flushing, abdominal or back pain, tightness in the chest or the throat, and respiratory distress. A potentially life-threatening acute hemolytic transfusion reaction in a patient who has received prior transfusions may differ clinically from an allergic, nuisance reaction only by its effects on the patient's pulse and blood pressure. One can safely treat an allergic reaction to leukocytes or plasma proteins causing hives, itching, fever, or chills by administering an antihistamine (but not into the blood infusion line) and stopping the transfusion.

When one encounters an increase in pulse rate, a decrease in blood pressure, respiratory symptoms, chest or abdominal discomfort, or the "sensation of impending doom," one must *stop* the transfusion *immediately* and must infuse normal saline to maintain blood pressure and urine output. Samples of urine and blood should be sent to the laboratory to verify the presence of free hemoglobin. The blood bank should also receive a clotted sample of blood to reassess the presence of any immune reaction. If the conclusion of the blood bank evaluation is that the reaction is a nonhemolytic allergic response, premedication with antihistamines (diphenhydramine or hy-

droxyzine) and antipyretics is indicated prior to the next transfusion. Alternatively, washed cells could be used.

The patient in whom a hemolytic transfusion reaction is suspected should be treated vigorously and promptly.[20] Most mortality and morbidity is secondary to hypotension and shock leading to cardiovascular instability, renal insufficiency, respiratory manifestations, or hemorrhagic complications of disseminated intravascular coagulation. The initial treatment is directed toward treating the hypotension by infusion of 5 per cent dextrose in saline or lactated Ringer's solution or vasopressors, if required. The volume and rate of infusion are determined by blood pressure response. Symptomatic treatment with acetaminophen, a warming blanket, epinephrine for bronchospasm or subglottic edema, or antipruritics or antihistamines is of secondary importance.

If an acute hemolytic transfusion reaction occurs, there may be some benefit from alkalinization of the urine with intravenous sodium bicarbonate, theoretically to prevent the precipitation of free hemoglobin. Forced diuresis with mannitol to maintain the urine output at 50 to 100 ml per hour has also been advocated. The benefit from alkalinization and diuresis in the prevention of acute renal shutdown is uncertain, although the use of these techniques is advocated by most texts.[8–10] When shock is controlled, an assessment of hemostasis, respiratory function, renal function, and cardiac function will help direct later therapy of the complications; disseminated intravascular coagulation may call for the administration of plasma, platelets, or fibrinogen, and acute tubular necrosis may dictate careful fluid management. Hemolytic transfusion reactions have become unusual. They are rarely fatal and are usually attributable to an error in identification (such as can result from the treatment of two "John Doe" patients simultaneously).

Delayed, or "late," hemolytic transfusion reactions may occur days, or even weeks, after transfusion of red cells. They are characterized by dropping hemoglobin levels, jaundice, hemoglobinemia, and indirect hyperbilirubinemia.[21] This complication is usually self-limited and is not life-threatening. Therapy is symptomatic, but future attempts at cross-matching for transfusions may be difficult because of the presence of red cell antibodies. Individuals so affected should wear identification tags or bracelets alerting medical personnel that prior transfusion reactions have occurred.

Conclusions

Upon the completion of a transfusion, an entry in the patient's record should be made to indicate the volume and nature of what was transfused and the presence or absence of any reaction. The progress note, the transfusion record sheet, or the transfusion laboratory slip can be used for this purpose and should be signed and dated by the physician or nurse, in accordance with hospital policies. The bag in which the blood was stored might be discarded or returned to the blood bank, as individual policies dictate.

The practitioner should emphasize to the patient and his family the critical importance of any blood transfusion in his care. It could then be suggested that the family consider arranging for replacement donations of units of blood, to afford other future patients the luxury of an ample, available supply of blood products.

1. Denis, J.: Philos. Proc. R. Soc. No. 32, 617, 1667–1668, cited in Mollison, P. L.: Blood Transfusion in Clinical Medicine, 6th ed. Oxford, Blackwell Scientific Publications, 1979, p. 1.
2. Cannan, R. K.: Foreword to "General Principles of Blood Transfusion." Transfusion 3:304, 1963.
3. The Medical Letter 21:00, 1979.
4. Milner, L. V., and Butcher, K.: Transfusion reactions reported after transfusions of red blood cells and of whole blood. Transfusion 18:493, 1978.
5. Blumberg, N., and Bove, J. R.: Un-cross-matched blood for emergency transfusion. JAMA 240:2057, 1978.
6. Dixon, J. L., and Smalley, M. G.: Jehovah's Witnesses: The surgical/ethical challenge. JAMA 246:2471, 1981.
7. Boral, L. I., and Henry, J. B.: The type and screen: A safe alternative and supplement in selected surgical procedures. Transfusion 17:163, 1977.
8. Cowley, R. A., and Dunham, M. (eds.): Shock Trauma/Critical Care Manual. Baltimore, University Park Press, 1982.
9. Walt, A. J., and Wilson, R. F. (eds.): Management of Trauma. Philadelphia, Lea & Febiger, 1975.
10. Zuidema, G. D., Rutherford, R. B., and Ballinger, W. F. (eds.): The Management of Trauma. Philadelphia, W. B. Saunders Co., 1979.
11. Counts, R. B., Haisch, C., Simon, L., et al.: Hemostasis in massively transfused trauma patients. Ann. Surg. 190:91, 1979.
12. Wilson, R. F., Mammen, E., and Walt, A. F.: Eight years of experience with massive blood transfusions. J. Trauma 11:275, 1971.
13. Shomer, P. R., and Dawson, R. B.: Transfusion therapy in trauma: A review of principles and techniques used in the MIEMS program. Am. Surgeon 45:109, 1979.
14. Clarke, J. R., Davidson, S. J., Bergman, G. E., and Geller, N. L.: Optimal blood ordering for emergency department patients. Ann. Emerg. Med. 9:1, 1980.
15. Murphy, R. J. C., Malhotra, C., and Sweet, A. Y.: Death following an exchange transfusion with hemoglobin SC blood. J. Pediatr. 96:110, 1980.
16. Herrera, A. J., and Corless, J.: Blood transfusions: Effect of speed of infusion and of needle gauge on hemolysis. J. Pediatr. 99:757, 1981.
17. Risberg, B. I., Hurley, M. J., Miller, E., et al.: Filtration characteristics of the polyester fiber micropore blood transfusion filter. South. Med. J. 72:657, 1979.
18. Snyder, E. L., Hezzey, A., Cooper-Smith, M., et al.: Effect of microaggregate blood filtration on platelet concentrates in vitro. Transfusion 21:427, 1981.
19. Ballance, J. II. W.: Equipment and methods for rapid blood transfusion. Br. J. Hosp. Med. 26:411, 1981.
20. Pineda, A. A., Brzica, S. M., and Taswell, H. F.: Hemolytic transfusion reaction: Recent experience in a large blood bank. Mayo Clin. Proc. 53:378, 1978.
21. Pineda, A. A., Taswell, H. F., and Brzica, S. M.: Delayed hemolytic transfusion reaction: An immunologic hazard of blood transfusion. Transfusion 18:1, 1978.

29

Autotransfusion (Autologous Blood Transfusion)

THOMAS B. PURCELL, M.D.
GARY P. YOUNG, M.D.

Introduction

Among the various afflictions that may jeopardize human life and well-being, traumatic injury has, in recent decades, been ravaging an ever-expanding proportion of men and women during their most productive years.[1] This fact, coupled with increasingly efficient and rapid emergency transportation systems, has resulted in growing numbers of these victims arriving at emergency facilities in potentially salvageable condition. The ensuing urgent demand for blood has often exceeded the immediately available supplies of homologous bank blood. Successful approaches to this problem have included earlier hemostasis (i.e., definitive surgery), use of blood substitutes (crystalloid, colloid), and autotransfusion.

Autotransfusion may be defined as "collection and reinfusion of the patient's own blood for volume replacement."[2] Emergency autotransfusion most often involves collection of shed blood from a major body cavity, usually the pleural space (hemothorax) and occasionally from the peritoneal space. Autotransfusion in the emergency department is generally limited to acute hemothorax with clinically significant hypovolemia. The following discussion will examine the advantages and potential complications of emergency autotransfusion, patient selection, equipment available, and procedural technique for one widely used device.

Background

Autotransfusion has a relatively extended tradition in the Western medical literature. The first report was published in 1818 by Blundell,[3] an obstetrician who salvaged and reinfused shed vaginal blood in 10 patients with severe postpartum hemorrhage. Highmore,[4] in 1874, espoused the use of autotransfusion after recounting his experience with a patient who succumbed to postpartum hemorrhage, and in 1886, Duncan[5] used the technique without notable ill effects while reinfusing blood shed during an amputation. In 1914, the use of the technique in ectopic pregnancies was popularized by Thies,[6] and 3 years later, Elmendorf[7] published a description of the first case of autotransfusion from traumatic hemothorax. Also in 1917, Lockwood[8] used the procedure for the first time in the United States during a splenectomy performed on a patient with Banti's syndrome. By 1922, Burch[9] was able to accumulate 164 cases for review from the world literature.

The discovery of ABO blood typing at the turn of the century and the institution of blood banks in the 1930's led to the almost exclusive use of homologous blood up to and following World War II. Interest in autotransfusion concomitantly declined, and only sporadic reports appeared in the literature during this period. During the 1960's and 1970's, cardiopulmonary bypass surgery generated extensive data regarding intraoperative retrieval of large quantities of blood for reinfusion. Concurrently, the Vietnam War created tremendous new demands for readily available blood in areas remote from conventional reserves of homologous bank blood. Thus, revitalized interest, coupled with growing experience, generated the early publications of such investigators as Dyer,[10] Klebanoff,[11, 12] and Symbas,[13, 14] which initiated the "new era" of autotransfusion.

Advantages

The advantages of autotransfusion over bank blood transfusion in patients who are hypovolemic from traumatic blood loss include the following:

1. Immediate availability to the patient (collection and initiation of reinfusion can be accomplished within minutes).

2. Blood compatibility, avoiding both untoward transfusion reactions and the problem of crossmatching uncommon blood types.

3. Immediate reinfusion of normothermic autologous blood and consequent lessening of life-threatening complications of hypothermia, created by the administration of room temperature fluids.[15]

4. Elimination of the risk of indirect patient-to-patient transmission of infectious diseases.

5. Levels of 2,3-DPG have been found to be significantly higher in autotransfused red blood cells than in stored homologous cells with an average 2,3-DPG shelf life of 4.2 days.[16]

6. No reported direct complications of metabolic acidosis, hypocalcemia, or hyperkalemia.[17–20]

7. Less risk of inadvertent circulatory overload.[21]

8. May be acceptable to those patients whose religious convictions prohibit transfusions with homologous blood.*

9. Autotransfusion lowers the cost of medical care. No blood drawing, typing, or crossmatching is required; thus, time, money, and personnel expenditures may be conserved. Davidson[23] reported the cost of autologous blood to be $12 per unit for the first three units and $8 per unit thereafter for emergency resuscitation compared with between $25 and $75 per unit of bank blood. Mattox[24] reported the autotransfusion of a total of 134 L of blood in 69 patients over a 2-year period. The total cost of the disposable equipment used was approximately $1500, which translated to a savings of $13,400 when compared with expenses for similar volumes of banked donor blood.

Indications and Contraindications
(Patient Selection)

In general, all victims of severe trauma, whether blunt or penetrating, should be considered potential candidates for autotransfusion. More specifically, Reul[20] has described three categories of patients for whom emergency autotransfusion is suitable. First, the ideal candidates are patients who have sustained blunt or penetrating chest trauma, with an acute chest tube collection of 1500 ml or more of blood. A second category consisted of patients with less than one whole body blood volume loss for whom no homologous blood, or only limited quantities, were available because of the urgency of the situation, bank blood shortage, or a difficult crossmatch. Under these circumstances, Reul used autotransfusion regardless of the type of injury or degree of contamination. A third category comprised patients with massive blood loss (over one whole body blood volume) for whom autotransfusion served as a supplement to homologous replacement. O'Riordan[18] adds a

---

*Techniques for intraoperative or extraoperative collection of autologous blood that involve blood storage or reinfusion of shed blood are objectionable to Jehovah's Witnesses. Nonetheless, salvage where extracorporeal circulation is uninterrupted may be acceptable to many members of that religion.[22]

fourth category: trauma patients who urgently require blood transfusion and whose religious convictions prohibit homologous transfusion. In a broader sense, it seems clinically reasonable to use autotransfusion in all suitable patients who have a hemothorax and will require even minimal blood replacement. In situations in which the need for homologous blood transfusion is borderline, autologous blood can be readily reinfused without the risk of complications associated with the use of bank blood.

In our own emergency department, we have simplified the *indications* for initiating collection for possible autotransfusion to the following:

1. Patients sustaining blunt or penetrating chest trauma with significant hemothorax (500 ml or more) as suggested on a chest film.

2. Multiple trauma patients with shock of uncertain etiology for whom immediate (prior to chest film) tube thoracotomy is contemplated.

3. Emergency thoracotomy.

4. Patients with hemothorax who urgently require blood and whose religious beliefs prohibit homologous transfusions.

Reul[20] also suggested the following four general *contraindications* to the use of emergency autotransfusion:

1. The presence of malignant lesions in the area of traumatic blood accumulation.

2. Known renal or hepatic insufficiency.

3. Wounds older than 4 to 6 hours (due to the theoretical problem of bacterial overgrowth).

4. Gross contamination of pooled blood, usually as a result of trauma of the gastrointestinal tract.

He added, however, that "the presence of any of these contraindications was occasionally overruled by the lack of available (bank) blood."

Several investigators believe that the reinfusion of possibly contaminated blood from the peritoneal cavity may be accomplished without unacceptable risk,[12, 20, 23, 25, 26] but the consensus is that exsanguinating hemorrhage is the only acceptable indication for autotransfusion when there is recognized intestinal contamination. Klebanoff,[27] on the other hand, believes that autotransfusion has "no place" where there is extensive fecal or urinary contamination of the pooled blood. Thus, the advisability of autotransfusing possibly contaminated blood from the peritoneal cavity remains controversial (see the section entitled Complications).

Equipment and Materials

AUTOTRANSFUSION UNITS

Symbas[13, 31, 32] described a simplified collection system using standard materials available in any emergency department. After insertion of a chest tube, drainage is established into a standard chest tube bottle containing 400 ml of normal saline, maintaining a suction of 12 to 16 torr.* If autotransfusion is required, the collected blood in the chest bottle is reinfused in one of two ways.

1. The chest bottle may be disconnected from the pleural drainage tube and simply inverted on an IV stand for reinfusion through a filter into the patient. During infusion, a second sterile chest bottle with saline is connected to the chest tube for continuing collection.

2. After disconnection from the pleural drainage tube, the chest bottle may be connnected to a standard blood collection bag and the salvaged blood is transferred to this bag for subsequent reinfusion in the conventional manner. Symbas reported more than 400 patients autotransfused by this method since 1966, with no adverse effects attributable to the procedure.

Von Koch and associates[28] reported their experience with the Sorenson unit in autotransfusing each of 30 trauma patients an average of 1000 ml of salvaged blood. They found this unit was quickly assembled and easily operated, and its use resulted in minimal air-blood interfacing (a source of hemolysis). They also described the unit as "efficacious, inexpensive, cost effective and safe." Davidson[23, 29] described in detail the step-by-step use of the Sorenson autotransfusion unit in the emergency department and characterized it as "probably the simplest and most practical device available for the emergency setting." The cost of this unit was less than $200 in 1980.[30] Autotransfusion using this device is explained in the following section.

The Haemonetics Cell Saver (Haemonetics Corp., Natick, MA) aspirates the patient's blood into a reservoir and brings the blood, after it has been anticoagulated, through a special suction line to a centrifuge. The centrifuge spins off the supernatant fluid consisting of plasma that contains hemolyzed cells, free hemoglobin, fat cells, electrolytes, anticoagulant, and contaminants. When the hematocrit of the remaining blood approaches 55 to 65 per cent, normal saline washes it clear of hemolyzed cells and the packed and washed cells are then reinfused. Major disadvantages of the device, in the opinion of Mattox,[33] are its complexity, requiring a specially trained technician for its operation, and its cost ($16,000 as of October 1980). Use of the Cell Saver system offers the theoretical advantage of avoiding reinfusion of "activated clotting factors." Brewster believes that this advantage is achieved "at the expense of an earlier dilutional decrease of coagulation factors, which are totally lost with discarded plasma and wash

---

*Many of the disposable plastic thoracostomy collection devices now have the ability to act as reservoirs for autotransfusion in case the need arises.

fluid."[34] Therefore, the system requires the use of fresh frozen plasma as well as additional colloid, such as albumin, to replace the discarded plasma volume.

Two autotransfusion devices that are off the market but may still be found in use are the Bentley ATS-100 (Bentley Laboratories, Inc., Santa Ana, CA) and the Pall Autotransfuser (Pall Corp., Glen Cove, NY). The former system consists of an aspirating segment that is activated by a roller pump, a reservoir that may be pressurized to augment return flow, and a delivery system.[27] The requirement of a specially trained technician plus the potential risk of massive air embolism makes this device less useful in the emergency department setting. The Pall autotransfusion device consists of two containers. While aspirating into one container, pressure can be applied on the other and blood can be given back to the patient. Mattox found "considerable hemolysis" associated with the device, as well as a filter that required changing after every two units of blood were collected.[33]

BLOOD FILTERS

Some form of in-line filtration is advisable during reinfusion of blood products in order to reduce the danger of microembolization and resulting pulmonary insufficiency.[24, 35] Drye[36] simply strained aspirated blood through eight layers of gauze into a bottle and reinfused directly into the patient without further filtration. He reported almost 100 cases, with only one case of morbidity, and in that case, the blood had not been strained. Controversy continues regarding the relation between microaggregates and the development of the respiratory distress syndrome;[37] however, most authors advise some form of micropore filtration during emergency autotransfusion. Pore size seems to be the only issue, and recommendations range from 170 microns[38] to 20 microns.[19] The preponderance of data appears to show that a pore size of 40 microns minimizes the risk of microembolization without undue elevations in filtration pressures.[2, 16, 17, 20, 24, 28, 39, 40]

VACUUM SUCTION

The amount of vacuum suction used should be limited to minimize red blood cell hemolysis.[34] Reul[20] found that 5 to 10 torr was well within the safe range. Von Koch and associates[28] used 10 torr, Davidson[23] used 20 to 40 torr, Noon[38] used 30 to 60 torr, and Brewster and colleagues[34] and Dyer and coworkers[10] found that levels below 100 torr kept hemolysis to a minimum.

Suction of 60 torr or less is preferred by most

authors for aspiration of hemothorax or hemoperitoneum,[20, 23, 28, 34, 38] but in the operating room, adequate suction to maintain a bloodless surgical field may require up to 100 torr or more.[10, 19]

ANTICOAGULATION

Anticoagulation of the aspirate during autotransfusion has been ensured using several different methods, including heparin both locally and systemically,[41] acid citrate dextrose (ACD),[12, 19] citrate phosphate dextrose (CPD),[17, 20, 24, 28, 41] and normal saline.[13, 31, 32] Local heparinization of tubing and reservoir may lead to the formation of platelet microaggregates on the filter,[13] and systemic heparinization could lead to further life-threatening hemorrhage in an already bleeding patient.[20, 24, 27] Therefore, the use of heparin as an anticoagulant during emergency autotransfusion of the trauma patient is discouraged by most investigators.[13, 16, 38, 42]

ACD was used as an alternative to heparin in several early reports.[32, 42, 43] Raines[19] found no clinical or laboratory evidence of intravascular coagulopathy after autotransfusion using ACD, even in patients who received more than 8000 ml of autologous blood. More recent studies report the use of CPD for extracorporeal anticoagulation. CPD avoids the complications of heparinization,[20] necessitates less volume as an anticoagulant, and results in less acidosis than does ACD.[48] Reul[20] found CPD to be well tolerated, even in large amounts.

Although reported volumes of citric acid and sodium citrate solution for each 500 ml of collected blood range up to 700 ml and 1800 ml, respectively,[17, 20, 24, 28, 44] most recent research has recommended lower levels, in the range of 25 to 30 ml, of CPD per 500 ml of collected blood.[17, 20, 24] A ratio of CPD to blood of 1:7 has also been suggested. This level compares favorably with the standard 67 ml of CPD per unit of bank donor blood.[20] Klebanoff[27] believes that CPD is currently the safest method of anticoagulation for autotransfusion and that use of CPD avoids the problem of clot formation on the blood filter, thus maintaining higher platelet counts in reinfused blood.

Davidson has noted that for the average chest wound, added anticoagulant may not be required,[23] because moderate rates of bleeding allow time for defibrination by contact with serosal surfaces (pleural surfaces) and by mechanical action of the heart.[23] Others[11, 13, 31, 32, 39, 45] report the same findings and recommend simple reinfusion through a filter without any coagulant. Nonetheless, wounds of the great vessels may bleed at a rate that allows coagulable blood to enter the collection reservoir and clot off the entire system.[23, 28] In such an instance, an anticoagulant,

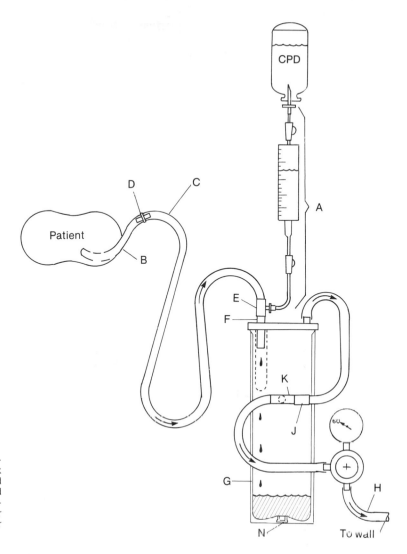

Figure 29–1. Collection Apparatus. *A*, Anticoagulant volume control burette; *B*, Chest tube; *C*, Latex drainage tubing; *D*, Male-to-male connector; *E*, End of drainage tubing with side port; *F*, Inlet port of red liner cap attached to collection canister; *G*, Collection liner bag; *H*, Downstream suction hose; *J*, Liner lid tubing connector; *K*, Canister tee; and *N*, Liner stem with protective cap.

specifically CPD, would be indispensable. Thus, accepted procedure includes the use of CPD, which itself undergoes such rapid metabolism that anticoagulation is, to a large degree, confined to blood in the autotransfusion apparatus. Rarely, with excessive use, CPD can cause citrate intoxication due to chelation of calcium and subsequent cardiac dysrhythmias. Use of insufficient or outdated CPD may result in clotting of collected blood.

Procedure Using the Sorenson Autotransfusion System

Mattox[33] set forth the properties of the ideal autotransfusion device: 1) easy and quick assemblage, 2) cost effectiveness, 3) easy operation, 4) in-line microfiltration, 5) minimization of air-fluid interfaces, 6) simple anticoagulation technique. The Sorenson device, which is currently in wide use, conforms to the above specifications and

therefore will be discussed in detail. The relatively low cost of the collection device allows one to prepare for possible autotransfusion in all patients requiring thoracostomy, with selective use of the system based on the subsequent clinical course.

The Sorenson autotransfusion system consists of a closed, rigid, nonsterile plastic canister into which a gas-autoclaved plastic bag is placed for blood collection. The canister is mounted on a movable support device (IV pole) and connected to a vacuum regulator valve for control of negative suction pressure. The collection bag is placed in-line with disposable collection tubing, which has a separate inlet valve for admixture of anticoagulant and aspirated blood. This inlet is connected via sterile tubing to a bottle of CPD (Fig. 29–1).

COLLECTION

1. To collect autologous blood from a hemothorax, first open the included "Trauma Drainage

Tubing Set'' containing one 36-French chest tube, latex drainage tubing (C) and a male-to-male connector (D). While tube thoracostomy is being performed in the usual manner, the burette set (A) is connected to the CPD bottle and the burette is filled with 150 ml of CPD.

2. Connect the yellow-tipped (E) end of the latex drainage tubing (the end with the side port) to the inlet port (F) of the red liner cap attached to the collection canister (Fig. 29–2). Then remove the protective cap from the side port and connect the anticoagulant (CPD) administration line (Fig. 29–3). Prime the liner with 50 ml of CPD from the burette.

3. Connect the downstream suction hose (H) to wall suction, and turn wall suction to maximum. Be sure that the regulator on the autotransfusion stand does not exceed the preset 60 torr during collection (100 torr Hg in special situations such as thoracotomy); otherwise, excessive hemolysis of red blood cells may result (see Fig. 29–1).

4. When the chest tube is in place, connect the latex drainage tubing and begin collection. During collection, stay ahead of the accumulating blood volume with the CPD in 50-ml increments. Always keep the ratio no less than one part CPD to 10 parts blood (1:7 ratio of CPD to blood is recommended by the manufacturer); otherwise the collected blood may clot, especially with massive ongoing hemorrhage. Do not overfill the liner bag; it will overflow, spilling blood into the regulator valve.

REINFUSION

1. Prepare a standard Y-type blood infusion line with a high capacity 40-micron in-line filter, prime the line and filter with normal saline, and connect it to a large bore intravenous access (14 gauge or larger) (see Fig. 29–7).

2. When the liner bag is full, temporarily clamp the chest tube, discontinue suction, and remove the yellow end of the latex drainage tubing (E) from the red liner lid. The liner lid tubing connector (J) is now removed from the canister tee (K) (Fig. 29–4) and connected to the inlet port (F) of the liner cap, thus sealing the top of the collection lid (Fig. 29–5).

3. Remove the liner assembly from the canister by pushing upward on the thumb tab (Fig. 29–5), lift out the liner bag, invert the bag, and unscrew the protective cap (N) over the bottom stem of the liner. Now insert the free recipient arm (L) of the Y-tube infusion line into the stem of the collection bag (Fig. 29–6), and hang the liner bag on the IV stand by the attached tab (M) (Fig. 29–7). Prior to infusion, briefly disconnect the liner lid tubing connector (J), *vent all air from the bag* (to eliminate the possibility of air embolism), then reconnect it to the inlet port.

4. Gravity flow, manual squeezing of the liner bag, or an in-line roller pump may be used to hasten reinfusion. Although some authors[23, 28] mention the use of encircling pneumatic blood pumps during reinfusion, the Sorenson Company[30] cautions that such devices may damage the pump or rupture the liner bag.

5. During reinfusion, autologous blood collection may be continued with a second liner bag. Be sure that the new liner bag is fully extended before placing it into the canister (Fig. 29–8). If the bag is crumpled at the top of the canister, blood may be sucked directly into the regulator valve. Insert the new liner into the canister, and snap the lid in place with the thumb tab directly over the

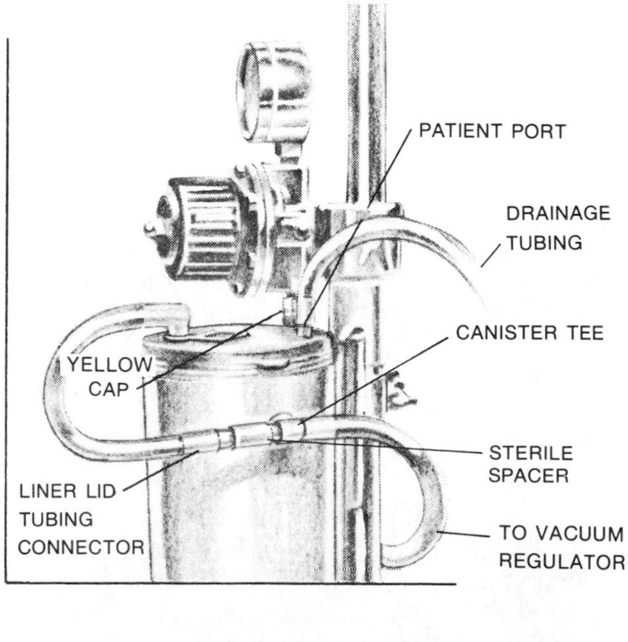

Figure 29–2. Collection Apparatus. Detail of canister connections prior to attachment of anticoagulant line. (From Receptal ATS Trauma. Sorenson Research Co., Salt Lake City, Utah, p. 5. Used by permission.)

PATIENT PORT

DRAINAGE TUBING

CANISTER TEE

YELLOW CAP

STERILE SPACER

LINER LID TUBING CONNECTOR

TO VACUUM REGULATOR

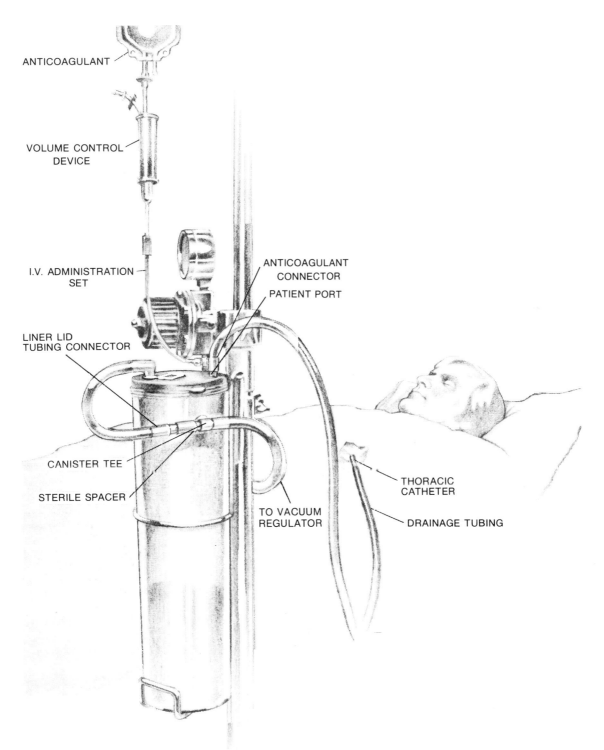

ANTICOAGULANT

VOLUME CONTROL
DEVICE

I.V. ADMINISTRATION
SET

LINER LID
TUBING CONNECTOR

CANISTER TEE

STERILE SPACER

ANTICOAGULANT
CONNECTOR

PATIENT PORT

TO VACUUM
REGULATOR

THORACIC
CATHETER

DRAINAGE TUBING

Figure 29–3. Collection Apparatus. Proper attachment of anticoagulant line. (From Receptal ATS Trauma. Sorenson Research Co., Salt Lake City, Utah, p. 5. Used by permission.)

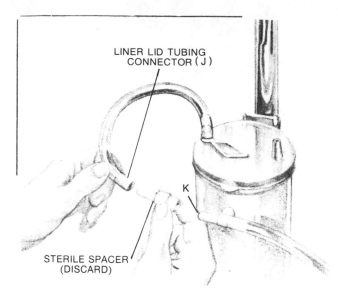

LINER LID TUBING
CONNECTOR (J)

K

STERILE SPACER
(DISCARD)

Figure 29–4. Preparation for reinfusion. Removal of liner lid tubing connector (J) from canister tee (K). (From Receptal ATS Trauma. Sorenson Research Co., Salt Lake City, Utah, p. 5. Used by permission.)

Figure 29–5. Preparation for reinfusion. Removal of liner assembly from the canister after connecting the liner lid tubing connector (J) to the inlet port of the liner cap. (From Receptal ATS Trauma. Sorenson Research Co., Salt Lake City, Utah, p. 6. Used by permission.)

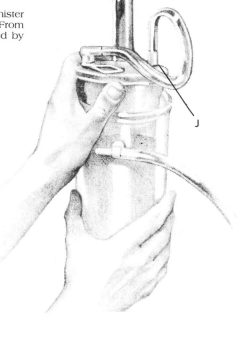

J

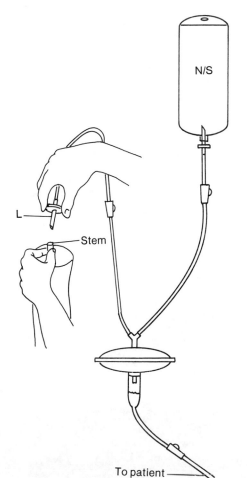

N/S

L

Stem

To patient

Figure 29–6. Preparation for reinfusion. Inserting the free recipient arm (L) of the prepared "Y"-type infusion line into the stem of the collection bag. (From Receptal ATS Trauma. Sorenson Research Co., Salt Lake City, Utah, p. 7. Used by permission.)

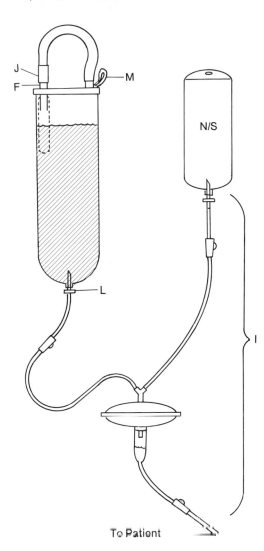

Figure 29–7. Reinfusion apparatus. *F*, Inlet port of liner cap; *I*, "Y"type blood infusion line with in-line 40 micron filter; *J*, Liner lid tubing connector; *L*, Liner bag connection with infusion line; *M*, Attached hanger tab at top of liner bag; and *N/S*, Normal saline intravenous fluid (for priming and maintaining patency of the system during liner bag changes).

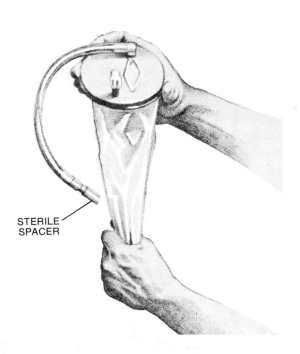

Figure 29–8. Straightening liner bag prior to insertion into canister. (From Receptal ATS Trauma. Sorenson Research Co., Salt Lake City, Utah, p. 3. Used by permission.)

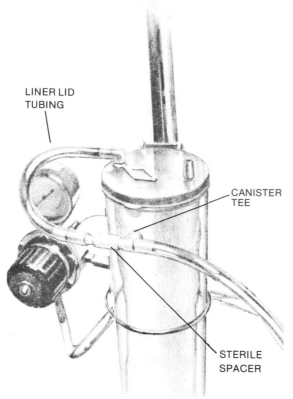

LINER LID
TUBING

CANISTER
TEE

STERILE
SPACER

Figure 29–9. Proper placement of liner bag lid on canister. (From Receptal ATS Trauma. Sorenson Research Co., Salt Lake City, Utah, p. 4. Used by permission.)

canister tee (Fig. 29–9). The unit is now ready for collection assembly as previously outlined.

ADDITIONAL INFORMATION

1. Use each liner bag only once.

2. After reinfusing a total of 3500 ml, or seven units, of autologous blood, one unit of fresh frozen plasma is required, and thereafter, one unit of fresh frozen plasma is required for every two units (1,000 ml) of autotransfused blood.[19]

3. To minimize risk from bacterial overgrowth, collected blood must not be allowed to stand for prolonged periods of time prior to reinfusion.[46] One source[47] advises a limit of no more than 4 hours between collection and reinfusion. On the other hand, Mollison[48] believes that "in temperate climates it is not essential to refrigerate blood until at least 8 hours after collection, since this period at room temperature has scarcely any adverse effect on red cell preservation, and partly because during a period of this duration the blood still contains viable phagocytes." The age of collected blood probably should be calculated from the time of injury, and reinfusion of blood older than 4 to 8 hours should be considered hazardous. Since one is performing the procedure for significant hypovolemia in the emergency department, the

collected blood is transfused as soon as the collection bag is full.

4. If some of or all the collected blood becomes clotted in the liner bag, the blood should be discarded.

5. The blood filter used during reinfusion is changed as needed (usually after each 1000- to 2000-ml transfusion).

Complications

Complications from autotransfusion are generally clinically insignificant if the proper technique is followed and if less than 3000 ml of blood is reinfused.

HEMATOLOGIC COMPLICATIONS

The complications of autotransfusion can be categorized as hematologic and nonhematologic (Table 29–1). The most reproducible hematologic consequence is thrombocytopenia (Fig. 29–10). Samples taken from collected autologous blood show low platelet counts; however, the number of platelets found in this blood was significantly greater than that found in bank blood.[39] Until patients receive more than 4000 ml of autologous blood, in vivo platelet counts do not decend below 60,000 per cu mm,[17, 19, 23, 31, 34] a level above which trauma surgery can be "performed satisfactorily."[50] Although those platelets collected from autotransfusion reservoirs function abnormally when tested in vitro by aggregation or serotonin uptake and release, postinfusion samples drawn from the patient aggregate normally.[19] Platelet counts should be followed, and significant thrombocytopenia can be remedied with platelet infusion.

The most common coagulation factor abnormality postautotransfusion is hypofibrinogenemia, especially when the volume of autologous blood

Table 29–1. POTENTIAL COMPLICATIONS OF AUTOTRANSFUSION

Hematologic
  Decreased platelet count
  Decreased fibrinogen level
  Increased fibrin split products
  Prolonged prothrombin time
  Prolonged partial thromboplastin time
  Red blood cell hemolysis
  Elevated plasma free hemoglobin
  Decreased hematocrit

Nonhematologic
  Bacteremia
  Sepsis?
  Microembolism
  Air embolism

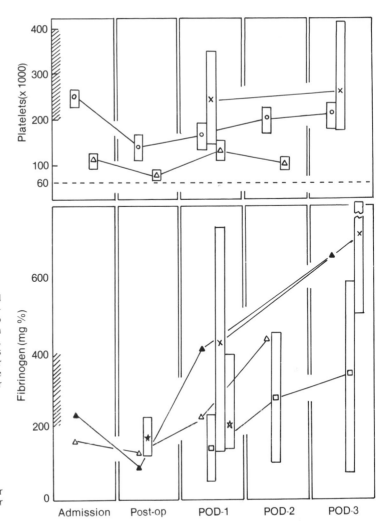

Figure 29–10. Representative platelet counts and serum fibrinogen levels in patients undergoing emergency autotransfusion. Samples were drawn prior to (Admission) and immediately after autotransfusion (Post-op) as well as on postoperative days (POD) one, two, and three. Normal ranges are represented as shaded areas along the ordinate. Points are coded for source identification (see Key) and designate average or mean values. Bars indicate standard deviations or ranges of reported data.

KEY

△ Broadic[45] 20 PTs—mean vol. 5535 ml
□ Mattox[24] 69 PTs—average vol. 2150 ml
☆ Reul[20] 25 PTs—average vol. 2104 ml
○ O'Riordan[18] 6 PTs—average vol. 4450 ml
× Symbas[13] 11 PTs—average vol. 1800 ml
▲ Stillman[51] (dog study)—150–300 ml/kg
(Sources from which data were extracted. The number of patients studied by each author and the average or mean blood volume autotransfused are noted.)

used exceeds 4000 ml.[13, 24, 39] Because of the liver's capacity to replenish fibrinogen rapidly (see Fig. 29–10), the low postautotransfusion levels have not proved to be clinically significant.[20, 23, 39] Yet some authors[20] believe that hepatic insufficiency is a relative contraindication to autotransfusion unless fibrinogen is supplemented.

Symbas[13, 14, 31, 32] extended his work with laboratory dogs to the clinical study of 11 victims of traumatic hemothorax. He found no clinical evidence of coagulopathy following autotransfusion in any patient as long as the volume collected and reinfused remained equal to or less than one half the patient's total blood volume. In those few patients who require a larger volume autotransfused, a proportional decrease in platelets and fibrinogen occurred, requiring subsequent correction with fresh frozen plasma and platelet packs. Other investigators[17, 23, 24] have confirmed these findings and have shown that there is a return to normal of both platelet and fibrinogen levels by 48 to 72 hours without replacement therapy. Similarly, elevations in prothrombin and partial thromboplastin times, which were encountered routinely, were not clinically significant. These coagulation abnormalities were self-corrected in 48 to 72 hours (Fig. 29–11).[20, 23, 34]

Raines and associates[19] studied 85 patients receiving autotransfusion and found no clinical or laboratory evidence of intravascular coagulopathy, even in patients receiving blood volumes in excess of 8000 ml. A dilutional coagulopathy was noted when volumes greater than 3500 ml were autotransfused. At least one unit of fresh frozen plasma was given for every two units of autotransfused blood beyond this 3500 ml limit.

Red blood cell hemolysis occurs with autotransfusion because of prolonged exposure of the cells to serosal linings of the traumatized body cavities.[51] Hemolysis may also result from mechanical factors during collection and reinfusion, such as high vacuum pressures during aspiration, roller pump trauma, or excess exposure to air-fluid interfaces.[20] An elevated plasma free hemoglobin is a consistent finding in patients receiving autotransfusions (Fig. 29–11).[20, 24, 25, 31, 32] For this rea-

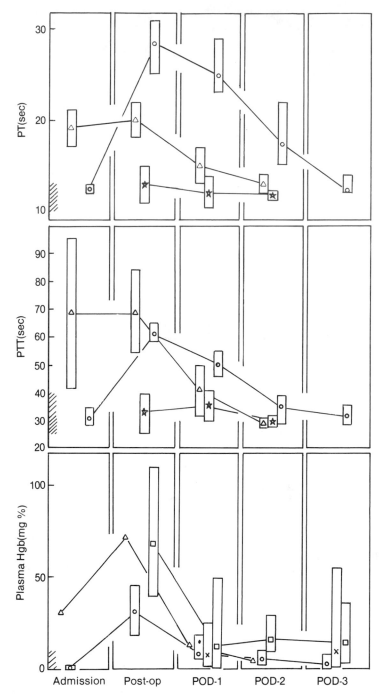

Figure 29–11. Representative prothrombin times (PT), partial thromboplastin times (PTT), and plasma free hemoglobin levels (Plasma Hgb) in patients undergoing emergency autotransfusion. Samples were drawn prior to (Admission) and immediately after autotransfusion (Post-op) as well as on postoperative days (POD) one, two, and three. Normal ranges are represented as shaded areas along the ordinate. Points are coded for source identification (see Key) and designate average or mean values. Bars indicate standard deviations or ranges of reported data.

KEY

△ Broadie[45] 20 PTs—mean vol. 5535 ml
☐ Mattox[24] 69 PTs—average vol. 2150 ml
☆ Reul[20] 25 PTs—average vol. 2104 ml
◯ O'Riordan[18] 6 PTs—average vol. 4450 ml
✕ Symbas[13] 11 PTs—average vol. 1800 ml
▲ Stillman[51] (dog study)—150–300 ml/kg
(Sources from which data were extracted. The number of patients studied by each author and the average or mean blood volume autotransfused are noted.)

son, any collected blood that clots must be discarded[20, 45] and pooled blood older than 4 to 6 hours also should not be autotransfused.[18, 20]

Most samples of blood from the autotransfusion reservoir have had free hemoglobin levels of less than 100 mg/dl.[20, 31] but some have been reported as high as 1388 mg/dl.[24] Plasma-free hemoglobin values immediately postautotransfusion range from 9 to 110 mg/dl., with most falling between 25 and 80 mg/dl.[20, 24, 25, 31, 32] When the binding capacity of haptoglobin is saturated and the

threshold of tubular resorption of hemoglobin is exceeded, hemoglobinuria is seen. This threshold corresponds to a free plasma hemoglobin concentration of 100 mg/dl.[52] It has been proposed that an isolated elevation of plasma-free hemoglobin increases the risk of acute tubular necrosis. The presumed nephrotoxicity of plasma-free hemoglobin and tubular obstruction by hemoglobin casts has been refuted by more recent evidence that indicates that acute renal failure following hemolytic transfusion reactions is primarily the result of renal ischemia secondary to antigen-antibody activated DIC (disseminated intravascular coagulation) and microcirculatory thrombosis.[53] Indeed, it has been shown that "massive hemoglobinuria may follow the transfusion of immunologically compatible hemolyzed RBCs with minimal symptoms and a benign outcome"[54] and that isolated free hemoglobin levels of between 1300 and 1800 mg/dl. may be tolerated without renal compromise.[54, 55] Even though renal failure as a direct consequence of autotransfusion has not been reported,[27] transient elevations in serum creatinine do occur,[18] and in the presence of shock and systemic acidosis, acute tubular necrosis remains a potential complication.[52] In fact, some authors[20] believe that renal insufficiency is only a relative contraindication to autotransfusion unless renal perfusion is at risk.

Finally, the hematocrit falls in direct proportion to the quantity of blood transfused, averaging an approximate drop of 10 to 20 per cent.[13, 20, 25, 31] Raines[19] studied RBC mass in each of 15 patients who were receiving an average of six units during autotransfusion and found that RBC mass fell by about 50 per cent, apparently as a result of a combination of irretrievable intraoperative losses, hemolysis, and hemodilution with priming solutions and other intravenous solutions. Nontraumatized RBC survival has been reported to be normal in all cases studied.[13, 19]

NONHEMATOLOGIC COMPLICATIONS

The theoretical risk of sepsis after the administration of potentially contaminated blood exists within the nonsterile surroundings of the typical emergency department resuscitation area. Experience has shown this risk to be minimal after competent autotransfusion of an isolated hemothorax,[12, 13, 17, 18, 20, 27, 56] and there is *no* evidence suggesting that routine prophylaxis with systemic antibiotics is beneficial in this situation.

The issue of whether or not to autotransfuse shed intraperitoneal blood, however, is somewhat more complex than in the case with hemothorax. Recovery and reinfusion of hemoperitoneum per se has proved to be relatively safe,[12, 17, 18, 20, 26, 56–58] and Klebanoff concluded that "for contaminant-free conditions at least, as in ruptured ectopic pregnancies, ruptured spleen and liver, traumatic hemothorax, and vascular surgery, autotransfusion can be performed readily to reduce the need for homologous blood replacement."[12]

Reinfusion of autologous blood with possible enteric contamination is still considered by most authors to be ill-advised in all but the most desperate of circumstances, such as in the patient who will exsanguinate *before* homologous blood can be made available. If contaminated blood is infused, systemic antibiotics should be used.[12, 17, 18, 24, 27, 58] At least 52 cases of collection and reinfusion of intestinally contaminated hemoperitoneum have been reported.[17, 26, 56–58] The overall mortality of this selected group was 16 per cent, not unexpectedly high considering the severity of the injuries involved. Experimental studies with dogs also show that autotransfusion of hemoperitoneum contaminated by intestinal contents, urine, or bile is tolerated.[12, 25] Nonetheless, when there is confirmed or suspected enteric contamination, autotransfusion should be considered only as a "last-ditch" lifesaving option.

Another complication, microemboli secondary to platelet microaggregation or fat emboli, has largely been eliminated by the use of micropore filters.[19, 20, 34] During reinfusion of collected blood, in most instances there is a mild increase in screen filtration pressures, indicating the formation of microemboli trapped by the filter.[34] There has been no clinical evidence of pulmonary insufficiency or unexplained elevation of the alveolar to arterial oxygen gradient that might be attributed to the passage of microemboli beyond the micropore filter systems.[20]

Air embolism has been reported sporadically as a complication of autotransfusion.[10, 17, 24, 35, 42, 56] This uncommon but often fatal complication has been associated, in all cases reviewed, with autotransfusion systems using automated roller pump units in which the aspirate reservoir was inadvertently allowed to run dry. Air embolism with gravity or with a manually assisted technique is rare.

Available data indicate that although autotransfusion is not free of complications, the risk/benefit ratio weighs heavily in its favor in the resuscitation of selected trauma victims. Klebanoff reviewed the evidence as of 1970 and determined that "in over 1000 documented cases of autotransfusion in the Western literature, not a single death or major complication was attributed directly to the transfusion."[12] Symbas[31] reported autotransfusing more than 200 patients with traumatic hemothorax without any significant morbidity related to the procedure. Mattox[17] reported autotransfusing 69 patients an average of 3.9 units each, with only one death (from air embolism) directly attributable to the procedure.

Conclusion

Autotransfusion, a technique with more than 165 years of experience, has become a subject of renewed interest in the emergency setting. The operation of a relatively simple system has been discussed in detail. The previously feared complications of hematologic or metabolic embarrassment and of sepsis have not proved to be of clinical significance when appropriate patient selection and careful technique are followed. In addition, the use of autologous blood has several advantages over the transfusion of stored homologous blood in the emergency patient, including ready availability of compatible blood, homeostasis of core temperature, higher levels of RBC 2,3-DPG, and cost effectiveness. A review of the literature reveals that, although the technique is not totally free of complications, the benefits to be gained from autotransfusing the selected trauma patient outweigh the relatively limited risk of the procedure. Complications are generally clinically insignificant when proper technique is followed and when less than 3000 ml of shed blood is reinfused.

1. Trunkey, D. D.: Trauma. Sci. Am. 249:28, 1983.
2. Schaff, H. V., Hauer, J. M., and Brawley, R. K.: Autotransfusion in cardiac surgical patients after operation. Surgery 84:713, 1978.
3. Blundell, J.: Experiments on the transfusion of blood. Medico Chir. Trans. 9:56, 1818.
4. Highmore, W.: Overlooked source of blood supply for transfusion in postpartum haemorrhage. Lancet 1:89, 1874.
5. Duncan, J.: On reinfusion of blood in primary and other amputations. Br. Med. J. 1:192, 1886.
6. Thies, H. J.: Zur behandlung der extrauterior graviditar. Zentralbl. Bynaek. 38:1190, 1914.
7. Elmendorf: Uber Wiedeninfusion nach Punktion eines frischern Haemothorax. Munch. Med. Wochenschr. 64:36, 1917.
8. Lockwood, C. D.: Surgical treatment of Banti's disease. Surg. Gynecol. Obstet. 25:188, 1917.
9. Burch, L. E.: Autotransfusion. Trans. South Surg. Assoc. 35:25, 1922.
10. Dyer, R. H., Alexander, J. T., and Brighton, C. T.: Atraumatic aspiration of whole blood for intraoperative autotransfusion. Am. J. Surg. 123:510, 1972.
11. Klebanoff, G.: Early clinical experience with a disposable unit for the intraoperative salvage and reinfusion of blood loss. Am. J. Surg. 120:718, 1970.
12. Klebanoff, G., Phillips, J., and Evans, W.: Use of a disposable autotransfusion unit under varying conditions of contamination. Am. J. Sug. 120:351, 1970.
13. Symbas, P. N., Levin, J. M., Ferrier, F. L., et al.: A study on autotransfusion from hemothorax. South Med. J. 62:671, 1969.
14. Symbas, P. N., et al.: Autotransfusion and its effects upon the blood components and the recipient. Curr. Top. Surg. Res. 1:387, 1969.
15. Mattox, K. L., Espada, R., Beall, A. C., et al.: Performing thoracotomy in the emergency center. JACEP 3:13, 1974.
16. Orr, M.: Autotransfusion: the use of washed red cells as an adjunct to component therapy. Surgery 84:728, 1978.
17. Mattox, K. L., Walker, L. E., Beall, A. C., et al.: Blood availability for the trauma patient—autotransfusion. J. Trauma 15:663, 1975.
18. O'Riordan, W. D.: Autotransfusion in the emergency department of a community hospital. JACEP 6:233, 1977.
19. Raines, J., Buth, J., Brewster, D. C., et al.: Intraoperative autotransfusion: equipment, protocols, and guidelines. J. Trauma 16:616, 1976.
20. Reul, G. J., Solis, R. T., Greenberg, S. D., et al.: Experience with autotransfusion in the surgical management of trauma. Surgery 76:546, 1974.
21. Rakower, S. R., and Worth, M. H.: Autotransfusion: perspective and critical problems. J. Trauma 13:573, 1973.
22. Dixon, J. L., and Smalley, M. G.: Jehovah's Witnesses: the surgical/ethical challenge. JAMA 246:2471, 1981.
23. Davidson, S. J.: Emergency unit autotransfusion. Surgery 84:703, 1978.
24. Mattox, K. L.: Autotransfusion in the emergency department. JACEP 4:218, 1975.
25. Smith, R. N., Yaw, P. B., and Glover, J. L.: Autotransfusion of contaminated intraperitoneal blood: an experimental study. J. Trauma 18:341, 1978.
26. Glover, J. L., Smith, R., Yaw, P. B., et al.: Autotransfusion of blood contaminated by intestinal contents. JACEP 7:142, 1978.
27. Klebanoff, G.: Intraoperative autotransfusion with the Bentley ATS–100. Surgery 84:708, 1978.
28. Von Koch, L., Defore, W. W., and Mattox, K. L.: A practical method of autotransfusion in the emergency center. Am. J. Surg. 133:770, 1977.
29. Davidson, S. J.: Correct use of autotransfusion in the emergency patient. ER Reports 2:73, 1981.
30. RECEPTAL. ATS Trauma. Salt Lake City, Sorenson Research Co., 1980.
31. Symbas, P. N.: Extraoperative autotransfusion from hemothorax. Surgery 84:722, 1978.
32. Symbas, P. N.: Autotransfusion from hemothorax: experimental and clinical studies. J. Trauma 12:689, 1972.
33. Mattox, K. L.: Comparison of techniques of autotransfusion. Surgery 84:700, 1978.
34. Brewster, D. C., Ambrosino, J. J., Darling, R. C., et al.: Intraoperative autotransfusion in major vascular surgery. Am. J. Surg. 137:507, 1979.
35. Dowling, J.: Autotransfusion: its use in the severely injured patient. Proceedings of the First Annual Bentley Autotransfusion Seminar. San Francisco, 1972, pp. 11–20.
36. Drye, J. C.: Discussion after Mattox, K. L., et al.: Blood availability for the trauma patient—autotransfusion. J. Trauma 15:663, 1975.
37. Burch, J. M.: Blood transfusion, microfiltration, and the adult respiratory distress syndrome. Curr. Concepts in Trauma Care. (Fall) 1983, pp. 16–21.
38. Noon, G. P.: Intraoperative autotransfusion. Surgery 84:719, 1978.
39. Bell, W.: The hematology of autotransfusion. Surgery 84:695, 1978.
40. Schaff, H. V., Hauer, J. M., Bell, W. R., et al.: Autotransfusion of shed mediastinal blood after cardiac surgery. A prospective study. J. Thorac. Cardiovasc. Surg. 75:632, 1978.
41. Second Annual Bentley Autotransfusion Seminar. Chicago, Bentley Laboratories, Inc., 1973.
42. Noon, G. P., Solis, R. T., and Natelson, E. A.: A simple method of intraoperative autotransfusion. Surg. Gynecol. Obstet. 143:65, 1976.
43. Oller, D. W., Rice, C. L., Herman, C. M., et al.: Heparin versus citrate anticoagulation in autotransfusion. J. Surg. Res. 20:333, 1976.
44. Johnston, B., Kamath, B. S., and McLellan, I.: An autotransfusion apparatus. Anaesthesia 32:1020, 1977.
45. Broadie, T. A., Glover, J. L., Bang, N., et al.: Clotting competence of intracavitary blood in trauma victims. Ann. Emerg. Med. 10:127, 1981.
46. Kluge, R. M., Calia, F. M., McLaughlin, J. S., et al.: Sources of contamination in open heart surgery. JAMA 230:1415, 1974.
47. Cowley, R. A., and Dunham, C. M. (ed.): Shock Trauma/Critical Care Manual. Baltimore, University Park Press, 1982, p. 40.
48. Mollison, P. L.: Blood Transfusion in Clinical Medicine. Oxford, Blackwell Scientific Publications, 1979, pp. 69, 638.
49. Mollison, P. L.: Blood Transfusion in Clinical Medicine. Oxford, Blackwell Scientific Publications, 1979, p. 652.
50. Cowley, R. A., and Dunham, C. M. (ed.): Shock Trauma/

Critical Care Manual. Baltimore, University Park Press, 1982, p. 38.

51. Stillman, R. M., Wrezlewicz, W. W., Stanczewski, B., et al.: The haematological hazards of autotransfusion. Br. J. Surg. 63:651, 1976.

52. Barbanel, C.: Hemoglobinuria and myoglobinuria. In Hamburger, J., Crosnier, J., and Grünfeld, J. P. (ed.): Nephrology. New York, John Wiley & Sons, Inc., 1979, pp. 185–189.

53. Goldfinger, D.: Complications of hemolytic transfusion reactions: pathogenesis and therapy. In Dawson, R. B. (ed.): New Approaches to Transfusion Reactions. Washington, American Association of Blood Banks, 1974, pp. 15–38.

54. Sandler, S. G., Berry E., and Zlotnick, A.: Benign hemo-

globinuria following transfusion of accidentally frozen blood. JAMA 235:2850, 1976.

55. Relihan, M., and Litwin, M. S.: Effects of stroma-free hemoglobin solution on clearance rate and renal function. Surgery 71:395, 1972.

56. Duncan, S. E., Klebanoff, G., and Rogers, W.: A clinical experience with intraoperative autotransfusion. Ann. Surg. 180:296, 1974.

57. Griswold, R. A., and Ortner, A. B.: Use of autotransfusion in surgery of serous cavities. Surg. Gynecol. Obstet. 77:167, 1943.

58. Boudreaux, J. P., Bornside, G. H., and Cohn, I.: Emergency autotransfusion: partial cleansing of bacteria-laden blood by cell washing. J. Trauma 23:31, 1983.

30

The Pneumatic Anti-Shock Garment (PASG)*

KENNETH FRUMKIN, M.D., Ph.D.

Introduction

The Pneumatic Anti-Shock Garment (PASG) is widely used, both by emergency medical technicians (EMTs) and paramedics in the prehospital care of hypotensive patients and by hospital emergency departments and critical care personnel. In the current commercially available forms,† the PASG resembles a pair of high-waisted men's trousers, constructed from two layers of an opaque, air-tight fabric sewn into three independently inflatable chambers (Figs. 30–1 and 30–2).

The device is easily applied, is considered "essential" equipment on ambulances, and is found in most emergency departments. In its most common use, for the patient who is hypotensive following trauma, it may provide a rapid improvement in blood pressure and may decrease the rate of internal or external bleeding. These devices have been called by many names: MAST (Military Anti-Shock Trousers, Medical Anti-Shock Trousers), PASG (Pneumatic Anti-Shock Garment), circumferential pneumatic compression device, shock pants, external counterpressure suit, air pants, MAST pants, MAST trousers, pressure pants, and G-suit.‡ Other terms have been used to refer to the *process* of applying external pressure to the body, regardless of the *device* used. Examples are external (or circumferential) pneumatic compression (EPC, CPC) and external counterpressure (ECP).[3]

Regardless of the name, the device has changed little in its design or application since 1903, when

G. W. Crile created a "pneumatic suit" from a double layer of rubber.[4] One or both legs or the abdomen could be inflated separately with a bicycle pump. Designed to manipulate blood pressure during head and neck surgery in the sitting position, the pneumatic suit also proved useful in trauma:

A cut-throat patient was admitted to the wards of Lakeside Hospital, exsanguinated and pulseless. Saline infusions and stimulants had been given in maximum amounts during twelve hours, but the circulation always relapsed, and at the time of the application of the rubber suit the pulse was barely perceptible, the respirations gasping, and the patient unconscious. On applying firm pneumatic pressure up to the costal borders the pulse became immediately better, the blood pressure rising to 110 mm of mercury, and consciousness was regained.[5]

Leaks in the material inhibited widespread use of the device, and the principle of external counterpressure lay dormant until its rediscovery by the military (allegedly at Crile's suggestion) during World War II.[6] Reincarnated as the G-suit, the

---

†MAST (David Clark Co., Inc., Worcester, Massachusetts) and Gladiator Antishock Pants (Jobst Institute, Inc., Toledo, Ohio).[1]
‡Authors writing on this subject have a plethora of terms from which to choose. Some of these names (e.g., MAST) are also registered commercial trademarks. Pneumatic Anti-Shock Garment (PASG) is the term adopted by the American College of Surgeons for its Advanced Trauma Life Support Course.[2] For convenience, that name will be used in this chapter to refer to the devices that are currently available.

*The opinions or assertions contained herein are the private views of the author and are not to be construed as official or reflecting the views of the Department of Defense or the Department of the Army.

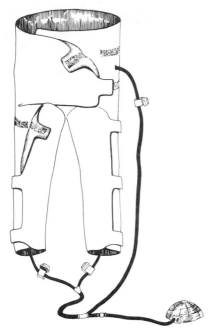

Figure 30–1. Assembled PASG and inflation pump. (Courtesy of the American College of Surgeons, Committee on Trauma.)

garment was used to provide momentary compression of up to 100 mm Hg to counteract the loss of consciousness and retinal ischemia that occurred during certain maneuvers in high-speed aircraft. Medical interest was renewed with investigations performed by Gardner and Dohn in 1956.[7] They used a homemade "G-suit" in patients who were likely to experience postural hypotension (neurosurgical patients in the sitting position, patients in whom spinal anesthesia had been administered, and those with severe diabetic neuropathy). Their device subsequently became commercially available (Curity) and consisted of a double-layered rectangular blanket wrapped completely around the patient from xiphoid to ankles. For the next decade or more, external counterpressure was used only in the hospital setting and usually as a

last resort in cases of uncontrollable postoperative hemorrhage (Table 30–1).

A successful trial by the military during the Vietnam War was the first recorded use of the external counterpressure principle in the preoperative stabilization of trauma patients.[8] The Army continued to develop the device until the current pants-like form (MAST) was achieved.[9] The inventor of the trousers (B. H. Kaplan) became the first to adapt them to their next area of extensive use: civilian prehospital application by paramedics and EMTs.[10]

Pelligra and Sandburg reviewed the clinical literature (174 cases over 75 years) and concluded that it was "unlikely that additional case studies will provide more documentation of the effectiveness of circumferential pneumatic compression."[3] Hypotensive patients have shown reliable, and often dramatic, improvement in blood pressure, pulse, mental status, a decrease in fluid and transfusion requirements, and probably an increased survival rate with the use of these devices.

In normal volunteers, predictable increases in central venous pressure (CVP),[11] intrathoracic blood volume,[11] total peripheral resistance (TPR),[12] blood pressure,[13] and cardiac index[13] have occurred following inflation of the PASG. In supine subjects, little or no change occurs in pulse[13, 14] or pulmonary compliance[11] with external counterpressure. Gaffney and coworkers found elevated blood pressure and peripheral resistance and decreased cardiac output and stroke volume with supine PASG application. In subjects tilted 60 degrees (head up), PASG produced only an elevation of stroke volume.[15]

Extensive data have been generated in dogs subjected to experimental hemorrhage and "treated" for their hypovolemia with external counterpressure. Most studies show that PASG applied to hypovolemic animals produces improvements in cardiac output,[6, 16, 17] stroke volume,[6] and blood pressure.[6, 16, 18] No significant changes in TPR were found in one study.[18]

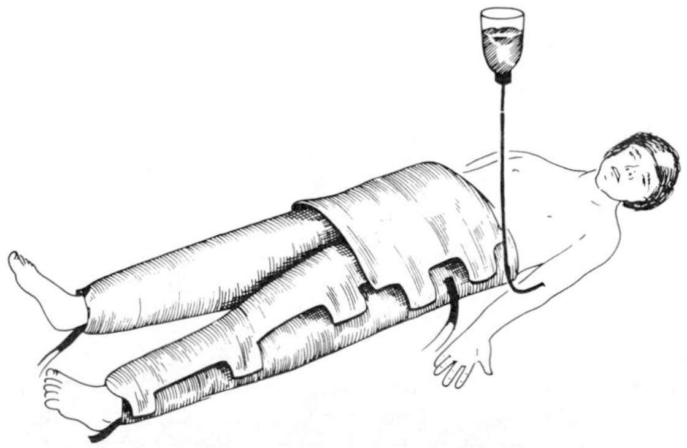

Table 30–1. EARLY USES OF THE G-SUIT COUNTERPRESSURE DEVICE

Retroperitoneal bleeding from massive pelvic trauma[34, 73]
Postoperative bleeding from hypocoagulation[35]
Postural hypotension[76, 82]
Spontaneous rupture of the liver[79]
Postoperative hemorrhage after:
   Abdominal procedures[56]
   Nephrectomy[63]
   Prostatectomy[63]
   Renal biopsy[63]
   Tubal ligation[81]
   Hysterectomy[78]
Leaking and ruptured abdominal aortic aneurysms[34, 53, 74, 77, 80]
Lower extremity fractures[80]
Placenta percreta[78]
Gastrointestinal bleeding[53]
Ruptured ectopic pregnancy[33, 53]

Figure 30–2. PASG applied to a patient and inflated. (Courtesy of the American College of Surgeons, Committee on Trauma.)

Mechanism of Action

In hundreds of reported cases, application of the PASG has resulted in elevation of blood pressure and control of bleeding.[3] A number of mechanisms have been proposed for each of these actions (Table 30–2).

BLOOD PRESSURE ELEVATION AND IMPROVED SUPRADIAPHRAGMATIC PERFUSION

Data appear to indicate that an increase in afterload (peripheral vascular resistance) rather than preload (autotransfusion) is principally responsible for increases in mean arterial pressure associated in the use of the PASG. Increased TPR would seem to be an invariable consequence of suit application. In normovolemic dogs and supine normovolemic humans, PASG application does increase TPR.[12, 19, 20] Yet, in dogs subjected to phlebotomy[18] and in human subjects tilted 60 degrees,[15] application of a pressure garment had no additional effect on the (already) elevated TPR. What most probably occurs in these subjects is a redistribution of blood flow. The increased lower extremity and abdominal resistance provides improved perfusion above the diaphragm, most commonly measurable as blood pressure elevation.

Nearly all researchers and clinicians working with external counterpressure devices have hypothesized that application results in an "autotransfusion" of blood from the venous system of the lower extremities and the splanchnic bed to the vital structures ("central circulation") above the diaphragm. The amount is usually quoted as 2 units (1000 ml) of blood.[21, 22] Yet experimental evidence to support this conclusion is very difficult to acquire, and no definite large autotransfusion effect has been experimentally verified. McSwain has remarked that "I have never seen any hard data on it, but in the papers that I have read, every one of them continued to quote this fig-

---

Table 30–2. PNEUMATIC ANTI-SHOCK GARMENT: PROPOSED MECHANISMS OF ACTION

Blood pressure elevation
    Increased total peripheral resistance
    "Autotransfusion"
Control of bleeding
    Direct pressure
    Fracture stabilization
    Coagulation
    Effects on bleeding vessels
        Decreased transmural pressure

---

ure."[23] A number of studies have shown increased central blood volumes in humans. These have been measured in various ways, including calculation from pulmonary circulation times,[13] changing lung density on repeated radiographs, and changing thoracic radioactivity after I^{131} albumin injection and PASG application.[11] Redistribution of blood flow centrally after suit application in dogs subjected to phlebotomy was demonstrated by Ferrario and associates. These investigators also found increased carotid blood flow in association with decreased flow in femoral vessels.[6] Changes in normovolemic subjects are most marked when venous pooling is increased by tilting.[13, 15] Attempts at quantification in humans using displacement of the center of gravity[24] or nuclear scanning after radioactive red blood cell injection[25] have resulted in estimates that 150 to 300 ml are "autotransfused." Animal experiments after phlebotomy and PASG inflation suggested an "autotransfusion" volume of 5 to 13 ml per kg.[26]

CONTROL OF BLEEDING

The PASG can serve as a pressure dressing over external bleeding sites. Acting as a pneumatic splint, the device prevents continued bleeding provoked by motion at fracture sites. This is particularly efficacious with long bone fractures and retroperitoneal bleeding from pelvic fractures.

The presence of a normal coagulation system contributes strongly to the ability of external counterpressure to control bleeding. Heparinized dogs bleeding from an aortic laceration cannot raise their intra-aortic pressure above the garment-produced intraperitoneal pressure. Nonheparinized animals, however, are able to do so.[27]

One puzzling question involves determining how external counterpressures that are considerably below the pressure within the bleeding blood vessel can reduce flow from a sizable defect while still allowing blood to circulate.[28] Much of the explanation derives from the physics involved.

La Place's law ($T = \Delta P \times R$) determines the wall tension (T) for a cylinder (Fig. 30–3). T is the force tangential to the circumference of the vessel that tends to pull apart the edges of a longitudinal laceration (*L* in Fig. 30–3). Transmural pressure (ΔP) is the difference between the intraluminal (P_I) and extraluminal (P_E) pressures ($\Delta P = P_I - P_E$). Increases in P_E are produced by the PASG, and the tendency to bleed (ΔP, T) declines. In addition, circumferential pressure causes the radius of the vessel (R) to decrease, limiting both of these contributions to the wall tension.

Bernoulli's principle takes more factors into account (Fig. 30–4). It relates the rate of flow from the injured vessel ($\dot{Q}$) to the surface area of the laceration site (A), transmural pressure (ΔP), den-

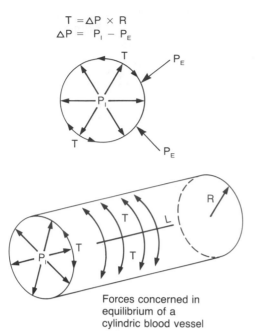

$$T = \Delta P \times R$$
$$\Delta P = P_I - P_E$$

Forces concerned in
equilibrium of a
cylindric blood vessel

Figure 30–3. Diagrammatic expression of the law of La Place. T refers to the wall tension, which is tangential to the circumference of the vessel and acts to pull the edges of a longitudinal laceration (L) apart. Transmural pressure (ΔP) is the difference between the intraluminal (P_I) and extraluminal (P_E) pressures and is decreased by external counterpressure. (Modified from Burton, A. C.: On the physical equilibrium of small blood vessels. Am. J. Physiol. 164:319, 1951.)

sity of the fluid medium (ρ), and V, the velocity of the fluid flowing through the vessel. In this model the major actions of the external counterpressure suits are to limit transmural pressure along with the surface area of the laceration (Fig. 30–5). A considerable number of animal studies have tested these relationships with *in vivo, in vitro,* and *ex vivo* models.[20, 27–31] Nearly all document decreased flow through lacerated vessels with external counterpressure and support one or the other of the equations listed, generally that of Bernoulli.

Clinical Application

The list of clinical applications for the external counterpressure device is modified frequently as

$$\dot{Q} = A \times \sqrt{\frac{\Delta P}{\rho} + V^2}$$

BERNOULLI'S PRINCIPLE

$\dot{Q}$ = RATE OF FLOW FROM INJURED VESSEL
A = SURFACE AREA OF LACERATION
P = TRANSMURAL PRESSURE ($P_I - P_E$)
ρ = DENSITY OF THE FLUID
V = VELOCITY OF THE FLUID IN THE VESSEL

Figure 30–4. Bernoulli's equation quantitates the rate of flow from an injured vessel.

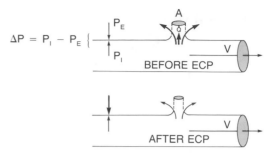

$$\Delta P = P_I - P_E$$

BEFORE ECP

AFTER ECP

Figure 30–5. Representation of flow through an injured blood vessel ($\dot{Q}$) before *(top)* and after *(bottom)* the application of external counterpressure (ECP). (Modified from Hall, M., and Marshall, J. R.: The gravity suit: A major advance in management of gynecologic blood loss. Obstet. Gynecol. 53:247, 1979.)

new suggestions appear in the literature. Many indications that were controversial in the past have changed as experience with these garments increases. There are few experimental data for some suggested indications. Obviously, specific therapy directed at the underlying cause is the mainstay of successful treatment of any condition that may respond initially to counterpressure.

INDICATIONS (Table 30–3)

Hypovolemic Shock. This is the most clear-cut indication for the use of PASGs. Most other clinical applications either have some degree of controversy attached or are supported by insufficient data. One widely published set of recommendations for application of the device (in the setting of trauma or other possible hypovolemia) includes:

1. all cases in which systolic blood pressure is 80 mm Hg or less, and

2. patients with systolic pressure less than 100 mm Hg with clinical signs of shock (cold and clammy skin, altered mental status, elevated pulse).[23]

There are a number of advantages of the PASG over massive fluid replacement alone in this setting. The device is quickly applied and offers some immediate response. Collapsed peripheral veins may become easier to cannulate after inflation. Less crystalloid may be required for fluid resuscitation, and the risk of subsequent pulmonary insufficiency is thereby decreased. Any decrease in blood requirements would also limit the complications associated with transfusion. PASGs can be applied in the absence of persons skilled in intravenous therapy, and the compressive effect to reduce flow from vessels that are bleeding internally cannot be duplicated by other means.[32, 33]

States of Relative Hypovolemia and Hypotension. Other causes of shock in which the pneumatic suit might be helpful but for which no data currently exist include neurogenic (spinal) shock, shock secondary to drug overdose, septic shock, and anaphylactic shock.

Table 30–3. INDICATIONS FOR PASG APPLICATION

Hypovolemic shock
Relative hypovolemia and hypotension
  Spinal shock
  Overdose
  Septic shock
  Anaphylaxis
Other uses
  "Prophylactic" use (gastrointestinal bleeding, aortic
    aneurysm)
  Stabilization of fractures
  Compression of external bleeding
  Postoperative hemorrhage
  Coagulation defects
New (investigational) uses
  Cardiogenic shock
  Cardiopulmonary resuscitation
  Paroxysmal supraventricular tachycardia

Other Uses. "Prophylactic" application (with or without inflation) may be helpful in potentially hypovolemic or hypotensive patients. Examples are trauma victims who are initially stable at the scene but who have a potential for developing hypotension, patients with gastrointestinal bleeding, or those with leaking abdominal aortic aneurysms.[34] In patients with leaking aneurysms, one should maintain the systolic blood pressure at approximately 100 mm Hg to avoid contributing to further rupture. Pelvic or lower extremity fractures are well stabilized by these devices, adding significantly to the patient's comfort. PASGs may serve as a compression dressing over external bleeding. Controlling postoperative intra-abdominal hemorrhage has been a classic indication.[3] Bleeding aggravated by coagulation defects has also been responsive to external counterpressure.[35]

NEW USES OF EXTERNAL COUNTERPRESSURE

The PASG is being investigated for use in a burgeoning number of situations. In most cases, the available data are sparse, and these applications should be considered investigational at best.

Cardiogenic Shock. Wayne has advocated the use of the PASG as a quickly "reversible fluid challenge" in patients with cardiogenic shock.[36] The intended use is to identify those patients in cardiogenic shock who might benefit from volume resuscitation and to continue with crystalloid infusions in these individuals. Pressor agents would be reserved for those patients who fail to improve or worsen with inflation. The complete "reversibility" of the effects of the device has not been well documented, particularly with a poorly functioning cardiovascular system. Normal subjects quickly compensate for PASG inflation. After 5 minutes, CVP, cardiac index, pulse, and central

blood volume return to preinflation values. With the release of pressure, cardiac index and central blood volume increase, and blood pressure and CVP fall.[13, 37] The changes after deflation are attributed to unmasking of the compensatory mechanisms (probably vasodilation) that had taken place during external counterpressure to normalize the patient's hemodynamics. Thus, mere removal of these devices after application does not necessarily restore the patient's cardiovascular system to a "baseline" state.

Cardiopulmonary Resuscitation (CPR). Interest in the use of external counterpressure devices during CPR is a result of recent changes in the way that blood flow is believed to occur during external chest compression.[38, 39] The heart is no longer thought to act as a pump, propelling blood as it is squeezed between the sternum and the spine. Instead, chest compression serves to raise intrathoracic pressures, and blood flows because of pressure gradients developed between intra- and extrathoracic vessels (see Chapter 16). External counterpressure from the PASG is believed to augment CPR in two ways: (1) by reducing diaphragmatic excursion and therefore increasing intrathoracic pressures during compression, and (2) by compressing the infradiaphragmatic vascular bed, producing selective perfusion of vital structures above and increased peripheral resistance below the diaphragm. Animal studies have demonstrated improvements in carotid blood flow and arterial pressures when abdominal compression or the PASG is added to standardized CPR.[40–42] Lilja and coworkers noted that PASG increased systolic blood pressure during CPR in seven of eight patients.[43]

Paroxysmal Supraventricular Tachycardia (PSVT). A number of word-of-mouth successes have been described with PSVT, attributed to reflex vagal excitation from increased aortic and carotid sinus pressure. At least one study is reported to be under way.[44]

CONTRAINDICATIONS (Table 30–4)

Pulmonary edema and congestive heart failure are the only current absolute contraindications to the use of external counterpressure devices. The increased venous return, decreased vital capacity, and elevation in pulmonary wedge pressures produced by these devices serve only to aggravate pre-existing pulmonary congestion.

Relative contraindications that have been proposed include pregnancy, evisceration of abdominal contents, the case of a foreign body impaled in the abdomen, lumbar spine injury, and lower extremity compartmental injury. Certainly, the leg chambers may be inflated without additional risk in patients without compartmental injuries, and

Table 30–4. CONTRAINDICATIONS TO PASG APPLICATION

Absolute contraindications
  Congestive heart failure
  Pulmonary edema
Relative contraindications
  Pregnancy
  Evisceration
  Impaled foreign body
  Lower extremity compartmental injury
  Lumbar spine instability

the relative risks and benefits of inflation of the abdominal binder can then be assessed.

CONTROVERSIAL APPLICATIONS
(Table 30–5)

There are a number of situations in which the use of PASG devices was advised against by early writers. Although no reported series addresses any of these circumstances, the authors with the most experience now recommend the judicious use of external counterpressure in those settings in which it was earlier felt not to be indicated.[32, 45]

Head Injuries. The only purely intracranial injury that can produce shock is transtentorial herniation. In the absence of this often fatal injury with its unique signs and symptoms, shock is usually the result of associated visceral injuries or spinal cord injury. Yet, fear that the PASG would increase cerebral edema and intracranial pressure has caused the manufacturers to interdict use of the device in head injury. A series of recent animal experiments has found no significant effects of PASG inflation in hypovolemic or normovolemic dogs with or without an intracranial "mass." The studies did document improvement in the cerebral perfusion pressure with PASG use.[46–48]

Intrathoracic Injuries. It was initially believed that external pressure applied below the diaphragm would merely increase the rate of blood loss from thoracic injuries. Most authors cite their clinical experience in noting no adverse effects of these devices in thoracic trauma.[22, 23, 49] Ransom and McSwain documented immediate blood pressure increases after PASG application in all eight of their patients with severe hemorrhage above the diaphragm and successful resuscitation in seven.[50]

Table 30–5. CONTROVERSIAL PASG APPLICATIONS

Head injuries
Intrathoracic injuries
Cardiac tamponade
Tension pneumothorax

Cardiac Tamponade and Tension Pneumothorax. Fluid infusion is a standard temporizing measure in cardiac tamponade. In one study of dogs with experimental cardiac tamponade, PASG inflation produced a doubling of mean arterial pressure and improved cardiac output.[51] The PASG may be lifesaving in this setting when persons skilled in definitive treatment are unavailable. Tension pneumothorax is a similar state of compromised venous return that might also respond temporarily to the redistributed fluid volume resulting from PASG application. Palafox and associates,[48] however, produced cardiac tamponade or tension pneumothorax in hypovolemic dogs and found a *decline* in arterial pressure and a rise in CVP when the abdominal binder was inflated above 80 mm Hg. This was believed to be caused by PASG-induced diaphragmatic elevation increasing intrathoracic pressures and further compromising venous return. Although cautious use of PASG in hypovolemic patients with cardiac tamponade or tension pneumothorax may be useful, a fall in blood pressure after full inflation should suggest the presence of one of these entities (if not previously suspected) and a reduction in inflation pressure.

Complications and Disadvantages
(Table 30–6)

HYPOTENSION

Clinical experience has shown that the major life-threatening complication resulting from the use of the PASG in hypovolemic patients has been the sudden and severe hypotension that results

Table 30–6. COMPLICATIONS AND DISADVANTAGES OF PASG APPLICATION

Hypotension after removal
Metabolic acidosis
Respiratory compromise
Decreased renal perfusion
Other (infrequent) complications
  Pulmonary edema, congestive heart failure
  Compartment syndromes
  Increased wound bleeding
  Urination, defecation, vomiting
  Skin breakdown
  Lumbar spine movement
Mechanical problems and disadvantages
  Limitation of diagnostic and therapeutic
    procedures
  Physical examination
  Urinary catheterization
  Peritoneal lavage
  Vascular access
Environmental influences
  Barometric pressure
  Temperature

from precipitous removal of the device in the absence of adequate fluid resuscitation (possibly from the sudden release of vasoactive chemicals pooled in the abdomen and the lower extremities).[4, 8, 33, 34, 45, 52-54] Although emergency department physicians and EMTs are well aware of the problem, many consultants are not. When faced with a patient encased in rubber from xiphoid to ankles, many have rapidly removed these devices, often with disastrous consequences. Recommended techniques for removal will be discussed later.

METABOLIC ACIDOSIS

Metatolic acidosis has been the most reproducible abnormality after application of external counterpressure. Wangensteen and associates first reported this "detrimental" effect of external counterpressure.[55] They noted acidosis (to a pH of 7.01) and an increased lactate/pyruvate ratio in hypovolemic dogs after 4 hours of external counterpressure. Hypovolemic dogs without external pressure had less of an acidosis and lived longer. Ransom and McSwain also found decreased central venous pH and increases in lactate and potassium in hypovolemic dogs wearing the PASG; these declines were more pronounced than those in hypovolemic dogs without counterpressure.[26] Although the treatment of hypovolemia with PASG alone without concomitant fluid replacement is an unusual situation, these results led McSwain to advise the earliest possible gradual release of pressure to prevent a bolus of lactate and potassium from the legs.[45] According to McSwain, 1 to 2 ampules of bicarbonate should be administered if the patient's systolic blood pressure has not been over 100 mm Hg during inflation. Inflation pressures less than the systolic pressure are felt to decrease the risk of acidosis. The limited data in humans have shown mild metabolic acidosis (pH 7.33 to 7.36), and many authors have given the impression that the acidosis is not a problem clinically.[34, 50, 56] Although metabolic acidosis may occur, close monitoring of arterial blood gases and correction with bicarbonate as needed should allow for the safe continued use of these devices.

RESPIRATORY COMPROMISE

Abdominal binding invariably has at least some subjective effects on respiration and alert patients may complain of shortness of breath when the abdominal compartment is inflated. Espinosa and Updegrove reported an 18 per cent decrease in vital capacity and a slight increase in respiratory rate in volunteers subjected to external counterpressure.[53] There were no changes in inspiratory and expiratory reserve volumes, maximum breathing capacity, or tidal volume. A more recent report using human volunteers with modern PASGs inflated demonstrated a 5 per cent reduction in vital capacity at an inflation pressure of 100 mm Hg.[84] Batalden found no pulmonary complications in ten patients with external counterpressure garments who underwent positive-pressure ventilation for 24 to 48 hours.[57] Yet, Burdick and colleagues found atelectasis, pulmonary edema, or pneumonia in 14 of 28 similar patients.[56] Cogbill and coworkers[58] demonstrated a mild impairment of pulmonary function in healthy individuals and those with airflow obstruction when the PASG was inflated. The impairment was restrictive rather than obstructive and was not clinically significant with inflation pressures less than 50 mm Hg. In hypotensive patients, Ransom and associates[50] failed to demonstrate impaired alveolar ventilation when the PASG was used. In general, authors concerned about respiratory compromise have recommended careful attention to arterial blood gases combined with controlled positive-pressure ventilation in those patients requiring prolonged external counterpressure.[21, 56, 59]

DECREASED RENAL PERFUSION

A number of reversible abnormalities in renal hemodynamics have been reported with external counterpressure. Normovolemic dogs in a PASG undergo a 40 to 50 per cent decline in renal blood flow and an elevation in renal vascular resistance.[60] Ten subjects in PASGs for 4 to 24 hours had no significant alterations in renal blood flow.[61] Normal human subjects experiencing increased abdominal pressure had 24 to 28 per cent declines in effective renal plasma flow and glomerular filtration rate (GFR), decreased urine output, elevated renal vein pressures, and increased urine specific gravity. These changes reversed after decompression.[62]

INFREQUENT COMPLICATIONS

A number of case reports document some infrequent but serious complications of the PASG.

Pulmonary edema and congestive heart failure have been attributed in isolated cases to increased pulmonary venous return and elevated pulmonary capillary wedge pressures.[3, 52, 56, 63]

Lumbar spine instability is another potential complication of the PASG. Older PASG designs included an abdominal bladder that inflated in the back as well as over the abdomen. Rockwell and coworkers[64] reported a case in which a lumbar spine injury was believed to have been aggravated by inflation of a circumferential abdominal bladder. They also demonstrated graphically on a volunteer the marked exaggeration of lumbar lordosis that is possible with the older-style garment. The recommendation of Rockwell and colleagues[64] that inflation be limited to the anterior aspect of the abdominal compartment, as is possible with the newer designs, should be heeded. The editors caution careful use of the abdominal portion of all designs of the PASG in patients who have possibly experienced trauma to the lumbar spine.

Lower extremity compartment syndromes have been reported, requiring fasciotomy in two cases[65, 66] and resulting in amputation in two others[67] (see also Chapter 75). Both patients requiring amputation had prolonged periods of hypotension prior to PASG application and significant lower extremity fractures. One patient who had sustained no lower extremity trauma developed bilateral compartment syndrome after only 140 minutes of PASG application.[66] Reversible peroneal nerve palsy has also been reported.[52]

Increased bleeding from lower extremity wounds after suit inflation was attributed in two cases to improvements in blood pressure.[8] The bleeding responded to rebandaging but required temporary deflation of the suit. Such bleeding may be hidden in bandages under the devices and should be considered in the differentiation of persistent hypotension from other conditions.

Stimulation of urination, defecation, and vomiting by suit inflation is noted as a complication and warned about by early authors.[32] McLaughlin and coworkers "know of one patient" without a nasogastric tube in place who died of aspirated vomitus after a PASG was applied.[34] Spontaneous defecation "has been a complication" in patients being treated for gastrointestinal bleeding with these devices.[53]

Skin breakdown at pressure points with prolonged use has prompted the suggestion to pad bony prominences.[52, 57, 68]

MECHANICAL PROBLEMS AND DISADVANTAGES

Limitation of Diagnostic Evaluation and Therapeutic Procedures. Physical examination of the lower extremities and the abdomen is limited by the counterpressure devices. This is a particularly difficult burden for the surgical consultant, who must nonetheless remember the devastating effects of precipitous removal. In a stable patient, one compartment at a time can be slowly deflated with careful monitoring of vital signs. If necessary, the compartment that has just been deflated may be reinflated before the next is approached. A method for cautious removal will be outlined later. Occasionally, the best way to remove the garment

is in the operating room after replacement of volume and administration of anesthesia. Similar problems exist with performing diagnostic peritoneal lavage. Urinary catheterization is challenging, particularly in female patients, even with the opening provided in the garments.

Vascular access can also be a problem. Lower extremity cutdowns are difficult to perform, and a pressure bag is required to produce flow of intravenous solutions. Access to the femoral artery and vein is also severely limited.

Environmental Influences on Device Pressures. Until recently, little attention had been paid to the role of the important environmental factors of pressure and temperature in modification of PASG inflation pressures.[69–71] With the current popularity and availability of helicopter ambulance transport, the role of Boyle's law (the volume of the gas is inversely proportional to its pressure) needs to be re-emphasized. As the helicopter rises, the air in the suit expands, increasing the trouser pressure. Decreasing altitude has the opposite effect. Temperature, too, has similar effects: As the temperature increases, trouser pressure rises, and vice versa. When the "optimal" inflation pressure is determined at the scene of the accident, changes produced by movement into the controlled climate of the ambulance or hospital need to be predicted and recognized.

Procedure (Fig. 30–6)

APPLICATION OF TROUSERS

Prior to application it is useful to inspect the device and to establish the proper orientation. Many find it helpful to mark the "up" side (inside) with paint or tape to aid in rapid correct application. The patient can be "logrolled" onto the opened trousers. Alternatively, with one person standing on either side and elevating the patient's legs, the trousers can be slid beneath to the buttocks. Then the patient's hips are elevated, and the upper border of the trousers is placed at the costal margin. The cervical spine must be stabilized in those at risk for cervical injury. The medial portion of each leg binder is brought between the legs, and the Velcro fasteners are closed over each leg and over the abdomen.

Many emergency departments prefer to keep the deflated PASG on the resuscitation table at all times. When patients arrive, they are placed on the garment so that it is immediately accessible should its use be required later during treatment. A recently suggested method involves assembling the trousers in advance. The operator places his arms through the pants legs from the bottom, sliding them completely onto his arms. He then

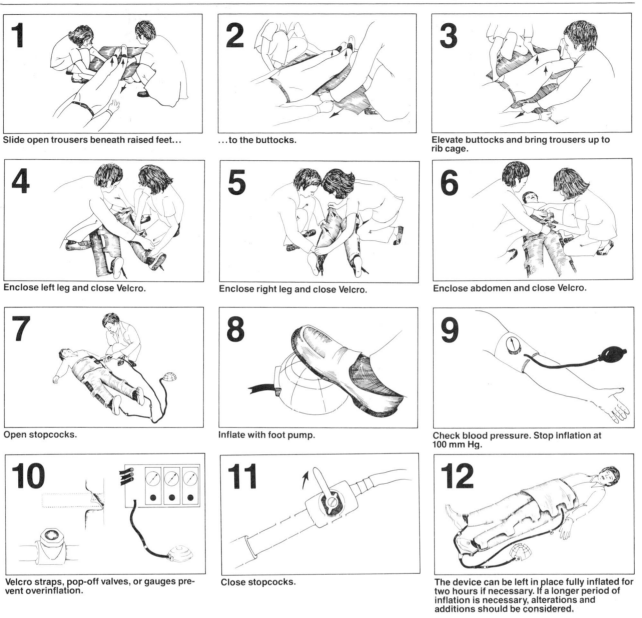

1 Slide open trousers beneath raised feet...

2 ...to the buttocks.

3 Elevate buttocks and bring trousers up to rib cage.

4 Enclose left leg and close Velcro.

5 Enclose right leg and close Velcro.

6 Enclose abdomen and close Velcro.

7 Open stopcocks.

8 Inflate with foot pump.

9 Check blood pressure. Stop Inflation at 100 mm Hg.

10 Velcro straps, pop-off valves, or gauges prevent overinflation.

11 Close stopcocks.

12 The device can be left in place fully inflated for two hours if necessary. If a longer period of inflation is necessary, alterations and additions should be considered.

Figure 30–6. PASG application. (Courtesy of the American College of Surgeons, Committee on Trauma.)

stands at the patient's feet, grabs the patient's toes, and lifts. An assistant pulls the trousers from the operator's arms and slides them over the patient, and the Velcro straps are retightened.[72] The foot-pump hoses are then attached to the stopcocks, and the foot-pump is used to inflate both legs first and then the abdomen. One can accomplish inflation faster if one initially fills the compartments by blowing into them. The lungs can provide more volume than the pump in a shorter period. After resistance to filling is met, the pump becomes more efficient at increasing trouser pressures.[72] Blood pressure and pulse should be continuously monitored during the pro-

cedure, and inflation should be stopped if the systolic blood pressure goes over 100 mm Hg.

Pediatric devices are available. In the absence of these smaller garments, one can effectively manage children by wrapping them in one leg of the adult-sized trousers. Inflation pressures should be titrated to a satisfactory pulse and blood pressure response.

The PASG alone can passively splint lower extremity fractures. Of the commonly available *traction* devices, only the Sager traction splint can be applied after the trousers are in place and inflated. The Sager splint can be used either inside or outside the device to splint one or both legs at the same time. The Hare traction splint and the Thomas splint are significantly more awkward to use with the PASG in operation. These seem to offer some risk of damage to the trousers themselves and result in an uneven application of circumferential pressure (see also Chapter 40).

INFLATION PRESSURE

Of the two major devices that are available, one has a pressure gauge (or gauges) for monitoring pants pressure (Jobst Gladiator). As with any such piece of equipment, gauges should be periodically checked for accuracy. The other device uses pressure-relief ("pop-off") valves that limit inflation pressures to 104 mm Hg. It is reasonable to assume that the side effects and complications of these devices are proportional to the pressure and duration of application. Both aspects of pressure application should be minimized as much as possible. Most animal experiments and some clinical studies in humans have suggested that hemorrhage control (presumably venous bleeding) in otherwise stable (often postoperative) patients is often acomplished with less than 40 mm Hg inflation pressure.[3] "Autotransfusion" and blood pressure elevations may require higher inflation pressures. McSwain has emphasized that the "only important pressure is the patient's blood pressure." The pants must be inflated until a "satisfactory" response (usually systolic blood pressure over 100 mm Hg) is obtained.[45] A recent study by Wayne and MacDonald suggests that most *prehospital* patients in shock will *not* respond with a blood pressure elevation with 30 mm Hg inflation pressure.[83]

DEFLATION

When? In the usual case, deflation may be considered when the combination of PASG and other resuscitative measures (fluids, hemorrhage control) has resulted in restoration of satisfactory vital signs. The gradual deflation procedure that will be outlined further on should be followed. The presence of any contraindications to continued use (congestive heart failure, renal disease, pulmonary disease) should also be considered. The presence of a coagulopathy may be a relative contraindication to removing the device.

Where? If emergency surgery is indicated, the operating table may be the best place to deflate the PASG. After all monitoring and venous lines have been started, the anesthesiologist is ready, and the surgeons are in attendance, the abdominal portion can be deflated (preferably slowly—see further on). The legs can be left inflated for an abdominal procedure until internal hemorrhage is better controlled.

How? Gradually! McSwain recommends 1 to 2 ampules of sodium bicarbonate if the patient's blood pressure has remained below 100 mm Hg with the trousers inflated,[45] although the use of periodic blood gas analysis to guide bicarbonate therapy is preferred. Deflation should begin with the abdominal binder. Small quantities of air are released, and the patient's blood pressure is rechecked. If no blood pressure drop occurs, further aliquots of air are released with repeated blood pressure measurement. If blood pressure falls more than 5 mm Hg, deflation should be halted and more fluids given until blood pressure is restored. After the abdominal binder is deflated, the legs should be deflated in a similar manner.

Conclusion

The Pneumatic Anti-Shock Garment is a useful adjunctive device in the care of the hypovolemic, hypotensive patient. When the garment is used, improvements in blood pressure and pulse are often dramatic, and bleeding is slowed. External counterpressure can "buy time" until definitive therapy is instituted. A major hazard is the profound hypotension that can result from the precipitous removal of the device by those who are unfamiliar with this possibility. As research and experience accumulate, the use of the PASG may expand to other areas.

1. Anti-shock trousers. Health Devices, vol. 6. Plymouth Meeting, PA, Emergency Care Research Institutes, 1977, pp. 265–277.
2. American College of Surgeons Committee on Trauma: Advanced trauma life support course.
3. Pelligra, R., and Sandberg, E. C.: Control of intractable abdominal bleeding by external counterpressure. JAMA 241:708, 1979.
4. Crile, G. W.: Blood Pressure in Surgery: Experimental and Clinical Research. Philadelphia, J. B. Lippincott Co., 1903, pp. 288–291.
5. Crile, G. W.: Hemorrhage and Transfusions: Experimental and Clinical Research. New York, D. Appleton and Co., 1909, pp. 137–145.
6. Ferrario, C. M., Nadzam, G., Fernandez, L. A., et al.: Effects of pneumatic compression on the cardiovascular dynamics in dogs after hemorrhage. Aerospace Med. 41:411, 1970.
7. Gardner, W. J., and Dohn, D. F.: The antigravity suit (G-suit) in surgery. JAMA 162:274, 1956.
8. Cutler, B. S., and Daggett, W.: Application of the g-suit to the control of hemorrhage in massive trauma. Ann. Surg. 173:511, 1971.
9. Kaplan, B. H.: Emergency autotransfusion medical pneumatic trouser. Disclosure of invention, Logbook Entry 21. Ft. Rucker, AL, U. S. Army Aeromedical Research Laboratory, June 1972, p. 6.
10. Kaplan, B. C., Civetta, J. M., Nagel, E. L., et al.: The

military anti-shock trouser in civilian pre-hospital emergency care. J. Trauma 13:843, 1973.

11. Bondurant, S., Hickam, J. B., and Isley, J. K.: Pulmonary and circulatory effects of acute pulmonary vascular engorgement in normal subjects. J. Clin. Invest. 36:59, 1957.

12. Eich, R. H., Smulyan, H., and Chaffee, W. R.: Hemodynamic response to g-suit inflation with and without ganglionic blockage. Aerospace Med. 35:247, 1966.

13. Gray, S., Shaver, J. A., Kroetz, F. W., et al.: Acute and prolonged effects of g-suit inflation on cardiovascular dynamics. Aerospace Med. 40:40, 1969.

14. Wood, E., and Lambert, E. H.: Some factors which influence the protection afforded by pneumatic anti-G-suits. J. Aviat. Med. 23:218, 1952.

15. Gaffney, F. A., Thal, E. R., Taylor, W. F., et al.: Hemodynamic effects of medical anti-shock trousers (MAST garment). J. Trauma 21:931, 1981.

16. Anderson, L. G., Selby, D. M., Wuerflein, R. D., et al.: Protective influences of external counterpressure after acute hemorrhage in dogs. Surg. Forum 15:4, 1964.

17. Shane, R. A., and Campbell, G. S.: Protective influence of external counterpressure in acute hemorrhagic hypotension in dogs. Am. J. Surg. 110:355, 1965.

18. Roth, J. S., and Rutherford, R. B.: Regional blood flow effects of g-suit application during hemorrhagic shock. Surg. Gynecol. Obstet. 133:637, 1971.

19. Shenansky, J. H., II, and Gillenwater, J. Y.: The renal hemodynamic and functional effects of external counterpressure. Surg. Gynecol. Obstet. 134:253, 1972.

20. Wangensteen, S. L., Ludewig, R. M., and Eddy, D. W.: Effect of external counterpressure on the intact circulation. Surg. Gynecol. Obstet. 127:253, 1968.

21. Abernathy, C., Dickinson, T. C,. and Lokey, H.: A Military Anti-Shock Trousers program in the small hospital. Surg. Clin. North Am. 59:461, 1979.

22. McSwain, N. E., Jr.: G-suits and shock: A non-invasive transfusion technique. J. Kans. Med. Soc. 77:438, 1976.

23. McSwain, N. E., Jr.: Pneumatic trousers and the management of shock. J. Trauma 17:719, 1977.

24. Tenney, S. M., and Honig, C. R.: The effect of the anti-g suit on the ballistocardiogram. J. Aviat. Med. 26:194, 1955.

25. Knopp, R. K.: Determination of anti-shock trouser autotransfusion volume by radioisotope scan. Paper presented to the University Association for Emergency Medicine 11th Annual Meeting, San Antonio, TX, April 15, 1981.

26. Ransom, K. J., and McSwain, N. E., Jr.: Metabolic acidosis with pneumatic trousers in hypovolemic dogs. JACEP 8:184, 1979.

27. Ludewig, R. M., and Wangensteen, S. L.: Effect of external counterpressure on venous bleeding. Surgery 66:515, 1969.

28. Eddy, D. M., Wangensteen, S. L., and Ludewig, R. M.: The kinetics of fluid loss from leaks in arteries tested by an experimental ex vivo preparation and external counterpressure. Surgery 64:451, 1968.

29. Gardner, W. J.: Hemostasis by pneumatic compression. Am. Surg. 35:635, 1969.

30. Gardner, W. J., and Storer, J.: The use of the g-suit in control of intra-abdominal bleeding. Surg. Gynecol. Obstet. 123:792, 1966.

31. Wangensteen, S. L., Ludewig, R. M., Cox, J. M., et al.: The effect of external counterpressure on arterial bleeding. Surgery 64:922, 1968.

32. Civetta, J. M., Nussenfeld, S. R., Row, T. R., et al.: Prehospital use of the military anti-shock trouser (MAST). JACEP 5:581, 1976.

33. Hall, M., and Marshall, J. R.: The gravity suit: A major advance in management of gynecologic blood loss. Obstet. Gynecol. 53:247, 1979.

34. McLaughlin, A. P., III, McCullough, D. L., Kerr, W. S., Jr., et al.: The use of the external counterpressure (g-suit) in management of traumatic retroperitoneal hemorrhage. J. Urol. 107:940, 1972.

35. Lewis, D. G., MacKenzie, A., and McNeill, I. F.: The use of the g-suit in the control of bleeding arising from hypocoagulation. Ann. R. Coll. Surg. Engl. 52:53, 1973.

36. Wayne, M. A.: The mast suit in the treatment of cardiogenic shock. JACEP 7:107, 1978.

37. Gray, S., Shaver, J. A., Kroetz, F. W., et al.: Acute and prolonged effects of g-suit inflation on cardiovascular dynamics. Circulation (Suppl. II) 36:125, 1967.

38. Babbs, C. F.: New versus old theories of blood flow during cardiopulmonary resuscitation. Crit. Care Med. 8:191, 1980.

39. Luce, J. M., Cary, J. M., Ross, B. K., et al.: New developments in cardiopulmonary resuscitation. JAMA 244:1366, 1980.

40. Bircher, N., Safer, P., and Stewart, R.: A comparison of standard "MAST"-augmented and open-chest CPR in dogs. Crit. Care Med. 8:147, 1980.

41. Lee, H. R., Wilder, R. J., Dorins, P., et al.: MAST augmentation of external cardiac compression: Role of changing intrapleural pressure. Ann. Emerg. Med. 10:560, 1981.

42. Rudikoff, M. T., Maughan, W. L., Effron, M., et al.: Mechanisms of blood flow during cardiopulmonary resuscitation. Circulation 61:345, 1980.

43. Lilja, G. P., Long, R. S., and Ruiz, E.: Augmentation of systolic blood pressure during external cardiac compression by use of the MAST suit. Ann. Emerg. Med. 10:182, 1981.

44. Hoffman, J. R.: External counterpressure and the MAST suit: Current and future roles. Ann. Emerg. Med. 9:419, 1980.

45. McSwain, N. E., Jr.: Pneumatic antishock trousers. Curr. Concepts Trauma Care 8, Summer 1980.

46. Cram, A. E., Davis, J. W., Kealey, G. P., et al.: Effects of pneumatic anti-shock trousers on canine intracranial pressure. Ann. Emerg. Med. 10:28, 1981.

47. Dannewitz, S. R., Lilja, G. P., and Ruiz, E.: Effect of pneumatic trousers on intracranial pressure in hypovolemic dogs with an intracranial mass. Ann. Emerg. Med. 10:176, 1981.

48. Palafox, B. A., Johnson, M. N., McEwen, D. K., et al.: ICP changes following application of the mast suit. J. Trauma 21:55, 1981.

49. Lilja, G. P., Batalden, D. J., Adams, B. E., et al.: Value of the counterpressure suit (MAST) in pre-hospital care. Minn. Med. 58:540, 1975.

50. Ransom, K., and McSwain, N. E., Jr.: Respiratory function following application of MAST trousers. JACEP 7:297, 1978.

51. Davis, J. W., McKone, T. K., and Cram, A. E.: Hemodynamic effects of military anti-shock trousers (MAST) in experimental cardiac tamponade. Ann. Emerg. Med. 10:185, 1981.

52. Bruining, H. A., Schattenkerk, M. E., De Vries, J. E., et al.: Clinical experience with the medical anti-shock trousers (MAST) in the treatment of hemorrhage, especially from compound pelvic fracture. Neth. J. Surg. 32–3:102, 1980.

53. Espinosa, M. H., and Updegrove, J. H.: Clinical experience with the g-suit. Arch. Surg. 101:36, 1970.

54. McSwain, N. E., Jr.: MAST pneumatic trousers: A mechanical device to support blood pressure. Med. Instru. 11:334, 1977.

55. Wangensteen, S. L., deHoll, J. D., Ludewig, R. M., et al.: The detrimental effect of the g-suit in hemorrhagic shock. Ann. Surg. 170:187, 1969.

56. Burdick, J. E., Warshaw, A. L., and Abbott, W. M.: External counterpressure to control postoperative intraabdominal hemorrhage. Am. J. Surg. 129:369, 1975.

57. Batalden, D. J., Wickstrom, P. H., Ruiz, E., et al.: Value of the g-suit in patients with severe pelvic fracture. Arch. Surg. 109:326, 1974.

58. Cogbill, T. H., Good, J. T., Moore, E. E., et al.: Pulmonary function after military antishock trouser inflation. Surg. Forum 32:302, 1981.

59. Elliott, D. P., and Paton, B. C.: Effect of oxygen pressure on dogs subjected to hemorrhagic hypotension. Surg. Forum 14:5, 1963.

60. Shenansky, J. H., II, and Gillenwater, J. Y.: The effects of

external abdominal counterpressure on renal function. Surg. Forum 21:528, 1970.

61. Cangiano, T. L., and Kest, L.: Use of a g-suit for uncontrollable bleeding after percutaneous renal biopsy. J. Urol. 107:360, 1972.

62. Bradley, S. E., and Bradley, G. P.: The effect of increased intra-abdominal pressure on renal function in man. J. Clin. Invest. 26:1010, 1947.

63. McCullough, D. L., McLaughlin, A. P., and Warshawsky, A. B.: The gravity suit: A useful device in complicated urologic hemorrhage. Urology 6:468, 1975.

64. Rockwell, D. D., Butler, A. B., Keats, T. E., et al.: An improved design of the pneumatic counter-pressure trousers. Am. J. Surg. 143:377, 1982.

65. Johnson, B. E.: Anterior tibial compartment syndrome following use of MAST suit. Ann. Emerg. Med. 10:209, 1981.

66. Williams, T. M., Knopp, R., and Ellyson, J. H.: Compartment syndrome after anti-shock trouser use without lower-extremity trauma. J. Trauma 22:595, 1982.

67. Maull, K. I., Capehart, J. E., Cardea, J. A., et al.: Limb loss following military anti-shock trouser (MAST) application. J. Trauma 21:60, 1981.

68. Reines, H. D., and Khoury, N. P.: Use of military antishock trousers in the hospital. Am. J. Surg. 139:307, 1980.

69. Dillman, P. A.: The bio-physical responses to shock trousers. J. Emerg. Nurs. 21, Nov.-Dec., 1977.

70. Sanders, A. B., and Meislin, H. M.: Alterations in MAST suit pressure with changes in ambient temperature. Cited in Sanders and Meislin.[71]

71. Sanders, A. B., and Meislin, H. M.: Effect of altitude change on MAST suit pressure. Paper presented at the 12th annual meeting of the University Association for Emergency Medicine, Salt Lake City, UT, April 16, 1982.

72. Dick, T.: Putting your pants on using the MAST suit. JEMS 7:22, 1982.

73. Brooks, D. H., and Grenvik, A.: G-suit control of massive retroperitoneal hemorrhage due to pelvic fracture. Crit. Care Med. 1:257, 1973.

74. Burn, N., Lewis, D. G., MacKenzie, A., et al.: The g-suit: Its use in emergency surgery for ruptured abdominal aortic aneurysm. Anaesthesia 27:423, 1972.

75. Burton, A. C.: On the physical equilibrium of small blood vessels. Am. J. Physiol. 164:319, 1951.

76. Burton, R. R.: Clinical application of the anti-g suit. Aviat. Space Environ. Med. 46:745, 1975.

77. Darling, R. C.: Ruptured arteriosclerotic abdominal aortic aneurysms: A pathologic and clinical study. Am. J. Surg. 119:397, 1970.

78. Gardner, W. J., Taylor, H. P., and Dohn, D. F.: Acute blood loss requiring 58 transfusions; the use of the anti-gravity suit as an aid in postpartum intraabdominal hemorrhage. JAMA 167:985, 1958.

79. Hibbard, L. T.: Spontaneous rupture of the liver in pregnancy: A report of eight cases. Am. J. Obstet. Gynecol. 126:334, 1976.

80. Lowe, R. R., Jr.: Emergency treatment of shock—use of medical antishock trousers (MAST). J. Miss. State Med. Assoc. 19:147, 1978.

81. Pelligra, R., Trueblood, W. H., Mason, R., et al.: Anti-g suit as a therapeutic device. Aerospace Med. 41:943, 1970.

82. Sieker, H. O., Burnum, J. B., Hickam, J. B., et al.: Treatment of postural hypotension with a counterpressure garment. JAMA 161:132, 1956.

83. Wayne, M. A., and MacDonald, S. C.: Clinical evaluation of the antishock trouser: prospective study of low-pressure inflation. Ann. Emerg. Med. 12:285, 1983.

84. McCabe, J. B., Seidel, D. R., and Jagger, J. A.: Antishock trouser inflation and pulmonary vital capacity. Ann. Emerg. Med. 12:290, 1983.

Introduction

Doppler ultrasound is an indispensable aid in the clinical evaluation of a wide variety of pathologic conditions encountered in the emergency department. Doppler ultrasound is commonly used to measure blood pressure in infants and in patients with low flow states and to detect fetal heart sounds in utero. With a basic knowledge of waveform analysis and blood flow characteristics, Doppler ultrasound can also help in assessing arterial injury, venous thrombosis, and arterial occlusive disease. The techniques are relatively easy to master, and the equipment is both inexpensive and portable.

Principles of Doppler Ultrasound

The phenomenon of the Doppler shift was first described by Christian Doppler in 1843, but it was not until the 1960's that the principle was applied to medical diagnosis. The Doppler phenomenon can be stated as follows: when sound waves are transmitted to and then reflected from a moving object, the waves will return to a stationary emitting source at a frequency that is different from the originally transmitted wave. The returning frequency will be higher if the object is moving toward the emitting source, lower if the object is moving away. The change in frequency (Doppler shift) between the transmitted and reflected sound wave can be quantitated and expressed as an index of the velocity of the target particle from which the sound wave was reflected. The major clinical application of Doppler ultrasound is the detection of blood flow where the target particle is a moving erythrocyte. The general formula used to determine the Doppler shift is

$$\Delta f = \frac{2f_T\,V \cos\theta}{c}$$

where Δf = frequency shift (Doppler shift); f_T = transmitting frequency (usually $2\text{--}10 \times 10^6$ cycles per second or 2–10 MHz); V = velocity of reflectors (erythrocytes); θ = angle between incident/reflected beam and the path of reflectors; and c = velocity of sound in tissue (about 1.5×10^5 cm per sec).

Medical Doppler devices couple an energy source to a transmitting piezoelectric crystal and a receiving crystal. Both crystals are placed adjacent to each other at the tip of a probe, which is held against the skin. The processing circuitry of the device transforms the Doppler shift to an audible sound that may be heard with the aid of a speaker or earphones. Some devices are equipped with gauges that quantitate the velocity of flow both

31

The Clinical Use of Doppler Ultrasound

THOMAS STAIR, M.D.

toward and away from the transmitting crystal and with a chart recorder to permanently record the waveform. Devices that can detect the direction of flow are termed *directional Dopplers,* but an audible pulse may be heard if the flow is either toward or away from the probe.

Figure 31–1 is a diagram of a basic Doppler ultrasound device. Figures 31–2 and 31–3 are two of the nonrecording, nondirectional Dopplers that are popular in the emergency department. Figure 31–4 is a recording directional Doppler. All Doppler devices detect only the *velocity*, not the volume, of blood flow. Therefore, the intensity of the audible signal or the height of the waveform on the print-out are representations of velocity, not of flow volume. Although the pitch of the audible signal may change as velocity changes, changes in the volume and clarity of the sound are related to technique, proximity of the artery, and the angle at which the vessel is studied. These facts are critical in the interpretation of the results of a Doppler examination.

Blood velocity must be at least 6 cm per second to be detected by currently available Doppler devices. This flow rate is normally seen in all arteries and most major peripheral veins, allowing both the arterial and venous system to be studied.

Smaller piezoelectric crystals are best for measuring flow velocity in small, superficial vessels, whereas larger crystals, approximately a centimeter square, are better for larger vessels and deeper fetal heart sounds. Lower frequency sound waves penetrate deeper tissues with less scatter, whereas higher frequencies provide better resolution of superficial vessels. Frequencies of 2 to 5 MHz are best for fetal heart sounds, 5 to 10 MHz are appropriate for limb arteries and veins, and 10 MHz are used for perivascular intraoperative probes. Doppler instruments are usually supplied with a fixed frequency; however, variable frequency devices are available.

An interface of acoustic gel (not to be confused with abrasive electrical conductive gel or electrocardiographic gel) must be used to couple the

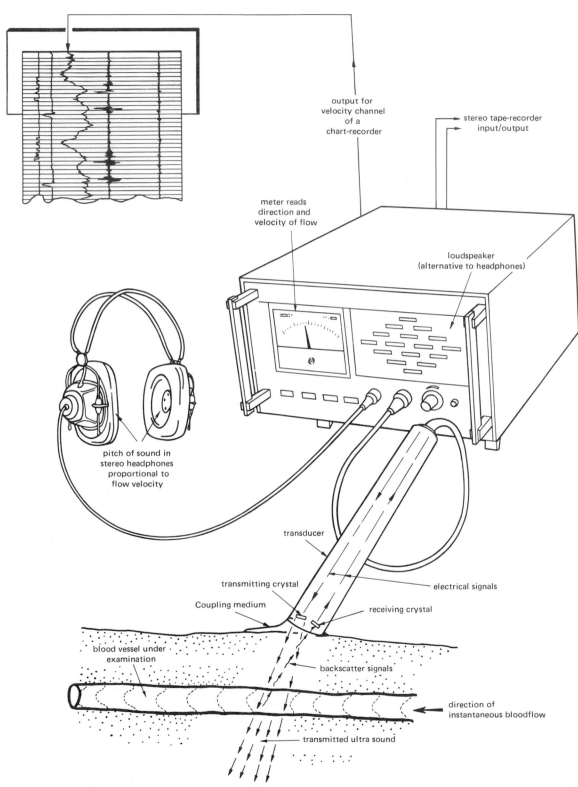

Figure 31–1. Schematic representation of a Doppler ultrasound device. (From Blood velocity waveforms and the physiological interpretation. Sonicaid, Inc., Fredericksburg, Virginia, p. 4. Used by permission.)

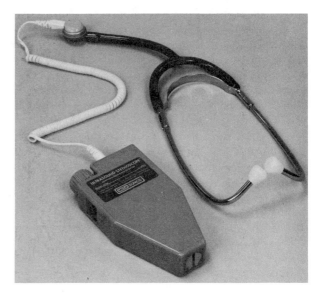

Figure 31–2. Pocket Doppler stethoscope (model BF4A, Medsonics, Inc., Los Altos, California).

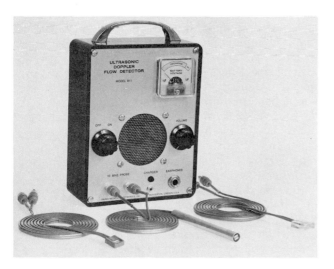

Figure 31–3. Ultrasonic Doppler Flow Detector with speaker and probes (model 811, Parks Electronics Labs, Beaverton, Oregon).

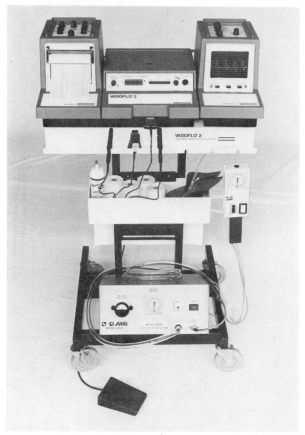

Figure 31–4. A recording directional Doppler device allows sophisticated wave form analysis.

piezoelectric crystals to the skin, both to protect the crystals and to reduce attenuation and reflection of the ultrasound signal. At every air-fluid interface, approximately 99.9 per cent of sound will be reflected and 0.1 per cent transmitted, a 30 dB decrease in volume. This attenuation by reflection is the basis of the Doppler ultrasound effect but limits its use in the anterior abdomen, chest, and skull.

After good acoustical contact with the skin has been made, the probe can be slowly angled in several directions until an optimum vascular flow signal is received. From the previous equation, because cos 0 equals 1, it is evident that frequency shifts will be greatest when the probe is pointed up or down the vessel using the most acute angle that allows good skin contact. In practice, this is usually about 45 degrees toward the axis of flow. Flow may often be detected by a probe that is held at right angles to the direction of flow; however, the amplitude of the signal will be increased by angling the probe.

Doppler flowmeters that are commonly used in the emergency department have a continuous output of sound waves. Pulsed or electronically gated ultrasound more accurately measures arterial flow

velocities, velocity profile, and vessel diameter. Coupled with a position-sensing transducer and a storage oscilliscope, these devices can even produce images of arterial flow in much the same manner as B-mode ultrasound imaging but are specific for moving blood and are comparable to arteriography. The devices that are discussed in this chapter, however, do not display an image on a screen.

Arterial Evaluation

WAVEFORMS AND FLOW CHARACTERISTICS

The audible signal and graphic waveforms obtained from Doppler devices are subject to analysis and detailed interpretation.[1] If the patient may possibly have arterial disease, from either trauma or occlusive disease, the waveform tracing and/or sounds from a potentially abnormal vessel should be compared with data from a normal vessel on the opposite side of the body.

The Doppler waveform of a normal pulse in most peripheral arteries, such as the brachial, femoral, dorsalis pedis, and radial arteries, consists of three components: late systolic forward flow, early diastolic reverse flow, and late diastolic forward flow (also termed *diastolic oscillation*). In a normal artery, one can always hear the first two components and, with practice, the third sound can usually be distinguished. The audible sound wave resembles a double ricochet sound. Various arterial waveforms are shown in Figure 31–5.

In the normal artery, late systolic forward flow is a sharp peak of increased frequency that is damped somewhat distally but remains the most prominent feature of the velocity waveform (Fig. 31–6). This phase is followed immediately by a negative deflection that is not quite as sharp and about half the amplitude, representing early diastolic reverse flow. This reverse flow and subsequent late diastolic oscillation are produced by elastic recoil of the arterial wall and thus will be reduced by extensive atherosclerosis, decreased peripheral vascular resistance, or vasodilatation.

Reverse flow and velocity oscillations are naturally damped distally and may normally be absent in the most distal arteries such as the digital arteries or dorsalis pedis artery (Fig. 31–7). Flow through collateral channels tends to lose the reverse phase, and loss of reverse flow may precede angiographically demonstrable arterial disease (Fig. 31–8).[2, 3]

ARTERIAL DISEASE

A Doppler device equipped with or without a graphic display can be helpful in the emergency

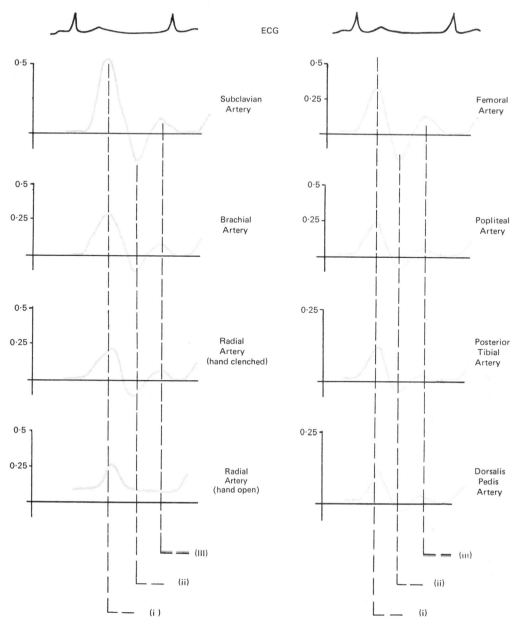

ECG

Subclavian
Artery

Brachial
Artery

Radial
Artery
(hand clenched)

Radial
Artery
(hand open)

Femoral
Artery

Popliteal
Artery

Posterior
Tibial
Artery

Dorsalis
Pedis
Artery

Figure 31–5. Normal waveforms of the peripheral system.

Figure 31–6. Femoral artery. Late systolic flow appears as a sharp peak. There is good reverse flow in early diastole. Clear oscillations are seen during diastole. The peak systolic velocity is about 30 cm/sec. (From Doppler evaluation of peripheral arterial disease: a clinical handbook. Sonicaid, Inc., Fredericksburg, Virginia. Used by permission.)

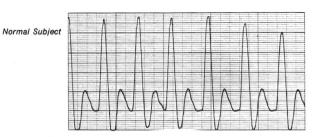

Normal Subject

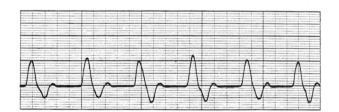

Figure 31–7. Dorsalis pedis artery. Although reduced in amplitude at this peripheral site, all characteristics of a healthy waveform persist. The peak systolic velocity is about 12 cm/sec. The zero flow at end-diastole is normal in the dorsalis pedis artery. (From Doppler evaluation of peripheral arterial disease: a clinical handbook. Sonicaid, Inc., Fredericksburg, Virginia. Used by permission.)

419

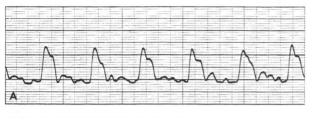

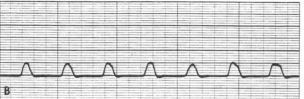

Figure 31–8. *A*, Absence of reverse flow in patient with extensive occlusions (femoral artery). *B*, Monophasic pulsatility. A monophasic pattern has a readily distinguishable systolic pulse but a lack of oscillatory activity during diastole. Such patterns demonstrate diminished arterial compliance. They may indicate a stenosis proximal to the examination site and/or low resistance in distal vessels. (From Doppler evaluation of peripheral arterial disease: a clinical handbook. Sonicaid, Inc., Fredericksburg, Virginia. Used by permission.)

department assessment of a patient with limb trauma by audibly and visually demonstrating the arterial blood flow waveforms of both the injured and uninjured limbs. Much information may be gained by listening to the flow, but in order to fully evaluate an artery, the print-out of the waveform is required. Although significant arterial injury may be present despite good distal pulses, damping of early systolic flow or loss of early diastolic reverse flow and late diastolic oscillations are much more sensitive signs of arterial injury or disease.[1, 2]

To evaluate a peripheral artery, place the probe at various sites over the distal artery and listen for the three-component sound while recording the waveform on the readout device. Arterial injury and disease (such as intimal damage, thrombosis, stenosis, external compression, and complete disruption) affect the peak velocity of blood flow and modify both the audible sound and the shape of the recorded waveform (Fig. 31–9). A normal Doppler evaluation of an artery is evidence against arterial pathology but is not always conclusive. Pathology should be suspected from even subtle changes in the flow characteristics or waveform analysis, especially if these changes are not seen on the opposite side. It must be stressed that *simply hearing the arterial flow with the Doppler device does not ensure a normal artery.*

Collateral blood flow, although minimal, may be enough to produce an audible pulse that can be detected with sensitive equipment. Collateral flow may even produce a measurable blood pressure despite significant pathology in the proximal artery. The three-component waveform analysis must be scrutinized in such situations. The waveform is also sensitive to vasoconstriction, hypovolemia or vasodilatation, temperature changes, and the normal aging process as well as to arterial injury or occlusion (Fig. 31–10). From a technical standpoint, one must keep these variables in mind. In addition, a 45 degree angle must be maintained between the probe and the skin.

BLOOD PRESSURE EVALUATION

Besides evaluating flow characteristics and waveform analysis of an artery, Doppler-assisted blood pressures should be taken to aid in the evaluation of any extremity.[4]

Because Doppler ultrasound is more sensitive and less suceptible to technical artifacts than auscultation by a stethoscope or detection of a pulse by palpation and because it detects flow rather than turbulence or pulsation, the Doppler device can be used to measure blood pressures that are not accessible for auscultation or palpation. Doppler readings of systolic blood pressure are accurate to as low as 30 mm Hg. (Diastolic pressures cannot be determined.) Such measurements can be of significant clinical value in obese patients, in newborns and in infants.

The probe is placed over a distal artery, such as the radial or ulnar artery at the wrist or the posterior tibial or dorsalis pedis artery at the ankle or foot, while a sphygmomanometer cuff is inflated proximally and slowly deflated. The pressure at which flow is first heard is recorded as the systolic pressure under the cuff. In addition to blood pressure determinations, segmental blood pressures can be measured to help document the level of arterial disease.[2, 3, 5–7] This is done with the cuff at four sites along each leg.

When evaluating peripheral vascular disease by the use of Doppler-assisted blood pressure determinations, compare the systolic pressure at the ankle and in the brachial artery (Fig. 31–11). Normally, the ankle systolic pressure (when supine) is higher than the brachial artery systolic pressure and the ankle/brachial index (ratio) is greater than 1. If the index is less than 1, it is suggestive of occlusive peripheral vascular disease in the leg (Fig. 31–12). If segmental pressures are taken, the area of occlusion may be predicted (Fig. 31–13). An exception may occur in diabetic patients who have calcified peripheral arteries. The rigid calcific vessels may be difficult to compress, and a systolic pressure in the range of 250 to 300 mm Hg will be obtained when there is severe vascular insufficiency.

CAROTID VESSEL EVALUATION

Occlusion or stenosis of the internal carotid artery may be assessed with a *directional* Doppler

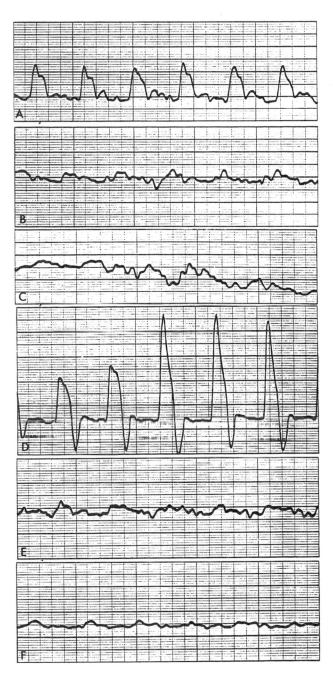

Figure 31–9. Patient with severe multilevel disease. This patient, age 64, exhibits symptoms of generalized atherosclerosis and also suffers from polycythemia.

A, Left femoral artery. Pulsatility is adequate, but the peak systolic velocity is only about 7 cm/sec. The systolic pulse is wide. There is no reverse flow. The diastolic portion exhibits some oscillation but less than is expected at the femoral site.

B, Left posterior tibial artery. At this level, pulsatility is essentially absent. The maximum velocity is about 7 cm/sec, suggesting a patent artery distal to an occlusion in which flow is virtually all derived from collaterals. The left leg ankle/brachial pressure index was determined to be .61, also consistent with severe occlusion.

C, Left dorsalis pedis artery. Pulsatility is entirely absent. The velocity is so low that it is at the lower limit of measurability by Doppler techniques. At times, an adjacent venous signal swamps the recording.

D, Right femoral artery. This side yields a much better waveform than the left femoral (*A*). Peak systolic velocity is about 30 cm/sec. There is good early diastolic reverse flow. The absence of diastolic oscillations suggests rigid, non-compliant arteries distally.

E, Right posterior tibial artery. The waveform is non-pulsatile, and the maximum velocity is only about 3 cm/sec. The right leg ankle/brachial pressure index was .58, even lower than the left leg.

F, Right dorsalis pedis artery. The completely non-pulsatile appearance of this waveform signifies collateral flow. Again, the maximum forward velocity is a barely measurable 3 cm/sec.

(From Doppler evaluation of peripheral arterial disease: a clinical handbook. Sonicaid, Inc., Fredericksburg, Virginia. Used by permission.)

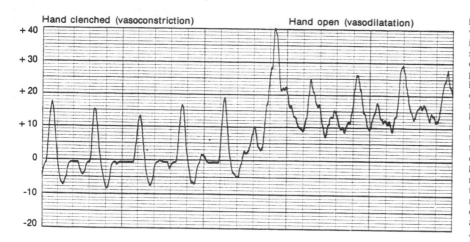

Hand clenched (vasoconstriction)   Hand open (vasodilatation)

Figure 31–10. Simulated effects of vasoconstriction and vasodilatation in the normal radial artery. Vasoconstriction of the lumen can mimic the effect of distal obstructions in the pathway. Vasodilatation, on the other hand, can partially mask evidence of occlusion. Therefore, it is necessary for the user of Doppler procedures to be aware of these phenomena. The rather dramatic difference in the patterns obtained during vasoconstriction and during vasodilatation can be easily simulated in the radial artery by performing the following experiment with a normal subject: Place the transducer over the radial artery and run a waveform with the fist tightly clenched to shut off the network of arteries and capillaries in the hand. As shown in the figure, the pattern obtained changes remarkably depending on whether vasoconstriction or vasodilatation is occurring. (From Doppler evaluation of peripheral arterial disease: a clinical handbook. Sonicaid, Inc., Fredericksburg, Virginia. Used by permission.)

Figure 31–11. Typical pressures in a normal subject. Findings, based on resting pressures, show no evidence of occlusive disease of the large- or medium-sized arteries.

Significant Findings (normal):

1. Ankle/brachial pressure index 1.0 or greater.
2. All pressure gradients less than 30 mm Hg.
3. Upper thigh pressure at least 40 mm Hg above brachial pressure.

(From Doppler evaluation of peripheral arterial disease: a clinical handbook. Sonicaid, Inc., Fredericksburg, Virginia. Used by permission.)

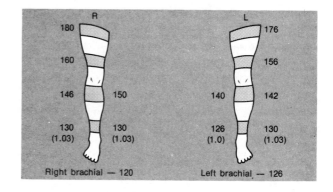

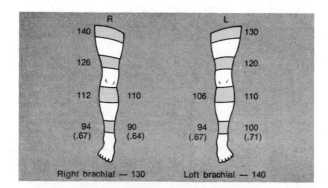

Figure 31–12. Typical pressures in a patient with obstruction of the abdominal aorta or aorta or bilateral iliac obstruction.

Significant Findings:

1. Ankle/brachial pressure index less than 1.0.
2. All segmental gradients less than 30 mm Hg.
3. Both upper thigh pressures low with respect to brachial pressure.

Findings are suggestive of severe aorto-iliac occlusive disease. (From Doppler evaluation of peripheral arterial disease: a clinical handbook. Sonicaid, Inc., Fredericksburg, Virginia. Used by permission.)

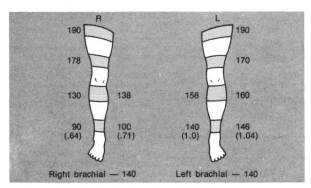

Figure 31–13. Typical pressures in a patient with obstruction of the popliteal or tibial arteries.

Significant Findings:

1. Ankle/brachial pressure index less than 1.0 in right leg.

2. Abnormally high gradient from ankle to below knee and again from below to above knee in right leg.

3. Upper thigh pressures are 50 mm Hg higher than brachial pressures, consistent with normal flow at the aorto-iliac level.

Findings are suggestive of a right popliteal occlusion and/or anterior and posterior tibial occlusion. (From Doppler evaluation of peripheral arterial disease: a clinical handbook. Sonicaid, Inc., Fredericksburg, Virginia. Used by permission.)

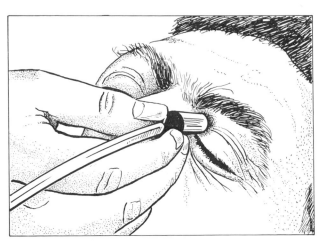

Figure 31–14. When evaluating the carotid system, the Doppler probe is placed on the inferior portion of the medial supraorbital ridge and aimed into the orbit. The probe is moved until a strong supraorbital pulse is noted.

device by noting the direction of flow in the supraorbital artery and by changes in the flow.[8–11] Place the probe over the supraorbital artery, just below the inferior margin of the medial supraorbital ridge, and angle it into the orbit (Fig. 31–14). The direction of flow, either toward or away from the probe, is noted by the waveform recording or by the directional gauges on the directional Doppler device. *Normally blood flow is pulsatile and out of the orbit toward the probe.* Greater than 50 per cent occlusion of the internal carotid artery on one side decreases flow forces enough to leave the supraorbital artery supplied by collaterals from the external carotid and the superficial temporal arteries. The net result is that flow is now *into* the orbit and *away* from the probe. Often, damped late diastolic oscillations and other changes in the waveform, which are the result of collateral circulation, can be noted. The opposite side is used for comparison.

Certain compression maneuvers may further elucidate this situation. Normally, compression of the ipsilateral superficial temporal artery will augment flow through the internal carotid system by reducing back pressure of the collaterals, and compression of this artery will increase flow out of the orbit and toward the probe (Fig. 31–15A). If the internal carotid artery is occluded, compression of the superficial temporal artery will decrease or stop flow in the supraorbital artery (Fig. 31–15B).[8]

Evaluation of the Venous System

Although Doppler ultrasound can be used to show varicose veins and postthrombotic valvular incompetency, its greatest clinical value is in demonstrating venous obstruction owing to deep vein thrombophlebitis.[12–16] History and physical examination alone are unreliable means of diagnosing deep venous thrombophlebitis. Iliofemoral thrombi are unlikely to produce clinical signs and symptoms, yet they often embolize to the lung. Other diagnostic tests are time consuming, expensive, and/or hazardous.

Although contrast phlebography or venography is the best technique for revealing deep venous thrombi, it is technically demanding and expensive and involves the risks of radiation exposure and dye allergy and may itself cause thrombophlebitis. Radionuclide scanning with ^{99m}Tc-labeled albumin is technically similar to venography, with less resolution but fewer hazards. Scanning with ^{125}I-labeled fibrinogen is sensitive for active thrombogenesis in the calf but is of little use for detecting established iliofemoral clot. Impedance plethysmography measures the decrease in diameter of the leg after a venous tourniquet is removed and, like Doppler ultrasound, is most sensitive for the iliofemoral thrombi.

Doppler ultrasound and impedance plethysmography share similar (80 to 90 per cent) published sensitivities and specificities in detecting deep venous thrombi. Both techniques can be carried out by a technician, both require calibration and semiportable equipment, and both produce hard-copy documentation. Doppler ultrasound, however, may also be used in another mode, particularly suited to the emergency department, in the form of a portable, battery-powered device with an audible output (see Figs. 31–2 and 31–3) to be used by the physician at the bedside to guide immediate clinical decision-making.

A patient who has leg pain with swelling, warmth, or discoloration has a differential diag-

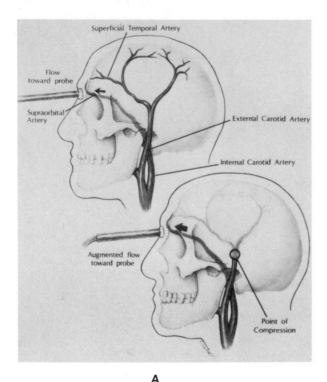

A

B

Figure 31–15. A, The normal direction of blood flow in the supraorbital carotid artery is toward the probe *(top)*. With compression of the superficial temporal artery, this flow is augmented *(bottom)*. B, With occlusion of the internal carotid artery, flow in the supraorbital artery is away from the probe *(top)*, because flow is mainly from the external carotid system. This flow is dimished by compression of the superficial temporal artery *(bottom)*. (From LoGerfo, F. W., and Mason, G. R.: Directional Doppler studies of supraorbital artery flow in internal carotid stenosis and occlusion. Surgery, 76:724, 1974. Used by permission.)

nosis that includes edema, cellulitis, hematoma, and thrombophlebitis. The clinician may, in 5 minutes at the bedside, perform a screening Doppler examination, guiding the subsequent choice of more invasive tests.

In the first 2 years of its use at the University of Iowa, Barnes compared Doppler ultrasound with 122 venograms. The results indicated both a sensitivity and specificity of 94 per cent.[13] Sumner summarized the results of 10 previous studies that had an overall accuracy of 88 per cent, and, in his own study, the results showed an overall accuracy of 94 per cent.[14] In a further study of 156 patients Doppler evaluation was 94 per cent sensitive and 90 per cent specific in detecting thrombi above the knee and 91 per cent sensitive and 84 per cent specific in detecting thrombi below the knee, with an overall accuracy of 92 per cent.[15]

VENOUS FLOW CHARACTERISTICS

Doppler flow characteristics of the venous system differ from those of the arterial system in several important aspects. Flow rates in the peripheral veins may be near the threshold of sensitivity of the instrument and may require various maneuvers to augment the flow velocity. Venous flow does not exhibit arterial-type waveforms, and the flow may be affected by several external variables, leading to false-positive examination results. Some peripheral veins may even be occluded by firm pressure with the Doppler skin probe. Because major arteries and veins often course together but in different directions, one must be able to differentiate flow patterns, either by a trained ear or by the use of directional flowmeters. The most striking difference from the characteristic pulsatile arterial pulse is the low-pitched, soft, blowing, and extended sound of venous flow. The sound of venous flow is best described as a "windstorm" sound.

When examining the venous system, assess both spontaneous venous flow and augmented venous flow. Spontaneous venous flow sounds can usually be heard in a normal peripheral vein. The absence of spontaneous flow is an indicator of disease, and the presence of spontaneous flow is a sign of a patent vein. Normal spontaneous flow is phasic with respiration and is *not continuous*. Continuous flow in a peripheral vein is a sign of venous disease. Holding one's breath will momentarily stop venous flow in the legs, but even normal inspiration will increase the intra-abdominal pressure enough to momentarily decrease (stop) venous flow. Expiration will release the pressure and allow venous flow to increase, producing the characteristic phasic flow during respiration. This phasic flow during respiration can be distinguished in most large peripheral veins, and its presence is a sensitive indicator of a normal vein.

Because spontaneous phasic venous flow is such a sensitive indicator of a normal vein, one must be certain not to produce false-positive examination results owing to technical errors. A false-positive test result may be produced by conditions and situations as subtle as patient anxiety, which tenses muscles; vasoconstriction owing to a cold room; hyperextension of the knee; elevation of the legs; the recent use of elastic support hose; or permitting the patient to raise his head to look at the examiner. Note that if positive-pressure ven-

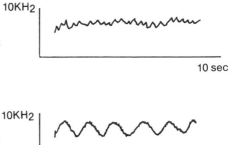

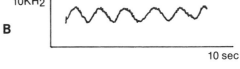

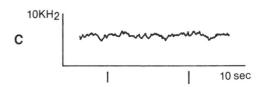

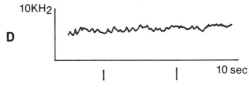

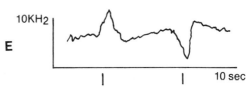

Figure 31–17. Abnormal findings in leg veins. A, Lack of respiratory variation. B, Pulsatile flow of congestive heart failure (normal in neck and proximal arm veins). C, No augmentation with distal compression (suggests obstruction). D, No decrease with proximal compression or augmentation with release (obstruction). E, Normal augmentation with distal compression, yet retrograde flow with release (suggests incompetent distal valves).

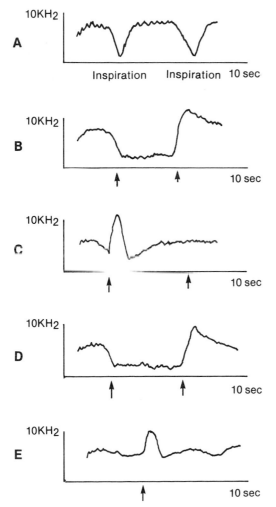

Figure 31–16. Normal Doppler ultrasound recording during examination of left veins. A, Normal respiratory variation at common femoral vein. Flow decreased with inspiration. B, Abolition of femoral vein flow with Valsalva maneuver and return with release. C, Augmentation of femoral vein flow with calf compression and no effect of release. D, Posterior tibial vein flow slowed by calf compression and augmented by release. E, Augmentation of saphenous flow by percussion (note damped respiratory variation).

tilation is used, the respiratory variation of venous flow is reversed.

Venous flow may be augmented by both compression distal to the site being examined and by releasing previous obstructing pressure at a site proximal to the area being examined. As with arterial flow, venous flow may be evaluated by its available characteristics and by the waveforms produced on a recorder (Figs. 31–16 and 31–17).

VENOUS EXAMINATION TECHNIQUE

In many sites, it is necessary first to locate the arterial flow signal and then the venous sound. Sigel termed the spontaneous flow sound, with its respiratory variation, the "S" sound and the brief rush of blood obtained by distal compression and other augmentation maneuvers the "A" sound.[12, 16] Six characteristics of venous flow that should be checked for at each examination are: patent vein, spontaneous flow, phasic flow (with respiration), augmented flow (with distal compression or release of proximal compression), competence of valves, and nonpulsatile flow.[13]

The standardized examination of venous flow in the legs described by Barnes[13] is as follows: With the patient in a supine position, the head of the bed should be elevated 30 degrees and the patient's legs should be rotated slightly externally and flexed at the hip and knee. The examiner first locates the flow signal of the posterior tibial vein, posterior to the medial malleolus. After generously applying acoustic gel, the probe is angled at about 45 degrees to the skin, being careful not to press so hard as to diminish flow in the vein. The examiner listens for respiratory variations in the venous flow, if present at this level; compresses the foot, which should augment flow; and then releases the foot, which should not affect flow (Fig. 31–18). Compression should be gentle but brisk. The machine is sensitive enough to identify

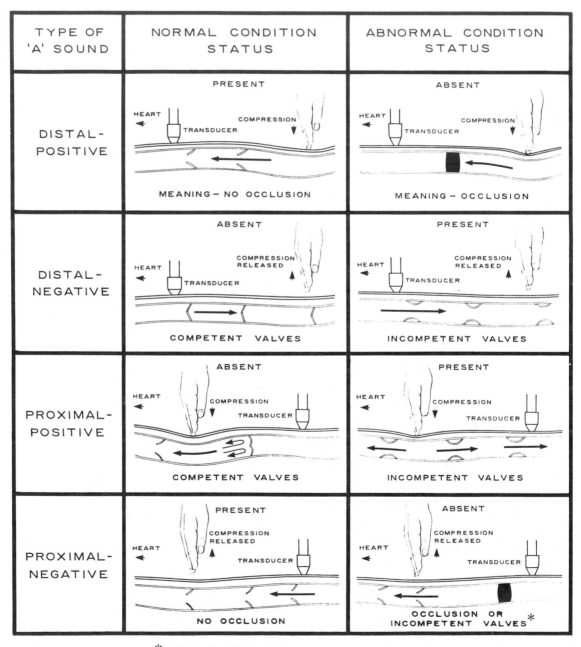

TYPE OF 'A' SOUND	NORMAL CONDITION STATUS	ABNORMAL CONDITION STATUS
DISTAL-POSITIVE	PRESENT HEART / TRANSDUCER / COMPRESSION MEANING – NO OCCLUSION	ABSENT HEART / TRANSDUCER / COMPRESSION MEANING – OCCLUSION
DISTAL-NEGATIVE	ABSENT HEART / TRANSDUCER / COMPRESSION RELEASED COMPETENT VALVES	PRESENT HEART / TRANSDUCER / COMPRESSION RELEASED INCOMPETENT VALVES
PROXIMAL-POSITIVE	ABSENT HEART / COMPRESSION / TRANSDUCER COMPETENT VALVES	PRESENT HEART / COMPRESSION / TRANSDUCER INCOMPETENT VALVES
PROXIMAL-NEGATIVE	PRESENT HEART / COMPRESSION RELEASED / TRANSDUCER NO OCCLUSION	ABSENT HEART / COMPRESSION RELEASED / TRANSDUCER OCCLUSION OR INCOMPETENT VALVES*

*USUALLY NOT TOTALLY ABSENT BUT ONLY DIMINISHED IF VALVES ARE INCOMPETENT.

Figure 31–18. The types of "A" sounds and their meaning when present or absent. (From Sigel, B., Popky, G. L., Mapp, E. M., et al.: Evaluation of Doppler ultrasound examination: its use in diagnosis of lower extremity venous disease. Arch. Surg. 100:535, 1970.)

changes with only light compression. Repeated compressions may drain the leg of blood for a few minutes. It is best to minimize the compressions to avoid false results.

The next site to examine in this position is the common femoral vein, in the femoral triangle, just inferior to the inguinal ligament and medial to the femoral artery, which can be located by palpating the pulse and hearing the characteristic arterial flow. As an aside, congestive heart failure may produce a pulsatile flow in the common femoral vein. In the femoral vein, there should normally be variations with respiration. Normally inspiration decreases venous flow, whereas expiration increases venous flow, as a result of diaphragmatic movement.

A sustained Valsalva maneuver should temporarily stop venous flow and produce an easily identifiable augmentation in flow when it is released. Lack of this augmentation may be a sign of iliofemoral occlusion, just as lack of respiratory variation or a decrease in flow would be to the other side.

Next, with the probe still over the common femoral vein, the examiner should compress the calf. This should produce augmentation of flow. Subsequent release of the calf should not alter the flow. Lack of augmentation on calf compression or an asymmetric effect suggests occlusion between the calf and the groin. Distal flow upon release suggests incompetent valves. Finally, the thigh should be compressed and released, resulting in the same results and interpretation as calf compression.

The next vein to examine is the superficial femoral vein, in the adductor canal at mid-thigh, alongside the superficial femoral artery. The examination is the same as that for the common femoral vein except that with the probe at mid-thigh it is pointless to compress the thigh.

To examine the popliteal vein, the patient must lie in the prone position with a pillow placed under his foot so that the knee is slightly flexed. The popliteal vein is usually best heard just lateral to the popliteal artery. After noting respiratory variations, the examiner can compress and release the thigh, which should slow or stop flow without reversing it but also produce a brief augmentation upon release of compression. Compression of the calf or dorsiflexion of the foot (as for Homans' sign) should produce augmentation of flow, and release should not reverse flow.

The test procedure and interpretation are summarized in Table 31–1. Normal and abnormal venous flows are diagrammed in Figure 31–18. By comparing both legs and noting any asymmetry in spontaneous and augmented flows, the examiner can usually deduce not only the presence but also the level of obstruction, as well as incompetent deep valves.

Incompetent perforating veins may be revealed by placing a loose venous tourniquet proximal to the probe and showing reverse flow produced by compression of the leg above the tourniquet. Flow and competence in the superficial veins may be tested in a similar manner, but rather than compressing and releasing a segment of leg to augment deep flow, the examiner can simply tap over the saphenous vein to augment superficial flow.

The Doppler device is best suited for examina-

Table 31–1. TEST PROCEDURE AND INTERPRETATION FOR DEEP VENOUS THROMBOSIS

Test Procedure Locate vein by using corresponding artery; perform following steps at each examination site*	Findings and Clinical Significance (Sounds usually graded as present, diminished, or absent)			
	Normal		Abnormal	
	Finding	Interpretation	Finding	Interpretation
Listen for spontaneous flow sounds	Present (may be absent at ankle)	No significant occlusions	Absent or diminished (at any site above ankle)	Significant occlusions present
Listen for effect of respiration	Sound phasic with respiration	Normal intra-abdominal pressure	Not phasic with respiration	High intra-abdominal pressure
Listen for pulsatility	Sound not pulsatile	Normal venous pressure	Sound pulsates with heart beat	High venous pressure—consider congestive heart failure
Apply compression distal to probe	Augmented sound present	No occlusion between site compressed and probe	Augmented sound diminished or absent	Occlusion between site compressed and probe
Release compression distal to probe	No Doppler sound	Competent valves	Augmented sound present	Incompetent valves
Apply compression proximal to probe	No Doppler sound	Competent valves	Augmented sound present	Incompetent valves
Release compression proximal to probe	Augmented sound present	No occlusion between probe and site compressed	Augmented sound diminished or absent	Occlusion between probe and site compressed

*Posterior tibial, common femoral, and superficial femoral veins normally examined in sequence with patient in a supine position; then popliteal vein is checked with patient in a prone position and with his leg flexed and supported at the calf.
(From Waxham, R. D.: Doppler ultrasound. Radiol. Today. April/May 1980.

tion of the lower venous system, but the veins of the thorax or the veins of the arms and neck may also be assessed. Velocity of blood flow in the internal jugular vein is pulsatile in a way that is approximately inverse to that of the familiar jugular venous pulses. Flow increases with inspiration and decreases but usually does not stop with expiration, although a Valsalva maneuver will stop flow. Flow in the subclavian, axillary, and brachial veins follows a similar pattern, although, in some people, inspiration may compress the subclavian vein and reduce flow. Flow in the brachial vein may also be tested with compression and release of the arm below to augment flow, as in the leg examination.

Other Applications

Fetal heart sounds may be heard with the Doppler stethoscope as early as the twelfth week of gestation, at a rate of 120 to 140 beats per minute and are audible through the sounds of placental flow. Their presence may aid in the diagnosis of pregnancy and the assessment of fetal distress after abdominal trauma or placental bleeding.

A Doppler probe may be used to provide instantaneous feedback on resuscitation and CPR, both in the hospital and in the field. A small probe may be taped over a radial artery and attached to a loudspeaker, allowing immediate correction of ineffective CPR or monitoring of a patient's pulse rather than cardiac rhythm. In addition to a sphygmomanometer cuff, also left in place for occasional inflation, such a monitoring probe can provide systolic blood pressure measurements without a stethoscope.[17]

A probe taped over the precordium has been described as a sensitive indicator of minute air emboli that may enter the right heart during surgery. The sound reflected by these bubbles has been described as a "squeak" or "chirp."[18]

Doppler ultrasound detection of intravascular bubbles has been suggested as a tool in the diagnosis of bends, or decompression sickness or in the guidance of hyperbaric therapy. Audible bubbles have been detected in the absence of symptoms and when standard decompression tables have been followed.[19]

Doppler examination may also be used to locate the tip of a catheter within a patient. The flow of intravenous fluid, devoid of cells or bubbles to reflect sound, will not be detectable, but, if the examiner withdraws and re-injects a few milliliters of blood or a few *tiny* bubbles, the to-and-fro velocity change along the catheter becomes evident.

Doppler ultrasound is also valuable in the differentiation between epididymitis and testicular torsion. In epididymitis, flow in the affected testicular artery is equal to or greater than that in the unaffected side of the scrotum, whereas in testicular torsion, there is a drop in testicular flow below the torsion. The Doppler evaluation of the acute scrotum is discussed in more detail in Chapter 61.

1. Felix, W. R.: Doppler ultrasound in the diagnosis of peripheral vascular disease. Semin. Roentgenol. 10:315, 1975.
2. Strandness, D. E., Schultz, R. D., Sumner, D. S., et al.: Ultrasonic flow detection: Am. J. Surg. 113:311, 1967.
3. Strandness, D. E.: The use of ultrasound in the evaluation of peripheral vascular disease. Prog. Cardiovasc. Dis., 20:403, 1978.
4. Felix, W. R., Jr.: Ultrasound measurements of arm and leg blood pressures. JAMA 226:1096, 1973.
5. Lennihan, R., Jr., and Mackereth, M. A.: Ankle pressures in vascular insufficiency involving the legs. J. Clin Ultrasound 1:120, 1973.
6. Yao, S. T., Hobbs, J. T., and Irvine, W. T.: Ankle systolic pressure measurements in arterial disease affecting the lower extremity. Br. J. Surg. 56:676, 1969.
7. Lennihan, R., Jr., and Mackereth, M. A.: Ankle pressures in arterial occlusive disease involving the legs. Surg. Clin. North Am. 53:657, 1973.
8. Barnes, R. W., Russell, H. E., Bone, G. E., et al.: Doppler cerebrovascular examination: improved results with refinements in technique. Stroke 8:468, 1977.
9. Brodie, T. E., and Ochsner, J. L.: Bilateral carotid stenosis: diagnosis by Doppler sonography. Vasc. Surg. 12:53, 1978.
10. Maroon, J. C., Campbell, R. L., and Dyken, M.: Internal carotid artery occlusion diagnosed by Doppler ultrasound. Stroke 1:122, 1970.
11. LoGerfo, F. W., and Mason, G. R.: Directional Doppler studies of supraorbital artery flow in internal carotid stenosis and occlusion. Surgery 76:723, 1974.
12. Sigel, B., Popky, G. L., Wagner, D. K., et al.: A Doppler ultrasound method for diagnosing lower extremity venous disease. Surg. Gynecol. Obstet. 127:339, 1968.
13. Barnes, R. W., Russell, H. E., and Wilson, M. R.: Doppler Ultrasonic Evaluation of Venous Disease, 2nd ed. Iowa City, University of Iowa Press, 1975.
14. Sumner, D. S.: Diagnosis of venous thrombosis by Doppler ultrasound. *In* Bergan, J. J., and Yao, J. S. (eds.): Venous Problems. Chicago, Year Book Medical Publishers, Inc., 1978, pp. 159–185.
15. Sumner, D. S., Lambeth, A.: Reliability of Doppler ultrasound in the diagnosis of acute venous thrombosis both above and below the knee. Am. J. Surg. 138:205, 1979.
16. Sigel, B., Popky, G. L., Mapp, E. M., et al.: Evaluation of Doppler ultrasound examination: its use in diagnosis of lower extremity venous disease. Arch. Surg. 100:535, 1970.
17. Grunau, C. F. V.: Doppler ultrasound monitoring of systemic blood flow during CPR. JACEP 7:180, 1978.
18. Michenfelder, J. D., Miller, R. H., and Gronert, G. A.: Evaluation of an ultrasonic device (Doppler) for the diagnosis of venous air embolism. Anesthesiology 36:164, 1972.
19. Gillis, M. F., Karagianes, M.T., and Peterson, P.O.: Detection of gas emboli associated with decompression using the Doppler flowmeter. J. Occup. Med. 2:245, 1969.

4

ANESTHESIOLOGY

32

Regional Anesthesia in the Emergency Department

LEVON M. CAPAN, M.D.
KATIE P. PATEL, M.D.
HERMAN TURNDORF, M.D.

Historical Background

Regional loss of pain sensation with the local anesthetic cocaine was first described by Koller in 1884.[1] He demonstrated that topical administration of cocaine on the conjunctiva results in anesthesia of the eye, allowing performance of painless surgery for glaucoma. Soon after this experience, Halsted and Hall were able to inject the drug into their own or each other's peripheral nerves and provide sufficient anesthesia to perform surgery.[2] It is interesting to note that as early as 1884 Hall predicted the wide applicability of this method for minor surgical procedures for outpatient surgery. One year later Halsted reported the successful use of this anesthetic method in more than 1000 minor surgical operations.[3] Both the acute and chronic adverse effects of cocaine, however, stimulated research concerned with finding other synthetic local anesthetic agents with more favorable therapeutic ratios. Benzocaine was synthesized in 1890 by Ritsert,[4] and procaine was synthesized in 1905 by Einhorn and Braun.[5, 6] Tetracaine and chloroprocaine were introduced into clinical practice in 1930 and 1952, respectively.[7, 8] All these local anesthetics were benzoic acid derivatives, and their major disadvantage was the causing of allergic reactions. In 1943, Löfgren synthesized lidocaine, an amide derivative of diethyl amino acetic acid.[9] This drug gained wide popularity, because unlike earlier benzoic acid ester derivatives, it lacked the property of causing allergic reactions. Since the synthesis of lidocaine, various amide-type local anesthetics (mepivacaine, prilocaine, bupivacaine, and etidocaine) have been introduced into clinical practice.

In the late nineteenth and early twentieth centuries, along with the development of anesthetic agents, techniques to block the conduction of pain impulses in various nerves were described.

Schleich described infiltration anesthesia in 1894.[10] Corning described spinal anesthesia in 1885,[11] Bier devised intravenous regional anesthesia in 1908,[12] Cathelin demonstrated epidural anesthesia by the caudal approach in 1901,[13] and Dogliotti described segmental peridural anesthesia in 1931.[14]

During recent decades, major developments in anesthesiology led to the refinement of techniques in regional anesthesia. A better understanding of neurophysiology and the pharmacology of local anesthetics has also resulted in an improvement in the prevention and treatment of associated complications. Although major nerve blocks should undoubtedly be performed by physicians who are specially trained in anesthesiology, minor nerve blocks can safely be administered by physicians who are trained in other specialties if they are familiar with the anatomic, physiologic, pharmacologic, and toxicologic aspects of these procedures. The availability of complete anesthetic and resuscitative equipment and a nursing staff familiar with these methods and their complications are also important requirements for the safe administration of these nerve blocks.

Regional block in the emergency department is usually performed for one or all of the following reasons: 1) to provide anesthesia for minor surgical procedures, 2) to provide analgesia and muscle relaxation enabling closed reduction of upper extremity fractures and dislocations, and 3) to treat acute pain states. The advantages of regional anesthesia given in the emergency department compared with general anesthesia administered in the operating room include less interference with preexisting diseases, decreased chance of pulmonary aspiration and postoperative nausea or vomiting, shorter postanesthetic nursing care requirements, and finally, shorter or no postoperative hospitalization requirements. An important disadvantage of regional ansthetic methods is the necessity of patient cooperation. Some patients, even in the presence of complete anesthesia, may not tolerate being awake during a surgical procedure. Small children rarely tolerate regional anesthesia. Additionally, in obese patients and in patients with anatomic deformities of the injection site, technical difficulties may arise in the administration of the blocks.

Pharmacologic Profile of Local Anesthetics

CHEMICAL STRUCTURE

Currently used local anesthetic agents can be divided into two main categories: amino-esters and amino-amides. Both groups of drugs have a common basic chemical structure that consists of an aromatic lipophilic group, an intermediate

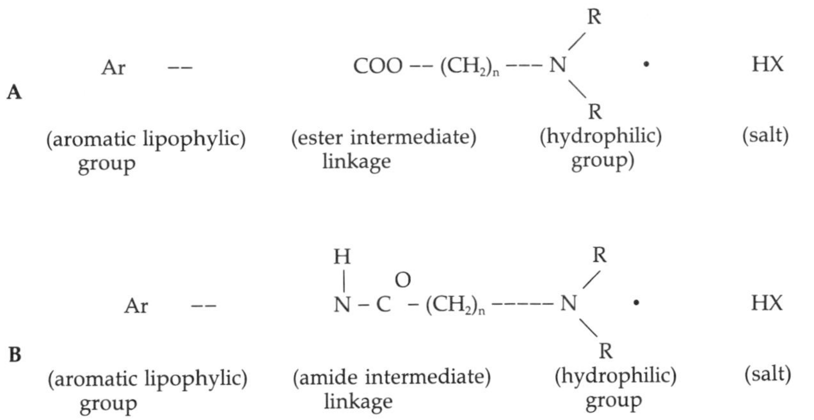

$$A \quad Ar \quad -- \quad COO -- (CH_2)_n --- N \overset{R}{\underset{R}{\diagup}} \quad \bullet \quad HX$$

(aromatic lipophylic) group   (ester intermediate) linkage   (hydrophilic) group)   (salt)

$$B \quad Ar \quad -- \quad \overset{H}{\underset{}{N}} - \overset{O}{C} - (CH_2)_n ----- N \overset{R}{\underset{R}{\diagup}} \quad \bullet \quad HX$$

(aromatic lipophylic) group   (amide intermediate) linkage   (hydrophilic) group   (salt)

Figure 32–1. Basic chemical structure of amino-ester (A) and amino-amide local anesthetics (B).

group of several carbon atoms (ester or amide linkage), and a hydrophilic group. Commercially, these weak bases (local anesthetic agents) are dispensed as salt of a weak acid, usually hydrochloric acid. The intermediate group that binds the aromatic lipophilic group to the hydrophilic group is an ester in amino-ester–type local anesthetics and an amide in amino-amide–type local anesthetics (Fig. 32–1). In a solution, the local anesthetics exist as both uncharged (non-ionized) molecules and positively charged (ionized) cations. The fraction of each form is closely dependent upon the pH of the medium (the vial or the injected site) and the pKa of the particular local anesthetic. Generally, in acidic solutions, the charged (ionized and water-soluble) fraction is increased, and in neutral or alkaline solutions, the

uncharged (non-ionized or lipid-soluble) fraction is increased.

Intrinsic potency, onset and duration of action, rate of degradation, and intrinsic anesthetic toxicity of local anesthetic agents are closely related to their structure.

Data relative to intrinsic potency are primarily based on in vitro and in vivo animal experiments. The in vitro and in vivo anesthetic potencies of various local anesthetics are shown in Table 32–1.[15] As can be seen from this table, the anesthetic potency determined by in vitro methods may differ from those of in vivo techniques. This difference may be related to factors such as vasodilation, which results in a different degree of vascular absorption. From a practical standpoint, however, it appears that procaine and chloroprocaine are the least potent anesthetics, whereas bupivacaine, etidocaine, and tetracaine are the most potent local anesthetics. Mepivacaine, prilocaine, and lidocaine are of intermediate potency levels.

Generally, onset and duration of the local anesthetic agents follow a similar pattern to their potency. The lower the potency of an agent, the faster the onset and the shorter the duration of its action. Onset and duration of a particular local anesthetic agent also differ according to the regional anesthetic method used.

During local field blocks, onset of anesthesia is very rapid (1 to 2 minutes) and similar for all local anesthetic agents. Nevertheless, the duration of action differs among various local anesthetics during local field block (Table 32–2). Procaine is a relatively short-acting drug. Lidocaine, mepivacaine, and prilocaine are of intermediate duration, and bupivacaine can produce up to 200 minutes of local anesthetic action. The addition of epinephrine certainly prolongs the duration of action; however, the effect of added epinephrine is greater on lidocaine than on procaine or bupivacaine (see Table 32–2). During minor peripheral nerve blocks, the onset of action of local anes-

Table 32–1. COMPARATIVE ANESTHETIC POTENCIES OF LOCAL ANESTHETICS (in vitro and in vivo animal data)

Agent	In Vitro Relative Potency*	Cm† Rat Sciatic Nerve	Cm‡ Cat Epidural Anesthesia
Procaine	1	1.0	4.0
Mepivacaine	2	0.5	2.0
Prilocaine	3	0.5	2.0
Chloroprocaine	4	1.0	2.0
Lidocaine	4	0.5	2.0
Bupivacaine	16	0.125	0.5
Etidocaine	16	0.125	0.5
Tetracaine	16	0.125	0.5

*In Vitro Relative Potency: Minimum local anesthetic concentration required to produce 50 per cent reduction in spike amplitude of a nerve fiber.
†Cm: Minimum concentration of local anesthetic required to produce nerve blockade in 50 per cent of animals.
‡Cm: Minimum concentration of local anesthetic required to produce nerve blockade in 50 per cent of animals.
Modified from Covino, B. G., and Vassallo, H. G.: Preclinical aspects of local anethesia. In Local Anesthetic Mechanisms of Action and Clinical Use. New York, Grune & Stratton, Inc., 1976, p. 49. Used by permission.

Table 32–2. DURATION OF ANESTHESIA
FOLLOWING INTRADERMAL INJECTION OF
VARIOUS LOCAL ANESTHETIC AGENTS

Agent	Concentration (%)	Duration Plain (min ± S.E. or range)	With Epinephrine 1:200,000
Procaine	0.5	20 (15–30)	56 (15–120)
Lidocaine	0.5	75 (30–340)	228 (60–435)
Lidocaine	1.0	127 ± 17	416 ± 26
Mepivacaine	0.5	108 (15–240)	240 (135–315)
Prilocaine	1.0	99 ± 19	289 ± 10
Bupivacaine	0.25	200 ± 33	429 ± 40

From Covino, B. G., and Vassallo, H. G.: Preclinical aspects of
local anesthesia. *In* Local Anesthetic Mechanisms of Action
and Clinical Use. New York, Grune & Stratton, Inc., 1976,
p. 63. Used by permission.

thetics takes longer than for local field blocks (4 to
8 minutes). The duration of anesthesia following
peripheral ulnar nerve block with various anesthetic agents is shown in Table 32–3.

During major peripheral nerve blocks (intercostal, brachial, sciatic, and femoral nerves), both the
onset and duration of all local anesthetic agents
are prolonged (Table 32–4). However, there are
differences between these blocks. For instance, the
onset and duration of action is longer during
brachial plexus block than during intercostal nerve
block (see Table 32–4). Complexity of anatomy in
the region of the brachial plexus is generally considered to be responsible for these findings.

The rate of degradation of local anesthetics differs significantly between the ester and amide
group of local anesthetic agents. The ester group
of agents is metabolized (hydrolysis) by plasma
cholinesterase.[16] Important differences also exist
within the ester group of local anesthetics relative
to their rate of hydrolysis. Chloroprocaine is hydrolyzed the fastest (4.7 μmol per ml per hour)
and tetracaine is hydrolyzed the slowest (0.31
μmol per ml per hour).[17] The hydrolysis rate for
procaine is intermediary (1.14 μmol per ml per

Table 32–3. DURATION OF ANESTHESIA WITH
VARIOUS LOCAL ANESTHETICS DURING
STANDARDIZED ULNAR NERVE BLOCK

Duration	Agents	Concentration (%)
Short (15–45 min)	Procaine	1.0
Moderate (60–120 min)	Lidocaine	1.0
	Mepivacaine	1.0
	Prilocaine	1.0
Long (400–450 min)	Bupivacaine	0.25
	Etidocaine	0.5

From Covino, B. G., and Vassallo, H. G.: Preclinical aspects of
local anesthesia. *In* Local Anesthetic Mechanisms of Action
and Clinical Use. New York, Grune & Stratton, 1976, p. 70.
Used by permission.

hour). There appears to be an inverse relationship
between the rate of hydrolysis and the duration
and toxicity of the ester type of local anesthetics.
Tetracaine is the longest acting and most toxic
agent in this group. Patients with pseudocholinesterase enzyme deficiency or those who have
abnormal pseudocholinesterase may theoretically
have less tolerance for and increased toxicity to
the ester type of local anesthetics. In clinical practice, however, this factor does not seem to be
important.

The amide group of local anesthetic drugs is
primarily metabolized by the liver.[18] Thus, a markedly decreased rate of degradation and higher than
usual blood levels resulting in a potential toxicity
may be seen in patients with advanced liver disease.[19, 20] Similarly, decreased hepatic blood flow
(congestive heart failure) may result in increased
blood levels. The metabolites of amide local anesthetic agents (glycinexylidide, methyl-glycinexyli-
dide) have little pharmacologic activity. Nonetheless, administration of these anesthetics for
prolonged periods, especially in the presence of
cardiac or renal failure, may result in a significant
metabolite-related toxicity.[21] The primary metabolite of prilocaine is toluidine blue O. This product
may result in methemoglobinemia, interfering
with the binding of oxygen to hemoglobin.[22]

MECHANISM OF ACTION

When deposited in the vicinity of a nerve, local
anesthetics interfere with the initiation and transmission of the impulse along the nerve fiber. In
order to understand the mechanisms of local anesthetic action, it is essential that one know the
physiology of impulse transmission in an intact
nerve. Detailed information on this subject can be
found in several monographs.[23, 24]

Like all other cells, axons are covered by a
lipoprotein membrane that separates axoplasm
from the extracellular fluid. Probably owing to the
selective permeability properties of the lipoprotein
membrane, the concentration of potassium ions in
the axoplasm at resting state is several tenfolds
higher than the potassium ion concentration in
the extracellular fluid. Conversely, the concentration of sodium ions in the extracellular fluid is
higher than that in the axoplasm. Because of a
concentration gradient and the relative permeability of the membrane to potassium ions, in the
resting state, potassium ions can diffuse from the
axoplasm to the extracellular fluid. Sodium ions
in this state, however, cannot move into the cell
because the membrane is impermeable to them.
As a result, the inside and outside of the membrane are polarized so that an electrical potential
exists across the membrane (transmembrane potential). In the resting state, this potential is be-

Table 32–4. ONSET AND DURATION OF VARIOUS LOCAL ANESTHETIC AGENTS
DURING INTERCOSTAL AND BRACHIAL PLEXUS BLOCK

Anesthetic Technique	Agent	Concentration (%)	Volume (ml)	Average Onset Time (min)	Average Duration of Sensory Analgesia (min)
Intercostal nerve block	A*	1.0	4/nerve	3–5	157–196
	B†	0.25–0.5	4/nerve	5–6	429–780
Brachial plexus block	A	1.0	40–50	14–17	195–245
	B	0.25–0.5	40–50	8–25	572–613

*A—includes lidocaine, mepivacaine, and prilocaine
†B—includes bupivacaine, tetracaine, and etidocaine
From Covino, B. G., and Vassallo, H. G.: Preclinical aspects of local anesthesia. *In* Local Anesthetic Mechanisms of Action and Clinical Use. New York, Grune & Stratton, Inc., 1976, p. 71. Used by permission.

tween −70 and −90 mv (the outside of the cell being positive relative to the inside of the cell). In the resting state, the extracellular fluid is charged positively.

When the impulse arrives at the nerve, depolarization takes place. This is accomplished by inward movement of sodium ions due to a transient increase in the permeability of the membrane. As a result, transmembrane potential becomes positive up to +40 mv (the outside of the cell being negative relative to the inside of the cell). Within a short period of time, the intracellular sodium ions are moved out of the cell by an active energy–consuming transport mechanism that brings the particular nerve segment into its initial polarized state. The transient depolarization of the nerve segment, however, is sufficient to electronically conduct the depolarizing impulse to the adjacent nerve segment. The entire cycle of depolarization and repolarization occurs within 1 msec. Depolarization consumes 30 per cent of this time. With successive sequential depolarization, the impulse spreads along the nerve up to its final destination.

Local anesthetics affect the impulse conduction along the nerve fibers by interfering with the membrane. They selectively prevent the opening of channels or pores of the nerve membrane, precluding the passage of sodium ions across the neural membranes.[25] They may also interfere with the membrane-bound Ca^{++} kinetics. Normally, an electrical impulse that reaches the nerve results in a release of membrane-bound Ca^{++}, allowing more ready access to sodium into the cell.[26] Local anesthetics seem to increase the binding of calcium to the membrane, preventing the opening of sodium channels and depolarization of the nerve.[27] Irrespective of the mechanism, when local anesthetics are deposited locally adjacent to the nerve, they progressively lower the action potential, reduce the rate of rise of the action potential, slow the velocity of impulse conduction, and prolong the refractory period. Ultimately, an impulse is unable to induce a normal change in transmem-

brane potential (action potential) and conduction blockade occurs.

The following sequence of events occurs in a stepwise manner during a local anesthetic blockade:

1. Binding of the local anesthetic agent to the reactor site
2. Blockade of the sodium channel, decreasing its conductance
3. Reduction of the rate of electrical depolarization
4. Failure to achieve threshold potential
5. Lack of propagated action potential
6. Conduction blockade

Factors that influence the quality of the conduction blockade include the distance between the nerve and the perineurally injected local anesthetic, adjacent tissue characteristics (pH, vascularity, fat content) size of the nerve to be blocked, and physicochemical characteristics of the local anesthetic.

For a successful nerve block, the drug should be deposited as close to the nerve as possible. Although the physician's anatomical knowledge and skill plays an important role in the success or failure of this action, methods devised to locate the nerve (eliciting paresthesia with a needle or being able to stimulate the nerve by the inserted needle with as little as 0.5 to 2 ma electrical current) may be extremely helpful in ensuring optimal drug deposition. During an attempted injection of local anesthetics to the closest proximity of the nerve, one should be certain to avoid intraneural injections. An anesthetic deposited perineually will diffuse into the nerve and exert its action. Because most nerves contain a tough outer sheath, direct intraneural injection may trap the solution and cause compression of the nerve fibers and blood vessels, resulting in nerve damage. Clinically, intraneural injection should be suspected if a patient complains of continuous pain during the injection of the local anesthetic and when the pain radiates to the distal sites innervated by the particular nerve. In these instances, it is prudent and advisable to withdraw the needle and repeat the block. Because of the risk of neural damage with intraneural injection, local anesthetic drugs should always be deposited around the nerve and *not directly into* the nerve.

The characteristics of adjacent tissue are also important factors in determining the onset of action and the quality of conduction blockade. An abundant vascular supply of the surrounding tissue leads to absorption of the local anesthetics and limits the drug availability to the nerve tissue. This situation can most effectively be counteracted by incorporating vasoconstrictor agents with local anesthetics. Almost every nerve in the body is surrounded by some fat tissue. Some local anesthetics are highly fat-soluble (bupivacaine and etidocaine). Injection of highly fat-soluble anesthetics at sites with extensive perineural fat tissue may result in an increase binding to the perineural fat tissue, limiting the drug availability to the nerve. Perineural tissue pH may also play a role in the availability of the drug to the neural tissue. Common physiochemical characteristics of local anesthetics are summarized in Table 32–5.

All local anesthetics are weak bases with pKa greater than 7.4. They are mostly available commercially as hydrochloride salts with a pH of 4.7. Consonant to the Hasselbach-Henderson equation, in such an acidic solution a large fraction of these drugs exist in a highly ionized form that is water-soluble. When these drugs are injected into the perineural tissue (extracellular fluid with a pH of 7.35 to 7.45), the dissociation occurs in such a way that the ionized fraction decreases and the non-ionized base fraction increases. The non-ionized base, unlike the ionized form, is lipid-soluble and can easily penetrate through the lipoprotein diffusion barriers of the nerve to reach the ultimate site of action (nerve fiber membrane). In a normal tissue (extracellular fluid), local anesthetics can easily dissociate into their lipid-soluble base forms. In infected tissues, however, because of the low pH of the tissues, the drugs exist in an ionized water-soluble form. Because the ionized water-soluble form cannot penetrate through the neural lipoprotein barrier, only a small amount of the injected local anesthetic is available for its ultimate site of action. As a result, local anesthetics injected into areas with a low pH (abscesses, cellulitis, and necrosis) cannot provide an adequate neural conduction blockade.

The larger the diameter of the nerve, the slower the onset of the conduction blockade is. This is because of the longer distance that local anesthetics must diffuse to reach the interior of large diameter nerves. An example of this can be clinically seen during epidural blockade. Whereas all other segments are easily blocked, the S1 route, because of its large diameter, may not be adequately blocked.[29] This problem can be overcome by using larger doses and higher concentrations of local anesthetics. Although this factor is not important during minor peripheral nerve blocks, blockade of the major peripheral nerves (brachial plexus) may be incomplete when small doses and low concentrations of local anesthetic solutions are used.

Although local anesthetics have pKa values greater than 7.4, this value differs significantly among various drugs (Table 32–6). For instance, procaine, chloroprocaine, and tetracaine have pKa values of 8.9, 8.7, and 8.5, respectively. This results in a very small percentage of lipid-soluble non-ionized (and hence diffusable) form to be present at physiologic pH, explaining the poor spreading qualities of these drugs. On the other hand, lidocaine, bupivacaine, and etidocaine, because of their relatively lower pKa values (7.7 to 8.1), result in a greater fraction of non-ionized (diffusable) free base at the site of injection at physiologic pH, which is capable of spreading through the lipoprotein nerve barrier.

Thus far, we have emphasized the importance of the lipid-soluble non-ionized form as a determinant of local anesthetic penetration into the nerve tissue. Equally important is the fact that after the penetration phase it is the ionized water-soluble fraction that actively blocks the nerve.[30] Normally, the pH values differ between intracellular and extracellular fluid. Therefore, once the drug enters into the cell, the ratio of the ionized and non-ionized forms are readjusted, usually in favor of the ionized form.

In addition to pKa, partition coefficients and protein binding of local anesthetics (see Table 32–6) are also important factors in determining the onset, spread, quality, and duration of anesthetic action during nerve block procedures.

Table 32–5. COMMON PHYSICOCHEMICAL CHARACTERISTICS OF LOCAL ANESTHETICS

Weak bases with pKa>7.4 (free base is poorly water-soluble).

Commercial form, hydrochloride salt, is acidic (pH 4–7), highly ionized, and thus water-soluble.

In a solution, the non-ionized, lipid-soluble (free base) and the ionized, water-soluble (cationic) forms exist as a mixture in equilibrium.

Body buffers raise the pH and therefore increase the amount of free base.

Lipid-soluble (free base) form crosses axonal membrane.

The water-soluble (cationic) form is the active nerve blocker for most agents.

From Tucker, G. T., and Mather, L. E.: Absorption and disposition of local anesthetics: pharmacokinetics. *In* Cousins, M., and Bridenbaugh, P. O. (eds.): Neural Blockade in Clinical Anesthesia and Management of Pain. Philadelphia, J. B. Lippincott Co., 1980, p. 45. Used by permission.

Table 32–6. PHYSICOCHEMICAL PROPERTIES OF COMMONLY USED LOCAL ANESTHETICS

Agent	Type	Molecular Weight (base)	pKa (25·C)	Partition Coefficient	Per cent Protein Binding	Equieffective Anesthetic Concentration	Anesthetic Duration on Rat Sciatic Nerve	Site of Metabolism
Procaine	Ester	236	8.9	0.02	5.8*	2	50	Plasma
Chloroprocaine	Ester	271	8.7	0.14	—	2	45	Plasma
Tetracaine	Ester	264	8.5	4.1	75.6*	0.25	175	Plasma
Lidocaine	Amide	234	7.9	2.9	64.3†	1	100	Liver
Bupivacaine	Amide	288	8.1	27.5	95.6†	0.25	175	Liver
Etidocaine	Amide	276	7.7	141	94†	0.25	200	Liver

*Nerve homogenate binding
†Plasma protein binding
(From Tucker, G. T., and Mather, L. E.: Absorption and disposition of local anesthetics: pharmacokinetics. In Cousins, M., and Bridenbaugh, P. O. (eds.): Neural Blockade in Clinical Anesthesia and Management of Pain. Philadelphia, J. B. Lippincott Co., 1980, pp. 48 and 49. Used by permission.)

TOXICITY

Local Neurotoxicity

Although animal studies have shown that muscle necrosis can occur with intramuscular injection of local anesthetics,[31, 32] neurological injury with clinically used concentrations of these drugs is rare. Recently, several case reports described acute paraplegia after accidental injection of chloroprocaine into the subarachnoid space.[33–35] Although inconsistent, the results of animal experiments tend to confirm the neurotoxic potential of intrathecally injected chloroprocaine.[36] There is some evidence to suggest that the preservative sodium bisulfite, used in commercial preparations, is responsible for such adverse reactions.[37] Nonetheless, there is no evidence to suggest that chloroprocaine is neurotoxic when used for peripheral nerve blocks. Thus, the drug appears to be safe for regional anesthetic procedures performed in the emergency department.

Systemic Toxicity

Hypersensitivity reactions, central nervous system (CNS) toxicity, and cardiovascular system toxicity may occur with local anesthetic agents.

Hypersensitivity Reactions. Less than 1 per cent of all reactions to local anesthetics appears to be due to an allergic mechanism.[38] Para-amino benzoic acid, the metabolite of the ester group local anesthetics, is primarily responsible for most reactions.[39] True allergic reactions to amide group local anesthetics are rare.[40] Methylparaben, the preservative in commercial ester and amide group products, may also induce hypersensitivity reactions.[39] Patients with a history of allergic reactions to this group of agents should be evaluated prior to the administration of regional anesthesia. Intradermal testing, though not totally reliable,[41–43] appears to be useful in evaluating possible hypersensitivity to these agents. However, considering the urgency of surgical procedures performed in the emergency department, such time-consuming testing methods may not be practical. The preferential use of amide-type local anesthetics (without preservative, if possible) should eliminate allergic reactions with a high degree of reliability in the emergency setting.

Central Nervous System Toxicity. Because local anesthetics can readily cross the blood-brain barrier, their CNS effects are closely related to their concentrations in the blood or plasma. Local anesthetics at *low* arterial blood concentrations actually have an *anticonvulsive* activity.[44, 45] In humans, the plasma concentrations of local anesthetics at which this anticonvulsive effect can be seen have not yet been determined. However, in cats at lidocaine blood levels of 0.5 to 4.0 μg per ml, an increase in convulsive threshold is observed when penicillin is injected intracortically.[46] At *higher* blood levels, local anesthetics have *convulsant* activity.

Knowledge of convulsive doses and blood levels of local anesthetics is primarily based on controlled studies carried out on monkeys[47] and isolated measurements of local anesthetic blood levels in patients who develop seizure after receiving local anesthetic agents.[48–50] In monkeys, during continuous intravenous infusion of local anesthetics, seizure activity begins at mean plasma concentrations of 4.3 μg per ml for etidocaine, 4.5 μg per ml for bupivacaine, and 18.2 μg per ml for lidocaine. These plasma concentrations can be obtained when etidocaine is administered at a mean dose of 5.4 mg per kg, bupivacaine 4.4 mg per kg, and lidocaine 22.5 mg per kg.

Human studies suggest that CNS toxicity in the form of CNS irritability (lightheadedness, slurred speech, circumoral numbness, and muscle twitches) occurs at much lower doses and plasma concentrations. For example, continuous intravenous infusion of lidocaine at a rate of 0.5 mg per kg per min results in convulsions in 12 minutes, indicating that its convulsive dose during slow infusion is about 6 mg per kg.[51] During slow infusion (10 to 20 mg per min), the intravenous dose of bupivacaine that causes CNS irritability is 1.6 mg per kg and that of etidocaine is about 3 to 3.5 mg per kg (Table 32–7).[52] In humans, the toxic arterial plasma concentrations for lidocaine are 5 to 10 μg per ml and 4 to 5 μg per ml for bupivacaine and etidocaine.

The following factors influence the CNS toxicity of local anesthetics:

Site of Injection. Injection of local anesthetics into vessels that supply blood flow to the brain results in convulsions at very low doses and low plasma concentrations. Accidental injection of doses as low as 2.5 mg (0.5 ml) of 0.5 per cent bupivacaine or 1.25 mg of bupivacaine and 5 mg of lidocaine mixture into the vertebral artery during a stellate ganglion block has produced generalized seizure activity.[53, 54] Similar CNS toxicity with much lower than usual toxic doses of local anesthetics can occur during intra-arterial injection in dentistry.[55, 56] Aldrete and associates showed that reverse arterial blood flow following a centripetal pathway may reach the brain and cause CNS local anesthetic toxicity when local anesthetics are accidentally injected into the arteries in the head and neck region.[56-58]

The site of injection is also important from the standpoint of the rate of vascular absorption. The local anesthetic absorption varies considerably depending upon the vascularity of the injected site. Tissues with rich vascular supply favor the absorption of local anesthetics, resulting in a higher plasma concentration with relatively lower doses. The same dose of local anesthetic agent results in a higher plasma concentration after intercostal block than after subcutaneous injection in the abdominal wall (Fig. 32–2).[59] Among the three

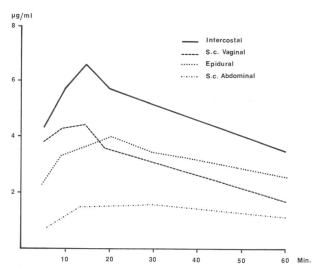

Figure 32–2. Plasma concentrations of lidocaine (400 mg) following intercostal, epidural, vaginal, and abdominal wall subcutaneous injection. (From Scott, D. B., Jebson, P.J.R., Braid, D. B., et al.: Factors affecting plasma levels of lignocaine and prilocaine. Br. J. Anaesth. 44:1040, 1972. Used by permission.)

major peripheral nerve blocks performed in the emergency department (intercostal, brachial, and femoral), intercostal blocks result in the highest plasma local anesthetic concentrations.[59, 60]

Local Anesthetic Agents. CNS toxicity of local anesthetics is closely related to their intrinsic potency.[52, 61-64] Procaine and chloroprocaine are the least potent and the least toxic agents. Lidocaine, mepivacaine, and prilocaine have intermediate potency with about four times the potency and toxicity of procaine. Bupivacaine, etidocaine, and tetracaine are the most potent and the most toxic agents.

pH and P_{CO_2}. Local anesthetics are more toxic to the CNS at a lower arterial pH and a higher arterial P_{CO_2}.[65, 66] Although the exact mechanism of this phenomenon is not known, increased cerebral blood flow at high levels of Pa_{CO_2} may play a significant role by delivering a greater amount of local anesthetics into the brain. Low pH may also be responsible for increasing the cerebral active cationic form of local anesthetics. Treatment of local anesthetic–induced seizures therefore requires a prompt correction of pH and Pa_{CO_2}.

Addition of Vasoconstrictors. Mixing local anesthetics with vasoconstrictors results in a decreased absorption and lower plasma local anesthetic levels.[67] The delay of absorption is particularly noticeable after injection of local anesthetics into tissues that have a high degree of vascularity. The use of epinephrine in conjunction with local anesthetics during intercostal nerve block provides significantly lower plasma local anesthetic concentrations and reduces toxicity.[68]

Cardiovascular Toxicity. Local anesthetics that reach very high plasma concentrations can cause myocardial depression. Like CNS toxicity, cardio-

Table 32–7. CNS TOXICITY THRESHOLD OF VARIOUS LOCAL ANESTHETIC AGENTS IN MAN

Agent	Threshold—CNS—Symptoms (Dose mg/kg)		
	Usubiaga*	Foldes	Scott
Procaine	18–55	19	—
Chloroprocaine	—	23	—
Lidocaine	6–9	6.4	>4
Mepivacaine	—	10	—
Prilocaine	—	—	>6
Bupivacaine	—	—	1.6
Etidocaine	—	—	3.4
Tetracaine	—	2.5	—

*Data from Usubiaga,[62] Foldes,[17] and Scott.[52]
Modified from Covino, B. G., and Vassallo, H. G.: Preclinical aspects of local anesthesia. *In* Local Anesthetic Mechanisms of Action and Clinical Use. New York, Grune & Stratton, Inc., 1976, p. 126. Used by permission.

Table 32–8. CARDIOVASCULAR AND CNS TOXICITY OF VARIOUS LOCAL ANESTHETICS

Agent	Convulsive Dose (mg/kg)	Lethal Dose (Dose/kg)	Cardio-vascular/CNS Toxicity Ratio
Tetracaine	3 ± 0.2	13 ± 1.2	4.3
Bupivacaine	3.4 ± 0.4	11 ± 1	3.2
Etidocaine	4.6 ± 0.4	22 ± 2	4.8
Lidocaine	11 ± 1	28 ± 1.2	2.5

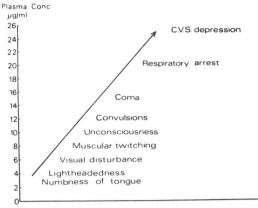

Figure 32–3. The clinical manifestations of lidocaine toxicity with different plasma concentrations. (From Scott, D. B., and Cousins, M.B.: Clinical pharmacology of local anesthetic agents. *In* Cousins, M. J., and Bridenbaugh, J. D. (eds.): Neural Blockade in Clinical Anesthesia and Management of Pain. Philadelphia, J. B. Lippincott Co., 1980, p. 113. Used by permission.)

vascular toxicity of local anesthetics also correlates well with the intrinsic potency of the agent.[69] Procaine and chloroprocaine cause myocardial depression at much higher plasma concentrations than tetracaine, lidocaine, bupivacaine and etidocaine.

The effect on peripheral vascular resistance is biphasic. At clinical concentrations, a slight vasoconstriction occurs.[70] Progressive increases in plasma concentrations result in peripheral vasodilation.[71] It is important to remember that cardiovascular toxicity of local anesthetics occurs at higher doses and plasma concentrations than those that cause convulsions. The cardiovascular and CNS toxicity of various local anesthetics is shown in Table 32–8. The lethal doses that cause cardiovascular collapse in animals are approximately three to four times greater than those capable of inducing seizure activity.

Recently, patients who were inadvertently receiving large doses of intravenous (IV) bupivacaine or etidocaine have been found to be resistant to all resuscitative measures.[72] The question of whether bupivacaine and etidocaine are more cardiotoxic than other local anesthetics has led to numerous studies. At present, available data suggest that bupivacaine and etidocaine in equipotent doses are no more myocardial depressive than is lidocaine.[73] Animal studies, however, suggest that at CNS toxic doses, these drugs are more dysrhythmogenic than is lidocaine.[74, 75] Dysrhythmias with bupivacaine may occur in the absence of hypoxemia and acidosis and at doses required to induce only convulsions.

Clinical manifestations of local anesthetic toxicity correlate well with the plasma concentrations of the drug (Fig. 32–3). At low blood levels, drowsiness, ringing of the ears, tongue and circumoral numbness, and metallic taste in the mouth can occur. As the plasma concentrations increase, double vision, nystagmus, fine tremors of the extremity muscles, and anxiety may be observed. At higher plasma concentrations, unconsciousness, convulsions, and coma may occur. When serum lidocaine levels reach 25 to 30 μg per ml, respiratory arrest and cardiovascular depression with various supraventricular and ventricular dysrhythmias occur. Preconvulsive manifestations of local

anesthetic toxicity should be carefully observed during injection of these drugs in the emergency department. If these signs and symptoms occur, the injection should be stopped immediately and oxygen via a face mask should be administered.

Treatment of local anesthetic–induced seizure activity should be promptly carried out in the following manner: First, administer oxygen and provide ventilation via a face mask.[77] Severe hypoxia and combined respiratory and lactic acidosis precede or occur concomitantly during convulsion induced by local anesthetic drugs.[78, 79] Second, attempt to abort the convulsions. Several drugs have been advocated for this purpose. Thiopental, even in small doses (50 to 100 mg), can usually terminate seizure activity. Diazepam, at a dose of 0.1 mg per kg IV, is a potent anticonvulsant agent and terminates the seizure activity within 20 to 30 seconds.[67] Diazepam may also be used preoperatively to raise the seizure threshold in order to prevent seizures induced by local anesthetics (dose 0.25 mg per kg P.O.).[80] Finally, succinylcholine, at a dose of 40 to 60 mg IV, will effectively abort the tonic clonic convulsions by blocking the neuromuscular junction; however, succinylcholine does not effect the seizure activity of the brain. Paralysis is helpful for controlling the airway and permitting mechanical ventilation. Furthermore, when the patient is paralyzed, lactic acid production due to muscle contraction is blocked. The third step in treatment is to secure the airway with an endotracheal tube. While adequate ventilation is provided, arterial blood samples should be drawn to measure pH, P_{O_2}, P_{CO_2}, and K^+. According to the results of these measurements, any metabolic acidosis should be corrected by appropriate doses of sodium bicarbonate. Hypotension and dysrhythmias, if present, should be treated by correction of hypoxia, administration of fluids, vasopressors, and antidysrhythmic agents. The use of vasopressors with both alpha and beta receptor activity (e.g., epinephrine) is theoretically preferred, because the hypotension is usually due to the combined effect of myocardial depression and peripheral vasodilation. Recently, clinical data from Moore and colleagues suggest that the use of 0.1 to 0.2 mg IV of epinephrine is effective when there is severe hypotension or cardiac arrest.[81]

Preparation for Regional Anesthesia

PATIENT PREPARATION

A brief medical history including systemic diseases, drug allergies, reactions to local anesthetic agents, and medications currently taken by the patient, should be taken and recorded. Patients with severe peripheral vascular diseases may develop persistent infections leading to abscess and ulcerations when needles are inserted into the ischemic distal parts of the extremities. Similarly, patients with hypertension or ischemic heart disease may show an increase in blood pressure or dysrhythmias when local anesthetics containing relatively large doses of vasoconstrictors are injected into highly vascular areas. Hematoma formation at the injection site may develop in patients with coagulation abnormalities and in those receiving anticoagulant agents. Current intake of monoamine oxidase (MAO) inhibitors precludes the injection of local anesthetics that contain a vasoconstrictor, because these patients may have exaggerated cardiovascular responses to these agents.

Almost all patients who are treated in the emergency department are assumed to have recent food ingestion. Although the existence of a full stomach does not preclude the use of minor nerve blockade, the decision to perform relatively major nerve blocks (brachial, femoral, or intercostal) should be carefully made by weighing the risks of possible toxic reactions leading to aspiration of gastric contents against the benefits and indications of the procedure. Toxic reactions during major peripheral nerve blockades are rare, provided that accidental intravascular injections of local anesthetics are avoided. Therefore, a full stomach should probably not prevent the use of major nerve blocks. Nonetheless, if the surgical procedure can be performed with a minor nerve block, the latter should be the preferred choice. Patients who have recently ingested alcohol or drugs may also receive regional nerve blocks, provided that they are able to cooperate.

All patients should be informed about the procedure as well as the extent of pain during the insertion of the needles. Usually, a simple preoperative explanation will help to reduce the patient's anxiety and fear, and will increase patient cooperation.[82]

EQUIPMENT PREPARATION

Two categories of functioning equipment—regional anesthesia equipment and resuscitation equipment—must be available in emergency departments that use regional anesthetic procedures.

Regional Anesthesia

The equipment needed for performing peripheral nerve blocks and local field blocks is listed in Table 32–9. Although some of the equipment may not be necessary for performing minor peripheral nerve blockade, this list is particularly useful for major nerve blocks. The equipment can be prepared in a tray and sterilized. In preparing these trays, meticulous care should be taken to prevent chemical and bacterial contamination; disposable, commercially prepared trays are more reliable and easier to use. Most commercially prepared trays incorporate a separate section for preparation of the field with antiseptic solutions, which prevents the needles and other equipment from being contaminated with antiseptic solutions.

Depending upon the anesthetic procedure and the desired onset and duration of action, various local anesthetic agents can be used. Recommended concentrations and doses of commonly used local anesthetics for local infiltration and minor and major nerve blocks are listed in Table 32–10.[83]

The use of a nerve stimulator capable of delivering currents within the range of 0.1 to 0.5 ma may be extremely helpful in locating the peripheral nerves to be blocked.[84-86] In Figure 32–4, one of these stimulators and its connection to the active

---

Table 32–9. EQUIPMENT NEEDED IN REGIONAL ANESTHESIA TRAYS

Sterile Prep Components

3 prep sponges
3 gauze sponges
4 towels
1 antiseptic-solution receptacle

Sterile Procedural Components

1 1-ml tuberculine syringe (used to measure vasoconstrictors)
1 3-ml syringe (used for skin wheal)
1 10-ml syringe (used for local anesthetic injection)
1 No. 25 or 27 gauge ⅝-inch (1.6 cm) skin wheal needle
1 No. 18 gauge 1½-inch (3.8 cm) needle (used to withdraw local anesthetic solution from the vial)
4 No. 22 gauge block needles of various lengths (1½ inch, 2 inch, 3 inch, and 4 inch or 3.8, 5.1, 7.7, and 10.2 cm)
1 No. 25 gauge 1½-inch (3.8 cm) block needle
1 local anesthetic solution receptacle (30 ml capacity)
1 narrow bore anesthesia extension set
1 three-way stopcock

Table 32–10. RECOMMENDED MAXIMUM DOSES AND CONCENTRATIONS OF THE VARIOUS LOCAL ANESTHETIC AGENTS FOR LOCAL FIELD AND MINOR AND MAJOR NERVE BLOCKS

Local Anesthetic Drugs	Maximum Dose* (mg/kg BW†)	Concentrations		
		Local Field Block (%)	Minor Field Block (%)	Major Nerve Block (%)
Procaine	10–12	0.5	1	2
Chloroprocaine	10–15	1	1	2
Lidocaine	7–8	0.5	0.5–1	1–1.5
Mepivacaine	7–8	0.5	0.5–1	1–1.5
Prilocaine	8	1	1–2	2–3
Tetracaine	2	0.05	0.1	0.15
Bupivacaine	3–4	0.25	0.25	0.5
Etidocaine	4–5	0.25–0.5	0.5	1

*Epinephrine-containing solutions. The maximum dose should be reduced by 25 per cent when epinephrine is not used.
†BW = body weight.
Modified from Kennedy, W. F.: Preparation for neural blockade: the patient, block equipment, resuscitation, and supplementation. *In* Cousins, M. J., and Bridenbaugh, J. D. (eds.): Neural Blockade in Clinical Anesthesia and Management of Pain. Philadelphia, J. B. Lippincott Co., 1980, p. 135. Used by permission.

Table 32–11. NECESSARY EQUIPMENT AND DRUGS FOR RESUSCITATION AND TREATMENT OF LOCAL ANESTHETIC TOXICITY

Oxygen source (central supply or a full tank)
Oxygen pressure regulator
Oxygen flowmeter
Ambu bag with a connecting tube to the flowmeter
Face mask connected to the Ambu bag
Suction apparatus with Yankauer suction tip
Oropharyngeal and nasopharyngeal airways (various sizes)
Laryngoscope
Cuffed endotracheal tubes (different sizes)
Endotracheal tube stylette
Thiopental (25 μg/ml), 10-ml syringe
Diazepam (Valium) (10 μg/ml), 2-ml syringe
Succinylcholine (20 μg/ml), 5-ml syringe
Atropine (0.4 μg/ml), 3-ml syringe
Epinephrine (0.1 mg/ml), 10-ml syringe

and indifferent electrode is shown. A special Teflon-coated insulated needle serves as both the stimulating electrode and the block needle. Except for the tip and the point of connection with the nerve stimulator cable, the entire length of the needle is electrically isolated. A separate EKG pad placed on the skin at a distance from the block needle serves as the indifferent electrode. When the tip of the active block needle is in reasonable proximity to the nerve that is to be blocked, the area supplied by the stimulated nerve twitches. Yasuda and associates demonstrated that 0.09 ma is the minimal stimulating current required to produce paresthesia and twitching of the fingers during supraclavicular brachial plexus block.[87] In our experience, occurrence of the twitch with a 0.1 to 0.5 ma current displayed on the stimulator

strongly suggests that the needle is in close proximity to the nerve. Although this method has not been commonly used for minor nerve blockade, it is extremely useful in performing brachial, femoral, and sciatic nerve blocks. It is important to remember that with greater currents, twitch will occur with direct stimulation of the adjacent muscles, leading to misinterpretation and failure in obtaining a successful block.

Resuscitation Equipment

Functioning resuscitation equipment must be made ready in a separate tray at the side of the patient's head. All resuscitation equipment should be checked prior to beginning the regional anesthetic procedure. A complete list of equipment for this purpose is given in Table 32–11.

Preparation for Asepsis

The use of an aseptic technique during a regional anesthetic procedure is important. With the exception of minor nerve blocks, all blocks should be performed using sterile gloves. There is probably no need to sterilize the vials, or ampules, of local anesthetic and vasoconstrictor agents. The skin can be satisfactorily prepared for asepsis using povidone-iodine solution.

Whether injection of local anesthetic agents and epinephrine solutions alter tissue defenses and increase the likelihood of wound infection clinically is not known. Stevenson and associates have identified several variables that seem to influence the development of wound infection in experimental animals subjected to local anesthetics.[88] They found a deleterious effect of high concentrations of epinephrine (1:100,000 or greater) when the drug was used in conjunction with lidocaine for local field block. The concentrated solutions

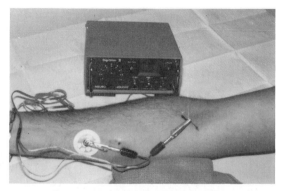

Figure 32–4. Nerve stimulator connected to the active and indifferent electrodes. The active electrode is the block needle that is insulated with a Teflon sheath except at its tip.

seemed to potentiate the wound infections in experimentally contaminated wounds, and the epinephrine caused ischemic necrosis of the tissue within healing wounds. Stevenson and colleagues suggested that concentrations of epinephrine no greater than 1:200,000 be used during routine local field blocks and that the vasoconstrictor be eliminated wherever possible. They also demonstrated experimentally that the passage of a needle through the cut edges of a contaminated wound will disseminate infection and that the preferred method of local anesthesia is injection through the intact skin at the periphery of the wound.

A 1 per cent solution of lidocaine is preferred to greater concentrations, and there is probably no clinical benefit to using concentrated solutions. Morris and associates have suggested the use of 0.5 per cent lidocaine during local field blocks, because even a 1 per cent solution of lidocaine resulted in a decrease in tensile strength of experimental wounds.[89] The validity of these experimental findings have not yet been substantiated with clinical studies.

Intraoperative and Postoperative Care

Intraoperatively, the patient's mental status, respiratory, and cardiovascular status should be monitored. Intermittent verbal contact; observation of the patient's color; and respiration, periodic blood pressure, and pulse measurement should be carried out to avoid serious complications.

Most patients may have residual sensory and motor blockade after surgery. Patients who have residual motor block should be kept in the emergency department until the block wears off. Those who have pure sensory block can be discharged; however, they should be informed about the numbness of the blocked area and strongly advised to avoid mechanical or thermal trauma to those areas until the numbness wears off. They should also be advised to contact the emergency department as soon as possible if such trauma occurs. Skin or deep tissue disintegration can occur with sustained trauma to the numb areas, because the withdrawal reflex is not functional. Delayed toxic reactions secondary to local anesthetic injection are rare and virtually do not occur 1 hour after the injection. After the nerve block wears off, most patients may develop pain at the site of surgery. Proper analgesic medication should be prescribed to alleviate the pain.

Postoperative peripheral nerve damage resulting in paresthesia, pain, and even motor dysfunction may occur after peripheral nerve blocks. Although this complication has not been shown to occur in all types of nerve blocks, the incidence

after brachial plexus block has been found to be as high as 5 per cent.[90] It is believed that transient neurologic deficit in these circumstances is partially caused by the trauma induced by the needle.[91] Compression of the nerves by local hematoma formation may also be responsible for transient nerve damage.[92] Careful follow-up and, if necessary, documentation with nerve conduction and electromyogram (EMG) studies may be helpful in preventing associated medicolegal problems.

Regional Anesthesia Methods

GENERAL CONCEPTS

Clinically, blockade of neural conduction can be performed by using several regional anesthetic methods. For practical purposes, these methods can be classified as infiltration or field blocks, peripheral nerve blocks, and central nerve blocks.

Infiltration or field blocks can be accomplished by simply injecting local anesthetic solutions into the tissues. With this method, only the small terminal branches of the nerves that supply the region are blocked. Intravenous regional anesthesia (Bier's block) can also be included in this category. During intravenous regional anesthesia, local anesthetics diffuse from the capillaries into the interstitial space of the tissues, where small nerve endings are located. Topical anesthesia is another modification of this type of blockade, because topically administered anesthetics block the small terminal branches of the nerves that lie at the surface of the mucous membranes. Peripheral nerve blockade can be divided into minor nerve blockade, as the blockade of a small single nerve, and major nerve blockade, as the blockade of multiple nerves or a nerve plexus. Central nerve blockade involves the spinal cord. Only local field blocks and peripheral nerve blocks can safely be performed in the emergency department. Major nerve blockades are associated with a higher incidence of complications and should not be performed by physicians who are not familiar with the technique and its complications. (See Chapter 33, Intravenous Regional Anesthesia, and Chapter 67, which contains a brief discussion of topical ocular anesthesia.)

UPPER EXTREMITY BLOCKS

Blockade at the Level of Axilla

Brachial plexus block provides complete anesthesia of the upper extremity, allowing almost any type of surgical procedure at the arm, forearm, and hand. When an adequate concentration and volume of local anesthetic is used, satisfactory muscle paralysis, allowing closed reduction of fractures and dislocations of the upper extremity, can also be obtained. Reduction of a shoulder dislocation, however, may not always be possible when an axillary approach is used, because the shoulder joint is supplied by the C5 spinal segment and local anesthetics injected at this level of the axilla may not be able to spread up to this level.[93] Brachial plexus blockade can also be used to provide pain relief in patients with upper extremity fractures or dislocations while awaiting surgery.

The brachial plexus can be approached and successfully blocked at various areas of the neck and upper extremity. Approaches that have been described to block this plexus include interscalene,[94] supraclavicular,[95] subclavian,[96] and axillary techniques.[97-100] The safest and most preferred method of blockade in the emergency department is the axillary approach. The supraclavicular approach, which at one time was commonly used, is now being performed rarely, because it is associated with a relatively high incidence of pneumothorax (1 per cent).[101, 102] The subclavian approach may also be associated with complications of pneumothorax and phrenic and laryngeal nerve blocks. The perivascular interscalene approach, when performed properly, produces a complete and satisfactory anesthesia of the upper extremity. Note that when this approach is performed by physicians who are not trained in anesthesia, serious complications may result. Inadvertent injections of local anesthetics into the vertebral vessels leading to convulsions, subarachnoid and epidural injections causing total spinal anesthesia, and phrenic nerve paralysis have been attributed to this approach.[103, 104] Although the technique for the axillary approach is the only technique described in this chapter, the important aspects of the entire brachial plexus anatomy are helpful in understanding the basic rationale for the various approaches.

Anatomy. The brachial plexus is formed by the anterior rami of C5–C8 and T1 nerves. These five nerves form three trunks (upper, middle, and lower) during their progression toward the clavicle. Three anterior and three posterior divisions arise from the trunks at the level of the clavicle. The divisions pass between the first rib and the clavicle toward the axillary fossa. Slightly above the axillary fossa, they form three cords (medial, posterior, and lateral), and at about the level of the axillary fossa, they divide into six main branches (musculocutaneous, radial, median, ulnar, medial cutaneous nerve of the arm, and medial cutaneous nerve of the forearm) that supply the entire arm (Fig. 32–5).[105]

The entire brachial plexus, from its origin at the neck to the upper portion of the main branches at the distal axilla, is wrapped by a fascia that is an

Figure 32–5. Formation of the brachial plexus and its anatomic relationship to the adjacent structures (From Galindo, A.: Illustrated regional anesthesia. Miami, Regional Master Co. Scientific Publications, 1982. Used by permission.)

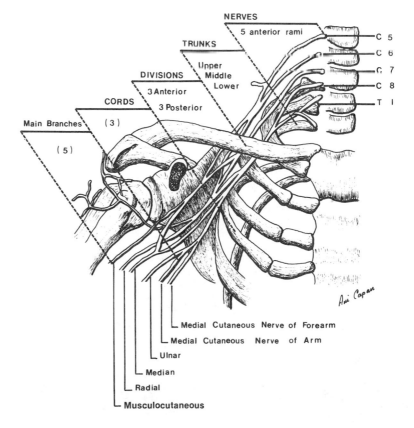

NERVES
5 anterior rami
TRUNKS
Upper
Middle
Lower
DIVISIONS
3 Anterior
3 Posterior
CORDS
(3)
Main Branches
(5)

C 5
C 6
C 7
C 8
T 1

└ Medial Cutaneous Nerve of Forearm
└ Medial Cutaneous Nerve of Arm
└ Ulnar
└ Median
└ Radial
└ Musculocutaneous

extension of the prevertebral fascia. Clinically, this is an important anatomical feature because the local anesthetic solution deposited into this perineural sheath at any level between the transverse processes of the cervical vertebra and the distal axilla can travel freely both distally and proximally in a continuous closed space, blocking the conduction of the nerves within the sheath. The cervical nerves arise between the anterior and posterior tubercles of the transverse processes of the cervical vertebrae. The anterior scalene muscle arises from the C3–C6 anterior tubercles of the transverse processes. The middle scalene muscle arises from the C3–C8 posterior tubercles of the transverse process. Both the anterior and middle scalene muscles distally attach to the superior surface of the first rib. The anterior scalene muscle is distally attached to the first rib medially and to the middle scalene muscle laterally. Because of this anatomical relationship, the brachial plexus at the level of the neck in its fascial cover lies between the anterior and middle scalene muscles until it reaches the first rib (Fig. 32–6).

After passing between the clavicle and the first rib, the plexus enters into the axillary fossa. At this level it is still enveloped in the fascial cover. It has been shown that the main branches perforate the perineural sheath at the level of the second portion of the axillary artery. The musculocutaneous nerve leaves the sheath at a higher level than the other branches, and anatomically, this nerve leaves the sheath at the level of the coracoid process or slightly below the inferior border of the pectoralis minor muscle (Fig. 32–7). Because of this anatomical relationship, insertion of the block needle into the axillary sheath at a relatively lower level may sometimes result in an inadequate blockade of the musculocutaneous nerve. Clinically, because the pectoralis minor muscle cannot easily be palpated as a landmark, the lower border of the pectoralis major muscle should be considered a landmark and the block needle should be advanced beyond this level. Note that using larger volumes of local anesthetic solution may provide adequate proximal spread to block the musculocutaneous nerve, even if the needle is inserted inferiorly.[106]

At the level of the axilla and the upper arm, the

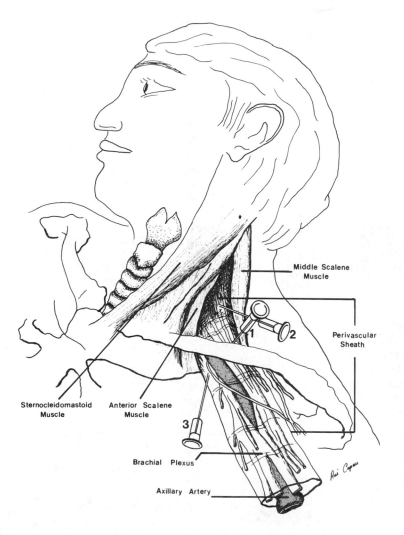

Figure 32–6. Anatomical relationship of the brachial plexus to the anterior and middle scalene muscles at the neck. *1,* Supraclavicular approach; *2,* Interscalene approach; and *3,* Subclavian approach for brachial plexus block.

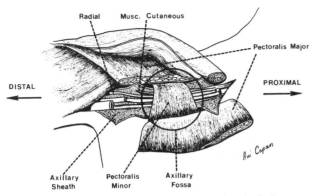

Figure 32–7. Anatomical relationship of the brachial plexus to the adjacent structures in the axillary fossa (circled). Note that musculocutaneous nerve perforates the axillary sheath slightly below the inferior border of the pectoralis minor muscle but proximal to the inferior border of the pectoralis major muscle.

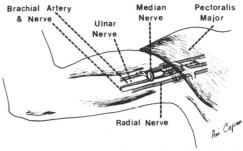

Figure 32–8. The location and the position of the block needle during axillary approach brachial plexus block. Note that the needle is inserted through the skin just below the inferior border of the pectoralis major muscle and advanced proximally underneath the muscle until its tip enters into the perivascular sheath.

axillary sheath contains the axillary artery, axillary veins, lymph nodes, and the main branches of the brachial plexus. Because of the complexity of this region, the following principles should be followed during the administration of this block: anesthetic agents should be injected into the sheath, insertion of the needle into the sheath should be as high as possible, and because the sheath also contains several vessels, care should be taken to avoid intravascular injections.

Technique. Prior to beginning the procedure, the patient is informed about the anticipated paresthesia and is asked to notify the operator when a shocklike sensation is felt at the hand and fingers. The patient is then placed in the supine position with the shoulder abducted 90 degrees and the forearm resting on a table, and both are flexed 90 degrees at the elbow and rotated externally. An axillary approach for brachial plexus block cannot be used in patients who are unable to abduct the arm. The inferior border of the pectoralis major muscle is located, and the axillary artery is palpated and followed proximally beyond the pectoralis major muscle. After location and stabilization of the artery by the fingers of the left hand (for a right-handed operator), a No. 22 gauge, 1.5 inch, short bevel needle is inserted through the skin over the artery at a 20-degree angle (Fig. 32–8). The needle is advanced at this angle until paresthesia that is reproducible by movement of the needle is obtained. The right hand is then removed from the needle while the left hand is kept in the original position, stabilizing the artery. During this maneuver, vigorous pulsation of the needle strongly suggests that its tip is in the axillary sheath. A nerve stimulator connected to an insulated block needle is extremely useful in locating the nerve during this block. A twitch of the hand produced by currents less than 0.5 ma strongly suggests that the needle tip is in the axillary sheath and in close proximity to the

plexus. The use of the nerve stimulator is also particularly helpful in locating the nerve in patients who are unreliable or unable to identify the paresthesia.

After location of the brachial plexus, careful attention should be paid to avoid displacement of the needle during its attachment to the local anesthetic syringe or during injection of the drug. This can best be avoided by connecting an anesthesia extension tubing–three-way stopcock–local anesthetic syringe assembly to the needle prior to its insertion through the skin.[107] The distal end of the extension tubing connects to the needle; the proximal end is connected to the syringe via a three-way stopcock. The use of this assembly eliminates the possibility of needle displacement, because there is no need to connect the local anesthetic syringe to the needle during the procedure and the drug is injected some distance away without undue pressure or traction being exerted on the block needle. After careful aspiration and having checked that the needle is not in a blood vessel, the local anesthetic solution is injected.

Injection of 40 ml of 2 per cent chloroprocaine provides a block of 45- to 60-minute duration. Onset of action with this agent occurs within about 5 minutes. Injection of 40 ml of 1 per cent lidocaine provides surgical anesthesia that lasts 200 to 250 minutes, with onset of action beginning 15 to 30 minutes after the injection. Thirty to 40 ml of 0.5 per cent bupivacaine results in at least 6 hours of anesthesia, with an onset of action 20 to 30 minutes after the injection. It is not uncommon to observe prolonged anesthesia lasting 24 to 36 hours when bupivacaine is used.

Immediately after the injection of the local anesthetic solution, the arm should be adducted and brought to the side of the patient. This maneuver prevents the obstruction of the perivascular space by the humeral head and allows the spread of the local anesthetic solution proximally. Finger pressure just distal to the injection site for 5 minutes also facilitates proximal spread.

During brachial plexus block, unlike other nerve blocks, the motor weakness either precedes sensory blockade or develops simultaneously.[108, 109] Characteristically, triceps muscle (forearm extensor) weakness develops first. This can be tested by asking the patient to lift up the arm and hold his nose. When the block is successful, the hand falls onto the face. Injury to the face can be prevented by the operator placing his hand between the patient's face and hand. Sensory block begins at the arm and gradually spreads over the forearm and the hand.[23] The early occurrence of motor block and the beginning of the sensory blockade at the proximal part of the limb are because the motor fibers of the upper extremity and the sensory fibers of the arm are located at the periphery of the plexus. Thus, the local anesthetic agents deposited around the plexus come in contact with these mantle fibers first. The diffusion of the local anesthetic agent to the center of the nerve, where the sensory nerve fibers of the forearm and the hand are located, takes some time, resulting in a delay of the block of these regions. Recovery of the block, however, follows a reverse order, so that motor block recovers after the sensory block. It is suggested that rapid vascular uptake of local anesthetic by the intraneural small vessels located close to the sensory core fibers is responsible for such findings during recovery.[109]

Puncture of the axillary artery may occur during brachial plexus block. In these circumstances, advancement of the needle until the blood return stops and injection of the local anesthetic after careful negative aspiration usually result in a successful block. Caution must be used, because a small amount of blood may enter the needle and clot the tip. This needle obstruction will yield a "negative" aspiration despite intravascular placement. Hence, care should be taken to ensure that the tip of the needle is not in the intravascular space during injection.

Even with properly performed brachial plexus blocks, the occurrence of a profound block and rapid onset of analgesia in one nerve distribution and partial or absent block in the other nerves is not uncommon. Traditionally, this phenomenon has been ascribed to the displacement of the needle outside the sheath after injection of local anesthetic into the sheath. Decreased proximal spread owing to obstruction of the perivascular sheath by the humeral head has also been suggested.[100] Recent studies of Thompson and Rorie of the functional anatomy of the brachial plexus sheaths offer a different explanation for the occurrence of this phenomenon.[110, 111] They showed that the connective tissue that forms the perineural sheath extends inward and forms septa between the components of the plexus. Thus, each nerve is covered by a separate connective tissue within the sheath, producing a potential barrier for the diffusion of the local anesthetic solution around the individual nerves.

Blocking of the spared nerve distally (at the level of the elbow or wrist) with a small amount of local anesthetic agents may overcome the problem of incomplete block. The upper medial aspect of the arm is supplied by the intercostobrachial nerve, which lies in the subcutaneous tissue outside the sheath. Deposition of 3 to 4 ml of local anesthetic to this area while the needle is being withdrawn provides adequate block of the intercostobrachial nerve.

Complications. Inadvertent intravascular injections may result in an immediate CNS or cardiovascular toxicity. If this occurs, prompt treatment, as described earlier, should be instituted. Also, vigorous exploration for paresthesia has been blamed for the relatively high incidence (0.3 to 5 per cent) of postblock neuritis.[90, 91]

Nerve Blocks at the Elbow

Nerve blocks at the elbow are rarely associated with complications and are relatively easy to perform. The ulnar, median, and radial nerves can be blocked individually at this level.

Blockade of the ulnar, median, and radial nerves at this level provides a satisfactory anesthesia at the forearm and the hand for various surgical procedures. Blockade of all three nerves at the elbow requires multiple insertion of needles and paresthesia of each nerve, causing undue patient discomfort. An axillary approach brachial plexus block using a single needle is a more comfortable technique for the patient requiring a block of all three nerves. The blocks at the elbow are most frequently performed to supplement inadequate anesthesia at the particular nerve distribution after a brachial plexus block. Also, blockade of a single nerve at the elbow may be useful for minor surgery performed within the region of that particular nerve's distribution.

Anatomy

Theoretically, the blockade of each nerve at the elbow should produce anesthesia at the regions of its distribution. In practice, however, because of an extensive overlapping among the nerves that supply the forearm and the hand, a predictable anesthesia may not always be produced.

Median Nerve. The median nerve is most superficial at the level between the two epicondyles. The nerve is located at the anteromedial aspect of the elbow and lies medial to the brachial artery. Anteriorly, the median nerve is covered by the aponeurosis of the biceps muscle. Two to 3 cm below the level of epicondyles, the nerve enters between the two heads of the pronator teres muscle (Fig. 32–9). The median nerve supplies the

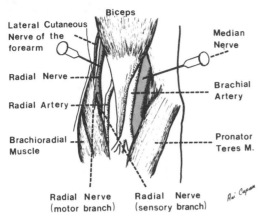

Figure 32–9. Anatomical relationships of the median, radial, and the lateral cutaneous nerve of the forearm with the adjacent structures at the elbow.

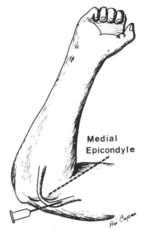

Figure 32–10. Relationship of the ulnar nerve with the adjacent structures at the elbow. Note that the tip of the block needle reaches the ulnar nerve slightly proximal to the ulnar groove of the medial epicondyle to prevent needle-induced ulnar nerve damage.

sensory innervation to the palm and to the lateral three and one half fingers at the palmar aspect. At the dorsal aspect, distal phalanges of the lateral three and one half fingers receive their sensory innervation from this nerve.

Radial Nerve. The radial nerve and the lateral cutaneous nerve of the forearm, (the sensory end branch of the musculocutaneous nerve) are located together at the anterolateral aspect of the elbow. At the level of the elbow, both nerves are located in a sulcus between the biceps muscle medially and the brachioradialis muscle laterally (Fig. 32–9). At this level the radial nerve contains both motor and sensory branches. Three or 4 cm below the level of the lateral epicondyle, at the level of the head of the radial bone, the motor branch enters into the extensor muscles of the forearm. The sensory branch continues distally with the radial artery along the medial edge of the brachioradialis muscle. The radial nerve and the lateral cutaneous nerve of the forearm supply the sensory innervation to the lateral aspect of the forearm and the dorsolateral aspect of the hand. The motor branch of the radial nerve supplies the extensor muscles of the forearm.

Ulnar Nerve. Block of the ulnar nerve is probably the easiest to perform because it is so superficial; in most patients, it can be palpated under the skin. The ulnar nerve at the elbow lies in the ulnar groove at the posterior aspect of the medial epicondyle (Fig. 32–10). It supplies the sensory innervation of the dorsal and palmar aspect of the hand, the fifth finger, and half of the fourth finger.

Techniques. Although blocks at the elbow are easy to perform, correct placement of the needle in the close vicinity of the nerves requires eliciting paresthesia. Reproduction of paresthesia to ensure correct needle placement is not without hazard. Stimulation of the particular nerve with small electrical currents provides characteristic movement of the hand and fingers for each nerve and

ensures adequate needle placement without significant damage to the nerve.[105] In the absence of a nerve stimulator, the physician must be guided by the development of appropriate paresthesias. Care must be taken to avoid neuronal damage produced by repeated needle trauma or injection of anesthetic agent into the perineural sheath. The following discussions will emphasize needle placement with the nerve stimulator. Needle placement using the paresthesia technique requires first eliciting a paresthesia with the needle, then retraction of the needle several mm to permit free flow of the anesthetic agent into the surrounding tissue.

Median Nerve Block. After the elbow joint has been placed in an extended position and the skin has been prepared with antiseptic solution, the brachial artery is palpated between the two epicondyles. An insulated 2.5-inch, No. 22 gauge needle attached to a nerve stimulator is inserted perpendicularly through the skin 0.5 cm medial to the brachial artery between the two epicondyles (see Fig. 32–9). Intermittent flexion of the hand and fingers with currents of less than 0.5 ma at 1 Hz frequency suggests that the block needle is in the immediate vicinity of the median nerve. The injection of 5 to 7 ml of 2 per cent chloroprocaine results in an immediate onset of the block, which lasts for 30 to 45 minutes. The same amount of 1 per cent lidocaine, mepivacaine, or prilocaine have an average onset time of 4 to 5 minutes and a duration of 60 to 120 minutes. Similar volumes of 0.1 to 0.2 per cent tetracaine and 0.5 per cent bupivacaine and etidocaine provide complete sensory analgesia within 7 to 8 minutes after the injection and last for 3 to 5 hours. It is important to avoid displacement of the needle during connection of the syringe to the needle. This can best be achieved by using an anesthesia extension set–stopcock assembly that is connected to the needle prior to the skin puncture.[107] If a satisfactory twitch with the nerve stimulator is not obtained, the needle should be withdrawn and inserted more medially or laterally to locate the nerve.[105, 112, 113]

Radial Nerve Block. The elbow joint is extended and placed on a table. The antecubital fossa is prepared with antiseptic solution. The lateral border of the biceps muscle and the medial border of the brachioradialis muscle are located at the elbow joint between the two epicondyles. Both the radial nerve and the lateral cutaneous nerve of the forearm lie in the groove between the biceps and the brachioradialis muscle at this level. An insulated 2.5-inch, No. 22 gauge needle attached to a stimulator is inserted perpendicularly through the skin in the groove 0.5 to 1 cm medial to the brachioradialis muscle (see Fig. 32–9). A twitch, characterized by the extension of the fingers and hand, with less than 0.5 ma at 1 Hz frequency suggests that the block needle is in close proximity to the nerve. Local anesthetic solution of the same strength and volume as that used for median nerve block is injected without displacing the needle.[105, 112, 113]

Ulnar Nerve Block. The patient is placed in a supine position and asked to abduct the shoulder joint to a 90-degree angle. The elbow is flexed to 90 degrees and externally rotated. After preparation of the medial aspect of the arm with antiseptic solution, the ulnar groove at the posterior aspect of the medial epicondyle is located. The ulnar nerve can usually be palpated in this groove without difficulty. Because the nerve is posteriorly supported by dense bone tissue, it can often be damaged between the block needle and the bone. To prevent this complication, the needle should be inserted 1 to 2 cm above the ulnar nerve groove, where the nerve is posteriorly supported by softer tissue (Fig. 32–10). A 1¼-inch, No. 25 gauge, short bevel needle connected to a 5- or 10-ml syringe filled with local anesthetic solution is inserted through the skin. It is best to direct the needle parallel to the nerve in either direction (proximal or distal) rather than to direct it perpendicularly; this prevents possible damage to the nerve. Injection of 5 to 10 ml of local anesthetic solution provides anesthesia at the ulnar nerve distribution. The use of a nerve stimulator is usually not necessary, because unsuccessful blocks are rare. When a stimulator is used, characteristic twitch of thumb adduction and flexion of the small and ring fingers can be seen with currents as low as 0.3 ma at 1 Hz frequency.[105, 112, 113]

Nerve Blocks at the Wrist

Individual nerve blocks at the wrist provide surgical anesthesia for minor procedures performed in the region of the distribution of the

blocked nerve. For relatively major procedures, a total wrist block involving all three nerves (median, radial, and ulnar) is preferred (Fig. 32–11).

Anatomy

Median Nerve. The median nerve at the wrist lies between the tendons of the flexor carpi radialis laterally and the palmaris longus medially (Fig. 32–11B). Both the tendons and the nerve are superficial at the anterior aspect of the wrist.

Radial Nerve. Approximately 7 to 10 cm superior to the wrist, the superficial sensory branch of the radial nerve perforates the superficial fascia of the forearm. The radial nerve emerges to the subcutaneous tissue at the dorsolateral aspect of the forearm (Fig. 32–12). Here it divides into several branches, supplying the dorsolateral aspect of the wrist and the hand.

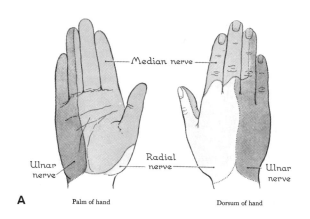

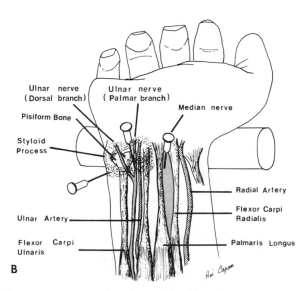

Figure 32–11. *A,* Distribution of the sensory nerves to the palm and dorsum of the hand. There may be considerable variation in the pattern of distribution, especially to the dorsum of the hand. (From Grant's Atlas, 7th ed. Baltimore, Williams & Wilkins, 1978. Used by permission.) *B,* Anatomical relationship of the median and ulnar nerves with the adjacent structures of the wrist. The dotted area at the medial aspect of the wrist represents the subcutaneous injection of the local anesthetic solution to block the dorsal branch of the ulnar nerve.

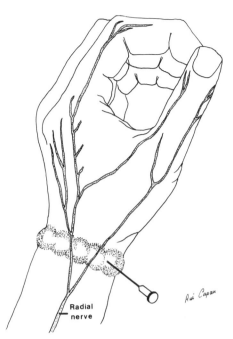

Figure 32–12. The antomy of the radial nerve at the wrist and its blockade by subcutaneous injection of local anesthetic solution in a semicircular manner.

Radial nerve

Ulnar Nerve. About 5 to 7 cm superior to the wrist, the ulnar nerve divides into two terminal branches, the dorsal and the palmar branches. Both branches run distally along the lateral aspect of the flexor carpi ulnaris. The dorsal branch enters the dorsal aspect of the hand and provides sensory innervation to this region. The palmar branch supplies the sensory innervation at the palmar aspect (Fig. 32–11B).

Technique
Median Nerve Block. The dorsal aspect of the forearm and the hand should be rested on a table with the palm facing the ceiling. The wrist is extended by placement of a roll of gauze between the table and its dorsal aspect. (This position is commonly used for the insertion of a radial artery catheter.)

The palmaris longus tendon is located at the level of the superior crease. The tendon becomes protuberant when the patient approximates the thumb and the little finger and flexes the wrist against resistance. This maneuver contracts both the palmaris longus and the flexor carpi radialis tendons and makes them palpable and visible. After the area has been prepared with an antiseptic solution, a 1½-inch, No. 23 gauge short bevel needle is inserted perpendicularly between the tendons of the palmaris longus and the flexor carpi radialis at the level of the superior crease of the wrist and advanced slowly. Within a distance of approximately 0.5 to 1.0 cm a "pop" may be felt, indicating that the flexor retinaculum is being pierced. The nerve lies underneath the retinaculum at a depth of approximately 0.5 to 1.0 cm. After obtaining paresthesia at the median nerve distribution, 2 to 5 ml of desired local anesthetic solution (2 per cent nesacaine; 1 per cent lidocaine, mepivacaine and prilocaine; or 0.5 per cent bupivacaine and etidocaine) is injected (see Fig. 32–11). The use of a nerve stimulator may be helpful in locating the nerve.

Some patients may not have a palmaris longus tendon. In such cases, the nerve is located between the flexor carpi radialis and the flexor digitorum superficialis tendons. The latter tendon may also be made easily palpable by having the patient make a fist and flex against a resistance.[114-116]

Radial Nerve Block. After the skin has been prepared with antiseptic solution, a 1½-inch, No. 25 gauge needle is inserted into the subcutaneous tissue immediately lateral to the radial artery at the level of the superior crease. Two ml of local anesthetic solution of choice of the same strength as described for median nerve block is deposited. The infiltration is then extended in the same tissue plane dorsolaterally to the midportion of the dorsal aspect of the wrist (see Fig. 32–12). A total injection of 10 to 12 ml of local anesthetic solution blocks all the sensory branches of the nerve.[117, 118]

Ulnar Nerve Block. Successful blockade of the ulnar nerve can be achieved by blocking its palmar and dorsal branches separately. The palmar branch runs distally lateral to the tendon of the flexor carpi ulnaris and medial to the ulnar artery. The tendon of the flexor carpi ulnaris is located at the level of the styloid process of the ulna. It attaches distally to the pisiform bone. Thus, identification of the pisiform bone is helpful in locating the flexor carpi ulnaris tendon. Having the patient flex and ulnarly deviate his wrist against resistance is also useful in locating the tendon.

After the tendon and ulnar artery have been located, a 1½-inch, No. 23 gauge needle is inserted perpendicularly between the tendon of the flexor carpi ulnaris and the ulnar artery at the level of the superior crease of the wrist (see Fig. 32–11). Because the nerve is located superficially above the flexor retinaculum, paresthesia should be sought in the subcutaneous tissue at a depth of 1 to 1.5 cm from the skin. The use of a nerve stimulator and obtaining twitch with less than 0.3 ma at 1 Hz frequency may also be helpful in locating the nerve. A characteristic thumb adduction with stimulation of the nerve ensures correct placement of the needle. Three ml of local anesthetic solution of choice of appropriate strength is then injected. The dorsal branch of the nerve is blocked by depositing 5 to 10 ml of local anesthetic solution subcutaneously from the lateral side of the flexor carpi radialis tendon to the midportion of the dorsal aspect of the wrist (see Fig. 32–11).[116, 118]

Nerve Blocks at the Base of the Fingers

Digital nerve block is one of the most frequently used anesthetic procedures in the emergency department. This procedure is relatively easy to perform and complications rarely occur. Indications include removal of a nail or repair of a nail bed, débridement or primary closure of finger lacerations, reduction of fractures and dislocations of the phalanges, skin closure of totally or partially amputated fingers, and drainage of infection.

Anatomy. Two sets of nerves supply sensation to the digits: the dorsal and the palmar digital nerves. One dorsal and one palmar digital nerve run along each side of each finger. The palmar digital nerve originates from the median nerve (supplying the thumb, index finger, middle finger, and the radial side of the ring finger) and the ulnar nerve (supplying the ulnar side of the ring finger and the fifth finger). The palmar digital nerves run distally with the digital vessels lateral to the flexor tendons (Fig. 32–13A). The palmar digital nerve (also called the *common digital nerve*) supplies the entire palmar surface of each finger and is sensory to the interphalangeal joints. The palmar branch alone supplies the entire distal portion of the middle three fingers, including the subungual area (Fig. 32–13B). Because of this innervation, only the palmar digital branch is blocked to obtain anesthesia of the entire distal middle three fingers or for the reduction of all interphalangeal dislocations of the fingers.

The dorsal digital nerves are smaller than the palmar digital nerves and are terminal branches of the superficial radial nerve or the dorsal branch of the ulnar nerve. The dorsal digital nerves are cutaneous nerves that are sensory to only the proximal dorsum of the three middle fingers yet supply much of the distal dorsum and subungual areas of the thumb and the fifth finger. Therefore, the dorsal branch must be blocked to obtain operating anesthesia of the distal dorsal area of both the thumb and the fifth finger (Fig. 32–13B).

Techniques. Both the palmar and the dorsal digital nerves may be blocked by injecting anesthetic solution at the base of the proximal phalanx (Fig. 32–14).

After the skin has been prepared with an antiseptic solution, a 1-inch, No. 25 gauge needle is inserted from the dorsal aspect to the base of the proximal phalanx about 2.5 mm lateral to the midline. The needle first contacts the base of the phalanx. The bone is passed by redirecting the needle laterally, and the needle is further advanced until a resistance created by the palmar skin is felt. One ml of local anesthetic solution of appropriate strength is deposited to block the palmar digital nerve. The needle is then withdrawn, and an additional 0.5 ml of local anesthetic solution is injected just under the point of entry

to block the dorsal digital nerve.[119] The procedure is then repeated on the other side of the finger.

The dorsal and palmar digital nerves can also be anesthetized separately by inserting needles from the respective sides of the finger. This, however, requires four separate needle insertions for each finger and may result in patient discomfort. Digital nerve block does not require eliciting paresthesia.

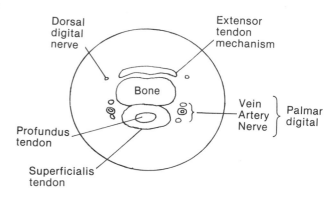

Dorsal surface

A

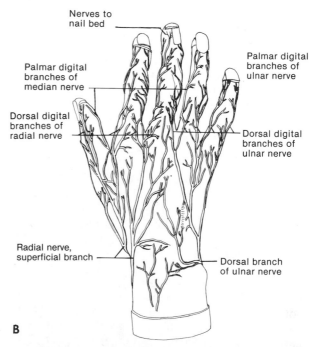

Palmar surface

B

Figure 32–13. A, Cross section of the proximal portion of the proximal phalanx demonstrating the relationship of the dorsal and palmar digital nerves to the digital artery and tendons. B, Digital nerve innervation of the fingers. Note that the palmar digital branches of the ulnar and median nerves curve around to the dorsum and alone supply the entire distal half of the three middle fingers, including the subungual area. The dorsal digital nerve must be blocked to obtain anesthesia of the distal dorsal portion of the thumb and fifth finger and the corresponding subungual area, whereas only the palmar branch needs to be blocked to obtain anesthesia of this area in the three middle fingers. (From Grant's Atlas, 7th ed. Baltimore, Williams & Wilkins, 1978. Used by permission.)

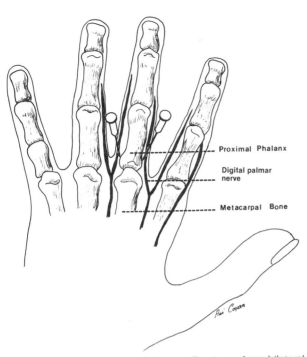

Figure 32–14. The position of the needles to perform bilateral digital nerve block at the base of the finger. Only the palmar digital nerves are shown. As the needle is withdrawn, the anesthetic is deposited to block the dorsal digital nerve.

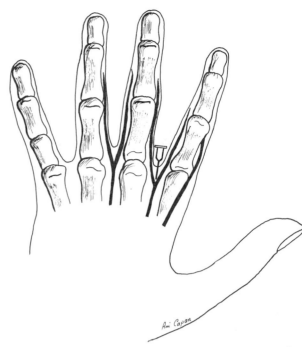

Figure 32–15. The location and position of the needle to perform palmar digital nerve block at the interdigital web space. The dorsal digital nerve will be blocked by diffusion of the anesthetic.

The fingers can also be anesthetized at the interdigital web space, where bifurcation of the palmar (common) digital nerve takes place. The fingers should be extended and widely abducted. A 1.5-cm, No. 25 gauge hypodermic needle is inserted into the web space 2 to 3 mm dorsally from the palm and is advanced in line to the fingers up to its hub (Fig. 32–15).[115] Two ml of local anesthetic solution is deposited. Gentle massage of the injected area may enhance the onset of the block by aiding diffusion of the anesthetic through the tissue to the nerves.

The web space block primarily anesthetizes only the palmar (common) digital nerve, but the terminal branches of the dorsal digital nerve are also blocked by diffusion of the anesthetic solution. As a result, satisfactory surgical anesthesia of the entire finger is usually obtained.

To obtain complete anesthesia of the thumb and the fifth finger, both the palmar and dorsal digital nerves must be blocked separately. This is easily accomplished by injecting the anesthetic solution circumferentially around the base of the proximal phalanx in the subcutaneous tissue.

A technique involving the insertion of a needle in the palm between the metacarpal bones below the level of the distal palmar crease has also been described.[119–121] This technique, however, is excessively painful, does not block the dorsal digital nerve, and does not offer any particular advantage over previous methods.

The total volume of the local anesthetic solution should not exceed 3 to 5 ml. The use of large volumes may result in vascular compromise to the fingers by exerting pressure on the digital vessels. Also, there is no need to use high concentrations of local anesthetic agents; adequate anesthesia can be produced by using lower concentrations of local anesthetic solutions (2 per cent nesacaine, 0.5 to 1 per cent lidocaine, and 0.25 per cent bupivacaine). The local anesthetic solutions should *not* contain vasoconstrictor agents. Vasoconstrictors may cause ischemia of the fingers.

Occasionally, immediately following a digital block, the finger may be cold and cyanotic, especially if the block was a bilateral injection of the sides of the finger at the base of the proximal phalanx. It is secondary to digital artery spasm and/or compression and is almost always a temporary condition, requiring no treatment and returning to normal in a few minutes with no sequelae. The problem can be avoided by using the web space block and keeping the amount of anesthetic solution to a minimum. It may take 2 to 5 minutes for a digital block to be effective; thus, the physician must be patient and not repeat the block if immediate anesthesia is not obtained.

LOWER EXTREMITY BLOCKS

Nerve Blocks at the Hip

Nerve supply to the lower extremity origi[n]ates mainly from the femoral, obturator, lateral fe[moral] cutaneous, and the sciatic nerves. The first three nerves arise from the lumbar plexus, and the sciatic nerves arise from the lumbosacral plexus. In the emergency department, blockade of the entire lower extremity is seldom necessary. The total dose of local anesthetic needed to block all the nerves that supply the lower extremity is relatively large. Thus, regional anesthetic methods are not usually chosen to provide surgical anesthesia of the lower extremity from this level. Isolated sciatic nerve block is also not indicated in most instances. In the emergency department, however, an indication to block the femoral nerve is to relieve pain and quadriceps muscle spasm caused by femoral shaft fractures.[122] Due to anatomical factors, blocking of the femoral nerve using Winnie's paravascular technique also provides simultaneous blockade of the obturator and lateral femoral cutaneous nerve blocks.[123]

Anatomy. The femoral nerve arises from the lumbar plexus, which also gives rise to the obturator and lateral femoral cutaneous nerves. The lumbar plexus is composed of the first three and the greater parts of the fourth lumbar nerves. Some additional fibers also enter into the lumbar plexus from the T12 nerve. The plexus, having been formed in front of the quadratus lumborum and behind the psoas muscles, gives rise to the lateral femoral cutaneous nerve, the femoral nerve, and the obturator nerve.

All three nerves are initially sandwiched between the quadratus lumborum and the psoas muscles and wrapped in a fascial sheath. At the level of L3 to L4, the lateral femoral cutaneous nerve leaves this fascial compartment and runs down in front of the iliac muscle (Figs. 32–16 and 32–17). The nerve passes under the inguinal ligament 1 cm medial to its attachment to the anterior superior iliac spine and gives sensory nerve supply to the entire lateral aspect of the thigh.

The obturator nerve leaves the fascial compartment at the level of L5 from the medial border of the psoas muscle (Figs. 32–16 and 32–17) and primarily supplies the adductor muscles of the thigh; however, it is also an important sensory supply to the anteromedial aspect of the thigh.

The femoral nerve leaves the fascial compartment from the lateral margin of the psoas muscle at about the level of the first and second sacral vertebrae (see Fig. 32–17). The femoral nerve anatomically differs from the obturator and the lateral femoral cutaneous nerves, because during its course distally, it is located in a sulcus between the psoas major and the iliacus muscles and is covered laterally by the iliacus fascia, medially by the psoas fascia, and anteriorly by the transversalis fascia. As the nerve runs under the inguinal ligament, it is covered posterolaterally by the fused psoas fascia, anteriorly by the inguinal ligament, inferiorly by the fascia lata, and medially

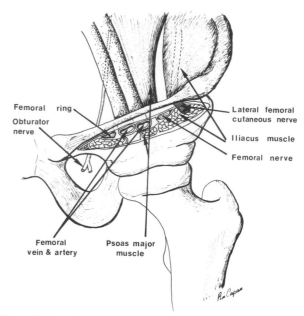

Figure 32–16. Diagram showing the anatomical relationship of the femoral, obturator, and lateral cutaneous nerves with the adjacent structures at the groin. (Modified from Winnie, A. P., Ramamurthy, S., and Durrani, Z.: The inguinal paravascular technique of lumbar plexus anesthesia: The "3 in 1 block." Anesth. Analg. 52:989, 1973. Used by permission.)

by the iliopectineal fascia (see Figs. 32–16 and 32–17). Thus, anatomically, the femoral nerve carries a tubular sheath from its origin at the lumbar plexus to a point 2 to 3 cm below the inguinal ligament where it can easily be blocked.

The obturator and lateral femoral cutaneous nerves also originate from the same plexus and

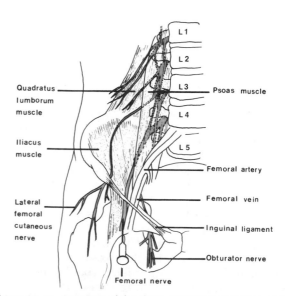

Figure 32–17. Anatomy of the three important branches of the lumbar plexus (femoral, obturator, and lateral femoral cutaneous nerves). The position of the block needle during Winnie's perivascular technique. (Modified from Winnie, A. P., Ramamurthy, S., and Durrani, Z.: The inguinal paravascular technique of lumbar plexus anesthesia: The "3 in 1 block." Anesth. Analg. 52:989, 1973. Used by permission.)

are sandwiched between the fascia of the psoas and the quadratus lumborum muscles. As these nerves emerge from the borders of the psoas muscle, they are still subfascial; therefore, an adequate amount of local anesthetic deposited into the perineural sheath of the femoral nerve travels proximally in the close perineural fascial space and blocks the conduction of all three nerves.[123]

Single Needle Technique. This technique is also called *3-in-1 block* and was developed by Winnie and colleagues in 1973 (see Fig. 32–17).[123]

The patient is placed in a supine position, and the skin is prepared with antiseptic solution. The physician stands on the side of the groin contralateral to where the block is to be performed. The femoral artery is palpated 1 cm below the inguinal ligament. An insulated 2 1/2-inch, No. 22 gauge needle with metal hub connected to a low-current nerve stimulator is inserted into the skin 0.5 to 1 cm lateral to the femoral artery. The needle is directed and advanced cephalad at a 45- to 60-degree angle to the skin until a distinct twitch of the quadriceps muscle is observed in response to the electrical stimulation. The nerve should be stimulated with no more than 0.5 ma at 1 Hz frequency. Because the nerve is covered with thick fascial layers, stimulation with greater currents indicates that the needle is above the fascia.[124] There may be a drop of as much as 2 ma of minimal stimulating current across the fascia. Care should be taken to avoid injecting the local anesthetic solution above the perineural fascia. After a satisfactory twitch has been obtained with minimal current (less than 0.5 ma), the finger palpating the femoral artery is removed and placed gently but firmly distal to the needle. A local anesthetic solution of choice (2 per cent nesacaine, 1 per cent lidocaine, mepivacaine, or prilocaine, and 0.5 per cent bupivacaine or etidocaine) is injected via the needle, and the needle is then removed. Distal pressure should be exerted on the skin by a finger for 5 minutes to allow the local anesthetic to diffuse proximally. Care should be taken to prevent displacement of the needle during injection. The use of an anesthesia extension set–three-way stopcock assembly is useful in providing an immobile needle.[107] The volume of the local anesthetic is also important. A total volume of at least 20 ml should be used in order to reliably block the conduction of all three nerves. Lower volumes (15 ml) block the femoral nerve but may not be enough to block the remaining two nerves.[123] The lateral cutaneous nerve is probably the most difficult nerve to be blocked using this method, because it originates the furthest from the site of injection.

At the inguinal region, the vascular and neural compartments are separated by thick fibrous fascial structures; therefore, intravascular injection is not common during femoral nerve block. When all three nerves are blocked, adequate anesthesia can be produced for the surgical repair of lacerations at the anterior aspect of the thigh. As previously mentioned, femoral nerve block in the emergency department can be used to control the acute pain caused by femoral shaft fractures.

The sciatic nerve originates from the fourth and fifth lumbar and from the first and second sacral nerves. Although the block of the sciatic nerve is not indicated in the emergency department, its terminal branches at the level of the ankle may be blocked to provide surgical anesthesia of the foot.

Nerve Blocks at the Knee

Two terminal branches of the sciatic nerve (tibial nerve and peroneal nerve) and one terminal branch of the femoral nerve (saphenous nerve) can be blocked at the level of the knee joint. In practice, however, this approach is rarely used, because any nerve block performed at the knee level provides anesthesia of the foot, which can be accomplished more easily by blocking these nerves at the ankle.

Blockade of the tibial nerve at the knee level is relatively difficult and painful. Because the nerve is in close proximity to the popliteal vessels, injury to the vessels may occur. Peroneal nerve block is a relatively simple procedure to perform. Injection of 5 ml of local anesthetic solution at the lateral aspect of the fibular bone 1 to 2 cm distal to its head provides adequate blockade. Vigorous attempts to elicit paresthesia may be associated with significant risk of postblock neuritis. The block of the saphenous nerve can be accomplished by 5 to 10 ml subcutaneous infiltration of local anesthetic solution (2 per cent nesacaine, 0.5 per cent lidocaine, mepivacaine, or prilocaine, and 0.25 per cent bupivacaine or etidocaine) at the medial side of the knee joint below the sartorious muscle in the area of the saphenous vein.

Nerve Blocks at the Ankle

Indications to perform ankle blocks include surgical procedures of the foot, removal of foreign bodies from the foot, débridement of burns, and repair of lacerations of the foot.

Anatomy

Posterior Tibial Nerve. This nerve is the larger terminal branch of the sciatic nerve. The smaller terminal branch is the common peroneal nerve. The sciatic nerve is divided into its terminal branches at the popliteal fossa (Fig. 32–18). After running distally in the calf muscles, at the distal two thirds portion of the leg the posterior tibial nerve turns medially and reaches the ankle at a location medial to the Achilles tendon. Here the nerve lies behind the posterior tibial artery and the tendons of the flexor digitorum longus and

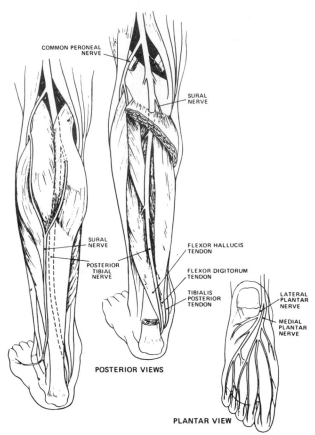

Figure 32–18. *Posterior views.* Anatomical relationship of the sciatic, posterior tibial, common peroneal, and the sural nerves with the adjacent structures at the posterior aspect of the leg and the foot. *Plantar view.* Nerve supply of the sole by the two terminal branches of the posterior tibial nerve; medial and lateral plantar nerves. (From Schurman, D. H.: Ankle-block anesthesia for foot surgery. Anesthesiology 44:348, 1976. Used by permission.)

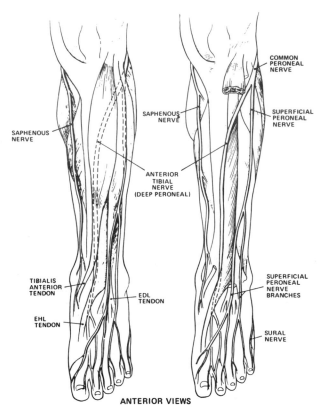

Figure 32–19. Anatomical relationship of the common peroneal, anterior tibial (deep peroneal), superficial peroneal, and the saphenous nerves with the adjacent structures at the anterior aspect of the leg and the foot. (EHL:Extensor Lalluci's longus, EDL: Extensor digitorum longus; From Schurman, D. H.: Ankle-block anesthesia for foot surgery. Anesthesiology 44:348, 1976. Used by permission.)

the flexor hallucis longus muscles, covered by the flexor retinaculum. The nerve then gives off the medial calcaneal branch to supply the inside of the heel and divides into the terminal branches, the medial and lateral plantar nerves, which supply the sole of the foot (see Figs. 32–18 and 32–21).

Anterior Tibial (Deep Peroneal) and Superficial Peroneal Nerves. After dividing from the sciatic nerve in the popliteal fossa, the common peroneal nerve runs laterally and winds around the fibular bone at about 1 to 2 cm distal to the fibular head (Figs. 32–18 and 32–19). Here, the nerve is superficial and can easily be palpated under the skin in people who are thin. After turning around the fibular bone, the common peroneal nerve reaches the anterolateral aspect of the leg and divides into two branches: the anterior tibial nerve (also called the *deep peroneal nerve*) and the superficial peroneal nerve (Fig. 32–20). The former runs distally anterior to the interosseus membrane of the leg between the anterior tibial muscle and the extensor hallucis longus muscle. At the ankle, the nerve

lies between the tendons of these two muscles (see Fig. 32–20). Anteriorly, it is covered by the extensor retinaculum. During its course, the nerve lies laterally to the anterior tibial artery and, upon reaching the ankle, crosses under the artery and becomes medial to it. This crossing occurs at the level of the extensor retinaculum. The nerve supplies motor branches to the short extensors of the toes and sensory branches to the skin of the lateral aspect of the big toe and the medial aspect of the second toe (Fig. 32–21).

The superficial peroneal nerve runs downward on the anterior leg and at two thirds of its distance, it perforates the crural fascia (see Fig. 32–19). It then divides into subcutaneous branches and supplies the dorsum of the foot (Fig. 32–21).

Sural Nerve. Just prior to turning around the fibular bone, the common peroneal nerve gives off a small branch that runs superficially in the calf muscles. This branch joins a superficial branch from the posterior tibial nerve and forms the sural nerve in the middle of the leg at the posterior aspect (see Fig. 32–18). The nerve then runs distally in the subcutaneous tissue and reaches the ankle behind and below the lateral malleolus. It

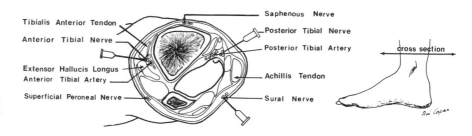

Figure 32–20. Cross section of the ankle showing the location of the nerves that supply the foot.

runs in close proximity to the short saphenous vein and provides the sensory supply to the skin of the heel and the outer margin of the foot (see Fig. 32–21).

Saphenous Nerve. After becoming superficial at the medial side of the knee joint, the saphenous nerve runs distally along the great saphenous vein. At the ankle, it is located anterior and medial to the medial malleolus and gives off sensory supply to the anteromedial aspect of the ankle (see Figs. 32–19 and 32–21).

Techniques. In order to obtain complete anesthesia, five nerves supplying the sensory innervation of the entire foot need to be blocked. Figure 32–20 shows the anatomic relationship of these nerves at the ankle, and Figure 32–21 shows their sensory distribution at the foot.

The patient is placed supine on the operating table. A bolster temporarily placed under the calf may facilitate the preparation of the foot with an antiseptic solution.[125, 126]

Posterior Tibial Nerve Block. This nerve can be blocked behind the medial malleolus. The posterior tibial artery is palpated, and a skin wheal is raised behind it, at the level of the upper border of the medial malleolus. A 2 1/2-inch, No. 23 or No. 25 gauge needle is inserted perpendicular to

the skin and moved gently in the mediolateral direction to elicit paresthesia in the sole of the foot. After paresthesia is obtained, 5 to 10 ml of a local anesthetic agent is deposited and the needle is withdrawn (Fig. 32–22). An injection of 10 to 12 ml of local anesthetic in a fanlike manner in this area, without attempting to elicit paresthesia, may also provide a successful nerve block. When paresthesia is not obtained, onset of anesthesia may take up to 30 minutes.

Anterior Tibial Nerve (Deep Peroneal) Block. A 2 1/2-inch, No. 23 or No. 25 gauge needle is inserted perpendicularly at the anterior aspect of the foot at the level of the malleoli. The insertion

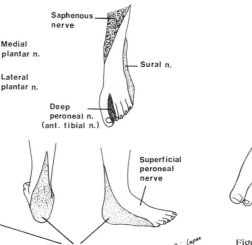

Figure 32–21. Regional distribution of the sensory nerve supply to the foot.

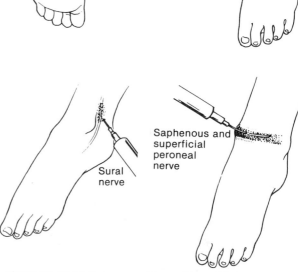

Figure 32–22. Technique used to perform ankle block. Saphenous and superficial peroneal nerve blocks (see text for detail). (From Schurman, D. H.: Ankle-block anesthesia for foot surgery. Anesthesiology 44:348, 1976. Used by permission.)

is made between the tendons of the anterior tibial and the extensor hallucis longus muscles (see Fig. 32–20). The hallucis longus tendon can be identified by having the patient dorsiflex the big toe while the physician pushes the remaining toes downward. The tendon at the ankle that moves synchronously with the big toe dorsiflexion is the tendon of the hallucis longus. Identification of the tendon of the anterior tibial muscle is difficult and unreliable. However, inserting the needle immediately medial to the tendon of the extensor hallucis longus usually locates the nerve. The needle is advanced toward the tibia. If paresthesia is elicited at the lateral aspect of the big toe and the medial aspect of the second digit, 5 ml of local anesthetic solution is injected. If paresthesia is not elicited, which is frequently the case, the needle is advanced until it comes in contact with the tibial bone. The needle is then withdrawn 2 or 3 mm, and 5 ml of local anesthetic solution is deposited (see Fig. 32–22).

Sural Nerve Block. The sural nerve is blocked by subcutaneous injection of local anesthetic agents just posterior to the distal fibula. A total injection of 5 to 8 ml of local anesthetic solution is needed to block this nerve (see Fig. 32–22). Subcutaneous injection from the Achilles tendon to the posterior border of the lateral malleolus may also provide adequate blockade of the sural nerve.

Saphenous and Superficial Peroneal Nerve Blocks. A total circumferential subcutaneous injection of 10 ml of 0.5 per cent lidocaine or 0.25 per cent bupivacaine without epinephrine is made at the level of the superior border of the malleoli. This injection anesthetizes the saphenous and superficial peroneal nerves as well as the small cutaneous branches of the sensory nerves that supply the foot (see Fig. 32–22).

Nerve Blocks at the Foot

Nerve blocks at the foot include metatarsal and digital blocks; they are usually performed to provide surgical anesthesia of the toes. Indications for anesthesia at this site are similar to those for the hand. Repair of toe lacerations and replantation of partially amputated toes, surgical intervention for nail bed injuries or infections, and removal of foreign bodies from the foot can be easily performed using this anesthetic method.

Anatomy. As in the hand, the terminal nerves in the foot are located at the dorsal and plantar aspect of the foot (Fig. 32–23). At the metatarsal level, the nerves pass through the intermetatarsal space, and at the toes, the nerves are located on both sides of the digits.

Techniques

Metatarsal Nerve Blocks. After the skin has been prepared with antiseptic solutions, skin wheals are raised on the dorsal aspect of the foot between the metatarsal bones. A 2-inch, No. 23 gauge needle is inserted through the skin wheal, and a local anesthetic solution (0.5 per cent lidocaine, mepivacaine or prilocaine or 0.25 per cent bupivacaine) is injected in a fanlike manner while the needle is advanced toward the sole. Care should be taken not to puncture the sole. A total injection of 5 ml of local anesthetic solution into each intermetatarsal space provides excellent anesthesia at the toes.

Digital Nerve Blocks. A 1-inch, No. 25 gauge

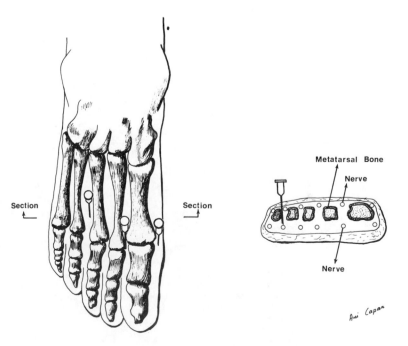

Figure 32–23. *Left.* The technique of the metatarsal and digital nerve block of the foot. *Right.* Distal transmetatarsal cross section showing the anatomical relationship of the metatarsal nerves with the adjacent structures.

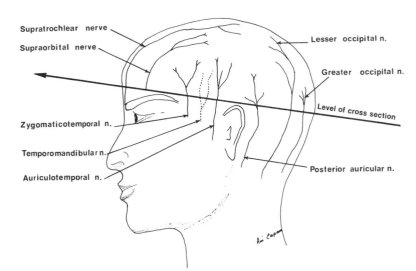

Figure 32–24. The sources of sensory nerve supply to the scalp.

needle is inserted through the skin from the dorsal aspect on the side of the toe and at the level of the proximal phalanx (see Fig. 32–23). Local anesthetic solution is injected while the needle is advanced in the plantar direction. The needle is then withdrawn and inserted from the opposite side of the toe, and the same steps are followed. During advancement of the needle, care should be taken to avoid piercing the plantar skin. There is no need to elicit paresthesia during digital nerve blocks. Total injected volume of local anesthetics should not exceed 2 ml. Addition of vasoconstrictor agents to local anesthetics should be avoided during metatarsal and digital nerve blocks.

The first (big) toe can be blocked by complete circumferential injection of local anesthetic solution at its base using a fine-gauge needle. A common but usually transient complication of digital nerve block is the development of ischemic changes of the toes, resulting from compression of digital vessels by the local anesthetic solution that is deposited in the close space.

BLOCKS OF THE HEAD

Scalp Block

Scalp blocks provide surgical anesthesia for the repair of scalp lacerations and satisfactory anesthesia for surgical decompression of the brain with burr holes.

Anatomy. (Figs. 32–24 and 32–25). The scalp receives its nerve supply from branches of the trigeminal nerve (5th cranial nerve) and the cervical plexus. The forehead is supplied by the supraorbital and supratrochlea nerves. Both nerves are branches of the opthalmic division of the trigeminal nerve. (See also Chapter 69). The temporal region receives its nerve supply from the zygomaticotemporal (the branch of the second

division of the trigeminal nerve), temporomandibular, and auriculotemporal nerves (the branches of the third division of the trigeminal nerve).

The posterior aspect of the scalp is innervated by the greater auricular and the greater, lesser, and least occipital nerves. The nerves that supply the posterior aspect of the scalp originate from the

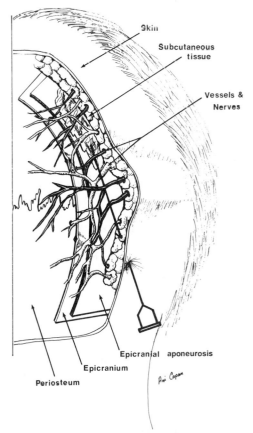

Figure 32–25. Topographic anatomy of the scalp taken above a line drawn from the upper border of the external ear to the occiput and the eyebrows.

cervical plexus. All the nerves become superficial above a line drawn from the upper border of the external ear to the occiput and the eyebrows and converge toward the vertex of the scalp (see Fig. 32–24).

Topographically, the nerves and vessels of the scalp are located in the subcutaneous tissue above the epicranial aponeurosis. From this level they divide into small branches that extend to the deeper layers (epicranium and periosteum). A section of the scalp from the skin to the skull shows the following layers: 1) skin; 2) subcutaneous tissue, rich in blood vessels and nerves; 3) epicranial aponeurosis; 4) epicranium; and 5) periosteum of the skull (see Fig. 32–25).[127]

Techniques. Scalp block can be accomplished by individually blocking each nerve that supplies the scalp, but this approach is time consuming, difficult, and cumbersome. Because the nerves on the scalp are superficially located, the scalp block can easily be performed by injecting local anesthetic agents into the subcutaneous tissue circumferentially around the area to be blocked. Injection of local anesthetic to the deeper levels is necessary only if bone is to be removed. Note that injection of local anesthetic agents only in the deeper layers without subcutaneous infiltration results in an unsuccessful block and a greater amount of bleeding during surgical intervention.[112, 128]

In preparation for the block, a band of hair may be shaved. (Some physicians prefer to shave the head, but this is of uncertain benefit.) Local anesthetics are injected in the shaved area. For small lacerations, a band 1-cm wide and 3 cm away from the lesion is shaved circumferentially. Larger lacerations require anesthesia either for the entire scalp or for half of it. For the former, a band of hair above the external ears and the occiput, comprising the entire circumference of the head, is shaved. If only one side of the scalp is to be anesthetized, a semicircumferentially shaved band around the scalp and extended over the vertex provides a circle for the injection.

The skin is prepared using an antiseptic solution, and a skin wheal is raised at any point of the shaved skin using a 1/2-inch, No. 25 gauge needle. A 3-inch, No. 22 gauge needle is inserted through the skin wheal into the subcutaneous tissue and advanced circumferentially following the previously shaved circular band. An injection of 0.5 to 1 per cent lidocaine or 0.125 to 0.25 per cent bupivacaine with epinephrine 1:200,000 is used. Epinephrine should be added to the local anesthetic agent to provide vasoconstriction and to prevent excessive blood loss and local anesthetic absorption. The total dose of the local anesthetic agents should not exceed the recommended dose for the particular agent. It may be useful to inject some local anesthetic solution into the temporalis muscle to prevent contraction of the muscle during surgery.

Recently, Colley and Heavner demonstrated that when bupivacaine is used, the peak plasma local anesthetic concentrations occur within 10 to 15 minutes after injection.[129] Thus, the first 10- to 15-minute period after the injection is the most critical period for the occurrence of local anesthetic toxicity. Colley and Heavner also found that despite its high vascularity, the absorption of local anesthetics from the scalp is not excessive. Using the upper limit of the recommended dose of bupivacaine without epinephrine (175 mg), they found that peak plasma bupivacaine concentrations were 0.8 µg per ml with a 0.125 per cent solution and 1.2 µg per ml with a 0.25 per cent solution. Considering that the toxic plasma threshold for bupivacaine is 4 µg per ml, these concentrations suggest that a scalp block using bupivacaine has a wide margin of safety even without the use of epinephrine. When epinephrine is used with bupivacaine, its effect on absorption becomes more pronounced with concentrations of 0.125 per cent than with those of 0.25 per cent. This is probably because at low concentrations (0.125 per cent), bupivicaine has a vasoconstrictor property.[130]

Greater and Lesser Occipital Nerve Block

This relatively simple block may be useful in the emergency department for treating occipital neuralgia and tension headaches.

Anatomy. The posterior aspect of the head is supplied by the posterior rami of the cervical nerves. Two important branches of these nerves are the greater and lesser occipital nerves. The greater occipital nerve becomes superficial on each side at the inferior border of the inferior obliques capitis muscle and runs superiorly toward the vertex over this muscle. The nerve is located medially to the occipital artery. The lesser occipital nerve is located approximately 2.5 to 3.5 cm lateral and 1 to 2 cm caudad to the greater occipital nerve (Fig. 32–26).[131]

Technique. It is not usually necessary to shave the scalp prior to performing greater and lesser occipital nerve blocks. The greater occipital nerve can best be blocked at the nuchal line, which is in the middle of the external occipital protuberance and the mastoid process. The nuchal line is located between the insertion sites of the trapezius muscle and the semispinalis muscles. At this site, the greater occipital nerve is just medial to the occipital artery.

The occipital artery is first palpated, and a 1½ inch, No. 22 gauge needle connected to a syringe that contains 5 ml of local anesthetic is inserted through the skin (see Fig. 32–26). After obtaining

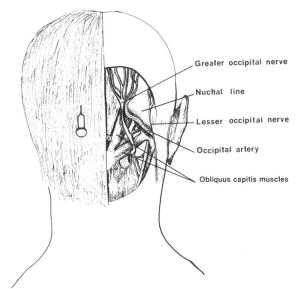

Figure 32–26. The right side of the figure shows the anatomical relationship of the greater and lesser occipital nerves and the adjacent structures at the posterior aspect of the head. The left side of the figure shows the point of entry of the needle for greater occipital nerve block.

paresthesia at the vertex, 5 ml of local anesthetic solution is injected. The lesser occipital nerve is blocked by a fanlike injection of a local anesthetic solution 2.5 to 3.5 cm lateral and 1 cm caudad to the point described for the greater occipital nerve.[131]

This procedure is not usually associated with any complication; however, intra-arterial injections should be avoided by careful aspiration.

NERVE BLOCKS OF THE TRUNK

Intercostal Nerve Block

This regional anesthetic method is commonly used in the emergency department to relieve chest and occasionally abdominal wall pain caused by rib fractures. Intercostal nerve block does not relieve the visceral pain produced by injuries to the thoracic and abdominal contents. Intercostal nerve block seems to improve the hypoventilation caused by pain-induced abdominal and chest wall splinting.[132, 133] Thus, especially in elderly patients and in those with limited respiratory reserve, intercostal nerve block may prevent further pulmonary complications. Whether this method offers any advantage over the administration of narcotics to relieve the pain in patients with acute chest injuries is a controversial issue. Almost all the studies performed to compare the effectiveness of these two methods were carried out on patients who have acute posthoracotomy pain. These studies suggest that the patients who receive intercostal nerve block after a thoracotomy or subcostal

laparatomy may have better results from pulmonary function tests, greater PaO$_2$, earlier return of arterial blood gases to normal, and earlier ambulation and discharge from the hospital.[132, 134, 135] However, the results of these studies may not necessarily apply to patients with acute chest injuries. Current data only suggest that intercostal nerve blocks in uncomplicated simple rib fractures appear to be more advantageous than the administration of large doses of narcotic agents.[136]

Anatomy. The intercostal nerves arise from the thoracic spinal nerves. After emerging from the intervertebral foramina, the spinal nerves divide into anterior and posterior primary rami. The intercostal nerves are the anterior primary rami of the thoracic spinal nerves. Prior to becoming the intercostal nerves, the anterior primary rami receive the grey rami and give off branches to the sympathetic chain via the white rami communicantes. Following this, the nerves run anteriorly along the inferior border of the ribs, giving off two important branches: the posterior cutaneous branch, which supplies the skin and the muscles of the paravertebral area, and the superficial lateral cutaneous nerve, which arises at the midaxillary line (Fig. 32–27). This branch sends cutaneous sensory supply to both the anterior and posterior aspects of the chest. After giving off these branches, the intercostal nerves run anteriorly. The upper six intercostal nerves penetrate the external intercostal and pectoralis muscles and supply the anterior aspect of the chest and the breasts. The lower six intercostal nerves terminate at the abdominal wall. They penetrate the abdominal rectus muscle at various levels from the subxyphoid region to the subumbilical area and provide

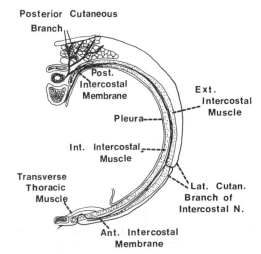

Figure 32–27. A horizontal section from the chest wall showing the anatomical relationship of the intercostal nerve to the adjacent structures along its course. Note that the lateral cutaneous branch is given off in the axillary line, and a block of the intercostal nerve anterior to this area will not provide cutaneous anesthesia.

both motor and sensory supply to the abdominal wall.

The intercostal nerves that are medial to the posterior angles of the ribs are in very close proximity to the pleura. Those that are lateral to the posterior angle of the ribs are located between the internal intercostal and the external intercostal muscles and thus, are relatively far from the pleura. At the inferior border of the ribs, the intercostal nerve is located in a groove. Here the nerve is accompanied by the intercostal vein and the artery. The nerve is always located caudal to the vessels.

Technique. The intercostal nerve block can be performed while the patient is in a sitting, a prone, or a lateral decubitus position. Regardless of the position of the patient, the scapula should be displaced laterally. This is especially important for blocks of the upper seven intercostal spaces. Scapular displacement can easily be accomplished by having the patient move the ipsilateral shoulder and arm anteromedially. This maneuver draws the scapula laterally and clears the space to be blocked.

The intercostal nerve blocks should not be attempted anterior to the midaxillary line. Because the nerve gives off the superificial lateral cutaneous nerve at around the midaxillary line, its blockade anterior to this line results in an incomplete and unsuccessful block. Horizontally from the paravertebral region to the midaxillary line, the nerves can be blocked successfully at any point. However, in practice, the sites most frequently used for intercostal block are the paravertebral region, the posterior angle of the rib, and the posterior or midaxillary line. In the paravertebral approach, the nerve is blocked approximately four finger breadths laterally from the spinous process. This point corresponds to the angle of the ribs, and the lateral border of the muscle mass of the erector spinae where the ribs are easily palpable (see Fig. 32–27).

The following step-by-step approach explains the technique of intercostal nerve blockade:

1. The area is prepared as usual with antiseptic solution.

2. An assistant is asked to pull the skin cephalad using a constant force. While the skin is being pulled cephalad, the inferior borders of the ribs are marked by the physician. The ribs are best identified by palpation with the fingertips.

3. A 3 to 4 cm, No. 22 gauge needle is inserted through the previously made marking perpendicular to all the planes of the skin until it comes in contact with the lower border of the rib. The depth of the needle required to contact the rib is marked.

4. The needle is withdrawn and reinserted slightly caudally. The direction of the needle should be parallel to the direction of the previous needle (Fig. 32–28). The tip of the needle is used

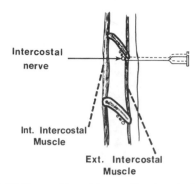

Figure 32–28. The position of the needle when the inferior border of the rib is being "walked" off. Note that the vessels are relatively protected by the rib and that the intercostal nerve is encountered immediately below the inferior portion of the rib.

to feel the rib. The needle should be "walked" caudally until the tip of it falls off the inferior portion of the rib. Cephalad traction of the skin is maintained during this maneuver.

5. At this point, the needle is advanced 2 to 3 mm and the assistant is asked to release the cephalad traction of the skin.

6. With the release of the traction, the needle takes a 45- to 60-degree angle to the skin. At this angle, the needle is again advanced 2 to 3 mm. The patient may describe paresthesia along the course of the intercostal nerve at this point.

7. A syringe containing 5 ml of local anesthetic solution of choice is tightly connected to the needle without causing needle displacement, and after careful aspiration for blood and air, its entire content is injected; the needle is then withdrawn.

This procedure is repeated to block the intercostal nerve above and below the fracture, because there is usually an area of surrounding pain. After the physician has had extensive experience with this procedure, an assistant may not be necessary. The skill of the physician determines the success of the block and the complication rate. Moore and Bridenbaugh reported a 98 per cent success rate in a series of 5000 intercostal nerve blocks.[137] The incidence of the most common complication, pneumothorax, was acceptably low in this series. Depending upon the experience of the physician, this complication has been reported at rates from 0.092 to 19 per cent. A chest film is not routinely obtained, but the patient should be observed for 15 to 30 minutes and instructed to return if problems arise. A coughing spasm during the procedure may indicate that the pleura has been penetrated and is a sign that further investigation or observation is necessary.

Intercostal nerve block is associated with high plasma concentrations of local anesthetics. *Thus, the dose of the local anesthetic agent should not exceed the recommended maximum dose of the particular local anesthetic used.* The upper limit of the recommended dose for bupivacaine is 175 mg without epinephrine and 225 mg with epinephrine. Note that this dose limit has been challenged by Moore and associates, who have injected larger than the recommended maximum dose of bupivacaine (400 mg total dose) without any toxic reactions.[49, 50, 136, 138]

Because of their long-lasting effects, bupivacaine and etidocaine are the most frequently used agents for intercostal nerve blocks. Bupivacaine can be used at concentrations of 0.25 and 0.5 per cent, whereas etidocaine is used at concentrations of 0.5 and 1 per cent. It is probably safer to use 0.25 per cent bupivacaine and 0.5 per cent etidocaine if multiple nerves are to be blocked. Epinephrine at a concentration of 1:200,000 should also be added to prevent excessive absorption and to prolong the duration of action of these local anesthetics.[68, 139] Epinephrine should not be used in patients with hypertension, cardiac disease, or thyrotoxicosis, or in those who are taking MAO-inhibitor medication.

Bupivacaine (total dose of 200 mg with epinephrine) provides analgesia for 8 to 12 hours. The block can be repeated every 12 hours without clinical evidence of toxicity.[140] Experience with etidocaine for repeated intercostal blocks has not been reported.

Although experience is limited, the intercostal nerve block may be used in children for the management of chest trauma.[141] When performing intercostal nerve blocks in children, two technical points should be carefully considered. First, the needles should not be inserted any deeper than 1 to 2 mm under the rib, because the pleura is in very close proximity to the skin. Second, the block should not be attempted medial to the angle of the rib, because the internal intercostal muscle does not exist in this region (see Fig. 32–27). The dose of bupivacaine is 2 to 4 mg per kg, and the concentration is 0.25 to 0.5 per cent. Recently, Rothstein and colleagues reported that the absorption of bupivacaine–epinephrine solution from the intercostal space is more rapid in children than that usually observed in adults.[142] This is probably due to the greater cardiac output in pediatric patients.

Complications. Complications of intercostal blocks include pneumothorax, intravascular injections, and subarachnoid injections (paravertebral approach). Pneumothorax may develop slowly and may be clinically evident several hours after the procedure. Patients should be informed about the symptoms of pneumothorax and should be advised to seek medical help if this complication occurs after discharge from the hospital. Both intravascular and subarachnoid injections result in immediate symptoms of CNS toxicity and total spinal blockade. Both complications should be

treated promptly to prevent fatality or organ damage. Treatment for local anesthetic toxicity was previously discussed. Total spinal anesthesia should be treated by adequate ventilation and oxygenation via a secure airway. Hypotension should be treated using fluids and vasopressors (5 to 10 mg of ephedrine intravenously).

OTHER BLOCKS

Regional nerve blocks are commonly used about the face. The principles for placement of regional nerve blocks on the face are the same as outlined in this chapter. Discussion of the technique of regional nerve blocks of the face is provided in Chapter 69 (Emergency Dental Procedures).

1. Koller, C.: On the use of cocaine for producing anaesthesia on the eye. Lancet 2:990, 1884.
2. Hall, R. J.: Hydrochlorate of cocaine. N.Y. Med. J. 40:643, 1884.
3. Halsted, W. S.: Practical comments on the use and abuse of cocaine; suggested by its invariably successful employment in more than a thousand minor surgical operations. N.Y. Med. J. 42:294, 1885.
4. Ritsert, E.: Benzocaine. Pharmaceutische Zeitung 37:427, 1892.
5. Einhorn, A., and Uhlfelder, E.: Ueber ester und alkaminester der m, p diaminobenzoe saure. Annalen Der Chemie 371:762, 1909.
6. Braun, H.: Ueber einige neue ortliche Anaesthetica (Stovain, Alypin, Novocain). Deutsh. Med. Worchscht. 31:1667, 1905.
7. Fussganger, R., and Schaumann, O.: Uber ein neues Lokalanasthetikum der Novokainreihe (Pantokain). Arch. Exp. Pathol. u Pharmakol. 160:53, 1931.
8. Foldes, F. F., and McNall, P. G.: 2-chloroprocaine: a new local anesthetic agent. Anesthesiology 13:287, 1952.
9. Löfgren, N.: Studies on local anesthetics. Xylocaine: a new synthetic drug. Stockholm, Hoeggstroms, 1948.
10. Schleich, C. L.: Zur Infiltrations ansathesie. Therapeutische Monatshefte, 8:429, 1894.
11. Corning, J. L.: Spinal anesthesia and local medication of the cord. N.Y. Med. J. 42:483, 1885.
12. Bier, A.: Ueber einen neuen weg local anasthesie an den Gliedmaassen zu erzeugen. Arch. Klin. Chir. 86:1007, 1908.
13. Cathelin, F.: Une nouvelle voie d'injection rachidienne—methodes des injections epidurales par le precede du canal sacre. Applications a l'homme. C. R. Soc. Biol. (Paris), 53:453, 1901.
14. Dogliotti, A. M.: Eine neue methode der regionarren Anasthesie: "Die peridurale segmentare Anasthesie." Zentralblott Chirurgie 58:3141, 1931.
15. Covino, B. G., and Vassallo, H. G.: Preclinical aspects of local anesthesia. In Local Anesthetic Mechanisms of Action and Clinical Use. New York, Grune & Stratton, Inc., 1976, p. 49.
16. Brodie, B. B., Lief, P. A., and Poet, R.: The fate of procaine in man following its intravenous administration and methods for the estimation of procaine and diethylaminoethanol. J. Pharmacol. Exp. Ther. 94:359, 1948.
17. Foldes, F. F., Davidson, G. M., Duncalf, D., et al.: The intravenous toxicity of local anesthetic agents in man. Clin. Pharmacol. Ther. 6:328, 1965.

18. Sung, C. Y., and Truant, A. P.: The physiological disposition of lidocaine and its comparison in some respects with procaine. J. Pharmacol. Exp. Ther. 112:432, 1954.

19. Aldrete, J. A., Homatas, J., Boyes, R. N., et al.: Effects of hepatectomy on the disappearance rate of lidocaine from blood in man and dog. Anesth. Analg. 49:687, 1970.

20. Selden, R., and Sasahara, A.: Central nervous system toxicity induced by lidocaine. Report of a case in a patient with liver disease. JAMA 202:908, 1967.

21. Strong, J. M., Parker, M., and Atkinson, A. J., Jr.: Identification of glycinexylidide in patients treated with intravenous lidocaine. Clin. Pharmacol. Ther. 14:67, 1973.

22. Hjelm, M., and Holmdahl, M. H.: Biochemical effects of aromatic amines. II cyanosis, methemoglobinemia and heinz-body formation induced by a local anesthetic agent (prilocaine). Acta. Anaesthesiol. Scand. 2:99, 1965.

23. de Jong, R. H.: Physiology and Pharmacology of Local Anesthesia. Springfield, Illinois, Charles C Thomas, Publisher, 1977.

24. Hille, B.: Ionic basis of resting and action potential. In Handbook of the Nervous System, Vol. 1 of Physiology Series. Baltimore, Williams & Wilkins, 1976.

25. Hille, B.: Common mode of action of three agents that decrease the transient change in sodium permeability in nerves. Nature 210:1220, 1966.

26. Goldman, D. E., and Blaustein, H. P.: Ions, drugs, and the axon membrane. Ann. N.Y. Acad. Sci. 137:967, 1966.

27. Blaustein, M. P., and Goldman, D. E.: Action of anionic and cationic nerve-blocking agents: experiment and interpretation. Science 153:429, 1966.

28. Tucker, G. T., and Mather, L. E.: Absorption and disposition of local anesthetics: pharmacokinetics. In Cousins, M., and Bridenbaugh, P. O. (eds.): Neural Blockade in Clinical Anesthesia and Management of Pain. Philadelphia, J. B. Lippincott Co., 1980, p. 45.

29. Galindo, A., Hernandez, J., Benavides, O., et al.: Quality of spinal extradural anaesthesia: the influence of spinal nerve root diameter. Br. J. Anaesth. 47:41, 1975.

30. Takman, B. H.: The chemistry of local anaesthetic agents: classification of blocking agents. Br. J. Anaesth. 47:183, 1975.

31. Benoit, P. W., and Belt, W. D.: Destruction and regeneration of skeletal muscle after treatment with a local anesthetic, bupivacaine (Marcaine). J. Anat. 107:547, 1970.

32. Benoit, P. W., and Belt, W. D.: Some effects of local anesthetic agents on skeletal muscle. Exp. Neurol. 34:264, 1972.

33. Ravindran, R. S., Bond, V. K., Tasch, M. D., et al.: Prolonged neural blockade following regional analgesia with 2-chloroprocaine. Anesth. Analg. 59:447, 1980.

34. Moore, D. C., Spierdijk, J., VanKleef, J. D., et al.: Chloroprocaine neurotoxicity: four additional cases. Anesth. Analg. 61:155, 1982.

35. Reisner, L. S., Hochman, B. N., and Plumer, M. H.: Persistent neurologic deficit and adhesive arachnoiditis following intrathecal 2-chloroprocaine injection. Anesth. Analg. 59:452, 1980.

36. Ravindran, R. S., Turner, M. S., and Muller, J.: Neurologic effects of subarachnoid administration of 2-chloroprocaine–CE, bupivacaine, and low pH normal saline in dogs. Anesth. Analg. 61:279, 1982.

37. Wang, B. C., Spielholz, N. I., Hillman, D. E., et al.: Subarachnoid sodium bisulfite (the antioxideant in nesacaine) causes chronic neurologic deficit. Anesthesiology 57:194, 1982.

38. Verrill, P. J.: Adverse reactions to local anesthetic and vasoconstrictor drugs. Practitioner 214:380, 1975.

39. Stoelting, R. K.: Allergic reactions during anesthesia. Anesth. Analg. 62:341, 1983.

40. Brown, D. T., Beamish, D., and Wildsmith, J. A. W.: Allergic reaction to an amide local anesthetic. Br. J. Anaesth. 53:435, 1981.

41. Fisher, M. M.: Intradermal testing in the diagnosis of acute anaphylaxis during anaesthesia—results of five years experience. Anaesth. Intensive Care 7:58, 1979.

42. Incando, G., Schatz, M., Patterson, R., et al.: Administration of local anesthetics to patients with a history of prior adverse reaction. J. Allergy Clin. Immunol. 61:339, 1978.

43. Aldrete, J. A., and Johnson, D. A.: Evaluation of intracutaneous testing for investigation of allergy to local anesthetic agents. Anesth. Analg. 49:173, 1970.

44. Berry, C. A., Sanner, J. H., and Keasling, H. H.: A comparison of anticonvulsant activity of mepivacaine and lidocaine. J. Pharmacol. Exp. Ther. 133:357, 1961.

45. French, J. D., Livingston, R. B., and Konigsmark, B.: Experimental observations on the prevention of seizures by intravenous procaine injections. J. Neurosurg. 14:43, 1957.

46. Julien, R. M.: Lidocaine in experimental epilepsy: correlation of anticonvulsant effect with blood concentrations. J. Neurophysiol. 34:639, 1973.

47. Munson, E. S., Tucker, W. K., Ausinsch, B., et al.: Etidocaine, bupivacaine, and lidocaine seizure thresholds in monkeys. Anesthesiology 42:471, 1975.

48. Moore, D. C., Balfour, R. I., and Fitzgibbons, D.: Convulsive arterial plasma levels of bupivacaine and the response to diazepam therapy. Anesthesiology 50:454, 1979.

49. Yamashiro, H.: Bupivacaine-induced seizure after accidental intravenous injection, a complication of epidural anesthesia. Anesthesiology 47:472, 1977.

50. Moore, D. C., Mather, L. E., Bridenbaugh, P. O., et al.: Arterial and venous plasma levels of bupivacaine following epidural and intercostal nerve blocks. Anesthesiology 45:39, 1976.

51. Foldes, F. F., Molloy, R., McNall, P. G., et al.: Comparison of toxicity of intravenously given local anesthetic agents in man. JAMA 172:1493, 1960.

52. Scott, D. B.: Evaluation of the toxicity of local anesthetic agents in man. Br. J. Anaesth. 47:56, 1975.

53. Kozody, R., Ready, L. B., Barsa, J. E., et al.: Dose requirement of local anesthetic to produce grand mal seizure during stellate ganglion block. Can. Anaesth. Soc. J. 29:489, 1982.

54. Peng, A. T. C., Bufalo, J., and Blancato, L. S.: Rare complication during stellate ganglion block. A case report. Can. Anaesth. Soc. J. 17:640, 1970.

55. Harris, S. C.: Aspiration before injection of dental local anesthetics. J. Oral Surg. 15:299, 1957.

56. Aldrete, J. A., Nicholson, J., Sada, T., et al.: Cephalic kinetics of intra-arterially injected lidocaine. Oral Surg. 44:167, 1977.

57. Aldrete, J. A., Romo-Salas, F., Arora, S., et al.: Reverse arterial blood flow as a pathway for central nervous system toxic responses following injection of local anesthetics. Anesth. Analg. 57:428, 1978.

58. Aldrete, J. A., and Usubiaga, L. E.: New concepts of toxicity for local anesthetic agents. Regional Anesth. 4:6, 1979.

59. Scott, D. B., Jebson, P. J. R., Braid, D. B., et al.: Factors affecting plasma levels of lignocaine and prilocaine. Br. J. Anaesth. 44:1040, 1972.

60. Tucker, G. T., Moore, D. C., Bridenbaugh, P. O., et al.: Systemic absorption of mepivacaine in commonly used regional block procedures. Anesthesiology 37:277, 1972.

61. Eriksson, E., and Persson, A.: The effect of intravenously administered prilocaine and lidocaine on the human electroencephalogram studied by automatic frequency analysis. Acta Chir. Scand. (Suppl.) 358:37, 1966.

62. Usubiaga, J. E., Wikinski, J., Ferraro, R., et al.: Local anesthetic-induced convulsions in man: an electroencephalographic study. Anesth. Analg. 45:611, 1966.

63. Munson, E. S., Martucci, R. W., and Wagman, I. H.: Bupivacaine- and lignocaine-induced seizures in rhesus monkeys. Br. J. Anaesth. 44:1025, 1972.

64. Munson, E. S., Gutnick, M. J., and Wagman, I. H.: Local

anesthetic drug-induced seizures in rhesus monkeys. Anesth. Analg. 49:986, 1970.

65. deJong, R. H., Wagman, I. H., and Prince, D. A.: Effect of carbon dioxide on the cortical seizure threshold to lidocaine. Exp. Neurol. 17:221, 1967.

66. Englesson, S., and Matousek, M.: Central nervous system effects of local anesthetic agents. Br. J. Anaesth. 47:241, 1975.

67. deJong, R. H.: Toxic effects of local anesthetics. JAMA 239:1166, 1978.

68. Moore, D. L.: Intercostal nerve block for postoperative somatic pain following surgery of the thorax and upper abdomen. Br. J. Anaesth. 47:284, 1975.

69. Stewart, D. M., Rogers, W. P., Mahaffey, J. E., et al.: Effect of local anesthetics on the cardiovascular system of the dog. Anesthesiology 24:620, 1963.

70. Jorfeldt, L., Lofstrom, B., Pernow, B., et al.: The effect of mepivacaine and lidocaine on forearm resistance and capacitance vessels in man. Acta Anesthesiol. Scand. 14:183, 1970.

71. Dhuner, K. G., and Lewis, D. H.: Effect of local anesthetics and vasoconstrictors upon regional blood flow. Acta Anaesthesiol. Scand. (Suppl.) 23:347, 1966.

72. Albright, G. A.: Cardiac arrest following regional anesthesia with etidocaine or bupivacaine. Anesthesiology 51:285, 1979.

73. Liu, P., Feldman, H. S., Covino, B. M., et al.: Acute cardiovascular toxicity of intravenous amide local anesthetics in anesthetized ventilated dogs. Anesth. Analg. 61:317, 1982.

74. Kotelko, D. M., Dailey, P. A., Brizgys, R. V., et al.: Bupivacaine cardiotoxicity in adult sheep. Anesth. Analg. 62:268, 1983.

75. deJong, R. H., Ronfeld, R. A., and DeRosa, R. A.: Cardiovascular effects of convulsant and supraconvulsant doses of amide local anesthetics. Anesth. Analg. 61:3 1982.

76. Scott, D. B., and Cousins, M. B.: Clinical pharmacology of local anesthetic agents. In Cousins, M. J., and Bridenbaugh, P. O. (eds.): Neural Blockade in Clinical Anesthesia and Management of Pain. Philadelphia, J. B. Lippincott Co., 1980, p. 113.

77. Moore, D. C.: Administer oxygen first in the treatment of local anesthetic induced convulsions. Anesthesiology 53:346, 1980.

78. Moore, D. C., Crawford, R. D., and Scurlock, J. E.: Severe hypoxia and acidosis following local anesthetic-induced convulsions. Anesthesiology 53:259, 1980.

79. Moore, D. C., Thompson, G. R., and Crawford, R. D.: Long-acting local anesthetic drugs and convulsions with hypoxia and acidosis. Anesthesiology 56:230, 1982.

80. deJong, R. H., and Heavner, J. E.: Diazepam prevents local anesthetic seizures. Anesthesiology 34:523, 1971.

81. Moore, D. C., and Scurlock, J. E.: Possible role of epinephrine in prevention or correction of myocardial depression associated with bupivacaine. Anesth. Analg. 62:450, 1983.

82. Egbert, L. D., Battit, G., and Turndorf, H.: The value of preoperative visit by an anesthetist. JAMA 185:553, 1963.

83. Kennedy, W. F.: Preparation for neural blockade: the patient, block equipment, resuscitation, and supplementation. In Cousins, M. J., and Bridenbaugh, P. O. (eds.): Neural Blockade in Clinical Anesthesia and Management of Pain. Philadelphia, J. B. Lippincott Co., 1980, p. 135.

84. Greenblatt, G. M., and Denson, J. S.: Needle nerve stimulator-locator: nerve blocks with a new instrument for locating nerves. Anesth. Analg. 41:599, 1962.

85. Koons, R. A.: The use of the block-aid monitor and plastic intravenous cannulas for nerve blocks. Anesthesiology 31:290, 1969.

86. Wright, B. D.: A new use for the block-aid monitor. Anesthesiology 30:236, 1969.

87. Yasuda, I., Hirano, T., Ojima, T., et al.: Supraclavicular brachial plexus block using a nerve stimulator and an insulated needle. Br. J. Anaesth. 52:409, 1980.

88. Stevenson, T. R., Rodeheaver, G. T., Golden, G. T., et al.: Damage to tissue defenses by vasoconstrictors. JACEP 4:532, 1975.

89. Morris, T., and Tracey, J.: Lignocaine: its effects on wound healing. Br. J. Surg. 64:902, 1977.

90. Selander, D., Dhuner, K. G., and Lundborg, G.: Peripheral nerve injury due to injection needles used for regional anesthesia. An experimental study of the acute effects of needle point trauma. Acta Anaesthesiol. Scand. 21:182, 1977.

91. Selander, D., Edshage, S., and Wolff, T.: Paresthesia or no paresthesia? Nerve lesions after axillary blocks. Acta Anaesthesiol. Scand. 23:27, 1979.

92. Wooley, E. G., and Vandam, L.: Neurological sequelae of brachial plexus nerve block. Ann. Surg. 149:53, 1959.

93. Lanz, E., Theiss, D., and Jankovic, D.: The extent of blockade following various techniques of brachial plexus block. Anesth. Analg. 62:55, 1983.

94. Winnie, A. P.: Interscalene brachial plexus block. Anesth. Analg. 49:455, 1970.

95. Kulen-Kampf, D.: Anesthesia of the brachial plexus. Zentral bl Chir. 38:1337, 1911.

96. Winnie, A. P., and Collins, V. J.: The subclavian perivascular technique of brachial plexus anesthesia. Anesthesiology 25:353, 1964.

97. Hirschel, G.: Die anasthesierung des plexus brachialis bei operationen an der oberen extremitat. Munch. Med. Wochenschr. 58:1555, 1911.

98. Burnham, P. J.: Regional block of the great nerves of the upper arm. Anesthesiology 19:683, 1958.

99. Eather, K. F.: Axillary brachial plexus block (correspondence). Anesthesiology 19:683, 1958.

100. Winnie, A. P.: The perivascular techniques of brachial plexus anesthesia. In Hershey, S. G. (ed.): Refresher Courses in Anesthesiology. Philadelphia, J. B. Lippincott Co., 1974, p. 149.

101. Moore, D. C.: Complications of regional anesthesia. Clin. Anesth. 7:217, 1969.

102. Bonica, J. J.: The Management of Pain. Philadelphia, Lea & Febiger, 1953.

103. Ross, S., and Scarborough, C. D.: Total spinal anesthesia following brachial plexus block. Anesthesiology 39:458, 1973.

104. Berry, F. R., and Bridenbaugh, L. D.: The upper extremity: somatic blockade. In Cousins, M. J., and Bridenbaugh, P. O. (eds.): Neural Blockade in Clinical Anesthesia and Management of Pain. Philadelphia, J. B. Lippincott Co., 1980, p. 296.

105. Galindo, A.: Illustrated regional anesthesia. Miami, Regional Master Co. Scientific Publications, 1982.

106. deJong, R. H.: Axillary block of the brachial plexus. Anesthesiology 22:215, 1961.

107. Winnie, A. P.: An immobile needle for nerve blocks. Anesthesiology 31:577, 1969.

108. Winnie, A. P., Lavallee, D. A., Sosa, B. P., et al.: Clinical pharmacokinetics of local anesthetics. Can. Anaesth. Soc. J. 24:252, 1977.

109. Winnie, A. P., Tay, C., Patel, K. P., et al.: Pharmacokinetics of local anesthetics during plexus blocks. Anesth. Analg. 56:852, 1977.

110. Thompson, G. E., and Rorie, D. K.: Functional anatomy of the brachial plexus sheaths. Anesthesiology 59:117, 1983.

111. Rorie, D. K.: The brachial plexus sheath. Anat. Rec. 187:451, 1974.

112. Capan, L. M.: Anesthesia outside the operating room. Emergency Medicine 14:103, 1982.

113. Lofstrom, B.: Nerve block at the elbow. In Eriksson E. (ed.): Philadelphia, W. B. Saunders Company, 1979, p. 86.

114. Poulton, T. J., and Mims, G. R.: Peripheral nerve blocks. Am. Fam. Phys. 16:100, 1977.

115. Adriani, J.: Local and regional anesthesia for minor surgery. Surg. Clin. North Am. 31:1507, 1951.
116. Simon, R. R., and Brenner, B. E.: Anesthesia and regional blocks. *In* Simon, R. R., and Brenner, B. E. (eds.): Procedures and Techniques in Emergency Medicine. Baltimore, Williams & Wilkins, 1982.
117. Bryce-Smith, R.: Local analgesia of the limbs. *In* Lee, J. A., and Bryce-Smith, R. (eds.): Practical Regional Anesthesia. New York, Elsevier Science Publishing Co., Inc., 1976.
118. Lofstrom, B.: Nerve block at the elbow. *In* Eriksson, E. (ed.): Illustrated Handbook in Local Anesthesia, 2nd ed. Philadelphia, W. B. Saunders Company, 1979, p. 90.
119. Soutworth, J. L., Hingson, R. A., and Pitkin, W. M.: Conduction anesthesia of the extremities. *In* Pitkin's Conduction Anesthesia. Philadelphia, J. B. Lippincott Co., 1953, p. 644.
120. Burnham, P. J.: Regional block anesthesia for surgery of the fingers and thumb. Industrial Med. Surg. 27:67, 1958.
121. Rank, B. K., Wakefield, A. R., and Hueston, J. T.: Surgery of Repair as Applied to Hand Injuries. Edinburgh, Livingstone, 1973, p. 88.
122. Berry, F. R.: Analgesia in patients with fractured shaft of femur. Anaesthesia 32:576, 1977.
123. Winnie, A. P., Ramamurthy, S., and Durrani, Z.: The inguinal paravascular technique of lumbar plexus anesthesia. The "3 in 1 block." Anesth. Analg. 52:989, 1973.
124. Galindo, A.: Lower extremity blocks. *In* Galindo, A. (ed.): Illustrated Regional Anesthesia. Miami, Scientific Publications, 1982, p. 98.
125. Schurman, D. H.: Ankle-block anesthesia for foot surgery. Anesthesiology 44:348, 1976.
126. McCutcheon, R. M.: Regional anesthesia for the foot. Can. Anaesth. Soc. J. 12:465, 1965.
127. Murphy, T. M.: Somatic Blockade. *In* Cousins, M. J., and Bridenbaugh, P. O. (eds.): Neural Blockade in Clinical Anesthesia and Management of Pain. Philadelphia, J. B. Lippincott Co., 1980, p. 410.
128. Bohm, E.: Local anesthesia of the scalp. *In* Eriksson, E. (ed.): Illustrated Handbook in Local Anaesthesia, 2nd ed. Philadelphia, W. B. Saunders Company, 1980, p. 25.
129. Colley, P. S., and Heavner, J. E.: Blood levels of bupivacaine after injection into the scalp with and without epinephrine. Anesthesiology 54:81, 1981.
130. Alps, C., and Reynolds, F.: The effect of concentration on vasoactivity of bupivacaine and lignocaine. Br. J. Anaesth. 48:1171, 1976.
131. Jenkner, F. L.: Greater (and lesser) occipital nerve block. *In* Jenkner, F. L. (ed.): Peripheral Nerve Block. Springer-Verlag, New York, Inc., p. 100.
132. Delikan, A. E., Lee, C. K., Young, W. K., et al.: Postoperative local analgesia for thoractomy with direct bupivacaine intercostal blocks. Anaesthesia 28:561, 1973.
133. Bergh, W. P., Dottori, O., Axisonhof, B., et al.: Effect of intercostal block on lung function after thoracotomy. Acta Anesthesiol. Scand. 24 (Suppl.):85, 1966.
134. Bridenbaugh, B., Du Pen, S. L., Moore, D. C., et al.: Postoperative intercostal nerve block analgesia versus narcotic analgesia. Anesth. Analg. 52:81, 1973.
135. Engberg, G.: Single dose intercostal nerve block for pain relief after upper abdominal surgery. Acta Anaesthesiol. Scand. 60 (Suppl.):43, 1975.
136. Gibbons, J., James, O., and Quail, A.: Relief of pain in chest injury. Br. J. Anaesth. 45:1136, 1973.
137. Moore, D. C., and Bridenbaugh, L. D.: Intercostal nerve block in 4333 patients: indications, technique, and complications. Anesth. Analg. 41:1, 1962.
138. Moore, D. C., Mather, L. E., Bridenbaugh, L. D., et al.: Arterial and venous plasma levels of bupivacaine following peripheral nerve blocks. Anesth. Analg. 55:763, 1976.
139. Dhuner, K. G., and Lund, N.: Intercostal nerve blocks with etidocaine. Acta Anaesthesiol. Scand. 60 (Suppl.):39, 1975.
140. Cronin, K. D., and Davies, M. J.: Intercostal block for postoperative pain relief. Anaesth. Intensive Care 4:259, 1976.
141. Schulte-Steinberg, O.: Neural blockade for pediatric surgery. *In* Cousins, M. J., and Bridenbaugh, P. O. (eds.): Neural Blockade in Clinical Anesthesia and Management of Pain. Philadelphia, J. B. Lippincott Co., 1980, p. 521.
142. Rothstein, P., Arthur, G. R., Feldman, H., et al.: Pharmacokinetics of bupivacaine in children following intercostal block. Anesthesiology 57:A426, 1982.

Introduction

The clinical use of intravenous regional anesthesia has been well established[1-3] as a safe, quick, and effective alternative to general anesthesia in selected cases requiring surgical manipulation of the upper and lower extremities. Although often relegated to the operating room, the procedure is readily applicable to outpatient use. The author has found it useful in the emergency department to obtain, quickly and easily, complete anesthesia, along with muscle relaxation and a bloodless operating field. The procedure is free from the troublesome side effects associated with other regional blocks, such as the axillary block. The procedure is easily mastered and has a very low failure rate, and consistently good results can be expected.

The first practical use of analgesia associated with intravenous injection of a local anesthetic agent was described by August Gustav Bier in 1908.[4] Colbern[5] has since proposed the eponym "Bier Block." Although the procedure has been in existence for more than 60 years, the need for special equipment and a safe anesthetic agent has limited its use. Only recently has it gained wide acceptance as a safe and effective procedure, and currently several papers extol its virtues.[6-9] Although complications do exist, no reported fatalities directly attributed to the use of the Bier block are found in the medical literature. In this chapter, the techniques and complications are discussed according to their application in the emergency department.

Indications

Indications for intravenous regional anesthesia include any procedure of the arm or leg that requires operating anesthesia, muscle relaxation, or a bloodless field. The author has used the procedure for the reduction of fractures and dislocations, repair of major lacerations, the removal of foreign bodies, the débridement of burns, and the drainage of infection. The procedure may be carried out on a patient of any age who is able to cooperate with the physician.

Equipment

The equipment required for intravenous regional anesthesia consists of the following:
1 per cent lidocaine (Xylocaine), without epinephrine—to be diluted to a 1/2 per cent solution.
Sterile saline solution as a diluent
50 ml syringe / 18 gauge needle
Pneumatic tourniquet (single or double cuff)
No. 18 and No. 20 plastic IV catheter or a No. 21 butterfly needle

33

Intravenous Regional Anesthesia*

JAMES R. ROBERTS, M.D.

Elastic bandage / Webrill padding
500 ml D₅W (5 per cent dextrose in water) and intravenous extension tubing.

Procedure

The procedure should be explained in advance to the patient. If the patient is extremely apprehensive, premedication with diazepam (Valium) or a narcotic may be helpful but need not be routinely used. The only painful portions of the procedure are the establishment of the infusion catheter and the exsanguination procedure. The procedure should not be done on patients who are intoxicated or obtunded or on those with a previous reaction to a local anesthetic.

The patient need not be free of oral intake (NPO) for a specific period of time prior to the procedure. As a precaution, a large bore open intravenous line of 5 per cent dextrose in water is established in the unaffected extremity. Resuscitation equipment, including anticonvulsant drugs and oxygen, should be readily available.

The dosage of lidocaine is 3 mg/kg, and it is injected as a 0.5 per cent solution (1 per cent lidocaine is mixed with equal parts of sterile saline in a 50-ml syringe). Lidocaine with epinephrine should *not* be used. Plain lidocaine is also available as a 0.5 per cent solution and can be used to avoid the necessity of diluting the stronger solution.

A pneumatic tourniquet with cotton padding to prevent ecchymosis under the cuff is applied proximal to the pathology (Fig. 33–1). *It is strongly advised that one not use a regular blood pressure cuff,* because they often leak or rupture and are not designed to withstand high pressures for any length of time. A specially designed portable double cuff pneumatic system, such as marketed by OEC Zimmer Corporation, is ideal (Fig. 33–2).

The anesthetic is pre-mixed in the syringe. The tourniquet is inflated and a No. 20 gauge plastic catheter or a metal butterfly needle is placed in the superficial vein, as close to the pathology as possible, and is securely taped in place (Fig. 33–3).

*Reprinted with permission from Roberts, J. R.: Intravenous regional anesthesia. J.A.C.E.P. 6:261, 1977.

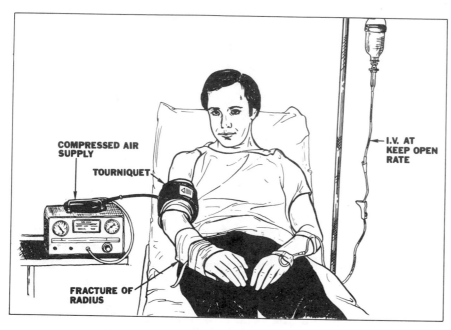

Figure 33–1. Preparation for induction of anesthesia in a patient with a fracture of the right radius. Note precautionary IV and deflated tourniquet in place. The procedure has been explained and pre-operative sedation or analgesia has been given if required. (From Roberts, J. R.: Intravenous Regional Anesthesia. JACEP 6:263, 1977. Used by permission.)

The hub remains on the catheter to avoid back bleeding or the syringe is attached to the butterfly tubing. This catheter will be the route of injection of the anesthetic agent.

The tourniquet is deflated, and the extremity is exsanguinated so that when the anesthetic agent is injected, it will fill the vascular system. Exsanguination may be accomplished by either of two methods. Simple elevation of the extremity for a few minutes may be adequate, but wrapping the extremity in a distal-to-proximal direction with an elastic bandage, being careful not to dislodge the infusion needle, will enhance the exsanguination (Fig. 33–4). Wrapping may be painful; this step can be eliminated if it causes too much anxiety to

the patient. If the wrapping procedure is not done, the extremity should be elevated for at least 3 minutes. During the wrapping procedure, care must be taken not to dislodge or infiltrate the infusion catheter.

With the extremity still elevated, the tourniquet is inflated to 250 mmHg, the arm is then placed by the patient's side, and the elastic exsanguination bandage is removed. In a child, the tourniquet is inflated to 50 mmHg above systolic pressure.

The 0.5 per cent lidocaine solution is then slowly injected into the infusion catheter at the calculated dose. Note that the solution is placed in the arm in which circulation is blocked, *not* in the precautionary keep-open IV on the unaffected side. At

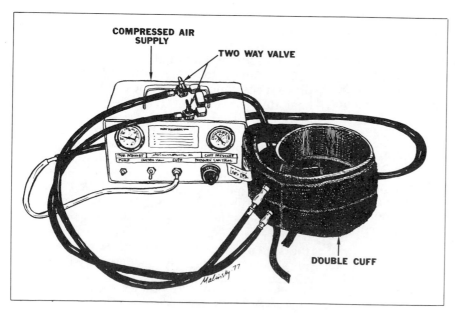

Figure 33–2. Double-cuff apparatus with two-way valves allows longer tourniquet time without pain. A standard blood pressure cuff should never be used. (From Roberts, J. R.: Intravenous Regional Anesthesia. JACEP 6:264, 1977. Used by permission.)

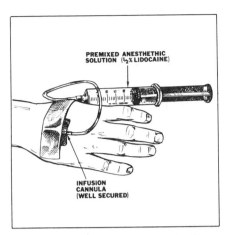

Figure 33–3. Infusion cannula securely taped in dorsum of hand. A butterfly needle is shown here, but a plastic catheter with the hub attached may also be used. (From Roberts, J. R.: Intravenous Regional Anesthesia. JACEP 6:263, 1977. Used by permission.)

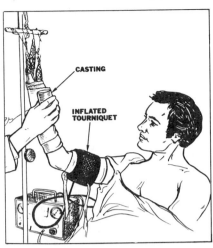

Figure 33–5. Cast is applied under anesthesia. Because the tourniquet is portable, post-reduction radiographs may be obtained without losing anesthesia. (From Roberts, J. R.: Intravenous Regional Anesthesia. JACEP 6:263, 1977. Used by permission.)

this point, blotchy areas of erythema may appear on the skin. This is not an adverse reaction to the anesthetic agent but merely the result of residual blood being displaced from the vascular compartment and it heralds success of the procedure.

In 3 to 5 minutes, the patient will experience paresthesia or warmth, beginning in the fingertips and traveling proximally, with final anesthesia occurring at the elbow. Complete anesthesia ensues in 5 to 10 minutes, followed by muscle relaxation. Then, the infusing needle is withdrawn and puncture site is tightly taped to prevent extravasation of the anesthetic agent. The surgical procedure or manipulation is performed, including postreduction x-ray films and casting or bandaging (see Fig. 33–5).

Anesthesia from a fingertip-to-elbow direction seems to occur irrespective of the site of anesthetic infusion, but selecting an injection site near the

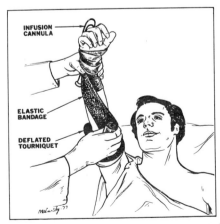

Figure 33–4. Exsanguination by elevation and elastic bandage. The tourniquet has yet to be inflated at this point. Care must be taken not to dislodge the infusion cannula. (From Roberts, J. R.: Intravenous Regional Anesthesia. JACEP 6:263, 1977. Used by permission.)

pathology will provide more rapid anesthesia at a lower dosage. If anesthesia is slow or inadequate, an extra 10–20 ml of *saline* solution may be injected to supplement the total volume of solution and to enhance the anesthesia. Additional anesthetic solution should *not* be infused.

Upon completion of the procedure, the deflation of the tourniquet is *cycled* to prevent a bolus effect of the lidocaine that may remain in the intravascular compartment. The cuff is deflated for 5 seconds and reinflated for 1 to 2 minutes. *This action is repeated three or four times.*

If the tourniquet has been in place for *less than 20–30 minutes*, it is dangerous to deflate it because adequate tissue fixation of the lidocaine probably has not occurred. This may result in a higher peak plasma lidocaine level with increased side effects. If the surgical procedure is completed rapidly, the tourniquet should remain inflated until a full 30 minutes has elapsed, and only then should it be deflated, using the cycling technique.

Sensation will return quickly when the tourniquet is removed, and in 5 to 10 minutes, the extremity will return to its preanesthetic level of sensation and function. After 20 minutes of observation, the patient is released (Table 33–1).

If the procedure takes longer than 20 or 30 minutes, many patients will complain of pain from the tourniquet because the tourniquet is not inflated over an anesthetized area. The use of a double-cuff tourniquet will alleviate the problem of pain under the cuff.

In the double-cuff system, there are two separate tourniquets placed side by side on the extremity. One is termed the *proximal cuff*, the other is called the *distal cuff*. The proximal cuff is inflated at the beginning of the procedure, and anesthesia is obtained under the deflated distal cuff. When

Table 33–1. IV REGIONAL ANESTHESIA—STEP-BY-STEP PROCEDURE

Begin intravenous line in uninvolved extremity.
Draw up 0.5 per cent lidocaine (3 mg/kg).
Place padded tourniquet, and inflate upper cuff.
Insert small plastic IV cannula near pathology, and secure.
Deflate tourniquet.
Elevate and exsanguinate extremity.
Inflate tourniquet (250 mmHg), and remove exsanguination device. Inflate the proximal cuff only, if a double-cuff system is used.
Infuse anesthetic solution.
Remove infusion needle, and tape site.
Perform procedure.
If pain is produced by the application of the tourniquet, first inflate the distal cuff, then deflate the proximal cuff.
After the procedure has been carried out, deflate the cuff for a few seconds, then reinflate it for 1 minute. Repeat three times. Do not deflate the cuff if total tourniquet time is less than 30 minutes.
Observe for possible reactions.

(From JACEP 6:264, 1977. Used by permission.)

the patient begins to feel pain under the proximal cuff, the distal cuff is first inflated over an already anesthetized area and the pain-producing proximal cuff is then deflated. One must be certain to inflate the distal cuff before the proximal cuff is released; otherwise, the anesthetic will rapidly diffuse into the general circulation.

Mechanism of Action

Some of the anesthesia is undoubtedly related to the ischemia produced by the tourniquet, but most of the anesthesia is secondary to the anesthetic agent itself. Although the exact mechanism by which anesthesia is produced is unknown, the site of action of the anesthetic may be at sensory nerve endings, neuromuscular junctions, or major nerve trunks.[10] Contrast studies have demonstrated that the anesthetic agent does not diffuse throughout the entire arm, yet anesthesia of the entire limb is obtained. For example, when the anesthetic agent is injected into the elbow and kept in that region with both distal and proximal tourniquets, anesthesia of the entire arm will develop.[11] Evidence indicates that the local anesthetic does not simply diffuse from the venous system into the tissue but travels via vascular channels directly inside the nerve. Regardless of where the anesthetic is infused, the fingertips are the first area to experience anesthesia, suggesting that the core of the nerve is in contact with the anesthetic agent initially. Following release of the tourniquet, a considerable amount of the drug still remains in the injected limb for at least 1 hour.[12] This would suggest that at least a portion of the anesthetic

leaves the vascular compartment and becomes tissue fixed.

Procedural Points

ANESTHETIC AGENT

One half per cent lidocaine at a dose of 3 mg/kg is the agent of choice. Other agents have been used without demonstrable benefits. In addition to lidocaine, bupivacaine, mepivacaine, prilocaine, etidocaine, chloroprocaine, and procaine have been used for the procedure.[13]

Dunbar and Mazze[7] showed that patients with intravenous regional anesthesia actually had significantly lower plasma–lidocaine concentrations than patients with axillary block or lumbar epidural anesthesia for similar procedures. Peak plasma concentrations are reached 2 to 3 minutes after deflation of the tourniquet, and side effects are minimal if the deflation is cycled following the surgical procedure.

Peak blood levels are directly related to the duration of vascular occlusion, to the concentration of the anesthetic, and to the specific agent used.[14, 15]

If the tourniquet is inflated for at least 30 minutes and the deflation–reinflation technique is used when the procedure is finished, plasma concentration of lidocaine should be approximately 2 to 4 mcg/ml, below the 5 to 10 mcg/ml level at which serious reactions occur.[7]

When equal amounts of lidocaine are used, the peak arterial plasma levels are 40 per cent lower when the 0.5 per cent solution is used than when the 1 per cent solution is used.[14] Some researchers have suggested that lower doses of lidocaine be used, but in my experience, anesthesia becomes less reliable and takes longer to take effect.

EXSANGUINATION

Exsanguination of the extremity prior to injection of the anesthetic agent is considered essential for success by many authors. Others do not believe that it is a critical factor. Exsanguination by simple elevation of the extermity should be done in all cases, but in certain cases, one should consider avoiding the painful wrapping of the extremity with an elastic or Esmarch bandage. A pneumatic splint, such as the type used for pre-hospital immobilization, is also a reasonable alternative to painful wrapping. The process of exsanguination is believed to allow for better vascular diffusion of the anesthetic.

SITE OF INJECTION

Anesthesia is usually obtained no matter where the local anesthetic is injected, but some evidence indicates that the procedure is more successful when the anesthetic is injected distally. For most cases, a vein in the dorsum of the hand or foot is most often used. If local pathology precludes the use of the hand, the antecubital fossa of the elbow is a good alternative.

Although most of the literature stresses the use of this technique on the upper extremity, it may also be used successfully in the leg. It cannot, however, be used for procedures above the knee. Tourniquet pain appears to be a limiting factor when the procedure is used on the leg. One must be certain to avoid damage to the peroneal nerve by using the tourniquet in the mid-calf area only.

Complications

Although intravenous regional anesthesia is both safe and simple, one should not be lulled into complacency, because complications do occur and are usually related to equipment failure or mistakes in the technique.

ANESTHETIC AGENT

Serious complications seldom occur if proper attention is paid to technique. Reactions to lidocaine are rare and are usually systemic reactions from high blood levels.[7, 16, 17] High levels may result from miscalculation of dosages, from too rapid release of the tourniquet before the anesthetic has become tissue-fixed ("bolus effect"), or rarely, from advancement of the infusion catheter proximal to the tourniquet, resulting in direct intravenous infusion.[16]

Generally, the central nervous system (CNS) effects of lidocaine are minor, resulting in mild reactions such as dizziness, lethargy, headache, or blurred vision. This should not occur in more than 2 to 3 per cent of patients and requires no treatment.[7] Convulsions may occur but are extremely rare.

In my experience, the most common complication relating to the anesthetic agent is systemic vascular absorption, which occurs when a blood pressure cuff explodes or slowly leaks, resulting in both loss of anesthesia and high blood levels.[18] Similar complications may occur if the cuff is deflated before 30 minutes following the induction of anesthesia. Both complications are the result of a bolus effect of the anesthetic, resembling an intravenous injection.

Van Neikerk[17] reported three seizures in a series of 1400 patients. Seizures are limited and are treated with oxygen and anticonvulsant drugs. Transient cardiovascular reactions, such as bradycardia and hypotension, are possible with large doses of lidocaine. Vasovagal reactions do occur. If resuscitation equipment is available and a precautionary intravenous line is started in the opposite arm, there should not be any serious side effects.

One case of cardiac arrest for 15 seconds, following the use of 200 mg of lidocaine was reported, but the actual clinical scenario may have described a vasovagal reaction rather than a true cardiac arrest.[19]

ADDITIONAL COMPLICATIONS

Thrombophlebitis can occur following intravenous administration of anesthetics, and the formation of insignificant amounts of methemoglobin with the use of prilocaine hydrochloride (Citanest) has been reported.[20]

A particularly bothersome problem has been the infiltration of the infusion catheter during exsanguination, resulting in tissue extravasation of the anesthetic agent. Also, there has been some back flow of anesthetic after the infusion needle has been removed. Both problems may result in poor anesthesia but may be minimized if a small, well-secured plastic infusion needle is used instead of a scalp vein needle and if the puncture site is tightly taped following withdrawal of the catheter.

This procedure cannot be used in manipulations or operations in which the pulse must be monitored as a guide to reduction, such as supracondylar fractures of the humerus, because the tourniquet occludes arterial flow. The use of the Bier Block in patients with sickle cell disease is not well documented in the medical literature. It should be used with caution until the ischemic effect of the tourniquet on the red blood cells of such patients has been clarified. In all patients the tourniquet time should not exceed 90 minutes. Ischemia for less than that amount of time is not associated with serious sequellae.

1. Holmes, C. M.: Intravenous regional analgesia: a useful method of producing anesthesia of the limbs. Lancet 1:245, 1963.
2. Bell, H. M., Slater, E. M., and Harris, W. H.: Regional anesthesia with intravenous lidocaine. JAMA 186:544, 1963.
3. Sorbie, C., Chacho, P. B.: Regional anesthesia by the intravenous route. Br. Med. J. 1:957, 1965.
4. Bier, A.: Ueber einen neuen weg Localanasthesia an den Gleidnassen zu erzevgen. Arch Klin Chir 86:1007, 1908.
5. Colbern, E. C.: Bier block. Anesth Analg 49:935, 1970.
6. Colbern, E. C.: Intravenous regional anesthesia: the perfusion block. Anesth Analg 45:69, 1966.
7. Dunbar, R. W., Mazze, R. I.: Intravenous regional anes-

thesia, experience with 779 cases. Anesth Analg 46:806, 1967.

8. Atkinson, P. I., Modell, J., and Moya, F.: Intravenous regional anesthesia. Anesth Analg 45:313, 1965.

9. Roberts, J. R.: Intravenous regional anesthesia—"Bier Block." Am. Fam. Phys. 17:123, 1978.

10. Raj, P. P.: Site of action of intravenous regional anesthesia. Regional Anesthesia 4:8, 1979.

11. Raj, P. P., Garcia, C. E., Burleson, J. W., et al.: The site of action of intravenous regional anesthesia. Anesth Analg 51:776, 1972.

12. Evans, C. J., Dewar, J. A., Boyes, R. N., et al.: Residual nerve block following intravenous regional anesthesia. Br. J. Anaesth. 46:668, 1974.

13. Katz, J.: Choice of agents for intravenous regional anesthesia. Regional Anesthesia 4:10, 1979.

14. Tucker, G. T., and Boas, R. A.: Pharmacokinetic aspects of intravenous regional anesthesia. Anesthesiology 34:538, 1971.

15. Covino, B. G.: Pharmacokinetics of intravenous regional anesthesia. Regional Anesthesia 4:5, 1979.

16. Clinical Anesthesia Conference. NY State J. Med. 66:1344, 1966.

17. Van Niekerk, J. P., de V, Tonkin, P. A.: Intravenous regional analgesia. S. Afr. Med. J. 40:165, 1966.

18. Roberts, J. R.: Intravenous regional anesthesia. JACEP 6:261, 1977.

19. Kennedy, B. R., Duthie, A. M., Parbrook, G. D., et al.: Intravenous regional anesthesia: an apprasial. Br. Med. J. 5440:954, 1965.

20. Mazze, R. I.: Methemoglobin concentrations following intravenous regional anesthesia. Anesth Analg 47:122, 1968.

34

Nitrous Oxide Analgesia

DAVID J. DULA, M.D.

an analgesic and anesthetic agent has gained support both in the operating room and in dental suites. Most recently, the gas has been used effectively in emergency departments in Great Britain and the United States as an analgesic agent. Within the last 10 years, nitrous oxide has also become popular in the prehospital care setting for relief of pain.[3] The emergence of nitrous oxide as an effective analgesic agent for use in the emergency department has been one of the most significant advances in pain control in some time.

Introduction

Pain control is an important aspect of emergency medicine. Patients often present to the emergency department because of pain, and many diagnostic and therapeutic maneuvers that are performed in the emergency department cause pain. A wide variety of analgesic agents are available, and the advantages and disadvantages of each agent should be considered. Ideally, an analgesic for emergency department use would be one that has a rapid onset of action and clears quickly when the drug is stopped. The drug should also be safe, effective, easy to use, and compatible with other analgesic agents. A drug with these characteristics would have the obvious benefit of relieving a patient's pain during the emergency department encounter while leaving the individual in a suitable state for safe discharge from the department, signing consent forms for surgery, or evaluation by other services without obtundation from the analgesic.

An agent that possesses all these characteristics is nitrous oxide.[1] This gas was first described by Humphrey Davey in 1797, who investigated its use for the control of tuberculosis.[2] Since the discovery of the gas, the use of nitrous oxide as

Pharmacology

Nitrous oxide has been used in the anesthesia suite for over 130 years and has proved to be an extremely safe agent. It is a colorless and slightly sweet-smelling gas. Nitrous oxide is highly soluble in plasma, approximately 30 times more soluble than nitrogen. Nitrous oxide does not bind to the hemoglobin molecule and does not produce sickling in sickle cell patients. The gas is not metabolized; it is excreted by the lungs. The effects of nitrous oxide on organ systems other than the central nervous system are quite limited. There are no known direct toxic effects of the gas on any tissue or organ system.

The heart and the cardiovascular system are not significantly affected by nitrous oxide analgesia. Data obtained during cardiac catheterization have shown that no clinically significant changes in cardiac output, heart rate, or cardiac rhythm occur during nitrous oxide administration.[4]

In the absence of underlying hypoxemia or hypercarbia, nitrous oxide does not produce any significant effects in blood pressure, venous pressure, peripheral vascular resistance, or blood volume. Minor cutaneous venous dilation may occur, producing a flushed appearance.[5,6]

The respiratory system is not directly affected by nitrous oxide. No change in bronchomotor tone occurs, secretions are not stimulated, and ciliary action is not depressed.

Inhalation of nitrous oxide produces a rapid effect on the central nervous system. Cortical function is rapidly depressed, and all modalities of sensation are affected, as evidenced by a decrease in the senses of hearing, taste, and smell and a decreased sensitivity to touch, temperature, pressure, and pain. Subcortical areas are affected to a less significant degree, and the body is still able to maintain normal temperature control and a normal respiratory drive. The sensitivity of the larynx is not significantly depressed, and the cough and gag reflexes are not notably altered. The risk of regurgitation from stimulation of the vomiting center is not clinically significant. Roberts and Wignal[7] recently demonstrated that children sedated with nitrous oxide for dental procedures maintained an intact laryngeal reflex and did not demonstrate aspiration during analgesia.

The effects on the central nervous system can vary from euphoria to early levels of anesthesia, depending upon the percentage of nitrous oxide delivered. Analgesic effects on skin and bone occur with concentrations of 35 to 80 per cent nitrous oxide.[8] The gas produces an effect on the central nervous system within 1 to 2 minutes.

Inhalation of 50 per cent nitrous oxide and 50 per cent oxygen has been reported to deliver an analgesic effect equal to that of 10 to 20 mg of intravenous morphine, although clinically all patients may not obtain this level of analgesia. Continued administration of the gas will not increase the analgesic effect, and in fact a mild tolerance may develop. Maximal analgesia is obtained within 5 minutes of continuous inhalation. In addition to its analgesic effect, nitrous oxide will produce an amnesic or dissociative effect, which may leave the patient unaware of any pain that he may have experienced while under the influence of nitrous oxide. A number of studies have shown that administration of 50 per cent nitrous oxide relieves pain completely 39 to 50 per cent of the time, partially in 35 to 36 per cent of patients, and not at all in 15 to 26 per cent of cases.[1,5,9,10] Because of the subjective nature of pain and accompanying anxiety, nitrous oxide may afford little or no relief in some patients while producing significant analgesia in others.

Danger to Medical Personnel. Measures to limit contamination of the emergency department with nitrous oxide are in order, since the side effects attributed to *chronic* exposure to nitrous oxide include increased risks of spontaneous abortion, liver ailments, and neurologic problems.[11–15]

For male dentists who were chronically exposed to low levels of nitrous oxide, the incidence of liver disease in one report[16] was increased 1.7-fold, that of kidney disease was increased 1.2-fold, and that of neurologic disease was elevated 1.9-fold. The incidence of spontaneous abortion was increased 1.5-fold among wives of male dentists exposed to nitrous oxide. In female dental assistants who were exposed to nitrous oxide, the incidence of liver disease was increased 1.6-fold, that of kidney disease was increased 1.7-fold, and that of neurologic disease was elevated 2.8-fold. The incidence of spontaneous abortions among chronically exposed female dental assistants was increased 2.3-fold. Layzer[17] reported a polyneuropathy in 15 patients exposed chronically to nitrous oxide.

Whereas these adverse effects of chronic exposure to low levels of nitrous oxide have been noted in operating suite and dental personnel, the incidence of harmful consequences should be lower in emergency department personnel because the gas is used less frequently in the emergency department. At high concentrations, some psychomotor effects may occur in persons administering or working around the gas. These effects are not usually a concern unless high levels of contamination (500 ppm or greater) are experienced by the workers. These side effects have encouraged the National Institute for Occupational Safety and Health (NIOSH) to establish guidelines for the safe use of nitrous oxide in the hospital setting. In the operating suite it is recommended that the spill-over of the gas not exceed 25 ppm; the recommended limit for dental suites is 50 ppm.[19,20] Guidelines for emergency department use have not been established; however, levels of 300 to 500 ppm have been noted in emergency department treatment rooms after 4 to 8 minutes of nitrous oxide use (Fig. 34–1).[21] With the current development of the scavenger device (a unit that vents expired nitrous oxide gas to the outside environment), levels in the emergency department can be kept as low as 10 ppm (Fig. 34–2).

Nitrous oxide analgesia during ambulance transport without an exhaust system for the cabin area results in nitrous oxide levels of 650 to 1700 ppm

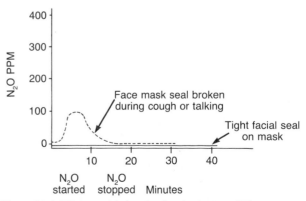

Figure 34–1. Nitrous oxide levels after 8 minutes of Nitronox use with scavenger in operation.

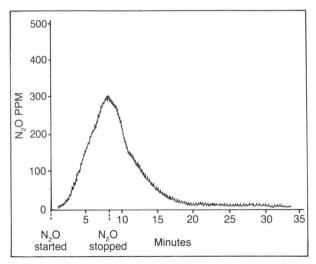

Figure 34–2. Nitrous oxide levels after 8 minutes of Nitronox use in a 16′ × 14′ × 10′ room without scavenger.

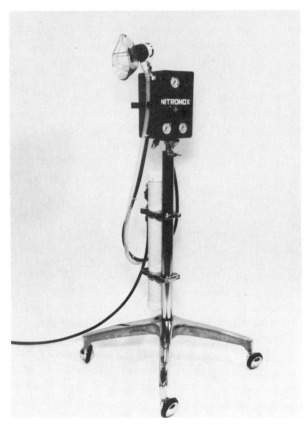

Figure 34–3. Nitronox unit.

with a top concentration of 7500 ppm. Use of a local exhaust system to vent expired gases to the outside environment, however, has reduced ambulance levels to less than 25 ppm.[22] Since nitrous oxide is heavier than air, it collects near the floor, making it more of a hazard in the ambulance than in a full-sized room.

Equipment

Two basic units are available for the administration of nitrous oxide analgesia in the emergency department. The Entonox machine (Canadian Oxygen Limited) is designed to administer nitrous oxide and oxygen from a single tank containing an equal mixture of oxygen and nitrous oxide. The concentration that is delivered is 50 per cent nitrous oxide and 50 per cent oxygen. There is one disadvantage to use of the Entonox in ambulances for prehospital care: Nitrous oxide is heavier than oxygen, and when the two gases are mixed in one tank, the nitrous oxide tends to settle at the bottom of the tank, especially in cold temperatures. When this occurs, the potential hazard is that the patient may breathe pure nitrous oxide when the tank is nearly empty. This is of concern only in cold environments and poses no significant threat when the device is used in the emergency department.

The other apparatus used to administer nitrous oxide is the Nitronox unit (Frazer Harlake Inc.—Fig. 34–3). This machine has two separate tanks that contain nitrous oxide and oxygen. The gases are mixed in a 50:50 concentration just before they are inhaled. The mixture can be delivered at up to 140 liters per minute.

The gas mixture in both machines is self-administered. The patient must create a tight seal between the face and the mask while inhaling to allow the demand valve to open and release the gas to the patient. Approximately 2 cm H_2O of negative pressure is required to open the delivery valve; the demand valve prevents continued escape of the gas when the patient is not inhaling. This allows patients who become overly sedated to break the tight seal and thus stop breathing the gas.

In the Nitronox machine, an oxygen fail-safe mechanism automatically stops the flow of nitrous oxide in the system when the oxygen supply is depleted. In the event of nitrous oxide depletion, the unit provides 100 per cent oxygen at a reduced maximum flow rate of 70 liters per minute. Oxygen reference pressure provides automatic oxygen enrichment at very shallow breathing rates. Dual diaphragms used throughout the system prevent internal mixing of gas in the event of diaphragm leakage. Connections for hookups to each gas supply are indexed to prevent improper mixing of oxygen and nitrous oxide tanks. A mixture pressure alarm provides an audible signal in event of valve seat leakage. With the development of a scavenger device, exhaled gases can be vented to the outside atmosphere, preventing the buildup of excessive levels of nitrous oxide in the emergency department (Figs. 34–4 and 34-5).

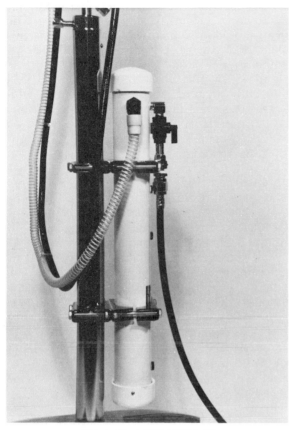

Figure 34–4. Scavenger unit.

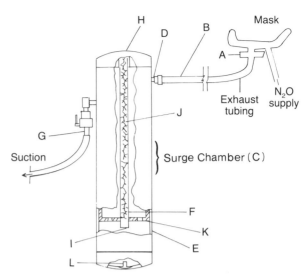

Figure 34–5. Schematic diagram of Nitronox scavenger.

1. All exhaled gases are diverted to the scavenger system by means of a special collector ring (A) fitted over the Nitronox demand valve.

2. Exhaled gases pass through the scavenger hose (B) and enter the scavenger surge chamber (C) at point D.

3. The surge chamber (C) is composed of a large-diameter outer tube (E) and a smaller-diameter inner tube (F).

4. The outer tube (E) is connected at point G to the central suction supply of the hospital.

5. The inner tube (F) is open at one end (H) to the atmosphere, and the other end (I) is open to the outer tube (E). The inner tube is filled with polyurethane cell foam (J) and is separated from the outer tube by a perforated disk (K).

6. In normal operation, exhaled gases enter the outer tube surge chamber at point D, and are exhausted through G. The surge chamber has a capacity of 1.6 liters. Should the exhaled gas rate be less than the suction rate applied to the surge chamber, atmospheric air will be entrained into the chamber through H. This atmospheric gas path, however, is through the foam (J), through the baffle (K), and then out through the outlet (G). Consequently, the preferential gas passage is always the path from patient inlet point (D) to outlet (G).

7. Any condensed water vapor is eliminated from the surge chamber through a drain valve (L).

Both of the units are available in an ambulance model for administration of nitrous oxide gas in the prehospital care setting. The in-hospital unit is available as either a portable model, which has a stand on wheels and uses "D" size cylinder tanks, or a wall-mounted unit, which is supplied by standard wall outlets for nitrous oxide and oxygen.

The maximum concentration of nitrous oxide that can be delivered with both Entonox and Nitronox equipment is 50 per cent for the sea level units and 65 per cent for the high-altitude models. At the maximum concentration, the patient may become slightly sedated but does not become unconscious. One must always administer nitrous oxide with at least 30 per cent oxygen to avoid hypoxia. Experience with nitrous oxide administered at higher elevations (specifically 5000 feet above sea level or higher) has indicated that a 50:50 mixture may be inadequate to produce a significant analgesic effect. For this reason, emergency department use at high altitudes may require a higher percentage of nitrous oxide. A 65 per cent nitrous oxide and 35 per cent oxygen mixture has been found to be effective at this higher altitude.[23]

Indications

There are many indications for nitrous oxide use in the emergency department. Any painful procedure or manipulation that requires the use of short-term analgesia would be ideal for nitrous oxide administration. Nitrous oxide can be used alone or as an adjunct to standard narcotic analgesics, such as meperidine or morphine, to provide an additive analgesic effect. When multiple analgesics are used, it is best to begin with nitrous oxide alone and judiciously add small increments of intravenous narcotics if necessary. Nitrous oxide may be supplemented with small doses of intravenous diazepam (Valium) in instances in which relaxation is required, such as for the reduction of a dislocated shoulder or hip. In addition to its use for clinical procedures, nitrous oxide may be administered for its clinical analgesic effect in cases of musculoskeletal trauma, myocardial infarction, or thermal burns.

Nitrous oxide is most useful in providing analgesia in clinical situations in which a consistent level of pain is present. The gas is less beneficial in instances in which acute pain is present for a short period. Therefore, the greatest benefit from nitrous oxide is obtained in the relief of pain from dressing changes, burn debridement, myocardial infarction, undiagnosed abdominal pain, skeletal and soft tissue trauma, thermal burns, and controlled orthopedic reductions. Nitrous oxide is useful, but to a lesser degree, in procedures that inflict acute pain for short periods, such as fracture reduction or abscess incision. The analgesia obtained with the gas is useful for anxiety reduction during culdocentesis, peritoneal lavage, or a painful pelvic examination. The gas is not a substitute for narcotic analgesia in instances such as renal colic or diagnosed acute appendicitis or biliary colic, nor is it designed to take the place of local anesthetics in suturing or abscess drainage. Patients may appear to be in pain during the use of nitrous oxide, but often they do not remember the procedure despite complaints of pain at the time.

Cautions

It is wise to have the nitrous oxide machine periodically inspected for leaks with a nitrous oxide analyzer. Leaking nitrous oxide gas may contaminate the emergency department even though the machine is not in use. Measures to limit the overuse of nitrous oxide in the emergency department are also important, since the longer the gas is administered the more contamination will occur. For this reason, we limit the use of the gas to a short period (10 to 15 minutes) in order to decrease the contamination of the emergency department.

Diffusion Hypoxia. During general anesthesia with high concentrations of nitrous oxide (greater than 50 per cent), some patients may become relatively hypoxic after the discontinuation of nitrous oxide administration. This is caused by an effect termed diffusion hypoxemia. The nitrous oxide diffuses from the blood stream into the alveolar spaces when the gas is discontinued. This results in a dilution of the oxygen content in the alveoli producing a relative hypoxic alveolar environment, which may be reflected as hypoxemia. In normal patients, this presents no significant hazard; however, in patients with underlying medical conditions that may predispose to a hypoxic state, diffusion hypoxia may be a potential cause of problems. One can prevent this situation from developing by providing 100 per cent oxygen to the high-risk patient for a few minutes after the nitrous oxide is discontinued. Diffusion hypoxia with a 50:50 mixture of oxygen and nitrous oxide

(which is used in the emergency department) may be of theoretic concern only, since 50 per cent oxygen should prevent any significant hypoxemia. Baskett and coworkers[24] demonstrated that the average arterial partial pressure of oxygen (Pa_{O_2}) with the 50:50 mixture is 210 mm Hg. This is significantly higher than the Pa_{O_2} obtained while the patient is breathing room air and even higher than is routinely obtained while the patient is breathing oxygen at 5 liters per minute through a nasal cannula.

Other Side Effects. Other minor side effects of nitrous oxide analgesia experienced by patients are tinnitus and vertigo (Table 34–1). These are self-limiting and resolve once the gas is discontinued. Some of the subjective effects, such as dizziness and paresthesias, may be partially related to hyperventilation. Some patients may experience unpleasant hallucinations, dysphoria, or a panic reaction. The patients with chronic obstructive pulmonary disease, who are carbon dioxide retainers, may experience hypercarbia if their hypoxic drive is diminished by the 50 per cent oxygen concentration delivered with the nitrous oxide. Nausea, giddiness, voice change, and laughing out loud are other minor side effects that are occasionally encountered.

Contraindications

When used properly, nitrous oxide is safe and is not accompanied by significant complications. In the emergency department, the gas is used in relatively low concentrations and for very short periods when compared with general anesthesia. Many of the contraindications discussed in this section (Table 34–2) are theoretic and have been gleaned from the anesthesia literature. There have been relatively few reports of serious side effects from Nitronox or Entonox in outpatient use.

Nitrous oxide analgesia is contraindicated in patients who are unable to hold the mask to their faces for self-administration of the gas because of facial trauma, obtundation, or musculoskeletal injury (Fig. 34–6). Patients with head trauma should not receive nitrous oxide, since there may be an

Table 34–1. SIDE EFFECTS OF NITROUS OXIDE ANALGESIA

Drowsiness
Giddiness
Nausea
Amnesia
Paresthesias
Dizziness or vertigo
Dysphoria or panic
Voice change
Laughing out loud

Table 34–2. CONTRAINDICATIONS TO
NITROUS OXIDE ANALGESIA

Head trauma
Facial trauma
Decreased level of consciousness
Pneumothorax
Intestinal obstruction
Middle ear pathologic condition
Combative patient
Patient too young to self-administer the gas
Significant obstructive lung disease
Pregnant patient or medical personnel
Conditions requiring prolonged or potent
  analgesia

increase in intracranial pressure associated with nitrous oxide use in patients with intracranial mass lesions. Furthermore, nitrous oxide should not be used for sedating an unruly patient, since such patients cannot self-administer the gas; hence, they may receive an excessive amount or their underlying injuries may be masked. Intoxicated patients also may become excessively obtunded from the gas.

Because nitrous oxide is so highly soluble, it will diffuse rapidly into any gas-filled structure until it reaches equilibrium with the inspired gas. Therefore, a pneumothorax or an intestinal obstruction may be increased in size if nitrous oxide is administered. It has been estimated that a pneumothorax may double in size in 10 minutes while the patient is breathing 70 per cent nitrous oxide, and intestinal gas may double in volume in 2 hours while the patient is breathing similar concentrations.[25] Recent reports indicate that the volume of air in a Swan-Ganz catheter balloon may double and pre-

dispose to balloon rupture if nitrous oxide is given during anesthesia.[26] Tympanic membranes have been reported to rupture (from a build-up of nitrous oxide in the middle ear with an occluded eustacian tube) following nitrous oxide anesthesia, and the gas should probably not be used in patients with a significant middle ear pathologic condition.[27] The high oxygen content associated with outpatient nitrous oxide analgesia makes significant obstructive lung disease a relative contraindication.

Fetal abnormalities have been detected in animals exposed to nitrous oxide. Although the exact effect on human pregnancy is unknown at this time, it is generally recommended that nitrous oxide not be given to pregnant patients, and pregnant medical personnel should not be exposed to the exhaled gas.

Patients who are too young to self-administer the gas should not be given this form of analgesia in the emergency department. Griffin and associates[28] describe a technique using a nasal inhaler for facilitating minor pediatric surgery. Such a technique requires a more elaborate system and continuous patient monitoring.

Although nitrous oxide is useful for supplemental analgesia, in cases of severe clinical pain, such as renal colic, a fractured hip, or biliary colic, it is best to opt for standard narcotic analgesics when the diagnosis is made and the patient is awaiting admission to the hospital or the operating suite.

Procedure

Nitrous oxide may be used routinely without the need for cardiac monitoring or a precautionary intravenous line. If adjunctive narcotics, muscle relaxants, or sedatives are used, resuscitation equipment should be available. The gas should be administered in a well-ventilated room or, preferably, with the use of a scavenger device. Both Entonox and Nitronox equipment are applicable to emergency department use. The features of the Nitronox apparatus are detailed here because this device is more popular in the United States.

The Nitronox machine is easily and quickly set up for use in the emergency department. The supply tanks of oxygen and nitrous oxide must be turned on (open pressure valve on the tanks) to allow a supply of gas to the machine. After this is done, one should check the pressure gauges to ensure that the nitrous oxide pressure line and the oxygen pressure line are reading in the green bands. This indicates proper pressure in the nitrous and oxygen lines. For models with a scavenger, the vacuum hose should be attached to wall suction.

The patient must be instructed on the use of the device and the effects that he will feel. The need

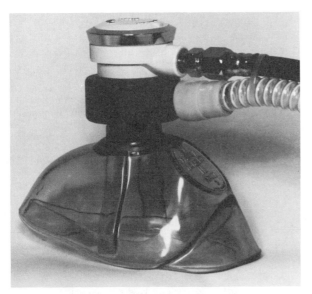

Figure 34–6. Example of face mask, which must be held in contact with the face by the patient.

to create and maintain a tight facial seal during both normal inspiration and normal expiration should be emphasized. The patient should be informed that in approximately 2 minutes he will begin to feel the effects of the gas. The effects are not unpleasant but make the patient feel a bit drowsy and will diminish the pain. One should explain to the patient that if at any time he becomes frightened or feels that he is receiving too much analgesic effect, he should simply remove the mask from his face and breathe room air. Within a minute or so he will begin to "lighten up" and feel normal. When the pain again becomes too severe, the patient should start to breathe the gas again. Thus, the patient can titrate the level of analgesia that he receives from the nitrous oxide. At no time should an assistant hold the mask to the patient's face; *the gas is always self-administered and self-titrated.* The physician or nurse should allow the patient to breathe the gas from approximately 1 to 3 minutes to ensure an appropriate analgesic effect before a clinical procedure is performed. When the procedure is completed, the patient should be instructed to stop breathing the nitrous oxide; within 1 to 3 minutes, the clinical effects of the gas will wear off. At this point, additional analgesics may be ordered if necessary.

Limitations of Nitrous Oxide Analgesia

Nitrous oxide can induce mild to moderate analgesia in the context of outpatient therapy. The gas does not produce the profound or prolonged analgesia required for pain relief in certain operative conditions or for such conditions as renal colic. The analgesia can be enhanced through the judicious use of adjunctive intravenous narcotics, but the addition of these agents negates some of the advantages of inhalation analgesia. One should not overestimate the analgesic potential of nitrous oxide nor eschew the more conventional use of local anesthetics or narcotic analgesics.

The portable machines are convenient, but explanation of the procedure is somewhat time-consuming. Reassurance and "verbal anesthesia" are required in many cases to enhance the analgesic effect. Although the gas is self-administered and self-titrated, patients should be kept under observation by emergency department personnel during its use. An empty stomach is not a strict requirement for nitrous oxide use, but the gas should not be given to a patient who has just eaten. There is a small but real potential for staff abuse of the gas, but the fact that the machine is kept in full view without the use of keys or storage cabinets minimizes the incidence. At this time the actual risk to medical personnel who are subject

to chronic low-dose exposure to nitrous oxide in the emergency department is unknown, but it is suggested that reasonable precautions to limit exposure be instituted.

1. Flomenbaum, N., and Gallagher, E. J.: Self administration of nitrous oxide in an analgesic. JACEP 8:95, 1979.
2. Rosenberg, H., Orkin, F. K., and Springstead, J.: Abusive nitrous oxide. Anesth. Analg. 58:104, 1979.
3. Amey, B. D., Ballinger, J. A., and Harrison, E. E.: Prehospital administration of nitrous oxide for control of pain. Ann. Emerg. Med. 10:247, 1981.
4. Wynne, J., et al.: Hemodynamic effects of nitrous oxide administered during cardiac catheterization. JAMA 243:1440, 1980.
5. Churchill-Davidson, H. C. (ed.): Wylie and Churchill-Davidson: A Practice of Anesthesia, 4th ed. Philadelphia, W. B. Saunders Co., 1978, pp. 240–247.
6. Collins, V. J.: Principles of Anesthesiology, 2nd ed. Philadelphia, Lea & Febiger, 1976.
7. Roberts, G. J., and Wignall, B. K.: Efficacy of the laryngeal reflex during oxygen–nitrous oxide sedation. Br. J. Anaesth. 54:1277, 1982.
8. Allen, G. D.: Dental Anesthesia and Analgesia, 2nd ed. Baltimore, Williams & Wilkins, 1979.
9. Thompson, P. L., and Lawn, B.: Nitrous oxide as an analgesic in acute myocardial infarction. JAMA 235:924, 1976.
10. Thal, E. R., et al.: Self-administered analgesia with nitrous oxide. JAMA 242:2418, 1979.
11. Virtue, R. W., Escobar, A., and Modell, J.: Nitrous oxide levels in the operating room air with various gas flows. Can. Anaesth. Soc. J. 26:313, 1979.
12. Nitrous oxide hazards. FDA Drug Bulletin, 10:15, 1980.
13. Nevins, M. A.: Neuropathy after nitrous oxide abuse. JAMA 244:2264, 1980.
14. Cohen, E. N., Brown, B. W., and Wu, M.: Anesthetic health hazards in the dental operatory. Anesthesiology 52:524, 1979.
15. Witcher, C., Zimmerman, D. C., and Piziali, R. L.: Control of occupational exposure to nitrous oxide in the oral surgery office. J. Oral Surg. 36:431, 1978.
16. Cohen, E. N., et al.: Occupational disease in dentistry and chronic exposure to trace anesthetic cases. J. Am. Dent. Assoc. 101:21, 1980.
17. Layzer, R. B.: Myeloneuropathy after prolonged exposure to nitrous oxide. Lancet 2:1227, 1978.
18. Ayer, W. A., Russel, E. A., Jr., and Burge, J. R.: Psychomotor responses of dentists using nitrous oxide-oxygen psychosedation. Anesth. Prog. 25:85, 1978.
19. Criteria for Recommended Standard, Occupational Exposure to Waste Anesthetic Gases and Vapors. U.S. Department of Health, Education and Welfare, Public Health Service, Centers for Disease Control, National Institute for Occupational Safety and Health, March 1977.
20. Whitcher, C.: Control of occupational exposure to nitrous oxide in the dental operatory. DHEW Publication 77–171. Cincinnati, U.S. Department of Health, Education and Welfare, Public Health Service, Centers for Disease Control, National Institute for Occupational Safety and Health, Division of Surveillance, Hazard Evaluation and Field Studies, April 1977.
21. Dula, D. J., Skiendzielewski, J. J., and Royko, M.: Nitrous oxide levels in the emergency department. Ann. Emerg. Med. 10:575, 1981.
22. Aucker, K., Halldeni, M., and Gothe, C. J.: Nitrous oxide analgesia during ambulance transportation. Acta Anaesthesiol. Scand. 24:497, 1980.
23. Nieto, J. M., and Rosen, P.: Nitrous oxide at higher elevations. Ann. Emerg. Med. 9:610, 1980.

24. Baskett, P. J. F., Eltringham, R. J., and Bennett, J. A.: An assessment of the oxygen tensions obtained with premixed 50 per cent nitrous oxide and oxygen mixture used for pain relief. Anesthesia 28:449, 1973.

25. Eger, E. J., and Saidman, L. T.: Hazards of nitrous oxide anesthesia in bowel obstruction and pneumothorax. Anesthesiology 26:61, 1965.

26. Eisenkraft, J. B., and Eger, E. I.: Nitrous oxide anesthesia may double the balloon gas volume of Swan-Ganz catheters. Mt. Sinai J. Med. (N.Y.) 49:430, 1982.

27. Perreault, L., Normandin, N., Plamondon, L., et al.: Tympanic membrane rupture after anesthesia with nitrous oxide. Anesthesiology 57:325, 1982.

28. Griffin, G. C., Campbell, V. D., and Jones, R.: Nitrous oxide–oxygen sedation for minor surgery: Experience in a pediatric setting. JAMA 245:2411, 1981.

5

GENERAL SURGERY

35

Principles of Wound Management

RICHARD L. LAMMERS, M.D.

Introduction

Nearly 10 million patients with traumatic wounds present to emergency centers in the United States each year.[1] To many physicians managing these injuries, the concept of wound care is synonymous with the technique of wound closure; it is assumed that healing will follow. Primary wound healing, however, is not an inevitable process. For centuries, victims of wounds commonly experienced inflammation, infection, and extreme scarring; in fact, these processes were considered part of normal wound repair. Only 100 years ago did surgeons first realize that sepsis could be separated from healing.[2]

The primary goal of wound care is not the technical repair of the wound; it is providing optimal conditions for the natural reparative processes of the wound to proceed.[2] Investigators have found that physicians' attempts to repair the wound are sometimes at odds with the body's attempt to heal the injury. Lister applied phenol to wounds as an antiseptic and in so doing caused extensive tissue necrosis and phenol poisoning.[3] As clinicians identify and abandon practices that retard wound healing, the treatment of traumatic wounds improves. The introduction of antiseptics and antibiotics, refinements in sterile procedure, and improvements in surgical materials and surgical technique have been major advances in the science of wound care.

The primary objectives in wound care are:
1. Preserving viable tissue,
2. Restoring tissue continuity,
3. Optimizing conditions for the development of wound strength,
4. Preventing excessive or prolonged inflammation,
5. Avoiding infection and other impediments to healing, and
6. Minimizing scar formation.

This chapter will review current strategies for achieving these goals.

SUMMARY OF WOUND HEALING

A general understanding of the process of wound healing is fundamental to successful management of wounds. Highlights of this complex phenomenon, as they relate to clinical decision making, will be reviewed.

Inflammation, epithelialization, fibroplasia, contraction, and scar maturation constitute the stages of scar formation, a nonspecific repair process that occurs in wounds extending beneath the epithelium.[2-7] Most traumatic wounds result in some tissue destruction, hemorrhage, and a breech in the epidermis through which bacteria and foreign materials enter. Inflammation is a beneficial response that serves to remove the bacteria, foreign debris, and devitalized tissue—a biological debridement. Increased vascular permeability follows, with an outpouring of plasma producing local swelling. Fibrin plugs arising from the plasma occlude lymphatic channels, limiting the spread of bacteria. For some time it was thought that any collection of blood and plasma in a wound serves as an ideal culture medium for bacteria and therefore must be minimized. Hohn and coworkers demonstrated that humoral factors in this fluid actually provide the wound with some protection against bacteria in the first week following injury.[8] Polymorphonuclear and mononuclear leukocytes concentrate at the site of injury and phagocytize dead and dying tissue, foreign material, and bacteria in the wound.

As the white blood cells die, their intracellular contents are released into the wound and, in large amounts, form the purulence characteristic of infected wounds. Some exudate is expected even in the absence of bacterial invasion; however, infection with the accumulation of pus will interfere with epithelialization and fibroplasia and thereby will impair wound healing. Wounds contaminated with significant numbers of bacteria or foreign material may undergo a prolonged or persistent inflammatory response and may remain unhealed. Granuloma formation surrounding retained sutures is an example of chronic inflammation.[4]

As white blood cells remove debris within the wound, epithelial cells at the surface of the wound begin to cover the tissue defect. In most sutured wounds, the surface of the wound develops an epithelial covering impermeable to water within 24 to 48 hours. The epithelium thickens and grows downward into the wound and along the course of skin sutures. Although there is initially some "adhesiveness" to the wound edges during the first few days, this is eliminated by fibrinolysis. By day 4 or 5, fibroblasts in the wound begin synthesizing collagen and protein polysaccharides, initiating the stage of scar formation known as fibroplasia.[5] In a wound healing by primary intention (following wound closure), the peak rate of collagen synthesis and the most rapid rate of increase in the tensile strength of the wound begin at approximately 5 to 7 days. The wound gains tensile strength as collagen fibrils are aligned in firm, parallel cords. Wound strength is a balance between the lysis of old collagen and the synthesis of new collagen "welding the wound edges."[2] The amount and organization of scar tissue are also influenced by physical forces acting across the wound, such as the stresses imposed on a wound oriented perpendicular to joint creases or a wrinkle line.[9]

Significant gains in tensile strength do not begin until approximately the fifth day following the injury. Strength increases rapidly for 6 to 17 days, more slowly for an additional 10 to 14 days, and almost imperceptibly for as long as 2 years (Fig. 35–1). The strength of scar tissue never quite reaches that of unwounded skin. Although the process of collagen formation is essentially completed within 21 to 28 days, collagen remodeling continues for up to 1 year. Scar widening occurs between the twenty-first and forty-ninth days. During the maturation phase of wound healing, collagen fibers reorient into a more organized pattern, and the scar changes in form, bulk, and strength.[4-7] Decisions regarding the optimal time for suture removal and the need for continued support of the wound with tape are influenced by (1) wound tensile strength, (2) the period of scar widening, and (3) the cosmetically unacceptable effect of epithelialization along suture tracks. Scars are quite red and noticeable at 3 to 8 weeks following closure, but the appearance of a scar should not be judged before the scar is well into its remodeling phase. Therefore, scar revision should be postponed until 6 to 12 months after injury.

Initial Examination

The approach to the management of a particular wound depends upon information gathered dur-ing history taking and on physical examination. The choice of cleaning techniques or the decision to debride a wound is determined by the mechanism of injury; the configuration, extent, and depth of the wound; and the amount and type of contamination present. The decision to close a wound immediately or after a period of observation is based not simply on wound age but on a variety of factors affecting the risk of infection. Identification of injury to underlying structures, such as nerves, vessels, tendons, joints, bones, or ducts, may lead the emergency physician to forgo wound closure and to consult a surgical specialist. It is crucial that the physician recognize wounds that may appear benign but, given the mechanism of injury, belie the extensive and devastating underlying tissue damage. The discovery that an extremity wound was produced by a roller or wringer device, by a high-pressure injection gun, by high-voltage electricity, by heavy and prolonged compressive forces, or by the bite of a human or a potentially rabid animal radically alters the overall management of the affected patient.

HISTORY

In the initial evaluation of a wound, the physician should ask the questions *how, when,* and *where* by inquiring about the mechanism of injury, the time of injury, and the environment in which the wound occurred.

Wound Age and the Golden Period

The fact that the infection rate in wounds increases in proportion to the time elapsed prior to definitive wound care has been well documented in the literature.[10-13] A delay in wound cleaning and closure may allow bacteria contaminating the wound to proliferate. During World War I, French investigators measured the growth of bacteria cultured from battlefield wounds. It was determined that approximately 12 hours after wounding, the

Figure 35–1. Graphic representation of the various phases of wound healing. Note that the tensile strength of scar tissue never reaches that of unwounded skin.

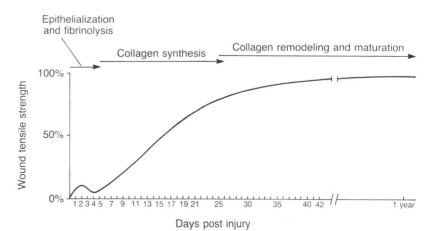

number of colonies of bacteria on the wound surface doubled. The conclusion was drawn that wound closure was safe before 12 hours had elapsed but dangerous after that time.[7]

Once the precise number of bacteria necessary to initiate a wound infection was established, investigators were able to demonstrate that a delay in treatment of a contaminated wound for as little as 3 hours could result in infection.[12, 14] Thus, the "golden period," the maximum time after injury that a wound may be safely closed without significant risk of infection, is not a fixed number of hours.[9] Peacock points out that "a clean razor slice of highly vascular skin of the face might be closed safely 48 hours after injury, whereas a stable-floor-nail penetration of the foot of an elderly person might not be closed safely one minute after injury."[7] All of the data accumulated in the initial evaluation, both historical and physical, must be used in the estimation of the golden period for a wound in a particular patient. In addition, the techniques of wound care in themselves may extend the golden period; a skillful clinician can often convert a dangerously contaminated wound into a clean wound that can be safely closed.[7] In the presence of normal tissue defenses and a relatively clean wound, an empiric guideline of primary closure, if the wound is less than 6 hours old, is often used.

Other Historical Data

Other factors affecting wound healing or the risk of infection include the patient's age and state of health. Patient age appears to be an important factor in host resistance to infection; those individuals at the extremes of age—young children and the elderly—are at greater risk.[15, 16] Infection rates are reported to be higher in patients with medical illnesses such as diabetes mellitus, immunologic deficiencies, malnutrition, anemia, uremia, congestive heart failure, cirrhosis, or malignancy, in obese patients, and in patients taking steroids or immunosuppressive drugs or those receiving radiation therapy. Shock, remote trauma, distant infection, bacteremia, and peripheral vascular disease also increase wound infection rates and slow the healing process.[15, 17–22]

Additional information pertinent to decision making in wound management includes:

Present medications (specifically, anticoagulants and immunosuppressive drugs),

Allergies (especially to local anesthetics, antiseptics, analgesics, antibiotics, and tape),

Tetanus immunization status,

Potential exposure to rabies (in bite wounds and mucosal exposures), and

Previous injuries and resultant deformities (especially in extremity and facial injuries).

PHYSICAL EXAMINATION

In his instructions for examining traumatic wounds, Edlich states that "the 11 most common causes of emergency department wound infections are the mouth and ten fingers of the examining physician."[1] A common error in wound management is to assume that a traumatic wound is already contaminated and then, in examining the wound, to proceed to contaminate it further. Despite the fact that all traumatic wounds are contaminated to some degree, one should always examine these injuries using aseptic technique. The examiner must wear sterile gloves and avoid droplet contamination from the mouth by maintaining distance or, preferably, by wearing a mask.[1]

Mechanism of Injury and Classification of Wounds

The magnitude and direction of the injuring force and the volume of tissue on which the force is dissipated determine the type of wound sustained. Three types of mechanical forces produce soft tissue injury: shear, tension, and compression forces. The resulting disruption or loss of tissue determines the configuration of the wound. Wounds may be classified into six categories:

Abrasions: Wounds caused by surface tensile stress—two forces of equal magnitude applied in opposite directions—and resulting in the loss of epidermis and possibly dermis (e.g., skin grinding against road surface).

Lacerations: Wounds caused by "shear forces of equal magnitude in opposite directions in two parallel planes separated by a small distance,"[15] producing a tear in tissues. Tensile and compressive forces also cause separation of tissue. Little energy is required to produce a wound by shear forces (e.g., a knife cutting a finger). Consequently, little tissue damage occurs at the wound edge, the margins are sharp, and the wound appears "tidy." The energy required to disrupt tissue by tensile or compressive forces (e.g., forehead impacting a dashboard) is considerably greater than that required for tissue disruption by shear forces because the energy is distributed over a larger volume. These lacerations have jagged, contused, "untidy" edges.

Crush wounds: Wounds caused by the impact of an object against tissue (a compressive force). These wounds usually contain contused or partially devitalized tissue.

Puncture wounds: Wounds with a small opening and whose depth cannot be entirely visualized. Puncture wounds are caused by a combination of forces.

Avulsions: Wounds in which a portion of tissue is completely separated from its base. Shear and tensile forces cause avulsions.

Combination wounds: Wounds with a combination of configurations. For example, stellate "lacerations" caused by compression of soft tissue against underlying bone create wounds with elements of crush and tissue separation; missile wounds involve a combination of shear, tensile, and compressive forces that puncture, crush, and sometimes avulse tissue.[1, 14, 15, 23]

Contaminants: Bacteria and Foreign Material

Numerous factors affect the risk of wound infection, but the primary determinants of infection are the amount of bacteria and the amount of dead tissue remaining in the wound.[24, 25]

Essentially all traumatic wounds are contaminated with bacteria to some extent. The number of bacteria remaining in the wound at the time of closure is directly related to the risk of infection. A critical number of bacteria must be present in a wound before a soft tissue infection develops. In experimental wounds produced by shear forces, an inoculum of $\geq 10^6$ aerobic bacteria per gram of tissue will in time inevitably produce wound infection. When the mechanism of injury involves a compressive force, the infective dose of bacteria is $\geq 10^4$ bacteria per gram of tissue. If bacterial counts after injury (or after wound management) are below this level, the wound has a very low probability of becoming infected.[10, 12, 14, 15, 26]

Surgical operations are categorized on the basis of the relative levels of bacterial contamination of the wounds as defined by the Committee on Trauma of the National Academy of Sciences National Research Council. Most traumatic wounds fall into one of two categories:

Contaminated wounds: Traumatic wounds less than 12 hours old.

Dirty wounds: Wounds heavily contaminated with pathogenic organisms, those with significant numbers of bacteria associated with large amounts of devitalized tissue, or traumatic wounds greater than 12 hours old.[27]

Infection rates in series of contaminated wounds of all types range from 5 to 21 per cent; rates in series of dirty wounds range from 29 to 38 per cent.[15, 16, 17, 24, 28, 29]

Most traumatic wounds that fit into the first category are usually described as "clean (traumatic) wounds"; those in the second category are called "heavily contaminated." This distinction between "clean" and "heavily contaminated" wounds is an important one for purposes of management, and any classification system based on wound age alone without consideration of other important factors is misleading. The nature and amount of foreign material contaminating the wound will often determine the type and quantity of bacteria implanted. The presence of undetected large foreign bodies in sutured wounds will almost guarantee an infection. Although bullet or glass fragments by themselves rarely produce wound infection, these foreign bodies may carry infection-potentiating particles of clothing, gun wadding, or soil into the wound. Minute amounts of organic or vegetative matter, feces, or saliva carry highly infective doses of bacteria. Fecal material contains bacteria in concentrations of 10^{11} bacteria per gram of feces. Bite wounds and intraoral wounds are heavily contaminated with facultative species and obligate anaerobes. Tooth plaque and debris found in gingival recesses also contain bacteria in the range of 10^{11} per gram wet weight.[14, 15] The bacterial inoculum from human bites often contains 100 million or more organisms per milliliter of saliva. At least 42 different bacterial species have been identified in human oral flora.[30]

Soil impairs the ability of a wound to resist infection. Rodeheaver and associates found that adding small quantities of sterile soil to wounds containing subinfective doses of microorganisms leads to infections in those wounds.[31, 32] Inorganic particulate matter, such as sand or road surface grease, usually introduces few bacteria into a wound and has little chemical reactivity; these contaminants are relatively innocuous. Soil containing a large proportion of clay particles readily potentiates infection. Presumably because of their marked chemical reactivity, clay particles damage local tissue defenses. These particles also react chemically with amphoteric (e.g., tetracycline) and basic (e.g., gentamicin) antibiotics, limiting their effectiveness in contaminated wounds. In contrast, acidic antibiotics, such as the cephalosporins and the penicillins, do not bind with these soil fractions and so maintain their antibacterial properties.[33]

Most wounds encountered in the practice of emergency medicine have low initial bacterial counts. If wound cleaning and removal of devitalized tissue is instituted before bacteria within the wound enter their accelerated growth phase, 3 to 12 hours following the injury, and if one uses aseptic technique in examining and managing these wounds, thereby avoiding iatrogenic contamination, bacterial counts will remain below the critical number needed to initiate infection.[10, 12, 15]

Wound Location

The anatomic location of the wound has considerable importance in the risk of infection. Areas with endogenous microflora in numbers sufficient to infect a wound (greater than 10^5 bacteria per cm^2) include the hairy scalp, the forehead, the axilla, the perineum, the foreskin of the penis, the vagina, the mouth, and the nails. In other regions, skin bacteria are sparse (10^2 to 10^3 per cm^2) and are not a source of infection.[1] Wounds in regions of high vascularity, such as the scalp and the face, more easily resist bacterial incursions. The high vascularity of the scalp probably accounts for low infection rates with scalp injuries, despite the large numbers of endogenous microflora. Distal extremity wounds, in contrast, are more at risk for the development of wound infections than are injuries of most other parts of the body.[11, 15, 16, 32, 34–36]

Devitalized Tissue

Identifying devitalized tissue is an important part of the examination of a wound.

Tissue damage lowers the resistance of the wound to infection. Devitalized or necrotic tissue potentiates infection in a wound by providing a culture medium in which bacteria proliferate, by inhibiting leukocyte phagocytosis, and by creating an anaerobic environment suitable for certain bacterial species.[1, 25]

Underlying Structures

The importance of detecting injury to underlying structures during the examination was mentioned previously. Procedures such as joint space irrigation, reduction and debridement of compound fractures, neurorrhaphy, vascular anastomosis, and flexor tendon repair are best accomplished in a controlled setting where optimal lighting, proper instruments, and assistance are available.[1]

Cleaning

After the initial evaluation of the wound has been completed, wound management may be undertaken. The cornerstones of wound care are cleaning, debridement, closure, and protection. Although most wounds are initially contaminated with less than an infective dose of bacteria, given time and the appropriate wound environment, bacterial counts may reach infective levels. The goals of wound cleaning and debridement are the same: (1) to remove bacteria and reduce their numbers below the level associated with infection, and (2) to remove particulate matter and tissue debris that would otherwise lengthen the inflammatory stage of healing or allow the growth of bacteria beyond the critical threshold.[20]

PREPARATIONS

Minimal aseptic technique requires the use of sterile gloves during the cleaning procedure. Thorough cleansing of bacteria, soil, and other contaminants from a wound cannot be accomplished without the patient's cooperation. Scrubbing most open wounds is painful, and the patient's natural response is withdrawal. Therefore, local or regional anesthesia often must precede the examination and cleaning of a wound.[15] Topical anesthetic solutions (e.g., tetracaine 0.5 per cent, epinephrine 1:2000, cocaine 11.8 per cent) are effective in providing anesthesia of small superficial wounds and are less painful than intradermal and subcutaneous injections of anesthetics.[37] There is a slight increase in wound infection when these solutions are used topically rather than using local anesthesia by injection.

Despite adequate anesthesia, the patient may be unable to cooperate because of apprehension. The physician should explain the wound-cleansing procedure to the patient and should provide the assurance that everything possible will be done to minimize any pain. In the majority of cases, reassurance will not alleviate the fears of young children, and both sedation and physical restraining devices must be used. One combination of medications used for sedation in children includes meperidine (Demerol), 1 to 2 mg per kg; promethazine (Phenergan), 0.5 to 1 mg per kg; and chlorpromazine (Thorazine), 0.5 to 1 mg per kg delivered intramuscularly in a single injection. Alternatively, diazepam (Valium) or morphine may be given by an intravenous route, titrated to achieve a drowsiness in the pediatric or adult patient. Nitrous oxide has also proved to be an effective analgesic. Several other methods of sedation are available. No more than one modality should be used in addition to local or regional anesthesia.

The two primary methods of wound cleaning are mechanical scrubbing and irrigation. The principle of soaking a wound in a saline or antiseptic solution prior to the arrival of a physician appears reasonable but is controversial and of unproven value. Little more can be said about this technique until definitive studies are performed. The methods of scrubbing and irrigation will be reviewed.

MECHANICAL SCRUBBING

Initially, a wide area of skin surface surrounding the wound should be scrubbed with an antiseptic solution in order to remove contaminants that in the course of wound management might be carried into the wound by instruments, suture material, dressings, or the physician's gloved hand. Much controversy surrounds the technique of scrubbing the internal surface of a wound. Scrubbing the wound with an antiseptic-soaked sponge does remove bacteria, debris, and loose devitalized tissue, thus debriding the wound and lessening the need to sacrifice tissue by excision. It is important to removal all nonabsorbable particulate matter; any such material left in the dermis may become impregnated in the healed tissue and result in a disfiguring "tattoo" effect.[4] Rodeheaver and co-workers, however, determined that scrubbing experimental traumatic wounds with a saline-soaked sponge did not decrease the incidence of infection. They concluded that tissue trauma inflicted by the sponge impairs the ability of that wound to resist infection, allowing residual bacteria to produce inflammation and infection.[38] Custer and associates found that experimental wounds scrubbed with a gauze sponge moistened with saline exhibited as much of an inflammatory response as did untreated wounds.[39] These experimental wounds were surgical incisions contaminated with bacteria rather than traumatic wounds containing particulate matter, cellular debris, and devitalized tissue in addition to bacteria. Other authors maintain that the importance of eliminating foreign material and nonviable tissue outweighs any concern about destroying viable tissue by excessive scrubbing.[40]

A reasonable compromise between these opposing views is to reserve mechanical scrubbing for "dirty" wounds contaminated with significant amounts of foreign material. If irrigation alone is ineffective in removing contaminants from a wound, the wound should be scrubbed. Since the amount of damage inflicted on tissues by scrubbing is correlated with the porosity of the sponge, a fine-pore sponge (e.g., Optipore sponge, Biosyntek, Inc.—90 pores per linear inch) should be used to minimize tissue abrasion.[38, 41] Detergents have an advantage over saline in that they minimize friction between the sponge and tissue, thereby limiting tissue damage during scrubbing. Detergents also solubilize particles, helping to dislodge the particles from the wound surface. Unfortunately, many of the available detergents are toxic to tissues.[38, 42]

IRRIGATION

Irrigation removes particulate matter, bacteria, and devitalized tissue loosely adherent to the edges of the wound and trapped within the depths of the wound. The effectiveness of irrigation is determined primarily by the hydraulic pressure at which the irrigant fluid is delivered.[43] Rodeheaver and colleagues studied the effect of irrigating experimental wounds contaminated with 20 mg of soil. Irrigating wounds with 400 ml of fluid at 1 pound per square inch (psi) removed 48.6 per cent of the soil, whereas increasing the pressure to 15 psi removed 84.8 per cent, reducing the infection rate from 100 per cent to 7 per cent.[31]

Significantly more force is required to rid the wound of particles with a small surface area (e.g., bacteria) than to remove particles with a large surface area (e.g., dirt, sand, or vegetation).[41] Bulb syringes or gravity flow irrigation devices deliver fluid at low pressures and as such are ineffective in ridding wounds of small particulate matter or in lowering wound bacterial counts. The flow rate of irrigation fluid delivered through intravenous (IV) tubing can be enhanced by inflation of a blood pressure cuff around a collapsible plastic IV bag, although this method provides considerably less irrigation pressure than can be delivered by a syringe. The maximum hydraulic pressure that can be delivered with a syringe varies with the force exerted on the plunger of the syringe and with the internal diameter of the attached needle. The pressure delivered by a simple irrigation assembly consisting of a 19 gauge plastic catheter or needle attached to a 35-ml syringe is 7 to 8 psi. This high-pressure irrigation system is sufficient to remove significant numbers of bacteria and a substantial amount of particulate matter from the wound surface (Fig. 35–2).[1, 41, 44] Commercial irrigation systems with a ring-handled syringe and a one-way valve that connects into a standard intravenous solution are available (Travenol pressure irrigation set, code no. 2D2113 or Irrijet, Ackrad Laboratories, Garwood, NJ).[14]

A number of investigators have compared pulsatile jet irrigation of wounds to wound irrigation with gravity flow and bulb syringe techniques. The pulsatile jet irrigation technique with pressures of 50 to 70 psi is significantly more effective in removing bacteria, foreign contaminants, and tissue fragments and in reducing infection rates.[45–50] Although the irrigation fluid penetrates

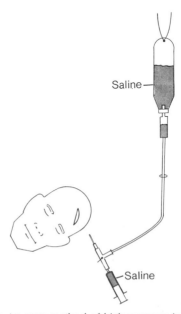

Figure 35–2. An easy method of high-pressure irrigation. Intravenous tubing with an in-line, one-way valve is attached to a bottle of sterile 0.9 per cent saline solution. The other end is connected to a stopcock. Saline solution is aspirated into the syringe. Maximal force is exerted on the plunger of the syringe, delivering the solution in a fine stream through an attached 19 gauge needle held close to the wound.

the wound tissues, predominantly in a lateral direction, high-pressure jet irrigation does not drive significant amounts of bacteria or surface contaminants into the soft tissues of the wound.[51-54] Although jet irrigation can damage tissue defenses,[54] Rodeheaver found the technique to be more effective in cleaning wounds, less traumatic to tissues, and less likely to produce edema than conventional scrubbing with a brush. Pulsatile and continuous irrigation, if delivered at the same pressures, are equally effective in removing bacteria.[31] The jet irrigation system used by many investigators was a Water Pik unit (Teledyne Aquatic Corp.) with a sterile tip nozzle held approximately 4 cm from the wound and delivering a 0.9 per cent saline solution at a pressure of approximately 50 psi. The irrigation pressures generated by this unit are considerably greater than those of the syringe system. Thus, pulsatile jet irrigation should generally be reserved for use in heavily contaminated wounds in which syringe irrigation proves to be ineffective.[41, 50, 54] Minimum recommended volumes of irrigation fluid vary, but for average-sized wounds, 200 to 300 ml should be used.[40, 41] Greater volumes may be required for larger or heavily contaminated wounds. Irrigation should continue until all visible, loose particulate matter has been removed.

ANTISEPTICS AND ANTIBIOTICS IN CLEANING

For many years, antiseptic solutions have been used for their antimicrobial properties in and around wounds. In the past decade, investigators have begun to consider the effects of these agents not only on the bacteria contaminating the wound but also on the tissues themselves. Intact skin can withstand strong microbicidal agents, whereas leukocytes and the exposed cells of the wound are very susceptible to further damage.[20]

The antiseptic agents most commonly used in wound care at present include:

Povidone-iodine solution (Betadine preparation)—iodine complexed with the carrier polyvinylpyrrolidone (PVP), a water-soluble organic complex; this combination is called an iodophor. Standard solutions of Betadine preparation are 10 per cent.

Povidone-iodine surgical scrub (Betadine scrub) —the iodophor PVP-I and an anionic detergent (pH 4.5).

pHisoHex—an emulsion of an anionic detergent, entsulfon, lanolin, cholesterols, petrolatum, and hexachlorophene (pH 5.5).

Hibiclens—chlorhexidine gluconate plus a sudsing base (pH 5.1 to 6.5).

Tincture of green soap—potassium oleate, isopropanol, potassium coconut oil, soap.

Hydrogen peroxide—an oxidizing agent.

Benzalkonium chloride (Zephiran)—a quaternary ammonium compound that works as a cationic surface active agent.[28, 39, 41]

Pluronic F-68 (Shur-Clens)—nonionic surfactant agent without antimicrobial activity (pH 7.1).[55]

Edlich and coworkers demonstrated in a 1969 study that *irrigation* of wounds with Betadine *solution* (preparation) provided significant protection against the development of infection in contaminated wounds.[3] In later studies, he and other investigators found that *scrubbing* experimental traumatic wounds with the detergents Betadine *scrub* or pHisoHex increased the incidence of infection.[39] They concluded that the deleterious effect of surgical scrub solutions was a consequence of their anionic detergent content and advised against the use of these agents inside wounds.[1, 39, 41]

In order to confirm the toxicity of antiseptic solutions, Faddis and associates injected these agents into the joints of rabbits. Betadine *scrub* and pHisoHex solutions each caused "severe gross and histologic damage to articular cartilage, synovia, and muscle." A 3 per cent hexachlorophene solution caused "moderate histologic damage" and "articular cartilage ground substance loss." Betadine *solution* (preparation) caused "only minimal gross and histologic damage, without any biochemical evidence of articular cartilage damage."[56] In vitro studies by Rodeheaver and colleagues illustrated the toxicity of antiseptics to the cellular components of blood. Exposure to Hibiclens destroyed all white blood cells and, to a lesser extent, red blood cells. Exposure to Betadine surgical scrub destroyed both.[55]

The tissue toxicity of some antiseptic solutions appears to be dependent upon their concentrations. Viljanto noted that in surgical (appendectomy) wounds sprayed with a 5 per cent povidone-iodine aerosol, the infection rate doubled—to a rate of 19 per cent compared with an infection rate in controls of 8.5 per cent. When a 1 per cent povidone-iodine aerosol was used, the infection rate dropped to 2.6 per cent.[20] Mullikan and coworkers studied the histologic effects of 1 per cent povidone-iodine solution in injuries and found that it did not decrease tensile strength in these healing wounds.[57] In contrast with Viljanto's results, Sindelar and Mason found that irrigation of the subcutaneous tissues of surgical wounds with a 10 per cent solution of povidone-iodine prior to closure reduced infections in contaminated wounds from a control rate of 26.1 per cent to 6.8 per cent and from 31 per cent to 8.3 per cent in dirty wounds. No selection of resistant organisms was reported.[28] These findings concur with other studies of surgical and traumatic wounds in which a 5 per cent povidone-iodine dry powder aerosol spray was used.[58-61] *It appears that the 1 per povidone-iodine solution is a relatively safe and effective antiseptic agent for use in contaminated traumatic wounds.* Whether higher concentrations are harmful or beneficial remains a debated issue. It should be noted that standard stock solutions of povidone-iodine are 10 per cent strength.

Quaternary ammonia compounds are less toxic to tissue but have a limited antimicrobial spectrum; gram-positive organisms are more susceptible to these solutions than are gram-negative bacteria. *Pseudomonas* has been known to proliferate in stored solutions.[41] Consequently, use of benzalkonium chloride has fallen into disfavor. Hydrogen peroxide is used by some clinicians for its effervescent effect in cleaning wounds. Gruber and associates found that hydrogen peroxide decreased healing time in experimental wounds, yet it also injured tissue.[62] Lau and colleagues found hydrogen peroxide irrigation of appendectomy wounds to be ineffective in reducing wound infection.[63] Because peroxide is hemolytic, it is best to use it only to clean reapproximated wound surfaces and surrounding skin encrusted with blood and coagulum or to soak off adherent blood-soaked dressings. Peroxide should not be used on granulation tissue, since oxygen bubbles lift newly formed epithelium off the wound surface.[62]

Another approach to wound cleaning involves the use of the nonantiseptic cleaning agent Pluronic F-68. In contrast with other antiseptic solutions, this preparation causes no tissue or cellular damage, leukocyte inhibition, or impairment in wound healing. The solution also causes no eye irritation or pain on contact with the wound. Pluronic F-68 is nontoxic, even when administered intravenously, and to date is nonallergenic. It has no antibacterial activity itself; the infection rate in wounds irrigated with Pluronic F-68 is equal to the rate in those irrigated with normal saline.[31] Nevertheless, when used on sponges to clean experimental wounds mechanically, Pluronic F-68 has resulted in lower infection rates than have been noted in controls scrubbed with saline solution, proving its ability to cleanse a wound effectively and atraumatically. Because of its lack of antibacterial activity, Rodeheaver and coworkers recommend that after scrubbing wounds with Pluronic F-68, systemic antibiotic therapy be given to patients with "infection-prone" wounds.[55]

Halasz reviewed the studies of several authors who analyzed the technique of irrigating wounds with antibiotic solutions. The antibiotics studied included ampicillin, a neomycin-bacitracin-polymyxin combination, tetracycline, penicillin, kanamycin, and cephalothin. Halasz concluded that "organisms in the wound can be exposed to adequate concentrations of antibiotics, and that the concentration of these drugs in the wound remains in the bactericidal range for long periods of time, far exceeding that obtainable by systemic administration." He recommended placing ampicillin sodium powder, 500 to 1000 mg, or kanamycin, 1 gm, in solutions used to irrigate clean and contaminated wounds.[64] Sher found topical cefazolin to be as effective as systemic cefazolin in preventing infections in wounds contaminated with *E. coli.*[65] Lindsay and associates demonstrated in a clinical trial that flooding traumatic lacerations with 10 ml of 5 per cent sodium benzyl penicillin significantly reduced wound infections when compared with treatment in controls.[66]

The use of antibiotics in irrigant solutions in lieu of antiseptic solutions avoids the tissue destruction of the antiseptics, but theoretically risks both topical sensitization of the patient to the antibiotic and the selection of wound-infecting organisms resistant to the antibiotic used. To date, there have been no reports of either complication. Within 3 hours of injury, a proteinaceous coagulum forms within the wound, surrounding bacteria and probably preventing their contact with topical or systemic antibiotics. Therefore, the wound should be scrubbed prior to irrigation with an antibiotic solution.[41, 67] Disruption of coagulum and clotted blood by the application of a proteolytic enzyme (e.g., Travase) also has been shown to prolong the effective period of antibiotic action in contaminated wounds when treatment is delayed for as long as 8 hours.[68-71] Since wound coagulum plays a positive role in defense against infection,[3, 34] its removal is not necessary in injuries for which antibiotics are not indicated.[68, 69] Rodeheaver and associates suggest that the use of enzymes is more effective than scrubbing the wound, but no comparison study has been performed. They agree that "the mechanism by which trypsin potentiates the effectiveness of antibiotics is, in part, its ability to facilitate removal of bacteria with the gauze sponge." The authors recommend that for maximum effectiveness the trypsin enzyme be in contact with the wound for a prolonged period (30 minutes). Repeated applications enhance its effectiveness. Proteolytic enzymes are ineffective in decreasing the infection rate if treatment is delayed more than 8 hours.[71] These enzymes also tend to cause considerable bleeding from the wound surface.

RECOMMENDATIONS

The prerequisites of any wound-cleaning technique are a calm or sedated patient, satisfactory local anesthesia, and a thorough scrub of the skin surface adjacent to the wound. The importance of effectively ridding the wound of major contaminants and infective doses of bacteria is unquestionable. Two strategies that will accomplish the goals of wound cleaning are apparent from this discussion. The contaminated or "dirty" wound can be irrigated or both scrubbed and irrigated with a 1 per cent povidone-iodine solution (*Betadine preparation*, not scrub). This should be followed by flushing with a 0.9 per cent saline solution. As an alternative, the wound can be scrubbed with Pluronic F-68 and irrigated with an antibiotic–normal saline solution. The use of proteolytic enzymes can be considered in extensive wounds that are heavily contaminated or that contain large amounts of crushed tissue, but enzymes should be used only as an adjunct to the usual methods of cleaning and debridement. All scrubbing should be performed with a fine-pore sponge; all irrigation should be accomplished with high-pressure techniques. The routine use of hydrogen peroxide on open wounds is discouraged.

The need for antibiotic solutions in cleaning relatively uncontaminated wounds is not entirely clear, although a decrease in wound infection can be demonstrated.[64–66] Gentle scrubbing with Pluronic F-68 and normal saline high-pressure irrigation both appear to be satisfactory methods for cleaning minimally contaminated wounds.

Débridement

Débridement is of undisputed importance in the management of the contaminated wound. With this technique, the physician can remove tissue impregnated with foreign matter, bacteria, and devitalized tissue that would otherwise impair the ability of the wound to resist infection and prolong the period of inflammation.[25] Debridement also creates a tidy, sharp wound edge that is easier to repair and results in a more cosmetically acceptable scar. Complete excision of grossly contaminated wounds, such as animal bites, will allow primary closure of such wounds with no greater risk of infection than in relatively uncontaminated lacerations.[14, 41]

PREPARATION

Prior to debridement (or wound closure), the wound must be prepared and draped, then anesthetized. Because of the trauma inflicted on the skin by a razor blade, the infection rate is greater in wounds that are shaved.[41, 72] For wounds in hair-bearing areas, hair should be removed by clipping or by shaving with a recessed blade razor only when the hair interferes with the procedure. Stubborn hairs that continually invade the wound during suturing can be coated with petrolatum jelly or water-soluble ointments to keep them out of the field. Eyebrows should not be shaved, since critical landmarks needed for exact approximation would be lost. Although shaved eyebrows will grow back in time, shaving produces an undesirable cosmetic effect.

The skin surface adjacent to the wound should be disinfected with a standard 10 per cent povidone-iodine solution. The solution is painted widely on the skin surrounding the wound but should not cover the interior of the wound itself. After brief handwashing, the physician and any assistants involved in the procedure must wear sterile gloves. Face masks are recommended—they are mandatory for any clinician with a bacterial upper respiratory infection. Since droplets of saliva may leak even from around the edges of a face mask, talking in proximity to the wound must be avoided.[73, 74]

A single fenestrated drape or multiple folded drapes are placed over the wound site. Instruments that may be required for debridement include two fine single- or double-pronged skin hooks, a scalpel with a number 15 blade, tissue scissors, hemostats, and a small tissue forceps (Fig. 35–3).

If the wound has not yet been anesthetized, anesthesia can be provided at this time. Epinephrine is often combined with lidocaine to overcome the vasodilatory effects of the latter, to provide vasoconstriction in wounds located in highly vascular areas, to decrease the systemic absorption of the anesthetic, and to prolong the duration of anesthesia by slowing the clearance of the anesthetic agent from tissues.[75] A drawback to the use of local anesthetics combined with vasoconstrictors, whether infiltrated intradermally or applied topically,[37] is the adverse effects of the vasoconstrictors on wound healing and infection rates.[41, 76–80] For this reason, the use of epinephrine in the anesthetic solution should be avoided whenever possible. If more prolonged anesthesia is desired, an alternative to lidocaine-epinephrine infiltrations is the long-acting anesthetic bupivacaine (Marcaine) or the combination of lidocaine

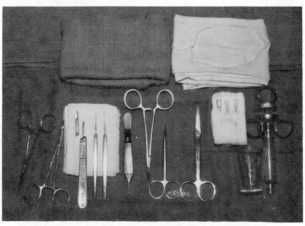

Figure 35–3. Materials for anesthesia and débridement.

and bupivacaine. The lidocaine-epinephrine mixture is useful for wounds in which multiple small vessel hemorrhage is a problem.

Many authors believe that the use of epinephrine in distally located tissues (digit, ear, nose, penis) is contraindicated. Vasoconstrictors may affect the end arteries supplying these regions and may cause irreversible ischemia and tissue necrosis. Scarlet and colleagues in reviewing the literature found no evidence to warrant this concern. They compared the blood perfusion in toes following digital anesthesia using 1 per cent lidocaine with and without epinephrine 1:100,000 and found a marked decrease in blood perfusion as measured by plethysmography only during the first 2 hours following the injection of epinephrine-containing solutions.[81] Kaplan and coworkers reported a series of 65,000 procedures involving toes in which epinephrine was used as a vasoconstrictor with no adverse effects.[82] Steinberg and associates reported similar results in a clinical study of over 200,000 digital injections.[83]

Nonetheless, during the 2-hour period of epinephrine-induced reduction in blood flow, marginally viable tissue in crush wounds, in stellate lacerations, or in flap lacerations might progress to necrosis. If vasoconstrictors are needed to create a bloodless operating field, their use should be restricted to healthy patients without peripheral vascular disease for the repair of simple lacerations.[84] In higher concentrations, lidocaine exerts a dose-related toxic effect on injured tissues; therefore, the lowest effective concentration (0.5 per cent to 1 per cent) should be used.[76, 85] Systemically, the toxic dose of lidocaine is 4.5 mg per kg; in lidocaine solutions containing epinephrine, the toxic dose is higher—7 mg per kg.[78]

There are other problems associated with the technique of local anesthesia. Though less painful than penetration of intact skin, the passage of a needle through the cut edges of a heavily contaminated wound can carry bacteria into uninjured tissue surrounding the wound.[78] Some of the harmful effects of lidocaine on wound healing are a consequence of injecting a volume of fluid into the skin and the subcutaneous tissue.[76] Local injection of anesthetic causes distention of tissues at the edges of a wound, which distorts landmarks and makes approximation of the wound edges more difficult. Much of the pain associated with the local infiltration of an anesthetic results from distention of tissues. All of these factors make regional anesthesia a preferred method of anesthetizing wounds. Regional nerve blocks should always be considered when heavily contaminated traumatic wounds are being anesthetized (see Chapter 32).[75]

The entire depth and the full extent of every wound should be explored in an attempt to locate hidden foreign bodies, particulate matter, bone fragments, and any injuries to underlying structures that may require repair. Lacerations through thick subcutaneous adipose tissue are treacherous in that large amounts of particulate matter can be totally obscured in deeper folds of tissue. Unless a careful search is undertaken, these contaminants may be left in the depths of a sutured wound and infection will almost inevitably follow.

Identifying devitalized tissue in a wound remains a challenging problem.[86] Some surgeons consider muscle to be nonviable if its color and consistency are abnormal; others refer to the absence of bleeding when cut. The most reliable criterion is the inability to contract when electrically stimulated, although rarely is this test necessary or practical in the emergency center setting.[25] Sometimes a sharp line of demarcation distinguishes devitalized skin and viable skin 24 hours after injury.[1] Since most wounds are examined earlier, there is usually only a subtle bluish discoloration. One author recommends the use of hydrogen peroxide in the wound (despite its cytotoxic effects) to produce a whitish discoloration of all necrotic tissue.[75]

EXCISION

If there is significant contamination in areas where there is a redundance or laxity of tissues and no important structures, such as tendons or nerves, lie within the wound, the entire wound may be excised.[7] This technique is the most effective type of débridement, since it converts the contaminated traumatic wound into a clean surgical wound (Fig. 35–4). Wounds of the trunk, the gluteal region, or the thigh are amenable to this technique. If necessary, the clinician can judge the adequacy of the excision by coloring the wound surface with a vital dye. One would then create a new wound by excising all dyed tissue.[25] Most traumatic wounds can be excised using the elliptic excision technique or a variation thereof. A lenticular configuration should be marked superficially around the wound with the blade of a number 15 scalpel, with only the epidermis cut. If a puncture wound is being excised, the axis of the excision should parallel a wrinkle, a skin line, or a line of dependency or facial expression, and the long axis should be three to four times as great as the short axis (Fig. 35–5). The clinician may plan this type of excision by premarking the skin with a surgical marking pen. Tension should be placed on the surrounding skin with a finger or a skin hook. With the clinician's hand steadied on the table or on the patient, the number 15 blade is used to cut through the skin at right angles or at slightly oblique angles to the skin surface (Fig. 35–6). If

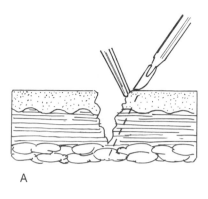

A

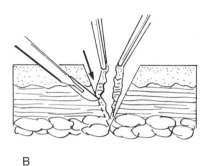

B

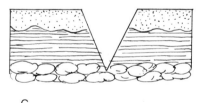

C

Figure 35–4. A–C, Complete excision of a wound. Grossly contaminated wounds may be excised and sutured primarily.

complete excision of the entire depth of the wound is not necessary, the tissue scissors may be used to cut the edge of the wound, following the path premarked in the epidermis by the scalpel blade. If a complete excision is desired, the incision on each wound edge should be carried past the deepest part of the wound (see Figure 35–4). In hair-bearing areas of the face, particularly through eyebrows, the incision should be angled parallel to the angle of hair follicles in order to avoid linear alopecia (Fig. 35–7). The wedge of excised tissue should be removed carefully, avoiding any contamination of the fresh wound surface.[87, 88]

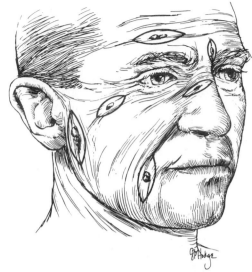

Figure 35–5. If a facial wound is grossly contaminated or too jagged for a cosmetic repair, the wound may be excised. Excisions of small wounds should be lenticular and parallel to skin creases. (From Grabb, W. C.: Basic techniques of plastic surgery. In Grabb, W. C., and Smith, J. W.: Plastic Surgery: A Concise Guide to Clinical Practice. Boston, Little, Brown & Co., 1979. Used by permission.)

SELECTIVE DÉBRIDEMENT

When there is a loss of tissue or insufficient skin elasticity or when the wound contains structures serving important functions (structures such as dura, fascia, nerves, or tendons), the technique of selective débridement must be used.[7, 25] Complete excision is impossible for most hand wounds. A simple excision of a wound of the palm or the dorsum of the nose would make approximation of the resulting surgical wound edges difficult. Contaminated bone fragments, nerves, and tendons are almost never removed. Every effort should be

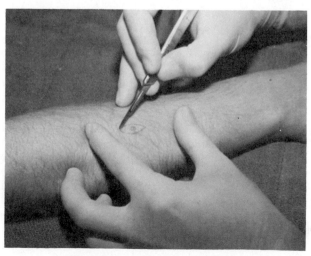

Figure 35–6. Technique of excision.

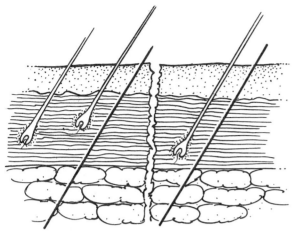

Figure 35–7. Excision through an eyebrow. (From Dushoff, I. M.: A stitch in time. Emerg. Med. 5(3):1, 1973. Used by permission.)

made to clean these structures and return them to their place of origin, since they may be functional later.[86] Selective débridement is more tedious and time-consuming, but it preserves more surrounding tissue. This technique involves sharp débridement of devitalized or heavily contaminated tissue in the wound piece by piece and eventual matching of one edge of the wound with the other.

In heavily contaminated wounds, especially those with abundant adipose tissue, all exposed fat and all fat impregnated with particulate matter should be removed. The subcutaneous adipose tissue attached to large flaps or to avulsed viable skin should be débrided prior to reapproximation of the wound; removal of this fatty layer will allow better perfusion of the flap or the graft.

Following débridement or excision, the wound should be irrigated again to remove any remaining tissue debris.

CONTROL OF HEMORRHAGE

Hemorrhage from a wound may be vigorous, and occasionally it requires control prior to examination, cleaning, or débridement. If minor bleeding is not a problem prior to débridement, it frequently becomes a complication once the wound edges are excised. Wound exploration or cleaning sometimes induces bleeding. Hemostasis is essential at any stage of wound care. Not only does persistent bleeding obscure the wound and hamper wound exploration and closure, but also hematoma formation in a sutured wound separates wound edges, impairs healing, and risks dehiscence or infection.

Several practical methods of achieving hemostasis are available to the emergency physician. Direct pressure with gloved fingers, gauze sponges, or packing material is always effective in immediately controlling a single bleeding site or a small number of sites. Sustained pressure on the wound for at least 5 minutes can effectively control capillary oozing, occluding capillaries until coagulation occurs. Arterial and arteriolar bleeding, although brisk initially, frequently subsides within minutes as the cut ends of these vessels constrict. Direct pressure on larger vessels minimizes blood loss until constriction occurs. Direct pressure is most effective when combined with elevation of the bleeding wound above the level of the patient's heart.

In a patient with multiple injuries and several urgent problems, hemorrhage can be controlled temporarily with a compression dressing. Several absorptive sponges are applied directly over the bleeding site, and these are secured in place with an elastic bandage (e.g., Ace wrap) or elastic adhesive tape (Elastoplast). Pressure is provided by the elasticity of the bandage. The bleeding part should be elevated. Wound care can then be deferred while the physician attends to more pressing matters.

Ligation of blood vessels with fine absorbable suture material is another method of achieving hemostasis. A common error, however, is to spend excessive time attempting to tie off small bleeding vessels while the patient slowly exsanguinates. In highly vascular areas, such as scalp, it is best to suture the laceration despite active bleeding; the pressure exerted by the closure will usually stop the bleeding.

Although simply crushing and twisting the end of a vessel with a hemostat avoids the introduction of suture material into the wound, this method provides unreliable hemostasis. Ligation of the vessel is preferred. Bleeding ends of vessels are clamped with fine-point hemostats, effecting immediate hemostasis. The tip of the hemostat should project beyond the vessel to hold a loop of a ligature in place (Fig. 35–8). While an assistant lifts the handle of the hemostat, a synthetic absorbable suture of size 5-0 or 6-0 is passed around the hemostat from one hand to the other (Fig. 35–9). The first knot is tied beyond the tip of the hemostat. Once the suture is securely anchored on the vessel, the hemostat is released.[79, 88, 89]

In actual practice, the emergency physician seldom has an assistant available for ligating vessels by this method. McDonald describes a technique that enables a single operator to maintain tension on the ligature while removing the hemostatic clamp. A needle holder is used to grasp one tail of the ligature; the other end is held by the third, fourth, and fifth fingers of the left hand. As the clamp held in the right hand is removed from the vessel, the needle holder is moved away from the left hand by extending the thumb and the index finger, maintaining tension on the ligature. The

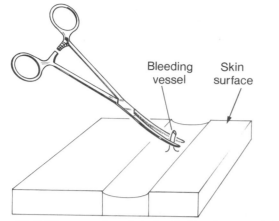

Figure 35–8. When one attempts to tie off a bleeding vessel, the tip of the hemostat should project beyond the clamped vessel.

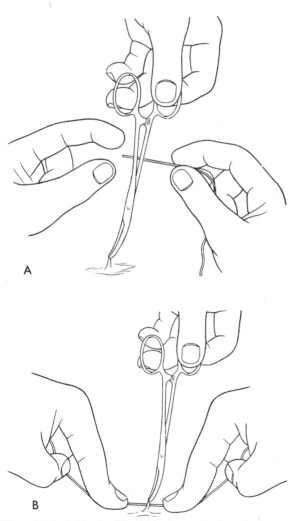

Figure 35–9. A, The handles of the hemostat have been raised by an assistant as a ligature is passed under them. B, The ligature thread stretched between the index fingertips is carried under the projecting tips of the hemostat. (From Kirk, R. M.: Basic Surgical Techniques. Edinburgh, Churchill Livingstone, 1978, pp. 50–51. Used by permission. © R. M. Kirk.)

right hand can discard the clamp, grasp the needle holder, and complete the tie (Fig. 35–10).[90] Three knots are sufficient to hold the ligature in place. The ends of the suture should be cut close to the knot in order to minimize the amount of suture material that is left in the wound.

Cut vessels that retract into the wall of the wound may frustrate attempts at clamping and ligation. Bleeding should be controlled first by downward compression on the tissue. A suture is passed through the tissue twice, using a figure-of-eight or horizontal mattress stitch, and then tied. The double thread will constrict the tissue containing the cut vessel (Fig. 35–11). The disadvantage of this method is that the tissue constricted by the ligature may necrose and leave devitalized tissue in the wound.

Vessels with diameters greater than 2 mm should be ligated. Those smaller than 2 mm that bleed despite direct pressure can be controlled by pinpoint electrocautery. A dry field is required for an effective electrical current to pass through the tissues; if sponging does not dry the field, a suction-tipped catheter should be used. Trauma is minimized by using fine-tipped electrodes to touch the vessel or by touching the active electrode of the electrocautery unit to a small hemostat or fine-tipped forceps gripping the vessel.[2] The power of the unit should be kept to the minimum level required for vessel thrombosis. Bipolar coagulation (such as that provided by the Bovie Unit) is preferred over monopolar coagulation because it produces approximately one third less tissue necrosis of surrounding tissue.[41] If the amount of tissue cauterized is kept to a minimum, wound healing is no more compromised by this technique than by ligation. Cauterization of medium- and small-sized vessels can quickly provide hemostasis.

Self-contained, sterilizable, battery-powered coagulation units are available. Vessels are cauterized by the direct application of a heated wired filament. These units may damage more surrounding tissue than electrocautery units; however, they are compact and simple and are therefore well suited for use in the emergency center (Fig. 35–12).

Epinephrine is an excellent vasoconstrictor. Topical epinephrine (1:100,000) can be applied to a wound on a moistened sponge to reduce the bleeding from small vessels.[88] Combined with local anesthetics, concentrations of 1:100,000 and 1:200,000 prolong the effect of the anesthetic and provide some hemostasis in highly vascular areas. As discussed previously, epinephrine used topically or intradermally will increase the risk of wound infection. Therefore, its use should be restricted to situations in which widespread small vessel and capillary hemorrhage in a wound is not controlled by direct pressure or cauterization.

Fibrin foam, gelatin foam, and microcrystalline

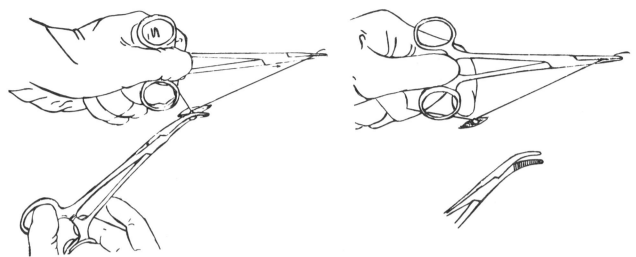

Figure 35–10. One maintains ligature tension with one hand by grasping one tail of the suture with a clamp and keeping its base between the thumb and the forefinger. As the pedicle clamp is removed with the other hand, the ligature is tightened by extension of the flexed thumb and index finger to the desired tension. The pedicle clamp is then discarded from the right hand, and further knots are applied in the usual fashion. (From MacDonald, R. T.: Maintenance of ligature tension by a single operator with simultaneous removal of a hemostatic clamp. Am. J. Surg. 143:770, 1982. Used by permission.)

collagen may be used as hemostatic agents. Their utility is limited in that vigorous bleeding will wash the agent away from the bleeding site. Their greatest value may be in packing small cavities from which there is a constant oozing of blood.[88] In most simple wounds with persistent but minor capillary bleeding, apposition of the wound edges with sutures will provide adequate hemostasis.

TOURNIQUETS

If bleeding from an extremity wound is refractory to direct pressure, electrocauterization, or ligation or if the patient presents with exsanguinating hemorrhage from the wound, a tourniquet can be used to control the bleeding temporarily.

Tourniquets are also helpful in examining extremity lacerations by providing a bloodless field; a partially lacerated tendon or joint capsule is easily obscured within a bloody wound. Tourniquets can cause injury in three ways:

1. They can result in ischemia in an extremity.

2. They can compress and damage underlying blood vessels and nerves.

3. They can jeopardize the survival of marginally viable tissue.

These injuries can be avoided (1) if there is a

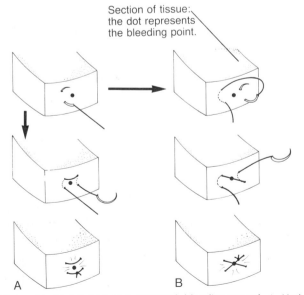

Figure 35–11. Ligation of a retracted, bleeding vessel. A, Horizontal mattress technique. B, Figure-of-eight technique.

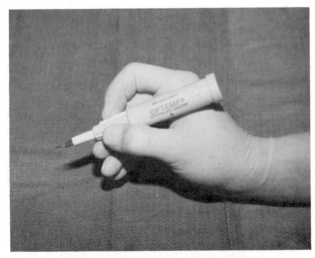

Figure 35–12. Battery-powered cautery.

limit placed on the total amount of time that an extremity is tourniqueted and (2) if narrow, band-like tourniquets are avoided.

A single cuff tourniquet (sphygmomanometer cuff) placed around an arm or a leg will effectively stop distal venous or arterial bleeding without crushing underlying structures. The length of time that a tourniquet may remain in place is limited by the development of pain underneath and distal to the tourniquet. This will occur within 30 to 45 minutes in a conscious patient, well within the limits of safety.[91, 92] In contrast, a narrow (less than 1 cm) rubber band serving as a finger tourniquet exerts a tremendous pressure over a small surface area at the base of the finger and thus risks pressure necrosis of digital vessels. Narrow rubber bands should not be used as tourniquets for digits. The maximum tourniquet time that is safe for a finger may easily be exceeded. Tourniquets can be used on digits, however, if the clinician strictly observes a time limit and uses a tourniquet that distributes pressure over a wide area (e.g., Penrose drain).

Prior to application of the tourniquet, the injured extremity should be elevated and then manually exsanguinated to prevent bothersome venous bleeding. An elastic bandage (e.g., Ace wrap or Esmark) may be wrapped circumferentially around the extremity, starting distally and moving in a proximal direction. A cuff placed around the arm proximal to the wound should be inflated to 250 to 300 mm Hg and the tubing clamped; the bandage is then removed and the extremity lowered.[92, 93] Other authors recommend a cuff pressure only slightly higher than the patient's systolic blood pressure.[94] It is recommended that the sphyngomanometer bulb be fully opened after the tube is clamped to permit rapid deflation of the cuff after the procedure. Because tourniquets impair circulation, their use in the emergency department should be limited to a 1 hour maximum.

A finger can be exsanguinated with a moistened piece of gauze. A piece of gauze measuring 4 inches × 4 inches is opened to its fullest length, folded in half longitudinally, moistened, and rolled tightly around the elevated finger from tip to base. A Penrose drain is stretched around the base of the finger and secured with a hemostat. The gauze is then removed. The maximum tourniquet time on a finger should not exceed 20 to 30 minutes.[93]

These techniques provide bloodless fields in which to examine, clean, and close extremity wounds. Débridement of questionably devitalized tissue in a wound is best accomplished *without* a tourniquet or pharmacologic vasoconstriction, since bleeding from tissues is often an indication of their viability.[86]

Closure

OPEN VERSUS CLOSED WOUND MANAGEMENT

Two of the objectives of wound care are prevention of excessive or prolonged inflammation and minimization of scar formation. Wounds that heal spontaneously (by "secondary intention") undergo much more inflammation, fibroplasia, and contraction than those whose edges are reapproximated by wound closure techniques.[4, 95] The process of contraction in wound healing serves to cover the defect of an open wound, yet it may have undesirable consequences—deformity (contracture) or loss of function. Left to itself, the healing process may be unable to close a defect completely in areas where surrounding skin is immobile, such as on the scalp or in the pretibial area.[4] An open wound of an extremity that exposes tendons, bone, nerves, or vessels may allow desiccation of these structures. If the patient is careless with an otherwise adequate dressing covering an open wound, the wound may be further contaminated.[96] The advantages of surgical closure of wounds are apparent—this procedure minimizes inflammation, fibroplasia, contracture, and scar width. Obviously, closed wounds are much less susceptible to contamination than are open wounds.

On the other hand, there are risks incurred when wounds are closed. Closure of contaminated wounds greatly increases the probability of wound infection, with impaired healing, dehiscence, and sepsis as possible complications. After cleaning and débridement, wounds left unsutured appear to have a higher resistance to infection than do closed wounds.[15, 16] Prusak found that inoculation of open wounds with 10^8 *Staphylococcus aureus* organisms resulted in minimal inflammatory response compared with that of uncontaminated wounds left to heal secondarily.[97] Sutures in themselves are detrimental to healing. Each suture inflicts an intradermal incision, damaging surface epithelium, dermis, subcutaneous fat, blood vessels, small nerves, lymphatics, and epithelial appendages—hair follicles, sweat glands, and ducts. These appendages, once divided and separated by a stitch, usually undergo inflammation and resorption.[5, 98] Bryant states that "each suture . . . should be regarded as another piece of foreign material that incites an inflammatory response."[4] Furthermore, when a suture is removed, bacteria that have settled on the exposed portion of the suture are pulled into the suture track and deposited there.[5]

Guidelines for deciding when to close wounds may be simply stated (but are poorly defined): If the wound is judged to be "clean" or is rendered "clean" by scrubbing, irrigation, and débridement, it may be closed. If the wound remains hopelessly contaminated despite the best of efforts, it must be left open to heal by secondary intention. If the status of the wound is uncertain, the practitioner can base the decision on clinical judgment (an educated guess based on past experience with similar wounds) or on quantitative bacteriologic analysis of the wound. Another option available is delayed primary closure.

QUANTITATIVE BACTERIOLOGIC ANALYSIS

The primary determinants of wound infection are the level of wound contamination and the amount of residual devitalized tissue. Also of importance is the ability of the patient's immune system to respond to bacterial invasion. Until recently, assessing these factors was a matter of clinical judgment. A number of investigators have demonstrated that quantitative analysis of samples of tissue from wound margins is accurately predictive of subsequent wound infection.

In most studies, 10^5 to 10^6 or more bacteria were needed to cause burn wound sepsis, wound infection, or pustule formation. In the presence of a single silk suture, considerably fewer bacteria were needed to initiate infection in any wound.[96, 99, 100]

A rapid slide technique (available within 20 minutes) has been used with 95 per cent accuracy in determining the safety of wound closure. Edlich showed that it was unsafe initially to close experimental wounds contaminated with 10^6 bacteria.[95] Robson found that greater than 10^5 bacteria prevented successful delayed surgical wound closure.[101, 102] A quantitative bacteriologic study of a wound thus makes the decision of wound closure a straightforward one. Using this laboratory method, if the number of bacteria per gram of tissue sampled after thorough cleaning and débridement is greater than 10^5, the wound should not be closed at that time.[96, 103] Unfortunately, very few emergency physicians have this test available to them, and it is impractical for routine use.

DELAYED CLOSURE

If there is a substantial risk that closure of a particular wound might result in infection, the decision to close or to leave the wound open can be postponed. The condition of the wound after 3 to 5 days will then determine the best strategy. Although cleaning and débridement should be accomplished as rapidly as possible, there is no

urgency in closing a wound. Edlich points out that "the fundamental basis for delayed primary closure is that the healing open wound gradually gains sufficient resistance to infection to permit an uncomplicated closure."[1] The concept of delayed closure is unfamiliar to many physicians who deal with outpatient wounds. Despite its effectiveness, delayed primary closure is a technique that is underused by most physicians.

Open wound management consists of the usual cleaning and débridement followed by packing of the wound with sterile, saline-moistened fine-mesh gauze. The packed wound is covered by a thick, absorbent, sterile dressing. Unless the patient develops a fever, the wound should not be disturbed for 4 days; unnecessary inspection risks contamination and infection. On the fourth postoperative day, the wound is re-evaluated. If there is no evidence of infection, the wound margins can be approximated (delayed primary closure) or the wound can be excised and then sutured (secondary closure) with minimal risk of infection (Fig. 35–13). It is important to note that since the wound is closed prior to the proliferative phase of healing, there is no delay in final healing, and the results are indistinguishable from those of primary healing. If available, quantitive microbiology can be used at the time of delayed closure to document further the safety of wound closure.[1, 13, 93, 104]

Certain wounds should almost always be managed open or by delayed closure. These include wounds contaminated by soil or organic matter, purulence, saliva, feces, or vaginal secretions (although primary repair of intraoral lacerations, surgical perineal wounds, and episiotomies is accepted). Also included in this category are wounds associated with extensive tissue damage (e.g.,

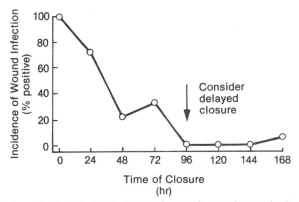

Figure 35–13. This graph depicts the incidence of wound infection over time when delayed closure is performed. Delayed closure is best accomplished on the fourth or fifth day to avoid infection. (From Edlich, R. F., Thacker, J. G., Rodeheaver, F. T., et al.: A Manual for Wound Closure. St. Paul, MN, Surgical Products Division/3M, 1979. Reproduced by permission of and copyright 1979 by Minnesota Mining and Manufacturing Company.)

high-velocity missile injuries, explosion injuries of the hand, or complex crush injuries) and most bite wounds. Various authors disagree as to which bite wounds may be closed initially. Most would suture cosmetically deforming injuries, including facial bites, and bite wounds that can be completely excised.[6, 41, 105] Others would suture nonextremity dog bites.[14] In severe soft tissue injuries, delayed closure will allow time for nonviable tissue to demarcate from uninjured tissue. Débridement can then be accomplished with maximal preservation of tissue.[96]

METHODS

Once the decision to close a wound has been made, the physician must select the closure technique that is best suited for the particular location and configuration of the wound.[15] Available techniques include suturing, taping, and metal stapling.

All emergency physicians should be skilled in the approximation of skin edges with surgical tape (Steri-strips, Shur-strips, Clearon). Tape is easy to apply and is preferable to sutures when the patient is frightened or uncooperative. Skin tape causes minimal skin reaction, results in no skin suture marks, and is associated with the lowest incidence of infection of any closure technique.[87, 106–109] Although tape will appose the edges of a superficial laceration without difficulty, the subcutaneous layer of a deep laceration must be sutured to prevent inversion of the skin edges by the tape.[87] Metal staples can be used to approximate a wound rapidly, but their use is limited to easily accessible, linear lacerations in noncosmetic areas.

In most situations, suturing is the method of choice. Detailed discussion of wound closure by tape and staples is provided in Chapter 36. The remaining discussion of wound closure will pertain to the use of sutures.

EQUIPMENT

Instruments

In addition to the instruments used for débridement (see Fig. 35–3), a needle holder and suture scissors are required for suturing. The size of the needle holder that is used should match the size of the needle selected for suturing—the needle holder should be large enough to hold the needle securely as it is passed through tissue, yet not so large that the needle is crushed or bent by the instrument. Instruments used to débride a grossly contaminated wound should be discarded and fresh instruments obtained for the closure of the wound. If the instruments are simply covered with coagulated blood, they can be cleansed with hydrogen peroxide and then used for suturing.

Suture Materials

There is a wide variety of suture materials available. For most wounds that require closure of more than one layer of tissue, the physician must choose sutures from two general categories—an absorbable suture for the subcutaneous layer and a nonabsorbable suture for skin closure.

Sutures can be described in terms of four characteristics:

1. chemical and physical properties,
2. mechanical performance and handling characteristics,
3. reactivity and absorption, and
4. retention of tensile strength.

Sutures are made from natural fibers (cotton, silk), from sheep submucosa or beef serosa (plain gut, chromic gut), or from synthetic materials, such as nylon (Dermalon, Ethilon, Nurolon, Surgilon), dacron (Ethiflex, Mersilene), polyester (Ti-Cron), polyethylene (Ethibond), polypropylene (Prolene, Surgilene), polyglycolic acid (Dexon), and polyglactin (Vicryl, coated Vicryl). Stainless steel sutures are rarely, if ever, useful in wound closure in the emergency center setting because of difficulty in handling, fragmentation, and harmful effects on tissues.[15, 110] Some sutures are made of a single filament (monofilament); others consist of multiple fibers braided together (Table 35–1).[111]

Desirable handling characteristics in a suture include smooth passage through tissues, ease in

Table 35–1. EXAMPLES OF SUTURE MATERIALS

Monofilament	
Absorbable Sutures	*Nonabsorbable Sutures*
Plain gut	Dermalon*
Chromic gut	Ethilon*
PDS‡‡	Prolene‖
	Silk
	Steel
	Surgilene‖
	Tevdek††

Multifilament	
Absorbable Sutures	*Nonabsorable Sutures*
Dexon¶	Ethibond§
Vicryl**	Mersilene†
Coated Vicryl**	Nurolon*
	Surgilon*
	Ti-cron‡

*Nylon.
†Dacron.
‡Polyester.
§Polyethylene.
‖Polypropylene.
¶Polyglycolic acid.
**Polyglactin.
††Teflon coated.
‡‡Polydioxanone.

knot tying, and stability of the knot once tied. Multifilament sutures have the best handling characteristics of all sutures, whereas steel sutures have the worst. In terms of performance and handling, significant improvements have been made in the newer absorbable sutures. Gut sutures have many shortcomings, including relatively low and variable strength, a tendency to fray when handled, and stiffness despite being packaged in a softening fluid.[112, 113] The newer, multifilament synthetic absorbable sutures are soft and easy to tie and have few problems with knot slippage. Polyglactin 910 (coated Vicryl) sutures have been improved with the application of an absorbable lubricant coating. The frictional "drag" of these coated sutures as they are pulled through tissues is less than that of uncoated multifilament materials, and the resetting of knots following the initial throw is much easier. This characteristic allows retightening of a ligature without knotting or breakage, and it allows smooth and even adjustment of suture line tension in running subcuticular stitches.[114] Synthetic monofilament sutures have the troublesome property of "memory"—a tendency of the filament to straighten, causing the knot to slip and unravel. Some nonabsorbable monofilament sutures are coated with polytetrafluorethane (Teflon) or silicone to reduce their friction. This coating improves the handling characteristics of these monofilaments but results in poorer knot security.[110, 113]

Thacker and coworkers found that when sutures were cut 3 mm from the ends of the knot, three square knots are required to secure a silk suture and five are needed for the Teflon-coated synthetic Tevdek.[115] Macht and associates warned that an excessive number of throws in a knot will weaken the suture at the knot. They recommended three square knots to secure a stitch with silk or other braided, nonabsorbable materials and four knots with synthetic, monofilament absorbable and nonabsorbable sutures.[116] With use of coated synthetic suture materials, attention to basic principles of knot tying is even more important. If the physician uses square knots (or a surgeon's knot on the initial throw followed by square knots) that lie down flat and are tied securely, knots will rarely unravel.[117]

Sutures that are rapidly degraded in tissues are termed "absorbable"; those that maintain their tensile strength for longer than 60 days are considered "nonabsorbable" (see Table 35–1). Plain gut may be digested by white blood cell lysozymes in 10 to 40 days; chromic gut will last 15 to 60 days. Remnants of both types of sutures, however, have been seen in wounds more than 2 years after their placement.[112, 116, 118] Vicryl is absorbed from the wound site within 60 to 90 days[110, 112, 116] and Dexon within 120 days.[119, 120] Wallace and colleagues report that when placed in the oral cavity, plain gut

disappears after 3 to 5 days, chromic gut after 7 to 10 days, and polyglycolic acid after 16 to 20 days.[121] In contrast, silk is absorbed within the skin in approximately 2 years.[116] The rate of absorption of synthetic absorbable sutures is independent of suture size.[119]

All sutures placed within tissue damage host defenses and provoke inflammation. Even the least reactive suture impairs the ability of the wound to resist infection.[122] The magnitude of the reaction provoked by a suture is related to the quantity of suture material (e.g., diameter and total length) present in the tissue and to the chemical composition of the suture. Among absorbable sutures, polyglycolic acid and polyglactin sutures are least reactive, followed by plain gut and chromic gut. The nonabsorbable polypropylene is less reactive than nylon or dacron.[113, 118, 123, 124] Significant tissue reaction is associated with silk and cotton sutures. Edlich and coworkers advise against the use of these highly reactive materials in contaminated wounds.[15] Adams found the "absorbable" polyglycolic acid sutures less reactive than "nonabsorbable" silk in the closure of wounds and noted that unlike silk, the polyglycolic acid suture does not require suture removal.[125] Based on this one report, if soft sutures are needed for skin closure in a highly mobile area (e.g., upper eyelids), it appears that Dexon or Vicryl sutures are preferable to silk sutures. If used for skin closure, the "absorbable" sutures should be removed from the skin surface at the usual time.

The chemical composition of sutures is an important determinant of early infection. The infection rate in experimental wounds when polyglycolic acid sutures are used is less than the rate when gut sutures are used. It is surprising that plain gut sutures elicit infection less often in contaminated wounds than do chromic gut sutures.[122] Lubricant coatings on sutures do not alter suture reactivity, absorption characteristics, breaking strength, or the risk of infection.[114, 122] Osterberg and Blomstedt found that in experimental wounds, multifilament sutures are more likely to produce infection than monofilament sutures if left in place for prolonged periods.[126, 127] Monofilament sutures elicit less tissue reaction than do multifilament sutures, and multifilament materials tend to wick up fluid by capillary action. Theoretically, bacteria can "hide" in the interstices of a multifilament suture and as a result can be inaccessible to leukocytes. Although Edlich and associates found no significant difference in the infective potential of these two configurations of sutures after a period of 4 days,[122] Sharp and colleagues found an increased degree of inflammation in wounds closed with multifilament sutures compared with wounds closed with monofilament sutures.[128]

Size of suture material (thread diameter) is a measure of the tensile strength of the suture; threads of greater diameter are stronger. The strength of the suture is proportional to the square of the diameter of the thread. Therefore, a 4-0 size suture of any type is larger and stronger than a 6-0 suture.[110] The correct suture size for approximation of a layer of tissue depends on the tensile strength of that tissue. The tensile strength of the suture material should be only slightly greater than that of the tissue, since the magnitude of damage to local tissue defenses is proportional to the amount of suture material placed in the wound.[1, 116, 129]

Of the absorbable types of sutures, a wet and knotted polyglycolic acid suture is stronger than a plain or chromic gut suture subjected to the same conditions.[113, 130] Polyglycolic acid and polyglactin sutures maintain tensile strength for 2 to 3 weeks, whereas the length of time that gut retains tensile strength is erratic.[112, 116] Gut sutures treated with chromium salts (chromic gut) have a prolonged tensile strength.[15, 110]

Some authors claim that silk maintains its tensile strength for approximately 1 year and nylon for greater than a year.[116] Others state that both silk and nylon lose their strength rapidly after the second month in a wound and may disintegrate within 6 months.[15] Polypropylene will remain unchanged in tissue for longer than 2 years after implantation.[15, 122] In comparison testing, Hermann and coworkers found that sutures made of natural fibers, such as silk, cotton, and gut, were the weakest; sutures made of dacron, nylon, polyethylene, and polypropylene were intermediate in tensile strength; and metallic sutures had the greatest strength.[113]

Synthetic absorbable sutures have made the older, natural suture materials obsolete. Polyglycolic acid (Dexon) and polyglactin 910 (coated Vicryl) have improved handling characteristics, knot security, and tensile strength. Their absorption rates are predictable and tissue reactivity is minimal.[6, 131] The distinct advantages of synthetic nonabsorbable sutures over silk sutures are their greater tensile strength, low coefficient of friction, and minimal tissue reactivity.[6, 122] They are extensible, elongating without breaking as the edges of the wound swell in the early postoperative period.[1, 6, 15] In contrast with silk sutures, synthetics can be easily and painlessly removed once the wound has healed.

The suture materials most useful to emergency physicians in wound closure are Dexon or coated Vicryl for subcutaneous layers and synthetic nonabsorbable sutures (e.g., nylon or polypropylene) for skin closure. Fascia can be sutured with either absorbable or nonabsorbable materials. In most situations, 3-0 or 4-0 sutures are used in the repair

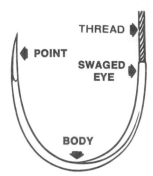

Figure 35–14. The eyeless, or "swaged," needle. (From Suture Use Manual: Use and Handling of Sutures and Needles. Somerville, NJ, Ethicon, Inc., 1977, p. 29. Used by permission.)

of fascia, 4-0 or 5-0 absorbable sutures in subcutaneous closure, and 4-0 or 5-0 nonabsorbable sutures in skin closure. The skin layer of facial wounds is repaired with 6-0 sutures, whereas 3-0 or 4-0 sutures are used when the skin edges are subjected to considerable dynamic stresses (e.g., wounds overlying joint surfaces) or static stresses (e.g., scalp).

Needles

The eyeless, or "swaged," needle is the type of needle used for wound closure in most emergency centers (Fig. 35–14). The traditional closed-eye needle requires additional handling in order to enable one to thread the needle with the suture. Since a closed-eye needle must carry a double strand of thread through its eye, it causes more damage in passing through tissue than does a swaged needle, whose diameter is nearly equal to that of the strand it carries.[110]

The selection of the appropriate needle size and curvature is based on the dimensions of the wound and the characteristics of the tissues to be sutured. The needle should be large enough to

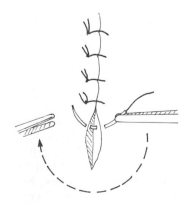

Figure 35–15. The needle should be large enough to pass through tissue and should exit far enough to enable the needle holder to be repositioned on the end of the needle at a safe distance from the point.

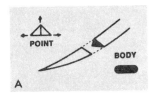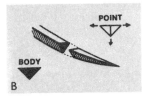

Figure 35–16. Types of needles. *A,* The conventional cutting needle has two opposing cutting edges with a third edge on the inside curvature of the needle. The conventional cutting needle changes in a cross-section shape from a triangular cutting tip to a flattened body. *B,* The reverse cutting needle is used to cut through tough, difficult-to-penetrate tissues, such as fascia and skin. It has two opposing cutting edges, with the third cutting edge on the outer curvature of the needle. The reverse cutting needle is made with the triangular shape extending from the point to the swage area, with only the edges near the tip being sharpened. (From Suture Use Manual: Use and Handling of Sutures and Needles. Somerville, N.J., Ethicon, Inc., 1977, p. 31. Used by permission.)

pass through tissue to the depth desired and to exit the tissue or the skin surface far enough that the needle holder can be repositioned on the distal end of the needle at a safe distance from the point (Fig. 35–15). In wound repair, needles must penetrate tough, fibrous tissues—skin, subcutaneous tissue, and fascia, yet the needles should slice through these tissues with minimal resistance or trauma and without bending. The type of needle best suited for closure of subcutaneous tissue is a conventional cutting needle. For percutaneous closure, a precision-point reversed cutting needle is preferred (Fig. 35–16).[1, 23, 110]

SUTURING TECHNIQUES

Skin Preparation

Prior to wound closure, the skin surrounding the wound is prepared with a povidone-iodine solution and covered with sterile drapes (see the section on débridement). Some surgeons do not drape the face but prefer to leave facial structures and landmarks adjacent to the wound uncovered and within view.[23] A clear plastic drape (Steri-Drape, 3M) can be used to provide a sterile field and a limited view of the area surrounding the wound. If no drapes are used on the face, the skin surrounding the wound should be widely cleansed and prepared. Wrapping the hair in a sheet prevents stray hair from falling into the operating field (Fig. 35–17).

Four principles apply to the suturing of lacerations in any location: (1) Minimize trauma to tissues; (2) relieve tension exerted on the wound edges; (3) close the wound in layers; and (4) accurately realign landmarks and skin edges.

Minimizing Tissue Trauma

The importance of careful handling of tissue has been emphasized since the early days of surgery.

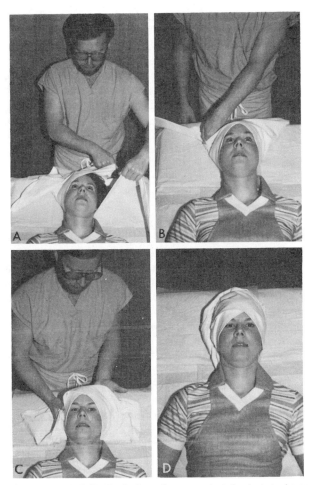

Figure 35–17. *A–D.* Technique for wrapping the hair to keep stray hair from falling into the operating field.

Skin and subcutaneous tissue that has been stretched, twisted, or crushed by an instrument or strangled by a suture that is tied too tightly may undergo necrosis, and increased scarring and infection may result. When the edges of a wound must be manipulated, the subcutaneous tissues should be grasped gently with a toothed forceps or skin hook, avoiding the skin surface.

When choosing suture sizes, the physician should select the smallest size that will hold the tissues in place. Skin stitches should incorporate no more tissue than needed to coapt the wound edges with little or no tension. Knots should be tied securely enough to approximate the wound edges but without blanching or indenting the skin surface.[23, 87]

Relieving Tension

Many forces can produce tension on the suture line of a reapproximated wound. Static skin forces that cause the edges of a fresh wound to gape will also continuously pull on the edges of the wound once it has been closed. Traumatic loss of tissue or wide excision of a wound may have the same effect. Muscles pulling at right angles to the axis of the wound impose dynamic stresses. Swelling following an injury creates additional tension within the circle of each suture.[15, 87] Skin suture marks result not only from tying sutures too tightly but also from failing to eliminate underlying forces distorting the wound. Tension can be reduced during wound closure in two ways: undermining of the wound edges and layered closure.

Undermining

Wounds subject to significant static tension require the undermining of at least one tissue plane on both sides of the wound in order to achieve a tension-free closure. Undermining involves the creation of a flap of tissue freed from its base at a distance from the wound edge equal to the width of the gap that the laceration presents at its widest point (Fig. 35–18). The depth of the incision can be modified, depending on the orientation of the laceration to skin tension lines and the laxity of skin in the area. A number 15 scalpel blade held parallel to the skin surface is used to incise the adipose layer or the dermal layer of the wound. The clinician can also accomplish this technique by spreading a scissors in the appropriate tissue

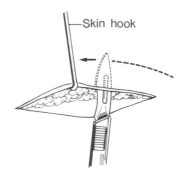

Figure 35–18. The technique of undermining.

plane. Undermining allows the skin edges to be lifted and brought together with gentle traction.[75, 98] Undermining will mobilize tissue without interrupting vascular supply.

Closing the Wound in Layers

The structure of skin and soft tissue varies with the location on the body (Fig. 35–19).[125] The majority of wounds handled in an emergency center require approximation of no more than three layers: fascia (and associated muscle), subcutaneous tissue, and skin surface (papillary layer of dermis and epidermis).[129, 132]

Closure of individual layers obliterates "dead space" within the wound that would otherwise

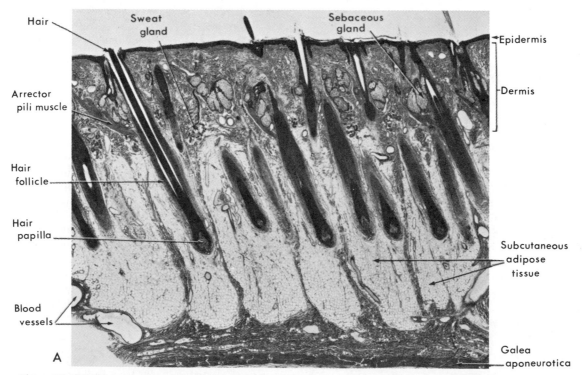

Figure 35–19. Variation in the structure of skin. *A*, Section of the skin of the scalp. ×15. (Courtesy of H. Mizoguchi.) *B*, Skin of the human fingertip, illustrating a very thick stratum corneum. Hematoxylin and eosin. ×65. *C*, Section of human sole perpendicular to the free surface. ×100. (After A. A. Maximow.) *D*, Section through human thigh perpendicular to the surface of the skin. Blood vessels are infected and appear black. Low magnification. (After A. A. Maximow.) (From Bloom, W., and Fawcett, D. W.: A Textbook of Histology, 10th ed. Philadelphia, W. B. Saunders Company, 1975. Used by permission.)

Illustration continued on opposite page

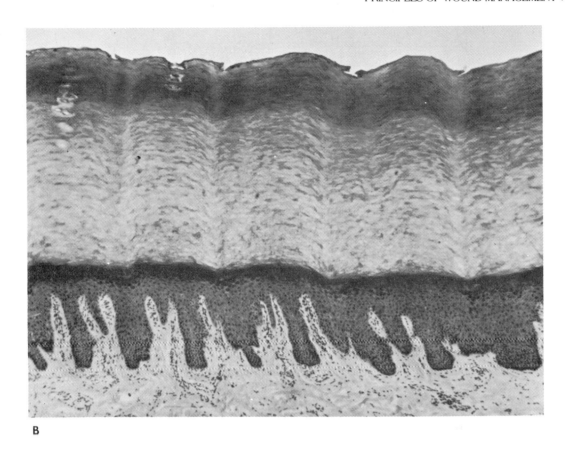

B

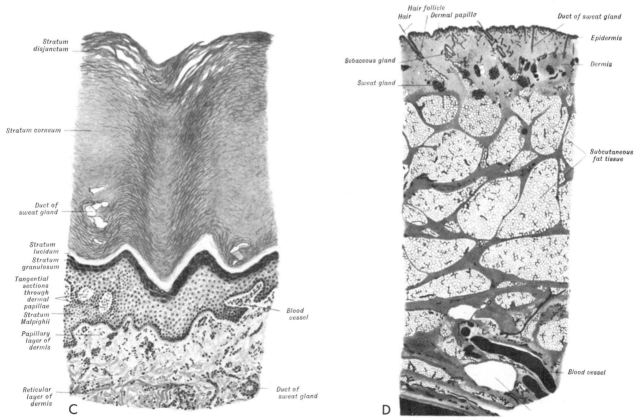

Stratum disjunctum

Stratum corneum

Duct of sweat gland

Stratum lucidum
Stratum granulosum
Tangential sections through dermal papilla
Stratum Malpighii
Papillary layer of dermis

Reticular layer of dermis

C

Blood vessel

Duct of sweat gland

Hair follicle
Hair
Dermal papilla
Duct of sweat gland
Epidermis

Sebaceous gland
Dermis

Sweat gland

Subcutaneous fat tissue

Blood vessel

D

Figure 35–19 (Continued).

fill with blood or exudate. DeHoll and associates demonstrated that the presence of dead space enhances the development of infection; however, it is not necessary to close the adipose layer of soft tissue with a separate stitch. A "fat stitch" is not necessary, since little support is provided by closure of the adipose layer, and the additional suture material that is required may potentiate infection.[107, 133, 134]

Separate approximation of muscle and subcutaneous layers hastens the healing and return of function to the muscle. *One should suture fascia, not muscle itself.* A divided muscle should be approximated in a stitch incorporating its fascial covering, since muscle tissue itself is too friable to hold a suture. Layered closure is particularly important in the management of facial wounds; this technique prevents scarring of muscle to the subcutaneous tissue and consequent deformation of the surface of the wound with contraction of the muscle. If a wound is closed without approximation of underlying subcutaneous tissue, a disfiguring depression may develop at the site of the wound. Finally, layered closure provides support to the wound and considerably reduces tension at the skin surface.

There are exceptions to the general rule of multilayered closure. Scalp wounds are generally closed in a single layer. For lacerations penetrating the dermis in fingers, hands, toes, and feet, a single-layer closure suffices.

Techniques of Suture Placement

Prior to suturing, the physician should ensure adequate exposure and illumination of the wound. The physician should assume a comfortable standing or sitting position, with the patient placed at an appropriate height. The best position for the physician is at one end of the long axis of the wound.

Subcutaneous Layer Closure. Once fascial structures are reapproximated, the subcutaneous layer is sutured. Although histologically the fatty and fibrous subcutaneous tissue (hypodermis) is an extension of (and continuous with) the reticular layer of the dermis,[135] suturing of these layers is traditionally referred to as a "subcutaneous" closure. Many authors recommend closing this layer in segments, placing the first stitch in the middle of the wound and bisecting each subsequent segment until the closure of the layer has been completed.[111] This technique is useful in the closure of wounds that are long or sinuous and is particularly effective in wounds with one elliptic and one linear side. The needle is grasped by the needle holder close to the suture end. Greater facility and speed in suturing is possible if the fingers are placed on the midshaft of the needle holder rather than in the rings of the instrument (Fig. 35–20).

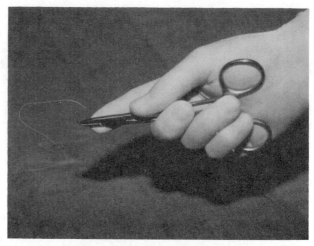

Figure 35–20. Technique of handling the needle holder.

The suture enters the subcutaneous layer at the bottom of the wound (Fig. 35–21A), or, if the wound has been undermined, at the base of the flap (Fig. 35–21B) and exits in the dermis. Once the suture has been placed on one side of the wound, it can be pulled across the wound to the opposite side (or the wound edges pushed together) to determine the matching point on the

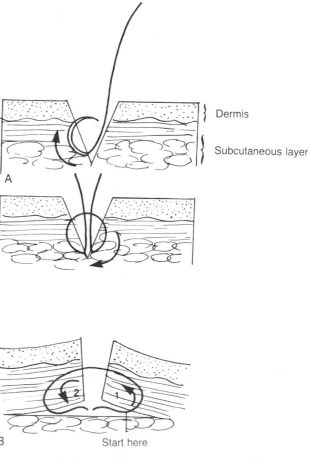

Figure 35–21. A and B, Inverted subcutaneous stitches.

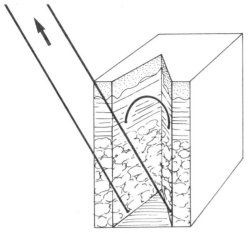

Figure 35–22. The two tails of the subcutaneous suture are pulled in the same direction, tightly apposing the edges of the wound.

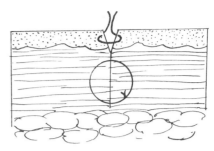

Figure 35–24. Horizontal dermal stitch.

opposite side. It is at this matching point along the opposite side of the wound that the needle is inserted. The needle should enter the dermis at the same depth as it exited from the opposite side, pass through the tissue, and exit at the bottom of the wound (or the base of the flap). One tightly opposes the edges of the wound by pulling the two tails of the suture in the same direction along the axis of the wound (Fig. 35–22). Some physicians place their subcutaneous suture obliquely rather than vertically to facilitate knot tying. When the knot in this subcutaneous stitch is tied, it will remain inverted, or "buried," at the bottom of the wound. Burying the knot of the subcutaneous stitch avoids a painful, palpable nodule beneath the epidermis and keeps the bulk of this foreign material away from the skin surface. The techniques of tying knots by hand and by instrument are well described and illustrated in various manuals.[15, 88] Once the knot has been secured, the tails of the suture should be pulled taut for cutting. The scissors are held with the index finger on the junction of the two blades. The blade of the scissors is slid down the tail of the suture until the knot is reached. With the cutting edge of the blade tilted away from the knot, the tails are cut. This technique prevents the scissors from cutting the knot itself and leaves a tail of 3 mm, which will protect the knot from unraveling (Fig. 35–23).[136] The entire subcutaneous layer is sutured in this manner.

After the subcutaneous layer has been closed, the distance between the skin edges indicates the approximate width of the scar in its final form. If this width is acceptable, percutaneous sutures can be inserted.[9] Despite undermining and placement of a sufficient number of subcutaneous sutures, on rare occasions a large gap between the wound edges may persist. In such cases, a horizontal dermal stitch may be used to bridge this gap (Fig. 35–24).

Skin Closure. The epidermis and the superficial layer of dermis are sutured with nonabsorbable synthetic sutures. The choice of suture size, the number of sutures used, and the depth of suture placement depend on the amount of skin tension remaining after subcutaneous closure. If the edges of the wound are apposed following closure of deeper layers, small sutures of size 5-0 or 6-0 can be used simply to match the epithelium of each side. If the wound edges remain retracted or if subcutaneous stitches were not used, a larger size of suture may be required. Skin closure may be accomplished with sutures placed in segments (Fig. 35–25) or from end to end. Either technique is acceptable.

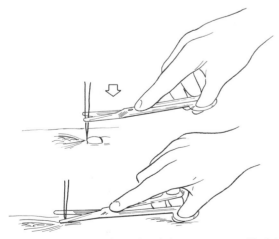

Figure 35–23. Cutting the tails of the suture. (Modified from Anderson, C. B.: Basic surgical techniques. *In* Klippel, A. P., and Anderson, C. B.: Manual of Outpatient and Emergency Surgical Techniques. Boston, Little, Brown & Co., 1979. Used by permission.)

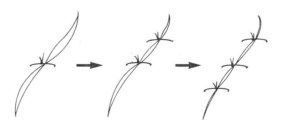

Figure 35–25. Closure of the surface of the wound in segments.

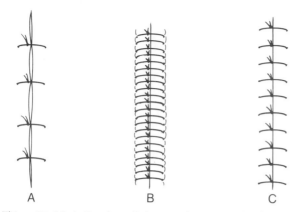

Figure 35–26. A, Too few stitches used. Note gapping between sutures. B, Too many stitches used. C, Correct number of stitches used for a wound under an average amount of tension.

"Sutures should be placed in a mirror-image fashion—the same depth and width on both sides of the incision unless uneven edges are encountered."[116] In general, the distance between each suture should be approximately equal to the distance from the exit of the stitch to the wound edge.[88, 111, 137] Grabb suggests that "the number of sutures used in closing any wound will vary with the case, location of the repair, and degree of accuracy required by the physician and patient. In an area such as the face, sutures would probably be placed between 1 and 3 mm apart and 1 to 2 mm from the wound edge."[87] Sutures act as foreign bodies in a wound, and any stitch may damage a blood vessel or strangulate tissue. Therefore, the physician should strive to use the smallest size and the least number of sutures that will adequately close the wound (Fig. 35–26).[4, 16, 122] Wounds with greater tension should have skin stitches placed closer to each other and closer to the wound edge; the technique of layered closure is of great importance in such wounds.[75] If sutures are tied too tightly around wound edges or if individual stitches are under excessive tension, blood supply to the wound may be impeded, increasing the chance of infection, and suture marks may form even after 24 hours.[116, 138, 139]

When suturing the skin, right-handed operators should pass the needle from the right side of the wound to the left.[88] The needle should enter the skin at an oblique angle in order to produce an everting, bottle-shaped stitch that is deeper than it is wide (Fig. 35–27). If the skin stitch is intended to produce some eversion of the wound edges, the stitch must include a sufficient amount of subcutaneous tissue.[75, 83] Yet encompassing too much tissue with a small needle is a common error. Forcefully pushing or twisting the needle in an effort to bring the point out of the tissue may bend or break the body of the needle. Using a needle of improper size will defeat the best suturing technique. One should drive the needle through tissue by flexing the wrist and supinating the forearm; the course taken by the needle should result in a curve that is identical to the curvature of the needle itself (Fig. 35–28). The angle of exit for the needle should be the same as its angle of entrance so that an identical volume of tissue is contained within the stitch on each side of the wound. Once the needle exits the skin on the opposite side of the wound, it is regrasped by the needle holder and is advanced through the tissue; care should be taken to avoid crushing the point of the needle with the instrument. Forceps are designed for handling tissue and thus should not be used to grasp the needle. The forceps should be used to hold the tissue through which the needle has just passed. Excess thread can be kept clear of the area being sutured by an assistant, or the excess can be looped around the fingers. If the point of the needle becomes dulled before all of the attached thread has been used, the suture should be discarded.[110]

If these techniques are applied to most wounds, the edges of the wound will be matched precisely in all three dimensions.

Eversion Techniques. If the edges of a wound invert or if one edge rolls under the opposite side, a poorly formed, deep, noticeable scar will result. Excessive eversion that exposes the dermis of both sides will also result in a larger scar than if the skin edges are perfectly apposed, but inversion produces a more visible scar than does eversion. Since most scars undergo some flattening with contraction, optimal results are achieved when the epidermis is very slightly everted (Fig. 35–29).[75, 87] Wounds over mobile surfaces, such as the extensor surfaces of joints, should be everted; in time, the scar will be flattened by the dynamic forces acting in the area.

A number of techniques can be used to achieve eversion of the edges of the wound. If the clinician angles the needle away from the laceration, percutaneous stitches can be placed so that their depth is greater than their width.[75, 98] Converse describes this method: "The needle penetrates the skin close to the incision line, diverging from the edge of the wound in order to encircle a larger amount of tissue in the lower depths of the skin than at the periphery."[140] The edge of the wound can be lifted and everted with a skin hook or fine-tooth forceps prior to insertion of the needle on each side (Fig. 35–30). Eversion can also be obtained simply by slight retraction of the wound with the thumb (Fig. 35–31) or with slight pressure on the wound edge with a closed forceps; each of these two methods also serves to steady the skin against the force of the needle.[88, 140] Vertical mattress sutures are particularly effective in everting the wound edges and can be used exclusively or

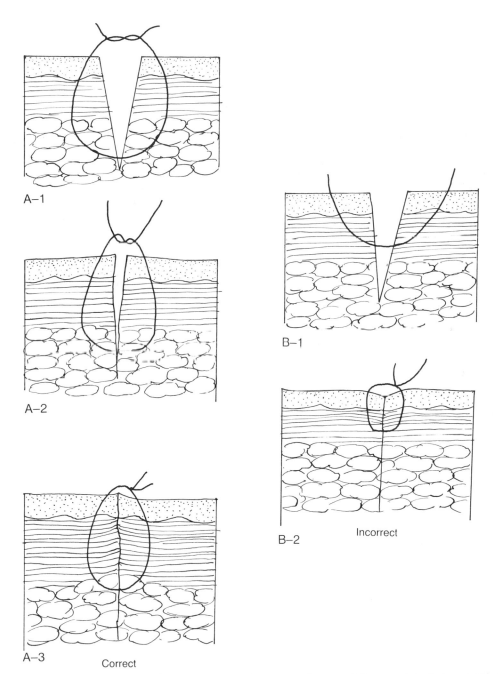

A–1

A–2

A–3   Correct

B–1

B–2   Incorrect

Figure 35–27. The stitch should be placed so that its depth is greater than its width *(A1–A3)*. A shallow, wide stitch *(B1–B2)* will invert the wound edges.

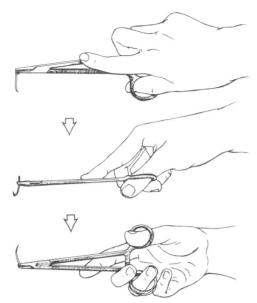

Figure 35–28. Motion of needle holder. (From Anderson, C. B.: Basic surgical techniques. In Klippel, A. P., and Anderson, C. B.: Manual of Outpatient and Emergency Surgical Techniques. Boston, Little, Brown & Co., 1979. Used by permission.)

can be alternated with simple interrupted sutures (Fig. 35–32).[110, 140] Walike states that in the repair of facial lacerations, the subcutaneous (dermal) stitch is a prerequisite to eversion of skin edges with a percutaneous stitch.[98] In wounds that have been undermined, a subcutaneous stitch placed at the base of the flap on each side can in itself evert the wound (Fig. 35–33).[23]

Interrupted Stitch. The simple interrupted stitch is the most frequently used technique in the closure of skin. It consists of separate loops of suture individually tied. Although the tying and cutting of each stitch is time-consuming, the advantage of this method is that if one stitch in the closure fails, the remaining stitches continue to hold the wound together (Fig. 35–34).[15, 110]

Continuous Stitch. In a continuous, or "running," stitch, the loops are connected; the stitch is tied at each end of the wound.[15] A continuous suture line can be placed more rapidly than a

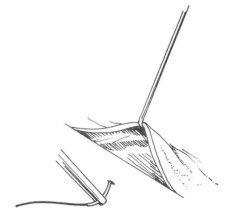

Figure 35–30. The use of a skin hook to evert the wound edge.

series of interrupted stitches. The continuous stitch has the additional advantages of strength (with tension being evenly distributed along its entire length), fewer knots (which are the weak points of stitches), and more effective hemostasis.[110] The continuous technique is useful as an epithelial stitch in cosmetic closures; however, if the underlying subcutaneous layer is not stabilized in a separate closure, the continuous surface stitch tends to invert the wound edges.

The continuous suture technique has some disadvantages. This technique cannot be used to close wounds overlying joints. If a loop breaks at one point, the entire stitch may unravel. Likewise, if infection develops and the incision must be opened at one point, cutting a single loop may allow the entire wound to fall open. There is a theoretical problem of impeded blood supply to the wound edges, particularly if the suture is

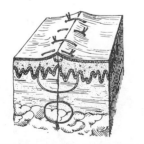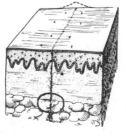

Figure 35–29. Skin edges that are everted will gradually flatten to produce a level wound surface. (From Grabb, W. C.: Basic technique of plastic surgery. In Grabb, W. C., and Smith, J. W.: Plastic Surgery: A Concise Guide to Clinical Practice. Boston, Little, Brown & Co., 1979. Used by permission.)

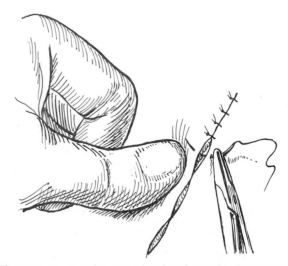

Figure 35–31. Eversion can often be obtained by slight thumb pressure. (From Converse, J. M.: Introduction to plastic surgery. In Converse, J. M.: Reconstructive Plastic Surgery: Principles and Procedures in Correction, Reconstruction, and Transplantation, 2nd ed., vol. 1. Philadelphia, W. B. Saunders Company, 1977. Used by permission.)

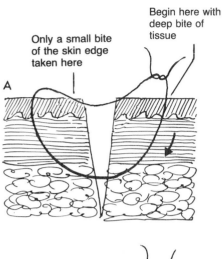

Only a small bite of the skin edge taken here

Begin here with deep bite of tissue

A

B

Figure 35–32. The vertical mattress suture is the best technique for producing skin edge eversion. A, Usual type of mattress suture for approximating and everting wound edges. B, "Tacking" type of vertical mattress suture, extending into deep fascia to obliterate dead space under wound. Note that only a small bite of skin is included on the inner suture. (Modified from Converse, J. M.: Introduction to plastic surgery. In Converse, J. M.: Reconstructive Plastic Surgery: Principles and Procedures in Correction, Reconstruction, and Transplantation, 2nd ed., vol. 1. Philadelphia, W. B. Saunders Company, 1977. Used by permission.)

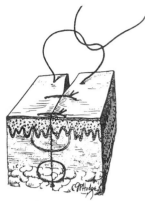

Figure 35–34. Simple interrupted stitch. Additional throws in partially tied knot are not shown. (From Grabb, W. C.: Basic techniques of plastic surgery. In Grabb, W. C., and Smith, J. W.: Plastic Surgery: A Concise Guide to Clinical Practice. Boston, Little, Brown & Co., 1973. Used by permission.)

interlocked.[116] Speer found that wounds closed with an interrupted stitch had 30 to 50 per cent greater tensile strength, less edema and induration, and less impairment in the microcirculation at the wound margin than did wounds closed with a continuous stitch. According to this study, wounds closed with interrupted stitches should have a smaller risk of infection than those closed with the continuous technique.[141] The simple continuous stitch has a tendency to produce suture marks if used in large wound closures and if left in place for more than 5 days.[87] If all tension on the wound can be removed by subcutaneous sutures, stitch marks are seldom a problem.

Among the variations of the continuous technique, the simple continuous stitch is the most useful to emergency physicians (Fig. 35–35). An interrupted stitch is placed at one end of the wound, and only the free tail of the suture is cut. As suturing proceeds, the stitch encircles tissue in a spiral pattern. After each passage of the needle, the loop is tightened slightly and the thread is held taut in the physician's non-dominant hand. The needle should travel perpendicularly across

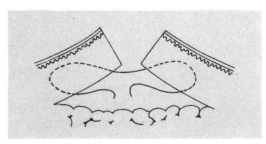

Figure 35–33. Deep dermis suturing technique. Suture enters base of flap, is brought up into dermis, and exits just proximally to wound edge along base of flap to be tied and cut. (From Stuzin, J., Engrav, L. H., and Buehler, P. K.: Emergency treatment of facial lacerations. Postgrad. Med. 71:81, 1982. Used by permission.)

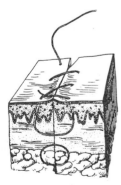

Figure 35–35. Simple continuous stitch. (From Grabb, W. C.: Basic techniques of plastic surgery. In Grabb, W. C., and Smith, J. W.: Plastic Surgery: A Concise Guide to Clinical Practice. Boston, Little, Brown & Co., 1979. Used by permission.)

the wound on each pass.[75] The last loop is placed just beyond the end of the wound, and the suture is tied with the last loop used as a "tail" in the process of tying the knot (Fig. 35–36). A locking loop may be used in continuous suturing in order to prevent slippage of loops as the suturing proceeds (Fig. 35–37). The interlocking technique allows the use of the continuous stitch along an irregular laceration.[98]

A continuous stitch is an effective method for closing relatively clean wounds that are under little or no tension and are on flat, immobile skin surfaces in patients without medical conditions that would impair healing.

Continuous Subcuticular Stitch. Nonabsorbable sutures used in percutaneous skin closure outlast their usefulness and must be removed. Some patients with wounds that require skin closure are unlikely or unwilling to return for suture removal. Some sutured wounds are covered by plaster casts. On occasion, the patient (child or adult) is likely to be as frightened and uncooperative for suture removal as for suture placement. The continuous subcuticular suture technique is ideal for these situations; the wound can be closed with an absorbable subcuticular stitch, obviating the need for later suture removal.[15] In patients prone to keloid formation, the subcuticular technique can be used in lieu of percutaneous stitches, and disfiguring stitch marks can thereby be avoided. (Because children's skin is under greater tension than adults', percutaneous sutures are more likely to produce stitch marks in children.) Because stitch marks are avoided, a nonabsorbable subcuticular suture can be left in place for a longer period than a percutaneous suture.[140]

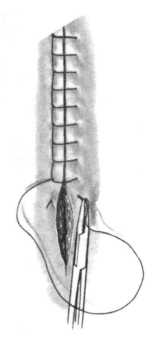

Figure 35–37. Continuous interlocking stitch. (Modified from Suture Use Manual: Use and Handling of Sutures and Needles. Somerville, NJ, Ethicon, Inc., 1977.)

Although this technique is commonly used in cosmetic closures, some authors believe that closure of the subcuticular layer alone does not alter the magnitude (width) of scar formation.[142] This technique does not allow for perfect approximation of the vertical heights of the two edges of a wound,[70] and in cosmetic closures it is often followed by a percutaneous stitch. With this technique, the large amount of suture material left in the wound would appear to increase the risk of infection and, once infection occurs, allows purulence to spread extensively along the suture line before infection is clinically apparent.[15] Other reports suggest a lower infection rate with the subcuticular technique because the skin microflora are not given an opportunity to invade the deeper tissues along percutaneous suture tracks.[142, 143]

The subcuticular stitch requires a 4-0 suture that is either made of absorbable material or is a nonabsorbable synthetic monofilament suture. An absorbable suture can be "buried" within the wound, whereas a nonabsorbable suture is used for a "pullout" stitch. A new absorbable synthetic monofilament suture called polydioxanone (PDS, Ethicon), is becoming available; it may pass through tissues as easily as nonabsorbable monofilament sutures, yet it will be absorbed if left in the wound by accident or by design. If PDS proves to have no undesirable characteristics, it may become the preferred suture material for this technique.

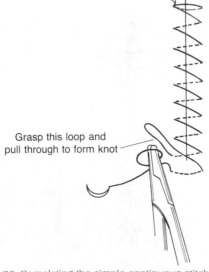

Grasp this loop and
pull through to form knot

Figure 35–36. Completing the simple continuous stitch. A series of square knots are tied using the loop as one of the ties.

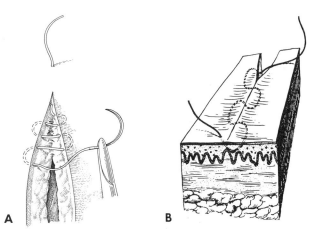

Figure 35–38. *A*, Pullout subcuticular stitch: The suture is introduced into the skin in line with the incision, approximately 1 to 2 cm away. (From Grimes, D. W., and Garner, R. W.: "Reliefs" in intra-cuticular sutures. Surgical Rounds 1:46, 1978. Used by permission.) *B*, By backtracking each stitch slightly, one can produce a straight scar. (From Grabb, W. C.: Basic techniques of plastic surgery. *In* Grabb, W. C., and Smith, J. W.: Plastic Surgery: A Concise Guide to Clinical Practice. Boston, Little, Brown & Co., 1979. Used by permission.)

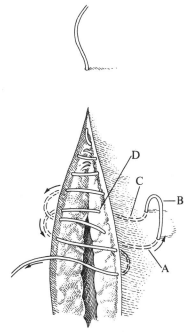

Figure 35–39. In construction of the relief, the suture is crossed to the opposite side, going into the subcuticular area beneath the skin for approximately 2 cm before exiting (*A*). The suture is then carried over the epidermis for approximately 2 cm (*B*), and then back under the dermis again (*C*). Re-entry is made into the wound area (*D* at approximately the same location as the next bite would have been placed had the relief not been used. (From Grimes, D. W., and Garner, R. W.: "Reliefs" in intra cuticular sutures. Surgical Rounds 1:47, 1978. Used by permission.)

Before the subcuticular stitch is placed, the subcutaneous layer should be approximated with interrupted sutures to minimize tension on the wound. The pullout subcuticular stitch is started at the skin surface approximately 1 to 2 cm away from one end of the wound. The needle enters and exits the dermis at the apices of the wound (Fig. 35–38). Bites through tissue are taken in a horizontal direction with the needle penetrating the dermis 1 to 2 mm from the skin surface. These intradermal bites should be small, of equal proportion, and at the same level on each side of the wound.[6, 140] Accidental interlocking of the stitch should be avoided. Each successive bite should be placed 1 to 2 mm *behind* the exit point on the opposite side of the wound so that when the wound is closed, the entrance and exit points on either side are not directly apposed (see Fig. 35–38). Small bites should be taken to avoid puckering of the skin surface.[87, 144] Some physicians prefer to place a fine (6-0) running skin suture in addition to the subcuticular suture for meticulous skin approximation. The skin suture is removed in 3 to 4 days to avoid suture marks.

If the subcuticular stitch is used on lengthy lacerations, it will be difficult to remove the suture. The placement of "reliefs" consisting of periodic loops through the skin during the length of the stitch facilitates later removal (Fig. 35–39). Reliefs should be placed every 4 to 5 cm. The suture is crossed to the opposite side and the needle is passed from subcutaneous tissue to the skin surface. The suture is carried over the surface for approximately 2 cm before re-entering the skin and subcutaneous tissue. The subcuticular stitch is then continued at approximately the point at which the next bite would have been placed had the relief not been used.[144]

At the completion of the stitch, the needle is placed through the apex to exit the skin 1 to 2 cm away from the end of the wound. One should tighten the stitch by pulling each end taut. If reliefs have been used, one can take up any slack in the stitch by pulling on the reliefs. The clinician can secure the two ends of the stitch by taping them to the skin surface with wound closure tape,[74] by placing a cluster of knots on each tail close to the skin surface, or by tying the two ends of the suture to each other over a dressing.[144] Laxity of the subcuticular stitch is often noted 48 hours after wound closure, possibly because of a decrease in tissue swelling. Some physicians will tighten the stitch when they re-examine the wound after 48 hours.

Stillman describes a technique using absorbable sutures that do not penetrate the skin. The closure is begun with a dermal or subcutaneous suture placed at one end of the wound and secured with a knot. After placement of the continuous subcuticular stitch from apex to apex, the suture is pulled taut and a knot is tied using a tail and a

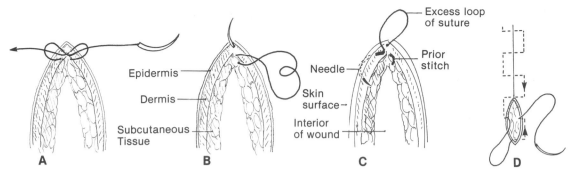

Figure 35–40. Subcuticular closure without epidermal penetration. *A*, The initial knot is secured in the dermal or subcutaneous tissue. *B*, The short strand is cut, and the needle is inserted into the dermis at the apex of the wound. *C*, Needle in dermis, close to the corner of the wound, and exiting the wound at the same horizontal level. *D*, After the subcuticular stitch has been completed, a knot is tied using the tail and the loop of the suture. (Modified from Stillman, R. M.: Wound closure: Choosing optimal materials and methods. ER Reports 2:43, 1981.)

loop of suture (Fig. 35–40). The final knot can be buried by insertion of the needle into deeper tissue; the needle exits several millimeters from the wound edge. If one pulls on the needle end, the knot will disappear into the wound.[6] The obvious advantage of this technique is that there are no suture marks in the skin. Another method that avoids penetrating the skin is the interrupted subcuticular stitch (Fig. 35–41).[140]

Nonabsorbable sutures can be left in place for 2 to 3 weeks, thus providing a longer period of support than percutaneous sutures without the problem of stitch marks.[87] If skin sutures are used in conjunction with the subcuticular stitch, they are removed in 3 to 4 days. A subcuticular closure in itself is stronger than a tape closure. If the subcuticular technique is used exclusively to approximate the skin surface, it is advisable to apply skin tape to correct surface unevenness and to provide a more accurate apposition of the epidermis.[15]

Mattress Stitch. The various types of mattress stitches are all interrupted stitches. The vertical mattress stitch is an effective method of ensuring eversion of the skin edges (Figs. 35–32 and 35–42).

The horizontal mattress stitch approximates skin edges closely while providing some degree of eversion (Fig. 35–43).[87] The half-buried horizontal mattress stitch, also called a mattress stitch with a dermal component, combines an interrupted skin stitch with a buried intradermal stitch (Fig. 35–44). It is effective in joining the edges of a skin flap to the edges of the "recipient site"; the dermal component is placed through the dermis of the flap.[140] The half-buried horizontal mattress stitch is also useful at the scalp-forehead junction when there is tension on the wound edges. This technique halves the number of suture marks in the skin and avoids necrosing the edge of a skin flap.

The half-buried horizontal mattress stitch is particularly useful in suturing the easily damaged apex of a V-shaped flap (Fig. 35–45). In the execution of the "corner stitch," the suture needle penetrates the skin at a point beyond the apex of the wound and exits through the dermis. The corner of the flap is elevated and the suture is passed through the dermis of the flap. The needle is then placed in the dermis of the base of the

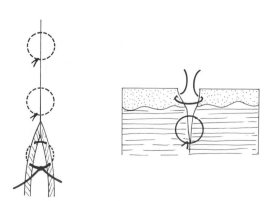

Figure 35–41. Interrupted subcuticular stitch (also called a "horizontal dermal stitch").

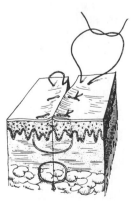

Figure 35–42. Vertical mattress stitch. (From Grabb, W. C.: Basic techniques of plastic surgery. *In* Grabb, W. C., and Smith, J. W.: Plastic Surgery: A Concise Guide to Clinical Practice. Boston, Little, Brown & Co., 1979. Used by permission.)

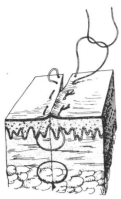

Figure 35–43. Horizontal mattress stitch. (From Grabb, W. C.: Basic techniques of plastic surgery. *In* Grabb, W. C., and Smith, J. W.: Plastic Surgery: A Concise Guide to Clinical Practice. Boston, Little, Brown & Co., 1979. Used by permission.)

wound and returned to the surface of the skin. All dermal bites should be placed at the same level. The suture is tied with a tension sufficient to pull the flap snugly into the corner without blanching the flap.[87, 89] If the tip of a large flap with questionable viability may be further jeopardized by postoperative swelling, a cotton stent can be placed underneath the knot of the corner stitch. The cotton will absorb the tension produced by swelling.[23]

Figure-of-Eight Stitch. The figure-of-eight stitch is useful in wounds with thin or friable tissue (Fig. 35–46). This stitch reduces the amount of tension placed on the tissue by the suture, allowing the stitch to hold in place when a simple stitch would tear through the tissue. One disadvantage of this technique is that more suture material is left in the wound. Dushoff recommends the figure-of-eight stitch for approximating muscle and fascial tissue, periosteum, and scalp lacerations.[129]

Cosmetic Closure of Facial Wounds. The ideal result in the repair of a facial laceration is an

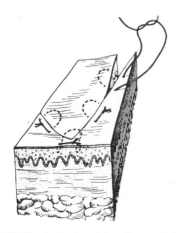

Figure 35–44. Half-buried horizontal mattress stitch. (From Grabb, W. C.: Basic techniques of plastic surgery. *In* Grabb, W. C., and Smith, J. W.: Plastic Surgery: A Concise Guide to Clinical Practice. Boston, Little, Brown & Co., 1979. Used by permission.)

extremely narrow, flat, and inapparent scar. In addition to basic wound management, a few additional techniques can be used to achieve this result. One of the factors that contributes to wide scars is necrosis of partially devitalized wound edges. On the other hand, skin with apparently marginal circulation may survive because of the excellent vascularity of the face. Subcutaneous fat, which in other locations may be débrided thoroughly, should be preserved if possible in facial wounds to prevent eventual sinking of the scar and to preserve normal facial contours. Therefore, débridement of most facial wounds should be conservative.[132, 145]

Converse pointed out that "precise approximation of skin edges without undue tension ensures primary healing with minimal scarring."[140] A layered closure is essential in the cosmetic repair of a facial wound. Approximation of the dermis with a subcutaneous stitch or a combination of subcutaneous and subcuticular stitches should bring the epithelial edges together or within 1 mm of apposition—close enough that the use of additional sutures seems unnecessary.[9] If a subcutaneous stitch is the only stitch used to close the deeper layers, it should pass through the dermal-epidermal junction or within 1 to 2 mm of the skin surface. The clinician must tie this stitch snugly, pulling the two ends of the suture in the same direction (see Fig. 35–22). Should the first subcutaneous stitch placed at the midpoint of a wound perfectly appose the skin edges, one can "protect" that stitch from disruption during further suturing by immediately placing a percutaneous stitch in the same location. If there is a slight gap in the wound edges after subcutaneous closure, the skin can be partially approximated with a few guide stitches. The first is placed at the midpoint of the wound, and subsequent stitches bisect the intervening spaces. Guide stitches allow the definitive epithelial sutures to be placed with little strain on each individual stitch, and they protect the subcutaneous stitches from disruption. Once the definitive stitches have been placed, the guide stitches, if slack, can be removed. Since a needle damages tissue with each passage through the skin, guide stitches should be used only when necessary.

The epithelial stitch should never be used to relieve the wound of tension; it serves only to match the epidermal surfaces precisely along the length of the wound. If there is a significant separation of the wound edges after closure of the subcutaneous layer, a 5-0 subcuticular suture can be used to eliminate the tension produced by this separation and to provide prolonged stability. Once the necessary near apposition of skin edges is produced, the epithelial stitch can be used to correct discrepancies in vertical alignment. A 6-0 synthetic nonabsorbable suture is an excellent ma-

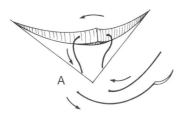

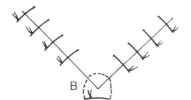

Figure 35-45. *A* and *B*, Approximation of a corner flap using a half-buried horizontal mattress stitch. Because of its applicability to this closure the stitch is often called a "corner stitch."

terial for this stitch, although some surgeons prefer 6-0 silk, trading greater reactivity for improved handling characteristics. A continuous stitch is preferable because it can be placed quickly, but interrupted stitches are acceptable. In a straight laceration, better apposition is achieved if the wound is stretched lengthwise by finger traction or by the use of skin hooks. When the needle is placed on one side of the wound, if that side is higher than the opposite side, a shallow bite is taken. The needle is used to depress the wound edge to the proper height, after which the needle "follows through" to the other side, "pinning" the two sides together. If the first side entered is lower, the needle is elevated to match the epithelial edges.

Grabb pointed out that "the closer the needle lies to the skin edge, the greater will be its effect in controlling the ultimate position of that edge."[87] Epithelial stitches should be spaced no more than 2 to 3 mm apart and should encompass no more than 2 to 4 mm of tissue.[98] If widely spaced, the sutures will leave marks.[9] Once skin closure is complete, final adjustments in the tension on the continuous suture line are made before the end of the stitch is tied. If any level discrepancies persist,

interrupted sutures or tape can be used to flatten these few irregularities.

Surgical tape is useful as a secondary support, protecting the epithelial stitch from stresses produced by normal skin movements (Fig. 35-47). Facial wounds have a tendency to swell and place excessive stretch on an epithelial stitch. This can be minimized by application of a pressure dressing and cold compresses to the wound following closure. Surgical tape can serve to a limited extent as a pressure dressing.

Correction of Dog-Ears. When wound edges are not precisely aligned horizontally, there will be an excess of tissue on one or both ends. This small flap of excess skin that bunches up at the end of a sutured wound is commonly called a dog-ear. This effect also occurs when one side of the wound is more elliptic than the opposite side or when an excision of a wound is not sufficiently elliptic—when it is either too straight or too nearly circular.[111, 140]

If a dog-ear is present, it can be eliminated on one side of the wound in the following manner: The flap of excess skin is elevated with a skin hook; an incision is carried at an oblique angle from the apex of the wound toward the side with

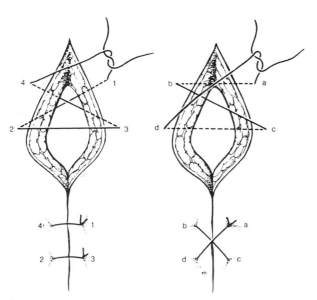

Figure 35-46. Figure-of-eight stitch—two methods. (From Dushoff, I. M.: About face. Emerg. Med. 6(1):1974. Used by permission.)

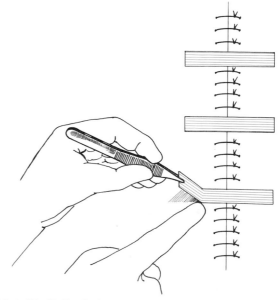

Figure 35-47. Surgical tape can be used to provide additional support while sutures are in place and after they are removed.

the excess skin. The flap is then undermined and laid flat. The resulting triangle of skin is trimmed, and the closure is completed (Fig. 35–48A).[7, 13, 75, 89] An alternative method consists of carrying the incision directly from the apex, in line with the wound. The flap of excess tissue is pulled over the incision while skin hooks retract the extended apex of the wound. Excess tissue is excised and the remainder of the wound is sutured.[140] If dog-ears are present on *both* sides of one end of the wound, the bulge of excess tissue can be excised in an elliptic fashion and the wound can be closed (Fig. 35–48B).[89]

V-Y Advancement Flap. If a corner stitch produces excessive tension on the tip of the flap, a V-Y closure can be used to approximate the edges without undue tension. An incision carried away from the apex of the wound converts it from a V to a Y configuration (Fig. 35–49). The newly formed wound edges are undermined, and the repair is completed. A half-buried mattress stitch is placed at the fork of the Y.[89]

Stellate Lacerations. The repair of a stellate laceration is a challenging problem. Usually a result of compression and shear forces, these injuries contain large amounts of partially devitalized tissue. The surrounding soft tissue is often swollen and contused. Much of this contused tissue cannot be débrided without creating a large tissue defect. Sometimes tissue is lost, yet the amount is not apparent until key sutures are placed. In repairing what often resembles a jigsaw puzzle, the physician can remove small flaps of necrotic tissue with an iris scissors; large, viable flaps can be repositioned in their beds and carefully secured with half-buried mattress stitches. If interrupted stitches are used to approximate a thin flap, small bites should be taken in the flap and larger, deeper bites in the base of the wound. A modification of the corner stitch can be used to approximate multiple flaps to a base (Fig. 35–50). The V-Y advancement flap technique is also useful. Thin flaps of tissue in a stellate laceration with beveled edges are often most easily repositioned and stabilized with a firm dressing.[87] Closure of stellate lacerations cannot always be accomplished immediately, especially if there is considerable soft tissue swelling. It may be best in some instances

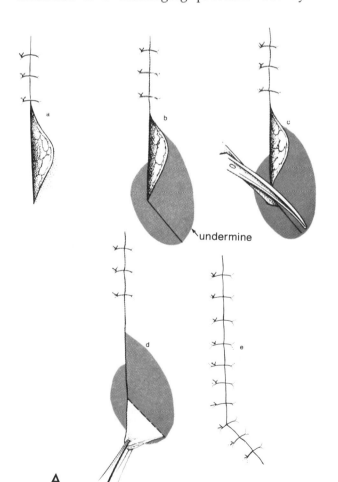

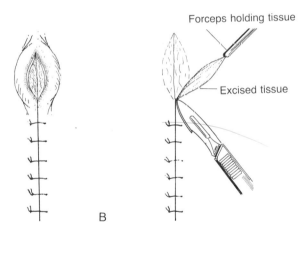

Figure 35–48. *A,* Correction of a "dog-ear." (From Dushoff, I. M.: A stitch in time. Emerg. Med. 5(3):1, 1973. Used by permission.) *B,* Excision of bilateral dog-ears.

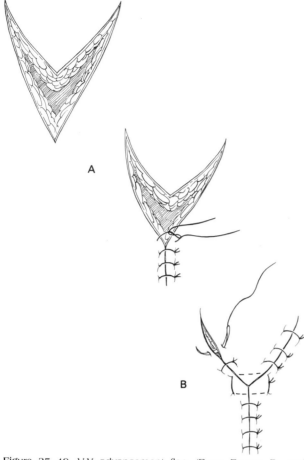

Figure 35—49. V-Y advancement flap. (From Rosen, P., and Sternbach, G.: Atlas of Emergency Medicine. Baltimore, Williams & Wilkins, 1979, p. 132. Used by permission.)

to consider delayed closure or revision of the scar at a later date. In complicated lacerations, inexact tissue approximation may be all that is possible initially.

Repair of Special Structures

Scalp. The scalp extends from the supraorbital ridges anteriorly to the external occipital protuberances posteriorly and blends with temporalis fascia laterally. There are five anatomic layers of the

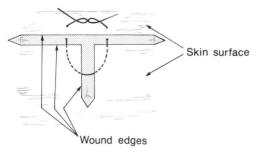

Figure 35—50. View from above stellate laceration, showing closure with half-buried mattress stitches.

scalp: skin, superficial fascia, galea aponeurotica, subaponeurotic areolar connective tissue, and periosteum (Fig. 35–51A). Surgically, the scalp may be divided into three distinct layers. The outer layer consists of the skin, superficial fascia, and the galea (the aponeurosis of the frontalis and occipitalis muscles). These three layers are firmly adherent and surgically are considered as one layer. The integrity of the outer layers is maintained by inelastic tough fibrous septae, which keep wounds from gaping open unless all three layers have been transversed. Wounds that gape open signify a laceration beneath the galea layer. The galea itself is loosely adherent to the periosteum by means of the slack areolar tissue of the subaponeurotic layer. The periosteum covers the skull. The periosteum is sometimes mistakenly identified as the galea, and vain attempts to suture the flimsy periosteum are made in the hope of "closing the galea."[146]

There are several unique problems associated with wounds of the scalp. The presence of a rich vascular network and the fact that severed scalp vessels tend to remain patent are both responsible for the profuse bleeding associated with scalp wounds. The tough, fibrous subcutaneous fascia hinders the normal retraction of blood vessels that have been cut, allowing for persistent or massive hemorrhage in simple lacerations. The subgaleal layer of loose connective tissue contains "emissary veins" that drain through diploic vessels of the skull into the venous sinuses of the cranial hemispheres. In scalp wounds that penetrate this layer, bacteria may be carried by these vessels to the meninges and the intracranial sinuses. Thus, a scalp wound infection can result in osteomyelitis, meningitis, or brain abscess.[147, 148] Careful approximation of galeal lacerations not only ensures control of bleeding but also protects against the spread of infection.

Shear-type injuries can cause extensive separation of the superficial layers from the galeal layer. Debris and other contaminants can be deposited several centimeters from the visible laceration.[129] Careful exploration and cleaning of scalp wounds is of obvious importance.

Because the scalp is so vulnerable to blunt trauma and because its superficial fascial layer is inelastic and firmly adherent to the skin, stellate lacerations are common in this region. Stellate lacerations not only pose additional technical problems in closure but also have a greater propensity toward infection. In the multiply injured patient, scalp wounds are easily overlooked; these are frequently numerous and hidden by a mat of hair.

When scalp wounds are débrided, obviously devitalized tissue should be removed, but débridement should be conservative, since closure of large defects is difficult on the scalp. When facing profuse bleeding, especially from extensive lacera-

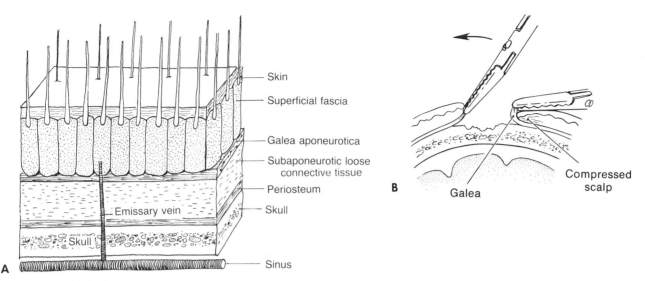

Figure 35–51. A, Anatomy of the scalp. B, Temporary control of bleeding from scalp lacerations by eversion of galea. (From Rosen, P., and Sternbach, G.: Atlas of Emergency Medicine. Baltimore, Williams & Wilkins, 1979, p. 128. Used by permission.)

tions, the physician should instruct an assistant to maintain compression around the wound during the closure rather than try to tie off bleeding vessels. Unless the vessels are large or few, ligation of individual scalp vessels seldom provides effective hemostasis, and considerable bleeding can occur during the attempt. The bleeding from scalp lacerations is best controlled by expeditious suturing.[89] The clinician may temporarily control bleeding in some cases by grasping the galea and the dermis with a hemostat and everting the instrument over the skin edge (see Fig. 35–51B). The disadvantage of this technique is that tissue grasped by the hemostat may be crushed and devitalized,[89] and if the subcutaneous tissue is also everted for a prolonged period, necrosis can occur. Without an assistant to apply direct pressure, the use of local anesthetics containing epinephrine is sometimes an effective method of controlling the persistent bleeding from small vessels in scalp wounds.

Prior to wound closure, the underlying skull should be palpated in an attempt to detect fractures. More small skull fractures are detected with the gloved finger than with radiographs. A common error is to mistake a rent in the galea or the periosteum for a fracture during palpation inside the wound. Direct visualization of the area should resolve the issue. In wounds exposing bone but not penetrating the skull, prolonged exposure may leave a nidus of dead bone that may develop osteomyelitis. Exposed bone that is visibly necrosed should be removed with ronguers until active bleeding appears.[89] Hair surrounding the scalp wound usually must be shaved or clipped far enough from the wound edge so that suturing can proceed without entangling the hair in knots or imbedding hair within the wound. Vaseline or

tape may be placed on stubborn hairs that persistently fall into the wound. Although shaving the scalp is not popular with some patients, failure to shave an area adequately is a common cause of improper preparation and closure of scalp wounds.

Unlike most wounds involving multiple layers of tissue, scalp wounds should be closed with a single layer of sutures, incorporating skin, subcutaneous fascia, and the galea. The periosteum need not be sutured. In order to minimize the chance of infection, subcutaneous deep sutures are avoided whenever possible. In superficial wounds, skin and subcutaneous tissue should be approximated with simple interrupted or vertical mattress stitches using a nonabsorbable 3-0 nylon or polypropylene suture. Smaller suture material tends to break while firm knots are being tied and should not be used. The ends of the tied scalp sutures should be left at least 2 cm long to facilitate subsequent suture removal. If the galea is also torn, one should include the galea in the skin stitch.[148] Some authors recommend a separate closure of the galea with an absorbable 3-0 or 4-0 suture, using an inverted stitch that "buries" the knot beneath the galea.[23, 89] Separate closure of the galea introduces additional suture material into the wound but in some circumstances allows a more secure approximation of this structure. Stellate lacerations or crush lacerations may be excised to produce elliptical incisions if the area involved is not extensive.

Large sections of skin avulsed from the scalp can, with microvascular techniques, be reimplanted. The emergency physician should use the same techniques in salvaging avulsed scalp as are used for amputated extremities.[148] (See chapter 42 for further discussion.)

Because of the extensive collateral blood supply of the scalp, most lacerations in this area heal without problems. Nonetheless, wound care must be careful and thorough if the devastating complication of scalp infection is to be avoided.

Sutured scalp lacerations need not be bandaged, and patients can wash their hair in 24 hours. If bleeding is persistent, an elastic bandage can be used as a compression dressing. Gauze sponges are placed over the laceration to provide direct local pressure beneath the elastic bandage.

Forehead. Although the forehead is actually a part of the scalp, lacerations in this region are treated as facial wounds. Vertical lacerations across the forehead are oriented 90 degrees to skin tension lines, and resulting scars are more noticeable than those from horizontal lacerations. Midline vertical forehead lacerations may result in cosmetically acceptable scars with standard closure techniques; those lacerations that are not centered often require S-plasty or Z-plasty techniques during the initial repair or during later revision of the scar.[129]

Superficial lacerations may be closed with skin stitches alone, but deep forehead lacerations must be closed in layers. The periosteum should be approximated before the closure of more superficial layers. If skin is directly exposed to bone, adhesions may develop that in time may limit the movement of skin during facial expressions. The frontalis muscle and adjacent fibrous tissue should be approximated as a distinct layer; if left unsutured, the retracted ends of this muscle will bulge beneath the skin. If the gap in a muscle belly is later filled with scar tissue, movement of the muscle will pull on the entire scar and will make it more apparent.[129, 132]

A U-shaped flap laceration with a superiorly oriented base poses a difficult problem. Immediate vascular congestion and later scar contraction within the flap produce the "trap-door effect," with the flap becoming prominently elevated (Fig. 35–52). This effect can be minimized by approximation of the bulk of subcutaneous tissue of the flap to a deeper level on the base side of the wound; the skin surfaces of the two sides are

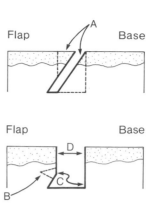

Figure 35–53. Repair of a U-shaped flap laceration with a superiorly oriented base. *A*, Excision of edges. *B*, Undermining. *C*, Approximation of subcutaneous tissue on the flap to subcutaneous tissue at a deeper level on the base. *D*, Skin closure.

apposed at the same level (Fig. 35–53). A firm compression dressing will help eliminate "dead space" and hematoma formation within the wound. Despite these efforts, secondary revision is sometimes necessary.[87] Often, swelling of the flap will resolve over a 6- to 12-month period. Because flap elevation can be quite disconcerting, the physician should forewarn the patient and family about a possible "trap-door effect."

When a forehead laceration borders the scalp and the thick scalp tissue must be sutured to thinner forehead skin, a horizontal mattress stitch with an intradermal component can be used (Fig. 35–54).[140]

Eyebrow and Eyelid Lacerations. Jagged lacerations through eyebrows should be managed with little, if any, débridement of untidy but viable edges. The hair shafts of the eyebrow grow at an oblique angle, and vertical excision may produce a linear alopecia in the eyebrow, whereas with simple closure the scar will remain hidden within the hair. If partial excision is unavoidable, the scalpel blade should be angled in a direction parallel to the axis of the hair shaft to minimize damage to hair follicles (see Fig. 35–7).[129]

Points on each side of the lacerated eyebrow should be aligned precisely; a single percutaneous stitch on each margin of the eyebrow should precede subcutaneous closure. The edges of the eyebrow serve as landmarks for reapproximation; therefore, the eyebrow must not be shaved or these landmarks will be lost. Shaved eyebrows grow back slowly and sometimes incompletely, and shaving them often results in more deformity than the injury itself. Care must be taken not to invert hair-bearing skin into the wound.[70]

The thin, flexible skin of the upper eyelid is relatively easy to suture. A soft, size 6-0 suture is recommended for closure of simple lacerations. Traumatized eyelids are susceptible to massive swelling; compression dressings and cold compresses can be used to minimize this problem.

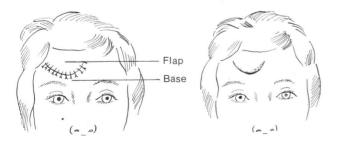

Figure 35–52. Elevation of a forehead flap—the "trap-door effect." (From Grabb, W. C., and Kleinert, H. E.: Technics in Surgery: Facial and Hand Injuries. Ethicon, Inc., 1980. Used by permission.)

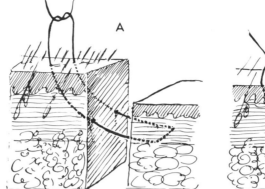 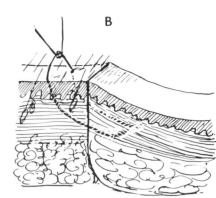

Figure 35–54. Horizontal mattress suture with an intradermal component. *A* and *B*, Eversion of thinner skin to obtain adequate approximation with thicker scalp tissue. (From Converse, J. M.: Introduction to plastic surgery. *In* Converse, J. M.: Reconstructive Plastic Surgery: Principles and Procedures in Correction, Reconstruction, and Transplantation, 2nd ed., vol. 1. Philadelphia, W. B. Saunders Co., 1977. Used by permission.)

It is essential that the emergency physician recognize complicated lid lacerations that require the expertise of an ophthalmologist. Lacerations that traverse the lid margin require exact realignment to avoid entropion or extropion. Injuries penetrating the tarsal plate frequently cause damage to the globe. A deep horizontal laceration through the upper lid that divides the thin levator palpebral muscle or its tendinous attachment to the tarsal plate will produce ptosis. If this muscle cannot be identified and repaired by the emergency physician, a consultant should repair the injury primarily. A laceration through the portion of the lower lid *medial* to the punctum frequently damages the lacrimal duct or the medial canthal ligament and requires specialized techniques for repair. If adipose tissue is seen within any periorbital laceration, one must assume that the orbital septum has been penetrated and the retrobulbar fat is herniating through the wound. The repair of lid avulsions, extensive lid lacerations with loss of tissue, and any of the other complex types of lid lacerations mentioned should be left to ophthalmologists.[129, 149]

Ear Lacerations. The primary goal in the management of lacerations of the pinna is expedient coverage of exposed cartilage. Cartilage is an avascular tissue, and when ear cartilage is denuded of its protective, nutrient-providing skin, progressive erosive chondritis will ensue. The initial step in the repair of an ear injury involves trimming away jagged or devitalized cartilage and skin. If the skin cannot be stretched to cover the defect, additional cartilage along the wound margin can be removed. Depending on the location, as much as 5 mm of cartilage can be removed without significant deformity. Cartilage should be approximated with 4-0 or 5-0 absorbable sutures initially placed at folds or ridges representing major landmarks. Sutures tear through cartilage; therefore, the anterior and posterior perichondrium should be included in the stitch. No more tension should be applied than is needed to touch the edges together.

In through-and-through ear lacerations, the posterior skin surface should be approximated next, using 5-0 nonabsorbable synthetic sutures. Once closure of the posterior surface is completed, the convoluted anterior surface of the ear can be approximated with 5-0 or 6-0 nonabsorbable synthetic sutures, with landmarks joined point by point. On the free rim, the skin should be everted if later notching is to be avoided. Care should be taken to cover all exposed cartilage. In heavily contaminated wounds of the ear (e.g., bite wounds) that already show evidence of inflammation, necrotic tissue should be debrided, the cartilage covered by a loose approximation of skin, and the patient placed on antibiotics.[74, 87, 129] After a lacerated ear has been sutured, it should be enclosed in a compression dressing.

Lacerations of the Nose. In the repair of lacerations of the nose, reapproximation of the wound edges is difficult because the skin is inflexible, and even deeply placed stitches will slice through the epidermis and pull out. When the wound edges cannot be easily coapted, absorbable sutures can be placed in the fibrofatty junction in a subcutaneous stitch prior to skin closure. Since it is difficult to approximate gaping wounds in this location, débridement must be kept to a minimum. Nasal cartilage is frequently involved in wounds of the nose, but it is seldom necessary to suture the cartilage itself.

The free rim of the nostril must be aligned precisely in order to avoid unsightly notching. As with ear lacerations, if the skin edges are not easily brought together, the edges of the divided cartilage can be slightly trimmed.

Many authors recommend early removal of stitches to avoid stitch marks, yet the oily nature of skin in this area makes it difficult to keep the wound closed with tape. A subcuticular stitch is recommended to provide support for a prolonged period.[129, 147, 150]

Lip and Intraoral Lacerations. Lip lacerations are cosmetically deforming injuries, but if the physician follows a few guidelines, these lacerations usually heal satisfactorily.

The contamination of all intraoral and lip wounds is considerable; they must be thoroughly irrigated. Regional nerve blocks are preferred to local injection, since the latter method distends tissue, distorts the anatomy of the lip, and obscures the vermilion border. Dushoff recommends converting all oblique lacerations through the vermilion border into incisions perpendicular to this line so that the wound remains parallel to skin tension lines (Fig. 35–55).[129] Losses of less than 25 per cent of the lip permit primary closure with little deformity; losses of greater than 25 per cent require a reconstructive procedure. Extensive lacerations directly through the commissure of the mouth also require surgical consultation in most cases.[23, 74, 129] Deep scars in the vermilion of the upper lip may produce a redundancy of tissue that requires later revision.[74, 132, 151]

Through-and-through lacerations of lip should be closed in three layers. The muscle layer is approximated using a 4-0 or 5-0 absorbable suture, with the stitch securely anchored in the fibrous tissue located anterior and posterior to the muscle. The vermilion-cutaneous junction of the lip is a critical landmark that, if divided, must be repositioned with precision; a 1-mm "step-off" is apparent and cosmetically unacceptable. The vermilion border should be approximated with a 5-0 or 6-0 nonabsorbable stay suture before any further closure to ensure proper alignment throughout the remainder of the repair (Fig. 35–56). The vermilion surface of the lip and buccal mucosa are then closed with interrupted stitches using an absorbable 4-0 or 5-0 suture. Finally, the skin is closed with 6-0 nonabsorbable sutures.[23, 152]

Small lacerations of the oral mucosa heal well without sutures. If a mucosal laceration creates a flap of tissue that falls between the occlusal surfaces of the teeth or if a laceration is extensive enough to trap food particles (e.g., a laceration approximately 2 to 3 cm or greater in length), it should be closed. Small flaps may be excised. Closure is easily accomplished with 4-0 Dexon or Vicryl using a simple interrupted suturing technique. These materials are soft and nonabrasive, whereas gut sutures become hard and traumatize adjacent mucosa. Muscle and mucosal layers should be closed separately. Sutures in the oral cavity easily become untied by the constant motion of the tongue. Each knot should be tied with at least four square knots. These sutures need not

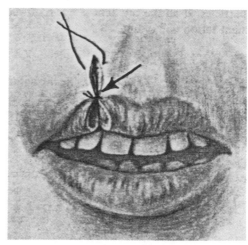

Figure 35–56. In the repair of lip lacerations, the first stitch should be placed at the vermilion-cutaneous border to obtain proper alignment. (From Grabb, W. C., and Kleinert, H. E.: Technics in Surgery: Facial and Hand Injuries. Somerville, NJ, Ethicon, Inc., 1980. Used by permission.)

be removed; they either will loosen and fall out within 1 week or will be rapidly absorbed.[132, 152, 153]

Tongue Lacerations. There is some controversy regarding when to suture tongue lacerations. Dushoff recommends suturing all lacerations of the tongue to prevent continuous bleeding.[129] Snyder suggests that only those lacerations that involve the edge or pass completely through the tongue, flap lacerations, and bleeding lacerations need to be sutured. There is no question that lacerations bisecting the tongue require repair.[147] Small flaps on the edge of the tongue may be excised. Large flaps should be sutured. Small tongue lacerations that are linear and involve the central portion of the tongue do well without suturing. Such lacerations are common in falls and during seizures. When peroxide mouth rinses and a soft diet are used for a few days, healing is rapid. Persistent bleeding from minor lacerations brings most patients to the hospital.

The repair of a tongue laceration in any patient is somewhat difficult, but in an uncooperative child the procedure may prove impossible under anything other than general anesthesia. A Denhardt side mouth gag aids in keeping the patient's mouth open. One may obtain anesthesia in a localized area of the tongue by covering the area with cocaine-soaked gauze or 4 per cent lidocaine-soaked gauze for 5 minutes. Large lacerations require infiltration anesthesia or a lingual nerve block. If the tip of the tongue has been anesthetized, a towel clip or suture can be used to secure the tongue. Further anesthesia and subsequent wound cleansing and closure are possible while an assistant applies gentle traction to the tongue.

Size 4-0 absorbable sutures should be used to close all three layers—inferior mucosa, muscle,

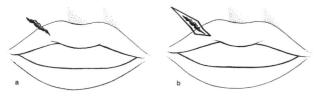

Figure 35–55. Dushoff's technique for lip lacerations. (From Dushoff, I. M.: About face. Emerg. Med. Nov. 1974. Used by permission.

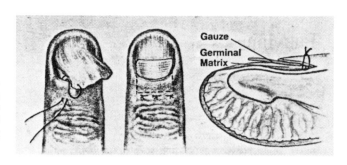

Figure 35–57. Avulsion of the nail leaving the matrix intact requires only a nonadherent dressing to separate the skin fold from the nail bed. If the germinal matrix is avulsed, it should be replaced with 6–0 plain absorbable surgical gut sutures. (From Grabb, W. C., and Kleinert, H. E.: Technics in Surgery: Facial and Hand Injuries. Somerville, NJ, Ethicon, Inc., 1980. Used by permission.)

and superior mucosa—in a single stitch[23] or the stitch should include one half of the thickness of the tongue, with sutures placed on the superior and inferior surfaces as well as on the edge of the tongue.[147] Sutures on the tongue frequently become untied. This problem can be avoided if the stitches are inverted.[132] Closure of the lingual muscle layer is usually sufficient to control bleeding and to return motor function to the lacerated tongue. Mucosal healing is rapid, and closure of the muscle layer only with a deep absorbable suture may be desirable when a surface suture is likely to be tugged at—as occurs with small children.

Nail Lacerations. Injuries to nails and nail beds are common problems in emergency medicine. If a nail is completely avulsed, no attempt should be made to reimplant it. If the nail bed has been lacerated, it is approximated with absorbable sutures. The nail bed should be protected by a light petrolatum gauze and a dry dressing for approximately 3 weeks.

One must be certain to maintain the proximal nail fold by gentle placement of the petrolatum gauze under the proximal cuticle overlying the germinal matrix (Fig. 35–57). If longitudinal scar bands are formed between the cuticle and the matrix, a split nail may result. Once the nail has been completely avulsed, the nail bed will become dry and less sensitive to pain.

A partially avulsed nail can be held in place as a temporary splint or "dressing" that protects the underlying nail bed. If the base of the nail is avulsed from the germinal matrix, it need not be forced back under the cuticle, since this may occasionally result in infection. Instead, the proximal portion of the nail can be removed and the distal part of the nail sutured in place.[86] Some authors believe that in children, replacement of the partially avulsed proximal nail into the nail fold is unlikely to lead to infection, although the injured nail may eventually be replaced by another. If the germinal matrix of the nail bed is avulsed, it should be reimplanted using a 5-0 or 6-0 absorbable suture in a mattress stitch (see Fig. 35–57).[132, 154]

If part of the nail bed has been lost, some authors recommend a split-thickness skin graft or

a matrix graft held in place with a stent dressing.[86, 132]

Lacerations through the nail bed should be sutured to prevent distortions in the new nail. The incidence of nail deformities following simple nail bed lacerations without an associated major crush injury is unknown. The desirability of nail removal prior to nail bed closure is also uncertain. Some authors recommend removal of the entire nail prior to nail bed closure. Dushoff recommends placement of stitches through a lacerated but attached nail.[92]

When repairing distal digit lacerations involving a nail, one should approximate the onychal fold first (Fig. 35–58). A sturdy needle attached to a

Suture the nail

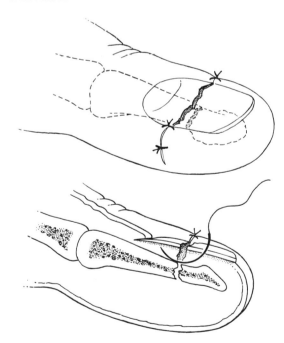

The nail seems to get neglected but it deserves better, particularly when it's cut through. First line up the onychal folds—your landmarks— tack them together, and do the requisite skin closure. Now put a stout reverse-cutting-edge needle, with 4-0 nylon, held halfway down so it doesn't bend, through the distal nail fragment, cross over the bone and up through the proximal nail. Two sutures should do the trick.

Figure 35–58. Repair of distal finger laceration involving the nail and the onychal fold. (From Dushoff, I. M.: Handling the hand. Emerg. Med. Oct. 1976, p. 111. Used by permission.)

4-0 thread is recommended for suturing lacerated nails. Needles seem to penetrate nails with the least difficulty when they enter at 90 degrees. The point of the needle carves a rigid path through the nail. Unless the entire length of the needle is allowed to follow this path as it passes through the nail, the needle is likely to bend or break. Alternatively, an electrical cautery instrument or a heated paper clip can be used to perforate the nail, thus permitting easy passage of the needle. Dushoff suggests that skin closure "consist of relatively few, accurately placed, wide and deeply spaced sutures, loosely tied in order to permit the free drainage of any fluid accumulation . . ."[92] The nail bed will heal in 2 to 3 weeks, and the nail is usually loose enough to be removed (if the patient desires) at that time.

Drains in Sutured Wounds

Drains do not prevent infection; they simply allow wounds to drain any collection of purulence or blood that may develop. When no infection exists and drains are used in soft tissue wounds "prophylactically," they are more harmful than beneficial. Edlich states that "drains act as retrograde conduits through which skin contaminants gain entrance into the wound. Furthermore, the presence of a drain impairs the resistance of the tissue to infection."[1] Magee found that drains placed in experimental wounds contaminated with subinfective doses of bacteria greatly enhanced the rate of infection, whether the drain was placed entirely within the wound or was brought out through the wound.[155] Drains behave as foreign bodies, provoking rather than preventing infection. If the wound is considered at high risk for infection, rather than suture the wound with a drain in place (in anticipation of disaster), the physician should leave the wound open and at a later time consider delayed primary closure, when the risk of infection is minimal. Furthermore, drains should not serve as substitutes for other methods of achieving hemostasis in traumatic wounds.

Protection

DRESSINGS

Wound dressings serve a variety of functions. They can be used to protect the wound from contamination and trauma, to absorb secretions from the wound, to immobilize the wound and the surrounding area, to exert downward pressure on the wound, and to improve the patient's comfort.[9, 156, 157] Occlusive dressings on burns or abrasions prevent painful exposure of the wound to the air and dehydration of the wound surface.[158]

Schauerhamer and coworkers demonstrated that sutured wounds are susceptible to infection from surface contamination during the first 2 postoperative days. Dressings effectively protect the wound from contamination during this vulnerable period. Taped wounds have a much higher resistance to infection than do sutured wounds.[159]

Stillman and associates found that the application of paint-on collodion dressing over a wound closed with a buried subcuticular stitch provided considerable resistance to infection compared with wounds closed by the same technique but with no dressing.[160] The use of collodion obviates the need for a gauze dressing, frequent dressing changes, and uncomfortable dressings in areas such as the groin, the axilla, and the neck.[6] The collodion, however, does not allow drainage of the wound and so is rarely used. Lawrence pointed out that wounds covered with permeable dressings, such as plain gauze, tend to dry out. Drying damages a shallow layer of exposed dermis, which can hinder healing, especially the healing of abrasions and burns.[157] On the other hand, occlusive dressings (e.g., Telfa pads, noncommercial occlusive dressings, polyurethane film) can macerate the skin surface beneath them and can allow bacterial growth, especially if they are not changed frequently.[157, 161]

One of the primary functions of a gauze dressing is to absorb the serosanguineous drainage that exudes from all wounds. Absorbent dressings also minimize the development of stitch abscesses to some extent. Surface sutures produce small indentations at their points of entrance; tiny blood clots and debris overlie these indentations, allowing bacterial growth at the site. Small "stitch abscesses" can develop; these are initially undetectable but are nevertheless destructive to epithelium. Stitch abscesses rarely infect the entire wound but can slightly increase the width of the scar and produce noticeable, punctate suture marks.[9]

A simple, dry dressing of sterile gauze held in place by adhesive tape is suitable for most wounds closed primarily. At the conclusion of the procedure, dried blood on the skin surface should be gently wiped away with gauze soaked in half-strength hydrogen peroxide. A nonadherent layer of petrolatum gauze (e.g., Adaptic, Xeroform, Aquaflo) can be applied next to the wound surface to prevent the wound from sticking to the dry gauze and to protect the regenerating epithelium. This material should always be used to cover skin grafts.[104]

Some authors advise using porous gauze dressing over wounds; when the gauze adheres to the wound surface, removal of the gauze "débrides" the wound. Unfortunately, new epithelium on the wound surface is also lost with this maneuver. It would seem that débridement of the wound with surgical instruments is more controlled and less traumatic to new tissue, yet as effective as débridement by dressing changes. Some authors use fine mesh gauze rather than petrolatum gauze on abrasions, especially on those wounds that are heavily contaminated, because removal of this type of dressing débrides only the small tufts of granulation tissue that become fixed in the mesh pores, leaving a clean, even surface. Once a healthy, granulating surface is present and re-epithelialization is proceeding, nonporous dressings can be used.[137] Fine mesh gauze is also used next to exposed tissue in wounds being considered for delayed primary closure; a protective and absorptive bulky dressing is placed on top of the wound.[104] In dressing wounds with considerable drainage, sufficient gauze should be used to cover the wound and to absorb all of the drainage. Dressings on such wounds can be changed daily, which is frequent enough to avoid bacterial overgrowth beneath the dressing.[4, 137] Once a dressing becomes moist, pathogens can pass through the dressing to the underlying wound.[157] Any dressing should be changed whenever it becomes soiled, wet, or saturated with drainage.

Dressings and bandages can serve as surface splints (as can surgical tape) by reducing mechanical stresses on the wound during the early phases of healing. Even when subcuticular stitches have been used, these "external splints" are useful in relieving tension across the wound. They are most needed between the seventh and forty-second days, the time of collagen synthesis and remodeling.[9] Stronger measures are required for wounds in mobile areas, such as around large joints, where rigid immobilization with plaster splints or braces is needed to protect the wound.

Compressive dressings may be helpful in preventing hematoma formation and eliminating dead space within a wound. They are particularly useful in wounds that have been undermined extensively and in facial wounds, where subcutaneous capillary bleeding and swelling can exert tension on fine skin sutures and jeopardize the skin closure (Fig. 35–59). Pressure dressings should be used to immobilize skin grafts. Surgical tape can serve as a pressure dressing in areas such

as fingertips, where bandages cannot be easily applied. Bryant points out that "because it has been amply demonstrated that the pressure beneath a dressing is maintained for only relatively short periods of time . . . a pressure dressing should not be used as a substitute for good hemostasis."[4]

Pressure dressings should be applied to all ear lacerations to prevent hematoma formation and the subsequent deformation and destruction of cartilage. The ear should be enveloped in the dressing so that pressure from the outer bandage is distributed evenly across the irregular surface of the pinna. Moistened cotton is packed into the concavities of the pinna until the cotton is level with the most lateral aspect of the helical rim. Square pieces of gauze cut to fit the curvature of the ear are placed *behind* (medial to) the pinna. Several more gauze squares are placed on the lateral surface of the ear; the packing is then secured in place with a circumferential head bandage. The bandage must not encompass the opposite ear, since it would just as easily cause pressure necrosis of that ear if left unprotected. Application of a pressure dressing for the ear is discussed further in Chapter 68.

Traumatic wounds are bandaged in order to compress or immobilize the wound or to secure and protect the underlying dressing. Most bandaging is performed on extremities, where dressings are difficult to secure with tape alone. Rolls of cotton (Kerlex, Kling) are well suited for this purpose. The bandage is wound around the extremity, advancing proximally with circular, overlapping turns. Care should be taken to avoid wrinkles in the bandage that later create pressure points or to make loose turns that "shorten the effective life of the dressing."[137] When joint surfaces are crossed, the cotton is anchored distally with several turns, unrolled obliquely across the joint several times in a figure-of-eight pattern, and anchored proximally by two complete turns. This process is repeated until the bandage is securely in place. The ends of the bandage are fastened to the skin by strips of adhesive tape.

Bandages over the forearm and the lower extremities are particularly prone to slippage because of the constant motion of these parts and because of the marked changes in extremity diameter over a short distance. The roll of bandage can be rotated 180 degrees after each circular turn, producing a reverse spiral and reducing its mobility (Fig. 35–60). A "tube" of elastic cotton netting (e.g., Surgifix, Tubex) pulled over the bandage or unrolled from a metal applicator frame will effectively stabilize the entire dressing in these areas. Another useful technique consists of placing strips of tape on opposite sides of the extremity, leaving the ends free. The bandage is wrapped around the dressing, covering the portions of the tape

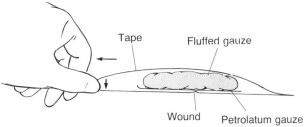

Figure 35–59. Compression dressing on the face. Adhesive tape is applied tightly over the dressing.

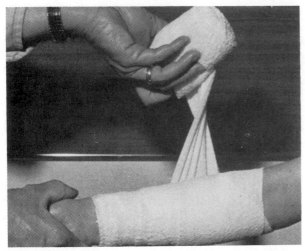

Figure 35–60. Snugness of the bandage is increased by rotation of the bandage roll 180 degrees after each circular turn to effect a reverse spiral. (From Norton, L. W.: Trauma. *In* Hill, G. J., II: Outpatient Surgery. Philadelphia, W. B. Saunders Company, 1980. Used by permission.)

that are attached to the skin. The free ends of tape are then incorporated in the bandage (Fig. 35–61).[162]

An elastic cotton roll (Kerlex) allows the bandage to conform to body contours, provides some mobility to bandaged joints, and permits the wound to swell without the circumferential bandage constricting the extremity. The inelastic Kling bandage better immobilizes the part.

Most scalp wounds do well when left uncovered. If a dressing is considered to be necessary, it must be held in place by a bandage. There are many techniques of bandaging heads. Stavrakis described the following method:

The assistant tightly holds a strip of bandage three inches wide and three feet long over the patient's head in a frontal plane [Fig. 35–62A]. While one person maintains tension on the first strip of bandage, the second person starts bandaging the head with the main bandage at the forehead level in a horizontal plane, using a full-length gauze bandage [Fig. 35–62B]. (The "Kling"-type bandage is preferred.) After several turns are made to stabilize the main bandage, it is passed near the patient's ear, then wrapped around the short strip of bandage in a full turn [Fig. 35–62C]. The main bandage is then taken across the front of the head, wrapped full-turn around the other side of the short bandage, then brought around the back of the head and wrapped around the first side again. This maneuver is repeated, alternating front and back until the head is covered by overlapping passes of bandage [Fig. 35–62D] . . . several turns of the bandage across the forehead in a horizontal plane stabilize the dressing. The dressing is . . . secured by tying the ends of the short strip under the chin [Fig. 35–62E]. Removal of this dressing can be accomplished easily by untying the chin straps and gently pulling both ends upward.[163]

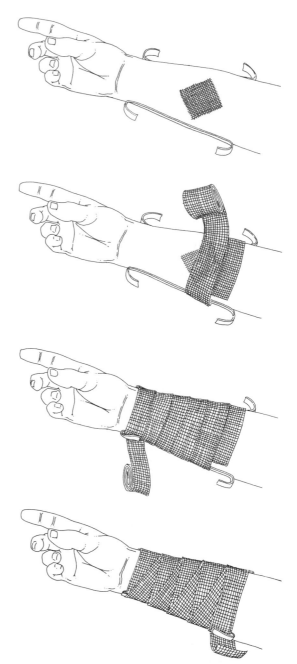

Figure 35–61. *A*, When you have to apply a Kling or Kerlex wrap to an area such as the forearm, start by putting a strip of tape on opposite sides of the arm, leaving the ends free. *B*, Wrap the bandage around the arm, covering the portions of the tape that are attached to the skin. *C*, After completing one layer of wrapping, tuck the free ends of the tape down so that the nonadhesive side faces the first layer of wrapping and the sticky side faces out. Place another layer of wrapping around the arm. *D*, After completing a second layer of wrapping, you will have a neat dressing that will not slip because it is adhered to itself as well as to the skin. (From Lazo, J.: Non-slip dressing technique. Res. Staff Phys. 22:103, 1976. Used by permission.)

Methods of bandaging wounds in other locations of the body are described in detail in other texts.[156]

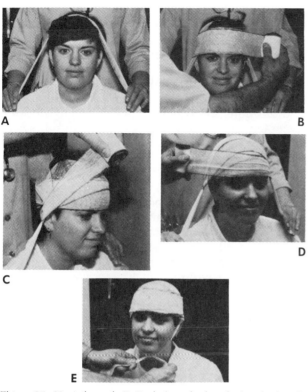

Figure 35–62. A through E, Technique for bandaging the head. (From Stavrakis, P.: A better head dressing. Res. Staff Phys. 26:88, 1980. Used by permission.)

SPLINTING AND ELEVATION

Immobilization of an injured extremity promotes healing by protecting the closure and by limiting the spread of contamination and infection along lymphatic channels. Wounds overlying joints are subjected to repeated stretching and movement, which delays healing, widens the scar, and could possibly disrupt the sutures.[1] Splints are almost always required for lacerations overlying joints and are frequently necessary for protection of wounds involving fingers, hands, wrists, the volar aspects of forearms, the extensor surface of elbows, the posterior aspect of legs, the plantar surfaces of feet, and on extremities where skin grafts have been applied. Splinting is often underused by the emergency physician in the treatment of lacerations. A reasonable axiom is that all *large* lacerations on the extremity should be splinted for the first few days of healing. Splinting may enhance the healing process and often adds to the comfort of the patient.

A plaster or aluminum splint may be incorporated into a bandage to reduce the mobility of the part. Splinting techniques for hand injuries are explained more fully in Chapter 45.

Elevation of injured extremities is important in all but trivial injuries. Elevation serves to limit edema formation, an expected sequela of trauma and inflammation, and allows more rapid healing.[1, 104] Elevation also reduces throbbing pain. Patients given this information are often more motivated to elevate the extremity as instructed. Slings can be used to elevate wounds involving the forearm or the hand.

OINTMENTS

The safety and efficacy of topical antibiotic preparations used on wound surfaces are still being debated. Norton claims that "topical antibiotics are of limited value and in some cases interfere with tissue regeneration."[137] Some authors warn of skin sensitization by preparations containing neomycin.[98] Leyden and Sulzberger report that with the use of a triple antibiotic preparation containing neomycin, bacitracin, and polymyxin, the wound is provided with a broad spectrum of protection against infection without systemic absorption and toxicity or the emergence of resistant strains of bacteria. These authors further state that unless this topical antibiotic ointment is used repeatedly or on inflamed skin, there is a relatively low risk of allergic sensitization. Unpublished experimental studies by Leyden demonstrate that this combination ointment is effective in preventing infection of experimental abrasions by *Staphylococcus aureus* and *Streptococcus pyogenes*.[164] Ayliffe and coworkers state that the topical use of antibiotics may result in the emergence of resistant strains of bacteria.[165] It has been shown in comparison with controls that the active agents in Neosporin ointment and Silvadene cream as well as their inert bases and vehicles improved wound healing.[158, 166, 167] USP petrolatum has been shown both to retard healing[166] and to have no effect on wound healing.[167] McGrath concluded that the beneficial effect of Silvadene cream placed on healing skin flaps was in its ability to provide a moist environment for the ischemic tissue rather than in its antibacterial activity. Knutson and associates reported the use of a granulated sugar (sucrose) povidone-iodine paste in a variety of open wounds. In this uncontrolled study, the combination of this paste, frequent dressing changes, and close follow-up resulted in rapid healing and reduced bacterial proliferation and tissue edema even in contaminated and infected wounds.[185]

Ointments are useful in minimizing the formation of a crust that covers and separates the edges of the wound. Lacerations surrounded by abraded skin are especially predisposed to coagulum formation. In such cases the patient can be instructed to cleanse the wound frequently and to follow the cleansing with an application of ointment during the first few days.[1, 23, 98] Ointments also prevent the dressing from adhering to the wound.[7] Some authors recommend the use of bacitracin applied in a thin coating not for protection against infection but for prevention of these mechanical problems.[98] The exact value of ointments in the treatment of wounds has yet to be determined.

SYSTEMIC ANTIBIOTICS

Most traumatic soft tissue injuries sustain a low level of bacterial contamination.[96] In a number of clinical studies of traumatic wounds, prophylactic antibiotics administered orally[16, 168] and intramuscularly[29, 168–170] in a variety of regimens proved ineffective in reducing the incidence of infection. In a small series of wounds caused by dog bites, Elenbaas and colleagues found that prophylactic oxacillin given orally had no effect on infection rates.[171] In a separate, small series, Callaham noted an improved outcome only in "high-risk" wounds, such as punctures and wounds of the hand.[172] From a limited study of *cat* bites (only 11 patients total studied), Elenbaas and coworkers suggest that oxacillin prophylaxis provides greater protection from infection than a placebo.[186]

In experimental models, the period after injury in which systemic antibiotics suppress infection is limited to 1 to 3 hours. Three hours after the injury, antibiotics have no therapeutic value.[27, 68, 69, 173] Edlich and coworkers found that delayed treatment with antibiotics was more effective in wounds closed immediately than in wounds closed 3 to 48 hours after injury. They concluded that the exudate filling the wound prevented the antibiotic from reaching the bacteria in the wound.[68]

As mentioned earlier, enzymatic débridement of the wound with Travase extends the period in which topical antibiotics are effective to at least 8 hours after injury. Travase also promotes the action of systemically administered antibiotics, but unfortunately the extent to which this enzyme prolongs the effective period for systemic antibiotics is unknown.[69] Studies to date suggest that systemic antibiotics are of no benefit to wounds débrided mechanically more than 3 hours after injury.

Most investigations into the use of antibiotics have omitted heavily contaminated wounds in their series. It remains common practice to administer antibiotics to patients with bite wounds; wounds involving tendons, bones, or joints; or wounds requiring extensive débridement in the operating room. Studies have shown that the therapeutic value of antibiotic treatment decreases as the number of bacteria in the wound increases. Edlich and associates state, "When the wound is contaminated with exceedingly large numbers of organisms (greater than 10^9 per gram of tissue), infection will develop despite antibiotic treatment. This circumstance is encountered when the wound surface is contacted by either pus or feces."[41] The necessity of systemic antibiotics for noncanine bite wounds and for intraoral lacerations is unstudied and for dog bites is incompletely studied.[172, 173]

Indications for antibiotics vary among authors, since few conclusions are based on sound, scientific data. Antibiotics are of no benefit in most soft tissue wounds, because the level of bacterial contamination after cleaning and débridement is below that necessary for infection. Antibiotics may be effective (perhaps only marginally effective) when the level of contamination is overwhelming or if the amount of questionably viable tissue left in the wound is considerable. Antibiotics should be considered for extremity bite wounds, puncture-type bite wounds in any location, intraoral lacerations that are sutured, wounds that cannot be satisfactorily cleaned or débrided, and highly contaminated wounds (e.g., those contaminated with soil, organic matter, purulence, feces, saliva, or vaginal secretions).[1] *If systemic antibiotics are considered necessary, they should be given intravenously or intramuscularly in the earliest stages of wound management.* Broad-spectrum antibiotics should be used—cephalosporins, penicillinase-resistant penicillins or, if allergy or cost precludes the use of these two groups, erythromycin.[14] If significant contamination with gram-negative or anaerobic organisms has occurred, an aminoglycoside and clindamycin should be considered.[1] Irrigation with topical antibiotics may be of benefit in these situations. In all cases, the use of antibiotics should remain subordinate to careful cleaning and débridement.

IMMUNOPROPHYLAXIS

Recommendations for tetanus prophylaxis have been changing during the past several years. The guidelines published by the Center for Disease Control should be reviewed (Table 35–2).[174] Treatment decisions are based on the differentiation between clean and contaminated wounds. Edlich and associates provide more precise definitions of these terms: "A clean, minor wound is a straight laceration due to shear forces that is less than six hours old since the time of injury and has *not* been contacted by feces, saliva, purulent exudate soil, or other infection-potentiating factions."[94] All other wounds are considered contaminated. Tetanus-prone wounds also include those with retained foreign bodies, devitalized or avascular tissue, penetrating abdominal wounds involving bowel, and deep puncture wounds. When patients are questioned about their tetanus immunization

Table 35–2. SUMMARY GUIDE TO TETANUS PROPHYLAXIS IN ROUTINE WOUND MANAGEMENT, 1981*

History of Tetanus Immunization (Doses)	Clean, Minor Wounds		All Other Wounds	
	Td‡	TIG	Td‡	TIG
Uncertain	Yes	No	Yes	Yes
0–1	Yes	No	Yes	Yes
2	Yes	No	Yes	No§
3 or more	No‖	No	No¶	No

*From Immunization Practices Advisory Committee, Center for Disease Control: Diphtheria, tetanus, and pertussis: Guidelines for vaccine prophylaxis and other preventive measures. Morbidity and Mortality Weekly Report 30:392–396, 401–407, August 1981. Used by permission.
†Important details are in the text. Td = tetanus and diphtheria toxoids (for adult use); TIG = human tetanus immune globulin.
‡For children less than 7 years of age, diphtheria and tetanus toxoids and pertussis vaccine adsorbed (diphtheria and tetanus toxoids adsorbed [for pediatric use], if pertussis vaccine is contraindicated) are preferred to tetanus toxoid alone. For persons 7 years of age and older, Td is preferred to tetanus toxoid alone.
§Yes, if wound is more than 24 hours old.
‖Yes, if more than 10 years since last dose.
¶Yes, if more than 5 years since last dose. (More frequent boosters are not needed and can accentuate side effects.)

status, it is not sufficient to ascertain only the interval of time since their "last tetanus shot." One should determine whether the patient has completed the primary immunization series, and if not, how many doses have been given.

Patients who have not completed a full primary series of injections may require both tetanus toxoid and passive immunization with tetanus immune globulin. The preferred preparation for active tetanus immunization in patients 7 years of age and older is 0.5 ml of tetanus toxoid (plus the lower, adult dose of diphtheria toxoid); the dose of tetanus immune globulin is 250 units given intramuscularly.[174]

When a wound results from the bite or scratch of a wild or domestic animal, prophylaxis against rabies also must be considered. Guidelines for the prevention of rabies are described in various references.[175–177]

Patient Instructions

Successful wound healing is partly dependent upon the care given to the wound once the patient leaves the emergency center. Therefore, the patient should receive thorough and understandable instructions.

The patient should be informed that no matter how skillful the repair, any wound of significance will produce a scar. Most scars deepen in color and become more prominent before they mature and fade. The final appearance of the scar cannot be judged before 6 to 12 months after the repair.[98, 116]

Since the wound edges are rapidly sealed by coagulum and bridged by epithelial cells within 48 hours, the wound is essentially impermeable to bacteria after 2 days.[9, 159, 178] The patient should be instructed to keep the wound protected by leaving the dressing undisturbed, clean, and dry for 48 hours. In this initial period the dressing should be changed only if it becomes externally soiled or soaked by exudate from the wound. If possible, the injured part should be kept elevated. There is a tendency on the part of most patients to avoid getting sutures wet. There is no proven harm in exposing sutured wounds to soap and tap water for short periods, and many physicians routinely allow patients to bathe after 48 hours. Some advise patients to wash wounds daily to remove dried blood and exudate, especially on areas such as the face or the scalp.

In 48 hours, it is reasonable to allow the patient to remove the dressing in uncomplicated wounds and to check for evidence of infection—redness, warmth, increasing pain, swelling, purulent drainage, or the "red streaks" of lymphangitis. If there is no sign of infection, the patient can care for the wound until it is time for removal of the sutures. A daily gentle washing with either hydrogen peroxide or a mild soap and water is beneficial. Generally, a wound should be protected with a dressing during the first week, and the dressing should be changed daily. If the wound is unlikely to be contaminated or traumatized, it may be left uncovered. Although it is generally recommended that uncovered scalp wounds can be washed after 1 to 2 days, a gentle shampoo in the first few hours after wound closure is unlikely to be harmful. Vigorous scrubbing of wounds should be discouraged.

Patients should be informed that sutures themselves do not cause pain. A very painful wound is often a sign of infection, and pain should prompt a wound check.

If an injured extremity or finger is being protected by a splint, it should generally be left undisturbed until the sutures are removed. Patients with intraoral lacerations should be instructed to use warm salt water or half-strength hydrogen peroxide mouth rinses at least three times a day.

Patients often ask about the efficacy of various creams and lotions (vitamin E, cocoa butter, and so forth) in limiting scar formation. At this time there are no data to support the use of these substances.

Secondary Wound Care

RE-EXAMINATION

Wounds should be examined in 3 to 4 days for signs of infection and sooner if the patient experiences increasing discomfort or develops a fever.[156] Bite wounds and other infection-prone wounds should be inspected in 2 days. Wounds being considered for delayed primary closure are evaluated in 4 to 5 days.[95]

If on examination of the wound a low-grade, localized cellulitis is discovered, as often occurs in wounds in which extensive dissection of subcutaneous tissue has been performed, it is rarely necessary to open the wound. The removal of one or two stitches may relieve some of the tension caused by mild swelling. With daily cleansing using water and a mild soap and with application of warm compresses, this type of wound reaction should subside within 24 to 48 hours.[156]

In most sutured wounds that become infected, the sutures must be removed to allow drainage. The presence of sutures in a contaminated wound considerably limits the activity of various antibiotics.[179] Infection around a suture can lead to the formation of a stitch mark.[87] Infected wounds should be treated with daily cleansing, warm compresses, and antibiotics. They should be left to heal by secondary intention, which involves wound contraction, granulation tissue formation, and epithelialization.[104]

SUTURE REMOVAL

Since wounds do not heal at a standard rate, there can be no strict guidelines for time of suture removal. At the time that suture removal is being considered, one or two sutures may be cut to determine if the skin edges are sufficiently adherent to allow removal of all the sutures.[7] Removing sutures too early invites wound dehiscence and widening of the scar, whereas leaving sutures in longer than necessary may result in epithelial tracts, infection, and unsightly scarring. Small stitch abscesses are common in wounds in which sutures have been left in place for longer than 7 to 10 days. Localized stitch abscesses generally resolve following removal of the suture(s) and with the application of warm compresses. There is usually no need for antibiotic therapy with stitch abscesses. The optimal time for suture removal varies with the location of the wound, the rate of wound healing, and the amount of tension on the wound. Certain areas of the body, such as the back of the hand, heal slowly, whereas facial or scalp wounds heal rapidly. Speed of wound healing is affected by systemic factors, such as malnutrition, neoplasia, or immunosuppression.

The amount and organization of scar tissue are influenced by the physical forces acting across the wound.[9, 180] Ordman and Gillman noted that "the earlier the suture is removed, the less aberrant and down-growing epithelium as well as foreign body granulation tissue will develop along the suture tract."[181] Stillman warns that "percutaneous sutures . . . provide a nidus for infection, establish a route for the entry of skin and sebaceous bacteria for 5–10 days, and provoke a foreign body reaction . . . Percutaneous sutures stimulate a granulomatous, then fibrous inflammatory reaction along the suture track."[6] Factors that determine the severity of stitch marks include the length of time skin stitches are left in place, skin tension, the relationship of the suture to the wound edge, the region of the body, infection, and tendency for keloid formation.[87, 182] The skin of the eyelids, palms, soles, and mucous membranes seldom shows stitch marks, unless the skin of the face is heavy with sebaceous glands (e.g., over the dorsum of the nose or the forehead). In contrast, oily skin and the skin of the back, the sternal area, the upper arms, and the lower extremities are likely to develop the permanent imprints of suture material on the skin surface.[15, 87, 129, 182]

Crikelair found that if sutures are removed within 7 days, no discernible needle puncture or stitch mark will persist.[182] In studying wound tensile strength, Meyers and coworkers found that incisions in which sutures were removed on the fourth day were stronger than those in which sutures were removed on the seventh day, suggesting that a moderate amount of tension on wounds enhances healing.[183] Yet at 6 days, the wound is held together by a small amount of fibrin and cells and has minimal strength (see Fig. 35–1).[5] The tensile strength of most wounds at this time is adequate to hold the wound edges together, but only if there are no appreciable dynamic or static skin forces pulling the wound apart.[7] Minimal trauma to an unsupported wound at this point could cause dehiscence. The physician should decide on the proper time of suture removal after weighing these various factors. If early suture removal is necessary, the strength of the closure may be maintained with strips of surgical skin tape. The key to wound tensile strength after suture removal is an adequate deep tissue layer closure.

Sutures on the face should be removed on the fifth day following the injury, or alternate sutures should be removed on the third day and the remainder on the fifth day. On the extremities and the anterior aspect of the trunk, sutures should be left in place for approximately 7 days to prevent wound disruption. Sutures on the scalp, the back, the feet, and the hands and over the joints must remain in place for 10 to 14 days, even though permanent stitch marks may result.[87] Some au-

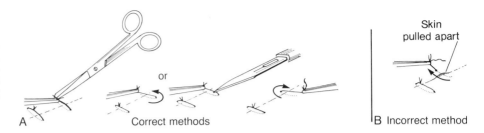

Figure 35–63. Technique for suture removal. Pull should be toward wound line (A) rather than away from it (B), which causes skin to tear apart. (Modified from Stuzin, J., Engrav, L. H., and Buehler, P. K.: Emergency treatment of facial lacerations. Postgrad. Med. 71:81, 1982.)

or

A   Correct methods   B Incorrect method

Skin pulled apart

thors recommend the removal of sutures in eyelid lacerations in 48 to 72 hours to avoid epithelialization along the suture tract with subsequent cyst formation.[184]

The technique of removing sutures is relatively simple. The wound should be cleansed, and any remaining crust overlying the wound surface or surrounding the sutures should be removed. The skin is wiped with an alcohol swab. Each stitch is cut with a scissors or the tip of a scalpel blade (number 11 Bard-Parker) at a point close to the skin surface on one side. The suture is grasped on the opposite side with forceps and is pulled across the wound (Fig. 35–63).[23] The amount of exposed suture that is dragged through the suture tract is thereby minimized. It is difficult to remove sutures with very short ends. At the time of suture placement, the length of the suture ends should generally equal the distance between sutures to permit easy grasping of the suture during subsequent removal, yet avoiding entanglement during the knotting of adjacent sutures.

Once the skin sutures are removed, the width of the scar will increase gradually over the next 3 to 5 weeks unless it is supported. Support is provided by previously placed subcutaneous stitches that brought the skin edges into apposition, by a previously placed subcuticular stitch, or by the application of skin tape (Fig. 35–64). A nonabsorbable subcuticular suture can be left in place for 2 to 3 weeks to provide continued support for the wound. Although complications from prolonged use of this stitch, such as closed epithelial sinuses, cysts, or internal tracts, can occur, they are unusual. These problems can be avoided by the placement of a buried subcuticular stitch using an absorbable suture.[6, 9]

If a subcuticular stitch with reliefs has been used, the suture is cut at the midpoint of the relief. Half of the suture is removed at the original point of entry into the skin and the other half through the original exit point (Fig. 35–65).[144] If a nonabsorbable subcuticular suture cannot be removed or a portion of it ruptures during removal, the protruding end should be grasped with a hemostat, pulled taut, and cut with a scissors as close to the skin as possible so that the end of the suture retracts under the skin.[140]

If the wound edges show signs of separating at the time of suture removal, alternate stitches can

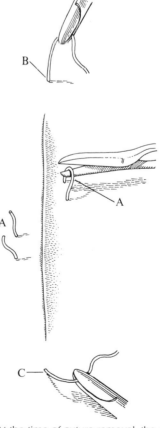

Figure 35–65. At the time of suture removal, the suture is cut at the midpoint of the relief (A). The proximal portion is removed at the point of original entry into the skin (B), and the distal portion is removed through the original exit point (C). (From Grimes, D. W., and Garner, R. W.: "Reliefs" in intra-cuticular sutures. Surgical Rounds Dec. 1978, p. 48. Used by permission.)

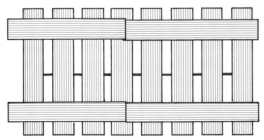

Figure 35–64. Support of the wound with surgical tape.

be left in place and the entire length of the wound supported by strips of adhesive tape. If time and effort has been invested in a cosmetic closure of the face, the repair should be protected with skin tape after the skin sutures have been removed. Wound contraction and scar widening continue for 42 days after the injury.[5] Since the desired result is a scar of minimal width, the tape should be used for 5 weeks following suture removal. "Skin tone" adhesive tape that is dyed the color of light skin is available. With exposure to sunlight, scars in their first 4 months will redden to a greater extent than surrounding skin. This should be prevented in exposed cosmetic areas with the use of a sunscreen containing para-amino benzoic acid (PABA) when prolonged exposure to the sun is anticipated.

Conclusion

The objective of traumatic wound management is the restoration of tissue continuity and strength in the least possible time, with maximal preservation of tissues and minimal scar formation, deformity, or loss of function.

Wounds fail to heal for a variety of reasons. Some of the impediments to healing include ischemia or necrosis of tissue, hematoma formation, prolonged inflammation caused by foreign material, excessive tension on skin edges, and immunocompromising systemic factors. In attempting to repair wounds, physicians sometimes inadvertently retard the healing process. Research has identified harmful practices that can be avoided, such as premature closure of contaminated wounds or the use of drains in uninfected wounds. With the development of new methods and solutions for cleansing wounds (or the discovery of the optimal concentrations of solutions currently in use), tissue-toxic antiseptic solutions can be abandoned. Better suture materials are replacing reactive sutures that often served as foreign bodies rather than supports. Future improvements in the materials used for dressing wounds will enhance wound healing.

One of the primary causes of delayed healing is wound infection. Wound cleaning and débridement, atraumatic and aseptic handling of tissues, and the use of protective dressings will minimize this complication. All new methods and materials used in wound management must be evaluated with respect to their potential for provoking or preventing infection.

The patient's actions affect wound healing. Delay in seeking treatment for an injury has a significant impact on the ultimate outcome of the wound. In the first few days following an injury, the patient must take responsibility for protecting the wound from contamination, further trauma, and swelling.

The final appearance of a scar is determined by several factors. Infection, tissue necrosis, and keloid formation will widen a scar. Wounds located in areas heavily concentrated with sebaceous glands or oriented 90 degrees to dynamic or static skin tension lines will result in wide scars. Inversion of the edges of a wound during closure produces a more noticeable scar, whereas skillful technique can convert a jagged, contaminated wound into a fine, inapparent scar. There are times when optimal wound management requires that the wound not be closed or instead closed at a later time, when the danger of infection has passed.

It is important that physicians adhere to the established, basic principles of wound care when cleaning, débriding, closing, and protecting wounds and continue to refine their management as further improvements in techniques and materials become available.

1. Edlich, R. F., Thacker, J. G., Buchanan, L., and Rodeheaver, G. T.: Modern concepts of treatment of traumatic wounds. Adv. Surg. 13:169, 1979.
2. Hunt, J. K., and Van Winkle, W.: Wound Healing: Normal Repair. Fundamentals of Wound Management in Surgery. South Plainfield, NJ, Chirurgecom, Inc., 1976.
3. Edlich, R. F., Custer, J., Madden, J., et al.: Studies in the management of the contaminated wound III. Assessment of the effectiveness of irrigation with antiseptic agents. Am. J. Surg. 118:21, 1969.
4. Bryant, W. M.: Wound healing. Clin. Symp. 29:1, 1977.
5. Ordman, L. J., and Gillman, T.: Studies in the healing of cutaneous wounds I. The healing of incisions through the skin of pigs. Arch. Surg. 93:857, 1966.
6. Stillman, R. M.: Wound closure: Choosing optimal materials and methods. ER Reports 2:41, 1981.
7. Peacock, E. E.: Wound healing and wound care. In Schwartz, S. I. (ed.): Principles of Surgery, 3rd ed. New York, McGraw-Hill, 1979.
8. Hohn, D. C., Granelli, S. G., Burton, R. W., et al.: Antimicrobial systems of the surgical wounds II. Detection of antimicrobial protein in cell-free wound fluid. Am. J. Surg. 133:601, 1977.
9. Peacock, E. E., and Van Winkle, W.: Surgery and Biology of Wound Repair. Philadelphia, W. B. Saunders Co., 1970.
10. Krizek, T. J., and Robson, M. C.: Evolution of quantitative bacteriology in wound management. Am. J. Surg. 130:579, 1975.
11. Sherman, R. T.: Infections. In Schwartz, S. I. (ed.): Principles of Surgery, 1st ed. New York, McGraw-Hill, 1969.
12. Robson, M. C., Duke, W. F., and Krizek, T. J.: Rapid bacterial screening in the treatment of civilian wounds. J. Surg. Res. 14:426, 1973.
13. Ogilvie, W. H.: Prevention and treatment of wound infection. Lancet 2:935, 1940.
14. Callaham, M. L.: Human and animal bites. Top. Emerg. Med. 4:1, 1982.
15. Edlich, R. F., Thacker, J. G., Rodeheaver, F. T., et al.: A manual for wound closure. St. Paul, MN, Surgical Products Division/3M, 1979.
16. Haughey, R. E., Lammers, R. L., and Wagner, D. K.: Use

of antibiotics in the initial management of soft tissue hand wounds. Ann. Emerg. Med. 10:187, 1981.

17. Cruse, P. J. E., and Foord, R.: A five-year prospective study of 23,649 surgical wounds. Arch. Surg. 107:206, 1973.

18. Doig, C. M., and Wilkinson, A. W.: Wound infection in a children's hospital. Br. J. Surg. 63:647, 1976.

19. Fekety, R. F., and Murphy, J. F.: Factors responsible for the development of infections in hospitalized patients. Surg. Clin. North Am. 152:1385, 1972.

20. Viljanto, J.: Disinfection of surgical wounds without inhibition of normal wound healing. Arch. Surg. 115:253, 1980.

21. Bierens, de Haas B., Ellis, H., and Wilks, M.: The role of infection on wound healing. Surg. Gynecol. Obstet. 138:693, 1974.

22. Burke, J. F.: Infection. Fundamentals of Wound Management in Surgery. South Plainfield, NJ, Chirurgecom, Inc., 1977.

23. Stuzin, J., Engrav, L. H., and Buehler, P. K.: Emergency treatment of facial lacerations. Postgrad. Med. 71:81, 1982.

24. Richards, V.: Simple wounds and simple incisions. J. Fam. Pract. 2:297, 1975.

25. Haury, B., Rodeheaver, G., Vensko, Jr., et al.: Debridement: An essential component of traumatic wound care. Am. J. Surg. 135:238, 1978.

26. Nylin, S., and Karlsson, B.: Time factor, infection frequency and quantitative microbiology in hand injuries. Scand. J. Plast. Reconstr. Surg. 14:185, 1980.

27. National Academy of Sciences–National Research Council: Post-operative wound infections: The influence of ultraviolet irradiation of the operating room and of various other factors. Ann. Surg. 160(suppl):1, 1964.

28. Sindelar, W., and Mason, G. R.: Irrigation of subcutaneous tissue with povidone-iodine solution for prevention of surgical wound infections. Surg. Gynecol Obstet. 148:227, 1979.

29. Hutton, P. A. N., Jones, B. M., and Low, D. J. W.: Depot penicillin as prophylaxis in accidental wounds. Br. J. Surg. 65:549, 1978.

30. Mann, R. J., Hoffeld, T. A., and Former, C. B.: Human bites of the hand: Twenty years of experience. J. Hand Surg. 2:97, 1977.

31. Rodeheaver, G. T., Pettry, D., Thacker, J. G., et al.: Wound cleansing in high pressure irrigation. Surg. Gynecol. Obstet. 141:357, 1975.

32. Rodeheaver, G., Pettry, D., Turnbull, V., et al.: Identification of the wound infection–potentiating factors in soil. Am. J. Surg. 67:140, 1980.

33. Roberts, A. H., Rye, D. G., Edgerton, M. I., et al.: Activity of antibiotics in contaminated wounds containing clay soil. Am. J. Surg. 137:381, 1979.

34. Morgan, W. J., Hutchison, D., and Johnson, H. M.: The delayed treatment of wounds of the hand and forearm under antibiotic cover. Br. J. Surg. 67:140, 1980.

35. Hutton, P. A. N., Jones, B. M., and Law, D. J. W.: Depot penicillin as prophylaxis in accidental wounds. Br. J. Surg. 75:549, 1978.

36. Rutherford, W. H., and Spence, R. A.: Infection in wounds sutured in the accident and emergency department. Ann. Emerg. Med. 9:350, 1980.

37. Pryor, G. J., Kilpatrick, W. R., and Opp, D. R.: Local anesthesia in minor lacerations: Topical TAC versus lidocaine infiltration. Ann. Emerg. Med. 9:568, 1980.

38. Rodeheaver, G. T., Smith, S. L., and Thacker, J. G.: Mechanical cleansing of contaminated wounds with a surfactant. Am. J. Surg. 129:241, 1975.

39. Custer, J., Edlich, R. F., Prusak, M., et al.: Studies in the management of the contaminated wound V. An assessment of the effectiveness of pHisoHex and Betadine surgical scrub solutions. Am. J. Surg. 121:572, 1971.

40. Ervin, M. E.: Minor surgical procedures. In Schwartz, G. R., et al. (eds.): Principles and Practice of Emergency Medicine. Philadelphia, W. B. Saunders Co., 1978, pp. 386–398.

41. Edlich, R. F., Rodeheaver, G. J., Thacker, J. G., et al.: Technical Factors in Wound Management. Fundamentals of Wound Management in Surgery. South Plainfield, NJ, Chirurgecom, Inc., 1977.

42. Rodeheaver, G., Turnbull, V., Edgerton, M. T., et al.: Pharmacokinetics of a new skin wound cleanser. Am. J. Surg. 132:67, 1976.

43. Madden, J., Edlich, R. F., Schauerhamer, R., et al.: Application of principles of fluid dynamics to surgical wound irrigation. Curr. Top. Surg. Res. 3:85, 1971.

44. Stevenson, T. R., Thacker, J. G., Rodeheaver, G. T., et al.: Cleansing the traumatic wound by high pressure syringe irrigation. JACEP 5:17, 1976.

45. Bhaskar, S. N., Cutright, D. E., Gross, A., et al.: Water jet devices in dental practice. J. Peridont. 42:658, 1971.

46. Gross, A., Bhaskar, S. N., Cutright, D. E., et al.: The effect of pulsating water jet lavage on experimental contaminated wounds. Oral Surg. 29:187, 1971.

47. Gross, A., Cutright, D. E., and Bhaskar, S. N.: Effectiveness of pulsating water jet lavage in treatment of contaminated crushed wounds. Am. J. Surg. 124:373, 1972.

48. Grower, M. F., Bhaskar, S. N., Horan, M. J., et al.: Effect of water lavage on removal of tissue fragments from crush wounds. Oral Surg. 33:1031, 1972.

49. Hamer, M. L., Robson, M. C., Krizek, T. J., et al.: Quantitative bacterial analysis of comparative wound irrigations. Ann. Surg. 181:819, 1975.

50. Brown, L. L., Shelton, H. T., Bornside, G. H., et al.: Evaluation of wound irrigation by pulsatile jet and conventional methods. Ann. Surg. 187:170, 1977.

51. Beasley, J. D.: The effect of spherical polymers and water jet lavage on oral mucosa. Oral Surg. 32:998, 1971.

52. Gross, A., Bhaskar, S. N., and Cutright, D. E.: A study of bacteremia following wound lavage. Oral Surg. 31:720, 1971.

53. O'Leary, T. J., Shafer, W. G., Swenson, H. M., et al.: Possible penetration of crevicular tissue from oral hygiene procedures—use of oral irrigating device. J. Periodontol. 41:158, 1970.

54. Wheeler, C. B., Rodeheaver, G. J., Thacker, J. G., et al.: Side effects of high pressure irrigation. Surg. Gynecol. Obstet. 143:775, 1976.

55. Rodeheaver, G. T., Kurtz, L., Kircher, B. J., et al.: Pluronic F-68: A promising new skin wound cleanser. Ann. Emerg. Med. 9:572, 1980.

56. Faddis, D., Daniel, D., and Boyer, J.: Tissue toxicity of antiseptic solutions: A study of rabbit articular and periarticular tissues. J. Trauma 17:895, 1977.

57. Mulliken, J. B., Healy, N. A., and Glowacki, J.: Povidone-iodine and tensile strength of wounds in rats. J. Trauma 20:323, 1980.

58. Gilmore, O. J. A., and Martin, T. D. M.: Aetiology and prevention of wound infection in appendectomy. Br. J. Surg. 61:281, 1976.

59. Gilmore, O. J. A., and Sanderson, P. J.: Prophylactic interparietal povidone-iodine in abdominal surgery. Br. J. Surg. 62:792, 1975.

60. Gosnold, J. K.: Prophylaxis of wound infection. The Practitioner 223:271, 1979.

61. Morgan, T. C. N., et al.: Prophylactic povidone-iodine in minor wounds. Injury 12:104, 1980.

62. Gruber, R. P., Vistnes, L., and Pardoe, R.: The effect of commonly used antiseptics on wound healing. Plast. Reconstr. Surg. 55:472, 1975.

63. Lau, W. Y., and Wong, S. H.: Randomized, prospective trial of topical hydrogen peroxide in appendectomy wound infection: High risk factors. Am. J. Surg. 142:393, 1981.

64. Halasz, N. A.: Wound infection and topical antibiotics: The surgeon's dilemma. Arch. Surg. 112:1240, 1977.

65. Sher, K. S.: Prevention of wound infection: The compar-

ative effectiveness of topical and systemic cefazolin and povidone-iodine. Am. Surg. 48:268, 1982.

66. Lindsay, D., Nava, C., and Marti, M.: Effectiveness of penicillin irrigation in control of infection in sutured lacerations. J. Trauma 22:186, 1982.

67. Edlich, R. F., Madden, J. E., Prusak, M., et al.: Studies in the management of the contaminated wounds IV: The therapeutic value of gentle scrubbing in prolonging the limited period of effectiveness of antibiotics in contaminated wounds. Am. J. Surg. 121:668, 1971.

68. Edlich, R. F., Smith, O. T., and Edgerton, M. T.: Resistance of the surgical wound to antimicrobial prophylaxis and its mechanisms of development. Am. J. Surg. 126:583, 1973.

69. Rodeheaver, G., Marsh, D., Edgerton, M. T., et al.: Proteolytic enzymes as adjuncts to antimicrobial prophylaxis of contaminated wounds. Am. J. Surg. 129:537, 1975.

70. Rodeheaver, G. T., Rye, D. G., Rust, R., et al.: Mechanisms by which proteolytic enzymes prolong the golden period of antibiotic action. Am. J. Surg. 136:379, 1978.

71. Rodeheaver, G., Edgerton, M. T., Elliott, M. B., et al.: Proteolytic enzymes as adjuncts to antibiotics prophylaxis of surgical wounds. Am. J. Surg. 127:564, 1974.

72. Seropian, R., and Reynolds, B. M.: Wound infections after preoperative depilatory versus razor preparation. Am. J. Surg. 121:251, 1971.

73. Haeri, G. B., et al.: The efficacy of standard surgical face masks: An investigation using "tracer particles." Clin. Orthop. 148:160, 1980.

74. Weatherley-White, R. C. A., and Lesavoy, M. A.: The integument. In Hill, G. J., (ed.): Outpatient Surgery. Philadelphia, W. B. Saunders Co., 1980, pp. 334–346.

75. Dushoff, I. M.: A stitch in time. Emergency Medicine 5:1, 1973.

76. Morris, T., and Appleby, R.: Retardation of wound healing by procaine. Br. J. Surg. 67:391, 1980.

77. Sturrock, J., et al.: Cytotoxic effects of procaine, lignocaine (lidocaine) and bupivacaine. Br. J. Anaesth. 51:273, 1971.

78. Stevenson, T. R., Rodeheaver, G. T., Golden, G. T., et al.: Damage to tissue defenses by vasoconstrictors. JACEP 4:532, 1975.

79. Barker, W., Rodeheaver, G. T., Edgerton, M. T., et al.: Damage to tissue defenses by a topical anesthetic agent. Ann. Emerg. Med. 11:307, 1982.

80. Roettinger, W., Edgerton, M. T., Kurty, L. D., et al.: Role of inoculation site as a determinant of infection in soft tissue wounds. Am. J. Surg. 126:354, 1973.

81. Scarlet, J. J., Walter, J. H., and Bachmann, R. J.: Digital blood perfusion following injections of plain lidocaine and lidocaine with epinephrine: A comparison. Journal of the American Podiatry Association 68(5):339-346, 1978.

82. Kaplan, E. G., Kashuk, K.: Disclaiming the myth of use of epinephrine local anesthesia in feet. Journal of the American Podiatry Association 61:335, 1971.

83. Steinberg, M. D., Block, P.: The use and abuse of epinephrine in local anesthetics. Journal of the American Podiatry Association 61:341, 1971.

84. Green, D., Walter, J., Heden, R., et al.: The effects of local anesthetics containing epinephrine on digital blood perfusion. J. Am. Podiatry Assoc. 69:397, 1979.

85. Morris, T., and Tracey, J.: Lignocaine: Its effects on wound healing. Br. J. Surg. 64:902, 1977.

86. Brown, P. W.: The hand. In Hill, G. J., II (ed.): Outpatient Surgery. Philadelphia, W. B. Saunders Co., 1980, pp. 643–686.

87. Grabb, W. C.: Basic techniques of plastic surgery. In Grabb, W. C., and Smith, J. W. (eds.): Plastic Surgery: A Concise Guide to Clinical Practice. Boston, Little, Brown & Co., 1979, pp. 3–74.

88. Kirk, R. M.: Basic Surgical Techniques. Edinburgh, Churchill Livingstone, 1978.

89. Rosen, P., and Sternbach, G.: Atlas of Emergency Medicine. Baltimore, Williams & Wilkins, 1979, pp. 125–133.

90. MacDonald, R. T.: Maintenance of ligature tension by a single operator with simultaneous removal of a hemostatic clamp. Am. J. Surg. 143:770, 1982.

91. Roberts, J. R.: Intravenous regional anesthesia. JACEP 6:261, 1977.

92. Dushoff, I. M.: Handling the hand. Emergency Medicine 8(10):26, 1976.

93. Wavak, P., and Zook, E. G.: A simple method of exsanguinating the finger prior to surgery (letter). JACEP 7:124, 1978.

94. Edlich, R. F., and Rodeheaver, G. T.: Scientific basis for emergency wound management. Emerg. Med. Annu. 2:1, 1983.

95. Edlich, R. F., Rogers, W., Kasper, G., et al.: Studies in the management of the contaminated wound I. Optimal time for closure of contaminated open wounds II. Comparison of resistance to infection of open and closed wounds during healing. Am. J. Surg. 117:323, 1969.

96. Marshall, K. A., Edgerton, M. T., Rodeheaver, G. T., et al.: Quantitative microbiology: Its application to hand injuries. Am. J. Surg. 131:730, 1976.

97. Prusak, M., Edlich, R. F., Payne, T. J., et al.: Studies in the management of the contaminated wound IX. Quantitation of the Evans Blue Dye content of open and primarily closed surgical wounds. Am. J. Surg. 125:585, 1973.

98. Walike, J. W.: Suturing technique in facial soft tissue injuries. Otolaryngol. Clin. North Am. 12:425, 1979.

99. Kriyek, T. J., and Robson, M. C.: Evaluation of quantitative bacteriology in wound management. Am. J. Surg. 130:579, 1975.

100. Elek, S. D.: Experimental staphylococcal infections in the skin of man. Ann. N. Y. Acad. Sci. 65:85, 1956.

101. Robson, M. C., and Heggers, J. P.: Delayed wound closures based on bacterial counts. J. Surg. Oncol. 2:379, 1970.

102. Robson, M. C., Lea, C. E., Dalton, J. B., et al.: Quantitative bacteriology and delayed wound closure. Surg. Forum 19:501, 1968.

103. Magee, C., Haury, B., Rodeheaver, G. T., et al.: A rapid technique for quantitating wound bacterial count. Am. J. Surg. 133:760, 1977.

104. Herrmann, J. B.: Open wounds. In Wolcott, M. W. (ed.): Ferguson's Surgery of the Ambulatory Patient, 5th ed. Philadelphia, J. B. Lippincott Co., 1974, pp.52–62.

105. Cramer, L. M., and Chase, R. A.: Hand. In Schwartz, S. I., et al. (ed.): Principles of Surgery. New York, McGraw-Hill, 1974, pp. 1895–1918.

106. Edlich, R. F., Tsung, M. S., Rogers, W., et al.: Studies in management of the contaminated wounds I. Technique of closure of such wounds with a note on a reproducible model. J. Surg. Res. 8:585, 1968.

107. Edlich, R. F., Rodeheaver, G. T., Kuphal, J., et al.: Technique of closure: Contaminated wounds. JACEP 3(6):375, 1974.

108. Carpendale, M. T. F., and Sereda, W.: The role of percutaneous suture in surgical wound infection. Surgery 58:672, 1965.

109. Conolly, W. B., Hunt, T. K., Zederfeldt, B., et al.: Clinical comparison of surgical wounds closed by suture and adhesive tapes. Am. J. Surg. 117:318, 1969.

110. Suture Use Manuel: Use and Handling of Sutures and Needles. Somerville, NJ, Ethicon, Inc., 1977.

111. Grossman, J. A.: The repair of surface trauma. Emergency Medicine 14(18):220, 1982.

112. Laufman, H., and Rubel, T.: Synthetic absorbable sutures. Surg. Gynecol. Obstet. 145:597, 1977.

113. Herrman, J. B.: Tensile strength and knot security of surgical suture materials. Am. Surg. 37:209, 1971.

114. Conn, J., and Beal, J. M.: Coated Vicryl synthetic absorbable sutures. Surg. Gynecol. Obstet. 150:843, 1980.
115. Thacker, J. G., Rodeheaver, G., Moore, J. W., et al.: Mechanical performance of surgical sutures. Am. J. Surg. 130:374, 1975.
116. Macht, S. D., and Krizek, T. J.: Sutures and suturing—current concepts. J. Oral Surg. 36:710, 1978.
117. Westreich, M., and Kapetansky, D. I.: Avoiding the slippery knot syndrome (letter). JAMA 236:2487, 1976.
118. Postlethwait, R. W., Willigan, D. A., and Ulin, A. W.: Human tissue reaction to sutures. Ann. Surg. 181:144, 1975.
119. Craig, P. H., Williams, J. A., Davis, K. W., et al.: A biologic comparison of polyglactin 910 and polyglycolic acid synthetic absorbable sutures. Surg. Gynecol. Obstet. 141:1, 1975.
120. Postlethwait, R. W.: Further study of polyglycolic acid suture. Am. J. Surg. 127:617, 1974.
121. Wallace, W. R., Maxwell, G. R., and Cavalaris, C. J.: Comparison of polyglycolic acid suture to black silk, chromic, and plain catgut in human oral tissues. J. Oral Surg. 28:739, 1970.
122. Edlich, R. F., Panek, P. H., Rodeheaver, G. T., et al.: Physical and chemical configuration of sutures in the development of surgical infection. Ann. Surg. 177:679, 1973.
123. Bergman, F., Borgstrom, S. J. H., and Holmund, D. E. W.: Synthetic absorbable surgical suture material (PGA). Acta Chir. Scand. 137:193, 1971.
124. Eilert, J. G., Binder, P., McKinney, P. W., et al.: Polyglycolic acid synthetic absorbable sutures. Am. J. Surg. 121:561, 1971.
125. Adams, I. W.: A comparative trial of polyglycolic acid and silk as suture materials for accidental wounds. Lancet 2:1216, 1977.
126. Osterberg, B., and Blomstedt, B.: Effect of suture materials on bacterial survival in infected wounds: An experimental study. Acta Chir. Scand. 145:431, 1979.
127. Blomstedt, B., Osterberg, B., and Bergstrand, A.: Suture material and bacterial transport: An experimental study. Acta Chir. Scand. 143:71, 1977.
128. Sharp, W. V., Belden, T. A., King, P. H., et al.: Suture resistance to infection. Surgery 91:61, 1982.
129. Dushoff, I. M.: About face. In Cohen, I. J. (ed): Back to Basics, EM Books, New York, 1979, pp. 341–364.
130. Howes, E. L.: Strength studies of polyglycolic acid versus catgut sutures of the same size. Surg. Gynecol. Obstet. 137:15, 1973.
131. Laufman, H.: Is catgut obsolete? Surg. Gynecol. Obstet. 145:587, 1977.
132. Grabb, W. C., and Klainert, H. E.: Techniques in Surgery: Facial and Hand Injuries. Somerville, NJ, Ethicon, Inc., 1980.
133. DeHoll, D., Rodeheaver, G., Edgerton, M. T., et al.: Potentiation of infection by suture closure of dead space. Am. J. Surg. 127:716, 1974.
134. Milewaki, P. J., and Thompson, H.: Is a fat stitch necessary? Br. J. Surg. 67:393, 1980.
135. Bloom, W., and Fawcett, D. W.: A Textbook of Histology, 10th ed. Philadelphia, W. B. Saunders Co., 1975, pp. 564–567.
136. Gant, T. D.: Suturing techniques for everyday use. Patient Care 13(14):45, 1979.
137. Norton, L. W.: Trauma. In Hill, G. J., II (ed): Outpatient Surgery. Philadelphia, W. B. Saunders Co., 1980, pp. 89–133.
138. Stephens, F. O., Hunt, T. K., and Dunphy, J. E.: Study of traditional methods of care on the tensile strength of skin wounds in rats. Am. J. Surg. 122:78, 1971.
139. Edlich, R. F., Rodeheaver, G. T., Thacker, J. G., et al.: Technical factors in wound management. In Hunt, T. K., and Dunphy, J. E. (eds.): Fundamentals of Wound Management. New York, Appleton-Century-Crofts, 1979, pp. 364–455.
140. Converse, J. M.: Introduction to plastic surgery. In Converse, J. M. (ed.): Reconstructive Plastic Surgery: Principles and Procedures in Correction, Reconstruction, and Transplantation, 2nd ed., vol. 1. Philadelphia, W. B. Saunders Co., 1977, pp. 3–68.
141. Speer, D. P.: The influence of suture technique on early wound healing. J. Surg. Res. 27:385, 1979.
142. Winn, H. R., Jane, J. A., and Rodeheaver, G.: Influence of subcuticular sutures on scar formation. Am. J. Surg. 133:257, 1977.
143. Stillman, R. M., Bella, F. J., Seligman, S. J., et al.: Skin wound closure: The effect of various wound closure methods on susceptibility to infection. Arch. Surg. 115:674, 1980.
144. Grimes, D. W., and Garner, R. W.: "Reliefs" in intracuticular sutures. Surgical Rounds 1(12):46, 1978.
145. Ryan, A. J.: Traumatic injuries: Office treatment of lacerations. Postgrad. Med. 59:259, 1976.
146. Roberts, J. R.: Pathophysiology, diagnosis and treatment of head trauma. Top. Emerg. Med. 1:41, 1979.
147. Snyder, C. C.: Scalp, face and salivary glands. In Wolcott, M. W. (ed.): Ferguson's Surgery of the Ambulatory Patient, 5th ed. Philadelphia, J. B. Lippincott Co., 1974, pp. 153–181.
148. Weinstein, P. R., and Wilson, C. B.: The skull and nervous system. In Hill, G. J., II (ed.): Outpatient Surgery. Philadelphia, W. B. Saunders Co., 1980, pp. 298–302.
149. Paton, D., and Emery, J.: Injuries of the eye, the lids, and the orbit. In Ballinger, W. F., Rutherford, R. B., and Zuidema, G. D. (eds.): The Management of Trauma. Philadelphia, W. B. Saunders Co., 1979, pp. 254–284.
150. English, G. M.: Ears, nose, throat and sinus. In Hill, G. J., II (ed.): Outpatient Surgery. Philadelphia, W. B. Saunders Co., 1980, pp. 369–459.
151. Edgerton, M. T.: Emergency care of maxillofacial and neck injuries. In Ballinger, W. F., Rutherford, R. B., and Zuidema, G. D. (eds.): The Management of Trauma. Philadelphia, W. B. Saunders Co., 1979, pp. 285–341.
152. Heintz, W. D.: Traumatic injuries: Dealing with dental injuries. Postgrad. Med. 61:261, 1977.
153. Horton, C.E., Adamson, J. E., Mladick, R. A., et al.: Vicryl synthetic absorbable sutures. Am. Surg. 40:729, 1974.
154. Wolcott, M. W.: Hands and fingers: Part I—soft tissues. In Wolcott, M. W. (ed.): Ferguson's Surgery of the Ambulatory Patient, 5th ed. Philadelphia, J. B. Lippincott Co., 1974, pp. 396–438.
155. Magee, C., Rodeheaver, G. T., Golden, G. T., et al.: Potentiation of wound infection by surgical drains. Am. J. Surg. 131:547, 1976.
156. Wolcott, M. W.: Dressings and bandages. In Wolcott, M. W. (ed.): Ferguson's Surgery of the Ambulatory Patient, 5th ed. Philadelphia, J. B. Lippincott Co., 1974, pp. 35–51.
157. Lawrence, J. C.: What materials for dressings? Injury 13:500, 1982.
158. McGrath, M. H.: How topical dressings salvage "questionable" flaps: Experimental study. Plast. Reconstr. Surg. 67:653, 1981.
159. Schauerhamer, R. A., Edlich, R. F., Panek, P., et al.: Studies in the management of the contaminated wound VI: Susceptibility of surgical wounds to postoperative surface contamination. Am. J. Surg. 122:74, 1971.
160. Stillman, R. M., Bella, F. J., Seligman, S. J.: Skin wound closure: The effect of various closure methods on susceptibility to infection. Arch. Surg. 115:674, 1980.
161. Bothwell, J. W., and Rovee, D. T.: The effect of dressings on the repair of cutaneous wounds in humans. In Harkiss, K. J. (ed.): Surgical Dressings and Wound Healing. London, Crosby-Lockwood, 1971, p. 78.

162. Lazo, J.: Non-slip dressing technique. Res. Staff Phys. 22(8):103, 1976.
163. Stavrakis, P.: A better head dressing. Res. Staff Phys. 26(9):88, 1980.
164. Leydon, J. J., and Sulzberger, M. B.: Topical antibiotics and minor skin trauma. Am. Fam. Physician 23:121, 1981.
165. Ayliffe, G. A. J., Green, W., Livingston, R., et al.: Antibiotic-resistant *Staphylococcus aureus* in dermatology in burn wounds. J. Clin. Pharmacol. 30:40, 1977.
166. Eaglstein, W. H., and Mertz, P. M.: ''Inert'' vehicles do affect wound healing. J. Invest. Dermatol. 74:90, 1980.
167. Geronemus, R., Mertz, P. M., and Eaglstein, W. H.: Wound healing: The effects of topical antimicrobial agents. Arch. Dermatol. 115:1311, 1979.
168. Grossman, J. A. I., Adams, J. P., and Kunec, J.: Prophylactic antibiotics in simple hand injuries. JAMA 245:1055, 1981.
169. Day, T. K.: Controlled trial of prophylactic antibiotics in minor wounds requiring suture. Lancet 4:1174, 1975.
170. Morgan, W. J., Hutchison, D., and Johnson, H. M.: The delayed treatment of wounds of the hand and forearm under antibiotic cover. Br. J. Surg. 67:140, 1980.
171. Elenbaas, R. M., McNabney, W. K., and Robinson, W. A.: Prophylactic oxacillin in dog bite wounds. Ann. Emerg. Med. 11:248, 1982.
172. Callaham, M.: Prophylactic antibiotics in common dog bite wounds: A controlled study. Ann. Emerg. Med. 9:410, 1980.
173. Burke, J. F.: The effective period of preventative antibiotic action in experimental incisions and dermal lesions. Surgery 50:161, 1961.
174. Immunization Practices Advisory Committee, Centers for Disease Control: Diphtheria, tetanus, and pertussis: Guidelines for vaccine prophylaxis and other preventive measures. Morbidity and Mortality Weekly Report 30:392–396, 401–407, 1981.
175. Public Health Service Advisory Committee on Immunization Practices: Rabies. Morbidity and Mortality Weekly Report 25:403, 1976.
176. Plotkin, L. A.: Rabies vaccination in the 1980's. Hosp. Pract. 15:65, 1980.
177. Davidson, S. J., and Lammers, R. L.: Soft tissues and joints (animal bite injuries). *In* Chipman, C. (ed.): Emergency Department Orthopaedics. Rockville, MD, Aspen Systems Corp., 1982, pp. 171–186.
178. Goldberg, H. M., Rosenthal, S. A. E., and Nemetz, J. C.: Effect of washing closed head and neck wounds on wound healing and infection. Am. J. Surg. 141:358, 1981.
179. Rodeheaver, G., Edgerton, M. T., Smith, S., et al.: Antimicrobial prophylaxis of contaminated tissues containing suture implants. Am. J. Surg. 133:609, 1977.
180. Peacock, E. E.: Control of wound healing and scar formation in surgical patients. Arch. Surg. 116:1325, 1981.
181. Ordman, L. J., and Gillman, T.: Studies in the healing of cutaneous wounds II. The healing of epidermal, appendageal, and dermal injuries inflicted by suture needles and by the suture material in the skin of pigs. Arch. Surg. 93:883, 1966.
182. Crikelair, C. T.: Skin suture marks. Am. J. Surg. 96:631, 1958.
183. Myers, M. B., Cherry, G., and Heinberger, S.: Augmentation of wound tensile strength by early removal of sutures. Am. J. Surg. 117:338, 1969.
184. Converse, J. M., and Smith, B.: The eyelids and their adnexa. *In* Converse, J. M. (ed.): Reconstructive Plastic Surgery: Principles and Procedures in Correction, Reconstruction, and Transplantation, 2nd ed., vol. 2. Philadelphia, W. B. Saunders Co., 1977, pp. 858–946.
185. Knutson, R. A., Merbity, L. A., Creekmore, M. A., et al.: Use of sugar and povidone-iodine to enhance wound healing: Five years' experience. South Med. J. 74:1329, 1981.
186. Elebaas, R. M., McNabney, W. K., and Robinson, W. A.: Evaluation of prophylactic oxacillin in cat bite wounds. Ann. Emerg. Med. 13:155, 1984.

36

Alternative Methods of Skin Closure

ALEXANDER TROTT, M.D.

WOUND STAPLES

Introduction

Automatic stapling devices have become commonplace for closure of surgically made incisions. They are of limited usefulness in traumatically induced wounds, however. In spite of the fact that stapling of lacerations can save time and can result in a lower wound infection rate than that produced by closure of wounds with standard superficial nylon sutures, there are several disadvantages.[1, 2] In experiments with guinea pigs, stapled lacerations developed significantly less tensile strength than did lacerations closed with nylon sutures.[3] Wound edges cannot be meticulously apposed, and the lack of apposition can lead to an undesirable cosmetic result. Staple removal is often painful. Use of stapling equipment requires careful training and practice. Wound closure with these devices should be performed by physicians and is best accomplished in an operating area or an emergency facility. It should be noted that current multiple-staple devices are approximately two to four times more expensive than a similar number of nylon sutures.

Use of stapling devices dates back to the early part of this century. Several Russian, Hungarian, and Japanese investigators pioneered various instruments, but it was not until the early 1960s that significant interest in the use of these devices developed in this country.[4, 5] Since that time, there has been a steady improvement in technology that includes the introduction of automatic and disposable devices, precocking mechanisms, and optimal staple configurations. Most recently, a new disposable single-staple instrument manufactured by 3M of St. Paul, Minnesota has been introduced. This apparatus has some promise for use in emergency departments.

Indications and Contraindications

Currently, the indications for stapling are limited to incisions created by a shearing force (i.e., knife wounds) and located on an extremity, the trunk, or the scalp. The most efficacious use would seem to be in the case of long, linear lacerations, in which time is crucial. Staples are contraindicated whenever good cosmetic results are important. *They should never be used on the face, the hands, or the feet.* They also are not to be placed in scalp wounds if computed tomography head scans are to be performed, because the metallic density will produce scan artifacts.

Equipment

The required equipment consists of standard wound care instruments as previously described in the section on wound preparation (see Chapter 35). Many devices are commercially available. According to Johnson and coworkers,[2] the stapling instrument with the most desirable features is the Premium, manufactured by the United States Surgical Corporation of Norwalk, Connecticut. The advantages of this instrument include an angle of placement of the staple that prevents it from being placed too deeply, a precocking mechanism that allows for precise positioning of staple points, an excellent view of the staple at the release point, and an automatic release mechanism that prevents binding of the staple to the device. The single-staple instrument previously mentioned appears to be useful for smaller lacerations not requiring more than three or four closure points.

Procedure

The wound is shaved and prepared in the standard manner. Whenever necessary, deep, absorbable sutures are used to close deep fasciae and to reduce tension of the superficial fascia and dermal layers. For best results, it is often preferable to

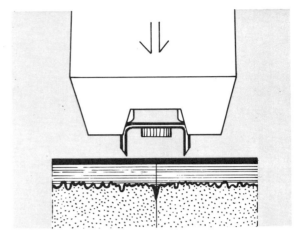

Figure 36–1. The skin edges must be approximated by hand or with forceps before they are secured with staples. (From Edlich, R. F.: A Manual for Wound Closure. 3M Co., 1979. Used by permission.)

have a second operator. This person precedes the operator along the wound and everts the wound edges with pickups. This technique allows the staple to be placed with greater precision and a smaller margin of error. Once the edges are held in eversion, the staple points are gently approximated to the skin surfaces (Fig. 36–1). By squeezing the stapler handle or trigger, one automatically advances the staple into the wound and bends it to the proper configuration (Figs. 36–2 and 36–3). One must take great care not to plunge too deeply, since this error will cause excessive wound ischemia (Fig. 36–4). Enough staples should be placed to provide proper apposition of the edges of the wound along its entire length.

Once the wound is stapled, a dry, sterile dressing is put in place. If necessary, the patient can remove the dressing and gently clean the wound in 72 hours. The length of time that staples are

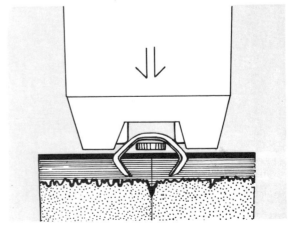

Figure 36–2. By squeezing the stapler handle, a plunger advances one staple into the wound margins. (From Edlich, R. F.: A Manual for Wound Closure. 3M Co., 1979. Used by permission.)

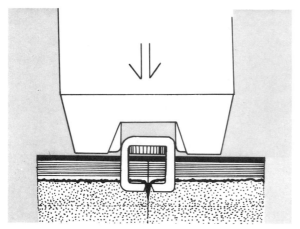

Figure 36–3. An anvil automatically bends the staple to the proper configuration. (From Edlich, R. F.: A Manual for Wound Closure. 3M Co., 1979. Used by permission.)

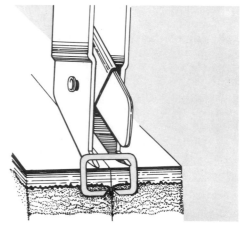

Figure 36–5. The lower jaw of the staple remover is placed under the crossbar of the staple. (From Edlich, R. F.: A Manual for Wound Closure. 3M Co., 1979. Used by permission.)

kept in place depends on the type and location of the wound. Occasionally, the staples are kept in longer than would be necessary for nylon sutures in recognition of the fact that wound tensile strength tends to be lower in stapled wounds.

Removal of staples requires a special instrument that is made available by each manufacturer of stapling devices. The lower jaw of the staple remover is placed under the crossbar (Fig. 36–5). One brings down the upper jaw by squeezing the handle (Fig. 36–6). This action compresses the crossbar, thereby releasing the staple points for easy removal (Fig. 36–7).

Complications

Complications can occur with staple closures, although the incidence is very low. In 1975, Len-

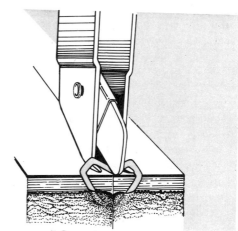

Figure 36–6. By squeezing the handle gently, the upper jaw compresses the staple. (From Edlich, R. F.: A Manual for Wound Closure. 3M Co., 1979. Used by permission.)

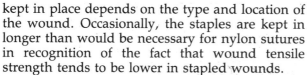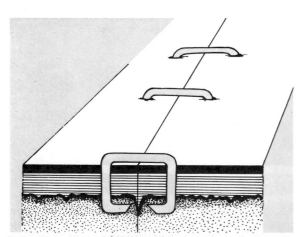

Figure 36–4. Care should be taken to ensure that a space remains between the skin and the crossbar of the staple. Excessive pressure created by placing the staple too deep will cause wound edge ischemia as well as painful removal. (From Edlich, R. F.: A Manual for Wound Closure. 3M Co., 1979. Used by permission.)

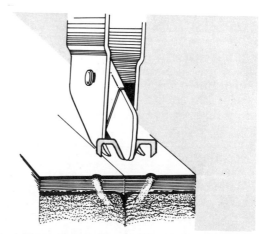

Figure 36–7. Compression of the crossbar allows the staple points to be withdrawn from the wound. (From Edlich, R. F.: A Manual for Wound Closure. 3M Co., 1979. Used by permission.)

nihan found that only 3 per cent of patients with surgical incisions closed by staples developed wound infection. Wound separation was seen in only 1 per cent of patients. Lennihan also reported significant erythema associated with the staples in 2 per cent of patients, but this complication was self-limited without treatment.[1]

Summary

Overall results are favorable when staples are used for surgical incisions. There are no data on staple use in traumatically induced wounds. Because of the increasing availability and versatility of stapling instruments, however, increased use in emergency departments can be anticipated.

1. Lennihan, R., and Mackereth, M.: A comparison of staples and nylon closure in varicose vein surgery. Vasc. Surg. 9:200, 1975.
2. Johnson, A., Rodeheaver, G. T., Durand, L. S., et al.: Automatic disposable stapling devices for wound closure. Ann. Emerg. Med. 10:631, 1981.
3. Harrison, I. D., Williams, D. F., and Cuschieri, A.: The effect of metal clips on the tensile properties of healing skin wounds. Br. J. Surg. 62:945, 1975.
4. Cooper, P., and Christie, S.: Development of the surgical stapler with emphasis on vascular anastomosis. Trans. N.Y. Acad. Sci. 25:365, 1963.
5. Steichen, F. M., and Ravitch, M. M.: Mechanical sutures in surgery. Br. J. Surg. 60:191, 1973.

WOUND TAPES

Introduction

The use of specially designed tape strips to close simple wounds has increased rapidly in recent years. Tape strips can be applied by health care personnel in many settings, including operating rooms, emergency departments, clinics, and first-aid stations. Advantages of tape strips include ease of application, reduced need for local anesthesia, more evenly distributed wound tension, no residual suture marks, no need for suture removal, superiority for some grafts and flaps,[6, 7] and suitability for use under plaster casts. One of the main advantages of wound tapes is their greater resistance to wound infection compared with standard sutures and wound staples.[8–10]

There are also disadvantages to tape closures. Tape does not work well on wounds that are under significant tension or wounds that are very irregular, on concave surfaces, or in areas of marked tissue laxity. In many cases, tape does not provide satisfactory wound edge apposition without underlying deep closures. Tape does not stick well to areas with copious secretions, such as in the axilla, the palms of the hands, the soles of the feet, and the perineum. Tape also has difficulty adhering to wounds that will have copious exudates. Tape strips can also be prematurely removed by young children.

Background

Tape closure of wounds has been reported since 1600 B.C.[11] It was not until the late 1950's, however, with the introduction of woven tapes and nonsensitizing adhesive, that tapes gained widespread acceptance in the United States.[12] Since then, there have been rapid advances in the manufacture of tapes with increased strength, improved adhesiveness, and presterilized packaging.

Currently, there are several brands of tapes with differing porosity, flexibility, strength, and configuration. Steri Strips* are microporous tapes with ribbed backing. They are porous to air and water, and the ribbed backing provides extra strength. Cover-Strips† are woven in texture and are claimed to have a greater degree of porosity. They allow not only air and water but also wound exudates to pass through the tape. Shur-Strip‡ is a nonwoven microporous tape, which, like the Cover-Strips and Steri-Strip is designed to permit the passage of gas and water through the tapes. Clearon§ is a synthetic plastic tape whose backing contains longitudinal parallel serrations to permit gas and fluid permeability. One of the latest developments is an iodoform-impregnated Steri-Strip tape,‖[6] intended to further retard infection without increased sensitization to iodine.

Comparison studies of the tapes have been limited. Koehn showed that the Steri-Strip tapes maintained adhesiveness approximately 50 per cent longer than Clearon tape.[13] Rodeheaver and coworkers[14] compared Shur-Strip, Steri-Strip, and Clearon tape in terms of breaking strength, elongation, shear adhesion, and air porosity. The tapes were tested in both dry and wet conditions. The

*3M Corporation, St. Paul, Minnesota
†Beiersdorf, South Norwalk, Connecticut
‡Deknatel, Inc., Floral Park, New York
§Ethicon, Inc., Somerville, New Jersey
‖Manufactured by 3M Corporation, St. Paul, Minnesota

Steri-Strip tape was found to have approximately twice the breaking strength of the other two tapes in both dry and wet conditions with minimal loss of strength in all tapes when wetted. The Shur-Strip tapes showed approximately 2 to 3 times the elongation of the other tapes at the breaking point (whether dry or wet). The shear adhesion (amount of force required to dislodge the tape when a load is applied in the place [angle = 0 degrees] of contact) was slightly better for the Shur-Strip tape than for the Steri-Strip tape and approximately 50 per cent better than for the Clearon tape. Although the application of benzoin to the skin prior to the application of the tapes increased the shear adhesion for all the tapes Day 1, the increase in shear adhesion was insignificant on subsequent days for the Shur-Strip and Steri-Strip tapes. There was a small, persistent improvement in shear adhesion for the Clearon tape up to Day 7 (last day tested). Air porosity was 10- to 20-fold better with the Shur-Strip tape than for the Steri-Strip or Clearon tapes when the tapes were tested dry. When tested wet, the Shur-Strip tapes remained twice as porous as the other tapes. Rodeheaver and coworkers[14] consider the increased porosity, greater shear adhesiveness, and greater potential for elongation (to reduce skin blistering under the tapes) of the Shur-Strip tapes as rationale for recommending the Shur-Strip tapes.

Indications

The predominant indication for tape closure is a superficial straight laceration under little tension. If necessary, tension can be reduced by undermining or placing deep closures. Areas particularly suited for tape closure are the forehead, chin, malar eminence, thorax, and non-joint areas of the extremities. They may also be preferred in children when painful suture placement and removal is not essential. Care must be taken to estimate the potential for premature tape removal by a child.

In an experimental study using guinea pigs, Edlich demonstrated that taped wounds inoculated with *Staphylococcus aureus* at various known concentrations resisted infection better than wounds closed with nylon.[9] Therefore, tape closures can be used on wounds with potential for infection when standard suture closure is not essential. Tape closures will work well under plaster casts when superficial suture closures cannot be used. Efron and Ger, in 1968, and Weisman, in 1963, demonstrated the efficacy of using tape to successfully hold flaps and grafts in place.[6, 7] Anatomical areas in which taping of grafts and flaps was useful included the fingers, the flat areas of the extremities, and the trunk. Tape closures can be applied to wounds that require early suture removal to reduce the chance of permanent suture mark scarring. Finally, because of the minimal skin tension created by tapes, they can be used on skin that has been compromised by vascular insufficiency or altered owing to prolonged use of steroids.

Contraindications

Tape closures are contraindicated in wounds that are irregular or under tension and in those that cannot be appropriately dried of blood or secretions. They are of little value on lax and intertriginous skin, on naturally moist areas, and in the scalp and beard areas.

Tapes should never be placed circumferentially around a digit, because they have no ability to stretch or lengthen. If placed circumferentially, the natural wound edema of an injured digit can make the tape act like a constricting band and can lead to ischemia and possible necrosis of the digit.

Equipment

For a simple tape closure, the required equipment includes forceps and tape of the proper size. Most taping can be done in the emergency department with 1/4 × 3-inch strips. In wounds larger than 4 cm, however, larger strips might be desirable. Most companies manufacture strips up to 1 inch wide and up to 4 inches in length. Standard suture instruments should also be available (see Chapter 35).

Procedure

Actual application of the tape must be preceded by proper wound preparation, irrigation, débridement, and hemostasis. Hair is removed, and the area of the tape application is thoroughly dried to ensure proper adhesion of the tapes. Benzoin can be applied initially to increase tape adhesion.[9] The physician should use sterile technique at all times. Wound tapes do not unduly adhere to surgical gloves, allowing the operator to maintain proper sterile technique. All tapes come in presterilized packages and can be opened directly onto the operating field.

After the wound has been dried (Fig. 36–8) and benzoin has been applied (Fig. 36–9), the tapes, with backing attached, are cut to the desired length (Fig. 36–10). Tapes should be long enough to allow for approximately 2 to 3 cm of overlap on each side of the wound. After the tape is cut to length, the end tab is removed (Fig. 36–11). The

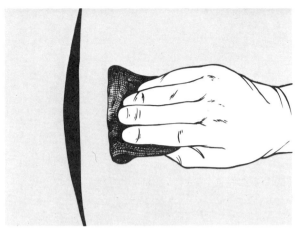

Figure 36–8. After wound preparation (and placements of deep closures, if needed), dry the skin thoroughly at least 2 inches around the wound.

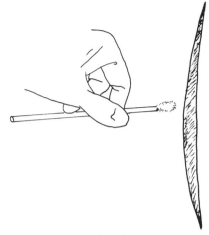

Figure 36–9. If desired, apply a very thin coating of tincture of benzoin around the wound.

tape is gently removed from the backing with forceps, by pulling straight back (Fig. 36–12). Do not pull to the side, because the tape will curl and be difficult to apply to the wound. One half of the tape is securely placed at the mid portion of the wound (Fig. 36–13). The opposite wound edge is gently but firmly apposed to its counterpart (Fig. 36–14). The second half of the tape is then applied. The wound edges should be as close together as possible and at equal height to prevent the development of a linear, pitting scar. Additional tapes are applied by bisecting the remainder of the wound (Fig. 36–15). Enough tapes should be placed so that complete apposition is provided but without totally occluding the wound edges (Fig. 36–16). Finally, additional cross tapes are placed to add support as well as to prevent blistering, which may be caused by unsupported tape ends (Fig. 36–17).[8]

Taped wounds should be left open, without occlusive dressings. Band-Aids and other dressings promote excessive moisture, which can lead to premature separation from the wound. Tapes may remain in place for approximately 2 weeks and, in some cases, longer. The desired time of application is a decision that varies with the requirements of each wound. The patient can be allowed to gently clean the taped laceration with a moist, soft cloth after 72 hours. If excessive wetting or mechanical force is used, however, premature separation may result.

Complications

As with any procedure, complications may arise. Fortunately, with tape closures, complications are rare. The infection rate is approximately 5 per cent in clean wounds closed with tape.[8] This rate compares favorably with other standard closures. Premature tape separation occurs in approximately 3 per cent of cases.[15] Other complications include skin blistering if the tape is not properly anchored with the cross-stay strip and wound hematoma if hemostasis is not accomplished.

Figure 36–10. Cut tapes to desired length before removing from backing.

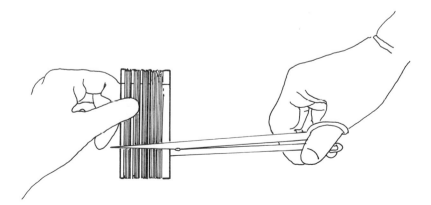

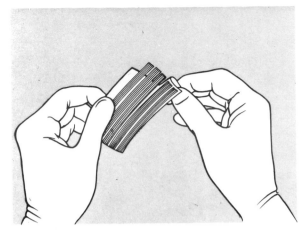

Figure 36–11. The tapes are attached to a card with perforated tabs on both ends. Gently peel the end-tab from the tapes.

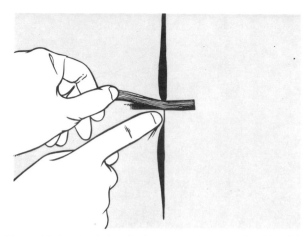

Figure 36–14. Gently but firmly appose the opposite side of the wound using the free hand or forceps.

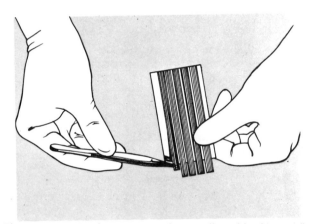

Figure 36–12. Use forceps to peel tape off card backing. Pull directly backward, not to the side.

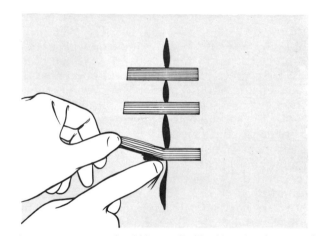

Figure 36–15. Tape should be applied by bisecting the wound until the wound is satisfactorily closed.

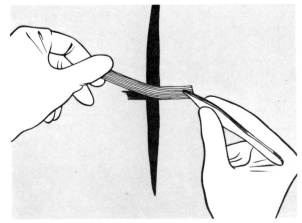

Figure 36–13. Place one half of first tape at the mid portion of the wound. Secure firmly in place.

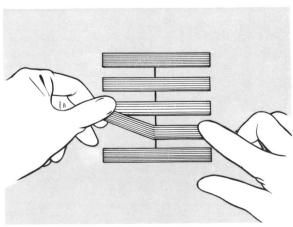

Figure 36–16. Wound margins are completely apposed.

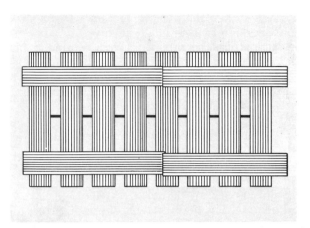

Figure 36–17. Additional supporting tapes are placed approximately 1 inch from the wound and parallel to the wound direction. Taping in this manner prevents skin blistering that may occur at tape ends.

When benzoin is used, it has to be applied very carefully, because increased wound infection has been noted if spillage occurs into the raw wound surface.[14] Benzoin vapors have also been known to cause patient discomfort when applied to the area of a wound that has not been anesthetized.

Conclusions

Most investigators believe that the results of proper tape closure are as successful as those of suture closure.[8, 11] Other investigators, however, believe that tape closure leads to inferior cosmetic results.[15] In the aggregate, however, modern tape products and techniques have earned a solid place in minor wound care management in emergency departments.

6. Efron, G., and Ger, R.: Use of adhesive tape (Steri-Strips) to secure skin grafts. Am. J. Surg. 116:474, 1968.
7. Weisman, P. A.: Microporous surgical tape in wound closure and skin grafting. Br. J. Plast. Surg. 16:379, 1963.
8. Connolly, W. B., Hunt, T. K., Zederfeldt, B., et al.: Clinical comparison of surgical wounds closed by suture and adhesive tape. Am. J. Surg. 117:318, 1969.
9. Edlich, R. F., Rodeheaver, G. T., Kuphal, J., et al.: Technique of closure: contaminated wounds. JACEP 3:375, 1974.
10. Johnson, A., Rodeheaver, G. T., Durand, L., et al.: Automatic disposable stapling device for wound closure. Ann. Emerg. Med. 10:631, 1981.
11. Emmett, A. J. J., and Barron, J. N.: Adhesive suture strip closure of wounds in plastic surgery. Br. J. Plast. Surg. 17:175, 1964.
12. Golden, T.: Nonirritating, multipurpose surgical adhesive tape. Am. J. Surg. 100:789, 1960.
13. Koehn, G. G.: A comparison of the duration of adhesion of Steri-Strips and Clearon. Cutis 26:620, 1980.
14. Rodeheaver, G. T., Halverson, J. M., and Edlich, R. F.: Mechanical performance of wound closure tapes. Ann. Emerg. Med. 12:203, 1983.
15. Panek, P. H., Prusak, M. P., Bolt, D., et al.: Potentiation of wound infection by adhesive adjuncts. Am. Surg. 38:343, 1972.
16. Ellenberg, A. H.: Surgical tape wound closure: a disenchantment. Plast. Reconstr. Surg. 39:625, 1967.

Successful removal of a foreign body is one of the most satisfying procedures in medicine. Carried out with skill and a minimum of discomfort to the patient, such a procedure can result in a grateful patient and a satisfied physician. In contrast, the unskillful attempt at removal of foreign material, particularly if the procedure has not been well thought out, may produce considerable discomfort and occasionally disastrous results. An extended search for an elusive foreign body may result in frustration to the physician and a dissatisfied patient. Improper setting, improper instrumentation, and insufficient time for the procedure are common pitfalls of foreign body removal.[1]

Guidelines for Approaching Foreign Bodies

Initially, the physician should take a history of the method of injury to quickly ascertain the specific characteristics of the foreign material and to formulate the best plan for judicious removal.

37

Soft-Tissue Foreign Body Removal

RICHARD C. BARNETT, M.D.

The history, physical examination, and localization techniques influence decisions about the time and place of foreign body removal. Some material such as wood should be removed immediately, because retained wood will surely lead to inflammation and infection. Other material such as glass or plastic may be removed on an elective basis, whereas innocuous metallic foreign bodies may often be permanently left imbedded in soft tissue. If localization is certain and if removal can be easily accomplished under local anesthesia within a manageable period of time (one hour is usually the upper limit of operative time using local anesthesia), removal is generally indicated on the initial visit. If, in contrast, the material is relatively inert and small (such as a BB) and located near no vital structures but is deeply imbedded in the subcutaneous tissues, the time, energy, and effort involved in the removal will probably be excessive compared with the possible adverse effects of the foreign material remaining in the soft tissue. The possibility of the foreign body migrating to involve vital structures is remote but should be reviewed in the decision of when and how to remove the foreign body.

All clinical decisions require an evaluation of the possibility of infection. Some foreign bodies produce infection in a few days, whereas with other objects, infection may be delayed for weeks or months, often flaring up for no apparent reason. If the foreign body carries dirt particles, pieces of clothing, or other sources of bacterial contamination with it, expeditious removal of the material may be necessary, even though the foreign body itself is relatively small and is not likely to cause a reaction. If some time has elapsed since the initial injury, careful review of the history of the type of foreign material and the method of introduction is warranted. One should not attempt a hasty exploration for foreign material that may not exist or that is best left alone. The initial history should also include any unusual medical problem that would preclude the use of adequate local anesthesia, such as allergy to local anesthetics, any bleeding diathesis, or any medical problems, including diabetes mellitus, uremia, or a compromised immune status, that might lead to unusual or more difficult wound management.

It is not uncommon to encounter a soft-tissue foreign body even though its presence has not been suggested by the history. Anderson and associates reported that physicians who initially treated a series of hand injuries did not diagnosis the presence of a foreign body in 75 of 200 consecutive cases.[2] The patient who experiences a sharp, sudden pain in the foot while walking barefoot across the carpet may have a sewing needle or toothpick imbedded in his foot, rather than the "sprained foot," which he complained about initially.

An abscess or cellulitis that recurs or does not heal as expected should always be investigated for an unsuspected retained foreign body. Finally, all metallic or foreign bodies that appear on the radiograph of a multiple trauma patient should be proven to be present on the radiograph table or clothing rather than being imbedded in the patient. Foreign objects, such as keys or coins, may be surreptitiously imbedded in a trauma patient and may easily be mistaken for artifact.

Radiographic Findings

With the introduction of radiographs, it was possible to localize radiopaque foreign bodies and to use the radiographic localization as a guide in the removal of the material. Therefore, it is important to decide whether the material involved is radiopaque. Formerly, it was thought that localization depended upon the lead content of the material, particularly glass. More recent information indicates that the visibility of foreign material in soft tissues is dependent upon its density (Fig. 37–1). In 1977, Pond and Lindsey revealed the ability to localize foreign fragments, including leaded and non-leaded glass, in an experimental phantom.[3] Tandberg subsequently demonstrated that, unless obscured by bone, virtually *all* glass is visible on a standard radiograph.[4] Pieces of glass as small as 0.5 mm are visible regardless of pigment content or source of the glass, including glass from automobile windshields, light bulbs, and laboratory equipment. Because almost all glass

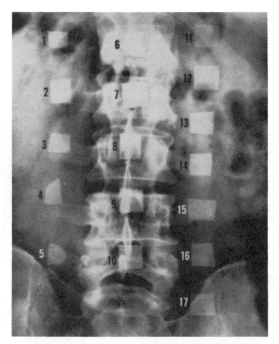

Figure 37–1. Samples of glass superimposed on abdomen and exposed to x-ray. (Reproduced with permission from Zatzkin, H. R.: The Roentgent Diagnosis of Trauma. Copyright © 1965 by Year Book Medical Publishers, Inc., Chicago.)

may be visible on radiographs, nonvisualization of glass suggests its absence but is not conclusive proof that it is not present if overlying radiopaque structures are visible. The identification of less dense foreign material such as splinters may be improved by the use of xeroradiography.[5, 6] The presence of some foreign bodies may be suspected by the accompaniment of soft-tissue gas, introduced with the foreign body, on the radiograph. It should be noted that even large pieces of wood are notoriously not visible on standard radiographs, although wood that is painted may be seen. Sea urchin spines may or may not be visible on plain radiographs. Pieces of cloth or clothing are not visible on radiographs. Fish bones are occasionally visible on radiographs because of their calcium content, but cartilaginous structures, such as spines and fins, are not.

After removing a radiopaque foreign body, it is prudent to take a postoperative radiograph to document that removal was complete (Fig. 37–2). A repeat radiograph may not be needed if the foreign body was a single object, such as a pin or needle, or if there is no evidence of fragmentation.

Foreign Body Reaction

Many soft-tissue foreign bodies have to be removed because of either infection or foreign body reaction. A purulent bacterial infection *may* develop in the presence of any foreign body but not in *all* cases. Karpman and associates revealed only a 15 per cent infection rate (*Staphylococcus aureus* and Enterobacteriaceae) in a series of 25 patients treated for cactus thorn injuries of the extremities.[7] Certain thorns (black thorn, rose thorns), redwood, toothpicks, hair, or sea urchin spines are noted for their ability to initiate chronic foreign body reaction. Sea urchin spines are covered with slime, calcareous material, and other debris that may initiate a foreign body granuloma. It has been speculated that the inflammatory reaction seen with cactus thorns may be an allergic reaction to fungus found on the cactus plant. Many foreign body reactions are thought to be due to the inflammatory response to organic material and may not be due to the introduction of bacteria at the time that the wound was incurred. Clinically evident reactions may be delayed for weeks or even years following injury (Fig. 37–3). The chronic infection or inflammatory reaction may not be accompanied by the production of pus, but it may be quite painful and may result in loss of function. Foreign bodies may also be associated with the formation of a chronic pseudotumor, development of a sinus tract, or evidence of osteomyelitis-like lesions of bone and soft tissue.[8] Organic material has also

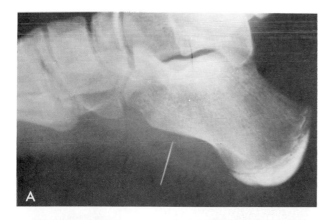

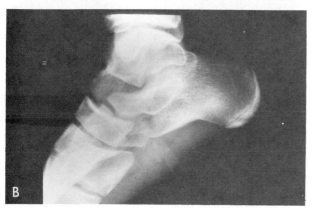

Figure 37–2. Preoperative (A) and postoperative (B) x-ray demonstrating complete removal of a metallic foreign body.

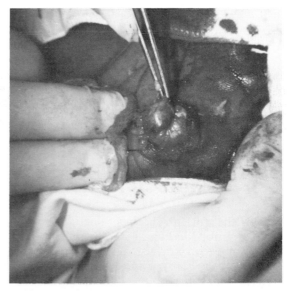

Figure 37–3. A foreign body granuloma developed after a foreign body was stable for 6 months in this laborer's hand. There was no gross infection, but the pain was quite bothersome. The foreign body and reactive tissue were excised under local anesthesia.

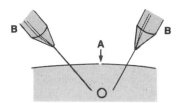

Figure 37–4. When a small entrance wound (A) is noted but the foreign body is not seen, noninvasive localization is preferable to blind probing. Metal markers taped to the skin or needles inserted close to the foreign body under local anesthesia (B) and radiographed at different angles will provide a guide to cutting down and extraction. (Reproduced from Hospital Medicine, January 1981, with permission of Hospital Publications, Inc.)

been noted to form a chronic tenosynovitis, chronic monoarticular synovitis, and chronic bursitis.

Rapidly traveling projectiles with considerable inherent heat are less likely to cause infection but are more apt to cause damage in the passage through the tissue. It is obvious, therefore, that one must judiciously evaluate each foreign body injury, and that one should not be dogmatic about exploration or benign neglect policies.

Guidelines for Foreign Body Removal

Following the initial history, examination, and *pre-operative and pre-anesthetic documentation of the neurovascular status of the patient*, a decision must be made as to the time and place of removal. If the foreign body is to be removed in the emergency department, it is wise to set a time limit of between 30 minutes and 1 hour and not to exceed that time allotment. Most simple foreign bodies can be successfully removed in 30 minutes to 1 hour, and more difficult procedures should be deferred. Note that many foreign bodies initially appear superficial, and the novice may mistakenly think that removal will be rapid and simple, only to find after prolonged searching that the elusive foreign body is yet to be found.

LOCALIZATION

Superficial foreign bodies, such as splinters, bullets, or imbedded glass may be palpated if they are near the skin surface. Deeper foreign bodies must be localized by other techniques. A metal probe may identify the foreign body by feel or sound. Glass is difficult to identify by sight in soft tissue but creates a characteristic grating sound when touched with metal. In larger wounds, a gloved finger may be carefully used to probe the wound for the presence of a foreign body.

Radiographs are the best method for estimating the general location, depth, and structure of foreign bodies. If one attaches a needle or paper clip to the skin surface at the wound entrance before taking a radiograph, the foreign body will be seen in relation to the entrance wound. This will also help to identify the path that leads to the foreign body. Needles at two angles may also be passed to help localize the foreign body (Fig. 37–4).

With the use of fluoroscopic image-intensifying equipment, it may be possible to follow the wound's entrance, to localize the material, and to grasp the foreign body and remove it without making a larger incision. A potential disadvantage of this proceudre is the excessive amount of radiation that may be required. Ariyan has described a technique in which two needles are placed in the soft tissue from opposite directions toward the foreign body.[9] The extremity is rotated while the physician watches the image under the image intensifier to obtain a three-dimensional effect. An incision is placed perpendicular to the plane of the needles, and the object is removed.

Some authors have suggested injecting the entrance wound with methylene blue to outline the tract of the foreign body.[10] (Excess methylene blue that spills onto the skin surface may be removed with ether.) The blue line is followed into the deeper tissues. This technique is of limited value, because the tract of the foreign body often closes tightly and does not allow the passage of the methylene blue.

EQUIPMENT

A standard suture tray with a scalpel is usually adequate equipment for removal of most simple foreign bodies. Tissue retractors, special pickups, and loupes may be added as needed. Good direct light is essential for success, and some physicians prefer to use a head lamp.

Local soft-tissue injection with lidocaine (1 per cent with epinephrine for other than digital blocks) is the recommended anesthesia for the removal of most soft-tissue foreign bodies. Intravenous regional anesthesia or axillary blocks may be useful for foreign body removal in the upper extremity. Children may require general anesthesia or sedation if they are unable to cooperate.

The use of an arterial tourniquet is essential to provide a bloodless field for the removal of a soft-tissue foreign body in an extremity. A blood pressure cuff or portable self-contained pneumatic cuff inflated above arterial pressure may be used on the upper arm, forearm, leg, or thigh. To limit back bleeding, the extremity is elevated and wrapped with an elastic bandage to exsanguinate the extremity before the tourniquet is inflated. In the digits, a

Penrose drain may be used as a tourniquet at the base of the finger or toes. Most patients can tolerate an ischemic tourniquet for 15 to 30 minutes, and it is safe to stop circulation to an extremity for this time period.

OPERATIVE TECHNIQUE

The specific technique for removal of a foreign body is tailored to each clinical situation. In general, foreign bodies should be removed only under direct vision. *Blind grasping into a wound with a hemostat in an effort to remove a foreign body should be avoided.* Blind grasping is especially dangerous in the hand, foot, or face, where vital structures may be easily damaged.

In most cases, one should enlarge the entrance wound with an adequate skin incision. Attempting to remove a foreign body through a puncture wound or an inadequate skin incision is both frustrating and self-defeating. Following a proper skin incision, the wound is explored by carefully spreading the soft tissue with a hemostat (Fig. 37–5). The foreign body can often be felt with an instrument before it can be seen. In an extremity that has been made ischemic by a tourniquet, the tract of the foreign body may be followed, although the tract frequently cannot be identified in muscle or fat.

If the foreign body is difficult to visualize (such as fiber glass or plastic) and if it is located in the superficial soft tissue, excision of a small block of tissue rather than removal of the foreign body alone may be necessary. Block excision is also required if the foreign body has contaminated the surrounding soft tissue. It must be noted that *excision of a block of tissue is done only under direct vision and after nerves, tendons, and vessels have been identified.*

If a foreign body such as a thorn or needle enters the skin perpendicularly, a linear incision may pass to one side of the foreign body and it will be difficult to determine where the foreign body lies in relation to the incision (Fig. 37–6A

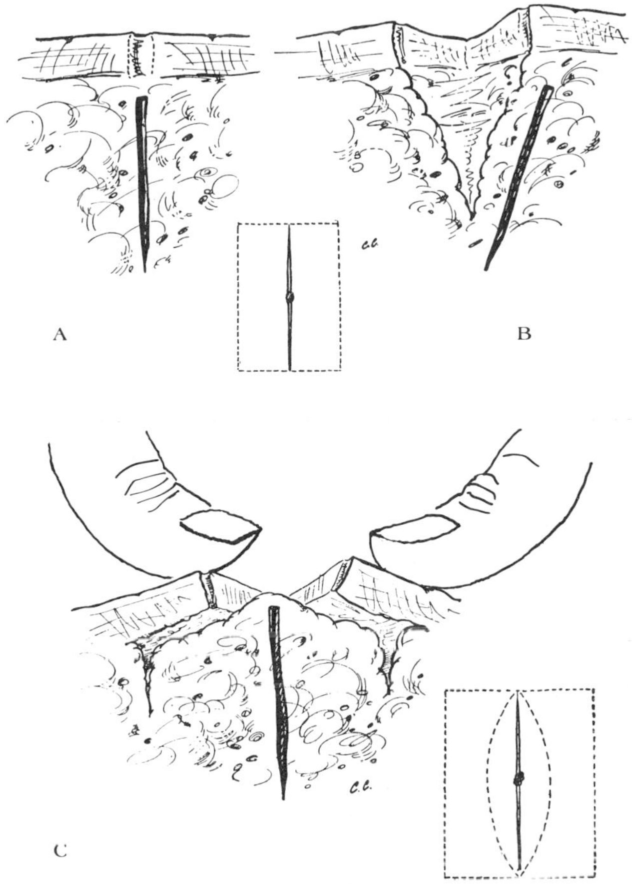

Figure 37–6. If a linear skin incision is used to locate a mobile foreign body that is perpendicular to the skin in the subcutaneous fat (A), the foreign body may be displaced (B). A modified elliptical incision is made (C), and the skin edges are undermined, displacing the foreign body into the middle of the wound. Pressure with the thumbs may be applied to the skin to force the foreign body into view. (From Rees, C. E.: The removal of foreign bodies: a modified incision. JAMA 113:35, 1939. Copyright 1939, American Medical Association.)

and B). The search must then be extended into the walls of the incision rather than through the skin.[11] In such cases, it is advisable to excise a small ellipse of skin and undermine the skin for 1/4 to 1/2 inch in all directions (Fig. 37–6C). The tissue is then compressed from the sides in hopes

Figure 37–5. A sewing needle completely embedded below the surface (A, B) is easily located by a radiograph. Following local anesthesia, a small incision over the superficial end will permit removal with a hemostatic forceps (C). The hemostat is introduced through an adequate incision, spread to open the tissue, and used to "feel" the foreign body as the hemostat is advanced. (Reproduced from Hospital Medicine, January 1981, with permission of Hospital Publications, Inc.)

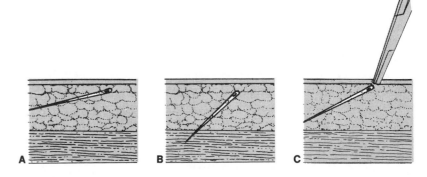

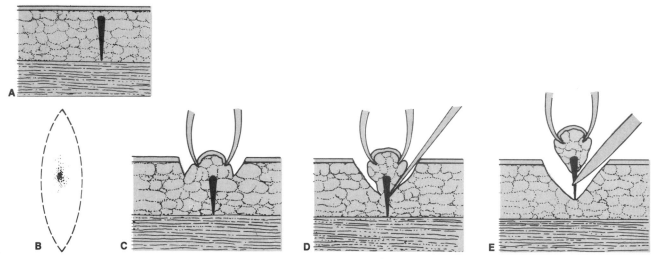

Figure 37–7. Foreign bodies in deep fat *(A)* may be approached by a small elliptical incision around the entry point *(B)*. The incision is then laterally undercut and grasped (without pulling) with an Allis clamp *(C)*. The ellipse is then further undercut until contact with the foreign body is made *(D)*. The foreign body may be grasped and removed along with the entry tract and the soiled local fat *(E)*. (Reproduced from Hospital Medicine, January 1981, with permission of Hospital Publications, Inc.)

that the foreign body will extrude and can be grasped with an instrument.

Following foreign body removal, the wound is irrigated under pressure with povidone-iodine. If a small incision has been made in a non-cosmetic area (such as the bottom of the foot), the incision is left open and is bandaged. The area may be soaked in hot water for a few days, and a return visit is necessary only if signs of infection develop. If a large incision has been created, the skin may be primarily sutured. In cases in which gross contamination has occurred, the wound should not be closed on the initial visit. The wound may be packed open, and the skin should be sutured in 3 to 5 days (delayed closure).

Traumatic Tattooing

Ground-in foreign material or tattooing of the skin is a troublesome problem, because foreign matter will permanently disfigure the skin. Many cases may be managed with adequate local anesthesia and meticulous débridement with a sponge, a scrub brush, or a toothbrush. If it is impossible to remove all the foreign material with these methods, careful consideration should be given to a secondary excision of the tattooed area, using primary closure and subsequent plastic surgery to repair the defect.

Foreign Bodies in Fatty Tissue

Foreign bodies located in the fatty tissues may be removed by making an elliptical incision surrounding the entrance wound, grasping the skin of the ellipse loosely with an Allis forceps, under-

cutting the incision until the foreign body is contacted, and removing the foreign body, skin, and entrance tract in one block (Fig. 37–7). In most instances, a small portion of subcutaneous fat should be removed along with the foreign body to minimize infection. Foreign bodies in fat are very mobile and probing may displace them even more. Foreign bodies that are imbedded in fat and that are perpendicular to the skin may also be removed as in Figure 37–6C.

Foreign Bodies in the Sole of the Foot

It is reasonable to assume that foreign matter is introduced into many wounds on the sole of the foot. This is particularly true if the wounds are caused by foreign material being driven into the foot such as occurs when one steps on a nail while wearing a shoe with a soft rubber sole. In cases of infected puncture wounds, exploration for a foreign body is mandatory, even when no foreign body is identified on a radiograph.

When exploring lesions on the sole of the foot, foreign material may often be located with the aid of a magnifying device. This enables the location of the sinus tract or the visualization of the tip of a splinter. *An ischemic tourniquet is mandatory when exploring the foot for a foreign body.* The persistence of a mass, a draining sinus, radiographic evidence of an exuberant inflammatory reaction, or a cyst or inflammation of adjacent bony structures should heighten suspicion that a retained foreign body has entered the foot and is now announcing its presence to the patient and physician by the continued efforts of the body to reject the foreign material. Cracchiolo reported three patients who

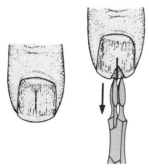

Figure 37–8. For foreign body deep in the nail bed, take as small a wedge of nail as will allow access to the proximal end of the splinter, then extract with splinter forceps. A digital nerve block may be necessary. (Reproduced from Hospital Medicine, January 1981, with permission of Hospital Publications, Inc.)

experienced recurrent pain and infection in the foot for a number of years.[12] The patients did not respond to antibiotics or to attempts at exploration. In each case, a toothpick (not seen radiographically) embedded in the sole of the foot was the cause.

Subungual Foreign Bodies

Special attention is required for subungual foreign bodies that are deeply imbedded in the nail bed.[13] In some instances, this may require removing a small portion of the nail with double-pointed heavy scissors and grasping the foreign material with the splinter forceps (Fig. 37–8). Occasionally, complete removal of the nail may be required. Obviously, a digital block is needed for techniques involving manipulation of the nail or nail bed. An interesting technique has been suggested in which a bent, at its tip, sterile hypodermic needle is slid under the nail and hooks the foreign body, allowing its withdrawal. Alternatively, a No. 19 gauge hypodermic needle can be slid under the nail to surround the splinter. The needle tip is then brought against the underside of the nail to secure the splinter. The needle and splinter are then removed as a unit. Wooden splinters are commonly imbedded under the fingernail. *Such foreign bodies must be completely removed because infection is certain*. The proximity of the distal phalynx to the

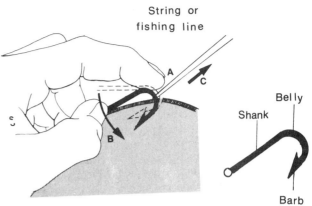

Figure 37–10. Method of removing embedded fish hook when anesthesia is unavailable or when the barb of the fish hook lies too deep to force out through a second wound without causing significant additional damage. Loop a piece of string (or thick suture material) around the belly of the hook and hold it down against the skin with the index finger of the left hand (A). Depress the shaft of the hook against the skin with the middle finger and thumb while applying light downward pressure with the index finger of the left hand to disengage the barb from the subcutaneous tissue (B), and pull *sharply* on the ends of the string with the right hand (C) to remove the hook through its entry wound. Bystanders should be out of the expected path of the hook. (Reproduced from Hospital Medicine, July 1980, with permission of Hospital Publications, Inc.)

subungual area is a constant concern for the development of osteomyelitis.

Fishhooks

There are several methods of removing a fishhook. The method that one uses depends upon the conditions under which the removal is to take place.[14–18] The traditional manner for removing small fishhooks requires local infiltration with 1 per cent lidocaine, forcing the barb through the anesthetized skin, clipping off the barb, and removing the rest of the hook along the direction of entry (Fig. 37–9). In the field or stream, removal of a fishhook may be accomplished without local anesthetic by following a technique that enables easy removal. The same technique may be used in the emergency department with 1 per cent lidocaine to facilitate removal. This "stream" technique (Fig. 37–10) is to loop a piece of string or fishing line around the belly of the hook at the

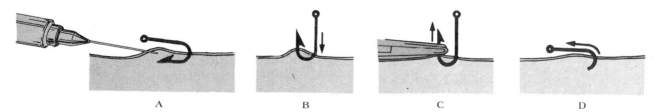

A   B   C   D

Figure 37–9. Method of removing embedded fish hook when anesthesia is available and when the point of the fish hook is close to the skin. A, Obtain local anesthesia overlying the point of the hook. B, Force the point through the anesthetized skin. C, Clip off the barb. D, Remove the rest of the hook by reversing the direction of entry. (Reproduced from Hospital Medicine, July 1980, with permission of Hospital Publications, Inc.)

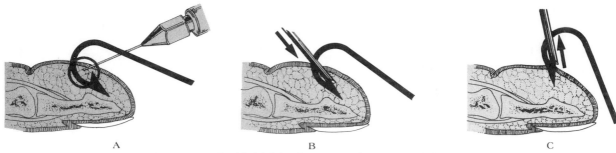

Figure 37–11. Method of removing embedded fish hook using aneshesia when the hook is large and not too deep in the skin. After anesthetizing the area with 1 per cent lidocaine (A), insert a short-bevel 18-gauge needle through the entry wound of the hook and attempt to sheath the barb of the hook within the needle (B). If this is done correctly, the hook and needle may then be backed out together (C). (Reproduced from Hospital Medicine, July 1980, with permission of Hospital Publications, Inc.)

point at which it enters the skin. Allow approximately 1 foot of string to be wrapped around the right hand to give strong traction. The shank of the hook should be held parallel to and in approximation with the skin by the index finger of the left hand. The thumb and middle finger of the left hand stabilize and depress the barb, which helps the index finger to disengage the barb from the subcutaneous tissue. When the barb has been disengaged, a *sharp* pull by the right hand removes the hook through the wound of entry. The hook often *flies* out of the patient. Care should be taken to keep bystanders out of the expected path of the hook.

If the hook is large and if it is not desirable to cause further trauma by pushing the pointed end through the skin, it may be possible to use an 18 gauge needle to cover the barb (Fig. 37–11). After adequate local anesthetic has been administered, the needle should be passed through the entrance wound of the hook parallel to the shank of the hook to sheath the barb and to allow the hook to be backed out while the barb is covered. An alternative to this procedure is to insert a No. 11 blade parallel to the shank of the hook down to the barb. Using the point of the blade, free the subcutaneous tissue that is engaged on the barb, sheath the barb with the point of the No. 11 blade,

and back the hook out, with the blade protecting the barb.

Wooden Splinters

Because of the potential for inflammation, *pieces of wood must be completely removed from soft tissue.* Simply grasping the end of a superficial protruding splinter may be adequate, but care should be taken not to leave small pieces of the foreign body in the wound (Fig. 37–12). Some splinters cannot be visualized at the point of entry but can be easily and readily palpated beneath the skin. In such cases, it is advisable to cut down on the long axis of the foreign body to remove it via a skin incision rather than through the entrance wound (Fig. 37–13). This method allows for thorough cleaning of the tract and removal of small pieces of the splinter that may otherwise remain. The linear skin incision may then be sutured. Particular mention should be made of certain wood splinters that are reactive and pliable, such as California redwood and Northwest cedar. Any wood that is easily fragmented requires meticulous care to ensure removal of all the material. Wood is not visible on a standard radiograph or xeroradiograph unless it is covered with lead paint.

Occasionally, the most expeditious method of

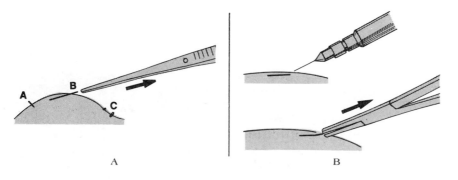

Figure 37–12. A, After local cleansing, superficial splinters (A, B) and other small foreign bodies (C) may be removed with sharp forceps and magnifier, usually without anesthesia. Avoid retention of fragments of long foreign bodies (B) by gentle withdrawal in the axis of entry. B, In tangentially embedded superficial splinters, careful teasing of the skin over the point of entry with the cutting edge of a fine hypodermic needle will often given access to the proximal end of the foreign body. (Reproduced from Hospital Medicine, January 1981, with permission of Hospital Publications, Inc.)

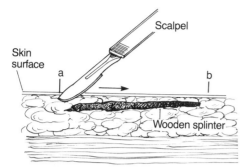

Figure 37–13. An imbedded wooden splinter is removed by cutting down on the foreign body from point *a* to point *b*. This allows one to open the tract and remove all pieces of wood. The resultant laceration may be sutured primarily if there is no gross infection.

removing wooden splinters is complete excision of the entrance tract and the foreign body en bloc, followed by a linear closure, resulting in a more cosmetic wound with less chance for infection.

Pencil Lead

Good judgment must be used in the removal of graphite from pencils when lodged in the skin. Because graphite invariably leaves a pigmented tattooing in the soft tissue, it is preferable to excise the material en bloc when pencil lead is found in a cosmetic area. The graphite specks cannot be irrigated or scrubbed off, and tattooing will result if they are not removed.

Metallic Fragments

High-velocity fragments, such as bullets, BB's, chips of wood-splitting mauls, or other metallic particles caused by metal striking metal, are easy to visualize radiographically and relatively simple to remove unless they are imbedded in areas that are anatomically difficult to approach. Prior to removal of the foreign material, the area in which the fragment is imbedded should be assessed in order to determine which structures are involved along the wound of entrance, which structures might be encountered in attempting to cut down on the foreign body, and which of those structures can be sacrificed to allow for adequate removal of the foreign material. It is preferable to defer the removal of deeply imbedded metallic foreign bodies unless symptoms or infection develop. The extensive treatment of high-velocity foreign bodies, such as modern military or sporting ammunition, is beyond the scope of this discussion, because high-velocity fragments frequently result not only in a foreign body but also cause severe trauma along its path. Retained metallic fragments are inert and rarely cause infection. They usually become encysted after a period of time. The value

of routine prophylactic antibiotic for metallic foreign bodies left in the soft tissue has not been proven.

Sea Urchin Spines

The spines of the sea urchin are often a problem of physicians who treat skin divers or abalone fishermen. Spines are reactive and may be contaminated with slime, debris, and calcareous material initially, causing an intensive foreign body reaction. They are almost colorless and very brittle, so attempts to remove them require the physician's greatest skill and the patient's patience. Retained sea urchin spines may produce significant morbidity and should not be taken lightly. In circumstances in which removal will be difficult, the easiest method may be to allow time for a reaction to take place. The wound is then opened and drained, all the foreign material is removed by curettage, and the wound is allowed to heal by secondary intention.

Postoperative Foreign Bodies

Foreign bodies in the form of non-absorbable suture material are frequently encountered in the postoperative period. The characteristic drainage, localized inflammatory reaction along the suture line, and localized pain and tenderness are characteristics of a retained foreign body (suture abscess). In this instance, probing the wound with a sterilized crochet hook or bent needle is frequently rewarding. Hooking the suture material through the sinus tract and removing it will allow the wound to heal over the tract.

Ring Removal

Frequently, a ring must be removed to prevent laceration of tissue or vascular compromise. If removal is not possible by thorough lubrication (a water-soluble lubricant, e.g., K-Y jelly) and circular motion with traction on the ring, it may be necessary to either cut the ring off or remove it by the string-wrap method.

String-Wrap Method (Fig. 37–14). A 15- to 20-inch piece of string, umbilical tape, or thick silk suture is passed between the ring and the finger. If there is marked soft-tissue swelling, the tip of a hemostat may be passed under the ring to grasp the string and pull it through the ring. The distal end of the string should be 10 to 15 inches long. The distal string is wrapped around the swollen finger (proximal to distal) to include the proximal interphalangeal (PIP) joint and the entire swollen finger. The wrapping is begun next to the ring. The wrap should be snug enough to compress the swollen tissue. The successive loops of the wrap

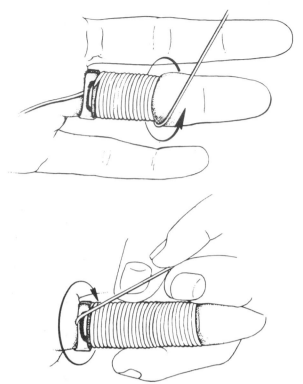

Figure 37–14. Remove a ring from a swollen finger by winding on a bit of string to compress the distal swollen tissues and then unwind the string and ring together. This string is passed under the ring prior to wrapping the finger. (From Emergency Medicine, September 15, 1982, p. 107.)

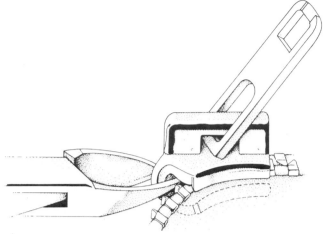

Figure 37–15. When loose skin is caught in the teeth of a zipper, one can release it quickly and without risk to the patient by cutting the diamond that holds the slider together with a bone cutter or a pair of wire clippers. (From Emergency Medicine, October 15, 1982, p. 215. Used by permission.)

are placed next to each other to keep any swollen tissue from bulging between the strands. When the wrapping has been completed, the proximal end of the string is carefully unwound, forcing the ring over that portion of the finger that has been compressed by the wrap. The PIP joint is the area that is most difficult to maneuver. Occasionally, one must re-wrap the finger if it was not carefully wrapped initially. The procedure may be painful and may require a digital block. Some non-anesthetized patients panic during the procedure because of increasing pain due to compression and unwinding.

Ring Cutter. A standard ring cutter should be used if the ring is not of high value or if there is excessive swelling. The ring cutter has a small hook that fits under the ring and serves as a guide to a saw-toothed wheel, which cuts the metal. The cut ends of the ring are spread using large hemostats (e.g., Kelley clamps), and the ring is removed. Cut rings may be repaired by a jeweler.

Obviously, it is preferable to remove all rings before the edema is extensive enough to cause pain or vascular compromise.

Zipper Injuries

The skin of the penis may become painfully entangled in the mechanism of a zipper. Unzip-ping the zipper frequently lacerates the skin and increases the amount of the tissue caught in the mechanism. Although the physician may anesthetize the skin and excise the entrapped tissue, a less invasive method may be useful.

The interlocking teeth of the zipper will fall apart if the median bar (diamond or bridge) of the zipper is cut in half (Fig. 37–15). The skin will subsequently be freed. A bone cutter or wire clippers and a moderate amount of force may be required to break the bar.

1. Barnett, R. C.: Removal of cutaneous foreign bodies. J. Hosp. Med. 97, Jan., 1981.
2. Anderson, A., Newmeyer, W. L., and Kilgore, E. S.: Diagnosis and treatment of retained foreign bodies of the hand. Am. J. Surg. 144:63, 1982.
3. Pond, G. D., and Lindsey, D.: Localization of cactus, glass, and other foreign bodies in soft tissues. Ariz. Med. 34:700, 1977.
4. Tandberg, D.: Glass in the hand and foot: will an x-ray film show it? JAMA 248:1872, 1982.
5. Bowers, D. G., and Lynch, J. B.: Xeroradiography for non-metallic foreign bodies. Plast. Reconstr. Surg. 60:470, 1977.
6. Carneiro, R. S., Okunski, W. J., and Heffernan, A. H.: Detection of a relatively radiolucent foreign body in the hand by xeroradiography. Plast. Reconstr. Surg. 59:862, 1977.
7. Karpman, R. R., Sparks, R. P., and Fried, M.: Cactus thorn injuries to the extremities; their management and etiology. Ariz. Med. 37:849, 1980.
8. Davis, L. J.: Removal of subungual foreign bodies. J. Fam. Pract. 11:714, 1980.
9. Ariyan, S.: A simple stereotactic method to isolate and remove foreign bodies. Arch. Surg. 112:857, 1977.
10. Bhavsar, M. S.: Technique of finding a metallic foreign body. Am. J. Surg. 141:305, 1981.
11. Rees, C. E.: The removal of foreign bodies: a modified incision. JAMA 113:35, 1939.
12. Cracchiolo, A.: Wooden foreign bodies in the foot. Am. J. Surg. 140:585, 1980.

13. Swischuk, L. E., Jorgenson, F., Jorgenson, A., et al.: Wooden splinter induced pseudo-tumor and osteomyelitis-like lesions of bone and soft tissue. Am. J. Roentgenol. Radium Ther. Nucl. Med. 122:176, 1974.
14. Barnett, R. C.: Removal of fishhooks. J. Hosp. Med. 56, July, 1980.
15. Barnett, R. C.: Three useful techniques for removing imbedded fishhooks. Hosp. Med. 72, July, 1982.
16. Editorial: A few ways to unsnag a fishhook. Emerg. Med. 13:222, 1981.
17. Friedenberg, S.: How to remove an imbedded fishhook in 5 seconds without really trying. N. Engl. J. Med. 284:733, 1971.
18. Rose, J. D.: Removing the imbedded fishhook. Austral. Fam. Phys. 10:33, 1981.

38

Skin Grafting in the Outpatient

SEUNG K. KIM, M.D.
LARS VISTNES, M.D.

Introduction

Skin grafting is one of the major techniques in the surgical armamentarium. It allows one to close a clean wound that cannot be closed primarily because of an insufficient skin cover. The wound could be traumatic or secondary to surgical excision or skin loss caused by a burn injury. The skin is a natural barrier between the body and the environment. Early coverage of an open wound and re-establishment of this barrier is essential in the restoration of the internal equilibrium and the prevention of further wound complications. In selected cases, minor skin grafting can be done easily in the outpatient setting with a minimum of equipment. When recipient site preparation, selection of the skin graft and dressing, and after-care of the graft are carefully performed with a knowledge of the physiology of skin grafting, one is amply rewarded with excellent results.

Types of Skin Grafts

The skin is composed of the epidermis and the dermis. Many of the skin appendages, such as hair follicles, sebaceous glands, and sweat glands, are located within the dermis (Fig. 38–1). A *full-thickness skin graft* contains the entire thickness of the epidermis and the dermis. As a result, if the graft is taken from a hair-bearing area, hair characteristic of the donor site may grow on the transplanted full-thickness skin graft. Other than for occasional use in resurfacing of the palmar aspect of the hand and the fingers, a full-thickness skin graft is rarely indicated in emergency situations.

A *split-thickness skin graft* includes the full thickness of the epidermis and a partial thickness of the dermis (see Fig. 38–1). Depending on the thickness, split-thickness skin grafts can be classified as thin, intermediate, and thick. A thin split-thickness skin graft is roughly 0.008 to 0.010 inches in thickness; an intermediate split-thickness skin graft is 0.012 to 0.014 inches. A thick split-thickness skin graft is usually from 0.015 to 0.025 inches thick. The numerical measurement of thickness is only a guide. The descriptive terminology of thin, intermediate, and thick split-thickness skin grafts is more applicable. Graft thickness can be judged by the appearance of the graft and the donor site. The thicker the grafts, the more opaque they are. The edges of the thicker graft tend to curl up more. The donor site for a thin split-thickness skin graft shows a velvety field of numerous very fine bleeding points. The bleeding pattern of a thick split-thickness skin graft donor site is much coarser. The punctate bleeding points are larger in size and fewer in number.

Once the skin grafts are harvested, they tend to shrink as a result of the inherent elasticity of the dermal element. The thicker the graft, the greater the potential for shrinking. A thin split-thickness skin graft barely shows evidence of shrinking, whereas the full-thickness skin graft shrinks markedly. As the skin grafts heal and undergo maturation, progressive contraction of the skin graft is evident. The degree of contraction again depends on the thickness of the graft. Thin split-thickness skin grafts contract the most, whereas full-thickness skin grafts show minimal evidence of contraction. Skin grafts acquire pigmentation as they mature. The degree of pigmentation is also dependent on the thickness of the skin graft. A thin split-thickness skin graft is more apt to develop a dark pigmentation than is a thicker split-thickness skin graft or a full-thickness skin graft. The problem of pigmentation is worse in skin grafts on sun-exposed areas of the body.

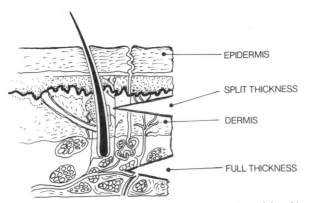

Figure 38–1. Schematic diagram of the cross section of the skin demonstrating the split-thickness and the full-thickness skin grafts.

EPIDERMIS

SPLIT THICKNESS

DERMIS

FULL THICKNESS

Graft Revascularization

A skin graft adheres to the recipient bed and is initially held by a fibrin network from the recipient bed. For the first 48 hours, survival of the skin graft is largely dependent upon serum imbibition. The endothelial channels of the skin graft become filled with serum-like fluid from the recipient bed. This is thought to be brought about by capillary action and diffusion within the skin graft. The nutritional supply and the metabolic exchange are carried out through this fluid medium.[1] Some believe that the main function of this phase of serum imbibition is to prevent the graft from drying and to keep the vessels open for later communication with the recipient vessels.[2]

During this early phase of serum imbibition, restoration of hemic circulation proceeds concurrently, evidenced by gradual change of the color of the graft from pale white to pink. There are three mechanisms that are believed to be responsible for revascularization: (1) end-to-end connection of the blood vessels between the recipient bed and the skin graft, known as *inosculation*,[3] (2) ingrowth of vessels from the recipient bed into the pre-existing endothelial channels of the skin graft, and (3) ingrowth of endothelial buds into the dermis of the skin graft.[4] Through these mechanisms, normal circulation is restored in the skin graft in anywhere from 4 to 7 days.[5]

The same mechanisms of graft survival and revascularization apply to split-thickness skin grafts and full-thickness skin grafts. A thin split-thickness skin graft, however, can be maintained longer on imbibition alone. This is attributed to the fact that thinner grafts have a shorter distance for diffusion and less cellular mass to be nourished. Revascularization of a thin split-thickness skin graft is also more rapid than revascularization of a thick split-thickness graft or a full-thickness graft for the same reason.[6]

Recipient Bed

Skin grafts can be placed on any exposed vascular surface. This includes all the musculoskeletal tissue and all the internal organs. Skin grafts do not survive on nonvascular surfaces, such as bare bone without periosteum, bare cartilage without perichondrium, and bare tendon without paratenon cover. A skin graft can bridge over a nonvascular area by vascularization through the graft edge, however. Up to 5 mm of skin graft from the edge can be vascularized. Hence, theoretically, a maximum of 10 mm of nonvascular area can be covered by bridging, provided that there is an adequate vascular rim of recipient bed at the perimeter of the skin graft.

One can best ensure that the graft will "take" by careful recipient bed preparation. All the nonviable tissue is removed surgically from the wound, creating a well-vascularized surface. Meticulous hemostasis of the recipient bed is also a key to a successful graft.

Donor Site Healing

The surface of the split-thickness graft donor site is a raw dermal surface with multiple openings into the remaining portions of the transected skin appendages, such as sweat ducts and glands, sebaceous glands, and hair shafts and follicles. These appendages are lined with squamous epithelium and are the source of epithelial cells for resurfacing of the exposed dermal surface. The epithelial cells proliferate, migrate out to the dermal surface, and spread radially until they become confluent and cover the entire raw surface. The dermal layer itself may become thicker with scar tissue but does not regenerate. As the thickness of the split-thickness skin graft becomes greater, fewer skin appendages are left in the donor surface. For this reason, the donor site of a thick split-thickness graft takes longer to heal than the donor site of a thinner split-thickness graft. Once the donor site is re-epithelialized, its appearance is again dependent on the graft thickness. A thin split-thickness skin graft donor site containing a thicker residual dermis and more of its skin appendages is closer to its surrounding skin in appearance and is less conspicuous than a thicker split-thickness graft donor site, which has a thin, scarred dermis with fewer remaining skin appendages.

Unfavorable Factors

Several factors adversely influence the outcome of skin grafting. They either interfere with the revascularization process or disturb the neovascular network that has already been formed.

1. *Hematoma and seroma.* A hematoma is the most common cause of skin graft failure. A hematoma under the skin graft causes separation of the skin graft from its bed. Consequently, revascularization of the graft is delayed or altogether prevented by the space-occupying effect of this intervening layer of blood or blood clot. The skin graft may survive for a short period on serum imbibition alone. If revascularization is delayed beyond this period of serum imbibition, however, the graft is doomed to fail. To prevent hematoma, one should obtain complete hemostasis of the graft bed prior to application of a skin graft. If complete hemostasis is not possible, the wound should be redressed, and skin grafting should be delayed for one to a few days. A seroma also prevents graft adherence and revascularization through a mechanism similar to that of a hematoma.

2. *Movement.* As discussed before, graft survival depends on reconstitution of the capillary vascular network between the recipient bed and the skin graft. It is easy to see how even the smallest motion of the skin graft relative to the recipient bed could disrupt and interfere with the formation of these fine, early vascular connections. Movement also promotes formation of a seroma or a hematoma. For these reasons, immobilization of the graft to its bed is essential in graft healing.

3. *Necrosis.* Any residual nonviable tissue left in the recipient bed will undergo necrosis and will lead to failure of the overlying graft. In particular, the vascularity of fatty tissue in a traumatic wound is often uncertain. Bits of fat may die and necrose. Again, it is very important to debride all the tissues of questionable vascularity before grafting. If the vascularity of the recipient bed is uncertain, it is best to delay skin grafting.

4. *Infection.* Despite its devastating effect on skin grafting, infection is the least common cause of graft failure. In addition to the obvious space-occupying effect of infection, a purulent collection actively separates the graft from its bed and destroys the newly formed vessels. The abundant proteolytic enzymes from inflammation and from the microorganisms are responsible for the lysis of the fibrin adhesion and the destruction of vascular connections. The most notable virulent organism that affects skin grafting is group A β-hemolytic streptococcus, which rapidly destroys the skin graft and literally melts it away. With prophylactic antibiotic coverage, this complication is seen less often.

Indication for Skin Grafting

Whether to close a wound or to leave it open to heal by secondary intention depends on the nature and the history of formation of the wound. Traumatic open wounds may be classified as either clean or contaminated. The majority of traumatic wounds can be considered clean, except for those resulting from bites, those made in a contaminated environment, and those that are 24 or more hours old. Of particular concern is wound contamination by microorganisms. Wounds that contain inorganic material, such as gravel, pieces of broken glass, metal, industrial lubricant, and the like, are not necessarily contaminated. As long as there is no suspicion of contamination by microorganisms, these wounds can be made clean by debridement and removal of foreign substances. Untidy wounds resulting from tearing, crushing, mangling, or explosive injuries with devitalized tissue debris can also be debrided and converted to clean, tidy wounds. In general, all clean wounds should be closed when possible, and most of the contaminated wounds should be left open.

When there is loss of full thickness of skin and the wound cannot be closed with local tissue alone, closure with a distant tissue is considered. Relatively superficial wounds are most often closed with split-thickness skin grafts. For those wounds in which graft color, texture match, and graft contraction are not of concern, a split-thickness skin graft is an ideal wound cover. In fact, a split-thickness skin graft is often used because of this propensity to undergo contraction. For instance, a split-thickness skin graft on a fingertip wound would contract, pulling the surrounding healthy pulp pad skin over the tissue defect, and would minimize the size of the wound. On the other hand, certain anatomic areas, such as the face and the flexion surface of the hand and the fingers, require coverage that produces minimal contraction. Facial wounds also demand color and texture match. These requirements are best met by full-thickness skin grafts. If deep structures, such as neurovascular bundle, tendon, bone, and joint, are exposed, some other means of distant tissue cover in addition to skin grafting may be considered.

Skin grafting of selected acute wounds in an outpatient setting is beneficial. Grafting affords early closure of the wound and obviates further wound complications, such as desiccation of exposed structures, repeated trauma to tissue, and infection. Grafting may decrease the degree and the length of morbidity significantly. For example, when grafted, a fingertip wound greater than 1 cm^2 in size would heal much sooner than a wound of equal size that is allowed to close by contraction and epithelialization. Grafted wounds are also more comfortable for the patient than open wounds.

Selection of Donor Site

In theory, one should be able to take a skin graft from anywhere on the body. Indeed, numerous donor sites are necessary when large areas need

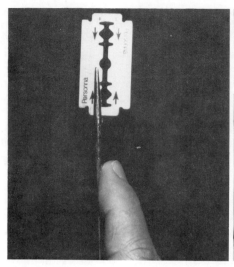
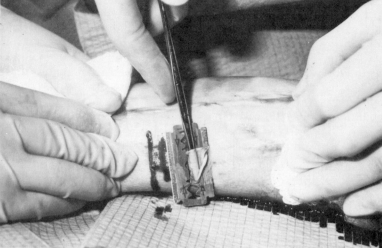

Figure 38–2. Regular double-edged razor blade used as a dermatome.

to be covered, as in a major burn injury. For smaller wounds, the functional and cosmetic quality of the skin graft at the recipient site and the resulting donor site deformity dictates the selection of the donor site.

A full-thickness skin graft is usually taken from a glabrous area of the body. There are many favored areas for taking full-thickness skin grafts. Among them, the hypothenar skin, the antecubital flexion creases, the wrist flexion crease, and the medial arm are most readily accessible and appropriate for emergency outpatient situations.

When a thin split-thickness skin graft is desired (as is the case for most emergency department skin grafting), the anteromedial aspect of the forearm is suitable. Some have expressed objections to this site, claiming obvious scarring in a frequently exposed area. Yet, in experienced hands, a very thin split-thickness skin graft from this area leaves minimal to no appreciable scarring.[7] The posterolateral aspect of the thighs, the buttocks, and the lower abdomen are also available for skin grafting. Relatively thicker skin grafts can be taken safely from these areas. In young women, the graft may be taken within the bikini line to conceal the donor site scar.

Dermatomes

There are many different types of dermatomes, varying from simple hand-held instruments to more complex mechanical devices. For outpatient use in an emergency facility, hand-held dermatomes are quite adequate. Only those that are useful for outpatient skin grafting will be described here.

Scalpel Blade. A scalpel blade is the simplest dermatome. A No. 10 or 20 blade is quite effective for taking a small split-thickness skin graft.

Razor Blade. A sterile, regular double-edged razor blade can be used to take a small skin graft. The razor blade is held with a straight clamp and is used in a freehand manner (Fig. 38–2). Varying thicknesses of split-thickness skin grafts can be cut with this dermatome. The thickness of the skin graft can be judged by the clarity with which the writing on the blade can be read through the skin graft. One can see through the usual thin and intermediate-thickness skin grafts quite readily.

Silver Dermatome. This dermatome consists of a handle and a platform at the oposite end that receives a regular, double-edged razor blade. The razor blade is fixed in place with a cover plate, which is secured with a wing nut. There is a roller just above and parallel to the blade edge. One can adjust the thickness of the graft by setting the distance between the roller and the blade, which one accomplishes by turning the knobs at the ends of the blade (Fig. 38–3). This is only a rough guide; the final product depends on the physician's touch and experience.

Goulian-Weck Knife. This is another freehand dermatome. The instrument consists of a handle with a metal slot at one end that receives a safety razor blade measuring 5.5 cm in length. Over this assembly, a blade guard is placed (Fig. 38–4). The blade guard determines the thickness of the skin graft. Three different blade guards with thicknesses of 0.008, 0.010, and 0.012 inches are available. Although these guards are made to cut skin grafts of fixed thicknesses, after repeated use they become sprung and are not very reliable. These blade guards should be used as rough guides to the thickness of the skin graft. The actual thickness should be controlled visually and by touch.

Humby Knife. This is the largest freehand dermatome available. The blade mechanism is similar to that of the Silver dermatome. The device uses a large, single-edged blade that is fixed to a han-

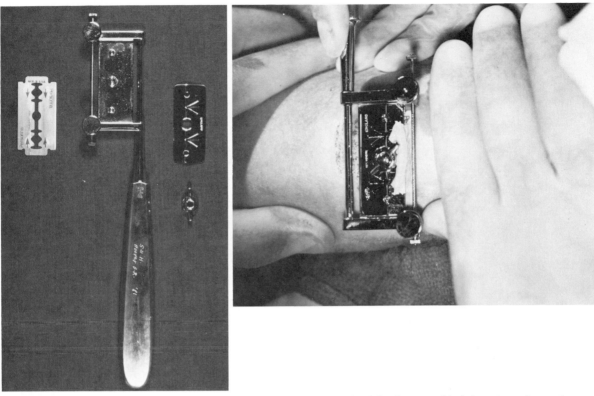

Figure 38–3. Components of the silver dermatome are shown on the left. The assembled dermatome in use is shown on the right.

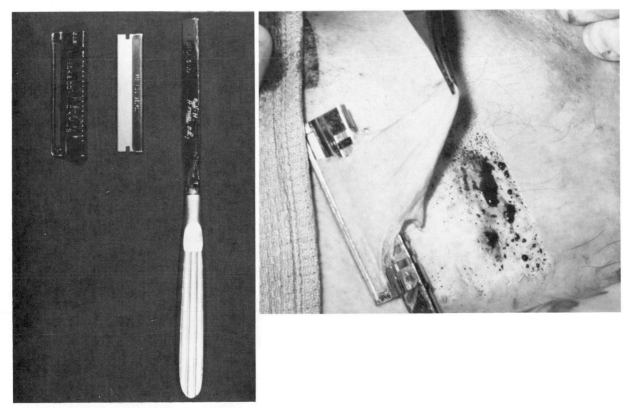

Figure 38–4. Components of the Goulian-Weck dermatome on the left and the assembled unit in use on the right.

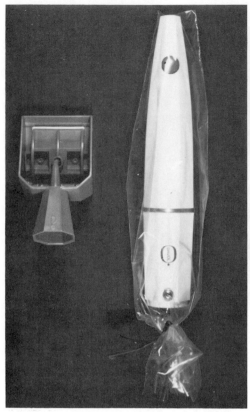

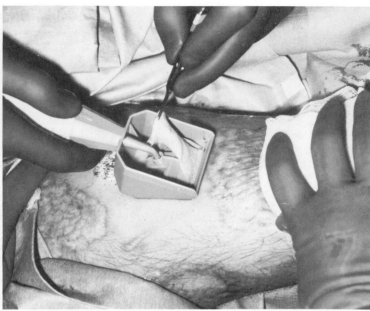

Figure 38–5. Davol disposable dermatome head driven by the battery-operated motor unit in the handle.

dle. An adjustable roller determines the thickness of the graft.

Davol Disposable Dermatome. A sterile, disposable blade unit that cuts a split-thickness skin graft of intermediate thickness and 3.5 cm in width is available from Davol.* This blade unit is driven by a battery-operated motor in an electric toothbrush handle unit (Fig. 38–5). The handle is placed in a sterile plastic bag. The blade unit is then pushed onto the handle, puncturing the plastic bag, and is attached to the handle. The device is operated by pressure placed on the button switch while the blade unit is kept lightly pressed against the skin with an equally light forward force to advance the dermatome. The battery in the handle is rechargeable through a recharging unit.

Harvesting of Skin Graft

The donor site is prepared with any of the number of surgical preparation solutions that are available. Local anesthetic (1 per cent or 0.5 per cent lidocaine [Xylocaine] and 1:100,000 or 1:200,000 epinephrine solution) is used for anesthesia and hemostasis. An area larger than the size of the desired graft is infiltrated. The plane of

anesthetic infiltration is in the deep dermis. The anesthetic solution is injected continuously while the needle is being passed back and forth in multiple parallel passes. A 25 or 27 gauge hypodermic needle 1.5 inches in length is used. This results in uniform infiltration of the entire area, forming an evenly elevated plateau (Fig. 38–6).

Full-Thickness Skin Graft. The size and the shape of the wound to be covered are measured on the donor site with a template made of any flat sheet of material that is available, such as glove

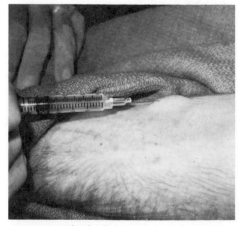

Figure 38–6. Infiltration of anesthetic in the donor site.

*Davol Inc., Providence, Rhode Island.

wrapping paper or a piece of foil from a suture package. A lenticular pattern of skin that contains the graft pattern is designed. One should plan carefully in order to orient the long axis of the pattern parallel to the adjacent skin creases; this will allow primary closure of the donor defect and will produce favorable orientation of the resulting scar. Using a scapel, one makes a skin incision along the lenticular pattern. One removes the full thickness of the skin by running the blade of the scalpel along the junction between the dermis and the subcutaneous fat. One then defats the graft by stretching it over a finger with the epithelial side down and snipping the bits of fat from the dermal surface with a pair of small scissors. The graft pattern is cut, and the skin graft is then ready for placement.

Often the patient will present to the emergency department with a portion of his fingertip, which has been removed in a slicing injury. The amputated tip, if relatively superficial, can be treated as a full-thickness skin graft. The tissue should be irrigated with saline to remove debris, defatted, and placed in saline soaked gauze while the recipient bed is being prepared. The thick epidermis of the fingertip is often cut five or six times with a scalpel to avoid separation of the graft and recipient bed as the fingertip dries. The graft is then attached by one of the techniques discussed in the following sections.

Split-Thickness Skin Graft. The skin graft donor site is first lubricated so that the dermatome can glide smoothly. This facilitates taking an even skin graft. Mineral oil, Vaseline, or any of the usual topical ointments can be used. The lubricant is applied thinly over the donor skin surface. The donor skin is stretched manually. One holds the skin proximally and distally to the graft donor site by firmly pressing the skin with either a wooden tongue blade or a piece of gauze. One applies traction by pulling away from the donor site in both directions (Fig. 38–7A). This usually requires two people. The surgeon's free hand should hold the traction toward the direction of the dermatome movement. An assistant applies the countertraction, and the surgeon cuts the skin graft toward his free hand.

The dermatome is held lightly with the fingers and the thumb. The upper extremity is relaxed with the wrist in a relatively fixed position. The motion is mainly at the elbow and the shoulder. The cutting motion consists of frequent to-and-fro strokes with a minimal forward pressure. Too much forward pressure may result in irregular thickness of the graft and possible interruption of graft continuity. The initial contact of the dermatome and the skin should be at an angle when the cut is begun. Once the cut is initiated, the dermatome is flattened out to effect tangential excision of the skin (Fig. 38–7B). The downward pressure on the dermatome determines the thickness of the skin graft. For the thin and intermediate-thickness skin grafts, the weight of the dermatome itself, without much additional external

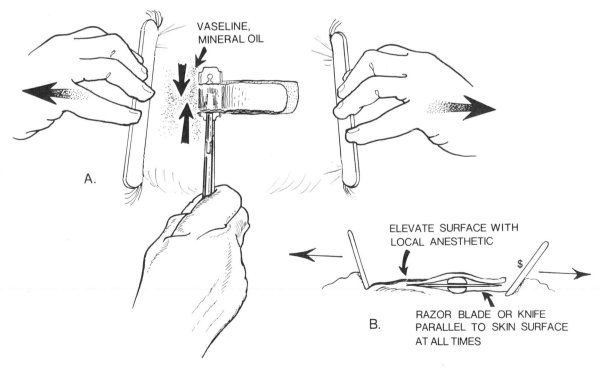

Figure 38–7. *A,* Cutting of a split-thickness skin graft with a double-edged razor blade held in a straight clamp. The skin is held taut by traction and countertraction. *B,* Tangential excision producing a skin graft of uniform thickness.

pressure, seems sufficient to cut the desired thickness. With experience, this procedure becomes quite natural.

Once harvested, the skin will curl and shrink immediately. One may think that the graft will not be large enough since it is now smaller than the area outlined at the donor site. The skin, however, will readily stretch when applied to the recipient bed. Uncurling the harvested graft on moist gauze will be helpful in keeping the graft flat. Furthermore, the graft should be kept moist between layers of wet gauze if it is not immediately applied to the recipient bed.

Application of Skin Graft

Full-Thickness Skin Graft. Following meticulous hemostasis of the recipient bed, the previously cut skin graft is laid on the recipient bed. Because of the inherent shrinkage of the full-thickness skin graft, even if the graft is cut to size, it is usually slightly smaller than the recipient defect. For this reason, the skin graft is sutured to the edge of the defect and is stretched to cover the defect. Several tacking sutures are placed in the periphery for proper fitting. These sutures are left long for a tie-over dressing. The remaining edges are sutured with a running circumferential suture. Sutures are easier to place if the needle is driven through the graft first and then through the skin edge of the recipient area.

Split-Thickness Skin Graft. The split-thickness skin graft is placed on the recipient bed with the dermal side down. The dermal side of the split-thickness skin graft is characterized by the wet, glistening sheen as opposed to the relatively dry, dull appearance of the epithelial surface. In addition, the edges tend to curl toward the dermal surface. If the recipient bed is larger than a single sheet of graft, several sheets of graft may be required. Any overlapping of skin grafts does not influence the graft take. On the other hand, it is very important to make sure that the free edges of the graft are fully uncurled so that it is not doubled over on itself. The epithelial surface of the graft must be adjacent to the recipient bed. Obviously, any curled portion will not get revascularized, and sectional failure of the graft will result.

The split-thickness skin graft should be laid in such a way that it follows all the hills and valleys of the wound and is in contact with the entire raw surface of the recipient bed. If the skin grafts tend to tent over a deep concavity, it is useful to tack down the tented portion to the base of the concavity using one or two through-and-through stitches; 4-0 or 5-0 chromic sutures can be used. This is supplemented by a conforming dressing.

The overhanging edges of the skin graft beyond the wound margin are trimmed. Suturing of the skin graft at the edges is not always necessary but may be desirable to offset the curling of the skin edges.

Dressings

Full-Thickness Skin Graft. A full-thickness skin graft is usually dressed with a tie-over bolster dressing. This dressing facilitates immobilization and affords moderate, even pressure to prevent collection of blood or serum under the skin graft. The skin graft is fixed in place with several interrupted sutures, usually 4-0 nylon, placed in a relatively evenly spaced pattern around the periphery of the skin graft and the recipient bed. The tails of the sutures are left long. The skin graft is covered with a single layer of nonadherent gauze, such as Xeroform or Vaseline gauze, which is cut larger than the grafted area. A bolster is formed using a wad of cotton, lamb's wool, gauze, or a polyurethane foam pad. The bolster is made to fit the size of the graft. The overhanging edges of the nonadherent gauze dressing are swept up to cover the rough edges of the bolster. The long tails of the sutures are tied, and the bolster is secured in place (Fig. 38–8). An additional soft dressing can be applied to protect the bolster dressing as necessary. If the skin graft is on an extremity and motion of the graft bed is a problem, immobilization of the parts involved with a loose plaster cast or a splint may be necessary.

Split-Thickness Skin Graft. There are numerous individual variations among physicians in dressing split-thickness skin grafts. These techniques are all quite functional, as long as they meet several basic requirements. The skin graft dressing should be nonadherent, absorptive, immobilizing, and protective. A split-thickness skin graft on a concave surface can be effectively immobilized by a tie-over bolster technique which

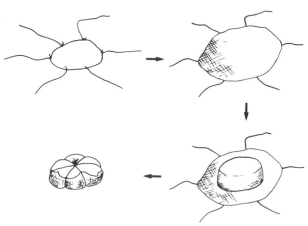

Figure 38–8. Method of tie-over bolster dressing application.

has been described previously. For uncomplicated small split-thickness skin grafts, there are much simpler and easier methods of applying dressings.

A small split-thickness skin graft on a flat surface can be secured with several strips of adherent porous closure strips without sutures (Fig. 38–9). The graft is then covered with a nonadherent petrolatum gauze to cover the entire extent of the wound closure strips. If the strips are not covered entirely by the greasy dressing, they may get lifted off as the dressing is removed and, in turn, may disrupt the skin graft. Next, a couple of layers of saline moistened gauze are applied. This layer of dressing aids in absorption of the early drainage through capillary action of the moist gauze fibers. The entire area is then covered with an oversized, thin sponge with an adhesive backing, such as a Reston pad.* The overhanging portion of the sponge is pressed and is allowed to adhere to the surrounding skin, which has been wiped dry.

If the adhesive sponge dressing is not available, the last step can be modified as follows: A surgical adhesive, such as tincture of benzoin or Acroplast, is applied to the skin surrounding the moist gauze dressing. An oversized dry gauze is applied over the entire area, and the edges are pressed to stick to the skin, which has been painted with surgical adhesive. The edges of the dressing can be reinforced with tapes if necessary. This last layer of dressing protects the graft from external shearing forces. The entire dressing and the whole graft-recipient unit may move, but the graft is not allowed to move relative to the recipient bed. This layer should not be occlusive. An occlusive layer, such as an adhesive plastic dressing, would prevent evaporation and would allow collection of drainage in the dressing and consequent maceration of the graft.

*Minnesota Mining and Manufacturing (3-M) Co., St. Paul, MN.

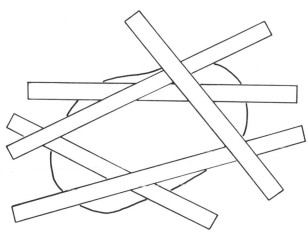

Figure 38–9. A method of graft fixation using multiple adherent, porous wound closure strips.

Contrary to common impression, a split-thickness skin graft on a fingertip wound is quite simple to dress. Fixing the skin graft with sutures is not necessary. This extra step is time-consuming and does not add to the outcome of the grafting. The skin graft is simply kept in place with several strips of petrolatum gauze that are placed across the skin graft and the adjacent skin in a criss-cross fashion. The strips should be narrower than the thickness of the finger, so that the gauze strips can be molded to the contour of the fingertip without folding or pleating. A thin layer of moist dressing gauze cut to size is placed next. Two strips of adhesive sponge foam pad are laid crossing each other over the fingertip. Dry gauze strips could be used in place of the foam pad. The entire assembly of dressing is then covered with a Tubegauze, if available. No more than two layers of Tubegauze should be used so that the dressing is not constricting.

The final step of skin graft dressing is immobilization of the graft site. External splinting is important for grafts that are on the parts of the body that normally go through motion, such as the extremities. The best way to splint an extremity with a skin graft is with a plaster cast. A cast may appear to be too much for a fingertip graft; however, in the long run, patients are more comfortable and can tolerate it well. Small individual finger splints that are taped on are not as reliable. These splints allow much motion and, hence, discomfort and graft disruption. With reinforcing strips of plaster in key areas, a relatively light cast that does the job can be fabricated.

The skin graft on the forearm can be splinted with a long arm cast including the wrist and the elbow. The wrist should be kept in 20 to 30 degrees of extension and the elbow in 90 degrees of flexion. A skin graft on a digit or the hand can be effectively immobilized with a short arm cast or bivalve plaster splint. Even if a single digit is injured, it is advisable to immobilize the fingers in groups, such as the index and middle fingers and the ring and little fingers. The thumb is immobilized with a thumb spica cast. The hand and the fingers are kept in the functional position. All casts should be generously padded with cast padding. The plaster roll should be applied loosely without constriction.

Care of Skin Graft

Large split-thickness skin grafts and grafts that are placed on a questionable recipient bed should be examined early. They should be examined in 2 days for possible infection, seroma, or hematoma. If no complications are apparent, the graft should be redressed and examined within a week.

Seromas and hematomas are drained by a small

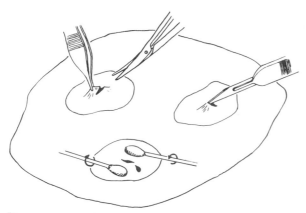

Figure 38–10. Techniques for draining a hematoma or seroma.

stab incision made in the overlying skin graft with a number 11 scalpel blade or a pair of scissors. The incision should be made directly over the center of the fluid collection. One then expresses the fluid by rolling two cotton swabs from the periphery to the center of the collection (Fig. 38–10). Each seroma or hematoma should be drained individually. If an attempt is made to drain a few of them through a single stab incision, the intervening portion of adherent skin graft may be lifted off the bed and disturbed. Following this, the skin graft is redressed and examined every day or two and is drained if necessary until the graft is fully taken. If there is gross infection, the involved portion of the skin graft is removed and appropriate dressing change is initiated.

Dressings on small split-thickness skin grafts (such as fingertip grafts) and tie-over bolster dressings on full-thickness skin grafts are left undisturbed for 5 to 7 days. Nonetheless, the patient should be seen a couple of days following the operation, and the area of the graft dressing should be examined for signs of infection. If the patient complains of pain and there is tenderness, warmth, and redness around the dressing, the graft should be exposed and examined in its entirety. Prophylactic antibiotics are *not* routinely used with outpatient skin grafts. The pain from a skin graft is usually minor and seldom requires narcotic analgesics.

Care of Split-Thickness Donor Site

The donor site is simply dressed with a piece of petrolatum gauze followed by a layer of moist gauze. The wet gauze is for absorption of early wound drainage. A layer or two of dry gauze is placed over this and is secured with tapes. In a day or two, the gauze dressing is removed, leaving the petrolatum gauze that is now adherent to the wound. The wound is then lightly dressed or left open to dry. The petrolatum gauze along with a thin layer of scab is gradually separated from the healed donor site in 10 to 14 days.

The impermeable adhesive plastic dressings (Op-site,* Tegaderm†) have been used successfully as donor site dressings. A sheet of the adhesive plastic dressing of a size considerably larger than the donor site itself is laid over the donor site area. Care is taken to dry the surrounding skin well so that there is good contact between the adhesive plastic sheet and the skin to form an occlusive dressing. Initially, a moderate amount of serosanguineous drainage may collect over the donor site, forming a blister under the plastic dressing. This need not be drained as long as there is no evidence of infection. With healing, the liquid component of the drainage is reabsorbed, leaving a thin layer of crust under the plastic dressing. The plastic layer is removed in 10 to 14 days when epithelialization is complete. In the case of infection, the plastic dressing is removed and dressing changes are started. Once gross infection is cleared, petrolatum gauze dressings may be applied and cared for as described previously.

*T.J. Smith & Nephew Ltd. Welwyn Garden City and Hull, England.
†Minnesota Mining and Manufacturing Co., St. Paul, MN.

1. Henry, L., Marshall, D. C., Friedman, E. A., Goldstein, D. P., and Dammin, G. J.: The rejection of skin hand grafts in the normal human subject. Part II. Histological findings. J. Clin. Invest. 41:420, 1982.
2. Clemensen, T.: The early circulation in split skin grafts. Acta Chir. Scand. 124:11, 1982.
3. Thiersch, C.: Ueber die feineren anatomischen veranderungen bei Aufheilung von Haut auf Granulationen. Arch. Klin. Chir. 17:318, 1874.
4. Smehel, J.: The revascularization of a free skin autograft. Acta Chir. Plast. 9:76, 1967.
5. Converse, J. M.: Reconstructive Plastic Surgery, Vol. 1. Philadelphia, W. B. Saunders Co., 1977, pp. 159–162.
6. Mir Y Mir, L.: Biology of skin graft; new aspects to consider in its revascularization. Plast. Reconstr. Surg. 8:378, 1951.
7. Newmeyer, W. L.: Primary Care of Hand Injuries. Philadelphia, Lea & Febiger, 1979, p. 97.

Introduction

The diagnosis of intraperitoneal injury, especially in children, pregnant women, and patients with altered mental status or multiple extra-abdominal injuries, has always been difficult. These clinical situations remain the classic indications for peritoneal lavage.

Clinical signs of serious visceral injury can be notoriously nonspecific, minimal, or absent even when life-threatening injury is present. This is true for both blunt and penetrating abdominal injuries. Likewise, many patients show signs and symptoms suggestive of intraperitoneal injury when none has occurred. The overall accuracy of the *initial* physical examination in diagnosing intraperitoneal injury in the traumatized patient is surprisingly low and has been variously reported to range from 16 to 45 per cent.[1-11] The physical examination is even less helpful in the patient with an altered mental status from head injury, intoxication, or drug ingestion.

It is interesting to note that even documented peritoneal penetration may *not* be associated with visceral injury in as many as 53 per cent of cases. Other laboratory tests and organ imaging techniques are generally selective and of limited value to the emergency physician. Likewise, if these imaging studies are undertaken in the acute situation to assess intra-abdominal trauma, valuable time may be lost, and the physician is often left with inconclusive results.[3, 7, 9-11]

Previously, the policy of selective or expectant observation was the rule to minimize the morbidity or mortality associated with negative exploratory laparotomy. Patients without obvious signs and symptoms of intra-abdominal injury were serially and frequently re-evaluated. If and when positive signs and symptoms developed, the patients underwent exploration. This delay in diagnosis was also associated with morbidity and mortality because of the development of sepsis or hemorrhagic shock, requiring multiple transfusions and causing prolonged recovery times. Operative delay has been reported to be associated with as many as 50 per cent of fatal cases and is directly responsible for as many as 17 per cent of these deaths. With combined head and trunk trauma, undiagnosed intra-abdominal injury has been found to be responsible for 20 to 40 per cent of deaths. Several authors demonstrated that expectant observation not only was significantly less accurate than peritoneal lavage in diagnosing intra-abdominal injury but also led to a delay that

The opinions or assertions contained herein are the private views of the author and are not to be construed as official or reflecting the views of the Department of Defense or the Department of the Army.

39

Abdominal Lavage

DIAGNOSTIC PERITONEAL LAVAGE

SAMUEL TIMOTHY COLERIDGE, D.O.

increased recovery time or resulted in increased deaths.[2, 4, 8, 11-15]

The use of catheter paracentesis and diagnostic peritoneal lavage as originally described by Root and coworkers in 1964 is now recognized as a rapid, effective means of facilitating diagnosis in problem cases. The procedure can be performed virtually anywhere, is quick, and requires little equipment.

Danto's review of 23 papers published since the initial report of Root and associates in 1964 describes a total of 9588 documented patients with both blunt and penetrating injuries; 4053 of these patients had a positive test and 5535 had a negative test.[16] The positive test was correct in 97 per cent of cases, resulting in negative celiotomies only 3 per cent of the time (3 per cent false positive rate). A negative test was correct in 98.7 per cent of cases (1.3 per cent false negative rate). These cases emphasize the high specificity of this test, which results in more false positives then false negatives. The significance of the negative test is emphasized by the finding that over half the authors cited in Danto's extensive review reported no false negative results.[16] The overall accuracy rate for paracentesis and diagnostic peritoneal lavage in these patients was 98 per cent. This was calculated as follows:

$$\text{Overall accuracy rate} = \frac{\text{True positive} + \text{true negative}}{\text{Number of tests}}$$

$$= \frac{(0.97)(4053) + (0.987)(5535)}{9588}$$

$$= 0.98$$

Peritoneal lavage can be used for other medical and surgical problems. The procedure allows retrieval of representative fluid early in the course of disease and offers an access for intraperitoneal fluid therapy or removal of unwanted or toxic chemicals through peritoneal dialysis.[3, 5, 6, 10, 12, 17-31]

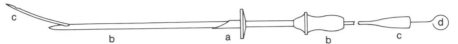

Figure 39–1. Original trocar with ureteral catheter used by Salomon in Berlin in 1906 to perform diagnostic abdominal paracentesis. a) Outer needle with guard to prevent deep tissue injury; b) stream-lined trocar device for penetration of peritoneum and guidance during catheter placement; c) ureteral catheter passed through the trocar; and d) wire stylet to aid catheter placement. (Modified from Salomon, H.: Die diagnostische Puncktion des Bauches. Berl. Klin. Wochenschr. 43:46, 1906.)

Ideally, the surgical consultant managing the trauma patient should perform the diagnostic peritoneal lavage, although often the emergency physician, pending arrival of the consultant, will be encouraged to perform this procedure in the multiple trauma patient.[32]

Background

In 1906, Saloman in Berlin reported the use of diagnostic paracentesis with a trocar and a ureteral catheter to assess diseases of the peritoneum.[27] His instrument (Fig. 39–1) was a modification of a device used by Adolf Schmidt, who was performing peritoneal lavage with normal saline or other nutritive substances to increase the resistance of the peritoneum to peritonitis. Fiedler is mentioned as the initiator of the technique. Saloman recognized that diagnostic paracentesis could be valuable in identifying peritonitis caused by gastric perforation or infectious and inflammatory disease as well as hemoperitoneum from a ruptured ectopic pregnancy. He recommended that the technique be used selectively and only to avoid exploratory laparotomy with its higher morbidity.

In 1922, Denzer proposed a method of abdominal puncture in infants and children using a trocar, a cannula, and a glass capillary tube.[33] This technique was improved upon by Neuhof and Cohen, who in 1926 used a lumbar puncture needle with stylet to perform paracentesis for diagnosis of acute abdominal conditions, including trauma, pancreatitis, and peritonitis of various causes. Their comprehensive study emphasized the usefulness as well as the limitations of this technique in diagnosing hemoperitoneum.[24] In 1941, Steinberg reported the first complete and organized analysis of peritoneal fluid in various abnormal and normal conditions.[29] Keith and others in 1950 added to this by reporting further peritoneal amylase values in acute pancreatic conditions.[12] Bronfin and coworkers in 1952 used a plastic cannula through their paracentesis needle to gain greater access to potential intra-abdominal fluid accumulations.[18]

In 1954, Thompson and Brown reported 300 cases of abdominal paracentesis used to rule out acute hemoperitoneum in multiple trauma patients, particularly in cases of blunt abdominal trauma associated with head injuries and crushing injuries to the chest. They used a number 22 spinal needle placed approximately 3 cm superior and medial to the anterior superior iliac spine and reported no complications.[34] In 1959, Williams and Zollinger reported a 79 per cent accuracy in diagnosing hemoperitoneum using the short-beveled spinal needle; however, abdominal tenderness was still a more sensitive indicator (86 per cent) in the conscious patient (although the peritoneal tap was more accurate if unconscious patients are included in the assessment).[11]

In 1960, Giacobine and Siler showed with dog studies that the accuracy of needle paracentesis alone is directly related to the amount of fluid in the peritoneal cavity. They commented that large fluid accumulations could exist in the pelvic gutters inaccessible to aspiration using the standard midline and four-quadrant approaches.[20] The natural extension of this finding came in 1964, when Root and coworkers reported the use of peritoneal lavage with normal saline to increase the volume of any abnormal intra-peritoneal fluids and thus to increase the likelihood of retrieving the irrigant fluid for examination.[35] They introduced an 18 French disposable catheter with multiple side holes overlying a trocar.

Root and associates' initial evaluation of peritoneal lavage used in 28 patients with blunt abdominal injury proved very accurate. The diagnosis was correct in all of the 16 cases of significant intraperitoneal injury. The important feature of this new technique was that there were no false negatives as well as no false positives. This accuracy in both ruling out and diagnosing injury was supported by numerous subsequent studies using this same technique rather than paracentesis alone.[3, 6, 7, 13, 25, 32, 36, 37]

Olsen and colleagues in 1972 established a simple bedside method of measuring the amount of blood in the lavage fluid without the aid of laboratory analysis.[25] Their technique, based on the ability to read newsprint through the intravenous tubing, remains a useful bedside test for distinguishing among patients with minimal or insignificant hemoperitoneum and those requiring prompt celiotomy.

Refinements of the blind thrust technique of Root were developed in hopes of minimizing complications and ensuring more meaningful results.

These included the open peritoneal lavage technique, or mini-lap, described by Perry in 1970,[38] the 14 gauge plastic-sheathed needle with side holes cut by a scalpel fashioned by Bivins for use in small children in 1976,[2] the periumbilical approach developed by Slavin in 1978,[39] the Lazarus-Nelson guide wire approach, introduced in 1979,[40] and the semi-open technique advanced by Myers and coworkers in 1981.[41]

Peritoneal Tap/Needle Paracentesis

Special note should be made of the difference between needle aspiration (peritoneal tap) and peritoneal lavage. The peritoneal tap, which uses a large needle on an aspirating syringe, has largely been replaced by the lavage method. A peritoneal tap is notoriously inaccurate in diagnosing hemoperitoneum; there is only a 20 per cent chance that 200 ml of free blood will be detected with needle aspiration and only an 80 per cent chance of detecting as much as 500 ml intraperitoneal blood.[20] The major problem with needle paracentesis is a false negative result, which may occur despite a significant hemoperitoneum. The so-called four-quadrant tap may detect a few more cases than a single aspiration attempt, but in general needle paracentesis for diagnosis of hemoperitoneum is outdated and inferior to the peritoneal lavage procedure. With the peritoneal tap, the return of *any free blood* has classically been termed a positive result and an indication for surgical exploration.

A general discussion of abdominal paracentesis for other indications is provided in this chapter following the discussion of diagnostic peritoneal lavage.

Indications for Peritoneal Lavage

Peritoneal lavage is a diagnostic procedure for recognizing intra-abdominal injury that necessitates immediate celiotomy. There need not be strong physical evidence for abdominal injury, since as many as 40 per cent of patients with unexplained hypotension will have a positive peritoneal lavage. Additionally, in the unconscious patient with head injury or altered mental status secondary to drug or alcohol ingestion, diagnostic peritoneal lavage is indicated to detect hemoperitoneum or other abnormal peritoneal fluid findings. As many as 25 per cent of patients who are unconscious from head injury will have a positive peritoneal lavage. In a patient with recent or pre-existing paraplegia, a positive peritoneal lavage may be the only objective finding in intra-abdominal injury. In patients with penetrating abdominal injuries or penetrating lower thoracic wounds located between the two anterior axillary lines but below the fifth ribs anteriorly, diagnostic peritoneal lavage is appropriate after aseptic local exploration of the abdominal stab wounds.[3-7, 9, 10, 13, 15, 30, 32, 34, 35, 37, 40, 42-46]

The indications for lavage in children are abdominal pain and tenderness or unexplained shock following trauma, altered sensorium, major thoracic injury, multiple trauma, and major orthopedic injury (such as a fractured pelvis, femur, or hip).[2, 5, 13, 47] The procedure is as accurate in the pediatric patient as in the adult.

In pregnant patients, the prompt diagnosis and treatment of abdominal injury is critical for fetal survival. The physiologic hypervolemia of pregnancy tends to ameliorate the natural response of the mother to blood loss; in contrast, the fetus suffers early anoxia as uterine flow decreases in response to maternal blood loss. Additionally, abdominal signs and symptoms are often diminished, delayed, or absent in pregnant women who have sustained blunt abdominal trauma.[6, 8] Peritoneal lavage is therefore useful in pregnancy, although the open technique (mini-cutdown) is mandated beyond the first trimester. Some authors prefer simple culdocentesis to peritoneal lavage in pregnant patients, relying on the presence of free blood to make a positive diagnosis. Another possibility is "culdage," a term applied to peritoneal lavage performed through the cul-de-sac.[48]

Peritoneal lavage has been used to diagnose acute pancreatitis in patients with a normal amylase level, since an elevated amylase concentration may persist in the peritoneal fluid for 3 to 5 days following pancreatitis. Primary peritonitis may also be diagnosed by the finding of pneumococci or staphylococci. Intestinal flora and debris found on Gram stain of lavage sediment may signify perforation of the gastrointestinal tract.[1, 4, 6, 12, 17, 19, 23, 24, 27, 29, 35, 36, 43]

Most surgeons would agree that no patient with significant abdominal injury or penetrating lower thoracic injury should be admitted for observation without a negative diagnostic peritoneal lavage.[3, 42]

Contraindications

There are no absolute contraindications for diagnostic peritoneal lavage other than obvious signs of intra-abdominal trauma necessitating celiotomy. Obvious signs of intra-abdominal trauma include blood in the gastrointestinal tract and free air on abdominal radiographs in addition to a distending abdomen or unexplained hypotension.[24, 30] Coagulopathy is not a contraindication to diagnostic peritoneal lavage, and the results are reliable even in these cases.[49]

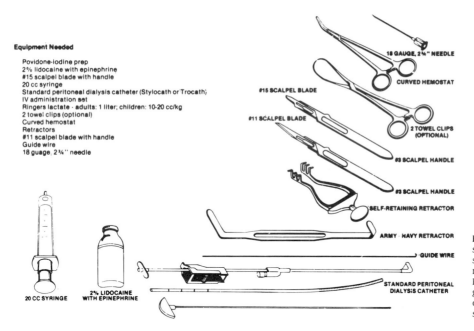

Equipment Needed

Povidone-iodine prep
2% lidocaine with epinephrine
#15 scalpel blade with handle
20 cc syringe
Standard peritoneal dialysis catheter (Stylocath or Trocath);
IV administration set
Ringers lactate - adults: 1 liter; children: 10-20 cc/kg
2 towel clips (optional)
Curved hemostat
Retractors
#11 scalpel blade with handle
Guide wire
18 guage, 2¾" needle

18 GAUGE, 2¾" NEEDLE

CURVED HEMOSTAT

#15 SCALPEL BLADE

#11 SCALPEL BLADE

2 TOWEL CLIPS (OPTIONAL)

#3 SCALPEL HANDLE

#3 SCALPEL HANDLE

SELF-RETAINING RETRACTOR

ARMY - NAVY RETRACTOR

GUIDE WIRE

STANDARD PERITONEAL DIALYSIS CATHETER

20 CC SYRINGE

2% LIDOCAINE WITH EPINEPHRINE

Figure 39–2. Peritoneal lavage tray; standard for all techniques described. Necessary equipment is noted. (From Honigman, B., Marx, J., Pons, P., and Rumack, B. H.: Emergindex. Englewood, CO, Micromedex, Inc., 1983. Used by permission.)

Relative contraindications to peritoneal lavage include a distended abdomen or scars from multiple previous abdominal surgeries, particularly pelvic surgery, in which one might anticipate adhesions or loculations that make lavage not only dangerous but also more likely to result in false negatives. Pregnancy and obesity should prompt consideration of alternative locations and techniques, such as the supraumbilical, periumbilical, and mini-lap approaches; likewise, inability to catheterize the bladder and distended loops of bowel might cause one to prefer the mini-lap approach for visualization.[8, 39, 48, 50, 51]

Equipment

The equipment included in the peritoneal lavage tray (Fig. 39–2) is more than sufficient for the guide wire, or Lazarus-Nelson, technique. The towel clips, number 15 scalpel, and self-retaining and Army-Navy retractors are not needed for this procedure; however, these additional instruments allow adequate resources for all other techniques, including the open mini-lap and the semi-open, infra- or supra-umbilical method as well as the periumbilical and closed percutaneous thrust technique, which is still used in many institutions.[52]

Procedure

The patient should be counseled regarding the purpose and sensitivity of this procedure and the importance of performing the technique as soon as possible to assess the need for immediate celiotomy or subsequent observation. A consent form

should be obtained from the patient if possible, and minimal but specific complications should be discussed (see the section on complications). Allergic reactions to lidocaine should be assessed and documented before the technique is begun.

If the abdomen is distended, lateral abdominal radiographs or, preferably, a left lateral decubitus or an upright chest radiograph may demonstrate free air, thus indicating that immediate celiotomy is mandated; later radiographs may reveal air introduced during the peritoneal procedure. If the abdomen is not distended, the benefits of radiographs are so small that lavage need not be delayed.[2, 7, 11, 16]

The guide wire, or Lazarus-Nelson, approach is recommended by the author because of its smaller number of complications; however, each procedure has its advantages and indications.[39–41, 47, 53–57]

GUIDE WIRE TECHNIQUE

The guide wire approach uses minimal sharp dissection to reach the peritoneal fascia. A relatively small-diameter 18 gauge needle is used to penetrate the peritoneum rather than the larger 9 to 11 French trocar that is normally used. The more time-consuming and meticulous dissection necessary for the infra/supra/periumbilical techniques and, particularly, for the mini-lap approach is thus avoided.

The site that is generally selected is the abdominal midline in the upper or middle third of the distance between the umbilicus and the symphysis pubis. The midline height can be adjusted upward for smaller patients and downward for larger patients to enable the catheter tip to reach the depth

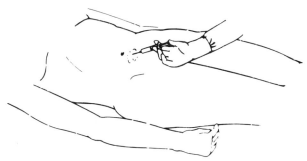

Figure 39–3. Anesthesia and bleeding control. The skin is infiltrated down to and including the fascia with lidocaine *with epinephrine* in the midline. The normal location is approximately 3 cm below or above the umbilicus, as circumstances dictate. (Note: Bladder and stomach should be decompressed by Foley catheter and nasogastric tube; abdomen should be prepared from above umbilicus to pubis, and the area should be draped.) (From Honigman, B., Marx, J., Pons, P., and Rumack, B. H.: Emergindex. Englewood, CO. Micromedex, Inc., 1983. Used by permission.)

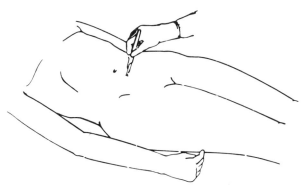

Figure 39–4. Skin incision for guide wire or Lazarus-Nelson technique (also for blind percutaneous approach): The physician makes a small nick with a number 11 scalpel through the anesthetized skin down to the fascia, palpating the fascia with the point of the scalpel. (From Honigman, B., Marx, J., Pons, P., and Rumack, B. H.: Emergindex. Englewood, CO, Micromedex, Inc., 1983. Used by permission.)

of the pelvic gutters and to minimize complications. The midline supraumbilical location can be used for the gravid uterus, in cases of lower abdominal surgical scars or lower intra-abdominal known masses, or in children.[5, 51]

The bladder and the stomach are decompressed with a Foley catheter and a nasogastric tube. It should be emphasized that *a Foley catheter and a nasogastric tube should be placed in all patients before lavage is performed,* and one should not view recent voiding or vomiting as an acceptable substitute. The abdomen is shaved and prepared with povidine-iodine solution and then draped with sterile towels. Soft wrist restraints are recommended for keeping the patient's hands to his sides and the surgical field sterile. Lidocaine with epinephrine is infiltrated deeply enough to include the fascia (Fig. 39–3); the anesthesia prevents patient splinting with consequent increase in intra-abdominal pressure, and the epinephrine helps prevent capillary oozing and false positives. One minute should pass before a skin incision is made; the

delay permits maximum vasoconstriction from the epinephrine.

The skin is then incised vertically with a number 11 blade (Fig. 39–4). The incision is carried through the subcutaneous tissue to the linea alba. The linea alba will produce a tough, gritty sensation when scraped with the scalpel. Alternatively, a larger incision (up to 2 to 3 cm) can be made to the linea alba in a search for the decussation of fibers in the avascular midline (Fig. 39–5). A syringe can be attached for support as the 18 gauge, 2 3/4-inch needle is used to "pop" through the peritoneum (Fig. 39–6).

At this point, the floppy end of the accompanying guide wire is passed through the needle into the peritoneal cavity. If the needle is directed inferiorly, the wire should fall easily into the abdomen toward the pelvis (Fig. 39–7). If this does not occur with ease, the needle should be advanced or redirected to ensure that the guide wire is not subsequently forced into a fascial plane. When approximately one half the wire is admitted,

Figure 39–5. (Alternative) skin incision for semi-open and mini-lap approach. The incision that is made is approximately 3 to 8 cm, depending on the abdominal fat pad, down to the decussating fibers of the preperitoneal fascia in the midline linea alba. (Modified from Honigman, B., Marx, J., Pons, P., and Rumack, B. H.: Emergindex. Englewood, CO, Micromedex, Inc., 1983. Used by permission.)

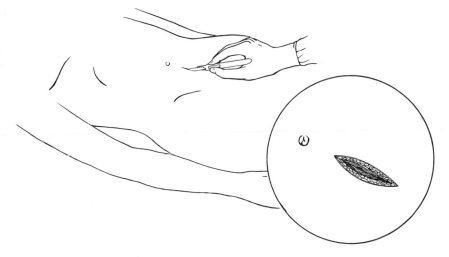

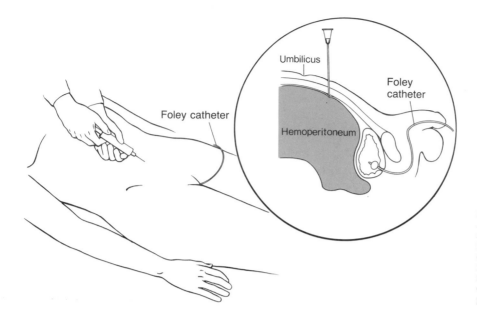

Figure 39–6. Peritoneal penetration. An 18 gauge, 2¾-inch needle is inserted through the fascia into the peritoneum. Note the mandatory Foley catheter in place. (Modified from Honigman, B., Marx, J., Pons, P., and Rumack, B. H.: Emergindex. Englewood, CO, Micromedex, Inc., 1983. Used by permission.)

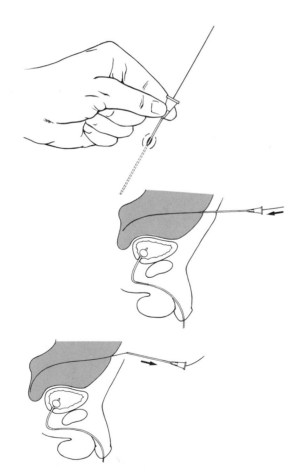

Figure 39–7. Guide wire insertion. The floppy end of the guide wire is inserted through the needle (easy passage suggests peritoneal entry). The needle is then removed, and the guide wire is left in place. A portion of the guide wire should always be held during its use. (Modified from Honigman, B., Marx, J., Pons, P., and Rumack, B. H.: Emergindex. Englewood, CO, Micromedex, Inc., 1983. Used by permission.)

the needle is removed and replaced with the lavage catheter. *A portion of the guide wire should always be held during its insertion and the subsequent needle removal to prevent inadvertent intra-abdominal wire migration.* The lavage catheter is twisted over the wire through the fascia, eased into the abdominal cavity, and directed toward one of the pelvic gutters (Fig. 39–8). The twisting motion is believed to minimize visceral or omental perforation and to aid in displacing abdominal contents en route to the inferior location of the catheter in the pelvis. Control of the guide wire must also be maintained during catheter placement.

For the blunt thrust, periumbilical, and semi-open techniques, once the trocar is popped through the fascia and the peritoneum, the lavage catheter is similarly advanced and twisted toward the pelvic gutter while the trocar is removed.

The abdominal cavity is next aspirated with a 10-ml syringe (Fig. 39–9). A free return of 10 ml or more of blood is considered a strongly positive result. If this occurs, the catheter can be removed and the area covered, since immediate celiotomy is required. Some authors view *any free blood return* as a positive tap and forgo lavage in lieu of surgical exploration.

If no blood is aspirated, the peritoneal cavity is lavaged with either lactated Ringer's solution or normal saline (Fig. 39–10). The normal amount is 1 L in adults or 10 to 20 ml per kg in children. When possible, after infusion the patient is rolled or shifted from side to side to increase mixing. The intravenous (IV) bag or bottle is placed on the floor (or below abdominal level), and the fluid is allowed to return. The fluid may not continue to return because of several factors. Some IV tubing

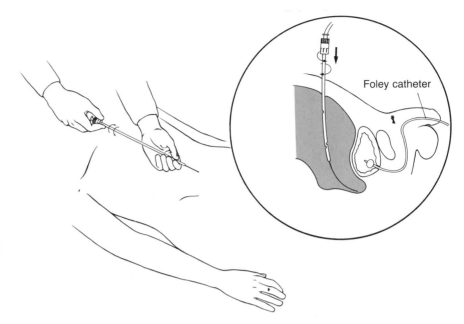

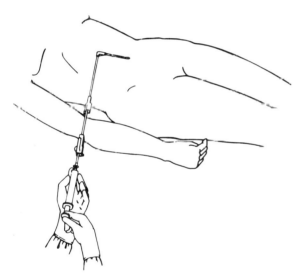

Figure 39–8. Lavage catheter insertion. A standard 9 French catheter with multiple side holes is inserted over the guide wire in a twisting and turning fashion and is advanced deeply into the pelvic gutter. The wire is then removed. (Modified from Honigman, B., Marx, J., Pons, P., and Rumack, B. H.: Emergindex. Englewood, CO, Micromedex, Inc., 1983. Used by permission.)

Figure 39–9. Paracentesis (aspiration). The operator attaches the syringe and aspirates for blood. If more than 10 ml of blood is aspirated, the study is positive. (From Honigman, B., Marx, J., Pons, P., and Rumack, B. H.: Emergindex. Englewood, CO, Micromedex, Inc., 1983. Used by permission.)

contains a one-way valve; this must be removed, and valveless tubing must be reinserted into the IV bag.[16] Another reason for poor return is inadequate suction. This can be corrected by insertion of a needle into the second opening at the bottom of the IV bag or the head of the IV bottle for aspiration of 10 ml of air. Alternatively, the catheter may be adherent to peritoneum. If so, relieving some of the pressure in the IV bottle or wiggling and twisting the catheter as well as applying abdominal pressure may aid flow return.

It is generally accepted that the return of 700 ml or more fluid in the adult is adequate for interpretation of findings. Some state that 10 to 20 per cent fluid return will give a representative sample for both gross and microscopic determinations.[16, 58] The dialysis catheter should be left in place whenever possible until the returned fluid is analyzed. The physician may wish to relavage when the initial results are borderline or an occult bowel perforation is suspected.

ALTERNATIVE TECHNIQUES

The percutaneous thrust technique using the standard 9 French peritoneal lavage catheter and an intraluminal trocar passed through a small 2- to 3-cm incision in the skin (see Fig. 39–4) is similar to the technique discussed previously. The larger-caliber stylet and blind penetration of the peritoneum do carry a higher complication rate, making this a less desirable technique, although in experienced hands this technique is more rapid and relatively safe. To decrease the likelihood of penetrating underlying viscera, some operators advocate holding the fingers low on the catheter/ trocar instrument such that upon entering the abdominal peritoneum the fingers will prevent deep penetration (Fig. 39–11). When a larger skin incision is made for the semi-open technique and the mini-lap procedure, the same midline location is used with cautious dissection and meticulous hemostasis through the loose subcutaneous fat until one reaches the tough, gritty preperitoneal fascia. This fascia can be grasped and lifted above the underlying viscera with hemostats, towel clips,

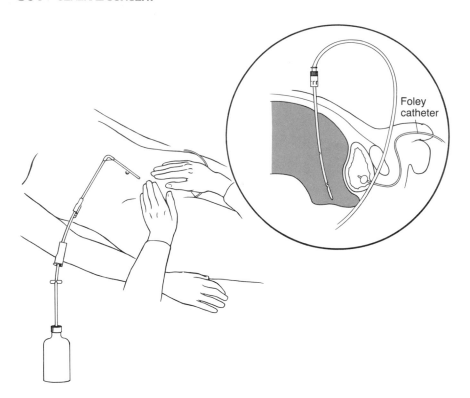

Figure 39–10. Lavage. If no blood is aspirated, the operator attaches intravenous tubing to a connector and runs 1 L of normal saline (or Ringer's lactate) into the abdominal cavity (10 to 20 ml per kg in children). The operator should gently rock the abdomen to distribute the fluid before lowering the intravenous bottle below the level of the patient in order to allow fluid to drain into the bottle from the abdominal cavity. Layered skin closure is preferred at the completion of the procedure when the lavage is negative; dressing without repair is preferred when the lavage is positive. (Modified from Honigman, B., Marx, J., Pons, P., and Rumack, B. H.: Emergindex. Englewood, CO, Micromedex, Inc., 1983.)

or self-retaining retractors (Fig. 39–12). The fascia can either be popped through with the trocar or carefully incised under direct visualization. When the latter procedure is performed, a purse-string suture of 0-polypropylene can be placed around the dialysis catheter to ensure hemostasis and, eventually, to close the peritoneum. The skin can likewise be aligned with 3-0 polypropylene suture if the lavage is negative. The direct vision, semi-open technique is quite safe and is the preferred method of some authors.[41] The periumbilical technique (Fig. 39–13) is a percutaneous insertion through the inferior portion of the umbilical ring. A gently curved incision is begun to one side of

the umbilicus at the level of the infraumbilical ring and is continued over the linea alba for approximately 4 cm. The incision is again extended through the loose subcutaneous tissue, and meticulous hemostasis is obtained. The fascia is elevated from underlying structures with towel clips before a 1-cm vertical incision is made through the linea alba at the level of the infraumbilical ring, exposing the preperitoneal fat. The pediatric peritoneal dialysis catheter is introduced through the peritoneum with the trocar in place. The trocar is then withdrawn, and the catheter is directed toward the pelvis. The principal advantages of this site are not only its avascularity and the absence of

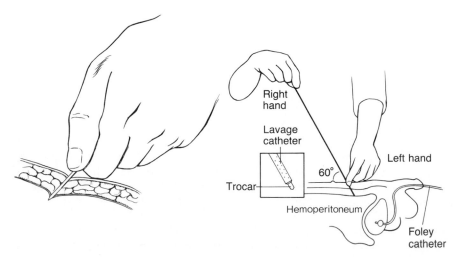

Figure 39–11. Blind percutaneous approach. The index finger and thumb of the left hand hold the trocar and resist the pressure applied by the right hand, thus preventing penetration too deeply into the peritoneal cavity. (Modified from Danto, L. A.: Paracentesis and diagnostic peritoneal lavage. In Blaisdell, F. W., and Trunkey, D. O.: Trauma Management, vol. 1. New York, Thieme-Stratton Inc., 1982 and Simon, R., and Brenner, B.: Procedures and Techniques in Emergency Medicine. Baltimore, Williams & Wilkins, 1982.)

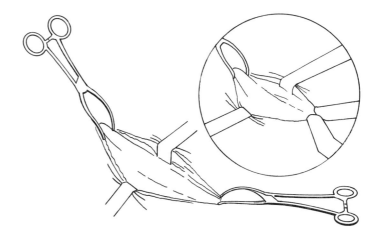

Figure 39–12. Mini-lap approach. A larger incision is made in the midline, and the fascia is grasped at each end with hemostats or towel clips and is lifted before an incision is made through the peritoneum. (Alternatively, a trocar can be popped through the elevated fascia in the standard approach.) (From Honigman, B., Marx, J., Pons, P., and Rumack, B. H.: Emergindex. Englewood, CO, Micromedex, Inc., 1983. Used by permission.)

subcutaneous fat but also a rigid adherence of the peritoneum to the cicatricial scar of the umbilicus, which expedites entry into the free peritoneal cavity. This technique is particularly useful in the obese patient.[39, 51, 56] Bivins discusses cutting side holes in a 14 to 16 gauge Angiocath of appropriate length as another alternative for infants (under 20 kg).[2]

Complications

Serious complications of peritoneal lavage are rare. Of the 9385 patients who had diagnostic peritoneal lavages reviewed by Danto, only 127 had complications, for an overall complication rate of 1.4 per cent. The rate in individual series ranges from 0 to 6 per cent. Minor complications include bleeding within the rectus sheath and at the puncture site with false positive results, rectus sheath

hematomas, retroperitoneal bladder penetrations, incisional hernia, wound infection, and wound separation.[3, 7, 9, 37, 39, 42, 50, 51, 54] Mechanical difficulties include lack of fluid return caused by intravenous tubing problems as mentioned in the section on procedure, kinking of the catheter or guide wire, and tearing of the catheter.

Major complications include trocar penetrations of the stomach, the small bowel, the colon, and the mesentery as well as lacerations of the mesenteric vessels and puncture of the abdominal aorta and the iliac artery and vein.[5, 7, 8, 19, 30, 50, 56] Because of these complications, the blind trocar technique is discouraged.

There has been no long-term morbidity associated with these complications, and no complication-related deaths have been reported. Virtually all complications result from errors in technique caused by inexperience or failure of the operators to follow standard precautions.[2, 16]

Interpretation

The main problem in interpretation of lavage aspirate is to decide how much blood indicates a positive lavage. Although some authors regard the immediate return of any free blood as a positive peritoneal tap, paracentesis is strongly positive for visceral injury if 10 ml or more of nonclotting blood is initially aspirated. This association has not changed since 1906, when it was demonstrated by Salomon. Both quantitative laboratory and visual determinations of lavage effluent have aided the diagnosis of hemoperitoneum and peritonitis of inflammatory and infectious etiology as well as suggested specific organ injury.[22, 27, 59]

Hemoperitoneum. Olsen's method for bedside quantitative determination of hemoperitoneum has been the most practical and is the most frequently used.[25] This technique can be performed in the majority of cases and divides the patients into three groups. In group I patients (clearly

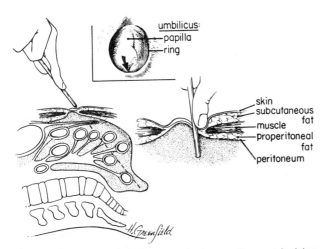

Figure 39–13. Periumbilical approach. A percutaneous incision is made through the inferior portion of the umbilical ring. The inset shows the surface anatomy of the umbilicus, with the arrow demonstrating the precise locus of puncture. (From Slavin, S. A.: A new technique for diagnostic peritoneal lavage. Surg. Gynecol. Obstet. 146:446, 1978. By permission of Surgery, Gynecology & Obstetrics.)

Table 39–1. CRITERIA FOR INTERPRETATION
OF PERITONEAL LAVAGE IN BLUNT
ABDOMINAL TRAUMA AND PENETRATING
ABDOMINAL STAB WOUNDS

Positive	
Free aspiration blood*	
Grossly bloody lavage return	
	Greater Than
RBCs	100,000/mm³
WBCs	500/mm³
Amylase	200 μ/dl
RBCs†	5000/mm³
Negative	*Less Than*
RBCs	50,000/mm³
WBCs	100/mm³
Amylase	75 μ/dl
Equivocal	
RBCs‡	50,000–100,000/mm³
WBCs	100–500/mm³
Amylase	75–200 μ/dl

*Some authors view any free blood as a positive result; others state that from 5 to 10 ml is necessary for surgical exploration.
†Criteria for interpretation of *penetrating wounds to the abdomen and lower chest trauma* (both stab wounds and gunshot wounds).
‡50,000 to 100,000 RBCs/mm³ is an inconclusive lavage and may be associated with a significant pathologic condition—cases must be handled selectively.

positive results), the lavage indicates greater than 25 ml of blood per liter of fluid in the abdomen. This is demonstrated by a bloody lavage aspirate that makes newsprint *unreadable* when IV tubing containing the lavage effluent is placed over newsprint and generally correlates well with the laboratory analysis of greater than 100,000 red blood cells (RBCs) per mm³ of fluid aspirate, a figure that is accepted by most as an *absolute* criterion for exploration. This analysis is dependent upon a minimum of 20 per cent fluid return from the lavage.[2, 16] Danto's review of 23 published papers using laboratory analysis as a criterion and documenting results in 9588 patients (both blunt and penetrating cases) revealed the test to be positive in 97 per cent of cases.

In group II patients (clearly negative results), clear lavage fluid is present in the IV tubing, and one can readily read newsprint through the effluent. In Danto's review of group II patients, the test was negative in 98.7 per cent of cases. Quantitatively, a negative test is associated with fewer than 50,000 RBCs per mm³ (Table 39–1). Even these low-risk patients should be appropriately observed, however.[8–10, 16, 17, 37, 42, 44, 47, 53, 55, 60, 61]

In group III patients (inconclusive results), lavage fluid is pink but one is able to read newsprint through the IV tubing. The RBC count is between 50,000 and 100,000 per mm³. This generally means that as little as 8 drops to 15 ml of blood per liter of peritoneal fluid may be present. (One ml of

blood in the peritoneal cavity represents approximately 4500 RBCs per mm³ of lavage effluent.[25, 50]) Some authors have suggested lowering the criterion for a positive result to 50,000 RBCs per mm³, and even less than 5,000 RBCs per mm³ has been termed positive if a penetrating injury has occurred.[64] There is ample evidence that a small number of significant injuries will be missed if one applies the strict criterion of greater than 100,000 RBCs per mm³ for a positive result. Therefore, patients with an "intermediate," or equivocal, lavage (between 50,000 and 100,000 RBCs per mm³) must be handled selectively. When the patient's condition is unstable as a result of an abdominal injury, celiotomy is obviously indicated, even in the case of an indeterminate RBC analysis. The stable patient should be observed, and a lavage sample should be sent to the laboratory for analysis of RBCs, WBCs, and perhaps amylase, alkaline phosphatase, and other enzymes or for a Gram stain, as desired. Weakly positive results can also be the result of extravasation of RBCs into the abdomen from retroperitoneal and pelvic hematomas as well as from isolated hollow viscus perforations.[10] Ultrasonography, computed tomography scans, or angiography might be considered for the stable patient with an indeterminant lavage. Repeated lavage with the peritoneal lavage catheter left in place may aid in further diagnosis.[7, 13, 25, 37, 50, 60]

Other Criteria. There is considerable controversy regarding the value of the other quantitative laboratory tests of peritoneal lavage effluent following blunt abdominal trauma. The majority of true positive tests are based on the presence of grossly bloody fluid. Quantitative cell counts require little time to perform (5 to 10 minutes)[17] and improve the sensitivity of the test, reducing the number of false negative results. Patients with a positive WBC count but a negative RBC count normally have sustained injury to the small bowel and, occasionally, to the colon.[4, 17, 32, 47, 60] Isolated small bowel injuries frequently do not produce hemoperitoneum. The contents of a perforated viscus normally produce an intense outpouring of leukocytes into the peritoneal cavity with insignificant hemoperitoneum.[4] *This response is normally delayed for 3 hours after injury,* thus limiting the value of the criterion of greater than 500 WBCs per mm³ for a positive lavage.[32, 35, 45] The lavage WBC count should be "corrected" in order to distinguish this peritoneal inflammatory response from the contribution of white cells from peripheral blood secondary to visceral hemorrhage into the peritoneal cavity. This corrected white blood cell count (Cwbc) equals the total lavage white blood cell count (Twbc) minus the white cells contributed by hemorrhage. (The Twbc is the laboratory WBC per mm³ count report for the peritoneal lavage aliquot.) One calculates the

Cwbc by multiplying the peripheral white blood cell count (Pwbc) by the ratio of the lavage red blood cell count (Lrbc) to the peripheral red blood cell count (Prbc) and subtracting this from the total lavage white blood cell count:

$$Cwbc = Twbc - Pwbc \times Lrbc/Prbc$$

The peritoneal lavage is considered positive if the Cwbc is greater than 500 per mm[3].[59] A recent study by the same authors, however, questions the results of their earlier quantitative studies on the basis of experimentally induced artifact.[62]

Elevation of amylase and the presence of bile or bacteria are late findings following bowel injury.[45] Most patients with a lavage amylase suggesting a positive result have a WBC count suggesting a positive lavage as well.[17] The measurement of amylase is time-consuming (25 to 45 minutes) and costly ($16 per test versus $9.50 for a WBC/RBC count)[3] and has a low yield.[17, 56] Only rarely is the amylase positive with negative RBC and WBC counts.[4, 12, 32] Nonetheless, when both the examination and laboratory results are equivocal, there is considerable value to these tests in the delayed or repeat lavage at 4 to 6 hours.[4, 7, 45, 60] Marx and coworkers noted an early elevation of lavage alkaline phosphatase (greater than 25 IU versus less than 5 IU) in small bowel injuries when all other quantitative tests are normal.[22] Burney and associates noted an elevation of liver enzyme levels in blunt hepatic trauma (but not in penetrating trauma) that appears to correlate with the severity of heptocellular disruption.[59]

False positive results are usually caused by bleeding at the catheter incision site or by omental or mesenteric laceration from the needle, the trocar, or the catheter. Proper technique with caution taken to elevate the abdominal fascia before puncture into the peritoneum as well as the judicious use of lidocaine with epinephrine in both the conscious and the unconscious patient should help to decrease the number of false positives.[51] Note should be made of possible false positive lavages in patients with a pelvic or retroperitoneal hematoma. Operations are generally not performed on such patients, but a lavage catheter inadvertently placed in the hematoma will result in a strongly positive (false) lavage.

False negative results are unusual but can be caused by misplacement of the catheter by the inexperienced operator, compartmentalization by adhesions, and retroperitoneal or bladder placement of the catheter.

Conclusions

Diagnostic peritoneal lavage has become one of the most common procedures performed in the emergency department to detect hemoperitoneum in the traumatized patient. Several techniques have been discussed, each involving minimal complications or false results in experienced hands. The results are highly accurate and can demonstrate significant intra-abdominal injury when the clinical examination is negative or equivocal, in the multiply traumatized patient with altered mental status or non-contiguous injuries above and below the abdomen, in penetrating lower thoracic or abdominal injuries, and in the difficult-to-examine traumatized obstetric or pediatric patient.

Peritoneal lavage can likewise prevent unnecessary celiotomy and allow safe observation of the stable patient with clinical signs of intra-abdominal injury. In some instances, serial peritoneal lavage may detect the unusual false negative initial lavage.[37, 42, 50, 60] Continuing interest in this procedure suggests that it may be useful in differentiating specific organs traumatized in blunt abdominal injuries.

1. Baker, W. N. W., Mackie, D. B., and Newcombe, J. F.: Diagnostic paracentesis in the acute abdomen. Br. Med. J. 3:146, 1967.
2. Bivins, B. A., Jona, J. Z., and Berlin, R. P.: Diagnostic peritoneal lavage in pediatric trauma. J. Trauma 16:739, 1976.
3. Danto, L. A., Thomas, C. W., Gorenbeim, S., and Wolfman, E. F.: Penetrating torso injuries: The role of paracentesis and lavage. Am. Surg. 43:164, 1977.
4. Engrav, L. H., Benjamin, C. I., Strate, R. G., and Perry, J. F.: Diagnostic peritoneal lavage in blunt abdominal trauma. J. Trauma 15:854, 1975.
5. Fischer, R. P., Beverlin, B. C., Engrav, L. H., Benjamin, C. I., and Perry, J. F.: Diagnostic peritoneal lavage fourteen years and 2,586 patients later. Am. J. Surg. 136:701, 1978.
6. Olsen, W. R., and Hildreth, D. H.: Abdominal paracentesis and peritoneal lavage in blunt abdominal trauma. J. Trauma 11:824, 1971.
7. Parvin, S., Smith, D. E., Asher, W. M., and Virgilio, R. W.: Effectiveness of peritoneal lavage in blunt abdominal trauma. Ann. Surg. 181:255, 1978.
8. Rothenberger, D. A., Quatteebaum, F. W., Zabel, J., and Fischer, R. P.: Diagnostic peritoneal lavage for blunt trauma in pregnant women. Am. J. Obstet. 129:479, 1977.
9. Thal, E. R.: Evaluation of peritoneal lavage and local exploration in lower chest and abdominal stab wounds. J. Trauma 17:642, 1977.
10. Thompson, J. S., Moore, E. E., Van Duzer-Moore, S., Moore, J. B., and Galloway, A. C.: The evaluation of abdominal stab wound management. J. Trauma 20:478, 1980.
11. Williams, R. D., and Zollinger, R. M.: Diagnosis and prognostic factors in abdominal trauma. Am. J. Surg. 97:575, 1959.
12. Keith, L. M., Zollinger, R. M., and McCleery, R. S.: Peritoneal fluid amylase determinations as an aid in diagnosis of acute pancreatitis. Arch. Surg. 61:930, 1950.
13. Powell, R. W., Smith, D. E., Zarius, C. K., Parvin, S., and Virgilio, R. W.: Peritoneal lavage in children with blunt abdominal trauma. J. Ped. Surg. 11:973, 1976.
14. Perry, J. F.: A five-year survey of 152 acute abdominal injuries. J. Trauma 5:53, 1965.
15. Yurko, A. A., and Williams, R. D.: Needle paracentesis in blunt abdominal trauma: A critical analysis. J. Trauma 6:194, 1966.
16. Danto, L. A.: Paracentesis and diagnostic peritoneal lavage.

In Blaisdell, F. W., and Trunkey, D. O.: Trauma Management, vol. I. New York, Thieme-Stratton Inc., 1982.

17. Alyono, D., and Perry, J. F.: Value of quantitative cell count and amylase activity of peritoneal lavage fluid. J. Trauma 21:345, 1981.

18. Bronfin, G. J., Liebler, J. F., and Katz, H. M.: A new method of abdominal paracentesis. Gastroenterology 21:426, 1952.

19. Denzer, B. S.: Abdominal puncture in the diagnosis of peritonitis in childhood. J. Pediatr. 8:741, 1936.

20. Giacobine, J. W., and Siler, V. E.: Evaluation of diagnostic abdominal paracentesis with experimental and clinical studies. Surg. Gynecol. Obstet. 110:676, 1960.

21. Lucas, C. E.: The role of peritoneal lavage for penetrating abdominal wounds. J. Trauma 17:649, 1977.

22. Marx, J. A., Moore, E. E., and Bar-Or, D.: Peritoneal lavage in penetrating injuries of the small bowel and colon: Value of enzyme determinations. Ann. Emerg. Med. 12:68, 1983.

23. Maetani, S., and Tobe, T.: Open peritoneal drainage as effective treatment of advanced peritonitis. Surgery 90:804, 1981.

24. Neuhof, H., and Cohen, I.: Abdominal puncture in the diagnosis of acute intraperitoneal disease. Ann. Surg. 83:454, 1926.

25. Olsen, W. R., Redman, H. C., and Hildreth, D. H.: Quantitative peritoneal lavage in blunt abdominal trauma. Arch. Surg. 104:536, 1972.

26. Press, O. W., Press, N. O., and Kaufman, S. D.: Evaluation and management of chylous ascites. Ann. Int. Med. 96:358, 1982.

27. Salomon, H.: Die diagnostische Punktion des Bauches. Berl. Klin. Wocheschr. 43:45, 1906.

28. Van Sonnenberg, E., Ferrucci, J. T., Mueller, P. R., Wittenberg, J., and Simeone, J. F.: Percutaneous drainage of abscesses and fluid collections: Technique, results and applications. Diag. Radio. 142:1, 1982.

29. Steinberg, B.: Peritoneal exudate: A guide for the diagnosis and prognosis of peritoneal conditions. JAMA, 116:572, 1941.

30. Veith, F. J., Webber, W. B., Karl, R. C., and Deysine, M.: Peritoneal lavage in acute abdominal disease: Normal findings and evaluation in 100 patients. Ann. Surg. 116:290, 1967.

31. Wright, K., Tarr, P. I., Hickman, R. O., and Gutherie, R. D.: Hyperbilirubinemia secondary to delayed absorption of intraperitoneal blood following intrauterine transfusion. J. Pediatr. 100:302, 1982.

32. Root, H. D., Keizer, P. J., and Perry, J. F.: The clinical and experimental aspects of peritoneal response to injury. Arch. Surg. 95:531, 1967.

33. Denzer, B. S.: Abdominal puncture in the diagnosis of peritonitis in childhood. Am. J. Med. Sci. 163:237, 1922.

34. Thompson, C. T., and Brown, D. R.: Diagnostic paracentesis in the acute abdomen. Surgery 15:916, 1954.

35. Root, H. D., Hauser, C. W., McKinley, C. R., La Fave, J. W., and Mendiola, R. P., Jr.: Diagnostic peritoneal lavage. Surgery 57:633, 1965.

36. Gumbert, J. L., Froderman, S. E., and Mercho, J. P.: Diagnostic peritoneal lavage in blunt abdominal trauma. Ann. Surg. 165:70, 1967.

37. Perry, J. F., Jr., and Strate, R. G.: Diagnostic peritoneal lavage in blunt abdominal trauma: Indications and results. Surgery 71:898, 1972.

38. Perry, J. F., Jr.: Blunt and penetrating abdominal injuries. *In*: Saegesser, F. (ed.): Current Problems in Surgery. Chicago, Year Book Medical Publishers, 1970.

39. Slavin, S. A.: A new technique for diagnostic peritoneal lavage. Surg. Gynecol. Obstet. 146:446, 1978.

40. Lazarus, H. M., and Nelson, J. A.: A technique for peritoneal lavage without risk or complication. Surg. Gynecol. Obstet. 149:889, 1979.

41. Myers, R. A. M., Agarwal, N. N., and Cowley, R. A.: A safe, semi-open procedure for diagnostic peritoneal lavage. Surg. Gynecol. Obstet. 153:739, 1981.

42. Soderstrom, C. A., DuPriest, R. W., and Cowley, R. A.: Pitfalls of peritoneal lavage in blunt abdominal trauma. Surg. Gynecol. Obstet. 151:513, 1980.

43. Talbert, J., Gruenberg, J. C., and Brown, R. S.: Peritoneal lavage in penetrating thoracic trauma. J. Trauma 20:979, 1980.

44. Thal, E. R.: Peritoneal lavage: State of the art. Ann. Emerg. Med. 10:84, 1981.

45. Thompson, J. S., and Moore, E. E.: Peritoneal lavage in the evolution of penetrating abdominal trauma. Surg. Gynecol. Obstet. 153:861, 1981.

46. Wright, L. T., and Prigot, A.: Traumatic subcutaneous rupture of the normal spleen. Ann. Surg. 39:551, 1939.

47. Drew, R., Perry, J. F., and Fischer, R. P.: The expediency of peritoneal lavage for blunt trauma in children. Surg. Gynecol. Obstet. 145:885, 1977.

48. Cantrill, S. V.: Emergency care records: The use of peritoneal lavage in the evaluation of penetrating abdominal trauma. J. Emerg. Med. 1:73, 1983.

49. Berry, T., Flynn, T. C., Miller, P. W., and Fischer, R. P.: Diagnostic peritoneal lavage in trauma patients with coagulopathy. Ann. Emerg. Med. 12:253, 1983.

50. Krausz, M. M., Manny, J., Ultsunomiya, T., and Hechtman, H. B.: Peritoneal lavage in blunt abdominal trauma. Surg. Gynecol. Obstet. 152:327, 1981.

51. Markovchick, V. J., Elerding, S. C., Moore, E. E., and Rosen, P.: Diagnostic peritoneal lavage. JACEP, 8:326, 1979.

52. Honigman, B., Marx, J., Pons, P., and Rumack, B. H.: Emergindex. Englewood, CO, Micromedex, Inc., 1983.

53. DuPriest, R. W., Rodriguez, A., Khaneja, S. C., Soderstrom, C. A., Maekawa, K. A., Ayella, R. J., and Cowley, R. A.: Open diagnostic peritoneal lavage in blunt trauma victims. Surg. Gynecol. Obstet. 148:890, 1979.

54. Hernandez, E. H., and Stein, J. M.: Comparison of the Lazarus-Nelson peritoneal lavage catheter with the standard peritoneal dialysis catheter in abdominal trauma. J. Trauma 22:153, 1982.

55. Moore, J. B., Moore, E. E., Markovchick, V., and Rosen, P.: Peritoneal lavage in abdominal trauma: A prospective study comparing the peritoneal dialysis catheter with the intracatheter. Ann. Emerg. Med. 9:190, 1980.

56. Moore, J. B., Moore, E. E., Markovchick, V. J., and Rosen, P.: Diagnostic peritoneal lavage for abdominal trauma: Superiority of the open technique at the infraumbilical ring. J. Trauma 21:570, 1981.

57. Roller, B., Adkinson, C., Bretzke, M., and Clinton, J. E.: Comparison of open and percutaneous wire guided closed peritoneal lavage. 12:252, 1983.

58. Bivins, B. A., Sachatello, C. R., Daugherty, M. E., Ernst, C. B., and Griffen, W. O., Jr.: Diagnostic peritoneal lavage is superior to clinical evaluation in blunt abdominal trauma. Am. Surg. 44:637, 1978.

59. Burney, R. E., Mueller, G. L., and Mackenzie, J. R.: Evaluation of experimental blunt and penetrating hepatobiliary trauma by sequential peritoneal lavage. Ann. Emerg. Med. 12:279, 1983.

60. Phillips, T. F., Brotman, S., Cleveland, S., and Cowley, R. A.: Perforating injuries of the small bowel from blunt abdominal trauma. Ann. Emerg. Med. 12:75, 1983.

61. Ward, R. E., Miller, P., Clark, D. G., Ben-Menachem, Y., and Duke, J. H.: Angiography and peritoneal lavage in blunt abdominal trauma. J. Trauma 21:848, 1981.

62. Mackenzie, J. R., Gundry, S. R., and Burney, R. E.: Animal model development in peritoneal lavage research: Pitfalls and prerequisites. J. Trauma 23:649, 1983.

63. Simon, R., and Brenner, B.: Procedures and Techniques in Emergency Medicine. Williams & Wilkins, 1982, pp. 12–29.

64. Oreskovich, M. R., et al: Stab wounds of the anterior abdomen: analysis of a management plan using local wound exploration and quantitative peritoneal lavage. Ann. Surg. 198(4):411, 1983.

Introduction and Background

Diagnostic peritoneal aspiration was originally described by Saloman in 1906.[1, 2] Saloman used a needle with a trocar to place a uretheral catheter into the peritoneal cavity.[3] In Saloman's day and until recently, paracentesis was frequently performed for therapeutic reasons (to remove excess peritoneal fluid). This indication has been largely replaced by medical therapy, and paracentesis is now an infrequent procedure because of the potential for rapid fluid shifts from the plasma into the peritoneal cavity, often leading to vascular collapse, hepatic coma, and renal failure.[4] In cases of tense ascites caused by malignancy, abdominal paracentesis to remove large volumes of ascitic fluid is still useful,[5] and the procedure has been recommended for the emergency relief of massive malignant ascites that may reduce respiratory capacity. Similarly, abdominal paracentesis can be performed in the cirrhotic patient with tense ascites that impairs respirations.

Present-day therapy of ascites consists mainly of medical management with excess salt and water restriction, diuretic therapy, potassium replacement and, possibly, the use of LaVeen shunting.[6] Needle paracentesis, or the "four-quadrant tap," was used in the diagnosis of hemoperitoneum before diagnostic peritoneal lavage became popular. It has been demonstrated that 200 ml of free blood in the peritoneal cavity may be detected only 20 per cent of the time with paracentesis, and 500 ml can be detected only 80 per cent of the time.[4] Because of these high false negative rates, needle aspiration of the abdomen for the diagnosis of hemoperitoneum is currently a technique of mainly historical interest. Abdominal paracentesis is now largely a diagnostic procedure for noninfectious ascites and peritoneal infections.

Indications

Before elective paracentesis, the presence of peritoneal fluid must be established. The abdominal cavity is divided into compartments according to mesenteric attachments, hence fluid may be localized.[7] These subdivisions are relatively difficult to appreciate by physical examination alone. Ultrasound and roentgenography are the procedures most frequently used in addition to physical examination to diagnose the presence of peritoneal fluid.[8–10] The differential diagnosis of ascites is given in Table 39–2.

When the presence of ascites is established, paracentesis is indicated to ascertain its cause. For practical purposes, the most worrisome entities causing ascites and those requiring most urgent therapy include bacterial peritonitis, tuberculous

ABDOMINAL PARACENTESIS

JONATHAN GLAUSER, M.D.

peritonitis, and pancreatic conditions.[11] For example, in a patient with known cirrhosis who presents with abdominal pain, leukocytosis, fever, hepatic encephalopathy, or rebound tenderness, the presence of bacterial peritonitis must be established or ruled out quickly. Spontaneous bacterial peritonitis may be very subtle and detectable only by the examination of peritoneal fluid. Paracentesis has been advanced as an aid in the diagnosis of ruptured ectopic pregnancy[4, 12] and bowel perforation,[13] but there are more accurate diagnostic procedures currently available. Hemoperitoneum due to trauma[1, 14] is best diagnosed by peritoneal lavage,[3, 15–22] and culdocentesis is accurate in detecting ruptured ectopic pregnancy in up to 95 per cent of cases. (See the chapter on culdocentesis.)

Precautions

Prior to performing a diagnostic peritoneal tap, careful preparation is mandatory. This is an invasive procedure, and many complications are pre-

Table 39–2. DIFFERENTIAL DIAGNOSIS OF ASCITES

Cirrhosis of any cause*
Tuberculosis*
Bacterial peritonitis
Pancreatic disease
Bile leakage
Congestive heart failure*
Tricuspid insufficiency
Constrictive pericarditis
Nephrotic syndrome, chronic renal disease
Hepatoma*
Myxedema
Vasculitis
Ascites associated with benign tumors of the ovary (Meig's syndrome)
Malignant tumor involvement of liver/peritoneum (ovary, stomach, pancreas, colon, breast, liver, bile duct, testes, various sarcomas, lymphomas)*
Ruptured hollow viscus
Intestinal infarction
Protein-losing gastroenteropathy
Budd-Chiari syndrome
Hepatic vein obstruction
Portal vein thrombosis
Ventriculoperitoneal shunt
Ureteroperitoneal fistula
Starch reaction (postsurgical)
Lymphatic obstruction with chylous ascites (thoracic duct trauma, filariasis, mediastinal tumors)

*Most common causes of ascites in North America.

ventable. The bladder must be emptied before paracentesis.[11, 23] If the patient is unable to void, a Foley catheter should be placed. Strict aseptic technique should be observed, including shaving, draping, preparation with iodophor or pHisoHex,[3] and the use of sterile gloves and a mask. Because of the risk of hemorrhage and because paracentesis is often performed in alcoholic cirrhosis patients, in whom platelet counts and clotting ability may be impaired, one should evaluate and correct the prothrombin time, the partial thromboplastin time, and the platelet count before proceeding with paracentesis.[11]

Some areas are unsuitable for needle insertion. The rectus muscle should be avoided because of the presence of the superior and inferior epigastric vessels.[24] It is also advisable to avoid the upper abdominal quadrants because of the frequency of undetected hepatosplenomegaly in the fluid-filled abdomen.[11] Visible collateral venous channels on the abdominal wall should be avoided. The preferred site is in the midline, a few centimeters below the umbilicus. Entering through the relatively avascular midline (linea alba) lessens the risk of hemorrhage (Fig. 39–14).[10] The right or left lower quadrants lateral to the rectus muscle are alternative sites for paracentesis.

There is a risk of intestinal perforation with abdominal paracentesis. Sites of surgical scars and known intra-abdominal adhesions must be avoided (Fig. 39–15).[1] The procedure should be withheld or performed with extreme caution in the presence of markedly distended bowel (e.g., in cases of bowel obstruction), since abnormally elevated intraluminal pressure may cause leakage of bowel contents following needle puncture.[11, 24] Although it has been shown that *mobile* loops of bowel are pushed away by the needle during

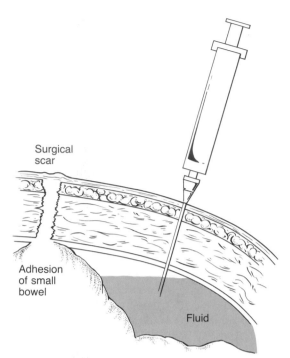

Figure 39–15. Sites of previous surgical incisions must be avoided, since adhesions may fix the bowel and predispose to bowel perforation. (Redrawn from Fisher, J. C.: Clinical Procedures: A Concise Guide for Students of Medicine. Baltimore, Williams & Wilkins, 1980.)

paracentesis and are difficult to penetrate with a needle,[3] adhesions or bowel obstruction may fix the bowel and may predispose to perforation. Mallory[11] reported two cases of bowel perforation that resulted in generalized peritonitis and abscess formation when paracentesis was performed on two patients who had previously undergone abdominal surgery. It is interesting to note that experimentally induced bowel punctures show no leakage until the intraluminal pressure reaches 260 mm Hg,[3] whereas intestinal pressure seldom rises above 20 mm Hg in the *nonobstructed* small or large bowel.[23] Moretz and Erickson found that bowel in dogs penetrated by a 13 to 20 gauge needle could withstand an intraluminal pressure of 120 mm Hg without leaking.[25] Although the risk of bowel perforation may seem small, areas of possible adhesions should be avoided, and distended bowel is at least a relative contraindication to the procedure.

Pregnancy is also a relative contraindication to paracentesis.[16] If the procedure is deemed necessary, one should choose a site above the umbilicus lateral to the midline. Alternatively, the Seldinger technique of catheter placement could be used. Ascitic fluid from patients whose serum is positive for hepatitis B surface antigen may be infectious and should be processed carefully.[26] Obviously, a needle should not be advanced through unmistakably infected skin or soft tissue. The procedure is more difficult in an uncooperative patient.

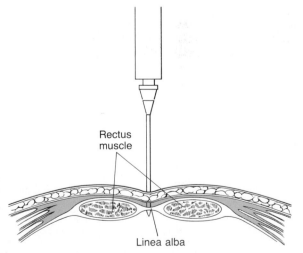

Figure 39–14. The avascular linea alba in the midline, a few centimeters below the umbilicus, is a commonly preferred site for paracentesis.

Technique

In general, 50 ml of ascitic fluid is required for adequate study,[10] although larger quantities of fluid (up to 500 ml), may be desired in some instances.[8, 23] In cases of tense ascites producing respiratory distress, the rapid removal of 1 to 3 L may be necessary to provide symptomatic relief.

The patient is usually supine during the procedure. Some physicians use the lateral decubitus position or have the patient stand. Standing may predispose to vagal fainting and is not recommended. Theoretically, if the patient is in the lateral decubitus position, the bowel floats upward and away from the midline. Sterile technique should be observed, and 1 per cent lidocaine is infiltrated subcutaneously down to the peritoneum.[3] The differences in technique generally involve location of aspiration and size and type of needle or catheter used. For simple diagnostic paracentesis, a needle and syringe are adequate. Following skin antisepsis, an 18 or 20 gauge short-beveled spinal needle is attached to a syringe and inserted through the abdominal wall. In patients with tense ascites, insertion of the needle at an oblique angle may help seal the needle tract after paracentesis, preventing persistent ascitic fluid drainage.[11] The needle is advanced while suction is applied until abdominal fluid return is noted; a "pop" may be felt upon penetration of the peritoneum when resistance diminishes.[1, 3] If large amounts of fluid are desired, one may use an 18 gauge Intracath or other suitable flexible catheter or a three-way stopcock and drain the fluid into a collection bag.

If fluid is not obtained by suction or if the initial flow stops, the needle or catheter may be advanced slowly with gentle suction. Rotation, angulation, or other manipulation of the needle or catheter may also remedy the problem. Turning the patient to a lateral decubitus position may help if the patient is initially supine.[3] If fluid is not readily obtained, the puncture site may be changed. A four-quadrant abdominal tap is still recommended by some. The suggested points of entry are in the right and left upper and lower quadrants of the abdomen, equidistant from the midline along the lateral border of the rectus muscle (Fig. 39–16).[24] Obviously, if a satisfactory amount of fluid is obtained at one site, the others need not be used. The four-quadrant method has a theoretic advantage in that the midline is avoided. It is speculated that, since air-filled bowel floats upward, the bowel will remain in the midline in a supine patient; with the use of physical and roentgenographic diagnosis and localization of ascites, one of the sites in a four-quadrant tap will almost always be successful if 200 ml or more exists in the peritoneal cavity. A number of alternative puncture sites have been proposed. The specific site is probably not important if proper attention is paid to technique and contraindications. Most authors prefer the lower abdominal sites. Aspiration may be successfully performed in either flank midway between the costal margin and the iliac spine.[24] Singh and coworkers[12] used sites approximately 1 inch medial to the anterior superior iliac spines. Rao and associates[23] used lumbar sites approximately 1½ to 2 inches lateral to the lateral border of the rectus muscle in the lumbar region, aspirating with a beveled 20 gauge, 5-cm-long needle. The lateral edge of either rectus muscle 4 cm below the umbilicus has been used.[18] Others claim that the specific location is not important as long as the site is lateral to the rectus sheath so that the inferior epigastric artery is avoided.[3, 22]

Gjessig and colleagues[27] describe a technique similar to that used for peritoneal dialysis. With the patient under local anesthesia, a small skin incision is made 3 to 5 cm below the umbilicus in the midline, and a trocar and a cannula are pushed through the parietal peritoneum (Fig. 39–17). The trocar is then removed, and a soft plastic dialysis catheter is inserted into the peritoneal cavity and gently manipulated into the pouch of Douglas. Fluid is then aspirated for examination. This technique may be preferred if the catheter is to remain in the peritoneal cavity for continued drainage. (See the detailed discussion under preceding sections on diagnostic periotoneal lavage.)

Analysis of Ascitic Fluid

A thorough discussion of the evaluation of ascitic fluid is beyond the scope of this chapter. Tables 39–3 through 39–6 offer a summary of

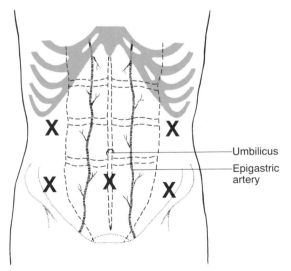

Figure 39–16. Standard landmarks for paracentesis include the four quadrants lateral to the rectus muscle and a few centimeters below the umbilicus in the midline. (Redrawn from Suratt, P. M., and Gibson, R. S.: Manual of Medical Procedures. St. Louis, C. V. Mosby Co., 1982, p. 217.)

Umbilicus

Epigastric artery

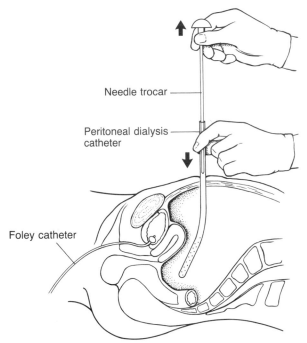

Figure 39–17. A needle trocar and a peritoneal dialysis plastic catheter may be used to perform paracentesis if continued drainage of fluid is required. The bladder *must* be emptied before this procedure is performed. (Redrawn from Suratt, P. M., and Gibson, R. S.: Manual of Medical Procedures. St. Louis, C. V. Mosby Co., 1982, p. 195.)

characteristics and specific parameters of ascitic fluid. These can be useful in selecting the proper laboratory test.

Potential Complications of Paracentesis

Serious intraperitoneal or abdominal wall hemorrhage has been reported following abdominal paracentesis. Although lacerations of major ves-

Table 39–3. STUDIES TO OBTAIN OR CONSIDER IN ASCITIC FLUID*

Protein concentration
Specific gravity
Gram stain
Acid-fast stain and culture
Culture for bacteria and fungi
Cytology
Amylase concentration
Total fat concentration
Polarized light for double refractile particles (if starch felt to be the cause)[35]
Sudan stain for fat[12]
Glucose
Ammonia[9]

*Data from Wintrobe, M. M., Thorn, G. W., Adams, R. D., et al. (eds.): Harrison's Principles of Internal Medicine, 9th ed. New York, McGraw-Hill Book Co., 1980 and Sleisenger, M. H., and Fordtran, J. S.: Gastrointestinal Disease, 2nd ed., vol. 2. Philadelphia, W. B. Saunders Co., 1978.

Table 39–4. CAUSES OF BLOODY ASCITES*

Malignancy, especially hepatoma or ovarian carcinoma
Tuberculous peritonitis
Spontaneous solid viscera injury (e.g., splenic rupture)
Trauma
Leaking ruptured abdominal aneurysm
Ruptured ectopic pregnancy[12, 13]
Strangulating bowel obstruction[13]
Ruptured mesenteric varix in cirrhosis[36]
Perforated duodenal ulcer[37]
Hepatic vein thrombosis[10]
Pancreatitis
Uncomplicated cirrhosis

*Data from Babb, R. R.: Diagnosing ascites—the value of abdominal paracentesis. Postgrad. Med. 63:219, 1978 and Sleisenger, M. H., and Fordtran, J. S.: Gastrointestinal Disease, 2nd ed., vol. 2. Philadelphia, W. B. Saunders Co., 1978.

sels are occasionally reported,[28] portal hypertension, clotting abnormalities, qualititative platelet defects, increased capillary fragility, and clotting factor deficiencies rather than major vessel injury are usually implicated as the cause of hemorrhage.[11, 29]

In a retrospective analysis of 242 consecutive diagnostic paracenteses in patients with liver disease,[11] only 4 cases of significant hemorrhage occurred. It was speculated that clotting abnormalities may have produced hemorrhage in all these patients.

A precipitous fall in blood pressure and a "shock-like" state may occur following rapid removal of large amounts of fluid from the peritoneal cavity. Usually over 1000 ml must be quickly removed[10] for this to occur. Although as much as 6 to 10 L removed over 10 to 15 minutes has been reported to be safe, if more than 1000 ml is to be removed *electively*, the rate should not exceed 1000 ml per 24 hours. Precipitation or aggravation of fluid or electrolyte imbalance may follow removal of large amounts of ascitic fluid. Baldus and Summerskill[30] reported the fatal complications of oliguric renal failure, hepatic coma, hyponatremia, and hypotension unresponsive to hypertonic saline infusion in a 56-year-old cirrhotic patient who had 20 L of ascitic fluid drained over a 36-hour period. Although some cases of hypotension following paracentesis may respond to intravascular fluid replacement, not all cases are reversible. The most commonly precipitated electrolyte disturbance is hyponatremia.

Table 39–5. CONDITIONS CAUSING AN ELEVATED PERITONEAL FLUID AMYLASE (OVER 100 U/100 ml)

Pancreatitis,[1, 10]
Pancreatic pseudocyst[8]
Mesenteric infarction[31]
Pancreatic duct tear
Small bowel perforation[19]
Perforated peptic ulcer

Table 39–6. CHARACTERISTICS OF ASCITIC FLUID BY ETIOLOGY*

Condition	Character	Total Protein	Amylase Concentration	Microscopic Findings (WBCs, RBCs)†	Cytology, Bacteriology, Total Fat
Uncomplicated cirrhosis	Clear, straw-colored	0.5 to 2.0 gm/dl		Usually < 1000 WBCs/mm³ (ref. 8)	
Malignant ascites	Bloody, chylous or straw-colored	> 2 to 3 gm/dl		Elevated RBCs > 10,000/mm³ in 20%	Malignant cells seen in 60 to 90% (refs. 9 and 10)
Tuberculous peritonitis	Fibrin clots, may be bloody or yellow	> 2 to 3 gm/dl		Mononuclear leukocytosis (> 1000 WBCs/mm³)	+ culture, acid-fast stain
Chylous ascites	Milky, turbid			Variable WBCs with lymphocytes	+ Sudan stain for fat
Bacterial peritonitis	Thick, cloudy, odoriferous	> 2 to 3 gm/dl	May be high if bowel perforation has occurred	Over 300 WBCs/mm³; over 25% polymorphonuclear leukocytes (ref. 38)	+ culture, Gram stain
Nephrotic syndrome	Clear, straw-colored or chylous	Low (< 2.0 gm/dl)		Usually < 250 WBCs/mm³; mononuclear, mesothelial	+ Sudan stain if chylous
Congestive heart failure	Clear, straw colored	Variable		Usually < 300 WBCs/mm³, mononuclear cells	
Pancreatitis	Variable	Over 3.0 gm/dl	High	Variable, may be bloody	

*Data from Sleisenger, M. H., and Fordtran, J. S.: Gastrointestinal Disease, 2nd ed., vol. 2. Philadelphia, W. B. Saunders Co., 1978; Cohn, E. M.: Ascites: Pathogenesis and differential diagnosis. In Bockus, H. L. (ed.): Gastroenterology, 3rd ed., vol. 4. Philadelphia, W. B. Saunders Co., 1976; and Wintrobe, M. M., Thorn, G. W., Adams, R. D., et al. (eds.): Harrison's Principles of Internal Medicine, 9th ed. New York, McGraw-Hill Book Co. 1980.

†Only typical figures are given; these vary widely in a given disease state. Use of the corrected WBC is recommended in peritoneal lavage effluent; this figure is more significant in evaluation of bacterial contamination, as from colonic or small bowel rupture. Corrected WBC = Total WBC × [peritoneal WBC × circulating RBC/peritoneal RBC].[39]

A number of other complications have been reported. Bowel puncture may be innocuous, but perforation of bowel followed by generalized peritonitis and abdominal wall abscess has been reported; catheter fragments have been sheared off and left in the peritoneal cavity,[11, 15] and mesenteric laceration has been reported.[18] In general, a major complication rate of less than 3 per cent has been reported.[11]

Minor complications, which are seldom of clinical importance, include scrotal edema, persistent ascitic fluid leakage,[31] hematoma of the anterior cecal wall and the adjacent mesentery following an iliac fossa tap,[23] and ovarian cyst laceration.[19] Persistent fluid leak may be remedied by placement of a suture around the puncture site.

Summary

Simple needle aspiration of ascitic fluid for diagnostic evaluation may be quickly, safely, and easily performed in the emergency department. The procedure is usually an elective one that can be performed at the bedside, but in cases of respiratory compromise or suspected bacterial peritonitis, abdominal paracentesis becomes an urgent or emergency procedure.

The complications of the procedure are usually minor and infrequent. With the refinement of the more accurate technique of peritoneal lavage, paracentesis should not be used for the diagnosis of hemoperitoneum.

1. Brown, Charles H. (ed.): Diagnostic Procedures in Gastroenterology. St. Louis, C. V. Mosby Co., 1967, pp. 284–286.
2. Saloman, H.: Die Diagnostische Punktion des Bauches. Berl. Klin. Wochenschr. 43:45, 1906.
3. McCoy, J., and Wolma, F. J.: Abdominal tap; indication, technic, and results. Am. J. Surg. 122:693, 1971.
4. Giacobine, J. W., and Siler, V. E.: Evaluation of diagnostic abdominal paracentesis with experimental and clinical studies. Surg. Gynecol. Obstet. 110:676, 1960.
5. Fischer, D. S.: Abdominal paracentesis for malignant ascites. Arch. Intern. Med. 139:235, 1979.
6. LaVeen, H. H., Christoudias, G., Ip, M., et al.: Peritoneovenous shunting for ascites. Ann. Surg. 180:580, 1974.
7. Meyers, M. A.: The spread and localization of acute intraperitoneal effusions. Radiology 95:547, 1970.
8. Babb, R. R.: Diagnosing ascites—the value of abdominal paracentesis. Postgrad. Med. 63:219, 1978.
9. Cohn, E. M.: Ascites: Pathogenesis and differential diagnosis. In: Bockus, H. L. (ed.): Gastroenterology, 3rd ed., vol. 4. Philadelphia, W. B. Saunders Co., 1976, pp. 48–55.
10. Sleisenger, M. H., and Fordtran, J. S.: Gastrointestinal Disease, 2nd ed., vol. 2. Philadelphia, W. B. Saunders Co., 1978, pp. 1949–1957.
11. Mallory, A., and Schaefer, J. W.: Complications of diagnostic paracentesis in patients with liver disease. JAMA 239:628, 1978.
12. Singh, A., and Kaur, B.: Paracentesis abdominis in ruptured ectopic pregnancy. J. Indian Med. Assoc. 73:54, 1979.
13. Root, H. D., Hauser, C. W., McKinley, C. R., et al.: Diagnostic peritoneal lavage. Surgery 57:633, 1965.
14. Manganaro, A. J., Pachter, H. L., and Spencer, F. C.: Experience with routine open abdominal paracentesis. Surg. Gynecol. Obstet. 146:795, 1978.
15. Caffee, H. H., and Benfield, J. R.: Is peritoneal lavage for the diagnosis of hemoperitoneum safe? Arch. Surg. 103:4, 1971.
16. Parvin, S., Smith, D. E., Asher, W. M., et al.: Effectiveness of peritoneal lavage in blunt abdominal trauma. Ann. Surg. 181:255, 1975.
17. McAlvanah, M. J., and Shaftan, G. W.: Selective conservatism in penetrating abdominal wounds: A continuing reappraisal. J. Trauma 18:206, 1978.
18. Veith, F. J., Webber, W. B., Karl, R. C., et al.: Diagnostic peritoneal lavage in acute abdominal disease: Normal findings in 100 patients. Ann. Surg. 166:290, 1967.
19. Engrav, L. H., Benjamin, C. I., Strate, R. G., et al.: Diagnostic peritoneal lavage in blunt abdominal trauma. J. Trauma 15:854, 1975.
20. Olsen, W. R., and Hildreth, D. H.: Abdominal paracentesis and peritoneal lavage in blunt abdominal trauma. J. Trauma 11:824, 1971.
21. Lamke, L., and Varenhorst, E.: Abdominal paracentesis for early diagnosis of closed abdominal injury. Acta. Chir. Scand. 144:21, 1978.
22. Civetta, J. M., Williams, M. J., and Richie, R. E.: Diagnostic peritoneal irrigation—a simple and reliable technique. Surgery 67:874, 1970.
23. Rao, R. N., and Ravikumar, T. S.: Diagnostic peritoneal tap. Int. Surg. 62:14, 1977.
24. Schwartz, S. I., Lillihei, R. C., Shires, G. T., et al. (eds.): Principles of Surgery, 3rd ed. New York, McGraw-Hill Book Co., 1979.
25. Moretz, W. H., and Erickson, W. G.: Peritoneal tap as an aid in the diagnosis of acute abdominal disease. Am. Surg. 20:363, 1954.
26. Cacciatore, L., Molinari, V., Guadagnino, V., et al.: Hepatitis B antigen in ascitic fluid in cirrhosis. Br. Med. J. 3:172, 1973.
27. Gjessing, J., Oskarsson, B. M., Tomlin, P. J., et al.: Diagnostic abdominal paracentesis. Br. Med. J. 1:617, 1972.
28. Thiel, E. R., and Shires, G. T.: Peritoneal lavage in blunt abdominal trauma. Am. J. Surg. 125:64, 1973.
29. Walls, W. J., and Losowsky, M. S.: The hemostatic defect of liver disease. Gastroenterology 60:108, 1971.
30. Baldus, W. P., and Summerskill, W. H. J.: The kidney in hepatic disease. Postgrad. Med. 41:103, 1967.
31. Quillen, C. G., and Polk, H. C., Jr.: The ascitic leak: A case presentation—management by paracentesis and saline-albumin infusion. Surgery 82:241, 1977.
32. Wilkins, E. J., Jr. (ed.): MGH Textbook of Emergency Medicine. Baltimore, Williams & Wilkins, 1978, p. 200.
33. Conn, H. O.: The rational management of ascites. In Popper, H., and Schaffner, F. (eds.): Progress in Liver Diseases, vol. 4. New York, Grune & Stratton, 1972, pp. 269–288.
34. Wintrobe, M. M., Thorn, G. W., Adams, R. D., et al. (eds.): Harrison's Principles of Internal Medicine, 9th ed., New York, McGraw-Hill Book Co., 1980.
35. Warshaw, A. L.: Diagnosis of starch peritonitis by paracentesis. Lancet 2:1054, 1972.
36. Rothchild, J. J., Gelernt, I., and Sloan, W.: Ruptured mesenteric varix in cirrhosis: Unusual cause for hemoperitoneum. N. Engl. J. Med. 278:97, 1968.
37. Bristow, J. D., and Medaed, N. E.: Hemorrhagic ascites due to perforated duodenal ulcer: Report of a case. Arch. Intern. Med., 105:105, 1960.

6

ORTHOPEDICS

40

Prehospital Splinting

THOM DICK, EMT–P

Cervical Spine

INTRODUCTION

The use of cervical extrication collars has been seriously questioned by the medical community. However, as an early adjunct in the sometimes complex process of immobilization and extrication of groups of trauma victims in the field, the cervical extrication collar has been of great value. There are several types of collars, varying in degree of comfort and support, but even the ones with the best combinations of these features provide less than adequate immobilization independently.

Choice of devices used in addition to extrication collars to ensure thorough immobilization depend upon a victim's position of origin and the complexity of the disentanglement process. If the victim is found in a sitting position, as in an automobile, some version of a short spine board is commonly used. The most effective of these are wraparound corset–type devices, designed both to immobilize the neck and to put "handles" on the patient.

Following the use of these intermediate, short immobilizers, the patient is usually fastened to a full-length spine board or a similar rigid appliance for transfer to a litter for transporting. This full-body immobilizer should incorporate lateral immobilization for the head, consisting either of sandbags and tape or a solidly attached pillow harness.

BACKGROUND

Since 1965, an entire industry aimed at the prehospital preservation of life has evolved. Specially manufactured spinal immobilizers were pioneered for field use during the late 1960's and early 1970's, with the development of devices that are still in use today. Many variations of these early devices have been further developed to solve specific prehospital problems.

In addition, new building materials evolved—more versatile plastics and stronger adhesives. Such materals were not available to the "pioneers" of the 1960's. Medical theory as it applied to spinal protection was also later incorporated into the rescue devices as the medical field became more involved in pre-hospital care.

It should be stressed that, although there seems to be widespread general agreement about the basic steps of spinal immobilization, pre-hospital care is a setting for people who can *adapt*. Because of the variety of circumstances that confront rescuers on a daily basis, there is little room for inflexible rules. An ambulance can carry only a limited number of tools.

The first widely distributed text to devote much attention to the role of a cervical extrication collar in early immobilization of the neck after injury was Grant and Murray's *Emergency Care*. This book was first published in 1971, and one of its principal contributors was J. D. Farrington, M.D., a consultant. Farrington's classic, "Death In A Ditch," was the first widely publicized reference concerning the use of a spine board and undoubtedly influenced rescue training programs worldwide.[1] Farrington had no faith in the cervical collars of his day; they were specifically designed for the post-hospital setting and were useless in the field. Farrington advocated the use of sandbags and tape, urging rescuers to maintain manual traction on the head and neck during extrication.[2] Manual traction, unfortunately, is a risky procedure to undertake during movement of the human body from a sitting to a supine position. In 1974, the "backyard" inventor, Glenn Hare, patented the first extrication-type collar that provided both comfort and support.

INDICATIONS

An extrication collar should be used as a primary adjunct in most cases that involve possible trauma to the head or neck. When such trauma is not obvious, it should be suspected unless it can be ruled out by careful questioning of both the victims and the witnesses involved. In any instance of doubt, it is best to immobilize and transport.

Commonly, patients who are both conscious and oriented are unaware of their own neck injuries in the field setting. The sensory impact of having one's automobile forcibly disassembled by fast-moving, shouting, and helmeted rescuers who are using modern rescue tools that produce noise in excess of 80 decibels may result in considerable distraction. Furthermore, one can never assume that a trauma victim who is under the influence of alcohol or other drugs will have sufficient self-awareness to recognize his own cervical spine injury.

The purpose of an extrication collar is to temporarily splint the head and neck either prophylactically or therapeutically in a normoflexed position as soon after the rescuers encounter the patient as possible. The collar is useful for the following reasons:

1. It provides substantial protection of the airway by limiting flexion in a patient whose position or mental status threatens airway patency.

2. It relieves stress on the basilar skull and cervical vertebrae when these structures have been injured.

3. It can free the hands of a rescuer, allowing him to participate in packaging, extrication, or other therapeutic procedures.

4. If properly chosen for size, it can provide enough traction to temporarily support the weight of the head while the patient is sitting and help to maintain the alignment of the cervical spine once the patient has been moved into a supine position. Furthermore, improper application of a collar may increase intracranial pressure in head injuries.

5. Once the patient has reached medical care, it can serve as a reminder that the integrity of the basilar skull and cervical spine are suspect because of the patient's mechanism of injury.

Serious cervical cord injuries may occur in the absence of demonstrable fracture, and permanent paralysis may result from spinal cord contusion in an intact bony milieu. Spinal cord injury is common in elderly patients with cervical spondylosis, and an arthritic osteophyte may sever a portion of the cord as permanently as a fracture-dislocation. In such cases, there may be little or no subjective pain.

The extrication collar does not constitute complete immobilization of the head and neck, even for the purpose of transportation. Complete immobilization is not possible until the patient has been properly secured to a long, backboard-type device. Nonetheless, the collar goes on first and remains in place.

CONTRAINDICATIONS

There are few circumstances that contraindicate the use of some type of extrication collar. The presence of a tracheal stoma, which is integral to the management of the patient's airway, is one such circumstance. In such a case, some of the best collars incorporate removable plugs. The plugs are approximately 5 cm in diameter and also serve to prevent compression of the thyroid cartilage during swallowing. With scissors, one can modify rigid collars to accommodate a stoma hole, although structural support should be ensured after modification. The presence of an invasive airway (i.e., cricothyroidotomy or needle tracheostomy) may similarly require modification of the cervical support.

A second circumstance that might preclude the use of a factory-made collar is cervical dislocation with field findings of fixed angulation. This situation is rarely encountered and can be managed with an improvised immobilizer, such as a version of a horse collar or prolonged manual-positioning without traction.

A third circumstance that could preclude the use of a collar is massive cervical swelling (i.e., secondary to hemorrhage or tracheal injury). The compressive effect of a collar may impede air exchange, decrease cerebral perfusion, or increase intracranial pressure. A penetrating foreign body such as knife, glass, or metal, would also make cervical spine immobilization difficult.

One must emphasize that *effect* is the determinant of the type of tool that should be used. Often, an improvised tool works better than one that is manufactured owing to the size and shape of the patient or the special circumstances involved in handling him. Adaptability is a function of well-trained and experienced field personnel.

EQUIPMENT[3]

There are two basic types of extrication collars, both of which currently appear in rigid and semirigid designs. Both types rely on the same support structures for the *bottom* of the collar, namely, the two trapezoid muscles posteriorly and the two clavicles anteriorly. These support structures constitute a four-point system. The collar types differ, however, in the way in which they come in contact with the head.

The first type is a relatively short collar that wraps rather tightly around the neck. Depending upon the collar's shape (usually fairly straight), it contacts the hyoid, the mastoids, and the occiput. Disadvantages of this type of collar are impingement on the thyroid cartilage and compression of the carotid sinuses and external neck veins. Thyroid cartilage restriction can affect airway management; carotid compression can be expected to decrease cerebral circulation; and jugular compression may increase intracranial pressures (Fig. 40–1).

The second type of collar design for supporting the head incorporates a higher collar with winglike flaps on its upper posterior edges that engage large areas of soft tissue on the posterior head. Anteriorly, this collar appears to be similar to the

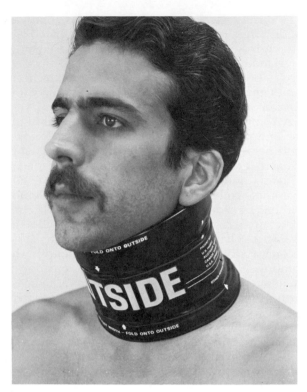

Figure 40–1. Loxley cervical collar. A low-style collar. Note the fact that it fits closer to the neck than other designs. Closer fitting collars tend to be less comfortable than other designs, offering less rotational stability. This one is constructed of plastic over cardboard. (Bound Tree Corporation, P. O. Box 401, Henniker, NH 03242; From Dick, T., and Land, R.: Spinal immobilization devices. Part I: Cervical extrication collars. J. Emerg. Med. Services 7:29, 1982. Used by permission.)

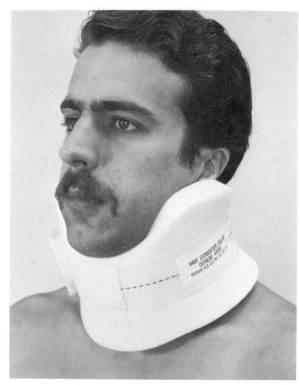

Figure 40–2. Hare cervical extrication collar. One of the earliest forms of extrication collar, this type provides anterior support via the mandible, posterior support by means of winglike flaps that engage the mastoids but not the occiput in most patients. When properly applied, it provides excellent support. A 5 cm soft insert over the thyroid protects that structure. (Dyna Med/Dyna Industries, 6200 Yarrow Drive, Carlsbad, CA 92008; From Dick, T., and Land, R.: Spinal immobilization devices. Part I: Cervical extrication collars. J. Emerg. Med. Services 7:29, 1982. Used by permission.)

lower-type collars, although this flaring design seems to prevent compression of some of those areas of the neck that were mentioned previously, even when the collars are applied firmly. The higher collars generally provide better rotational stability, although some allow more extension than those that are tighter fitting. Properly sized, they can provide respectable traction. Some are equipped with expansion plugs to accommodate the thyroid cartilage. In addition, one new style of collar uses the sternum as a fifth, thoracic support point (see Figs. 40–2 through 40–6).

There is an important trade-off among field collars, between those that have a rigid and those that have a soft design. A rigid collar can provide excellent support but only for a narrow range of neck sizes. A soft collar, on the other hand, will generally fit a wider range of sizes but at the cost of support.

In addition, comfort is extremely important from the standpoint of patient compliance. Some rigid collars, regardless of proper sizing and despite their support characteristics, are useless because of patient discomfort. Some relatively comfortable collars serve little more than a decorative function and are probably responsible for the fact that some physicians do not support the use of any collars.

Aprahamian and associates,[4] in 1982, studied the impact of various airway maneuvers, with and without two types of collars, on a fresh cadaver with surgically induced cervical instability at C5 to C6. They concluded that a collar's primary value may be only that of a warning device to call attention to possible cervical injury. Podolsky and colleagues[5] compared neck movements in 25 volunteers who were in the supine position, immobilized with various collars. They concluded that of the four collars used none were effective immobilizers except for the Philadelphia-style device and that all collars should be used in conjunction with sandbags and tape. Podolsky and colleagues also concluded that sandbags and tape actually did more to limit motion of people in a supine position than any collar whose effectiveness had been examined (Table 40–1).

Of course, trauma patients in the field are not often encountered in the supine position. As of this printing, I am not aware of any scientific analysis that studies the effectiveness of specific

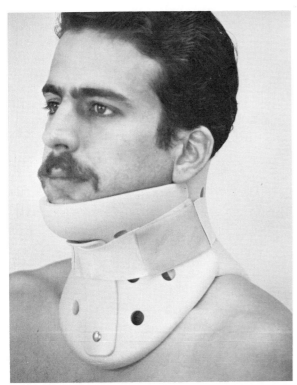

Figure 40–3. Philadelphia collar. This is a two-piece, high-type collar that comes in 17 sizes. The collar supports the head in a dish-shaped contour, formed when the front and rear halves are velcroed together. Properly sized for a patient, this collar provides excellent support. Applied too tightly, it tends to force the mandible backward and in some patients can cause thyroid compression. It is extremely comfortable. (Armstrong Industries, 3660 Commercial Ave, P.O. Box 7, Northbrook, Il. 60062; From Dick, T., and Land, R.: Spinal immobilization devices. Part I: Cervical extrication collars. J. Emerg. Med. Services 7:29, 1982. Used by permission.)

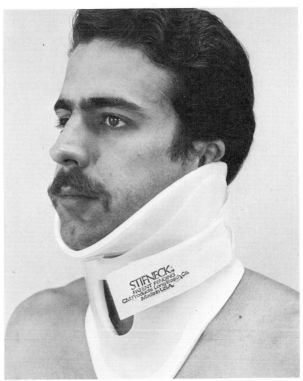

Figure 40–4. Stifneck collar. This collar is a radically different type of high-design collar, made of high-density polyethylene (a hard material) padded with semi-flexible foam margins. It provides probably the best overall support of all field collars, considering the adaptability of a single collar to several patient sizes. Note the low reaching anterior panel, which contacts the sternum. (California Medical Products, 334 Colorado Place, Long Beach, CA 90814; From Dick, T., and Land, R.: Spinal immobilization devices. Part I: Cervical extrication collars. J. Emerg. Med. Services 7:29, 1982. Used by permission.)

collar types on human subjects in more realistic positions of origin after trauma.

Dick and Land published a subjective, matrix-type analysis based on 14 criteria that compared the effectiveness of 13 extrication-type collars with that of an ideal model (Table 40–2). They outlined the following characteristics of a good extrication collar:

1. It should support the weight of the head in normoflexion.

2. It should provide and maintain traction on the neck and should prevent lateral, rotational, and anteroposterior movement of the head.

3. It should be comfortable, x-ray translucent, and compact enough to fit into a standard paramedic equipment box without undergoing deformity.

4. It should be able to be applied reliably by a single trained technician and an untrained bystander.

5. It should be capable of sustaining repeated sanitation.

6. Its price should be such that it can be carried in sufficient numbers in various sizes by any ambulance.

7. It should not interfere with the position of function of important airway structures, nor adversely affect cerebral circulation in any way.

8. Simplicity of design should permit its application by two technicians in less than 60 seconds, in darkness, rain, and cold weather, without manipulation of the head or neck.

9. It should be available in as few sizes (that adapt to and properly immobilize as many patients) as possible. Proper application is assumed.

Figures 40–1 through 40–6 illustrate representative devices that are commonly used for in-field cervical immobilization and provide the unique features of each.

Procedure

Application of an extrication collar is a straightforward procedure. A collar should be treated as a splint. The normal axiom in splinting is to

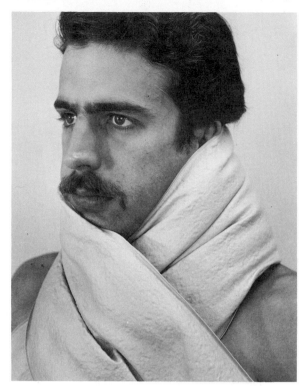

Figure 40–5. Vac-Pac vacuum-type cervical collar. Although expensive, this is a vacuum splint designed for the neck. Vacuum splints are similar to pneumatic devices in their ability to conform to anything while avoiding inward pressure. This device is a phenomenal immobilizer, although it will not maintain traction. The vinyl cover is filled with polystyrene beads, which act as a form when the splint is evacuated with a suction device. (Olympic Medical Corporation, 4400 Seventh Ave. South, Seattle WA 98108; From Dick, T., and Land, R.: Spinal immobilization devices. Part I: Cervical extrication collars. J. Emerg. Med. Services 7:29, 1982. Used by permission.)

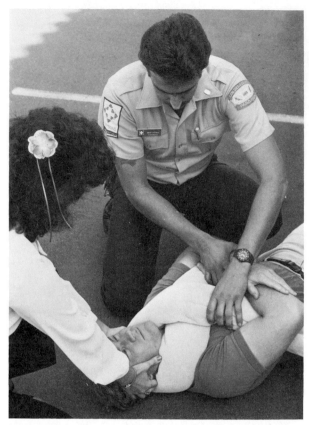

Figure 40–6. Horse collar. Most extrication collars are available in three to five factory sizes. If a collar is not sized properly to fit a particular patient, it performs no function. Patients with extremely long necks or especially short ones can be immobilized by means of a horse collar, fashioned from a bulky rescue blanket. The blanket is rolled to thickness desired, slid under the victim's neck while a bystander applies traction; the ends of the blanket are then brought across the victim's anterior chest. The victim's forearms are fastened as shown to stabilize the "tails" of the collar. Emergency medical technicians must be able to adapt to a wide range of possible patients and environmental circumstances. (From Dick, T.: Tricks of the trade: horse sense, immobilizing necks that don't fit collars. J. Emerg. Med. Services 7:23, 1982. Used by permission.)

immobilize joints above and below the areas of injury. Because no currently marketed collar performs this function perfectly, a rescuer should be charged with maintaining traction on the head in a normoflexed position until the patient can be fully immobilized in a corset-type immobilizer or on a full backboard. Continuous manual traction is not alway possible under field conditions. A collar (like any splint) requires one person to stabilize the neck in its position of function and a second person to apply the hardware. The rescuers' intentions should be thoroughly explained to the patient throughout the procedure.

The neck should be examined prior to application of a collar. Once the collar is in place, a conscious patient should be cautioned repeatedly against movement of the head until all equipment has been removed on arrival at a hospital. Any persistent complaints of pain or dyspnea by the patient should be investigated by removal and possible replacement of the device while manual traction is *continuously* maintained.

In cases in which a factory-manufactured collar of the proper size for a given patient is not avail-

able, an improvised device should be made from available materials (see Fig. 40–6).

Once the patient is in supine position on the backboard, lateral stabilization should be added, either in the form of sandbags and tape or by means of a factory-made pillow harness.

COMPLICATIONS

Improper application of an extrication collar generally occurs in one of two ways: either the wrong size or type of device is used, or too little care is exercised in its placement. The best means of preventing either error is strong physician involvement in the training and continuing education of rescue crews, together with vigorous feedback in cases of correct and incorrect application.

A collar that is too small for a patient may be

Table 40-1. MEAN DEGREES OF MOVEMENT ± STANDARD DEVIATION OF SIX CERVICAL IMMOBILIZATION METHODS AND NO IMMOBILIZATION IN 25 NORMAL VOLUNTEERS

	No Immobilization	Soft Collar (Howmedica)	Extrication Collar (Hare)	Hard Collar (Orthopedic Systems)	Philadelphia Collar (Philadelphia Collar Company)	Tape and Sandbags	Tape, Sandbags, Philadelphia Collar
Flexion	35.7 ± 5.1	34.2 ± 6.4	26.4 ± 6.4	25.8 ± 6.0	24.2 ± 7.8	0.1 ± 6.0	0.1 ± 0.4
Extension	21.0 ± 5.8	18.1 ± 5.8	16.4 ± 6.7	15.4 ± 5.3	12.0 ± 7.0	15.0 ± 6.9	7.4 ± 5.5
Lateral	21.2 ± 5.4	21.1 ± 4.6	15.4 ± 4.9	14.2 ± 6.3	17.4 ± 5.0	1.8 ± 1.7	1.4 ± 1.5
Rotary	75.8 ± 6.5	67.4 ± 11.7	48.9 ± 11.6	49.9 ± 15.3	49.9 ± 14.2	2.5 ± 2.2	4.0 ± 3.0

(Adapted from Podolsky, S., Baraff, L. J., Simon, R. R., et al.: Efficacy of cervical spine immobilization methods. J. Trauma 23:461, 1983.)

Table 40-2. COLLAR EVALUATION CHART*

Category	Ferno-Washington	FP Extrication	FP Standard	Hare	Immobilizer	Loxley	Philadelphia	Quic-kollar	Rapid-Form	Stif-neck	Stubbs	Thomas	Vac-Pac
Support	+1‡	+1	-1‖	+2†	+2	+2	+2	0§	+1	+2	+2	+2	+2
Traction	0	0	-2¶	+2	+2	+2	+2	-1	0	+2	+2	+2	0
Lateral	+1	+1	-2	+2	+2	+2	+2	0	+2	+1	+2	+1	+2
Rotational	+1	+1	-2	+1	+2	-2	+2	-2	+2	+2	+1	+2	+2
Flex-extension	+1	+1	+2	+2	-1	+1	-2	+1	+1	+2	+1	+1	+2
Comfort	+2	+2	+1	+1	-2	-2	+2	-1	-2	+2	+1	-2	+2
Compactness	+1	+2	+1	+2	+1	-2	0	+2	+1	0	+1	+2	-1
Simplicity	+2	+2	0	+2	+2	-2	+1	+2	+1	0	+1	0	+1
Cleaning	+2	+2	+2	+2	+2	+2	+2	+2	+1	+2	-2	+2	+2
# Sizes	+1	+1	+2	+1	+1	+2	0	+2	+2	+1	+1	+1	+2
Circulation	+1	+2	+2	+2	-2	-1	+2	0	-2	+2	+2	-1	+2
Ease of application	+2	+2	+1	+2	+2	+2	+1	+2	+1	+2	+1	+1	+1
Airway	+1	+1	-1	+2	+2	0	-1	+1	+1	+2	+2	+2	+2
Price	+2	+1	+2	+2	+2	+2	0	+2	+1	+1	+2	0	-2

*This chart compares 13 collars to an imaginary "perfect" extrication collar. Although x-ray and cold weather performance are important considerations, the collars were not evaluated for these factors. Please note that rigid collar designs are likely to accommodate only narrow ranges of neck sizes, whereas firm but flexible designs tend to be more adaptable while still providing good immobilization.

† +2 = performance is ideal.
‡ +1 = performance is good, but not ideal.
§ 0 = performance is about adequate or marginal.
‖ -1 = performance is mildly unsatisfactory.
¶ -2 = performance is highly unsatisfactory.
**The collars are presented in alphabetical order.
(Adapted from Dick, T., and Land, R.: Spinal immobilization devices, Part I: cervical extrication collars. J. Emerg. Med. Services 7:29, 1982. Used by permission.)

either too tight for the girth of the neck (with obvious complications) or too short to provide adequate immobilization. Too large a collar commonly results in hyperextension, which can exacerbate any pre-existing injury.

Improper application can result from not removing the patient's shoulder clothing prior to application of the hardware; this should be done by cutting if necessary, in every case. Insistence upon taking spinal precautions whenever the mechanism of injury even mildly suggests cervical injury will ensure high competence levels among rescuers as well as a comfortable margin of safety.

One final complication should be mentioned. The patient who, for whatever reason, actively resists placement of an extrication collar should not be forced to wear it or any other splint that he resists. Immobilization of the resisting patient cannot be accomplished without considerable muscular exertion not only by rescuers but also by the patient. If fractures do exist, it is possible that this kind of struggling can cause further damage. If such fractures involve the cervical spine, this could be fatal. If the patient will permit manual traction, this should be maintained as an alternative.

CONCLUSIONS

The competent use of a good cervical extrication collar has proven itself to be important as an early immobilizer in the field, prior to disentanglement of the traumatized patient, although it is less valuable in a hospital environment. The cervical collar should not be relied upon for total immobilization. The latter can only be provided in the field by means of a full backboard and lateral immobilization of the head and neck.

Thoracolumbar Spine

INTRODUCTION

Adequate full-body thoracolumbar spinal immobilization in the field, like good cervical spinal immobilization, is probably best done by means of a full-length spine board (also called a *backboard*). Full-body spinal immobilization should incorporate early application of a good extrication collar, lateral immobilization of the head and neck, and ample belting of the entire body. The last measure is important in cases in which the backboard will have to be used to carry the patient for any distance or when there is likelihood of emesis, as in the patient with probable head injuries or ingestion of depressants such as alcohol.

Transference of a victim from a location and position of origin to a backboard may require the use of an intermediate immobilizer. Until recently, this meant using a short spine board to which a patient's head, neck, and torso were fastened by belts. Currently, devices that resemble corsets are preferred. Such devices have extensions that engage the head and neck and are equipped with weight-bearing loops that enable the rescuers to handle the patient more easily. Intermediate immobilizers or extrication splints are indicated either when a patient must be removed from a confined environment in which he is found in the sitting position or under any circumstances that require movement in or from a sitting position.

When extrication is not required by a patient's location, position of origin, or route of egress, the patient is most often found lying at ground level. With an extrication collar in place and with manual traction maintained on the neck until stabilization is complete, he may then be logrolled onto a backboard.

Visual inspection of the back and possibly percussion of the flanks should be carried out during the logrolling process as the body is kept in a single plane.

An optional but effective means of moving a patient from the ground is provided by a type of stretcher that breaks apart longitudinally and can be slid beneath a victim without disturbing his position. The *scoop stretcher*, as this device is called, facilitates movement and eliminates the need for immediate examination of the back, a factor that should not be considered a limitation of the equipment. One definite advantage to using the scoop stretcher is its shape. Its halves are anatomically contoured, not only enhancing its comfort but also limiting lateral movement of the immobilized patient.

A third means of both immobilizing and moving a trauma victim consists of a specially designed full-body splint, complete with factory-made straps or harnesses. There are several such immobilizers, most of which are highly effective and provide good lateral stability as well as anatomic conformity.

BACKGROUND

As recently as 1965, the principle of "rapid transportation above all" held widespread acceptance among rescuers who had little or no orthopedic training and among physicians whose emergency care experience, by modern standards, was just as limited. The most commonly agreed upon means of getting a sitting patient out of a wrecked automobile was to use some version of a chair-carry. If the victim originated in a position other than the sitting position, he was first placed into a sitting position and *then* moved by means of a chair-carry, or he was simply dragged out bodily.

In fact, one respectable source of the period says that rescuers rarely found a victim in his car unless he was trapped there; civilians had usually dragged him out,[6] or, conditioned by the number of accidents involving higher-octane fuels and a lack of safety-capping systems, the victim was just as likely to flee for his life.[7] He may also have been thrown out of the vehicle, without the benefit of safety belts.

Colonel Louis Kossuth, Commander of the U.S. Air Force's Medical Service School at Gunter Air Force Base in Alabama, made note of several auto accidents at the scenes of which he thought patients were handled very roughly by civilians who were trying to be of help. He searched, to no avail, the medical literature of that time for references that might show how these victims should be packaged and handled. He questioned several hundred accident victims who had sustained major fractures to determine how they had been removed from their automobiles. Most said that they had been grabbed under the shoulders and dragged, often in terrible pain, from their vehicles.

Kossuth experimented with a torso version of the Timmons splints, a set of canvas splints reinforced with semi-rigid steel stays as slats, similar to the modern Kendrick Extrication Device (K.E.D. or Ked Sled). In addition, Kossuth probably developed the first modern-type spine board.[2]

In 1967 and 1968, J. D. Farrington, M.D., authored two classic articles (filled with detailed illustrations) that showed the use of a type of extrication collar, spinal traction, 9-foot webbing straps, and both long and short spine boards similar to modern designs to remove people in every position from automobiles.[1, 2] Much of today's extrication theory is essentially as Farrington taught it.

In 1967, the Committee on Trauma of the American College of Surgeons listed the minimum amounts of and types of equipment that should be carried in an ambulance. The list included both short and long spine boards, with accessories.[8] A similar document published the following year by the National Academy of Sciences' Division of Medical Sciences also provided a list of medical requirements for ambulance equipment and also recommended long and short spine boards.[7]

In 1969, St. Louis surgeons Allen P. Klippel and Marshall B. Conrad described the use of a full-length spine board that was capable of being broken down into separate components for the upper and lower halves of the body. The lower portion included a simple traction device that could accommodate right- or left-sided lower extremities of various lengths.[9] By 1971, both of the

first recognized texts for emergency medical technicians referred to the use of the short spine board as a widespread practice.[10, 11]

INDICATIONS

Generally, the application and maintenance of spinal precautions in the field setting depend upon the rescuers as well as the receiving emergency physicians being well educated and experienced in the mechanics of injury.

Any mechanism capable of injury to the cervical spine should prompt rescuers to immobilize not only the head and neck but also the entire body. The motion of any vertebral joint is impossible to isolate. In order to immobilize the head and neck, they both must be fastened into a common plane with the thorax. Extrication devices (such as short spine boards) can be made to do this to an extent, although movement of the lower extremities causes movement of the pelvis, which in turn results in lumbar movement. Movement of the lumbar spine in turn induces some thoracic movement, although the extent has not been quantified. Considering the fact that the most feasible position for transport is the supine position, full-body immobilization is easily achieved on a long spine board. In the absence of deterrent factors, supine full-body immobilization is a reasonable choice.

Mechanisms that arouse suspicion of direct injury to the thoracolumbar spine should also suggest full-body spinal immobilization. Very generally, they include: 1) most penetrating injuries to the thorax and abdomen, including all missile-related incidents; 2) blunt trauma involving high-energy impact in any area of the body; 3) blunt trauma involving moderate energy impact to the posterior truncal surfaces; and 4) blunt trauma involving localized impact of any energy level in the posterior thoracic, abdominal, or pelvic spinal areas.

The mechanism of injury should dictate both suspicion of injury and immobilization of potential spinal injuries from a field standpoint, even when no neurological signs are present. In many cases, this should result in immobilization despite the absence of pain if the mechanism is suggestive enough. In such cases, the possibility of occult fractures are best ruled out by a physician.

It should be emphasized that in any case in which spinal injury is plausible, rescuers should take vigorous measures to immobilize the spine prior to transport, leaving diagnosis to the receiving physician. The physician, in turn, should not permit in-hospital removal of immobilizers until rescuers have reported on the mechanism of injury.

CONTRAINDICATIONS

Essentially, the only known contraindication to the use of commonly recognized means to immobilize the spine of a patient whose mechanism of injury suggests spinal injury, is *the existence of a greater threat*. Recognizing such circumstances and taking appropriate action when they arise are the functions of a competent rescuer. The threat to a patient's life may exceed the threat of *possible* spinal injury under the following circumstances.

Hazards on the Scene. Problems with traffic control in the direct vicinity of the patient's location such that the patient, along with rescuers or other patients, is likely to be further injured suggest urgent extrication. Such hazardous situations include fuel or other flammable substances leaking at the scene (these should be assumed to be in immediate danger of ignition, with possible ensuing explosions); fire on the scene; hostile crowds or persons on the scene; and physically unstable environments, such as partially collapsed structures or unstable vehicles that cannot be stabilized quickly.

Ongoing Gunfire at the Scene. Gunfire is usually considered an indication for rescue personnel to stay away from a scene. A rescuer who finds himself confronted with a patient *and* gunfire is considered fortunate if he can extricate himself and the victim from such a situation in any way possible.

Overwhelming Casualties. Rescuers may have to improvise in cases in which casualties might exceed available resources. In such cases, proper spinal immobilization may merit a lower priority than usual.

Weather Extremes. Under conditions of extremely adverse weather, the urgency of the movement of victims may supersede the priority of normal treatment, including immobilization.

Patient Noncompliance. One cannot overemphasize that if a patient cannot be persuaded to tolerate the placement of any immobilizer it is better not to use the device. A competent rescuer can do much to make a device comfortable by means of padding and reassurance. If this fails, however, immobilization that is applied by force is worse than no immobilization at all.

EQUIPMENT

Cervical Extrication (CE) Splints

There are almost as many variations of short spine boards as there are sizes of victims who will use them. A recently published study analyzed the performance of eight short spine boards and concluded that many were non-analogous to one another and that strict comparison would be impossible.[12] However, some reasonable expectations of a good cervical extrication splint, considering its role in the field, can be specified.

During Application. The device should not produce jostling of a patient or change the position of the head, neck, shoulders, or torso during application by two rescuers who are competent in its use.

After Application. Used in conjunction with a good extrication collar that has been properly applied, a CE splint should *immobilize* the head and neck while the patient is being removed from the area in which he was found and until the patient can be fastened to an auxillary stretcher, such as a long spine board, for further movement. This immobilization should effectively limit the lateral, flexion and extension, and rotational motions of the head and neck.

Once applied, a CE splint should not cause most patients to be uncomfortable. If a patient is uncomfortable, he is likely to resist its placement, thus defeating its use in the first place. In addition, an extrication device is apt to be left on a patient for up to 2 hours after arrival in an emergency department.

If necessary, a CE splint should be removable from one patient *at the scene* for use in extricating another. Properly immobilized by means of a good collar, lateral stabilizers such as sandbags and tape, and a full-body spine board, a patient should be able to tolerate this procedure in the supine position without adverse changes in position.

The device should be x-ray translucent, visible but not obstructive. Simplicity of design should allow placement of the device by two technicians in less than 3 minutes in any situation, including darkness and rain, without causing manipulation of the head or neck.

General. The CE splint should take up as little space as possible around a patient, enabling rescuers to apply it in as many types of extrication situations as possible. Cost should be reasonable enough so that at least one device can be carried in every ambulance. Finally, it should be capable of repeated sanitation, whether by wiping with a disinfectant or by laundering in hot water and detergent.

There are two devices that meet all these criteria, the Kendrick Extrication Device (KED) and the XP–1 (Extrication Plus One) (Figs. 40–7 and 40–8).

Kendrick Extrication Device (KED). This snug-fitting, highly adaptable descendant of the military Neil-Robertson stretcher and the Timmons splints is truly designed around the principle of packaging a patient. The KED was developed by EMT-firefighter Rick Kendrick, of El Cajon, California, as a result of the frustration of rescuers with the difficulty of the removal of victims from wrecked race cars.

Properly applied, the KED is a phenomenal

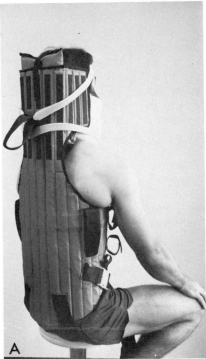
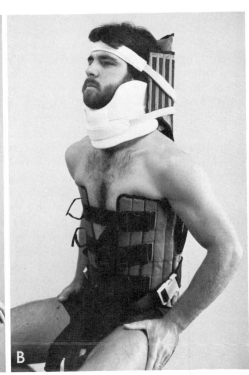

Figure 40–7. The Kendrick Extrication Device (K.E.D.). Note the presence of a cervical collar, applied prior to the K.E.D. (Medi-ked, 1946 John Towers Ave., El Cajon, CA 92020; From Dick, T., and Land, R.: Spinal immobilization devices. Part II: Cervical extrication devices. J. Emerg. Med. Services 8:25, 1983. Used by permission.)

immobilizer that can be used under even the most adverse circumstances. Part of its anterior thoracic panels can be folded backward to accommodate the obese, pregnant, or pediatric patient.

The nylon loop behind the patient's head is continuous with the pelvic support straps; the loop can be attached to the hook on a wrecker crane for vertical lifts, although this would rarely be necessary. All five 2–inch belt buckles are made of polycarbonate plastic. The device is made of two layers of nylon mesh impregnated with plastic; these layers are sewn over ⅜-in. plywood slats, which act as stays.

XP–1. This device is very similar to the KED,

Figure 40–8. The XP-One (Extrication Plus One). The device is designed to be used with its own Philadelphia-type collar. (Med-spec, 4911 Wilmont Road, Charlotte, NC 28208; From Dick, T., and Land, R.: Spinal immobilization devices. Part II: Cervical extrication devices. J. Emerg. Med. Services 8:25, 1983. Used by permission.)

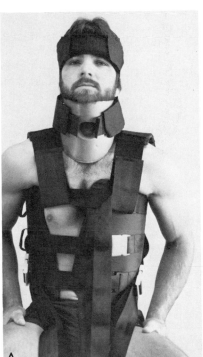
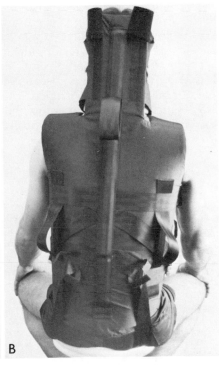

but it is designed to be used in conjunction with its own two-piece, Philadelphia-type, foam collar. The collar is velcroed into place by means of a pair of flaps that are part of the splint itself, providing an additional margin of rotational stability. A pair of velcro shoulder straps engage the top thoracic strap, keeping the thoracic panels snug in the axillae, an important weight-bearing concept, although most of the patient's weight during lifting is borne by the pelvic straps.

The device is slightly more flexible vertically than the KED, to allow easier placement on patients in bucket seats; this flexibility disappears when the splint is wrapped around the patient's thorax. Two layers of ballistic nylon are sewn over an inner layer of ⅜-in. reinforced polyethylene foam.

Full-Body Spinal Immobilizers[13]

There are three basic classes of full-body spinal immobilizers, each with advantages and disadvantages. It should be stressed that in the field it is more important for a rescuer to achieve results than to be particular about using one specific piece of equipment to do a given job, such as to immobilize the spine. This flexibility requirement is due to the immense variety of circumstances that can be encountered in the field; it necessitates a rescuer who understands both the anatomy of patients and the capabilities and limitations of rescue equipment.

Full-Body Spine Boards (Backboards)

There are probably as many different kinds of backboards (Fig. 40–9) as there are rescuers who know how to operate a power saw. Basically, backboards are either rectangular or tapered (like a coffin lid). The tapered, or Ohio type, is preferred by most rescuers, because it takes up less horizontal room when angled into narrow doorways (such as that of an automobile). In addition, the slight narrowing of these boards on either end

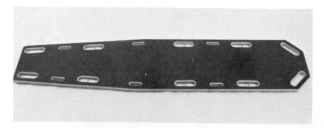

Figure 40–9. The Bound Tree spine board. An example of a commercial plywood back board. (Bound Tree Corporation, EMS Products Division, P.O. Box 401, Henniker, NH 03242; From Dick, T., and Land, R.: Spinal immobilization devices. Part III: Full spinal immobilizers. J. Emerg. Med. Services 8:34, 1983. Used by permission.)

of the recumbent patient tends to enhance the effectiveness of lateral immobilization via strapping.

Many boards also feature hardwood runners, usually about 1 inch thick, on their undersides. These serve both as stiffeners and as spacers. They "lift" the board slightly off the ground so that rescuers can get their fingers under the board during lifting. The runners limit the effectiveness of a board when a patient lying on a hard surface for reasons of space must be slid lengthwise onto the board rather than logrolled onto it.

Advantages of boards over full-body immobilizers are their ease of storage, their low cost and ready availability, and their extreme versatility. No single piece of rescue equipment can be used in as many ways. A victim can be slid out of an automobile onto a backboard (its most common application). Also, several boards can be used in conjunction with one another to form a chute to facilitate this process. They can even be used in conjunction with shoring jacks to help prevent cave-in when the patient is found in a ditch. Boards make good ramps in mud, good insulation against many electrical hazards, and improvised shelter during extrication in bad weather.

Disadvantages of boards as immobilizers are few, but two in particular are important. Boardlike splints, as a class, are the least comfortable of all immobilizers. Discomfort can be overcome by means of appropriate use of padding (e.g., small rolled towels), especially in the occipital area. A further disadvantage of the backboard as an immobilizer, ironically, is one of its advantages: it is slippery and by itself provides only one-dimensional immobilization. For this reason, the backboard is an unstable carrying device and must be used cautiously with the addition of lateral support straps. Furthermore, when the immobilized patient must be carried, a backboard is normally used in conjunction with a stretcher; otherwise, it is not used at all.

Scoop Stretchers

If a trauma victim has to be slid out of a tight location, a smooth backboard is probably the best immobilizer. If the victim is not in a tight location, the scoop stretcher is an ideal field immobilizer (Fig. 40–10). The scoop stretcher is comfortable, rigid, and adaptable to patients of various lengths and provides unobstructed radiographic transparency of the entire spine. If necessary, it can be almost instantly applied or removed without disturbing the position of the victim. The stretcher provides good lateral stability owing to the trough-like shape of its top surface. The device is also stable enough to be used for carrying purposes.

The scoop interferes slightly with the ischial ring of a half-ring traction splint but works well

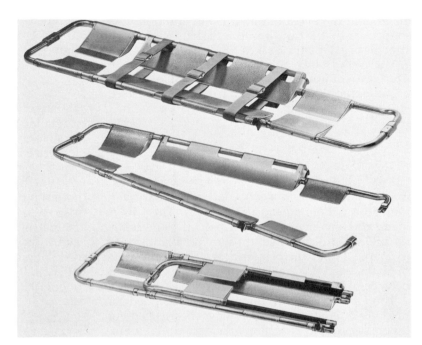

Figure 40–10. The Ferno-Washington Model 65 orthopedic (scoop) stretcher. (Ferno-Washington, Inc., 70 Weil Way, Wilmington, OH 45177; From Dick, T., and Land, R.: Spinal immobilization devices. Part III: Full spinal immobilizers. J. Emerg. Med. Services 8:34, 1983. Used by permission.)

in conjunction with the Sager traction splint. The scoop has no adverse effect on any other immobilizers, however, or on cardiopulmonary resuscitation (CPR). In fact, it is probably the best way to move a CPR patient in the field. The Ferno-Washington Model 65 Scoop is the most widely accepted stretcher of this type.

Full-Body Splints

There are various devices that take the concept of full-body immobilization one step further than the spine board. One such device, designed by

Los Angeles County Fire Department paramedic Larry Miller in the mid-1970's, is a narrow spine board shaped like the human body, with handles on both long edges and a system of harnesses to provide immobilization. The Miller Body Splint, as it is called, consists of a polyethylene shell injected with a closed-cell foam that provides buoyancy in water and also acts as a stiffener (Fig. 40–11). The full-body splint features a removable head harness, a thoracic harness, and pelvic and lower extremity belts, all with ample amounts of velcro as closures. The space between its "lower extremities" facilitates wrapping with bandage

Figure 40–11. The Miller Body Splint. (BP Systems, Inc., 2 Faraday St., Irvine, CA 92714–4198; From Dick, T., and Land, R.: Spinal immobilization devices. Part III: Full spinal immobilizers. J. Emerg. Med. Services 8:34, 1983. Used by permission.)

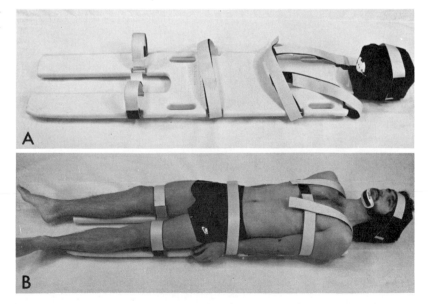

material in the event of fractures. In addition, it is shaped so that it can fit into a basket-type rescue stretcher such as the Stokes.

The Miller Body Splint is an excellent immobilizer; it is comfortable, firm and adaptable, as well as radiographically translucent. It can also be used as a water-rescue stretcher.

Pillow Harnesses

The Bashaw Cervical Immobilizer Device, or CID, is a pillow harness designed to be fastened quickly and easily to a scoop or spine board and then to a patient's head (Fig. 40–12). The CID is made of Herculite nylon and polyethylene foam; its pillows are fastened to a nylon platform by means of large velcro interfaces. The platform is then fastened to the stretcher, either by elastic belts or by non-elastic belts with buckled closures.

The CID is a superb immobilizer, designed for field use. Sandbags, which have been used for this purpose for years, are an adaptation of an in-hospital immobilizer. They work well on table tops but not in the field, although most rescuers use sandbags (or IV bags) and tape with a supine patient because of their lower cost.

COMPLICATIONS

In general, complications are more likely to occur as a result of *non*-immobilization of spinal injuries prior to movement than from immobilization. When complications do arise as a result of

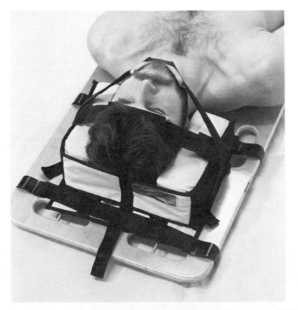

Figure 40–12. The Bashaw Cervical Immobilizer Device (CID). (Bashaw Medical, Inc., 4909-B Mobile Highway, Pensacola, FL 32506; From Dick, T., and Land, R.: Spinal immobilization devices. Part III: Full spinal immobilizers. J. Emerg. Med. Services 8:34, 1983. Used by permission.)

the type of care, however, it is probably related to improper choice or use of equipment and/or ignorance of concomitant problems.

Improper Choice (or Use) of Equipment

Emergency medical technicians who are trained by qualified instructors to understand the pathophysiology of forces in trauma rather than to memorize rules of treatment are the best guarantee *against* complications involving equipment. Implicit in the former type of training is gaining a thorough grasp of the capabilities and weaknesses of specific types of rescue equipment rather than an algorhythmic approach to treatment, such as is used in cardiac resuscitation. The wide variation of situations that are encountered routinely in the field call for a practical-sense approach to orthopedics, more than any other branch of field care.

Ingorance of Concomitant Problems

Immobilization of the victim's spine can impair the rescuer's ability to manage or recognize other priorities such as airway patency, comfort, or body position. Transport is also made more difficult.

Ideally, a spine board is kept waxed to aid in sliding patients onto or off of it. This does impair its effectiveness as a litter, and for reasons of slipperiness, backboards are not usually used as litters to carry victims long distances. Victims are generally excessively belted in place on a spine board to prevent sliding during transport. If too few straps are used or if the straps are loosely applied, transport becomes a problem. On the other hand, patients who are strapped too firmly in place have expressed extreme discomfort and even panic.

Once strapped into place, an unresponsive patient who vomits can be protected from aspiration in one of two ways. The traditional means is to logroll the patient, board and all, onto the left side and suction vigorously. No amount of strapping can keep this patient immobilized, however, and what actually takes place is that the spinal precautions are abandoned in favor of the airway. Another means is to quickly raise the foot end of the board so that vomitus drains into the pharynx. If the patient takes a breath while in this position, assuming incomplete filling of the pharynx, he can inspire without aspirating. Meanwhile, suction can be used to remove any emesis from the pharynx. Spinal precautions are not usually affected with this head-down tilt maneuver.

PROCEDURE

Once an extrication collar is in place, further spinal immobilization may be either difficult or relatively easy, depending upon the situation in which rescuers find the patient and the equipment available. For purposes of discussion, we shall assume ideal circumstances.

Despite the presence of an extrication collar, if room permits, it would be advisable to have a rescuer maintain manual cervical traction until the patient is fully immobilized, either in an extrication splint or on a full-body splint (such as a backboard). From that point onward, rescue procedures depend upon the patient's position of origin.

Sitting Position

The sitting patient is placed in an extrication splint by two (or possibly more) rescuers. He is then rotated into a position from which he can be laid in a supine position on a spine board, lateral immobilization can be applied, and he can be slid out of his environment onto a waiting cot that has been elevated to an appropriate level.

Prior to use, the extrication splint should be stored in such a way that its straps are secured in their individual retainers. This reduces the likelihood of their becoming tangled during application. When used, the device is opened up, butterfly-style, and gently slid behind the victim, with a rocking motion. If necessary, the rescuer who has been maintaining manual traction can gently rock the patient forward a few degrees, thus facilitating movement of the splint.

Once behind the victim, the splint's pelvic support straps should be freed from their retainers and allowed to dangle at the patient's sides. These straps would otherwise be trapped by the splint. Next, the lateral thoracic panels are brought forward beneath the patient's shoulders, and, grasping these panels, a rescuer *slides the splint upward until the top edges of the panels firmly engage the patient's axillae.*

Now the thoracic straps can be used to secure the splint, beginning with the middle strap, then the bottom strap, and lastly, the top strap. The straps should be fastened snugly but not tightly; all straps will be tightened slightly before the patient is moved.

Next, the head is fastened. When using the KED, the head panels are wrapped snugly around the head and neck by one rescuer while another rescuer applies the diagonal head straps. The forehead can be used as a point of engagement for one strap, and the cervical collar itself can be used for the other. The XP–1, on the other hand, has broad velcro straps that are fastened to the splint and are stored rolled up. The bottom pair of straps directly engages the mating velcro surfaces on the collar; these straps should be secured first. Next, the top pair of straps engage a removable forehead pad, which is velcroed into place.

In using either device, the pelvic support straps are those that are fastened next. They can be slipped, one at a time, beneath the patient's lower extremities, and *using a back-and-forth sawing movement, they can be brought directly beneath the pelvis.* This is a key point. If the pelvic straps are *not* applied in this way, they will allow considerable slippage when the patient is lifted. The free end of each of these straps mates with a buckle located approximately at the patient's hip on the outside of the splint. Once a strap is ready to be buckled, it can be attached either to the buckle on its own side or moved across the patient's lap and engaged with the opposite buckle. The latter method is preferred by most people, because it allows the patient's knees to remain together without discomfort to the patient. It should be noted that both methods work well.

Lastly, all buckles should be tightened until the entire splint seems to be firmly in place. (It may be necessary to leave the top strap untightened if the patient has any respiratory discomfort.)

The patient can now be moved. Neither the KED or XP–1 is designed specifically for lifting, although lifting is an accepted means of using the splints to get a patient out of a vehicle. If the patient is to be lifted from a vehicle, the ambulance cot, with a spine board on it (all belts and blankets having been removed) is brought as close as possible to the patient. One rescuer then supports the patient by the patient's knees while the other rescuer uses the handholds on the splint, which are located beneath and slightly behind the axillae (on the outside surface of the splint).

It is usually preferable to rotate the patient if possible, then lay him supine onto a backboard before removing him from the vehicle. Before the patient's hips are unflexed, the pelvic straps should be loosened or undone, because they tighten when the patient's thighs return to their anatomic positions.

With the patient now in a supine position on a board, he can be slid carefully out of his location and onto a waiting cot. Some type of lateral immobilizer may be applied, although both the KED and XP–1 provide substantial lateral support for the head and neck. The body should, however, be belted into place on the board.

If for any reason rescuers strongly believe that the patient should be transported in a Fowler's position, the long board may be waived and the patient placed on the cot without it. If the extrication splint causes the patient respiratory discomfort, the thoracic straps may be loosened or undone. In addition, if the splint is needed to extricate another patient, it can be removed from the first patient, with manual traction applied to the neck until the first patient is fully immobilized on the spine board. Furthermore, if the patient has a flail segment of the chest wall, firm application of the splint may reduce discomfort, although adequate respirations must be ensured. (The splint may be fully unfastened and left beneath a patient to facilitate examination of the chest.)

In the course of any extrication maneuver, special care should be taken to examine the lower extremities to ensure that instability in those areas is not overlooked in the interest of spinal protection.

Recumbent Position

A patient who is found in a recumbent position should be placed in a supine position , if he is not already in one. If such repositioning is necessary, it would be worthwhile to examine the back in the process, if possible, eliminating having to do so at a later time. Generally, having the victim in a supine position makes physical examination easier, makes transport more comfortable, and lends itself well toward the goals of immobilization and airway management.

Patients who are found lying in a supine position generally do not require the use of an intermediate immobilizer for the spine, such as an extrication splint. They should, however, receive initial immobilization by means of manual cervical traction and an extrication collar. After that, they are usually fastened to a full-body spinal immobilizer, such as a scoop stretcher, a backboard, or a full-body splint.

Scoop Stretcher. A patient who is in a supine position should be moved by means of a scoop stretcher if one is available and if there are no limitations of space. This device is easily applied, is comfortable once in place, and provides more lateral support for the torso than any other device. Additional means will be necessary to immobilize the head laterally. A scoop stretcher may be removed from beneath the patient, without disturbing the patient's position, after transport has taken place.

A scoop is applied as follows: Rescuers first explain to the patient that they are about to apply a scoop-type stretcher beneath him, that the stretcher may be cold to the touch initially, and that it is important that he not move. One rescuer applies manual cervical traction, even with a collar in place. Another rescuer places the scoop on the ground next to the patient and opens the latches that regulate its length. The length should be adjusted so that approximately 2.5 cm or more of space is allowed at the patient's head and feet.

The latches that regulate the length of the device should then be engaged. Two more latches are located at either end of the stretcher; these should be released next, enabling rescuers to separate the two halves of the stretcher. One half is placed on each side of the patient. Next, one rescuer gently pushes half the stretcher under one side of the patient, making allowances at the head and feet, while another rescuer gently rocks the patient, not more than about 1-cm elevation. Then the latch at the head end of the device is engaged. The same procedure takes place with the opposite half of the scoop until both halves are nearly beneath the patient. Now the foot-end latch can be engaged, completing the integrity of the stretcher. The patient can finally be strapped into place, his head immobilized with a pair of sandbags and tape or a pillow harness. The scoop stretcher is then lifted as a cot is rolled beneath the stretcher.

Whenever possible, a patient should be moved on wheels rather than be carried, regardless of whether he is in the bed of a pickup truck, on a cot, or in an ambulance. This minimizes the possibility of a rescuer slipping in an oil spot or tripping on glass or other debris commonly found at accident scenes. The scoop stretcher should *not* be used when the patient is in an automobile or other cramped environment and must be slid out.

Full-Body Spine Boards (Backboards). A cramped environment from which the patient must be slid out is precisely the circumstance in which a backboard works best. There are three means of getting a patient onto a spine board; the method used depends upon the amount and configuration of space available around the patient.

If a patient can only be moved lengthwise, as from an automobile seat, he may be slid, either footfirst or headfirst. Special care must be taken to ensure that rescuers move him by *pulling*, not by *pushing*. Traction minimizes the possibility that a spinal injury will accidentally be compressed.

The procedure should be explained to the patient. A cot is then brought as close to the vehicle as possible, in line with the move, at a level as close to or slightly below that of the patient. Oncoming traffic should be halted or kept at least two lanes away from the scene. One rescuer sits on the cot and keeps the end of the board from moving off the seat or doorsill of the automobile while another rescuer (preferably two rescuers) apply traction on the patient's body and slide the body onto the board. If the patient is being moved footfirst, a third rescuer should be inside the car directing the rate of movement and managing the head and neck in a normoflexed postion. Once the patient is completely on the board, the board is slid outward until it comes to rest on the cot.

If a patient is recumbent on the ground and a board is chosen as the means of movement, the patient can be logrolled onto it by at least two rescuers. The rescuers decide which way to roll the patient, and one rescuer takes a position at the patient's head. In addition to applying manual traction, it will be this person's responsibility to oversee the move, watching the patient's overall body position. The other rescuer takes a position on the side that the patient will be rolled *away* from and places the board within an arm's reach. He then raises the patient's knee that is on his side, extends the patient's arm that is on his side across the patient's chest, and grasps the patient by that elbow. Then, pushing the patient away from him, he brings the patient into a laterally recumbent position and uses one hand to grasp the patient by the hip and maintain the patient's position. He then uses his other hand to slide the board into place, being certain that the top edge of the board is flush with the top of the patient's head. Finally, both rescuers roll the patient back onto the board, center his body on it, and fasten him firmly in place. The board is then lifted while a cot is rolled beneath it.

A patient who is recumbent on the ground can also be slid sideways onto a spine board; this is usually an improvised means and requires three or four rescuers, one of whom can maintain control of the patient's head and neck.

CONCLUSIONS

The wide variety of circumstances in which a traumatized patient is likely to be involved mandates the need for many approaches to full-body spinal immobilization, before and during disentanglement. In general, however, an overall goal of rescuers is to fasten the victim to a boardlike full-body immobilizer. After early application of an effective cervical extrication collar, this process involves the following steps:

1. Application of a cervical extrication device that serves to immobilize the cervical and thoracic spine as well as put the patient into a "package" for removal from the scene. This sort of device is used when the patient is first encountered in a confined environment, such as a wrecked automobile or a bathtub. The device may have to be used for several patients.

2. Placement of the patient on a full-body spine board (also called a backboard), a scoop stretcher, or a factory-designed full-body immobilizer.

3. Application of lateral immobilization for the head. Traditionally, this has been done by means of sandbags placed on either side of the head, then taped in place. Currently, there are factory-manfactured devices that are comfortable, lightweight, and much more effective in the field setting.

4. Use of straps to fasten the patient securely to the stretcher or splint. These straps may best be applied diagonally, rather than transversely, to provide longitudinal immobilization against forces acting on the victim during acceleration and deceleration of the transporting vehicle.

5. Placement of the immobilized victim into a rescue litter, such as a Stokes basket stretcher, if

it is necessary to move him by foot, helicopter, or other special means prior to loading in an ambulance.

6. Clear, careful communication by rescuers to the receiving physician about the mechanism of injury, surrounding circumstances, and initial status of the patient, both prior to and following the disentaglement/immobilization process.

It should be remembered that rescuers may have to improvise or adapt extensively to circumstances that they encounter. The primary measure of success in field orthopedics is, therefore, the overall result, not the choice of equipment used or the rules that are followed in the process.

Lower Extremity Traction Splints

INTRODUCTION

Since World War I, when the Thomas Full-Ring (later to become a half-ring) Traction Splint was popularized for pre-hospital use, extremity traction for femur fractures has been an important aspect of pre-hospital orthopedic care. In fact, the splint devised by Sir Hugh Owen Thomas was credited with decreasing the mortality rate associated with fractures of the femur from 80 to 14 per cent during that period. Since then, several modifications of the traction splint have appeared. These earlier, modified traction splints carry the names of their inventors (Glenn Hare, Joseph Sager, and Dr. Allen Klippel) and have encouraged further refinements.

INDICATIONS AND CONTRAINDICATIONS

Application of a lower extremity traction splint is indicated whenever a fractured mid-shaft to distal femur is encountered, provided that the device can offer stabilization of the injury. Traction also minimizes the potential space for accumulation of blood in the thigh with a femur fracture. A femur fracture is clinically suspected when there is shortening, angulation, thigh-swelling, or thigh-ecchymosis of the injured extremity accompanied by pain on movement in the awake patient or creptitus in the unconscious or drug-altered patient. Traction splints may also be used for splinting proximal tibia fractures.

There is some controversy regarding the merit of applying traction to an open femur fracture. Concern has been expressed that standard traction will retract the bone fragments back into the tissue before adequate operative débridement can be accomplished. One workable philosophy is to use the traction device to apply sufficient traction to provide stabilization without actually retracting the bony fragments into the tissues. Alternatively, a vacuum (bean bag splint) could be substituted to immobilize the bony fragments in the position of presentation. In any case, stabilization of the fracture site to prevent further hemorrhage, neurovascular damage, and soft-tissue injury should take precedence over the theoretical risk of increased contamination, which would subsequently be managed surgically.

Another potential contraindication would be to use the traction splint on infants and very small children who can be satisfactorily splinted with a vacuum splint, arm board, or metal splint.

DEVICES

This discussion will be limited to several of the popular types of lower extremity traction splints. A comparison of these traction splints is provided in Figure 40–13.[14] With the exception of the Sager splint, the traction splints produce flexion at the hip joint because of their half-ring design. This flexion of up to 30 degrees will not allow complete fracture alignment unless the patient is in a reclining position or the lower extremity is elevated.[15] Furthermore, the Sager splint can be applied to the outside of the injured extremity using the supplied straps, thus making it more readily applied and more comfortable (especially for men).

PROCEDURE

The application of a traction splint device to an extremity with a femur fracture requires careful attention to associated soft-tissue injuries. In particular, the presence of distal pulses and capillary refill must be assessed prior to and following the application of the device. The loss of pulses or an increase in capillary refill time associated with the application of a traction splint requires that the position of strap application and the amount of applied traction be reassessed.

Whenever possible, the splinting procedure should be explained to the patient. There is always pain associated with the application of the traction splint, but the patient should be reassured that the resultant stabilization of the fracture is usually associated with diminished pain. When possible, the area of injury should be exposed. Open fractures should be managed as discussed in the section entitled Indications and Contraindications. If the injured leg is markedly deformed, it should first be straightened using manual traction and maintained in that position by an assistant.

If the splint has an adjustable bar, the non-injured extremity can be used for length adjustment. The splint will need to be approximately 10–15 cm longer than the heel. With the extremity slightly elevated, the half-ring splint is placed under the injured leg and brought firmly against the ischial tuberosity. The Sager device is either placed against the symphysis pubis or positioned laterally against the greater trochanter of the femur. When the padded end of the splint is placed in the crotch of male patients, care should be taken to move the genitalia out of the way. The thigh strap is now firmly secured.

An ankle harness is then placed about the ankle above the medial and lateral malleoli. The harness is attached to the distal end of the traction device, and traction is applied gradually. For the Sager device, the inner shaft of the splint is extended by opening the shaft lock and pulling the inner shaft out until the desired amount of traction is noted on the calibrated wheel at the distal end of the splint (Fig. 40–14). Approximately 10 per cent of body weight to a maximum of 22 to 25 pounds (10 to 12 kg) is adequate traction. The Hare traction splint uses a ratchet mechanism to apply traction to the ankle strap. The Klippel Pulsion splint uses a foot plate to strap the foot down; traction is applied by adjusting the length of the splint. After application of traction, distal neurovascular status should be rechecked. Prior to transport, supportive straps about the thigh, knee, and distal leg should be applied to vertically stabilize the extremity.

Removal of a traction splint should be performed in reverse order of application and should follow basic stabilization of the patient. The traction splint should be replaced by definitive stabilization of the fracture at that time.

SPECIAL CONSIDERATIONS

The traction splints in common usage can be applied prior to application of the Pneumatic Anti-Shock Garment (PASG). Except for the Sager splint, however, the application of a PASG over a traction splint is awkward and associated with an uneven pressure distribution under the PASG. The Sager splint has the additional advantage that it can be applied *after* application of the PASG as well as before PASG application.

Unless the patient is found in a hazardous environment (e.g., extremely cold surroundings), the shoe on the injured extremity should be removed prior to splinting so that pulses can be evaluated. Furthermore, change in color, temperature, and pulses distal to the injury can subsequently be monitored enroute to the hospital. The shoe can be removed by cutting only the shoelace, then simply pulling forward on the tongue of the shoe. The underlying sock can be removed with scissors. Exposure of the noninjured foot permits comparison of the extremities.

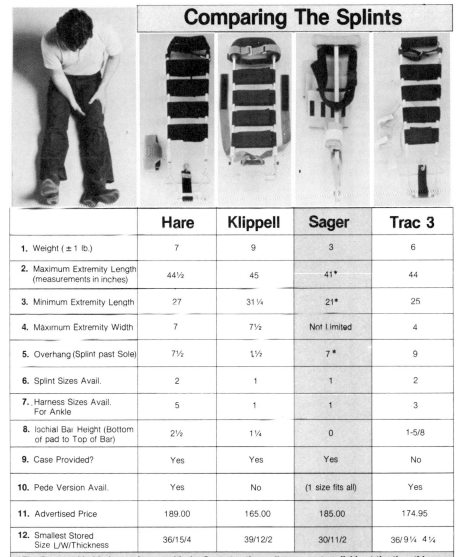

Comparing The Splints

	Hare	Klippell	Sager	Trac 3
1. Weight (± 1 lb.)	7	9	3	6
2. Maximum Extremity Length (measurements in inches)	44½	45	41*	44
3. Minimum Extremity Length	27	31¼	21*	25
4. Maximum Extremity Width	7	7½	Not Limited	4
5. Overhang (Splint past Sole)	7½	1½	7*	9
6. Splint Sizes Avail.	2	1	1	2
7. Harness Sizes Avail. For Ankle	5	1	1	3
8. Ischial Bar Height (Bottom of pad to Top of Bar)	2½	1¼	0	1-5/8
9. Case Provided?	Yes	Yes	Yes	No
10. Pede Version Avail.	Yes	No	(1 size fits all)	Yes
11. Advertised Price	189.00	165.00	185.00	174.95
12. Smallest Stored Size L/W/Thickness	36/15/4	39/12/2	30/11/2	36/9¼ 4¼

*The Sager ankle hitch now in use with the Sager traction splint was not available at the time this study was made. The new adjustable ankle hitch changed the following figures: *Maximum Extremity Length 46" *Minimum Extremity Length 18½" *Overhang of splint past sole, 5½" at 15 lbs. traction.

Figure 40–13. Comparison of traction splints. (From Dick, T.: Traction splinting: a comparative look at the tools of the trade. J. Emerg. Med. Services 6:26, 1981. Used by permission.)

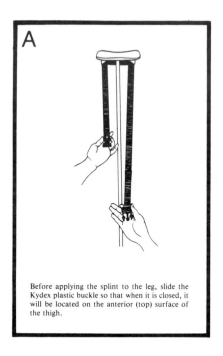

Before applying the splint to the leg, slide the Kydex plastic buckle so that when it is closed, it will be located on the anterior (top) surface of the thigh.

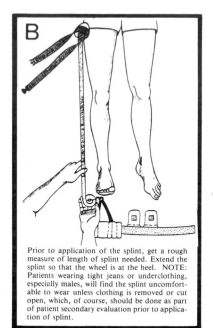

Prior to application of the splint, get a rough measure of length of splint needed. Extend the splint so that the wheel is at the heel. NOTE: Patients wearing tight jeans or underclothing, especially males, will find the splint uncomfortable to wear unless clothing is removed or cut open, which, of course, should be done as part of patient secondary evaluation prior to application of splint.

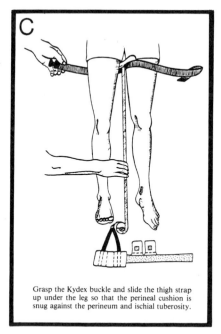

Grasp the Kydex buckle and slide the thigh strap up under the leg so that the perineal cushion is snug against the perineum and ischial tuberosity.

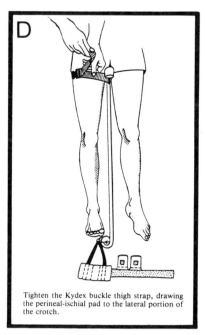

Tighten the Kydex buckle thigh strap, drawing the perineal-ischial pad to the lateral portion of the crotch.

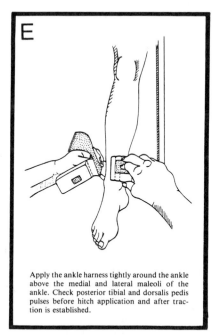

Apply the ankle harness tightly around the ankle above the medial and lateral maleoli of the ankle. Check posterior tibial and dorsalis pedis pulses before hitch application and after traction is established.

Figure 40–14. Application of the Sager Emergency Traction Splint. *A–J,* Standard application; *K–N,* Application on outside of leg; *O–Q,* Application of the bilateral splint.

Illustration continued on opposite page

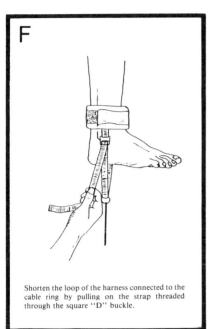

F

Shorten the loop of the harness connected to the cable ring by pulling on the strap threaded through the square "D" buckle.

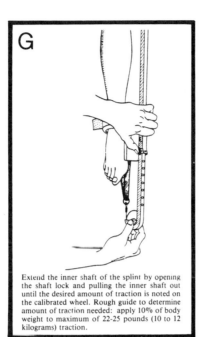

G

Extend the inner shaft of the splint by opening the shaft lock and pulling the inner shaft out until the desired amount of traction is noted on the calibrated wheel. Rough guide to determine amount of traction needed: apply 10% of body weight to maximum of 22-25 pounds (10 to 12 kilograms) traction.

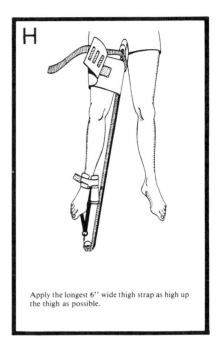

H

Apply the longest 6'' wide thigh strap as high up the thigh as possible.

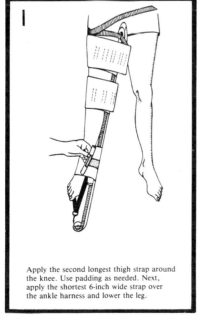

I

Apply the second longest thigh strap around the knee. Use padding as needed. Next, apply the shortest 6-inch wide strap over the ankle harness and lower the leg.

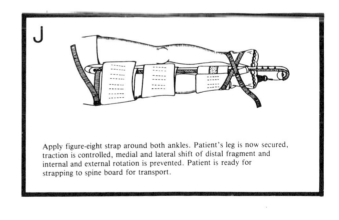

J

Apply figure-eight strap around both ankles. Patient's leg is now secured, traction is controlled, medial and lateral shift of distal fragment and internal and external rotation is prevented. Patient is ready for strapping to spine board for transport.

Figure 40–14 (Continued).

Illustration continued on following page

APPLICATION
ON THE OUTSIDE OF THE LEG

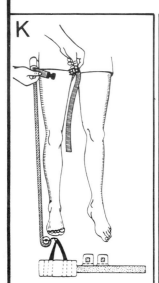

K

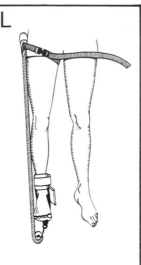

L

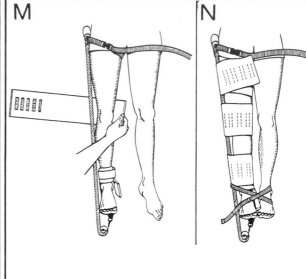

M

N

Application of Sager Splint on the outside of thigh is appropriate if perineal injuries or pelvic fractures are encountered. Carry out steps 1 and 2, then apply the splint on the outside of the leg as noted.

Leave the Kydex buckle thigh strap loose so that it makes a sling around the upper thigh and forms an angle of about 55 degrees with the shaft of the splint. Pad the strap as needed.

Apply the thigh straps in sequence, adding figure-eight strap as last step prior to securing the patient on the sping board.

APPLICATION OF THE BILATERAL
SPLINT

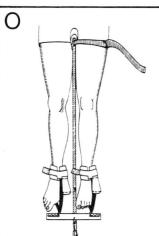

O

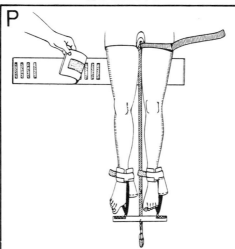

P

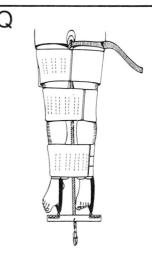

Q

Application of double splint is accomplished in same manner as with the single splint. Modify step 2 by lengthening splint so that the harness bar is adjacent to the patient's heels.

Apply the 6'' wide thigh straps, hooking together more than one thigh strap to give you a proper length to wrap strap around both thighs.

Apply all three sections of leg strapping to secure the legs together. A figure-eight strap may be used around ankles and feet, if needed.

Figure 40–14 (Continued).

COMPLICATIONS

Complications are generally the result of incorrect application of the device. If the neurovascular status is checked frequently, ischemia should not result from use of the splint. The key to traction application is stabilization of the fracture. Once the fracture site is stabilized, additional traction is unnecessary and potentially dangerous.

1. Farrington, J. D.: Death in a ditch. Bull. Am. Coll. Surg. 3:121, 1967.
2. Farrington, J. D.: Extrication of victims—surgical principles. J Trauma 8:493, 1968.
3. Dick, T., and Land, R.: Spinal immobilization devices. Part I: cervical extrication collars. J. Emerg. Med. Serv. (2):29, 1982.
4. Aprahamian, C., Thompson, B. M., and Finger, W. A.: Experimental cervical spine injury model: evaluation of airway management and splinting techniques. Presented at the 1982 Annual Meeting of the University Association for Emergency Medicine. April 15–17, 1982. Salt Lake City, Utah.
5. Podolsky, S., Baraff, L. J., Simon, R. R., et al., Efficacy of cervical spine immobilization methods. J. Trauma 23:461, 1983.
6. Kossuth, L.: Removal of injured personnel from wrecked vehicles. J. Trauma 5:704, 1965.
7. Committee On Emergency Medical Services, Division of Medical Sciences, National Academy of Sciences. Medical Requirements For Ambulance Design and Equipment. Pamphlet. (September, 1968).
8. Committee On Trauma, American College of Surgeons: Minimal Equipment for Ambulances. Bull. Am. Coll. Surg. 3:92, 1967.
9. Klippel, A., and Conrad, M.: A compact multipurpose spine board. Bull. Am. Coll. Surg. Nov.–Dec. 1969, pp. 1–4.
10. Grant, H., and Murray, R.: Emergency Care. Bowie, Maryland, Robert J. Brady Co./Prentice-Hall, Inc., 1971.
11. Committee On Injuries, American Academy of Orthopaedic Surgeons. Emergency care and transportation of the sick and injured. Menasha, Wisconsin, George Banta Company, 1971.
12. Dick, T., and Land, R.: Spinal immobilization devices. Part II: cervical extrication devices. J. Emerg. Med. Serv. 8:25, 1983.
13. Dick, T., and Land, R.: Spinal immobilization devices. Part III: full spinal immobilizers. J. Emerg. Med. Serv. 8:34, 1983.
14. Dick, T.: Traction splinting: a comparative look at the tools of the trade. J. Emerg. Med. Serv. 6(3):26, 1981.
15. Borschneck, A. G., and Wayne, M. A.: Sager emergency traction splint: a new splinting device for lower limb fractures. EMT J. 4:42, 1980.

41

Helmet Removal

JERRIS R. HEDGES, M.D.

Introduction

Although originally developed for protection of the head during combat, helmets are most commonly seen on injured football players and motorcyclists. The modern helmet is designed to tightly conform to the head. Interestingly, the modern helmet has protected the cranium so well that some football players have adopted the ill-advised technique of "spearing" an opponent with their helmets. This practice has been associated with cervical spine injuries.[1]

Careless removal of the helmet may exacerbate a pre-existing cervical spine injury. In 1980, the American College of Surgeons endorsed the helmet removal technique that is discussed in this chapter.[2]

Indications and Contraindications

Helmet removal in the pre-hospital area is rarely needed. Removal *is* indicated when the following conditions cannot be met with the helmet in place: airway control, cervical spine stabilization, and control of hemorrhage. Most motorcycle helmets have detachable or movable face masks that permit airway access in normal situations. Extrication bolt cutters (or preferably a screwdriver, if time permits) can be used to remove the "cage" face guard from football helmets. Cervical spine immobilization can usually be adequately maintained with the helmet in place using tape, sandbags (or intravenous bags), and a backboard, although some of the newer immobilization devices (e.g., CID-Cervical Immobilization Device) require prior removal of the helmet. Uncontrollable hemorrhage within the helmet cavity is rarely a problem because of the helmet's intrinsic protection of the cranium.

In the emergency department, removal of the helmet is indicated for a thorough head and neck examination, radiologic (including computed tomography) examination of the head and neck, and application of cervical tongs for traction. Obviously, when the helmet does not interfere with

Helmet Removal from Injured Patients

1

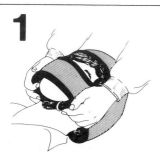

One rescuer applies inline traction by placing his or her hands on each side of the helmet with the fingers on the victim's mandible. This position prevents slippage if the strap is loose.

2

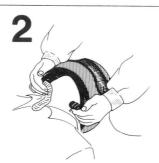

The rescuer cuts or loosens the strap at the D-rings while maintaining inline traction.

3

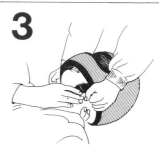

A second rescuer places one hand on the mandible at the angle, the thumb on one side, the long and index fingers on the other. With his other hand, he applies pressure from the occipital region. This maneuver transfers the inline traction responsibility to the second rescuer.

4

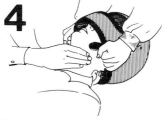

The rescuer at the top removes the helmet. Three factors should be kept in mind.

• The helmet is egg-shaped, and therefore must be expanded laterally to clear the ears.
• If the helmet provides full facial coverage, glasses must be removed first.
• If the helmet provides full facial coverage, the nose will impede removal. To clear the nose, the helmet must be tilted backward and raised over it.

5

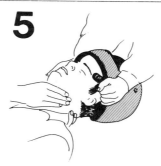

Throughout the removal process, the second rescuer maintains inline traction from below in order to prevent head tilt.

6

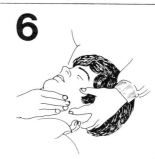

After the helmet has been removed, the rescuer at the top replaces his hands on either side of the victim's head with his palms over the ears.

7

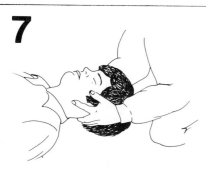

Inline traction is maintained from above until a backboard is in place.

Summary
The helmet must be maneuvered over the nose and ears while the head and neck are held rigid.
• Inline traction is applied from above.
• Inline traction is transferred below with pressure on the jaw and occiput.
• The helmet is removed.
• Inline traction is re-established from above.

American College of Surgeons Committee on Trauma, July 1980

Figure 41–1. Helmet removal technique. (From McSwain, N.: Bull. Am. Coll. Surg. 65:20, 1980. Used by permission.)

airway management, neck stabilization, or control of hemorrhage, removal of the helmet can be delayed by the emergency physician until the primary trauma survey and initial resuscitative measures have been undertaken.

Contraindications to helmet removal are lack of familiarity with the technique of removal, insufficient assistance (at least two persons are needed), and the need to provide higher priority tasks. As the rapid transport of injured patients from the pre-hospital phase to the hospital is stressed, the desirability of helmet removal in the pre-hospital situation will receive greater scrutiny.

Procedure[2]

The key to helmet removal is cervical immobilization. At the outset, prior to releasing the patient's chin strap, longitudinal traction should be applied to the neck (Fig. 41–1). The neck is then further stabilized by an assistant who places one hand on the anterior neck to support the mandible and the other hand posterior to the neck. The assistant can maintain an open airway by using the jaw thrust maneuver. The physician, situated cephalad to the patient, releases the chin strap while applying longitudinal traction on the base of the helmet. The helmet base is simultaneously spread apart, and the lateral aspects are sequentially pulled over each ear to remove the helmet while traction is continued. The helmet may also need to be tilted backward to clear the nose. After helmet removal, the spine is again immobilized

while the assistant maintains the manual cervical traction.

Complications

Although no controlled studies have proven this technique of helmet removal to be superior over other techniques, this technique is consistent with the current consensus policy of maintaining continuous in-line cervical traction when cervical spine injury is suspected. Furthermore, the lateral flexion/extension motion that is common with patient-initiated helmet removal is minimized.

Conclusions

Helmet removal is a skill that is easily learned. As more rapid transport from the pre-hospital area to the hospital is emphasized, more emergency physicians will be confronted with the helmeted patient. Helmet removal is necessary for a thorough examination, although initial resuscitative measures may take precedence over helmet removal.

1. Torg, J. S., Truox, R., Jr., Quedenfeld, T. C., et al.. The national football head and neck injury registry JAMA 241:1477, 1979.
2. McSwain, N. E., Jr.: Techniques of helmet removal from injured patient. Bull. Am. Coll. Surg. 65:19, 1980.

Introduction

"Injury occurs to the hand more frequently than to any other part of the body and the first person caring for an injured hand will probably determine the ultimate stage of its usefulness."[1] The rapid and proper primary care of a patient with an amputated part are crucial to salvage and preservation of function.

Amputations may be partial or complete. Injuries with interconnecting tissue between the distal and proximal portions, even if there is only a small piece of bridging skin, are technically considered incomplete, or partial, amputations. Complete amputations are replanted, whereas partial amputations are revascularized. This distinction is arbitrary, and for emergency physicians, treatment for both injuries is very similar. The prognosis and outcome of partial and complete amputations are similar, although partial amputations often have better venous and lymphatic drainage, and if there

42

Management of Amputated Parts

WILLIAM DALSEY, M.D.

is little anatomic damage, functional recovery may be more complete.

The peak incidence of traumatic amputations occurs between the ages of 20 and 40 years,[2, 3] and men predominate over women at a ratio of 4:1. Local crush injuries are the most common mechanism of injury, and guillotine amputations are the least common.[4-7] Partial amputations occur as often as total amputations.[8] Power saws and lawn mowers are frequently the instruments of destruction.[8] Proximal amputations are less common than distal amputations.

The media has somewhat exaggerated the success of replantation and has often generated unrealistic expectations from the public. The technical limitations of successfully repairing vessels less than 0.3 mm in diameter usually precludes replantation of digits distal to the distal interphalangeal (DIP) joint.[9] Successful revascularization of amputated parts often ensures viability, but neurologic, osseous, and tendinous healing are critical for ultimate function. If there is incomplete neurologic recovery, limited range of motion and cold intolerance, the replanted part may have little functional value for the patient. Rehabilitation from replantation surgery may be prolonged, often requiring in excess of a year and repeated surgical procedures. The emergency physician should be aware of the limitations of replantation surgery and should not encourage unrealistic expectations in injured patients or their family.

Historical Background

The possibility of restoring viability and function to traumatically severed parts has fascinated physicians for centuries. Physicians have attempted replanting parts with little more than a few sutures and secure bandaging, with an occasional spectacular result. One of the earliest medical reports is by Fiorvanti, who in 1570 reported the successful replantation of a soldier's nose, which was severed by a saber, after first cleansing it with urine and then carefully bandaging it.[10, 11] In 1814, Dr. Balfour reported the successful replantation of a finger, which was severed by a hatchet,[12] using only meticulous alignment and secure bandaging. The ability to consistently replant amputated parts awaited the development of modern microvascular surgical techniques. The first reported successful upper limb replantation was by Malt and McKhann in 1962.[13] Later that year, a successful replantation of a hand and arm was reported by Chen Zhang Wei.[14] Developments in microsurgical techniques, advanced optics, and microsurgical instruments have created the ability to consistently replant amputated parts with a high degree of success. Since 1965, when Kleinert and Kasdan reported the first successful microvascular anastomosis of a digital vessel,[15] there have been several large series of replantations, with success rates ranging from 70 to 90 per cent.[4, 8, 16-28] To the original pioneers in replant surgery, survival of the replanted tissue was the criterion for success, but with further refinements, today's surgeons emphasize functional recovery as well as viability.

The replantation of a part that will be painful or useless or that interferes with function is a disservice to the patient and is less desirable than early restoration of function without replantation.

Indications

Preservation of the amputated part is generally indicated when replantation or revascularization is a potential therapeutic modality for care of the injured part. Revascularization and reanastomosis of partially and completely amputated parts should be provided when there is hope of preservation or restoration of function. Aesthetic considerations, avocations, and occasionally religious or social customs may also influence the decision to proceed with surgery.[29-31] Ultimately, the decision must be reached by both the operating microsurgical team and the patient after a rational explanation of potential results and successes.

Indications for replantation of fingers and hands have been proposed and are generally accepted, though they should not be rigidly applied to all circumstances. Successful functional recovery is more likely in distal than in proximal amputations.[32, 33] Usually, multiple digit amputations, single digit thumb amputations, and transmetacarpal amputations are indications for replantation (Table 42–1).

Successful replantations have been reported in patients from the age of 1 year to 84 years.[34, 35] There are no fixed age limits for replantations, although particularly good results have been reported in children owing to their regenerative capacity and adaptability to rehabilitation.[3, 36-40] The decision to replant is made on a case-by-case

Table 42–1. REPLANTATION OF THE AMPUTATED EXTREMITY

Indications
Young stable patient
Thumb
Multiple digits
Sharp wounds with little associated damage
Upper extremity (children)

Absolute Contraindications
Associated life threats
Severe crush injuries
Inability to withstand prolonged surgery

Relative Contraindications*
Single digit, unless thumb
Avulsion injury
Prolonged warm ischemia (12 hr or more)
Gross contamination
Prior injury or surgery to part
Emotionally unstable patients
Lower extremity

*If the victim is a child or if there are multiple losses, salvage replantations are attempted and the relative contraindications are ignored.

basis by the microsurgical team, who must weigh all the factors involved.

Contraindications

There is no contraindication to managing the amputated part and stump as though replantation was to occur, even when replantation is considered unlikely by the emergency physician. The care of the whole patient must take precedence over the amputated part, although the requirements of the amputated part and stump can often be handled by ancillary personnel during resuscitation and transportation of the patient. Contraindications to replantation are listed in Table 42–1 and are discussed in the following sections. Note than even when replantation is contraindicated, tissue (skin, bone, tendon) from the amputated part may be useful in restoring function to other damaged parts.

General Considerations

MECHANISM OF INJURY

The potential for successful replantation in terms of survival as well as useful function is directly related to the mechanism of injury. Guillotine injuries, which are sharp, are the least common but have the best prognosis owing to the limited area of destruction. Crush injuries, which are the most common, produce more tissue injury and therefore have a poorer prognosis. The avulsion injury has the worst prognosis, because a significant degree of vessel, nerve, tendon, and soft-tissue injury invariably occurs.[3, 4, 6–8]

ISCHEMIA TIME

The time that an amputated part can survive prior to replantation is as yet undetermined. After 6 hours, additional delay may decrease the success rate of revascularization and lead to diminished function. Skin, bone, tendons, and ligaments tolerate ischemia much better than do muscle and connective tissue. Therefore, as a general rule, the more proximal the amputation, the less ischemia time the amputated part can tolerate. Attempts to extend viability during ischemia have shown that the most important controllable factor is the *temperature* of the amputated part. Warm ischemia may be tolerated for 6 to 8 hours.[41] When cooled properly to 4°C, 12 to 24 hours of ischemia may be tolerated with distal amputations.[3, 6–8, 16–28, 42] There is a report of successful digital replantation after 33 hours of cold ischemia.[42] The way in which hypothermia protects tissue from ischemia is cur-

rently under investigation. It has been theorized that hypothermia may limit metabolic demand, thereby preserving intracellular energy.[43–46] Other recent investigations suggest that the effect is due to the retardation in development of an acidotic pH.[47] Hypothermia may also prevent the no–reflow phenomenon that can follow low flow states.[48]

Delay in replantation of proximal arm and leg amputations with significant amounts of muscle tissue can lead to the build-up of toxic products. In such cases, when blood supply is restored, the absorbed toxic products have been reported to cause respiratory failure, renal failure, cardiovascular collapse, and even death.[49–56]

Perfusion techniques such as those used in organ transplants to extend anoxic time have not yet been developed. In the past, surgical teams used intraoperative perfusion as a technique to help cool the amputated part. The benefits of intraoperative perfusion with cold hypertonic solutions are currently being investigated. Perfusion should not be attempted by emergency physicians. The risk of damage to vessels and the potential delay in care and rapid transport of the patient and the amputated part override the theoretical benefits of emergency department cold perfusion at this time.[49, 57]

Special Considerations

HAND FUNCTION

Hand function is often determined in part by pinch and grasp functions. If the index finger is removed, the pinching function of the index finger is adequately provided by the middle finger. Power in grasping and gripping is mainly considered an ulnar function of the 4th and 5th digits. Effective grip that provides the ability to hold a variety of objects is a central function of the ring and middle fingers. In addition to its function in pinching, the thumb is the major opposing force for successful grip and grasp. The thumb is the most important digit for adequate hand function, and its loss results in 40 to 50 per cent disability. Such disability requires aggressive attempts to replant amputated thumbs. If this is impossible or unsuccessful, pollicization of other digits or toe transfers are secondary alternatives.[58–62]

LOWER EXTREMITY AMPUTATIONS

There are few reports of replantation of amputated parts of the lower extremity.[63, 64] Indications for replantation of amputated parts of the lower extremity are different than those for replantation of amputated parts of the upper extremity. The goal of all replantations is improved function. If this cannot be achieved, a patient is substantially better off with a prosthesis.

The lower extremity is primarily used for weight-bearing, thus providing the ability to ambulate. Lower limb prostheses, especially those used below the knee, are well tolerated and functional. Prostheses provide a secure stance and the ability for locomotion. Lower extremity replantation generally requires skeletal shortening, and distal nerve regeneration is often imperfect. Both deficits may produce dysfunction. A patient with a replanted lower extremity with significant shortening and without sensation would function better with a prosthesis. This is not necessarily true of an upper extremity replant. For these reasons, lower limbs are not generally replanted except under ideal circumstances, usually in children, although there are documented cases of successful lower extremity replantation in adults.[63, 64] The final decision regarding replantation should be left to the replantation team.

FINGERTIP AMPUTATION

Proper treatment of distal fingertip injuries is controversial. Fingertip amputations can heal by normal wound contracture, but this may result in loss of functional ability to palpate. In distal amputations in which the wound area is less than 10 mm,[2] this is not a problem (Fig. 42–1). The challenging problem of fingertip injuries is when there is significant loss of volar tissue. Volar skin is unique in its combination of toughness and sensitivity. Whereas small distal wounds or larger dorsal wounds heal well by secondary intention, wounds with significant volar tissue loss require additional treatment. Children, with their regen-

erative capacity, often progress very well when significant volar wounds are allowed to heal primarily. For older people and in amputations that involve a more significant amount of the distal digit, a wide variety of techniques for managing the injured fingertip have been advocated, including partial thickness skin grafts, full thickness skin grafts, VY, Kutler, Kleinert, and Island advancement flaps, as well as a variety of local and distal flap coverage techniques. Each of these procedures has its own indications, complications, and limitations.[65–69] Discussion of these procedures is beyond the scope of this chapter. Most of these techniques are best performed by a specialist in the operating room as primary procedures under ideal circumstances or as delayed procedures when necessary.

PENIS/EAR/NOSE AMPUTATIONS

Replantation of the penis, ear, and nose generally results in better function and cosmesis than a prosthesis or reconstructive surgery. The amputated parts and wounds should be handled as they are for digital replantations.

Penile amputations are an uncommon problem. Most cases result from self-inflicted trauma in patients who are severely psychologically disturbed. Successful replantation has been reported using microsurgical techniques. Preservation or reconstruction of the urethra to maintain a competent urinary stream is critical for success.[70–72]

Ears and noses are frequently partially amputated and are occasionally totally amputated. Whenever possible, these body parts should be replanted unless they are severely traumatized and there is gross contamination. These wounds frequently heal well, with a high survival rate and a low incidence of total necrosis. Replantation of these parts requires good suture technique and careful placement but does not necessarily require microsurgical techniques.[70, 71, 73]

Assessment of the Patient

The initial care and treatment of the patient who has had a part of his body amputated are the same as those for any trauma patient. The physician must not be distracted by the amputated extremity or the excitement of others from assessing and stabilizing the patient's airway, breathing, and circulation. Amputations are generally not life-threatening injuries, and other potentially more serious injuries must first be assessed and treated. Hemorrhage from amputated limbs is often limited by the retraction and spasm of severed vessels. Therefore, partial amputations may result in more serious hemorrhage than if the vessels were totally

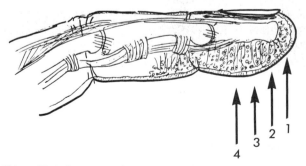

Figure 42–1. Successive levels of fingertip amputation. (1) Skin loss only at the tip responds nicely to simple dressing treatment. (2) Exposure of bone and a moderately severe loss of skin and soft-tissue padding. This can heal secondarily, but the result may not be ideal. (3) Loss of the entire convex soft-tissue fingertip pulp. Secondary healing will be marginal at best, and this should be repaired surgically. (4) Major loss of the entire fingertip in which severe fingernail deformity is anticipated. The choice is between major flap repair and disarticulation of the distal joint. (From Gaul, S. J., Jr.: Management of acute hand injuries. Ann. Emerg. Med. 9:139, 1980. Used by permission.)

severed. Usually, hemorrhage can be adequately controlled with direct pressure and elevation. *Vascular clamps and hemostats have no role in the emergency department management of these injuries and may cause additional injury, which may make replantation impossible.* A proximally placed blood pressure cuff inflated 30 mm Hg above systolic pressure can be used for short periods of time (30 minutes) to control severe bleeding, if necessary.

After initial primary assessment and treatment with subsequent stabilization of the patient, care of the stump and amputated part can safely be initiated. In addition to the general history obtained from all trauma patients, particular attention should be focused on the exact mechanism of injury, the time and duration of injury, handedness, allergies, medications, illnesses, prior injury to the affected part, care of the stump and amputated part prior to arrival, occupation, avocations, and tetanus history. In addition to radiographs of the amputated part and proximal stump to the level of at least one joint proximal to an extremity injury, preoperative laboratory studies should also be obtained. Tetanus prophylaxis and broad spectrum (e.g., cephalosporins) systemic antibiotic therapy should be initiated. Analgesic medications may be necessary, especially with crushing injuries, for managing patient discomfort. Some authors recommend the early use of aspirin and/or low molecular weight dextran for amputation patients, but such attempts to maintain small-vessel perfusion are controversial and have not been proven efficacious in preoperative treatment.

Amputation patients often experience denial, shock and disbelief, and feelings of hopelessness and helplessness about their injury;[6, 67] some people have even become suicidal. Amputation patients should be treated with supportive and realistic assurance, but unrealistic medical promises should be avoided.

Examination of the stump may be brief and should primarily be an assessment of the degree of damage to the surrounding tissue. Gross contamination can be removed by irrigation with normal saline. Local antiseptics, especially hydrogen peroxide or alcohol, *should not be used*, because they may damage viable tissues. Similarly, tissues should not be manipulated, clamped, tagged or further traumatized in any way. It is important to assess the degree of contamination, the level of injury, and any concomitant injury, such as crushing or multiple levels of injury or amputation.

The neurologic status of the stump or distal extremity in partial amputations should be assessed by pin prick and with two-point discrimination tests. The presence of sweat may indicate autonomic–neurologic functioning. Vascular competence can be assessed by noting the color, temperature, capillary refill, and presence of pulses. An Allen's test at the wrist or a modified Allen's test at each digit can aid in determining the existence of an arterial injury (see Chapter 26). The neurovascular status should be carefully and clearly documented in the medical record. Motor and tendon function should be evaluated immediately. The regional resource center should be contacted as soon as possible to arrange transportation and to provide adequate time for mobilization of the replantation team.

Care of the Stump and Amputated Part (Table 42–2)

The stump can be evaluated and primary care can be rendered during the secondary assessment of the trauma victim. If replantation is proposed, the goals of the initial care include control of hemorrhage and prevention of further injury or contamination. The stump should be irrigated with normal saline to remove gross contamination. Débridement and dissection should await the specialist. The stump wound should then be covered with a *saline-moistened* sterile dressing to prevent further contamination and to limit damage from desiccation. The stump should be splinted for protection and to prevent further injury from concomitant fractures or compromise of blood flow owing to a change in position. All jewelry should be removed. Splinting and elevation may reduce the extent of edema.

Care of the amputated part follows the same general guidelines as that for the stump. Gross contamination can be eliminated by irrigation with saline. All jewelry should be removed. The amputated part should be handled minimally to prevent further damage, and it should be wrapped in a saline-moistened sterile dressing. Direct immersion in hypotonic fluids should be avoided, because it may cause severe maceration of tissue and may make replantation more difficult technically. The amputated part should be cooled as soon as possible. The ideal temperature is 4°C. Care must be taken to prevent the freezing of tissues. Amputated parts should not be placed

Table 42–2. AXIOMS FOR CARE OF AMPUTATIONS

Do's	Don't's
Splint and elevate	Apply dry ice or freeze tissue
Apply pressure dressing	Place tags on tissue
Protect from further trauma or injury	Place sutures in tissue
Protect from further contamination	Sever skin bridges
Provide analgesia	Initiate perfusion of amputated part
Supply tetanus prophylaxis and antibiotic	Place tissue in formalin or water
Obtain radiographs	

directly on ice, because this may cause freezing of the tissue that is lying in direct contact with the ice. Currently, the recommended method for cooling amputated parts is to place the part, which is wrapped in saline-moistened gauze, in a watertight plastic bag and immerse the bag in a container with ice and water (Fig. 42–2). Cooling coils and refrigeration devices have occasionally been used but are generally not available and offer no significant advantages. The tissue containers should be labeled with the patient's name, the amputated part contained within, the time of the original injury, and the time that cooling began.

Treatment for partial amputations with vascular compromise is the same as that just described. Clean the wound with normal saline irrigation. Place a saline-moistened sponge on the open tis-

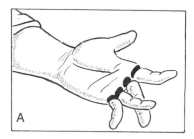

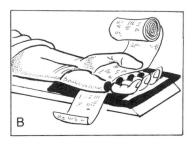

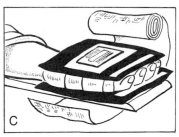

Figure 42–3. For a partial amputation *A*, rinse with saline, place part(s) in a functional position, apply dry sterile dressing *B*, splint and elevate *C*. Apply coolant bags to the *outside* of the dressing. *Do not scrub or apply antiseptic solution to wound.* Control bleeding with pressure. If a tourniquet is necessary, place it close to the amputation site. (From Hand Trauma: Emergency Care. Maryland Emergency Services.)

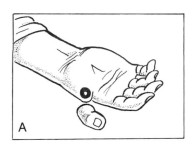

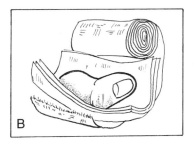

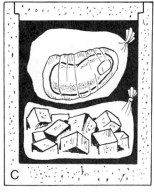

Figure 42–2. *A*, Evaluate the patient's condition to ensure that he does not need to be resuscitated before transfer. *B*, The wound should be rinsed with saline solution. *Do not scrub or apply antiseptic solution to the wound.* Apply dry sterile dressing, wrap in kling or kerlix for pressure, and elevate. *C*, The amputated part should be rinsed with saline. *Do not scrub or apply antiseptic solution to the amputated part.* Wrap it in moist sterile gauze or a towel, depending upon size, and place in a plastic bag or plastic container. The part is then put in a container, preferably Styrofoam, and cooled by separate plastic bags containing ice. (From Hand Trauma: Emergency Care. Maryland Emergency Services.)

sue, and wrap the injury in a sterile dressing, incorporating a splint to protect it from further injury. Ice packs or commercial cold packs should be applied over the dressing to cool the devascularized area (Fig. 42–3).

Complications

The care of amputated parts should not lead to avoidable complications if the aforementioned principles are followed. Improper management of the parts or stump with subsequent additional injury of the tissue from overzealous hemostasis or cleansing should be avoided. Furthermore, desiccation, maceration, or freezing of tissue from improper storage should not occur. The physician must consider expediting the preoperative workup of the patient and immediate notification of the replantation team as crucial factors in the patient's care.

Despite optimal initial care, replantation itself may be associated with acute or long-term complications. There is the usual risk of anesthesia and protracted surgery. Postoperative complications include vascular thrombosis, hemorrhage, infection, and reaction to accumulated toxins. It is not unusual for emergent second and third operations to be required to re-establish adequate blood flow. Patients are often placed on anticoagulants, which create an additional risk. Toxins accumulate in ischemic amputated parts despite cooling. The amount of toxins is directly proportional to the amount of muscle mass and the duration of ischemia. Reports of significant pulmonary failure, electrolyte disturbance, and even death have been reported in replantation efforts.

Later complications include a significant percentage (60 per cent) of patients with cold intolerance, limited function, anesthesia, pain, paresthesias, malunions, and nonunions. Repeated operative procedures may be required to obtain a functionally useful result. To minimize the morbidity from amputations, proper initial care is essential and may be the most important determining factor in the patient's eventual outcome.

1. Kleinert, H. E., and Raber, R. M.: Compendium on hand surgery. 19, 1973.
2. Tamai, S.: Digit replantation: analysis of 163 replantations in an 11-year period. Clin. Plast. Surg. 5:195, 1978.
3. May, J. W., and Gallico, G. G.: Upper extremity replantation, current problems in surgery. 17:634, 1980.
4. Weiland, A. J., et al.: Replantation of digits and hands: analysis of surgical techniques and the fusal results in 71 patients with 86 replantations. J. Hand Surg. 2:1, 1977.
5. Morris, R. L., et al.: Assessment of viability in transplanted tissue-electromagnetic flowmeter. Microsurgical Composite Tissue Tranplantation. St. Louis, The C. V. Mosby Co., 1979, p. 208.
6. Morrison, W. A., O'Brien, B. M., and MacLeod, A. M.: Evaluation of digital replantation—a review of 100 cases. Orthop. Clin. North Am. 8:295, 1977.
7. Morrison, W. A., O'Brien, B. M., and MacLeod, A. M.: Digital replantation and revascularization: a long-term review of one hundred cases. Hand 10:125, 1978.
8. Kleinert, H. E., et al.: Digital replantation—selection technique and results. Orthop. Clin. North Am. 8:309, 1977.
9. Kleinert, H. E., and Tsai, T. M.: Microvascular repair in replantation. Clin. Orthop. 133:205, 1978.
10. Fiorvanti, L.: In Tesoro della vita Humana. Venetia, Appresso gli heredi di M. Sessa, 1570.
11. Gibson, T.: Early free grafting: the restitution of parts completely separated from the body. Br. J. Plast. Surg. 18:1, 1965.
12. Balfour, W.: Two cases, with observations, demonstrative of the powers of nature to reunite parts which have been, by accident, totally separated from the animal system. Edinburgh Med. Surg. J. 10:421, 1814.
13. Malt, R. A., and McKhann, C. E.: Replantation of severed arms. JAMA 189:716, 1964.
14. Chen, C. W., and Pao, Y. S.: Salvage of the forearm following complete traumatic amputation; report of a case. Clin. Med. J. 82:633, 1963.
15. Kleinert, H. E., and Kasdan, M. L.: Anastomoses of digital vessels. J. Kentucky Med. Assoc. 63:106, 1965.
16. Yoshizu, I., et al.: Replantation of untidily amputated finger, hand, and arm. J. Trauma 18:194, 1978.
17. Sclenker, J. D. et al.: Methods and results of replantation following traumatic amputation of the thumb in 64 patients. J. Hand Surg. 5:63, 1980.
18. O'Brien, B. M.: Replantation surgery. Clin. Plast. Surg. 1:405, 1974.
19. O'Brien, B. M.: Replantation and reconstructive microvascular surgery. Ann. Roy. Coll. Surg. 58:87, 1976.
20. O'Brien, B. M., et al.: Clinical replantation of digits. Plast. Reconstr. Surg. 52:490, 1973.
21. O'Brien, B. M., and Miller, G. D.: Digital reattachment and revascularization. J. Bone Joint Surg. 55A:714, 1973.
22. Tsai, T. M.: Experimental and clinical application of microvascular surgery. Ann. Surg. 2:169, 1975.
23. Biemer, E., et al.: Results of 150 replantations on the upper extremity with microvascular surgery. Paper at Third Composium Eur. Sect. I.V.P.R.S. The Hague, Netherlands, May 1977.
24. May, J. W., et al.: Digital replantation distal to the PIP joint. J. Hand Surg. 7:161, 1982.
25. Kleinert, H. E., et al.: An overview of replantation and results of 347 replants in 245 patients. J. Trauma 20:390, 1980.
26. Urbaniak, J. R., et al.: Experimental evaluation in microsurgical techniques in small artery anastomosis. Orthop. Clin. North Am. 8:249, 1977.
27. Bancke, H. J., et al.: Replantation surgery in China. Plast. Reconstr. Surg. 52:476, 1973.
28. Zhang-Wei, Chen, et al.: Present indications and contraindications for replantation as reflected by long-term functional results. Orthop. Clin. North Am. 12:849, 1981.
29. Buncke, H. J., et al.: Replantation surgery in China. Report of the American Replantation Mission to China. Plast. Reconstr. Surg. 52:476, 1973.
30. Beasley, R. W.: General considerations in managing upper limb amputations. Orthop. Clin. North Am. 12:743, 1981.
31. Wilson, C. S., et al.: Replantation of the upper extremity. Clin. Plast. Surg. 10:85, 1983.
32. Malt, R. A., and Smith, R. J.: Limb replantation: selection of patients and technical considerations. Vascular Surgery. Philadelphia, W. B. Saunders Company, 1978.
33. Lendway, P. G.: Replacement of the amputated digit. Br. J. Plast. Surg. 26:398, 1973.
34. Ping-Chung, L.: Hand replantation in an 83-year-old woman—the oldest replantation? Plast. Reconstr. Surg. 64:416, 1929.
35. Sekiguchi, J., and Ohmdri, K.: Youngest replantation with microsurgical anastomosis: a successful replantation of a finger on an infant, aged 12 months and 15 days, by microsurgical repair is reported. Hand 11:64, 1979.
36. Van Beek, A. L., et al.: Microvascular surgery in young children. Plast. Reconst. Surg. 63:457, 1979.
37. Stelling, F. H.: Surgery of hand in children. J. Bone Joint Surg. 45A:623, 1963.
38. Wakefield, A. R.: Hand injury in children. J. Bone Joint Surg. 45A:1226, 1964.
39. Green, D. P.: Hand injury in children. Ped. Clin. North Am. 24:4, 1977.
40. Jaeger, S. H., et al.: Upper extremity replantation in children. Orthop. Clin. North Am. 12:897, 1981.
41. Berger, A., et al.: Replantation and revascularization of amputated parts of extremities: a three-year report from the Viennese replantation team. Clin. Orthop. 133:212, 1978.
42. Sixth People's Hospital, Shanghai: Reattachment of traumatic amputations. A summing up of experience. Chinese Med. J. 1:392, 1967.
43. Hayhurst, J. W., et al.: Experimental replantation after prolonged cooling. Hand 6:134, 1974.
44. Lapchinsky, A. G.: Recent results of experimental transplantation of preserved limbs and kidneys and possible use of this technique in clinical practice. Ann. N.Y. Acad. Sci. 87:539, 1960.
45. Levy, M. N.: Oxygen consumption and blood flow in hypothermic perfused kidney. Am. J. Physiol. 197:1111, 1959.
46. Tsai, Tsu Min, et al.: The effect of hypothermia and tissue

perfusion on extended myocutaneous flap viability. Plast. Reconst. Surg. 70:444, 1982.

47. Osterman, A. L.: Hypothermic muscle ischemia: a bio-energetic study using 31p nuclear magnetic resonance spectroscopy. J. Trauma 23:654, 1983.

48. May, J. W., et al.: The no–reflow phenomenon in experimental free flops. Plast. Reconstr. Surg. 61:256, 1978.

49. Razaboni, R., and Shaw, W. W.: Preservation of tissues for transplantation and replantation. Clin. Plast. Surg. 7:211, 1980.

50. Cooney, W. P., et al.: Replantation of above-elbow traumatic amputations. J. Trauma 23:631, 1983.

51. Ferreira, M. C., et al.: Limb replantation. Clin. Plast. Surg. 5:211, 1978.

52. Wilson, C. S., et al.: Replantation of the upper extremity. Clin. Plast. Surg. 10:85, 1983.

53. Chen, C. W., et al.: Extremity replantation. World J. Surg. 2:513, 1978.

54. Matsuda, M., et al.: Long-term results of replantation of 10 upper extremities. World J. Surg. 2:603, 1978.

55. Tamai, S., et al.: Major limb, hand, and digital replantation. World J. Surg. 3:17, 1929.

56. O'Brien, B. M., et al.: Major replantation surgery in the upper limb. Hand 6:217, 1974.

57. Harashina, T., and Buncke, H. J.: Study of washout solutions for microvascular replantation and transplantation. Plast. Reconstr. Surg. 56:54, 1975.

58. Strauch, B.: Microsurgical approach to thumb reconstruction. Orthop. Clin. North Am. 8:319, 1977.

59. O'Brien, B. M., et al.: Hallux to hand transfer. Hand 7:128, 1975.

60. Buck-Gramcko, D.: Thumb reconstruction by digital transposition. Orthop. Clin. North Am. 8:329, 1977.

61. Bunnel, S.: Physiologic reconstruction of a thumb after total loss. Surg. Gynec. Obstet. 52:245, 1931.

62. Little, J. W.: On making a thumb: one-hundred years of surgical effort. J. Hand Surg. 1:35, 1976.

63. Morrison, W. A., et al.: Major limb replantation. Orthop. Clin. North Am. 8:343, 1977.

64. Jupiter, J. B.: Salvage replantation of lower limb amputation. Plast. Reconstr. Surg. 69:1, 1982.

65. Flatt, A.: The Care of Minor Hand Injuries. St. Louis, The C. V. Mosby Co., 1959.

66. Illingworth, C. M.: Trapped fingers and amputated fingertips in children. J. Pediatr. Surg. 9:853, 1974.

67. Cowley, R. A.: Hand–emergency care including replantation. Collected papers in EM Surgery and Traumatology. May 9, 1976.

68. Schwartz, G. R., et al.: Principles and Practice of Emergency Medicine. Philadelphia, W. B. Saunders Company, 1978, pp 725–726, 759–760, 208.

69. Simon, R. R., and Carter, P. R.: Symposium on trauma. 1982 Scientific Assembly, San Francisco, California.

70. Strauch, B., et al.: Replantation of amputated parts of the penis, nose, ear, and scalp. Clin. Plast. Surg. 10:115, 1983.

71. Grabb, W. C., and Dingman, R. O.: The fate of amputated tissues of the head and neck following replacement. Plast. Reconstr. Surg. 49:28, 1972.

72. Best, J., and Angelo, J.: Complete traumatic amputation of the penis. J. Urol. 87:134, 1962.

73. Mohler, L. R., et al.: Replantation and revascularization replant potentiality. Ohio State Med. J. 75:395, 1979.

43

Management of Common Dislocations

JOHN L. LYMAN, M.D.
MICHAEL E. ERVIN, M.D.

Introduction

Joint dislocations are frequent presenting complaints of patients evaluated in emergency departments. At times, a dislocation is seen in association with other more dramatic problems in which case the dislocation may not be the chief complaint. Emergency physicians must be able to recognize a variety of dislocations as well as direct their management.

This chapter addresses the diagnosis and management of common dislocations. With most dislocations, there are a variety of reduction techniques, many of which have been called "the best" by different authors. This chapter will not describe all techniques; rather, it presents one or two methods that are relatively safe and easy to perform to accomplish reduction. The emphasis of this chapter is on isolated dislocations, not fracture-dislocations. Major fracture-dislocations may require slightly different principles of management, and as a general rule, most fracture-dislocations require prompt orthopedic consultation.

Analgesia

Recommendations for types and quantities of analgesics and muscle relaxants vary greatly, and each physician has his own favorite regimen. Selection of such agents is based on several factors, including the type of injury, the patient's allergy history, the patient's age and underlying medical condition, and the physician's familiarity with the drugs available. Whereas some dislocations will require high doses of intramuscular (IM) or intravenous (IV) analgesic and muscle relaxant agents to facilitate reduction, others require a minimum of such medication.

Often, the key to a successful reduction is adequate analgesia and muscle relaxation. The judicious use of analgesics results in a smooth, less traumatic, and less painful procedure. A variety of narcotic analgesics are available. These agents can be administered either intramuscularly or intravenously, with the onset of action and the time to peak effect being somewhat quicker with intravenous administration. Useful parenteral medications include meperidine (Demerol) 1 to 2 mg/kg IM (adult and pediatric populations), morphine sulfate 0.1 to 0.2 mg/kg IM or IV, fentanyl (Sublimaze) titrated IV (up to 0.002 mg/kg), and hydromorphone (Dilaudid) 1 to 2 mg IV (not recommended for pediatric population). These medications may be readily reversed with naloxone. Titration to effect while observing cardiovascular and respiratory function is mandatory when using these agents.

The drug of choice for muscle relaxation is diazepam (Valium) 5 to 10 mg IV (adult) or 0.1 to 0.2 mg/kg IV (pediatric). Intramuscular diazepam is of little value for acute reductions. Furthermore, diazepam should be used with caution in the very young and the very old, and respiratory support should be available for all patients. A combination of narcotics and diazepam may also be used quite effectively. A reasonable regimen is to use narcotics intramuscularly initially while awaiting radiographs, then supplement them with diazepam intravenously for the actual reduction. Dislocations that must be reduced quickly may mandate the concomitant use of intravenous narcotics and diazepam. A common pitfall is to underuse analgesics in acute reductions, thereby making the procedure more painful for the patient and more difficult for the physician.

Some joints can be adequately anesthetized with nerve blocks or injection of a local anesthetic. The digits are particularly amenable to nerve blocks, for example a proximal interphalangeal (PIP) joint dislocation of the hand can often be reduced after a digital block. A metacarpophalangeal dislocation of the thumb may be more readily reduced with local lidocaine injection. See Chapter 32 for a description of local and regional anesthesia.

In some incidences, general anesthesia will be required. Those dislocations that may require general anesthesia will be indicated.

All procedures should be explained to the patient prior to their initiation. Patients like to know what is going to happen and what to expect; they do not appreciate surprises. Some of the reduction techniques require an extensive amount of time to accomplish. During the reduction procedure, the physician should talk to the patient in a calm manner, explain the procedure, and attempt to relax the patient. This has been referred to as *vocal anesthesia*.

General Principles of Management

1. Dislocations are often associated with fractures that may not be evident on physical examination. For this reason, radiographs should be obtained for joint dislocations prior to and following reduction. Exceptions to this may be made when vascular embarrassment is present and when there may be some delay in obtaining a radiograph. Some cases of radial head subluxation in children do not require films. Some fractures will not be evident until a postreduction film has been taken.

2. Joint dislocations are described in terms of where the distal articulating surface ends up relative to the proximal articulating surface. For example, in an anterior shoulder dislocation, the humeral head (distal articulating surface) takes a position anterior to the glenoid fossa (the proximal articulating surface).

3. A subluxation ("partial dislocation") occurs when there is a joint disruption but the articulating surfaces are maintained in some degree of apposition.

4. Acute dislocations may reduce spontaneously or be reduced by direct patient intervention prior to presentation in the emergency department. If the physician suspects that a dislocation has been reduced prior to examination in the emergency department, the joint injury should be treated as if a dislocation or subluxation did in fact occur.

5. Once a dislocation has been reduced, postreduction films should be taken, both to verify and document reduction and to evaluate for subtle fractures. It is important to immobilize the joint prior to having radiographs taken, because the joint may be unstable and may redislocate with minimal movement.

6. Inability to relocate a dislocated joint does not necessarily mean that an improper technique has been used. Some dislocations are irreducible by a closed technique, most commonly because of the interposition of soft tissue. Persistent attempts at relocation when soft tissue is interposed lead to further trauma of the joint and surrounding tissue. After one or two unsuccessful attempts at relocation, appropriate referral for possible open reduction or an attempt at closed reduction under general anesthesia should be made.

7. A properly reduced joint dislocation not only will relieve pain but also will relieve stress on the surrounding soft tissues. The corollary to this statement is that the sooner a joint is reduced, the sooner the stress on the neurovascular bundles is relieved.

8. The neurovascular and circulatory status of the affected extremity should be checked imme-

diately upon the patient's presentation to the emergency department. Any compromise of these structures indicates that prompt action should be taken. The neurovascular status must also be reassessed and documented after reduction.

9. Three keys to successful reduction are 1) knowledge of the anatomy and reduction manuever, 2) use of proper analgesia, and 3) proceeding in a slow and gentle manner.

10. The physician must understand the importance of a complete and appropriate patient history, including the mechanism of injury and any previous injuries to the joint.

11. The physician should know common associated musculoskeletal injuries. For example, knee injuries in a motor vehicle accident should alert the physician to the possibility of a posterior hip dislocation. Also, when there is a fracture of the proximal ⅓ of the ulna, the physician should be aware of the possibility of a radial head dislocation (Monteggia's fracture).

12. The postreduction treatment is as important as the reduction itself. Following reduction, the joint must be properly splinted. *An acute joint dislocation is not a minor injury.* Because there is always concomitant muscular, ligamentous, or other soft-tissue disruption with any dislocation, disability is often the end result. Because soft-tissue swelling and muscle spasm may initially obscure joint instability or disability, proper follow-up is mandatory.

13. It is imperative that the physician understand the complications and possible sequelae of the various types of dislocations.

14. Before attempting a reduction, the physician must be properly prepared in terms of adequate assistance.

Shoulder Dislocations

The shoulder is designed for a large range of motion, with a large humeral head resting on a shallow glenoid fossa. This anatomical arrangement allows for a wide range of motion, but there is a relative lack of stability. Most shoulder dislocations are anterior; the humeral head comes to rest in a position anterior to the glenoid fossa. The next most common shoulder dislocation is the posterior dislocation. Inferior (luxatio erecta), superior, and intrathoracic dislocations are rarely seen. Although anterior dislocations are usually relatively apparent on clinical examination, posterior dislocations may be difficult to appreciate clinically and radiographically. Posterior dislocations are the most commonly overlooked dislocation in the emergency department. Such dislocations may occur during a grand mal seizure or as the result of an electric shock. Shoulder

dislocations are uncommon in young children. In this age group, the most common major joint dislocation is the elbow.

When a shoulder is dislocated, there is, necessarily, some surrounding soft-tissue trauma. Despite proper reduction and follow-up care, some people are left with weakness in the surrounding soft tissue of the shoulder, which allows recurrent dislocations. Often these recurrent dislocations are the result of minor joint-positioning, such as raising one's arm over the head to comb the hair or rolling over in bed. Although recurrent dislocations can be reduced by the techniques described, surgical intervention may be needed to prevent subsequent dislocations.

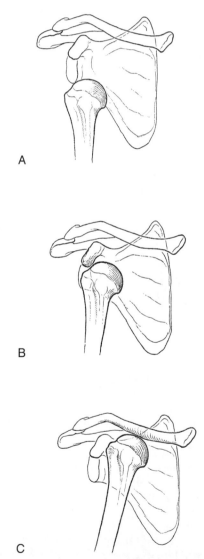

Figure 43–1. Types of anterior dislocations. All types of anterior dislocations should receive the same treatment. *A*, Subglenoid dislocation (rare type); *B*, subcoracoid dislocation (most common type); and *C*, subclavicular dislocation (rare type). (From DePalma, A. F.: Management of Fractures and Dislocations: An Atlas. Philadelphia, W. B. Saunders Company, 1970, p. 617. Used by permission.)

ANTERIOR SHOULDER DISLOCATIONS

Anterior shoulder dislocations are the most common major joint dislocations in adults. They account for most of the shoulder dislocations seen in the emergency department. An anterior shoulder dislocation is usually the result of forceful abduction and external rotation of the humerus. A direct blow to the posterior aspect of the humeral head may also result in an anterior dislocation.

There are three subtypes of anterior dislocations that are named according to where the humeral head lies. The humeral head may lie in a position beneath the clavicle (subclavicular), beneath the coracoid process (subcoracoid, most common), or anterior and inferior to the glenoid fossa (subglenoid) (Fig. 43–1). All these anterior dislocations can be reduced in the same manner.

Typically, when the patient presents, he is supporting the injured extremity in some manner and is resisting any movement of the shoulder (Fig. 43–2). The shoulder is usually held in slight abduction. If trauma was minimal or if the patient has minimal pain in the joint area, the dislocation is probably recurrent rather than an initial injury. Physical examination will usually reveal a loss of the deltoid contour of the shoulder when compared with the normal side. The dislocated humeral head may be palpable, although this is often not possible due to soft-tissue swelling. Manipu-

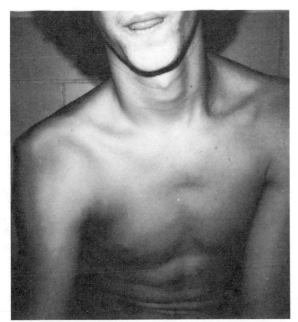

Figure 43–2. Typical presentation of an anterior shoulder dislocation. The shoulder is very painful; thus, the patient resists movement. The outer round contour of the shoulder is flattened, and the displaced humeral head may be appreciated in the subcoracoid area. Often the patient will slightly abduct the arm, bend the torso toward the injured side, and support the flexed elbow on the injured side with the other hand.

lation of the shoulder is not indicated until radiographs have demonstrated the pathology and associated fractures have been identified. The need for prereduction radiographs in the patient who suffers a *recurrent* dislocation in the *absence* of trauma must be individualized. In all cases, postreduction films are essential.

It is extremely important that the neurovascular status of the affected extremity be assessed early in the evaluation. Circulatory status can be quickly checked by comparing peripheral pulses. The neurologic status should include evaluation of all the major nerves of the arm (Fig. 43–3). The axillary nerve is the most commonly injured nerve in anterior shoulder dislocations. Injury of this nerve may produce an area of anesthesia on the upper lateral aspects of the arm (Fig. 43–4) and can result in paralysis of the deltoid muscle. Deltoid function is often difficult to evaluate in the acutely painful shoulder, but sensory evaluation can be accomplished without difficulty. Usually axillary nerve injuries are transient and resolve with time. The presence of an axillary nerve injury does not change the initial treatment of an anterior shoulder dislocation.

Radiographs

Radiographic evaluation of suspected shoulder dislocations should include at least two views of the shoulder. True anteroposterior (AP) and true lateral radiographs are the films of choice in shoulder trauma (Figs. 43–5 and 43–6). The true AP view is shot at right angles to the scapula, not at right angles to the coronal plane. This requires the rotation of the patient 30 to 40 degrees as shown in Figure 43–5. The true lateral view is shot tangential to the scapula. The resultant film clearly delineates the relation of the humeral head to the glenoid fossa (see Fig. 43–6).

Postreduction films should include a true AP film view, the true lateral view, and preferably an axillary view. The axillary view may reveal an impaction fracture of the humeral head, known as *Hill Sacks lesion*. When the patient is sent for postreduction films, the shoulder should be properly immobilized. To prevent redislocation, manipulation of the shoulder should be gentle and minimal.

Reduction

Many methods have been proposed for reducing anterior shoulder dislocations. Successful reduction is usually quite obvious, as indicated by a marked reduction in pain, by the practitioner or patient feeling the shoulder slip back into place, and by regaining the normal roundness of the shoulder contour. Following reduction, the shoulder may be gently manipulated through a small

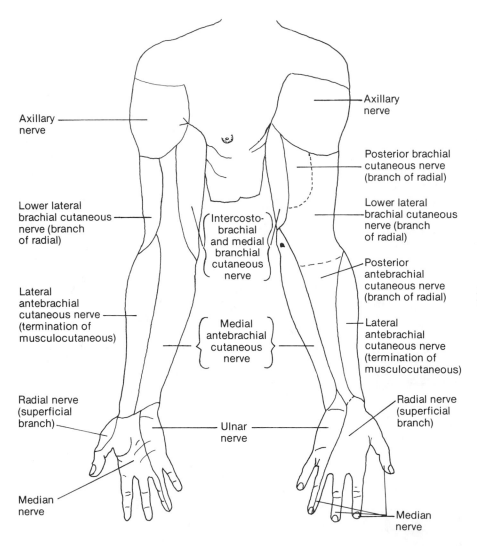

Axillary
nerve

Axillary
nerve

Posterior brachial
cutaneous nerve
(branch of radial)

Lower lateral
brachial cutaneous
nerve (branch
of radial)

Lower lateral
brachial cutaneous
nerve (branch
of radial)

Intercosto-
brachial
and medial
branchial
cutaneous
nerve

Posterior
antebrachial
cutaneous nerve
(branch of radial)

Lateral
antebrachial
cutaneous nerve
(termination of
musculocutaneous)

Medial
antebrachial
cutaneous
nerve

Lateral
antebrachial
cutaneous nerve
(termination of
musculocutaneous)

Radial nerve
(superficial
branch)

Ulnar
nerve

Radial nerve
(superficial
branch)

Median
nerve

Median
nerve

Anterior (palmar) aspect

Posterior (dorsal) aspect

Figure 43–3. Sensory innervation of
the upper extremity.

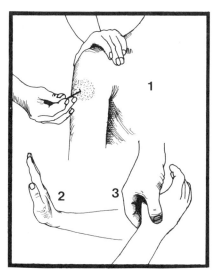

Figure 43—4. Evaluation of the upper extremity with a shoulder dislocation. Axillary (circumflex) nerve palsy is the most common neurological complication. Test for integrity of the nerve by assessing sensation to pin prick (1) in its distribution over the "regimental badge" area. (The shoulder is usually too painful to assess deltoid activity with certainty.) Look for other (rare) involvement of the radial portion of the posterior cord (2) and involvement of the axillary artery (3). (From McRae, R.: Practical Fracture Treatment. Edinburgh, Churchill Livingstone, 1981, p. 84. Used by permission.)

10- to 15-degree range of motion to ensure that normal integrity has been achieved. If reduction has been successful, such passive range of motion is not particularly painful or dangerous and it ensures proper reduction.

In this section, the three methods that are relatively safe, atraumatic, and easy to master are discussed. The key to a successful shoulder reduction is a slow, yet steady, approach with adequate analgesia and muscle relaxation.

Stimson Maneuver (Fig. 43—7). In this technique, the patient is placed in the prone position on a bed or cart with the affected shoulder toward one side of the cart. The arm should hang down but not touch the floor. A small weight (10 to 20 lb) is strapped to the wrist or attached above the elbow to produce steady traction. A bucket of water or a sand bag may also be used. The weight is left in place for 20 to 30 minutes or until the shoulder is reduced. This is not a particularly painful reduction, but some analgesia is recommended. If no reduction is noted after 30 minutes, gentle internal and external rotation with manual traction may help to relocate the shoulder.

This method is often successful, because it allows gravity, with the help of weights, to gradually overcome the associated muscle spasm and permit reduction without the use of excessive analgesics. Care must be taken to secure the patient to the stretcher or table, especially if the patient is intoxicated or sedated.

External Rotation Method (Fig. 43—8). With this technique, the patient is placed in a supine position and the affected arm is adducted to the side. The elbow on the affected side is flexed to 90 degrees, and then, very slowly, the physician externally rotates the arm using the forearm as a lever. The external rotation should be slow and gentle. No traction is applied, and the rotation is halted as pain is produced. It should take about 10 minutes for the forearm to go from a sagittal plane to a coronal plane. Usually the shoulder is reduced by the time the coronal plane is reached. This method is often successful and requires only one physician and little exertion or strength.

Traction/Countertraction (Fig. 43—9). Using this method, the patient is placed in a supine position on a cart and a sheet or a strap is wrapped around

Figure 43—5. A and B, Trauma series includes two views of the shoulder made perpendicular and parallel to the scapular plane. The advantage is that roentgenograms may be obtained without moving the patient or removing the arm from the sling. (From Heppenstall, R. B.: Fracture Treatment and Healing. Philadelphia, W. B. Saunders Company, 1980, p. 374. Used by permission.)

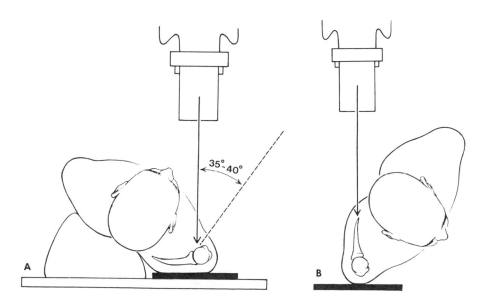

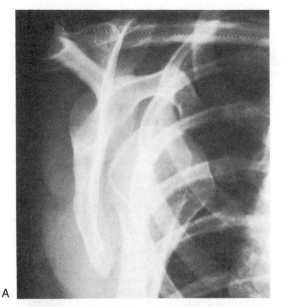

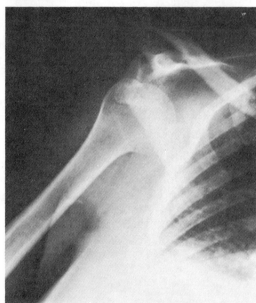

Figure 43–6. *A*, Lateral roentgenogram of the trauma series demonstrating a definite anterior dislocation. Note the humeral head in a subcoracoid location anterior to the glenoid fossa. *B*, Anteroposterior projection of the same shoulder. (From Heppenstall, R. B.: Fracture Treatment and Healing. Philadelphia, W. B. Saunders Company, 1980, p. 392. Used by permission.)

the upper chest under the axilla of the affected shoulder. An assistant holds the ends of this sheet and applies countertraction. Alternatively, the strap may be attached to the stretcher itself. The physician applies in-line traction to the affected extremity, holding the extremity at the wrist or elbow with both hands. Such steady in-line traction will help overcome the associated muscle spasm and dislodge the humeral head. Slight external rotation can be helpful after the application of traction although *the application of rotation with traction has been associated with humeral neck*

fractures in the elderly. If relocation does not occur, slight lateral traction applied to the upper arm by a second assistant with the aid of a sheet may help. If necessary, the physician can adduct the arm *across the midline* during these maneuvers.

This method requires stamina on the part of the physician, because traction must be maintained for several minutes. Adequate analgesia and muscle relaxation are essential with this method, because it may be difficult to overcome muscle spasms with traction alone. It is best if the physician holds the patient's upper extremity and leans backward, using the body to give continuous traction rather than attempting to pull on the patient's arm by using the power of the biceps. Some physicians prefer to wrap a strap around their backs, looping it over the patient's flexed elbow. The physician can then support the flexed elbow in his hands while gradually applying traction by leaning away from the patient. With this method, the reduction can be readily palpated.

Other Methods. The use of the Hippocratic technique (physician's foot placed on the chest wall to provide countertraction) is discouraged. Although the Hippocratic technique is often successful, it is dangerous and associated with complications. Uncomplicated dislocations should be easily reduced with the aforementioned methods.

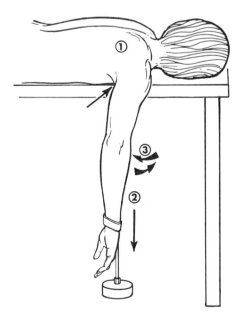

Figure 43–7. Stimson technique. This technique should be tried first, because it is the least traumatic if the patient can relax his shoulder muscles. *1*, The patient is prone on the edge of the table. One must be careful so that the drugged or intoxicated patient does not fall off the table. Belts or sheets can be used to secure the patient to the stretcher. *2*, 10-kg weights are attached to the arm, and the patient maintains this position for 20 to 30 minutes, if necessary. *3*, Occasionally, gentle external and internal rotation of the shoulder with manual traction aids reduction. (From DePalma, A. F.: Management of Fractures and Dislocations: An Atlas. Philadelphia, W. B. Saunders Company, 1970, p. 618. Used by permission.)

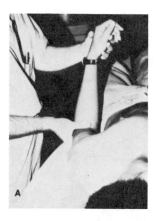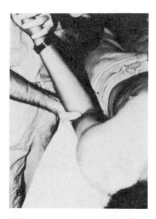

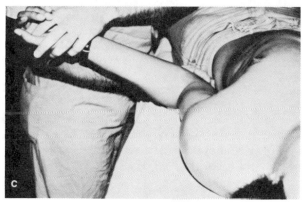

Figure 43–8. External rotation method. A, Arm is adducted to patient's side. In one hand, elbow is held flexed at 90 degrees while other hand grasps wrist. B, Slowly and gently, the forearm is used as a lever to rotate the arm externally. C, Usually by the time the forearm has reached the coronal plane, the shoulder will have been reduced. (From Mirick, M. J., et al.: External rotation method of shoulder dislocation reduction. JACEP 8:529, 1979. Used by permission.)

If these methods fail, general anesthesia or orthopedic consultation is recommended.

Postreduction Care

Following reduction the shoulder should be immobilized with a sling and swath or shoulder immobilizer or similar method that keeps the arm abducted in neutral rotation. One must avoid abduction and external rotation of the humerus. The circulatory states of the shoulder should be reassessed and the integrity of the axillary nerve should be rechecked. Postreduction films should be taken. If relocation has occurred and if no fractures are noted on the postreduction film, the patient can be discharged from the hospital with a shoulder immobilizer or a similar immobilization device. The patient should be given instructions for follow-up, with a physician of choice, in 2 to 3 days. If any fractures are noted on the postreduction film, orthopedic consultation is required.

The length of time that the uncomplicated anteriorly dislocated shoulder is immobilized de-pends upon the age of the patient and associated injuries. Generally, the shoulder is immobilized for 3 weeks in younger patients, followed by 3 weeks of gentle, active range-of-motion exercises. Older patients may have considerable stiffness and other disabilities following dislocation; thus, mobilization may be begun sooner to avoid complications such as a frozen shoulder. Orthopedic follow-up is recommended in all such cases.

POSTERIOR SHOULDER DISLOCATIONS

Posterior shoulder dislocations account for a small percentage of all acute shoulder dislocations and can be very difficult to diagnose both clinically

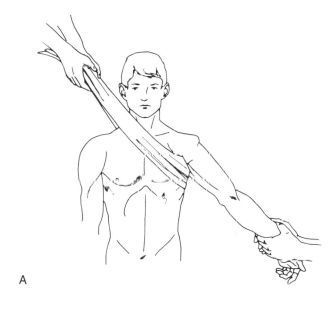

A

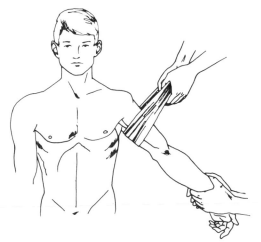

B

Figure 43–9. A, Traction–countertraction technique for reducing anterior shoulder dislocations. B, Traction–lateral traction technique for reducing anterior shoulder dislocations. An additional sheet should be wrapped around the chest (A), and traction should be applied. (From Simon, R., and Koenigsknecht, S.: Orthopedics in Emergency Medicine. New York, Appleton-Century-Crofts, 1982, p. 343. Used by permission.)

and radiographically. Consequently, a posterior shoulder dislocation is the most frequently undiagnosed major joint dislocation seen in the emergency department. The causal mechanism for posterior dislocations is usually abduction and internal rotation, although occasionally posterior dislocations result from direct anterior forces. A common etiology of posterior dislocations is seizures, when muscular forces can cause tremendous internal rotation. It should be noted that during seizure activity bilateral posterior dislocations can occur.

The patient may present with complaints of shoulder pain, having sustained a mechanism of injury compatible with posterior dislocation. The arm will be adducted and internally rotated, and resistance to any movement will be noted. Physical examination will reveal a shoulder that has a loss of contour compared with the other shoulder (beware of a bilateral dislocation), and passive or active external rotation will not be possible. Neurovascular deficits are infrequent following posterior dislocations.

Radiographs

As with anterior dislocations, a true AP and a true lateral shoulder film should be obtained. The AP view may appear deceptively normal, although close examination will usually reveal a slight distortion of the normal elliptical overlap of the humeral head on the glenoid rim (Figs. 43–10 and 43–11). The true lateral (transscapular) view will

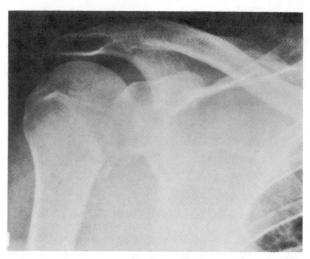

Figure 43–11. Posterior dislocation of the humeral head. This anteroposterior view shows medial displacement of the humeral head and an abnormal overlap with the glenoid rim. A fracture fragment of the lesser tuberosity is superimposed upon the inferior rim of the glenoid. (From Greenbaum, E. (ed.): Radiology of the Emergency Patient. New York, John Wiley & Sons, Inc., 1982, p. 511. Used by permission.)

reveal the humeral head to be located posterior to the glenoid fossa (Fig. 43–12).

Treatment

Posterior dislocations can usually be reduced with gentle in-line traction. With the patient in a

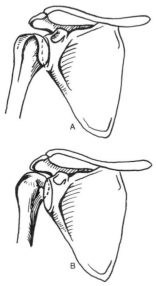

Figure 43–10. A, Note the normal elliptical pattern of overlap produced by the head of the humerus and the glenoid fossa. B, In the patient with a posterior dislocation, this pattern is lost and there is also internal rotation of the greater tuberosity. (From Simon, R., and Koenigsknecht, S.: Orthopedics in Emergency Medicine. New York, Appleton-Century-Crofts, 1982, p. 344. Used by permission.)

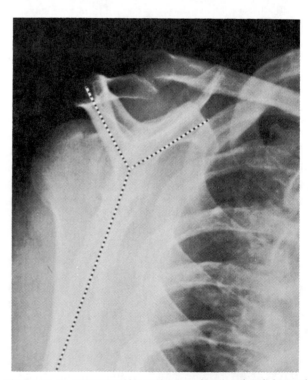

Figure 43–12. Transscapular projection showing the dislocated humeral head, posterior in relationship to the intersecting limbs of the "Y." (From Greenbaum, E. (ed.): Radiology of the Emergency Patient. New York, John Wiley & Sons, Inc., 1982, p. 512. Used by permission.)

supine position, in-line traction is applied to the arm. Countertraction is supplied in the same manner as described for anterior dislocations. The physician should maintain gentle in-line traction for 10 to 15 minutes, holding the affected extremity at the wrist or elbow and leaning backward. If the humeral head does not relocate with in-line traction, the physician may apply direct pressure over the humeral head to gently manipulate the head around the glenoid rim and into the glenoid fossa. After the shoulder has been reduced, the arm can be gently internally and externally rotated without difficulty.

Postreduction Care

Following shoulder reduction, the neurovascular status should be reassessed and postreduction films should be taken. If the shoulder joint is grossly stable, a shoulder immobilizer may be used to immobilize the shoulder. If the shoulder appears to be grossly unstable, a spica cast with the humerus in external rotation is usually required. Such unstable shoulder dislocations should be promptly referred to an orthopedist.

Because posterior dislocations are uncommon injuries, early orthopedic consultation and referral are suggested.

SUMMARY

1. The neurovascular status must be checked both pre- and postreduction.

2. Failure to reduce a dislocation may indicate entrapment of soft tissue or a fracture fragment in the joint space. If the dislocation does not reduce readily, it should not be assumed that it is because the wrong technique is being used and/or that not enough force is being applied.

3. The shoulder should be immobilized when postreduction films are being taken.

4. Posterior dislocations can occur bilaterally, especially when the etiology is a major motor seizure.

5. Although recurrent dislocations can be reduced by the aforementioned methods, surgical intervention may eventually be necessary and early orthopedic referral is strongly recommended.

6. Usually successful reduction is obvious to both the patient and the physician, but prior to the patient being discharged from the hospital, it should be ascertained that complete reduction has been achieved. The physician may be misled by a partial reduction if he only relies on feeling motion during the reduction maneuver.

Elbow Dislocations

The elbow is the second most frequently dislocated joint in adults and is the most commonly dislocated joint in children younger than 10 years of age. The elbow is a relatively stable joint. Dislocation often involves severe disruption of associated ligaments and other soft tissues. Frac-

Figure 43–13. Classification of elbow dislocations. (From Simon, R., and Koenigsknecht, S.: Orthopedics in Emergency Medicine. New York, Appleton-Century-Crofts, 1982, p. 333. Used by permission.)

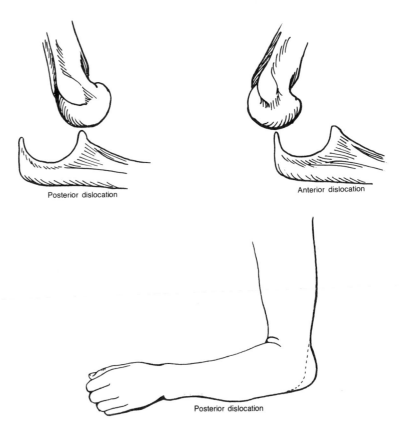

Posterior dislocation

Anterior dislocation

Posterior dislocation

tures frequently accompany elbow dislocations, especially those involving the coronoid process, radial head, capitulum, or olecranon. An avulsion fracture of the medial epicondyle of the humerus may be seen in children with elbow dislocations. The radius and ulna frequently displace as a unit, and elbow dislocations are classified according to the relationship between the proximal ulna and radius and the distal humerus. For example, in a posterior dislocation, the ulna and radius are displaced backward and lie behind the humerus (Fig. 43–13).

One of the feared consequences of elbow dislocations is damage to the neurovascular bundles that cross the elbow. The various forces applied to the elbow during dislocation can cause severe damage to the brachial artery or to the ulnar and median nerves. It is vitally important that an adequate neurologic assessment of the major nerve trunks distal to the elbow be carried out prior to, as well as after, reduction. The same is true for the circulatory status of the forearm. Compromise of the vascular status of the forearm demands immediate radiographs and urgent reduction of the elbow. Elbow dislocations may result in marked soft-tissue swelling of the elbow and forearm even after reduction. The swelling itself may cause embarrassment of the neurovascular bundles of the forearm, a type of compartment syndrome. For this reason, it it advised that all patients with elbow dislocations be admitted to the hospital for ongoing evaluation of the neurovascular status of the forearm for a period of 24 hours. Traumatic myositis ossificans of the brachialis muscle or ossification of a subperiosteal hematoma may be seen following an elbow dislocation. Stiffness, especially in elderly patients, is also a common sequela.

ANALGESIA

Elbow dislocations are usually quite painful, and inadequate analgesia will make reduction difficult. Intramuscular and intravenous regimens of analgesia and muscle relaxant agents as described previously can be used. Nitrous oxide may also be helpful. Axillary blocks or intravenous regional anesthesia (see Chapters 32 and 33) may also be used.

If none of these methods are applicable or available, general anesthesia may be necessary.

RADIOGRAPHS

Two radiographic views, including a lateral and an AP view (Fig. 43–14), should be obtained.

POSTERIOR DISLOCATIONS

This is the most common type of elbow dislocation. In a posterior dislocation, the olecranon assumes a position posterior to the distal humerus (Fig. 43–15). The mechanism of injury is a fall on an outstretched arm held in extension. The patient usually presents with the arm held to the side with the elbow in moderate flexion of about 30 to 40 degrees. Physical examination will reveal an unusually prominent olecranon process, although the severe swelling sometimes seen with elbow dislocations may make palpation of the olecranon difficult.

Reduction of Posterior Dislocation of the Elbow

Reduction of a posterior elbow dislocation can be a relatively simple procedure (Fig. 43–16). When extremity muscle spasm is severe, an axillary nerve block may be needed to obtain adequate muscle relaxation. Once muscle relaxation is attained, the patient is placed in a supine position. An assistant then stabilizes the humerus by holding it with both hands. The physician holds the wrist of the affected extremity with one hand and applies slow and gentle, yet steady, in-line traction. It is important to supinate the patient's wrist and to maintain the elbow in slight flexion, avoiding hyperextension. A clunk can be heard or felt as the elbow is reduced. One may gently flex the forearm as traction is maintained if reduction is not easily achieved by traction alone.

If the elbow does not reduce using this technique, the physician may need to apply downward pressure at the proximal forearm or apply pressure behind the olecranon while, at the same time, maintaining in-line traction. This downward force may help to "unlock" the coronoid process, which may be trapped in the olecranon fossa. At times, reduction can be best accomplished with the shoulder abducted and the distal humerus resting on the back of a chair. In this position, the olecranon can be pushed up and away from the distal humerus by the physician while an assistant applies gentle longitudinal downward traction on the flexed forearm. When reduction does occur, gentle flexion and extension of the elbow will be possible and should be performed to confirm anatomical reduction and stability.

ANTERIOR DISLOCATIONS

Although uncommon, anterior dislocations are the second most common elbow dislocations seen in the emergency department. The mechanism of injury is a fall on the flexed elbow with a direct force displacing the olecranon anteriorly so that it

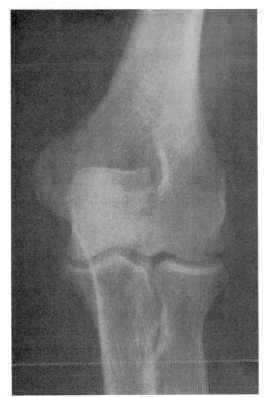
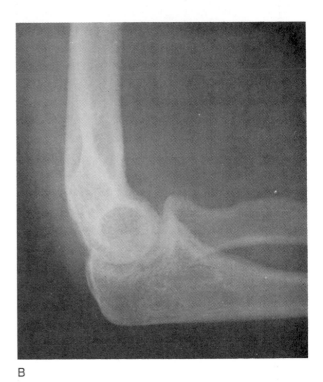

Figure 43–14. Routine anteroposterior *(A)* and lateral *(B)* radiographs of a normal adult elbow. In the frontal projection, note the relationship between the articulating surface of the radius and the capitellum and the articulating surface of the coronoid process and the trochlea. Note, also, in the frontal projection, the normal smooth concave cortical sweep from the radial neck to the radial head. In the lateral projection *(B)*, note that the image of the coronoid process is superimposed upon the image of the radial head and that the soft-tissue density around the elbow is homogeneous. (From Harris, J. H., Jr., and Harris, W. H.: Radiology of Emergency Medicine, 2nd ed. Baltimore, Williams & Wilkins Co., 1981, p. 203. Used by permission.)

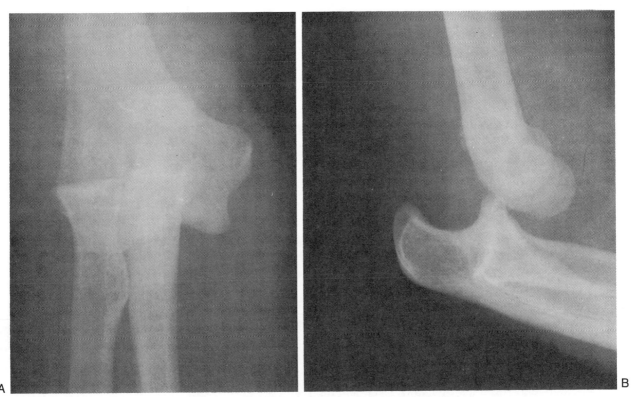

Figure 43–15. *A* and *B,* Complete posterior dislocation of the elbow. (From Harris, J. H., Jr., and Harris, W. H.: Radiology of Emergency Medicine, 2nd ed. Baltimore, Williams & Wilkins Co., 1981, p. 208. Used by permission.)

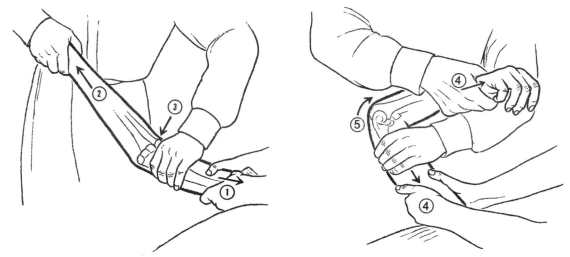

Figure 43–16. Manipulative reduction of posterior elbow dislocation. While an assistant holds the arm and makes steady countertraction (1), Grasp the wrist with one hand, and apply steady traction on the forearm in the position in which it lies (2). While traction is maintained, correct any lateral displacement with the other hand (3). While traction is maintained (4) gently flex the forearm (5). *Note* that with reduction, a click is usually felt and heard as the olecranon engages the articular surface of the humerus. (From DePalma, A. F.: Management of Fractures and Dislocations: An Atlas. Philadelphia, W. B. Saunders Company, 1970, pp. 793 and 794. Used by permission.)

comes to rest in a position anterior to the distal humerus. Great forces are required to cause such a dislocation, and consequently such dislocations are often associated with fractures, especially about the olecranon process.

Injuries to the neurovascular bundles are seen more frequently with anterior dislocations than with posterior dislocations. Again, it is imperative that the neurovascular status of the forearm be adequately assessed as soon as possible during the evaluation process.

On physical examination, the elbow joint will be markedly disrupted. Because there is nothing overlying the elbow except skin, one may be able to palpate the olecranon anterior to the distal humerus. The elbow itself is generally held in full extension, and the patient usually resists any attempt at flexion or extension of the elbow.

Reduction of Anterior Dislocation of the Elbow

After adequate analgesia, the patient is placed in a supine position (Fig. 43–17). An assistant stabilizes the humerus with two hands while the physician applies steady in-line traction by holding the wrist with one hand while the second hand applies a downward force at the proximal radius and ulna. This downward force helps to lift the olecranon process over the distal humerus.

RADIAL HEAD SUBLUXATION

This is a common elbow subluxation seen in children between the ages of 1 and 4 years. The injury is referred to as a *pulled elbow* and *Nursemaid's elbow*.

The proximal head of the radius articulates with the proximal ulna, and this joint is stabilized by the annular ligament. In children, the lip of the radial head is not fully developed and sudden traction may cause the radial head to slip out from the confines of the annular ligament. The mechanism of injury for this radial head subluxation is sudden traction of the forearm that extends and

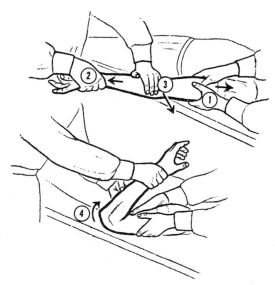

Figure 43–17. Manipulative reduction of anterior elbow dislocation. Reduction is performed with the patient under local or general anesthesia. *1*, An assistant grasps the arm and makes countertraction. *2*, The operator grasps the wrist with one hand and makes traction in the line of the arm, and with the other hand makes firm, steady pressure downward and backward on the upper end of the forearm (3). A click usually indicates that reduction is achieved. *4*, The arm is flexed to 45 degrees beyond a right angle. (From DePalma, A. F.: Management of Fractures and Dislocations: An Atlas. Philadelphia, W. B. Saunders Company, 1970, p. 796. Used by permission.)

pronates the elbow. Such sudden traction often occurs when a child is pulled up from the wrist.

A child usually presents with the forearm pronated and hanging to the side and refuses to use the arm. As long as the arm is not being used or moved, there is minimal pain, but as soon as any attempt is made to flex the elbow or supinate the arm, the child expresses intense pain. Parents often think that the elbow is sprained and delay medical care for 24 to 36 hours. There is no associated soft-tissue swelling, ecchymosis, or neurovascular deficit.

Radiographs

Radiographic findings of the radial head subluxation will be normal but are frequently required to rule out any associated fractures. Ossification of the radial head does not occur until age 3 or 4 years. There will be no excess joint fluid and therefore no positive fat pad signs. With a straightforward history and clinical presentation or with recurrences, the physician may wish to treat the patient without radiographic films. If radiographs are obtained, a standard AP and lateral film will be sufficient.

Reduction

Reduction can usually be accomplished without anesthesia. The physician sits facing the child and cups the affected elbow with his opposite hand (e.g., using the left hand if the right elbow is injured). The physician then places the thumb of the supporting hand over the radial head area. The forearm is flexed and *supinated* with the physician's other arm, using the supporting thumb as a fulcrum. Slight longitudinal traction is often helpful prior to and during elbow flexion (Fig. 43–18). A palpable click is usually noted, although the child may continue to refuse to use the elbow for a few minutes. Giving the child a popsicle or a balloon to play with will usually confirm the success of the reduction. No immobilization is required if the child is able to use the arm without pain. If the child does not use the arm in a normal manner within 10 to 15 minutes, it should be suspected that reduction was not accomplished. If the physician is assured that reduction has occurred but pain persists, a posterior splint and sling are indicated, with instruction to have the child rechecked within 24 hours.

POSTREDUCTION CARE

Patients with anterior or posterior elbow dislocations (except radial head subluxation in children) should be admitted to the hospital for 24 hours for elevation of the injured extremity and neuro-

vascular monitoring. Splints should be used as follows: Posterior dislocations should be splinted with a posterior splint to include the wrist with the elbow in 90 degrees of flexion and the wrist in neutral position. Anterior dislocations should be splinted with a posterior splint with the elbow in 45 degrees of flexion. As noted previously, radial head subluxations do not usually require splinting, but if splinting is required, a posterior splint with the elbow in 90 degrees of flexion can be applied.

It should be emphasized that elbow injuries can result in marked swelling of the elbow and the forearm. For this reason, circumferential casts are contraindicated initially.

SIGNIFICANT POINTS

1. The physician must have a high index of suspicion of associated fractures.
2. Circulatory compromise can occur by direct injuries to the brachial artery as well as secondary to post-traumatic swelling.
3. Compartment syndrome can develop secondary to elbow dislocations. The physician must have a high index of suspicion to diagnose and prevent progression of this dreaded complication. The classic end result of this syndrome, if untreated, is development of forearm ischemic contracture (Volkmann's contracture).
4. Another known complication of elbow dislocations is traumatic myositis ossificans. This is a localized intramuscular ossification that develops secondary to a hematoma in an injured muscle. The most common ossifying muscle involved in an elbow injury is the brachial muscle.

Thumb Dislocations

The thumb is involved in many hand functions. This activity, in conjunction with the fact that the thumb is the first digit of the hand, makes it particularly susceptible to joint injuries. Dislocations and subluxations of the thumb joints are commonly seen in the emergency department. These injuries occur in spite of the strong ligamentous support of the thumb.

METACARPOPHALANGEAL (MCP) JOINT INJURIES OF THE THUMB

One of two mechanisms usually serve to subluxate or dislocate this joint. With marked hyperextension of the MCP joint, dorsal dislocation may result. In this most common type of dislocation, the proximal phalanx takes the position dorsal to the first metacarpal (Fig. 43–19). The second mech-

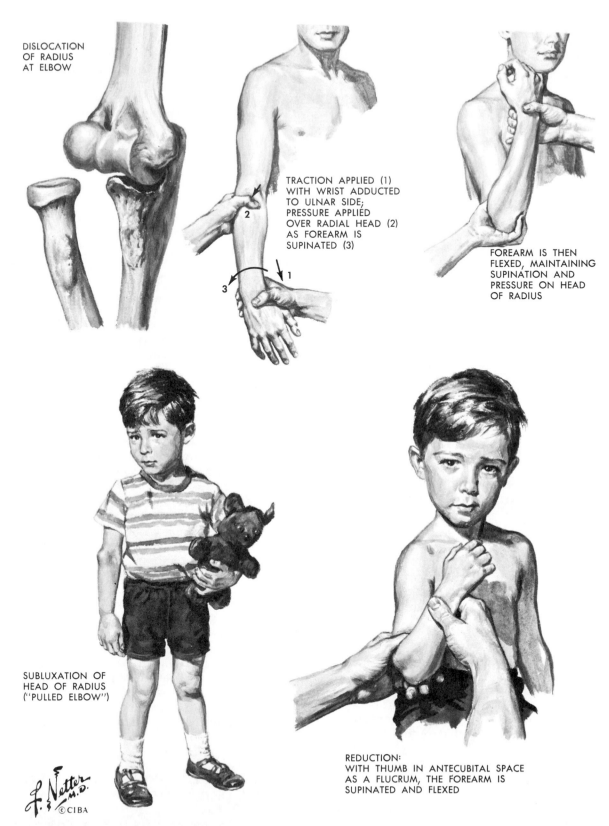

DISLOCATION
OF RADIUS
AT ELBOW

TRACTION APPLIED (1)
WITH WRIST ADDUCTED
TO ULNAR SIDE;
PRESSURE APPLIED
OVER RADIAL HEAD (2)
AS FOREARM IS
SUPINATED (3)

FOREARM IS THEN
FLEXED, MAINTAINING
SUPINATION AND
PRESSURE ON HEAD
OF RADIUS

SUBLUXATION OF
HEAD OF RADIUS
("PULLED ELBOW")

REDUCTION:
WITH THUMB IN ANTECUBITAL SPACE
AS A FLUCRUM, THE FOREARM IS
SUPINATED AND FLEXED

Figure 43–18. Reduction of radial head subluxation. Traction applied (1) with wrist adducted to ulnar side. Pressure is applied over the radial head (2) as the forearm is supinated (3). The forearm is then flexed, maintaining supination and pressure on the head of the radius. (Copyright 1969, CIBA Pharmaceutical Company, Division of CIBA–GEIGY Corporation. Reprinted with permission from Clinical Symposia, illustrated by Frank H. Netter, M.D. All rights reserved. Legend adapted.)

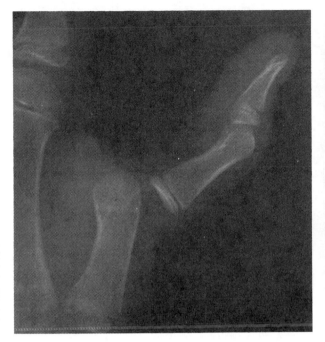

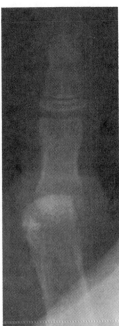

Figure 43–19. Complete dorsal dislocation at the metacarpophalangeal joint of the thumb. There is neither associated fracture nor epiphyseal separation. (From Harris, J. H., Jr., and Harris, W. H.: Radiology of Emergency Medicine, 2nd ed. Baltimore, Williams & Wilkins Co., 1981, p. 239. Used by permission.)

anism that may cause subluxation or dislocation of the MCP is severe valgus strain, resulting in a rupture of the ulnar collateral ligament (Fig. 43–20).

Both the MCP and interphalangeal joints are stabilized by a joint capsule comprised of a collateral ligament–volar plate apparatus (Fig. 43–21). On the lateral surfaces, the two collateral ligaments span each side of the joint space to provide

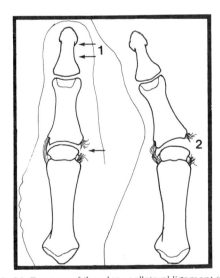

Figure 43–20. Rupture of the ulnar collateral ligament (Gamekeeper's thumb). 1, This injury is caused by forcible abduction. If unrecognized and untreated, there may be progressive MCP subluxation (2) with interference during grasp, causing significant permanent disability. Suspect this injury when there is complaint of pain in this region. Look for tenderness on the medial side of the MCP joint. (From McRae, R.: Practical Fracture Treatment. Edinburgh, Churchill Livingstone, 1981, p. 162. Used by permission.)

stability. The dorsal surface has no collateral ligaments, and on the volar (anterior) surface, the collateral ligament is replaced by a fibrocartilaginous (hence radiolucent) volar plate.

When a joint becomes completely dislocated, at least two of the three supporting structures (two collateral ligaments, one volar plate) tear. The clinical significance of this anatomical disruption is twofold. First, the volar plate may become interposed in the joint space and prevent reduction. Second, a complete tear of the capsule means that the joint is unstable, requiring prolonged immobilization or, occasionally, surgery in order to mend. In the thumb, the volar plate is attached more firmly to the base of the phalanx, and more loosely to the base of the metacarpal. Thus, in a dorsal dislocation, the volar plate may become avulsed from the metacarpal and dislocate with the phalanx, and hence become interposed in the MCP joint space (Fig. 43–22).

There are primarily two types of dorsal dislocations of the thumbs, simple and complex. The importance of distinguishing between these two types of dislocations is that a simple dislocation can be reduced with a closed technique whereas a complex dislocation can be reduced only with an open technique. In a complex MCP dislocation, the volar plate is avulsed during the dislocation and becomes interposed between the articulating surface of the joint. The volar plate is not visible on a radiograph, but the presence of a sesamoid bone, which dislocates with the volar plate in the joint space, may indicate volar plate interposition between the two bones (Fig. 43–23). Closed reduction of this dislocation is impossible. If the dislocation is complex, repeated attempts at reduction

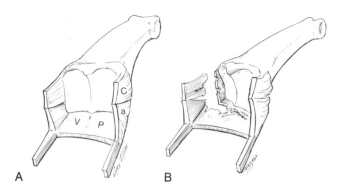

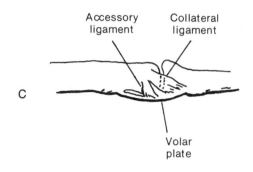

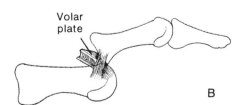

Figure 43–21. *A* and *B*, The collateral ligament–volar plate relationship. The metacarpal-phalangeal and interphalangeal joints derive their strength from a combination of the two collateral ligaments and the volar plate. Dislocations of these joints require tear of at least two parts of this three-part structure. (From Carter, P. (ed.): Common Hand Injuries and Infections. Philadelphia, W. B. Saunders Company, 1983, p. 114. Used by permission.) *C*, Lateral view, demonstrating collateral ligament–volar plate relationship. (Redrawn from Eaton, R. G.: Joint Injuries of the Hand. Springfield, Ill. Charles C Thomas, 1972.)

of the MCP can lead only to discomfort for the patient as well as an increased risk of damage to the surrounding soft tissue and the neurovascular bundles. In simple dislocations, the volar plate is not entrapped in the joint space. Because there is no tissue interposition, closed reduction is usually possible in these injuries.

It may be difficult to differentiate the complex from the simple dislocation on clinical grounds. In the complex dislocation, the proximal phalanx often lies parallel to the metacarpal, whereas in the simple dislocation, the proximal phalanx usually sits at a right angle to the metacarpal (see Fig. 43–22). If it is not possible to reduce a supposed simple dislocation in one or two attempts, a presumptive diagnosis of a complex dislocation should be made and the patient should be referred appropriately.

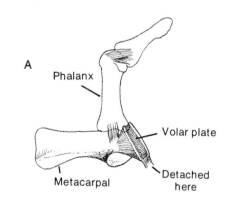

Figure 43–22. *A*, In a simple dorsal MP joint dislocation (note right angle between phalanx and metacarpal), the volar plate remains in front of the metacarpal head, although it is detached from its weaker metacarpal insertion. *B*, In a complex dislocation (note more parallel alignment between phalanx and metacarpal), the volar plate becomes entrapped in the joint and results in an irreducible reduction by closed methods. (From DePalma, A. F.: Management of Fractures and Dislocations: An Atlas. Philadelphia, W. B. Saunders Company, 1970, p. 1177. Used by permission.)

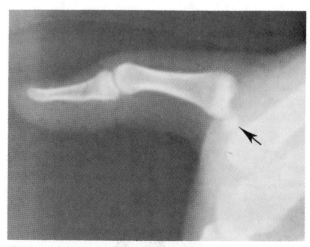

Figure 43–23. Irreducible MP joint dislocation of the thumb. Note the sesamoid bone (arrow) indicating volar plate interposition between the two bone ends, which may prevent reduction. (From Carter, P. (ed.): Common Hand Injuries and Infections. Philadelphia, W. B. Saunders Company, 1983, p. 115. Used by permission.)

The second most common injury to the thumb MCP joint is a *rupture of the ulnar collateral ligament* (see Fig. 43–20). Years ago, this type of injury was most commonly seen in gamekeepers as a result of breaking rabbits' necks with the webbed space between the thumb and index finger and acquired the interesting name of *Gamekeeper's thumb*. Today, the injury most commonly results from catching one's thumb on a ski pole and therefore is known as *Skier's thumb*.

The diagnosis of this injury requires a high degree of suspicion. The patient usually presents with pain and soft-tissue swelling at the base of the thumb, especially at the ulnar side of the MCP joint, without obvious bony deformity. The ulnar collateral ligament itself may rupture, or the ligament may remain intact while the ligament avulses a small fragment of bone. Standard film findings will be normal unless there is an associated avulsion fracture. The diagnosis of this injury requires an understanding of the mechanism of injury and stress films. An improperly treated ulnar collateral ligament injury may lead to significant dysfunction of the thumb and may especially compromise one's strength for pinching with the thumb and index finger.

Radiographs

A true AP view, a true lateral view, and one oblique view should be obtained in MCP joint injuries (Fig. 43–24). The fingernail can be used as a guide to proper positioning. It is important that the radiology technician obtain a true lateral film and be instructed to cone down on the injured joint.

To properly identify an ulnar collateral injury, stress radiographs of the thumb must be obtained. It is difficult to document instability by clinical examination alone. Following anesthesia, the stability of the ulnar ligament is checked with the thumb in full extension (Fig. 43–25). If the joint "opens," it may be compared with the other hand, both clinically and with stress radiographs (Fig. 43–26). If there is greater than 20 degrees instability when compared with the other hand, open repair may be required.

Anesthesia

Proper anesthesia for MCP joint injury is local infiltration or a combined median and radial nerve block at the wrist.

Reduction

A simple dorsal dislocation of the thumb usually reduces quite easily. If the reduction is not done in the proper manner, however, a simple dislocation may be converted to a complex dislocation. To facilitate reduction, the thumb of the patient and the hand of the physician are wrapped with gauze, thereby increasing the gripping strength and decreasing the risk of the hand slipping off the thumb. Wearing dry surgical gloves is also helpful for maintaining a good grip. The phalanx is then hyperextended on the metacarpal bone to greater than 90 degrees. As the phalanx is hyperextended, in-line traction is applied to the phalanx. While hyperextending the phalanx and applying in-line traction, pressure can be applied to the surface of the proximal phalanx, in a sense "pushing" rather than "pulling" the joint to a reduced position. The MCP can then be gently flexed as reduction occurs (Fig. 43–27).

Postreduction Care

Following reduction, ligamentous stability of the joint must be assessed with stress testing, as noted previously. The thumb should then be splinted in a position of function, with the MCP and the IP joints flexed at approximately 45 degrees. The thumb is usually splinted or placed in a cast for 3 to 4 weeks. Unstable injuries after reduction or complex dislocations should be considered for surgical treatment.

Minor strains of the ulnar collateral ligament should be splinted with a plaster splint or thumb spica cast for 3 to 4 weeks and re-examined for stability. Unstable sprains or complete ruptures of the ulnar collateral ligament often require surgery and should be referred to an orthopedic surgeon. One should be cautious of making the diagnosis of a simple sprain of the thumb, and the splinting of even minor soft-tissue injuries of the thumb should be routine.

INTERPHALANGEAL (IP) JOINT DISLOCATION OF THE THUMB

IP joint dislocations are less common than MCP dislocations of the thumb. When they do occur, they are often open. Most commonly, the distal phalanx is dislocated dorsally with respect to the proximal phalanx, although lateral dislocations do occur.

The joint capsule of the IP joint is relatively strong and resistant to rupture. Although the avulsion of the volar plate on the distal phalanx can occur, it is rare. When it does occur, it is the result of an open injury, and it can become interposed in the joint space. The reduction of such a joint dislocation is impossible by the closed technique.

Radiographs

An AP view, a lateral view, and an oblique view usually reveal any associated fractures or other bony injuries.

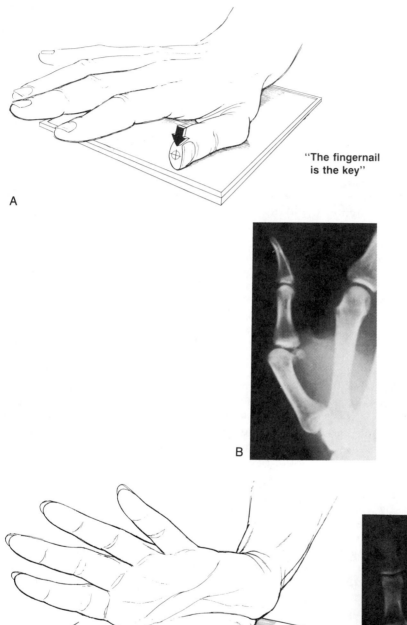

"The fingernail
is the key"

A

B

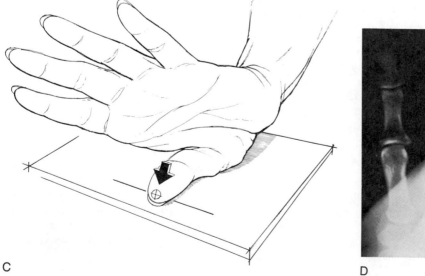

C

D

Figure 43–24. *A* and *B*, Thumb lateral radiograph. Use the thumbnail as a landmark. Do not take an AP film of the hand and expect a lateral of the thumb. *C* and *D*, Thumb AP radiograph. Use the thumbnail as a landmark. (From Carter, P. (ed.): Common Hand Injuries and Infections. Philadelphia, W. B. Saunders Company, 1983, p. 79. Used by permission.)

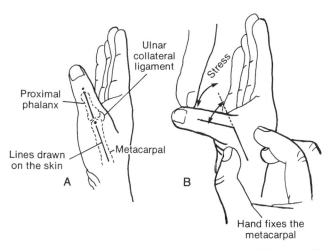

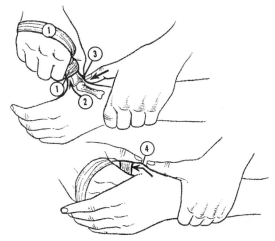

Figure 43–25. Stress testing of the ulnar collateral ligament of the thumb. This is done both clinically and with an AP radiograph. A line is drawn on the skin with a pen (A). The line is along the long axis of the metacarpal and the proximal phalanx. Deviation of the straight line during stress indicates instability (B). The metacarpal is fixed with the physician's other hand.

Figure 43–27. If a simple thumb MCP dislocation is treated with traction alone, the forces will often interpose the volar plate and result in a nonreducible complex dislocation. The proper technique for reduction includes (1) a good hold on the patient's distal thumb, (2) initial hyperextension of the dislocated phalanx, (3) pushing the base of the dislocated phalanx rather than traction alone, and (4) flexing of the thumb. (From DePalma, A. F.: Management of Fractures and Dislocations: An Atlas. Philadelphia, W. B. Saunders Company, 1970, p. 1178. Used by permission.)

Anesthesia

A digital block is usually sufficient.

Reduction

The thumb of the patient and the hand of the physician should be wrapped with gauze to prevent slippage. With mild hyperextension of the distal phalanx and in-line traction, the joint should reduce easily. If it does not reduce easily, the volar plate may be interposed and further attempts should not be made.

Postreduction Care

Following reduction, ligamentous stability of the joint should be assessed and postreduction films should be obtained. The joint should be splinted

in slight flexion of 30 to 45 degrees for a minimum of three weeks. Follow-up examination is required.

Finger Dislocations

Dislocations of the fingers are relatively common injuries seen in the emergency department. Most finger dislocations involve the proximal interphalangeal (PIP) joint, followed in frequency by dislocations of the distal interphalangeal (DIP) joint and then the relatively rare MCP joint dislocations. When MCP joint dislocations do occur, they usually occur en bloc and are complex irreducible dislocations that require open reduction.

Most often PIP dislocations are posterior (dorsal), with the middle phalanx taking a position dorsal to the proximal phalanx. The mechanism of injury is usually hyperextension of the PIP joint. Because of the hyperextension, there is either simple rupture of the junction between the volar plate and the middle phalanx or avulsion of a small bone fragment together with the volar plate (Fig. 43–28). Usually the volar plate does not interpose in the joint space, and therefore closed reduction is possible.

Lateral dislocations can also occur secondary to adduction or abduction stress at the joint. Complete lateral dislocation is not possible unless both the volar plate and one of the collateral ligaments are torn. Volar dislocations are rare but are associated with either extensor tendon rupture (leading to a later boutonnière deformity) or an irreducible dislocation, because the condyle of the

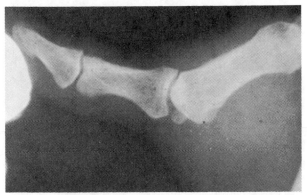

Figure 43–26. Radiograph of ulnar collateral ligament with instability greater than 45 degrees. (From Heppenstall, R. B.: Fracture Treatment and Healing. Philadelphia, W. B. Saunders Company, 1980, p. 573. Used by permission.)

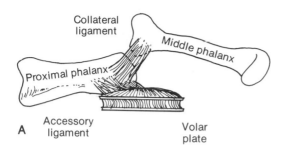

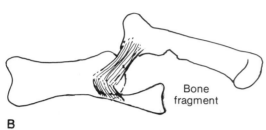

Figure 43–28. A dorsal PIP joint dislocation may involve rupture of the volar plate itself (A) or may involve an avulsion of varying amounts of bone from the middle phalanx (B). If a large fragment of bone is avulsed from the base of the phalanx, the dislocation is unstable after reduction. The collateral ligaments will tear in varying degrees and should be assessed with stress-testing following reduction.

proximal phalanx "buttonholes" itself through the extensor mechanisms and becomes trapped.

DIP joint injuries, although less common than PIP joint injuries, are frequently seen in the emergency department. In DIP dislocations, the direction of the dislocation is usually volar and the mechanism of injury is usually hyperflexion of the distal phalanx. If there is an avulsion of the extensor tendon and it is not treated appropriately, the distal phalanx will be pulled in an unopposed direction by the flexor tendon. The long-term consequences will be a distal phalanx that cannot be extended and must be held in a stance of continuous flexion. This is known as a *mallet* or *baseball finger* (Fig. 43–29). Extensor tendon injuries are discussed in detail in Chapter 44.

RADIOGRAPHS

Three views of all joint injuries of the fingers should be obtained: a true AP view, a true lateral view, and an oblique view. A film of the injured joint should be ordered, not a film of the hand in general. If a general hand film or insufficient views are ordered, the extent of joint injury may be difficult to discern secondary to overlapping structures (Fig. 43–30). Small avulsion fractures are often not seen until the postreduction film has been taken (Fig. 43–31).

ANESTHESIA

Joint injuries to the fingers are particularly amenable to digital blocks (see Chapter 32).

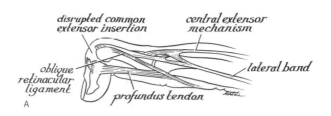

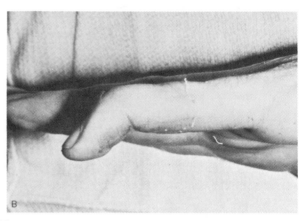

Figure 43–29. A, The mallet finger injury. B, This mallet deformity was caused by a laceration, but the appearance in profile is the same as that of a closed mallet injury. (From Newmeyer, W. L.: Primary Care of Hand Injuries. Philadelphia, Lea & Febiger, 1979, p. 142. Used by permission.)

PROXIMAL INTERPHALANGEAL (PIP) DISLOCATIONS

PIP dislocations usually reduce quite easily unless a complex dislocation is present, in which case they do not reduce at all. After a digital block has been administered and the injured digit of the patient and the hand of the physician have been wrapped with gauze (as pictured in Fig. 43–27), gentle in-line traction should be applied to the digit with slight hyperextension of the joint (Fig.

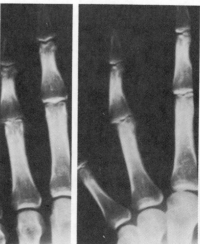
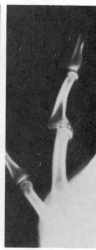

Figure 43–30. This fracture dislocation is only fully appreciated on the true lateral film. (From Carter, P. (ed.): Common Hand Injuries and Infections. Philadelphia, W. B. Saunders Company, 1983, p. 113. Used by permission.)

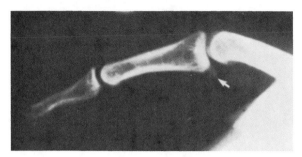

Figure 43–31. A small fragment of bone was avulsed with the volar plate. This frequently will be appreciated only with the postreduction film in a true lateral projection. (From Carter, P. (ed.): Common Hand Injuries and Infections. Philadelphia, W. B. Saunders Company, 1983, p. 113. Used by permission.)

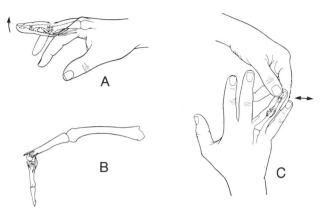

Figure 43–33. Postreduction stress of PIP dislocation. A, If the volar plate has been completely disrupted, the PIP joint will hyperextend with both passive and active motion. B, An inability to actively extend the PIP joint indicates a rupture of the central slip of the extensor tendon. C, Passive lateral stress is performed to check integrity of collateral ligaments. (From DePalma, A. F.: Management of Fractures and Dislocations: An Atlas. Philadelphia, W. B. Saunders Company, 1970, pp. 1203 and 1204. Used by permission.)

43–32). The injured hand should be held by the physician's other hand for countertraction. If the dislocation does not easily reduce, it should be assumed that it is a complex dislocation and proper orthopedic referral should be initiated.

Postreduction Care

Following reduction, the PIP joint should be examined for instability in extension, indicating a volar plate tear (Fig. 43–33). Lateral instability is also tested to document collateral ligament integrity. Inability to fully extend the PIP joint may indicate an extensor tendon avulsion. One cannot adequately test a PIP joint that is acutely painful; thus, a digital block is usually required. Instability of a PIP joint following reduction mandates orthopedic referral.

If there are no associated fractures or instability, simple PIP joint dislocations that have been adequately reduced should be splinted with the PIP joint in flexion of 15 to 20 degrees for 7 to 10 days.

A dorsal foam-padded splint is preferred to a volar splint, because it affords better immobilization and patient acceptance. "Buddy taping" may also be done in simple dislocations (Fig. 43–34). Gentle range-of-motion exercises can usually be initiated 7 days after injury.

All complicated PIP joint dislocations, or those associated with even small avulsion fractures, should be considered complex injuries and require proper referral. Even seemingly minor PIP joint injuries may produce significant or permanent disability, and *injuries to this joint should not be taken lightly.* Lateral and volar dislocations should be considered complicated.

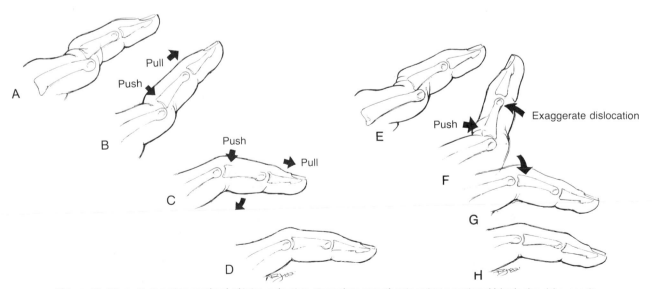

Figure 43–32. A–D, Traction method of joint reduction. Complete anesthesia using a regional block should precede reduction attempts. E–H, Exaggeration of existing deformity method. First, exaggerate the deformity that is present, then in addition to steady traction, push the joint back into position. (From Carter, P. (ed.): Common Hand Injuries and Infections. Philadelphia, W. B. Saunders Company, 1983, pp. 109 and 110. Used by permission.)

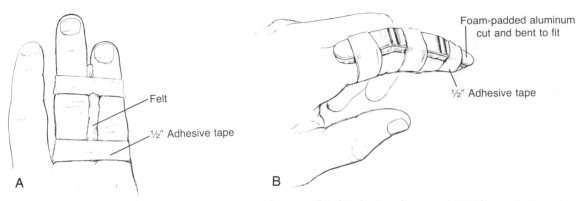

Figure 43–34. *A,* Buddy tape technique. By taping between the digital joints, the normal neighboring finger can protect the collateral ligament of its injured neighbor. *B,* Dorsal aluminum foam splint. The bone is subcutaneous dorsally. Splints here result in better immobilization of the digit. The dorsal splint also allows preservation and use of the tactile sense, which encourages function and better splint acceptance by the patient. (From Carter, P. (ed.): Common Hand Injuries and Infections. Philadelphia, W. B. Saunders Company, 1983, p. 85. Used by permission.)

DISTAL INTERPHALANGEAL (DIP) DISLOCATIONS

DIP dislocations usually reduce easily with in-line traction. The hand of the physician and the fingertip of the patient should be wrapped with gauze to reduce slippage. The injured hand should be stabilized by the physician's other hand. Occasionally, soft-tissue interposition in the joint space will not allow proper reduction and an open technique is required. In any case, orthopedic referral is suggested for all DIP dislocations and is a necessity if there is any avulsion fracture associated with the dislocation.

Postreduction Care

DIP joint dislocations may be splinted with a splint that holds the joint in full extension (Fig. 43–35). Splints should be designed to hold the DIP in full extension while allowing full range of motion in the PIP joint; padded dorsal splints are also used.

SUMMARY

1. If dislocations in the digits are not reduced easily, there may be interposition of soft tissue in the joint. Repeated attempts at relocation are not indicated and may increase the amount of damage already done to the joint.

2. All fingers should be splinted in a position of function, the MCP's and IP's are flexed and the thumb webbed space is open.

3. Injuries at the PIP joint can result in damage to the extensor mechanism at this joint. If the extensor mechanism is damaged, the lateral bands may stretch to a position that is volar to the axis of the PIP joint. These lateral bands, which are normally extensors of the PIP joint, then become

flexors of this joint. The result is a digit that is hyperflexed at the PIP joint and hyperextended at the DIP joint. This is referred to as a *boutonnière* deformity and is not always obvious on initial examination. All PIP joint injuries require proper orthopedic referral.

Hip Dislocations

The hip is a very stable joint. The head of the femur fits deeply into the hip socket and is well supported by the surrounding ligaments and muscular attachments. Because of this inherent stability of the hip, dislocations are rare and when they do occur they are the result of major forces. Because great forces are involved in traumatic hip dislocations, associated fractures are common.

The blood supply to the femoral head is rather tenuous and is often disrupted with hip dislocations. For this reason a dislocated hip should be reduced as soon as possible. One of the feared complications of hip dislocations is avascular necrosis of the femoral head. Even with early reduction and proper management, this complication can be seen. With delayed reduction, the incidence of avascular necrosis increases significantly.

As might be expected, sciatic nerve injuries are also seen with hip dislocations, especially posterior hip dislocations. Although early reduction will not repair damage that has already been done to the sciatic nerve, such action will prevent further damage from occurring by minimizing traction or compression of the nerve.

Most hip dislocations seen in the emergency department are of the posterior variety. In this injury, the femoral head comes to rest in a position posterior to the acetabulum (Fig. 43–36). A small percentage of hip dislocations are anterior, wherein the femoral head comes to rest in a position anterior to the acetabulum. In an anterior

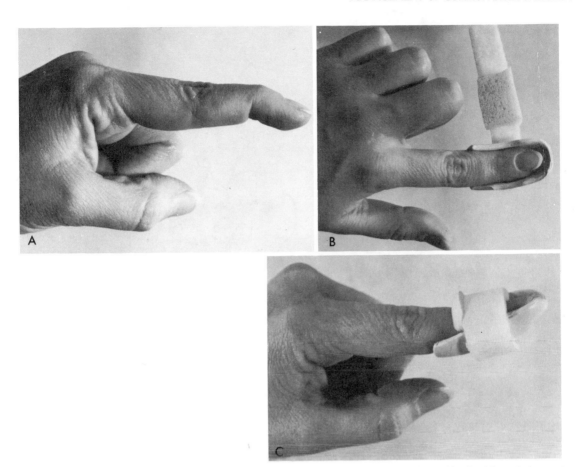

Figure 43–35. A, Mallet finger. B and C, Conservative treatment of mallet finger splint, with distal interphalangeal joint held straight. (From Heppenstall, R. B.: Fracture Treatment and Healing. Philadelphia, W. B. Saunders Company, 1980, p. 567. Used by permission.)

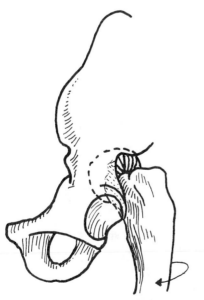

Figure 43–36. Posterior dislocation of the hip. (From Simon, R., and Koenigsknecht, S.: Orthopedics in Emergency Medicine. New York, Appleton-Century-Crofts, 1982, p. 366. Used by permission.)

dislocation, the femoral head usually comes to rest in one of three locations: within the obturator canal, in front of the pubic symphysis, or beside the iliac bone (Fig. 43–37).

Hip dislocations are frequently associated with other major trauma and, as a result, are sometimes overlooked, because attention is focused to more critical aspects of the patient's management. The physician must maintain a high index of suspicion for hip injuries in major trauma; most physicians recommend that pelvic films be taken of all seriously injured patients. Although hip dislocations are not life-threatening entities, delay in reduction or delay in proper management greatly increases the morbidity.

RADIOGRAPHS

The suspected hip injury should be assessed radiographically with at least two different views. A standard AP view, as well as an oblique view, is required. Both of these film views can be ob-

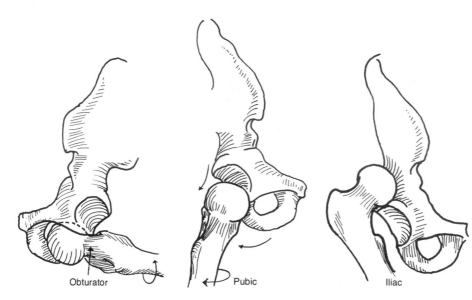

Figure 43–37. Anterior dislocations of the hip: obturator, pubic, and iliac. (From Simon, R., and Koenigsknecht, S.: Orthopedics in Emergency Medicine. New York, Appleton-Century-Crofts, 1982, p. 367. Used by permission.)

tained without moving the patient by placing a cassette under the patient and rotating the x-ray machine from an anterior to an oblique position.

ANALGESIA

Most authorities recommend either spinal or general anesthesia for the proper reduction of hip dislocations. In circumstances in which reduction must be performed under less than ideal circumstances, an attempt can be made to relocate the dislocated hip in the emergency department. Depending upon the condition of the patient and associated injuries, parenteral narcotics and diazepam, either alone or in combination, may be used.

POSTERIOR DISLOCATIONS

A posterior dislocation is usually the result of forces applied to a flexed knee with a hip in flexion, such as seen in a motor vehicle accident when the knee strikes the dashboard during deceleration. Forces are transmitted down the femur to the hip joint, and the femoral head is forced out of the acetabulum. The femoral head comes to rest in a position posterior to the acetabulum. Such dislocations are commonly associated with a fracture of the acetabulum (Fig. 43–38).

Reduction

There are two methods of reduction of posterior dislocations. The first is the Stimson technique, in which the patient is placed in a prone position on the table with his hips at the edge and the affected extremity hanging over the edge of the table. While an assistant stabilizes the pelvis, the knee of the affected extremity is flexed at 90 degrees

and the physician applies steady downward traction at the proximal calf for 10 to 15 minutes (Fig. 43–39). While this downward traction is maintained, an assistant may apply pressure over the greater trocanter and gently push it into the acetabulum.

The second method of reduction is the Allis technique. With the patient in the supine position, the pelvis is again stabilized by an assistant (Fig. 43–40). The hip and knee of the affected extremity are flexed at 90 degrees, maintaining the extremity in adduction with slight internal rotation. Upward traction is then applied at the proximal calf, thereby lifting the head of the femur into the acetabulum. During this maneuver, the physician may stand on the stretcher above the patient.

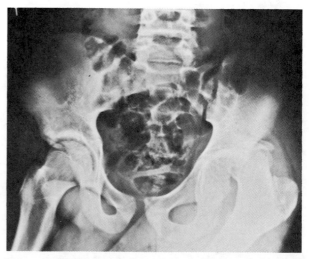

Figure 43–38. Posterior dislocation of the hip. The femur is adducted, internally rotated, and superiorly displaced, with an associated posterior acetabular fracture. A Malgaigne fracture of the pelvis is also present, with diastasis of the pubic symphysis and left sacroiliac joint. (From Greenbaum, E.: Radiology of the Emergency Patient. New York, John Wiley & Sons, Inc., 1982, p. 563. Used by permission.)

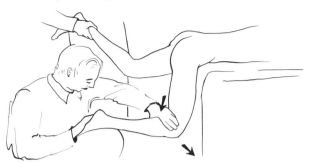

Figure 43–39. Stimson method of reduction for posterior dislocation of the hip (see text for description). This is the preferred method. (From Heppenstall, R. B.: Fracture Treatment and Healing. Philadelphia, W. B. Saunders Company, 1980, p. 672. Used by permission.)

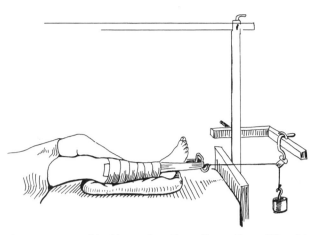

Figure 43–41. Buck's skin traction. (From Simon, R., and Koenig-sknecht, S.: Orthopedics in Emergency Medicine. New York, Appleton-Century-Crofts, 1982, p. 369. Used by permission.)

Forceful rotation should be avoided, because it may result in a fracture of the femoral neck.

After reduction has been accomplished, the leg should be placed in longitudinal traction, such as Buck's traction (Fig. 43–41). The leg should be maintained in slight abduction and slight external rotation. Alternatively, a pillow may be placed between the knees to prevent adduction, and the legs may be tied together. As with other dislocations, postreduction films are needed to ensure proper reduction and realignment and to rule out the possibility of associated fractures.

ANTERIOR DISLOCATIONS

Anterior hip dislocations are usually the result of forced abduction such as may occur in a fall or a motor vehicle accident. The forced abduction

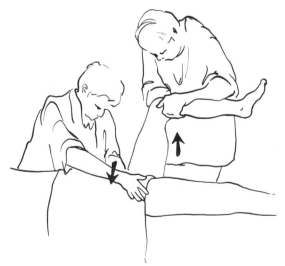

Figure 43–40. Allis method of reducing posterior dislocation of the hip (see text for description). (From Heppenstall, R. B.: Fracture Treatment and Healing. Philadelphia, W. B. Saunders Company, 1980, p. 672. Used by permission.)

results in a levering of the femoral head out of the acetabulum and through a rent in the anterior capsule. If the hip is in flexion when the forced abduction occurs, the femoral head will come to rest in the obturator canal. If the hip is in extension, the femoral head will come to rest anterior to the pubic symphysis or iliac spine. Obturator dislocations are slightly more common than the other two types of anterior hip dislocations. These three types of anterior dislocations can be managed in the same way.

Reduction

For reduction of anterior dislocations, the patient should be placed in a supine position and the pelvis should be stabilized by an assistant putting pressure on the iliac spine (Fig. 43–42). The hip and knee should be greatly flexed to 90 degrees and the femur should be rotated to a neutral position. The physician should then apply steady in-line traction while applying upward traction at the proximal calf, which serves to lift the femoral head into the acetabulum. Gentle internal rotation may aid in this reduction. Do not forcefully adduct the femur, because this may fracture the femoral head or neck. Postreduction treatment includes applying in-line traction with Buck's traction as well as obtaining postreduction films.

SUMMARY

1. Hip dislocations are usually caused by great forces and as such are often associated with fractures or severe trauma of soft tissue.

2. If attempts at closed reduction are not successful, open reduction is mandatory.

3. All hip dislocations require hospitalization with bed rest and traction.

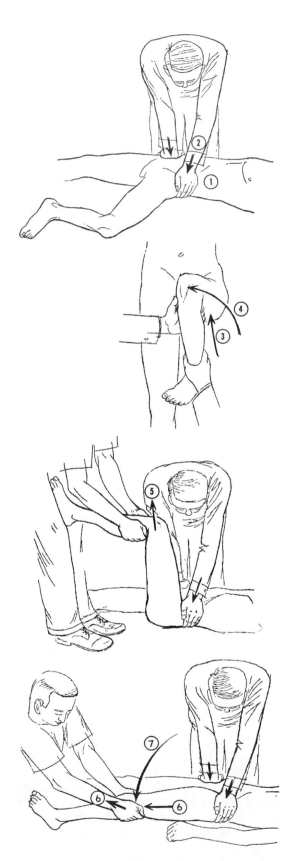

Figure 43–42. Reduction of obturator (anterior hip) dislocation. This procedure should be done under general anesthesia and with adequate muscle relaxation, although occasionally simply positioning the hip for radiographs will reduce the dislocation. *1*, The patient is placed on the floor in a supine position. *2*, An assistant makes downward pressure on the anterosuperior iliac spines. *3*, Grasp the affected limb and flex the hip and knee to a right angle. *4*, Rotate the limb to a neutral position. (This position converts an anterior dislocation to a posterior dislocation.) *5*, Make steady traction on the leg directly upward, lifting the head of the femur into the acetabulum. *Note:* Do not adduct the hip until it is reduced in the acetabulum; otherwise, a fracture of the femoral head or neck may occur. *6*, While upward traction is maintained, lower the thigh to the floor to the extended position *(7)*. (From DePalma, A. F.: Management of Fractures and Dislocations: An Atlas. Philadelphia, W. B. Saunders Company, 1970, p. 1319. Used by permission.)

Knee Dislocations

Dislocations of the knee (with the exception of patellar dislocations) are rare and require a great deal of force in order to occur. This force may be of either a direct or an indirect nature. The knee is a stable joint, the stability being enhanced by strong ligaments. For knee dislocations to occur, these ligamentous attachments must be disrupted by varying degrees. For complete dislocation, both the anterior and posterior cruciate ligaments must be ruptured.

The incidence of damage to the neurovascular structures that cross the knee as a result of dislocation is high. Dislocations may produce both neurologic and vascular embarrassment. For this reason, a knee dislocation must be reduced as soon as possible and, once reduced, continuous observation is essential.

Dislocations of the knee are classified with respect to the position of the tibia in relation to the femur. The most common dislocation is anterior, in which the tibia takes the position anterior to the distal femur. Knee dislocations can also be posterior, lateral, medial, or rotary (Fig. 43–43). Any of these dislocations implies severe damage to the knee joint, and although definitive therapy requires surgical intervention, immediate therapy involves reduction of the dislocation. Often, the extensive ligamentous damage accompanying the dislocation renders the knee extremely unstable. Frequently, prehospital personnel will have reduced the dislocation during the process of splint application.

The patient with a knee dislocation will usually present to the emergency department with a grossly deformed knee. As with any joint injury, distal neurovascular bundles must be assessed immediately and subsequently at appropriate intervals.

RADIOGRAPHS

AP and lateral views are necessary, with additional views as required for clarification. Radiographs of the pelvis and hip should also be considered to rule out the possibility of associated injuries.

ANALGESIA

General anesthesia is the analgesia of choice for reduction of a knee dislocation when the knee is fixed in the dislocated position. If general anesthesia is not available or if for some reason the patient is unable to be given it, analgesia with parenteral narcotics and muscle relaxant agents may be attempted.

REDUCTION

Reduction of a rigidly fixed dislocated knee is probably best accomplished with a closed technique under general anesthesia. Attempts at reduction in the emergency department will usually prove to be unrewarding and, for this reason, should not be undertaken unless there is vascular compromise and no immediate orthopedic referral is available. In this instance, an attempt at reduction is warranted; otherwise, immediate orthopedic referral should be sought with an eye toward the definitive therapy of reduction under general anesthesia.

As with other dislocations, traction, countertraction, and manipulation (and at least two persons) are required if reduction is to be attempted. While an assistant stabilizes the distal femur, in-line traction is applied by the physician with the knee in extension (Fig. 43–44). For anterior dislocations, in which the proximal tibia lies anterior to the distal femur, the assistant attempts to lift the distal femur into a reduced position while in-line traction is applied by the physician. This lifting of the distal femur into position should not occur with pressure over the popliteal space, because such pressure would increase the chance of injury to the structures that traverse this space. For posterior knee dislocations in which the tibia is located posterior to the distal femur, the tibia is gently lifted into a reduced position while in-line traction is maintained. Again, avoidance of pressure over the popliteal fossa is indicated.

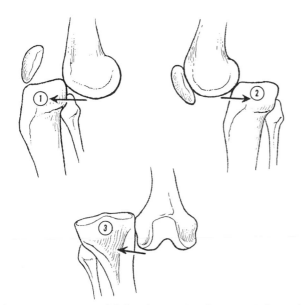

Figure 43–43. Types of dislocations. 1, Anterior, 2, posterior, and 3, lateral. (From DePalma, A. F.: Management of Fractures and Dislocations: An Atlas. Philadelphia, W. B. Saunders Company, 1970, p. 1621. Used by permission.)

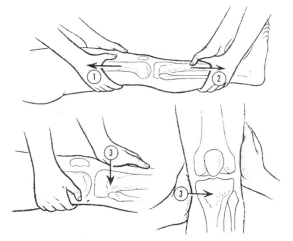

Figure 43–44. Manipulative reduction of a knee dislocation. *1,* An assistant fixes and makes countertraction on the thigh. *2,* Another assistant makes straight traction on the leg (this usually reduces the dislocation). *3,* The physician puts direct pressure over the displaced bones. (From DePalma, A. F.: Management of Fractures and Dislocations: An Atlas. Philadelphia, W. B. Saunders Company, 1970, p. 1623. Used by permission.)

Lateral and medial dislocations can also be reduced with stabilization of the distal femur and in-line traction. Lateral dislocations may benefit from flexion of the knee approximately 90 degrees to relax the hamstrings.

POSTREDUCTION CARE

After the knee has been relocated, the neurovascular status of the lower extremity must be reassessed at appropriate time intervals. Any vascular compromise following reduction demands further evaluation, including arteriography. If the neurovascular status seems to be intact, the knee should be immobilized and postreduction films should be taken. Following reduction of a dislocated knee and after postreduction films have indicated proper alignment without fractures, the stability of the knee joint must be evaluated. This is best accomplished while the patient remains under general anesthesia, because this allows for the evaluation of the ligamentous structures of the knee without resistance from the patient.

All patients with dislocated knees should be hospitalized. Evidence of vascular compromise may be delayed.[13] Close observation and immediate vascular evaluation at the first sign of vascular compromise are indicated.[14] The knee should be immobilized in a slight flexion of approximately 20 to 30 degrees. No weight-bearing is allowed initially. Surgical intervention is eventually required for repair of the damaged ligamentous structures and other associated knee injuries.

SUMMARY

1. Knee dislocations require a great deal of force.

2. There is a high incidence of associated neurologic and/or vascular embarrassment.

3. If vascular embarrassment is present, attempts at reduction in the emergency department are warranted. Otherwise, the knee should be reduced in the operating room under general or spinal anesthesia.

4. Hospitalization is usually required for knee dislocations.

PATELLAR DISLOCATIONS

Patellar dislocations are rather common injuries, especially in adolescents, particularly in girls. Patellar dislocations occasionally result from direct trauma to the patella, although more commonly the mechanism of dislocation is sudden flexion and external rotation of the tibia on the femur with concomitant contraction of the quadriceps, as might occur with the twisting of the knee in a golf swing. These indirect forces cause the patella to ride over the lateral condyle of the femur.

Patellar dislocations are described by indicating where the patella is located in relation to the knee joint. By far, the most common dislocation is a lateral dislocation, with the patella lateral to the knee (Figs. 43–45 and 43–46). Uncommon patellar dislocations include superior, medial, and the very rare intercondylar dislocations.

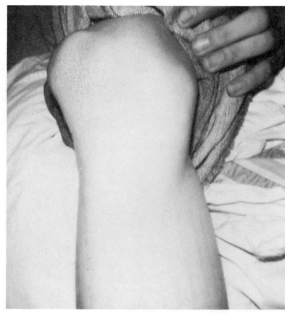

Figure 43–45. Lateral dislocation of the patella.

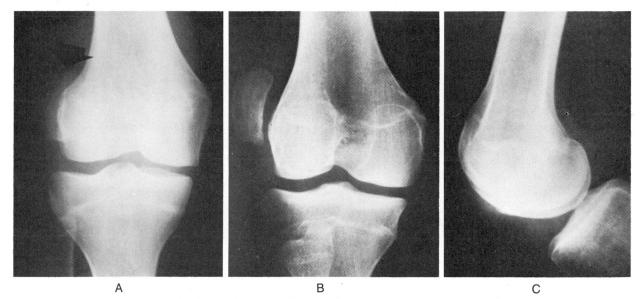

A B C

Figure 43–46. A–C. Complete lateral dislocation of the patella. (From Harris, J. H., Jr., and Harris, W. H.: Radiology of Emergency Medicine, 2nd ed. Baltimore, Williams & Wilkins Co., 1981, p. 575. Used by permission.)

Patellar dislocations often reduce spontaneously, and the physician may not note any obvious abnormalities of the knee when the patient presents to the emergency department. In this case, when the patient's history is consistent with a patellar dislocation, films should be obtained and the knee should be treated as if a patellar dislocation did in fact occur. Patients with recurrent dislocations will usually know their diagnosis.

The patient with a dislocated patella is unable to bear weight and usually presents with the affected knee held in slight flexion. Pain is a significant element of this injury, and there may be some associated swelling or mild hemarthrosis. Even if the patella has reduced spontaneously, the patient usually exhibits some mild apprehension when examination of the patella is attempted, especially lateral movement. Any lateral motion of the patella will generally elicit a reaction (apprehension sign) from the patient, such as a grasp for the examiner's hand and stating that it feels as if the patella is going to dislocate again.

Radiographs

Initially, AP and lateral views of the knee are sufficient to indicate the type of dislocation as well as to rule out the possibility of associated fractures. Postreduction films should again include AP and lateral views (see Fig. 43–46) as well as a sunrise view, that is, a view in which the patella is isolated on the film, allowing the under surface of the patella to be examined (Fig. 43–47).

Analgesia

In most instances, the patella may be reduced without parenteral analgesia. Occasionally however, parenteral analgesia is required.

Reduction

Lateral dislocations are usually easily reduced using a closed technique. The patient should be placed in a supine position, and the knee should be gently flexed and supported, followed by gentle extension of the knee to 180 degrees. Extension alone may suffice to reduce the patella. If the knee is fully extended and the patella does not reduce, slight anteriorly directed pressure over the lateral aspect of the patella will aid in moving the patella over the lateral condyle and back into its normal anatomical position (Fig. 43–48).

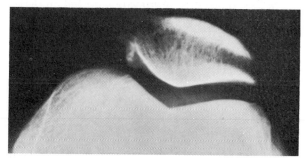

Figure 43–47. Dislocated patella. The fracture of the medial aspect of the patella, seen with this "skyline" view, was the only evidence of a previous traumatic patellar dislocation. (From Greenbaum, E.: Radiology of the Emergency Patient. New York, John Wiley & Sons, Inc., 1982, p. 575. Used by permission.)

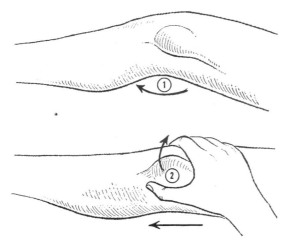

Figure 43–48. Manipulative reduction. *1*, Extend the knee gradually while medially directed pressure is applied upon the patella *(2)*, pushing it over the lateral femoral condyle. (From DePalma, A. F.: Management of Fractures and Dislocations. Philadelphia, W. B. Saunders Company, 1970, p. 1665. Used by permission.)

The other types of knee dislocations (superior, medial, and intra-articular) are usually resistant to reduction with closed techniques. For this reason, orthopedic consultation is recommended and no attempt at closed reduction is made in the emergency department.

Postreduction Care

Postreduction care for lateral displacements includes postreduction films and the placement of the knee in a knee immobilizer. The patient should be instructed not to bear weight, and orthopedic referral is made for 1 to 2 days postreduction. Hospitalization is not usually required for lateral dislocations.

Ankle Dislocations

The ankle joint is comprised of the distal fibula and tibia, which are firmly attached to one another by the interosseous membrane, and the talus bone of the foot. The ankle is a stable joint with strong ligamentous support. Dislocations of the ankle are the result of great forces applied to the ankle, and they are often associated with fractures.

Dislocations are classified according to the description of the talus in relation to the distal tibia and fibula. In a posterior dislocation, the talus is found in a position posterior to the distal tibia and fibula. An anterior dislocation places the talus in a position anterior to the distal tibia and fibula (Fig. 43–49).

Posterior dislocations are the most common type of ankle dislocations. They are most often the result of a forced plantar flexion, which might be seen with a fall on a plantar-flexed foot. Such

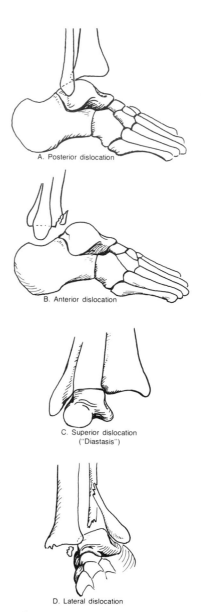

Figure 43–49. The types of dislocations of the ankle. (From Simon, R., and Koenigsknecht, S.: Orthopedics in Emergency Medicine. New York, Appleton-Century-Crofts, 1982, p. 419. Used by permission.)

dislocations are often accompanied by malleolar fractures or fractures of the posterior tibia (Fig. 43–50). The patient will usually present with a markedly swollen ankle, unable to bear weight, and resistant to any attempt at dorsiflexion. Although the fact that the patient has had a serious ankle injury will be obvious to the examiner, clinical diagnosis without radiologic confirmation of a dislocation is rather difficult. Attempts at manipulation of the ankle should be kept to a minimum until radiographic films are obtained. Neurovascular injury to the foot should be ascertained prior to the taking of radiographs.

Anterior dislocations of the ankle are usually the result of forced dorsiflexion of the foot, al-

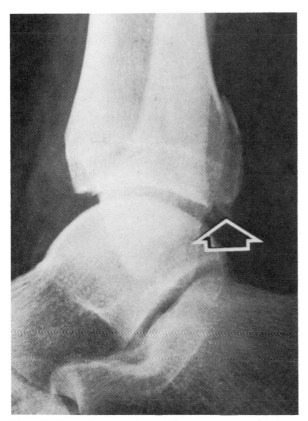

Figure 43–50. Isolated posterior tibial lip fracture (open arrow), seen after reduction of posterior ankle dislocation. (From Harris, J. H., Jr., and Harris, W. H.: Radiology of Emergency Medicine, 2nd ed. Baltimore, Williams & Wilkins Co., 1981, p. 629. Used by permission.)

though a direct blow to the heel with the foot in dorsiflexion may also produce an anterior dislocation. The most common causes of such dislocations are the deceleration injuries seen in motor vehicle accidents with forced dorsiflexion. Anterior dislocations are also associated with malleolar fractures (Fig. 43–51). The third type of dislocation of the ankle is an upward dislocation of the talus. In this type of dislocation, the talus is driven upward, disrupting the syndesmotic tibiofibular joint (see Fig. 43–49). This type of injury most commonly results when a person falls from a distance and lands on his feet. The force is directed upward and drives the talus into the tibiofibular joint. This type of dislocation requires open reduction and internal fixation. Lateral dislocations of the joint can also occur and are most often the result of marked inversion of the foot. Lateral dislocations are always associated with fractures of the malleoli and are often open and require surgical correction.

Any indication of vascular compromise demands expeditious reduction. One complication of dislocations of the ankle is avascular necrosis of the talus, and a delay in reduction increases the risk of this complication.

RADIOGRAPHS

The minimal films required for evaluation of an ankle injury are AP, lateral, and oblique views.

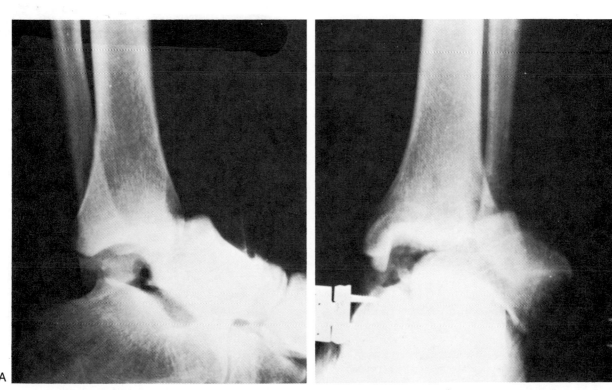

A   B

Figure 43–51. A and B, Anterior dislocation of the talus. (From Harris, J. H., Jr., and Harris, W. H.: Radiology of Emergency Medicine, 2nd ed. Baltimore, Williams & Wilkins Co., 1981, p. 629. Used by permission.)

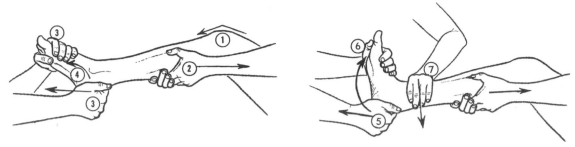

Figure 43–52. Manipulative reduction of a posterior ankle dislocation. *1*, The knee is flexed. *2*, The assistant makes countertraction on the leg. *3*, Grasp the forefoot with one hand and the heel with the other hand. *4*, The foot is slightly plantar flexed. *5*, Make straight downward traction on the plantar-flexed foot, then pull the foot forward *(6)* while a second assistant makes counter pressure on the front of the lower leg *(7)*. (From DePalma, A. F.: Management of Fractures and Dislocations. Philadelphia, W. B. Saunders Company, 1970, pp. 1916 and 1917. Used by permission.)

Additional views may be obtained as needed to more clearly delineate fractures and anatomical relationships.

ANALGESIA

Although these reductions can be performed using parenteral analgesia and muscle relaxants when vascular compromise is evident, general anesthesia or spinal anesthesia is preferred.

REDUCTION

For posterior dislocations, the patient is placed in supine position and the knee of the affected extremity is flexed 30 to 45 degrees. The physician should than grasp the foot with both hands, one hand holding the heel and the other hand holding the forefoot. While traction is applied to the foot, an assistant should hold the calf and apply countertraction (Fig. 43–52). While traction and countertraction are being steadily maintained, a second assistant should apply downward pressure on the distal calf. At the same time, the physician should lift the foot anteriorly and gently dorsiflex the foot. When the relocation occurs, dorsiflexion will be accomplished without resistance.

For anterior dislocations, the patient is placed in a supine position and the knee is slightly flexed. While an assistant applies countertraction to the calf, the physician should grasp the foot with both hands as previously described and apply traction to the foot. The foot, which is in mild dorsiflexion secondary to the dislocation, may need to be dorsiflexed to a greater degree in order to disengage the talus. With traction being maintained on the foot, a second assistant should apply pressure in an anterior direction at the posterior calf at the same time that the physician pushes the foot in a posterior direction (Fig. 43–53). It is important that in-line traction be maintained during this maneuver. When the ankle is reduced, gentle plantar flexion will be possible without resistance.

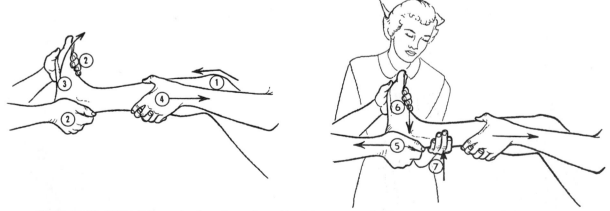

Figure 43–53. Manipulative reduction of anterior ankle dislocation. *1*, The knee is flexed. *2*, The physician grasps the forefoot with one hand and the heel with the other hand. *3*, Dorsiflexion of the foot is slightly increased (to disengage the talus). *4*, An assistant makes countertraction on the leg. *5*, Straight longitudinal traction is made, then the foot is pushed directly backward *(6)* while a second assistant makes countertraction on the back of the lower leg *(7)*. (From DePalma, A. F.: Management of Fractures and Dislocations. Philadelphia, W. B. Saunders Company, 1970, pp. 1918 and 1919. Used by permission.)

POSTREDUCTION CARE

Postreduction care includes hospitalization for 24 to 48 hours, with the ankle splinted in a neutral position. In 24 to 48 hours, the splint can be replaced with a circular plaster cast below the knee. No weight-bearing should be allowed for at least 6 weeks.

SUMMARY

1. The ankle joint has strong ligamentous support; thus, dislocations are usually the result of great forces.

2. The reduction of ankle dislocations is best carried out under general or spinal anesthesia.

3. All patients with ankle dislocations require hospitalization.

1. Carter, P.: Common Hand Injuries and Infections. A Practical Approach to Early Treatment. Philadelphia, W. B. Saunders Company, 1983.
2. Connolly, J.: DePalma's The Management of Fractures and Dislocations, 3rd ed. Philadelphia, W. B. Saunders Company, 1980.
3. Conwell, H.: Injuries to the elbow. Clin. Symp. 21:35, 1969.
4. Greenbaum, E. (ed.): Radiology of the Emergency Patient. An Atlas Approach. New York, John Wiley & Sons, Inc., 1982.
5. Harris, J., and Harris, W.: The Radiology of Emergency Medicine, 2nd ed. Baltimore, Williams & Wilkins, 1981.
6. Heppenstall, R.: Fracture Treatment and Healing. Philadelphia, W. B. Saunders Company, 1980.
7. McRae, R.: Practical Fracture Treatment. New York, Churchill Livingstone, 1981.
8. Mirick, M., Clinton, J., and Ruiz, E.: External rotation method of shoulder dislocation reduction. JACEP 8:528, 1979.
9. Newmeyer, W.: Primary Care of Hand Injuries. Philadelphia, Lea & Febiger, 1979.
10. Rockwood, C.: Fractures. Philadelphia, J. B. Lippincott Co., 1975.
11. Simon, R., and Koeningsknecht, S.: Orthopedics in Emergency Medicine. The Extremities. New York, Appleton-Century-Crofts, 1982.
12. Wilson, J. (ed.): Fracture and Joint Injuries. New York, Churchill Livingstone, 1982.
13. Lefrak, E. A.: Knee dislocation: an illusive cause of critical arterial occlusion. Arch. Surg. 111:1021, 1976.
14. Dart, C. H., and Braitman, H. E.: Popliteal artery injury following fracture or dislocation at the knee: diagnosis and management. Arch. Surg. 112:969, 1977.

Introduction

Extensor tendons are more superficial than flexor tendons; they are covered for most of their course by only skin and very thin fascia (Fig. 44–1). The mechanism of action of extensor tendons in the digits is complex and little understood by most physicians. Extensor tendons are more subject to *closed* injury than flexor tendons, and closed injuries are usually more difficult to diagnose than open ones. Extensor tendon injuries can often be definitively treated in a well-equipped outpatient setting if the treating physician is conversant with the pathophysiology involved.

44

Extensor Tendon Injuries in the Hand and Wrist

WILLIAM L. NEWMEYER, M.D.

Surgical and Functional Anatomy

There are twelve extrinsic extensor musculotendinous units, all innervated by the radial nerve in the upper dorsal forearm. Four of these tendons insert at the wrist level. The most radial of these is the abductor pollicis longus (APL) tendon, which arises deep on the lateral side of the forearm from the radius, the interosseous membrane, and the ulna. The APL tendon passes deep to the other extensors and inserts into the base of the first metacarpal. The APL tendon acts as a radial wrist deviator and stabilizes the base of the first metacarpal. The extensor carpi radialis longus (ECRL) and the extensor carpi radialis brevis (ECRB) arise from the lateral epicondyle and insert into the bases of the second and third metacarpals, respectively. The ECRL is a powerful wrist extensor and, to some extent, a radial wrist deviator, whereas the ECRB is a powerful wrist extensor (Fig. 44–2). The fourth wrist extensor is the extensor carpi ulnaris (ECU), which also arises from the lateral epicondyle and inserts into the base of the

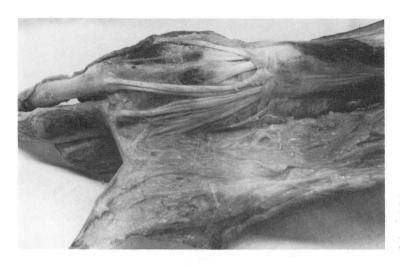

Figure 44–1. The first 10 figures show a cadaver dissection of the dorsal hand to illustrate important facets of extensor anatomy. In this figure, the very thin cover of skin and dorsal fascia is demonstrated, and it can be seen that the tendons have sheaths only at wrist level.

fifth metacarpal, acting as a wrist extensor and an ulnar wrist deviator (Fig. 44–3). Wrist extension is critical to hand function because the finger flexors cannot work with force unless the wrist is extended (dorsiflexed).

Fibro-osseous tendon sheaths are present *only* at wrist level on the dorsal or extensor surface (Fig. 44–4). There are six synovial lined tendon sheaths, some with one or more subdivisions. The APL passes through the first dorsal compartment, the ECRL and ECRB through the second dorsal compartment, and the ECU through the sixth. These sheaths, collectively referred to as the dorsal retinaculum, are necessary to prevent the tendons from bowstringing when the wrist is extended. Distal to the wrist the tendons lie in loose areolar tissue beneath the thin dorsal skin and very thin dorsal fascia.

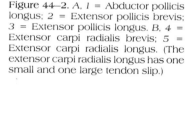

Figure 44–2. A, 1 = Abductor pollicis longus; 2 = Extensor pollicis brevis; 3 = Extensor pollicis longus. B, 4 = Extensor carpi radialis brevis; 5 = Extensor carpi radialis longus. (The extensor carpi radialis longus has one small and one large tendon slip.)

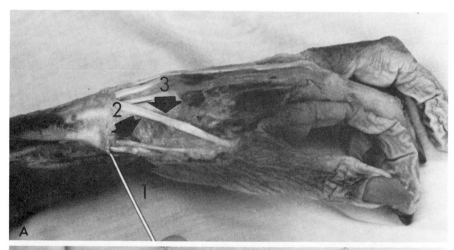

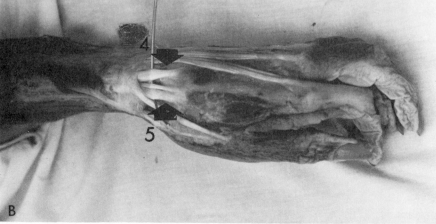

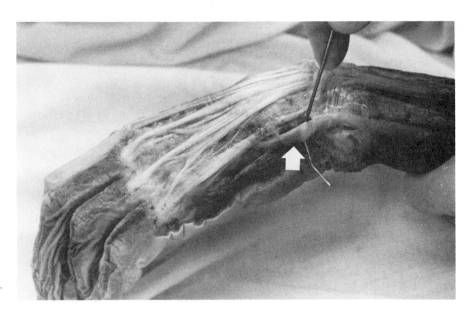

Figure 44–3. The extensor carpi ulnaris tendon (*arrow*).

There are eight digital extensor tendons. The thumb has two, the extensor pollicis brevis (EPB) and the extensor pollicis longus (EPL) (see Fig. 44–2). The EPB arises with the APL and passes through the first dorsal compartment with it. The first dorsal compartment actually has two or more subcompartments for these two tendons. (In fact, the APL may have three or four slips, each with its own compartment.) The EPL passes through the third dorsal compartment, which is just on the ulnar side of Lister's tubercle, a bony prominence on the radial side of the distal dorsal radius. The EPL crosses directly over the two radial wrist extensors and pursues a radial-distal direction to its ultimate insertion on the distal phalanx of the thumb (see Fig. 44–2). The EPB inserts on the proximal phalanx of the thumb. The EPL is the only extrinsic digital extensor that has its primary insertion and function on an interphalangeal (IP) joint.

There are six tendons to extend the other four

digits; their primary action is at the metacarpal phalangeal (MCP) joints. Each digit has its own extensor digitorum communis (EDC) tendon. The index and little fingers each have an independent extensor, the extensor indicicis proprius (EIP) for the index finger and the extensor digiti quinti minimi (EDQM) for the little finger. The four EDC tendons and the EIP pass together through the fourth dorsal compartment, but the EDQM has its own compartment the fifth (Fig. 44–5A and B).

On the dorsum of the hand at the level of the distal metacarpals the six tendons are interconnected with oblique tendinous bands, called juncturae tendineae (Fig. 44–6). These juncturae can give an examiner a false sense of security because they may allow weak active digital extension even if the main tendon is cut.

The six digital extensors to these four digits (i.e., the second to fifth digits) have a fibrous insertion distal to the MCP joints and act primarily at this site (Fig. 44–7), but each digit also has a dorsal

Figure 44–4. The dorsal retinaculum with a probe passing through the fourth dorsal compartment.

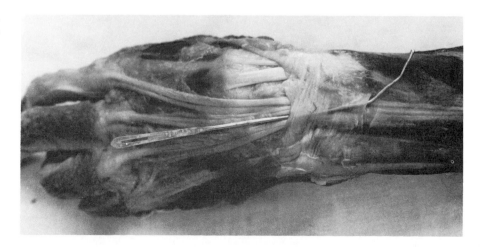

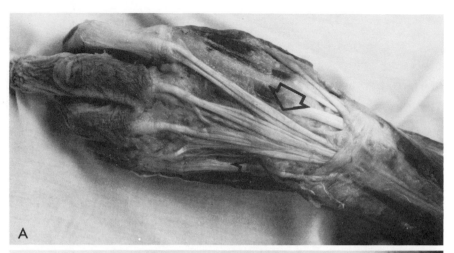

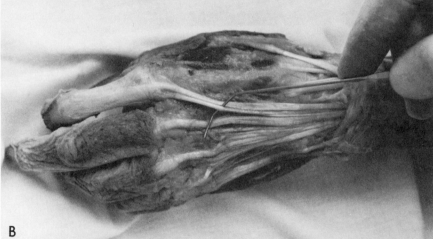

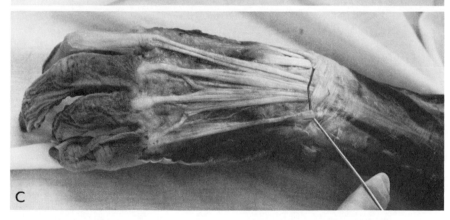

Figure 44–5. *A,* The digital extensor tendons (*between the arrows*). *B,* The extensor indicicis proprius. *C,* The extensor digiti quinti minimi.

extension along the proximal phalanges to a final bony insertion on the dorsal proximal lip of the middle phalanx (Fig. 44–8). The central intrinsic muscles (i.e., the four lumbricals and the seven interossei) have tendons known as lateral bands (Fig. 44–9), which act as flexors of the MCP joints but then move dorsally to become extensors of the IP joints. They are connected to the extrinsic extensor tendon by a broad, flat sheet of fascia known as the sagittal fibers. This troika of the central slip and lateral bands is known as the extensor mechanism of the digit. Beyond the level of the PIP joint these entities fuse into a tendon known as the terminal extensor mechanism (TEM) (Fig. 44–10). The TEM has its insertion on the dorsal lip of the proximal portion of the distal phalanx. It is very important to understand this mechanism if one is to diagnose and treat extensor tendon injuries—especially in the fingers.

It is obvious to all that tendons function by

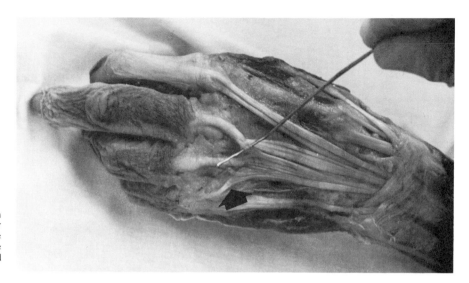

Figure 44–6. The arrow points to an interconnecting band of the extensor tendons on the dorsum of the hand—a juncturae tendineae. The probe is lifting up another such band of tendons.

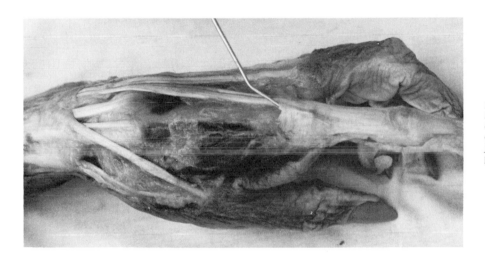

Figure 44–7. The mainly fibrous insertion of an extrinsic extensor tendon on the proximal phalanx just distal to the metacarpal phalangeal joint with a probe inserted under its proximal edge.

Figure 44–8. The extensor mechanism on the dorsum of a finger. Arrows point to the radial and ulnar lateral band portions of the extensor mechanism. The thinner central portion is the central extensor mechanism, and the probe lifts the entire structure up off the phalanx.

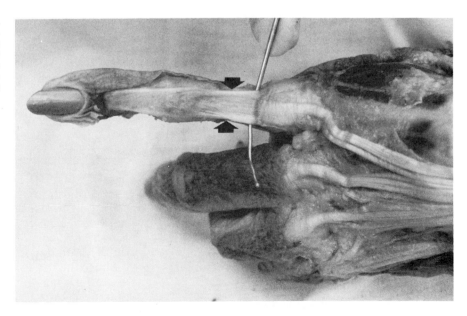

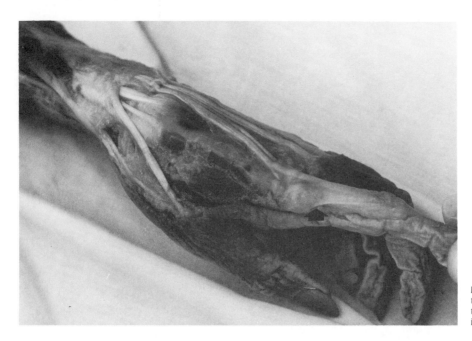

Figure 44–9. The proximal portion of the lateral band (*arrow*), in this case the one arising from the first dorsal interosseous muscle.

moving. This movement, which varies in degree according to several factors (including how close the tendon is to its insertion), is known as amplitude, or glide. If a tendon is lacerated in an area of large amplitude and it is not otherwise fixed, the proximal (and, to some extent, the distal) ends

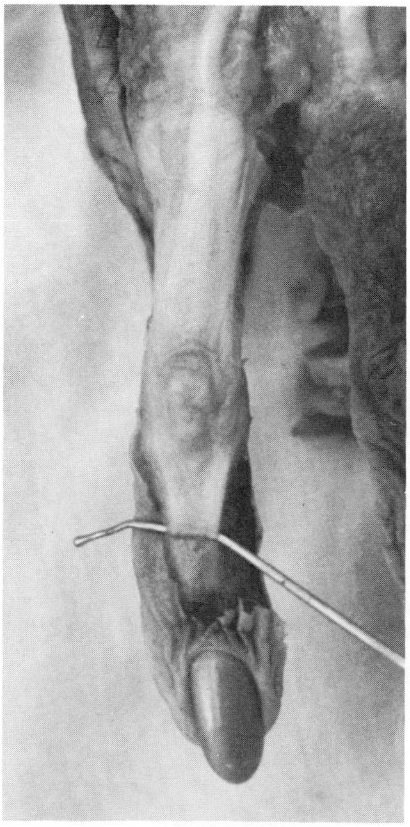

Figure 44–10. The terminal extensor mechanism.

will retract and retrieval may be a major problem. This may occur on the dorsum of the hand, especially as the site of injury becomes more proximal. This is a significant problem at the wrist level with the complicating factor of having to deal with a synovial lined sheath (as discussed earlier). Fortunately, on the distal dorsal hand and especially on the fingers not only is the amplitude small but also the extensor mechanism is a broad flat sheet, that is seldom cut in its entirety, and therefore, retrieval is usually not a problem.

Pathophysiology of Extensor Injuries

Whereas most (but not all) flexor tendon injuries are open injuries, closed injuries of the extensors, especially in the fingers, are very common. Injuries may occur from closed trauma that may appear to be trivial. One must be aware of this because it is more difficult to diagnose closed injuries than open ones. With injuries at the distal or middle joint level (DIP or PIP), a fracture may be a key part of the problem, and it is usually advisable to obtain a radiograph. This is particularly true of closed injuries.

Extensor tendons of the hand and the wrist are very superficial. Therefore, it is difficult *not* to have at least a partial tendon injury in all but the most superficial wounds in that area. Thus, *all dorsal wrist, hand, and digital lacerations should be approached with the thought that there is a partial or total tendon laceration in their depth.* The techniques for determining and repairing these lacerations are outlined in the following sections. Partial tendon lacerations may not be obvious, since function will initially be normal. Therefore, one must inspect all wounds visually and examine the wound while putting the fingers and wrist through a range of motion if partial lacerations are to be discovered. If an injury occurred with the fist closed, the injured area of the tendon may not be visualized in the wound if the hand is examined in full extension. In the case of an open injury, the tendon may be either partially or completely divided. Partial division is the most usual situation on the dorsal finger, whereas on the hand and the wrist total division is much more common. Completely divided tendons, obviously, must be repaired. If a tendon is partially lacerated one must consider the location and extent of the laceration in deciding whether or not to repair it. If the partial laceration is 10 per cent of the total tendon bulk or less it may be safely left alone. If it is greater than 10 per cent, it should be repaired either with a running 5–0 nylon suture or in a manner similar to that for complete laceration (see later).

Open Injury Treatment Prerequisites

If one is to undertake the repair of open extensor tendon injuries in the outpatient setting, certain principles must be rigorously adhered to or disaster is sure to follow. These include the following:

1. The procedure must be performed in a relatively clean room with the necessary supplies readily available in the room. This area must be out of the traffic pattern of both hospital personnel and patients.

2. The patient should always be supine on a stretcher or a gurney. The hand should be supported on a firm platform that allows access from either side.

3. There should be good overhead lighting.

4. Plastic surgery–type instruments should be available. These should include a Webster needle holder; two small double-pronged skin hooks; two small right-angled (Ragnell) retractors; one pair of small curved sharp (Iris) scissors (for cutting tissue); one pair of small blunt-nosed scissors (for cutting sutures); several small hemostats, both curved and straight; one pair of small single-toothed (Adson) forceps; and one larger pair of blunt-nosed scissors for cutting the dressings to proper size.

5. Proper suture material with a needle of appropriate size should be used. Monofilament nylon (Ethilon from Ethicon or Dermalon from Davis & Geck) is an excellent material. Some surgeons like to use a material that is not as slippery as monofilament nylon. Either braided nylon (Surgilon) or Dacron (Ticron) is satisfactory. Four-zero is the best size, although 5-0 may serve in some cases. *Silk should never be used.* Absorbable sutures may dissolve before the tendon ends have healed together. Plastic needles should be used, such as the P-3 from Ethicon and PRE-2 from Davis & Geck.

6. An arm tourniquet *must* be used. It is not possible to identify and repair small structures in the hand in a pool of blood. An ordinary blood pressure cuff may be used. The cuff is placed on the mid- to upper arm with the tube or tubes pointing cephalad. The cuff is wrapped with two or three layers of cast padding after it has been placed on the arm. This is to prevent its unwrapping when the cuff is put to working pressure. Blood pressure cuffs are not designed for the pressures used and will unwrap in the middle of the procedure if padding is not used. When all else is ready, the arm is exsanguinated by gravity for 1 minute, the cuff is elevated to 260 to 280 mm Hg, and the tube or tubes are *clamped* to maintain the pressure. If this is not done the manometer will steadily lose its pressure with a resultant venous tourniquet and a very bloody field. After the tubes are clamped the pressure obviously can no longer be monitored. The assistant should be advised of this so that he or she does not fuss with the inflating bulb. In fact, it is advisable to open the bulb screw and to let the monitor go to zero, since it is now separated from the cuff by the clamp. At the conclusion of the procedure, releasing the clamp will let the pressure go immediately to zero, but if the bulb is still under pressure a rather awkward situation may result with a persistent venous tourniquet effect until all realize what is going on. This tourniquet is well tolerated by a conscious, alert patient for approximately 15 to 20 minutes. This time duration serves as a good cutoff point, because anything that takes longer than that is probably more than can be comfortably tackled in an outpatient setting. It is a good idea for a physician who is going to be using a tourniquet on conscious patients to try it out on himself or herself for 20 minutes just to see how it feels.

7. Anesthesia must be used when tendons are explored and repaired. The easiest thing to use on the dorsum of the hand is a field block of 1 per cent plain lidocaine placed through the already cut skin edges using a 1½-inch, number 27 needle. One should always remember to anesthetize not only the area of the wound but also a proximal area if the wound has to be extended. (For further details on local and limited regional anesthesia, consult Chapter 32 or reference #1.) The anesthesia should always be in place and set *before* the tourniquet is inflated. Tourniquet time must be used for exploration and operating and *not* for ancillary procedures that can be performed without a tourniquet.

8. Exposure must be adequate and can be a problem in the repair of extensor tendon lacerations. One should not hesitate to extend the

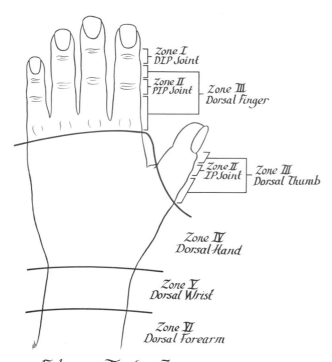

Extensor Tendon Zones

Figure 44–11. Extensor tendon zones. (From Newmeyer, W. L.: Primary Care of Hand Injuries. Philadelphia, Lea & Febiger, 1979. Used by permission.)

wound proximally (the usual area in which more exposure is needed) or distally.

9. The most important principle is that the practitioner must have adequate knowledge. It should be noted that the tendons do not look the same in the living hand as they do in the illustrations. Reference #2 is a valuable, inexpensive anatomic reference for all outpatient emergency treatment center libraries. Tendon repair should not be attempted unless the physician performing the repair has had some instruction by a surgeon with hand experience. It is an excellent idea to do a cadaver dissection of the dorsal hand before undertaking repairs on a living hand. The only thing lacking in the cadaver hand is the tendon amplitude, which can stymie the uninitiated. (Also, exposure is easier in cadaver hands.)

Extensor Tendon Zones

It is helpful to divide extensor tendon injuries into zones (Fig. 44–11) and to consider open and closed injuries in each zone. These zones are somewhat arbitrary but are functionally useful. They are:

Zone I: The area over the DIP joint. An injury at this area is known as a mallet finger.

Zone II: The area over the PIP joint. An injury at this level results in the so-called boutonniere deformity.

Zone III: This is the area on the dorsal finger between the joints. The tendon in this area is a broad, flat sheet of fascia-like tissue and is seldom totally divided.

Zone IV: In this area tendons look like tendons rather than broad bands of fascia. Especially in the proximal part of this zone, retraction of the cut tendon end can be a major problem.

Zone V: This is the area of the dorsal retinaculum. Injuries in this area require treatment in the operating suite under high regional or general anesthesia.

Zone VI: This is above the retinaculum. The problems of exposure and the operative requirements are similar to those for Zone V.

ZONE I INJURIES

Injuries at this level may be the result of closed trauma with attenuation or rupture of the terminal extensor insertion on the distal phalanx, a laceration of the terminal extensor tendon, or a fracture avulsion of the bony insertion of the TEM.

The most common injury is the closed avulsion of the tendon. The trauma that causes this is often rather mild. The patient usually complains of a painless droop of the distal phalanx, and a radiograph shows only the flexed distal phalanx. The best treatment for the common condition of mallet finger is splinting in full extension for 8 weeks. The splint should be one that holds the DIP joint in extension while allowing easy motion of the PIP joint (Fig. 44–12). The patient should be advised to change the splint at least once a day to make sure there are no pressure spots under the splint. During the splint change the patient should be advised to avoid flexing the DIP joint and to hold it in full extension either with the other hand or by placing the palmar surface of the finger on a hard table. It is useful to give the patient several extra splints. The patient should be advised to leave the splint in place during bathing and to change the wet splint afterward. In most instances, if the splint is worn faithfully for 8 weeks (and then for 4 more weeks at night) a good result can be expected. If the result is not satisfactory to the patient, there are various tendon reconstructive procedures that can be considered, but none of these are uniformly satisfactory. The joint can always be fused if instability is a major problem.

If the deformity is the result of a fracture one should consider operative fixation of the fragment if a significant portion of the articular surface is involved (over 30 to 40 per cent) and especially if there is volar subluxation of the distal phalanx upon the middle phalanx (Fig. 44–13). Unfortunately, operative fixation of this tiny fragment is often quite difficult, and some degree of joint injury often results with less than full restoration

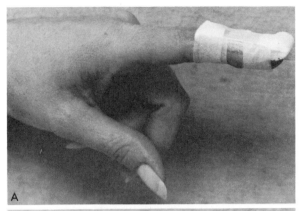

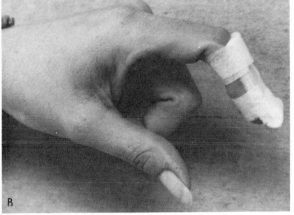

Figure 44–12. A proper mallet finger splint (A). It should allow easy active motion of the distal interphalangeal joint (B).

of DIP function. If the fracture fragment is small and there is minimal or no distal phalangeal subluxation, treatment is the same as that outlined for the closed mallet deformity.

Open mallet injuries caused by a laceration that severs the terminal extensor mechanism should be treated by suture fixation of the tendon. In most instances it is advisable to splint the DIP joint internally with a Kirschner wire (0.035-inch size). The internal splint should be left in place for at least 6 weeks and preferably for 8 weeks. This is a procedure that can be performed in the outpatient setting but is easier if performed in an oper-

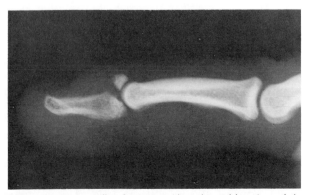

Figure 44–13. A mallet fracture with volar subluxation of the distal phalanx.

ating suite, although neither general nor high regional anesthesia is required. Passing a K wire through the distal phalanx and into the middle phalanx is not as easy as it looks. A powered drill simplifies the task. The power may be supplied by either air or electricity; electric drills may be battery- or wall-powered. There are several battery-powered drills on the market that can readily be used in the outpatient setting. Some physicians use a number 19, 1½-inch disposable needle as a fixation wire. A syringe is used as the "driver." Usually, the top of the needle bends in the course of this maneuver, causing a fair amount of trauma. Although this may be satisfactory in some cases, it is not advised if a more conventional fixation wire is available.

ZONE II INJURIES

Injuries at this level may also be either open or closed. Open injuries are usually straightforward in that they are easy to recognize. Treatment consists of suturing the tendon with a running 4-0 nylon and supporting the joint with an external or internal splint for approximately 4 to 6 weeks. The internal splint, if used, is a K wire or some equivalent (0.035- or 0.045-inch size). The problems of placing this are similar to those outlined in the preceding section for the DIP joint.

The closed injuries cause problems because they are difficult to diagnose, and if they are *not* recognized the so-called boutonniere deformity that results is often difficult to correct surgically. To understand this deformity one has to recall the normal anatomic patterns as discussed previously. If there is an injury to the central extensor mechanism (CEM) over the PIP joint function may initially be normal, because extension is still possible via the lateral bands. With time the central support for the lateral bands collapses and they sink, lying on the volar side of the axis of flexion of the PIP joint (Fig. 44–14). The joint more or less herniates, or buttonholes, through the extensor mechanism (hence the name of the deformity). It is obvious that the lateral bands are then in the paradoxical position of being flexors of the joint they are supposed to extend. As this occurs they pull on and tighten the *terminal* extensor mechanism, causing the DIP joint to go into hyperextension. If the finger gets fixed in this position, a great deal of function is lost, and it is very difficult to get things back to normal or even back to good function. As with so many other injuries, the best treatment is prevention.

When one treats a patient who complains of blunt trauma to a finger and has swelling around the PIP joint, the first step is to obtain a radiograph and rule out a fracture. The patient's usual presenting complaint is, "I jammed my finger." The second step is to assume that there may be at least

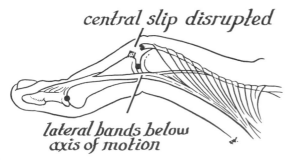

central slip disrupted

lateral bands below axis of motion

Figure 44–14. Diagrammatic explanation of a boutonniere deformity. (From Newmeyer, W. L.: Primary Care of Hand Injuries. Philadelphia, Lea & Febiger, 1979. Used by permission.)

a potential boutonniere deformity (even if initial function is normal) and to treat accordingly. The treatment consists of splinting the PIP joint in full extension, leaving the MCP and DIP joints free to move (Figure 44–15). The patient should be followed at fairly frequent intervals in order for the status of the injury to be assessed. Usually, splinting for 4 weeks is sufficient.

ZONE III INJURIES

Injuries in this zone, which is the area between the MCP and PIP joints and between the PIP and

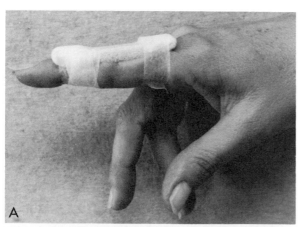

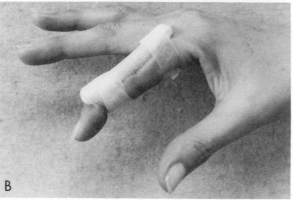

Figure 44–15. A, Boutonniere splint. B, This allows active flexion at the metacarpal phalangeal and distal interphalangeal joints.

DIP joints, are virtually always open but with only a partial laceration of the tendon. The only way to make the diagnosis is by exploration of the wound. The lacerated tendon should be closed with a running 4-0 or 5-0 suture. The degree of splinting required will depend on the amount of the tendon lacerated. If the laceration is a small one, a finger guard (see Chapter 45) for 7 to 10 days is all that is necessary. If the laceration is a large one, a full forearm-hand-wrist-digit splint for 3 weeks is required. When exploring wounds in this area, one should remember that the only thing that can be cut between skin and bone is tendon.

ZONE IV INJURIES

This is the area between the distal end of the dorsal retinaculum (the six dorsal sheaths) and the area over the MCP joints, where the extensor mechanism of the digits begins. In this area the tendons are discrete structures with interconnecting bands (juncturae tendineae—see earlier). One should assume that any laceration on the dorsum of the hand has a lacerated tendon in its depths; it is up to the treating physician to disprove this thesis. This means that the wound must be explored with tourniquet, anesthesia, and a suitable sterile preparation and field.

The biggest problem in fixing tendons in this zone is retrieving the proximal stump, which almost always retracts to some extent. The more proximal the laceration, the greater the retraction. Recovery of this stump can be quite difficult for the uninitiated, and if the proximal stump cannot be readily found, the attempt should be postponed. The wound should be closed and dressed, and arrangements should be made for repair in an operating suite under high regional or general anesthesia. One can almost always bring the distal stump into view by simply passively bringing the involved digit into full extension.

Because proximal stump retrieval is a problem, it is a good idea to extend the traumatic wound proximally along the course of the divided tendon before even making the effort of locating it. This is done from one corner of the traumatic wound, with care taken to avoid veins and sensory nerves. Often, if the physician will lift up the edge of the skin flap created by wound extension and look proximally under the flap, a tunnel with blood staining will be seen. This is the clue to the location of the proximal stump, and if one carefully puts a small hemostat or tooth forceps up this "canal," the stump can be grasped and drawn into the wound. As will be understood from a reading of the anatomy section, this is not a synovial sheath (unless one is at wrist level) but rather a pseudocanal. A 4-0 nylon suture should be already loaded, and as one grasps the proximal stump with forceps or clamp tip, the suture is placed as far proximally in the retrieved tendon stump as possible. This acts as a holding suture while the repair is accomplished.

Tendon repairs in this area are performed as shown in Figure 44–16. Basically, these are horizontal mattress sutures placed so that the knot lies between the cut tendon ends. In fair, thin-skinned persons it is a good idea to use clear rather than colored 4-0 nylon, because the colored material may show through the skin and upset the patient, although it does no physical harm. Because there is no tendon sheath on the extensor surface except at the wrist level, there need be no worry about repairing or not repairing the sheath on the dorsal hand and digits. Virtually without exception, extensor tendon lacerations at wrist level require surgical repair in an operating suite under high regional or general anesthesia. The exposure required and the length of time needed for repair at this level are beyond the capacity of local anesthesia.

Following repair, a forearm-wrist-hand-digit splint is used. The wrist is extended 30 degrees, the MCP joints are in approximately 10 to 20 degrees of flexion, and the IP joints are nearly straight. It is wise to splint the adjacent digit or digits, except in the case of the thumb, which is splinted alone. The splint is worn for 3 weeks; however, it may be changed at approximately 10 days for wound inspection and removal of sutures. There is always a question of when to give antibiotics with open trauma. Many hand surgeons (the author included) like to err on the side of giving rather than withholding them. If there is the least suspicion of a contamination from the trauma, antibiotics should be given. Erythromycin, 250 mg every 6 hours, is satisfactory. A penicillinase-resistant penicillin or an oral cepha-losporin is also satisfactory. Ampicillin is not a very useful drug for hand wounds.

ZONE V AND VI INJURIES

Extensor tendon injuries in these zones are not amenable to repair in the outpatient setting, even by experienced hand surgeons. The structures are too deep and their anatomic arrangement too complex for this. The injury should be diagnosed, the skin closed, and the wound dressed and splinted. The patient should be given antibiotics (erythromycin is good), and arrangements should be made for surgical repair. This repair need not be performed as an emergency procedure but should be accomplished within a week or so after injury. Management following the repair is similar to that described for Zone IV injuries.

Complications

The problems that may follow treatment of extensor tendon injuries include the general category of wound complications (e.g., infection and wound breakdown with disruption of the repair), disruption of the repair without wound problems, and adhesions at the site of repair that prevent full excursion of the tendon.

Wound infections can be minimized by careful observance of sterile technique at the time of wound treatment and, even more important, by the gentle handling of the tissues. When tissues are not handled gently there is an increase in post-traumatic swelling, which leads to venous congestion and lowered tissue oxygenation. This is the ideal setup for a wound infection. The principles of wound preparation are discussed in Chapter 35. The use of antibiotics may also lower the incidence of wound infection, but careful tissue handling and wound preparation are by far the most important steps in preventing soft-tissue infections following surgical repair of injuries.

Tendon disruption will occur if the sutures are ill-placed or if the surgical knot is not well tied. With nylon this means *at least five throws* placed to create *square* knots. If nylon is not laid down flat and squarely, it will untie. Some surgeons prefer to use a less "slippery" material, such as Dacron or braided nylon; this is acceptable, but square knots are still important. The other cause of disruption is inadequate immobilization. Three weeks of *complete immobilization* followed by another week or two of "protection" are advised. "Protection" means that the patient should not be using the hand with full force. If these steps are observed the incidence of disruption will be very low.

Adhesions are fairly common after tendon repair but are less of a problem with extensors than with

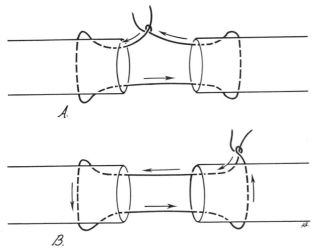

Figure 44–16. A satisfactory scheme for extensor tendon repair. (From Newmeyer, W. L.: Primary Care of Hand Injuries. Philadelphia, Lea & Febiger, 1979. Used by permission.)

flexors. Usually, the adhesions will loosen up with time. Very occasionally, an extensor tendolysis will be required.

Aftercare

Usually, the patient can recover good function after extensor tendon injuries by just doing activities of daily living. If the patient is having trouble or needs help, arrangements can be made for hand therapy. Occasionally there may be skin adherence to a tendon repair for months or even permanently. This is of little functional significance, and a lysis can be performed if the condition is very troubling to the patient.

1. Newmeyer, W.L.: Primary Care Of Hand Injuries. Philadelphia. Lea & Febiger, 1979.
2. Lampe, E. W.: Surgical anatomy of the hand with special reference to infections and trauma. Clin. Sympos. 21:66, 1969.

45

Dressings and Splints for Injured Hands

WILLIAM L. NEWMEYER, M.D.

Introduction

The purpose of a dressing is to protect an injured part from the outside world until that part has recovered sufficiently to function, if not normally, at least without harm. In the hand there is another dimension to the dressing: to protect the part against ill-advised use by its owner. Overuse of an injured hand results in swelling, circulatory stasis, a decrease in useful function, a delay in healing, and an increase in·the chance of infection. Furthermore, in many patients, unless the dressing makes use of the injured part difficult or impossible, the person will continue to use the part and then wonder why his or her problems are increasing rather than decreasing. Not all hand injuries require a large dressing, but a large dressing with or without splint supplementation will often speed recovery. Most patients and many physicians are not aware of the potential benefit of splinting "minor" hand injuries. One should always remember that it is much easier to prevent swelling or infection in the hand than it is to treat it. In the long run, a few days of enforced inactivity is a sound investment.

The usual hand dressing consists of a *core* portion and a *shell* portion. In some situations only one or the other is desirable or necessary. The core is the soft portion that is applied to the wound, and the shell is the rigid splint that protects the core and holds the hand or digit in the proper position. A list of materials used in dressing a hand is provided in Table 45–1.

The Core Dressing

Before any dressing is put in place, all constrictive or potentially constrictive items, such as clothing or rings and other jewelry, should be removed. The layer that is placed directly on the wound should consist of a nonadherent type of gauze. Since all gauze sticks to a wound to some extent, this layer is really semi-adherent. Xeroform gauze, which is commercially available in sterile packages of various sizes, has proved itself over the years to be an excellent material to apply to a wound. This is not a proprietary type of gauze and can be made up by the practitioner. Other types of gauze that can be used include Adaptic, Vaseline gauze, and Telfa. New types are being marketed, and the reader need only consult the advertisements in any journal with a surgical orientation to learn their names. This innermost first layer should be applied in one or two thicknesses in such a way that it overlaps the wound by a considerable margin (Fig. 45–1). This overlap makes it far easier to remove at the time of a dressing change, because a sterile instrument can be slipped under the free edge and the dressing teased off the wound. The second layer of the core should consist of several layers of moistened sterile gauze of approximately the same dimensions as the first layer (Fig. 45–2). This wet gauze serves to encourage the egress of blood and other tissue fluids out of the wound and into the dressing. Sterile water or sterile saline may be used to wet the gauze, but

Table 45–1. TRADE NAMES OF MATERIALS USED

1. Xeroform. Various sizes, but 1″ × 8″ is most useful. Petrolatum dressing (3% bismuth tribromphenate in petrolatum blend). Chesebrough Pond's Inc., Greenwich, CT 06830.

2. Adaptic. Nonadherent dressing, various sizes. Johnson & Johnson Products, Inc., New Brunswick, NJ 08903.

3. Vaseline Gauze. Nonadherent dressing, various sizes. Chesebrough Pond's, Inc., Hospital Products Division. Greenwich, CT 06830.

4. Telfa. Nonadherent dressing, various sizes. Kendall Co., Hospital Products Division, Boston, MA 02101.

5. Reston. Self-adhering foam roll, #1563. 3M Medical Products Division, St. Paul, MN 55101.

6. Kling. Stretch roller gauze, various sizes. Johnson & Johnson Products, Inc., New Brunswick, NJ 08903.

7. Elastomull. Distributed by Beiersdorf Inc., South Norwalk, CT 06854.

8. Tubegauze. (Use Double Seal.) Scholl Inc., Hospital Products Division, Memphis TN 38151.

9. Betadine. Brand of povidone-iodine. Purdue Frederick Co., Norwalk, CT 06856.

10. Silvadene. (1% silver sulfadiazine). Marion Laboratories, Inc., Kansas City, MO 64137.

11. Zinc Oxide Ointment. Topical astringent. Pharmaderm, Inc., Hicksville, NY 11802.

12. Scarlet Red Ointment 5%. Eli Lilly and Co., Indianapolis, IN 46285.

13. Cutter Cast. Cutter Biomedical, Emeryville, CA 94608. This and other fiberglass materials come in splints (also called casting tape by the manufacturers) and rolls of various sizes. The tapes are used for the purposes described in this chapter.

14. Scotchcast. 3M Orthopedic Products, St. Paul, MN 55144.

15. Delta-Lite. Fabric and fiberglass casting tape. Johnson & Johnson Products, Inc., Orthopaedic Division, New Brunswick, NJ 08903.

16. Four-pronged finger splints. (Crushed finger splints in three sizes: #16–0730, 16–0731, and 16–0732.) Richards Mfg. Co., Memphis, TN 38116.

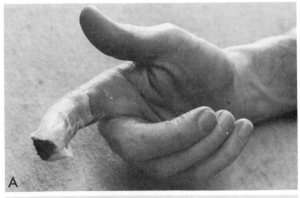

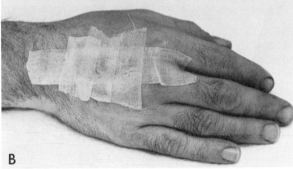

Figure 45–1. A, Xeroform gauze in 1-inch-wide strips is criss-crossed over a digit with a finger pad injury. Note that there is a wide overlap proximal to the wound. This substance is commercially available in sterile wraps of 1- × 8-inch strips from Cheseborough-Ponds. B, The same principle of wound dressing is seen on a dorsal hand injury.

I have used hundreds of outpatient dressings wetted with tap water with no ill effects.

Two thicknesses of dry gauze are placed over the wet gauze. A piece of Reston foam material is placed over this (Fig. 45–3), and the layers are held in place with an elasticized roller bandage, such as Kling or Elastomull. This bandage is applied with just enough force to hold the dressing in place, with great pains taken to prevent constriction (Fig. 45–4A). In the case of a digit it is often useful to hold this dressing on with two or three layers of a circular elasticized gauze (Tubegauze) applied with a metal applicator (Fig. 45–4B). Reston is a unique material in that it has one adherent and one nonadherent surface (which makes for ease of application) and does not deteriorate when it comes in contact with body fluids. The dressing may be autoclaved or gas-sterilized. Reston is manufactured by the 3M Company and comes in several thicknesses. The type that is most suitable for hand dressings is 5 mm thick and comes in rolls. The thicker varieties that come in large sheets are too bulky for use in the hand.

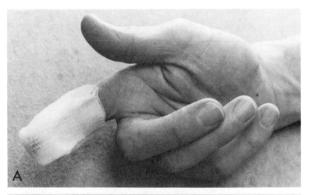

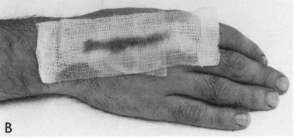

Figure 45–2. A and B, The second, or wet, gauze layers of the same dressings seen in Figure 45–1 A and B.

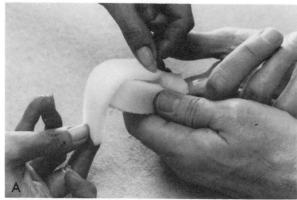

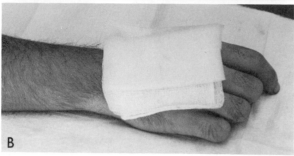

Figure 45–3. *A,* Two strips of Reston are placed along the injured digit at right angles to each other. Gauze should underlie the Reston because otherwise the sticky layer will stick to skin and its removal is painful, especially on hair-bearing areas. *B,* A single piece of Reston is applied to a dorsal hand wound.

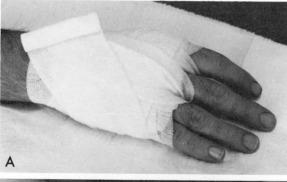

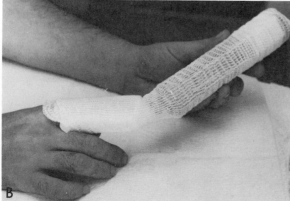

Figure 45–4. *A,* An elasticized gauze (Elastomul in this case) is applied over the Reston with gentle compression but never so tightly as to cause constriction. *B,* In the digit this next layer is conveniently applied with Tube gauze or an equivalent material.

If the dressing is being applied to multiple digits or to the hand, the principles are the same as those outlined earlier for a single digit. In this case it is a wise idea to put a small amount of sterile wet gauze between the digits (Fig. 45–5) to prevent interdigital maceration. Great care must be taken not to pack too much gauze between the fingers, because this will lead to constriction and will do much more harm than good.

Ointments and Other Substances Applied Directly to the Wound

PROS AND CONS

A number of substances are available for direct application to a wound for various purposes. In general their use is unnecessary, but in some specific instances they may have a place. The factors most important in wound healing are immobilization and prevention of swelling, both of which encourage good tissue perfusion. In a few instances, however, an ointment or other substances may have a use.

Substances that should definitely be avoided in hand wounds are ones that stop bleeding by some type of thrombotic mechanism. These generally result in a sticky mess at the time of the first dressing change. The way to stop bleeding in the hand is by elevation, the use of a tourniquet (see Chapter 44), and the application of a layered dressing. Occasionally in a wound with excessive granulation tissue a silver nitrate stick may be applied for cauterization, but this is not very effective in stopping active bleeding. Battery-powered disposable cautery devices, if available, are useful for hemostasis. The area must be anesthetized prior to the use of these instruments.

A good substance for preparation of a wound is povidone-iodine (Betadine) solution (not scrub) applied with pressure irrigation or gentle rubbing.

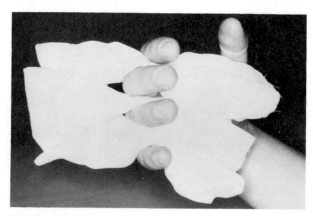

Figure 45–5. The placement of interdigital gauze when multiple digits are included in the dressing.

Unless a protective ointment is needed in a healing but still tender burn or other wound, antibiotic ointments are not indicated. With fresh burns that are small enough for outpatient treatment, silver sulfadiazine cream (Silvadene) is recommended for its antibacterial effect. This cream must be reapplied daily after washing of the wound. Close follow-up is recommended.

Zinc oxide ointment, which acts as a "soakless soak," is very useful in certain situations in which soaking the wound is desirable. Zinc oxide can be very helpful in loosening wound debris and aiding in the drainage of small abscesses that have been incised. Zinc oxide ointment is applied generously directly onto the wound (Fig. 45–6). Its use is *not* recommended for every wound, only for those in which warm water soaks would be of benefit. Zinc oxide has the advantage over soaks in that the wound can be dressed occlusively; this is far easier and more convenient for the patient. Zinc oxide is a hygroscopic agent that causes the skin to wrinkle as it does with soaking. Maceration is not a problem in short-term (3 to 5 days) use.

Large superficial wounds with a partial-thickness skin loss may be treated with the application of scarlet red ointment either directly onto the wound or on the gauze. This substance helps to dry the wound and to promote healing. Abrasions are usefully treated by application of this substance. A thin layer of a petrolatum-based antibiotic ointment may be applied once or twice a day to a wound that is healing and clean but is still tender.

The Shell Dressing

The purpose of the shell is twofold: to protect the core and to hold the hand in a proper position. The usual substance used to make a shell dressing is plaster, but there are now several water-activated fiberglass polymers that are fairly easy to use and that result in splints and casts that are lighter, stronger, more durable, and impervious to water. These materials are more expensive than plaster but, because they are more durable, are generally more cost-effective. Examples include Cutter Cast, made by the Cutter Company; Scotchcast, made by the 3M Company, and Delta-Lite, made by Johnson & Johnson. Also available are ready-made forearm-wrist-hand splints. As is true of many ready-made appliances, the patient must adapt to these splints, which may be too large or too small or not correct for the injury in question. It is much better to adapt a splint to a patient than to make a patient fit into a splint. The splint that fits everyone does not fit anyone very well. The use of ready-made forearm-wrist-hand splints is therefore strongly discouraged. Ready-made finger splints, however, may be quite useful; their use will be discussed later. Circular plaster or fiberglass is not bad per se. Rather, casts are often poorly or totally incorrectly applied, which has given them a bad name. It is certainly easier to release a too-tight splint than to release a too-tight cast; for this reason alone, a splint is the best shell dressing in the acute situation.

Designing the Shell. The first thing that must be decided is what needs to be immobilized and in what position the hand should be placed. All other things being equal, the intrinsic plus position (also called the position of protection) is the best one to strive for (Fig. 45–7). If a hand that is put in this position were to become irretrievably stiff, some function could still be salvaged. The position to be *avoided* is that of rest-injury (Fig. 45–8). If a hand becomes stiff in this position all is lost, because little or no useful function can be salvaged.

In designing the splint the first step is to cut out a pattern (Fig. 45–9A). This is usually done with 5-mm Reston, but cast padding can be used.

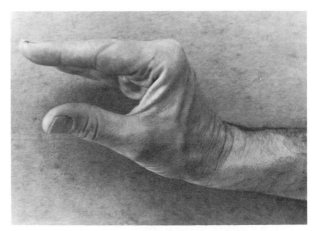

Figure 45–7. The intrinsic plus position (also known as the protected position). Note that the wrist is extended (dorsiflexed), the metacarpophalangeal joints are flexed, and the interphalangeal joints are in nearly full extension while the thumb web is open.

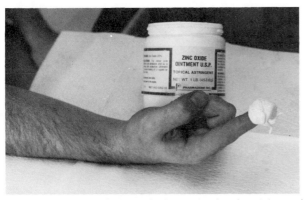

Figure 45–6. Zinc oxide is applied generously when it is used (see text). The ointment is messy to handle but very useful.

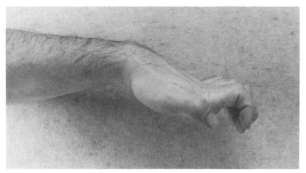

Figure 45–8. This is the position of rest-injury and should be avoided. A hand frozen in this position is useless.

In making a splint it is better to use a flat, non-yielding cast padding, such as Webril. A pattern for the thumb is shown in Figure 45–9B, one for the long and ring fingers is depicted in Figure 45–9C, and a pattern for the ulnar three digits is pictured in Figure 45–9D

If Reston is being used, the next step is to remove the backing (Fig. 45–10A). A double layer of cast padding is laid on so that one layer of the padding adheres to the Reston (Fig. 45–10B). This is cut generously to overlap the Reston just a little bit. Application of the plaster or fiberglass material is next. The plaster or fiberglass material is also cut to fit the pattern but should be a bit shy of the edges so that the scratchy plaster or fiberglass

does not come in contact with the skin (Figure 45–10C and D shows plaster and Figure 45–10E and F depicts fiberglass, in this case Cutter Cast). If plaster is used, warm water will speed up the curing time, but hot water should be avoided because it may cause a burn. A keel may be made in the plaster to give more strength (see Fig. 45–10B). Usually 10 to 12 thicknesses of plaster are required for a splint, but somewhat more or less can be used. For fiberglass splints one must be careful to use *cold* water, because this material hardens with release of considerable heat and if warm or hot water is used, the heat may be great enough to burn the patient. One package of 4" × 30" fiberglass material is usually sufficient for a splint. On occasion a 3" × 15" package is enough.

At this point the plaster splint is applied to the injured area and wrapped with a dry Ace wrap or bias-cut stockinette (Fig. 45–11A); the shell is now complete. The hand should always be wrapped from a distal to a proximal direction to avoid distal venous engorgement. If fiberglass is used, it should be wrapped with a cool, wet elastic gauze to take up some of the heat produced and to conform the splint to the extremity. When the splint has set, the wet wrap is removed and replaced by a dry wrap (Fig. 45–11B and C). The dry wrap should be put on tightly enough to hold the splint in place but not so tightly that there is impedance of vascular flow (especially venous

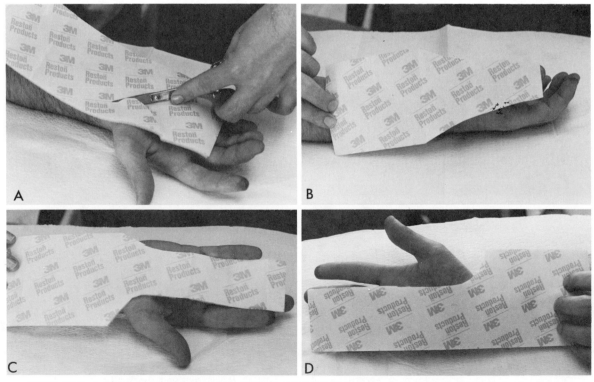

Figure 45–9. A, The method of designing a splint. B, For a thumb (e.g., for de Quervain's disease). C, For digits III and IV (e.g., for a bad laceration). D, For digits III, IV, and V (e.g., for a fourth metacarpal fracture).

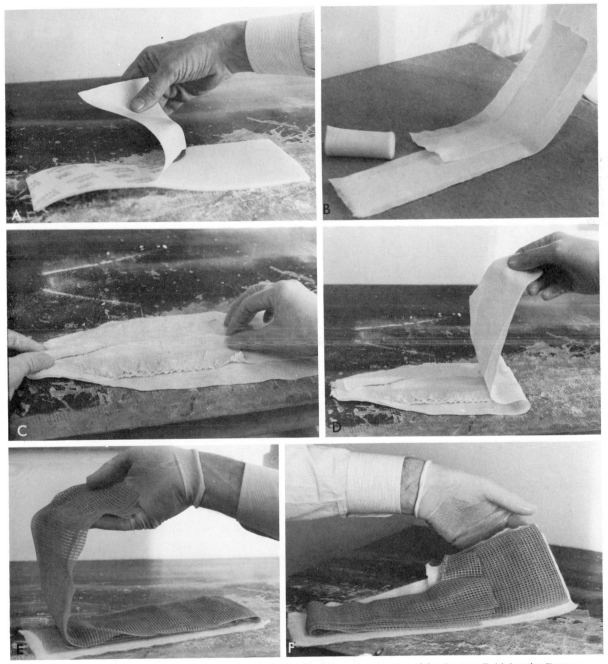

Figure 45–10. *A*, The protective backing is peeled away from the adherent part of the Reston. *B*, Lining the Reston pattern with cast padding. *C* and *D*, Using plaster for the splint. *E* and *F*, Using fiberglass for the splint.

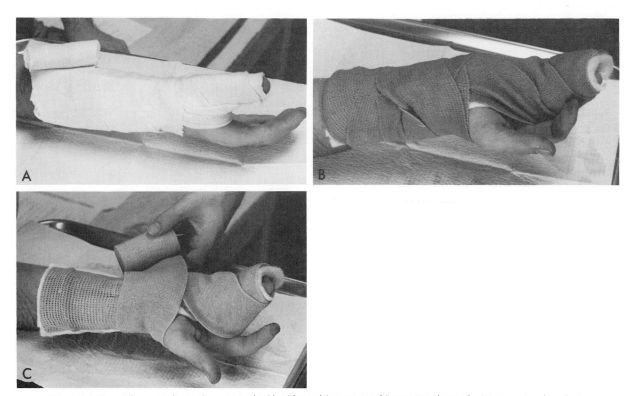

Figure 45–11. *A*, The wet plaster is wrapped with either a bias cut stockinette (as shown here) or an Ace bandage. *B*, A fiberglass splint is wrapped with a wet elastic bandage until it has set. *C*, The wet wrap is then replaced with a dry one.

drainage). The real advantage of the fiberglass splint becomes apparent only after a week or so of use. At this point plaster splints have often cracked or broken, whereas those made of fiberglass are still firm and strong. If wear of the splint is to be continued, the Reston lining, which by this time is usually quite soiled, is removed and a new liner of same material is put in (Fig. 45–12).

Elevation of the Injured Extremity

It is important that the injured extremity be kept elevated. Patients usually learn that an elevated hand hurts less than a dependent one. It is very important to emphasize this to patients and to assist them with elevation. A variety of slings is available. Many of these are very elaborate but do not allow adequate elevation of the hand, which should be at or above heart level. The old-fashioned muslin triangular sling used as shown in either Figure 45–13*A* or Figure 45–13*B* is the best. The situation shown in Figure 45–13*C* is to be avoided because the hand is too low and is hanging out of the sling. At night a pillow wrapped around the hand (Fig. 45–14) will help the patient keep it satisfactorily elevated.

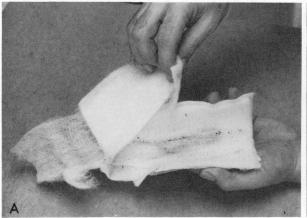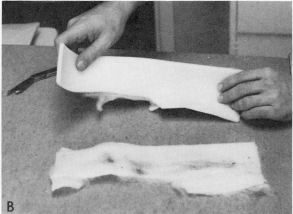

Figure 45–12. One of the main advantages of a fiberglass splint is that the old soiled Reston is easily removed and replaced with a clean one (see Figure 45–11*B*).

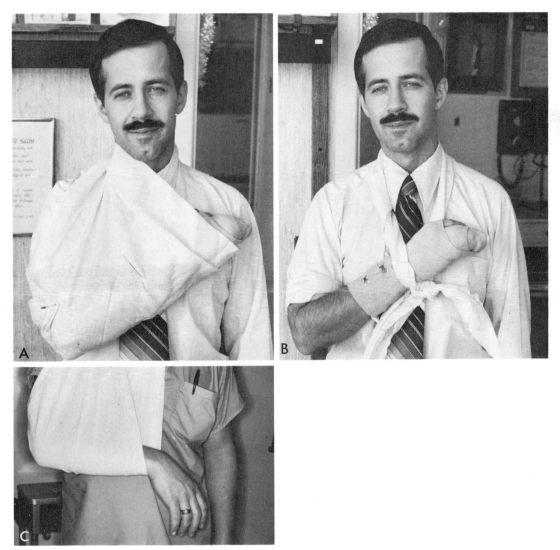

Figure 45–13. A triangular muslin sling can be used either as shown in *A* or as seen in *B*. The sling shown in *C* is *too low* and the hand is hanging out—a *very poor arrangement.*

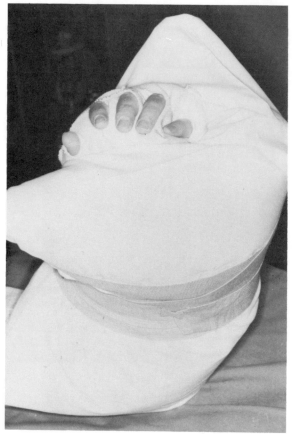

Figure 45–14. The "pillow" method of elevation for use while in bed. This can be easily set up by the patient and his family and is very useful.

Finger Splints

In certain finger injuries it is not necessary to apply a hand-wrist-forearm splint. If the metacarpal phalangeal joint needs to be immobilized, a larger splint is necessary. The use of a long, foam-lined piece of aluminum that extends from fingertip to wrist is discouraged. Mallet fingers, potential boutonniere fingers, fingertip injuries, and some local wounds, however, are well treated by a splint limited to the finger alone. These splints come in two types: (1) flat splints that are applied to one surface and (2) finger guards that are applied to two or more digital surfaces.

One-Surface Splints. These are commercially available with either aluminum or plastic wire backing (Fig. 45–15A) or can be made from Reston and a tongue blade cut to size (Fig. 45–15B through E). This third type involves approximately one tenth the cost of the other two. The commercially available finger splints with numerous fancy curves are unnecessary. They are expensive, excessively elaborate, and generally not appropriate.

One device that is particularly to be discouraged is the "Freddy the frog" splint (Fig. 45–16). This splint is designed to hold the distal interphalangeal joint hyperextended while holding the PIP joint flexed. This is an almost intolerable position even in a normal finger, and the patient will take it off or loosen it, which negates what it was designed to do.

The previously mentioned finger splints may be used on either the palmar or the dorsal surface of the digits but are usually more effective when applied dorsally. They are especially useful in mallet fingers and boutonniere deformities (see Chapter 44).

Finger Guards. Either padded or unpadded finger guards (Fig. 45–17A and B) are very useful in protecting a sore or healing distal finger tip. The Richards Company of Memphis, Tennessee makes a very useful padded guard (Fig. 45–17A) that can have its prongs bent, clipped, or otherwise adapted to fit a finger. (One should remember the principle "fit the splint to the patient, not the patient to the splint.") In making and modifying finger splints and guards, it is very useful to have a pair of tin snips (available for a nominal sum at any hardware store) to cut the aluminum or wood. Even heavy-duty scissors will be ruined when used for this purpose. Breaking the aluminum off by bending it back and forth usually leaves a sharp edge that may cut the patient.

Pitfalls of Hand Dressings and Splints

The two most common problems with hand dressings are putting them on too tightly and leaving them on too long. One must be especially careful to avoid wrapping elastic bandages too snugly. The patient should be instructed to loosen an elastic bandage if it feels too tight. Symptoms of a too-tight bandage include throbbing pain and numb, blue, or swollen fingers. The patient should always have access to emergency follow-up care. There is a tendency to leave dressings and, particularly, splints in place for too long. Some suggested times of immobilization are listed in Table 45–2. It is very important to note that these times are not written in stone. Each patient must be considered as an individual. It is often advisable to start patients on early protected motion. This means that the patient removes the splint for a specified period, does a prescribed exercise, and then replaces the splint. A splint is not an all-or-none device, and generally the patient will be weaned slowly away from it before it is discarded entirely. One should keep in mind that a stiff hand is a nonfunctional one and that stiffness is often a consequence of overlong immobilization.

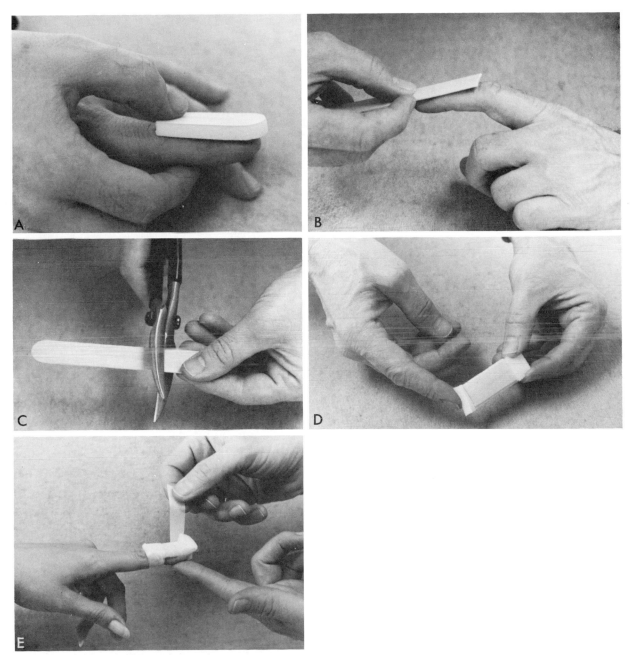

Figure 45–15. Types of digital splints. *A,* Wire- and plastic-backed splint. *B* through *E,* The steps for making a digital splint from a tongue blade and Reston.

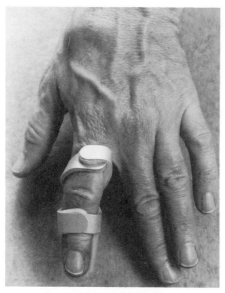

Figure 45–16. A "Freddy the frog" splint, which is considered suboptimal by the author.

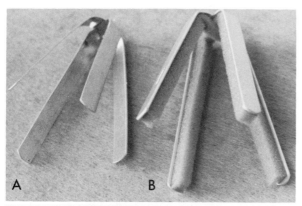

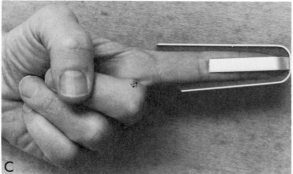

Figure 45–17. Unpadded (A) and padded (B) four-prong finger guards. C, A padded guard cut to allow finger motion at the proximal interphalangeal joint.

Table 45–2. USEFUL ESTIMATES OF SPLINT TIMES FOR VARIOUS HAND PROBLEMS

Injury	Splint Type	Immobilization Time*
Mallet finger	FIN†	8 weeks
Boutonniere deformity	FIN	6 weeks
Distal phalanx—soft tissue	FIN	2 to 3 weeks
Extensor tendon	DHWF‡	3 weeks
Sprain-strain§		
Interphalangeal joint	FIN	1 to 2 weeks
Wrist	DHWF	1 to 2 weeks
Hand burn	DHWF	5 to 7 weeks
Infection		
Digit	DHWF	5 to 7 days
Hand	DHWF	5 to 7 days
Severe hand contusion	DHWF	5 to 7 days
Fracture		
Distal phalanx	FIN	2 to 3 weeks
Mid phalanx	FIN	2 to 3 weeks
Proximal phalanx	DHWF	2 to 3 weeks
Metacarpal	DHWF	2 to 3 weeks
Carpal tunnel	DHWF	Night only
De Quervain's disease	DHWF	2 to 3 weeks
Trigger finger	FIN	Night only

*These are average times only. Every patient is treated as an individual when a splint is used. Clinical judgment is critical.
†Finger splint.
‡Digit-hand-wrist-forearm splint.
§The diagnosis of a sprain should be made only after a thorough effort has been made to rule out a fracture or a dislocation. This is particularly true in the wrist.

It is very important that the patient be made aware of his or her responsibility for the injured hand.

Conclusion

The purpose of the hand dressing that was stated at the outset of this chapter should always be kept in mind. The reader is encouraged to modify and adapt his or her own dressings, but only if the principles of a good dressing are followed. These are: (1) to maximize protection, (2) to minimize patient discomfort (on application, wearing, and removal), and (3) to maximize long-term good results by avoiding bad hand positions that lead to swelling, causing stiffness and long-term disability.

46

Injection Therapy of Bursitis and Tendinitis

DAVID H. NEUSTADT, M. D.

Introduction

Bursitis and tendinitis are terms frequently used to describe a variety of regional musculoskeletal conditions that are characterized chiefly by pain and disability at the site involved. Bursitis of the shoulder may be considered as the prototypical disorder. All too often in ill-defined regional soft tissue rheumatic problems, the designation "bursitis" or "tendinitis" is used as a "wastebasket" diagnosis. For purposes of this chapter, in consideration of the accurate diagnosis that is necessary to institute appropriate therapy, the terms will be reserved for well-defined specific clinical entities.

General Anatomic Considerations of Bursae and Tendon Sheaths

Bursae are potential spaces or sacs, subcutaneous or deep, that develop in relation to friction and are provided to facilitate the gliding motion of tendons and muscles. There are approximately 78 bursae on each side of the body. These were well described in the classic atlas of anatomy by Monro[1] in 1788 and were later elaborated in greater detail in the atlas of Spalteholz.[2]

The normal bursal wall is lined with a thin layer of synovial cells that appear to be similar to those of joint synovial membrane when examined by electron microscopy.[3] When a bursa becomes subacutely or chronically inflamed, the normally thin surface of sparse cells may become thickened to 1 to 2 mm. The cause of bursitis may be trauma, infection, crystal deposition, chronic friction, or a systemic inflammatory arthropathy. In addition, so-called adventitial bursae may form in response to abnormal shearing stress at sites subjected to chronic pressure, such as the "bunion" over the head of the first metatarsal bone of the great toe.

Involvement of the synovial lining of bursae and tendon sheaths may also result from underlying systemic diseases, including rheumatoid arthritis, ankylosing spondylitis, psoriatic arthropathy, and gout. The most common bursal lesions in these systemic inflammatory arthropathies involve the olecranon at the elbow and the trochanter region of the hip. Smaller bursae, especially those around the Achilles tendon, also may be affected.

Recently, attention has been called to an increased rate of occurrence of *septic bursitis*.[4] Bacterial infection usually affects the superficial bursae, such as the olecranon and the prepatellar regions. Factors that predispose to infected bursa include trauma, steroid therapy, uremia, diabetes mellitus, and alcoholism.[5] Tuberculosis may affect any bursa but is rare, whereas other types of mycobacteria, such as *Mycobacterium kansasii*, are occasionally reported.[6] Another uncommon cause of involvement of superficial bursae and tendon

sheaths is sporotrichosis, which can be contracted by gardeners and farmers. In addition, tendon sheaths at the hands, the wrists, and the ankles may be affected by acute bacterial infections, such as gonorrhea.

Tendinitis and *tenosynovitis* are useful terms that describe inflammatory reactions in tendons and tendon sheaths. Tendon sheaths are relatively long and tubular, whereas bursae are round and flat. Except for their shape, however, the structures are similar.

Flexor tenosynovitis, ("trigger," or "snapping," finger) is a frequent extra-articular manifestation of rheumatoid arthritis and occasionally may be the presenting symptom.

In *calcareous* (or calcific) tendinitis of the shoulder, there is a calcific deposit in and about one of the rotator cuff tendons (commonly the supraspinatus). The musculotendinous rotator cuff is composed of the supraspinatus, infraspinatus, teres minor, and subscapularis muscles, which insert as the conjoined tendon into the greater tuberosity of the humerus. The bursae in relation to the greater tuberosity and the subdeltoid (subacromial) bursa are the most common sites of calcific deposits. The nidus of the pathologic process is considered to be the calcific deposit (hydroxyapatite) within the substance of one or more of the involved tendons. The process has been likened to a chemical furuncle, or the so-called calcium boil. Calcific tendinitis may be hyperacute or acute, and release of the pressure from the inflammatory edema with rupture into the contiguous bursa (for example, the subacromial bursae) provides prompt relief.

Bursitis and tendinitis embrace a variety of conditions that may be grouped together on a regional basis for the sake of a simple and convenient classification (Table 46–1).

Rationale for Steroid Injections

The management of pain resulting from bursitis and tendinitis may be greatly enhanced by the

Table 46–1. CLASSIFICATION OF BURSITIS AND TENDINITIS (REGIONAL)

Upper Extremity Disorders
Elbow
  Radiohumeral bursitis, olecranon bursitis, epicondylitis
Shoulder
  Bicipital tendinitis, calcareous tendinitis (subacromial, subdeltoid bursitis), rotator cuff tendinitis
Wrist and Hand
  Stenosing tenosynovitis ("trigger" finger syndrome), de Quervain's syndrome
Lower Extremity Disorders
Hip
  Trochanteric bursitis, ischiogluteal bursitis
Knee
  Prepatellar, suprapatellar, and anserine bursitis
Ankle, Foot, and Heel
  Ankle tendinitis, bunion bursitis, calcaneal bursitis (with heel spur)

proper selection and administration of local injections. The successful application of local injection and intrasynovial therapy requires an understanding of the diagnosis, accurate localization of the pathologic condition, and the choice of suitable injection techniques. Not infrequently, injections of lidocaine or corticosteroid preparations provide the additional aid that alone or as an adjunct to the management program overcomes the refractory pain.

Although local injection intrasynovial therapy is essentially palliative, it may provide striking and lasting relief. Restoration of function may follow a single injection, especially in a self-limited painful soft tissue condition. The precise mechanism of the lasting analgesia and the beneficial therapeutic effects have not been clarified. Explanations that have been considered include induction of local hyperemia, relaxation of reflex muscle spasm, generalized response from systemic absorption, pain relief allowing controlled activity or rest, favorable influence on local tissue metabolism, and mechanical benefit. The increased mobility permitted as a result of pain relief certainly accelerates recovery and restoration of function. Finally, the "power of suggestion" of the needle must not be underestimated (placebo therapy). Some observers believe the pain relief may result from stimulation and release of the patient's endorphins.

Some physicians prefer to follow local injection with a short course of salicylates, oral corticosteroids, or nonsteroidal anti-inflammatory medications. Others prefer to prescribe simple analgesics and to evaluate the response to injection. Cases must be individualized according to the specific pathologic condition and patient variables.

Indications for and Contraindications to Injection Therapy

Local injection therapy with corticosteroids or local anesthetics may provide valuable aid in a variety of acute or subacute bursitides and other painful soft tissue conditions. Abolition of symptoms would confirm the localization of the involved site or structure even if the response were not lasting. Visceral disease must be ruled out as a source of referred pain. Appropriate injection therapy is indicated when there are local accessible signs that are likely to respond to direct therapeutic infiltration. Acute localized bursitis or tendinitis warrants immediate direct injection for rapid relief.[7,8]

Contraindications are relative and include infections either local or in the vicinity of the site of involvement and hypersensitivity to any preparation or substance that might be injected. The procedure is also contraindicated in patients receiving anticoagulants or those with any bleeding disorder. The patient with a pre-existing tendon injury may be subject to tendon rupture that can inhibit full activity when the corticosteroid injection removes pain. Hence, partial tendon rupture is a relative contraindication.[9] Poorly motivated "needle-shy" and severely neurotic patients obviously are considered poor subjects for this type of treatment. Herpes simplex infection and tuberculosis are generally considered absolute contraindications.

Hazards and Complications

Local anesthetics are often mixed with a corticosteroid preparation to increase volume and to decrease postinjection pain. Local anesthetics may also be used prior to injection of the corticosteroid. The major hazards in the use of local anesthetics are hypersensitivity and accidental intravenous or intra-arterial introduction. Serious (possibly even fatal) hypersensitivity to procaine and other regional anesthetic compounds is encountered very rarely; the possibility is usually suggested by a history of previous reactions. "Have you ever had any trouble from the numbing injection used in the dentist's office?" should be a routine question prior to the performance of any injection procedure. Lidocaine or one of the newer "caine" derivatives may be used to avoid sensitivity reactions to procaine. If a past history of a reaction is suggested, one should proceed cautiously and use small dilute anesthetic solutions. When there is a definite history of sensitivity, it is wise to avoid the use of anesthetic agents during injection therapy.

In the event of accidental intravenous injection of a "caine" drug or if symptoms of hypersensitivity arise from these compounds (a significant slowing of the pulse rate, or even a seizure, is an indication of a major reaction to intravenous administration), one of the soluble barbiturate preparations, such as sodium pentothal or the anticonvulsant diazepam, should be readily available and should be given promptly in accordance with the reaction and response. In addition, a clear airway should be maintained and oxygen should be administered.[10] Severe reactions from accidental vascular injection of these drugs in the doses usually given are very rare.

A repository corticosteroid given intravenously by accident has been reported but has not been observed by us.[11] To my knowledge, no serious reaction to a depot corticosteroid preparation given intravenously has been reported. The possibility of an allergic reaction caused by corticosteroids is highly unlikely. A recent report, however, has described an unusual skin rash following an intra-articular methylprednisolone injection that would appear consistent with a delayed type of hypersensitivity.[12]

Minor reactions occasionally seen after injection of "caine" preparations include lightheadedness or dizziness, pallor, weakness, sweating, nausea, and (rarely) fainting and tachycardia. These symptoms usually disappear within a few minutes after the injection and rarely require any treatment except reassurance and a cold compress to the forehead of the patient. Often it is difficult to decide whether the symptoms are the result of sensitivity to the drug or a fright reaction (vasovagal). Preferably, the patient should be supine, prone, or seated in a reclining position during the injection to minimize the effect of any vasovagal reaction.

The obvious precautions against entering a blood vessel are for the physician to be aware of the local anatomy and to aspirate after every 1 to 2 ml of solution is injected. Penetration into or striking of a nerve may cause sharp pain or paresthesias, and the patient should be warned of this possibility in advance.

Complications are listed in Table 46–2. Although the possibility of introducing infection is the most serious potential complication, in a review of our extensive experience and that of others we have found that infections occurring as an aftermath of intrasynovial injections are extremely rare.[13–16] I do not recommend routine prophylactic antibiotic administration unless the patient has had a significant recent systemic infection. Although with meticulous attention to aseptic technique the problem of infection is usually avoided, the patient should be cautioned to report the development of any significant pain, redness, or swelling after any local injection.

Local undesirable reactions are usually minor and reversible. A postinjection "flare" may begin within a few hours after steroid injection and usually tends to subside spontaneously in up to 24 hours. Rarely, it can continue for as long as 72 hours. This transient increase in inflammation is considered to represent a true "crystal-induced synovitis" caused by precipitation of the microcrystalline steroid ester suspension.[17] Usually, the reaction is mild and adequately controlled with application of ice or cold compresses and analgesics as needed. Rarely, "after-pain" lasting for a few to several hours may occur following injections. Although the cause is obscure, this phenomenon may result from the trauma of needle insertion, penetration of inflamed tissue, or pressure on adjacent nerves from local swelling or bleeding. After-pain usually is relieved by application of moist or dry heat and analgesics until the pain abates.

Occasional subcutaneous bleeding at the site of injection may occur with penetration of a venule, an arteriole, or a capillary. The patient should be warned that this may occur and should be reassured that the discoloration or hematoma will disappear spontaneously. Ice packs or cold compresses to the involved area for the first 24 hours are commonly advised.

Another relatively minor complication is localized subcutaneous or cutaneous atrophy at the site of the injection.[8,18] This problem is chiefly of cosmetic concern and is recognized as a small depression in the skin frequently associated with depigmentation, transparency and, occasionally, the formation of telangiectasia. These changes in the skin occur when injections are made near the surface and some of the injected steroid leaks back along the needle track. The depression usually recedes and the skin returns to normal with time when the crystals of the steroid have been completely absorbed. Careful technique (avoiding the leaking of the steroid suspension to the skin surface) will prevent this complication. A small amount of lidocaine or normal saline can be used to flush the needle of the suspension prior to removal of the needle.

The potential danger of "spontaneous" tendon rupture (especially of Achilles tendons) following local corticosteroid injections in the Achilles bursal area must be given serious consideration. Cautious administration with infiltrations around and beneath the tendons to keep any of the material from entering the substance of the tendon will minimize the occurrence of this complication.[9,19] In general, *the injection of major stress-bearing tendons*, such as the Achilles and patellar tendons, *should be avoided in the emergency department.* Treatment with oral anti-inflammatory medications and splinting is preferred.

Table 46–2. COMPLICATIONS OF INJECTION THERAPY

Infection
Postinjection flare
Afterpain
Bleeding (local)
Cutaneous atrophy (local)
Tendon rupture

Table 46–3. INJECTABLE CORTICOSTEROIDS

Intrasynovial Preparations	Trade Name	Strength per ml	Range of Usual Dosage
Hydrocortisone tebutate	Hydrocortisone TBA	50 mg	12.5–75 mg
Prednisolone tebutate	Hydeltra TBA	20 mg	5.0–30 mg
Methylprednisolone acetate	Depo-Medrol*	20 mg	4.0–30 mg
Triamcinolone acetonide	Kenalog-40	40 mg	4.0–40 mg
Triamcinolone diacetate	Aristocort Forte	40 mg	4.0–40 mg
Triamcinolone hexacetonide	Aristospan	20 mg	4.0–25 mg
Betamethasone acetate and disodium phosphatate	Celestone Soluspan	6 mg†	1.5–6.0 mg
Dexamethasone acetate	Decadron-La	8 mg	0.8–4.0 mg

*Supplied in 20 mg per ml, 40 mg per ml, and 80 mg per ml preparations.
†Available as 3 mg acetate, 3 mg phosphate.

Available Preparations and Choice of Compound

Hydrocortisone and a variety of available corticosteroid repository preparations are described in Table 46–3. Local anesthetics, such as lidocaine or mepivocaine, can be mixed with the corticosteroid preparation in the same syringe. All corticosteroid suspensions, with the exception of cortisone and prednisone, can produce a significant and rapid anti-inflammatory effect (in synovial spaces). Unfortunately, soluble corticosteroids are absorbed and dispersed too rapidly, having only a brief duration of action locally. The tertiary butyl acetate (TBA) ester prolongs the duration of local tissue effect because of decreased solubility. The decreased solubility probably causes dissociation of the corticosteroid by enzymes to proceed at a delayed rate.

No single steroid agent has demonstrated a convincing margin of superiority, with the exception of triamcinolone hexacetonide.[20,21] Prednisolone tebutate, however, simply by virtue of price advantage and long-term usage, is generally the drug of choice. Triamcinolone hexacetonide is the least water-soluble preparation currently available. Triamcinolone hexacetonide is two and one half times less soluble in water than prednisolone tebutate, providing the longest duration of action. There is minimal systemic absorption, or "spillover," with this preparation, but because of its high potency and higher cost it is usually reserved for use in conditions in which prednisolone tebutate or one of the other compounds has shown an inadequate response.

Dosage and Administration

The dose of any corticosteroid suspension used for intrasynovial injection must be arbitrarily selected. Factors that influence the dosage and expected response include the size of the affected area, the presence or absence of synovial fluid or edema, the severity and extent of any synovitis, and the steroid preparation selected for injection.

A useful guideline for estimating dosage follows: For relatively large spaces, such as subacromial, olecranon, and trochanteric bursae, 20 to 30 mg of prednisolone tebutate or equivalent; for medium- or intermediate-sized bursae and ganglia formation at the wrists, the knees, and the heels, 10 to 20 mg; for tendon sheaths, such as flexor tenosynovitis of digits and the abductor tendon of the thumb (de Quervain's disease), 5 to 15 mg. Sometimes, it may be necessary to give larger doses for optimal response. Intrabursal therapy of the elbow (olecranon) or knee (prepatellar) bursae containing considerable fluid may require 30- to 40-mg doses.

Unlike intra-articular injections for synovitis in chronic joint disease, repeat infiltrations for soft tissue conditions, such as bursitis and tendinitis, frequently will not be required. If only a partial response occurs or if recurrence develops, however, a single repeat injection can be given; the length of the interval between injections should not be a source of undue concern. In contrast with intra-articular injections, in which the hazard of "overworking" an injected joint is usually not a problem, following intrasynovial injection we recommend a reduction in activity with rest or splinting of the involved extremity. Limiting motion also delays somewhat the systemic absorption of the steroid. Anecdotal evidence suggests that those patients with inflammatory soft tissue lesions who follow a postinjection modified rest regimen obtain a more rapid and lasting resolution of the painful disorder. Frequency of injections will be considered further in the discussion of techniques for the specific entities.

Preparation of Site

Preparation of the site before injection requires meticulous adherence to aseptic technique. Anatomic "landmarks" are outlined with a black or red skin pencil. Tincture of iodine or Merthiolate applied with a sterile swab can be used in place of the skin pencil. The point of entry is cleansed with pHisoHex or an equivalent detergent or with povidone-iodine (Betadine), and then alcohol is sponged over the area. Sterile drapes and gloves are not generally considered necessary, especially after sufficient skill and experience with the procedure has been acquired. Sterile gauze-pads are useful for drying the area.

Techniques

GENERAL CONSIDERATIONS

Materials required for local injection procedures include needles, syringes, and items for preparation of the injection site. Disposable needles and syringes are convenient and sterile. For those who give many injections it is a great convenience to have a sterile aspiration-injection tray prepared and ready (Fig. 46–1). The tray should contain items needed to inject almost any site. The usual sizes of needles for various approaches are:

Intracutaneous skin wheal	0.5", 25 gauge
Tendinitis in elbow and shoulder inflammation	1.5 to 2.0", 22 gauge
Digital tenosynovitis	7/8", 25 gauge
Bursitis with fluid	1.0 to 1.5", 20 gauge
Possible septic bursitis	1.0 to 1.0", 18 gauge
Deep gluteal bursitis	3.0 to 4.0", 20 gauge

Table 46–4. ASPIRATION-INJECTION TRAY

Sterile tray (13 × 9 × 1 inches)
Syringes, preferably Luer-Lok
  10 ml. (3)
   2 ml. (3)
Needles
  0.6", 25 gauge (3)
  1.5", 22 gauge (3)
  2.0", 22 gauge (3)
  2.0", 18 gauge (2)
  2.5", 20 gauge (3)
  2.5", 22 gauge (3)—security type with safety bead
  4.0", 20 gauge (3)—security type with safety bead
Towels, gauze pads, and cotton-tipped applicators
Hemostat or forceps
Tubes for culture and synovial fluid analysis (EDTA, 5 mg, or heparin, 1 or 2 drops, is a satisfactory anticoagulant)

Table 46–4 lists the contents of the tray illustrated in Figure 46–1. Table 46–5 lists appropriately sized needles for various injection sites.

Once the point of entry has been determined and the site is prepared, either a superficial skin wheal is made with 1 per cent lidocaine (Xylocaine) or 1 per cent procaine (Novocain) or the skin is sprayed with a refrigerant, such as Frigiderm. Another vapor coolant, ethyl chloride, is not recommended because it may potentially cause general anesthesia if inhaled. Ordinarily, preanesthesia is not necessary, but occasionally in highly nervous or agitated individuals, it may be advisable to give diazepam (Valium), 5 mg intravenously, or to administer a nitrous oxide/oxygen mixture prior to the procedure. Thus, an anxiety-

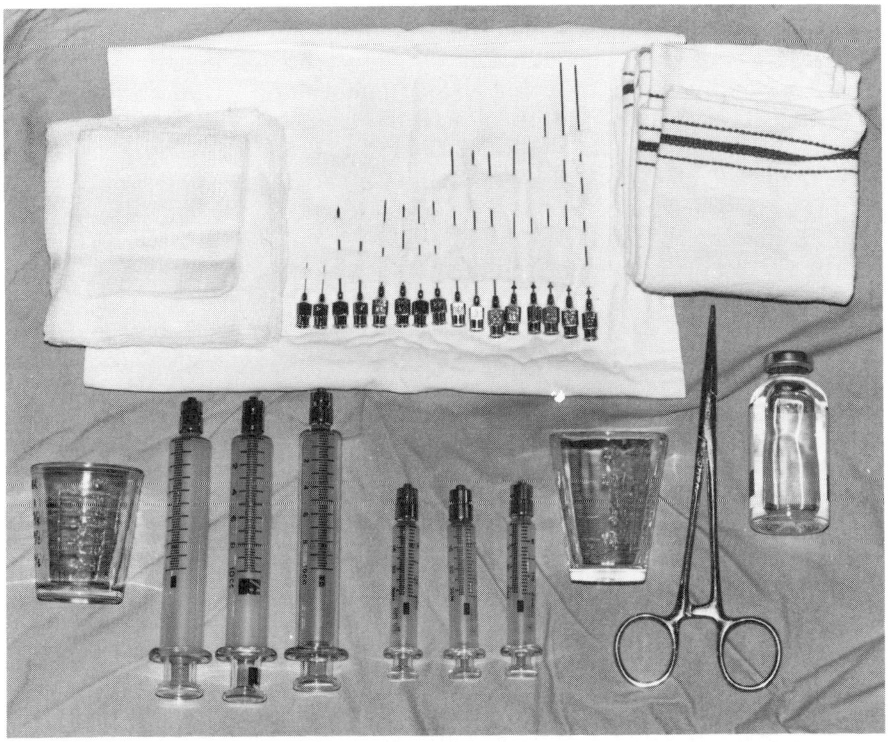

Figure 46–1. Aspiration-injection tray contents (see Table 46–4). (From Steinbrocker, O., and Neustadt, D. H.: Aspiration and Injection Therapy in Arthritis and Musculoskeletal Disorders: A Handbook on Technique and Management. Hagerstown, MD, Harper & Row, 1972. Used by permission.)

Table 46–5. A GUIDE FOR NEEDLE SIZE AND DOSAGE FOR
INJECTION OF COMMON REGIONAL DISORDERS

Disorder or Injection Site	Needle Size: Inches and Gauge	Usual Dosage of Prednisolone Tebutate
Bicipital tendinitis	1.5"–2.0", 22 gauge	20–30 mg
Calcareous tendinitis	1.5"–2.0", 22 gauge	20–40 mg
Subacromial bursitis		
Radiohumeral bursitis	1.5", 22 gauge	20–30 mg
Epicondylitis		
Olecranon bursitis	1.0"–1.5", 20 gauge	15–30 mg
Ganglia on wrist	1.0", 18 gauge	10–15 mg
de Quervain's syndrome	7/8", 25 gauge	10–20 mg
Carpal tunnel syndrome	1.0"–1.5", 22 gauge	20–40 mg
Digital flexor tenosynovitis	7/8", 25 gauge	5 mg
Trochanteric bursitis	1.5"–2.0", 20–21 gauge	20–40 mg
Prepatellar bursitis	1.0"–1.5", 20–21 gauge	15–20 mg
Anserine bursitis	1.0"–1.5", 22 gauge	20–40 mg
Bunion bursitis	1.0", 20 gauge	5–10 mg
Calcaneal bursitis	1.0", 22–23 gauge	10–20 mg

provoking injection can be carried out with patient cooperation.

Local injections can be administered with corticosteroids and local anesthetics mixed together in the same syringe, or the local anesthetic can be given alone. Generally, when injecting synovial spaces we introduce the steroid without anesthetic but often change syringes and follow with lidocaine to flush out the needle, frequently injecting and depositing several milliliters of the local anesthetic. When injecting a painful soft tissue structure directly, we are more apt to administer a mixture of corticosteroid and anesthetic. This both relieves pain immediately and confirms the accuracy of the injection. The duration of action of lidocaine is approximately 100 minutes, whereas that of procaine is approximately 50 minutes. In our experience the long-acting anesthetic agents, such as bupivacaine (Marcaine) and etidocaine (Duranest), serve no additional useful purpose. The patient should be cautioned that the local anesthetic effect may "wear off" within a couple of hours and the beneficial effects of the corticosteroid may be delayed.

The most important aspect of a successful technique is accurate positioning of the needle. The needle must "hit the mark" or the results will be disappointing. Injecting an inflamed synovial space, such as a bursitis-containing fluid, may be as simple as puncturing a balloon. Aspiration of the fluid confirms that the needle has correctly entered the sac. On the other hand, injecting directly into a painful soft tissue lesion requires additional skill that can be acquired only with experience. When a bursa is injected, as much fluid as possible is aspirated prior to instillation of the corticosteroid suspension in order to reduce the dilution factor. Sometimes it is advisable to reaspirate and reinject several times within the barrel of the syringe, so-called *barbotage*, to obtain heterogeneous mixing and maximal dispersion of the steroid throughout the synovial cavity.

It should be emphasized that most painful, localized disorders of the musculoskeletal system are of mild traumatic, irritative (possibly transient) inflammatory origin. Often they are self-limiting or responsive to medical and physical measures, including analgesics, nonsteroidal anti-inflammatory drugs, regulated rest, and applications of heat and cold. Our main concern is with conditions that are acute and require rapid relief and with the less severe but still bothersome discomfort and disability that persist in spite of conventional therapy. Some acute disorders practically demand immediate medical intervention by local injection. These include acute calcareous tendinitis of the shoulder, tense painful swollen bursitis, acute tenosynovitis, and similar disturbances of the locomotor system. Many uncomfortable musculoskeletal disorders will need a combination of local injection and basic measures.

SPECIFIC REGIONS AND CLINICAL ENTITIES

Table 46–1 lists the areas of involvement by region. In addition, certain nonarticular disorders that may require local injection will be included.

Upper Extremity Regions

The Shoulder Region. Pain associated with disability may result from any of the intrinsic shoulder disorders, including bicipital tendinitis, calcareous tendinitis, and subacromial bursitis. These areas are frequently injected because of the consistently good response to therapy and the danger of persistent inflammation resulting in a "frozen shoulder."

Bicipital Tendinitis (Tenosynovitis). This is a nonspecific low-grade inflammation or irritation of the long head of the biceps tendon sheath.[22] The tendon courses through the joint and along the bicipital (intertubercular) groove. Pain at the shoulder is accompanied by restricted motion and disturbed scapulohumeral rhythm. Efforts to elevate the shoulder, reach the hip pocket, or pull a back zipper all aggravate the symptoms. "Rolling" the bicipital tendon produces localized tenderness (Lipman's test), and Yergason's test may be positive. Yergason's test elicits pain along the bicipital groove when the patient attempts supination of the forearm against resistance, holding the elbow flexed at a 90-degree angle against the side of the body. Radiographs are normal.

TECHNIQUE. The point of maximal tenderness of the bicipital tendon is located. Entry is made with a 22 gauge, 1.5- to 2.0-inch needle through a lidocaine skin wheal (Fig. 46–2). The needle is brought in along the side of the tendon aimed at one border of the bicipital groove to give a peritendinous infiltration. One third of the injection is administered at this point. The needle is then withdrawn slightly but is kept subcutaneous. It is redirected upward approximately 1 inch for another one third of the injection, withdrawn again, and redirected downward, touching the bicipital border gently; the remainder of the drug is deposited at this point. Usually the corticosteroid suspension, 1 to 1.5 ml of prednisolone tebutate, is instilled at the maximum area of tenderness and the lidocaine is injected along the upper and lower borders of the tendon. Two to four repeat injections may be required at 1- to 2-week intervals.

Calcareous Tendinitis, Supraspinatus Tendinitis, and Subacromial Bursitis. These are so similar that their symptoms and signs are difficult to distinguish. The acute irritative inflammation of the bursa is a secondary reaction produced by the calcific tendinitis of the supraspinatus or one of the other rotator cuff tendons. After the calcific material ruptures into the subdeltoid bursa, spontaneous relief usually is obtained within a few days. During the acute or hyperacute stage, the patient holds the arm in a protective fashion against the chest wall. Pain may be incapacitating, and all ranges of motion are disturbed, with internal rotation markedly limited. Tenderness is often diffuse over the perihumeral region. Constitutional symptoms are rare, but sometimes in the hyperacute form actual swelling may be visible, and even fever and an accelerated sedimentation rate may develop. When shoulder radiographs demonstrate a calcific deposit, the shadow appears "hazy" with lightening of the periphery caused by the pressure of inflammatory edema. Night pain may be intolerable, requiring narcotics for control.

TECHNIQUE. In calcific tendinitis or supra-

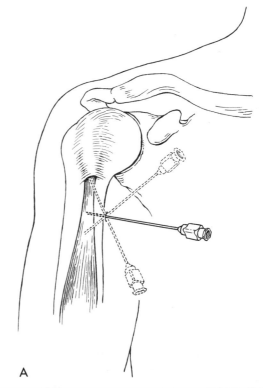

A

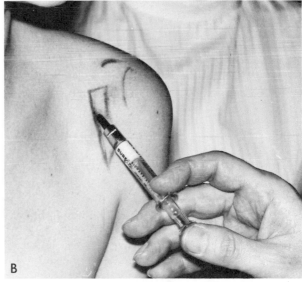

B

Figure 46–2. A, Fan-wise method of infiltration of bicipital tendon sheath. B, Actual injection of bicipital tendinitis; patient seated with arm in lap and externally rotated. (From Steinbrocker, O., and Neustadt, D. H.: Aspiration and Injection Therapy in Arthritis and Musculoskeletal Disorders: A Handbook on Technique and Management. Hagerstown, MD, Harper & Row, 1972. Used by permission.)

spinatus tendinitis without calcification, the injection is given by the anterior (subcoracoid) or lateral approach, below the acromion (Fig. 46–3). If the tenderness is not localized, a point is selected over the depression that is palpable between the anterolateral or anteromedial border of the acromion and the head of the humerus.

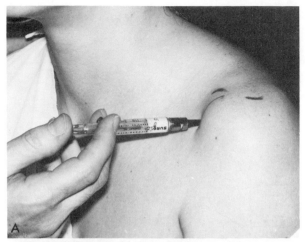

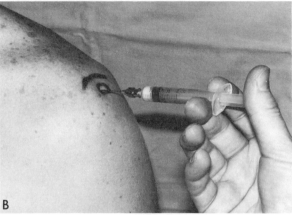

Figure 46–3. *A,* Anterior approach to subacromial bursa or supraspinatus tendon. *B,* Lateral approach to subacromial bursa or supraspinatus tendon. (From Steinbrocker, O., and Neustadt, D. H.: Aspiration and Injection Therapy in Arthritis and Musculoskeletal Disorders: A Handbook on Technique and Management. Hagerstown, MD, Harper & Row, 1972. Used by permission.)

TECHNIQUE. With the patient sitting and the lower part of the extremity resting on the lap, a lidocaine skin wheal is made at a posterolateral point under the acromion (Figs. 46–3 and 46–4). A 1.5- to 2.0-inch, 22 gauge needle is then directed toward the center of the head of the humerus upward at an angle of approximately 10 degrees. After the site has been penetrated 0.75 to 1.25 inches, aspiration is carried out for any fluid or calcific material. One then removes the syringe, leaving the needle in position. Another syringe containing 20 to 40 mg of prednisolone suspension or equivalent is attached, and the medication is instilled. This injection can be followed with 1 to 5 ml of 1 per cent lidocaine, or 1 to 2 ml of lidocaine can be given combined with the steroid in the same syringe. A single treatment will relieve the majority of acute disorders, but occasionally it may have to be repeated once or twice.

Sometimes a painful reaction may follow when the analgesic has worn off. To avoid severe pain the patient should be warned about this possibility

and given codeine or meperidine to take in such an event.

Acromioclavicular Joint Inflammation. Pain arising in the acromioclavicular joint is frequently an aftermath of an acute injury. With this injury, all ranges of motion of the shoulder cause pain, and the joint is tender and rarely swollen.

TECHNIQUE. Entry is made through a cutaneous lidocaine wheal over the interosseous groove at the point of greatest tenderness (Fig. 46–4). The joint line is relatively superficial, and a ⅞-inch or 1-inch, 22 gauge needle is adequate. One to 1.5 ml of lidocaine and 5 to 10 mg of a prednisolone suspension are injected. It is not necessary to advance the needle beyond the proximal margin of the joint surface.

The Elbow Region. The elbow is subject to frequently occurring characteristic extra-articular disorders. These include radiohumeral bursitis, epicondylitis ("tennis" and "golfer's" elbow), and olecranon bursitis ("barfly's" elbow).

Radiohumeral Bursitis. This occurs at the juncture of the radial head and the lateral epicondyle of the elbow. Radiohumeral bursitis is commonly found in combination with lateral epicondylitis. The symptoms of the two adjacent problems are indistinguishable, but tenderness in bursitis overlies the site of the radiohumeral groove, whereas tenderness in "tennis" elbow occurs chiefly at the lateral epicondyle. A clinical sign supporting the diagnosis of "tennis" elbow is the provocation of pain when the patient attempts elevation of the middle finger against resistance with the wrist and the elbow held in extension.

TECHNIQUE. The entry site is the point of maxi-

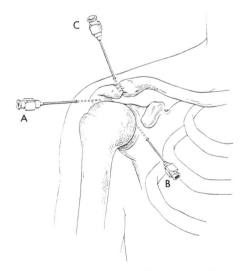

Figure 46–4. Injections at the shoulder. *A,* Lateral approach to the subacromial bursa or supraspinatus tendon. *B,* Anterior approach to the glenohumeral joint (see chapter on arthrocentesis). *C,* Approach to the acromioclavicular joint. (From Steinbrocker, O., and Neustadt, D. H.: Aspiration and Injection Therapy in Arthritis and Musculoskeletal Disorders: A Handbook on Technique and Management. Hagerstown, MD, Harper & Row, 1972. Used by permission.)

mal tenderness, usually found at a point slightly distal to the lateral epicondyle. The radial head can be palpated and confirmed by rotation of the patient's forearm (Fig. 46–5). The injection enters through a skin wheal with a 1.5-inch, 22 gauge needle, depositing 20 to 30 mg of prednisolone mixed with lidocaine. Alternatively, the steroid is followed with 1 to 3 ml of the local anesthetic. Part of the repository preparation may be instilled into the radiohumeral bursa and part at the lateral epicondyle (Fig. 46–6). Generally, it is wise to limit repeat injection attempts to two or three. In medial epicondylitis ("golfer's" elbow), a similar technique can be used, but it is important to remember to avoid the ulnar nerve, which lies in a groove behind the medial epicondyle.

Olecranon Bursitis. "Student's" elbow, or "miner's beat" elbow, is a common condition that is frequently idiopathic or provoked by trauma.[4, 23] The bursa also can be involved in rheumatoid arthritis and gout. Although most cases of olecranon bursitis are sterile, the olecranon bursa is the most frequent site of septic bursitis. The diagnosis of olecranon bursitis is obvious when the elbow is inspected and examined during flexion and extension. Occasionally in rheumatoid arthritis and gout, nodules, or tophi, may be readily palpated within the bursal sac. The olecranon bursa that is most commonly involved lies between the skin and the olecranon process. Motion at the elbow joint remains complete and painless unless there is also "true" elbow joint involvement. Olecranon bursitis often does not cause discomfort and may resolve spontaneously unless there has been bleeding into the bursa or the effusion is extremely tense. When the bursa is large and subject to

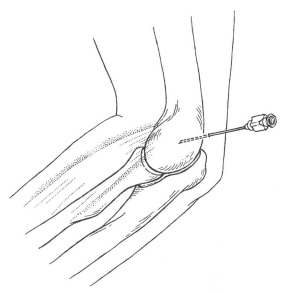

Figure 46–6. Injection at lateral epicondyle. (Redrawn from Steinbrocker, O., and Neustadt, D. H.: Aspiration and Injection Therapy in Arthritis and Musculoskeletal Disorders: A Handbook on Technique and Management. Hagerstown, MD, Harper & Row, 1972.)

trauma or tender and inflamed, provided that infection is excluded, aspiration and a steroid injection will expedite resolution. Aspiration without injection is often followed by recurrence in a few days or weeks. Fluid may be aspirated for analysis and culture to help distinguish a noninflammatory process from an inflammatory or septic bursitis. Clear or serosanguineous fluid is seen with a sterile bursitis, whereas cloudy fluid should suggest a septic process. *Septic bursitis should not be treated by injection with a corticosteroid.* Rarely, a cholesterol crystal synovitis develops, and this may mimic a suppurative bursitis.

TECHNIQUE. A 1.0- to 1.5-inch, 20 gauge needle is introduced at a dependent aspect of the bursal sac through a skin wheal, Frigiderm spray, or unanesthetized skin. After *all* the fluid is aspirated, 15 to 30 mg of prednisolone tebutate or equivalent preparation is injected. If infected or inspissated fluid is anticipated, a 16 to 18 gauge needle may be necessary for aspiration of the viscous contents. In frank septic bursitis, especially with thickening of the bursal wall, open incision with drainage may be required, with possible subsequent excision of the bursa.

The Wrist and Hand

Ganglia. These are cystic swellings occurring frequently on the hands and the feet, especially on the dorsal aspect of the wrist. The cystic structures are attached or may arise from tendon sheaths or near the joint capsule. They contain a clear gelatinous or mucoid fluid of great density. The material in the cyst may sometimes represent almost pure hyaluronic acid. Spontaneous regression is common. When the ganglion is painful or

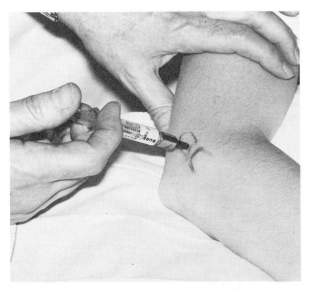

Figure 46–5. Actual injection of radiohumeral bursitis. (From Steinbrocker, O., and Neustadt, D. H.: Aspiration and Injection Therapy in Arthritis and Musculoskeletal Disorders: A Handbook on Technique and Management. Hagerstown, MD, Harper & Row, 1972. Used by permission.)

tender, aspiration with a 1-inch, relatively large gauge needle (17 to 18 gauge) and introduction of 10 to 15 mg of corticosteroid suspension is generally a satisfactory approach. Surgical excision may become necessary if this technique is unsuccessful.

de Quervain's Disease. This is a stenosing tenosynovitis of the short extensor (extensor pollicis brevis) and long abductor tendon (abductor pollicis longus) of the thumb. Although occasionally associated with rheumatoid arthritis, the disorder more often occurs following repetitive use of the wrist, especially with a wringing motion. The syndrome has been called "washerwoman's sprain." Tenderness and, occasionally, palpable crepitation is elicited just distal to the radial styloid process. A useful specific clinical examination is Finkelstein's test. One conducts the test by adducting the patient's thumb into the palm of the hand and folding the fingers over the thumb. Forcible ulnar deviation at the wrist is then carried out, provoking severe pain at the site of the affected tendon sheaths when the test is positive. It should be noted that gonococcal tenosynovitis of the wrist may mimic de Quervain's disease.

TECHNIQUE. A 7/8-inch, 25 gauge needle is introduced at the most tender point (just distal to the radial styloid) through a skin wheal, and 10 to 20 mg of prednisolone suspension is deposited in the tendon sheath with or followed by lidocaine (Fig. 46–7). The injection may be repeated one or two times at 7- to 14-day intervals if needed. A lightweight splint for wrist support and protection may be used at night for several weeks after the injection.

Carpal Tunnel Syndrome. Carpal tunnel syndrome (CTS) is a common nerve entrapment caused by median nerve compression. CTS is characterized by pain at the wrist that sometimes radiates upward into the forearm and is associated with tingling and paresthesias of the palmar side of the index and middle fingers and the radial half of the ring finger. Typically, the patient wakes during the night with burning or aching pain,

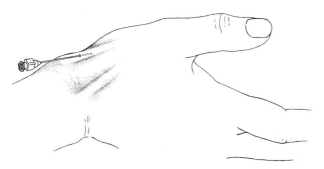

Figure 46–7. Injection of abductor tendon sheath (de Quervain's disease). (From Steinbrocker, O., and Neustadt, D. H.: Aspiration and Injection Therapy in Arthritis and Musculoskeletal Disorders: A Handbook on Technique and Management. Hagerstown, MD, Harper & Row, 1972. Used by permission.)

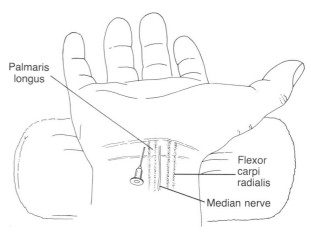

Figure 46–8. Injection of the median carpal tunnel with the wrist dorsiflexed over a rolled towel. To avoid direct injection of the median nerve, the needle is introduced just medial (ulnar) to the palmaris longus tendon. (Redrawn from Steinbrocker, O., and Neustadt, D. H.: Aspiration and Injection Therapy in Arthritis and Musculoskeletal Disorders: A Handbook on Technique and Management. Hagerstown, MD, Harper & Row, 1972.)

numbness, and tingling and shakes the hand outside the bed in order to try to obtain relief and restore sensation. Occasionally the discomfort is extremely severe, causing the patient to seek emergency aid. Clinical signs supporting the diagnosis include a positive Tinel's sign, in which one reproduces the tingling and paresthesias by tapping (with a reflex hammer) over the median nerve at the volar crease of the wrist.[24] Additionally, one can perform wrist flexion maneuvers (Phalen's sign) in an effort to provoke the symptoms in the median nerve distribution.[25] Severe muscle atrophy of the thenar eminence may develop in advanced or neglected cases. Causes of carpal tunnel syndrome include rheumatoid arthritis (sometimes as the presenting manifestation), pregnancy, hypothyroidism, diabetes, and acromegaly, but in many cases the disturbance is idiopathic without a recognizable underlying cause.

TECHNIQUE. When injecting the carpal canal, one should insert the needle through a skin wheal at a site just medial or ulnar to the palmaris longus tendon and proximal to the distal crease at the wrist (Fig. 46–8). Injecting medial to the palmaris longus is preferred because it avoids direct injection of the median nerve and superficial veins. A 1.0- to 1.5-inch, 22 gauge needle is directed at an angle of approximately 60 degrees to the skin surface, pointing toward the palm. The needle is advanced 1 to 2 cm, and 20 to 40 mg of prednisolone suspension with or without lidocaine is injected along the track and into the tissue space. Up to 2 weeks may be required for the symptoms to abate significantly. A lightweight wrist splint may hasten recovery. Repeat injections may be given, but if response is not successful or lasting after two or three injections, decompressive sur-

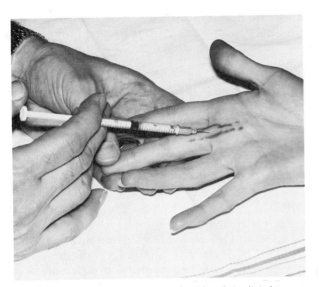

Figure 46–9. Injection of flexor tendon sheath in digital tenosynovitis. (From Steinbrocker, O., and Neustadt, D. H.: Aspiration and Injection Therapy in Arthritis and Musculoskeletal Disorders: A Handbook on Technique and Management. Hagerstown, MD, Harper & Row, 1972. Used by permission.)

gery should be considered. Nerve compression should be confirmed by nerve conduction studies before surgery.[26]

Digital Flexor Tenosynovitis. A "trigger," or "snapping," finger is characterized by a stenosed tendon sheath on the palmar surface over the base of the metacarpal head. Tenderness is usually confined to this site. The area of stenosis leads to intermittent catching of the enclosed tendon. Locking occurs when the offending digit is in flexion and is especially bothersome when the patient awakens in the morning. The common causes are trauma and rheumatoid arthritis. A nodule or fibrinous deposit may form at a point in the tendon sheath at the site where the snapping occurs.

TECHNIQUE. The technique for injecting flexor tenosynovitis includes locating and marking the tendon point at the involved metacarpal base and instilling 0.25 ml of any corticosteroid suspension subcutaneously with a ⅞-inch, 25 gauge needle into the involved tendon sheath (Fig. 46–9). Frigiderm can be used to numb the skin before entry of the needle. Resistance should not be encountered on injecting. Similar injections can be administered to the base of the thumb metacarpal for a "snapping" thumb. Up to four repeat injections may be given at 6- to 8-week intervals. If relapses are frequent or the clinical response is not satisfactory, then surgical release is indicated.

Lower Extremity Regions

Painful lower extremity disorders that deserve consideration for local injection procedures include affected bursae at the hip, knee, and heel regions.

The Hip Region
Trochanteric Bursitis. Trochanteric bursitis may simulate hip joint disease and sciatica.[27] The principal bursa lies between the gluteus maximus and the posterolateral prominence of the greater trochanter. The chief locus of the pathologic condition is in the abductor mechanism of the hip. Pain occurs near the greater trochanter and may radiate down the lateral or posterolateral aspect of the thigh. Pain is provoked by lying on the side of the hip, stepping from curbs, and descending steps. Tenderness may be elicited over and adjacent to the greater trochanter. In contrast with true hip involvement, the Patrick (fabere) sign may be negative, and there is a relatively painless complete passive range of motion. Active abduction when the patient lies on the opposite side typically intensifies the discomfort, and sharp external rotation may accentuate the symptoms. Hip radiographs may demonstrate a calcific deposit adjacent to the trochanter.[27] Trochanteric bursitis is a fairly frequent complication in rheumatoid arthritis.[28]

TECHNIQUE. Intrabursal injection uses the site of maximum tenderness for the entry point. A 1.5- to 2.0-inch, 20 or 21 gauge needle is advanced until the needle tip reaches the trochanter. The needle is then withdrawn slightly and the site is infiltrated fairly widely with 3 to 10 ml of lidocaine and 20 to 40 mg of prednisolone tebutate or equivalent. The condition usually improves following one or two local injections.

Ischiogluteal Bursitis. "Weaver's bottom" is a painful disorder characterized by pain over the center of the buttocks with radiation down the back of the leg.[29] This condition is rarely diagnosed, but when recognized a skillful intrabursal injection coupled with a few days' rest usually relieves the extreme pain. The bursa is adjacent to the ischial tuberosity and overlies the sciatic and posterior femoral cutaneous nerves. Pain is provoked by sitting on hard surfaces. Tenderness is present over the ischial tuberosity.

TECHNIQUE. The usual technique for injection requires that the patient lie in a prone position. A 2-inch, 20 to 22 gauge needle is inserted through a skin wheal and is advanced cautiously in an effort to avoid the sciatic nerve, which lies at a depth of approximately 2.5 to 3 inches. Paresthesias occur on striking the nerve, and if this occurs the needle should be withdrawn from the nerve. Generally, 5 to 10 ml of lidocaine and 20 to 40 mg of prednisolone suspension are introduced into the bursa.

The Knee Region. Of the numerous bursae in the region of the knee, only the prepatellar, suprapatellar, and anserine commonly are considered for injection.

Prepatellar Bursitis. "Housemaid's," or "nun's," knee is characterized by swelling with effusion of the superficial bursa overlying the lower pole of the patella. Passive motion is fully preserved, and pain is generally mild, except during extreme knee flexion or direct pressure. Although the disorder is usually caused by pressure from repetitive kneeling on a firm surface ("rug cutter's" knee), rarely it can develop after direct trauma and occasionally is a manifestation of rheumatoid arthritis. The prepatellar bursa is also a common site of septic bursitis.

TECHNIQUE. Aspiration often yields a surprisingly scant amount of clear, serous fluid, owing to the fact that the prepatellar bursa is a multilocular structure rather than the usual single cavity. The instillation of 1 to 2 ml of lidocaine with 15 to 20 mg of a prednisolone suspension with a 1-inch 20 to 21 gauge needle is usually sufficient to cause the swelling to abate. In some cases one may need to repeat the procedure a couple of times to obtain a lasting result. The provocative activity should be discontinued.

Suprapatellar Bursitis. Suprapatellar bursitis usually is associated with synovitis of the knees. On occasion the bursa is largely separated from the synovial cavity with only a very minor communication, and the swelling and effusion are chiefly confined to the suprapatellar area. This may be traumatic in origin or may be an associated manifestation of an inflammatory arthropathy.

TECHNIQUE. The procedure for aspiration and injection of the suprapatellar area is similar to that for the knee (see chapter on arthrocentesis).

Anserine Bursitis. "Cavalryman's" disease now mainly occurs in heavy women with disproportionately large thighs in association with osteoarthritis of the knee. The bursa is on the anteromedial side of the knee, inferior to the joint line at the site of the insertion of the conjoined tendons of the sartorius, semitendinous, and gracilis and superficial to the medial collateral ligament. The entity is characterized by a relatively abrupt onset of knee pain with localized tenderness and a puffy sensation in the vicinity of the anserine bursa.

TECHNIQUE. An injection of 2 to 4 ml of lidocaine with or followed by approximately 20 to 40 mg of a corticosteroid suspension is given at the point of greatest tenderness from an anterior or medial approach with a 1.0- to 1.5-inch, 22 gauge needle. Prompt symptomatic relief frequently is obtained, but the duration of benefit is variable and probably correlates with the patient's weight-bearing activities.

The Ankle, Foot, and Heel Region

Ankle Tendinitis. This is a relatively uncommon condition. It may result from unusual repetitive activity or, rarely, from acute trauma. Crepitant swollen tendon sheaths commonly occur in rheumatoid arthritis. The disorder is differentiated from ankle joint involvement by the lack of pain or restricted motion during passive flexion and extension of the ankle. Active flexion and extension of the toes does produce pain. Local tenderness is elicited along the flexor and extensor tendons. Injection of the tendonsheaths is useful, producing considerable relief of symptoms.

TECHNIQUE. A 1.0- to 1.5-inch, 20 or 21 gauge needle is used. One makes a tangential entry to the enlarged tendon sheath, distending the sheath with approximately 2 to 4 ml of a mixture of corticosteroid and lidocaine and instilling 20 to 40 mg of prednisolone tebutate. It may be necessary to repeat the injection after several months.

"Bunion" Bursitis. A common condition is "bunion" bursitis overlying the first metatarsophalangeal joint at its medial surface on the great toe. On occasion, tense swelling occurs and decompression is required. Aspiration with culture of the fluid should be performed.

TECHNIQUE. If no infection is present, the bursa is injected with 5 to 10 mg of prednisolone suspension with a 1-inch, 20 gauge needle. Special shoes or an orthopedic correction will be needed if the swelling recurs.

Heel Pain. "Talalgia" may be caused by Achilles tendinitis, calcaneal bursitis, or plantar fasciitis. The bursae of clinical significance around the heel include the space between the skin and the Achilles tendon, the retrocalcaneal bursa, and the subcalcaneal bursa. Achilles tendinitis or bursitis may be traumatic in origin but is more apt to be part of a systemic disease, such as rheumatoid or gouty arthritis. Although the normal Achilles tendon is thick and strong, when affected by an inflammatory arthropathy it is predisposed to degeneration, and since the Achilles tendon is not invested by a full synovial sheath, it is more vulnerable to intratendon instillation. *Because of the potential hazard of tendon rupture after local steroid injection, it is wise to avoid infiltration of steroids into this area.*[30] It is preferable to treat Achilles tendinitis with rest, splinting, and oral medication. The major injectable condition in this region is calcaneal bursitis (plantar fasciitis), which is frequently associated with painful heel spurs ("policeman's," or "soldier's," heel). If orthopedic shoe corrections and aids are not effective, injection of the painful heel is sometimes beneficial.

TECHNIQUE. At the spot of maximal tenderness a 1.0-inch, 22 to 24 gauge needle enters the plantar surface at 90 degrees, sliding into the space at the midpoint of the calcaneus. The tip of the needle lies in the aponeurosis of the attachment to the os calcis (Fig. 46–10). One ml of lidocaine and 10 to 20 mg of prednisolone tebutate are instilled. The injection may need to be repeated once or twice at an interval of 6 to 8 weeks.

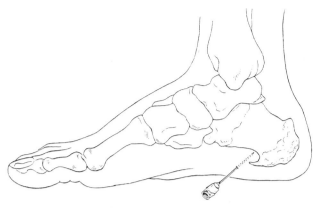

Figure 46–10. Injection of calcaneal bursitis with heel spur. (Redrawn from Steinbrocker , O., and Neustadt, D. H.: Aspiration and Injection Therapy in Arthritis and Musculoskeletal Disorders: A Handbook on Technique and Management. Hagerstown, MD, Harper & Row, 1972.)

Septic Bursitis

Occasionally, bursitis may be caused by an acute bacterial infection of the bursal fluid and surrounding soft tissue.[5, 31] Septic bursitis is most common in the olecranon and prepatellar bursae, whereas infection of other bursae is exceedingly rare.[31] The infection is probably secondary to acute trauma that results in direct penetration of the bursa by common skin pathogens rather than by hematogenous spread. The patient frequently reports a history of minor trauma or is engaged in an occupation associated with sustained pressure on the knees or the elbows.

Septic bursitis is not associated with septic arthritis of the underlying joint, although rarely, adjacent bone may become involved.[32] Many patients have an underlying predisposition to infection (e.g., diabetes mellitus, alcoholism, uremia, or gout). Rarely, an infection may follow a bursal injection of corticosteroids.

In most cases, the diagnosis of septic bursitis is obvious. The onset of pain and swelling may be quite rapid (over 8 to 24 hours) as compared with the more prolonged onset of aseptic bursitis. The bursa is tense and swollen and is very painful. Pitting edema and classic cellulitis of the peribursal soft tissue may be present. In some cases it may be difficult to distinguish septic bursitis from trauma or other acute inflammatory disorders, such as acute gout or tenosynovitis. In questionable cases it is prudent to aspirate and culture the fluid and to treat with antibiotics and oral nonsteroidal anti-inflammatory medications. Corticosteroid injection is withheld pending negative bacteriologic findings.

One confirms the diagnosis by culturing bacteria from the bursal aspirate. Fluid is usually easily obtained from the tense bursa and (in the case of an advanced infection) is cloudy or grossly purulent. The white blood cell count of the fluid is 50,000 to 100,000 cells per mm^3 or greater, and polymorphonuclear cells usually exceed 90 per cent. Gram-positive organisms may be seen on Gram stain. The infecting organism is usually penicillin-resistant *Staphylococcus aureus*, but streptococcal organisms may be isolated. The treatment of septic bursitis includes the use of antibiotics directed against penicillinase-producing staphylococcus, splinting, hot soaks, and drainage of the bursa. Drainage may be adequately performed with one or more needle aspirations, but open incision and drainage may be required. Corticosteroid injections should not be performed in infected tissue. Outpatient therapy with oral antibiotics is generally acceptable.

Concluding Comments

Local injection therapy for painful nonarticular rheumatic disorders is a relatively simple, safe, and effective form of treatment. The patient may experience rapid relief of pain and swelling, and on occasion may return to work after a single injection. The response may be long-lasting as well as very gratifying. An additional benefit of injection therapy is that it may avoid surgical intervention in such soft tissue problems as carpal tunnel syndrome, digital tenosynovitis (de Quervain's disease and "trigger" finger), and ganglia.

The local introduction of a corticosteroid suspension should be carried out with due regard for any coexisting disease, such as diabetes mellitus and peptic ulcer. It is highly unlikely that these diseases would be provoked or aggravated after a single intrasynovial injection in usual therapeutic dosage, however. Systemic "spill-over" and absorption may occur, depending on the size of the dose and the solubility of the preparation injected. Transient adrenal suppression may develop but rarely lasts longer than a few days.

1. Monro, A. S.: A Description of All the Bursae Mucosae of the Human Body. Edinburgh, Elliott, 1788.
2. Spateholz, W.: Hand Atlas of Human Anatomy, Vol. 2, 6th ed. Philadelphia, J. B. Lippincott Co., 1932.
3. Bywaters, E. G. L.: Lesions of bursae, tendons and tendon sheaths. Clin. Rheum. Dis. 5:883, 1979.
4. Neustadt, D. H.: Bursitis and tendinitis. In Conn, H. F., and Conn, R. B. (eds.): Current Diagnosis^6 Philadelphia, W. B. Saunders Co., 1980, p. 964.
5. Canoso, J. J., and Sheckman, P. R.: Septic subcutaneous bursitis. J. Rheum. et al, 6:96, 1979.
6. Parker, M. D., and Irwin, R. S.: Tendinitis due to *Mycobacterium kansasii*. J. Bone Joint Surg. 57A:557, 1975.
7. Finder, J. C., and Post, M.: Local injection therapy for rheumatic diseases. JAMA 172:2021, 1960.
8. Steinbrocker, O., and Neustadt, D. H.: Aspiration and Injection Therapy in Arthritis and Musculoskeletal Disorders: A Handbook on Technique and Management. Hagerstown, Md, Harper & Row, 1972, p. 16.
9. Halpern, A. A., Horowitz, B. G., and Nagel, D. A.: Tendon

ruptures associated with corticosteroid therapy. West, J. Med. 127:378, 1977.

10. Bonica, J. J.: The Management of Pain. Philadelphia, Lea & Febiger, 1953, p. 234.

11. Murnagham, G. F., and McIntosh, D.: Hydrocortisone in painful shoulder. A controlled trial. Lancet 2:798, 1955.

12. Konttinen, Y. T., Friman, C., Tolvanen, E., et al.: Local skin rash after intraarticular methylprednisolone acetate injection in a patient with rheumatoid arthritis. Arthritis Rheum. 26:231, 1983.

13. Hollander, J. L.: Intrasynovial corticosteroid therapy in arthritis. Md. State Med. J. 19:62, 1972.

14. Gray, R. G., Tenenbaum, J., and Gottlieb, N. L.: Local corticosteroid injection treatment in rheumatic disorders. Semin. Arthritis Rheum. 10:231, 1981.

15. Fitzgerald, R. H.: Intrasynovial injection of steroids. Uses and abuses. Mayo Clin. Proc. 51:655, 1976.

16. Gottlieb, N. L., and Riskin, W. G.: Complications of local corticosteroid injections. JAMA 243:1547, 1980.

17. McCarty, D. J., and Hogan, J. M.: Inflammatory reaction after intrasynovial injection of microcrystalline adrenocorticosteroid esters. Arthritis Rheum. 7:359, 1964.

18. Cassidy, J. T., and Bole, G. G.: Cutaneous atrophy secondary to intra-articular corticosteroid administration. Ann. Intern. Med. 65:1008, 1966.

19. Neustadt, D. H.: Tendon rupture and steroid therapy (letter to the editor). South. Med. J. 73:271, 1980.

20. Neustadt, D. H.: Chemistry and Therapy of Collagen Diseases. Springfield, IL, Charles C. Thomas, 1963, p. 52.

21. Bain, L. S., Baleh, H. W., Wetherly, J. M. R., et al.: Intraarticular triamcinoline hexacetonide: Double-blind comparison with methylprednisolone. Br. J. Clin. Pract. 26:559, 1972.

22. Steinbrocker, O., Neustadt, D. H., and Bosch, S. J.: Painful shoulder syndromes. Med. Clin. North Am. 39:1, 1955.

23. Thompson, M.: Joints and their diseases. The elbow. Br. Med. J. 3:399, 1969.

24. Sonntag, V. K. H.: Tinel's sign. N. Engl. J. Med. 291:263, 1974.

25. Sheon, R. P., Moskowitz, R. W., and Goldberg, V.: Soft Tissue Rheumatic Pain: Recognition, Management and Prevention. Philadelphia, Lea & Febiger, 1982, p. 107.

26. Wakefield, G.: The entrapment neuropathies. Clin. Rheum. Dis. 5:941, 1979.

27. Leonard, M. H.: Trochanteric syndrome. JAMA 168:175, 1958.

28. Raman, D., and Haslock, I.: Trochanteric bursitus—a frequent cause of "hip" pain in rheumatoid arthritis. Ann. Rheum. Dis. 41:602, 1982.

29. Swartout, R., and Compere, E. L.: Ischiogluteal bursitis. JAMA 227:551, 1974.

30. Neustadt, D. H.: Complications of local corticosteroid injections (letter to the editor). JAMA 246:835, 1981.

31. Ho, G., Tice, A. D., and Kaplan, S. R.: Septic bursitis in the prepatellar and olecranon bursae. Ann. Intern. Med. 89:21, 1978.

32. Simonelli, C., Zoschke, D., Bankhurst, A., et al.: Septic arthritis. Ann. Intern. Med. 89:575, 1978.

47

Trigger Point Therapy

ANDERS E. SOLA, M.D.

Introduction

Myofascial pain is probably the most common pain problem faced by physicians. It may be the primary complaint or may be a crippling adjunct to any number of other problems and is often accompanied by either local or generalized fatigue. Myofascial pain is a very common complaint in the emergency department, and affected patients often present with torticollis, headache, or lower back pain. For many years, highly localized, exquisitely sensitive areas that are usually found within or near the painful region have been recognized as a common feature of myofascial pain. Pressure on these areas, known as trigger points, will cause local pain, referred pain or both.[1-9]

The local or referred pain associated with trigger points may not follow segmental neurologic patterns and therefore may not present with a well-defined dermatome distribution. Actions taken at the trigger points, such as application of heat or cold, electrical stimulation, injection with local anesthetic or saline, or simply stimulation of the sensitive point with a needle, have proven the trigger points to be, in many cases, the key to control of the painful experience. A somewhat similar needling effect is associated with acupuncture points (many of which are located in areas in which trigger points are commonly found).[10-12] The exact mechanisms by which trigger points are involved in and contribute to myofascial pain as well as the response to intervention at trigger points indicate a continuous, cyclic relationship between trigger point activity and the pain phenomenon.

Background

The trigger point phenomenon has its western origin in Germany, the Scandinavian countries, and Great Britain (the "rheumatic" countries).[3, 4] The Germans first reported on these painful muscular problems (Muskel schmerzen) and "hard" muscles in the mid-nineteenth century. Most of the investigations were directed at the microscopic findings of these "hard nodules," or so-called rheumatic lesions of muscle. These sensitive areas in muscle caused local pain or tenderness on palpation with or without a predictable pain reference away from the local point of maximal tenderness. The British followed with similar studies and failed to determine the faulty microanatomy and pathophysiology of these elusive pain problems—these conditions were referred to as fibrositis, myalgia, and nonarticular rheumatism. Gower introduced the term *fibrositis* at the turn of the century, and it became fixed in the English literature when Llewellyn and Jones' massive text was published in 1915.[13, 14] Despite intensive investigation, no satisfactory explanation of the mechanisms of (muscular) pain was discovered to resolve the controversy.

Kraus published an innovative study on the use of the ethyl chloride spray technique to relieve myofascial pain in 1937.[15] This was followed by the studies of Travell, who has done extensive research and has published works on the trigger point problem over many years. She has carefully plotted the pain patterns most commonly encountered and has emphasized the use of procaine injections and the coolant spray, Flouri-Methane (Gebaur Chemical Co., Cleveland, OH), instead of the more dangerous ethyl chloride.

Dr. Travell has described a trigger point caused by acute or chronic overload of a muscle as a palpable, firm, tense band in the muscle. The trigger point is characterized by a local twitch response to tapping of the muscle, restricted range of motion, weakness without atrophy, and no neurologic deficit. Subjectively, the patients complain of pain in a predictable pattern, stiffness and fatigue, and deep tenderness at the trigger point.[9]

In addition to muscular overload, a variety of stress-inducing stimuli—emotional or physical—may be implicated in the onset of myofascial pain (Fig. 47–1). The power of these stressors to induce pain in a particular individual is moderated by the genetics, personality, conditioning, and physiologic state of that individual. Once established, however, a painful event may sustain itself in spite of control or elimination of the initiating stimuli through a characteristic internal cyclic process of self-stimulus and response. Furthermore, the painful trigger point itself may become the stressor that involves other muscles in the event. Thus, trigger points may act both as translators of stress to pain and, secondarily, as stressors that perpetuate pain.[16]

Trigger points can occur in any muscle or muscle group in the body. Since the stresses involved in the onset of myofascial pain can commonly affect not only single muscles but also whole muscle groups, trigger points tend to cluster. In the upper trunk, a common trigger point cluster involves the muscles of the neck and the shoulder area—the

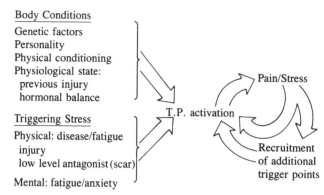

Figure 47–1. Stress and body conditions. A variety of stress-inducing stimuli may be implicated in the onset of myofascial pain. The power of these stimuli to induce pain in a particular individual is moderated by the genetics, personality, conditioning, and physiologic state of that individual. Once established, however, a painful event may sustain itself in spite of control or elimination of the initiating stimuli. (From Sola, A. E.: Myofascial trigger point therapy. Resident and Staff Physician 27(8): 1981. Used by permission.)

trapezius, the levator scapulae, and the infraspinatus. In the lower trunk, a group of muscles that is often involved includes the quadratus lumborum, the gluteus medius, and the tensor fasciae latae. As individuals age there is an increase in the potential for nerve root irritation problems and subsequent pain. Although nerve root irritation cannot be alleviated by treatment of trigger points, myofascial disturbances that may arise as a result of the irritation may be reduced through such treatment.

Painful trigger points in a given muscle often affect all other muscles innervated from the same spinal segments, and treatment is usually directed at those muscles innervated by both the *posterior* branch of the spinal nerve(s) and the *anterior* spinal branch (Fig. 47–2). Therefore, the search for trigger points and subsequent treatment should be di-

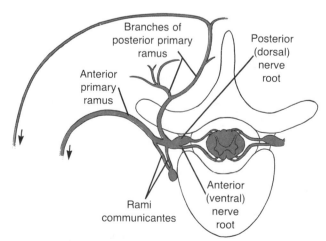

Figure 47–2. Cross section of a typical spinal nerve showing anterior and posterior divisions. The posterior segment innervates the erector spinae, whereas the anterior segment innervates the remaining muscles supplied by the spinal nerves.

rected at both spinal nerve divisions. Pain may be felt in a muscle innervated by an anterior spinal nerve, whereas little or no pain may be initially felt in muscles innervated by the posterior branch of the same spinal nerves. Palpation of the muscles innervated by the posterior branch, however, may reveal evidence of active trigger points: hypersensitive areas, or, more important, a tight band-like local spasm plus hypersensitivity.

Trigger points in a given muscle may affect not only the anterior and posterior branch of the specific segmental spinal nerve but also spinal nerves related by common musculature for several segments above and below the major trigger point. Thus, muscles in the erector group in the cervical area can be the source of noxious impulses that can cause pain to be transmitted as far as the midthoracic area (Fig. 47–3).[17]

Furthermore, the presence of trigger points in the gluteal or lumbar muscles may often be related to hypersensitivity in the muscles of the upper trunk group. Therefore, a patient who is suffering muscle tension headaches on one side should be checked not only for trigger points in the ipsilateral upper trunk muscles but also for hypersensitive areas (trigger points) in the gluteal and lumbar musculature. If trigger points are found, they should be treated to reduce both the hyperactivity in the lower segment and the sensitivity of the upper muscle group. If hyperactive trigger points are ignored in the lumbar and (especially) the gluteal region, treating only the cervical trigger

points can precipitate a painful low back spasm. This may be severe enough to cause another trip to the emergency department.

Both the longevity and the spread of myofascial pain may be caused by cycles of physiologic responses that involve one or more trigger points. These may include such well-defined pathways as motor reflexes, less well-known autonomic feedback cycles and, quite probably, a number of as yet ill-defined interrelationships that include changes in the microenvironment of the tissues in the area. Frequently seen autonomic concomitants of trigger points include decreased electrical skin resistance, pilomotor reactions in the reference area, and vasodilation with dermatographia and skin temperature changes.[9] I have also noted hypoesthesia in the involved extremity (and, when upper and lower muscle groups are involved, in the affected side), local and general fatigue, fine tremor, and weakness.

The exact physiologic mechanism of trigger points has not been defined. Trigger points may be considered as "weak points" within the muscle or fascia that are particularly sensitive to stress-induced change. In the absence of stress, the trigger point may remain quiescent, only to become activated by a number of positive-feedback cycles that involve sensory motor reflexes, autonomic responses, vascular changes, and numerous other ill-defined events ultimately leading to muscle tension, fatigue, and pain.

The initiating stress may also be soft tissue trauma, such as a muscular strain or contusion, causing prolonged pain that is more intense, out of proportion, or of excessively long duration, given the initial injury. Such may be the case with a worker who suffers a relatively minor injury on the job but has persistent disability or impairment long beyond the expected period of disability for that particular injury.

Therefore, one can consider trigger points as contributing two aspects to the etiology and prolongation of myofascial pain: (1) a primary role (Fig. 47–4) as a translator of stimuli to the pain response, and (2) a secondary role (Fig. 47–5) of pain intensification when pain is a component of the initial stress.

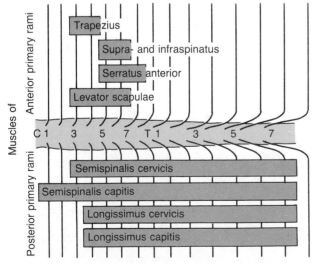

Figure 47–3. This schematic illustration gives examples of upper extremity muscles supplied by the anterior primary rami of the cervical spine. Note the length of the muscles supplied by the posterior rami shown for the same cervical region. Activation of trigger points that exist along the entire length of a muscle can cause or intensify pain felt in muscles supplied by any common nerve segment. Therefore, pain experienced along a muscle such as the semispinalis capitis can contribute to shoulder pain. Injection treatment of posterior primary rami muscles beginning at T-6 is indicated if hypersensitive trigger points are found in the muscles.

Patient Profile

Patients commonly attribute their symptoms to overuse of muscles, sitting in drafts, or a "cold" in the muscle. Many myofascial syndromes are short-lived and respond well to initial therapy, but many require repeated visits and long-term therapy that is not available in many emergency departments.

Patients with prolonged or debilitating myofascial pain syndromes may present to the emergency

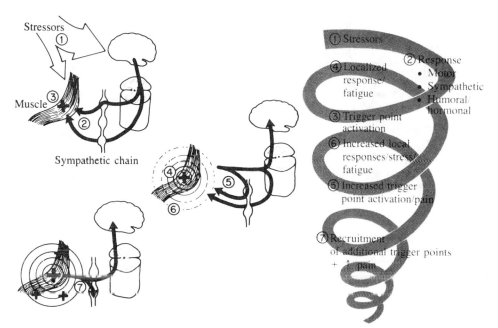

Figure 47–4. The primary role. The individual, subjected to the physical and emotional stresses of daily living *(1)*, responds with defense mechanisms that include various physiologic changes, such as splinting and bracing of muscles, vasomotor changes, increased sympathetic discharge, and hormonal and other humoral changes in the plasma and extracellular fluids *(2)*. A particular point in a braced, stressed muscle or fascia that is more sensitive than the surrounding tissue—perhaps because of previous injury or genetic mandate—fatigues and begins to signal its distress to the central nervous system *(3)*. There are a number of responses that may result. The most readily understood involves the motor reflexes. Various muscles associated with the trigger point become more tense and begin to fatigue. Sympathetic responses lead to vasomotor changes within and around the trigger point. Local ischemia following vasoconstriction or increased vascular permeability following vasodilation may lead to changes in the extracellular environment of the affected cells, release of algesic agents (bradykinins, prostaglandins), osmotic changes, and pH changes, all of which may increase the sensitivity or activity of nociceptors in the area. Sympathetic activity may also cause smooth muscle contraction in the vicinity of nociceptors, thus increasing their activity *(4)*. Increased nociceptor input contributes to the cycle by increasing motor and sympathetic activity, which in turn leads to increased pain *(5)*. The pain is shadowed by growing fatigue, which adds an overall mood of distress to the patient's situation and feeds back to the cycle *(6)*. As tense muscles in the affected area begin to fatigue in an environment of sympathetic stimulation and local biochemical change, latent trigger points within these muscles may also begin to fire, thus adding to the positive feedback cycle and spreading the pain to these adjacent muscle groups. Finally, the stress of pain and fatigue, coupled with both increased muscle tension and sympathetic tone throughout the body (conceivably with ipsilateral emphasis through the sympathetic chain), may lead to flare-ups or trigger points in other muscles remote from the initial area of pain *(7)*. (From Sola, A. E.: Myofascial trigger point therapy. Resident and Staff Physician 27(8):39, 1981. Used by permission.)

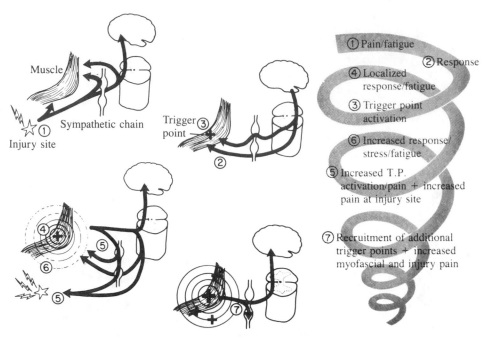

Figure 47–5. The secondary role. Myofascial pain generated secondarily to other painful stimuli, such as trauma, ligamental injury, facet lesions, or nerve root lesions, follows much the same course as myofascial pain generated due to nonpainful stress stimulators. In this situation, fatigue, muscle tension and, perhaps, splinting, sympathetic activation, and extracellular fluid changes in response to the painful stimulus lead to the initial myofascial pain. Subsequent events duplicate the primary course. In addition, the cyclic responses accompanying trigger point involvement may feed back on the initial pain stimulus. Conditions such as phantom pain, painful scars, or trauma to peripheral tissues may often stimulate trigger points in the segment and may subsequently be affected by these same trigger points. Thus, conditions such as increased stimulation and increased levels of algesic agents in the blood may act with the increased emotional stress to the individual to prolong and intensify the pain and dysfunction of the site of injury. (From Sola, A. E.: Myofascial trigger point therapy. Resident and Staff Physician 27(8):41, 1981. Used by permission.)

department after becoming frustrated with unsuccessful visits to numerous other physicians. They may have consulted chiropractors; tried home remedies or vitamin therapy; or received treatment with a variety of muscle relaxants, anti-inflammatory medications, or potent analgesics. Their physicians may have dismissed them as chronic complainers or neurotics because there has been no radiographic or laboratory confirmation of their complaints, or their symptoms may have been given the vague diagnosis of chronic bursitis, arthritis, or sciatica. The patients describe the pain as deep and aching. Physical examination fails to elicit any neurologic deficits or atrophy, although there may be some weakness of the involved muscle groups.

Examination for Trigger Points

Any treatment of myofascial syndromes must be preceded by a history and physical examination to rule out other causes of apparent myofascial pain. Once this is accomplished, a systematic search for trigger points is carried out, with special emphasis placed on the painful muscles and their segmental associates. Trigger point areas should be compared with the contralateral counterparts as a guide to their relative sensitivity. The most reliable method of locating trigger points is by searching in the painful area with the tip of the finger. Pressure applied to the hypersensitive area in the muscle will reproduce or accentuate the pain. This is usually accompanied by an involuntary "wince" by the patient. The hypersensitive area may feel rope-like, indurated, or tight, depending on which muscle is examined. The muscles should be examined in both relaxed and stretched positions. Although there may be a halo area or a surrounding zone of tenderness, one should search for the area of maximal tenderness or response.

In sedentary populations, trigger points are common and are usually associated with chronic strain and stress. They tend to occur with great regularity in the same areas. In my clinical experience, trigger points are less common in laborers and athletes and, when present, are usually the result of overuse or injury rather than chronic strain or stress. This suggests that regular exercise is of therapeutic value.

Although the pain reference pattern may help to isolate the hypersensitive area, one should remember that the pattern differs according to severity and longevity of the trigger point injury, body build, state of health, gender, and degree of injury or weakness.

When searching for trigger points, one should carefully examine the entire area of all muscles that may be involved. For example, in treating torticollis, one should check the levator scapulae, trapezius, sternocleidomastoid, and posterior strap muscles (supplied by the posterior spinal ramus), especially the splenius and semispinalis muscles. The muscles are often innervated from many vertebral segments—for instance, innervation of the splenius starts at the C-2 vertebral level and reaches to the midthoracic level. Thus, hypersensitivity at one level may readily involve other muscles with overlapping segmental innervation. When treating neck pain problems, one must look for tender trigger points along the entire spinal insertion of these muscles. The same principle of extended search is also especially important in the treatment of myofascial shoulder pain, headache pain, and pain in the lumbar sacral region.

Indications

Treatment of sensitive trigger points by injection is often quite effective for pain relief when the trigger point is the primary source of myofascial pain. Such treatment may reduce pain and may speed recovery at sites of trauma in the same segment. Treatment of trigger points that flare up secondarily to other painful stimuli, such as nerve root lesions and nerve compression, is never more than moderately successful in relieving pain. Nonetheless, is often difficult to ascertain the source of the stress that leads to the myofascial involvement until trigger point injection has been tried. Therefore, in many cases, the response to injection treatment may also be an element of the diagnosis.

Under certain conditions, injection treatment not only may be ineffective but also may precipitate a medical or emotional crisis. Contraindications to injection treatment include the presence of a systemic illness (especially with fever), high anxiety or emotional stress levels (including "needle" anxiety, manifestations of psychosis, and abuse of drugs or alcohol), and a history of hypersensitive or syncopal reactions to injections. If there is doubt concerning the diagnosis of myofascial pain caused by trigger point involvement as opposed to such possible causes as a nerve root lesion, one should not inject the patient but should have the patient return for further studies. Although the possibility of injection treatment may discourage some malingerers, it is less effective as a screening tool than is acute observation of the "too-perfect" account of symptoms often given by these patients.

Equipment

Little equipment is necessary for the injection procedure. A simple tray may contain a 5-ml syringe, a 25 or 26 gauge needle, an antiseptic preparation, and a local anesthetic (1 per cent lidocaine, 0.25 per cent bupivacaine, or 1 per cent procaine hydrochloride) or physiologic saline for injection. Some physicians use a repository corticosteroid preparation, such as hydrocortisone or prednisolone tebutate, methylprednisolone acetate, or triamcinolone acetonide or hexacetonide (see Chapter 46, Table 46–2).

General Procedure

Injection of the hypersensitive trigger point often provides dramatic pain relief. There is a body of evidence that indicates that at least a portion of the benefit is derived from the stimulation of the trigger point by the needle regardless of the substances injected. Although local anesthetics are often used, I have used normal physiologic saline for many years with good results.[18–21] In one controlled study, Frost and coworkers[19] actually demonstrated better results when plain saline was used in comparison with the local anesthetic mepivacaine.

When injection therapy is performed in patients with moderate to severe pain in the emergency department, the supplemental use of a local anesthetic is advised for immediate relief, although good results have been obtained even in severe pain with saline injection alone. Local injection should be used in conjunction with appropriate oral analgesics and muscle relaxants. Some clinicians routinely inject small doses of a long-acting steroid preparation into painful trigger points in conjunction with saline or a local anesthetic. Although steroids are of proven value in the treatment of inflammatory conditions, their usefulness in trigger point therapy is unknown. A therapeutic trial of steroids may be warranted if proper precautions concerning the side effects are observed.

It is wise to inject patients who are in a supine position in order to minimize syncopal reactions. If the upper back, the neck, or the shoulder is being injected, a pillow is placed under the hips.

The hypersensitive point is located by palpation, and the area for injection is prepared in the usual manner. The point of entry should be in the area of maximal tenderness. One inserts the needle and injects 0.5 to 2 ml of fluid using a "fanning" technique, in which the needle is repeatedly withdrawn part of the way and redirected (Fig. 47–6). This ensures maximal coverage of the area of the trigger point. In most cases, a short series of two to five injections over a period of days to weeks

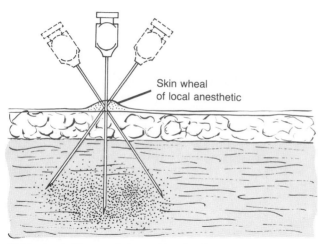

Figure 47–6. The needle is used in a fan-like motion to distribute the solution throughout the trigger point.

is enough to rule out myofascial pain caused by muscle strain or injury. After injection, a moist pack applied to the area relieves the temporary discomfort of the injection. It has been my experience that younger patients are more responsive to trigger point injection than are older individuals. In younger patients, trigger points are more easily located and are less complicated in their pain reference patterns. As people age, muscle weakness and shortening and the effects of degenerative processes frequently confuse the pain reference pattern.

Follow-up treatment for patients with myofascial pain may include one or more of the following: repeated injection therapy, adjunctive physical therapy, and special techniques, including intermittent cervical or lumbar traction, relaxation techniques, ultrasound, electrical stimulation, massage (especially deep friction) and application of coolant sprays or ice packs, and, routinely, therapeutic exercise.

Complications

Some patients are hyper-reactors. These individuals may respond to even an injection of saline by fainting if sitting upright and may have an excessive flare-up of pain after treatment (that night). I always ask about an allergic history (e.g., allergies to foods and drugs and sensitivity to the sun). It has been my experience that patients with red or auburn-colored hair and certain fair-skinned, blue-eyed blondes are more likely to faint. I also monitor patients with the back of my hand, touching their skin to detect excessive sweating.

If complications occur, one should stop injecting. Some physicians inject as much as 5 to 10 ml of fluid at a given trigger point. I have found that

this is excessive. The patient frequently develops a flu-like syndrome, characterized by malaise and myalgias, the next day. I have experienced few complications using saline with a normal pH. Some patients have fainted, but these individuals were seated rather than supine. The use of local anesthetics, a standard procedure in emergency departments, increases the risk very little if "caine" allergies, excessive drug quantities, and intravenous injections are avoided.

Particular care must be used in injecting the neck, the intercostal muscles, and the periscapular area, since these areas contain many large vessels and nerves and the pleura is in close proximity to the injection sites. This is complicated if the patient is agitated or young or is in a state of confusion.

Emergency Department Treatment of Common Presentations of Myofascial Pain

SHOULDER DISORDERS

A painful shoulder will frequently have trigger points located in the posterior scapular muscles. Other muscles that are often involved include the supraspinatus, the infraspinatus, and the pectoralis major. Less commonly, the teres, the deltoid, and the triceps are involved. Trigger points in the splenius, the semispinalis, and the gluteal muscles may also contribute to shoulder pain and should be treated if found in conjunction with myofascial shoulder pain. Such pain often prompts the diag-

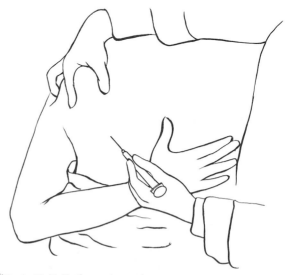

Figure 47–7. Surface view of serratus anterior muscle. The internally rotated arm is slid across the back toward the midline, bringing the inferior angle of the scapula into a "winged" position. The needle is slipped in anteriorly to the edge of the angle of the bone.

nosis of bursitis, which is usually a catchall or insurance diagnosis and is often not correct. Patients may have had numerous unsuccessful treatments with muscle relaxants and potent anti-inflammatory medications.

When injecting the scapular and periscapular muscles, one should take extreme care to stabilize the scapula. The patient should lie on a bed with his arms along his sides and a pillow under his chest to round the shoulders and to facilitate injection. A small pillow may be used to rest the forehead. The boundaries (borders) should be noted before injection, and the patient should be warned not to move his shoulder. If the lower portion of the scapula moves, one can easily miss the muscle and pierce the pleura. Therefore, one should "fix the scapula" before injecting and should always double-check. I frequently hook my thumb on the medial border while injecting trigger points in the infraspinatus muscle.

Myofascial pain is commonly associated with a number of muscles at the medial border of the scapula. These include the rhomboids, the serratus anterior, the subscapular muscles and, at the superior edge, the levator scapulae muscle. It is best to inject the levator at an oblique angle to the muscle, since patients frequently flinch during injection, and the needle could puncture the pleura.

If the painful areas are on the lower medial border, then the patient should place his hand behind his back. This causes a winging of the scapula, allowing easier and safer injection. A tangential laterally directed needle will reach much of the scapular undersurface (Fig. 47–7). The rhomboids and the serratus anterior are easily treatable with this maneuver. On occasion, the subscapularis muscle is involved, and the only complaint besides poorly localized scapular pain may be a sensation of "sleeping on a marble." When injecting along the lateral border (teres major and minor and lateral dorsi), one should fix the scapula and should warn the patient not to move.

HEADACHES

Trigger points are a frequent cause of the muscle component of any type of headache. These are usually found in the sternocleidomastoid, levator scapulae, and trapezius muscles and, not infrequently, in the scalp and facial muscles. In addition, the posterior strap muscles are often involved, particularly the semispinalis and splenius muscles (Fig. 47–8). When preparing to treat a patient with headache, one should carefully examine the entire back for hypersensitive areas, paying special attention to the paraspinal muscle

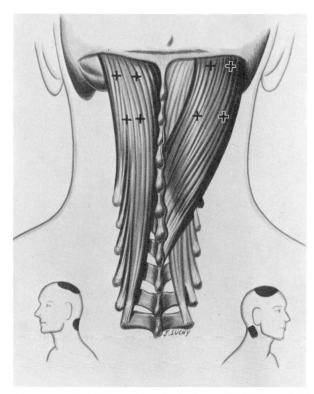

Figure 47–8. Splenius and semispinalis capitis. Pain resulting from involvement of these muscles may be located over the muscles themselves. Both the splenius and the semispinalis can mediate pain to the head and the face, and both are commonly involved in headache. Occasionally, dizziness will accompany involvement of these muscles. Because trigger points are difficult to pinpoint in these muscles, patient cooperation in pointing out positions of maximal tenderness is extremely helpful. (From Sola, A. E.: Myofascial trigger point therapy. Resident and Staff Physician 27(8):44, 1981. Used by permission.)

group. As previously discussed, trigger points located in the quadratus lumborum and the gluteus medius may contribute to headache problems. These muscles seem to have particular significance if the headache is unilateral.

BACK PAIN

Unilateral back pain is usually responsive to trigger point injection. The trigger points are most commonly found in the quadratus lumborum, gluteus medius, and tensor fasciae latae muscles. Hip pain caused by gluteal trigger points may mimic trochanteric bursitis, and by far the most frequently diagnosed syndrome, sciatica, is often caused by gluteal trigger points (Fig. 47–9).

The lumbosacral muscles are commonly involved in lower back pain. Here the trigger points are frequently secondary to vertebral or nerve root irritation, and treatment may be of only temporary benefit. Affected patients, if no better after treatment, should be referred for further evaluation and treatment.

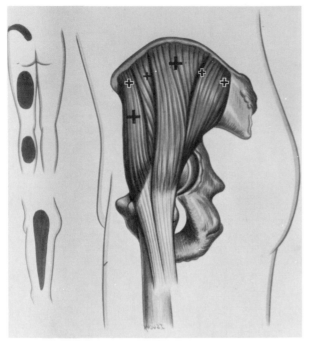

Figure 47–9. Trigger points about the hip. These muscles are easy to examine, and it is easy to locate the common trigger points that are present in the muscle bellies. Pain is usually referred to the lateral aspect of the thigh as far as the knee. (From Sola, A. E.: Myofascial trigger point therapy. Resident and Staff Physician 27(8):44, 1981. Used by permission.)

TORTICOLLIS

Torticollis usually is a simple problem involving one to three muscles. The trapezius, sternocleidomastoid, and levator scapulae are the main offenders. A careful search of the posterior strap muscles, however, may reveal exquisite tenderness of the splenius and the semispinalis muscles. If the trapezius is involved, particular care must be taken with the injection technique (Fig. 47–10).

The apical pleura in some individuals is much higher than normal. If there is a sudden upward flinch of the shoulder during injection, the pleura could be punctured. If possible, one should inject transversely with the trigger point located between index finger and thumb.

Some of the muscles that are commonly involved in pain problems are listed in the following paragraphs. Although the pain reference sites are fairly consistent, they may differ because of involvement of more than one muscle.

Levator Scapulae. Painful sensitive foci may occur at the origin on the superior medial aspect of the scapula, along the entire flat muscle belly, or on the insertions on the transverse processes of the first four cervical vertebrae (Fig. 47–11). Invariably, the levator scapulae muscle is involved in chronic cervical conditions as well as in torticollis. The pain is usually referred to the posterior cervical region, the posterior scalp, and the area around the ear.

Infraspinatus. This muscle, a prominent member of the rotator cuff, is usually involved in many types of shoulder lesions (Fig. 47–12). Careful palpation is necessary to locate trigger areas. It is useful to search the entire muscle along the length of the muscle bundles as well as across the "grain" of the muscle. Related pain is usually located on the posterior and lateral aspect of the shoulder and, occasionally, may return to the anterior chest. All of the scapular muscles are frequently involved either singly or in concert with each other.

Quadratus Lumborum. Travell has referred to this muscle as "the joker" in the lower back syndrome, and it deserves this title.[22] It is a hip hiker and a lateral flexor of the spine, and in addition it assists respiratory function by anchoring the twelfth rib for the pull of the diaphragm. It frequently signals its distress on deep inspiration with twelfth-rib pain. Pain can be local or it can

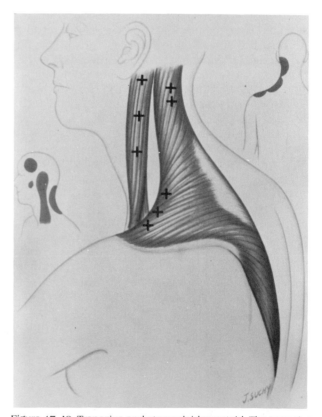

Figure 47–10. Trapezius and sternocleidomastoid. The trapezius is a frequent source of muscle pain and headache, especially at the angle of the neck or at the occipital insertions of the muscle, where trigger points are most commonly located. When injecting trigger points at the angle of the neck, one must take care to avoid the apical pleura. The sternocleidomastoid muscle also is often the source of neck pain and headache. In addition, dizziness and ipsilateral ptosis, lacrimation, and reddening of the conjunctiva have been reported in association with involvement of this muscle. Trigger points are most commonly located at the occiput insertion in the upper two thirds of the muscle and frequently on its sternal and clavicular origins. The pain pattern may involve the muscle or may be referred to the ear region, the face, and the frontal area. (From Sola, A. E.: Myofascial trigger point therapy. Resident and Staff Physician 27(8):45, 1981. Used by permission.)

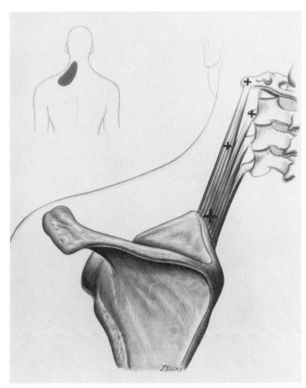

Figure 47–11. Levator scapulae. Painful sensitive foci may occur at the origin of the superior medial aspect of the scapula, along the entire flat muscle belly, or on the insertions on the transverse processes of the first four cervical vertebrae. Invariably, the levator scapulae is involved in chronic cervical conditions as well as in torticollis. The pain is usually referred to the posterior cervical region, the posterior scalp, and the area around the ear. (From Sola, A. E.: Myofascial trigger point therapy. Resident and Staff Physician 27(8):43, 1981. Used by permission.)

and maximus muscles from the sacroiliac joint to the anterior superior spine) may contain painful trigger points. It is estimated that 10 per cent of the population have legs that differ in length by at least 1 cm. This can cause unilateral back pain and trigger points of the gluteus, erector spinae, and quadratus lumborum muscles.

Tensor Fasciae Latae. This muscle is easy to examine, and it is also easy to locate the common trigger points that are present in the muscle belly. Pain is usually referred to the lateral aspects of the thigh as far as the knee (see Fig. 47–9).

Anterior Tibialis. Pain in the anterior ankle is usually experienced when the trigger points of this muscle flare up, although in severe cases the entire muscle may be painful. Trigger points are most commonly found in the upper one third of the muscle, and pain is referred to the anterior portion of the leg and into the dorsal portion of the ankle (Fig. 47–14).

Gastrocnemius/Soleus. Myofascial pain related to this muscle group is felt behind the knee, over the muscle bellies, and along the achilles tendon near the heel. Trigger points are usually found on the medial and lateral margins of the muscle group

be referred to the anterior abdominal wall. This may accentuate postoperative pain or painful abdominal scars over the lower quadrant. Trigger points occur on the twelfth rib, on the iliac crest, and along the lateral border of the entire muscle (Fig. 47–13).

Gluteus Medius. The trigger points in the gluteus medius may well be the most critical in the lower extremity. Activity of these trigger points often involves activation of trigger points in the quadratus lumborum, the tensor fasciae latae, and the other gluteal muscles, thus inducing widespread lower back discomfort (see Figs. 47–9 and 47–15). There is also an interaction between the trigger points of the gluteus medius and those in the cervical area, sometimes involving this remote muscle in cervical pain and headache. Although this muscle seldom causes pain without involving other muscles, the pain pattern most often attributed to the gluteus medius is along the iliac crest and into the posterior thigh and calf. It is a frequent cause of hip pain in the later stages of pregnancy and simulates sciatica. The trigger points most commonly are found along the iliac shelf and, with extensive involvement, the entire gluteal ridge (including also the gluteus minimus

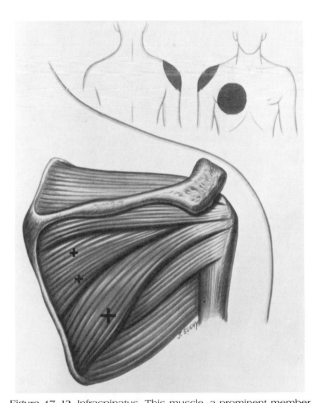

Figure 47–12. Infraspinatus. This muscle, a prominent member of the rotator cuff, is usually involved in many types of shoulder lesions. Careful palpation is necessary to locate trigger areas. It is useful to search the entire muscle along the length of the muscle bundles as well as across the "grain" of the muscle. Related pain is usually located on the posterior and lateral aspects of the shoulder and, occasionally, may return to the anterior chest. All of the scapular muscles are frequently involved, either singly or in concert with each other. (From Sola, A. E.: Myofascial trigger point therapy. Resident and Staff Physician 27(8):43, 1981. Used by permission.)

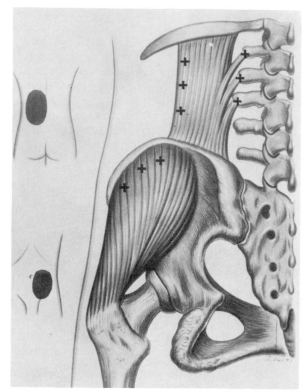

Figure 47–13. Quadratus lumborum and gluteus medius. The quadratus lumborum has been referred to as the "joker" in the lower back syndrome, and it deserves this title. It is a hip hiker and a lateral flexor of the spine. In addition, it assists respiratory function by anchoring the twelfth rib for the pull of the diaphragm and frequently signals its distress on deep inspiration with twelfth-rib pain. Pain can be local or can be referred to the anterior abdominal wall. This may accentuate postoperative pain or painful abdominal scars over the lower quadrant. Trigger points occur on the twelfth rib and the iliac crest and along the lateral border of the entire muscle. The trigger points in the gluteus medius may well be the most critical in the lower extremity. Activity of these trigger points often involves activation of trigger points in the quadratus lumborum, the tensor fasciae latae, and the other gluteal muscles, thus inducing widespread lower back discomfort. There is also an interaction between the trigger points of the gluteus and those in the cervical area, sometimes involving the remote muscle in cervical pain and headache. Although this muscle seldom causes pain without involving other muscles, the pain pattern most often attributed to the gluteus medius is along the iliac crest and into the posterior thigh and calf. It is a frequent cause of hip pain in the later stages of pregnancy and simulates sciatica. The trigger points most commonly are found along the iliac shelf, and with extensive involvement the entire gluteal ridge, including the gluteal minimus and maximus muscles from the sacroiliac joint to the anterior superior spine, may contain painful trigger points. (From Sola, A. E.: Myofascial trigger point therapy. Resident and Staff Physician 27(8):43, 1981. Used by permission.)

and along the midline of the group. These trigger points often flare up when a patient is experiencing vascular problems of the lower extremities. One report has suggested injecting these trigger points for the relief of pain associated with intermittent claudication.[23] The pain is referred to the achilles tendon and the heel (Fig. 47–15).

Splenius Capitis/Semispinalis Capitis. Pain resulting from involvement of these muscles may be located over the muscles themselves. Both the splenius and the semispinalis can mediate pain to the head and the face, however, and both are commonly involved in headache. Occasionally, dizziness will accompany involvement of these muscles. Because trigger points are difficult to pinpoint in these muscles, patient cooperation in pointing out positions of maximal tenderness is extremely helpful (see Fig. 47–8).

Rectus Abdominis. These muscles are frequent sites of anterior abdominal wall pain. The trigger points are best located with the patient in the supine position and with his head and neck flexed so his abdominal rectus muscles are under tension. These trigger points frequently flare up after abdominal surgery and can be one of the chief constituents of postoperative pain. The trigger points are most commonly found in the upper three segments of abdominal rectus muscle, and the pain is usually localized over the muscle (Fig. 47–16).

Pectoralis Major/Pectoralis Minor. The pectoralis major muscles are a frequent site of myofascial pain in the area of the muscle insertion on the

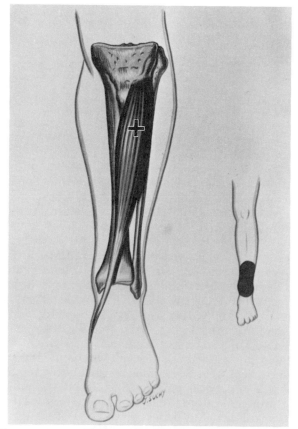

Figure 47–14. Anterior tibialis. Pain in the anterior ankle is usually experienced when the trigger points of this muscle flare up, although in severe cases the entire muscle may be painful. Trigger points are most commonly found in the upper one third of the muscle, and pain is referred to the anterior portion of the leg and into the dorsal portion of the ankle. (From Sola, A. E.: Myofascial trigger point therapy. Resident and Staff Physician 27(8):44, 1981. Used by permission.)

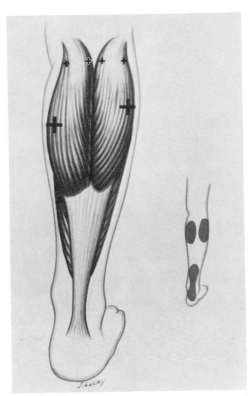

Figure 47–15. Gastrocnemius/soleus. Myofascial pain related to this muscle is felt behind the knee, over the muscle bellies, and along the Achilles tendon near the heel. Trigger points are usually found on the medial and lateral margins of the muscle group and along the midline of the group. These trigger points often flare up when a patient is experiencing vascular problems of the lower extremities. A recent report suggests injecting these trigger points for the relief of pain associated with intermittent claudication.[23] (From Sola, A. E.: Myofascial trigger point therapy. Resident and Staff Physician 27(8):44, 1981. Used by permission.)

anterior medial shoulder. The inferior belly of the muscle is a common area of trigger points; however, the entire muscle must be searched diligently. The clavicular portion of this muscle usually refers pain to the uppermost part of the muscle. On occasion, there is some referral into the arm (Figs. 47–16 and 47–17).

Intercostals. One should examine the intercostals for chest pain routinely by palpating the intercostal spaces with the fingers. The intercostals are frequently involved after any chest surgery or trauma. In treating chest pain when intercostal blocks are not successful, one must take care on injection to avoid entry into the pleural space. Pain from the exterior intercostal muscle is usually localized near the site of the trigger point and is emphasized during inspiration (see Fig. 47–17).

Trapezius. The trapezius is a frequent source of muscle pain and headache, especially at the angle of the neck or at the occipital insertions of the muscle, where trigger points are most commonly located. When injecting trigger points at the angle of the neck, one must take care to avoid the apical pleura (see Fig. 47–10).

Sternocleidomastoid. This muscle is often the source of neck pain and headache. In addition, dizziness and ipsilateral ptosis, lacrimation, and reddening of the conjunctiva have been reported in association with the involvement of these muscles.[24] Trigger points are most commonly located at occiput insertion in the upper two thirds of the muscle and frequently on its sternal and clavicular origins. The pain pattern may involve the muscle or may refer to the ear region, the face, and the frontal area (see Fig. 47–10).

Conclusion

In summary, trigger points may be involved in any painful event. They may play either a primary role (translating stress to pain) or a secondary role

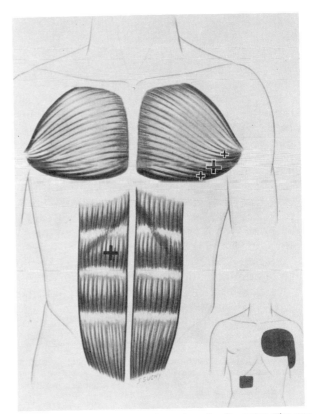

Figure 47–16. Rectus abdominis and pectoralis major. The rectus abdominis muscles are frequent sites of anterior abdominal pain. The trigger points are best located with the patient in the supine position with the head and the neck flexed so the abdominal rectus muscles are under tension. These trigger points are frequently flared up after abdominal surgery and can be one of the chief constituents of postoperative pain. They are commonly found in all segments of the abdominal rectus muscle, and the pain is usually localized over the involved site of the muscle. The pectoral major muscles are a frequent site of myofascial pain in the area of the muscle insertion on the anterior medial shoulder. The inferior belly of the muscle is a common area of trigger points; however, the entire muscle must be searched diligently. The clavicular portion of this muscle usually refers pain to the uppermost part of the muscle. On occasion, there is some referral into the arm. (From Sola, A. E.: Myofascial trigger point therapy. Resident and Staff Physician 27(8):45, 1981. Used by permission.)

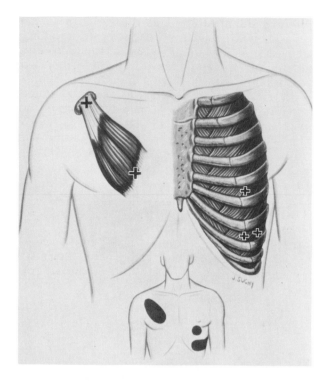

Figure 47–17. Pectoralis minor and intercostal muscles. In the pectoralis minor, pain is usually deep and sharply circumscribed over the outline of the muscle when involved. Trigger points are most commonly found near the origin and insertion of the muscle. One should examine the intercostals for chest pain routinely by palpating the intercostal spaces with the fingers. The intercostals are frequently involved after any chest surgery or trauma. In treating chest pain when intercostal blocks are not successful, one must take care on injection to avoid entry into the pleural space. Pain from the exterior intercostal muscle is usually localized near the site of the trigger point and is emphasized during inspiration. (From Sola, A. E.: Myofascial trigger point therapy. Resident and Staff Physician 27(8):45, 1981. Used by permission.)

(supporting and intensifying a painful stimulus). They can complicate any type of pain and may mimic underlying visceral disorders. Obviously, interventions that directly affect the trigger point will have a much greater chance for complete pain control if the trigger point is acting in the primary role of translator than if it is acting in the secondary role of pain intensifier. Even in the secondary role, however, there is the potential for benefit from properly administered treatment. Treatment considerations in addition to trigger point injection include administration of muscle relaxants, anesthetics, and analgesics; referral for physical therapy; reduction of stress; and prescription of therapeutic exercise following resolution of the event.

1. Bonica, J. J.: Management of myofascial pain syndromes in general practice. JAMA 164:732, 1957.
2. Cooper, A. L.: Trigger point injection: Its place in physical medicine. Arch. Phys. Med. 43:704, 1961.
3. Simons, D. G.: Muscle pain syndromes: Part I. Am. J. Phys. Med. 54:289, 1975.
4. Simons, D. G.: Muscle pain syndromes: Part II. Am. J. Phys. Med. 55:15, 1976.
5. Sola, A. E., Kuitert, J. H.: Quadratus lumborum myofascitis. Northwest Med. 53:1003, 1954.
6. Sola, A. E., and Kuitert, J. H.: Myofascial trigger point in the neck and shoulder girdle. Northwest Med. 54:980, 1955.
7. Travell, J.: Myofascial pain syndrome masquerading as temporomandibular joint pain. Oral Surg. 43:11, 1977.
8. Travell, J.: Myofascial Trigger Points in Advances in Pain Research and Therapy. New York, Raven Press, 1976.
9. Travell, J., and Rinzler, S. H.: The myofascial genesis of pain. Postgrad. Med. 11:425, 1952.
10. Melzack, R., Stillwell, D. M., and Fox, E. J.: Trigger points and acupuncture points for pain: Correlations and implications. Pain 3:2, 1977.
11. Lawrence, R. M.: New approach to the treatment of chronic pain: Combination therapy. Am. J. Acupuncture 6:59, 1978.
12. Gunn, C. C.: Prespondylosis and some pain syndromes following denervation supersensitivity. Spine 5:185, 1980.
13. Gower, W. R.: Lumbago: Its lesions and analogues. Br. Med. J. 1:117, 1904.
14. Llewellyn, L. J., and Jones, A. B.: Fibrositis. London, Heinemann, 1915.
15. Kraus, H.: Behandlung akuter Muskelharten. Wien. Klin. Wochenschr. 50:1356, 1937.
16. Sola, A. E.: Myofascial trigger point therapy. Resident and Staff Physician 27:38 August, 1981.
17. Edagawa, N., and Friedmann, L. W.: The Treatment of Disordered Function. Smithtown, NY, Exposition Press, 1981.
18. Sola, A. E., and Williams, R. L.: Myofascial pain syndromes. Neurology 6:91, 1956.
19. Frost, F. A., Jeason, B., and Siggaard-Anderson, J.: A controlled, double-blind comparison of mepivacaine injection versus saline injection for myofascial pain. Lancet 1:499, 1980.
20. Tfelt-Hansen, P., et al.: Lignocaine versus saline in migraine pain. Lancet 1:1140, 1980.
21. Bray, E. A., and Sigmond, H.: The local and regional injection treatment of low back pain and sciatica. Ann. Intern. Med. 15:840, 1941.
22. Travell, J.: Personal correspondence, 1955.
23. Dorigo, B., Swintak, E. F., Schriver, W. R., et al.: Fibrositic myofascial pain in intermittent claudication effect of anesthetic block of trigger points on exercise tolerance. Pain 6:183, 1979.
24. Travell, J.: Referred pain from skeletal muscle. N. Y. State J. Med. 55:331, 1955.

Recommended Reading

Travell, J. G., and Simons, D. G.: Myofascial Pain and Dysfunction: The Trigger Point Manual. Baltimore, Williams & Wilkins, 1983.
Sola, A. E.: Upper extremity pain. In Wall, P. D. and Melzack, R. (eds.): Textbook of Pain. Edinburgh, Churchill Livingstone (in press).

48

Arthrocentesis

MARC KOBERNICK, M.D.

Introduction

Arthrocentesis, the puncture and aspiration of a joint, is an acknowledged, useful procedure that is easily performed in the emergency department. It has been established as both a diagnostic and a therapeutic tool for a variety of clinical situations. Many physicians are wary of joint fluid aspiration because of a lack of experience and because of the fear of introducing infection. When performed properly, however, the procedure offers a wealth of clinical information and is associated with very few complications. In the emergency department it is almost impossible to make an accurate assessment of an acutely painful and swollen joint without performing arthrocentesis.

Indications

The indications for arthrocentesis include:[1]
1. Diagnosis of nontraumatic joint disease by synovial fluid analysis (septic joint or crystal-induced arthritis).
2. Diagnosis of ligamentous or bony injury by confirmation of the presence of blood in the joint. Arthrocentesis may be required to differentiate a traumatic joint effusion from an inflammatory process.
3. Establishment of the existence of an intra-articular fracture by the presence of blood with fat globules in the joint.
4. Relief of the pain of an acute hemarthrosis or a tense effusion. Although a minor hemarthrosis need not be drained, arthrocentesis not only will reduce pain in large effusions but also will facilitate examination of an injured joint.
5. Local instillation of medications in acute and chronic inflammatory arthritides. The instillation of lidocaine into an injured joint will also make the initial examination of a traumatic injury much easier.
6. Obtaining of fluid for culture, Gram stain, and cell count in cases of suspected joint infection.

Contraindications

The most important contraindication to arthrocentesis is the presence of infection in the tissue overlying the site to be punctured, e.g., an abscess or a frank cellulitis. Inflammation with warmth, swelling, and tenderness may overlie an acutely arthritic joint, and this may mimic a soft tissue infection. Once convinced that a cellulitis does not exist, one should not hesitate to obtain the necessary diagnostic joint fluid. A relative contraindication to joint puncture is the presence of a bacteremia. Not all joint infections following arthrocentesis are the result of poor antiseptic technique, since the hematogenous spread of bacteria into the joint, with or without hemorrhage, in a bacteremic patient may also lead to infection.

Bleeding diatheses may at times be a relative contraindication, but arthrocentesis to relieve a tense hemarthrosis in bleeding disorders, such as hemophilia, is an accepted practice following infusion of the appropriate clotting factors. Arthrocentesis is also relatively contraindicated in a patient receiving anticoagulants or in the presence of a joint prosthesis, unless the procedure is being performed to rule out infection.

Articular Versus Periarticular Disease

Periarticular disease, such as tendonitis, bursitis, contusion, cellulitis, or phlebitis, may mimic articular disease and suggest the need for arthrocentesis. Therefore, it is desirable to differentiate the pain and inflammation that arise from periarticular structures from those secondary to joint disease.

If swelling is secondary to joint effusion or inflammation, the entire articular capsule is inflamed and distended and one can often palpate fluid within the joint. In articular disease there is tenderness on all sides of the joint. Movement of the joint in all directions is limited, and both active and passive motion produce pain. The pain arising from a pathologic condition involving a joint may be diffuse or clearly localized to the joint or it may radiate. Hip pain, for example, frequently radiates into the groin or down the front of the thigh into the knee. Shoulder joint pain will also commonly radiate into the elbow or the neck.

In contrast, pain from a periarticular process is often more localized, and tenderness can be elicited only with certain specific movements or at specific points around the joint. In periarticular inflammation one can often passively lead a joint through a range of motion with minimal discomfort, yet pain is significant when the patient attempts active motion. Crepitus may be elicited in tendonitis or the pain may be traced along the course of a specific tendon.

Septic Arthritis

Acute monoarticular arthritis is a common problem in emergency medicine. Although there are many causes of acute monoarticular arthritis, the one most requiring urgent diagnosis and treatment is septic arthritis. Infectious arthritis is still relatively frequent, and suspicion of a septic process in the joint is the first step in appropriate management; confirmation requires arthrocentesis and synovial fluid culture. Although repeated arthrocentesis may be needed when treating a septic joint, such therapy is only performed on an inpatient basis.

Gonococcus, staphylococcus, and streptococcus are the most frequently identified etiologic agents.[2] Gonococcus is the most common organism causing septic arthritis among adolescents and young adults.[3, 4] Patients over 40 and those with other medical illnesses are more likely to have staphylococcus joint infection, whereas infants aged 6 months to 2 years show a higher incidence of *Hemophilus influenzae*. In neonates, staphylococci and *Escherichia coli* predominate.[5] Intravenous drug abusers may develop staphylococcal or *Pseudomonas* infections.

Although precise incidences for nongonococcal septic arthritis have not been established, predisposing factors have been described. These include chronic debilitating disease; prior antibiotic or immunosuppressive medications; a previous history of joint damage, such as from rheumatoid arthritis or degenerative joint disease; and prosthetic joints.[6, 7] In a study by Sharp and coworkers, 19 per cent (22 of 113) of patients with septic arthritis had other arthritides, the most common being rheumatoid arthritis.[2] Elderly patients with a debilitating arthritis and minor skin infections seem to be the most susceptible; the infection may be overlooked and the patient's findings thought to be an exacerbation of the rheumatoid arthritis.[8]

The simultaneous occurrence of gout and septic arthritis may be more common than generally recognized. One should not allow the establishment of a diagnosis of crystal-induced disease to shut off a thorough search for infection.[9]

Because gonococcus is the most common organism causing septic arthritis, gonococcal arthritis deserves special mention. The incidence in men is increasing, but the majority of disseminated gonococcal infections occur in women with asymptomatic anogenital infections. Dissemination usually occurs during menstruation or pregnancy.[3, 10]

A useful context in which to view gonococcal arthritis was presented by Gelfand and coworkers.[11] Three *sequential* stages with associated clinical subgroups have been described, although in practice fewer than 50 per cent of patients will fit classically into one of the three stages. Patients in the first group (hematogenous phase) have constitutional symptoms (high fever and chills), polyarthralgias-polyarthritis (but with very little effusion), tenosynovitis, and dermatitis. They then enter a second transitional phase with skin lesions, positive blood cultures and, occasionally, positive joint fluid cultures in a developing arthritis with effusion. Those in the third stage (joint localization phase) do not have systemic symptoms or skin lesions. The infection settles into one or two large joints, yielding a purulent arthritis.[11]

Whereas gonococcus-infected joint fluid is usually "septic" in character, the yield of positive synovial fluid cultures has ranged from 25 to 60 per cent.[12] It is rare to find simultaneously positive joint fluid cultures and blood cultures.[3] A positive Gram stain is immediately diagnostic of septic arthritis. A Gram stain will be positive in approximately 65 per cent of cases of septic arthritis. Certainly a negative Gram stain does not rule out an infectious process. A white blood cell count and a synovial fluid glucose evaluation may give confirmatory data.

Equipment

Necessary materials for arthrocentesis include skin preparation solution (usually povidone-iodine followed by alcohol); sterile gloves and a drape; 1 per cent lidocaine and a 3- to 5-ml syringe with a 25 gauge needle; various syringes for aspiration with 18 to 22 gauge, 1½-inch needles or intravenous catheter and needle set; a three-way stopcock; and sterile specimen tubes. Fluid for cell count should be collected in a tube with anticoagulant; however, glucose and viscosity determinations do not require anticoagulants. One should immediately examine fresh synovial fluid in its unadulterated form for crystals. Calcium oxalate and lithium heparin anticoagulants have been reported to introduce artifactual crystals into the fluid. If one is culturing for *Neisseria gonorrhoeae*, the fluid should be immediately placed on proper medium and stored in a low oxygen environment in the emergency department.

General Arthrocentesis Technique

Joint fluid may be obtained even when there is little clinical evidence of an effusion. Although one may successfully aspirate where the joint bulges maximally, certain landmarks are important. The most crucial part of arthrocentesis is spending adequate time in defining the joint anatomy by palpating the bony landmarks as a guide.

These are described in detail later in this chapter. A puncture site and an approach to the joint should be selected; tendons, major vessels, and major nerve branches should be avoided. In most instances, the approach will be via the extensor surfaces of joints, since most major vessels and nerves are found in flexor surfaces. Also, the synovial pouch is usually more superficial on the extensor side of a joint.

The overlying skin is cleansed and sterilized. A double preparation of povidone-iodine and alcohol is suggested. Using sterile gloves, the clinician raises a skin wheal with anesthetic. A new bottle of local anesthetic is recommended to avoid the risk of introducing a contaminated anesthetic into the joint space. Deeper injection of anesthetic along the expected track of the aspirating needle then follows. With appropriate local anesthesia, arthrocentesis should be a relatively painless procedure; without anesthesia it may be quite painful and distressing to the patient. The synovial membrane itself has some pain fibers associated with blood vessels, and the articular capsule and bone periosteum are richly supplied with nerve fibers and are very sensitive. The articular cartilage has no intrinsic pain fibers. It is important to have the patient relax during the procedure. Tense muscles will narrow joint spaces and will make the procedure more difficult, requiring repeated attempts at aspiration, or will result in inadequate drainage. Distraction of the joint may enhance the target area, especially in areas such as the wrist and the finger joints. Traction not only will increase the chance of entering the joint but also will lessen the chance of scoring the articular cartilage with the needle.

An 18 to 22 gauge needle or intravenous catheter and needle set of appropriate length attached to a syringe is inserted at the desired anatomic point through the skin and subcutaneous tissue into the joint space. The largest needle that is practical is used to avoid obstructing the lumen with debris or clot. In large joints such as the knee, which can accommodate large effusions, it is suggested that one use a 30- to 55-ml syringe, since it may be difficult to change a syringe when the needle is within the joint cavity. A three-way stopcock placed between the needle and syringe is an option for draining large effusions. If the syringe must be changed during the procedure, the hub of the needle should be grasped with a hemostat and held tightly while the syringe is removed. If the intravenous catheter and needle set is used, the needle is removed leaving the outer atraumatic plastic catheter in the joint space. The syringe is now attached to the catheter for aspiration. Now manipulation of the joint or catheter can occur with little threat of injury.

Aspiration of synovial fluid and the easy injection and return of fluid indicate intra-articular placement of the needle tip. As a general rule, *one should completely remove all fluid or blood.* If the fluid stops flowing, this is a sign that the joint has been drained completely, the needle tip has become dislodged, or debris or clot is obstructing the needle. One should slightly advance or retract the tip of the needle, rotate the bevel, or ease up on the force of aspiration. Occasionally, reinjecting a small amount of fluid back into the joint space will confirm the needle placement and may clear the needle. If fluid flows freely back into the joint and is easily reaspirated, one has probably removed all the fluid. If resistance is met, the needle has probably been jarred from the joint space and is lodged in the soft tissue. In some instances minor changes in the flexion or extension of the joint may allow the fluid to flow more freely. Scraping or shearing the articular cartilage with the needle should be avoided, since this may produce permanent cartilage damage. One should enter the joint in a straight line and avoid unnecessary side-to-side motion of the syringe. After aspiration, the needle is removed and a sterile dressing is applied over the puncture site.

Synovial fluid should be sent for studies as indicated by the clinical situation. Studies usually obtained include cell count with differential, crystal analysis, Gram stain, bacterial culture and sensitivity analysis, and synovial fluid sugar measurement. Less frequently obtained studies include synovial fluid protein measurement, rheumatoid factor analysis, lupus erythematosus (LE) cell preparation, viscosity analysis, mucin clot, fibrin clot, fungal and acid-fast stains, fungal and tuberculous culture, and synovial fluid complement analysis. If the arthrocentesis is performed for the relief of a hemarthrosis, the fluid need not be sent for analysis. One should be selective in ordering tests. There is no need to order a large battery of tests routinely on all fluids.

Complications

Significant complications are rare with arthrocentesis. They include:

1. *Infection.* Skin bacteria may be introduced into the joint space during needle puncture. One can, of course, prevent this complication by maintaining rigorous sterile technique and avoiding inserting the needle through obviously infected skin or subcutaneous tissue. The chance of introducing infection with arthrocentesis through a noninfected area is minimal if proper attention is paid to technique. Various studies report the incidence of infection following routine arthrocentesis to be in the range of 1 per 10,000 aspirations.[13] Joint aspiration in the presence of a bacteremia has been discussed previously.

2. *Bleeding.* Bleeding with subsequent hemar-

throsis is rarely a complication, except in the patient with a bleeding diathesis. If a patient has a bleeding diathesis, such as hemophilia, arthrocentesis should be delayed until clotting competence has been enhanced by the infusion of specific clotting factors.

3. *Allergic reaction.* Hypersensitivity to the local anesthetic that is used can usually be prevented by thorough history taking. Fainting during the procedure is not uncommon and is the result of vasovagal influences.

4. *Corticosteroid-induced complications.* (see section on intra-articular corticosteroid injections.)

HEMARTHROSIS

Isolated nontraumatic hemarthrosis may occasionally be seen by the emergency physician. An inflammatory reaction may follow an intracapsular bleed, and the proliferative reaction and hyperplastic synovium formed may predispose to recurrent hemorrhage in that joint, especially in patients with bleeding diatheses. The knee is the most commonly affected joint (whether the cause is hemophilia or oral anticoagulants), followed by the foot and the ankle.[4]

The most common cause of intra-articular hemorrhage in the setting of no trauma or minor trauma is a hereditary clotting factor deficiency, as in hemophilia. Hemarthrosis is an infrequent complication of oral anticoagulant therapy and may occur even with prothrombin times within the normal range.[14] Chronic arthritis does not appear to be a long-term complication in patients with intra-articular bleeds from oral anti-coagulant therapy. Hemarthrosis may also be a complication of sickle cell anemia, pseudogout, amyloidosis, pigmented villonodular synovitis, synovial hemangioma, rheumatoid arthritis, and infection.[4]

Management of acute hemarthrosis depends on the cause. Studies by Jaffer and Schmid and Wild and Zvaifler showed that the synovitis associated with oral anticoagulant therapy will improve only after the oral anticoagulant is discontinued and the prothrombin time returns to normal.[14, 15]

Hemarthrosis following trauma is a frequent occurrence. It is most common in the knee and often denotes significant internal damage. In an otherwise healthy joint that is subjected to a single traumatic event, even a relatively large hemarthrosis will be spontaneously resorbed without significant sequelae. Therefore, there is no pressing need to drain all cases of hemarthrosis. A large, tense traumatic effusion is quite painful, however, and its presence precludes proper evaluation of an injured joint. Therapeutic arthrocentesis to drain a symptomatic traumatic effusion is a well-accepted practice. The source of blood following trauma is a tear in a ligamentous structure,

knee capsule, or synovium or a fracture. Cruciate (especially anterior) ligament injury is the most common cause of significant hemarthrosis following trauma to the knee. Cartilage is avascular, and an isolated meniscal injury (rare) will not produce a hemarthrosis. A joint effusion that develops 1 to 5 days following trauma may be secondary to a slow hemorrhage or a reinjury, but the swelling is often caused by a nonhemorrhagic irritative synovial effusion.

Occasionally, one will diagnose an occult fracture or a fat pad injury by the presence of fat globules in the arthrocentesis blood. If a history of trauma is vague, arthrocentesis may be required to differentiate hemorrhage from other causes of joint effusion. Following therapeutic arthrocentesis for a hemarthrosis, it may be desirable to inject 10 to 15 ml of a local anesthetic into the joint to facilitate examination or to provide temporary symptomatic relief.

Intra-articular Corticosteroid Injections

Hollander and coworkers in 1951 first demonstrated that intra-articular corticosteroid injections were useful for symptomatic relief in patients with severe rheumatoid arthritis.[16] The use of steroids has proved to be a dependable method for providing rapid relief from pain and swelling of inflamed joints, although it is strictly local, usually temporary, and rarely curative.[17]

The most serious complication is intra-articular infection. Conversely, steroids should never be injected into a joint if there is any suspicion of a joint space infection. Repeated injections into one joint carry the risk of necrosis of juxta-articular bone with subsequent joint destruction and instability. Other complications include local soft tissue atrophy and calcification, tendon rupture, intra-articular bleeding, and transient nerve palsy.[18] Deposition of steroid crystals on the synovium may give rise to a transient, self-limited flare-up of a synovitis.[19]

It is always important to ascertain if local corticosteroid therapy has been used previously, not only to consider the array of clinical conditions associated with steroid use but also because crystalline corticosteroid material can hinder proper interpretation of crystals found in synovial fluid.[19]

Specific Arthrocentesis Techniques

FIRST CARPOMETACARPAL JOINT (Fig. 48–1)

Landmarks: The radial aspect of the proximal end of the first metacarpal is the arthrocentesis land-

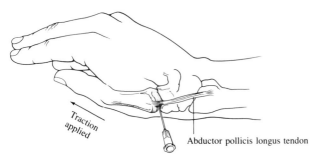

Figure 48–1. Landmarks for arthrocentesis of first carpometacarpal joint (see text). (From Akins, C. M.: Aspiration and injection of joints, bursae, and tendons. *In* Vander Salm, T. J., et al.: Atlas of Bedside Procedures. Boston, Little, Brown & Co., 1979. Used by permission.)

mark for this joint. The abductor pollicis longus tendon is located by active extension of the tendon.

Position: The thumb is opposed against the little finger so that the proximal end of the first metacarpal is palpable. Traction is applied to the thumb in order to widen the joint space between the first metacarpal and the greater multangular.

Needle insertion: A 22 gauge needle is inserted at a point proximal to the prominence at the base of the first metacarpal, on the palmar side of the abductor pollicis longus tendon.

Comments: Degenerative arthritis commonly affects this joint. Arthrocentesis is of moderate difficulty. The anatomic "snuff box" (located more proximally and on the dorsal side of the abductor pollicis longus tendon) should be avoided, since it contains the radial artery and superficial radial nerve. A more dorsal approach may also be used.

INTERPHALANGEAL AND METACARPOPHALANGEAL JOINTS
(Fig. 48–2)

Landmarks: The landmarks are on the dorsal surface—the prominence at the proximal end of the proximal phalanx for metacarpophalangeal joints and the prominence at the proximal end of the middle or distal phalanx for interphalangeal joints. The extensor tendon runs down the midline.

Position: The fingers are flexed to approximately 15 to 20 degrees and *traction is applied.*

Needle insertion: A 22 gauge needle is inserted into the joint space dorsally, just medial or lateral to the central slip of the extensor tendon.

Comments: Synovitis will cause these joints to bulge dorsally. Normally, it is unusual to obtain fluid in the absence of a significant pathologic condition.

RADIOCARPAL JOINT (WRIST) (Fig. 48–3)

Landmarks: The dorsal radial tubercle (Lister's tubercle) is an elevation found in the center of the dorsal aspect of the distal end of the radius. The extensor pollicis longus tendon runs in a groove on the radial side of the tubercle. The tendon can be palpated by active extension of the wrist and thumb.

Position: The wrist should be positioned in approximately 20 to 30 degrees of flexion. *Traction is applied to the hand.*

Needle insertion: The needle is inserted dorsally, just distal to the dorsal tubercle and on the ulnar side of the extensor pollicis longus tendon. The anatomic "snuff box" located more radially should be avoided.

RADIOHUMERAL JOINT (ELBOW)
(Fig. 48–4)

Landmarks: The lateral epicondyle of the humerus and the head of the radius are the arthrocentesis landmarks for the radiohumeral joint. With the elbow extended, the depression between the

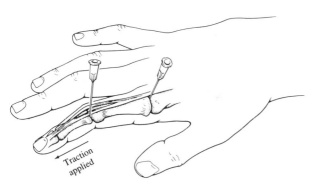

Figure 48–2. Landmarks for arthrocentesis of interphalangeal and metacarpophalangeal joints (see text). (From Akins, C. M.: Aspiration and injection of joints, bursae, and tendons. *In* Vander Salm, T. J., et al.: Atlas of Bedside Procedures. Boston, Little, Brown & Co., 1979. Used by permission.)

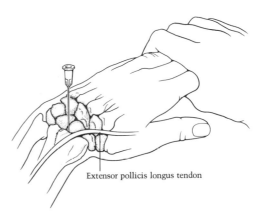

Figure 48–3. Landmarks for arthrocentesis of the radiocarpal joint (see text). (From Akins, C. M.: Aspiration and injection of joints, bursae, and tendons. *In* Vander Salm, T. J., et al.: Atlas of Bedside Procedures. Boston, Little, Brown & Co., 1979. Used by permission.)

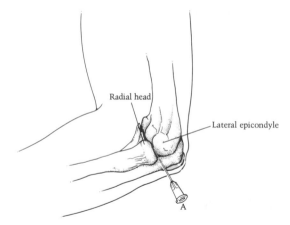

Figure 48–4. Landmarks for arthrocentesis of the radiohumeral joint (see text). (From Akins, C. M.: Aspiration and injection of joints, bursae, and tendons. *In* Vander Salm, T. J., et al.: Atlas of Bedside Procedures. Boston, Little, Brown & Co., 1979. Used by permission.)

radial head and the lateral epicondyle of the humerus is palpated.

Position: With the palpating finger still touching the radial head, the elbow is flexed to 90 degrees. The forearm is pronated and the palm is placed down flat on a table.

Needle insertion: The needle is inserted from the lateral aspect just distal to the lateral epicondyle and is directed medially.

Comments: Effusions in the elbow joint may bulge and be readily palpated. Often the effusion will present inferior to the lateral epicondyle. The bulge can then be aspirated from a posterior approach on the lateral side. A medial approach should not be used, because the ulnar nerve and the superior ulnar collateral artery may be damaged. This is a common joint for gout or septic arthritis. A small hemarthrosis need not be aspirated.

GLENOHUMERAL JOINT (SHOULDER)

Anterior Approach (Fig. 48–5)
Landmarks: The coracoid process medially and the proximal humerus laterally are palpated anteriorly.

Position: The patient should sit upright with his arm at his side and his hand in his lap.

Needle insertion: The needle is inserted at a point inferior and lateral to the coracoid process and is directed posteriorly toward the glenoid rim.

Comments: Arthrocentesis of this joint is of moderate difficulty. Other approaches have been suggested but are less well accepted.

KNEE JOINT

Anteromedial Approach (Fig. 48–6)
Landmarks: The medial surface of the patella at the middle or superior portion of the patella is the landmark for the knee joint.

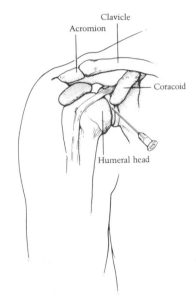

Figure 48–5. Landmarks for arthrocentesis of glenohumeral joint (see text). (From Akins, C. M.: Aspiration and injection of joints, bursae, and tendons. *In* Vander Salm, T. J., et al.: Atlas of Bedside Procedures. Boston, Little, Brown & Co., 1979. Used by permission.)

Position: The knee is fully extended as far as possible. Relaxation of the quadriceps muscle greatly facilitates needle placement.

Needle insertion: An 18 gauge needle or catheter and needle set is inserted at the midpoint or superior portion of the patella approximately 1 cm medial to the anteromedial patella edge. The needle is directed between the posterior surface of the patella and the intercondylar femoral notch. The patella may be grasped with the hand and elevated.

Comments: If the patient is tense, contraction of the quadriceps will greatly hinder entering the joint. The knee is probably the easiest joint to

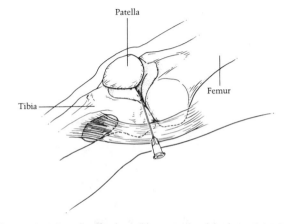

Figure 48–6. Landmarks for arthrocentesis of the knee joint (see text). (From Akins, C. M.: Aspiration and injection of joints, bursae, and tendons. *In* Vander Salm, T. J., et al.: Atlas of Bedside Procedures. Boston, Little, Brown & Co., 1979. Used by permission.)

enter, however. Removal of a tense hemarthrosis will relive pain and facilitate examination for ligamentous injury. If fluid stops flowing, one should *squeeze the soft tissue area of the suprapatellar region to "milk" the suprapatellar pouch of fluid.* The knee can easily accommodate 50 to 70 ml of fluid, and the clinician should therefore be prepared to change syringes during the procedure. The knee is a common site for septic arthritis (especially gonococcal) and various inflammatory or degenerative diseases. An anterolateral approach can be accomplished in a similar manner if the patella is approached laterally.

TIBIOTALAR JOINT (ANKLE) (Fig. 48–7)

Landmarks: The medial malleolar sulcus is bordered medially by the medial malleolus and laterally by the anterior tibial tendon. The tendon can be easily identified by active dorsiflexion of the foot.

Position: With the patient lying supine on the table, the foot is plantar flexed.

Needle insertion: The needle is inserted at a point just medial to the anterior tibial tendon and is directed into the hollow at the anterior edge of the medial malleolus. The needle will have to be inserted 2 to 3 cm to penetrate the joint space.

Comments: If the joint bulges medially, one may use an approach that is more medial than anterior, entering at a point just anterior to the medial

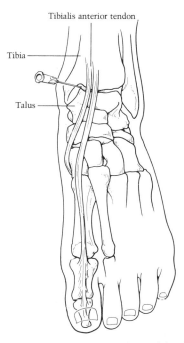

Figure 48–7. Landmarks for arthrocentesis of the tibiotalar joint (see text). (From Akins, C. M.: Aspiration and injection of joints, bursae, and tendons. *In* Vander Salm, T. J., et al.: Atlas of Bedside Procedures. Boston, Little, Brown & Co., 1979. Used by permission.)

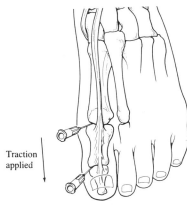

Figure 48–8. Landmarks for metatarsophalangeal and interphalangeal joints (see text). (From Akins, C. M.: Aspiration and injection of joints, bursae, and tendons. *In* Vander Salm, T. J., et al.: Atlas of Bedside Procedures. Boston, Little, Brown & Co., 1979. Used by permission.)

malleolus. The needle may have to be advanced 1 to 1½ inches with this approach.

METATARSOPHALANGEAL AND INTERPHALANGEAL JOINTS (Fig. 48–8)

Landmarks: For the first digit, landmarks are the distal metatarsal head and the proximal base of the first phalanx. For the other toes, the landmarks are the prominences at the proximal interphalangeal and distal interphalangeal joints. The extensor tendon of the great toe can be located by active extension of the toe.

Position: With the patient supine on the table, the toes should be flexed 15 to 20 degrees. *Traction is then applied.*

Needle insertion: The needle is inserted on the dorsal surface at a point just medial or lateral to the central slip of the extensor tendon.

Synovial Fluid Interpretation

Synovial fluid examination is essential for the diganosis of septic arthritis, gout, and pseudogout. Inflammatory joint disease of unknown etiology can often be diagnosed precisely by synovial fluid studies. Joint fluid is a dialysate of plasma that contains protein and hyaluronic acid. Normal fluid is clear enough to allow newsprint to be read through it and will not clot. Normal fluid is straw-colored and flows freely with the consistency of motor oil. Normal fluid produces a good mucin clot and gives a positive "string" sign (see later). The uric acid level of joint fluid approaches that of serum, and the glucose concentration is normally at least 80 per cent that of serum. A normal joint contains only a few milliliters of fluid. Clarity of fluid reflects the leukocyte count. High leukocyte counts result in opacity, the degree of which generally correlates with the degree of elevated synovial fluid leukocytes.

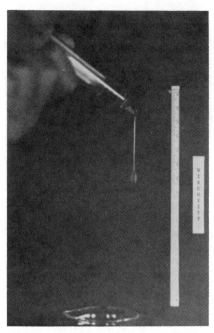

Figure 48–9. Ability of normal synovial fluid to form a long tenacious string. (From Schmid, F. R., and Ogata, R. I.: Synovial fluid evaluation in joint disease. Med. Clin. North Am. 49:165, 1965. Used by permission.)

Viscosity correlates with the concentration of hyaluronate in the synovial fluid. Any inflammation degrades hyaluronate, characteristically resulting in low-viscosity synovial fluids. The "string" sign is a simple test for assessing viscosity. The practitioner measures the length of the "string" formed by a falling drop extruded from a syringe of synovial fluid. Normal joint fluid will produce a "string" of 5 to 10 cm (Fig. 48–9). If viscosity is reduced, as in inflammatory conditions, the synovial fluid will form a shorter "string" or will fall in drops.

The mucin clot test also corresponds to viscosity and inflammation. Therefore, the greater the inflammatory response, the poorer the mucin clot and the lower the viscosity. The mucin clot test is useful to define the degree of polymerization of hyaluronate. Mucin clots are produced by mixing 1 part joint fluid with 4 parts 2 per cent acetic acid. A good clot indicates a high degree of polymerization and correlates with normal high viscosity. In inflammatory synovial fluid, the mucin clot is poor.

A leukocytosis consisting predominantly of neutrophils is usually seen with inflammatory arthritides; a white blood cell count greater than 50,000 per mm^3 is highly suggestive of a septic joint. Joint fluid glucose usually decreases as inflammation increases, but a proper interpretation requires a simultaneous blood glucose evaluation. A ratio of joint fluid to serum glucose of less than 50 per cent suggests a septic joint.

No synovial fluid analysis is complete until the fluid has been examined under a polarizing light microscope for crystals. Heparin should be the anticoagulant used, because crystalline anticoagulants may appear as crystals under the microscope. Clear nail polish may be used to seal the cover slip over a specimen used for crystal analysis. This procedure will preserve the slide and arrest fluid motion. Items found in synovial fluid that can be confused with sodium urate (Fig. 48–10) or calcium pyrophosphate crystals (Fig. 48–11) include collagen fibrils, cartilage fragments (Fig. 48–12), cholesterol crystals (Fig. 48–13), metallic fragments from prosthetic arthroplasty, and corticosteroid esters.[19] One may also identify fat globules (Fig. 48–14). Note that rare cases of uric acid spherulites in gouty synovia have been reported.[20] The spherulites are birefringent and do not take up fat stains.

Table 48–1 summarizes synovial fluid features for the joint diseases commonly encountered and studies commonly performed in the emergency department.

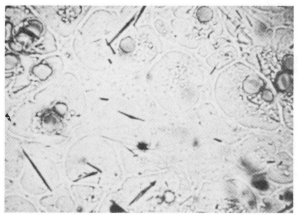

Figure 48–10. Synovial fluid with uric acid crystals. (From ER Reports 4:40, 1900. Used by permission.)

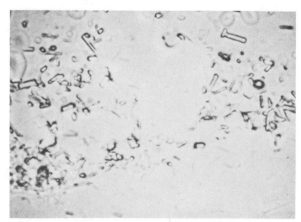

Figure 48–11. Synovial fluid with calcium pyrophosphate crystals. (From ER Reports 4:41, 1900. Used by permission.)

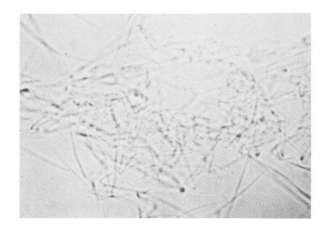

Figure 48–12. Appearance of cartilage fragments. (From ER Reports 4:42, 1900. Used by permission.)

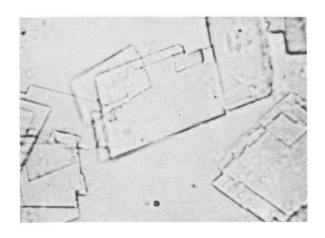

Figure 48–13. Appearance of cholesterol crystals. (From ER Reports 4:41, 1900. Used by permission.)

Figure 48–14. Appearance of fat globules in synovial fluid. (From ER Reports 4:42, 1900. Used by permission.)

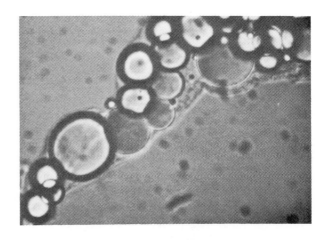

Table 48–1. SYNOVIAL FLUID INTERPRETATION

Diagnosis	Appearance	WBCs/mm³	% Polymorphonuclear Leukocytes	Glucose: % Blood Level	Crystals Under Polarized Light	Culture
Normal	Clear	< 200	< 25	95 to 100	None	Negative
Degenerative joint disease	Clear	< 4000	< 25	95 to 100	None	Negative
Traumatic arthritis	Straw-colored, bloody, xanthochromic, occasionally with fat droplets	< 4000	< 25	95 to 100	None	Negative
Acute gout	Turbid	5000 to 50,000	> 75	80 to 100	Negative birefringence;* needle-like crystals	Negative†
Pseudogout	Turbid	5000 to 50,000	> 75	80 to 100	Positive birefringence;* rhomboid crystals	Negative
Septic arthritis	Purulent/turbid	> 50,000	> 75	< 50	None	Positive (usually)
Rheumatoid arthritis/ seronegative arthritis (Reiter's disease, psoriatic arthritis, ankylosing spondylitis, inflammatory bowel disease)	Turbid	5000 to 50,000	50 to 75	~ 75	None	Negative†

*Negative birefringence means that crystals appear yellow when lying parallel to the axis of the slow vibration of light of the first-order red compensator. With the same orientation to the compensator, positive birefringence crystals appear blue. When the crystals lie perpendicular to the axis, the opposite is true; that is, negative birefringence crystals are blue, positive ones are yellow. A polarizing microscope is necessary for this distinction to be made.
†May be coexisting infection.

1. Gilliand, B. C., and Mannik, M.: Approach to disorders of the joints. *In* Isselbacher, K. (ed.): Harrison's Principles of Internal Medicine. New York, McGraw-Hill, 1980.
2. Sharp, J. T., Lidsky, M. D., Duffy, J., and Duncan, M. W.: Infectious arthritis. Arch. Intern. Med. 139:1125, 1979.
3. Brandt, K. D., Cathcart, E. S., and Cohen, A. S.: Gonococcal arthritis: Clinical features correlated with blood, synovial fluid, genitourinary cultures. Arthritis Rheum. 17:503, 1974.
4. Hume, R. L., Short, L. A., and Gudas, C. J.: Hemarthrosis: A review of the literature. J. Podiatry Assoc. 70:283, 1980.
5. Wolski, K. P.: Staphylococcal and other Gram-positive coccal arthritides. Clin. Rheumatic Dis. 4:181, 1978.
6. Goldenberg, D. L., Brandt, K. D., Cathcart, M. D., et al.: Acute arthritis caused by gram-negative bacilli: A clinical characterization. Medicine 53:197, 1974.
7. Goldenberg, D. L., and Cohen, A. S.: Acute infectious arthritis. Am. J. Med. 60:369, 1976.
8. Rimoin, D. L., and Wennberg, J. E.: Acute septic arthritis complicating chronic rheumatoid arthritis. JAMA 196:109, 1966.
9. Hamilton, M. E., Parris, T. M., Gibson, R. S., and Davis, J. S.: Simultaneous gout and pyarthrosis. Arch. Intern. Med. 140:917, 1980.
10. Holmes, K. K., Counts, G. W., and Beaty, H. N.: Disseminated gonococcal infection. Ann. Intern. Med. 74:979, 1971.
11. Gelfand, S. G., Masi, A. T., and Garcia-Kutzbach, A.: Spectrum of gonococcal arthritis: Evidence for sequential stages and clinical subgroups. J. Rheumatol. 2:83, 1975.
12. Rodnan, G. P., McEwan, C., and Wallace, S. L.: Primer on the rheumatic diseases. JAMA 224(Suppl.):661, 1973.
13. Katz, W. A.: Diagnosis of monoarthritis, polyarthritis and monoarticular rheumatic disorders. *In* Katz, W. A. (ed.): Rheumatic Diseases, Diagnosis and Treatment. Philadelphia, J. B. Lippincott Co., 1977, pp. 192–197.
14. Jaffer, A. M., and Schmid, R.: Hemarthrosis associated with sodium warfarin. J. Rheumatol. 4:215, 1977.
15. Wild, J. J., and Zvaifler, N. J.: Hemarthrosis associated with sodium warfarin therapy. Arthritis Rheum. 19:98, 1976.
16. Hollander, J. L., Brown, E. M., Jessar, R. A., et al.: Hydrocortisone and cortisone injected into arthritic joints: Comparative effects of and use of hydrocortisone as a local antiarthritic agent. JAMA 147:1629, 1951.
17. Anastassiades, T. P., Dwosh, I. L., and Ford, P. M.: Intra-articular steroid injections: A benefit or a hazard? CMA Journal 122:389, 1980.
18. Cohen, S. H.: Regional corticosteroid therapy. *In* Katz, W. A. (ed.): Rheumatic Diseases: Diagnosis and Management. Philadelphia, J. B. Lippincott Co., 1977, p. 910.
19. Kahn, C. B., Hollander, J. L., and Schamacher, H. R.: Corticosteroid crystals in synovial fluid. JAMA 211:807, 1970.
20. Fiechtner, J. J., Simkin, P. A.: Urate spherulites in gouty synovia. JAMA 245:1533, 1981.

49

Low Back Exercises

SAMUEL TIMOTHY COLERIDGE, D.O.
LOREN H. REX, D.O.

Therapeutic exercise should be prescribed as if it were a patent drug, in correct dosage and of suitable quality.

HANS KRAUS, M.D.

Introduction

Backache is among the most common of all human disabilities. In Anderson's British study of 2688 men, it was found that 30 per cent had backache and 76 per cent of these had lumbar pain.[2] A similar study of Israeli workers in eight different jobs reported a backache prevalence rate of 6.4 to 21.6 per 100 men and women.[3] Ikata reported sciatica in 5.2 to 22.4 per cent of 1110 Japanese workers in 10 jobs,[4] and Hult in Sweden reported that 60 per cent of 1193 persons with varied jobs had suffered backache.[5] Rowe in New York City reported low back pain to be second only to upper respiratory infections in terms of work time lost because of illness.[6] According to Benn and Wood, men in Great Britain missed an average of 32.6 work days in 1969–70 because of low back pain.[7] Another British study showed that one man out of 25 changes his work there because of back pain.[8]

Swedish studies based on National Health Insurance data indicate that the average absence period caused by backache is 36 days—the highest of any disease group.[9] In the United States, impairments of the back and the spine were the most frequent cause of activity limitation in persons under 45 years of age and the third most frequent cause of those 45 to 64 years of age. In 1963–65, backache was the diagnosis in 10 per cent of all patients with chronic conditions.[10]

Probably the most common cause of backache is both degenerative and mechanical change within the intervertebral disk. Activities of daily living, faulty posture, previous trauma, occupation, muscle strength, physical fitness, age and sex, and social and psychological factors have also been blamed for contributing to the high incidence of acute, chronic, and intermittent backache in

Western society.[9, 11, 12] Kraus reports that over 83 per cent of patients with backache show no pathologic condition except for muscle problems.[13] Williams believes that the forward tilt of the sacral table when a human is in the standing position is the main cause of posterior marginal stress on the lower lumbar intervertebral discs and thus the primary cause of disc degeneration at this site.[12] His therapeutic exercise program, similar to the one presented here, is directed toward reducing the angle that the sacral table forms with the horizontal plane, i.e., inducing lumbar flexion and hence decreasing lumbar lordosis. Williams noted that patients' symptoms diminish with standing lumbar flexion, walking in a stooped or flexed-forward position, or lying in the fetal position. Hyperextension of the lumbar spine while the patient is walking erect or lying supine is generally uncomfortable.[14]

The lumbosacral facets are gliding joints exposed to stresses approximately 100 times greater per square inch than those encountered in the knee. Slippage is restrained by the joint ligaments, including the intraspinal, sacrospinal, and anterior longitudinal ligaments and the ligamentum flava.[15]

The muscles of the lumbar area are massive. The erector spinae muscles and the hip flexors, including taut fasciae and ligaments, are the principal extensors of the lumbosacral spine and act as firm stabilizers of the trunk over the pelvis. The abdominal and gluteus maximus muscles are the main flexors and prevent overextension (Fig. 49–1). Therapeutic exercises should be directed toward reducing lumbosacral extension, thus shifting the center of gravity forward and thereby relieving the posterior pressure in the lumbosacral spine. To accomplish this it is necessary to strengthen the flexors of the lumbosacral spine actively and to stretch the contracted extensor apparatus passively to develop a balance between opposing postural muscles.[11, 12, 14, 16, 17]

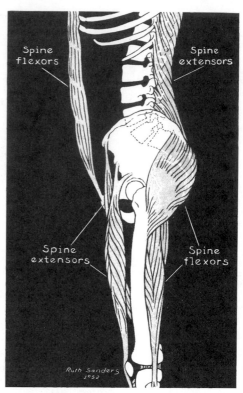

Figure 49–1. Schematic drawing demonstrating principal muscle groups concerned in flexion and extension of the lumbosacral spine in the weight-bearing position. (From Williams, P.C.: The Lumbosacral Spine. New York, McGraw-Hill, 1965. Used by permission.)

Indications and Contraindications

Low back exercises are indicated for musculoskeletal back pain as an adjunct to common medical therapy. Physical examination should help identify patients with back pain caused by a ligamentous sprain, a muscle strain, or disc disease.[18] Patients with these acute injuries are most likely to benefit from therapeutic exercises. Conditions such as aortic dilatation/dissection, chronic pancreatic disease, carcinoma of the pancreas, and renal disease as well as prostatic and pelvic disease may be associated with muscle weakness and complaints that may temporarily improve with therapeutic exercise. Therefore, *therapeutic* exercises should not be used for *diagnostic* purposes, since progression of life-threatening disease might occur as a result of delay in proper diagnosis.

Other contraindications to exercises include inflammation, fractures, ligamental tears, or tumors of the axial skeleton. Furthermore, activities that produce pain, extreme fatigue, syncope, or respiratory distress should be avoided. Finally, patients with advanced cardiovascular disease or those who are emotionally unstable are unlikely to follow the exercise program.[13]

General Instructions

The original flexor exercises were described by Williams in 1937;[12] most therapeutic exercise programs are merely modifications of Williams' flexor exercises. We recommend that the exercises be performed on a carpeted floor one to three times daily; the repetitions should vary with the ability and age of the individual. Elderly patients might begin with as few as five to six repetitions, whereas adolescents may begin with as many as 20 to 40 repetitions. Seldom have we had a patient begin with more than 12 to 15 repetitions. Exercises involving many repetitions should be avoided, because they fatigue and tighten muscles.[13] We prefer that the patient increase the *frequency* of performing the exercise rather than the number of repetitions.

In planning an exercise program for the low back, one must have an understanding of the effect of the principal muscle groupings upon the lumbar spine (see Fig. 49–1). To meet the individual needs of the patient, the physical examination should include assessment of the patient's postural impairment, the strength and flexibility of the principal muscle groups, the special action that each exercise imposes upon the principal muscle groups, and the patient's limitations as a result of his disability.[13, 14]

The exercise program is begun as soon as rest and medical therapy sufficiently reduce pain and permit activity; usually, this occurs within 2 weeks after the acute insult.[14, 16, 19] Injury-induced muscle spasm can often be relieved with local ice or moist heat. Applying an ice pack will often do more to relieve muscle spasm than will administering potent analgesic medication to interrupt the cycle of pain-induced muscle spasm; ice inhibits the gamma-efferent portion of the reflex arc, markedly reducing muscle spasm of central or peripheral origin.[20] Other modalities of treatment include trigger point therapy (see Chapter 47); whirlpool bath; short-wave and microwave diathermy and ultrasound; transcutaneous electrical nerve stimulation (TENS); splinting with corsets; and sufficient analgesic and anti-inflammatory medications plus muscle relaxants, tranquilizers, and spinal manipulation.[14, 16, 17, 19, 21] Each can be used alone or in combination with therapeutic exercise.

The schedule of performing exercises three to four times daily (usually associated with meals and bedtime or before and after work as well as before bedtime) is easily remembered by the patient. Daily psychic stresses from family and work problems may generate emotional tension and aggravate low back pain involving muscle spasm, much as does the muscle contraction or tension headache common to many of us.

The low back program should begin with relaxation and limbering exercises. Finneson has described two such exercises:[14] (1) While lying on the floor, the patient raises his arms slowly over his head as he inhales deeply and then exhales as he allows his arms to return slowly to the floor and his entire body to become flaccid. This is repeated 10 times. (2) The patient breathes deeply again and contracts all his muscles by squeezing the arms against the body and the legs together tightly, making tight fists and tightening the muscles of the buttocks. Then, with each exhalation, he allows all the muscles to relax and the extremities to drift away from the body. If performed properly, each succeeding repetition will become more relaxing and hypnotic, thereby producing total physical and mental relaxation prior to the beginning of the low back exercises.

The exercises that will be discussed are basically adopted from Finneson (Figs. 49–2 and 49–3);[14] these are programmed into three phases. The physician should withhold those exercises that he does not consider to be indicated or those that might exacerbate the patients' symptoms because of the muscle groups involved. The exercises are arranged so as to allow modification in the number of repetitions. The purpose of each exercise is included with the instructions in order to help the physician to decide which exercises he may wish to exclude on the basis of the physical examination. It is recommended that patients bring their exercise sheet with them on follow-up visits and document exercises that they find to increase symptoms instead of help them. Generally, one should begin with five repetitions for each exercise to treat the acute episode of low back pain; this is particularly true for the middle-aged, nonathletic individual. One might begin with a larger number of repetitions for the adolescent and move from phase 1 to phase 2 in 1 to 2 weeks instead of the 3 to 4 weeks that are normally suggested. The normal progression for phase 1 is five repetitions of each exercise for the first week, seven for the second week, and ten for the third and fourth weeks. The recreational exercises in phase 3 are normally deferred until those in phase 2 are partially or totally completed, when the patient is less likely to exacerbate his symptoms. We should mention that selected exercises from both phase 1 and phase 2 need to be continued *indefinitely* to maintain muscle elasticity and strength but can be performed *less often* as time goes by (e.g., 3 times per week or when low back pain symptoms recur as a result of acute sprain or strain or emotional stress).

Phase 1 (see Fig. 49–2)

The exercises in phase 1 are prescribed for the athletic patient with acute muscle strain or the nonathletic patient who has recently recovered from an episode of moderate to severe low back pain. The nonathletic patient should be *pain-free* prior to undertaking these exercises.

Exercise 1. As noted in Figure 49–2, the patient begins supine on a carpeted floor with the knees flexed. The patient slowly allows his legs to fall to the ground in the extended position (limp and relaxed). The purpose of the exercise is to promote relaxation and mentally prepare the patient for the next exercises. Additionally, it strengthens the abdominal muscles and promotes hamstring and lumbar elasticity. This exercise should be repeated five to ten times as needed to "relax" the patient;

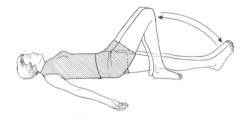

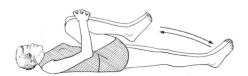

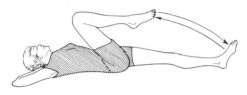

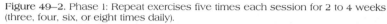

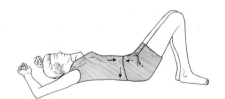

Figure 49–2. Phase 1: Repeat exercises five times each session for 2 to 4 weeks (three, four, six, or eight times daily).

Exercise 1: Allow knees to drop limply to floor, relaxed, repeat ×5. Purpose: Relaxation; to promote lumbar elasticity and abdominal muscle strength.

Exercise 2: Flex knees to chest, then pull knees toward chest and hold for 10 seconds. Return to starting position. Repeat ×5. Purpose: To promote lumbar and hamstring elasticity and increase abdominal muscle strength.

Exercise 3: With hands behind the head, raise one knee toward chest and hold 10 seconds, then return to floor. Repeat with opposite leg (×5). Purpose: To promote lumbar, hamstring, and iliopsoas elasticity and to increase abdominal muscle strength.

Exercise 4: With hands above the head, flatten low back against the mat and tighten abdominal muscles for 10 seconds, repeat ×5. Purpose: To increase lower and upper abdominal muscle and gluteal muscle strength.

Exercise 5: From sitting position, drop head between legs and touch floor for 3 seconds. Purpose: To promote lumbar and hamstring elasticity and to increase low back muscle strength.

(Modified from Finneson, B.E.: Low Back Pain, 2nd ed. Philadelphia, J.B. Lippincott Co., 1980.)

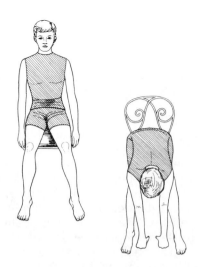

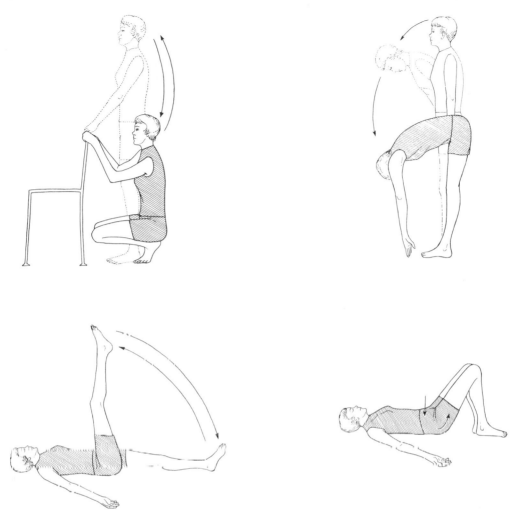

Figure 49–3. Phase 2: Repeat exercises 5, 10, or 15 times each session (one, two, or three times daily).
    Exercise 1: Squat from erect position and straighten up again while touching chair, repeat ×5. Purpose: To increase quadriceps and abdominal muscle strength.
    Exercise 2: Alternate raising one leg as far as possible without pain and slowly lowering to ground, repeat ×5. Purpose: To promote lumbar, hamstring, and iliopsoas elasticity.
    Exercise 3: Slowly bend forward from hips with knees straight, repeat ×5. Purpose: To promote lumbar and hamstring elasticity.
    Exercise 4: "Pelvic uptilt." Press lumbar spine to floor and elevate buttocks, uptilting the pelvis for 10 seconds, repeat ×10. Purpose: To increase gluteus muscle and abdominal muscle strength.
    (Modified from Finneson, B. E.: Low Back Pain, 2nd ed. Philadelphia, J. B. Lippincott Co., 1980.)

it requires the least amount of effort of all those in phase 1.

Exercise 2. Lying supine again with knees flexed, as in exercise 1, the patient brings both knees up to his chest; clasping the knees with his hands, he pulls them to his chest with the legs spread and the knees in the axillae. He holds the position for 10 seconds and then returns to the extended leg position. The grip on the knees should not be released during flexion. Maintaining the head on a pillow prevents a rocking action. The aim of the exercise is to lift the buttocks off the floor, but not so far that the knees are pulled over the shoulder. This limits the flexion to the lumbosacral level; the erector spinae and contracted fasciae and the ligaments of the posterior structures are passively involved.

Exercise 3. Lying on his back with his legs extended and his hands locked behind his neck, the patient raises one knee as high as his chest (if possible) for 10 seconds. He returns the flexed leg to the extended position and repeats with the opposite leg five times. The purpose of this exercise is to promote lumbar, hamstring, and iliopsoas elasticity and to increase abdominal muscle strength.

Exercise 4. Lying on his back with his arms above his head and his knees bent, the patient flattens his back against the floor and contracts the abdominal muscles for 10 seconds. He relaxes for 10 seconds and repeats five to ten times. The purpose of this exercise is to increase the strength of the abdominal lumbar flexors and to decrease the lumbar lordosis. This exercise provides satisfying symptomatic relief during periods of acute low back strain and can be used in conjunction with exercise 1 when all others are too painful to try.

Exercise 5. Sitting in a chair, the patient drops his head down between his legs and places his hands on the floor. He maintains this stretched position for 3 seconds and then resumes the sitting position. He relaxes for 5 seconds and then repeats five times. Clasping the left ankle to stretch the right erector spinal group and returning to the sitting position before stretching the opposite erector spinal group is an adaptation of this exercise. This modification should be offered to the patient with residual soreness in the erector spinae when the exercises in phase 1 are discussed. This will show the patient that the physician is attempting to "individualize" his therapeutic exercise program and is not just blindly handing him an impersonal "do-it-yourself kit."

The exercises in phase 1 should be performed two to three times daily for a period of 2 to 4 weeks. If at that time the patient is still pain-free during exercise, he may begin phase 2 of the program. If the patient is not improving, the frequency of exercise should be increased to four, six, or eight times per day; only five repetitions should be performed during each session.

Phase 2 (see Fig. 49–3)

These exercises are either added to the phase 1 program at the end of 2 to 4 weeks or substituted for those exercises when the patient can easily perform them without discomfort. The patient should no longer require ice massage or analgesic medication in order to do his exercises. Again, certain exercises may be temporarily omitted if the history or physical examination suggests that symptoms are exacerbated by these activities.

Exercise 1. Standing erect and using the back of a chair or the edge of a table for balance, the patient squats down and then straightens up again. The aim here is mainly to increase quadriceps strength.

Exercise 2. From the supine position, the patient raises one leg as far as possible without producing pain, keeping the leg straight. After lowering it slowly to the floor, he repeats the exercise, alternating with the opposite leg 5 to 15 times. The goal is to stretch the lumbar, hamstring, and iliopsoas muscles.

Exercise 3. Standing erect, the patient slowly flexes the head and bends slowly from the hips with the knees straight while attempting to touch the floor with his fingers. This is repeated five to ten times. The idea is to promote lumbar and hamstring elasticity. Obviously, caution should be

advised for elderly patients or those prone to orthostatic symptoms.

Exercise 4. The "pelvic uptilt" is similar to the isometric exercise 4 in phase 1 but goes a bit further by having the patient elevate the buttocks off the floor while maintaining pressure of the lumbar spine against the floor with the knees flexed. The most common patient error in this exercise is to elevate the entire lumbar spine to a position of increased lumbar lordosis instead of the desired accentuated lumbar flexion. The strengthening of the abdominal and quadriceps muscles developed from this exercise aids in maintaining a decreased lumbar lordosis and, hence, less posterior vertebral body compression at the lumbosacral levels. This exercise may be performed two to four times per day in lieu of the other exercises with 10 to 20 repetitions. As this exercise becomes easier to perform with increased repetitions, the patient may try it in the upright position with the feet approximately 12 inches from the wall, attempting to "flatten" the lumbar spine against the wall. Lumbar flexion may be accentuated if this is begun in a doorway with the extended arms providing counterpressure against the door frame as the patient presses his lumbar spine against the opposite door frame. Eventually, the feet can be moved progressively closer to the wall or the door frame until the heels are touching. This upright "pelvic uptilt," together with exercises 1 and 3 of phase 2, can be easily accomplished at work several times a day when the patient feels sore after prolonged sitting.

Phase 3

This is the maintenance program. It is extremely important to sustain adequate muscle balance with strong and elastic spine flexors (the hamstring, gluteus, and abdominal muscles) to counter the normally well-developed spine extensors (the iliopsoas, quadriceps, and erector spinae).[12–14, 17, 22, 23] One can maintain muscle balance by continuing any of the aforementioned exercises three times per week or performing suitable recreational activities. As the memory of back pain fades, so does the inclination to maintain an exercise program. Proper exercises continued for many months may well prevent the recurrence of the strain, since strain results from using a muscle beyond its capacity. Hence, the greater the capacity, the less likely that the back muscles will be strained.[16, 24] One must consider recreational activities or an exercise program that can be maintained throughout the year despite the weather and can be tailored to the age and physical condition of the patient.[13, 25]

Bicycle riding with the lumbar spine flexed is

optimal; swimming might exacerbate symptoms if the patient increases his lumbar lordosis doing the breast stroke. Tennis, golf, and bowling each cause considerable torsion of the lumbar spine. Tennis is usually more easily tolerated. Jogging, horse-back riding, and weightlifting normally increase symptoms.[14] For the adolescent or young adult who wishes to lift weights, we recommend O'Shea's book, which discusses the muscle groups involved with each weightlifting technique.[26] His standing dumbbell swing is the only weightlifting exercise that is appropriate during the latter half of phase 2. During phase 3, a complete, balanced weightlifting exercise program may be enjoyed if it is performed with an understanding of the muscle groups involved.[26, 27]

Naturally, at first one must perform any recreational activity less strenuously than before the onset of low backache; the activity may be gradually increased.[24] Shuman's statement is as true today as it was 30 years ago: "There's no question that walking—simple pick-'em-up-and-lay-'em-down walking—is the greatest exercise ever developed."[28]

When prescribing a therapeutic exercise program, the physician must provide patient education regarding daily posture when sleeping, sitting, standing, lifting, and performing daily household or occupational activities.[12, 14, 22, 25, 29]

Williams and MacNab offer general instruction sheets to remind patients of these important changes in their posture. Modification of posture can prevent relapses as well as promote proper muscle strengthening (Table 49–1).[12, 29]

A limited activity program prohibits any heavy lifting, prolonged forward bending, excessive stooping, or long automobile trips. One should eliminate prolonged standing, extensive walking, and frequent stair climbing. A firm mattress or a supporting 3/4-inch plywood sheet between the mattress and the bedsprings is optimal.[14]

The proper bed rest position is one affording slight lumbar flexion with the head elevated and the knees flexed. One can best achieve this by lying on the side with the hips and the knees flexed or by applying a rolled blanket under the mattress at the knee level to create the flexed-knee position.

When lifting, the patient should inhale deeply to increase intrathoracic and intra-abdominal pressure, which in turn decrease intradisk pressure. Likewise, strong abdominal muscles also help to decrease intradisk pressures.[11]

Complications

Complications of a therapeutic exercise program generally result from misinterpretation of the pro-

Table 49–1. POSTURAL INSTRUCTIONS

Exercises are essential to maintaining proper muscle balance, but correct posture is acquired only through conscious effort.

General Observations
Do not lift weights above the head.
Do not move furniture by pulling it in front of you; push it instead.
Do not push windows up; lift them upward while standing close to the window.
Do not put on weight.
Do not get overtired.
Do not maintain any one position for a prolonged period.
Do not reach for objects above your head; use a footstool.
All equipment should have long handles to prevent frequent stooping forward.
Avoid wearing high heels as much as possible.

Sleeping
Your mattress should be firm or a board should be placed beneath it.
Sleep on your side with the hips and the knees bent.
When rising from bed, roll to your side, swing your legs over the side of the bed, and push with your arms to the sitting position instead of sitting up and twisting the body.

Sitting
When driving a car, the seat should be as close to the steering wheel as possible, thereby allowing you to flex the knees and hips.
Avoid prolonged automobile trips.
Adjust your chair such that you sit with your knees higher than your hips; otherwise, elevate your feet on a stool or cross your legs.
Sit with your buttocks "tucked under" so that the hollow in the low back is eliminated.
Chair arm supports enhance your opportunity to change body positions without stressing your back.

Getting Up from Sitting
Do not arch your back when standing from a chair; flex forward and use your hands if necessary to rise.

Standing/Walking
Elevate one foot on a stool or like object when standing.
Avoid prolonged standing.
Never bend backward.
Try to form a crease across the upper abdomen by holding the chest up and forward while elevating the front of the pelvis; walk as if you are going up an incline.

Lifting
When lifting or squatting to pick up an object from the floor, bend the hips and the knees while keeping the spine straight, then hold the object as close to the body as possible when standing—lift with the legs, not the back.
Never hold heavy objects more than 2 feet from the body.
Inhale deeply before lifting.

---

cedures for performing the exercises, overzealous repetition, or continuation of specific exercises that increase symptoms despite the pain.[11, 16, 21, 22] If certain exercises increase pain, they should be stopped and discussed at the next follow-up visit. It is possible that certain exercises may be reintroduced later in the exercise phase, when greater muscle elasticity or strength develop.

Noncompliance with any exercise regimen, premature return to recreational activities, or inclusion of those sports causing more stress upon the disk, rather than the prescribed exercise program, is often the cause of acute exacerbations.

Interpretation

When the patient returns to the physician's office and can explain or perform the exercises properly yet continues to show no improvement, one must seriously question the efficacy of the therapeutic exercise program. Normally, increased muscle strength and a decreased lumbar lordosis should be noted if a patient is maintaining his program. This is sometimes difficult to assess on physical examination in the obese patient with a protuberant abdomen who is a frequent sufferer of low back pain because of his compensatory lumbar lordosis. Standing radiographs for objective documentation of progress can be useful, despite the voluntary splinting by the patient that is possible.[24]

Conclusion/Comment

A therapeutic exercise program is an inexpensive, effective treatment modality for acute and chronic low back pain. This program is generally used for chronic pain but can be initiated in cases of acute low back pain after ice massage analgesia in acute mild strains. Complete restoration of muscle function with respect to strength and total elasticity is promoted by the exercises and helps to prevent reinjury.

Patient adherence to an exercise regimen is dependent upon the individual's perception that it is worth the invested time and effort. Often, this is indicated by the physician's enthusiasm or his assessment that his physician truly believes that the exercises will work, that exercises are not just a ploy to avoid giving medications, and that the exercises will work this time even if they have not been successful in the past. One should explain to the patient how and why exercises work. If exercises were used in the past, the physician must ask which exercises were performed and for how long. The physician can enhance patient confidence and increase patient compliance (which is the main goal) by using a handout exercise sheet, demonstrating how a few of the exercises are performed, circling the ones that he personally prefers, or scratching out the ones that he suspects will increase symptoms, based on the physical examination. Likewise, tailoring the number of repetitions by circling the appropriate number is time-efficient for the physician and indicates to the patient that his treatment is individualized despite the standard "handout exercise program."

All treatment programs have a significant placebo effect, and it is important to use this to the best advantage of the patient.[14]

Follow-up is mandatory, whether by telephone to discuss with the patient which exercises exacerbate the symptoms or by return appointment in several weeks to assess if the exercises are being performed appropriately, if there is a change in the patient's condition, or whether revision of the exercise program is indicated.[22] The therapeutic exercise program that is generally suggested is successful for patients with mechanical joint dysfunction if they are indeed convinced to continue with the program long enough to obtain relief, if they change their postural habits, and if they maintain a preventative exercise program. One must stress to the patient that he is the one responsible for the success of the treatment program and that the physician is only assisting him.

1. Kraus, H.: Clinical Treatment of Back and Neck Pain. New York, McGraw-Hill, 1970.
2. Anderson, J. A. D.: Rheumatism in industry: A review. New York, Br. J. Ind. Med. 28:103, 1971.
3. Magora, A., and Tanstein, I.: An investigation of the problem of sick-leave in the patient suffering from low back pain. Ind. Med. Surg. 38:298, 1969.
4. Ikata, T.: Statistical and dynamic studies of lesions due to overloading on the spine. Skikoka Acta Med. 40:262, 1965.
5. Hult, L.: The Munkfors investigation. Acta Orthop. Scand. (Suppl.) 17:16, 1954.
6. Rowe, M. L.: Disc surgery and chronic low-back pain. J. Occup. Med. 7:196, 1965.
7. Benn, R. T., and Wood, P. H. N.: Pain in the back: An attempt to estimate the size of the problem. Rheumatol. Rehabil. 14:121, 1975.
8. Taylor, D. G.: The costs of arthritis and the benefits of joint replacement surgery. Proc. R. Soc. Med. 192:145, 1976.
9. Andersson, G. B. J.: Epidemiologic aspects on low-back pain in industry. Spine 6:53, 1981.
10. Kelsey, J. L., White, A. A., Pastides, H., and Bisbee, G. E., Jr.: The impact of musculoskeletal disorders on the population of the United States. J. Bone Joint Surg. 61A:959, 1979.
11. Jensen, G. M.: Biomechanics of the lumbar intervertebral disk: A review. Phys. Ther. 60:765, 1980.
12. Williams, P. C.: The Lumbosacral Spine. New York, McGraw-Hill, 1965, pp. 80–98.
13. Kraus, H.: Muscle pain: Non-invasive therapy. Part II. Medical Times 110:33, 1982.
14. Finneson, B. E.: Low Back Pain, 2nd ed. Philadelphia, J. B. Lippincott Co., 1980, pp. 199–243.
15. Wallace Pharmaceuticals, Cranberry, NJ: Musculoskeletal Resumes, Chapter 7, 1970.
16. O'Donaghue, D. H.: Treatment of Injuries to Athletes, 3rd ed. Philadelphia, W. B. Saunders Co., 1976, pp. 452–458.
17. Burton, C., Mida, G., Ray, C., and Heithoff, K.: Treating low back pain in the elderly. Geriatrics, 33:61, 1978.
18. Hoppenfeld, S.: Physical Examination of the Spine and Extremities. New York, Appleton-Century-Crofts, 1976, pp. 237–249.
19. Merck, Sharpe & Dome: Back Pain: Diagnosis and Treatment for Primary Care Physicians. May 1981, West Point, PA.

20. Dawson, E. G.: You can help patients with acute low back pain. Consultant 20:11, 1980.
21. Hoehler, F. K., Tobis, J. S., and Buerger, A. A.: Spinal manipulation for low back pain. JAMA 245:1835, 1981.
22. Cailliet, R.: Low Back Pain Syndrome. Philadelphia, F. A. Davis Co., 1968, pp. 58–77.
23. Hasue, M., Fujiwara, M., and Kikuchi, S.: A new method of quantitative measurement of abdominal and back muscle strength. Spine 5:143, 1980.
24. Curry, H. B., Dawson, E. G., Dunsker, S. B., Fisher, J. V., Fitzgerald, C. E., Jr., Friedman, L. W., Henry, J. T., Longmire, W. T., and Ward, R. C.: Round table: Key to treating acute back or neck pain. Patient Care 10:18, 1976.
25. Kagen, L. J.: Musculoskeletal syndromes of the elderly. Drug Therapy 5:64, 1981.
26. O'Shea, J. P.: Scientific Principles and Methods of Strength Fitness, 2nd ed. Reading, MA, Addison-Wesley Publishing Co., 1976, pp.54–59.
27. Paulsen, E.: Back muscle strength and weight limits in lifting burdens. Spine 6:73, 1981.
28. Shuman, D., and Staab, G. R.: Your Aching Back and What You Can Do About It. Gramercy Publishing Co., 1960, p. 165.
29. MacNab, I.: Backache. Baltimore, Williams & Wilkins, 1978, pp. 154–155.

7

OBSTETRICS AND GYNECOLOGY

50

Emergency Childbirth

LYNNETTE A. DOAN, M.D.

Introduction

Since ancient times, midwives, specialists of the obstetrical art, have supervised the labor of women and the delivery of babies. Physicians did not become involved in this practice until the end of the eighteenth century.

With improved prenatal and obstetrical care, the perinatal death rate has fallen by almost 50 per cent in the past 25 years; the maternal death rate has decreased from 582 per 100,000 live births in 1935 to 9.2 per 100,000 live births in 1980.[1, 2]

From the viewpoint of safer care during labor, the outstanding advance of the past 40 years has been the great increase in the proportion of in-hospital deliveries. As recently as 1940, fewer than 60 per cent of births took place in hospitals. For those women in the middle and upper socioeconomic classes, this figure now exceeds 99 per cent.[1] In-hospital births have not only the advantage of better facilities but also care by individuals who are specially trained in obstetrics and perinatology.

The degree to which the emergency physician interacts in the process of labor and delivery varies among institutions, depending upon the availability and readiness of inpatient obstetrical services. The role of the emergency physician may be only to determine that the patient is indeed in active labor and to order transport directly to the labor and delivery area. In a hospital with little or no obstetrical services, the emergency physician may alternatively be called upon to manage a complicated delivery and neonatal resuscitation until transfer to another hospital is possible.

To this end the emergency physician must be able to assess the stage and timing of labor, aid the mother in delivery of the infant, and provide initial stabilization of the neonate.

Labor

Labor is defined as the coordinated effective sequence of involuntary uterine contractions that result in progressive effacement and dilatation of the cervix. This, coupled with the voluntary bear-ing-down efforts of the mother, terminates in delivery, the actual expulsion of the products of conception.

Labor is normally divided into three stages. The first stage begins when uterine contractions reach sufficient force to cause cervical effacement and dilatation and ends when the cervix is completely dilated. The average duration of the first stage of labor is 6 to 8 hours in multiparous patients and is 8 to 12 hours in primiparous patients.[3] The second stage of labor begins when dilatation of the cervix is complete and ends with delivery of the infant. This stage may vary from several minutes to 2 hours. In general, if the second stage lasts more than 2 hours, abnormal labor has developed.[1, 3] The third stage of labor begins after delivery of the infant and ends after delivery of the placenta. Infrequently, a fourth stage of labor is described as that period during which myometrial contractions and vessel thrombosis occur (usually lasting approximately 1 hour), effectively controlling bleeding from the former placental implantation site.[1, 3]

IDENTIFICATION OF LABOR

True vs False Labor

Before the establishment of true or effective labor, women may experience so-called false labor. Quite common in late pregnancy, false labor is characterized by irregular, brief contractions of the uterus, usually with discomfort confined to the lower abdomen and groin. The contractions, commonly referred to as *Braxton Hicks contractions*, are typically irregular in timing and strength; there is no change in the cervix and no descent of the fetus.

True labor, on the other hand, is characterized by a regular sequence of uterine contractions, with progressively increasing intensity and decreasing intervals between contractions. The discomfort produced by the uterine contractions of true labor begins in the fundal region and radiates over the uterus into the lower back. The uterine contractions of true labor are accompanied by effacement and dilatation of the cervix, with descent of the presenting part of the fetus.

False labor is most common in late pregnancy and in parous women. Although false labor usually stops spontaneously, it may convert rapidly to the effective contractions of true labor (Table 50–1). True labor contractions generally occur at intervals of 10 minutes or less following the onset of labor.[4]

Show

A rather dependable sign of the approach of labor is the "show" or "bloody show." Occasion-

Table 50–1. CHARACTERISTICS OF CONTRACTIONS OF TRUE VERSUS FALSE LABOR. (Adapted from Taylor, E. S.: Obstetrics and Fetal Medicine, 2nd ed. Baltimore, Williams & Wilkins, 1977. Used by permission.)

False Labor	True Labor
Occur at irregular intervals	Occur at regular intervals
Intervals remain long	Intervals gradually shorten
Intensity remains same	Intensity gradually increases
Discomfort mainly in lower abdomen	Discomfort in back and upper to mid-abdomen
Cervix does not dilate	Cervix dilates
Usually relieved by sedation	Not stopped by sedation

ally preceding the onset of labor by as much as 72 hours, show consists of a small amount of blood-tinged mucous discharged from the vagina. Show represents extrusion of the mucous plug that filled the cervical canal during pregnancy and is evidence of cervical dilatation and effacement.[1, 3, 4] *Bloody show must be distinguished from more active third trimester bleeding,* which is classified as a true emergency and in which vaginal examination is *contraindicated.*

Rupture of the Membranes

Spontaneous rupture of the membranes usually occurs during the course of active labor, although it may occur prior to the onset of labor in approximately 10 per cent of cases.[3] Rupture of the membranes is typically manifested by a sudden gush of a variable amount of clear or slightly turbid fluid. Rupture of the membranes can be verified if amniotic fluid is extruding from the cervical os or is found in the vaginal fornix upon sterile speculum examination.

Differentiation of amniotic fluid from vaginal fluid may be made by testing a drop of the fluid with *nitrazine paper*. Amniotic fluid has a pH of 7.0 to 7.5 and will turn the paper blue-green to deep blue. In the presence of vaginal secretions only, with a pH of 4.5 to 5.5, nitrazine paper will remain yellow.[1, 5, 6]

Because of its neutral pH, blood may cause a false-positive nitrazine reading in women who have intact membranes and an unusually large amount of bloody show.[1, 6] Abe found the nitrazine test to be positive in 98.9 per cent of women with known rupture of the membranes and negative in 96.2 per cent of women with intact membranes.[5] In clinical practice, however, the test is less reliable, because it is frequently used in cases of questionable rupture in which the amount of amniotic fluid is small and therefore more subject to pH changes from admixed blood and vaginal secretions.[1]

A less frequently used method to test for amniotic fluid is *ferning*. A drop of fluid from the cervical os or vaginal fornix is placed on a clean glass slide. Owing to the high sodium-chloride content of amniotic fluid, a fern pattern will be seen through the microscope as amniotic fluid dries. Blood may interfere with ferning, causing a false-negative result.[4]

Documentation of rupture of the membranes is significant for three reasons. First, if the presenting part is not already fixed in the pelvis, the possibility of prolapse of the cord with cord compression and subsequent fetal distress is increased. Second, labor may be imminent. Finally, if labor does not begin within 24 hours after rupture of the membranes, the pregnancy must be considered to be complicated by prolonged premature rupture of the membranes with an increased chance of intrauterine infection.[1, 3] If rupture of the membranes is documented in the emergency department, the patient's obstetrician should be notified and hospital admission of the patient should be considered.

EVALUATION OF LABOR

When a woman presents in labor, the general condition of the fetus and mother must be quickly ascertained by means of the patient history and physical examination. Inquiry is made as to the onset and frequency of contractions, the presence or absence of bleeding, the possible loss of amniotic fluid, and the prenatal care and condition of the mother and fetus. In the absence of active vaginal bleeding, the position, presentation, and lie of the fetus are determined by abdominal palpation and sterile vaginal examination. Staging of labor is assessed by vaginal examination. Fetal well-being is monitored by auscultation of fetal heart tones, particularly immediately following a uterine contraction.

Lie, Presentation, and Position

In the latter months of pregnancy, the fetus assumes a characteristic posture within the uterus, usually forming an ovoid mass that corresponds roughly to the shape of the uterine cavity. Typically, the fetus becomes folded or bent upon itself in such a way that the back becomes markedly convex, with the head, thighs, and knees being sharply flexed. Usually the arms are crossed over the thorax and are parallel to the sides of the body. The umbilical cord lies in the space between the arms and the lower extremities. This characteristic posture is due in part to the mode of growth of the fetus and is also a result of accommodation to the uterine cavity.

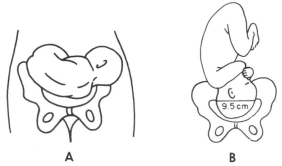

Figure 50–1. A, Transverse lie with shoulder presentation. B, Longitudinal lie with vertex presentation. (From Romney, S., et al. (eds.): Gynecology and Obstetrics: The Health Care of Women. New York, McGraw-Hill, Inc., 1975. Used by permission.)

Lie refers to the relation of the long axis of the fetus to that of the mother. Lie is either longitudinal or transverse (Fig. 50–1). Longitudinal lies occur in more than 99 per cent of pregnancies at term.[1]

The *presentation,* or presenting part, refers to that portion of the body of the fetus that is nearest to or foremost in the birth canal. The presenting part is felt through the cervix on sterile vaginal examination. In longitudinal lies, the presenting part is either the fetal head or the buttocks or the feet. In transverse lie, the shoulder is the presenting part.

Cephalic presentations are classified by the relation of the fetal head to the body of the fetus (Fig. 50–2). Ordinarily, the head is sharply flexed so that the occipital fontanel is the presenting part. This is referred to as the *vertex* or *occiput presentation.* Less commonly, the neck is fully extended and the face is foremost in the birth canal; this is termed *face presentation.* Occasionally the fetal head assumes a partially flexed or partially extended position, resulting in sinciput and brow presentations, respectively. Sinciput and brow presentations, associated with preterm infants, are almost always unstable and convert to either the occiput or face presentation as labor progresses.

Breech presentations are classified as frank, complete, and footling or incomplete (Fig. 50–3).

When the fetus presents with the hips flexed and the legs extended over the anterior surfaces of the body, this is termed *frank breech.* Flexion of the fetal hips and knees results in complete breech presentation. When one or both of the feet or knees are lowermost in the canal, an incomplete or footling breech results.

At or near term, the incidence of the various presentations is approximately 96 per cent for vertex, 3.5 per cent for breech, 0.3 per cent for face, and 0.4 per cent for shoulder.[1]

Position refers to the relation of the presenting part to the birth canal and may be either left or right. The occiput, chin, and sacrum are the determining parts in vertex, face, and breech presentations, respectively. The presentation and position of the fetus are initially determined by abdominal palpation using Leopold's maneuvers.

Abdominal Palpation (Leopold's Maneuvers). Abdominal palpation may be performed throughout the latter months of pregnancy and during labor in the intervals between contractions. The findings from abdominal palpation provide information about the presentation and position of the fetus and the extent to which the presenting part has descended into the pelvis (Fig. 50–4). The mother should be placed on a firm bed or examining table with her abdomen bared. For the first three of the four maneuvers, the examiner stands at the side of the bed facing the patient. During the first maneuver (Fig. 50–4A), the upper abdomen is gently palpated with the fingertips of both hands to determine which fetal pole is present in the uterine fundus. The fetal breech gives the sensation of a large, nodular body, whereas the fetal head is hard, round, and freely moveable.

During the second maneuver, the examiner places his hands on either side of the abdomen, exerting deep, gentle pressure (Fig. 50–4B). On one side, the hard, resistant back is felt; on the other side, the fetal extremities or small parts are felt. By noting whether the back is directed anteriorly, posteriorly, or transversely, fetal orientation or lie is determined.

The third maneuver is performed by grasping the lower portion of the maternal abdomen just

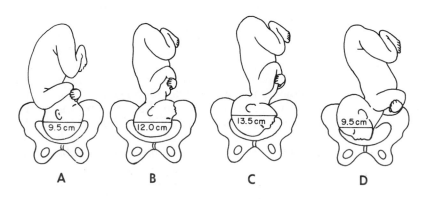

Figure 50–2. Cephalic presentations—deflexion attitude of fetal head: A, vertex; B, sinciput; C, brow; and D, face. Diameter of the presenting fetal head is shown for each of the attitudes. (From Romney, S., et al. (eds.): Gynecology and Obstetrics: The Health Care of Women. New York, McGraw-Hill, Inc., 1975. Used by permission.)

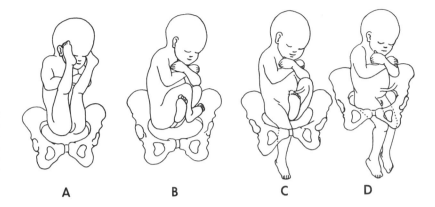

Figure 50–3. Fetal attitude in breech presentations. *A,* frank; *B,* complete; *C,* single footling—incomplete; and *D,* double footling—incomplete. (From Romney, S., et al. (eds.): Gynecology and Obstetrics: The Health Care of Women. New York, McGraw-Hill, Inc., 1975. Used by permission.)

above the symphysis pubis with the thumb and forefinger of one hand (Fig. 50–4C). If the presenting part is not engaged, the position of the head in relation to the back and extremities is ascertained. If the cephalic prominence is palpated on the same side as the small parts, the head must be flexed and therefore a vertex or occiput presentation exists. If the cephalic prominence is on the same side as the back, the head must be

extended. If the presenting part is deeply engaged in the pelvis, the findings from this maneuver indicate that the lower pole of the fetus is fixed in the pelvis. The details of presentation and position are then defined by the fourth maneuver.

To perform the fourth maneuver, the examiner changes position and faces the mother's feet. With the tips of the first three fingers of each hand, the examiner exerts deep, gentle pressure in the di-

Figure 50–4. Abdominal palpation (four maneuvers of Leopold). *A,* Determination of the fetal part occupying the uterine fundus. *B,* Palpation of fetal small parts and back. *C,* Determination of part occupying the lower uterine segment. *D,* Determination of the cephalic prominence. (From Romney, S., et al. (eds.): Gynecology and Obstetrics: The Health Care of Women. New York, McGraw-Hill, Inc., 1975. Used by permission.)

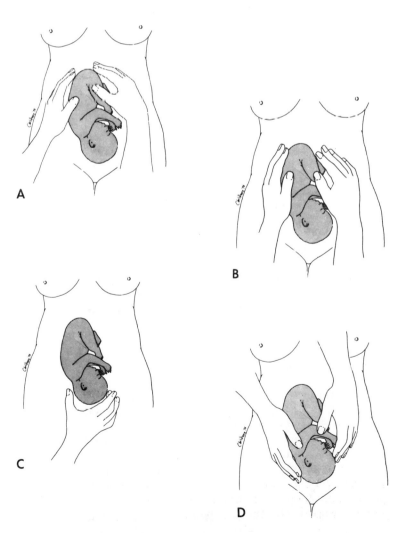

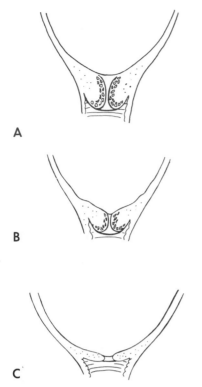

Figure 50–5. Effacement of cervix: *A*, none; *B*, partial; and *C*, complete. (From Romney, S., et al. (eds.): Gynecology and Obstetrics: The Health Care of Women. New York, McGraw-Hill, Inc., 1975. Used by permission.)

rection of the axis of the pelvic inlet (Fig. 50–4*D*). When the head is the presenting part, one examining hand will be stopped sooner than the other by a rounded body, the cephalic prominence, while the other hand continues more deeply into the pelvis. The cephalic prominence is felt on the same side as the small parts in vertex presentations and on the same side as the back in face presentations. In breech presentations, the information obtained from this maneuver is less precise.[1]

Vaginal Examination. Unless there has been bleeding in excess of a bloody show, a manual (not speculum) vaginal examination should be performed to identify fetal presentation and position and to assess the progress of labor.

First the vulva and perineal area are prepped with an antiseptic solution such as povidone-iodine. The woman is placed on a bedpan with her legs widely separated. Scrubbing is directed from anterior to posterior and away from the vaginal introitus; each sponge should be discarded after it passes over the anal region. A dry sponge placed on the introitus will prevent contaminated solution from running into the vagina.

Following preparation of the vulvar and perineal regions, the examiner uses the thumb and forefinger of a sterile-gloved hand to widely separate the labia to expose the vaginal opening; this prevents

the examining fingers from coming into contact with the inner surfaces of the labia. The index and second fingers of the other hand are then introduced into the vagina to perform the examination. Cervical effacement, dilatation, and fetal station are assessed. Fetal presentation and position are confirmed.[1]

Effacement of the cervix is the process of cervical thinning that occurs before and during the first stage of labor (Fig. 50–5). The degree of cervical effacement is assessed by palpation and is determined by the palpated length of the cervical canal compared with that of the uneffaced, or normal, cervical canal. Effacement is expressed as a percentage from 0 per cent, or totally uneffaced, to 100 per cent, or completely effaced. The completely effaced cervix is usually less than 0.25 cm thick.[3]

Cervical dilatation is determined by estimating the average diameter of the cervical os. The examining finger is swept from the cervical margin on one side across the cervical os to the opposite margin. The diameter transversed is expressed in centimeters. Ten cm constitutes full cervical dilatation. A diameter of less than 6 cm can be measured directly. For a diameter greater than 6 cm, it is frequently easier to determine the width of the remaining cervical rim and subtract twice that measurement from 10 cm. For example, if a 1-cm rim is felt, dilatation is 8 cm.

Station refers to the level of the presenting fetal part in the birth canal (Fig. 50–6). The ischial spines are used as the reference point. Zero station is used to denote that the presenting part is at the level of the ischial spines. When the presenting part lies above the spines, the distances are stated in negative figures, for example, −1 cm, −2 cm, −3 cm, and floating. If the presenting part is below the spines, the distances are stated in pos-

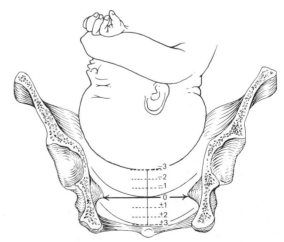

Figure 50–6. Station of the fetal head. (From Benson, R. C. (ed.): Current Obstetric and Gynecologic Diagnosis and Treatment, 3rd ed. Los Altos, California, Lange Medical Publications, 1980. Used by permission.)

itive figures, for examples, + 1 cm, + 2 cm, and + 3 cm. Determination is made by simple palpation.

Progressive cervical dilatation with no change in fetal station suggests fetopelvic disproportion.[1, 7]

Position and presentation of the fetus may be inconclusive before labor, because the presenting parts must be palpated through the lower uterine segment. After dilatation and effacement of the cervix, however, further delineation of presentation and position of the fetus may be made by vaginal examination.

After the perineal area has been appropriately prepped, as previously described, three maneuvers are used to determine fetal presentation and position. In the first maneuver, two fingers of the examiner's gloved hand are introduced into the vagina and advanced to the presenting part, differentiating face, vertex, and breech presentations. In vertex presentations, the examiner's fingers are carried up behind the symphysis pubis and then swept posteriorly over the fetal head toward the maternal sacrum, identifying the course of the sagittal suture. The positions of the two fontanels, located at opposite ends of the sagittal sutures, are then defined by palpation. The anterior fontanel is diamond-shaped; the posterior fontanel is triangular in shape (Fig. 50–7).

In face and breech presentations, the various parts are more readily distinguished. In breech presentations, the fetal sacrum is the point of reference; in face presentations, the easily identifiable fetal chin is used.

Auscultation. Auscultation of fetal heart tones is necessary to determine fetal well-being. The heart rate of the fetus can be identified with a stethoscope, a fetoscope, or a doppler placed firmly on the maternal abdominal wall overlying the fetal thorax and repositioned until fetal heart tones are heard. When a doppler is used, a conducting gel should be applied to the abdominal wall, interfacing with the doppler receiver. To avoid confusion of maternal and fetal heart sounds, the maternal pulse should be palpated as the fetal heart rate is auscultated.

Normal baseline fetal heart rate is 120 to 160 beats per minute. Changes in the fetal heart rate that are indicative of fetal distress are usually evident immediately after a uterine contraction. During labor, fetal distress is suspected if the fetal heart rate repeatedly drops below 120 beats per minute immediately following a contraction. If prolonged monitoring of labor is necessary in the emergency department, fetal heart sounds should be assessed immediately after a contraction at 15-minute intervals during the first stage of labor and at 5-minute intervals during the second stage of labor.[1]

Management of Fetal Distress. If fetal distress

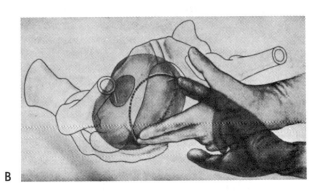

A

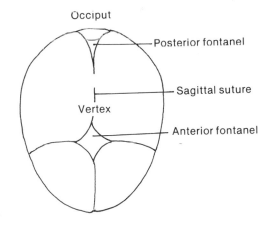

B

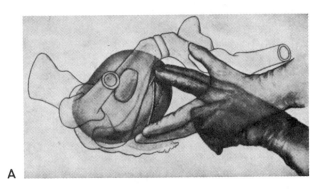

Occiput — Posterior fontanel

Vertex

Sagittal suture

Anterior fontanel

C

Figure 50–7. Locating the sagittal suture (A) and fontanels (B) on vaginal examination. C, Diagram of fontanels and sutures. (From Pritchard, J. A., and MacDonald, P. C.: William's Obstetrics, 16th ed. New York, Appleton-Century-Crofts, 1980. Used by permission.)

is suspected on the basis of fetal heart tones, changing of maternal position, typically into the left lateral recumbent position, may be beneficial. Maternal oxygen should be administered to improve fetal oxygenation. In the absence of bleeding, a vaginal examination should be performed to rule out the possibility of prolapse of the umbilical cord. The definitive therapy for fetal distress is delivery of the infant, either vaginally or by cesarean section.[3, 4]

Cord prolapse usually occurs at the same time as rupture of the membranes and is diagnosed by palpation of the umbilical cord on vaginal examination or by visualization of the cord protruding through the introitus. The incidence of cord prolapse in labor is approximately 0.5 per cent and most often occurs when the fetal presenting part does not completely fill the lower uterine segment during labor or when there is unusual mobility of the cord.[4] Cord prolapse is frequently encountered with breech presentation, multiple pregnancies, prematurity, and premature rupture of the membranes.

The management of cord prolapse is directed at sustaining fetal life until delivery is accomplished. Unless immediate delivery is feasible or the fetus is known to be dead, preparations should be made for an emergency cesarean section. Compression of the umbilical cord should be minimized by exerting manual pressure through the vagina to lift and maintain the presenting part away from the prolapsed cord. The patient should be placed in the knee-chest or deep Trendelenburg position. This position should be maintained until delivery is accomplished.[3]

With cord prolapse, the fetal prognosis is dependent upon presentation, gestation, and the timing of diagnosis and management. The perinatal mortality rate is approximately 25 per cent, with the associated high incidence of prematurity contributing to this rate.[4]

VAGINAL BLEEDING DURING THE THIRD TRIMESTER

Bleeding during the third trimester should always be considered an emergency. Profound shock secondary to exsanguinating hemorrhage may occur within minutes. Although bleeding may result from local vaginal and cervical lesions, genital lacerations, circumvallate placenta, vasa previa, or rupture of the uterus, placenta previa and premature separation of the placenta account for one half to two thirds of all cases.[8] *Placenta previa* refers to implantation of the placenta in the lower uterine segment with varying degrees of encroachment upon the cervical os. Occurring in 0.1 to 1.0 per cent of all pregnancies, placenta previa is characterized clinically by vaginal bleeding with little or no abdominal or pelvic pain. Premature separation of the placenta, or *abruptio placenta*, refers to separation of the placenta from its site of implantation in the uterus before delivery of the fetus and occurs in 0.2 to 2.4 per cent of all pregnancies. In contrast to placenta previa, abruptio placenta is associated with varying degrees of abdominal pain and uterine irritability. The degree of clinical shock may be out of proportion to the amount of apparent hemorrhage. Consumptive coagulopathy occurs in 20 to 38 per cent of all cases of abruptio placenta.[8]

As noted previously, third trimester vaginal bleeding should always be considered an emergency. Stabilization should be initiated with at least two large-bore intravenous lines. In addition to routine laboratory work-up and the taking of blood for type and cross-matching, clotting studies, including a fibrinogen level, should be drawn. Vaginal examination is *contraindicated* in the emergency department because of the possibility of tearing or dislodging a placenta previa, which may result in profuse, potentially fatal hemorrhage.[1] The patient should be immediately transferred to the care of her obstetrician for further evaluation. Definitive diagnosis via the "double set-up" examination has generally been replaced by localization of the placenta by ultrasound.[9, 10]

Delivery

Full dilatation of the cervix signifies the second stage of labor, heralding delivery of the infant. Typically, the patient begins to bear down and, with descent of the presenting part, develops the urge to defecate. Uterine contractions may last 1½ minutes and recur after a myometrial resting phase of less than 1 minute.

The mechanism of labor in vertex and breech presentations consists of engagement of the presenting part, flexion, descent, internal rotation, extension, external rotation or restitution, and expulsion (Fig. 50–8). The mechanism of labor is determined by the pelvic dimensions and configuration, the size of the fetus, and the strength of uterine contractions. Essentially, the fetus will follow the path of least resistance by adaptation of the smallest achievable diameters of the presenting part to the most favorable dimensions and contours of the birth canal.

The sequence of movements in vertex presentations is as follows:

1. **Engagement.** Usually occurring in the last 2 weeks of pregnancy in the primiparous patient and at the onset of labor in the multiparous patient, engagement refers to the mechanism by which the greatest transverse diameter of the head, the biparietal diameter in occiput presentations, passes through the pelvic inlet.

2. **Flexion.** Flexion of the head is necessary to minimize the presenting cross-sectional diameter of the head during passage through the smallest diameter of the bony pelvis. In most cases, flexion is necessary for both engagement and descent.

3. **Descent.** Descent is gradually progressive and is effected by uterine and abdominal contractions as well as by straightening and extension of the fetal body.

4. **Internal Rotations.** Internal rotation occurs with descent and is necessary for the head or presenting part to traverse the ischial spines. This

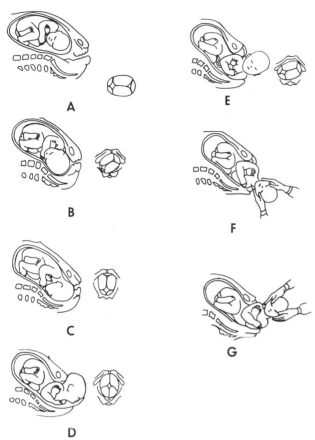

Figure 50–8. Mechanism of labor for cephalic presentation. A, Prior to labor. B, Engagement, flexion, and descent. C, Internal rotation extension. D, Extension to delivery of head. E, External rotation (restitution). F, Delivery of anterior shoulder. G, Delivery of posterior shoulder. Note that the head is being supported and guided in F and G. Traction is to be minimized. (From Romney, S., et al. (eds.): Gynecology and Obstetrics: The Health Care of Women. New York, McGraw-Hill, Inc., 1975. Used by permission.)

descend in a path similar to that traced by the head, rotating anteroposteriorly for delivery. First, the anterior shoulder is delivered beneath the symphysis pubis, followed by the posterior shoulder across the perineum. Expulsion of the remainder of the fetal body occurs with ease.

The mechanism of the labor for breech presentations varies (Fig. 50–9). Usually the hips engage in one of the oblique diameters of the pelvic inlet. As descent occurs, the anterior hip generally descends more rapidly than the posterior hip. Internal rotation occurs as the intertrochanteric diameter assumes the anteroposterior position. Lateral flexion occurs as the anterior hip catches beneath the symphysis pubis, allowing the posterior hip to be born first. The infant's body then rotates, allowing for engagement of the shoulders in an oblique orientation. There is gradual descent, with the anterior shoulder rotating to bring the shoulders into the anteroposterior diameter of the outlet. The anterior shoulder follows lateral flexion to appear beneath the symphysis, with the posterior shoulder delivered first as the body is supported. The head tends to engage in the same diameter as the shoulders. Subsequent flexion and descent of the head occurs, following the path of the shoulders. Internal rotation occurs toward the hollow of the sacrum.

Delivery of the infant will usually occur spontaneously. The role of the physician or attendant is principally to provide control of the birth process, preventing forceful, sudden expulsion or extraction of the infant with resultant fetal and maternal injury.

MANAGEMENT OF DELIVERY

Equipment (Fig. 50–10)

OB pack (sterile)
  1 large basin (for placenta)
  1 pair of scissors
  2 medium Kelly clamps or umbilical tape
  1 bulb syringe or DeLee suction trap*
  1 double grip cord clamp
  3 small sterile towels
  1 package of gauze sponges
  1 baby blanket
  2 pairs of sterile gloves
  Sterile tubes for placental blood collection
Optional
  Infant resuscitation tray
  Warm blankets
  Name bands
  Heated isolette or Sterile Infant Swaddler†

*Argyle Manufacturing Company, St. Joseph, Missouri
†American Hospital Supply Company, McGaw Park, Illinois

movement is essentially a turning of the head such that the occiput gradually moves from its original, more transverse position, anteriorly toward the symphysis pubis or, less commonly, posteriorly toward the hollow of the sacrum.

5. **Extension.** Following internal rotation, the sharply flexed head reaches the anteriorly directed vulvar outlet, undergoing extension. With increasing distention of the perineum and vaginal opening, an increasingly larger portion of the occiput appears gradually. The head is born by further extension as the occiput, bregma, forehead, nose, mouth, and finally chin pass successively over the anterior margin of the perineum.

Immediately after its birth, the head drops downward such that the chin lies over the maternal anal region.

6. **External Rotation.** External rotation or restitution follows delivery of the head as it rotates to the transverse position that it occupied at engagement. Following this movement, the shoulders

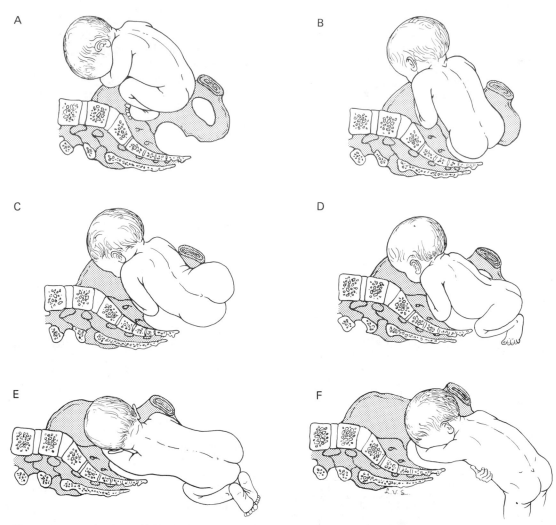

Figure 50–9. Mechanism of labor for breech presentation. *A,* Prior to labor. *B,* Engagement of the buttocks, internal rotation. *C,* Lateral flexion of the trunk, delivery of the buttocks. *D,* External rotation of the buttocks, engagement of the shoulders. *E,* Internal rotation of the shoulders, delivery of the posterior shoulder. *F,* Lateral flexion of the trunk, delivery of the anterior shoulder. (From Benson, R. C. (ed.): Current Obstetric and Gynecologic Diagnosis and Treatment, 3rd ed. Los Altos, California, Lange Medical Publications, 1980. Used by permission.)

Figure 50–10. OB pack.

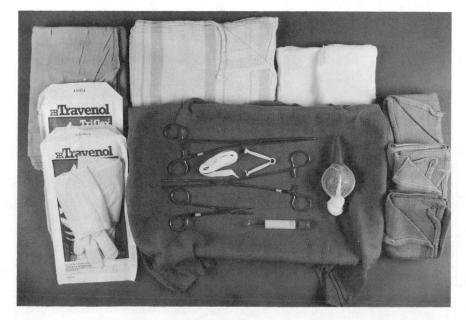

Technique

Owing to the high bacterial content of the vagina and perineum, complete sterility is not a priority.[11] When time permits, however, sterile technique should be used. The hands should be cleansed and sterilely gloved. The perineum should be cleansed as described for vaginal examination and draped such that only the immediate area about the vulva is exposed. Care should be taken to avoid fecal contamination of the infant. Equipment in the OB pack should be sterile.

General Considerations. The patient should be positioned on a stretcher with her hips and knees partially flexed, the thighs abducted, and the soles of the feet placed firmly on the stretcher. The delivery position may be enhanced by placing the patient's buttocks on the underside of a sterile bedpan, providing up to 5 inches of additional space between the bed and the perineum.[11]

Vertex Delivery. Spontaneous delivery of the vertex-presenting infant is divided into three phases: delivery of the head, delivery of the shoulders, and delivery of the body and legs.

Delivery should be anticipated when the presenting part reaches the pelvic floor. With each contraction, the perineum bulges increasingly and the vulvovaginal opening becomes more and more dilated by the fetal head. Just prior to delivery, "crowning" occurs; the head is visible at the vaginal introitus, and the widest portion, or biparietal diameter, of the head distends the vulva.

Gentle, gradual, controlled delivery is desirable. As the fetal head becomes progressively more visible, one palm of the physician's hand is placed over the occipital area, providing gentle pressure to control delivery of the head. *Explosive delivery of the head should be avoided.* The other hand, preferably draped with a sterile towel to protect it from the anus, may exert forward pressure on the chin of the fetus through the perineum just in front of the coccyx in a modified Ritgen maneuver (Fig. 50–11). This maneuver will extend the neck at the proper time, thereby protecting the maternal perineal musculature.

The head is gently supported during subsequent delivery of the forehead, face, chin, and neck.

After the head has been delivered, the infant's face and mouth should be quickly wiped and the oral cavity and nares should be suctioned with a bulb syringe. This will minimize the chance of aspiration of amnionic fluid, debris, and blood, which may occur with inspiration during delivery of the thorax.

With delivery of the neck, a finger should be passed around the neck to determine whether it is encircled by one or more coils of the umbilical cord (Fig. 50–12). If a cord is felt, it should cautiously be loosened and gently slipped over the infant's head. If this cannot be done easily, the cord should be doubly clamped and cut and the

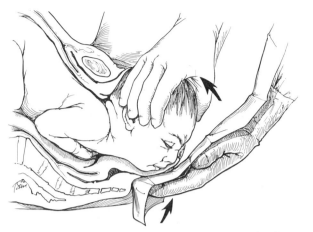

Figure 50–11. Modified Ritgen maneuver. (From Pritchard, J. A., and MacDonald, P. C.: William's Obstetrics, 16th ed. New York, Appleton.-Century-Crofts, 1980. Used by permission.)

infant should be delivered *promptly*. In approximately 15 to 20 per cent of deliveries, the umbilical cord is around the infant's neck but is rarely tight enough to cause fetal hypoxia.[1]

Just prior to external rotation, the head usually falls posteriorly, bringing it almost into contact with the anus. As rotation occurs, the head assumes a transverse position and the transverse diameter of the thorax or bisacromial diameter rotates into the anteroposterior diameter of the pelvis. In most cases the shoulders are born spontaneously. Delivery may be aided by grasping the sides of the head and exerting *gentle* downward (posterior) traction until the anterior shoulder appears beneath the symphysis pubis. The head is then *gently* lifted upward to aid the delivery of the posterior shoulder (see Fig. 50–8).[6, 7] The remainder of the body usually follows without difficulty.

Delivery may be assisted by *gentle* traction on the head after the shoulders have been freed. Hooking the fingers in the axilla during delivery

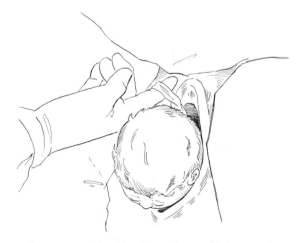

Figure 50–12. Checking for cord around infant's neck.

may result in brachial plexus injury, hematoma of the neck, or fracture of the clavicle; thus, it should be avoided. Furthermore, traction should always be exerted in the direction of the long axis of the child; if applied obliquely, traction may cause bending of the neck and excessive stretching of the brachial plexus.[1, 3, 11, 12]

As soon as the infant is delivered, it should be held with the head lower than the body, at an angle of not greater than 15 degrees to facilitate drainage of accumulated mucus and bronchial secretions in the airway. The infant's airway should be thoroughly suctioned. Although some controversy exists as to the optimal position of the infant in relation to the mother during this stage, most authorities recommend that the infant be placed at or below the level of the vaginal introitus for 30 seconds before the cord is clamped.[1, 13] This will allow up to 100 ml of blood to be transfused from the placental circulation into the infant.[1]

The umbilical cord should be cut 30 to 60 seconds after delivery. Blood samples from the placental end of the cord should be collected for determination of infant serology, including rhesus factor (Rh) studies. Two sterile clamps should be placed several inches apart, and the cord between the clamps should be cut with sterile scissors. A sterile cord clamp or cord tie of umbilical (cloth) tape is then placed around the cord, approximately 1 centimeter distal to the skin edge of the cord insertion site (navel).[1, 3, 11]

Immediately following the cutting of the umbilical cord, the infant should briefly be evaluated and, if necessary, resuscitation should be initiated. Because of the relatively large surface area of the neonate, attention should be directed toward maintaining body temperature by placing the neonate in a heated isolette, Sterile Infant Swaddler, or using warm blankets.[1, 3]

Delivery of the Placenta. Placental separation usually occurs within 5 minutes following delivery of the infant and may be recognized by the following signs:

1. The uterus becomes globular and firmer as it contracts.
2. The uterine fundus rises in the abdomen.
3. There is a sudden gush of blood.
4. The umbilical cord protrudes further out of the vagina, indicating placental descent.

Intra-abdominal pressure produced by the mother may be enough to effect complete expulsion of the placenta. If maternal force alone is insufficient to expel the placenta, it may be recovered by the Brandt–Andrews maneuver as follows (Fig. 50–13): One hand is placed on the abdomen just above the symphysis pubis. Pressure is used to elevate the uterus into the abdomen while the placenta is expressed into the vagina. The cord is kept slightly taut to help guide the placenta out of the birth canal. As the placenta passes through the introitus, fundal pressure is stopped and the placenta is gently lifted away from the introitus. Membranes that are adherent to the uterine lining should be grasped with a clamp or ring forceps and removed by *gentle* traction. Traction should never be used to pull the placenta out of the uterus, since traction may result in uterine inversion. The placenta should be examined for completeness and saved for later evaluation by the obstetrician.[1]

The uterus should be palpated and elevated when the third stage of labor has been completed.

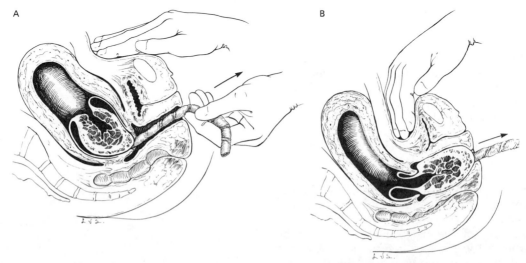

Figure 50–13. Delivery of the placenta using the Brandt-Andrews maneuver. A, The uterus is elevated into the abdomen as gentle traction is exerted on the cord. B, Pressure is exerted between the uterine fundus and the symphysis, forcing the uterus upward and the placenta outward. (From Benson, R. C. (ed.): Current Obstetric and Gynecologic Diagnosis and Treatment, 3rd ed. Los Altos, California, Lange Medical Publications, 1980. Used by permission.)

Firm compression of the uterus may express clots and stimulate the uterus to contract, reducing total blood loss. If there is persistent bleeding from a flaccid uterus, gentle massage and oxytocics may be used as necessary.[1, 3] Oxytocics should not be used prior to placental delivery during the third stage of delivery, because the resultant uterine contraction may entrap the placenta within the uterus. Use of oxytocics before delivery of an undiagnosed second twin may prove fatal to the entrapped fetus.

Oxytocin (Pitacin) is the most commonly used oxytocic and is usually given by intravenous infusion. Twenty units of oxytocin are added to 1 L of normal saline and are given at a rate of 10 ml per minute for several minutes until the uterus remains firmly contracted and bleeding is controlled. The infusion rate is then reduced to 1 to 2 ml per minute. If an intravenous line is not available, 5 to 10 IU (0.5–1.0 ml) of oxytocin may be given intramuscularly. An injection of 0.2 mg methylergonovine maleate (Methergine) may be given intramuscularly as an alternative. Because methylergonovine may cause serious hypertension and seizures, it is contraindicated in patients with hypertension and preeclampsia.[1]

Occasionally, the placenta may fail to separate completely, resulting in a retained placenta or placental fragments, with persistent uterine bleeding. Manual removal of the placenta, exploration of the uterine cavity for retained products, and, occasionally, hysterectomy are indicated. These procedures are beyond the scope of emergency department care and should be left to the obstetrician. The patient should be supported with intravenous fluid, blood, and fresh frozen plasma as indicated until definitive therapy is available. Constant firm *uterine massage* can lessen hemorrhage and may be lifesaving.

Shoulder Dystocia

The term *shoulder dystocia* refers to impaction of the fetal shoulders in the pelvic outlet occurring after delivery of the head in vertex presentations. Occurring more commonly with large infants, shoulder dystocia is a serious and at times fatal complication. Swartz sites an overall incidence of 0.15 per cent, increasing to 1.7 per cent in infants weighing nore than 4000 g.[14] Impaction of the fetal shoulders and thorax in the maternal pelvis prohibits adequate respiration; compression of the umbilical cord frequently compromises fetal circulation.

Management. General anesthesia is desirable but is seldom available in the emergency department. A wide episiotomy will reduce the incidence of major perineal lacerations and provide additional space for manipulation. Frequently, placing the mother in the extreme lithotomy position with her hips completely flexed, allowing the knees to rest upon her chest, will cause the fetal shoulders to engage appropriately and will allow delivery to progress.[15, 16] If this simple change in maternal position fails to effect delivery, the infant should immediately be examined. The examiner's hand is inserted as far within the birth canal as possible to rule out the possibility of a fetal tumor or anomaly as the cause of obstruction. If no anomaly is found, two maneuvers are commonly used to effect delivery (Fig. 50–14). In the first maneuver, rotation of the shoulder girdle into one of the oblique pelvic diameters may be accomplished by applying pressure to the infant's posterior scapula, rotating it upward and anteriorly. When the bisacromial diameter has been dislodged from the anteroposterior diameter of the pelvis, fundal pressure alone may result in advancement of the anterior shoulder. If advancement does not occur, Wood's "screw principle" may be used. Rotation of the shoulders is continued anteriorly in a screw-like motion until the posterior shoulder passes beneath the symphysis pubis and is delivered as an anterior shoulder.[1, 14, 17]

If rotation is unsuccessful, delivery of the infant's posterior arm may be used to effect delivery. The physician's hand is passed into the uterus along the hollow of the sacrum, bringing down the entire posterior arm by flexing the elbow, looping a finger around the forearm, and delivering it. Frequently, the anterior shoulder usually follows without difficulty. If the anterior shoulder cannot be delivered, rotation of the shoulder girdle into one of the oblique diameters of the pelvis will aid delivery.[1, 18] This maneuver is highly effective but may result in uterine rupture and other serious lacerations of the maternal perineum.[3]

Cleidotomy, division of the clavicles to reduce the bulk of the shoulder girdle, is the ultimate solution for cases of shoulder dystocia but should be done only under the direct supervision of the obstetrician.

Breech Delivery

When compared with cephalic presentations, the breech delivery is associated with a greater incidence of prematurity, prolapsed cord, low implantation of the placenta, uterine and congenital abnormalities, multiple pregnancies, and increased perinatal morbidity and mortality rates.[1, 3, 9, 19] The incidence of breech presentation varies inversely with gestational age and weight. At term, the incidence of breech presentation is 3 to 4 per cent; from 28 to 38 weeks, 17 per cent; and at less than 28 weeks gestation, 40 per cent.[20]

Although increased rates of prematurity and congenital anomalies associated with breech presentation account for much of the perinatal loss, when these factors are excluded, the perinatal

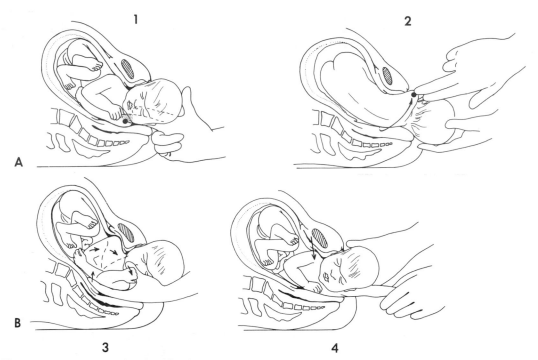

Figure 50–14. Maneuvers for shoulder dystocia. *A*, Rotation: 1. Rotation of the posterior shoulder; 2. Delivery of the rotated shoulder. *B*, Delivery of the posterior arm: 3. Flexion of the posterior arm. 4. Delivery of the posterior arm to permit delivery of the anterior shoulder. (From Romney, S., et al. (eds.): Gynecology and Obstetrics: The Health Care of Women. New York, McGraw-Hill, Inc., 1975. Used by permission.)

mortality rate for breech remains three to four times that for vertex presentations.[21, 22] Fetal distress also occurs more frequently. Whereas umbilical cord prolapse occurs in only 0.3 to 0.5 per cent of vertex presentations, the incidence rate increases to 3.8 to 5.2 per cent in breech presentations.[20] Prolapse occurs more commonly with footling and incomplete presentations than with frank breech. Frank breech is the most frequent type of breech presentation, occurring in approximately 65 per cent of the cases; complete breech occurs in about 10 per cent of the cases and footling or incomplete breech occurs in about 20 per cent.[3]

The increased use of cesarean section has greatly decreased the morbidity and mortality associated with breech delivery. Although cesarean section is now recognized as the standard of care, vaginal delivery may be the method of choice in carefully selected cases.[22, 23] The emergency physician will seldom, if ever, be called upon to make the decision as to the most appropriate means of delivery but, rather, could be faced with the imminent vaginal delivery of the breech infant. Breech delivery is most appropriately performed with both a physician and an assistant present.

Types. There are three types of vaginal breech delivery.

Spontaneous Breech. This type of delivery is that in which the infant is delivered spontaneously without any manipulation or traction other than supporting the infant. Although this form of de-

livery is rare with term infants, there is little associated traumatic morbidity.

Partial Breech Extraction. In this type of delivery, the infant is delivered spontaneously as far as the umbilicus; the remainder of the body is extracted.

Total Breech Extraction. The entire body of the infant is extracted by the physician in total breech-extraction.

Delivery is easier and perinatal morbidity and mortality are reduced when the breech is born spontaneously to the level of the umbilicus.[1, 24] If fetal distress develops before this time, however, a decision must be made whether to perform a total breech extraction or prepare for cesarean section. Total breech extraction is indicated only if there is a definite diagnosis of fetal distress and cesarean section cannot be performed promptly. To perform any vaginal breech delivery, the birth canal must be sufficiently large to allow passage of the fetus without trauma and the cervix must be completely effaced and dilated. If these conditions do not exist, a cesarean section is indicated. To ensure full cervical dilatation in the footling or complete breech, it is important that the feet, legs, and buttocks advance through the introitus to the level of the fetal umbilicus before the physician intervenes in delivery and further extraction is attempted. *The mere appearance of the feet through the vulva is not in itself an indication to proceed with delivery.*

Technique. If fetal distress is documented and

total extraction is deemed necessary, the following procedures are carried out. The physician's hand is introduced into the vagina, and both feet of the fetus are grasped, with the index finger placed between the fetal ankles. Gentle traction is applied until the feet are pulled through the vulva (Fig. 50–15). At this point, a wide episiotomy is usually made. Because the legs are slippery and difficult to hold owing to vernix caseosa, they should be wrapped in a sterile towel as they emerge through the vulva. Downward gentle traction is continued as successively higher portions of the legs and thighs are grasped (Fig. 50–16). When the breech appears at the vulva, gentle traction is applied until the hips are delivered. As the buttocks emerge, the fetal back usually rotates anteriorly. The thumbs of the physician are then placed over the sacrum while the fingers are placed over the hips, and gentle downward traction is continued (Fig. 50–17). As the scapulas emerge, the infant usually rotates back to its original position, with the back directed laterally.

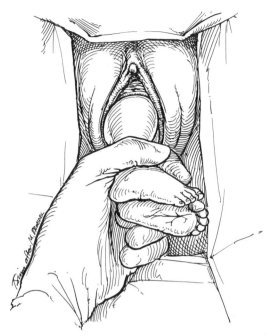

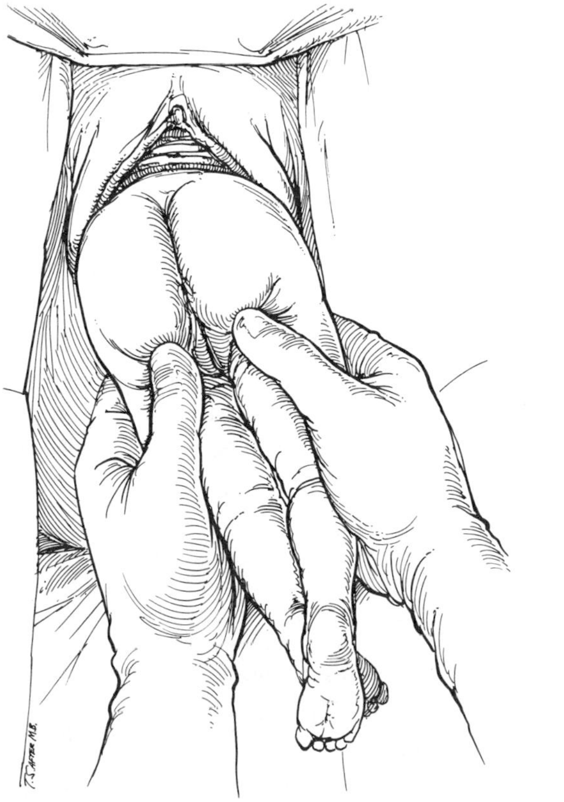

Figure 50–15. Breech extraction. Traction of the feet and ankles. Note that the index finger is placed between the ankles. (From Pritchard, J. A., and MacDonald, P. C.: William's Obstetrics, 16th ed. New York, Appleton-Century-Crofts, 1980. Used by permission.)

Figure 50–16. Breech extraction. Traction of the legs and thighs. (From Taylor, E. S.: Obstetrics and Fetal Medicine, 2nd ed. Baltimore, Williams & Wilkins, 1977. Used by permission.)

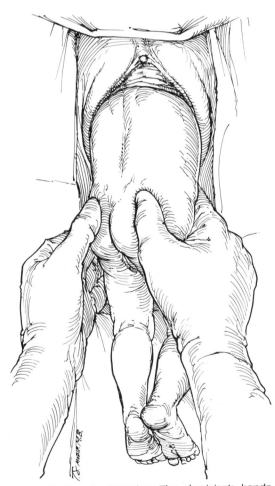

Figure 50–17. Breech extraction. The physician's hands are placed over the infant's sacrum to deliver the body. (From Taylor, E. S.: Obstetrics and Fetal Medicine, 2nd ed. Baltimore, Williams & Wilkins, 1977. Used by permission.)

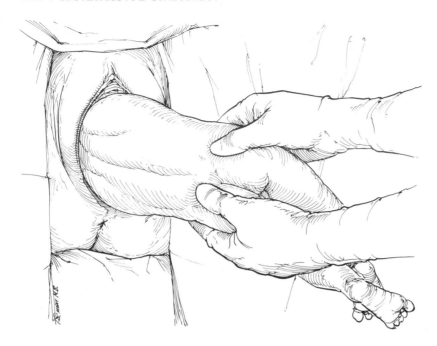

Figure 50–18. Breech extraction. Rotation occurs as the scapulae emerge. (From Taylor, E. S.: Obstetrics and Fetal Medicine, 2nd ed. Baltimore, Williams & Wilkins, 1977. Used by permission.)

If spontaneous rotation does not occur, slight rotation should be added to the traction to bring the bisacromial diameter of the fetus into the anteroposterior diameter of the pelvis (Fig. 50–18). Delivery of the shoulders should not be attempted until the lower halves of the scapula are delivered outside the vulva and the axilla becomes visible at the introitus. Two methods of shoulder delivery are commonly used. In this first method, with the scapulas visible, the trunk is rotated such that the anterior arm and shoulder appear at the vulva and can be easily released and delivered. The body of the fetus is then rotated in the reverse direction to deliver the other shoulder and arm beneath the symphysis pubis. In the second method, if trunk rotation is unsuccessful, the posterior shoulder must be delivered first. The feet are grasped in one hand and drawn upward over the mother's groin. In this manner, leverage is exerted on the posterior shoulder, which slides out over the perineal margin, usually followed by the arm and hand. The anterior shoulder, arm, and hand are then delivered beneath the symphysis pubis by downward traction on the fetal body (Fig. 50–19).

Occasionally, spontaneous delivery of the arm and hand will not follow delivery of the shoulder. If this occurs, upward traction of the fetal body should be continued after delivery of the posterior shoulder. Two fingers of the physician are then passed along the fetal humerus until the fetal elbow is reached. The fingers are used to splint the fetal arm, which is then swept downward and delivered. The anterior arm may then be delivered by depression of the fetal body alone. In some cases it may be necessary to sweep the anterior arm down over the thorax using two fingers as a splint.

After the shoulders appear, the head usually occupies one of the oblique diameters of the pelvis, with the chin directed posteriorly. The head may then be extracted using the Mauriceau maneuver. With the fetal body resting upon the physician's palm and forearm, the index and middle finger of the hand are placed over the infant's maxilla, flexing the fetal head. Two fingers of the other hand are hooked over the fetal neck, and, grasping the shoulders, downward traction is applied until the suboccipital region appears under the symphysis pubis (Fig. 50–20). As the body of the fetus is then elevated toward the mother's abdomen, the fetal mouth, nose, brow, and eventually occiput successively emerge over the perineum. Suprapubic pressure applied by an assistant is helpful in delivery of the head. If delivery of the head is not effected by the Mauriceau maneuver, forceps delivery may be necessary. Forceps application is beyond the scope of this text.

At times, delivery of a frank breech may be necessary. Facilitated by an episiotomy, the breech should be allowed to deliver spontaneously as far as possible. Moderate traction may be exerted by a finger placed in each fetal groin (Fig. 50–21). Once the knees appear outside the birth canal, the legs may be slowly flexed to assist delivery, which usually occurs without trauma.

Complications. Traumatic morbidity associated with breech presentations is approximately twelve times that of vertex presentations and is directly related to the manipulations used to effect delivery and the relationship of fetal size to that of the maternal pelvis.[25] One of the most significant features of breech delivery is that progressively increasing diameters and less distensible fetal parts must traverse the maternal pelvis.

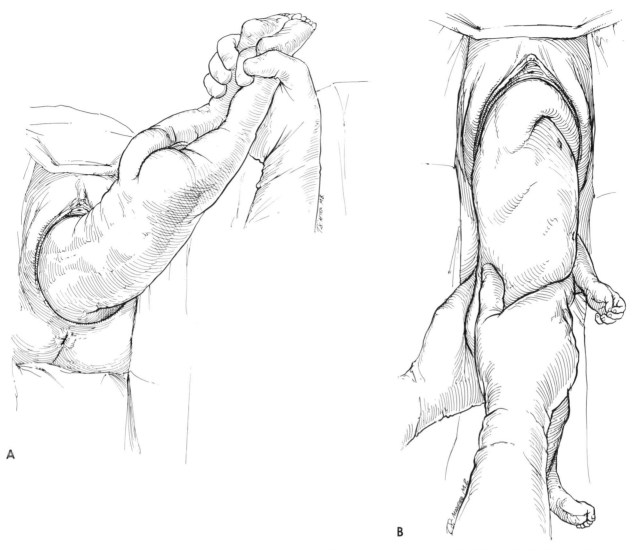

50–19. Breech extraction. *A*, Delivery of the posterior shoulder by upward traction on the fetal body. *B*, Delivery of the anterior shoulder beneath the symphysis by downward traction. (From Taylor, E. S.: Obstetrics and Fetal Medicine, 2nd ed. Baltimore, Williams & Wilkins, 1977. Used by permission.)

Figure 50–20. Mauriceau maneuver: delivery of the aftercoming head. While suprapubic pressure is applied by an assistant, the head is gently flexed by pressure on the mandible. (From Taylor, E. S.: Obstetrics and Fetal Medicine, 2nd ed. Baltimore, Williams & Wilkins, 1977. Used by permission.)

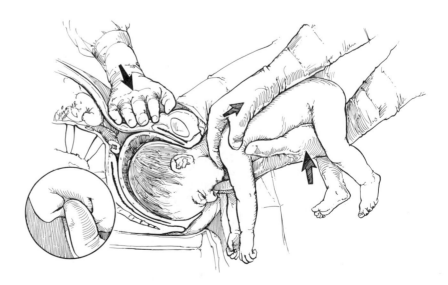

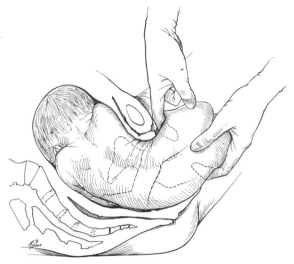

Figure 50–21. Extraction of a frank breech by moderate traction exerted with a finger in each groin. (From Pritchard, J. A., and MacDonald, P. C.: William's Obstetrics, 16th ed. New York, Appleton-Century-Crofts, 1980. Used by permission.)

If cephalopelvic disproportion is not diagnosed until the fetal body has been delivered and if the fetal head will not descend, the prognosis is grave. In addition, whereas in vertex presentations, in which moulding the fetal head is gradual, occurring over the course of hours, in breech presentation, moulding is abrupt, subjecting the delicate supporting tissues of the aftercoming head to sudden and often violent stresses. Intracranial hemorrhage is the most frequent cause of death in breech delivery, with injury to the spinal cord, liver, adrenal glands, and spleen occurring in decreasing order of frequency.[1, 26]

Both assisted breech delivery and breech extraction involve a change in motive powers for delivery, substituting traction from below for pressure from above and inreasing the probability of occurrence of unilateral or bilateral nuchal arms or hyperextension of the fetal head. Decomposition and extraction of a frank breech infant carry significantly increased fetal risks and impose additional maternal risks because of intrauterine manipulation. The fact that manipulation does indeed correlate with traumatic morbidity was illustrated by Ravinsky and coworkers, who found that, whereas spontaneous breech delivery was associated with no traumatic complications, increasing degrees of obstetric manipulation corresponded to progressive elevations of the traumatic morbidity rate.[25] The highest traumatic maternal morbidity rate, 8.3 per cent, which is ten times the rate for assisted breech delivery and four times the rate for breech extraction, occurred with breech decomposition and extraction.

Episiotomy

An episiotomy is an incision of the posterior vaginal wall and a portion of the pudenda, which is made to enlarge the vaginal introitus to permit easier passage of the fetus and to prevent perineal lacerations of the mother, preserving the structure and function of the vaginal introitus. An episiotomy helps to minimize compression and trauma of the fetal head; facilitates the second stage of labor by removing the resistance of the pudendal musculature; substitutes a straight surgical incision for the ragged laceration that frequently results from tearing of the musculature; and reduces the incidence of subsequent symptomatic cystocele, rectocele, and uterine prolapse. It is generally recommended that an episiotomy be performed for most breech deliveries; for deliveries in primiparous patients when possible; to facilitate delivery of premature infants; and when a perineal tear is imminent.[3]

Although both the median and mediolateral episiotomy are commonly described (Fig. 50–22), the median episiotomy is usually preferred.[4, 27, 28] A median incision is the easiest type of episiotomy to perform and repair, results in the least amount of blood loss, and heals rapidly with minimal discomfort. The only disadvantage to the median incision is occasional accidental extension of the incision through the anal sphincter or through the sphincter into the rectum, resulting in third and fourth degree lacerations, respectively. There is minimal morbidity if laceration of the rectal sphincter is recognized early and is properly repaired. Failure to repair the sphincter, however,

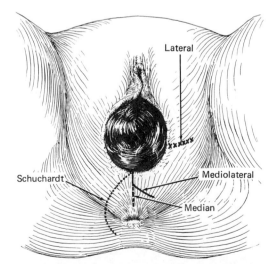

Figure 50–22. Types of episiotomy. Median and mediolateral are those most commonly performed. (From Benson, R. C. (ed.): Current Obstetric and Gynecologic Diagnosis and Treatment, 3rd ed. Los Altos, California, Lange Medical Publications, 1980. Used by permission.)

often leads to incontinence and a rectovaginal fistula. Although a mediolateral episiotomy seldom results in extension through the anal sphincter, with this type of episiotomy blood loss is generally greater, it is more difficult to repair, and painful healing and postpartum dyspareunia often result.

PROCEDURE

Equipment

Tissue scissors or scalpel (with tongue blade)
3-0 or 2-0 absorbable suture on atraumatic needle (e.g., chromic catgut or polyglycolic acid)
Needle holder
Suture scissors
Gauze pack

Technique

The episiotomy should be timed so that it precedes trauma to the maternal tissues and fetus but avoids excessive maternal blood loss before delivery. With vertex presentations, the episiotomy should be performed when the fetal head begins to distend the perineum and the caput becomes visible to a diameter of 3 to 4 cm during a contraction.[1, 28] With breech delivery, the episiotomy is usually performed as the fetal buttocks distend the vulva but occasionally may not be necessary until delivery of the head.[4] Anesthesia for episiotomy in the emergency department is usually limited to local infiltration of the perineum with 1 or 2 per cent lidocaine.

The episiotomy is a simple incision that extends through the skin and subcutaneous tissues, the vaginal mucosa, the urogenital septum, the superior fascia of the pelvic diaphragm, and, if the episiotomy is mediolateral and deep, through the lowermost fibers of the puborectalis portion of the levator ani muscles. The incision may be made with either a scissors or a scalpel. When using a scalpel, a tongue blade is placed between the infant's head and the maternal perineum as the perineum is incised. For the median episiotomy, the incision is made through the median raphe of the perineum almost to the anal sphincter (Fig. 50–23). For the mediolateral episiotomy, the incision is directed downward and outward in the direction of the lateral margin of the anal sphincter and may be either to the right or to the left (see Fig. 50–22).

Following delivery of the infant and placenta, the episiotomy is repaired. The goals of episiotomy repair are to restore anatomy and achieve adequate hemostasis with a minimum of suture material. It is preferable to perform the closure after delivery

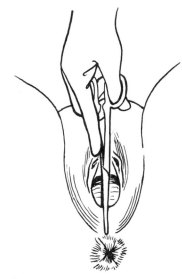

Figure 50–23. Midline episiotomy. (From Romney, S., et al. (eds.): Gynecology and Obstetrics: The Health Care of Women. New York, McGraw-Hill, Inc., 1975. Used by permission.)

of the placenta and following inspection and repair of the cervix and upper vaginal canal. The same principles of repair are followed for both the median (Fig. 50–24) and mediolateral (Fig. 50–25) episiotomy.

Because there is minimal tension on the closed wound, most authorities recommend the use of 3-0 or 2-0 chromic catgut or polyglycolic acid on a large, atraumatic needle. The first step is to close the vaginal mucosa using a continuous suture from the apex of the incision to the mucocutaneous junction, reapproximating the margins of the hymenal ring. Burying the closing knot in the incision, not at the hymenal ring, will minimize the amount of scar tissue and prevent tenderness and dyspareunia. All large actively bleeding vessels should be separately ligated during closure with separate absorbable suture ligatures. Next, the perineal musculature is reapproximated with three or four interrupted sutures. Closure of the superficial layers may be accomplished by one of two methods. In the first method, a continuous suture is used to close the superficial fascia from the mucocutaneous junction outward and is then continued upward as a subcuticular skin closure, returning to and ending at the mucocutaneous junction. Alternatively, several interrupted sutures may be placed through the skin and subcutaneous fascia and loosely tied. This last method of skin closure avoids burying two layers of suture in the more superficial layers of the perineum.

Alternatively, one continuous suture may be used to close the entire episiotomy in three layers. First, the vaginal mucosa is sutured as previously described. The suture is then inverted below the hymenal ring and continued outwardly, reapprox-

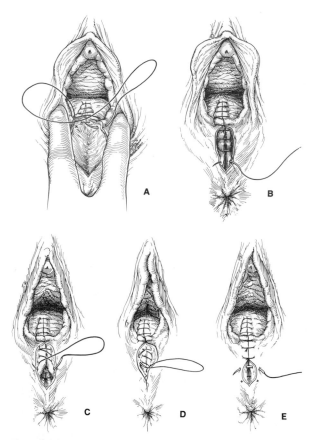

Figure 50–24. Closure of median episiotomy. A, Closure of mucosa and hymenal ring with continuous suture. B, Approximation of perineal musculature with interrupted sutures. C, Continuous suture to unite superficial fascia. D, Completion of repair by carrying continuous suture upward as a subcuticular stitch. E, Alternatively, closure of the superficial fascia and skin (C and D) may be accomplished by a series of loosely tied interrupted sutures. (From Pritchard, J. A., and MacDonald, P. C.: William's Obstetrics, 16th ed. New York, Appleton-Century-Crofts, 1980. Used by permission.)

imating the deep tissue. The skin and subcutaneous fascia are closed with a continuous subcuticular stitch carried upward and ending at the hymenal ring.

During episiotomy closure, it is helpful to maintain a dry field by inserting a large gauze pack in the vagina, leaving a tail or portion of the pack outside the vagina to aid in removal after the repair.

The most common complication of episiotomy is hematoma formation owing to inadequate hemostasis; a hematoma is treated by evacuation and drainage. Occasionally, large bleeding vessels will require delayed ligation. Postpartum episiotomy pain can usually be controlled by analgesics and local heat or sitz baths. Infection is a rare complication and responds readily to adequate drainage and appropriate antibiotic therapy.

Immediate Postpartum Hemorrhage

Postpartum hemorrhage, defined as maternal blood loss greater than 500 ml during the 24 hours following delivery, is the most common cause of serious obstetrical hemorrhage and accounts for up to 25 per cent of obstetrical deaths caused by hemorrhage.[1] Postpartum hemorrhage is conventionally divided into immediate hemorrhage occurring within 12 to 24 hours of delivery and delayed hemorrhage occurring more than 24 hours after delivery.

Postpartum hemorrhage is frequently characterized by steady moderate bleeding that persists until serious hypovolemia develops rather than by sudden massive hemorrhage. Because of the relative hypervolemia that occurs during normal preg-

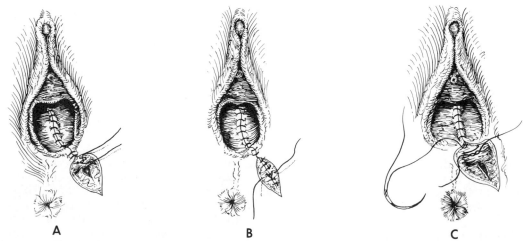

Figure 50–25. Closure of mediolateral episiotomy. A, Continuous suture for closure of vaginal mucosa and hymenal ring. B, Approximation of levator ani and perineal musculature. C, Closure of skin. (From Benson, R. C. (ed.): Current Obstetric and Gynecologic Diagnosis and Treatment, 3rd ed. Los Altos, California, Lange Medical Publications, 1980. Used by permission.)

nancy, blood loss may exceed 1500 ml before significant clinical changes in pulse and blood pressure become manifest.[29] Careful observation for blood loss, including evaluation of uterine size and consistency, is therefore mandatory during the early postpartum period.

The most common causes of immediate postpartum hemorrhage, in order of frequency, are uterine atony, lacerations of the vagina and cervix, and retained placenta or placental fragments. Less commonly, coagulation disorders, uterine rupture, uterine inversion, and paravaginal vessel laceration result in postpartum blood loss.[3, 30]

MANAGEMENT

Management of postpartum hemorrhage consists of replacement of intravascular volume with crystalloid and blood products as needed, as well as therapy directed toward the cause of hemorrhage. The diagnosis of uterine atony, the most common cause of bleeding, is made when uterine palpation reveals a soft "boggy" uterine corpus. Although the diagnosis may be suspected on the basis of abdominal examination alone, bimanual pelvic examination is frequently necessary to confirm the diagnosis.

Uterine atony is managed by manual massage of the uterine fundus (Fig. 50–26). One hand of the physician is used to compress and massage the posterior aspect of the uterus through the abdominal wall while the knuckles of the other sterile gloved hand are used to gently massage the anterior aspect of the uterus through the vaginal wall. Oxytocics should be administered in con-

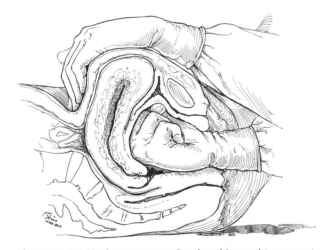

Figure 50–26. Uterine massage. One hand is used to massage the posterior aspect of the uterus through the abdominal wall. The other hand, inserted in the vagina, compresses the anterior uterus. (From Pritchard, J. A., and MacDonald, P. C.: William's Obstetrics, 16th ed. New York, Appleton-Century-Crofts, 1980. Used by permission.)

junction with massage. Packing the uterus, formerly a common procedure, is contraindicated in the immediate postpartum period and may result in uterine dilatation with concealed, potentially fatal hemorrhage.[1]

If vaginal bleeding persists despite uterine massage and a firmly contracted uterus, a cause other than uterine atony should be suspected. The labia, vagina, and cervix should be carefully inspected for lacerations. Bleeding from lacerations may be controlled by direct pressure or, in the case of cervical lacerations, by gentle application of the ring forceps to the bleeding point. Absorbable sutures may be used to control bleeding from easily accessible lacerations. Because adequate visualization of the cervix and upper vagina is difficult and repair of extensive lacerations frequently requires general anesthesia, repair of these lacerations is often better left to the obstetrician.

Although rare, occurring in approximately 1 in 4000 to 5000 deliveries, *uterine inversion* usually manifests with dramatic hemorrhage and shock occurring in 27 to 39 per cent of the patients.[28] Diagnosis is made by visualization and palpation of the soft, pear-shaped fundal wall near the cervical os or extending through it. On abdominal examination, no mass representing the uterine corpus can be palpated above the symphysis pubis. Treatment is aimed at maintaining cardiovascular stability through the use of intravenous fluids and immediate repositioning of the uterine corpus. Unless already completely separated, the placenta should be left attached during repositioning.[4, 28, 29] Repositioning may be accomplished by inserting one hand into the vagina and extending the fingers to identify the margins of the cervix; the uterine corpus is allowed to rest in the palm of the hand. Gentle pressure exerted with the fingers on the edges of the uterus closest to the cervix in the direction of the umbilicus is followed by gradual replacement of the corpus (Figs. 50–27 and 50–28). Pressure should not initially be exerted centrally on the fundus, because this will cause the uterus to be compressed, forcing more "layers" of the uterus to simultaneously lie within the relatively tight cervical ring. Once the uterus has been repositioned, the placenta may be removed. Because traction on the cord of an adherent placenta is one of the principal causes of uterine inversion, this procedure may be deferred until the obstetrician arrives. Although replacement of the inverted uterus can usually be accomplished by vaginal manipulation, occasionally a dense cervical contraction ring is present, preventing repositioning. General anesthesia and laparotomy may be necessary for uterine repositioning.

Management of refactory postpartum hemorrhage requires specialized care and should be left to the obstetrician. Fluid replacement and the

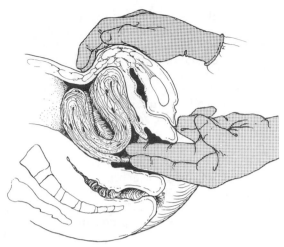

Figure 50–27. Replacement of a partially inverted uterus. (From Benson, R. C. (ed.): Current Obstetric and Gynecologic Diagnosis and Treatment, 3rd ed. Los Altos, California, Lange Medical Publications, 1980. Used by permission.)

application of the pneumatic antishock garment are used to stabilize the patient in the interim.[30]

The Neonate

Evaluation of the neonate begins before delivery with assessment of maternal well being, gestational age, ease and type of previous deliveries, and the recognition of fetal distress as evidenced by meconium staining of the amniotic fluid, fetal bradycardia, or evidence of cord prolapse. Care of the newborn begins with delivery of the head while the mouth and nares are suctioned. Following delivery and cutting of the umbilical cord, the infant should immediately be placed in a supine position with the head lowered and turned to the side to prevent aspiration. Becuase of the relatively large surface area of the infant, temperature drops rapidly immediately after birth, with subsequent chilling, which produces shivering and increased oxygen demand. Care must be taken, therefore, to maintain body temperature by placing the infant in warm blankets, a Sterile Infant Swaddler, or a heated isolette, or if resuscitation is necessary, under a radiant warmer.

EVALUATION

Traditionally, the *Apgar Scoring System,* applied at one and five minutes after birth, is the standard of neonatal evaluation (Table 50–2).[1, 3, 31] In general, the higher the score, the better the condition of the infant. The 1-minute Apgar Score reflects the need for immediate resuscitation. A score of 7 to 10 indicates that the infant is in excellent condition, requiring no aid other than nasopharyngeal

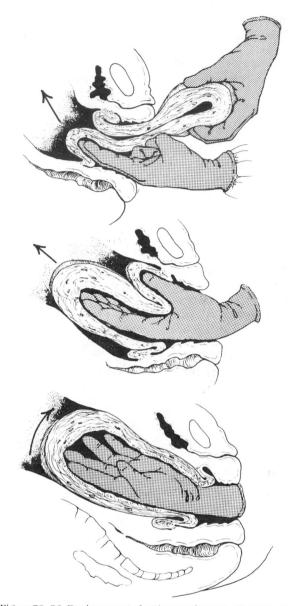

Figure 50–28. Replacement of an inverted uterus. (From Benson, R. C. (ed.): Current Obstetric and Gynecologic Diagnosis and Treatment, 3rd ed. Los Altos, California, Lange Medical Publications, 1980. Used by permission.)

suctioning. A moderately depressed infant with depressed respirations, flaccidity, and pallor or cyanosis usually scores 4 to 7 and may require resuscitation. A score of 0 to 4, indicating a severely depressed infant, mandates immediate resuscitation. The 5-minute Apgar Score is an indicator of neonatal and long-term prognosis; a low score suggests increased risk of subsequent infant morbidity and mortality.[1, 3, 31]

Although the Apgar Score is the traditional standard for neonatal evaluation, the decision to resuscitate and the infant's response to resuscitation can be more accurately assessed by evaluating the heart rate, respiratory activity, and neuromuscular tone of the infant.[31]

Table 50–2. APGAR SCORING SYSTEM

Sign	0	1	2
Heart rate	Absent	Slow(<100)	>100
Respiratory effort	Absent	Slow, irregular	Good, crying
Muscle tone	Flaccid	Some flexion of extremities	Active motion
Reflex irritability	No response	Grimace	Vigorous cry
Color	Blue, pale	Body pink, extremities blue	Completely pink

Normally, the newborn takes its first breath within a few seconds of birth and cries within 30 seconds.[1] Apnea is the most common initial manifestation of depression in the neonate and unless reversed may lead to progressive hypoxemia, hypercarbia, and acidosis. Hypoventilation quickly leads to cardiovascular depression with subsequent slowing of the heart rate, the most sensitive indication of infant distress. A heart rate of less than 100 beats per minute is considered abnormal.[31]

STABILIZATION

Equipment

Bulb syringe or DeLee suction trap*
Oral airways (size 0, 00, and 000)
Suction catheters (size 5, 6, and 8F)
Endotracheal tubes (size 2.5 mm, 3.0 mm, and 3.5 mm)
Endotracheal tube stylet (optional)
Laryngoscope
Laryngoscope blade (straight; sizes 0 and 1)
Resuscitation bag
Face masks (sizes 0 and 1)
Wall suction
Wall oxygen
Radiant warmer

Technique

If neonatal respirations are infrequent or absent, suctioning the mouth and pharynx with a bulb syringe or DeLee suction trap and stimulating the infant by lightly slapping the soles of the feet and rubbing the back may serve to stimulate breathing. If necessary, the airway should be gently suctioned with an 8-French Foley suction catheter, using negative pressures not exceeding 30 cm of water. Because the neonate is an obligate nose breather, it is advisable to suction once through each nostril to ensure patency of the upper airway. Failure to establish effective respirations indicates either marked central nervous system depression, mechanical obstruction, or an intrinsic lung abnormality and demands active resuscitation.

*Argyle Manufacturing Company, St. Joseph, Missouri

If signs of airway obstruction, that is, decreased chest expansion and sternal and intercostal retractions are present and persist after suctioning, the larynx should be directly visualized with a laryngoscope. Suctioning of the larynx should be done under direct vision. For obstruction distal to the glottic opening, it is advisable to intubate the infant and suction through the endotracheal tube. Appropriate size of the endotracheal tube varies with the size of the neonate from 2.5 mm for those weighing 1000 g or less to 3.5 mm for the term infant.

Because *meconium aspiration* is a major cause of neonatal morbidity and mortality, its prevention deserves special mention. Up to 60 per cent of neonates with meconium staining of the amniotic fluid will aspirate; approximately 20 per cent of these neonates will later develop pulmonary complications.[31] In order to prevent aspiration, neonates born with meconium staining of the amniotic fluid require thorough suctioning of the hypopharynx prior to the completion of delivery and the initiation of respiration. Tracheal intubation and suctioning of the lower airway may be necessary to adequately clear the airway of meconium.

Bag and mask ventilation should be initiated as soon as it is recognized that tactile stimulation is not sufficient to establish spontaneous ventilation or that ventilation is not adequate to maintain a heart rate of greater than 100 beats per minute.

The heart rate should be monitored during the course of neonatal evaluation and stabilization with either direct ausculation over the chest or by palpating the pulse at the base of the umbilical cord. A readily discernible heart beat of 100 or more beats per minute is acceptable. If the heart rate drops to less than 80 beats per minute and does not immediately respond to effective ventilation and oxygenation, chest compression should be instituted while ventilation is continued. The two-handed method of chest compression is preferred. The hands encircle the chest with the fingers placed over the back, and the thumbs are placed over the midportion of the sternum to provide compression. The sternum is compressed 1/2 to 3/4 inches at a rate of 100 compressions per minute. Ventilation is interposed after every fifth compression. If there is no response in heart rate, an intravenous or umbilical line should be placed

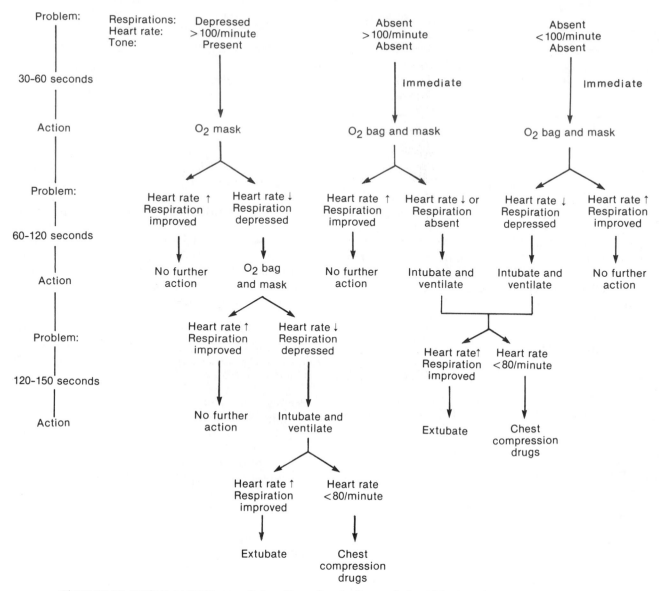

Figure 50–29. Guide to neonatal resuscitation. (Reproduced with permission of the American Heart Association.)

and appropriate drug therapy should be instituted. A general guide to neonatal resuscitation is outlined in Figure 50–29.

1. Pritchard, J. A., and MacDonald, P. C.: William's Obstetrics, 16th ed. New York, Appleton-Century-Crofts, 1980.
2. Monthly Vital Statistics Report, Volume 34, Washington, D.C., National Center for Health Statistics, August 11, 1983.
3. Benson, R. C.: Current Obstetrics and Gynecological Diagnosis and Treatment. Los Altos, California, Lange Medical Publications, 1980.
4. Romney, S. L., Gray, M. J., Little, A. B., et al.: Gynecology and Obstetrics: The Health Care of Women. New York, McGraw-Hill, Inc., 1975.
5. Abe, T.: The detection of the rupture of fetal membranes with nitrazine indicator. Am. J. Obstet. Gynecol. 39:400, 1940.
6. Baptisti, A.: Chemical test for the determination of ruptured membranes. Am. J. Obstet. Gynecol. 35:688, 1938.
7. Friedman, E. A.: The graphic analysis of labor. Am. J. Obstet. Gynecol. 68:1568, 1954.
8. Abdul-Karim, R. W., and Chevli, R. N.: Antepartum hemorrhage and shock. Clin. Obstet. Gynecol. 10:533, 1976.
9. Wheeler, A. S., and Francis, M. J.: Anesthesia for complicated obstetrics. J. Am. Assoc. Nurse Anesth. 47(3):300–308, 1979.
10. Booher, D., and Little, B.: Vaginal hemorrhage in pregnancy. N. Engl. J. Med. 290:611, 1974.
11. Jennings, B.: Emergency delivery: how to attend one safely. Maternal Child Nursing 4:148, 1979.
12. Schrader, K., and Budassi, S. A.: Emergency childbirth. J. E. N. 5:45, 1979.
13. Yao, A. C., and Lind, J.: Placental transfusion. Am. J. Dis. Child 127:128, 1974.
14. Swartz, D. P.: Shoulder girdle dystocia in vertex delivery: clinical study and review. Obstet. Gynecol. 15:194, 1960.
15. Gonik, B., Stringer, C. A., and Held, B.: An alternative

maneuver for management of shoulder dystocia. Am. J Obstet. Gynecol. 145:882, 1983.

16. Hunt, A. B.: Problems of delivery of the oversized infant. Am. J. Obstet. Gynecol. 64:559, 1952.

17. Woods, C. E.: A principle of physics as applicable to shoulder delivery. Am. J. Obstet. Gynecol. 45:796, 1943.

18. Mazzanti, G. A.: Delivery of the anterior shoulder. Obstet. Gynecol. 13:603, 1959.

19. Brenner, W. E., Bruce, R. D., and Hendricks, C. H.: The characteristics and perils of breech presentation. Am. J. Obstet. Gynecol. 118:700, 1974.

20. James, F. M.: Anesthetic considerations for breech or twin delivery. Clin. Perinatol. 9:77, 1982.

21. Morley, G. W.: Breech presentation—a 15-year review. Obstet. Gynecol. 30:745, 1967.

22. Collea, J. V., Rabin, S. C., Weghorst, G. R., et al.: The randomized management of term frank breech presentation: vaginal delivery vs. cesarean section. Am. J. Obstet. Gynecol. 131:186, 1978.

23. Johnson, C. E.: Breech presentation at term. Am. J. Obstet. Gynecol. 106:865, 1970.

24. Hall, J. E., Kohl, S. G., O'Brien, F., et al.: Breech presentation and perinatal mortality. Am. J. Obstet. Gynecol. 91:665, 1965.

25. Rovinsky, J. J., Miller, J. A., and Kaplan, S.: Management of breech presentation at term. Am. J. Obstet. Gynecol. 115:497, 1973.

26. Tank, E. S., Davis, R., Holt, J. F., et al.: Mechanisms of trauma during breech delivery. Obstet. Gynecol. 38:761, 1971.

27. Beynon, C. L.: Midline episiotomy as a routine procedure. The Journal of Obstetrics and Gynaecology of the British Commonwealth 81:126, 1974.

28. Herbert, W. N. P.: Complications of the immediate puerperium. Clin. Obstet. Gynecol. 25:219, 1982.

29. Watson, P.: Postpartum hemorrhage and shock. Clin. Obstet. Gynecol. 23:985, 1980.

30. Kelly, J. V.: Postpartum hemorrhage. Clin. Obstet. Gynecol. 19:595, 1976.

31. McIntyre, K. M., and Lewis, A. J.: Textbook of Advanced Cardiac Life Support. American Heart Association, 1981.

51

Examination of the Female Rape Victim

G. RICHARD BRAEN, M.D.

Introduction

Rape is reported to be the fastest growing violent crime in the United States,[1] and it has been estimated that one of six women will be the victim of a rape or an attempted rape in her lifetime.[2] The victims of rape can experience extensive trauma (both physical and psychological), can be exposed to disease, and can become pregnant. The physicians and nurses dealing with a rape victim have a professional, ethical, and moral responsibility to provide the best medical and psychological care possible while simultaneously collecting and preserving the proper medicolegal evidence that is unique to the evaluation of rape cases.

The emergency department is the most common place to which rape victims are brought by police. This occurs for several reasons but is mainly a matter of logistics—the peak hours for this crime are from 8:00 P.M. to 2:00 A.M.,[3] and the most common days on which it occurs are weekends. In many localities, the only available physician at these times is the emergency physician, and it is often his or her responsibility to perform the evaluation and treatment. Emergency personnel can help change the impact of rape. Through proper care of the victim, careful and thorough acquisition of evidence, and cooperation with the law and the legal process, emergency department staff can help the victim toward recovery from the assault and can aid society in improving the prosecution and conviction rates.[4]

Management of the Adult Female Rape Victim

An important aspect of performing a rape evaluation is preparation. This includes the establishment of a protocol and the assembly of appropriate forms and equipment. All of this must be accomplished through a cooperative effort with the police, the crime laboratory, the hospital laboratory, rape crisis volunteers, and the emergency department clerical, social service, nursing, and physician staffs. Careful step-by-step planning concerning the way in which a victim will be handled in the emergency department and in follow-up will help both to ensure the best care for the victim and to aid in the prosecution and conviction of assailants.

Major provisions in the emergency department protocol should include patient privacy and the designation of a separate area for the care of rape victims. Emergency personnel should know the appropriate steps for evaluation and treatment of the victim, follow-up care, and maintenance of evidence. Rape examination kits should be available in the emergency department, and the staff should be familiar with them. A list of the contents of the kits should be kept in the department (Table 51–1). The kits save a tremendous amount of nursing and physician time when a victim comes to the department. A "check list for rape examinations" (Table 51–2) should be included in the kits. This will serve as a reminder of all of the medicolegal procedures to be completed.

Even though this chapter is devoted to the evaluation of the adult female rape victim, a guideline to the evaluation of the adult male sexual assault victim, the female child victim, the male child victim, and the accused rapist is provided in Table 51–3. Each of these individuals has special needs, and separate protocols should be developed in the emergency department for them.

CONSENT

Consent for treatment of a victim of sexual assault is mandatory. The victim has undergone an experience in which her right to grant or deny consent was taken from her,[5] and obtaining consent for medical treatment and for the gathering of evidence has important psychological and legal implications. The victim has the right to refuse medicolegal examination and even medical treatment. She should, however, be encouraged to have physical evidence collected in the event that she later decides to seek prosecution. Witnessed, written, informed consent therefore should be obtained before evaluation and treatment are begun. If the victim refuses any part of the examination, her wishes should be honored, and the refusal should be noted in the hospital record.

When the court orders an examination but the victim does not want to be examined, the physician must realize that an uncooperative victim (who indeed has the right to refuse examination) can make a thorough examination impossible. This would add additional trauma to the victim's psychological state, and the examining physician should discuss the situation with the authority that issued the court order before proceeding.

Table 51–1. BASIC RAPE EXAMINATION KIT*

Contents	Purpose
Paper bags	Clothing collection
Two urine containers	Urine for pregnancy test and drug screen
Fingernail file and envelope	Fingernail scrapings
Forceps, scissors, envelope	Pubic hair trimming
Plastic comb, large paper towel, envelope	Pubic hair combing
Vaginal speculum, aspiration pipette, red-topped test tube and stopper	Aspiration of vaginal contents
Two glass slides (one frosted at one end), two cotton-tipped swabs, red-topped test tube and stopper, pencil for marking slide	Swabbing of vagina
10 ml of saline, aspiration pipette and bulb, test tube	Vaginal washing
Cervical scraper, slides, Pap smear fixative	Pap smear
Thayer-Martin plates or Transgrow media, cotton-tipped swabs	Gonorrhea culture
Three cotton-tipped swabs and a test tube or an envelope	Saliva for secretor status
Three red-topped test tubes, tourniquet, nonalcohol swab to prepare skin, syringe and needle	Blood samples
Appropriate laboratory forms, rape examination forms, labels for samples, camera and film (optional)	
5 ml of toluidine blue dye	Vaginal laceration examination

*From Braen, G. R.: Sexual assault. In Rosen, P., et al. (eds.): Emergency Medicine, Concepts and Clinical Practice. St. Louis, The C. V. Mosby Co., 1983. Used by permission.

Table 51–2. CHECK LIST FOR RAPE EXAMINATIONS

General
____ Photographs

Urine
____ Pregnancy test
____ Urine drug screen

Blood
____ VDRL test
____ β-hCG test
____ Ethanol or complete drug screen, or both
____ Red-topped test tube for blood typing

Pelvic Examination Specimens
____ Pap smear
____ Three vaginal swabs
____ Potassium hydroxide slide
____ Normal saline slide
____ Dry mount slide
____ Thayer-Martin plates (gonococcal culture)

Buccal Specimens
____ Three buccal swabs

Pubic Hair
____ Combed hair
____ Cut or plucked hair

Fingernails
____ Scrapings from under nails

Clothes
____ Panties and any other articles requested by police

Table 51–3. SEXUAL ASSAULT EXAMINATION PROTOCOL FOR MEDICAL PERSONNEL

	Female Adult Victim	Female Child Victim (Prepubertal)	Male Adult Victim	Male Child Victim	Male Suspect
I. History					
A. History of the event					
1. Time, date, place	*	*	*	*	*
2. Use of force, threats of force	*	*	*	*	
a. Type of violence	*	*	*	*	
b. Threats of violence	*	*	*	*	
c. Use of restraints	*	*	*	*	
d. Number of assailants	*	*	*	*	
e. Use of alcohol or drugs	*	*	*	*	
f. Loss of consciousness	*	*	*	*	
3. Type of assault	*	*	*	*	
a. Fondling	*	*	*	*	
b. Vaginal penetration (or attempt)	*	*	*	*	
c. Oral penetration (or attempt)	*	*	*	*	
d. Anal penetration (or attempt)	*	*	*	*	
e. Ejaculation—where on or in body	*	*	*	*	
f. Was condom used?	*	*	*	*	
g. Use of lubricant	*				*
B. Sexual history					
1. Use of birth control	*	I.A.	*	I.A.	
2. Last voluntary intercourse or sexual activity	*	I.A.	*	I.A.	*
3. Gravidity, parity	*				
4. Recent gynecologic surgery	*	I.A.	*	I.A.	*
5. Recent venereal disease	*	I.A.	*	I.A.	
C. Medical history					
1. Current medications	*	*	*	*	*
2. Tetanus immunization status	*	*	*	*	*
3. Allergies	*	*	*	*	*
D. History of douching, bathing, urination, defecation, or enema use following the assault	*	*	*	*	*
II. Physical Examination					
A. Rapid survey for airway, breathing, circulation	*	*	*	*	*
B. Inspection of clothing for signs of violence or other evidence, such as feces, semen, blood (retain appropriate evidence, consider photographs)	*	*	*	*	*
C. Examination of all areas of skin for signs of violence, foreign material (retain appropriate evidence, consider photographs)	*	*	*	*	*
D. Examination of extremities for fractures, sprains, and so forth	*	*	*	*	*
E. Examination of oral cavity for signs of trauma, infection	*	*	*	*	*
F. Examination of breasts for trauma	*	*	*	*	*

Table continued on following page

Table 51-3. SEXUAL ASSAULT EXAMINATION PROTOCOL FOR MEDICAL PERSONNEL (*Continued*)

	Female Adult Victim	Female Child Victim (Prepubertal)	Male Adult Victim	Male Child Victim	Male Suspect
G. Genital/rectal examination					
1. Male genitalia	*	*	*	*	*
a. Examination for signs of trauma to penis, dried semen, infection, and so forth			*	*	*
b. Examination of shaft of penis for lubricant, feces, blood			*	*	*
c. Examination for signs of trauma to testicles, scrotum			*	*	*
d. Examination for vasectomy scars					*
2. Female genitalia					
a. Wood's light (filtered ultraviolet) to detect seminal stains on perineum	*	*			
b. Inspection of vulva for signs of trauma or semen	*	*			
c. Inspection of introitus	*	*			
d. Inspection of hymen	*	*			
i. By speculum examination	*	I.A.			
ii. By separating vulva manually	I.A.	*			
e. Inspection of vaginal vault for trauma and foreign bodies	*	I.A.			
f. Inspection of cervix	*	I.A.			
i. For parity	*	I.A.			
ii. For signs of pregnancy	*	I.A.			
iii. For menstruation	*	I.A.			
iv. For trauma	*	I.A.			
v. For signs of infection	*	I.A.			
g. Refer to Section III: H, I, J, K, L of this protocol	*	*			
h. Bimanual pelvic examination	*				
i. Palpation of uterus per rectum	*	*			
3. Anal and perianal area	*	*	*	*	
a. Inspection for signs of trauma	*	*	*	*	
b. Inspection for signs of lubricant, semen, blood, foreign material, pre-established infection	*	*	*	*	
c. Digital rectal examination for trauma, foreign bodies	*	*	*	*	
d. Refer to Section III: L, M, N of this protocol	*	*	*	*	
III. *Laboratory*					
A. Photography (optional)					
1. Signs of trauma (patient clothed)	*	*	*	*	*
2. Signs of restraint (patient clothed)	*	*	*	*	*
3. Signs of trauma (patient unclothed)	*	*	*	*	*
4. Signs of restraint (patient unclothed)	*	*	*	*	
B. Clothing collection (for secretions, blood, semen, signs of violence, and so forth)	*	*	*	*	*
C. Removal of dried seminal or blood stains from skin	*	*	*	*	*

Procedure					
D. Fingernail scrapings for foreign material	*	*	*	*	*
E. Combings from pubic hair	*	I.A.	*	I.A.	I.A.
F. Plucked or trimmed pubic hair	*	I.A.	*	I.A.	I.A.
G. Plucked or trimmed head hair	*	*	*	*	*
H. Vaginal pool aspiration					
1. Sperm motility and morphology	*	I.A.	I.A.	*	*
2. Acid phosphatase	*	I.A.	I.A.	*	*
3. Blood group antigens	*	I.A.	I.A.	*	*
4. Sperm precipitin test	Optional	Optional			
I. Swab of posterior vaginal fornix (same tests as previously described if vaginal aspirate not available)	*	I.A.	*	*	*
J. Vaginal washing with 10 ml saline solution (same tests as described previously if vaginal aspirate not available)	*	I.A.	*	I.A.	
K. Pap smear from cervix and vaginal wall	*	*	*	*	
L. Gonorrhea cultures					
1. Cervix	*	I.A.	I.A.	I.A.	I.A.
2. Rectum	*	*	I.A.	I.A.	I.A.
3. Oropharynx	*	*	I.A.	I.A.	
M. Collection of foreign material from perianal area (especially lubricant)	*	*	*	I.A.	I.A.
N. Rectal washing					
1. Sperm motility and morphology	I.A.	I.A.	I.A.	I.A.	I.A.
2. Acid phosphatase	I.A.	I.A.	I.A.	I.A.	I.A.
O. Saliva for secretor status	See Note 1	See Note 1	See Note 1	See Note 1	See Note 1
P. Blood samples					
1. VDRL test	*	*	*	*	*
2. Drug and alcohol screen	I.A.	I.A.	I.A.	I.A.	I.A.
3. Blood typing	*	*	*	*	*
4. Pregnancy test (β subunit of hCG)	See Note 2	I.A.	I.A.	I.A.	I.A.
Q. Urine samples					
1. Pregnancy test	I.A.	I.A.	I.A.	I.A.	I.A.
2. Drug screen	I.A.	I.A.	I.A.	I.A.	I.A.
R. Penile shaft swabs					
1. For vaginal epithelium		I.A.	I.A.	I.A.	*
2. For fecal stains		I.A.	I.A.	I.A.	*
S. Penile urethral swab					
1. Gram stain for gonorrhea	I.A.	I.A.	I.A.	I.A.	*
2. Culture for gonorrhea	I.A.	I.A.	I.A.	I.A.	*
T. Radiographs for trauma	I.A.	I.A.	I.A.	I.A.	I.A.
IV. Consolidation of Evidence	*	*	*	*	*
V. Initiation of "Chain of Evidence"	*	*	*	*	*

I.A. = If appropriate
* = indicated

Note 1: Collection of saliva for secretor status is appropriate only if samples from the body, clothing, or crime scene potentially containing antigens that could link the victim with the suspect or suspects have been or will be obtained.

Note 2: The β-hCG serum pregnancy test is more sensitive and quantitative but is not readily available in some hospitals.

HISTORY

It should be emphasized that the rape victim is actually a patient whose physical stability takes priority over all else (e.g., if she is in physical danger from hemorrhage, shock, or respiratory difficulty, treatment of these conditions takes precedence).

The history appropriate to a rape case basically is divided into three categories: history of the event, gynecologic history, and medical history. The history of the event should include only those elements necessary for the physician to complete a thorough physical examination and collection of evidence. Questions beyond this, such as a description of the assailant, should be left to the police investigators. Limiting the history not only will shorten the evaluation in the emergency department but also will help prevent discrepancies between the emergency department history and the official police investigation report. Discrepancies could weaken the case if it comes to trial. For the sake of time, the medical history may be obtained by a nurse and expedited by the use of a checklist, which is then reviewed by the physician.

The history of the event should include the time, date, and place of the rape and a description of the use of force or threats of force and the type of assault. Elements of force include the type of violence used, threats of violence, the use of restraints, the number of assailants, the use of alcohol or drugs (forcedly or willingly) by the victim, and any loss of consciousness experienced by the victim. Elements of the type of assault include fondling; vaginal, oral, or anal penetration or attempted penetration; ejaculation on or in the body; the use of a condom; and the insertion of foreign bodies into the vagina or the anus. The use of force or violence is partly a police matter, but from a medical standpoint it is desirable to correlate the physical examination with a description of any force, restraint, or violence.

A basic gynecologic history should be obtained in preparation for treatment plans regarding venereal disease and pregnancy. For example, it might be medicolegally important to know of any recent gynecologic surgical procedure that could be misinterpreted as local trauma. The gynecologic history therefore includes the use of birth control prior to the attack (with information regarding any missed birth control pills), last normal menstrual period, last voluntary intercourse, gravidity and parity, recent gynecologic surgery, and recent venereal disease. Some points of the gynecologic history are optional—for example, a history of birth control methods would be inappropriate for a 72-year-old rape victim.

The medical history should include current medications, tetanus immunization status, and allergies. One should note whether the victim douched, bathed, urinated, defecated, used a mouthwash, or brushed her teeth following the rape. Each of these can alter the recovery of seminal specimens and other rape evidence. In addition, any nonperineal or nonoral trauma should be reassessed when the medical history is taken.

Several elements of the history taken together can help the physician decide which samples to obtain. For example, sperm remain motile in the cervix for up to 5 days and remain motile in the vagina for 6 to 12 hours.[6] If the victim had voluntary intercourse 48 hours prior to examination and was raped 3 hours prior to examination, the physician should obtain samples from both the vagina and the cervix, keeping the two separate.[7] By taking a careful history, the physician is able to perform an appropriate examination given these two events.

PHYSICAL EXAMINATION

The physical examination of the rape victim is an extension of the history. The purpose of the examination is twofold: to aid in the proper medical evaluation of the patient and to gather samples and observations that might serve as evidence. The findings on physical examination help the physician and the court to answer the following questions: (1) Is or was the victim capable of consenting to intercourse? (2) Was force used? (3) Did vulvar, oral, or anal penetration occur? (4) Is there collectable physical evidence from the rapist in or on the victim's body? A number of standardized rape kits have been developed to assist the physician in gathering evidence in a systemic fashion. Each kit should be reviewed for completeness as it applies to the local legal protocol.

Consent is an important issue in determining rape. Consent here refers to the victim's ability or inability to agree to having intercourse. If consent is denied, or if the victim is unable to give consent because of mental retardation, immaturity, or the influence of drugs, this is important in a legal sense.

Photographs should be considered, particularly if the victim is still wearing the clothing worn during the attack. Some institutions take their own photographs; others use police photographers. Patient consent should be obtained for photographs taken by hospital personnel, and a chain of evidence should be maintained. Self-developing film that can be permanently labeled (subject, date, details of pictured injury, and so forth) should be used. The photographs should be labeled immediately and may be added to the legal evidence. These photographs may serve as evidence or may simply refresh the examiner's memory at the time of the trial. After the victim has been photographed, she should remove her own clothing, piece by piece, placing each item in a separate *paper* bag. If semen, blood, or other foreign material is present, it will dry in a paper bag, whereas it could become moldy if placed in a plastic bag.

At this time the entirety of the patient's body, excepting the pelvic, anal, and oral areas, should be examined for signs of trauma and foreign bodies. Important areas for evaluation are the back, the thighs, the breasts, and the wrists, and the ankles (particularly if restraints were used). Even in the absence of ecchymoses, tender contusions should be reported. Leaves, grass, sand, and so forth can occasionally be found in the hair or on the skin and should be retained as evidence. Areas of trauma should be documented and further evaluated (e.g., with radiographs) as indicated by the type and extent of injury. Up to 30 per cent of rape victims show external evidence of trauma.[3] This evidence may range from abrasions to multiple major blunt and penetrating trauma. In addition, dried semen stains may be visible on the hair or the skin of the victim. These appear as lightly crusted, flaking areas that can be removed by saline-moistened swabs; the swabs are then air-dried and preserved as evidence. Not only the skin but also the fingernails can contain hidden bits of evidence. Rape victims may have bits of the assailant's skin, blood, or facial hair or other foreign material from the rape site beneath their fingernails, fingernail scrapings thus should be routinely obtained.

Following this initial examination, the patient should be placed in a lithotomy position for the pelvic examination. The thighs and the perineum should be inspected for signs of trauma and for foreign materials, such as seminal stains. An ultraviolet light used in a darkened room can aid in the search for external seminal stains. Any such stains should be removed and preserved as previously described. The pubic hair should then be combed for foreign material, particularly pubic hairs from the assailant. These combings can be placed directly into a large paper envelope; the samples are submitted along with the comb. Foreign pubic hairs can help identify race and hair color, but generally there are not enough individual characteristics in hair to enable one to state positively that a hair of unknown source came from a particular person to the exclusion of all others.[8] In the future, crime laboratories may be able to perform enzyme typing of hair roots. Currently, sufficient phosphoglucomutase activity can be found in plucked hair roots to enable typing of individual roots by starch-gel electrophoresis.[9] This capability may some day be extended to hair roots collected by brushing.

The pelvic examination includes careful evaluation of the vulva and the introitus for signs of trauma, foreign material, and degree of maturity or senility. The internal examination should be done with a water-lubricated speculum.[10] The hymen should be inspected and one of the four following conditions noted: (1) that the hymen is present, intact, and free of evidence of trauma; (2) that the hymen is present and intact and shows old scarring; (3) that the hymen is present and recently ruptured; or (4) that the hymen is absent. A recently ruptured hymen is associated with bleeding or fresh clots.

The vaginal wall should be inspected for lacerations. These appear near the introitus in younger, sexually inexperienced females; in older, sexually active females they appear higher, particularly in the right fornix.[11, 12] The cervix should be inspected for signs of pregnancy, menstruation, trauma, and pre-existing infection.

After the inspection of the introitus, the vagina, and the cervix, the following samples should be obtained:

1. Any vaginal tampon that may have been inserted prior to or after the assault.

2. Any foreign body. (I have found condoms, a bar of soap, and a handkerchief).

3. Vaginal swabs from pooled secretions in the posterior fornix. (These may contain acid phosphatase or sperm[6, 13, 14]). A wet mount of one swab may reveal motile sperm if the examiner has ready access to a microscope. One swab can be used to make a dry mount for the crime laboratory, and one or two swabs can be air-dried for submission to the crime laboratory. If there are no pooled secretions, a vaginal washing using 5 ml of sterile (but not bacteriostatic) water can be obtained with a syringe. The washing can be examined for sperm and acid phosphatase.

4. A Papanicolaou (Pap) smear to determine sperm and cervical mucosa morphology. Occasionally, the Pap smear may detect sperm when other tests do not.

5. A separate swab from the cervix for sperm and acid phosphatase. Dried specimens for acid phosphatase need not be refrigerated, but liquid specimens require refrigeration.

6. A cervical culture for gonorrhea.

Each sample should be separately labeled; the label should include the area from which the specimen was collected. Some physicians also obtain cervical chlamydial cultures.

After these samples have been obtained, a bimanual pelvic examination should be performed to assess uterine size and to identify adnexal masses and tenderness.

A new test that can be performed for rape victims is the toluidine blue dye test for traumatic intercourse. This test involves the application of toluidine blue to the vaginal mucosa. Tears in the mucosa expose superficial nuclei of underlying cells. These nuclei have an affinity for the toluidine blue, and lacerations (minute and large) become stained. In one study, 70 per cent of nulliparas and 40 per cent of the total number of patients examined within 48 hours after complaint of sexual assault demonstrated toluidine blue–positive lacerations.[15] Toluidine blue is primarily used in gynecology for outlining cervical neoplasia.[16] The dye is applied with cotton-tipped applicators; all excess is wiped off with cotton balls until no further dye can be removed. Lacerations will retain the dye. The authors of the report on the use of toluidine blue in rape cases suggest that it be applied to the external genitalia before the insertion of a speculum, because the speculum itself may cause small lacerations.[15] Because of the spermicidal activity of toluidine blue, the examiner must decide on a case-by-case basis when to perform this test.

The anorectal area should be examined for traces of foreign material (particularly lubricants) and trauma. Because of a reluctance of some victims to admit to anal or oral sodomy, an examination of these areas should be performed in all cases. Anorectal swabs should be obtained for gonorrhea culturing and sperm and acid phosphatase testing. If the patient admits to anal penetration, one can perform a rectal washing by injecting 5 to 10 ml of normal saline with a syringe and a small plastic intravenous catheter, aspirating and preserving the fluid as evidence. This washing can be examined for sperm and acid phosphatase, even though acid phosphatase determination has been of little value from samples taken from the anal canal and the rectum.[17]

The mouth, particularly if oral sodomy is reported, should be inspected for signs of trauma. These can include bruises about the mouth, a torn frenulum of the lower lip, a torn frenulum beneath the tongue, and contusions or lacerations of the tonsilar pillars or the posterior pharyngeal wall. The examiner tests for acid phosphatase and sperm in the oral cavity by swabbing between the teeth with cotton-tipped applicators. The acid phosphatase test is seldom positive, but spermatozoa have been identified in oral smears up to 6 hours after the attack despite tooth brushing, using mouthwash, and drinking various fluids.[17] In addition, saliva samples (two to three saliva-soaked swabs) should be obtained so that one can assess the victim's secretor status of blood group antigens if foreign blood group antigens are found in the vagina. Eighty per cent of people secrete blood group antigens in saliva, semen, and so forth. Culturing of the pharynx for gonorrhea should also be performed.

Blood tests in rape victims may include the following: drug and alcohol testing, blood typing, a serologic test for syphilis, and, if available and appropriate, a pregnancy test using the β subunit of human chorionic gonadotropin (hCG).[18, 19] If this pregnancy test is positive within a few hours

or days of the assault, the victim was probably already pregnant at the time of the rape. If the test is negative at the initial examination but positive at a 2-week follow-up visit, it can be assumed that the victim became pregnant at or near the time of the rape.[7]

Motile and immotile sperm may be found microscopically in wet mounts of vaginal aspirates and in vaginal, oral, and rectal swabs. The samples should be examined microscopically immediately after the physical examination. The forensic pathologist may not be able to examine the samples for several hours, days, weeks, or months after they are collected, when sperm motility (a very good sign of recent intercourse) has been lost. The absence of sperm does not rule out sexual assault. The assault may have been without penetration, there may have been coitus interruptus, and the assailant may have used a condom or have had a vasectomy.

Samples and other evidence must be given to the police, a crime laboratory, or a forensic pathologist. Each sample must be labeled with the patient's name, the hospital number, the date and time of collection, the area from which the specimen was collected, and the collector's name. These specimens should then be packaged and transferred to the next appropriate official (police officer, pathologist, or other individual) along with a written "chain of evidence" that includes a list of the specimens, the signature of each person who provided them, and the signature of each person who received them. If this chain is broken, important evidence may become worthless in the courtroom.

TREATMENT

The factors of venereal disease, pregnancy, psychological distress, and follow-up should be considered in the treatment of a rape victim.

Rape victims are reported to have a 1 in 30 chance of developing gonorrhea and a 1 in 1000 chance of developing syphilis.[3] Depending on patient reliability and other factors, a physician may choose to treat a rape victim as if she had been exposed to a known case of gonorrhea or may choose to rely on cultures. (When cultures are obtained from the cervix, the pharynx, and the rectum, 90 per cent of gonorrhea cases can be diagnosed at a single visit.[20]) Gonorrhea resulting from a rape may possibly be culturable within hours of the attack but should be almost always culturable at a 2-week follow-up visit. Syphilis is generally treated only if it is discovered at a 4- to 6-week follow-up visit. Intramuscular penicillin administered for gonorrhea will also treat incubating syphilis.[21] Data concerning other venereal diseases (herpes, chlamydia, and so forth) in rape

Table 51–4. ALTERNATIVE DRUG REGIMENS FOR PREGNANCY PREVENTION IN RAPE VICTIMS*†

Oral diethylstilbestrol in a dose of 25 mg twice daily for 5 days

Intravenous conjugated estrogen (Premarin) in a dose of 50 mg once daily for 2 days

Oral conjugated estrogen (Premarin) in a dose of 30 mg once daily for 5 days

Oral ethinyl estradiol in a dose of 5 mg once daily for 5 days

*From Rosen, P., Baker, F. J., Braen, G. R., et al.: (eds.): Emergency Medicine: Concepts and Clinical Practice. St. Louis, C. V. Mosby, 1983, p. 1236. Used by permission.
†All should be begun within 24 hours of the rape. All of these preparations may cause nausea and vomiting. Note that treatment is started only after pregnancy has been ruled out.

cases are not currently available. Some physicians will empirically treat with tetracycline to cover potential exposure to chlamydial organisms. A negative pregnancy test is a prerequisite for this therapy.

Pregnancy occurs in approximately 1 per cent of rape victims. The examiner must be very careful to determine that pregnancy did not exist prior to the attack, and pregnancy tests should be obtained before any postcoital therapy is offered. The greater sensitivity of the serum pregnancy test using β-hCG makes it the preferred test. This test is sensitive at 5 days after implantation of the products of conception. Newer urine tests are being developed that have a greater sensitivity than the old tests. These may be acceptable in the future. Rape victims should be offered pregnancy prevention as outlined in Table 51–4.

Rape precipitates a psychological crisis for the patient, and psychological care should begin when the patient first arrives in the emergency department.[22, 23] The victim often develops a post-traumatic stress disorder, manifested by numbed responsiveness to the external world, sleep disturbances, guilt feelings, memory impairment, avoidance of activities, and other symptoms.[24] The rape victim is particularly vulnerable to this stress disorder because of the following characteristics of rape: (1) it is sudden, and the victim is unable to develop adequate defenses; (2) it involves intentional cruelty or inhumanity; (3) it makes the victim feel trapped and unable to fight back; and (4) it often involves physical injury.[25] The initial psychological care of the rape victim in the emergency department is fundamental (Table 51–5). One can learn the methods for proper psychological care with a minimum of training.

Follow-up for rape victims is essential. A 2-week follow-up examination conducted by a physician should be arranged; medical (venereal disease and pregnancy) and psychological re-evaluation is performed at this time. Further evaluations can be performed at 4 and 6 weeks at the discretion of the physician following the patient. In addition, local volunteer support groups can be of immense

Table 51–5. STEPS FOR INITIAL PSYCHOLOGICAL CARE BY THE PHYSICIAN*

Introduction of self
Reassurance that patient is safe
Empathetic listening to the patient about her ordeal
Informing the patient of her current physical condition in a supportive way
Involvement of the patient in procedures and decision making
    Allowing patient to determine rate of questioning
    Obtaining permission from patient for steps in examination and informing her of what is being done and why
    Involving patient in decisions regarding treatment (e.g., use of prophylactic antibiotics or pregnancy prevention)
    Involving patient in decisions regarding medical and psychological follow-up
    Involving patient in decisions regarding contacting and giving information to husband, boyfriend, or family
Brief discussion of the psychological sequelae of rape with the patient or contact with someone trained in rape crisis intervention
Arrangements for supportive follow-up

*From Martin, C. A., Warfield, M. C., and Braen, G. R.: Physician's management of the psychological aspects of rape. JAMA 249:501, 1983. Used by permission.

assistance to a rape victim, and contact with such a group should be offered to each victim of sexual assault.

1. Hicks, D. J.: Rape: Sexual assault. Obstet. Gynecol. Annu. 7:447, 1978.
2. Nelson, C.: Victims of rape: Who are they? In Warner, C. G. (ed.): Rape and Sexual Assault: Management and Intervention. Rockville, MD, Aspen Publications, 1980.
3. Schiff, A. F.: A statistical evaluation of rape. Forensic Sci. 2:339, 1973.
4. Braen, G. R.: Sexual assault. In Rosen, P., et al. (eds.): Emergency Medicine, Concepts and Clinical Practice. St. Louis, C.V. Mosby, 1983.
5. Burgess, A. W., and Holstrom, L. L.: The rape victim in the emergency department. Am. J. Nurs. 73:1741, 1973.
6. Gomez, R. R., et al.: Qualitative and quantitative determinations of acid phosphatase activity in vaginal washings. Am. J. Clin. Pathol. 64:423, 1975.
7. Braen, G. R.: Physical assessment and emergency medical management for adult victims of sexual assault. In Warner, C. G. (ed.): Rape and Sexual Assault: Management and Intervention. Rockville, MD, Aspen Publications, 1980.
8. Don't miss a hair. F.B.I. Law Enforcement Bulletin 9, May 1976.
9. Twibell, J., and Whitehead, P. H.: Enzyme typing of human hair roots. J. Forensic Sci. 23:356, 1978.
10. Togatz, G. E., Okagaki, T., and Sciarra, J. J.: The effect of vaginal lubricants on sperm motility in vitro. Am. J. Obstet. Gynecol. 113:88, 1972.
11. Fish, S. A.: Vaginal injury due to coitus. Am. J. Obstet. Gynecol. 72:544, 1956.
12. Rush, R., and Milton, P. J. D.: Injuries of the vagina. S. Afr. Med. J. (Suppl.) 47:1325, 1973.
13. McCloskey, K. L., et al.: Prostatic acid phosphatase activity in the postcoital vagina. J. Forensic Sci. 21:630, 1975.
14. Rupp, J. C.: Sperm Survival and prostatic acid phosphatase activity in victims of sexual assault. J. Forensic Sci. 14:177, 1968.

15. Lauber, A. A., and Souma, M. L.: Use of toliudine blue for documentation of traumatic intercourse. Obstet. Gynecol. 60:644, 1982.
16. Richart, R. M.: A clinical staining test for the in vivo delineation of dysplasia and carcinoma in situ. Am. J. Obstet. Gynecol. 86:703, 1963.
17. Enos, W. F., and Beyer, J. C.: Spermatozoa in the anal canal and rectum and in the oral cavity in female rape victims. J. Forensic Sci. 23:231, 1978.
18. Hayman, C. R.: Serologic tests for syphilis in rape cases. JAMA 228:1227, 1974.
19. Saxena, B. B., et al.: Radio-receptorassay of human gonadotropin: Detection of early pregnancy. Science 184:793, 1974.
20. U.S. Department of Health, Education and Welfare: VD Fact Sheet 1975 (32nd ed.). DHEW Pub. No. (CDC) 76–8195. Atlanta, Center for Disease Control, 1975.

21. Schroeter, A. L., et al.: Therapy for incubating syphilis: Effectiveness of gonorrhea treatment. JAMA 218:711, 1971.
22. Burgess, A. W., and Holstrom, L. L.: Rape trauma syndrome. Am. J. Psychiatry 131:981, 1974.
23. Martin, C. A., Warfield, M. C., and Braen, G. R.: Physician's management of the psychological aspects of rape. JAMA 249:501, 1983.
24. American Psychiatric Association Committee on Nomenclature and Statistics: Diagnostic and Statistical Manual of Mental Disorders, 3rd ed. Washington, D.C., American Psychiatric Association, 1980.
25. Andreasen, N. C.: Post-traumatic stress disorder. In Kaplan, H. I., Freedman, A. M., and Sadock, B. J. (eds.): Comprehensive Textbook of Psychiatry III, Vol. 2. Baltimore, Williams & Wilkins, 1980, pp. 1517–1525.

52

Culdocentesis

G. RICHARD BRAEN, M.D.

Introduction

There are a number of conditions in which the clinician must sample the intraperitoneal fluid for confirming a diagnosis or for microbial culturing. This fluid can be obtained from the peritoneal cavity in a number of ways. Culdocentesis involves the introduction of a hollow needle through the vaginal wall into the peritoneal space. Culdocentesis is a simple, rapid, and safe procedure. The technique has several indications, but it is used primarily for diagnosing ruptured ectopic pregancies and ruptured ovarian cysts and for obtaining fluid to aid in the culture diagnosis of pelvic inflammatory disease (PID).

Anatomy

Before a culdocentesis is attempted, the clinician must be familiar with the anatomy of the rectouterine pouch (pouch of Douglas) and the vagina. In the adult female, the vagina is approximately 9 cm long. From its inferior to its superior aspect, the posterior wall of the vagina is related to the anal canal by way of the perineal body, the rectum, and the peritoneum of the rectouterine pouch.[1] The rectouterine pouch and the posterior wall of the vagina are adjacent only at the upper quarter (approximately 2 cm) of the posterior vaginal wall. The vaginal wall in this area is less than 5 mm thick. The uterus lies nearly at a right angle to the vagina.

The blood supply of the upper vagina comes from the uterine and vaginal arteries, which are branches of the internal iliac artery. The area is drained by a vaginal venous plexus that communicates with the uterine and vesical plexuses. The vagina has its greatest sensation near the introitus, and there is little sensation in the area adjacent to the rectouterine pouch.

The rectouterine pouch is formed by reflections of the peritoneum, and it is the most dependent intraperitoneal space in both the upright and the supine positions. Blood, pus, and other free fluids in the peritoneal cavity will pool in the pouch because of its dependent location. This pouch separates the upper portion of the rectum from the uterus and the upper part of the vagina. The pouch often contains small intestine and normally a small amount of peritoneal fluid.

Indications

Culdocentesis is indicated in any adult female when fluid aspirated from the rectouterine pouch will help confirm a clinical diagnosis.[2] Analysis of peritoneal fluid is a reliable method of differentiating inflammatory from hemorrhagic pelvic pathologic conditions. Conditions in which a culdocentesis may be of diagnostic value include a ruptured viscus (particularly a ruptured ectopic pregnancy or corpus luteum cyst), pelvic inflammatory disease (PID), and other intra-abdominal infections (particularly appendicitis with rupture or diverticulitis with perforation), intra-abdominal injuries to the liver or the spleen, and ruptured aortic aneurysms.[3]

Ectopic Pregnancy. Ectopic pregnancy is often one of the most difficult gynecologic lesions to diagnose.[4] In a series of 300 consecutive cases of ectopic pregnancy, 50 per cent of patients received medical consultation at least two times before the correct diagnosis was made.[5] In 11 per cent of the patients in this series, the diagnosis was not made until the third medical visit. Because of the severe consequences of a ruptured ectopic pregnancy, an early, accurate diagnosis is essential. Ectopic pregnancy is the leading cause of maternal death in the first trimester of pregnancy.[6]

The clinical picture of ectopic pregnancy may include vascular collapse, pelvic pain, amenorrhea or abnormal menses, shoulder pain, syncope, cervical or adnexal tenderness, an adnexal mass, and anemia and leukocytosis. There is often a history of salpingitis, use of an intrauterine contraceptive device, or tubal ligation. No combination of these signs, symptoms, or historical data is diagnostic for an ectopic pregnancy. To confuse the diagnosis further, a normal menstrual history and a negative urine pregnancy test are found in approximately 50 per cent of patients with ectopic pregnancy.[7] The greater sensitivity of the serum hCG-β subunit radioreceptor assay and urine hemagglutination inhibition tests, coupled with the development of pelvic ultrasound and laparoscopy, has increased the chances for early diagnosis of *unruptured* ectopic pregnancy.[8] Culdocentesis, however, continues to play an important role in the diagnosis of *ruptured* ectopic pregnancy, with an accuracy rate of 85 to 95 per cent.[5, 9, 10] Although a culdocentesis is most often positive in the presence of a frankly ruptured ectopic pregnancy, it may be diagnostic even in the nonruptured case when bleeding has been slow or intermittent. It is useful to note that many ectopic pregnancies will leak varying amounts of blood for days or weeks prior to rupture.

Pelvic Infection. Acute PID has a polymicrobial etiology.[11–13] It has been common practice to define the etiology of PID by isolation of pathogens from the endocervix. The etiology is probably better defined by examination of the tubal flora. In fact, there is little correlation between cul-de-sac cultures and cervical cultures in PID.[14] Some medical centers routinely use aspirates obtained through culdocentesis to aid in determining the microbial agents causing the PID.[15] As the microbiology of PID becomes more complex and as the causative organisms develop resistance to antimicrobial agents, culdocentesis may evolve as one of the prime methods of obtaining meaningful micro-

biological cultures that will dictate appropriate therapy.

Blunt Abdominal Trauma. Although diagnostic peritoneal lavage remains a popular and valuable technique, the use of culdocentesis to detect hemoperitoneum has been advocated.[3, 16] Because small amounts of blood tend to collect in the rectouterine pouch, the aspiration of clear peritoneal fluid is of great potential value in *excluding* hemoperitoneum. The procedure may be more advantageous than peritoneal lavage in some instances, because there is less risk of urinary bladder perforation or bowel injury. In addition, previous abdominal surgery is not a contraindication to culdocentesis, as it is with peritoneal lavage.[17]

Contraindications

The contraindications to culdocentesis are relatively few and include a pelvic mass detected on bimanual pelvic examination, a nonmobile retroverted uterus, and coagulopathies. Pelvic masses may include tubo-ovarian abscesses, appendiceal abscesses, ovarian masses, and pelvic kidneys. It has been suggested that "the only major risk with the procedure is that of rupturing an unsuspected tubo-ovarian abscess into the peritoneal cavity. This can be avoided by careful bimanual pelvic examination to exclude patients with large masses not affixed to the cul de sac."[14] In a review of many reports on culdocentesis, I found no reference to the age of patients in whom culdocentesis may be safely performed. I contend that a culdocentesis should be limited to patients who are beyond puberty, because after the pubertal stage the vagina has begun to lengthen and mature. This limitation is suggested on the basis of anatomy and with the consideration that the procedure is difficult to perform through a small, prepubertal vagina.

Equipment

The equipment required for culdocentesis is listed in Table 52–1. Either an 18 gauge spinal

Table 52–1. EQUIPMENT FOR CULDOCENTESIS

Adjustable examination table with stirrups
Bivalve vaginal speculum
Uterine cervical tenaculum
No. 19 gauge butterfly needle or 18 gauge spinal needle
No. 25 gauge needle (for local anesthetic infiltration)
Ring sponge forceps
Syringes (20 ml)
Surgical preparation (iodinated, such as Betadine)
Sterile water, cotton balls, 4 × 4 gauze sponges
Cocaine (10 per cent solution) or lidocaine (1 per cent) with epinephrine
Culture media or test tube without anticoagulant

needle or a 19 gauge butterfly needle held by ring forceps is acceptable. It is also acceptable to anesthetize the posterior vaginal wall at the site of the puncture using 1 to 2 per cent lidocaine with epinephrine through a 25 gauge needle. Some physicians use a cocaine-soaked cotton ball to anesthetize the mucosa prior to infiltration with a local anesthetic. Although local anesthesia is often unnecessary (since the puncture of the posterior vaginal wall at the upper one fourth of the vagina is relatively painless), there may be some advantage to local anesthesia, since multiple attempts at culdocentesis are occasionally required. In addition, the epinephrine may produce vasoconstriction and may reduce bleeding associated with the needle puncture. Although culdocentesis is not usually very painful, it may be stressful to the patient, and all attempts should be made to render the procedure as painless as possible.

Technique

A culdocentesis is an invasive procedure that, in many hospitals, requires a written, witnessed, and signed consent form from the patient, parent, or guardian when the patient's condition permits. Once this consent is obtained, the patient is placed in a lithotomy position with the head of the table slightly elevated (reverse Trendelenburg position) so that intraperitoneal fluid will gravitate into the rectouterine pouch. The patient's feet are placed in stirrups. In selected patients, some physicians prefer to premedicate with intravenous narcotics, such as meperidine (Demerol), or sedatives, such as diazepam (Valium). The administration of nitrous oxide analgesia is also an accepted practice. Although pain may not be an overriding aspect of culdocentesis, the judicious use of analgesia and sedation will make the procedure easier for both physician and patient.

Radiographs when indicated in the stable patient are taken *prior* to culdocentesis to avoid possible confusion if a pneumoperitoneum is detected following the procedure.

A bimanual pelvic examination must be performed prior to culdocentesis to rule out a fixed pelvic mass and to assess the position of the uterus. The examiner then inserts the bivalve vaginal speculum and opens it widely by adjusting both the height and the angle thumbscrews. The *posterior* lip of the cervix is grasped with the toothed uterine cervical tenaculum, and the cervix is elevated (Fig. 52–1). This maneuver will elevate a retroverted uterus from the pouch, expose the puncture site, and stabilize the posterior wall during the needle puncture. Some physicians prefer

to use longitudinal traction on the cervix to produce the same result. Pain is often felt by the patient when the cervix is grasped with the tenaculum, and the patient should be forewarned of a possible sharp pain during this part of the examination. The vaginal wall adjacent to the rectouterine pouch will be tightened somewhat between the inferior blade of the bivalve speculum and the elevated posterior lip of the cervix. This tightening of the vaginal wall will expose the puncture site and will keep it from moving away from the needle when the wall is punctured.

After the tenaculum is applied and the posterior lip of the cervix is elevated or traction is applied, the vaginal wall in the area of the rectouterine pouch should be swabbed with surgical preparation followed by a small amount of sterile water. Local anesthesia may be administered at this point. Anesthesia may be injected with a separate No. 25 gauge needle or by the spinal needle to be used for the culdocentesis. A cotton ball soaked in cocaine solution can also be used for topical anesthesia of the posterior vaginal wall prior to infiltration with a local anesthetic. The needles used for both the local anesthetic and for the puncture should be attached to a 20-ml syringe. A smaller syringe may not be long enough to allow adequate control of the needle, and the physician's hand may block the view of the puncture site if a smaller syringe is used.

Following local anesthesia the syringe and the spinal needle to be used for the culdocentesis are advanced parallel to the lower blade of the speculum. It is helpful to fill the syringe with 2 to 3 ml of air or saline (nonbacteriostatic) before puncture. Following needle puncture, the free flow of the air or fluid from the syringe confirms that the needle tip is in the proper position and is not lodged in the uterine wall or the intestinal wall. Saline (rather than air) is preferred, because if air is used, one must be careful in interpreting the presence of free peritoneal air on subsequent radiographs. To avoid the need to change the syringe during the procedure, lidocaine (Xylocaine) may be used for both anesthesia and confirmation of proper needle placement, but the bacteriostatic property of this agent precludes its use if the procedure is performed to obtain fluid for culture.

The vaginal wall should be penetrated in the midline 1 to 1½ cm posteriorly (inferiorly) to the point at which the vaginal wall joins the cervix (Fig. 52–2).[18] The needle should penetrate a total of 2 to 2½ cm.[18, 19] Suction is then applied with the syringe while the needle is slowly withdrawn. It is important for the physician to avoid aspirating any blood that has accumulated in the vagina from previous needle punctures or from cervical bleed-

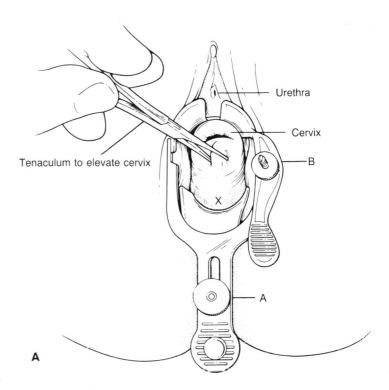

Tenaculum to elevate cervix

Urethra

Cervix

B

X

A

A

Figure 52-1. A, Preparation for culdocentesis. Note that one opens the speculum widely by using both the height (A) and the angle adjustments (B). The cervix is grasped on the posterior lip with a toothed tenaculum. X marks the site for puncture of the vaginal wall. (From Vander Salm, T. J., et al.: Atlas of Bedside Procedures. Boston, Little, Brown & Co., 1979.) B, This diagram demonstrates the use of a butterfly needle for culdocentesis. The needle is inserted 1 cm posterior to the point at which the vaginal wall joins the cervix. (From Webb, M. J., Culdocentesis. J.A.C.E.P., 7:452, 1978.)

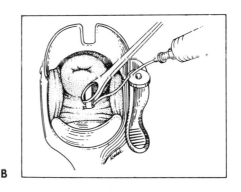

B

ing, since this may give the false impression of a positive tap. Bleeding from the puncture site in the vaginal wall is minimized if epinephrine is added to the local anesthetic.

Blood or fluid may be obtained immediately but may also be obtained just before the needle is withdrawn from the peritoneal cavity. Therefore, it is important to aspirate throughout the gradual withdrawal procedure. Because small clots may clog an 18 gauge needle, some physicians prefer using a larger gauge needle (e.g., 15 or 16 gauge), which will permit easier aspiration of small clots.[4] These needles are rarely required, however. If no fluid is aspirated, the needle should be reintroduced and directed only slightly to the left or right of the midline. Directing the needle too far laterally may result in puncture of mesenteric or pelvic

vessels. It is important to note that if no fluid is obtained on the first attempt, the procedure should be repeated.

Some physicians prefer the use of a No. 19 gauge butterfly needle held with a ring forceps (Fig. 52–3).[2] This technique offers a built-in guide to needle depth and allows for good control of the needle during puncture. An assistant must aspirate the tubing while the physician controls positioning and withdrawal of the needle.

Fluid that is aspirated may be old, nonclotting blood, bright red blood, pus, exudate, or a straw-colored and serous liquid. Any fluid that is not blood should be submitted for Gram staining, aerobic and anaerobic culture, and cell counts. Blood should be observed for clotting. Blood should also be sent for a hematocrit determination.

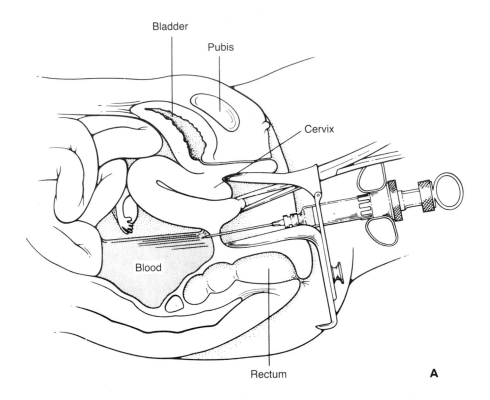

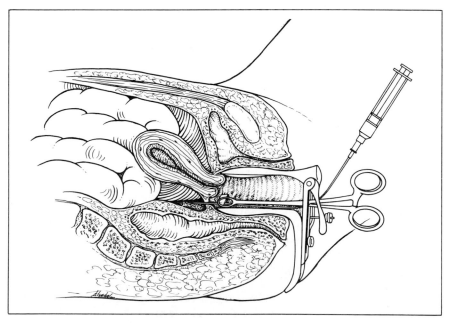

Figure 52–2. The needle is advanced parallel to the lower blade of the speculum. Aspiration is continued throughout the gradual withdrawal of the needle. Figure A demonstrates the use of a spinal needle and Figure B demonstrates the use of a butterfly needle and ringed forceps. (A, From Vander Salm, T. J., et al.: Atlas of Bedside Procedures. Boston, Little, Brown & Co., 1979. B, From Webb, M. J.: Culdocentesis. J.A.C.E.P., 7:452, 1978.)

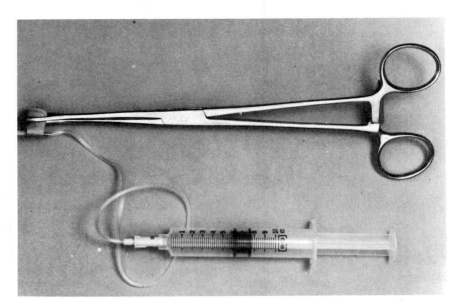

Figure 52–3. Culdocentesis may be performed with a 19 gauge butterfly needle held with ring forceps. (From Webb, M. J.: Culdocentesis. JACEP 7:451, 1978. Used by permission.)

Interpretation of Results

An interpretation of the results of a culdocentesis depends primarily on whether or not any fluid was obtained. In the absence of a pathologic condition, one will often aspirate a few milliliters of clear, yellowish peritoneal fluid. When there is no return of fluid of any type (a so-called dry tap), the procedure has *no diagnostic value*. Since a dry tap is nondiagnostic, it should not be equated with normal peritoneal fluid. In addition, when less than 2 ml of clotting blood is obtained, this is also considered to be a nondiagnostic tap, since the source of this small amount of blood may be the puncture site on the vaginal wall. Such blood will

Table 52–2. INTERPRETATION OF CULDOCENTESIS FLUID

Aspirated Fluid	Condition and Suggested Differential Diagnosis
Clear, serous, straw-colored (usually only a few milliliters)	Normal pelvic fluid
Large amount of clear fluid	Ruptured ovarian cyst (fluid may be serosanguineous) Ascites Carcinoma
Exudate with polymorphonuclear leukocytes	Pelvic inflammatory disease Gonococcal salpingitis Chronic salpingitis
Purulent fluid	Bacterial infection Tubo-ovarian abscess with rupture Appendicitis with rupture Diverticulitis with perforation
Bright red blood*	Ruptured viscus or vascular injury Recently bleeding ectopic pregnancy* Bleeding corpus luteum Intra-abdominal injury Liver Spleen Other organs Ruptured aortic aneurysm
Old, brown, nonclotting blood	Ruptured viscus Ectopic pregnancy with intraperitoneal bleeding over a few days or weeks Old (days) intra-abdominal injury (e.g., delayed splenic rupture)

*Note: The hematocrit of blood from a ruptured ectopic pregnancy is usually greater than 15 per cent (97.5 per cent of cases)[5]

usually clot. Over 2 ml of *nonclotting blood* is certainly suggestive of a hemoperitoneum. There is no particular significance to larger amounts of blood, since this may be related to the needle position or the rate of bleeding. Brenner and coworkers[5] reported no blood from culdocentesis in 5 per cent of patients with proven ectopic pregnancies, even when rupture had occurred.

Since the culdocentesis is usually used to diagnose an ectopic pregnancy, a "negative tap" is one that yields pus or clear, straw-colored peritoneal or cystic fluid. A large amount of clear fluid (greater than 10 ml) indicates a probable ruptured ovarian cyst, ascites, or possibily carcinoma. The significance of these fluids is outlined in Table 52–2.

A "positive tap" is one in which nonclotting blood is obtained. Blood will remain unclotted for days in the syringe as a result of the defibrination activity of the peritoneum. This finding is indicative of hemoperitoneum caused by conditions such as a ruptured ectopic pregnancy, a hemorrhagic ovarian cyst, or a ruptured spleen. The return of a serosanguineous fluid also suggests a ruptured ovarian cyst. The hematocrit of blood from active intraperitoneal bleeding is greater than 10 per cent. In one series, the hematocrit of blood from a ruptured ectopic pregnancy was at least 15 per cent in 97 per cent of cases.[5]

Complications

Culdocentesis is one of the safest procedures performed in the emergency setting, and there are probably fewer complications with this technique than with peripheral venous cannulation. Complications have been reported, however, and include the rupture of an unsuspected tubo-ovarian abscess.[18] This is the most common of the serious complications. Others include perforation of the bowel, perforation of a pelvic kidney, and bleeding from the puncture site in patients with clotting disorders. Since the most common complications result from the puncture of a pelvic mass, careful bimanual examination of the patient should help prevent this problem. Puncture of the bowel and the uterine wall occurs relatively frequently, but this occurrence does not generally result in serious morbidity. Obviously, penetration of the gravid uterus has greater potential for harm. Occasionally, one will aspirate air or fecal matter, confirming inadvertent puncture of the rectum. Although this may be disconcerting, it is seldom of serious clinical concern and requires no immediate change in therapy.

Conclusion

In the emergency setting, culdocentesis is a very helpful diagnostic procedure. It is used mainly in the evaluation of ruptured ectopic pregnancy but should also be considered as a diagnostic aid in the evaluation of PID and in abdominal trauma. This is a safe, simple procedure that every physician who deals with the emergency evaluation of women, *particularly women of the childbearing age,* should know and use. It is the most reliable, and certainly the most rapid, way to perform a definitive evaluation of the unstable patient with suspected ruptured ectopic pregnancy.

1. Ellis, H.: Clinical Anatomy, A Revision and Applied Anatomy for Clinical Students, 5th ed. Oxford, Blackwell Scientific Publications, 1972, pp. 129–131.
2. Webb, M. J.: Culdocentesis. JACEP 7:451, 1978.
3. Clarke, J. M.: Culdocentesis in the evaluation of blunt abdominal trauma. Surg. Gynecol. Obstet. 129:809, 1969.
4. Capraro, V. J., Chuang, J. T., and Randall, C. L.: Cul-de-sac aspiration and other diagnostic aids for ectopic pregnancy. Int. Surg. 53:4, 1970.
5. Brenner, P. F., Roys, S., and Mishell, D. R.: Ectopic pregnancy. A study of 300 consecutive surgically treated cases. JAMA 243:673, 1980.
6. National Center for Health Statistics: Final Mortality Statistics, 1975. Washington, D.C., U.S. Government Printing Office, 1977.
7. Kistner, R. W.: The oviduct-tubal ectopic pregnancy. *In* Kistner, R. W. (ed.): Gynecology: Principles and Practice, 2nd ed., Chicago, Year Book Medical Publishers, 1971, pp. 304–308.
8. Chung, S. J.: Review of pregnancy tests. South. Med. J. 74:11, 1981.
9. Hall, R. E., and Tod, W. D.: The suspected ectopic pregnancy. Am. J. Obstet. Gynecol. 81:1220, 1969.
10. Webster, H. D., Barclay, D. L., and Fischer, C. K.: Ectopic pregnancy: A seventeen-year review. Am. J. Obstet. Gynecol. 92:23, 1965.
11. Thompson, S. E., III, and Hager, W. D.: Acute pelvic inflammatory disease. Sex. Transm. Dis. 4:105, 1977.
12. Eschenbach, D. A.: Epidemiology and diagnosis of acute pelvic inflammatory disease. Obstet. Gynecol. 55:142S, 1980.
13. Monif, G. R. G.: Significance of polymicrobial bacterial superinfection in the therapy of gonococcal endometritis-salpingitis-peritonitis. Obstet. Gynecol. 55:154S, 1980.
14. Chow, A. W., Malkasian, K. L., Marchall, J. R., et al.: The bacteriology of acute pelvic inflammatory disease, value of cul-de-sac cultures and relative importance of gonococci and other aerobic or anaerobic bacteria. Am. J. Obstet. Gynecol. 122:876, 1975.
15. Eschenbach, D. A., Buchanan, T. M., Pollock, H. M., et al.: Polymicrobial etiology of acute pelvic inflammatory disease. N. Engl. J. Med. 293:166, 1975.
16. Generelly, P., Moore T. A., and LeMay, J. T.: Delayed splenic rupture: Diagnosed by culdocentesis. JACEP 6:369, 1977.
17. Olsen, W. R.: Peritoneal lavage in blunt abdominal trauma. JACEP 2:271, 1973.
18. Webb, M. J.: Culdocentesis. JACEP 7:12, 1978.
19. Lucas, C., Hassim, A. M.: Place of culdocentesis in the diagnosis of ectopic pregnancy. Br. Med. J. 1:200, 1970.

53

IUD Removal

SAMUEL TIMOTHY COLERIDGE, D.O.

Introduction

Intrauterine contraceptive devices (IUDs) are the third most popular method of temporary contraception used by married couples in the United States and second only to oral contraceptives in effectiveness in preventing pregnancy.[1] It is generally accepted that the mechanism of action of the IUD is the production of a local sterile inflammatory reaction caused by the presence of a foreign body in the uterus. The addition of copper increases this inflammatory reaction. Copper ions as well as the locally released high levels of progesterone probably also act to prevent the normal process of implantation.[2, 3] Upon removal of an IUD, the inflammatory process rapidly disappears, although controversy exists as to whether the mechanism of resumption of fertility is the same as that following discontinuation of mechanical methods, such as the condom or the diaphragm.[4]

In general, with IUDs the pregnancy rate is approximately 2 per cent, the rate of expulsion is 10 per cent, and the rate of removal for medical reasons is 15 per cent. The major reasons for removal are uterine bleeding or lower abdominal pain during the first year of use. The incidence of each complication diminishes in subsequent years.[3, 5, 6] The complications of IUDs include an increased odds ratio of 1.9 to 12.3 of developing pelvic inflammatory disease (PID),[3, 4, 7–15] a 4.4 to 8.9 per cent increased risk of extrauterine pregnancy if the patient with an IUD should get pregnant,[3, 7, 10–12, 16–24] and increased incidence of uterine perforation and uterine bleeding.[6, 25] In pregnant patients who fail to remove the IUD, there is an increased risk of spontaneous and septic abortion with both increased mortality and increased morbidity,[1, 3, 7, 10, 17, 26–29] a higher incidence of abruptio placenta and placenta previa,[7] and a possible increased risk of prematurity in IUDs containing copper.[3] Keith and coworkers noted an increased incidence of actinomycosis infections with prolonged IUD usage,[10] and Misenhimer and Garcia-Bunuel noted an association between intrauterine fungal contamination and neonatal death in two case reports.[30] There is no evidence to suggest that IUDs are associated with an increased incidence of congenital anomalies.[3, 10]

Several long-term studies have indicated that IUDs are not associated with an increased incidence of carcinoma of the cervix or the endometrium.[3] It is estimated, however, that among IUD users mortality is 3 to 5 deaths per million females annually, mainly as a result of infection. The IUD is as safe as or safer than other methods of contraception, including sterilization, and safer than no contraception, regardless of age group.

Over the past 7 years there has been a gradual decrease in the number of IUDs used, especially in the United States. In 1977, the Conception Control Subcommittee of the Panel on Review of OB/GYN Devices of the United States Food and Drug Administration recommended that IUD labeling include the statement, "IUD use is associated with a 3- to 5-fold increase in infection rate."[3] It has been estimated that 5 to 6 per cent of patients using an IUD will have it removed because of minor or major sepsis.[14] Gonococcal endometritis/salpingitis is increased by a factor of 2.8 in IUD users, whereas the risk of nongonococcal endometritis/salpingitis is increased by a factor of 6.5.[4, 9] The nullipara seems to be especially prone to pelvic infection with an IUD in place and should therefore be discouraged from using this type of contraceptive.[4, 13, 14, 31]

Among current IUD users, those using an IUD 25 months or more are 2 to 6.5 times more likely to have an ectopic pregnancy than are short-term users (those less than 25 months).[20, 23, 24] This difference between long- and short-term users persists for 1 year after removal of the IUD and then declines.[20]

Several authors have found that women with an IUD in place at the estimated time of conception are three to eight times more likely to experience second trimester fetal loss than are women who conceive without an IUD in place.[26, 28, 29] If the IUD is removed during the first trimester, there is little increase in the risk of second trimester fetal loss over patients who conceive without an IUD in place. The observed 20.3 per cent incidence of second trimester fetal loss is similar to the 17 per cent incidence of spontaneous abortion among nonusers of IUDs. In contrast, the estimated relative risk of fetal loss for women with an IUD in place at conception that was not removed in the first trimester is 10.3 per cent higher than the risk in nonusers.[16, 17, 26]

The relative risk for septic second trimester fetal loss in patients with IUDs versus nonseptic losses in this group ranges from 2- to 13-fold.[26, 28] There is no association between IUD use in the recent past (less than 1 year) or in the remote past (greater than 1 year) and second or third trimester fetal loss, provided that there is no IUD in situ at conception. The type of IUD does not affect the risk of fetal loss.[7, 9, 26] The clinical features of the febrile spontaneous abortion in IUD users and in nonusers are similar; both groups of patients experience mainly localized symptoms, such as pelvic pain, uterine cramping, and vaginal hemorrhage.[28] This differs from the generalized symptoms that have been reported with maternal deaths. The clinical course of an IUD-associated maternal death from spontaneous abortion begins with generalized symptoms of septicemia, which precede the abortion. Fever was the presenting sign in 13 of 17 women who died with IUDs in place in Cates' study. No maternal deaths from an IUD in situ occurred during the first trimester; however, the risk of maternal death was 50 times greater in women who continued their pregnancy with an IUD in situ than in those who did not.[17]

Uterine perforation, although not common, is a potentially serious complication. *Perforation usually occurs initially at insertion* and is related to the shape of the IUD and the amount of force needed during insertion.[6, 32] During the months following insertion, continued uterine contractions may be responsible for either partial or complete perforation through the uterine musculature.[6, 32] Eisenberg describes the "widened Lippe's loop" on plain AP roentgenograms of the pelvis to definitively diagnose perforations of this type of IUD. He describes the distance from the bullous tip at the end of the loop to the second loop as approximately 1 cm in every case (normal controls were usually 2 or 3 mm and never greater than 5 mm).[33] Contiguous organs can become involved, particularly the rectosigmoid colon, the small bowel, and the bladder. In addition, problems can occur in more esoteric locations (e.g., fistulas to the abdominal wall).[6] The detailed discussion and classification of uterine perforations by Zakin, Stern, and Rosenblatt is recommended for a discussion of the multiple possibilities involved and for an explanation of why gentle traction for removal with or without sonography, radiography, or hysterography is indicated rather than repeated forceful attempts at removal (Fig. 53–1).[6, 25]

Indications for IUD Removal

If a woman with an IUD in situ becomes pregnant, it is advisable to remove her IUD as soon as the pregnancy is recognized in order to give her pregnancy the optimal chance of progressing to term and to eliminate the possibility of maternal death in the second or third trimester from sepsis. The IUD can usually be easily withdrawn by the physician if the string is visible. If the IUD cannot be removed, interruption of the pregnancy should be offered as an option. If the patient elects to

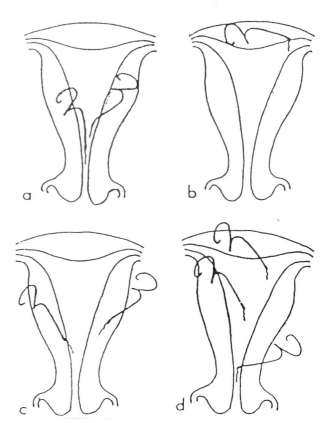

Figure 53–1. Types of partially perforated IUDs. For schematic purposes, the underlined number indicates the preponderant compartment involved; however, all degrees of perforation are possible. Uterine perforation has occurred with all types of IUDs; the IUD represented here is a stylized version. The string of the IUD is shown as missing at the external os because this is most often the case. *a,* Type 1–2; type 1–2. IUD present in compartments 1 (uterine cavity) and 2 (myometrium). *b,* Type 2. IUD present in compartment 2. *c,* Type 2–3; type 2–3. IUD present in compartments 2 and 3 (peritoneal cavity). *d,* Type 1–2–3; type 1–2–3; type 1–2–3. IUD present in compartments 1, 2, and 3. (From Zakin, D., Stern, W. Z., and Rosenblatt, R.: Complete and partial uterine perforation and embedding following insertion of intrauterine devices I. Classification, complications, mechanism, incidence, and missing string. Obstet. Gynecol. Surv. 36:335, 1981. Used by permission.)

maintain her pregnancy with the IUD in place, she should be warned of the increased risk of sepsis and should be closely followed for signs of septicemia.[1, 3, 16, 26, 28]

Likewise, the shortened or invisible IUD string suggests uterine perforation and merits attempted IUD removal.[6, 10] The presence of endometritis in a patient with an IUD in place is also an indication for IUD removal. Although the issue is controversial, the consensus is that the IUD may act as a foreign body and may prohibit eradication of the bacterial infection with antibiotics alone.[14, 15, 34] It is generally advised that broad-spectrum antibiotics be given for 7 to 14 days after IUD removal if PID is diagnosed. Antibiotics are not required if IUD removal is accomplished in the absence of infection.

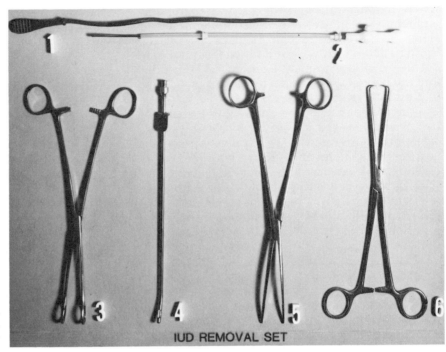

Figure 53–2. IUD removal tray. *1,* Uterine sound. *2,* IUD extractor device. *3,* Sponge (ring) forceps. *4,* Novak curette. *5,* Bozman forceps. *6,* Tenaculum.

Equipment

Equipment useful for simple IUD removal is depicted in Figure 53–2. A tray containing the uterine sound, a tenaculum, and Bozman forceps (numbers 1, 6, and 5, Fig. 53–2) is often adequate. Included on the tray should be a Novak curette, sponge forceps and, possibly, the IUD extractor device (numbers 4, 3, and 2, Fig. 53–2).

Procedure

Prior to removal of the IUD, a consent form should be signed by all patients, particularly the pregnant patient. The patient should be given instructions regarding the procedure, the probable side effects of mild uterine cramping and spotting for a few days, and the possible complications of uterine perforation and induced abortion if she is pregnant. The patient should be cautioned to return immediately if fever develops.

Removal of the IUD during menses is somewhat easier, although this is not always possible. Swabbing the cervix with a povidone-iodine or soap solution is recommended prior to the insertion of any instrument in the uterine cavity. Slow removal of the IUD by gentle, constant traction with the Bozman forceps is usually successful. A sudden jerking movement may cause the string to break. If the IUD does not dislodge easily, sounding the uterus and gently probing the device may facilitate removal. If this is not adequate, then progressive

dilation of the cervix is appropriate. A tenaculum to steady the cervix or to straighten the ante- or retroverted uterus may be useful. A paracervical block of anesthesia is indicated when significant patient discomfort exists.[6, 18]

When the string is not visible at the cervical os, pregnancy must be excluded before any exploration of the uterine cavity. After pregnancy has been ruled out, the cervix is grasped with a tenaculum and the uterine cavity is explored with a sound to locate the IUD. After the presence and the position of the device have been noted, an IUD extractor, as described by Landesman (number 4, Fig. 53–2),[35] or a Novak curette is passed beyond the IUD and is withdrawn. Likewise, Husemeyer and Gordon advocate use of the "Mi-Mark Helix" (Simpson/Basye Inc.) device, originally designed to obtain endometrial mucus, as an IUD extractor similar to Landesman's device.[36] With repeated gentle passes of either instrument, the string will become visible or the device itself will be visible at the external cervical os. Once visualization is assured, a Bozman or sponge (ring) forceps can be used to grasp the IUD and to complete the extraction. Avoidance of winding or angulating the thread about the jaws of the instrument is important.

If the device is not felt, a radiograph can be obtained. The uterine sound should be inside the uterine cavity to demonstrate the cavity position in both posteroanterior and lateral films.[6, 18, 25] Practitioners in some institutions may prefer to use sonography to determine location.[3, 6, 37] If the IUD is outside the uterus, referral in a routine but timely manner to a gynecologist for laparoscopy and removal is indicated to prevent potential adhesions and bowel obstruction. Similarly, the Majzlin Spring IUD (which was withdrawn from the market in 1973) is extremely likely to be embedded and the patient with this device should be referred to a gynecologist for removal.[38]

If the patient is pregnant and wishes to maintain her pregnancy, she should be thoroughly counseled that removal will statistically improve the chances for a successful outcome but that a spontaneous abortion may also occur. Removal of the IUD with a visible string should be accomplished with gentle traction. The patient should be told to return should bleeding, cramping, or signs of infection occur.

Complications

As previously stressed, removal of IUDs from the uterine cavity—whether diagnosed as free, embedded, or partially perforated (see Fig. 53–1)—should be accomplished cautiously and in a tentative fashion. It should be predetermined that attempts at removal will be stopped if undue resistance to instrumental traction is encountered. Complications of severe continuous or delayed bleeding, uterine cramping, or signs of sepsis suggest uterine perforation, and no further attempts at extraction in the emergency department are appropriate if these are present.[6, 25] Urgent referral to a gynecologist after telephone consultation is necessary. If uterine perforation occurs, the patient should be started on broad-spectrum antibiotics and typed for possible blood transfusion if hemorrhage is present.

Intravenous or oral antibiotics for 1 to 2 weeks in the symptomatic patient with PID are mandatory *with* IUD removal to prevent bacteremia/septicemia. Some physicians recommend antibiotic therapy be initiated *prior* to IUD removal. Although extended therapy prior to removal has been recommended by some, a 30-minute delay following intravenous antibiotics in the noncompromised patient (without valvular heart disease) should be adequate in the patient *without* uterine perforation. If the device is removed because of persistent cramping or uterine bleeding in the absence of infection, prophylactic antibiotics are not routinely given. It must be stressed, however, that low-grade endometritis is often difficult to exclude in the presence of pain and bleeding in the IUD user, and a course of antibiotics is justified in borderline cases.

Generally, only mild analgesia, if any, need be prescribed following the extraction. Alternative means for future birth control should be advocated for the patient who experiences an IUD-related complication.

Summary

Voluntary removal of the IUD is generally a simple procedure when the device is indeed intrauterine. In the pregnant patient, removal is both recommended and generally safe in the first trimester. When the IUD string of a nonpregnant patient cannot be seen, appropriate investigation for its location by radiographs with an intrauterine sound in place or by sonography is indicated if cervical dilation with gentle, unhurried, and careful endocervical and intrauterine probing is unsuccessful. If the IUD is not easily found or if gentle, constant traction is ineffective in removing the IUD, then one should consider uterine perforation. Referral to a gynecologist is appropriate for further investigation; hysteroscopy, laparoscopy, or laparotomy may be required. Removal can be difficult and even hazardous, depending on the degree of myometrial penetration or the extrauterine location.

1. Cates, W., Jr., Ory, H. W., and Tyler, C. W.: Publicity and the public health: The elimination of IUD-related abortion deaths. Fam. Plann. Perspect. 9:138, 1977.
2. Beerthuizen, R. J., Van Wijck, J. A., Eskes, T. K., Vermeulen, A. H., and Vooijs, G. P.: IUD and salpingitis: A prospective study of pathomorphological changes in the oviducts in IUD-users. Eur. J. Obstet. Gynecol. Reprod. Biol. 13:31, 1982.
3. Mischell, D.: Intrauterine devices. Clin. Obstet. Gynecol. 6(1):27, 1979.
4. Eschenbach, D. A.: Do IUDs increase relative risk of infection? Contemporary OB/GYN 14:93, 1979.
5. Chaudhury, R. R.: Current status of research on intrauterine devices. Obstet. Gynecol. 34:333, 1980.
6. Zakin, D., Stern, W. Z., and Rosenblatt, R.: Complete and partial uterine perforation and embedding following insertion of intrauterine devices I. Classification, complications, mechanism, incidence, and missing string. Obstet. Gynecol. 36:335, 1981.
7. Burkman, R. T.: Association between intrauterine device and pelvic inflammatory disease. Obstet. Gynecol. 57:269, 1981.
8. Edelman, D. A.: Pelvic inflammatory disease and the intrauterine device: A causal relationship. Int. J. Gynecol. Obstet. 17:504, 1980.
9. Eschenbach, D. A., Harnisch, J. P., and Holmes, K. K.: Pathogenesis of acute pelvic inflammatory disease: Role of contraception and other risk factors. Am. J. Obstet. Gynecol. 8:838, 1977.
10. Keith, L. G., Berger, G. S., and Edelman, D. A.: Clinician's guide to using IUD's—safely. Contemporary OB/GYN 19:159, 1982.
11. Malhotra, N., and Chaudhury, R. R.: Current status of intrauterine devices II. Intrauterine devices and pelvic inflammatory disease and ectopic pregnancy. Obstet. Gynecol. Surv. 37:1, 1982.
12. Oser, S., Liedholm, P., Gullberg, B., and Sjoberg, N. O.: Risk of pelvic inflammatory disease among intrauterine device users irrespective of previous pregnancy. Lancet 1:386, 1980.
13. Vessey, M. P., Yeates, D., Flavel, M., and McPherson, K.: Pelvic inflammatory disease and the intrauterine device: Findings in a large cohort study. Br. Med. J. 282:855, 1981.

14. Westrom, L., Bengtsson, L. P., and Mardh, P. A.: The risk of pelvic inflammatory disease in women using intrauterine contraceptive devices as compared to non-users. Lancet 2:161, 1976.
15. Westrom, L.: The risk of pelvic inflammatory disease in women using intrauterine contraceptive devices as compared to non-users. Lancet 2:221, 1974.
16. Alvior, G.: Pregnancy outcome with removal of intrauterine device. Obstet. Gynecol. 41:894, 1973.
17. Cates, W., Jr., Ory, H. W., Rochat, R. W., and Tyler, C. W.: The intrauterine device and deaths from spontaneous abortion. N. Engl. J. Med. 295:1155, 1976.
18. Hatcher, R. A., and Stewart, G. K.: Contraceptive Technology. Irvington Publishing Inc., 1981, pp. 72–97.
19. McMorries, K. E., Lofton, R. H., Stinson, J. C., and Cummings, R. V.: Is the IUD increasing the number of ovarian pregnancies? Contemporary OB/GYN, 13:165, 1979.
20. Ory, H. W.: Ectopic pregnancy and intrauterine contraceptive devices: New perspectives. Obstet. Gynecol. 57:137, 1981.
21. Pagano, R.: Ectopic pregnancy: A seven-year survey. Med. J. Aust. 2:526, 1981.
22. Progestasert IUD and ectopic pregnancy in patients using IUDs. FDA Drug Bulletin 8:37, 1978.
23. Tatum, H. J., and Schmidt, F. H.: Contraceptive and sterilization practices and extrauterine pregnancy: A realistic perspective. Fertil. Steril. 28:407, 1977.
24. Vessey, M. P., Yeates, D., and Flavel, R.: Risk of ectopic pregnancy and duration of use in an intrauterine device. Lancet 2:501, 1979.
25. Zakin, G., and Lindgren, S.: Influence of an intrauterine device on the course of an acute salpingitis. Contraception 24:199, 1981.
26. Foreman, H., Stadel, B. V., and Schlesselman, S.: Intrauterine device usage and fetal loss. Obstet. Gynecol. 58:669, 1981.
27. Kelaghan, J., Rubin, G. L., Ory, H. W., and Layde, P. M.: Barrier-method contraceptives and pelvic inflammatory disease. JAMA 248:184, 1982.
28. Kim-Farley, R. J., Cates, W., Jr., Ory, H. W., and Hatcher, R. A.: Febrile spontaneous abortion and the IUD. Contraception 18:561, 1978.
29. Shine, R. M., and Thompson, J. F.: The in-situ IUD and pregnancy outcome. Am. J. Obstet. Gynecol. 119:124, 1974.
30. Misenhimer, H. R., and Garcia-Bunuel, R.: Failure of intrauterine contraceptive device and fungal infection in the fetus. Obstet. Gynecol. 34:368, 1969.
31. Gray, R. H.: Pelvic inflammatory disease and the IUD. Lancet 1:718, 1980.
32. Vessey, M. P., Johnson, B., Doll, R., and Peto, R.: Outcome of pregnancy in women using an intrauterine device. Lancet 1:495, 1974.
33. Eisenberg, R. L.: The widened loop sign of Lippe's loop perforations, A.J.R. 116:847, 1972.
34. Soderberg, G., and Lindgren, S.: Influence of an intrauterine device on the course of an acute salpingitis. Contraception 24:199, 1981.
35. Landesman, R.: An intrauterine device. Obstet. Gynecol. 37:618, 1971.
36. Husemeyer, R. P., and Gordon, H.: Retrieval of contraceptive-device threads from within the uterine cavity. Lancet 1:807, 1979.
37. McArdle, C. R.: Ultrasonic localization of missing intrauterine contraceptive devices. Obstet. Gynecol. 51:330, 1978.
38. Weiss, B. D.: The Majzlin spring revisited. Am. Fam. Phys. 26:123, 1982.

8

GASTROENTEROLOGY

54

Nasogastric Intubation

JONATHAN M. GLAUSER, M.D.

Introduction and Background

The first written account of the use of a stomach tube appeared in a 1790 publication by John Hunter, in which he described the use of a fresh eel skin stretched over a whalebone to feed a patient with paralysis of deglutition. In 1813, a Philadelphia surgeon named Physick described gastric lavage by means of a urethral catheter used to treat a case of morphine poisoning.[1]

In this century, stomach tubes were originally used to treat postoperative ileus and secondary gastric distention. When a patient vomited or when the stomach became distended, a large stomach tube with a metal basket was passed through the mouth, the stomach contents were aspirated, and the tube was then removed. Nasogastric tubes of modern design were first used in the 1920s. In 1921, Dr. Levin described the tube that bears his name, and in 1924 Dr. Matas introduced the concept of prophylactic nasogastric drainage in prevention of postoperative distention. Paine and Wangensteen popularized this concept in the 1930s.[2] By the mid-1930s, postoperative mortality and morbidity related to gastric distention and perforation were greatly reduced.[3] In 1934, Miller and Abbott introduced the long balloon-tipped intestinal tube that bears their names. The length of the tube made a suction apparatus mandatory. Subsequently, the concept of suction drainage in prevention of gastric distention became widespread.

The first nasogastric tubes were made of soft rubber. More recently, devices made of Silastic and polyethylene compounds have been shown to elicit less of an inflammatory tissue reaction than do soft rubber tubes.[3] Other than the aforementioned change in tube composition from rubber of use to plastics, little change occurred in the methods of use or design of gastrointestinal suction equipment until the 1960s.

In the early 1960s, manufacturing advances facilitated development of a double-lumen sump tube. The theoretic advantages to this type of tube were the prevention of the gastric mucosal damage and flow blockage that were seen with single-lumen tubes. At this time, the two prototypes of nasogastric tubes are the double-lumen Salem Sump tube and the single-lumen Levin tube.[2]

Tube Design

The two common types of nasogastric tubes in use today, the Levin tube and the Salem Sump, are different in certain fundamental respects (Fig. 54–1). The Levin tube is a single-lumen tube and is not radiopaque. The Salem Sump tube is a radiopaque double-lumen tube. In addition to the drainage lumen, it contains a smaller secondary tube that is open to the atmosphere and permits continuous airflow when suction is applied (Fig. 54–2). The Levin tube is perfectly adequate for instillation of material into the stomach or for diagnostic aspiration. When continual suction is desired, the Salem Sump is preferred.

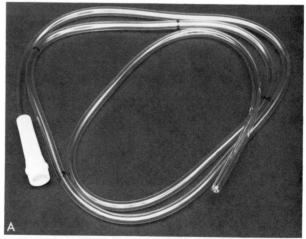

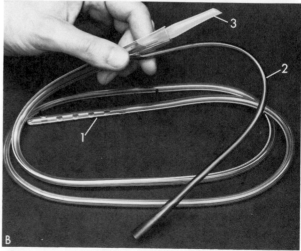

Figure 54–1. A, Standard Levin tube. This tube has a single lumen and is best used for instilling material into the stomach and for diagnostic stomach aspiration. B, Salem Sump tube. This double-lumen tube is preferred for continuous gastric suction. 1, Gastric end with suction eyes. 2, Pigtail extension of the air vent lumen. 3, "5-in-1" connector.

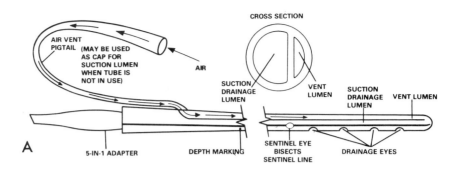

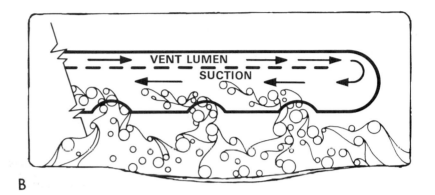

Figure 54–2. Diagram of the Salem Sump tube. A, General design. B, Diagram of double-lumen principle for suction. (Courtesy of the Argyle Division of Sherwood Medical, St. Louis, Missouri.)

Both tubes have multiple drainage openings, or eyes, at the distal gastric end. Each tube also has graduated markings so that the length of insertion can be measured.[4] The single lumen of the Levin tube is smaller than the double lumen of the Salem Sump. The latter has a blue "pigtail," which is an extension of the vent lumen.

The major advantage of a double-lumen tube is that the constant airflow allows for a controlled suction force at the drainage eyes.[5] Suction applied to a single-lumen tube may pull gastric mucosa into the drainage eyes. The tube may become occluded with tissue, and excessive negative pressure during suctioning may cause ulceration or damage to the gastric mucosa. Development of a suction force above 25 mm Hg, the commonly cited level of capillary fragility, is more apt to occur with Levin tubes for this reason. Suction is inversely proportional to flow, so the less flow through the tube, the higher the level of suction in the tube. If one end of the tube is blocked, the level of suction inside the tube increases rapidly, even though suction is still being applied at the same level as before. The tube may even collapse if the suction is great enough. As long as flow is maintained, a single-lumen tube can rid the stomach of air, liquid, and small particles. Ultimately, as the stomach is emptied of air and liquid, flow cannot be maintained, and the mobile gastric mucosa is drawn into the drainage eyes of the Levin tube.[2]

Levin tubes are usually attached to intermittent suction pumps. Intermittent suction pumps, such as the Gomco, work in cycles. When an intermittent pump is used at a high setting (usually 120 mm Hg) the initial suction applied is at a safe level, or approximately 20 mm Hg. As the drainage eyes of the Levin tube become invaginated and occluded with tissue, flow stops. The intermittent pump will then move in stages toward successively higher suction settings until full suction is reached (approximately 120 mm Hg). The amount of suction reaching the patient's tissue at the drainage eyes of a Levin tube thus can be unsafe even with an intermittent pump.

When the eyes of a Levin tube are obstructed, flow resumes only when fluid again builds up in the stomach or when tissue is pulled away from the tip of the tube. Although irrigation of the Levin tube will initially correct the problem, occlusion recurs as soon as the irrigant is evacuated from the stomach. Therefore, suction proceeds on a cyclic basis with frequent periods of invagination and possibly harmful suction levels. The fundamental disadvantage of a Levin tube is that there is no way of controlling the amount of suction reaching the gastric mucosa.[2]

The larger lumen of the Salem Sump tube is designed for suction drainage, whereas the smaller vent lumen allows outside air to be drawn into the stomach, permitting continuous flow through the tube regardless of the gastric content at the time. This design reduces tissue grabbing and minimizes the suction applied to the mucosa in comparison with the single-lumen tubes. The vent of the double-lumen tube communicates with the suction lumen through a perforation in the septum separating the two lumens at the distal end of the tube (see Fig. 54–2). Ideally, the constant flow of atmospheric air moderates the amount of suction in the tube, keeping it at a maximum of 20 mm Hg (below 25 mm Hg in any case).[2]

In practice, however, vacuum can be applied at levels exceeding the venting capacity of the second lumen. In that case, the sump is overpowered, and the same traumatic suction levels can develop as occur with Levin tubes.[5] The ratio of the area of the air vent lumen to the suction drainage lumen determines whether the sump will be overpowered as well as limiting the capability of suction and drainage.[2] Occasionally, personnel who are unfamiliar with the tube may inadvertently clamp the venting pigtail and defeat the purpose of the design of the tube.

Indications and Contraindications

Indications for use of nasogastric tubes fall into two broad categories. The first is aspiration of stomach contents for either diagnostic or therapeutic reasons.[6] Aspiration is mandatory in the assessment and management of upper gastrointestinal bleeding.[5] Nasogastric suction is indicated in the prevention and treatment of paralytic ileus, acute gastric dilation, and intestinal obstruction. Nasogastric tube placement is indicated in management of the patient with multiple injuries and in the assessment of possible gastrointestinal trauma. Gastric tubes are also indicated for gastric lavage in the case of overdose. In general, an orogastric tube is indicated for drug overdose because of the larger bore, which is required for pill fragment removal. The list of nonemergency uses for nasogastric suction is longer yet and includes such procedures as pentagastrin testing and postoperative intubation to protect gastric suture lines.[5]

The second indication for nasogastric tubes is for feedings or for the administration of therapeutic substances, e.g., medications, antacids, or activated charcoal in drug overdose cases. For the most part, nasogastric tubes are placed for aspiration, although the emergency physician may be required to replace a feeding tube or to assess tube placement.[7]

Contraindications to nasogastric tube placement include the following clinical situations: facial fractures with suspected cribriform plate injuries, which would permit intracranial intubation; esophageal strictures or a history of alkali ingestion, which would increase the possibility of esophageal perforation; comatose patients with unprotected airway, increasing the risk of aspiration; and penetrating cervical wounds in the awake trauma victim whose gagging efforts could stimulate hemorrhage.

Equipment

In preparing for nasogastric tube insertion, the following equipment is useful: towel (for covering the patient's gown), tissues, emesis basin, number 14 or number 16 nasogastric tube, glass of water with drinking straw, water-soluble jelly, stethoscope, hypoallergenic tape (in strips 4 inches in length), safety pin, rubber band, urethral or bulb syringe, drainage collection bottle, topical anesthetic jelly or ointment, and vasoconstrictor nasal spray.[4, 5, 8]

Depending on the indication, other equipment may be needed (for example, saline for irrigation or Magill forceps in an uncooperative or anesthetized patient). The equipment in the aforementioned list is adequate for the typical elective intubation in an adult.

Preparation

In preparing for the insertion, one should observe simple hygiene; this, of course, cannot be a sterile procedure. The head of the bed should be raised so that the patient is in a high Fowler's position. A towel is placed over the patient's chest to protect the gown, and an emesis basin should be available on the patient's lap.[9]

The largest possible tube for the nostril size of the patient should be selected. A large tube is less likely to become blocked during use or to curl back on itself during insertion. One should select a 16 French gauge or larger tube for an adult and should curve the end of it by coiling the first 6 inches. The curved end will be pointing down on insertion.

The nasogastric tube should be lubricated with a water-soluble jelly (K-Y or other) for 3 to 4 inches over its distal end. It has been recommended that lidocaine gel (2 per cent) or a similar topical anesthetic be applied to the nose to facilitate passage,[6] especially if the tube does not pass on the first attempt. The patient is asked to inhale through the nose so that the physician may select the more open passageway. The more patent nostril may also be identified by examination with a flashlight and a nasal speculum. If there is significant nasal congestion, one should apply a spray of a topical vasoconstrictor, such as ephedrine, phenylephrine hydrochloride (Neo-Synephrine), or cocaine. Cocaine is a good selection because of its additional local anesthetic properties. Some prefer to have the patient sip 2 per cent viscous lidocaine (Xylocaine) to numb the pharynx and esophagus and thus help prevent gagging. Cetacaine spray applied to the pharynx is another option for anesthetizing the throat and reducing gagging.

Procedure

The procedure may be divided into two phases. The first phase involves passage into the nasopharynx; the second phase consists of passage down the esophagus. With the patient sitting and the head supported to prevent reflex withdrawal, the lubricated tube is introduced along the floor of the nose. The tube should not be directed toward the bridge of the nose, but rather toward the floor (Fig. 54–3). If one nostril is narrowed by a deviated septum, the other side may be used, although often even the narrowed side will accommodate the tube below the inferior turbinate along the floor of the nose.[6] If difficulty persists, a smaller tube may be tried. If resistance is severe, the other nostril may again be tried, or insertion may ultimately be attempted through the mouth. At no time should the tube be forced. Failure to advance the tube is more often caused by abutment of the tip against a sensitive structure than by a nasal opening that is too small.

Resistance will be felt as the tip of the tube reaches the nasopharynx; this is the most uncomfortable part of the procedure for the patient and may cause nasal bleeding. Often the patient can aid this phase of tube passage by taking a sip or two of water through the straw. A slight twisting motion applied to the tube can also be helpful. Once the tube is in the nasopharynx, the physician should pause a few seconds and allow the patient to regain composure.

Reflex gagging may direct the tip of the tube into the mouth as one attempts passage into the esophagus. If this occurs, one of the following may be tried:

1. Repeating the attempt by withdrawing the tip of the tube into the nasopharynx and advancing again until it passes.

2. Removing the tube and cooling the tip for 20 minutes in a container of ice to stiffen it so that it becomes less likely to coil when tube passage is retried.

3. Observing the tube with the aid of a tongue depressor as it passes through the posterior pharynx and then using Magill forceps or a tongue blade to guide the tube down the esophagus.[6, 10]

4. Applying a topical anesthetic to the oropharynx (Cetacaine, viscous lidocaine) and reattempting passage.

There is usually no need to visualize the larynx during the procedure; as long as the tube passes along the posterior pharyngeal wall, it should enter the esophagus. If the tube twists in the mouth or kinks during passage, it should be withdrawn to the level of the nasopharynx but not completely removed. Flexion of the patient's neck when cervical injury is not present will help guide the tube into the esophagus.

The cooperation of the patient facilitates passage and should be encouraged by the inserter. The patient should be asked to continue swallowing from a glass of water through a straw once the tube has passed the nasopharynx while the inserter continues to advance the tube.[5] Passage down the esophagus should be accomplished without resistance. If a stricture or a pharyngeal pouch is present, causing obstruction, a general anesthetic and direct vision may be required for tube placement. The tube should be passed fairly quickly; hesitation by the inserter serves to prolong the patient's discomfort.[9] Inadvertent intubation of the trachea is usually quickly recognized in the conscious patient by coughing and panic. Inability to speak is also a characteristic sign of tracheal passage. It should be stressed that incorrect passage is not so easily identified in the unconscious patient, and one must be cognizant of this fact when passing a nasogastric tube in an obtunded or unconscious individual.

The gastroesophageal junction is reached typically at 40 cm in the adult. If no measurement has been taken beforehand, nasogastric tubes are typically inserted to the second or third black marking in adults. The Salem Sump tube is 48 inches long, for example, and has markings at 18, 22, 26, and 30 inches (approximately 45, 55, 65, and 75 cm, respectively).

Alternatively, the desired insertion distance may be obtained beforehand in the following manner: The tip of the tube is placed on the patient's nose. The tube is then extended to the tip of the patient's ear lobe on the same side and from there to the end of the xiphoid process. This total distance approximates that required for insertion, and the spot is marked with adhesive tape prior to insertion.[5, 9] The nose-ear-xiphoid length (NEX) has been modified to give the following formula for recommended length of insertion (in centimeters):[11]

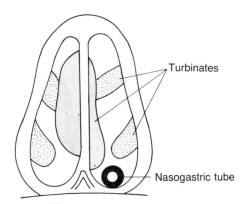

Figure 54–3. The nasogastric tube is directed along the *floor* of the nose, not toward the bridge. The tube often slides through the tunnel beneath the inferior turbinate.

$$\frac{NEX - 50}{2} + 50$$

Omitting the measurement of needed tube length prior to tube passage is a common error that may result in esophageal placement or inserting multiple coils of the tube into the stomach.

CONFIRMATION OF TUBE PLACEMENT

Once the tube has been passed, confirmation of correct placement must be obtained as soon as possible. There are several ways of checking tube placement:

1. The suction lumen is aspirated gently. The presence of stomach contents implies that the tube is in the stomach.[8] The patient may have to be placed in a left lateral decubitus position to maximize the return. The aspiration of food may give a false impression of location if lower esophageal obstruction exists. Blue litmus paper may be used to test the aspirate for acid.[6]

2. The patient may be asked to hum or talk. If this is not possible, the tube should be withdrawn, since it may have passed through the larynx. The mouth should be inspected under direct vision for coiling of the tube.

3. A 60-ml syringe filled with air is connected to the suction lumen of the nasogastric tube. The examiner auscultates the stomach while an assistant empties the syringe slowly. A "whooshing" sound of borborygmi is produced by only 10 to 20 ml of air if the tube is in the stomach. The patient may belch upon injection of air if the tube is in the esophagus.[8, 9] Alternatively, injection of air in the esophagus may produce typical borborygmi, but in a delayed fashion.

4. The open end of the tube may be placed in a glass of water. Escaping air bubbles imply that the tube is in a bronchus or in the trachea and should be removed immediately.[5] Crackling noises

heard when the end of the tube is held up to the inserter's ear also suggest location in a bronchus.

5. If the tube is radiopaque, as in the case of a Salem Sump, radiographic confirmation of tube location can be obtained.[5, 8] If one is considering films of the abdomen for other diagnostic purposes, it is best to pass the nasogastric tube prior to obtaining the radiographs so that the position of the tube may be confirmed.

SECURING THE TUBE

Once the correct position of the tube is determined, the tube is anchored to the nose with hypoallergenic tape, either in a butterfly fashion around the tube or with vertical taping over the nose and the tube. Tincture of benzoin may help to secure the tape. One should attempt to tape the tube so it rests in the middle of the nasal opening and does not lie directly in contact with the skin. A rubber band is then looped in a slip knot around the nasogastric tube and is pinned to the patient's gown.[9] This prevents slippage of the tube or tugging on the patient's nose during movement. To prevent pressure necrosis to the nose, the tube should never be taped to the patient's forehead[5] and should not rest against the nostril for long periods.

When a Salem Sump tube is used, the blue pigtail should be kept above the level of fluid in the patient's stomach. This prevents reflux of gastric contents into the vent lumen. If the pigtail is below the patient's midline, the vent lumen acts as a siphon, allowing gastric contents to flow out the lumen, possibly blocking the sump.[2, 5] When dealing with sump tubes, one should place the collection trap below the patient's midline to prevent reflux (Fig. 54–4). Otherwise, gastric contents

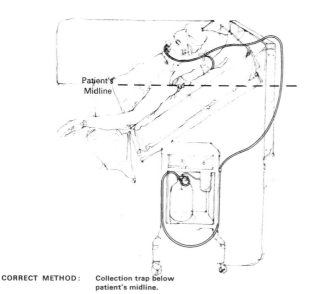

Figure 54–4. Correct position of the collection trap below the patient's midline. Note that the pigtail vent lumen is kept above the patient's midline. (Courtesy of the Argyle Division of Sherwood Medical, St. Louis, Missouri.)

CORRECT METHOD: Collection trap below patient's midline.

will flow out the vent lumen. Increasing the suction may cause fluids to be lifted the entire length of the tube, but increasing the suction simply for this purpose is ill-advised. Once the tube is devoid of fluid, the full force of suction will be applied to an empty tube and could overpower the sump.[2, 5]

Ambulation is possible with a nasogastric tube in place. The suction-drainage system is disconnected and, in the case of a Salem Sump, the blue pigtail is placed in the 5-in-1 connector. Alternatively, for either the Levin tube or the Salem Sump tube, a syringe can be placed into the suction-drainage lumen and taped to the patient's gown so that it does not pull on the tube.

PLACEMENT IN THE UNCONSCIOUS PATIENT

Levin claimed that a nasogastric tube could be easily introduced even when the patient was under anesthesia.[12] This is not always the case, and several methods have been suggested for accomplishing nasogastric intubation in a patient who is unable to swallow.

In an unconscious patient, the nasogastric tube may be placed initially through a naris into the oropharynx. The tip of the tube is then visualized with a laryngoscope, grasped with Magill forceps, and pulled out of the mouth. An endotracheal tube with an internal diameter that is slightly larger than the external diameter of the nasogastric tube is selected and is slit along its lesser curvature from its proximal end to a point 3 cm from its distal end. The slit endotracheal tube is then passed through the mouth into the esophagus. Passage is facilitated by the stiffness of the larger endotracheal tube and does not require active swallowing. The tip of the nasogastric tube is then threaded into the endotracheal tube and advanced into the stomach (Fig. 54–5). One removes the slit endotracheal tube from the esophagus by separating the nasogastric tube from the endotracheal tube through the slit. When the distal part of the endotracheal tube is in the mouth, the unslit 3-cm distal part is slit as well. The endotracheal tube is removed, and the nasogastric tube remains in place.[13]

A very similar method had previously been described by Cohen and Fox.[10] They recommended insertion of an esophageal stethoscope through a plastic slit endotracheal tube to make the nasogastric tube easier to insert into the esophagus. The passage of the nasogastric tube through the nose with later insertion through the endotracheal tube is much the same as in the method discussed previously.

Others have advocated simply guiding the nasogastric tube with one's fingers once it has been

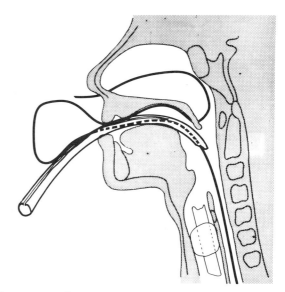

Figure 54–5. Diagrammatic representation of the separation of the nasogastric tube from the endotracheal tube through the slit in the endotracheal tube. The introducing endotracheal tube has been removed from the esophagus prior to separation from the nasogastric tube. Note the prior placement of an endotracheal tube in the trachea (partially shown). (From Sprague, D.H., and Carter, S.R.: An alternate method for nasogastric tube insertion. Anesthesiology 53:436, 1980. Used by permission.)

passed through the nose. This has been deemed unreliable by some.[10]

Ultimately, if all other methods fail, a flexible fiber optic bronchoscope or esophagoscope can be placed under direct vision into and through the esophagus. A guide wire is threaded into the stomach. The nasogastric tube can be placed over the guide wire into the stomach; the guide wire is then removed.[15]

SUCTION SETTINGS

Levin tubes are usually attached to intermittent low-suction or straight-bag drainage. When a Salem Sump is used, the following guidelines are recommended: If intermittent suction from a thermotic pump is used, suction should be set on high (80 to 120 mm Hg). This intermittent suction allows airflow during the closed cycle.[5] Intermittent suction from a central suction source should be set at a low level (30 to 40 mm Hg), and suction should be increased either until there is fluid flow or until bubbling is observed in the Salem Sump. When continual suction is used, it should be set at a low level and increased until fluid flow or bubbling is observed in the Salem Sump.[2] At all times, the vent should be kept open; closing the vent of the Salem Sump tube may cause mucosal damage similar to that encountered with single-lumen tubes. A functioning Salem Sump makes a hissing sound, which may be misinterpreted as an air leak or as a malfunction by those who are not familiar with the design.

USE OF THE TUBE

Nasogastric tubes may be used for feeding or lavage as well as for suction. Anything instilled into a nasogastric tube, such as activated charcoal, antacids, or medications, must be in liquid form. The plug or Hoffman clamp is removed from the nasogastric tube, and the desired material is instilled with either a bulb syringe or a 50-ml piston syringe. As always, the position of the tube should be confirmed *prior* to instillation of liquid. It is preferable to let the medication or charcoal flow by gravity if at all possible rather than by the use of force; the tube may need to be flushed with 30 to 50 ml of water at intervals.[4] After any feeding or administration of antacids or medication, suction should be discontinued for 15 to 20 minutes.

Irrigation of a Salem Sump tube may be performed through either the vent lumen or the suction-drainage lumen. When irrigating the vent lumen, one need not interrupt the suction. Any irrigation should be followed by injection of air through the sump lumen to ensure its patency. During irrigation of the main lumen, the Salem Sump tube is disconnected from the suction source, and the 5-in-1 connector is removed from the main lumen. An irrigating syringe is inserted, and irrigation is carried out with approximately 30 ml of saline. If gastric drainage is particularly viscous, drainage may have to be carried out at frequent intervals.[2, 4]

Complications

Serious complications from nasogastric tube placement are uncommon, and almost all complications are minor. More serious complications may develop in comatose patients or in those with underlying nasal, cervical, esophageal, or gastric pathologic conditions.

Epistaxis is a frequent occurrence but often can be prevented if the tube is not forced during insertion. Inability to pass the tube is common as well and may be related to the creation of a false passage,[6] the presence of an esophageal stricture, a gagging or uncooperative patient, or repetitive coiling of the tube in the mouth or the esophagus.

Perforation of the esophagus has been reported but is rare in the absence of esophageal disease.[6] If choking is noted, the tube should be assumed to be in the trachea until proved otherwise.

One should exercise extreme caution when passing a nasogastric tube in a patient with a suspected or proven facial or skull fracture. Intracranial penetration of nasogastric tubes inserted in patients

with head injuries has been reported (Fig. 54–6).[16, 17] One can readily appreciate the consequences of suction or irrigation of a tube placed in the cranium. Trauma to the cribriform plate of the ethmoid bone is the speculated anatomic injury. Inadvertent central nervous system penetration may be prevented by prior insertion of a lubricated number 34 Davol Silastic nasopharyngeal airway into the nose; the nasogastric tube is subsequently passed through the nasopharyngeal airway. Because of its preformed curve, the Silastic airway will presumably be directed away from the cribriform plate.[16] Perhaps it is safer to pass the nasogastric tube through the mouth in such cases or to observe passage of the tube into the pharynx by direct vision with a laryngoscope. Inadvertent passage of a nasogastric tube into the cranium may occur more frequently than previously appreciated.[17]

Hemorrhage from a penetrating neck wound may develop if passage of the nasogastric tube induces gagging in the awake stab wound victim. The trauma victim with a cervical spine injury may also be further traumatized if motion of the neck is used during tube passage.

Several laryngeal injuries have been reported from nasogastric tube usage; often these involve tubes that have been in place for a long time. Hoarseness and pharyngodynia have occurred with long-term use.[1] Cricoid chondritis, arytenoid edema, and bilateral vocal cord paralysis have been reported with long-term use of nasogastric tubes.

Nasal alar necrosis occurs but should be largely preventable if one does not tape the nasogastric tube to the patient's forehead and if one pins the tube to the patient's gown to prevent pressure necrosis.

A multitude of respiratory tract complications from nasogastric tubes have been reported. Pneumonia has occurred from a tube placement into a patient's right lower lobe bronchus (Fig. 54–7).[16] Hydropneumothorax has resulted from a bronchially placed nasogastric tube.[18] Bronchopleural fistula and empyema developed in this case. Malpositioned nasogastric tubes in the lung have been described even with cuffed endotracheal tubes in place.[18, 19] Air injected to check the position of the tube may over distend the alveoli and cause a pneumothorax.[20] One study concluded that routine use of nasogastric tubes postoperatively caused a higher incidence of pneumonia when compared with management without the tubes.[21] The authors of the study postulated that the nasogastric tube may have hindered coughing, causing accumulation of mucous plugs in the bronchial tree. Gastrointestinal bleeding may occur from mucosal damage caused by the tube, although this complication is unlikely to be seen immediately after passage of tubes in the emergency department.

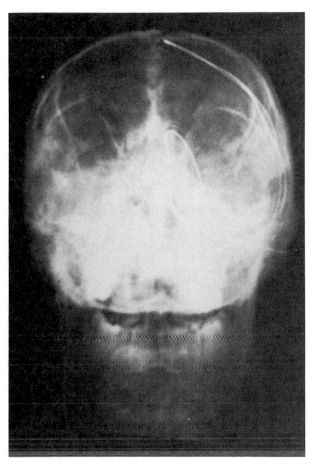

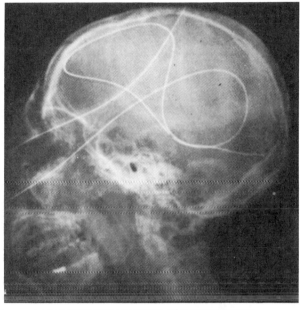

Figure 54–6. Anteroposterior and lateral skull radiographs demonstrating intracranial insertion of a nasrogastric tube in a patient with multiple skull fractures. (From Johnson, J. C.: Letter to the Editor: Back to basics for morbidity-free nasogastric intubation. JACEP 8:289, 1979. Used by permission.)

Figure 54–7. Levin tube inadvertently placed in the right main stem bronchus; An alveolar infiltrate consistent with early pneumonia is also shown. (From Johnson, J. C.: Letter to the editor: Back to basics for morbidity-free nasogastric intubation. JACEP 8:289, 1979. Used by permission.)

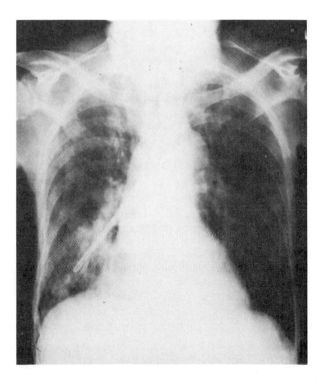

Others do not favor routine use of nasogastric tubes because of patient discomfort. Clearly, nasogastric suction has the potential to produce fluid and electrolyte imbalance. There does not seem to be any evidence that increased nasal resistance occurs in adults when a nasogastric tube is in place, but this has been reported in infants.[22]

If Magill forceps are used in nasogastric tube insertion, there is the potential for damage to the uvula, the soft palate, or the pharyngeal mucosa.

As a final note, it should be stressed that a nasogastric tube may inadvertently be passed into a number of undesirable and potentially dangerous places in the unconscious patient. It is incumbent upon the physician to verify the correct passage by direct vision in all obtunded patients.

1. Sofferman, R. A., and Hubbell, R. N.: Laryngeal complications of nasogastric tubes. Ann. Otol. 90:465, 1981.
2. Clinical Considerations in the Use of the Argyle Salem Sump Tube. St. Louis, MO, Argyle Division of Sherwood Medical, 1979, pp. 1–16.
3. Friedman, M., Baim, H., Shelton, V., et al.: Laryngeal injuries secondary to nasogastric tubes. Ann. Otol. 90:469, 1981.
4. Jackson, E. W.: Nursing photobooks: Giving medication through a nasogastric tube. Nursing '80 71, 1980.
5. McConnell, E. A.: Ensuring safer stomach suctioning with the salem sump tube. Nursing '77, 1977.
6. Tucker, A., and Lewis, J.: Passing a nasogastric tube. Br. Med. J. 10:1128, 1980.
7. McGuirt, W. F., and Strout, J. J.: Securing of intermediate duration feeding tubes. Laryngoscope 90:2046, 1980.
8. Jackson, E. W.: Performing GI Procedures: Nursing Photobook. Horsham, PA, Intermed Communications, 1981, pp. 44–70.
9. Volden, C., Grinde, J., and Carl, D.: Taking the trauma out of nasogastric intubation. Nursing '80 64, 1980.
10. Cohen, D. D., and Fox, R. M.: Nasogastric intubation in the anesthetized patient, Anesth. Analg. 42:578, 1963.
11. Hanson, R. L. New approach to measuring adult nasogastric tubes for insertion. Am. J. Nurs. 1334, July 1980.
12. Levin, A. L.: A new gastroduodenal catheter. JAMA, 76:1007, 1921.
13. Sprague, D. H., and Carter, S. R.: An alternate method for nasogastric tube insertion. Anesthesiology, 53:436, 1980.
14. Ohn, K. C., and Wu, W. H.: A new method for nasogastric tube insertion. Anesthesiology 51:568, 1979.
15. Lee, T. S., and Wright, B. D.: Flexible fiberoptic bronchoscope for difficult nasogastric intubation. Anesth. Analg. 60:904, 1981.
16. Johnson, J. E.: Back to basics for morbidity-free nasogastric intubation. JACEP 8:289, 1979.
17. Bouzarth, W. F.: Nasogastric intubation. Ann. Emerg. Med. 9:49, 1980.
18. Culpepper, J. A., Veremakis, C., Guntupalli, K. K., et al.: Malpositioned nasogastric tube causing pneumothorax and bronchopleural fistula. Chest 81:389, 1982.
19. Sweatman, A. J., Tomasello, P. A., Loughhead, M. G., et al.: Misplacement of nasogastric tubes and esophageal monitoring devices. Br. J. Anaesth. 50:389, 1978.
20. Holliman, P. W., and McFee, A. S.: Pneumothorax attributable to nasogastric tube. Arch. Surg. 116:970, 1981.
21. Argov, S., Goldstein, I., and Barzilai, A.: Is routine use of the nasogastric tube justified in upper abdominal surgery? Am. J. Surg., 139:849, 1980.
22. Stocks, J.: Effect of nasogastric tubes on nasal resistance during infancy. Arch. Dis. Child. 55:17, 1980.

55

Gastric Lavage in the Poisoned Patient

DAN TANDBERG, M.D.
WILLIAM G. TROUTMAN, Pharm.D.

Introduction

More than 2 million cases of accidental and intentional poisoning occur each year in the United States. As many as 5000 of these patients die, and many who survive are left with permanent disability.[1] In one report, approximately 1 per cent of all patients seen in an emergency department were suffering from acute drug overdose;[2] in another series, self-poisoned patients represented 20 per cent of all adult hospital admissions.[3] The diagnosis and management of acute poisoning in children and adults is a common problem and requires that physicians caring for these patients be expert in the procedures used in their management.

After initial stabilization of the acutely poisoned patient, most authorities recommend that attempts be made to diminish further absorption of any ingested toxin from the gastrointestinal tract.[4–10] Methods for accomplishing this include ipecac-induced emesis, gastric lavage, administration of activated charcoal, and administration of cathartics. This chapter will focus on gastric lavage and will discuss its development, its indications and contraindications, the technical aspects of the procedure, and its complications.

Historical Development

The use of a hollow tube to evacuate poison from a patient's stomach dates from the early 1800s and has been thoroughly reviewed by Major.[11] In 1810, Dupuytren demonstrated that a rubber tube could be used to remove opium from the stomach of poisoned dogs. Phillip Syng Physick, the father of American surgery, used a long, flexible, hollow tube to remove accidental overdoses of laudanum (opium in alcohol) from the stomachs of two infants suffering from whooping cough and reported his results in 1812. A dramatic demonstration of the efficacy of gastric lavage in adults took place in 1822 when Edward Jukes, an English surgeon, tested the procedure on himself after purposefully ingesting a potentially lethal dose of laudanum. He used an elastic gum rubber catheter 25 inches long and ½ inch in diameter attached to an elastic bottle. Warm water was introduced into his stomach and was then removed. Jukes became somewhat nauseated and slept deeply for 3 hours afterward but suffered no serious aftereffects.

Kussmaul, who is commonly credited with inventing gastric lavage for the treatment of poisoning, did much to popularize its use after his 1869 publication.[12] During the next 75 years, gastric lavage was widely held to be the most effective procedure for emptying the stomach of an acutely poisoned patient.

The safety and efficacy of gastric lavage were called into question after the investigative work of Harstad and coworkers was published in 1942.[13] These investigators studied 80 patients suffering from severe poisoning with unknown quantities of phenobarbital or other sedative drugs. They found that in only 5 of their 80 cases could more than 500 mg of drug be recovered in the gastric washings. In addition, they reported that in some of the patients who died, particles of previously administered activated charcoal could be found in the respiratory tract, suggesting that aspiration of gastric contents had occurred. It was concluded that gastric lavage was relatively ineffective and potentially unsafe. Unfortunately, there were a number of methodologic problems with this study: The size of the stomach tube was not specified, the assay methods were crude and nonquantitative (crystallization), and the positioning of the patient may not have been optimal. In addition, the airway was often unprotected. As a result of this study, the procedure fell into some disrepute and was thereafter performed less often at many medical centers.[14, 15] This was accompanied by a growing interest in the use of induced emesis as a means of evacuating the stomach in poisoned patients.

Some sources have advocated mechanically induced emesis, but this was shown to be relatively ineffective by Dabbous and associates.[16] In their study of 30 children poisoned with various substances, gagging the patient with a finger or a tongue blade resulted in emesis in only 4 of the 30. The use of hypertonic saline to induce emesis fell into disfavor after reports of multiple cases of severe hypernatremia and several deaths in children.[17–21]

Copper sulfate was advocated as an emetic in poisoning and was shown to induce vomiting in over 90 per cent of patients treated.[22] The corrosive complications of this agent together with the possibility of systemic absorption, however, resulted in its being rejected as an emetic agent.[23–26]

Apomorphine has been shown to be an effective emetic in children and adults.[27, 28] MacLean, however, found that many patients treated with apomorphine developed central nervous system depression and concluded that this represented an unnecessary risk.[29] This problem, together with the fact that ipecac syrup could be administered in the home and did not require parenteral administration, resulted in the widespread acceptance of ipecac syrup as the emetic of choice in acute poisoning.[30–35]

The 1950s saw the beginning of a controversy regarding the relative efficacy of gastric lavage versus ipecac-induced emesis that persists to this day.[36, 37] In 1959, Arnold and his colleagues administered sodium salicylate tablets to dogs and found that ipecac-induced emesis produced an average recovery of 45 per cent, whereas lavage recovered only 38 per cent of the administered dose.[38] Unfortunately, lavage was carried out with a 16 French gastric tube, and positioning of the dogs may not have been optimal in this study. Abdallah and Tye repeated this experiment in dogs using barium sulfate as a tracer.[39] They found that 62 per cent of the barium could be recovered with immediately administered ipecac, whereas 54 per cent was recovered with immediate lavage. In a third animal study, six mongrel puppies were given barium sulfate in gelatin capsules and were then treated with gastric lavage, ipecac syrup, or apomorphine.[40] Lavage resulted in a recovery rate averaging 29 per cent compared with a 19 per cent recovery rate in the animals treated with ipecac-induced emesis. Again, the diameter of the tube, the positioning of the dogs, and the use of a nonparticulate tracer impair the usefulness of the study. Furthermore, there is some question concerning whether syrup of ipecac has comparable efficacy in dogs and in humans. Thus, animal evidence does not conclusively show superiority of one method over the other.

Boxer and colleagues studied the ipecac versus lavage problem in children who had ingested aspirin overdoses.[41] Their 17 patients were randomized either to be treated with ipecac-induced emesis followed by gastric lavage or to undergo gastric lavage followed by ipecac-induced emesis. The relative quantities of drug retrieved by each method were then compared for each patient, and a ratio was established. More drug was apparently removed by induced emesis than by lavage, but the precise details of the lavage technique used in this study were not specified. Particularly important omissions from the report included specification of gastric tube diameter, patient position, and lavage solution volume.

Matthew and associates showed that carefully performed gastric lavage could remove clinically significant amounts of ingested drug in a series of 259 severely poisoned patients.[42] Since the actual ingested dose was never known for certain, however, the true efficacy of gastric lavage could not be precisely determined. Burke performed careful gastric lavage in 10 volunteer adults undergoing general anesthesia for elective bronchoscopy.[43] There is good radiographic evidence from this study that water-soluble radiopaque dye can be effectively removed from the stomach if a large gastric tube is used and careful attention is paid to lavage technique and to positioning of the patient. Burke reported an 84 per cent recovery rate but, unfortunately, did not present enough quantitative data to substantiate this figure.

Many clinicians and many authorities have strong opinions regarding the superior effectiveness of gastric lavage or ipecac-induced emesis, and these have found their way into textbooks. In view of the difficulty in interpreting the experimental data, the question remains unsettled.

Editorial note: Ipecac-induced emesis has proven value in the prehospital setting. When gastric lavage has been used following ipecac-induced emesis, lavage will at times recover significant amounts of ingested drug, even though emesis was considered successful. Therefore, it is prudent to consider lavage *in addition to emesis* if a particularly toxic ingestion has occurred or if one suspects that emesis may have been ineffective. If, for example, a patient states that he took 100 adult aspirin tablets and only minimal drug is recovered by emesis, lavage is mandatory.

Indications and Contraindications

The decision as to whether to use ipecac-induced emesis or gastric lavage in a given patient should be based on the clinical condition and the history of what was ingested. There are, however, many conflicting opinions in the medical literature regarding the relative indications and contraindications for induced emesis and gastric lavage.

Most authorities agree that gastric emptying should be avoided in patients with a clear history of ingestion of an inconsequential amount of drug or other toxic substance. Attempting to administer ipecac syrup to agitated or uncooperative patients is not likely to be successful and merely delays eventual gastric lavage. One should not waste an inordinate amount of time attempting to cajole an uncooperative patient into drinking ipecac. Occa-

sionally, demonstrating the lavage tube to the patient does wonders for compliance.

The patient's level of consciousness is the most important factor in deciding whether to carry out induced emesis or gastric lavage. Patients who are not alert enough to hold the medicine cup unaided should undergo gastric lavage rather than induced emesis. Ipecac-induced emesis should be avoided in patients likely to have diminished airway-protective reflexes; gastric lavage with a cuffed endotracheal tube in place should be carried out instead. Such patients include those with depressed sensorium, depressed gag reflex, absent lid reflex,[44] or seizures. In addition emesis should not be induced in conscious patients who have ingested drugs that are likely to produce coma or seizures rapidly (rapid-acting barbiturates, cyanide, camphor, strychnine, and so forth). In no instance should ipecac be forced down the throat of an obtunded (or *soon to become obtunded*) patient.

Ipecac-induced emesis has traditionally not been recommended in cases of poisoning with phenothiazine or other antiemetics because it was thought that the antiemetic effects of these drugs would make induced emesis ineffective. It has since been shown, however, that approximately 95 per cent of patients treated with ipecac will vomit even after antiemetic poisoning.[45, 46] Ipecac-induced emesis should be used cautiously in patients poisoned with phenothiazines, however, because of the risk of dystonic reactions involving the face and the neck, which can produce vomiting against a tightly clenched jaw with subsequent pulmonary aspiration of gastric contents. This risk has led one major phenothiazine manufacturer to include a warning against the use of ipecac-induced emesis in its product literature.[47]

The delay between ingestion of the poison and initiation of gastric emptying is also an important consideration. For rapidly absorbed drugs, such as the barbiturates, there is good evidence that attempts at gastric emptying after more than 4 hours have elapsed is not likely to be of much clinical value.[42] Most authorities teach that ipecac-induced emesis or gastric lavage carried out after 3 to 6 hours rarely yields significant quantities of ingested drug. Many drugs, however, delay gastric emptying and may be retrieved later than 4 hours after ingestion. Gastric emptying is especially likely to be delayed in patients with diminished or absent bowel sounds or radiographic evidence of poison in the stomach or in those with a history of ingestion of drugs with anticholinergic properties or drugs such as aspirin, glutethimide, or ethchlorvynol.[42, 48, 49] A meal immediately preceding the ingestion may further delay gastric emptying. Certain drugs, such as phencyclidine, may also be re-excreted into the stomach and trapped there because of the low pH. *Continued* gastric lavage may be of value in such instances. Since the account of when the ingestion occurred is often inaccurate, it is best to err on the side of caution and to perform lavage whenever the possibility of significant recovery exists.

Another consideration is the possibility that semisolid masses of drug will form in the stomach and remain there for long periods. These may sometimes be removed by repeated gastric lavage with a large-bore tube following abdominal massage, but in some cases endoscopy, or even gastrotomy, may be required.[50-53]

The possible ingestion of strong alkalis is also a contraindication to both induced emesis and gastric lavage. The esophageal and gastric burns associated with alkali ingestion occur within minutes, and attempts at gastric intubation or the forceful vomiting produced by ipecac syrup may result in serious esophageal injury, or even perforation.[54]

On the other hand, the ingestion of strong acids rarely produces severe esophageal injury but subsequently may cause deep burns to the stomach and the duodenum. This burning continues for as long as 90 minutes in experimental animals[55] and suggests that rapid removal of the ingested acid should be beneficial. Since no esophageal perforation has ever been reported in acid-poisoned patients treated with gastric lavage, this would seem to be the procedure of choice until further evidence is available.[56]

The management of patients who have ingested a hydrocarbon chemical is complicated by the broad range of compounds covered by that label and by the significant controversy that surrounds the selection of a treatment technique. A hydrocarbon product that also contains other toxic chemicals (pesticides, heavy metals, halogenated aromatic compounds, camphor) mandates prompt removal from the gastrointestinal tract. Similarly, there is little evidence supporting the removal of very viscous and relatively nontoxic hydrocarbon products, such as petroleum jelly, grease, paint, or motor oil. The major debate centers on what to do with ingestions of products falling between these two extremes, such as gasoline, kerosene, turpentine, and charcoal lighter fluid.

The most serious complication of hydrocarbon ingestion is the development of a chemical pneumonitis. This complication is much more likely to occur with low-viscosity hydrocarbons. Obviously, one would expect pneumonitis to result from aspiration of the product, but for some time it was believed that hydrocarbons could also produce pulmonary toxicity by reaching the lungs through the blood stream.[57] This assumption placed a high priority on the evacuation of hydrocarbons from the gastrointestinal tract. More recent findings indicate that pulmonary toxicity is highly unlikely unless aspiration occurs[58] and that aspiration may pose a threat that is more than 100 times greater than uncomplicated ingestion.[59-61]

In the past, the decision to remove a hydrocarbon from the stomach was based on an arbitrary cut-off value of 1 ml per kg. This value was established subjectively,[62] and recent animal data suggest that as much as 20 times this amount can safely be tolerated.[58] Most recent review publications have abandoned the arbitrary 1 ml per kg figure.[63]

Gastric lavage has long been recognized as having little effect on the clinical outcome in hydrocarbon ingestion cases.[64] Ipecac-induced emesis would be expected to have a comparable impact. Ng and coworkers found a higher incidence of pulmonary radiographic changes in cases of hydrocarbon ingestion treated with gastric lavage than in cases treated with ipecac-induced emesis.[65] but this report, unfortunately, lacks certain methodologic details (e.g., efforts that were made to protect the airway) that are necessary to permit the drawing of significant conclusions.

The usual quantities of hydrocarbons ingested by patients seen in the emergency department generally need not be removed from the stomach unless the product is a particularly toxic one. The regional poison control center can aid in the recognition of these particularly toxic compounds.

Equipment and Procedure

If the decision is made to perform gastric lavage, then careful attention to the details of the procedure will result in increased safety for the patient and more effective removal of the ingested poison.

Prior to initiation of the procedure, the airway should be protected with a cuffed endotracheal tube if there is depression of the level of consciousness or diminution of the patient's airway-protective reflexes. A reliable way to test the gag reflex is to stimulate the posterior pharynx with a tongue blade or a cotton-tipped applicator. The absence of a strong gag reflex in an otherwise awake and alert patient, however, does *not* preclude emesis. Many people have a subdued gag reflex normally. Fully conscious and alert patients may be lavaged without prior tracheal intubation.

The position in which the patient is lavaged is very important. All patients should be lavaged in the left lateral decubitus position with the head down. The left lateral decubitus position diminishes the passage of gastric contents into the duodenum during lavage; this has been well documented by fluoroscopy during the procedure. (Fig. 55–1).[43] In addition, positioning the patient's body with the head lowered approximately 15 degrees downward decreases the risk of pulmo-

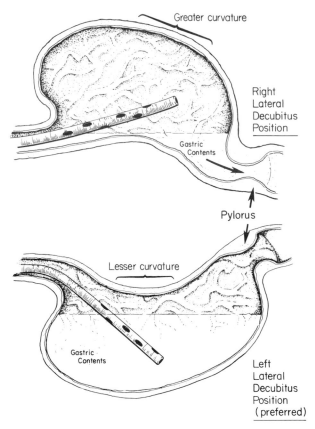

Greater curvature

Right
Lateral
Decubitus
Position

Gastric
Contents

Pylorus

Lesser curvature

Gastric
Contents

Left
Lateral
Decubitus
Position
(preferred)

Figure 55–1. The effect of patient positioning on gastric lavage.

nary aspiration of gastric contents should vomiting or retching occur.

Large-diameter gastric hoses with extra holes cut near the tip should be used for gastric lavage (Fig. 55–2). There are no human data to refute or support this recommendation, and one study of a small number of dogs failed to show any difference in efficacy with lavage through a 32 French tube compared with a 16 French lavage tube.[66] Nevertheless, it is logically held that large-diameter nasogastric or orogastric tubes (greater than 1 cm) are more likely to retrieve particulate matter suc-

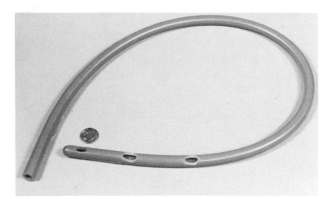

Figure 55–2. A large-diameter gastric tube. Note the extra side holes that have been cut near the tip.

cessfully. A 32–40 French tube is usually recommended for adults. Prior to passage, one should estimate the length of tube required to enter the stomach by approximating the distance from the nose to the mid-epigastrium. This avoids curling and kinking of excess hose in the stomach.

The gastric tube should be passed gently to avoid damage to the nose or the posterior pharynx. If the nonintubated patient begins to vomit with the tube in place, the tube should be removed immediately to allow for unobstructed emesis. The tube may be passed through either the nose or the mouth. Tubes larger than 36 French should not be forced through the nose of an adult male. Even this size may produce mucosal or turbinate injury. Passage through the mouth is generally more comfortable for the patient, but the inserter is in danger of being bitten when this technique is used. In addition, orogastric tubes tend to be chewed on and occluded by stuporous or combative patients. These problems may be minimized by the concomitant use of a bite block or an oral airway. Nasogastric intubation with large-diameter tubes can be more easily carried out if lubricating jelly is used; shrinkage of the nasal mucosa with phenylephrine (Neo-synephrine) should be performed first for additional patient comfort. One can facilitate passage of the tube into the esophagus once the pharynx has been entered by putting the patient's chin on his chest. Should cough, stridor, or cyanosis occur, the tube has entered the trachea; it must be withdrawn immediately and passage reattempted. Once the tube is passed, its intragastric location should be confirmed by auscultation of the stomach during injection of air with a 50-ml syringe. If this step is omitted, one may occassionally end up irrigating the esophagus from a tube that has doubled back during passage.

A large fraction of the gastric contents can subsequently be removed by careful gastric aspiration prior to gastric irrigation with repeated repositioning of the tube tip. Only after the stomach has been thoroughly "vacuumed" should gastric lavage be carried out, since aspiration may be the most effective part of the procedure.[42, 43, 48]

The aliquots of lavage fluid may be introduced using a syringe or a funnel. The use of a Y connector and clamp makes the procedure even easier (Fig. 55–3). This arrangement can be purchased ready-made (Travenol, Ethox, and others) or can be made up from readily available components. The equipment turns a messy and difficult task into an efficient procedure that can be performed by one technician.

Lavage is performed by clamping the drainage arm of the Y and running 200 to 300 ml of fluid into the stomach from a reservoir. The reservoir arm of the Y is then clamped, and the drainage arm is opened to permit gravity drainage of the stomach contents. The procedure is then repeated

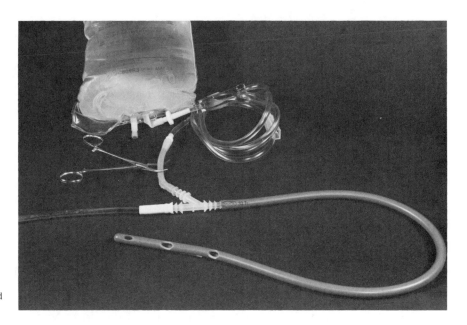

Figure 55–3. One convenient method for instilling lavage solution. See text.

as below. Some resistance is produced by the Y connector and tubing. Suction can be applied intermittently to the drainage tubing to enhance stomach emptying. Rudolph has developed a device (Autovage, Armstrong Industries, Inc., Northbrook, IL 60062) that performs this task automatically.[68] Severe dilutional hyponatremia has occurred in children lavaged with tap water; physiologic saline is therefore generally recommended.[67] Tap water appears to be a safe lavage solution in adults but may produce measurable decrements in the serum sodium and potassium in some patients.[67] The use of prewarmed (45°C) lavage fluid increases the solubility of most substances, delays gastric emptying, and theoretically should increase the effectiveness of the procedure.[69, 70] In addition, the use of prewarmed fluid diminishes the risk of lowering the patient's body temperature. Small aliquots of lavage solution should be repeatedly introduced into the stomach and removed. The size of each aliquot is subject to some dispute in the literature, but most recommendations generally are fairly close to 300 ml in adults and 10 ml per kg in children. Larger amounts theoretically increase the risk that the

gastric contents will be washed into the duodenum, and much smaller amounts are not clinically practical because of the dead space in the tubing (approximately 50 ml in the 36 French hose) and the increase in time that is required. The amount that is returned is always slightly less than the amount that is introduced. The fluid should flow in freely and drain easily by gravity. If this does not occur, the tube is usually malpositioned or kinked in the stomach. Manual agitation of the patient's stomach prior to removal of each aliquot may increase recovery and is recommended.[70]

We recommend continuation of lavage for at least 1 to 2 liters after the returns seem clear. No careful study in humans regarding the optimal total volume of lavage solution to be used exists, and there is considerable difference in recommendations regarding this question in the literature.

There is in vitro and some anecdotal clinical evidence supporting the use of specific substances in the solution used to lavage patients who have been poisoned with certain substances (Table 55–1).[71, 72] These "specific" lavage solutions may convert the poison to an insoluble complex or may change it to a less toxic compound. The clinical

Table 55–1. EXAMPLES OF SPECIAL LAVAGE SOLUTIONS

Substance Ingested	Special Lavage Solution	Remarks
Ferrous salts	1.5% sodium bicarbonate	Forms insoluble ferrous carbonate complex; phosphate lavage is no longer recommended.
Fluorides	15 to 30 gm per L calcium gluconate	Forms insoluble calcium fluoride precipitate.
Formaldehyde	10 mg per L ammonium acetate	Forms methenamine (much less toxic).
Iodine	80 gm per L cornstarch	
Oxalic acid	15 to 30 gm per L calcium gluconate	Forms calcium oxalate precipitate.

efficacy of these modes of therapy is generally unproven, but they are widely used.

Perhaps the best accepted example is the use of a 1.5 per cent sodium bicarbonate lavage solution in iron salt–poisoned patients.[73] Patients poisoned with strong acids or bases should not be lavaged with "neutralizing" solutions, since heat is produced and further tissue damage may result.[54, 56]

After gastric aspiration and lavage have been completed, a slurry of activated charcoal (from 30 to 120 gm) should be administered through the gastric tube. Unfortunately, not all substances are well absorbed by activated charcoal; major exceptions include strong alkalis, boric acid, cyanide, DDT, ferrous sulfate, mineral acids, lithium, and carbamate insecticides.[74] After adsorption of the poison by activated charcoal, most authorities recommend the use of a cathartic, but few clinical data have been published supporting the efficacy of this.[75] Activated charcoal is generally withheld in cases of acetaminophen poisoning until the need for N-acetylcysteine therapy is determined.[76, 77] The gastric tube should be pinched or clamped during its removal to avoid "dribbling" fluid into the airway. One should not remove the endotracheal tube quickly in the intubated patient following lavage. Emesis is not uncommon following lavage, and the airway is often still unprotected at the completion of the lavage.

Complications

Complications of gastric lavage therapy can be broadly subdivided into those associated with the placement of the tube and those resulting from the lavage fluid.

Skillful hands and adequate practice will allow the physician to place a large gastric tube with minimal trauma. If the nasal route is selected, care must be exercised if the delicate nasal turbinates are not to be damaged. Rubber tubes are preferred, since they seem to be less traumatic than plastic ones. Once the tube has been placed, it is important to make sure that it is in the stomach and not in the lungs, since inadvertent placement of the tube in the lungs can be fatal.[78] A second major concern during gastric lavage is the risk of perforation of the stomach or the lower esophagus. This is most commonly encountered in cases in which substantial damage had already been done to these tissues. Alkaline-corrosive ingestions represent a situation in which significant esophageal damage can occur and the risk of perforation is high.[79] Preexisting esophageal strictures also make tube passage more hazardous.

The lavage fluid itself is a potential source of problems. The large amounts of fluid used during a lavage procedure can potentially produce fluid and electrolyte disturbances in the patient; these have been reported with both hypertonic[80, 81] and hypotonic[67] lavage fluids. These problems appear to be encountered most commonly in children. Adults are more resistant to lavage-induced electrolyte disturbances.[67] Rudolph was unable to document electrolyte changes in tap water–lavaged patients aged 2 to 94 years.[68] Hypothermia is another possible pediatric complication of gastric lavage, leading many pediatricians to warm the lavage fluid after the first liter.

The use of large aliquots of lavage fluid (greater than 300 ml per wash in adults, 10 ml per kg in children) has the potential to force the gastric contents through the pylorus and into the upper small intestine, where more rapid absorption may take place.[82]

Pulmonary aspiration of gastric contents or lavage fluid poses a potential risk during lavage, although with properly performed lavage, this should be very low. In their series of 259 lavaged patients, Matthew and coworkers showed that both emesis and gastric lavage increased the incidence of pulmonary radiographic changes in patients who had ingested petroleum distillates or turpentine.[64]

Conclusions and Summary

Gastric lavage is an old and accepted emergency procedure commonly used by physicians for minimizing the absorption of ingested poisons. A major problem in determining the exact value of gastric lavage in poisoned patients is the difficulty in interpreting the available literature evaluating the procedure. The "definitive" study of gastric lavage has yet to be performed.

Often lost in the discussion of gastric lavage techniques is the determination of whether the procedure needs to be performed at all. Although the risks associated with properly conducted gastric lavage appear slight, they are measurable, and no patient should undergo gastric lavage unless it is likely that more good than harm will result. These considerations hold true for ipecac-induced emesis as well.

The performance of careful gastric aspiration and lavage requires a great deal more staff and physician time than does ipecac-induced emesis, and in a busy emergency department this consideration often plays a major part in the choice of method. Small children are rarely severely poisoned and are particularly difficult to lavage effectively unless they are obtunded; thus, in most instances ipecac-induced emesis is used.

If the physician decides to perform gastric aspiration and lavage in the management of a severely poisoned patient, then careful attention to the techniques used in carrying out the procedure will ensure that it is safely done and clinically beneficial to the patient.

1. Arena, J. M.: The treatment of poisoning. Clin. Symp. 30:3, 1978.
2. Schernitzki, P., et al.: Acute drug intoxication at a University hospital: An epidemiological study. Vet. Hum. Toxicol. 22:235, 1980.
3. Smith, A. J.: Self-poisoning with drugs: A worsening situation. Br. Med. J. 4:157, 1972.
4. Cashman, T. M., Shirley, H. C.: Emergency management of poisoning. Pediatr. Clin. North Am. 17:525, 1970.
5. Easom, J. M., and Lovejoy, F. H.: Efficacy and safety of gastrointestinal decontamination in the treatment of oral poisoning. Pediatr. Clin. North Am. 26:827, 1979.
6. Ariens, E. J., et al.: Introduction to General Toxicology. New York, Academic Press, 1976, pp. 192–193.
7. Schwartz, H. S.: Toxicologic Emergencies In Wilkins E. A., Dineen, J. J., and Moncure, A. C. (eds.): MGM Textbook of Emergency Medicine. Baltimore, Williams & Wilkins Co., 1978, p. 305.
8. Schwartz, G. R.: Emergency toxicology and general principles of medical management of the poisoned patient. In Schwartz, G. R., et al. (eds.): Principles and Practice of Emergency Medicine. Philadelphia, W. B. Saunders Co., 1978, pp. 1322–1323.
9. Rosen, P., and Sternbach, G. L.: Atlas of Emergency Medicine. Baltimore, Williams & Wilkins Co., 1979, p. 77.
10. Rumack, B. H., and Peterson, R. G.: Poisoning: Prevention of absorption. Top. Emerg. Med. 1:13, 1979.
11. Major, R. H.: History of the stomach tube. Ann. Med. History 6:500, 1934.
12. Kussmaul, A.: Ueber dia Behandlung der Magenerweiterung durch eine neue Methoda, mittelst der Magenpumpe. Dtsch. Arch. Klin. Med. 6:455, 1869.
13. Harstad, E., Moller, K. O., and Simesen, M. H.: The value of gastric lavage in the treatment of acute poisoning. Acta Med. Scand. 112:478, 1942.
14. Editorial: Value of gastric lavage in treatment of acute poisoning. JAMA 133:545, 1947.
15. Louw, A.: Treatment of acute barbituric acid poisoning: Ten years' experience at the centre for the treatment of poisoning in Copenhagen. Dan. Med. Bull. 5:137, 1958.
16. Dabbous, I. A., et al.: The ineffectiveness of mechanically induced vomiting. J. Pediatr. 66:952, 1965.
17. Ward, D. J.: Fetal hypernatremia after a saline emetic. Br. Med. J. 2:432, 1963.
18. Laurence, B. H., and Hopkins, B. E.: Hypernatremia following a saline emetic. Med. J. Aust. 1:1301, 1969.
19. DeGenaro, F., and Nyhan, W. L.: Salt—a dangerous antidote. J. Pediatr. 78:1048, 1971.
20. Robertson, W. O.: A further warning on the use of salt as an emetic agent. J. Pediatr. 79:877, 1971.
21. Barer, J., et al.: Fatal poisoning from salt used as an emetic. Am. J. Dis. Child. 125:889, 1973.
22. Mellencamp, F.: Copper sulphate as an emetic. Appl. Therap. 8:233, 1966.
23. Chuttani, H. K., et al.: Acute copper sulfate poisoning. Am. J. Med. 39:849, 1965.
24. Karlsson, B., and Norén, L.: Ipecacuanha and copper sulphate as emetics in intoxications in children. Acta Paediatr. Scand. 54:331, 1965.
25. Mellenkamp, F.: Copper sulfate as an emetic. Appl. Therap. 8:233, 1966.
26. Holtzman, N. A., and Haslam, R. H. A.: Evaluation of serum copper following copper sulfate as an emetic. Pediatrics 42:189, 1968.
27. Berry, F. A., and Lambdin, M. A.: Apomorphine and levellorphan tartrate in acute poisonings. Am. J. Dis. Child. 105:160, 1963.
28. Corby, D. G., et al.: Clinical comparison of pharmacologic emetics in children. Pediatrics 42:361, 1968.
29. MacLean, W. C. Jr.: A comparison of ipecac syrup and apomorphine in the immediate treatment of ingestion of poisons. J. Pediatr. 82:121, 1973.
30. Thoman, M. E.: The use of emetics in poison ingestion. Clin. Toxicol. 3:185, 1970.
31. Shirkey, H. C.: Ipecac syrup. Its use as an emetic in poison control. J. Pediatr. 69:139, 1966.
32. Abramowicz, M.: Ipecac syrup and activated charcoal for treatment of poisoning in children. Med. Lett. Drugs Ther. 21:70, 1979.
33. Manno, B. R., and Manno, J. E.: Toxicology of ipecac: A review. Clin. Toxicol. 10:221, 1977.
34. Robertson, W. O.: Syrup of ipecac—a slow or fast emetic? Am. J. Dis. Child. 103:136, 1962.
35. Ilett, K. F., et al.: Syrup of ipecacuanha as an emetic in adults. Med. J. Aust. 2:91, 1977.
36. Matthew, H.: Gastric aspiration and lavage. Clin. Toxicol. 3:179, 1970.
37. Meester, W. D.: Emesis and lavage. Vet. Hum. Toxicol. 22:225, 1980.
38. Arnold, J. A., et al.: Evaluation of the efficacy of lavage and induced emesis in treatment of salicylate poisoning. Pediatrics 23:286, 1959.
39. Abdallah, A. H., and Tye, A.: A comparison of the efficacy of emetic drugs and stomach lavage. Am. J. Dis. Child. 113:571, 1967.
40. Corby, D. G., et al.: The efficiency of methods used to evacuate the stomach after acute ingestions. Pediatrics 40:871, 1967.
41. Boxer, L., et al.: Comparison of ipecac-induced emesis with gastric lavage in the treatment of acute salicylate ingestion. J. Pediatr. 74:800, 1969.
42. Matthew, H., et al.: Gastric aspiration and lavage in acute poisoning. Br. Med. J. 1:1333, 1966.
43. Burke, M.: Gastric lavage and emesis in the treatment of ingested poisons: A review and a clinical study of lavage in ten adults. Resuscitation 1:91, 1972.
44. Collins, V. J.: General anesthesia—clinical signs. In Collins, V. J. (ed.): Principles of Anesthesiology, 2nd ed. Philadelphia, Lea & Febiger, 1976, pp. 253–264.
45. Thoman, M. E.: Ipecac syrup in antiemetic ingestion. JAMA 196:147, 1966.
46. Manoguerra, A. S., and Krenzelok, E. P.: Rapid emesis with high-dose ipecac syrup in adults and children intoxicated with antiemetics or other drugs. Am. J. Hosp. Pharm. 35:1360, 1978.
47. Thorazine. In Physicians Desk Reference, 36th ed. Oradell, NJ, Medical Economics Co., 1982, pp. 1815–1818.
48. Sharman, J. R., et al.: Drug overdoses: Is one stomach washing enough? N. Z. Med. J. 81:195, 1975.
49. Jenis, E. H., et al.: Acute meprobamate poisoning. A fatal case following a lucid interval. JAMA 207:361, 1969.
50. Schwartz, H. S.: Acute meprobamate poisoning with gastrotomy and removal of a drug-containing mass. N. Engl. J. Med. 295:1177, 1976.
51. Bartecchi, C. E.: Removal of gastric drug masses. N. Engl. J. Med. 296:282, 1977.
52. Sogge, M. R., et al.: Lavage to remove enteric-coated aspirin and gastric outlet obstruction. Ann. Intern. Med. 87:721, 1977.
53. Marsteller, H. J. and Gugler, R.: Endoscopic management of toxic masses in the stomach. N. Engl. J. Med. 296:1003, 1977.
54. Kirsh, M. M., and Ritter, F.: Caustic ingestion and subsequent damage to the oropharyngeal and digestive passages. Ann. Thorac. Surg. 21:74, 1976.
55. Ritter, F. N. et al.: A clinical and experimental study of corrosive burns of the stomach. Ann. Otol. Rhinol. Laryngol. 77:830, 1968.
56. Penner, G. E.: Acid ingestion: Toxicology and treatment. Ann. Emerg. Med. 9:374, 1980.

57. Diechmann, W. B., et al.: Kerosene intoxication. Ann. Intern. Med. 21:803, 1944.
58. Dice, W. H., et al.: Pulmonary toxicity following gastrointestinal ingestion of kerosene. Ann. Emerg. Med 11:138, 1982.
59. Richardson, J. A., and Pratt-Thomas, H. R.: Toxic effects of varying doses of kerosene administered by different routes. Am. J. Med. Sci. 221:531, 1951.
60. Gerarde, H. W.: Toxicological studies on hydrocarbons V. kerosene. Toxicol. Appl. Pharmacol. 1:462, 1959.
61. Gerarde, H. W.: Toxicological studies on hydrocarbons. IX. The aspiration hazard and toxicity of hydrocarbons and hydrocarbon mixtures. Arch. Environ. Health 6:329, 1963.
62. Mofenson, H. C., and Greensher, J.: The new correct answer to an old question on kerosene ingestion. Pediatrics 59:788, 1977.
63. Hydrocarbons. In Poisindex. Denver, CO, Micromedex, 1982.
64. Subcommittee on Accidental Poisoning: Co-operative kerosene poisoning study: Evaluation of gastric lavage and other factors in the treatment of accidental ingestion of petroleum distillate products. Pediatrics 29:648, 1962.
65. Ng, R. C. et al.: Emergency treatment of petroleum distillate and turpentine ingestion. Can. Med. Assoc. J. 111:537, 1974.
66. Fane, L. R., et al.: Physical parameters in gastric lavage. Clin. Toxicol. 4:389, 1971.
67. Peterson, C. D.: Electrolyte depletion following emergency stomach evacuation. Am. J. Hosp. Pharm. 36:1366, 1979.
68. Rudolph, J. P.: Automated gastric lavage and a comparison of 0.9 normal saline solution and tap water irrigant. Submitted for publication.
69. Ritschell, W. E., and Erni, W.: The influence of temperature of ingested fluid on stomach emptying time. Int. J. Clin. Pharmacol. 15:172, 1977.
70. McDougal, C. B., and McLean, M. A.: Modifications in the technique of gastric lavage. Ann. Emerg. Med. 10:514, 1981.
71. Arena, J. J.: Poisoning: Toxicology-Symptoms-Treatments. Springfield, IL, Charles C Thomas, 1976, pp. 51–54.
72. Skoutakis, V. A.: Clinical Toxicology of Drugs: Principles and Practice. Philadelphia, Lea & Febiger, 1982, p. 12.
73. Czajka, P. A.: Iron poisoning: An in vitro comparison of bicarbonate and phosphate lavage solutions. J. Pediatr. 98:491, 1981.
74. Greensher, J., et al.: Activated charcoal update. JACEP 8:761, 1979.
75. Riegel, J. M., and Becker, C. E.: Use of cathartics in toxic ingestions. Ann. Emerg. Med. 10:254, 1981.
76. Klein-Schwartz, W., and Oderda, G. M.: Adsorption of oral antidotes for acetaminophen poisoning (methionine and N-acetylcysteine) by activated charcoal. Clin. Toxicol. 18:283, 1981.
77. North, D. S., et al.: Effect of activated charcoal administration on acetylcysteine serum levels in humans. Am. J. Hosp. Pharm 38:1022, 1981.
78. Fioria, A., Cecchetti, G., and Giusti, F. V.: A lethal complication of gastric lavage leading to malpractice suit: A case report. Forensic Sci. 11:47, 1978.
79. Knopp, R.: Caustic ingestions. JACEP 8:329, 1979.
80. Carter, R. F., and Fotheringham, B. J.: Fatal salt poisoning due to gastric lavage with hypertonic saline. Med. J. Aust. 1:539, 1971.
81. Bachrach, L., et al.: Iron poisoning: Complications of hypertonic phosphate lavage therapy. J. Pediatr. 94:147, 1979.
82. Rumack, B. H.: Management of acute poisoning and overdose. In Rumack, B. H., and Temple, A. R. (eds.): Management of the poisoned patient. Princeton, Science Press, 1977, pp. 250–280.

56

Balloon Tamponade of Gastroesophageal Varices

JONATHAN M. GLAUSER, M.D.

Background

The first reported successful control of variceal hemorrhage by tamponade was achieved by Westphal in 1930.[1, 2] He used a Gottstein sound distended with water.[3] In 1950, Sengstaken and Blakemore[4] reported the technique of double-balloon tamponade, a method still widely used. The Sengstaken-Blakemore tube (Davol, Inc.) is a triple-lumen rubber tube (Fig. 56–1). Two of the lumens are used to inflate a gastric balloon and an esophageal balloon, and the third lumen is used for nasogastric suction.

In 1953, a single-balloon tube with only a gastric suction lumen was introduced by Linton; this device was refined in 1955 by Nachlas.[5] The Linton-Nachlas tube contains two lumens for suction—one for the stomach and one for the esophagus.[6] The Linton-Nachlas tube has a single gastric balloon that is larger than the gastric balloon of the Sengstaken-Blakemore tube. The Linton-Nachlas tube probably works through compression of the cardioesophageal junction, cutting off blood flow to the esophageal varices.

In 1962, Boyce introduced a modification of the original Sengstaken-Blakemore tube (Fig. 56–2). The modification consisted of a standard nasogastric tube sutured to the Sengstaken-Blakemore tube, with the tip of the nasogastric tube positioned just proximally to the esophageal balloon.[7] A silk suture was placed through the wall of the nasogastric tube and was tied around the Sengstaken-Blakemore tube. The purpose of the Boyce

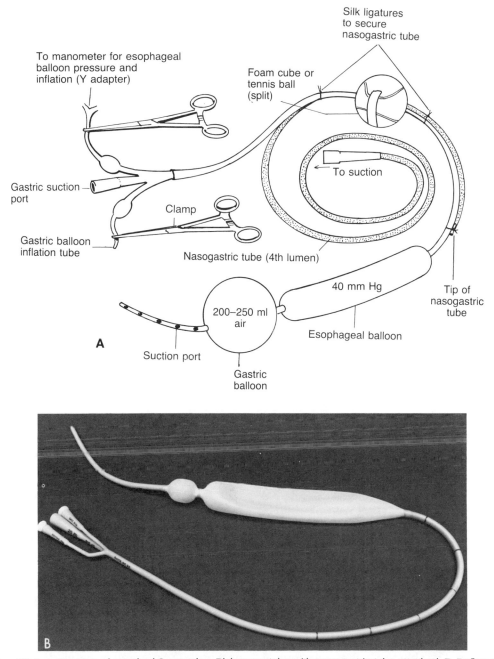

Figure 56–1. A, Diagram of standard Sengstaken-Blakemore tube with nasogastric tube attached. B, Deflated tube.

modification was to enable oropharyngeal secretions to be suctioned from above the balloons, which (it was hoped) would prevent aspiration. Edlich[8] has introduced a commercial Sengstaken-Blakemore–type tube with a fourth lumen that is designed to provide suction just proximally to the esophageal balloon, eliminating the need for a separate nasogastric tube. Some believe that the lumen of this device may be too small to permit effective suctioning.[2] Advances in technology have provided a clear tube that can accommodate a fiber-optic endoscope to permit direct examination of the esophageal and gastric mucosa through the main lumen of the core tube.[9] Lower inflation pressures may be required with this method, but it is not widely used on an emergency basis. Most clinical situations can be managed with either the Sengstaken-Blakemore tube or the Linton-Nachlas tube. Although these tubes are infrequently used today, they may be lifesaving, and a thorough knowledge of their structure and function is necessary should the need for their use arise.

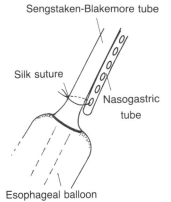

Figure 56–2. The Boyce modification of the original Sengstaken-Blakemore tube is a standard nasogastric tube sutured to secure the tip of the suction tube just proximal to the esophageal balloon.

Indications

The indications for use of a Sengstaken-Blakemore tube or a Linton-Nachlas tube are not standardized, but in general they include:

1. "Severe" variceal bleeding that cannot be controlled with other measures.

2. Moderate or persistent variceal bleeding requiring transfusion of more than 2000 ml of blood over a 24-hour period.[10]

3. Traumatic longitudinal tears of the esophagogastric mucosa (Mallory-Weiss syndrome) that do not stop bleeding spontaneously.

Since the use of balloon tamponade is associated with serious and potentially lethal complications, several caveats are in order. Endoscopy should be performed as soon as possible to document that an upper gastrointestinal bleed is actually variceal in origin. Endoscopy is most helpful after blood and clots have been evacuated by a Ewald tube.[3, 6, 11–16] It is demanded by some authors that bleeding varices be endoscopically visualized before a Sengstaken-Blakemore tube is inserted,[17, 18] but in patients with a massive hemorrhage, the endoscopist may not be able to see the exact source of bleeding. In such cases, angiography or a therapeutic trial with a Sengstaken-Blakemore tube may be necessary.

Use of Balloon Tamponade

Thirty per cent of patients with cirrhosis of the liver will hemorrhage at least once from gastroesophageal varices; the mortality is 30 to 80 per cent. The initial stabilization of these patients is often complex and difficult and involves more than balloon tamponade. Although definitive treatment is often surgical, it is generally agreed that mortality from any surgical procedure is reduced if the procedure is performed electively,[3, 16, 19] and balloon tamponade may be required to stabilize the patient before elective surgery. The risk of complications from balloon tamponade must be weighed against the chances of death from exsanguination. Since major complications occur with balloon tamponade in up to 10 per cent of patients, the procedure is not usually a first-line treatment. Iced nasogastric lavage,[13, 20] treatment of shock with fluids and fresh blood,[9, 14, 15] intravenous vasopressin,[21–24] central venous pressure monitoring, platelet transfusions,[22, 25] vitamin replacement,[13, 14] fresh frozen plasma infusion,[21, 22, 24, 25] and methods to lower serum ammonia levels and to prevent hepatic coma (lactulose, neomycin) may all be used before balloon tamponade. One study reports that it is very unusual for either a Sengstaken-Blakemore or a Linton-Nachlas tube to be inserted within 6 hours of the onset of variceal bleeding.[26]

To reinforce the limits of balloon tamponade, it is emphasized that a Sengstaken-Blakemore tube is used, quite simply, for temporary bleeding control. Balloon tamponade has failed to improve measurably the mortality associated with bleeding esophageal varices in the past three decades.[13] The procedure often does not control hemorrhage definitively. Most studies report that the Sengstaken-Blakemore tube provides initial hemostasis in 80 to 90 per cent of patients who are bleeding from esophageal varices,[2, 5, 27] although a rate of initial hemostasis as low as 40 per cent has been reported.[26] The tube may be used on all patients regardless of the results of hepatic function studies.[20]

Bleeding recurrences after initial balloon tamponade are common. One of the following definitive procedures must be performed after stabilization: sclerotherapy of varices by endoscopic injection,[3, 12, 18, 28–33] percutaneous transhepatic obliteration of varices[3, 21, 22, 24, 31, 34, 35] laser obliteration of varices,[15] gastroesophageal transection with a staple gun,[23, 31, 32, 35] transthoracic ligation of the esophageal varices,[14, 20, 35] porta-azygous disconnection,[14, 35] emergency or elective portasystemic shunting,[2, 21, 22, 34] or even varix obliteration using electric current passed through longitudinal electrodes placed on a Sengstaken-Blakemore tube.[36]

The Sengstaken-Blakemore tube is used more frequently than the Linton-Nachlas tube. One study has reported that the Sengstaken-Blakemore tube may be more effective than the Linton-Nachlas tube for achieving permanent hemostasis in esophageal bleeding, whereas the Linton-Nachlas tube may be more effective in managing gastric varices.[37] When a hiatal hernia exists, the Sengstaken-Blakemore tube may be more liable to displacement than the Linton-Nachlas tube. Also, if bleeding is from fundic varices, the Sengstaken-Blakemore tube may be less effective than the

Linton-Nachlas tube because of the smaller gastric balloon size.

There are generally two sources of blood in bleeding varices. Submucosal vessels of the stomach traverse the cardioesophageal junction and anastomose with periesophageal veins, and periesophageal veins provide perforating branches through the wall of the esophagus. There may also be distinct gastric varices, usually near the cardioesophageal junction or fundus. For these anatomic reasons, bleeding from esophageal varices may often be controlled with inflation of the gastric balloon alone.

It is interesting to question whether it is the pressure transmitted to the esophageal varices by the esophageal balloon that actually stops the hemorrhage. It has been demonstrated that barium will freely pass both inflated balloons of a well-positioned and properly inflated Sengstaken-Blakemore tube.[27] The actual transmitted pressure to the esophageal wall is less than one half of the balloon pressure; a balloon inflation pressure of 100 mm Hg maintains an esophageal pressure of 40 mm Hg. A sustained Valsalva maneuver can cause a pressure rise of as much as 195 mm Hg in the varices; this is far greater than any pressure that can be transmitted to the esophageal wall by an intraluminal balloon. At recommended inflation pressures, the average esophageal balloon diameter is 27 mm, and further increases in inflation pressure cause only minor variations in the diameter of the balloon. Although it has been questioned whether the esophageal varices are actually being compressed adequately to control bleeding,[27] in many cases inflation of both balloons does provide more effective hemostasis in bleeding esophageal varices than is provided by a single-balloon Linton-Nachlas tube.[37]

Preparations And Precautions

The patient must be in an intensive care area,[10] since patients with a balloon tube in place require considerable nursing care. This includes airway and cardiac monitoring, pharyngeal suction,[20, 38] and frequent measurement of vital signs.

Aspiration and airway obstruction from use of the Sengstaken-Blakemore tube have been reported so frequently (especially in obtunded patients) that some authors favor definitive airway management with either endotracheal intubation, cricothyroidotomy, or tracheotomy before balloon tamponade is used.[6] Although intubation is usually not required in the alert patient, tracheal suction apparatus and intubation equipment should be readily available at all times.[2, 39]

Because of the danger of airway occlusion from gastric balloon deflation and slippage of an esophageal balloon forward into the pharynx, scissors should always be readily available to transect the tube.[31] Cutting the entire tube in cross section ensures balloon deflation for rapid removal.[17] If respiratory distress occurs with the Sengstaken-Blakemore tube in place, the tube should be grasped at the mouth. The tube is cut just above the grasping hand (but below the entrance of the three-channel inlets of the Sengstaken-Blakemore tube) and then is removed immediately.

Only new tubes should be used. One should check all balloons for leakage by inflating them underwater in a basin.[2, 6, 38, 39] In a Sengstaken-Blakemore tube, the esophageal balloon should be tested to a pressure of 50 mm Hg, and the gastric balloon should be tested with 250 ml of air. Patency of all lumens, both for suction and for balloon inflation, should be confirmed before tube insertion.

Local anesthesia of the nose may be appropriate, but the pharynx should not be anesthetized for tube passage in order for the patient's gag reflex to be preserved.[2] The head of the bed should be raised 6 to 10 inches to prevent hiccups or vomiting.[17] Some very short patients are not suitable for Sengstaken-Blakemore tube insertion, because the esophageal balloon may be inflated in the throat.[38] Although aspiration pneumonia is frequently a complication of balloon tamponade, prophylactic antibiotics are not recommended.

Technique

It should be noted that passage of balloon tubes is not a simple procedure. Even under the best circumstances, passage is difficult and complicated. In the combative or obtunded patient, the procedure is even more difficult, and one must be thoroughly familiar with the function of the various balloons and lumens before passage is attempted.

Before passage of the Sengstaken-Blakemore tube, a standard nasogastric tube is placed alongside of the Sengstaken-Blakemore tube to premeasure the distance for subsequent insertion of the nasogastric tube. The tip of the nasogastric tube should lie just above the proximal portion of the esophageal balloon. A piece of tape is wrapped around the proximal end of the nasogastric tube as a marker for proper positioning of the nasogastric tube to evacuate oropharyngeal secretions. Alternatively, a 14 to 16 gauge nasogastric tube can be sutured to the Sengstaken-Blakemore tube with silk sutures before passage, as described by Boyce.[7] Using the method of Boyce, the Sengstaken-Blakemore and nasogastric tubes are passed as a unit rather than sequentially.

Prior to the procedure, the stomach is emptied of blood and clots with a Ewald tube to decrease the chance of aspiration during passage of the

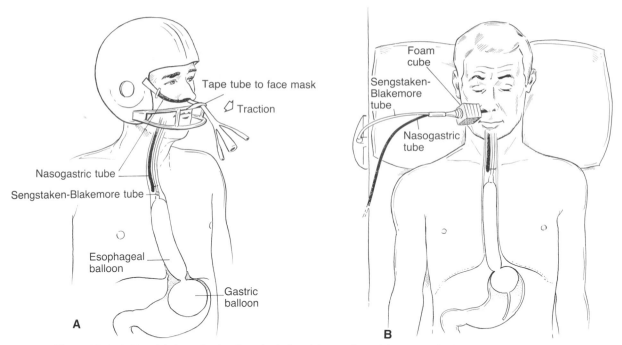

Figure 56–3. A, Traction is maintained on the inflated Sengstaken-Blakemore tube by taping the proximal end to the face mask of a football helmet. B, An alternative is to split a foam cube in half and run the tube through the center.

balloon tube. The balloons should be evacuated of all air with a syringe and then twisted around the tube to facilitate passage.[31] The Sengstaken-Blakemore tube is then well lubricated and passed nasally. While the patient swallows some water through a straw, the tube is passed through the esophagus.[2] In some circumstances, it may be necessary to resort to oral passage, although nasal passage is preferred. Flexion of the neck slightly may enhance esophageal entry.

The tube is passed to 50 cm, and gastric contents are aspirated. This procedure must be followed to reduce the risk of esophageal perforation by a misplaced gastric balloon. Some authors recommend initial inflation of the gastric balloon with only 50 ml of air followed by radiographic confirmation of the position of the balloon below the diaphragm.[3] Once gastric placement is ensured, the gastric balloon is inflated with 200 to 250 ml of air,[2, 6] and the intake lumen is double-clamped with a rubber-protected surgical clamp. No more than 300 ml of air should be used.[10, 26] It is emphasized that only *air* should be used to inflate the balloons. If water or contrast material is used, rapid emergency deflation may not be possible. Very gentle hand traction is applied until the gastric balloon is felt to be lodged at the gastroesophageal junction. It is the pressure of the gastric balloon that produces the majority of the hemostasis.

If a Linton-Nachlas tube is used, the balloon is inflated with 600 ml of air (no more than 750 ml), the intake lumen is double clamped,[39] and the proximal end of the tube is pulled gently against the gastroesphageal junction. Gentle traction at a maximum of 1 to 2 lbs is applied to produce the tamponade effect. With either tube, a follow-up radiograph is mandatory. The radiograph should be portable to avoid disaster in the radiology department.

There are several acceptable ways of providing traction to the tube (Fig. 56–3). Tubes can be taped to the mouthpiece of a football helmet,[2, 3, 10] or to eye goggles.[38] Some advocate pulley traction with 1 to 2 lbs of weight,[20] but pulley traction should be avoided in the emergency department because of the higher risk of airway obstruction and aspiration.[3] In addition, disoriented or obtunded patients can quickly become entangled in pulley set-ups. Traction can be maintained with a split tennis ball or a cube of foam rubber. The tube is inserted between the two halves, and the ball or the cube is placed against the nose and firmly strapped to the tube to maintain tamponade at the gastro-esophageal junction.[18] Some authors prefer to avoid traction and simply fix the tube with tape at the corner of the patient's nose.[17]

With the tube in place, the stomach is lavaged with cold water until the aspirate is clear.[6, 20] If the bleeding is not controlled, the esophageal balloon is inflated to 30 to 40 mm Hg.[2, 39]

The pressure in the esophageal balloon must be carefully calibrated (Fig. 56–4). To inflate the esophageal balloon, the operator inserts one end of a Y connector into the correct lumen opening. A mercury manometer is attached to the other end

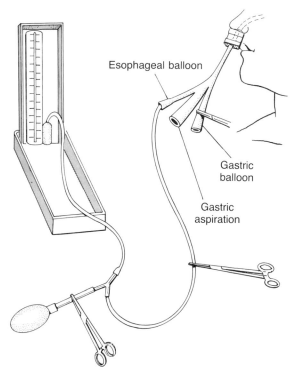

Figure 56–4. The pressure in the esophageal balloon should be calibrated frequently with a manometer and should not exceed a baseline of 40 mm Hg.

of the Y connector, and the balloon is inflated until a reading of 30 to 40 mm Hg is attained. The esophageal tubing is then double-clamped.[39]

The pressure in the esophageal balloon will vary with respiration. Esophageal spasm and intermittent variations of up to 30 mm Hg above the baseline are acceptable, as long as the pressure returns to 30 to 40 mm Hg in the steady state.

At this point, if the original version of the Sengstaken-Blakemore tube is being used (without the Boyce adaptation) a 14 to 16 French nasogastric tube is passed through the other external nares into the esophagus until it is felt to abut the upper portion of the esophageal balloon.[16] The nasogastric tube should be measured against the Sengstaken-Blakemore tube before either tube is inserted to ensure that the nasogastric tube is placed above the esophageal balloon.[31] The nasogastric tube is attached to intermittent suction. Oral, nasal, and pharyngeal secretions in excess of 1500 ml per day make suction proximal to the esophageal balloon mandatory in preventing aspiration. The nasogastric tube should be passed even if the esophageal balloon is not inflated, because the gastric balloon does not allow the patient to swallow secretions. Obviously, with either a Linton-Nachlas tube or the Boyce modification of the Sengstaken-Blakemore tube, no extra nasogastric tube is needed.

Once passed, the tube is not disturbed for 24 hours. During this time, adjunctive therapy and work-up are instituted. If bleeding does not abate,

other methods must be considered. It is difficult for most patients to tolerate these tubes for more than a few hours without narcotics or other forms of sedation. Meperidine sedation is acceptable, but one should be careful not to induce respiratory depression. Soft restraints may be needed to prevent the patient from dislodging the tube.

Complications

The complications from the use of the Sengstaken-Blakemore and Linton-Nachlas tubes are numerous and will be listed as major or minor. Major complications are airway obstruction, aspiration, and esophageal injury. The incidence of major complications from use of the Sengstaken-Blakemore tube generally ranges from 8 to 16 per cent.[2, 14, 20, 26] The mortality directly related to use of the Sengstaken-Blakemore tube is generally listed at 3 to 3.7 per cent,[14, 20] although one study claims that the tube was a direct cause of death in 22 per cent of the patients on whom it was used.[6] Bleeding from esophageal varices carries a 50 to 80 per cent mortality overall.[3, 22] The best marker of long-term survival seems to be an early stabilization.[40] The quality of emergency care is therefore critical in these patients.

Aspiration pneumonitis is the most frequent major complication. Aspiration may result from secretions accumulating in the esophagus or from regurgitation of gastric contents.[2, 10, 20, 26, 29] Death has been reported from aspiration of bloody gastric contents,[2, 17, 38] and the stomach should be emptied before passage of the balloon tube is attempted.[2, 17] Other major complications include esophageal laceration caused by overinflation of a misplaced gastric balloon[6, 10, 11, 17, 38] (especially in the distal esophagus),[26] esophageal rupture[2, 6] with mediastinitis,[26] and esophageal necrosis caused by excessive or prolonged pressure by the esophageal balloon.[10] One may prevent esophageal necrosis by intermittently deflating the balloons at 6-hour intervals. Death from hemorrhage at the site of esophageal erosion has been reported.[2] Injuries to the esophagus occur more frequently after 24 hours of tamponade.

Airway obstruction can occur with dislodgement of an underinflated gastric balloon and can produce asphyxiation.[2, 15] If this happens, one should divide the tube immediately and extract it. Inadvertent slow deflation or rupture of the gastric balloon may make it possible for the esophageal balloon to slip proximally until it obstructs the airway at the oropharynx or the larynx.[5, 38]

The tubes may fail to control the bleeding.[2] Correctable causes for this include misplaced balloons, inadequate tamponade, and misdiagnosis of the site of bleeding (e.g., duodenal ulcer).[3, 10, 38] Uncommon complications of concern are bilateral hemothorax, jejunal rupture with a Sengstaken-Blakemore tube placed in the efferent jejunal limb of a gastrojejunostomy (rare),[41] and innominate vein obstruction by esophageal tamponade.[42]

Minor complications include retrosternal discomfort and chest pain,[26, 29] agitation,[26] gastric erosion, ulcerations at the cardioesophageal junction,[26] epistaxis,[38] deep erosions of the pharynx,[38] and submucosal esophageal hemorrhage. Other minor complications are the inability to pass the Sengstaken-Blakemore tube because of local swelling or muscle spasm, or because the patient will not cooperate;[38] coiling of the tube in the stomach or the esophagus;[38] hiccups;[17] and temporary balloon deflation.[17]

The diaphragm may relax following placement, allowing the tube to become dislodged. It is necessary to reassess the position of the tube at frequent intervals to ensure proper and safe use.

Summary

Gastroesophageal balloon tamponade is an effective way to control hemorrhage from gastric or esophageal varices. Both single- and double-balloon tubes are useful in conjunction with a method to control oropharyngeal secretions.

Because of the high incidence of serious complications, the procedure should be used only when there is a high risk of exsanguination and when more conservative methods to control hemorrhage have failed.

1. Westphal, K.: Ueber eine Kompressionsbehandlung der Blutungen aus Oesophagusvarizen. Dtsch. Med. Wochenschr. 56:1135, 1930.
2. Bauer, J. J., Kreel, I., and Kark, A. E.: The use of the Sengstaken-Blakemore tube for immediate control of bleeding esophageal varices. Ann. Surg. 179:273, 1974.
3. Hanna, S. S., Warren, W. D., Galambos, J. T., et al.: Bleeding varices: Emergency management. CMA Journal 124:29, 1981.
4. Sengstaken, R. W., and Blakemore, A. H.: Balloon tamponade for the control of hemorrhage from esophageal varices. Ann. Surg. 131:781, 1950.
5. Burcharth, F., and Malstrom, J.: Experiences with the Linton-Nachlas and the Sengstaken-Blakemore tubes for bleeding esophageal varices. Surg. Gynecol. Obstet. 142:529, 1976.
6. Conn, H. O., and Simpson, J. A.: Excessive mortality associated with balloon tamponade of bleeding varices: A critical reappraisal. JAMA, 202:587, 1967.
7. Boyce, H. W., Jr.: Modification of the Sengstaken-Blakemore balloon tube. N. Engl. J. Med. 267:195, 1962.
8. Edlich, R. F., Lande, A. J., Goodale, R. L. et al.: Prevention of aspiration pneumonia by continuous esophageal aspiration during esophagogastric tamponade and gastric cooling. Surgery 64:405, 1968.
9. Idezuki, Y., Hagiwara, M., and Watanabe, H.: Endoscopic balloon tamponade for emergency control of bleeding esophageal varices using a new transparent tamponade tube. Trans. Am. Soc. Artif. Intern. Organs 23:646, 1977.
10. Schwartz, G. R., Safar, P., Stone, J. H., et al. (eds.): The Principles and Practice of Emergency Medicine. Philadelphia, W. B. Saunders Co., 1978, pp. 1024–1026.
11. Joelsson, B., Borjesson, C., Carlsson, C., et al.: Acute treatment of bleeding oesophageal varices: A retrospective study of 88 patients. Scand. J. Gastroenterol. 16:81, 1981.
12. Johnson, A. G.: Injection sclerotherapy in the emergency and elective treatment of oesophageal varices. Ann. R. Coll. Surg. Eng. 59:497, 1977.
13. Orloff, M. J.: Emergency treatment of variceal hemorrhage. Can. J. Surg. 22:550, 1979.
14. Schiff, L., and Schiff, E. R.: Diseases of the Liver, 5th ed. Philadelphia, J. B. Lippincott Co., 1982, pp. 894–902.
15. Butler, M. L.: Variceal hemorrhage: A review. Milit. Med. 145:766, 1980.
16. Holman, J. M., and Rikkers, L. F.: Success of medical and surgical management of acute variceal hemorrhage. Am. J. Surg. 140:816, 1980.
17. Pitcher, J. L.: Safety and effectiveness of the modified Sengstaken-Blakemore tube: A prospective study. Gastroenterology 61:291, 1971.
18. Terblanche, J.: Treatment of Esophageal Varices by Injection Sclerotherapy. Chicago, Year Book Medical Publishers, 1981, pp. 257–267.
19. Fischer, J. E.: Portal hypertension and bleeding esophageal varices. Am. J. Surg. 140:337, 1980.
20. Hermann, R. E., and Traul, D.: Experience with the Sengstaken-Blakemore tube for bleeding esophageal varices. Surg. Gynecol. Obstet. 130:879, 1970.
21. Nabseth, D. C., Johnson, W. C., Widrich, W. C., et al: Bleeding esophageal varices: Treatment by embolization and shunting. Jpn. J. Surg. 11:8, 1981.
22. O'Donnell, T. F., Jr., Gembarowicz, R. M., Callow, A. D. et al.: The economic impact of acute variceal bleeding: Cost-effectiveness implications for medical and surgical therapy. Surgery 88:693, 1980.
23. Sägar, S., Harrison, I. D., Brearley, R. et al.: Emergency treatment of variceal hemorrhage. Br. J. Surg. 66:824, 1979.
24. Gembarowicz, R. M., Kelly, J. J., O'Donnell, T. F., et al: Management of variceal hemorrhage: Results of a standardized protocol using vasopressin and transhepatic embolization. Arch. Surg. 115:1160, 1980.
25. Osborne, D. R., and Hobbs, K. E. F.: The acute treatment of hemorrhage from oesophageal varices: A comparison of oesophageal transection and staple gun anastomosis with mesocaval shunt. Br. J. Surg. 68:734, 1981.
26. Chojkier, M., and Conn, H. O.: Esophageal tamponade in the treatment of bleeding varices: A decadal progress report. Dig. Dis. Sci. 25:267, 1980.
27. Agger, P., Andersen, J. R., and Burcharth, F.: Does the oesophageal balloon compress oesophageal varices? Scand. J. Gastroenterol. 13:225, 1978.
28. Hennessy, T. P., Stephens, R. B., and Keane, F. B.: Acute and chronic management of esophageal varices by injection sclerotherapy. Surg. Gynecol. Obstet. 154:375, 1982.
29. Barsoum, M. S., Bolous, F. I., El-Rooby, A. A., et al.: Tamponade and injection sclerotherapy in the management of bleeding oeosophageal varices. Br. J. Surg. 69:76, 1982.
30. Terblanche, J., Yakoob, H. I., Bornman, P. C., et al: Acute bleeding varices: A five-year prospective evaluation of tamponade and sclerotherapy. Ann. Surg. 194:521, 1981.
31. Jamieson, G. G., Faris, I. B., and Ludbrook, J.: A selective approach to bleeding esophageal varices. Henry Ford Hosp. Med. J. 28:210, 1980.
32. Johnston, G. W.: Bleeding oesophageal varices: the management of shunt rejects. Ann. R. Coll. Surg. Eng. 63:3, 1981.
33. Smith, P. M., and Jones, D. B.: Control of oesophageal variceal bleeding (letter). Lancet 747, 1980.
34. Johnson, W. C., Nabseth, D. C., Widrich, W. C., et al.: Bleeding esophageal varices: Treatment with vasopressin, transhepatic embolization and selective splenorenal shunting. Ann. Surg. 195:393, 1982.

35. Matory, W. E., Sedgwick, C. E., and Rossi, R. L.: Non-shunting procedures in management of bleeding esophageal varices. Surg. Clin. North Am. 60:281, 1980.
36. Taylor, T. V., and Neilson, J. M.: "Currents and clots"—an approach to the problem of acute variceal bleeding. Br. J. Surg. 68:692, 1981.
37. Teres, J., Cecilia, A., Bordas, J. M., et al.: Esophageal tamponade for bleeding varices: A controlled trial between the Sengstaken-Blakemore tube and the Linton-Nachlas tube. Gastroenterology 75:566, 1978.
38. Conn, H. O.; Hazards attending the use of esophageal tamponade. N. Engl. J. Med. 259:701, 1958.
39. Jackson, E. W.: Nursing Photobook: Performing GI Procedures. Horsham, PA, Intermed Communications, 1981, pp. 33–37.
40. Smith, J. L., and Graham, D. Y.: Variceal hemorrhage: A critical evaluation of survival analysis. Gastroenterology 82:968, 1982.
41. Goff, J. S., Thompson, J. S., Pratt, C. F., et al.: Jejunal rupture caused by a Sengstaken-Blakemore tube. Gastroenterology 82:573, 1982.
42. Juffe, A., Tellez, G., Eguaras, M. G., et al.: Unusual complication of the Sengstaken-Blakemore tube. Gastroenterology 72:724, 1977.
43. Idezuki, Y., Hagiwara, M., and Watanabe, H.: Endoscopic balloon tamponade for emergency control of bleeding esophageal varices using a new transparent tamponade tube. Trans. Am. Soc. Artif. Intern. Organs 23:646, 1977.

57

Abdominal Hernia Reduction

JONATHAN M. GLAUSER, M.D.

Introduction

The emergency physician is often called upon to diagnose abdominal hernias. Once the diagnosis has been made, the physician must reduce the hernia sac or properly refer the patient for definitive care. Although by definition a hernia represents a weakness or defect in supporting structures through which an organ may protrude, or herniate, the emergency physician is rarely consulted by the patient unless the hernia is considered irreducible (incarcerated) by the patient or family. The challenge of the emergency physician is thus to differentiate the incarcerated hernia from other forms of swelling and to achieve reduction before ischemia of the incarcerated hernia (strangulation) occurs. Strangulation is believed to result from progressive venous and lymphatic congestion causing tissue edema and subsequent compromise of perfusion.

Although the exact prevalence of hernias is unknown, Zimmerman and Anson estimate that approximately 5 per cent of the total adult male population is afflicted.[1] Hernias in general are over five times more common in males. The most common hernia for both sexes is the indirect inguinal hernia. Direct hernias are unusual in females, whereas femoral hernias occur more commonly in females then in males. Indirect inguinal hernias and umbilical hernias are common in children. They occur more frequently in boys than in girls (9:1 ratio) and are often associated with prematurity or developmental defects.

Classification of Abdominal Hernias

Detailed discussions of the historical development of the treatment of hernias including recognition, preoperative management, and operative repair can be found elsewhere.[1-3]

Since a hernia can be defined as a potential weakness in the abdominal wall, the defect will permit protrusion of peritoneum and abdominal contents. If a contained viscus can be returned from the defect in the abdominal wall to the abdominal cavity, the hernia is defined as *reducible*. When the contents of the hernia sac cannot be reduced, the hernia is considered *incarcerated*. For the purposes of this chapter, a hernia will be defined as incarcerated when the patient, family, or physician on initial evaluation (prior to medication and other techniques described later) is unable to reduce the hernia sac. When there is ischemia of the contents of the hernia sac, the herniated tissue is said to be *strangulated*. A *sliding* hernia occurs when a portion of the wall of the hernia sac is composed of an organ (e.g., the cecum). If only a portion of the antimesenteric wall of the bowel is incarcerated or strangulated, the hernia is called a *Richter's* hernia.[4, 5]

Groin hernias can be categorized as femoral or inguinal hernias; the inguinal hernias can be either direct or indirect (Figs. 57–1 and 57–2).

Direct Inguinal Hernia. A direct inguinal hernia represents a weakening of the abdominal wall (transversalis fascia) that will permit protrusion of

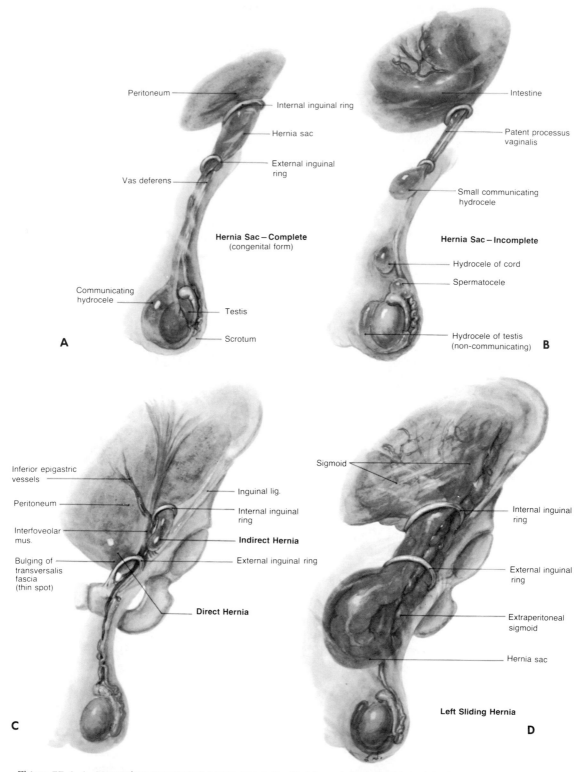

Figure 57–1. *A,* A complete (congenital) hernia sac extending through both the internal and external inguinal rings with communication to a hydrocele in the scrotum. *B,* An incomplete hernia sac with a small communicating hydrocele distal to the external ring. Also shown are noncommunicating hydroceles of the cord and testis and a spermatocele. *C,* Detailed illustration of the anatomical orgins of a direct hernia and an indirect hernia. Note the location of the inferior epigastric vessels medial to the internal inguinal ring. *D,* A sliding hernia with the bowel shown traversing both the internal and external rings. (From Schlossberg, L., and Zuidema, G. D.: Surgical Anatomy of the Abdomen and Pelvis: A Series of Translucent Plates in Color. Philadelphia, W. B. Saunders Company, 1972. Used by permission.)

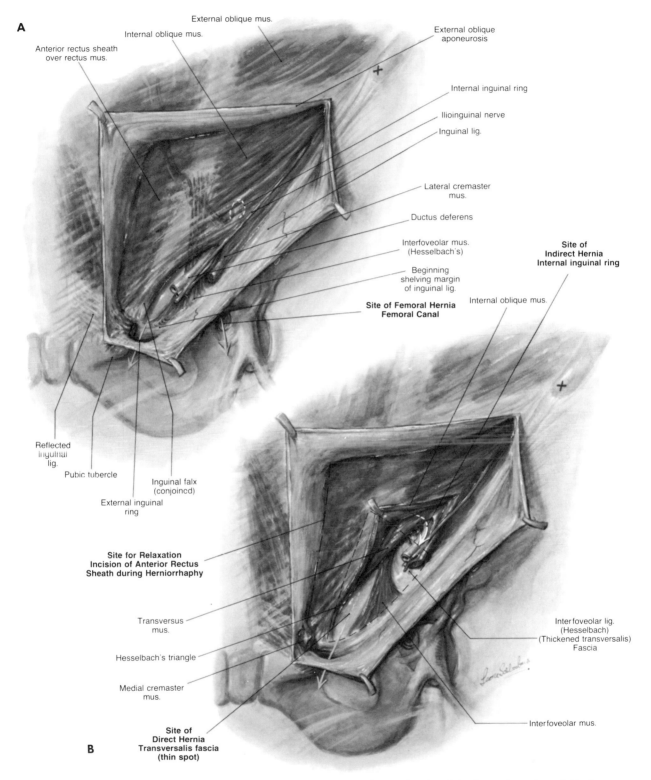

A, External oblique mus.
Internal oblique mus.
Anterior rectus sheath over rectus mus.
External oblique aponeurosis
Internal inguinal ring
Ilioinguinal nerve
Inguinal lig.
Lateral cremaster mus.
Ductus deferens
Interfoveolar mus. (Hesselbach's)
Beginning shelving margin of inguinal lig.
Site of Indirect Hernia Internal inguinal ring
Site of Femoral Hernia Femoral Canal
Internal oblique mus.
Reflected inguinal lig.
Pubic tubercle
Inguinal falx (conjoined)
External inguinal ring

Site for Relaxation Incision of Anterior Rectus Sheath during Herniorrhaphy
Transversus mus.
Hesselbach's triangle
Medial cremaster mus.
Interfoveolar lig. (Hesselbach) (Thickened transversalis) Fascia
Interfoveolar mus.
Site of Direct Hernia Transversalis fascia (thin spot)
B,

Figure 57–2. *A,* Layers of abdominal wall about the inguinal canal. Note the site of the femoral canal medial to the femoral vessels but lateral to the external inguinal ring. *B,* Hesselbach's triangle and sites of direct and indirect herniation. (From Schlossberg, L., and Zuidema, G. D.: Surgical Anatomy of the Abdomen and Pelvis: A Series of Translucent Plates in Color. Philadelphia, W. B. Saunders Company, 1972. Used by permission.)

peritoneal contents through Hesselbach's triangle. The triangle is bounded laterally by the inferior epigastric artery, inferiorly by the inguinal ligament, and medially by the lateral margin of the rectus sheath. The key to diagnosis of a direct inguinal hernia is the observation that the hernia does not traverse the inguinal canal. In the rare situation in which the hernia sac enters the scrotum, the hernia sac must pass through the external ring separate from and behind the spermatic cord. In contrast with the other groin hernias, the direct hernia represents a diffuse weakness of the abdominal wall. The absence of a narrow neck to the direct hernia sac makes incarceration unusual. When incarceration does occur, it is usually associated with the rare entrapment of the hernia sac at the external ring.

Indirect Inguinal Hernia. The indirect inguinal hernia represents the passage of the hernia sac (peritoneum and contents) through the internal ring (because of weakness in the transversalis fascia and the transversus abdominis)—a variable distance down the inguinal canal or all the way into the scrotum. The internal ring is defined medially by the inferior epigastric artery. Thus, indirect hernias frequently are associated with scrotal swelling, and incarceration can develop as a result of swelling at either the internal or the external ring.

Femoral Hernia. The weakness in the transversalis fascia that causes a femoral hernia is similar to the weakness that causes a direct inguinal hernia but is inferiorly directed rather than anteriorly directed. The peritoneum and contents herniate beneath the inguinal ligament in a small potential space medial to the femoral vein. The resulting hernia sac has a small neck, although once the sac enters the subcutaneous tissue of the thigh, it may enlarge considerably and even double back on top of the external oblique aponeurosis, thus masquerading as an inguinal hernia. The narrow neck makes incarceration common with this type of hernia and makes preoperative reduction unlikely.

Ventral Hernia. Ventral hernias are frequently caused by postincisional weakness of the anterior abdominal wall. Umbilical hernias represent another common ventral hernia and rarely pose a problem. An *epigastric* hernia may penetrate through a defect in the linea alba above the umbilicus. The *Spigelian* hernia is a rare defect located at the inferior one third of the rectus abdominis where the arcuate line meets the lateral border of the rectus muscle.

Other Hernias. Lateral abdominal wall hernias are uncommon but may develop following renal surgery. A rare site of abdominal weakness and herniation is *Petit's triangle*. Petit's triangle is bounded anteriorly by the external oblique muscle, inferiorly by the iliac crest, and posteriorly by the muscle. Other hernias that will not be discussed further include perineal hernias through the levator ani or through the sciatic foramina, obturator hernias into the medial thigh through the obturator foramen, diaphragmatic hernias, and internal hernias (e.g., bowel herniation through the foramen of Winslow).

Differential Diagnosis of Groin Masses in Children

Although groin lumps are often hernias, an inguinal mass may in fact be something else. An enlarged inguinal lymph node, a lipoma, a hydrocele of the cord, a saphenous varix, a psoas abscess, or an incarcerated ovary can appear as a groin mass.[6]

Lymph nodes are usually multiple and are found *distal* to the groin crease. If a contributory lesion on a lower extremity can be found, differentiation of a lymph node from a hernia is made easier. Ulceration of the urethral meatus can rarely cause adenopathy about the inguinal ligament, so the genitalia must also be examined. Lymphatics in the anal canal below the pectineal line also drain to the superficial inguinal nodes. In most circumstances, however, inguinal nodes are *unusual* in the anterior abdominal wall immediately superficial to the inguinal ligament. Lymph nodes in general are equally mobile in all directions, unlike (for example) femoral hernias, which tend to have decreased mobility in the transverse direction.

Lipomas in the subcutaneous fat can usually be separated from the underlying fascia and are not associated with a hernia sac neck extending under the inguinal ligament. A saphenous varix may reduce with pressure and may protrude when the patient coughs or stands upright but has a very soft consistency. Furthermore, as the varix enlarges and displaces subcutaneous fat it appears bluish beneath the skin.

If an infant has a tender, hard bulge at his external ring, the differentiation between incarcerated inguinal hernia and acute hydrocele of the cord may be difficult. The internal inguinal ring can be palpated with an examining finger in the rectum and the other finger over the cord. If the mass is an incarcerated hernia, bowel can be felt entering and exiting the internal ring.

A hydrocele of the cord is not necessarily benign. If the mass is tense and the hydrocele is contained within the rigid walls of the inguinal canal, testicular infarction can occur. This condition can mimic torsion of the testis if the testicle is tender, although the hydrocele may transilluminate. In the case of torsion the cord should also be shortened on the affected side. Although ultrasound and radionuclide scan examinations may be helpful (see Chapter 61), surgical exploration is often necessary to differentiate these conditions. In general, an acute hydrocele of the cord should be treated as an incarcerated hernia unless the emergency physician can definitively conclude otherwise by examination. Acute hydroceles within the scrotum rarely become as hard or painful as those within the inguinal canal and can generally be dealt with electively. Psoas abscesses are uncommon and are only rarely confused with a femoral hernia. The margins of the abscess are softer and more ill-defined than those of a hernia. Furthermore, psoas abscesses lie in a position lateral to the femoral artery, whereas hernias are medial.

Patient Presentation

Incarcerated hernias are common in infancy and are seen most frequently in children under 1 year of age. Usually the hernia has gone unnoticed by the child's parents and is first noted at the time of incarceration. In a small infant, irritability may be the main parental concern, and the physician must be certain to examine the groin to evaluate the child for a potential hernia. Very large infant hernias containing several loops of bowel almost never incarcerate and even more rarely strangulate. Aside from the visible lump, incarceration of the hernia is occasionally associated with minor discomfort caused by stretching of nerve endings during tissue dissection when the hernia sac first expands.

In female infants, the ovary is the organ most likely to herniate into the inguinal canal. The herniated ovary is usually palpable as a mobile nodule measuring 1 × 2 cm. Although unusual, infarction of the herniated ovary may occur as a result of torsion or compression of the pedicle. This condition may mimic inflamed lymphadenopathy, although the location is atypical for adenopathy. In the case of testicular feminization, the gonad in the inguinal canal is a testicle, although the patient is an "apparent female."

Incarceration occurs in approximately 10 per cent of indirect inguinal hernias and 20 per cent of femoral hernias. Since prolonged incarceration is often associated with intestinal obstruction and strangulation, early attempts at hernia sac reduction are indicated. Another advantage of reduction of an incarcerated hernia is that it permits the inflammatory response in and around the hernia to subside, allowing a delayed, controlled, elective repair.

Incisional hernias infrequently incarcerate and strangulate. Reduction of these hernias is generally routine or spontaneous, although sedation may be required. Incarceration in these cases usually results from adhesions of the contents of the sac either to each other or to the sac itself. Occasionally, feces within the loops of bowel in the hernia prevent reduction. Often, after a reduction attempt only a small piece of omentum or properitoneal fat will remain incarcerated. Although this incarcerated fat is not associated with significant morbidity, there may be considerable pain, requiring operative reduction and subsequent repair of the abdominal wall defect.

If strangulation occurs, most commonly the clinical picture is one of intestinal obstruction. The patient experiences severe pain, vomiting, distention, and obstipation. The patient may be febrile and may have a leukocytosis. There may be no impulse transmitted to the hernia sac upon coughing, and the overlying skin often becomes inflamed and edematous. These features may be less marked if only omentum is contained within the sac. Ultimately gangrene of the bowel or the omentum occurs if strangulation is not relieved, and the involved gut will perforate into the sac.

The presentation and differential diagnosis of hernias in adults are similar to those of hernias in children, although adults are generally more cooperative in an examination and can provide more extensive historical information. Nonetheless, unusual conditions (such as Richter's hernias, which may mimic a groin abscess because of the absence of bowel obstruction symptomatology,[7] and traumatic abdominal wall hernias,[8, 9] which may mimic a hematoma following injury[10]) may be confusing.

Indications and Contraindications

Whenever possible, incarcerated hernias should be reduced. Reduction minimizes inflammation and tissue edema, thus preventing strangulation. Some clinicians state that it is impossible to reduce a strangulated hernia because of the extensive inflammation, edema, and tenderness. Fortunately, most patients present early following incarceration, and the question of whether strangulation has occurred is rarely an issue. In most cases, the patient will present within hours of the incarceration without fever, leukocytosis, or other evidence of generalized toxicity. In that circumstance reduction of the hernia is indicated.

A femoral hernia presents a special problem in that the small neck present in the femoral canal and the usual generous overlying subcutaneous tissue make a complete reduction virtually impossible. Therefore, femoral hernias are best referred on an emergency basis to a surgical consultant for evaluation and consideration of operative reduction and simultaneous hernia repair. Attempts at reduction are best deferred until that consultation has been obtained. Similarly, an incarcerated ovary or an undescended testis in an inguinal hernia represents an indication for surgical reduction.

Peritonitis or other clinical evidence of strangulation (fever, marked leukocytosis, toxic appearance) are contraindications to an attempt at a nonsurgical reduction of an incarcerated hernia. In addition, immediate surgical repair of a traumatic hernia is recommended both for prevention of delayed morbidity from herniation and for evaluation of underlying organ injury.[8]

Procedure

When clinically indicated, gentle reduction of incarcerated hernias should be attempted. Adequate sedation must be given to allay anxiety and to minimize discomfort. For infants, meperidine (Demerol) in the dose of 1 mg per lb intramuscularly can be given, whereas for older children morphine sulfate in the dose of 0.1 mg per lb can be administered intramuscularly. Chloral hydrate or phenobarbital may also be effective. Adults often require 50 to 100 mg of meperidine given with 25 to 50 mg hydroxyzine (Vistaril) to potentiate the analgesic effects and to reduce the emetic properties of meperidine. The judicious use of analgesia or sedation is the key to successful reduction of an incarcerated hernia.

Following sedation, the patient is placed in a head-down tilt of approximately 20 degrees for groin hernias (no tilt when other hernias are treated). A pillow may be placed under the buttocks. For infants, the legs should be swaddled and secured to prevent slippage. This technique is successful in spontaneously reducing 80 per cent of pediatric incarcerated hernias over a 2-hour period without taxis. In addition, the light application of a cold pack or a padded ice bag to reduce local blood flow and to diminish intraluminal gas pressure is helpful while the analgesic is taking effect.

If after 20 to 25 minutes spontaneous reduction has not occurred, gentle taxis can be added to the aforementioned method. For inguinal hernias the physician positions the thumb and index finger of one hand along the inguinal canal and presses gently on the incarcerated hernia just distal to the external inguinal ring. Simultaneous massage of the inguinal region in the level of the internal and external rings is used as the other thumb and index finger slowly funnel the incarcerated viscera toward the rings. These maneuvers, if successful, often result in a "gurgle" signifying hernia sac reduction. A slow, steady, atraumatic manipulation is preferred. Repeated forceful attempts at reduction are contraindicated.

Reduced bowel almost certainly will not be strangulated. Rectal examination may confirm re-

duction. Once reduction occurs, corrective surgery can be performed 1 week later, after local edema has subsided. If reduction cannot be achieved, emergency surgery is indicated after dehydration and electrolyte imbalances are corrected. Nasogastric suction is indicated if obstruction is present. Reduction of other abdominal wall hernias is accomplished in a fashion similar to that described for inguinal hernias.

Complications

An attempt at manual reduction of a hernia may be unsuccessful or only partially successful. The physician must recognize a partial reduction and obtain appropriate consultation. Persistent attempts at reduction produce patient discomfort and may delay operative intervention for relief of bowel obstruction or organ ischemia. Testicular or ovarian rupture may be caused by overzealous attempts to reduce a hernia associated with an undescended or ectopic gonad.

Conclusions

By far the greatest challenge in the immediate management of groin lumps is the differential diagnosis of conditions that may mimic a groin hernia. Reduction of groin and other abdominal wall hernias is usually straightforward, as has been discussed. Once the hernia is reduced, the patient and family must be instructed that straining at stool, urination, or coughing may produce another prolapse of the hernia sac. The patient or family should rapidly reduce any recurrent herniation to avoid recurrent incarceration and the need for a return to the emergency department. A demonstration of the reduction technique to be used by the patient or family will usually aid in cooperation. The emergency physician should not overlook the need to evaluate and treat potentially complicating conditions, such as urinary tract infections, bladder outlet obstruction, constipation, and respiratory infections that may increase intra-abdominal pressure and produce recurrent herniation. Appropriate referral for these related problems and subsequent care of the reduced hernia is recommended.

Finally, the emergency physician must be aware that to the patient the development of hernia symptoms is often associated with employment-related activities. Although physical exertion can certainly exacerbate a pre-existing weakness in the abdominal wall and can lead to frank herniation, most frequently the abdominal wall defect is congenital in origin. Therefore, to minimize confusion in workmen's compensation cases, the physician should be careful to note that the patent's hernia became symptomatic during an activity rather than stating that the hernia was the result of an activity.

1. Zimmerman, L. M., and Anson, B. J.: The Anatomy and Surgery of Hernia. Baltimore, Williams & Wilkins, 1953.
2. Carlson, R. I.: The historical development of the surgical treatment of inguinal hernia. Surgery 39:1031, 1956.
3. Koontz, A. R.: Hernia. New York, Appleton-Century-Crofts, 1963.
4. Gillespie, R. W., Glas, W. W., Metz, G. H., et al.: Richter's hernia: Its etiology, recognition, and management. Arch. Surg. 73:590, 1956.
5. Richter, A. G.: Abhandlung von der Bruchen. Gottingen, Germany, Dietrich, 1785, pp. 596–597.
6. Fallis, J.: Hernias. In Vaughan, V. C., III, and McKay, R. J. (eds.): Nelson Textbook of Pediatrics. 11th ed. Philadelphia, W. B. Saunders Co., 1979, pp. 1107–1109.
7. Doubleday, L. C.: A colocutaneous fistula in the inguinal area. JAMA 247:2407, 1982.
8. Malangoni, M. A., and Condon, R. E.: Traumatic abdominal wall hernia. J. Trauma. 23:356, 1983.
9. Clain, A.: Traumatic hernia. Br. J. Surg. 51:549, 1964.
10. Jones, T. W., and Merendino, K. A.: The deep epigastric artery: Rectus muscle syndrome. Am. J. Surg. 103:159, 1962.

Introduction

Desormeaux in 1853 first devised an endoscopic instrument to look into the rectum. He used a reflecting mirror and a lamp burning a mixture of alcohol and turpentine as a light source.[1]

Sigmoidoscopes have classically been subdivided into those with distal lighting and those with proximal lighting. Originally, the devices with distal illumination (for example, the early Strauss pattern) used light carried on the distal end of a long wire attachment that projected inside the tube. If there were either liquid feces or mucus in the bowel, the light was submerged, and the instrument had to be removed for cleansing and reinsertion.[2] Sigmoidoscopes with proximal illumination therefore became popular. More recently, sigmoidoscopes have been developed with distal illumination, which is obtained by incorporation of fiber optic fibers in the wall of the tube to convey light from a bulb at the proximal end.[2, 3] The fiber optic cold light can be attached proximally to either an anoscope or a rigid sigmoidoscope (Fig. 58–1).

Equipment

The sigmoidoscope itself is a hollow, rigid tube that may be metal or plastic and clear or black.[4] The length may vary but typically is 25 cm. The device can therefore be inserted for a distance of approximately 21 cm above the anal verge. The barrel of the sigmoidoscope is calibrated in centimeters, so that the distance of any lesion from the anal verge can be noted.

The window of the Welch-Allen sigmoidoscope, the most commonly used model, magnifies two times.[2] The internal diameter should be measured before insertion so that the size of any lesions that

58

Sigmoidoscopy/ Anoscopy

JONATHAN M. GLAUSER, M.D.

SIGMOIDOSCOPY

are seen can be estimated. This diameter typically is 12 to 19 mm[1] and in general can be tolerated by infants and children as well as adults.

Accessory materials for proctosigmoidoscopy are listed in Table 58–1.[5]

Indications

It has been claimed that proctosigmoidoscopic examination is indicated in almost all patients with complaints related to bowel.[4] Specifically, the procedure is indicated in the following cases: recent occurrence of constipation or diarrhea or a change in either symptom;[3] bright red blood per rectum or mixed in stool;[3, 6, 7] pain or difficulty in defecation;[7] rectal discomfort; involuntary seepage of stool;[3] pencil-sized stools resulting from a lesion in the anal area or a stenosing process in the rectum;[3] and lesions around the anal opening (characterized by abscesses, fistulae, discharge, ulcers, external piles, or pruritus). The procedure is also indicated in conjunction with examination

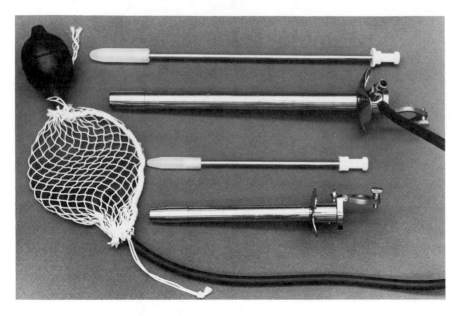

Figure 58–1. Standard rigid sigmoid-oscope. Two sizes are shown here, with obturator and insufflation balloon.

Table 58–1. ACCESSORY MATERIALS FOR PROCTOSIGMOIDOSCOPY

Rectal gloves
Lubricant
Paper towels, sheets
Glass microscope slides and cover slips for examination of stool as indicated
30-cm rectal cotton swabs (alternatively, long 35-cm alligator forceps for gripping pledgets of wool can be used in swabbing out the bowel lumen)
Suction tube
Waste basket
Guaiac material to test for fecal occult blood
Probes for examination of fistulae

and speciment collection for suspected parasitic infestation;[7] biopsy of colorectal lesions; and reduction of a sigmoid volvulus.[8]

Contraindications

There are few contraindications to the procedure. Imperforate anus is the only absolute contraindication.[4] Various relative contraindications have been reported, including the following: pain on examination (examination of some patients with regional enteritis or carcinoma may require general anesthesia), excessive angulation of the rectosigmoid colon, a grossly uncooperative patient,[3] acute peritonitis, rectal abscess, and acute inflammatory bowel disease (e.g., toxic megacolon, acute diverticulitis, fulminant ulcerative colitis). Patients with coronary artery disease can be examined, although caution is advised in these cases, since coronary ischemia or dysrhythmias can be precipitated.

Preparation

Preparation for sigmoidoscopy is often unnecessary, since the rectal ampulla is normally empty.[4] Some recommend a 4- to 4½-oz enema 30 to 60 minutes prior to examination.[9–11] Plain saline or a commercially available phosphate solution (Fleet's enema) in such cases is acceptable and generally cleans to the level of the splenic flexure.

There are drawbacks to enema administration. The enema tube tip may leave a superficial linear abrasion on the anterior rectal wall.[4] The soap in an enema is irritating to the mucosa and causes a discharge of mucus. This mucus, along with the retained enema solution, may interfere with vision and may obscure abnormalities.[7] As a rule, fluid feces are harder to remove for proctoscopic examination than are solid feces.[2] Furthermore, in ulcerative colitis the characteristic bloody purulent mucosa is better recognized without any preparation.[3] Enemas should certainly be avoided if brisk diarrhea is present or if ulcerative colitis is suspected.

Sedation with diazepam (Valium), 5 to 10 mg intravenously, has been recommended by some[3, 12] but is not generally necessary. Nitrous oxide analgesia is also appropriate.

In general, no specific bowel preparation is required. Although some authors recommend bowel preparation for 24 to 48 hours with liquid diet, stool softeners, cathartics, and suppositories,[12, 13] such a regimen is clearly impractical for an emergency procedure.

Positioning

Three positions are generally accepted for sigmoidoscopy. These are the lateral decubitus (or Sims) position, the knee-chest position, and the dorsal lithotomy position. All three will be described here, although the first two are preferred (Fig. 58–2).

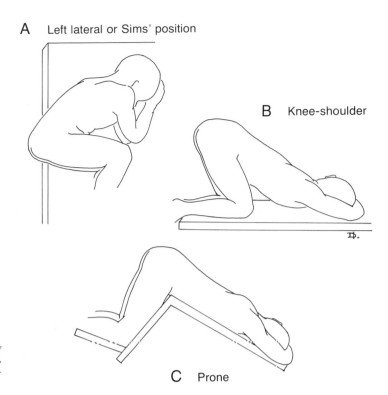

A Left lateral or Sims' position

B Knee-shoulder

C Prone

Figure 58–2. Positions for performing sigmoidoscopy or anoscopy. (From Hill, G. J., II: Outpatient Surgery, 2nd ed. Philadelphia, W. B. Saunders Company, 1980. Used by permission.)

The lateral decubitus position is generally performed with the patient on his or her left side. The lower back is extended, with the buttocks positioned just over the edge of the table or bed.[2, 4, 10] With the lumbar spine extended, the axis of the rectal canal is easier to follow along the rectum. The knees and the hips are flexed, with the patient's trunk obliquely across the table. Optionally, one may move the patient's right shoulder and buttocks slightly forward, perhaps by placing a sandbag under the left hip.

The left lateral decubitus position is preferable for right-handed physicians and is more comfortable for the patient than are the other positions. The major disadvantage is that the examiner's freedom of motion is rather limited; passage of the instrument above the pelvic floor is frequently difficult.

The knee-chest position can be used either on an examination table or, preferably, on a tilt table. If the sigmoidoscopy is performed on an examination table or in bed, the patient is positioned with the knees drawn up, the hips flexed, and the buttocks elevated. The chest is angled down, and the patient lies with the head on upward-folded arms.[5]

If a tilt table is available, the patient is arched with the knees on the step of the table and the chest lying against the flat surface. The platform on which the patient's knees are resting must be kept high enough to extend the lower spine. Flexion of the lumbar spine and resting the abdomen on the table should be avoided.[10] The arms are extended above the head, and the physician then adjusts the forward tilt of the table.[5]

The advantage of this position is that it affords good visualization of the anorectal region. The abdominal contents fall cephalad, the sigmoid colon stretches, and air insufflation is generally unnecessary. The drawbacks to the knee-chest position concern the patient's discomfort. This position is unacceptable for examinations of long duration and may be unsatisfactory for ill or elderly patients.[3] In experienced hands, sigmoidoscopy takes less than 5 minutes and, if tolerated, the knee-chest position is the one of choice for this procedure.

For completeness, the dorsal lithotomy position will be mentioned. This is currently not a popular position for sigmoidoscopy, although it is comfortable for the patient. Another advantage is that a gynecologic examining table, which is necessary for the lithotomy position, is almost always present in physicians' offices, clinics, and emergency departments. The major drawback to the dorsal lithotomy position is that the abdominal contents lie on top of the sigmoid colon and compromise the lumen of the bowel. This necessitates frequent air insufflation to maintain an open lumen.

Anatomy

A general review of the relevant anatomy is suggested for those without extensive experience in sigmoidoscopy (Fig. 58–3).

The distal large bowel is divided into three anatomic areas: the anal canal, the rectum, and the sigmoid colon. As one proceeds proximally from the anus, the first 3 to 4 cm constitute the

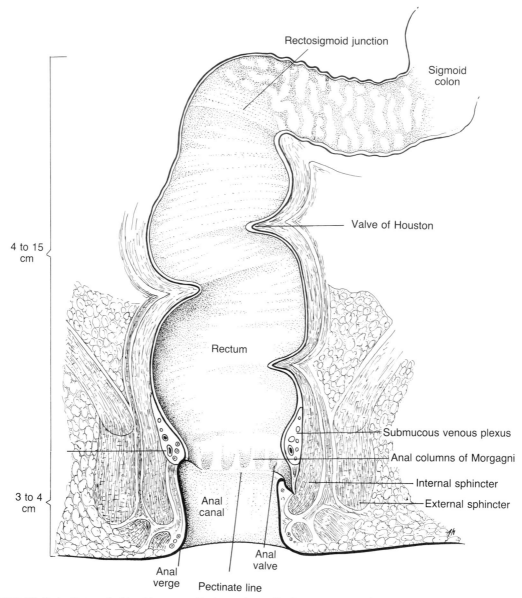

Figure 58–3. Anatomy of sigmoidoscopy. (Redrawn from Abrahams, P. H., and Webb, P. J.: Clinical Anatomy of Practical Procedures: A Guide for Nurses, Students and Junior Doctors. New York, Beekman Publishers Inc., 1975.)

anal canal. The area 4 to 15 cm proximal to the anus is the rectum. At the junction of the anal canal and the rectum is the pectinate line. At the pectinate line the distal vertical folds of the rectal mucosa form the anal columns, which terminate as the anal valves. The rectum is approximately 12 cm long and has a smooth, plum-colored mucosa. Lateral reflections of the bowel wall in the rectum form the valves of Houston. The rectum is dilated inferiorly to form the ampulla.

At approximately 15 cm in depth, the rectum joins the sigmoid colon at the rectosigmoid. The sigmoid colon is recognized through the sigmoidoscope at this point by its circular mucosal rings.

There are two areas of sharp angulation of the distal bowel. As one proceeds with a sigmoidoscopic examination, one encounters the first sharp angle at approximately 15 cm in depth at the rectosigmoid. Here the bowel takes a turn to the patient's left at almost a right angle. This area of extreme angulation is the section that is the most difficult to negotiate with the scope and is the most frequent site of perforation. Four to 8 cm proximal to the rectosigmoid, the colon makes another sharp angle and proceeds cephalad. From this point proximally the anatomy varies considerably.

Technique

Before insertion of either the sigmoidoscope or the anoscope, a rectal examination with a lubricated gloved finger must always be performed.[7]

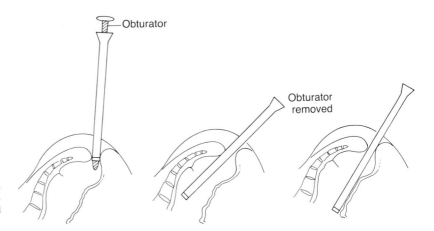

Figure 58–4. Various positions of the sigmoid-oscope during examination. Note that the obturator is withdrawn after entry into the anal canal.

This will determine the presence or absence of fecal impaction, rectal tumor, enlarged prostate, or stricture. The angle of the anal canal can also be determined by rectal examination.[4]

The sigmoidoscope, with obturator in place and light source removed, is warmed and well lubricated. It is inserted into the anus and passed initially toward the umbilicus. For the first 3 to 4 cm, the initial direction of the tip of the scope is down (anteriorly) and forward into the anal canal (Fig. 58–4). A right-handed examiner holds the head of the sigmoidoscope with the right hand and assists the tip through the anal sphincter with the left hand (Fig. 58–5).[14] A left-handed examiner reverses the hand positions. Insertion is accomplished by gentle pressure; the patient should be warned that there may be a transient sensation of a bowel movement but that this is an artificial sensation.

If the examiner feels muscle spasm of the sphincters, insertion should be delayed until muscle relaxation occurs.[2] A double "give" of both external and internal sphincters may be felt. Asking the patient to "bear down" in a manner similar to a bowel movement will help relax the sphincter.

Once the sigmoidoscope is within the anal canal, the obturator is removed and the instrument is advanced under direct vision (Fig. 58–6). The obturator is never replaced, and the sigmoidoscope is advanced only under direct visualization of the bowel lumen. The proximal end of the sigmoidoscope carrying the glass window, the light, and the bellows is now firmly attached.[2] After the initial entry into the anal canal, the tip of the scope is directed posteriorly (the eyepiece is moved anteriorly) to follow the curvature of the sacrum. One may move the scope from side to side to negotiate the valves of Houston in the rectum. Usually, there is little need for distention of the colon until the instrument nears the sharp turn at the pelvic floor (10 to 12 cm). The hand holding the tip of the sigmoidoscope may rest on the patient's buttocks for steadiness. Once the level of the rectosigmoid is reached at approximately 15

cm, one must follow the anterior and leftward curve of the bowel lumen. The tip of the scope is directed anteriorly and to the patient's left (the eyepiece is swung posteriorly and to the patient's right). If the rectosigmoid is successfully passed, one now simply follows the lumen of the bowel, since the anatomy is variable at this point.

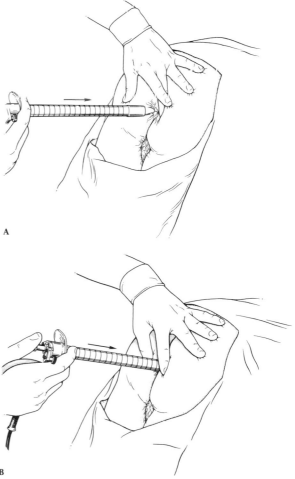

A

B

Figure 58–5. Insertion of the sigmoidoscope with obturator in place. The left hand is used to aid in spreading the buttocks and to stabilize the scope. (From Vander Salm, T. J., et al.: Atlas of Bedside Procedures. Boston, Little, Brown & Co., 1979. Used by permission.)

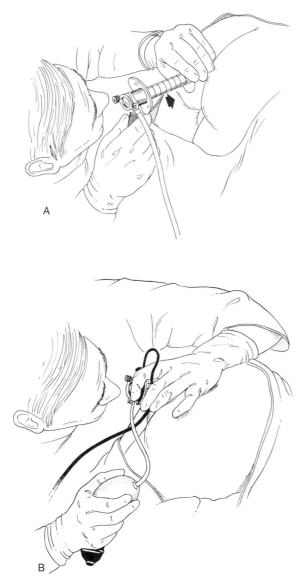

Figure 58–6. The sigmoidoscope is advanced under direct vision (A). Insufflation may be required (B). Detailed examination is performed upon withdrawal of the sigmoidoscope. Suction should be available. (From Vander Salm, T. J., et al.: Atlas of Bedside Procedures. Boston, Little, Brown & Co., 1979. Used by permission.)

For the beginning examiner, the greatest difficulty is in following the lumen. When a "dead end" or "blind pouch" is reached, the edge of the lumen is inspected in a circumferential manner. In this way, the edge of a valve of Houston may be found to hide a turn in the canal. The free edge should be displaced toward the direction of the lumen, so that the central position is open and passage is continued.[10] If the lumen is lost, it is helpful to withdraw the instrument a few centimeters, because the tip may be in a pouch of bowel.

The sigmoidoscope is advanced gently and slowly. Fine scrutiny of the mucosa is generally left until the withdrawal phase of the examina-

tion.[1, 4] Once the device has been inserted 10 cm or more, changes in the axis of the instrument may stretch the peritoneum and cause crampy discomfort. Females may undergo more discomfort than males if the uterus anteriorly increases the leverage necessary for full insertion of the scope.[2] The examiner should anticipate the flexures and should direct the sigmoidoscope accordingly. Major changes in direction and displacement should be made slowly to lessen patient discomfort.

For an adequate study, the sigmoidoscope should be advanced to at least 15 cm. A barium enema is sufficiently accurate to define abnormalities at this level and above. As a rule, one should insert the instrument as far as possible, with careful scrutiny of each square centimeter of mucosa on withdrawal.[1, 4]

Intermittent insufflation of gas (either air or carbon dioxide) may be essential for effective intubation.[14] Since excessive insufflation of gas is uncomfortable for the patient, use of this technique should be minimized.[2] Insufflation may also stretch adjacent limbs of a redundant loop of sigmoid, causing an unnecessary additional acuteness in the angle to be negotiated.[14] Some authors are completely against insufflation.[1, 4]

If the lumen is not easily seen, the instrument may need to be withdrawn until the examiner can see the lateral wall of the true lumen. Rotation of the leading end of the sigmoidoscope may help locate the lumen. Some side-to-side movement may be necessary for negotiation of the instrument, especially past the lower and middle valves of Houston.

Suction should be provided only with a guarded tube. Pledgets are preferable, either with long, pledget-holding forceps to clean the mucosa[7] or with rectal swabs long enough to extend the length of the sigmoidoscope.[5]

The mucous membrane is inspected for color, texture, and mobility. Normal rectosigmoid mucosa is intact, smooth, pink, and glistening. Erosions, ulcers, polyps, blood, pus, or the raised edge of a carcinoma should be sought. The distance in centimeters and position of any lesions that are found should be noted when findings are reported (e.g., 16-cm level at 10 o'clock, with 12 o'clock representing a true dorsal location).[4]

It should be noted that one may see clusters of petechiae on the posterior wall at the rectosigmoid junction where the tip of the sigmoidoscope superficially contused the mucosal membrane as it was impinged on the sacrum. A linear scratch on the anterior rectal wall, caused by an enema tube, may be visible. This minor trauma may also result in a false positive test for occult blood in the stool.

Some areas are difficult to see, although effort should be made to view them. The examiner may have to describe a wide arc with the proximal end of the sigmoidoscope in order to see the entire rectal circumference. The upper surfaces of the valves and the posterior rectal wall require special care to visualize.

Full insertion to 25 cm has been reported to be possible in only 42 per cent of patients.[4] In one study, 966 of 1000 sigmoidoscopies were successful in visualizing the sigmoid to 15 cm, the cutoff for accuracy of a barium enema.

Complications are generally few and minor. Perforation is considered the most catastrophic and was reported as early as 1912.[15] A comprehensive survey performed in 1946 found 46 known cases of perforation. A later study reported a perforation rate from colonoscopy and sigmoidoscopy of 0.2 per cent.[3] Another report claimed a much lower incidence even than this: 5 perforations in 172,351 sigmoidoscopic examinations in one study, 4 perforations in 350,000 cases in another.[4] Perforation of the sigmoid mandates prompt surgical exploration. Perforation usually occurs at 10 to 15 cm on the anterior portion of the bowel, where the sigmoid makes its first sharp turn. This complication is usually quite obvious, but recognition may be delayed, with serious consequences. Rarely, perforation may occur in the rectum, in which case the scope enters the retroperitoneal space. Whitish discoloration of the mucosa (blanching) occurring when the bowel wall slides by and accompanied by patient discomfort should be taken as a warning that excessive pressure is possibly being applied to the wall and that perforation may be imminent. Under these circumstances, the instrument must be rapidly withdrawn. Occasionally, perforation is accompanied by bleeding or the appearance of peritoneal fluid or omentum in the lumen.

Forcible insufflation of air causes abdominal cramping and may be a factor in perforation, especially if diverticulae are present. If there is any question of perforation, one should immediately take an upright chest radiograph following the procedure to look for free air under the diaphragm. If perforation occurs in the rectum, one may see retroperitoneal air along the shadows of the psoas on an abdominal film. Persistent pain, fever, or bleeding after the procedure should raise the possibility of occult perforation. The incidence of deaths attributed to postoperative complications following laparotomy necessitated by perforation is 0.03 per cent.[3]

Proper positioning, a well-cleansed colon, and proper technique should reduce the incidence of perforation. Swabs and suction devices should be used with caution. If unusual angulation of the bowel is present, if the patient is uncooperative, if vision is hampered by stool or blood, or if adhesions from pelvic surgery or past infection make it impossible to negotiate a rectosigmoid angle, the examination should be terminated.

Transient bacteremia in as many as 10 per cent of cases (usually enterococcal organisms) has been reported during sigmoidoscopy.[10, 16] This is generally believed to be of no clinical significance. In the past, some authors have advocated prophylactic antibiotic coverage for patients with valvular heart disease,[17] but current thinking is that this is unnecessary.

Pain can be severe enough to cause termination of the examination. In one study, 12 per cent of sigmoidoscopies were terminated for this reason,[11] although 88 per cent of patients undergoing the procedure experienced some discomfort.[18]

Sigmoidoscopy has its limitations. The sigmoidoscope does not provide as good a view of the anal canal as does the anoscope.[7, 10] Colonoscopy[19] and flexible sigmoidoscopy provide greater accuracy in diagnosis.[11, 18, 20–23] Furthermore, there is increasing evidence that colonic malignancies today are more proximal than in the past.[6, 18] Although the rigid sigmoidoscope was once thought to be able to diagnose 75 per cent of large bowel malignancies, it cannot reach such a high proportion of colonic malignancies today. The average lengths of insertion in two studies were only 18.6 cm[19] and 20 cm.[18]

Although some authors suggest using the sigmoidoscope to reduce acute sigmoid volvulus, the procedure is not definitive treatment and is not generally an emergency department practice.

ANOSCOPY

Introduction

Anoscopy is an easily performed outpatient procedure for evaluating the anal orifice and the anal canal. The procedure is not adequate to evaluate all rectal pathologic conditions, since only the most distal portion of the rectum may be visualized with this procedure. The indications for the procedure are the same as for sigmoidoscopy, except that the area to be examined is much smaller.

Equipment

The anoscope has two basic designs: (1) a conical tube, and (2) a "slotted" tube with a side opening, or "slot," at the distal end. This latter design

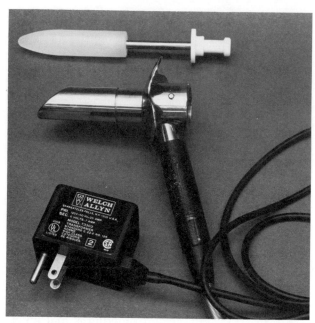

Figure 58–7. Standard anoscope. An instrument with its own light source is preferred.

For patients with painful anal lesions or with some degree of anal spasm or stenosis, a narrower instrument is necessary. The anal canal of a child is quite distensible and generally is capable of admitting an adult-sized anoscope.

Anoscopy, like sigmoidoscopy, should be attempted only after digital examination has been performed to detect tenderness or a mass and to determine the axis of the anal canal.[10] No other preparation is necessary.[2, 10] A light source is needed. In addition, the examiner should have long, nontoothed forceps (such as Emmett's 20-cm forceps) and cotton balls for swabbing out the lumen[2, 7] and appropriate culture material, if needed.

Preparation and Positioning

The examination can be performed with the patient in either the Sims lateral decubitus position or the knee-chest position, as was described in the section on sigmoidoscopy. Anal stenosis or severe pain on digital examination is a contraindication to the passage of an anoscope. Some authors advocate the use of topical anesthetic gels or ointments to produce anesthesia in very painful examinations. Others believe that the agents are not needed, since they do not produce profound anesthesia and have the potential to produce contact dermatitis or mucosal irritation. Although the slow and gentle passage of the instrument is the key to success, the judicious use of parenteral sedation and analgesia is justified in selected cases.

allows a portion of the side wall of the anus or the rectum to prolapse within the lumen of the anoscope.[10] Variations affect the length, caliber, and shape (conical versus cylindric) of the tube; the possession of side slits, grooves, or sliding attachments; and the method of illumination.[2] Instruments that incorporate their own light source are desirable and eliminate the need for an assistant (Fig. 58–7).

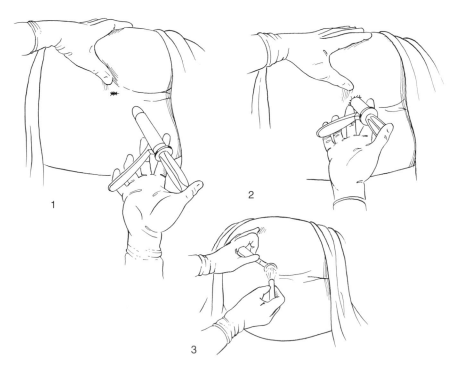

1

2

3

Figure 58–8. Anoscopy. Initially, the anoscope is directed toward the umbilicus, and the obturator is not withdrawn until the scope has been passed to the hilt. Detailed examination is performed upon withdrawal of the instrument. A pen light is used in this illustration for illumination.

Procedure

The instrument is well lubricated. The obturator is inserted completely in the anoscope, and the device is placed at the anal verge.[2] As the patient bears down, the instrument is advanced initially in line with the axis of the anal canal (in general, with the anoscope pointing toward the umbilicus).[10] The instrument initially follows an inward, downward (anterior), and forward course (Fig. 58–8).

Once beyond the level of the sphincter, the anoscope should be directed backward to avoid abutment of the prostate gland and to follow the axis of the rectum along the curve of the sacrum. If the instrument is gripped by the anal sphincters, gentle pressure should be maintained in the long axis of the canal until the muscles gradually relax (generally within 60 seconds).[2] Passage of the instrument to its shoulder is usually accomplished without difficulty until the outer flange impinges against the anal verge.

The obturator must be kept fully engaged in the anoscope during insertion to avoid nipping the anal mucosa and causing pain.[7] For the same reason, the obturator should not be reinserted except when the entire instrument is withdrawn from the patient. As with the sigmoidoscope, examination of the rectum is performed during gradual withdrawal of the anoscope.

The anoscope is then stabilized, and the obturator is removed. A small (1 cm^2) area of ecchymosis or abrasion of the mucosa frequently is found where the obturator has rested.[10] The light source is shined into the lumen, and forceps with cotton balls are used as necessary for swabbing to visualize the anorectum.[7] A proper examination cannot be performed without adequate lighting.

Normal mucosa is pink and smooth and glistens. The instrument is angled so that the distal lumen of the rectum is seen. The anoscope is then slowly withdrawn and moved in a circular fashion so that the entire wall is inspected.[1, 10]

As one approaches the zone above the sphincters, one should take care to detect the presence of enlarged hemorrhoids.[7] To help demonstrate these structures, the patient is asked to bear down. Enlarged hemorrhoids will protrude into the lumen and will be easily seen. The Valsalva maneuver should be repeated several times until the instrument passes beyond the pectinate line.[10]

If the patient has much discomfort during the terminal portion of the examination, reflex spasm of the anal sphincter may expel the instrument quickly. For this reason, the examiner may be unable to obtain an adequate view. Anoscopy may be repeated several times if necessary.

The following pathologic conditions should also be searched for: anal fistulas and fissures, sentinel tag, thickened or prolapsed anal papillae, tumors, and thrombosed or edematous hemorrhoids.[1] The stool is examined for blood or pus.

The mucous membrane is observed for thickening and granularity. The examiner can check for contact bleeding by rubbing the mucosa gently with a swab or forceps;[2] contact bleeding is an important sign of mucosal inflammation. Pinworms may also be seen writhing in the lower rectum.

1. Brown, C. H. (ed.): Diagnostic Procedures in Gastroenterology. St. Louis, C. V. Mosby Co., 1967, pp. 213–240.
2. Goligher, J. C., Duthie, H. L., Nixon, H. H., et al. (ed.): Surgery of the Anus, Rectum, and Colon, 4th ed. London, Balliere Tindall, 1980, pp. 52–68.
3. Otto, P., and Klaus, E.: Atlas of Rectoscopy and Colonoscopy. Berlin, Springer-Verlag, 1979, pp. 1–16, 23–27.
4. Bockus, H. L. (ed.): Gastroenterology, vol. 2, Philadelphia, W. B. Saunders Co., 1976, pp. 836–843.
5. Schapiro, M., and Kuritsky, J.: The Gastroenterology Assistant: A Lab Manual. Springfield, IL, Charles C Thomas, 1972, pp. 70–73.
6. Leicester, R. J., and Hunt, R. H.: Letter. Br. Med. J. 283:1607, 1981.
7. Ellis, D. J., and Bevan, P. G.: Proctoscopy and sigmoidoscopy. Br. Med. J. 281:435, 1980.
8. O'Connor, J. J.: Reduction of sigmoid volvulus by flexible sigmoidoscopy (letter). Arch. Surg. 114:1092, 1979.
9. Marino, A. W. M., Jr.: Looking ahead: Types of flexible sigmoidoscopes and preparation of the patient. Dis. Colon Rectum 20:91, 1977.
10. Christian, R. L.: Anorectal disorders. In Branch, W. T. (ed.): The Office Practice of Medicine. Philadelphia, W. B. Saunders, Co., 1982, pp. 664–678.
11. Marks, G., Boggs, H. W., Castro, A. F., et al.: Sigmoidoscopic examinations with rigid and flexible fiberoptic sigmoidoscopes in the surgeon's office. Dis. Colon Rectum 22:162, 1979.
12. Stone, R. V.: Proctoscopy and sigmoidoscopy (letter). Br. Med. J. 281:682, 1980.
13. Devadhar, D. S. C.: Preparation for sigmoidoscopy (letter). N. Z. Med. J. 93:394, 1981.
14. Coller, J. A.: Technique of flexible fiberoptic sigmoidoscopy. Surg. Clin. North Am. 60:465, 1980.
15. Andresen, A. F. R.: Perforations from proctoscopy. Gastroenterology 9:664, 1947.
16. Adami, B., Eckhardt, V. F., Suermann, R. B., et al.: Bacteremia after proctoscopy and hemorrhoidal injection sclerotherapy. Dis. Colon Rectum 24:373, 1980.
17. Engeling, E. R., and Eng, B. F.: Bacteremia after sigmoidoscopy: Another view (letter). Ann. Intern. Med. 94:77, 1981.
18. Winnan, G., Bergi, G., Panish, J., et al.: Superiority of the flexible to the rigid sigmoidoscope in routine proctosigmoidoscopy. Engl. J. Med. 302:1011, 1980.
19. Talbott, T. M.: Looking ahead: Evaluation of new flexible sigmoidoscopes. Dis. Colon Rectum 20:89, 1977.
20. Foster, G. E., Vellacott, K. D., Balfour, T. W., et al.: Outpatient flexible fiberoptic sigmoidoscopy, diagnostic yield, and the value of glucagon. Br. J. Surg. 68:463, 1981.
21. Record, O., Bramble, M. G., Lishman, A. H., et al.: Flexible sigmoidoscopy in outpatients with suspected colonic disease. Br. Med. J. 283:1291, 1981.
22. Bohlman, T. W., Katon, R. M., Lipshutz, G. R., et al.: Fiberoptic pansigmoidoscopy: An evaluation and comparison with rigid sigmoidoscopy. Gastroenterology 72:644, 1977.
23. Vellacott, K. D., and Hardcastle, J. D.: An evaluation of flexible fiberoptic sigmoidoscopy. Br. Med. J. 283:1583, 1981.

59

Thrombosed External Hemorrhoids

JONATHAN M. GLAUSER, M.D.

Introduction

The treatment of hemorrhoids has been of interest to surgeons since Babylonian times.[1] In 1869, Morgan initiated the modern era of hemorrhoid management when he described injection therapy.[2] Whereas recent literature discusses various techniques in the management of internal hemorrhoids, the treatment of thrombosed external hemorrhoids has not changed in recent years.

Hemorrhoids are varicosities of the venous plexus that lie in the wall of the anal canal (Fig. 59–1). The varicosities may be internal or external. *Internal hemorrhoids* lie above the pectinate line in the submucosal space of the upper anal canal and are covered with columnar epithelium. Internal hemorrhoids are usually asymptomatic, but the salient symptoms are bleeding or prolapse. Prolapse out of the rectum may occur during defecation, but when the hemorrhoids are large enough, they may prolapse with coughing or walking. Internal hemorrhoids commonly bleed. The blood is bright red because of the presence of arterioles, capillaries, and arteriovenous fistulas in the area. Most of the bleeding is not from the hemorrhoid itself but from the traumatized mucous membrane that overlies it. Bleeding may occur during defecation or spontaneously; prolapsed hemorrhoids may produce a mucous discharge. The internal hemorrhoids may be painful when they become thrombosed or remain prolapsed. The treatment of internal hemorrhoids will not be covered in this chapter.

External hemorrhoids may be pruritic or may be noticed by the patient when they become enlarged. When thrombosed, external hemorrhoids become more symptomatic. A thrombosed external hemorrhoid appears as a purplish mass external to the pectinate line[3] and is usually easily visible when the patient spreads the buttocks (Fig. 59–2). Because it is covered by skin and not colonic mucosa, a thrombosed external hemorrhoid tends to be extremely painful, especially when direct pressure is applied. The bluish color of the contained clot can generally be appreciated through the tense, stretched skin.

The patient typically reports the sudden development of a painful lump at the anus, often relating its onset to an episode of constipation or straining at stool.[4] The pain is continuous but is aggravated by defecation and by sitting.[5] The pain and swelling may subside spontaneously, but frequently thrombosis requires surgery. An insignificant amount of bleeding may occur as a result of rupture of the hematoma, but simple thrombosed external hemorrhoids do not usually bleed.

The term "thrombosed external hemorrhoid" implies clotted blood in the veins of the subcutaneous external hemorrhoidal plexus. What occurs more commonly is a rupture of one of the external veins during straining at defecation with escape of blood into the subcutaneous tissues, where it

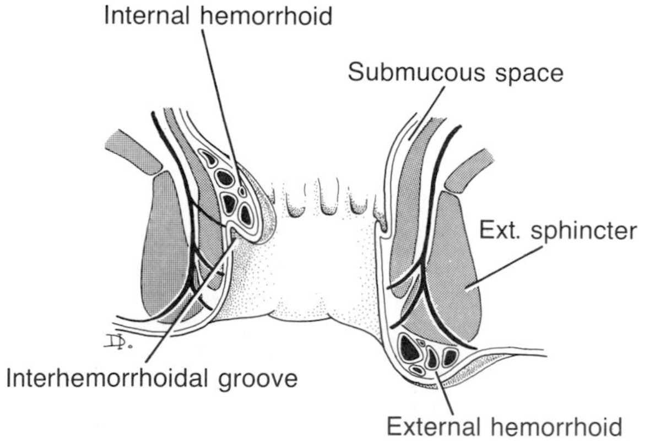

Internal hemorrhoid

Submucous space

Ext. sphincter

Interhemorrhoidal groove

External hemorrhoid

Figure 59–1. Anatomic location of internal and external hemorrhoids. (From Hill, G. J., II: Outpatient Surgery, 2nd ed. Philadelphia, W. B. Saunders Company, 1980. Used by permission.)

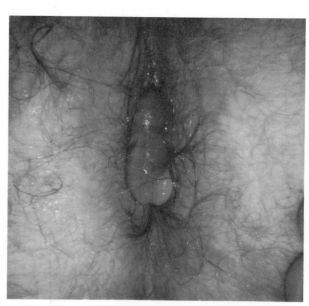

Figure 59–2. Large thrombosed external hemorrhoid.

clots and forms a tense, painful swelling. This clinical condition is therefore more accurately referred to as anal hematoma[4, 6] or external anal thrombosis.[3]

In the early stages, the swelling is very tender, but after a few days the tenderness tends to diminish markedly. After 1 week the swelling may be painless.[4] As the process subsides without specific treatment, the overlying skin becomes wrinkled, leaving a residual skin tag when the mass diminishes in size. Spontaneous resolution over the course of weeks generally occurs, with gradual subsiding of pain and swelling.

Spontaneous rupture of the hematoma occasionally occurs and may be followed by complete extrusion of the clot. More often, the clot is only partially extruded through the overlying skin and has to be expressed manually. A residual skin tag frequently remains following rupture. Multiple hematomas may be present. They can occasionally present as a conglomerate and cause swelling of most or all of the anal circumference.[4]

Almost immediate relief can be obtained by surgery if the thrombosis is confined to a well-defined mass or masses.[7] Treatment consists of evacuation of the clot under local anesthesia or of excision of the thrombosed segment of vein.

Indictions and Contraindications

Although most thrombosed external hemorrhoids will resolve spontaneously, many patients cannot tolerate the pain associated with an acute thrombosis, even when oral narcotic analgesia is available. Excisional therapy of the thrombosed hemorrhoids should be considered in such painful situations, although a patient with a small tolerable thrombosed external hemorrhoid or anal hematoma can often be managed satisfactorily with conservative therapy consisting of oral analgesics, sitz baths, and stool softeners.

Patients with coronary disease that may predispose them to myocardial ischemia or dysrhythmias should receive conservative therapy for their hemorrhoids whenever possible. When surgical therapy is necessary, the cardiac patient should be treated in a closely monitored setting with an intravenous line, cardiac medications at the bedside, and continuous rhythm monitoring. Emergency department treatment is contraindicated in the uncooperative or overly anxious patient. Treatment under general anesthesia in the operation suite should be considered for these more challenging patients.

Procedure

The patient is placed prone on a stretcher, and the buttocks are taped open to expose the anus

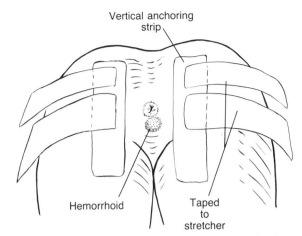

Figure 59–3. Taping the buttocks to gain exposure for the surgical excision of a thrombosed external hemorrhoid.

(Fig. 59–3). Tape adherence is enhanced by the application of benzoin to each buttock followed by a longitudinal anchoring layer of tape. Strips of cloth adhesive tape are subsequently run from the anchoring strips laterally to the sides of the stretcher. A scalpel and a standard suture tray or incision and drainage tray provide sufficient instruments. The operator infiltrates the area surrounding the thrombosed external hemorrhoid subcutaneously using lidocaine with epinephrine or bupivacaine (Marcaine) (Fig. 59–4).

The anesthesia is often delivered in a fan-shaped distribution, with the apex of the fan at the lateral aspect of the hemorrhoid. Superficial and deep (up to 5 mm) placement should be used. Occasionally, the medial (anal) aspect of the hematoma will need to be injected. This injection procedure is rather painful but provides complete anesthesia.

Apprehension and the initial pain of infiltration of the local anesthetic may be lessened with intravenous meperidine (Demerol) or diazepam (Valium). The judicious use of analgesia and sedation makes the procedure easier for both the patient and the physician.

When anesthesia is achieved, the skin is elevated with forceps, with tension away from the anal orifice. An elliptic incision is made around the clot and is directed radially (Fig. 59–5).[7] The incision can be made either with scissors or with

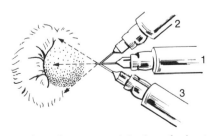

Figure 59–4. The subcutaneous injection of a long-acting local anesthetic provides complete anesthesia.

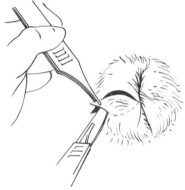

Figure 59–5. An unroofing technique uses an ellipitic or triangular incision that removes a piece of overlying skin. A simple linear incision should not be used.

a number 15 scalpel blade. The flap of skin is then picked up and excised to expose the underlying clot or the thrombosed vein. With Allis forceps placed on each lip of the incision, other clots or thrombosed veins are sought and excised. Clots are usually easily removed with forceps, and blunt dissection may expose deeper clots (Fig. 59–6). At all times, the incision should not extend under the cutaneous layer; this is a simple unroofing procedure. An alternative to the elliptical incision is to remove a triangular piece of overlying skin. Bleeding is usually minor. A small piece of surgical foam (such as Gelfoam) is placed directly in the wound, and the area is covered with a vaginal pad or sterile gauze. The foam promotes hemostasis; the elliptic or triangular incision prevents any recurrence of pain by eliminating increased tissue pressure during hemostasis. A less desirable alternative method is to use a very short incision, approximately 1 cm long, placed radially over the clot. The physician then evacuates the thrombus by squeezing between the thumb and the index finger.[4] It has been claimed that this method causes a higher incidence of infection than does an unroofing procedure because the skin edges fall together,[7] and this technique is therefore not

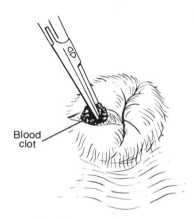

Blood clot

Figure 59–6. Blood clots are removed with forceps.

recommended. Most authorities generally prefer to unroof the hemorrhoid by removing at least some overlying skin as opposed to using a linear incision. The site is not sutured but is left open to drain.

When marked edema is present, conservative treatment with hot, moist dressings or sitz baths is preferred until the inflammation has subsided, at which time a definitive procedure, such as wide excision of the hemorrhoidal mass, can be performed. Wide excision is not an emergency department procedure.[7]

Postoperative Care

Postoperative care includes warm sitz baths[8, 9] at frequent intervals—at least four times a day for 30 minutes during the first 2 days. A dry cotton vaginal pad or rolled gauze dressing may be placed over the anal region for a few days.[4] Bleeding seldom persists for more than 2 to 3 days.

The buttocks can be taped together over the vaginal pad or gauze dressing for 6 to 12 hours to apply pressure to the incision site. Pain may be mild to severe after the local anesthetic has worn off, and the patient should be given adequate oral analgesia, usually narcotics. A stool softener is generally prescribed for 3 to 4 days to avoid the constipation associated with narcotic analgesic agents. Straining at stool can prolong bleeding in the postoperative period. Patients are instructed to avoid prolonged walking or sitting for a few days. Following a bowel movement, the patient is instructed to wash the anal area with soap and water in the shower and to avoid toilet paper for a few days. Antibiotics are not indicated in the absence of an obvious infection following the procedure.

Measures that have been proposed to prevent chronic straining at stool and possible further hemorrhoidal problems generally include the use of stool softeners[8] and a high-residue diet,[5, 9] but these are of questionable value in preventing recurrence.

Complications

Complications of thrombosed external hemorrhoids are rare, although if the clot remains exposed, or even if it is completely evacuated, infection may occur with resulting abscess or fistula formation.[4] Occasionally, a clot may re-form in a few days, in which case it may be easily removed under direct vision at the first postoperative visit. Actual bacterial infection is rare. At least one or two postoperative checks are required, and the first one should preferably occur within two to four days. It is possible that the area may become thrombosed again at some future date, and the patient should be warned of possible recurrence. In general, however, the procedure is curative for hemorrhoids in the area in question.

1. Jeffery, P. J., Ritchie, S. M., Miller, W., et al.: The treatment of hemorrhoids by rubber band ligation at St. Mark's Hospital. Postgrad. Med. J. 56:847, 1980.
2. Corman, M. L. (ed.): Classic articles in colonic and rectal surgery: John Morgan's varicose state and saphena veins, erectile tumour of the forehead, external haemorrhoids treated successfully by the injection of tincture of persulphate of iron. Dis. Colon Rectum 24:491, 1981.
3. Branch, W. T.: Office Practice of Medicine. Philadelphia, W. B. Saunders, Co., 1982, p. 671.
4. Goligher, J. C., Duthie, H. L., Nixon, H. H., et al. (eds.): Surgery of the Anus, Rectum, and Colon, 4th ed. London, Balliere Tindall, 1980, pp. 130–131.
5. Dworken, H. J.: Gastroenterology: Pathophysiology and Clinical Applications. Boston, Butterworth Publishers, 1982, pp. 511–513.
6. Kaufman, H. D.: Hemmorhoids. Gastrointest. Dis. 7:47, 1981.
7. Wolcott, M. W. (ed.): Ferguson's Surgery of the Ambulatory Patient, 5th ed. Philadelphia, J. B. Lippincott, Co., 1974, pp. 248–250.
8. Medical Letter 17:7, 1975.
9. Dandapat, M. C.: Management of haemorrhoids. J. Indian Med. Assoc. 74:234, 1980.

Introduction

Rectal prolapse is a rare condition in which some or all of the layers of the rectum protrude through the external anal sphincter. The definitive treatment of complete prolapse is usually surgical, but the acute prolapse may be reduced in the emergency department. The condition, although not usually serious, is very distressing to the patient or parent and occasionally is painful. Failure to reduce a prolapse may result in eventual gangrene of the bowel. Rectal prolapse may be partial or complete (procidentia).

Diagnosis

The condition is divided into three different types of prolapse. False procidentia, or type 1 prolapse, involves protrusion of redundant colonic mucosa only. The mucosa is seen extruding in radial folds.[1] Generally, this false prolapse is associated with hemorrhoids, and protrusion is only 1 to 3 cm.

Type 2 procidentia is a true intussusception of all layers of the rectum through the anal canal without an associated cul-de-sac sliding hernia (Fig. 60–1). Type 3 prolapse is basically a sliding hernia of the cul-de-sac. The pouch of Douglas is viewed as the hernial sac, which presses on the anterior wall of the rectum and forces the anterior wall into the rectal lumen to produce an intussusception within the rectum and the anal canal with protrusion through the anus (Fig. 60–2).[2] Although there is disagreement among authorities concerning whether procidentia is a sliding hernia or an intussusception, the condition gives the appearance that the rectum has been turned inside out, as is seen when one removes a surgical glove (Fig. 60–3).

60

Rectal Prolapse

JONATHAN M. GLAUSER, M.D.

In complete or true prolapse, the bowel lumen lies posteriorly because of the greater thickness of the anterior part of the prolapse from the pouch of Douglas. The protrusion is seldom more than 3½ to 4 inches, even in its fully developed form.[3]

The diagnosis of partial (mucosal) prolapse can generally be made by digital examination. A finger is inserted into the lumen of the bowel, and palpation of the prolapse between the examiner's finger and thumb reveals that there is no muscular wall within it.[4, 5] In addition, the presence of prolapse restricted to the left lateral, right anterior, and right posterior positions combined with normal anal sphincter tone is highly suggestive of hemorrhoidal, and not true rectal, prolapse.[6]

Conditions that must be differentiated from true rectal prolapse include a mass of hemorrhoidal tissue, a large rectal or sigmoidal polypoid lesion prolapsing through the anus and, possibly, a higher intussusception coming through the normally positioned anus. These will each be discussed briefly.

Prolapsed hemorrhoidal tissue tends to be lobular, with a definite sulcus between the masses of tissue down to the level of the anal skin. A false impression that the entire rectal wall is protruding may be obtained if such hemorrhoids become

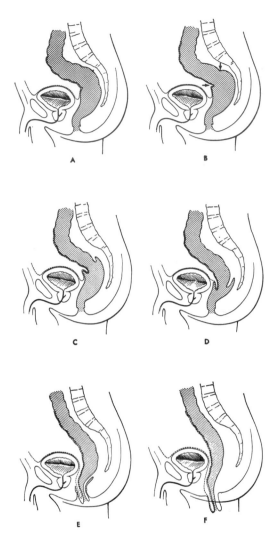

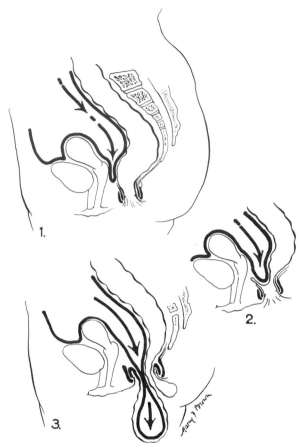

Figure 60–2. Diagrammatic sagittal sections of the pelvis to demonstrate the anatomy of complete rectal prolapse conceived as a sliding hernia of the pouch of Douglas. (From Goligher, J. C.: The treatment of complete prolapse of the rectum by the Roscoe Graham operation. Br. J. Surg. 45:323, 1958. Used by permission.)

Figure 60–1. A, Normal relationship of rectum to pelvic structures. B, Earliest stage of intussusception (prolapse) just proximal to the uppermost normal fixed point of rectum. C, Fixed point lowers. Upper rectum separated from sacrum. Intussusception commencement assumes lower position. Sigmoid mesentery elongates. Pseudomesorectum may develop. Rectosigmoid begins to straighten. D, Further lowering of fixed point. Previous changes become exaggerated. E, Cul-de-sac deepens. Rectum may or may not protrude. F, Final stage of intussusception (prolapse). Commencement occurs at mucocutaneous border. Deep cul-de-sac (may contain small bowel). Elongated sigmoid mesentery. Straight rectosigmoid. Rectum and sacrum separated. Rectum protruded completely. (From Theuerkauf, F. J., Beahrs, O. H., and Hill, J. R.: Rectal prolapse: Causation and surgical treatment. Ann. Surg. 171:819, 1970. Used by permission.)

thrombosed and the tissue becomes bluish, firm, and edematous. True rectal prolapse occurs with concentric radial folds; a deep sulcus between each tissue mass definitely establishes the diagnosis of hemorrhoids.[7] Polypoid lesions protruding through the anus can generally be diagnosed by digital examination and proctoscopic visualization after replacement of the mass. The mobile mass is felt separately from the lower rectum and the anal canal, which are felt to be in their normal posi-

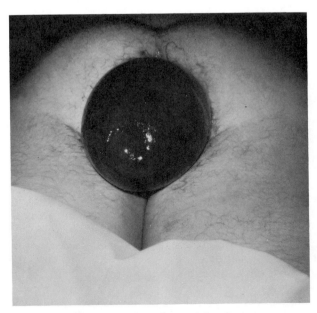

Figure 60–3. Complete rectal prolapse.

tions. In addition, polypoid tissue appears grossly granular and quite different from rectal mucosa. Finally, the pedicle itself can be visualized endoscopically to confirm the diagnosis.

An intussusception coming through the anus is suggested when there is a sulcus around the entire protruding mass. In this case, a finger can be inserted into the anal canal between the wall of the canal and the projecting mucosa-covered swelling, whereas in rectal prolapse no such crevice exists.[3]

In addition to the presence of a protruding mass, the patient with rectal prolapse may have other presenting complaints. These include a bloody or mucous discharge from the rectum, diarrhea, constipation, fecal incontinence with a patulous anus, or vague perineal pain with a constant urge to defecate.[5, 8]

Etiology and Epidemiology.

The epidemiology and etiology of rectal prolapse vary with the population studied but deserve some discussion because of related diseases that should be searched for and treated. In Western society the condition is most prevalent in debilitated elderly patients and in young children.[2, 9] Elderly women are affected more than elderly men.[4, 8, 10, 17] In countries with poor sanitation, young men are most frequently afflicted, with amebiases, schistosomiasis, and *Ascaris* infestation noted as inciting factors.[11, 12]

Idiopathic rectal prolapse in developed nations is most common in children aged 1 to 3 years and coincides with toilet training. There may be a history of constipation or of prolonged stays on the potty. Occasionally, a child with cystic fibrosis presents with frequent or persistent rectal prolapse. A measurement of sweat chloride will confirm the underlying diagnosis.[13] Prolapse resulting from a severe bout of pertussis generally resolves with conservative treatment.

Children with myelomeningocele or other causes of paraplegia may have rectal prolapse.[12] Various lesions of the cauda equina have been mentioned as causing rectal prolapse as well.[7, 3] Affected patients generally require surgical correction of the problem, unlike most children who have no obvious underlying neurologic cause of rectal procidentia.

Many possible causes and associated factors have been listed for rectal prolapse in adults. The condition has been associated with mental retardation, organic brain syndrome, poliomyelitis, cerebral thrombosis, and tabes dorsalis, among other psychiatric and neurologic conditions.[2, 13] There is a higher rate of procidentia among institutionalized patients.[1] Some authorities have postulated other factors predisposing to rectal prolapse, including pregnancy, hemorrhoidal disease, poor bowel habits, diarrhea, and wasting disease in general.[1, 2]

Anatomically, it is widely held that intussusception of the rectosigmoid is the true underlying pathologic condition.[6, 8, 10, 14, 15] The intussusception pulls the rectosigmoid from its attachments, and, with repeated straining, the rectum pulls away distally. The starting point of the intussusception has been listed from 6 to 8 cm above the anal verge[6] to the rectosigmoid junction.[15] Eventually, the bowel protrudes from the anus, producing stretching and paralysis of the external sphincter.[2, 15]

The concept that rectal prolapse is a sliding hernia was advanced as early as 1912.[7] By this theory, the pouch of Douglas slides through a defect in the pelvic diaphragm, invaginating the anterior wall of the rectum.[1] Today, many doubt that rectal prolapse is a sliding hernia.[16, 17]

Indications

Cases of rectal prolapse should be referred for surgical evaluation, but the acute prolapse should be reduced in the emergency department. Management of rectal prolapse in children and in adults with type 1 (false) procidentia is generally nonsurgical. Reduction of the acute prolapse is usually quite easy; the bowel slips back as one starts to examine it,[3] or it may be easily replaced with gentle pressure on the mass.

Procedure

In children with a prolapse that is difficult to reduce, sedation with chloral hydrate or phenobarbital may be required. Then, with the child prone on the mother's lap, gentle but firm compression is applied to the prolapsed part for 5 to 15 minutes. A gloved finger wrapped in gauze may be placed into the rectal lumen, and gentle force is applied to reverse the direction of the prolapse. Following reduction, a pressure dressing is applied, and the child can be sent home with a stool softener prescribed.[9] The condition in children is self-limited as a rule. Increased bulk in the diet may help in order to prevent constant straining at stool.[4]

There are other adjunctive modes of treatment in children. Some consideration may be given to advising defecating in the lateral recumbent position to prevent straining; toilet training may have to be abandoned for several months. The parents should be taught to reduce the prolapse promptly, because otherwise it may become so edematous that replacement is difficult.

For the outpatient management of recurrent

prolapse, taping may be useful. First, one should place wide, vertical strips of adhesive tape on both buttocks. A wad of Vaseline gauze is placed over the anus, and a bulky, dry dressing is placed between the buttocks. The gauze and dressing are then taped securely in place with transverse strips to prevent recurrent rectal prolapse.[13] After each bowel movement, the dressing must be replaced, with the vertical strips of tape left in place on the buttocks. In this way, excoriations from frequent dressing changes are avoided. Later, if necessary, the child can be treated with 5 per cent phenol injected locally as a sclerosant.[7]

Reduction of a complete prolapse in an adult may be more difficult. The patient is placed at bed rest in a prone position, and moist compresses are applied. Steady, gentle compression to the area is applied, starting at the least prolapsed part.[9] The bowel wall may be slippery and difficult to grasp. It is helpful to place two gauze pads on the prolapsed part at 3 and 9 o'clock. The thumbs are placed near the bowel lumen, and the fingers grasp the exterior wall. Then, with pressure placed on the thumbs into the lumen, the sides are gently rolled inward to force the prolapse back through the anus (Fig. 60–4). It may be necessary to sedate the patient for this procedure, since straining hinders reduction. Reduction is best accomplished with a slow and gentle (yet deliberate) approach. Definitive repair may be accomplished at a later date.

Reducible protrusions of less than 3 to 4 cm can be managed on an outpatient basis. For incomplete or mucosal prolapse, treatment can be accomplished either by rubber band ligation or by injection of sclerosing agents, as for internal hemorrhoids.[7, 18]

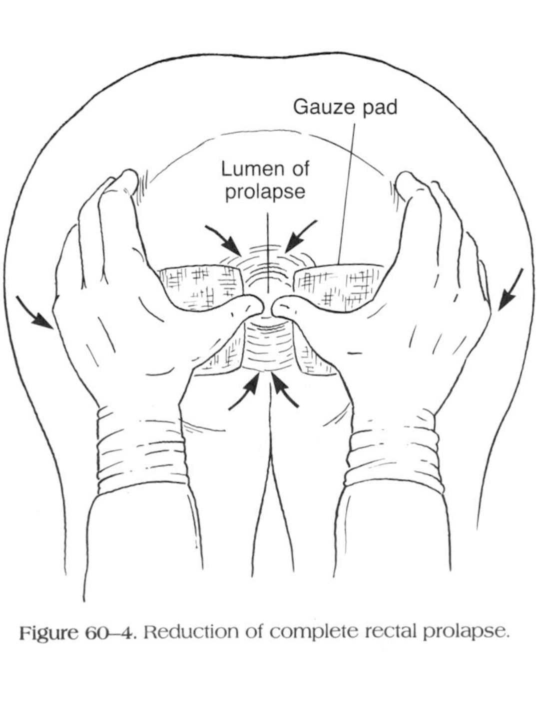

Definitive treatment of rectal prolapse in adults is surgical and is not performed as an emergency procedure. Well over 50 different surgical procedures to cure rectal prolapse have been described since the report of Moschcowitz in 1912.[2, 10, 19] These operations are based on one or more of the following six general principles:[2, 3, 8, 20]

1. Resection of the prolapsed and redundant bowel.
2. Reduction of the size of the anus.
3. Plastic reconstruction or reinforcement of the perineal floor.
4. Abdominal suspension or fixation of the prolapsed bowel to the sacrum or to other pelvic structures.
5. Obliteration of the cul-de-sac.
6. Repair of the perineal sliding hernia.

A description of the various fascial or Teflon slings, wire sutures, perineal floor reconstructions, and Ivalon-sponge placements is beyond the scope of this text and may be found elsewhere.[1, 2, 5, 7, 10, 11] Surgical complications include fecal impaction, sepsis, pelvic abscess, presacral hemorrhage, fistula, stricture, and impotence.[5]

Complications of the rectal prolapse itself include ulceration and, rarely, bleeding. Irreducibility occurs as well, with gangrene as a possible complication. If the prolapsed bowel is gangrenous, the patient should be admitted and observed for evidence of intraperitoneal extension or systemic signs. If this appears to be a danger, colostomy may be required with resection of the non-viable tissue.

Figure 60–4. Reduction of complete rectal prolapse.

1. Schwartz, S. I., Lillehei, R. C., Shires, G. T., et al. (eds.): Principles of Surgery, 3rd ed. New York, McGraw-Hill, 1977, pp. 1246–1247.
2. Altemeier, W. A., Culbertson, W. R., Schowengerdt, C., et al: Nineteen years' experience with the one-stage perineal repair of rectal prolapse. Ann. Surg. 173:993, 1971.
3. Goligher, J. C.: Prolapse of the rectum. In Nyhus, L., and Condon, R.: Hernia, 2nd ed. Philadelphia, J. B. Lippincott Co., 1978, pp. 463–477.
4. Ellis, H. and Calne, R. Y.: Lecture Notes in General Surgery. London, Blackwell Scientific Publications, 1977, p. 233–234 and 253–255.
5. Failes, D., Killingback, M., Stuart, M., et al.: Rectal prolapse. Aust. N.Z. J. Surg. 49:72, 1979.
6. Henry, M. M.: Rectal prolapse. Br. J. Hosp. Med. 302, Oct. 1980.
7. Nigro, N. D.: Procidentia of the rectum. Surg. Clin. North Am. 58:539, 1978.
8. Goldberg, S. M.: Procidentia of the rectum: A symposium. Dis. Colon Rectum 18:457, 1975.
9. MacLeod, J. H.: A Method of Proctology. Hagerstown, MD, Harper & Row, 1979, pp. 119–122.
10. Eisenstat, T. E., Rubin, R. J., and Salvati, E. P.: Surgical treatment of complete rectal prolapse. Dis. Colon Rectum 22:522, 1979.
11. Aboul-Enein, A.: Prolapse of the rectum in young men: Treatment with a modified Roscoe Graham operation. Dis. Colon Rectum 22:117, 1979.
12. Armstrong, A. L., Bivins, B. A., and Sachatello, C. R.:

Rectal prolapse: A brief review. J. Ky. Med. Assoc. 76:329, 1978.

13. Hill, G. J., II: Outpatient Surgery, 2nd ed. Philadelphia, W. B. Saunders Co., 1980, pp. 1199–1203.

14. Miller, R. L., Thomas, J. M., and O'Leary, J. P.: Ripstein procedure for rectal prolapse, Am. Surg. 45:531, 1979.

15. Theuerkauf, F. J., Beahrs, O. H., and Hill, J. R.: Rectal prolapse: Causation and surgical treatment. Ann. Surg. 171:819, 1970.

16. Ryan, P.: Observations upon the etiology and treatment of complete rectal prolapse. Aust. N.Z. J. Surg. 50:109, 1980.

17. Bates, T.: Rectal prolapse after anorectal dilatation in the elderly. Br. Med. J. 2:505, 1972.

18. Dutta, B. N., and Das, A. K.: Treatment of prolapsed rectum in children with injections of sclerosing agents. J. Indian Med. Assoc. 69:275, 1977.

19. Uhlig, B. E., and Sullivan, E. S.: The modified Delorme operation: Its place in surgical treatment for massive rectal prolapse. Dis. Colon Rectum 22:513, 1979.

20. Moore, H. D.: The results of treatment for complete prolapse of the rectum in the adult patient. Dis. Colon Rectum 20:566, 1977.

9

UROLOGY

61

Emergency Urologic Procedures*

IVAN ZBARASCHUK, M.D.
RICHARD E. BERGER, M.D.

Urethral Catheterization

INTRODUCTION

Urethral catheterization seems a simple task—insertion of a tube into a larger tube. Nonetheless, many difficulties may arise. Patients often remember catheterization—either painfully, as a reflection on the institution's personnel, or with admiration for the fine coordination of expertise, confidence, and gentleness that marks the catheterist of skill.

Patients are often apprehensive about catheterization. If the physician shows concern regarding position and exposure, the patient will be reassured of the competence and kindness of the catheterist. A moment should be spent in making sure a patient is positioned comfortably and appropriately for the procedure. Although adequate exposure may be obtained from a frog-legged position, the use of a table with stirrups may be helpful with female catheterization. Support under the knees will make the patient (male or female) more comfortable.

Preparation of all materials necessary for a smooth catheterization will reassure the patient that he is in the hands of a competent person. It is frustrating for the catheterist to hunt for a missing item and upsetting to the patient to be told "not to move or touch anything" while the search is made. Most catheterizations are performed with the use of a "cath tray." The trays usually contain most of the needed equipment. Our uniform practice is to go through the tray with sterile gloves and to arrange every item from the tray on the sterile paper around it. Only when every item has been considered and the tray is empty is the preparation complete. When a tray is not used, the catheterist should mentally go through the procedure, trying to visualize all the items he will need and then make them available before he starts.

BACKGROUND

Catheterization of the bladder has been widely practiced at least since the time of Hippocrates. Paul of Aegina (625–690 A.D.) described in detail the mechanics of male catheterization, which are largely used today. Phazes (c. 850–923 A.D.) described malleable catheters made of lead as well as the first catheter guide and stylet. In 1853, Reybards invented the self-retaining catheter, which is the prototype of today's Foley catheter.

INDICATIONS/CONTRAINDICATIONS

Urinary catheterization and instrumentation can be a direct cause of urinary infection. Therefore, catheterization needs to be limited only to clinical situations in which the benefits outweigh the risk. The following are usually considered to be indications for urinary catheterization:

1. acute urinary retention with inability to void,
2. urethral or prostatic obstruction leading to hydronephrosis and decreased renal function,
3. urine output monitoring in the critically ill, unstable patient,
4. collection of an uncontaminated urine specimen for diagnostic purposes,
5. intermittent bladder decompression in patients with neurogenic bladders, and
6. urologic study of the anatomy of the urinary tract.

Although there are few absolute contraindications to urethral catheterization, the procedure should be avoided when other less invasive methods may obtain the same information. The only absolute contraindication to urethral catheterization is in the case of the trauma patient with suspected urethral injury as evidenced by blood at the ureteral meatus, prostatic displacement on rectal examination, or perineal hematoma.

EQUIPMENT

The equipment listed in Table 61–1 must be at hand prior to catheterization attempts. Most of this equipment is available in prepackaged catheterization kits. The catheterist should check the list of contents on the kit *before* catheterization, however, since some kits do not include certain items. For most routine adult catheterizations, an 18 French Foley device is adequate. In infants or neonates, a 5 French feeding tube taped in place will produce the least ureteral trauma. In older boys, a 5 to 12 French retention catheter may be

*Special acknowledgment to Janice J. Schroeder and Helen P. Faulkner for typing.

Table 61–1. STERILE EQUIPMENT REQUIRED FOR URETHRAL CATHETERIZATION

Sterile tray
Sterile drapes
Sterile gloves
Sponges (5 to 10)
Antiseptic solution
Water-soluble lubricant for catheter
Sterile specimen cup with lid
Forceps
Foley catheter of appropriate size
10-ml syringe of sterile water
Sterile drainage bag with tubing

used. An 18 French coudé catheter should be used in a male patient with a known enlarged median lobe of the prostate or after unsuccessful passage of a straight retention catheter in such a patient. If a coudé catheter is not available, a 22 to 24 French catheter should be used. In a male patient with a urethral stricture, insertion of a silicone catheter of 12 to 14 French may be attempted prior to the use of filiforms and followers.

ANATOMIC CONSIDERATIONS

Female Catheterization

The female urethra is short (approximately 4 cm), straight, and usually of wide caliber. Yet this urethra must be approached between double labia, and its meatus is often not obvious (in contradistinction to that of most males). If the patient nervously adducts her legs, success is most uncertain (Fig. 61–1).

Because the urethra is so short, urine may start to come through the catheter before the balloon has disappeared into the meatus. Since the female urethra is approximately 4 cm in length and the balloon and tip portions of the catheter add up to another 4 cm, it is clear that approximately half the total length of the catheter will have to be inserted before it is safe to inflate the balloon.

The urethral meatus may be difficult to find. If the operator is uncertain of its location, he may resort to hunting for the meatus with the catheter tip—an unsettling experience for both the patient and the catheterist. The urethra is a narrow tube lying on top of a larger tube—the vagina. The urethral meatus is an anteroposterior slit with rather prominent margins that is situated directly anterior to the opening of the vagina and approximately 2.5 cm posterior to the glans clitoris.[1] Occasionally, the meatus has receded into the vagina either because of surgical procedures or for other reasons and is not immediately visible. In such cases, if the index finger is gently advanced into the vagina in the superior midline, the meatus will usually be found as a soft center surrounded by a firmer ring of supporting tissue. Rarely, the meatus will have receded so far that it cannot be visualized at all, and the catheterization must be carried out in conjunction with a speculum examination or by palpation alone. From the meatus (if the patient assumes a supine position), the urethra proceeds slightly upward as it advances toward the bladder just behind the symphysis pubis. Trying to push the catheter down will force the tip into the sensitive wall of the floor of the urethra. In women with a urethrocele in whom the urethra or the bladder sags into the vagina, the course will be more posterior, but the relation-

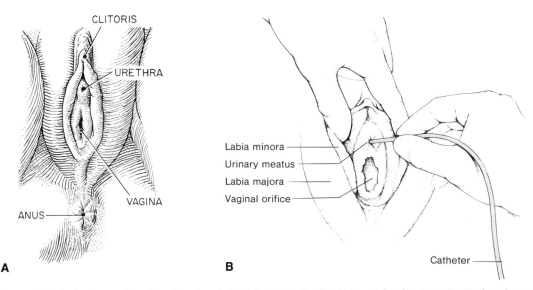

Figure 61–1. A, Anatomy of the female external genitalia. (From Flocks, R. H., and Culp, D. A.: Surgical Urology: A Handbook of Operative Surgery, 4th ed. Chicago, Yearbook Medical Publishers, Inc., 1975, p. 357. Used by permission.) B, Uncomplicated catheterization in the female. (From Brunner, L. S., and Suddarth, D. S.: Lippincott Manual of Nursing Practice, 1st ed. Philadelphia, J. B. Lippincott Co., 1974, p. 465. Used by permission.)

ship of urethra to vagina does not change. If the anterior vaginal wall bulges into the introitus, the catheter must be proportionately redirected according to the degree of prolapse.

Male Catheterization

In males, because the urethral meatus is usually evident, it may seem a simple matter to insert a catheter.[2] Yet catheterization of the male involves more hazards than does catheterization of the female. The normal male urethra is approximately 20 cm long from the external meatus to the internal meatus at the bladder neck (Fig. 61–2). The prostatic uretha is approximately 3.5 cm long, and the external sphincter is 4 cm from the bladder neck. The catheter must be inserted at least 24 cm in males before it is safe to inflate the balloon. At the first return of urine from the catheter, the balloon is just passing through the membranous portion of the urethra. The catheter still has 3 cm or more to go before clearing the bladder neck. In practice, it is customary to insert the catheter to the "hilt" (balloon-inflating sidearm channel) before inflating the balloon.[3]

The male urethra is relatively fixed at the level of the symphysis pubis; traction downward will kink the urethra at the level of the penile suspensory ligament and will create a point of obstruction, through which the catheterist will have to pass the catheter (Fig. 61–2B). One should place the distal urethra on a slight stretch straight up to straighten the urethra. The catheter then needs to make only a single curve rather than a complex S curve on its way into the bladder.

GENERAL PROCEDURE

Following exposure of the external urethra in the female and the penile urethra in the male, an antiseptic solution (e.g., povidone-iodine) is used to cleanse the exposed uretha and the surrounding tissue. An appropriately sized catheter (10 French is adequate for small children, whereas 16 French is commonly used in adults) that has been prelubricated is gently passed into the urethra using sterile technique. The patient should be forewarned of urethral discomfort and the urge to void. During passage, one should be aware of the anatomic considerations, as discussed previously. A catheter that inadvertently enters the vagina should not be reused. After passage into the bladder, the balloon should be *gradually* inflated with 5 ml of saline. Resistance or the complaint of discomfort upon balloon inflation should signal incomplete passage of the catheter. If resistance is met or pain is felt, the balloon should be immediately deflated, and passage of the catheter "to

the hilt" should again be assessed prior to reinflation. After successful passage and inflation of the balloon, one gently pulls the catheter distally until the balloon contacts the bladder neck. The catheter is connected to a sterile closed-drainage system. The catheter is secured to the thigh or the abdomen (preferred with males) with adhesive tape.

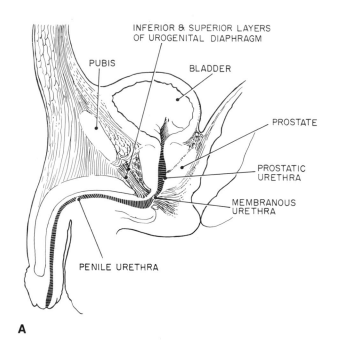

A

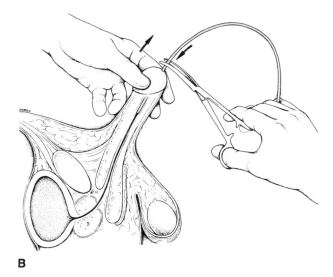

B

Figure 61–2. A, Anatomy of the male urethra. (From Flocks, R. H., and Culp, D. A.: Surgical Urology: A Handbook of Operative Surgery, 4th ed. Chicago, Yearbook Medical Publishers, Inc., 1975, p. 359. Used by permission.) B, Proper uncomplicated male catheterization with upward traction on the penis. (From Brunner, L. S., and Suddarth, D. S.: Lippincott Manual of Nursing Practice, 1st ed. Philadelphia, J. B. Lippincott Co., 1974, p. 465. Used by permission.)

DIFFICULTIES IN CATHETERIZATION OF MALES

Phimosis. The foreskin, especially in diabetics, is susceptible to recurrent infections and inflammation. A scarred, contracted ring of foreskin may result and may be difficult to retract. Inability to retract the foreskin because of a narrowed ring of foreskin is termed *phimosis*. Phimosis precludes optimal cleansing, resulting in a consequent increased risk of infection. Occasionally, the phimotic ring is so tight that the meatus cannot be visualized, even for a nonsterile catheterization. If the patient truly needs to have a catheter, it will probably be necessary to make a dorsal slit in the foreskin to expose the glans sufficiently for cleansing and for catheterization. This procedure is discussed elsewhere in this chapter.

Edema of the Foreskin. Patients with anasarca or with significant lymphatic obstruction from irradiation or cancer may have marked edema of the foreskin, so that the glans is totally buried in several centimeters of boggy foreskin. Since these patients often require careful fluid monitoring, they may need a catheter. The physician's problem is to retract enough foreskin to enable location of the meatus.

Two separate methods of visualizing the glans are available to the physician.[4] The simplest method is to compress the foreskin between opposing cold packs or with the hand in an attempt to reduce the amount of edema. In less severe cases, this is often successful, and no further maneuvers are required. In the more severe cases, the foreskin may be swollen to several inches in diameter. In such cases, the least traumatic way to visualize the glans is to use a pediatric-sized vaginal speculum. The outer surfaces of the speculum are lubricated, and the speculum is inserted into the edematous foreskin. It is possible to tell when the glans has been reached by palpation. The operator then opens the speculum gently and visualizes the glans as he would a cervix between the leaves of the speculum. Cleansing and catheterization must be performed with instruments. A ring forceps is a helpful tool for advancing the catheter, although we have accomplished catheterization with only the plastic forceps in the catheterization tray.

Meatal Stenosis. The meatus may be either congenitally or secondarily narrowed by scarring. The narrowing may prevent a normal-sized catheter from being introduced. If the meatus will admit a small-caliber tube (i.e., 5 French pediatric feeding tube or larger), this may be all that is required for short-term use. It should be remembered that the inner diameter of the drainage tube is the effective diameter for drainage. A smaller, single-lumen tube may provide better drainage than will a larger, double-lumen tube.

Should a larger-caliber catheter or a self-retaining catheter be required, a meatotomy or meatal dilation may be performed.[5] Meatal dilation is accomplished by the use of progressively larger meatal dilators or urethral sounds. This procedure should be performed with local or topical anesthesia.

A meatotomy may be performed in men in whom long-term catheterization is required. Using a 27 gauge needle, one infiltrates the ventral midline of the glans with local anesthesia from the corona to the edge of the meatus. A straight hemostatic clamp is then gently applied, with one jaw inside the meatus and the other on the anesthetized midline of the glans. After the hemostat has been applied for 1 or 2 minutes, it is removed. The crushed tissue is then cut with scissors. Some physicians place a chromic 4-0 suture through the apices of the skin and urethral incisions to prevent re-formation of the stricture. A catheter left indwelling for several days may also prevent re-formation of the stenosis.

Urethral Stricture. Obstruction met proximal to the prostate (less than 20 cm) during catheterization may be a result of urethral strictures.[5] *Force should never be used to bypass strictures.* Force will merely cause false passages, bleeding, and increased difficulty in subsequent catheterization.

Stricture that cannot be easily passed with the catheter may require dilation with filiforms and followers. Filiforms are very narrow, flexible, solid catheters usually not exceeding 4 French in caliber. Each filiform has a female-threaded coupling into which a male follower may be threaded. Under topical anesthesia with the penis stretched upward, the filiform is passed through the narrow strictured portion of the urethra (Fig. 61–3A). Filiforms are *not* dilators and have the sole function of finding the true urethral passage through the stricture. Filiforms should not be used to overcome any resistance as they are advanced into the urethra. Resistance represents the edge of the stricture or a fold of urethral mucosa. Any undue pressure on the filiform may result in perforation of the urethra and creation of a false passage along the urethra and under the bladder. Our practice, therefore, is to advance the filiform with the gentlest of pressure. If the filiform meets resistance, it is partially withdrawn, rotated slightly, and advanced again. If resistance is met at the same location again, the first filiform is left in place (to block that particular obstructing point) and a second is advanced alongside it. A third and a fourth may be necessary before one of them slips easily through the narrowed stricture into normal urethra and bladder. The sine qua non of success is *effortless passage of the filiform* into the bladder. Pigtail filiforms (with a corkscrew-shaped tip) may be helpful in advancing over an abrupt urethral edge (Fig. 61–3D). Once through the stricture, the

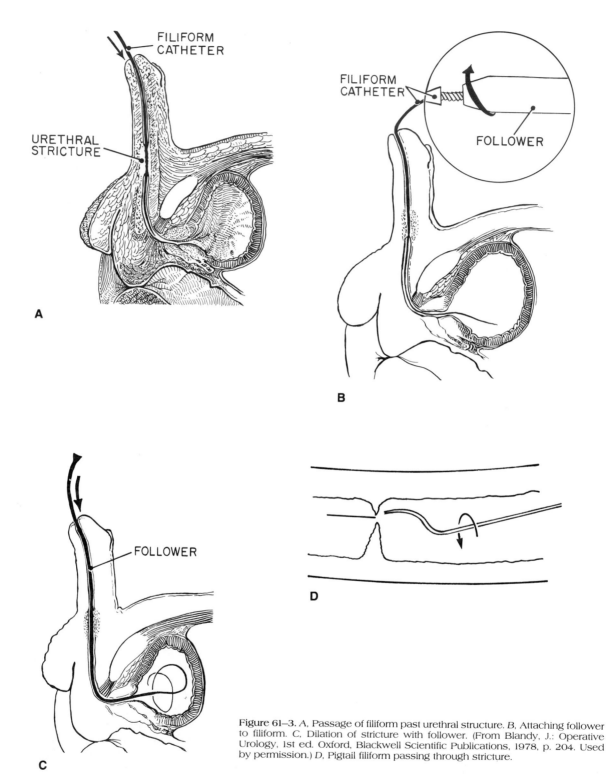

Figure 61–3. *A,* Passage of filiform past urethral structure. *B,* Attaching follower to filiform. *C,* Dilation of stricture with follower. (From Blandy, J.: Operative Urology, 1st ed. Oxford, Blackwell Scientific Publications, 1978, p. 204. Used by permission.) *D,* Pigtail filiform passing through stricture.

filiform is advanced until the tip is in the bladder or until the threaded coupling is near the glans. Since filiforms are very pliable, they must be held securely in place. One can best accomplish this by stabilizing the penis just proximal to the glans between the fourth and ring fingers and holding the filiform at the glans with the index finger and the thumb.

A follower of the smallest caliber (usually 8 French) is selected, lubricated, the threaded onto the filiform. When it has been threaded on completely (no threads showing), it is advanced into the urethra with the penis on stretch to straighten the urethra (Fig. 61–3B and C). Stretching the penis prevents kinking of the filiform in a telescoped urethra. The follower is advanced into the bladder until some urine escapes through the inner channel, guaranteeing the successful passage of the follower through the stricture and into the bladder. The same procedure is repeated with larger followers until one size larger than the catheter proposed for retention is introduced. Occasionally, the urethral course is so irregular that it is not possible to pass a catheter, even after dilation. The filiform with follower may be then left in place to provide bladder drainage. Occasionally, a stricture may be so dense that only a single follower can be introduced. The follower may be taped in place for 1 or 2 days until the stricture "softens" enough for a larger tube to be passed.

The following procedure is used to secure the follower in place. After wiping excess lubricant from the tube and from the penile glans and shaft, one may apply tincture of benzoin to the tube and to the unbroken skin of the penile shaft (not to the glans). When the benzoin is dry, strips of paper tape ½ inch in width are placed on the penile shaft without overlapping and then are wrapped around the tube. These longitudinal strips will securely keep the tube in place. It is important not to have a circumferential strip of tape over the penis, since the tape may constrict venous and lymphatic return sufficiently to produce a paraphimosis.

Dilation with filiforms and followers should be neither bloody nor excessively uncomfortable for the patient. Should the procedure be bloody or uncomfortable or should no urine be returned despite advancement of the follower for at least 24 cm, the physician should consider that the filiform may not be in the urethra, but instead be in a false passage. In such a situation, it may be better to place a suprapubic cystostomy tube rather than persist with an unsuccessful dilation.

Spasm in External Urethral Sphincter. The male patient may voluntarily or involuntarily contract the striated urethral sphincter at the apex of the prostate. (This is especially true of men with neurologic dysfunction and pelvic floor spasms.) The catheterist will meet a resistance at approxi-mately 16 cm. Because increased abdominal pressure causes reflex contraction of the external sphincter, the patient should be encouraged to lie flat and to take slow, deep breaths through his mouth. Plantar flexing of the toes also aids in relaxation of the pelvic floor. Because the external sphincter is composed of striated muscle and will fatigue within a few minutes, gentle but steady pressure should be exerted on the catheter. If these maneuvers do not result in passage of the catheter, the catheterist may be confronting a rigid stricture that will require dilation.

High Bladder Neck. Occasionally, when a man has an enlarged prostate with a high bladder neck, the tip of the catheter will hit against the posterior lobe of the prostate and will not slip up through the bladder neck. Resistance is usually encountered after the catheter has been passed 16 to 20 cm into the urethra. Slow injection of 20 to 30 ml of sterile lubricating jelly by syringe into the urethra may allow the catheter to slip over the prostate and into the bladder. If this fails, a coudé catheter (elbow catheter) may be inserted. This catheter has a bend in the tip, and one will almost always be able to maneuver it gently into the bladder (Fig. 61–4). If the catheter is still unable to be advanced, a scarred, fixed narrowing at the bladder neck may be present. Such a contracture is usually secondary to scarring from a previous prostatectomy and is often very difficult to pass. The insertion of a suprapubic catheter or direct visualization of the obstruction by a urologist may be required.

CATHETERIZATION IN THE PATIENT WITH PELVIC TRAUMA

The patient with pelvic trauma or a straddle injury presents special problems in urinary management. He may often be in shock from blood loss into the pelvis or from associated injuries. Accurate minute-to-minute monitoring of urinary output, requiring bladder catheterization, may be of assistance in the initial resuscitation. Furthermore, radiographic evaluation of the degree of urinary injury will require a cystogram, which usually necessitates catheterization.

The hazard of catheterization in the patient with pelvic trauma is the potential exacerbation of urethral injuries that are often associated with such trauma. The crucial finding on physical examination suggesting such an injury is *blood at the urethral meatus.* This most often results from injury of the membranous urethra just above the pelvic diaphragm, where the prostate is displaced from its attachments to the pubic bone (puboprostatic ligaments) during the pelvic fracture. A partial urethral disruption may heal with little or no scarring. On the other hand, a complete disruption of the

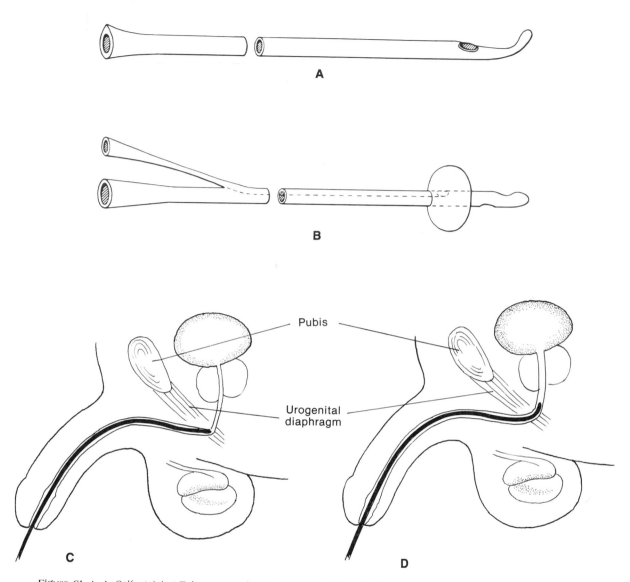

Figure 61–4. *A,* Self-retaining Foley-type catheter. *B,* Self-retaining Coudé catheter (also is available in a non-self-retaining model). *C,* Straight catheter may not pass over the rise in the prostate. *D,* Coudé catheter will pass more easily over enlarged median lobe.

urethra will usually result in a significant urethral stricture. The danger of urethral catheterization in this situation therefore is that a partial injury may be converted to a complete injury, which will result in a stricture requiring extensive surgical repair. Successful atraumatic placement of a urethral catheter, however, could obviate the need for open cystostomy placement in the patient who does not otherwise require laparotomy.

All patients with significant abdominal or pelvic trauma or permanent injuries should be examined for blood at the urinary meatus. Blood present at the urinary meatus and a "high-riding" or absent prostate on rectal examination almost always indicate complete urethral disruption. A retrograde cystourethrogram (see Chapter 62) should be per-

formed prior to catheterization and, preferably, prior to an excretory urogram. In the unlikely event that contrast flows easily from the urethra into the bladder with little or no extravasation, an attempt to pass an 18 French Foley catheter should be made. If *any* resistance to passage is encountered, the attempt should be immediately aborted. If passage is successful, relatively clear urine will usually be found in the patient's bladder. A cystogram can now be performed to rule out bladder rupture (see Chapter 62). If required, an excretory urogram can also be performed to rule out renal or ureteral injury. If the urethrogram shows extravasation, no further attempt at urethral catheterization should be made. If possible, an excretory urogram should be performed to identify renal or ureteral injuries and to identify the condition and the position of the bladder. In total disruption, the bladder is often higher than usual in the abdomen and may be laterally placed because of an asymmetrically expanded hematoma. Once identified, the position of the bladder may be confirmed by placement of a 22 gauge spinal needle into it. Further contrast may be introduced through the needle. Once the bladder is identified and is adequately filled, a Cystocath may be placed into the bladder alongside the spinal needle. Clear urine is obtained if no damage to the bladder or the kidneys has occurred. (The Cystocath can later be exchanged for a larger tube after the patient's condition has clinically stabilized.) If the patient is not stable enough to undergo an excretory urogram, he will probably require exploratory laparotomy, and an open cystostomy tube may be placed at that time.

COMPLICATIONS OF URETHRAL CATHETERIZATION

Although urethral catheterization performed by skilled personnel in appropriate circumstances has an acceptable complication rate, untoward sequelae of catheterization are not unusual.

The frequency of bacteriuria after a single catheterization in a healthy outpatient population is probably less than 1 per cent.[6] On the other hand, in hospitalized, elderly, debilitated, or postpartum patients, the rate may be considerably higher. Urinary catheterization is the leading cause of nosocomial urinary tract infections. The mortality in patients with nosocomial urinary tract infection is approximately three times that in patients not acquiring infection.[7] Of patients catheterized for 2 to 7 days with a closed system, 8 to 10 per cent will have significant bacteriuria once the catheter is removed.[8] Patients with catheters in place longer than 10 days almost always acquire an infection. Infection from the urethra and the bladder may spread to cause epididymitis, pyelonephritis, and sepsis.

In addition, complications may occur during the act of catheterization. False channels may be established even with soft latex catheters in either the pendulous urethra or the posterior urethra when force is placed on the catheter. In an uncircumcised patient, negligence in replacing the retracted foreskin over the glans penis after catheterization may lead to painful paraphimosis and even gangrene of the penis.

Leaving a catheter in place too long or using a catheter that is too large will lead to poor drainage of the periurethral glands and to urethritis and periureteral abscess, which in time may lead to urethral stricture. Likewise, in chronic catheterization concretions may form around a catheter balloon and may lead to the formation of bladder stones, which will require removal.

Phimosis and Dorsal Slit

INTRODUCTION

Subsequent to injury, the foreskin reacts (as do other tissues) by forming scar tissue. The normally highly pliable foreskin can therefore develop sufficient scar tissue to make retraction difficult. This is especially true if the end of the foreskin is injured, such as in zipper injuries, in toilet seat or other crush injuries (known as the Tristram Shandy syndrome, named after the well-known literary character who had a window sash fall on him while he was urinating out of the window), or in chronic irritation and superficial infection, such as often occurs in diabetes.[9] Occasionally, a tight phimosis and accompanying poor hygiene can lead to abscesses of the foreskin, which may result in further contracture.

Asymptomatic phimosis does not ordinarily call for any emergency treatment but may prevent sterile (or even unsterile) catheterization. In such situations, the phimosis may be relaxed by a dorsal slit of the foreskin. This minor operative procedure is similar to the relaxing incision in treating irreducible paraphimosis and can be performed with local anesthesia in the cooperative patient.

BACKGROUND

Phimosis has existed since ancient times. Models of phimotic foreskin have been found near the altars of Hygeia and Aesendopius in ancient Greece. Orikosius (325–403 A.D.) was the first to describe the treatment of phimosis by incision.

INDICATIONS/CONTRAINDICATIONS

The dorsal slit is used to allow urethral catheterization in an emergency situation in which phimosis is present. The technique should not be used in a nonemergency situation in which circumcision could be performed.

EQUIPMENT

The equipment needed is listed in Table 61–2.

PROCEDURE

After cleansing the penis using sterile technique and draping it with sterile towels, one infiltrates

Table 61–2. EQUIPMENT NEEDED TO PERFORM DORSAL SLIT FOR THE EMERGENCY TREATMENT OF PHIMOSIS

1 per cent lidocaine (Xylocaine) without epinephrine
5-ml syringe
27 gauge needle
1 straight Crile clamp
1 straight scissors
1 needle holder
4-0 chromic catgut suture

1 per cent local anesthetic *without* epinephrine into the dorsal midline of the foreskin along the course of the proposed slit, starting proximally and proceeding distally (Fig. 61–5). After an appropriate duration, the foreskin is tested for anesthesia with a forceps. The operator should be certain that the inner surface of the foreskin is also anesthetized. If it is not, a more circumferential infiltration of the skin around the base of the penis may need to be made (Fig. 61–6).[10, 11]

After adequate anesthesia, the operator takes a straight hemostatic or Crile forceps and advances one jaw carefully under the foreskin but *not* into the glans or the urethra (Fig. 61–7). After the forceps has been positioned correctly, the instrument is closed. The forceps are allowed to remain in place for a few minutes. When the forceps are removed, the serrated, crushed skin should be cut lengthwise with scissors. Normally little bleeding occurs, and often there is no separation of the skin edges. Nonetheless, to prevent bleeding and to keep the cut edges of the foreskin from separating, a 4-0 chromic suture is used to close the edge of the incision (Fig. 61–8A and B).

After suturing the slit open, the operator may retract the foreskin for cleansing and for completing the procedure that necessitated the dorsal slit.

After a dorsal slit procedure, a delayed elective

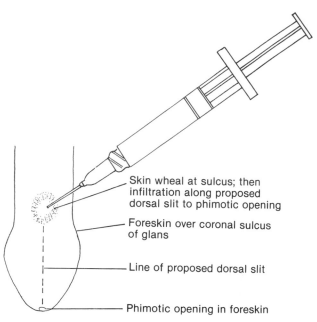

Figure 61–5. Technique for obtaining anesthesia before performing dorsal slit.

- Skin wheal at sulcus; then infiltration along proposed dorsal slit to phimotic opening
- Foreskin over coronal sulcus of glans
- Line of proposed dorsal slit
- Phimotic opening in foreskin

circumcision will often be required. A dorsal slit alone produces a "beagle-eared" deformity by transposing all the foreskin to a ventral position. The patient may complain about the appearance and the inconvenience during urination (Fig. 61–8C).

COMPLICATIONS

Injury to the meatus and the glans penis may occur if the hemostat or scissors is introduced into the urethra. Bleeding may occur if the hemostat has not adequately crushed the tissue or the incision made lateral to the crushed area.

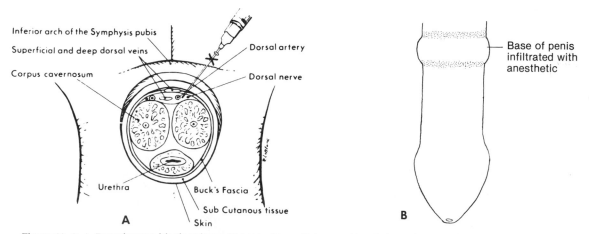

Figure 61–6. *A*, Dorsal nerve block at base of penis. (From Solomon, Magdi G., et al.: Nerve blocks of the penis for postoperative pain relief in children. Anesth. Analg. 57:496, 1978. Used by permission.) *B*, Subcutaneous infiltration for field block at base of penis providing anesthesia to entire distal penis.

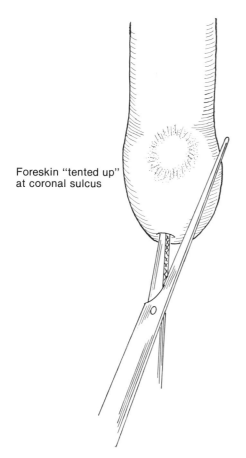

Foreskin "tented up" at coronal sulcus

Figure 61–7. Placement of forceps for treatment of phimosis. Foreskin "tented up" in this manner proves that the tip of the forceps is not in the urethra or under the glans.

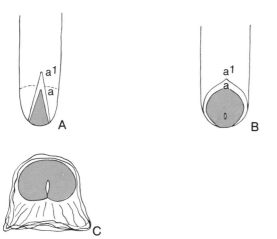

Figure 61–8. Treatment of phimosis. A, Dorsal slit in phimotic foreskin. Exposed glans is shaded. A single (dorsal) lengthwise incision has been made through crushed tissue. (a^1 = outer layer of foreskin; a = inner layer of foreskin). B, Cut edges of foreskin drawn back around glans penis. First, a^1 is sutured to a, then the remainder of the cut edges are sewn together for hemostasis. C, Final "beagle-ear" deformity of ventral transposed foreskin after the dorsal slit procedure has been completed.

Paraphimosis

Paraphimosis is secondary retraction of a phimotic foreskin causing painful swelling in the glans penis. The constricting ring interferes with venous and lymphatic return, precipitating swelling. The swelling then prevents reduction of the retracted foreskin. When left untreated, a paraphimosis may progress from tissue anoxia to skin ulceration and infection or penile gangrene.[12] Paraphimosis may occur if the foreskin is left retracted over the glans after the patient has cleansed under the foreskin (even in as benign a procedure as penile cleaning) or with catheterization.

Reduction of the edematous foreskin is a temporary measure to relieve discomfort and edema and to permit resolution of more serious effects—skin ulceration and infection—until a definitive treatment (circumcision) can be performed.

BACKGROUND

Paraphimosis has probably existed ever since the first retraction of the foreskin. Today, the most common cause is iatrogenic—the catheterist forgets to replace the foreskin after urethral instrumentation.

INDICATIONS

Reduction of a paraphimotic foreskin is indicated whenever the condition is present. There are no contraindications.

EQUIPMENT

The equipment needed for reduction of paraphimotic foreskin is listed in Table 61–3.

Table 61–3. EQUIPMENT NEEDED FOR REDUCTION OF PARAPHIMOSIS

For Nonoperative Emergency Reduction of Paraphimosis
1 per cent lidocaine (Xylocaine) jelly
Crushed ice
Size 8 latex surgical glove
6 to 8 Babcock clamps

For Operative Reduction of Paraphimosis
Sterile preparation solution
1 per cent lidocaine (Xylocaine) without epinephrine
5-ml syringe
27 gauge needle
No. 15 surgical knife with handle
Needle holder
4-0 chromic catgut suture

METHODS OF REDUCTION

Manual Reduction.[12, 13] A non-irritating lubricant is applied to the foreskin and the glans to reduce friction. A topical anesthetic lubricant jelly will decrease the considerable discomfort of the procedure. The foreskin is then manually compressed for several minutes to reduce edema as much as possible. Injection of hyaluronidase[16] has also been reported to reduce edema but is unnecessary.

The glans penis is then gently but persistently pressed through the phimotic constricting ring with both thumbs until it slips through. At the same time, an attempt is made to draw the foreskin back down over the glans with the index and middle fingers. The physician must determine that the glans has truly passed through the ring, since the proximal foreskin may easily hide the glans and may give a false appearance of reduction.

Assisted Manual Reduction ("Iced-Glove" Method[14] **or Babcock Clamp Method**[15]**).** If the constricting ring cannot be brought down over the glans easily, additional measures may be tried. In the "iced-glove" method,[14] cold compression is used to reduce foreskin swelling and to induce vasoconstriction in the glans. A large latex glove is half filled with crushed ice and water, and the cuff end is securely tied. The thumb of the glove is invaginated by the operator and then is drawn over the lubricated paraphimotic penis. The thumb of the glove is held securely in place over the penis for 5 to 10 minutes. The combination of cooling and compression usually decreases the edema sufficiently to permit full reduction of the foreskin. If the constricting ring cannot be brought down over the glans after this maneuver, it may be necessary to be more forcible. Six or eight Babcock clamps (*not* Allis clamps, which are serrated and intolerably painful for the patient) are used to grasp the phimotic ring circumferentially.[15] The clamps are then slowly levered forward over the glans. With gentle, slow traction, the ring is brought over the glans (Fig. 61–9).

Dorsal Slit.[10] This procedure is indicated when other methods are not successful or when skin ulceration and infection are present. Should manual or assisted reduction not be successful, a dorsal slit may be required.[17–19] Although it is usually recommended that this procedure be performed in the operating suite, it may be undertaken with local anesthesia in the emergency department.

The penis is cleansed and draped with sterile towels. Using a 1 per cent solution of local anesthetic *without epinephrine*, one infiltrates the foreskin at 12 o'clock, making sure to infiltrate proximally and distally as well as into the constricted ring (Figs. 61–10 and 61–11).

The skin, the edematous subcutaneous layer,

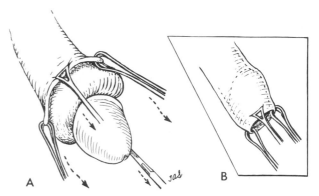

Figure 61–9. *A*, Application of Babcock clamps to reduce paraphimosis. *B*, Foreskin reduced. (From Skoglund, R. W., and Chapman, W. H.) Reduction of paraphimosis. J. Urol. 104:137, 1970. Used by permission.)

and the constricting ring are then incised with a knife. One should take care not to injure the penile shaft below the dartos fascia or the glans. The skin on the penile shaft should not be incised too proximally, because a tethered or hidden penis may result. When the constricting ring is incised completely, the foreskin edges will relax laterally and produce a diamond-shaped defect, which is then ready for suturing.

Using 3-0 or 4-0 chromic sutures, the two apices of the dorsal slit (labeled *a* and *b* in Figure 61–11) are approximated. The two wings of the slit are then sutured in interrupted or continuous fashion to ensure hemostasis and rapid healing.

Few patients with a dorsal slit will be satisfied with the "beagle-eared" appearance of their foreskin after the edema resolves, and a circumcision will be needed to complete the treatment of the paraphimosis. (Circumcision is elective, however, and should be delayed until edema, inflammation, and ulceration have cleared.)

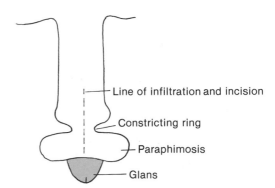

Figure 61–10. Anesthetizing the penis for surgical treatment of paraphimosis. Line of infiltration of local anesthesia used before performing dorsal slit.

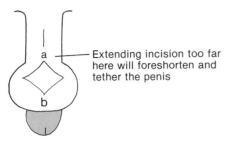

Figure 61–11. Incision for paraphimosis. Diamond-shaped defect resulting from incision of foreskin. The two apices of the dorsal slit (a and b) are approximated.

a — Extending incision too far here will foreshorten and tether the penis

b

COMPLICATIONS

In reduction of paraphimosis with Babcock clamps, if traction is applied asymmetrically or too vigorously, tearing of the skin may result. If tearing occurs, operative reduction using a dorsal slit should be performed.

Removing the Nondeflating Catheter

INTRODUCTION

The self-retaining balloon of the Foley-type catheter obviates cumbersome taping or suturing of the catheter to keep it in place. Occasionally, however, a self-retaining balloon will not deflate. Needless to say, this problem has challenged and frustrated physicians who encounter it and has produced a number of solutions. The usual cause of the nondeflating catheter balloon is the presence of a flap-type valve in the inflating lumen of the catheter, which allows fluid to enter the balloon of the catheter but prevents fluid removal (Fig. 61–12).[20] The ideal solution is one that will resolve the problem—getting the balloon to deflate—without creating a second problem (for example, unnecessary irritation of the bladder or fragmentation of the balloon). Of the methods used to deflate catheter balloons, the only technique that approaches the ideal is treatment of this flap valve

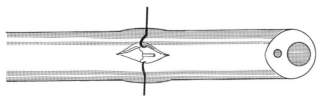

Figure 61–12. A flaplike defect in the inflating channel of a balloon catheter being raised by a wire stylet passed down the inflating channel to deflate the balloon. (From Eichenberg, H. A., Amin, M., and Clark, J.: Non-deflating Foley catheters. Intern. Urol. Nephrol. 8:171, 1976. Used by permission.)

deformity. Other methods of deflation often produce secondary problems and therefore should be avoided when possible.

TECHNIQUES

One method of catheter removal is inflation of the catheter balloon with water or air until the balloon is overstretched to the point of rupture. Up to 200 ml of fluid can be injected before a 5-ml balloon will rupture.[20, 21] Adding volume to the empty bladder may not be a problem. Unfortunately, this solution may produce unacceptably painful bladder distention for the patient whose catheter is blocked and whose bladder is distended to the point of discomfort. An even more compelling reason not to use this method of balloon deflation is the disconcerting frequency of balloon fragmentation. In an experimental study of 100 catheters (50 of which were overdistended with water and 50 of which were overdistended with air), all 100 catheter balloons ruptured into fragments.[20] Consequently, fragments of balloon may be left in the bladder to become nidi for calculus formation. Cystoscopy to inspect the bladder and to remove any fragments is indicated if this method of balloon deflation is used.

A second method of balloon deflation involves injecting an erosive substance into the balloon. This will cause the balloon to deflate after part of the wall has been eroded. Organic compounds that will attack the latex polymers are often used. Ether, acetone, mineral oil, and even petrolatum ointment have been used. In general, the more volatile the substance, the more rapidly it will rupture the balloon. Rupture of the balloon may be partly a result of the rapid expansion that some of these volatile substances—especially ether—undergo at body temperature. Ether was reported to rupture 58 of 60 catheter balloons within 2 minutes of injection into the balloon. Unfortunately, in 56 of the catheters, a free fragment of the balloon was ruptured off. Mineral oil, which works more slowly, was associated with fragment production in 95 of 100 catheters tested.[21] When released into the bladder, organic substances often produce a very symptomatic chemical cystitis.

A third method of deflating the balloon is to pierce it with a sharp instrument. With gentle traction, the balloon is drawn against the bladder neck and is punctured with a thin spinal needle transvesically, transvaginally, or transperineally. This may be done either blindly[22] or with the help of some system of visualization. Fluoroscopy with the bladder filled with contrast media,[21] ultrasonography,[23] and cystoscopy[21] have been used. In women, the spinal needle may be gently introduced along the catheter transurethrally. Fragmentation during rupture has frequently been reported with this method.[24]

The most rational way to deflate a nondeflating balloon is to attack the valve-like defect in the inflate-deflate channel that prevents the removal of the inflating fluid. Cutting the catheter may result in rapid deflation if the valve-like defect happens to be present in the part of the catheter that is cut off. A cut catheter with a more proximal valve-like defect can often be left for 24 hours with frequent slow deflation,[23] but this maneuver leaves the problem of managing an unconnected catheter. Devising a waterproof and aseptic method of collecting urine from the cut balloon may require use of a ureteral catheter drainage bag or another ingenious invention.

It is often helpful to insert a very thin, rigid item into the lumen of the inflating channel in an effort to deform the valve defect sufficiently to allow the inflating fluid to escape from the balloon. A stainless steel wire suture of 3-0 or 4-0 gauge is the thinnest suitable material.[25] The wire stylet from an angiographic catheter,[20] stylets from ureteral catheters,[27] and very small, well-lubricated ureteral catheters[23] have all been reported to achieve success. When a ureteral catheter stylet was used in one series, 34 of 39 balloons were deflated without fragmentation. In the five unsuccessful cases, a needle rupture was required.[15]

Our recommended method is to use a stepwise series of maneuvers. If the balloon will not deflate, we remove the syringe adaptor plug from the inflating channel. This rules out a malfunction of the adaptor. If the inflating water does not escape, we next insert one angiographic catheter stylet into the inflating channel and rotate it. Usually, the water from the balloon will flow along the wire. If it does not, we cut the catheter short and wait for 24 hours before trying to puncture the balloon. The shortened catheter is firmly attached to a drainage system to avoid intravesicular migration and to collect drained urine.

Once a problem balloon has been deflated, it is mandatory to inspect the balloon portion carefully for missing fragments. Should a piece of the balloon be missing, it will be necessary to arrange for cystoscopy to remove the fragment.

Suprapubic Aspiration of the Bladder

INTRODUCTION

One of the problems of interpreting voided urine samples is that the urine from the bladder passes through a progressively more contaminated urethral conduit. In the female, the perineum is a site where bacteria are seemingly eager to be swept along into the sterile cup and onto the agar plate. To avoid this dilemma of interpretation, physicians have devised maneuvers to minimize contaminating organisms. Male patients are instructed to retract the foreskin, cleanse the meatus, discard the first portion of urine, and catch the midstream urine. Female patients are asked to perform even more difficult maneuvers to avoid the bacterial contamination: hold the labia apart with one hand, cleanse the periurethral skin blindly with the other, then reach for the cup, initiate voiding, and catch the midstream urine—all the while holding the labia apart and maintaining a precarious position on the commode. Some experts[28] have women void in the lithotomy position while an assistant retracts the labia, cleanses the perineum, and then catches the midstream urine.

In transurethral bladder catheterization, even with sterile materials, the catheter must traverse the contaminated urethra and may introduce contaminating bacteria into the specimen and into the bladder of the patients, resulting in infection. In addition, the procedure is often uncomfortable.

Suprapubic aspiration of the bladder, first reported as a method of collecting urine for bacteriologic study in 1956,[29] offers the physician a relatively simple means for obtaining uncontaminated bladder urine. Urethral contamination is successfully avoided, and positive results always represent true bacteriuria.

INDICATIONS

In the neonate or the young child who cannot collect a reliably clean-catch urinary specimen, suprapubic aspiration can provide the physician with a sample that is useful for bacteriologic interpretation.[29-31]

For adult patients, the indications for suprapubic aspiration are more limited, since these patients usually can cooperate with the physician. Men with condom catheters or phimosis, however, may require suprapubic aspirate to minimize contamination. Aspirate cultures may be needed to rule out contamination in patients with asymptomatic bacteriuria on routine urine collection. In infections caused by organisms that in other circumstances are often discounted as contaminants (e.g., staphylococci or *Candida albicans*) suprapubic aspiration may be required in order to confirm the significance of such pathogens.

In patients in whom the possibility of infravesicular infection must be evaluated (e.g., in those with chronic infections of the urethra or the periurethral glands), suprapubic aspiration helps to separate "bladder urine" from "urethral urine."

METHOD

The physician should first locate the bladder. A full, palpable, percussable bladder is most helpful, but even a partially filled bladder may be aspirated. The point of entry in the skin should be 1 to 2 cm cephalad to the upper edge of the symphysis. The angle of needle advancement toward the bladder through the intervening tissues is vertical in children and somewhat caudad in adults (Figs. 61–13 and 61–14).

Once the prepared skin has been draped and the point of entry has been chosen, a skin wheal of local anesthetic agent is raised to reduce discomfort. When the skin has been anesthetized, a longer, larger-caliber needle (usually 22 gauge, 1½ to 3½ inches in length) is advanced through the skin and quickly into the bladder. We prefer to advance the needle attached to a syringe, with minimal aspiration during advancement. As soon as the bladder is entered, urine will enter the syringe. A short needle is adequate for virtually all pediatric patients. Aspiration is commenced as soon as the bladder is entered. A child may start voiding as soon as the bladder is irritated by the needle. Prior placement of a perineal collection bag ("wee bag") may assist urine collection. After the urine has been collected, the syringe and the needle are withdrawn. Usually, no further care is needed.

In most patients, a urine sample will be obtained with the first needle pass. If the needle points too caudad, in order to avoid entering the peritoneum, it is possible to enter the retropubic space, skimming the bladder muscle and never penetrating

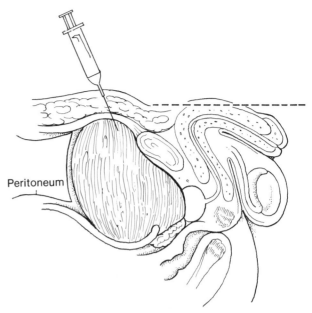

Figure 61–14. Peritoneum pushed cephalad by filled bladder during suprapubic aspiration in adult. Needle is directed slightly caudad.

the bladder mucosa. After the urine has been collected, the syringe and the needle are withdrawn. Usually, no further care is needed.

COMPLICATIONS

Stamey has performed several thousand aspirations without complications.[28] Bowel penetration has occurred in children who had "distended" abdomens from gastrointestinal disturbances.[32] The combination of gaseous distention of bowel and relative hypovolemia may displace and flatten the relatively empty bladder against the pelvic floor. Even when the large bowel has been penetrated, the patient has recovered uneventfully. Pathologic examination of a clinically penetrated bowel wall was performed in a single postmortem case (the patient died of an already established peritonitis); no entry "needle track" could be found in the deceased. A simple penetration of the bowel with a needle is considered an innocuous event and requires no specific treatment.

Doppler Diagnosis of Testicular Blood Flow

INTRODUCTION

Diagnosis in the patient with acute scrotum can at times be difficult. The condition most easily

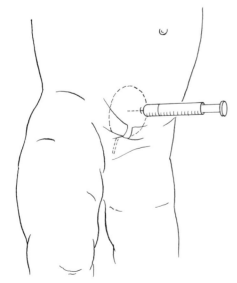

Figure 61–13. Suprapubic aspiration in the neonate.

confused with acute epididymitis is torsion of the testicle. The prompt diagnosis and differentiation of this condition is crucial to the patient's care. The treatment of acute epididymitis requires appropriate antimicrobial and supportive therapy. On the other hand, treatment of torsion of the testicle requires that de-torsion be performed within 4 to 6 hours in order to obtain an acceptable testicular salvage rate.[33]

Torsion of the testicle is the most frequent cause of acute testicular pain in boys and in men under the age of 30. In men over the age of 30, torsion is less common, although it may occur into the seventh decade.[34] In contrast, epididymitis is an *uncommon* condition in children and a frequently occurring problem in older men.[35] In men under the age of 30, epididymitis is commonly associated with either coliform urinary tract infections or gonococcal or nongonococcal (e.g., chlamydial) urethritis; signs and symptoms of infection may be minimal when the patient is first examined.[36] Since urethritis may easily go unnoticed if the patient has recently urinated, evidence of infection may be lacking. The presence of genitourinary infection may, however, provide an important clue to the diagnosis of epididymitis. Furthermore, if one makes the clinical diagnosis of epididymitis, one should have some objective confirmation, since the misdiagnosis of torsion as epididymitis means the destruction of the testicle.

Since blood flow to the testicle is increased with the inflammation of epididymitis and decreased in torsion of the testicle, the Doppler ultrasound stethoscope can provide objective information that may aid in the differential diagnosis. Although the accuracy of the Doppler examination has been challenged and there have been reports of both false negative and false positive results, the advantage of Doppler ultrasound examination is that it can be performed (in the outpatient setting) by anyone familiar with its use.

BACKGROUND

In 1974, Milleret and Liaras reported the use of the Doppler ultrasound stethoscope in two cases of torsion of the testicle.[37] Levy[38] in 1975 reported seven more cases. Pederson and coworkers in 1975 used the Doppler stethoscope to examine 45 patients. Levy,[38] Perri,[39] and Pederson and associates[40] reported 100 per cent accuracy in the diagnosis of torsion of the testicle. Caution was, however, advised by Perri,[41] Thompson and colleagues,[42] Rodriquez and coworkers,[43] and Brereton,[44] who found false positive and negative results. The most common error was the false impression of blood flow in the twisted testicle.

INDICATIONS/CONTRAINDICATIONS

Testicular blood flow determination by Doppler ultrasonography should be used to *confirm* the diagnosis of epididymitis in men of the age group in which torsion may commonly occur. This would include any male under the age of 30. Because epididymitis is extremely rare in children, the diagnosis of torsion in boys with acute scrotum should be presumed, and surgical exploration for de-torsion should be undertaken. In postpubertal men in the absence of convincing evidence of urethritis or urinary tract infection, torsion should also be presumed and exploration should be performed promptly. Radioisotope scans may also be useful for the differential diagnosis but are beyond the scope of this chapter.[41, 43, 45] In young men in whom the diagnosis of epididymitis is suggested both by findings on physical examination and by the presence of genitourinary inflammation (pyuria), Doppler ultrasound may be used to confirm the diagnosis by showing that there is blood flow to the testicle. This will help prevent one from making the tragic mistake of misdiagnosing a torsion of the testicle. Doppler ultrasound should not be relied upon as the sole diagnostic indicator in the differentiation of torsion from acute epididymitis. Clinical history, physical signs, and examinations of the genitourinary tract for signs of infection should be used to suggest the diagnosis and Doppler used to confirm it. Most errors in diagnosis could have been prevented if the physicians had not overrelied on the Doppler technique.

EQUIPMENT

The directional Doppler operating on a 5.3- to 10-mHz transducer is often used. See Chapter 31 for a detailed discussion of Doppler ultrasound physics. A pencil transducer is the most appropriate; the Model 806 Directional 10-mHz Doppler (Park Electronics Laboratory, Beaverton, Oregon) and the Medtronics 8-mHz Model BF5A are acceptable devices. The Doppler response may be transmitted over a loudspeaker, copied on a measuring device, or transmitted through a stethoscope to the physician. The higher the megahertz, the narrower the beam and the less distance of transmission through the tissues.[13] In this respect, a 10-mHz transducer may be more appropriate for examination of the testicle.

PROCEDURE

Since scrotal tenderness often precludes adequate examination, proper anesthesia must be obtained. We perform a cord block using 1 per cent lidocaine (Xylocaine) at the external ring.[46] The skin is first prepared with an iodophor solution. The cord can usually be grasped between thumb and forefinger, and 10 ml of 1 per cent lidocaine can be directly injected. If the cord is also swollen or if the testicle is very high in the scrotum (so as to preclude grasping), the cord may be palpated as it passes over the pubis and the lidocaine injected at this point. The patient will often thank the physician for this anesthetic procedure after the pain in his testicle acutely subsides. At this time, adequate examination of the testicle may be performed and the area of maximum swelling determined. An aqueous transmission gel is then placed over the scrotum. Holding the testicle in one hand and the Doppler probe in the other, one displaces as much of the scrotal wall as possible between the skin and the underlying testicle. The Doppler probe should be placed in the center of the testicle, pointing slightly caudally so that one does not pick up pulsations in the cord (Fig. 61–15). (Firm probe pressure will "focus" the ultrasound waves deep to the scrotum into the testis.) The pulsation in the ipsilateral testicle is then compared with that in the contralateral testicle. Decreased or absent flow to the ipsilateral testicle is most surely a result of torsion. Increased flow to the ipsilateral testicle may be a result of epididymitis, inflamed scrotal tissue, a false signal from either the cord or the patient's fingers,[43] or a false comparison with a contralateral partial torsion of the testis.[41–45] The *funicular compression test* as described by Pederson and associates[40] is then performed. If the increased signal lessens on compression of the patient's spermatic cord, then the signal is most probably coming from the patient's testicle and not from inflamed scrotal tissues. If there is no change in

the signal on adequate cord compression, the increased flow may be originating in inflamed scrotal tissue, and torsion should still be suspected.

If the diagnosis of torsion is made, the Doppler stethoscope may be used to monitor manual detorsion of the testicle.[47, 48] The testicle is rotated first one way and then the other in an attempt to untwist the testis. After the testicle has been untwisted, the evaluation of the Doppler will show that blood flow has been re-established. Manual detorsion may save valuable time while the operating suite is being prepared for the patient. It should not be allowed to delay operative preparations.

SOURCES OF ERROR

There are several sources of error in the performance and interpretation of Doppler ultrasound of the testicle. An understanding of these errors will lead to better use and assessment of the procedure. Errors include failing to detect blood flow when it is present and falsely attributing flow from vessels other than the testicular artery as testicular perfusion.

The use of Doppler probes with low-megahertz transducers (less than 10 mHz), which are used for large arteries, is not proper for medium-sized arteries, such as are found in the testes. These probes are able to pick up adjacent arteries in the cord or in the examiner's finger, which may produce positive flow signals.[45] False positive signals from secondarily inflamed scrotal vessels may be heard. This results from inadequate compression of the skin of the scrotum with the transducer because of pain in an inadequately anesthetized testis. Failure to perform the funicular compression test may lead to the mistaking of scrotal blood flow for testicular blood flow. As the testis liquefies, it may act as a blob of tissue-sonic jelly, and a false positive signal may be heard from the opposing examining finger. With a partial twist of the testicle, one may also hear an arterial pulse in the testicle with an early partial torsion. For these reasons, it should be evident that one cannot rely entirely on the Doppler ultrasound examination.[44] False positive flow signals may also be heard if the Doppler is directed upward instead of slightly downward, thus picking up a pulse in the cord above the testicle. A partial twist of the contralateral testicle may also serve as a falsely low standard for arterial blood flow in the rare patient with bilateral torsion.[44]

A false negative signal may be obtained if the testicular artery in the cord is inadvertently manually compressed by the examiner while he holds the testicle.[44] Hydrocele may also create false neg-

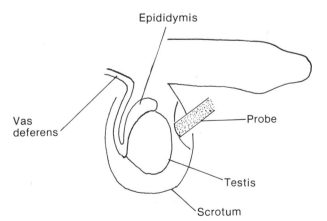

Figure 61–15. Proper position of the Doppler probe in the examination of the acute scrotum. Note caudal orientation of the probe.

ative results. If these pitfalls are kept in mind and the Doppler ultrasound examination of testicular blood flow used only as one clinical parameter in the management of patients with acute scrotal pain, many errors in diagnosis may be avoided.

Percutaneous Suprapubic Cystostomy

BACKGROUND

Although suprapubic cystostomy was described as early as four centuries ago, the safety of the procedure was first demonstrated by Garson and Peterson in 1888. The first modern method was Campbell's trocar set, described in 1951.[50, 51] Campbell used a sharp trocar passing through a sheath. The sheath had a longitudinal portion of its wall missing to permit a balloon-type retention catheter to be passed into the bladder. The Campbell trocar is a large-diameter instrument, accepting up to a 20 French catheter. It is thus probably unsuitable for use under local anesthesia in a non–surgical suite setting.

Subsequently, a wide variety of smaller suprapubic cystostomy devices were reported: large-gauge intravenous Teflon catheters,[52–54] thin polyethylene catheters inserted through large gauge needles,[55] and spinal needles.[56] Although it is true that all of these may have a useful role in the management of bladder and urethral problems, their small caliber makes them prone to obstruction and applicable only for short-term use.

The development of punch thoracostomy tube sets suggested their use as modified cystostomy tubes. This led to the invention of medium-caliber cystostomy tubes, which were easier to insert than the Campbell trocar but provided more satisfactory drainage than adaptations of intravenous infusion sets.[58, 59] Ingram's trocar catheter is perhaps the best known of these tubes. It has three lumina: one for inflating the retention balloon and the other two for drainage or irrigation. The Ingram catheter is available in a 12 or 16 French size. Stamey's suprapubic catheter is another variation of this type, but it uses a four-wing Malecot-type retention device rather than an inflatable balloon.

Perhaps the most widely known and frequently used trocar cystostomy tube is the Cystocath.[60] It is available in 8 and 12 French sizes. The latter is more commonly used for adult patients. The Cystocath is packaged as a self-contained set supplying virtually everything needed for insertion. The device is easy to insert and may be satisfactory for relatively long periods of trouble-free use if the patient is given conscientious nursing care.

A major difficulty with cystostomy tubes of all designs has been securing them to the patient's skin. Those with retention balloons, such as the regular Foley urethral catheter or the Ingram catheter, are most secure and need tape only to provide a "safety factor" security. Virtually all other systems depend on tape or skin adhesive to hold either the tube or the appliance in place. With the development of newer adhesives and secure taping of the tubing to the urinary drainage bag, these devices may also be securely maintained. As with all tubing, these urinary drainage devices require awareness and care on the part of all personnel involved.

INDICATIONS

In general, any patient who would require a urethral catheter but in whom a catheter cannot be passed needs a suprapubic cystostomy tube. In emergency situations, the majority of these patients will be men with urethral or prostatic disease. Dilation can usually be performed in patients with urethral strictures using filiforms and followers. If there is any difficulty with the passage of either filiforms or followers, a cystostomy tube is prudent and will prevent further injury to an already diseased urethra. Patients who present with acute urethral trauma may also need a cystostomy tube either to prevent further trauma to the urethra or to bypass a completely transected urethra. Complete urethral transection associated with a pelvic fracture is an indication for emergent suprapubic cystostomy. Many affected patients need laparotomy because of associated injuries, and a large tube can be placed at surgery. On the other hand, if the patient does not require laparotomy, a percutaneous urinary diversion will allow urologic surgery to be delayed until the patient is clinically stable.

Patients with lower genitourinary infection deserve special care before urethral instrumentation. The risk of inciting an episode of sepsis with urethral catheterization is considerable. Suprapubic drainage should be considered in these patients. In men with acute prostatitis or epididymitis who require drainage, a suprapubic catheter will allow both urinary drainage and unobstructed drainage of prostatic, seminal vesicular, and urethral secretions.

Neurologically disabled patients (e.g., quadriplegics or paraplegics) who have been maintained on a program of intermittent catheterization occasionally have difficulties with urethral catheter passage. In such patients, especially high paraplegics and quadriplegics, suprapubic cystostomy can be a rapidly effective method of relieving bladder distention. Catheter passage in the dysreflexic, profusely perspiring, hypertensive quadriplegic in "sympathetic crisis" or "autonomic dysreflexia" is perhaps the most dramatic example of suprapubic cystostomy tube placement as a truly emergency procedure.

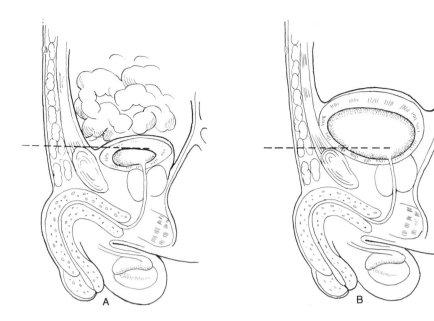

Figure 61–16. Cytostomy tube placement. Relation of peritoneum to bladder with bladder empty and full. *A*, With an empty bladder or a peritoneum scarred down into the pelvis from previous surgery or radiation, the peritoneal reflection may descend below the top of the symphysis pubis and thus "close the window" for passing the trocar along the dotted line (arrow). *B*, As the bladder fills, it lifts the peritoneum above the symphysis pubis and "opens the window" for safe trocar insertion (arrow).

Suprapubic catheterization is *not* recommended for a patient who is merely voiding poorly from lower tract obstruction. Such a person, although symptomatic, is better off without instrumentation. Patients with uninfected chronic retention should not be introduced to the hazards of catheter drainage prior to definitive surgical correction. A sterile residual urine is less of a hazard to the patient than an offense to the physician. Patients with idiopathic retention, typically young females with psychosocial or emotional problems, can often be managed by intermittent urethral self-catheterization.

CONTRAINDICATIONS

Since placement of a suprapubic tube involves some risk, patient selection is important. The procedure should not be performed in a patient whose bladder is not definable. Although no absolute reported minimum bladder volume has ever been established, there must be enough urine in the bladder to allow the trocar to penetrate the bladder dome fully without immediately exiting through the base. There also must be enough urine in the bladder to push the bowels free from the anterior surface of the bladder and the entrance of the trocar (Fig. 61–16). If there is doubt about the bladder limits, ultrasound guidance may be used to place the catheter.

Individuals who have a lower abdominal scar and a history of intraperitoneal surgery or irradiation may have adhesions of bowel to the anterior bladder and are at risk for bowel injury during percutaneous cystostomy tube placement. Blind suprapubic cystostomy tube placement in these patients should be avoided. The absence of a lower abdominal scar or irradiation history unfortunately does not totally protect the patient from the risk of bowel or intraperitoneal injury.

Patients with bleeding disorders are at relatively greater risk for postinsertion bleeding either into the bladder or into the retropubic space.

EQUIPMENT

The equipment needed for Cystocath placement is listed in Table 61–4.

PROCEDURE

The comments that follow describe the use of the Cystocath set, although with modifications, they are applicable for any type of suprapubic tube.

Preparing the Patient

Having decided that a particular patient is a suitable candidate for the procedure, we prepare him for placement of the device. If necessary, the

Table 61–4. MATERIALS FOR CYSTOCATH
PLACEMENT (AUTHORS' METHOD)

Cystocath set
Urinary cath tray (without catheter)
1 per cent lidocaine (Xylocaine)
10-ml syringe with 22 gauge, 1½″ or 22 gauge, 3½″ spinal needle
Scalpel blade (no. 11)
Urinary collection bag
Cloth or plastic tape
Benzoin (for increasing tape adherence)

lower abdomen is shaved. Povidone-iodine skin preparation or another suitable bactericide is used to cleanse the area. The extra liquid is then wiped off, and the skin is allowed to dry. Next, a 1-ml syringe is half filled with 1 per cent lidocaine, and a 22 gauge, 3½-inch spinal needle is attached. A skin wheal in the proposed site (approximately 2 to 3 cm above the pubic symphysis) is raised, and the subcutaneous tissue and the fascia of the rectus abdominis muscle are infiltrated at a 10- to 20-degree angle toward the pelvis. By the time the rectus fascia has been infiltrated, the syringe is empty (Fig. 61–17).

With the same needle, an attempt is next made to *find* the bladder. Our experience has been that when one can find the bladder with the smaller needle rather than the trocar, success is virtually assured and complications of placement are eliminated.

One finds the bladder by advancing the needle in the prescribed direction while pulling back on the syringe plunger. When the bladder is entered, urine is easily aspirated. The operator should then make a mental note of the angle and the depth of entry. The needle may be left in place. Care should be taken not to advance the needle into the prostatic fossa under the pubis in the male with a large prostate.

Placing the Tube

Having found the bladder, the operator now makes final preparation of the Cystocath apparatus. First, the face plate is inspected and the central hole is enlarged with a scalpel or a scissors. We have found that this is necessary because the trocar insertion will be restrained by the small hole in the face plate and will increase the pressure required to advance the trocar. Enlarging the opening also facilitates cleaning of the entry site.

Next, if the patient's pubic hair line (even after shaving) interferes with satisfactory placement of the face plate hole over the anesthetized skin wheal, part of the lower half of the face plate may be trimmed off. The adhesive bottle is opened, and both the face plate and the patient's skin are covered with adhesive and allowed to dry.

While the adhesive is drying, the tubing is "customized." The bladder end of the tubing has only two side openings supplied by the manufacturer. We always make four or five extra side openings using a scalpel or a scissors. This reduces the possibility of blockage of the tube.

By the time the tubing has been prepared, the face plate is ready for positioning. We position the face plate with the flanges at the 10 and 4 o'clock positions rather than at 9 and 3 o'clock (Fig. 61–18). Positioned in this manner, the tubing will approach the face plate from above the iliac crest, not over it, and will be much more comfortable

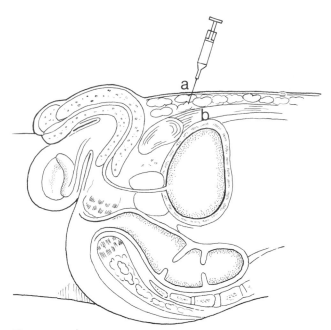

Figure 61–17. Cystostomy tube placement. Anesthetizing the trocar track. After the skin wheal (a) is raised, the suprapubic track for the trocar is anesthetized, including the rectus fascia (b). Anesthetizing until the bladder is penetrated will ensure total comfort for the patient during trocar insertion.

for the patient (see Fig. 61–22). In addition, the iliac crest will "protect" the tubing if the patient turns on his side.

The faceplate is then carefully placed on the skin with the central opening over the skin wheal. When the faceplate is well adhesed, we use the scalpel to make a stab wound in the skin at the entry site. In thin patients, we also incise the previously anesthetized rectus fascia. Incising the

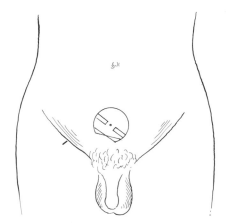

Figure 61–18. Cystostomy tube placement. Faceplate orientation. If the faceplate is rotated with the flange in the 10:00–4:00 o'clock position, the tubing will pass above the iliac crest and be protected by it. We also trim the lower edge of the faceplate to permit placement lower on the abdomen.

skin and the fascia with the scalpel reduces the resistance to the trocar and allows the operator's fingers to sense the layers of the abdominal wall and the bladder without having to "discount" the resistance of the skin and the rectus fascia.

Using the angle of approach and depth of penetration already known from the earlier needle search, one advances the trocar into the bladder (Fig. 61–19). The characteristic release of resistance when the trocar penetrates the bladder muscle and mucosa is an indication of success, but the sine qua non is return of urine through the trocar sheath. After urine is obtained, we advance the trocar another 2 to 3 cm to make sure that the trocar *sheath* as well as the trocar *point* is in the bladder, since urine may escape along the trocar point and into the sheath even if the sheath is not well into the bladder (Fig. 61–20).

The trocar is then withdrawn. Escape of urine is prevented by a finger over the trocar sheath end, and tubing is advanced into the sheath. We always advance the tubing until the black midway mark is inside the trocar sheath. Then the trocar sheath is withdrawn while the tubing is gently advanced. The soft Silastic tubing easily coils in the bladder (Fig. 61–21).

With the trocar sheath withdrawn, the tubing is connected to the three-way urine bag adaptor. The *adaptor* is then positioned in the groove of the face plate flange.

After the urine collection bag has been attached and the three-way stopcock has been opened, the urine may be allowed to drain freely. The puncture

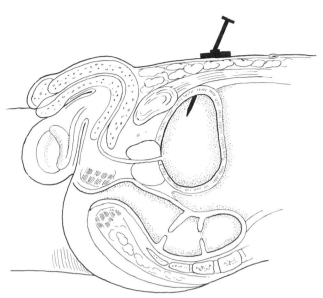

Figure 61–20. Cystostomy tube placement. Trocar position. The trocar should be advanced until its sheath, as well as the point, is fully in the bladder.

site is cleaned, and antimicrobial ointment is placed over the tube entry site. The face plate adhesive may be reinforced with tape at this time.

The tubing of the urine bag *must* be taped to the patient so that the flange and the adaptor do not hold the urine bag up, since they are not designed for this purpose (Fig. 61–22).

COMPLICATIONS

A wide variety of complications have been reported and serve as reminders that suprapubic

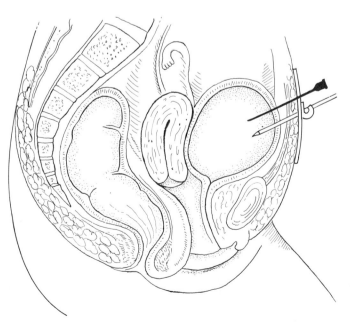

Figure 61–19. Cystostomy tube placement. Needle localization of the bladder. A spinal needle may be used even during trocar insertion to locate the bladder.

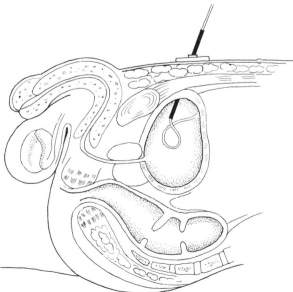

Figure 61–21. Cystostomy tube placement. Tubing position. Enough tubing should be inserted so that it will not pull out of the bladder when the bladder empties.

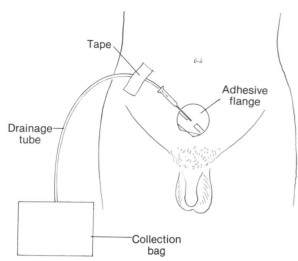

Figure 61–22. Cystostomy tube placement. Urine bag taped firmly to the patient.

cystostomy is not innocuous. Occasionally, despite the best intentions, the tube cannot be positioned or maintained successfully without untoward sequelae (Table 61–5).

The most serious complications involve perforation of the peritoneum or the intraperitoneal contents. Any condition that might fix the anterior peritoneum so low that the filled bladder cannot lift the peritoneum cephalad may result in either transperitoneal bladder puncture or possible perforation of the small or large bowel (Fig. 61–23).[61]

The cystostomy tube that merely traverses the peritoneum may produce a mild ileus, serve as a route for peritoneal infection, or drain the bladder contents into the peritoneum. The last situation should be expected if one of the extra holes of the tubing opens into the peritoneal cavity. Through-and-through bladder penetration with associated rectal, vaginal, or uterine injury is also possible, although the consistent use of small gauge bladder needles and the judicious advancement of the trocar should reduce the incidence.

We believe that our practice of finding the bladder with a small gauge needle helps to reduce bowel injury, but we are cognizant of the fact that even in the most apparently successful bladder punctures a complication may result.

Occasionally, the physician is tempted to continue with suprapubic cystostomy when the bladder is not palpable and has not been found with the needle. Injury of adjacent organs is much more frequent in such circumstances. If the physician reminds himself that the bladder will eventually refill, he will find waiting much more tolerable. If the bladder cannot be found with the trocar at the first pass, one should resist the inclination to "look for" it with the trocar. It is better to backtrack, using the small gauge needle to find the bladder again, and then to advance the trocar alongside the spinal needle (see Fig. 61–19). If one finds a small bladder with the needle only, one may fill it by putting saline into the bladder through the needle. If a catheter can be passed, the bladder may be filled by way of the catheter. Rarely, the Cystocath tubing will end up in a ureteral orifice or in the urethra.[62] By aspirating on the tubing gently while retracting it, one can usually reposition it correctly. Fluoroscopy may be helpful in such circumstances. Since the Cystocath tubing comes coiled up and may still be slightly curled, inserting the tube with the coil pointing posteriorly or laterally will allow the tube to enter the bladder away from the urethra.

Tube drainage may cease for several reasons. A small blood clot or mucus may obstruct the tubing. The tubing may kink in or outside of the bladder.

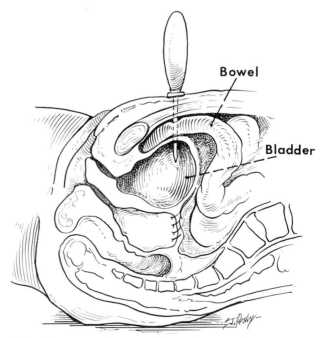

Figure 61–23. Bowel injury in suprapubic cystostomy. Previous injury, radiation, or even an empty bladder may result in the peritoneal reflection dipping below the symphysis pubis and allowing intraperitoneal contents to be interposed into the trocar track. (From Noller, K. L., et al.: Bowel perforation with superpubic cystostomy. Obstet. Gynecol. 48:695, 1976. Used by permission.)

Table 61–5. REPORTED COMPLICATIONS OF SUPRAPUBIC CYSTOSTOMY

Bowel perforation
Intraperitoneal extravasation (without a prior history of surgery)
Extraperitoneal extravasation
Infection of space of Retzius
Ureteral catheterization
Obstruction of tubing by blood, mucus, or kinking
Tubing comes out
Face plate not secure
Hematuria

When kinked, the tube can be irrigated easily, although no fluid can be aspirated.

The catheter tubing may be inadvertently pulled partially out of the bladder, causing extravasation out one of the tubing holes. One can often prevent this problem by inserting enough tubing into the bladder so that minor dislocation will not alter drainage.

Infection may occur at the skin puncture site or anywhere along the course of the tube.[63] Use of antimicrobial ointment daily with cleaning of the tube entry site will reduce purulence around the tube. Deeper infections may result from infected urine or from a superficial infection spreading along the tube to a hematoma at the bladder, rectal, or fascial level. Parenteral antibiotics may be required, although open drainage is rarely needed.

Hematuria is rarely more than a temporary problem.[64] After insertion, bladder irrigation may occasionally be required.

1. Warwick, R., and William, P.L.: Gray's Anatomy, 35th British Edition. Philadelphia, W. B. Saunders Co., 1973, p. 1336.
2. Blandy, J.P.: Acute retention of urine. Br. J. Hosp. Med. 19:109, 1978.
3. Sellett, T.: Iatrogenic urethral rupture due to preinflation of a urethral catheter. JAMA 21:1518, 1971.
4. Walden, T.B.: Urethral catheterization in anasarca. Urology 13:82, 1979.
5. Blandy, J.P.: Urethral stricture. Postgrad. Med. J. 56:383, 1980.
6. Turck, M., Goffe, B., and Petersdorf, R.G.: The urethral catheter and urinary tract infections. J. Urol. 88:834, 1962.
7. Platt, R., Polk, B.F., Murdock, B.S., and Rosner, B.: Mortality associated with nosocomial urinary tract infection. N. Engl. J. Med. 357:637, 1982.
8. Gulhan, P.D., Bayley, B.C., Metzger, W., et al.: The case against the Foley catheter. Initial report. J. Urol. 101:909, 1969.
9. Chapra, R., Fisher, R.D., and French, R.: Phimosis and diabetes mellitus. J. Urol. 127:1101, 1982.
10. Goulding, F.J.: Penile block for postoperative pain relief in penile surgery. J. Urol. 126:337, 1981.
11. Soliman, M.G., and Trumble, N.A.: Nerve block of the penis for postoperative pain relief in children. Anesth. Analg. 57:495, 1978.
12. Campbell, M., and Harrison, J.H. (Eds.): Urology, Vol. 3, 2nd ed. Philadelphia, W. B. Saunders Co., 1963.
13. Schenck, G.F.: The treatment of paraphimosis. Am. J. Surg. 8:329, 1930.
14. Houghton, G.R.: The "iced-glove" method of treatment of paraphimosis. Br. J. Surg. 60:876, 1973.
15. Skoglund, R.W., and Chapman, W.H.: Reduction of paraphimosis. J. Urol. 104:137, 1970.
16. Ratcliff, R.K.: Hyaluronidase in treatment of paraphimosis. JAMA 156:746, 1954.
17. Cletsoway, R.W., and Lewis, E.L.: Treatment of paraphimosis. U.S. Armed Forces J. 8:361, 1957.
18. Cumston, C.G.: The correct operation for paraphimosis. Int. Clinic 2:47, 1920.
19. Barry, C.N.: A simple method for reduction of paraphimosis. J. Urol. 71:450, 1954.
20. Eichenberg, H.A., Amin, M., and Clark, J.: Non-deflating Foley catheters. Int. Urol. Nephrol. 8:171, 1976.
21. Moisey, C.A., and Uiamus, W.: Self-retained balloon catheter—a safe method for removal. Br. J. Urol. 52:67, 1980.
22. Reammon, R.O.: Balloon catheters which will not deflate: Simple method of puncturing balloon. J. Urol. 84:438, 1960.
23. Blandy, J.P.: How to catheterize the bladder. Br. J. Hosp. Med. 26:58, 1981.
24. Lewis, G.J.: Problems with a Foley catheter. J. R. Soc. Med. 73:305, 1980.
25. Sun, A.U.: If the catheter won't deflate after catheterization. Patient Care. 6:69, 1972.
26. Brookes G.: (Urology technician, Harborview Medical Center, Seattle, Washington): Personal communication, 1981.
27. Sood, S.C., and Sabsta, H.: Removing obstructed balloon catheter. Br. Med. J. 4:735, 1972.
28. Stamey, T.A.: Pathogenesis and Treatment of Urinary Tract Infections. Baltimore, Williams & Wilkins, 1980.
29. Huze, L.B., and Beeson, P.B.: Observations on the reliability and safety of bladder catheterization for bacteriologic study of the urine. N. Engl. J. Med. 255:474, 1956.
30. Pryles, P.V.: Percutaneous bladder aspiration and other methods of urine collection for bacteriologic study. Pediatrics 36:128, 1965.
31. Nelson, J.D., and Peters, P.C.: Suprapubic aspiration of urine in term infants. Pediatrics 36:132, 1965.
32. Weuthers, W.T., and Wenzl, J.E.: Suprapubic aspiration. Perforation of the viscus other than the bladder. Am. J. Dis. Child. 117:590, 1969.
33. Deluillar, R.G., Ireland, G.W., and Cass, A.S.: Early exploration in acute testicular conditions. J. Urol. 108:887, 1972.
34. Barker, K., and Raper, R.P.: Torsion of the testis. Br. J. Urol. 36:35, 1964.
35. Dolittle, K.H., Smith, J.P., and Saylor, M.L.: Epididymitis in the prepubertal boy. J. Urol. 108:987, 1972.
36. Berger, R.E., Alexander, E.R., Harnisch, J.P., et al.: Etiology, manifestations, and therapy of acute epididymitis: Prospective study of 50 cases. J. Urol. 121:750, 1979.
37. Milleret, R., and Liaras, H.: Ultrasonic diagnosis and therapy of torsion of the testes. J. Urol. 107:35, 1974.
38. Levy, B.: The diagnosis of torsion of the testicle using the Doppler stethoscope. J. Urol. 113:63, 1975.
39. Perri, A., Slacha, G., Feldman, A., Kendall, A.R., and Karafin, L.: The Doppler stethoscope and the diagnosis of the acute scrotum. J. Urol. 116:598, 1976.
40. Pederson, J.F., Holm, H.H., and Huld, T.: Torsion of the testes diagnosed by ultrasound. J. Urol. 113:66, 1975.
41. Perri, A.J., Rose, J., Feldman, A.E., Parker, J., Karafin, L., and Kardull, A.R.: An evaluation of the role of the Doppler stethoscope and the testicular scan in the diagnosis of torsion of the spermatic cord. Invest. Urol. 15:275, 1978.
42. Thompson, I., LaTourette, H., Chadwick, S., Ross, G., and Licht, E.: Diagnosis of testicular torsion using Doppler ultrasonic flowmeter. Urology 6:706, 1975.
43. Rodriquez, D.D., Rodriquez, W.C., Rivera, J.J., Rodriquez, S., and Otero, A.C.: Doppler ultrasound versus testicular scanning in the evaluation of the acute scrotum. J. Urol. 125:343, 1981.
44. Brereton, R.J.: Limitation of the Doppler flow meter in the diagnosis of the "acute scrotum" in boys. Br. J. Urol. 53:380, 1981.
45. Blackshear, W.M., Phillips, D.J., and Strandness, D.E.: Pulsed Doppler assessment of normal human femoral artery velocity patterns. J. Surg. Res. 27:73, 1979.
46. Smith, D.P.: Treatment of epididymitis by infiltration at spermatic cord with procaine hydrochloride. J. Urol. 46:74, 1941.
47. Nazrallah, P.F., Murzone, D., and King, L.R.: Falsely negative Doppler examinations in testicular torsion. J. Urol. 118:194, 1977.
48. King, L.M., Sekasan, S.K., and Schwantker, F.N.: Untwisting in delayed treatment of torsion of the spermatic cord. J. Urol. 112:217, 1974.
49. Frazier, W.J., and Bucy, J.G.: Manipulation of torsion of the testicle. J. Urol. 114:415, 1975.

50. Campbell, M.: A new fenestrated trocar for introduction of balloon catheter in cystostomy, nephrostomy and pyelostomy. J. Urol. 65:160, 1951.
51. Hodgkinson, C.P., and Hodari, H.: Trocar suprapubic cystostomy for postoperative bladder drainage in the female. Am. J. Obstet. Gynecol. 96:773, 1966.
52. Simon, G., and Berdon, W.E.: Suprapubic bladder puncture for voiding cystourethrography. J. Pediatr. 81:555, 1972.
53. Cameron, E.: Urinary retention managed without urethral catheterization. Lancet 2:606, 1963.
54. Sinha, A.K.: Intracath in suprapubic cystostomy. Lancet 2:1160, 1971.
55. Mattingly, R.: Commentary on #51. Am. J. Obstet. Gynecol. 96:782, 1966.
56. Hey, H.W.: Asepsis in prostatectomy. Br. J. Surg. 33:415, 1945.
57. Ingram, J.M.: Suprapubic cystostomy by trocar catheter. Am. J. Obstet. Gynecol. 113:1108, 1972.
58. Tinckler, L.F.: Intracath in suprapubic cystostomy. Lancet 2:206, 1971.
59. Mitchell, J.P., and Gingell, J.C.: Intracath in suprapubic cystostomy. Lancet 1:206, 1972.
60. Greene, W.R., McLeod, D.G., and Mittemeyer, B.R.: Nonoperative suprapubic urinary drainage. Am. Fam. Phys. 16:136, 1977.
61. Noller, K.L., Pratt, J.H., and Symonds, R.E.: Bowel perforation with suprapubic cystostomy. Obstet. Gynecol. 48 (Suppl. 1): 67s, 1976.
62. McLeod, W.L. Commentary on #57. Am. J. Obstet. Gynecol. 113:1112, 1972.
63. Langley, I.I.: Suprapubic cystostomy. Postgrad. Med. 50:171, 1972.
64. Wolf, H., Olsen, S., and Madsen, P.O.: Suprapubic trocar cystostomy with balloon catheter. Scand. J. Urol. Nephrol. 1:66, 1967.

62

Radiologic Procedures for the Evaluation of Urinary Tract Trauma

GEOFFREY E. HERTER, M.D.
MARTIN SCHIFF, JR., M.D.

Trauma to the urinary tract is frequently seen in emergency departments. The signs of genitourinary (GU) trauma are not usually subtle, and the injury often can be thoroughly evaluated in the emergency department setting. Radiologic imaging of the entire urinary tract can be performed quickly and easily, yielding valuable information to the physician prior to any surgical intervention. The timing of the radiologic evaluation may be challenging to the emergency physician when faced with a critically ill patient with multiple-systems trauma. Nonetheless, rarely during resuscitation is a patient not in the emergency department long enough for at least a minimal but critical diagnostic GU evaluation. The extent of such an evaluation, of course, must be determined by the physicians involved in each situation.

Indications for Evaluation

The urinary tract includes the kidneys, ureters, bladder, and urethra. The primary indications for radiologic evaluation of these structures after trauma are hematuria, blood at the urethral meatus, pelvic fracture in the male, and a high index of suspicion.

HEMATURIA

Gross hematuria is an absolute indication for further diagnostic work-up. An intravenous pyelogram (IVP) is definitely indicated, and retrograde cystourethrography should also be considered when significant pelvic or lower abdominal trauma is suggested. In the authors' series, the degree of hematuria corresponded to the severity of injury in the lower urinary tract. In a recent review of 234 patients with traumatic pelvic fractures, no single major lower tract injury was seen in the absence of gross hematuria.[1] Nonetheless, this association may not always be true, and any degree of hematuria after *major* trauma should be considered significant and should be evaluated with an IVP.

Approximately 8 to 10 per cent of *blunt* abdominal trauma is associated with urinary tract injuries.[2] Seven per cent of gunshot wounds and 5.9 per cent of stab wounds to the abdomen resulted in *penetrating* wounds to the kidney in one large series.[3] A few patients with significant urinary tract trauma present without red cells in the urine. Approximately 25 per cent of renal pedicle disruptions may not even have microhematuria, and complete ureteral transection may also be present without hematuria.[4] Although these injuries should always be considered in the setting of flank contusion, transverse process or lower rib fractures, penetrating flank trauma, or other similar localized flank injury in the absence of hematuria, they are relatively rare.

Even in *minor* blunt trauma to the flank, urinalysis is routinely indicated. Microhematuria is a relatively frequent occurrence following seemingly minor injuries, and treatment may vary in different medical centers. The authors have arbitrarily designated greater than 20 red cells per high-powered field on a spun specimen as an indication for an IVP following *minor* blunt trauma. If the IVP is normal, the patient is sent home for bed rest or decreased activity, with repeat urinalysis in 24 to 48 hours. If, on the other hand, the urinalysis shows less than 20 red blood cells per high-powered field and if the patient is otherwise totally stable, he is usually sent home without an IVP and a repeat urinalysis is obtained in 24 to 48 hours. If any red cells are present in the urine at this time, an IVP is performed. Additionally, we believe that microhematuria in the presence of any parenchymal abnormality on IVP requires admission to the hospital, with bed rest, until the urine is cleared of blood.

BLOOD AT THE URETHRAL MEATUS (URETHRAL INJURY)

When there is evidence of major trauma, placement of a Foley catheter has become the standard method of monitoring urine output. Blood at the urethral meatus, however, may mean partial or complete urethral disruption. Great care should be taken with any urethral instrumentation. We believe that monitoring urine output during *initial* resuscitation of the critically injured patient is rarely used clinically, and the hemodynamic stability of the patient can readily be ascertained by monitoring vital signs and central venous pressure until a retrograde urethrogram can be performed. A urethrogram can easily be done in the emergency department or on the operating room table if the patient needs immediate surgical intervention for other life-threatening injuries. The patient suffers a disservice if a partial urethral tear is converted to a complete disruption of the urethra by the attempted passage of a catheter. Therefore, we consider urethral instrumentation to be *contraindicated* if blood is seen at the meatus prior to retrograde urethrography. If the patient is able to void easily, it is unlikely that he has a urethral injury but the presence of blood at the meatus still mandates urethrography before catheterization. Patients should not be forced to void, however, because extravasation of urine is undesirable.

The posterior male urethra, which includes the membranous portion and the prostatic urethra, is injured more frequently than the anterior urethra. The urogenital diaphragm fixes the membranous urethra; the prostate and prostatic urethra are firmly attached to the posterior surface of the symphysis pubis by the puboprostatic ligaments. Blunt trauma and pelvic fractures (especially if the bladder is full) may result in shearing forces that partially or completely avulse portions of the firmly fixed posterior urethra. Usually the bladder and prostate gland are sheared from the membranous urethra, resulting in a complete urethral disruption (Fig. 62–1). The female urethra is short and relatively mobile and generally escapes injury in blunt trauma. Occasionally, a significant pelvic

Figure 62–1. A common posterior urethral injury is disruption of the membranous urethra. In this case, a distended bladder and attached prostate gland are sheared from the fixed membranous urethra. Note the development of a perivesical hematoma and the presence of a "high-riding" prostate gland.

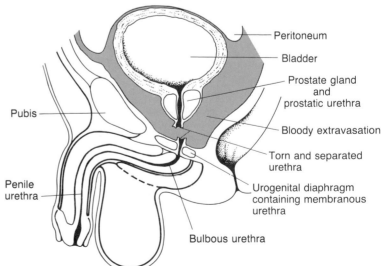

Peritoneum

Bladder

Prostate gland and prostatic urethra

Bloody extravasation

Torn and separated urethra

Urogenital diaphragm containing membranous urethra

Pubis

Penile urethra

Bulbous urethra

fracture will result in avulsion of the female urethra at the bladder neck. Direct injuries to the female urethra may also occur secondary to penetrating trauma of the vagina or perineum.

Contusions or lacerations of the anterior male urethra usually occur when the bulbous urethra is compressed against the inferior surface of the symphysis pubis. This happens most commonly as a result of straddle injuries in males but may result from any blunt perineal trauma. Significant trauma to the penile urethra is rare when there are no penetrating injuries or urethral instrumentation. Anterior urethral injuries may result in extravasation of blood or urine into the penis, scrotum, perineum, or anterior abdominal wall. This is in contrast to posterior urethral injuries, in which blood and urine extravasate into the pelvis (Fig. 62–2).

The rectal examination is used by some physicians for the evaluation of urethral disruption. If the prostate is clearly high-riding or if a hematoma can be felt, one should be suspicious of a posterior urethral injury, and a retrograde urethrogram should be performed prior to attempted catheterization. Nonetheless, a normal rectal examination alone should never be considered definitive evidence of an intact urethra when other clinical signs indicate that further evaluation is necessary.

PELVIC FRACTURE IN THE MALE

Pelvic fracture in the male is an indication for retrograde urethrography with cystography. Urethral injuries from pelvic fractures in the female are extremely rare and thus are seldom of concern. The incidence of lower-tract injuries in males with pelvic fractures ranges from 7.5 to 25 per cent. Approximately 80 per cent of all urethral injuries are associated with pelvic fractures.[1] Because of the severity of late complications, that is, severe stricturing that requires difficult surgical correction, it is paramount that these injuries are not overlooked initially.

HIGH INDEX OF SUSPICION

A high index of suspicion of urinary tract injury is an indication in itself for further diagnostic study. Flank tenderness, abrasions, hematoma of the flank or upper quadrant, hypotension without obvious cause, penetrating flank trauma, or external genitalia trauma should lead one to suspect urinary tract injury. We believe that erring on the side of excessive diagnostic tests is preferable to overlooking a significant injury.

Contraindications

There are few contraindications to performing an IVP or a retrograde cystourethrogram. Known previous reaction to intravenous contrast material is the most obvious contraindication, and in such cases, when the patient is hemodynamically stable, a renal scan or computed tomography (CT) scan may be obtained to demonstrate the integrity

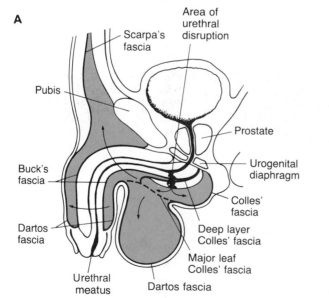
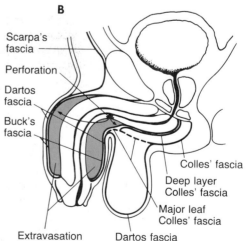

Figure 62–2. *A*, Disruption of the anterior urethra (bulbous urethra) occurs with straddle-type injuries in the male. There may be extravasation of urine and blood into the perineum, scrotum, or anterior abdominal wall. Note that Buck's fascia has been penetrated in this diagram. *B*, Anterior urethral injury in which Buck's fascia remains intact. In this diagram, extravasation will result in a swollen and ecchymotic penis. Such an injury may occur with instrumentation of the anterior urethra.

of the renal pedicle and cortical outline. CT scanning is becoming increasingly available as a 24-hour-a-day emergency study. As yet, our personal experience is limited, but there is no question that renal detail and evidence of extravasation are well outlined by the CT scan. Another advantage of CT is that multiple organs can be evaluated simultaneously. In the past, our policy was to use arteriography when there was total or partial nonvisualization of the kidney. Several studies have been done in which CT scans were found to be helpful in evaluating renal trauma.[2, 5] In the future, as wider experience in CT scanning becomes available, it may assume a greater role in the work-up of renal trauma.

Technique

Kidney, ureter, and bladder (KUB). The plain film of the abdomen taken in such a way as to include the kidneys, ureters, bladder, and full pelvis is essential for diagnostic purposes as well as for comparison of all future contrast films. Important diagnostic signs that may alert the physician to the possibility of urinary tract injury include the following:

1. Loss of one or both psoas shadows secondary to blood in the retroperitoneum.
2. Spinal curvature secondary to splinting—concave to the side of the injury.
3. Lower rib or transverse process fractures, both of which may be close to the kidney.
4. Pelvic fracture. The KUB should never be omitted, because radiopaque shadows seen on the plain film must be differentiated from extravasation on later contrast films.

IVP. Although formal intravenous pyelography with computed tomography can and should be performed in the radiology department on stable trauma patients, valuable time should not be lost if the patient is unstable and likely to require immediate surgery. We have found that an abbreviated IVP with one or two post-contrast injection films can provide critical information concerning the kidneys and ureters and can be performed with ease in the emergency department. As part of our trauma room equipment, two 50-ml syringes filled with 60 per cent Renografin are always ready for injection. These syringes are kept available in the same place in the trauma room, and we have found that this saves time during resuscitation of the critically injured patient. As soon as plain films have been taken, 100 ml of contrast material is injected intravenously through either a central or peripheral line. The injection should be performed quickly over 30 to 60 seconds. The physicians may continue with other resuscitative measures while the radiology technicians prepare for additional films. We routinely take a single 10-minute KUB initially, followed by a 30-minute film if necessary and if the patient is still in the emergency department. These films are examined for the following:

1. Bilateral and symmetrical nephrograms indicating the integrity of the renal pedicles.
2. Evidence of major parenchymal disruption (Fig. 62–3).
3. Evidence of major urinary extravasation (Fig. 62–4).
4. Presence of two kidneys and their position within the retroperitoneum. There may indeed be contrast outlining the bladder at the time of the 10-minute or 30-minute film. This abbreviated IVP should never be used as the definitive examination of the bladder. A formal cystogram should always be performed if bladder injury is suspected.

Urethrogram. Several techniques have been used to perform the retrograde urethrogram, two of which will be described. The choice of technique is not as important as attention to a few critical details. First, a plain film must be taken prior to injection of contrast material. For the injection film, we prefer to oblique the patient's pelvis slightly on a foam wedge under one hip. This position enables a better view of the entire urethra and prevents the double image of the proximal pendulous and bulbar urethra from being superimposed. Second, after sterile preparation, an 8-French Foley catheter is placed into the urethral meatus and the balloon is inflated in the fossa navicularis or further up the pendulous urethra with approximately 2 to 3 ml of sterile water or saline. Inflation of the balloon, when performed slowly, causes minimal discomfort to the patient. Third, approximately 10 to 15 ml of suitable contrast material is then *slowly* injected into the Foley catheter (Fig. 62–5). Forceful injection may cause intravasation of contrast material into the venous drainage of the urethra. We routinely use diluted solutions of either 50 per cent Hypaque, Cystografin 40, or Renografin 60. Note that all materials are diluted to less than a 10 per cent solution using a sterile saline for the diluent. For example, Renografin 60 is a 60 per cent solution, so it is diluted slightly more than 4:1 with saline to produce a dilute solution. Likewise, Cystografin 40 is a 40 per cent solution and Hypaque 50 is a 50 per cent solution; both are diluted similarly. Fourth, during the injection, a film is taken.

An alternative to this method is to take a sterile irrigating-tipped piston syringe with the contrast material drawn up and place the lubricated tip directly into the urethral meatus. A tight seal is made by compression of the glans around the tip of the syringe with one hand, while injection is accomplished with the other (Fig. 62–6).

The extravasation of contrast material from a tear in the urethra appears as a flamelike area outside the urethral contour. Figure 62–7A–C

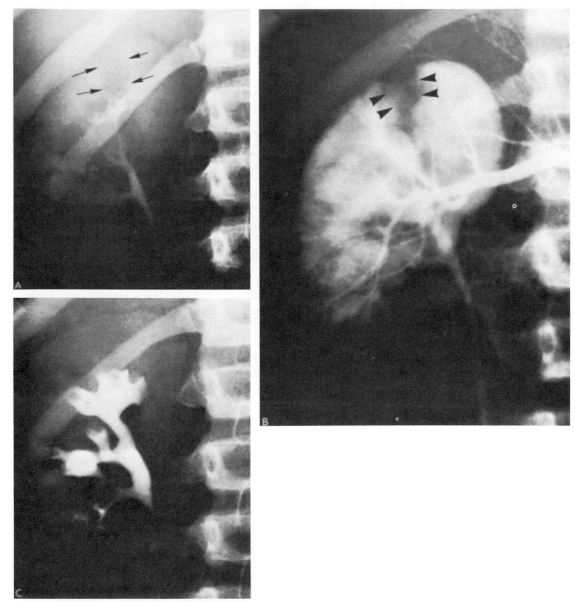

Figure 62–3. *A,* IVP delineates a defect on a nephrogram in the right superior pole (arrows) of the kidney in an 11-year-old boy who fell from a tree. *B,* Arteriogram substantiates a sharply demarcated laceration (between arrows). *C,* Delayed film after arteriogram, showing intact pelvicalyceal system. (From Richter, M. W., Lytton, B., Myerson, D., and Grnja, V.: Radiology of genitourinary trauma. Radiol. Clin. North Am. XI(3):600, 1973.)

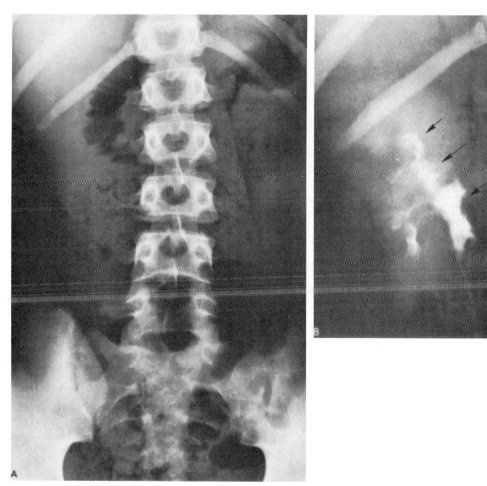

Figure 62–4. This 15-year-old girl presented with right flank pain and gross hematuria after falling down a flight of stairs. *A*, Scout film shows scoliosis, concavity toward the injured kidney, and loss of psoas and renal outlines. *B*, Excretory urography shows extravasation of contrast (arrows) from a tear in the pelvicalyceal system.

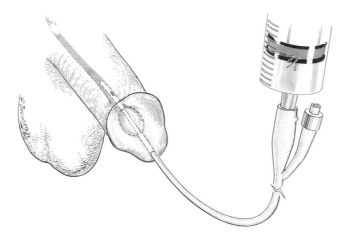

Figure 62–5. Urethrogram using a Foley catheter (8F). Slowly inflate the balloon with 2 ml of sterile fluid; then slowly inject 10 ml of a 10 per cent solution of contrast material through the catheter lumen (see text).

shows examples of urethral injuries diagnosed by urethrography. If contrast material is seen within the bladder along with extravasation, it is said that the urethral injury may be partial in nature rather than a complete disruption. Occasionally, contrast material can be seen in the venous drainage of the periurethral area (Fig. 62–8). Sometimes it is mistaken for extravasation; however, it is of no consequence.

If a Foley catheter has been successfully placed into the bladder and yet a partial urethral injury is still suspected, the injury can be easily seen without removing the catheter. The lubricated end of a pediatric feeding tube is placed into the pendulous urethra beside the existing Foley catheter. A seal can once again be obtained with compression of the glans using one hand and injecting contrast material via a Luer-Lok syringe with the other (Fig. 62–9). In this way, extravasation can be easily detected. It should be noted, however, that successful placement of a Foley catheter obviates the need for further work-up of a possible urethral tear in the emergency setting,

because an indwelling catheter alone is appropriate initial management for this type of injury.

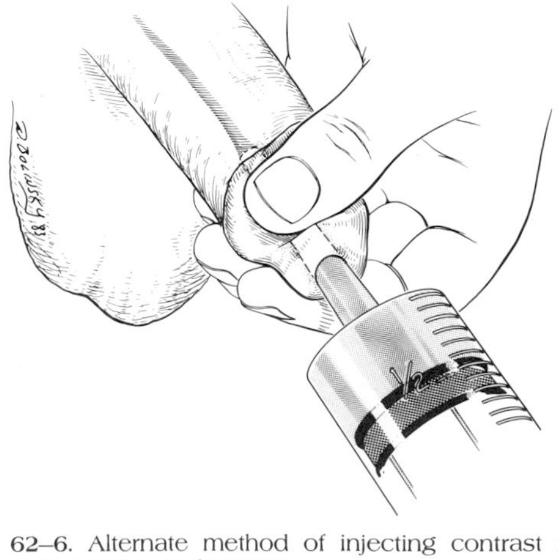

Cystogram. A cystogram is performed with a Foley catheter in place. Again, a plain film of the pelvis is taken so that it can be used as a comparison for all further films. After this film has been taken, we routinely obtain two other films, a fill-up film and a drain-out film. The technique involves gravity drainage of contrast material into the bladder, performed by attaching a 60-ml catheter-tip syringe to the Foley catheter and holding it above the level of the patient's bladder. The contrast material is then poured into the syringe and allowed to drain by gravity into the bladder. Again, we use a *dilute solution of contrast material* in the event of extravasation. It has been our policy when performing both urethrograms and cystograms to use less than a 10 per cent concentration of the contrast materials previously mentioned, because extravasation into periurethral or perivesical tissues may cause considerable reaction with higher concentrations. See the discussion in the section entitled Urethrogram for preparation of the solutions. We have never found that this dilute mixture compromises the quality of the study. Optimally, the bladder should be filled to approximately 400 ml and the catheter should then be occluded with a Kelly clamp. Volumes of 250 ml or less have been associated with false-negative retrograde cystograms.[6] An anteroposterior film of the pelvis is taken with the Foley clamped. At times, the patient may have difficulty cooperating due to head injuries or pain, and, if severely injured, he may have involuntary bladder contractions, causing contrast material to back up into the syringe. If this is the case, one may have to be satisfied with somewhat less than adequate films. Care must be taken to ensure that the contrast material is not spilled on the patient during the procedure. If this does happen, it can lead to spurious findings on the fill-up film. Once

Figure 62–6. Alternate method of injecting contrast material before performing a urethrogram.

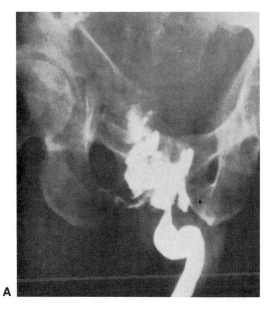

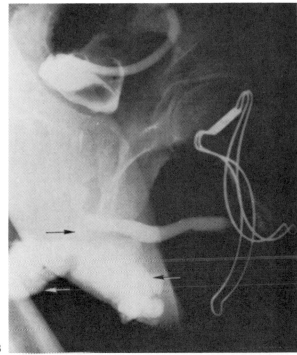

Figure 62–7. *A,* Retrograde urethrogram. Urethrogram in case of supramembranous rupture. Dye extravasation is typical of that seen with this type of injury. (From Morehouse, D. D., and MacKinnon, K. J.: Posterior urethral injury: etiology, diagnosis, initial management. Urol. Clin. North Am. 4(3):74, 1977.) *B,* Rupture at proximal bulbous urethra into scrotum (arrows). *C,* Residual contrast material within perineum and scrotum. (From Richter, M. W., Lytton, B., Myerson, D., and Grnja, V.: Radiology of genitourinary trauma. Radiol. Clin. North Am. XI(3):627, 1973.)

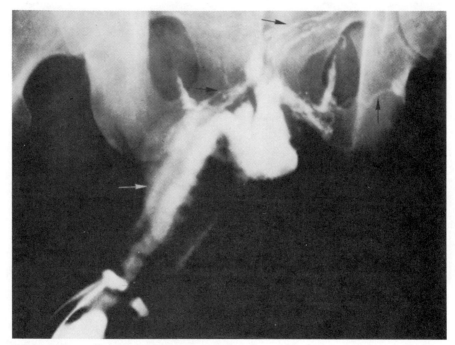

Figure 62–8. Venous intravasation (arrows) during forceful retrograde urethrogram. This may mimic a urethral injury, but its presence is benign. (From Richter, M. W., Lytton, B., Myerson, D., and Grnja, V.: Radiology of genitourinary trauma. Radiol. Clin. North Am. XI(3):626, 1973.)

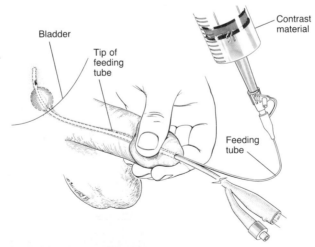

Figure 62–9. Evaluation of a urethral injury with a Foley catheter in place. A lubricated pediatric feeding tube has been advanced into the urethra beside the indwelling Foley catheter.

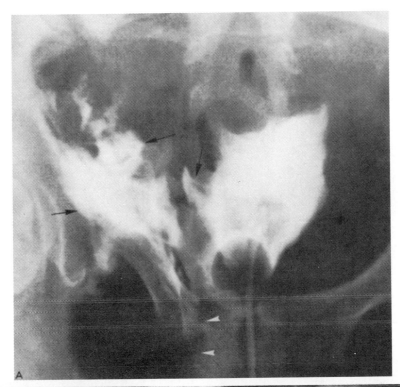

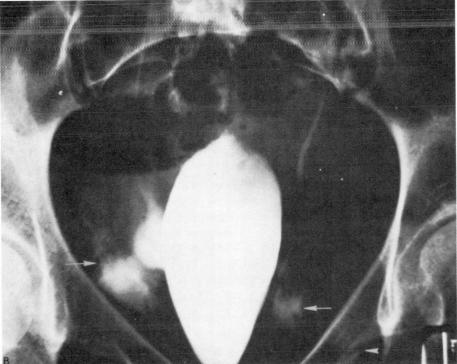

Figure 62–10. Examples of extraperitoneal bladder rupture. *A,* Note amorphous extravasation of contrast material within perivesical space (arrows) in a patient with right pelvic fracture (arrowheads). *B,* Second patient with pelvic fracture (arrowhead) and perivesical hematoma shows tear-drop shape of deformed bladder and extraperitoneal extravasation (arrows). (From Richter, M. W., Lytton, B., Myerson, D., and Grnja, V.: Radiology of genitourinary trauma. Radiol. Clin. North Am. XI(3):623, 1973.)

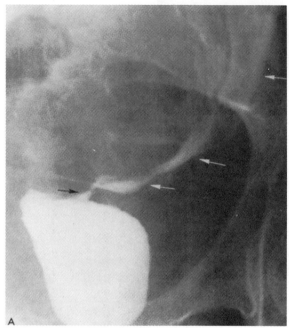

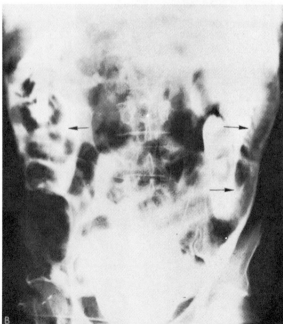

Figure 62–11. Intraperitoneal bladder rupture. *A,* 22-year-old pedestrian hit by an automobile. Note extravasation of contrast material beginning at dome and tracking up left paracolic gutter (arrows). *B,* This 57-year-old man had exfulguration of a tumor at the bladder dome and sustained perforation. A cystogram dramatically demonstrates contrast extravasation outlining bowel loops (arrows) and the paracolic gutters. (Courtesy of Morton A. Bosniak, M. D., New York, New York.) (From Richter, M. W., Lytton, B., Myerson, D., and Grnja, V.: Radiology of genitourinary trauma. Radiol. Clin. North Am. XI(3):623, 1973.)

the fill-up film has been taken, we unclamp the Foley catheter and allow the contrast material to drain out of the bladder. A drain-out film is then taken. This allows visualization of any posterior extravasation that may have been hidden by the distended bladder during the fill-up phase. Extravasation from an injured bladder may be intraperitoneal, extraperitoneal, or both. Extraperitoneal extravasation is usually seen as flamelike areas of contrast material lateral to the bladder into the pelvis (Fig. 62–10). If the contrast material is extravasated intraperitoneally, there is usually an outline of intraperitoneal structures, particularly the bowel, by the contrast material (Fig. 62–11).

Complications

Several possible problems in the diagnosis of urinary tract injury should be emphasized. First, the IVP cystogram should never be used as the definitive examination for a bladder injury. We have been fooled more than once by accepting the normal-appearing cystogram on the IVP, only to find extreme injury to the bladder wall at the time of laparotomy for other injuries. Second, occasionally, during vigorous fluid administration for hypotension or after Mannitol administration for head injury, a brisk diuresis may ensue. We have occasionally seen nonvisualization of both kidneys on a 10- and 30-minute IVP film in these cases, but, later, the patient had normal renal arteriograms. This is probably due to extreme dilution of

contrast material in the former instance or to the brisk clearance of contrast material in the latter. Third, we cannot overemphasize the importance of performing all GU diagnostic studies in the emergency department setting, if possible. Although all studies can be performed intraoperatively, we have always found intraoperative films to be less adequate and more difficult to interpret.

Summary

Trauma to the GU tract is commonly seen in the emergency department. The kidneys, ureters, bladder, and urethra may be involved. By performing any or all three of the basic radiologic tests: the IVP, cystogram, or retrograde urethrogram, the physician can simply, quickly, and accurately assess the status of the urinary tract.

1. Antoci, J. P., and Schiff, M., Jr.: Bladder and urethral injuries with pelvic fractures. J. Urol. 128:25, 1982.
2. McAninch, J. S.: The injured kidney. Monogr. Urol. 4:46, 1983.
3. Carlton, C. E., Scott, R., Jr., and Goldman, M.: The management of penetrating injuries of the kidney. J. Trauma 8:1071, 1968.
4. Stables, D. P., et al.: Traumatic renal artery occlusion. J. Urol. 115:229, 1976.
5. Sandler, C. M., and Toombs, B. D.: Computed tomographic evaluation of blunt renal injuries. Radiology 141:461, 1981.
6. Cass, A. S.: False-negative retrograde cystography with bladder rupture owing to external trauma. J. Trauma 24:168, 1984.

10

NEUROLOGY AND
NEUROSURGERY

63

Insertion of Cervical Traction Devices*

ROBERT G. R. LANG, M.D.

Introduction

Caliper traction devices or "skull tongs" are important not only to immobilize the cervical spine and prevent further injury but also to reduce a fracture-dislocation. Return of vertebral elements to their anatomic position can be associated with marked improvement of a neurologic deficit if spinal cord transection has not occurred.

Skull tongs are inserted to provide steady traction by means of weights attached to the tongs by a cord. The weight of the body provides counter traction. Insertion of skull tongs can be easily carried out in the emergency department using only local anesthetic.

Cervical immobilization should begin in the prehospital care phase of trauma management. Inline manual traction is often required while awaiting radiographs if an unstable cervical fracture is suggested by clinical and historical (mechanism of injury) findings. Caliper traction should complement the more rapidly introduced techniques of cervical immobilization discussed in Chapter 40.

Historical Background

Until the early 1930's, skeletal traction was accomplished by halter, casts, or rings with turnbuckles.[1] These devices were often unsatisfactory because the patient was in a recumbent position and had adjacent injuries, encroachment of the anterior surface of the neck, pain, and pressure sores.

Skeletal skull traction was first described by Crutchfield in 1933.[1] His first case was a woman severely injured in an automobile accident. In addition to a complete fracture-dislocation of the

axis, she had multiple facial lacerations and a compound fracture of the mandible. Ordinary methods for reduction of the cervical fracture could not be used; so, on the suggestion of Dr. Coleman, burr holes were drilled through the outer table in the parietal eminences, Edmonton extension tongs were inserted, and traction was applied.

In the same year, Neubeiser described the use of No. 8 Kirby fishhooks, with the barbs removed, inserted under the zygomatic processes.[2] A device with blunt hooks was later developed by Selmo, but it resulted in disfiguring incisions for insertion under the zygomatic processes.[3] In 1940, Peyton used No. 5 fishhooks, with the barbs removed, inserted under the zygomatic arches percutaneously.[4] This traction device left minimal, if any, scars after removal, and the hooks could be easily maintained while in place.

In 1935, Crutchfield developed small skull tongs,[5] but an unfortunate error in construction made many of the initial instruments almost worthless.[6] For proper application, the maximum spread of the tongs had to be at least 10 cm, whereas many of the defective tongs had spreads less than 7 cm.

Over the years, a variety of skull traction devices were developed, each bearing the name of its developer. Barton, Blackburn, and Vinke are among the better known types. The correctly constructed small tongs of Crutchfield were perhaps the most popular of their time and indeed are still in use in many institutions.

In 1973, Gardner described spring-loaded points for cervical traction.[7] His "skull traction tong" gained popularity very quickly and is now the principal device in use. The spring-loaded points require no skin incision for insertion and can be inserted in minutes. When properly inserted, they rarely pull out and can be left in place for prolonged periods of time. They will readily tolerate up to 65 lb of traction.

In recent years, there has been a tendency toward more aggressive early surgical stabilization of cervical fracture dislocations. The development of the Halo brace has allowed earlier ambulation of patients with unstable cervical spine injuries.[8] Patients who previously remained in tongs on spinal frames for 16 to 20 weeks are now frequently up within 1 to 2 weeks after injury.

Indications

Skull tongs should be inserted in all patients with unstable cervical spine injuries and in those with stable subluxations that need to be reduced prior to immobilization, including fracture-dislocations, subluxations, unilateral and bilateral

*I would like to thank Edean Berglund, Medical Librarian at St. Peter Hospital, for her assistance in obtaining the reference material and my secretary, Teresa Edwards, for typing the manuscript.

locked facets in the lower cervical region (C3 to C7), hangman's fracture (C2 pedicles) with and without subluxation, fractures of the odontoid process, and possibly Jefferson's fracture (ring of the atlas). A pure, severe ligamentous injury, often associated with a teardrop fracture, may also be unstable and require traction.

Insertion of skull tongs by emergency physicians should be carried out without delay in patients who have obvious fracture-dislocations and neurologic deficits when neurosurgical consultation is not rapidly available. Early reduction can sometimes result in a dramatic reversal of neurologic deficit.

Skull tongs are *not* indicated for stable compression fractures of the vertebral bodies or fractures of cervical spinous processes (clay-shovelers' fracture) unless they are associated with severe ligamentous disruption. Skull tongs are also not indicated for thoracic or lumbar fracture-dislocations. Placement of tongs directly over skull fractures is to be avoided.

If instability or if the extent of injury is uncertain despite quality cervical radiographs, the patient's neck should be immobilized in a Philadelphia collar and the patient should be admitted to the hospital and kept at bed rest until muscle spasm resolves. Flexion extension views, with the physician in attendance, can then be carried out under fluoroscopy to determine whether instability is present. Tomography (both standard and computed) should also be considered.

Equipment

Insertion of Gardner-Wells Tongs
Disposable safety razor
Povidone-iodine (Betadine) soap and solution
One per cent lidocaine (Xylocaine) with 1 per 100,000 epinephrine
12-ml syringe
19 gauge 1½-inch needle
27 gauge 1½-inch needle
Gardner-Wells skull tongs
Suitable bed or frame with pulleys and weights for establishing cervical traction
Insertion of Crutchfield Tongs
Disposable safety razor
Povidone-iodine (Betadine) soap and solution
One per cent lidocaine (Xylocaine) with 1 per 100,000 epinephrine
12-ml syringe
19 gauge 1½-inch needle
27 gauge 1½-inch needle
Scalpel handle with No. 11 blade
Sterile metal ruler
Blue marking pen
Twist drill

Twist drill bit with 4-mm point-fixed guard
Crutchfield tongs with minimum spread of 10 mm point to point
Suitable bed or frame with pulleys and weights for establishing cervical traction

Technique

INSERTION OF GARDNER-WELLS TONGS

The scalp is shaved above both ears for a diameter of about 5 cm. The skin is then scrubbed with povidone-iodine soap and painted with povidone-iodine solution.

The tongs are inserted above and slightly behind the ears and below the "equator" of the skull. The points should be located just below the temporal ridges, about 5 cm above the mastoid bone (Figs. 63–1 and 63–2). Placing the tongs directly above the external canals distributes the pulling force too far anterior.

Infiltration of 1 per cent lidocaine with epinephrine is least painful when carried out with a No. 27 gauge 1½-inch needle. It is important to raise a large wheal in the skin and then infiltrate subcutaneous tissue, muscle, and especially the sensitive pericranium. Approximately 4 ml of local anesthetic should be infiltrated on each side.

One side of the tongs has a spring-loaded point to indicate when proper "squeeze pressure" has been achieved. As pressure increases, the indica-

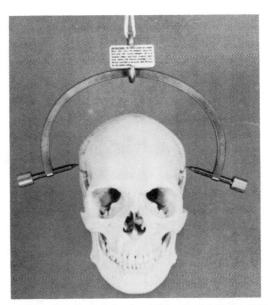

Figure 63–1. Insertion of Gardner-White tongs. The points are applied above the ears and below the "equator." Flexion or extension of the head is determined by height of the pulley. Note that the instructions attached to the tong always face anteriorly. (From Gardner, W. J.: The principle of spring-loaded points for cervical traction. Technical note. J. Neurosurg. 39:543, 1973. Used by permission.)

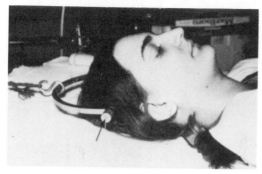

Figure 63–2. When the outer end of the spring-loaded point barely protrudes beyond the flat surface, the spring is fully compressed. (From Gardner, W. J.: The principle of spring-loaded points for cervical traction. Technical note. J. Neurosurg. 39:543, 1973. Used by permission.)

tor begins to emerge. The tongs are inserted by simply applying the points to the infiltrated skin and then tightening each side alternately until the spring indicator on the spring-loaded point barely protrudes from the flat surface of the knurled end (see Fig. 63–2). A protrusion of 1 mm or a distance equal to the thickness of the associated lock washer is generally recommended. This indicates that the spring is fully compressed and is exerting 30 lb of "squeeze" between the points. The tong is tilted (rocked) back and forth to ensure proper seating and is then re-tightened if the indicator has recessed. Traction is now applied. The tightness of the tongs should be checked after 24 hours to ensure that the indicator is flush with the outer flat surface of the screw assembly. The depth of penetration is self-limited by a gradual lessening of spring tension accompanied by an exponential increase in the surface area of contact between the tapered points and the bone.

The skin should be cleaned daily with peroxide around the pin sites. Povidone-iodine solution for cleaning is avoided, because it can cause corrosion of the pins.

INSERTION OF CRUTCHFIELD TONGS

The scalp is shaved for 6 cm on each side of the sagittal midline in line with the mastoid tips. The Crutchfield tongs are opened so that the distance between the tips is 11 cm. The sagittal midline is marked with a sterile blue marking pen, and the tips of the opened tongs are applied to the skin equidistant from the midline (Fig. 63–3). The point at which the tips touch the skin is marked with the pen and then infiltrated with 1 per cent lidocaine with 1 per 100,000 epinephrine. A skin wheal is raised, and approximately 3 ml should be infiltrated at each site down to and including the pain sensitive pericranium. Stab wounds, just large enough to permit entry of the drill bit so that the pins will fit snugly and limit bleeding, are then

made in the skin with a No. 11 blade. A 4-mm point with a fixed guard is used to drill the holes on each side of the skull to a depth of 4 mm. The skull must be drilled to the full depth of the guard or else the points of the tongs may later slip out. After each hole has been drilled, its depth should be checked by slipping the drill point from the edge to the depth of the hole and observing the distance through which it passes.

When drilling is completed, the points of the tongs are slipped into the holes and the instrument is tightened and locked. The tongs should be checked every 2 or 3 days and tightened only when necessary. Pin sites are cleaned with peroxide daily.

APPLICATION OF TRACTION

Traction should be applied in the plane of the articulating facets in order to eliminate an uneven pull on muscles and tendons (Fig. 63–4A). Tongs are frequently applied too far forward on the skull (Fig. 63–4B). The tips of the traction device should be directly perpendicular to the mastoid tips. The minimal corrective pull varies according to the level of injury and the position of the patient while in traction. Weights listed in Table 63–1 are only an approximation for various levels of cervical spine injury with the head of the patient's bed

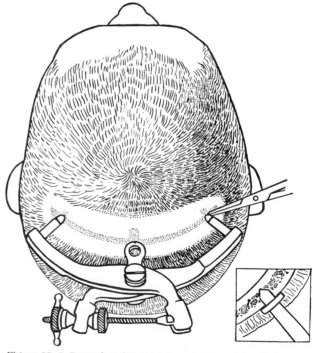

Figure 63–3. Procedure for correct application of the skull tongs developed by Crutchfield. Lines are painted on the scalp to indicate the midline of the skull and the approximate plane of the cervical articulations (through mastoid tip). (From Crutchfield, W. G.: Skeleton traction in treatment of injuries to the cervical spine. JAMA 155:29, 1954. Used by permission.)

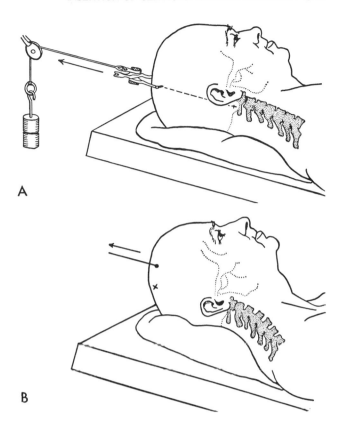

A

B

Figure 63–4. A, Traction correctly applied in the plane of the articulating facets. B, Ineffective traction applied in a plane anterior to that of the articulating facets, which may even increase the deformity in cases of anterior displacement of the upper segment. (From Crutchfield, W. G.: Skeletal traction in treatment of injuries to the cervical spine. JAMA 155:29, 1954. Used by permission.)

elevated no more than 20 degrees. No effort should be made to bring about a rapid reduction. Force sufficient to accomplish this may injure soft tissues and endanger the spinal cord. A minimal corrective pull that provides immediate protection for the spinal cord and begins the reduction that may be complete within 1 hour should be applied. When a very strong pull is used, portable radiographs should be carried out every 15 minutes until it is shown that the force is not too strong. Overdistraction must be avoided at all costs. In some cases, the spinal ligaments are so badly torn that traction considerably widens the intervertebral space and additional serious injury may occur to the spinal cord or cervical nerves. If follow-up radiographic examination does not show complete

reduction and if there is no wide gap between the bodies of the affected vertebrae, additional weight is added gradually. After the vertebrae have been pulled sufficiently apart for them to slip back into position, no additional weight should be added, even though some deformity is present. The same amount of pull or even less pull usually brings about complete and satisfactory reduction within a few days. Analgesia and sedatives may be required to keep the patient comfortable while traction is being applied. As soon as satisfactory alignment has been obtained, the pull for holding the corrected position is reduced to a minimum (5 to 7 lb).

Complications

The potentially most serious complication with application of skull tongs for cervical traction is overdistraction and worsening of the patient's neurologic condition. This complication has been reported in several cases.[9] Simple traction on the patient's shoulders for visualization of lower cervical vertebrae during a portable cervical radiograph has also resulted in distraction.[10] Immediate follow-up radiographs are needed after application of tongs, after the addition of any weight, and at regular intervals while the patient is in traction. Muscle relaxants such as diazepam (Valium) and analgesics will significantly reduce the amount of weight required for reduction and maintenance of

Table 63–1. SUGGESTED WEIGHTS FOR THE TREATMENT OF FRACTURES AND DISLOCATIONS AT VARIOUS LEVELS IN THE CERVICAL SPINE

Level	Minimum Weight (lb)	Maximum Weight (lb)
1st	5	10
2nd	6	10–12
3rd	8	10–15
4th	10	15–20
5th	12	20–25
6th	15	20–30
7th	18	25–35

(From Crutchfield, W. G.: Skeletal traction in treatment of injuries to the cervical spine. JAMA 155:31, 1954.)

position; overdistraction is likely to occur if the amount of weight is not adequately reduced during a procedure.

Skull tongs may pull out if they are not checked periodically for tightness, and perforation of the inner table has been reported with both types of tongs.[1, 11] Inner-table penetration can be prevented by correct application of the tongs and by not overtightening them. Periodic tangential views of the skull will provide early identification of inner-table perforation and may prevent secondary complications, such as intracranial bleeding or brain abscess. Infection around the pin sites is another frequent problem. Most infections are localized cellulitis and can be prevented by regular cleaning with hydrogen peroxide and by keeping the pin sites shaved. Osteomyelitis and brain abscess have been reported infrequently.[12]

Conclusions

Skull traction devices are an effective way to reduce fracture-dislocations and stabilize the cervical spine.

Ease of application of Gardner-Wells tongs makes them preferable for use in the emergency department, but Crutchfield tongs are better tolerated by the patient when prolonged traction is anticipated.

Application of skull tongs for cervical traction to reduce a fracture-dislocation is best done under the care of a neurosurgeon or orthopedic surgeon who has had training in spinal injuries. In circumstances in which these specialists are not immediately available, early reduction of a fracture-dislocation prior to transfer may improve a patient's neurologic deficit by relieving pressure on the spinal cord and its vascular supply. Adequate precautions against overdistraction must always be taken.

1. Crutchfield, W. G.: Skeletal traction for dislocation of the cervical spine. South. Surg. 2:156, 1933.
2. Neubeiser, B. L.: A method of skeletal traction for neck extension. J. Missouri Med. Assoc. 30:495, 1933.
3. Selmo, J. D.: Traction on the zygomatic process for cervicovertebral injuries. Am. J. Surg. 46:405, 1939.
4. Peyton, W. T., Hall, H. B., and French, L. A.: Hook traction under zygomatic arch in cervical spine injuries. Surg. Gynecol. Obstet. 79:311, 1944.
5. Crutchfield, W. G.: Further observations on treatment of fracture dislocations of cervical spine with skeletal traction. Surg. Gynecol. Obstet. 63:513, 1936.
6. Crutchfield, W. G.: Skeletal traction in treatment of injuries to the cervical spine. JAMA 155:29, 1954.
7. Gardner, W. J.: The principle of spring-loaded points for cervical traction. Technical note. J. Neurosurg. 39:543, 1973.
8. Nickel, V. L., Perry, J., Garrett, A., et al.: The Halo. A spinal skeletal traction fixation device. J. Bone Joint Surg. 50:1400, 1968.
9. Fried, L. C.: Cervical spinal cord injury during skeletal traction. JAMA 229:181, 1974.
10. Kaufman, H. H., Harris, J. H., Jr., Spencer, J. A., and Kopanisky, D. R.: Danger of traction during radiography for cervical trauma (letter). JAMA 247:2369, 1982.
11. Feldman, R. A., and Khayyat, G. F.: Perforation of the skull by a Gardner-Wells tong. J. Neurosurg. 44:119, 1976.
12. Weisl, H.: Unusual complications of skull caliper traction. J. Bone and Joint Surg. 54B:143, 1972.

Introduction

Head injury, termed the *silent epidemic* by the National Head Injury Foundation, disables 30,000 to 50,000 people a year in the United States,[1] and in most published trauma series, it accounts for approximately half the fatalities.[2] Although up to 60 per cent of deaths from head injury occur before people are admitted to the hospital,[3] an intracranial hematoma will be present in about 40 per cent of unconscious patients with head injuries who arrive in the emergency department.[4] The mortality rate of these patients has been quoted at a staggering 45 to 90 per cent.[4]

If we assume that tentorial herniation is an emergency condition that becomes more profound with time, early decompression should result in better survival with less neurologic deficit. Indeed, few medical conditions require more urgent care. Clearly, there is a large group of patients who might benefit from emergency burr holes or twist drill trephination when other conservative measures for lowering intracranial pressure have failed.

Intracranial Anatomy and Pathophysiology

An understanding of the basic pathophysiology of transtentorial herniation is essential for everyone who treats head injured patients. The cranial cavity is surrounded by a rigid nondistendable structure, the skull, and divided into compartments by the semi-rigid densely fibrous folds of dura mater: the falx cerebri and tentorium cerebelli (Fig. 64–1). There are three components within the cranial cavity: cerebrospinal fluid (CSF), blood, and semigelatinous brain. If there is any addition to the volume of the intracranial cavity by hematoma, pus, edema, or tumor, there must be a corresponding decrease in the volume of one or more of the three original components; otherwise, intracranial pressure rises. Compensation does indeed occur when CSF is expressed from the ventricles and subarachnoid cisterns, when blood is expressed from the collapsible veins, and, in cases of slow growing tumors, when a certain amount of interstitial fluid is squeezed from the brain itself. Once the volume of the mass exceeds the compensating capacity of the intracranial components, pressure rises very rapidly, often within minutes, and brain shift occurs from one compartment to another. Because of the attachment of cranial nerves and delicate blood vessels, the brain tolerates shift very poorly. In the case of an expanding temporal epidural hematoma, the most medial part of the brain, the uncus, will begin to pass into the tentorial notch (uncal herniation) and the cingulate gyrus will pass under the falx (subfalcine

64

Emergency Neurosurgical Procedures*

ROBERT G. R. LANG, M.D.

EMERGENCY DRAINAGE OF TRAUMATIC INTRACRANIAL HEMATOMAS

herniation) (Fig. 64–2). The herniating uncus commonly exerts pressure on the oculomotor nerve in the tentorial notch, resulting in pupillary dilation on the side of the hematoma (Fig. 64–3). Pupillary dilation is the most reliable sign for determining the side of the hematoma but is accurate in only 80 per cent of the cases.[5] When pupillary dysfunction does occur contralateral to the mass lesion, it is often due to direct pressure of the tentorium cerebelli on the displaced oculomotor nerve contralateral to the mass. As brain shift continues, the opposite cerebral peduncle can also be forced against the free edge of the tentorium, producing extremity paralysis on the same side of the hematoma (Kernohan's notch) (see Fig. 64–2). Direct pressure on the ipsilateral cerebral peduncle by the mass can likewise produce contralateral paralysis. Thus, paralysis is not as accurate a localizing sign as is pupillary dilation and can be present on the same or opposite side of the hematoma. Further herniation and shift of the midbrain will result in tearing of delicate perforating vessels and the characteristic midbrain hemorrhages of Duret (Fig. 64–4). At this point, irreversible damage has occurred. Damage to the midbrain reticular formation results in deep unconsciousness and cessation of eye movements, and the pupils become fixed at midposition.

The infratentorial compartment is much smaller than the two supratentorial compartments; compensatory mechanisms are exhausted much more quickly, and volumes tolerated are much smaller. Patients with initial symptoms of drowsiness, in-

*I would like to thank Edean Berglund, Medical Librarian at St. Peter Hospital, for her assistance in obtaining the reference material and my secretary, Teresa Edwards, for typing the manuscript.

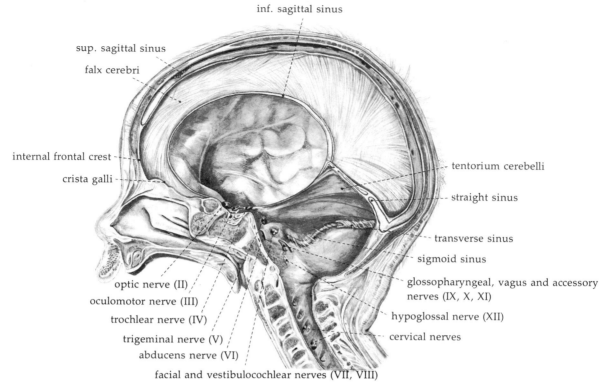

Figure 64–1. Folds of the dura mater. (From Grant, J.C.B.: An Atlas of Anatomy, 5th ed. Baltimore, Williams & Wilkins, 1962. Used by permission.)

coordination, ataxia, and nystagmus will suddenly become deeply unconscious, apneic, and decerebrate. Bradycardia and wide pulse pressure from direct brainstem pressure are more common with infratentorial masses. There can be upward herniation through the tentorial notch or downward herniation of cerebellar tonsils through the foramen magnum (tonsillar herniation) (Fig. 64–5). Infratentorial hematomas are difficult to diagnose without computed tomography. If a fracture is

seen extending through the occipital bone to the foramen magnum, one should suspect an infratentorial hematoma.

Historical Background

Successful evacuation of traumatic intracranial hematomas has been carried out since ancient times. Neolithic skulls more than 4000 years old have been found with fractures and manmade defects that suggest surgical removal of bone (Fig.

Figure 64–2. Intracranial shifts from supratentorial lesions. The drawing on the left shows the relationships of the various supratentorial compartments as seen in a coronal section. The drawing on the right illustrates herniation of the cingulate gyrus under the falx (1), herniation of the temporal lobe into the tentorial notch (2), compression of the opposite cerebral peduncle against the unyielding tentorium, producing Kernohan's notch (3), and downward displacement of the brain stem through the tentorial notch (4). (From Plum, F., and Posner, J.B.: The Diagnosis of Stupor and Coma, 2nd ed. Philadelphia, F.A. Davis Co., 1972. Used by permission.)

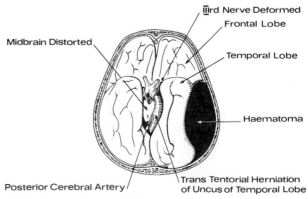

Figure 64–3. Lateral tentorial herniation. A view of the undersurface of the cerebrum shows the distortion produced by a hematoma in the right temporal region. (From Jennett, B., and Teasdale, G.: Management of Head Injuries. Philadelphia, F.A. Davis Co., 1980. Used by permission.)

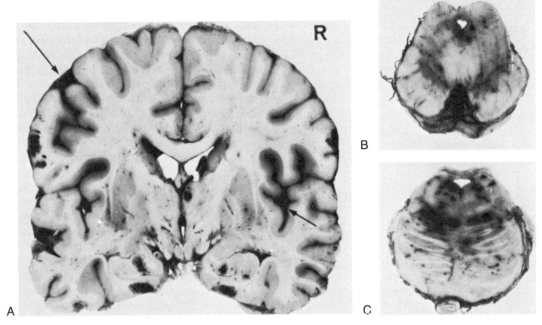

Figure 64—4. Multiple fractures of both sides of the skull in a 47-year-old man. *A.* Coronal section of the brain. Note the contusions in the right and left parietal regions and in the parahippocampal gyri (related to the edge of the tentorium cerebelli). Hemorrhages are present in the hippocampi and in the right thalamus. Subarachnoid blood *(arrows)* and a little intraventricular blood are also seen. *B.* Midbrain. There are several hemorrhages. *C.* Pons. Numerous hemorrhages are present in the floor of the fourth ventricle and in the tegmental region. (From Blackwood, W., Corsellis, J.A.N., and McMenemy, W.H.: Greenfield's Neuropathology, 3rd ed. Chicago, Year Book Medical Publishers, 1976. Used by permission.)

64–6). Bony proliferation around the edges suggests that the patients survived not only their injury but also the surgery.[6] Implements made of stone (flint), obsidian, shell, and even sharks' teeth were used in various parts of the world,[7] and techniques for trephination included scraping, sawing, and boring. The ancient Egyptians may have used trephining for the treatment of migraine and epilepsy,[8] but it is not mentioned as a treatment for head injuries in Breasted's translation of the Edwin Smith papyrus.[9]

Greek and Roman surgeons were more concerned with the skull fracture itself than with intracranial hematomas. Trephination was practiced by the Hippocratic school, but its rationale was not clearly stated by Hippocrates. It seems that the elimination of blood was not a primary consideration, because the operator often left a thin shell of bone intact.[6] It appears that trephination was practiced more as a prophylactic measure to allow the products of suppuration to escape than as a method of relieving pressure. Later, in approximately 30 B.C., Celsus recommended trephining for meningeal hemorrhage.[10] The important conclusion that pressure on the brain rather than the skull fracture itself was the most significant factor in head injury was not reached, however, until the time of Rhazes, an Arabic physician, who lived about A.D. 900.[11] Unfortunately, Arabic

surgeons of Rhazes' era apparently had lost the art of trephination.[12]

Gradually, a better understanding of the pathophysiology of head injury evolved. The significance of the dilated pupil cannot be attributed to any one author, but Jean Louis Petit, in the mid-eighteenth century, recognized that a history of unconsciousness after head injury, followed by a lucid period, and then progressive lethargy, was indicative of an extradural hemorrhage. He recommended trephination in all cases of scalp wound with fracture—"Not only to elevate the bone and remove splinters but to give exit of blood effused between the dura and the bone."[12] Hill and Petit operated on subdural hematomas to allow extravasated blood to escape.[6]

Trephination became unpopular during the early nineteenth century because of the high incidence of sepsis, but, after the introduction of the antiseptic technique by Lister in 1867, this rapidly changed. Diagnostic burr holes became so popular in the early twentieth century that they were often done without clear indications; thus, the term *woodpecker surgery* was coined.

The introduction of cerebral angiography reduced the need for "diagnostic" burr holes, but the importance of immediate decompression when rapid neurologic deterioration occurs has increasingly been recognized in recent neurosurgical lit-

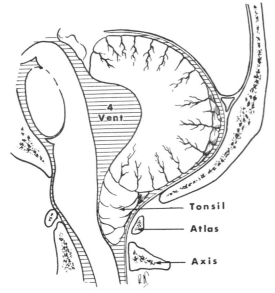

Figure 64–5. Cerebellar tonsils driven between the posterior arch of the atlas and the medulla, which is compressed. (From Jennett, B.: An Introduction to Neurosurgery, 3rd ed. Chicago, Year Book Medical Publishers, 1977. Used by permission.)

erature. Jamieson (1968) reported that epidural hematomas were usually found under the most prominent fractures and that angiography was an unnecessary delay.[13] He reported a mortality rate of 8 per cent with early evacuation.

There have been, however, infrequent reports of trephination in the emergency department. Burton and Blacker (1965) reported on the use of a compact hand drill for emergency decompression.[14] They found this to be most useful for chronic subdural hematomas that were liquefied and that could easily be evacuated by subsequent needle puncture through the trephine hole. The use of the compact hand drill for trephination was only of occasional assistance in the management of acute head injuries in which epidural or subdural hematomas often consisted of clotted blood, which made aspiration through a needle difficult. Mahoney (1981) reported better results with emergency twist drill trephination.[11] Twist drill trephinations were performed in patients with signs of brain herniation and in whom there was no time for diagnostic studies. Although twist drill holes are easier to place than burr holes, the problem of inadequate decompression remains.

At Cook County Hospital, an emergency burr hole tray is kept ready for use in the emergency department. If a trauma patient with a dilated pupil does not respond to mannitol within 10 to 15 minutes, a low temporal burr hole is placed on the side of the large pupil (or first pupil to dilate) and is enlarged to a small craniectomy.[15] If extradural or subdural hematoma is present, it exudes under pressure. The last pupil to dilate often becomes smaller. When a hematoma is not found on the side of the dilated pupil, the patient's head is turned and a burr hole is placed on the opposite side. The patient is then taken to the operating room for a thorough fronto-temporo-parietal craniotomy.

The advent of computed tomography (CT) has made diagnosis much more rapid. CT scanners are frequently located in close proximity to emergency departments, and an accurate diagnosis can be established in a matter of minutes. Unfortunately, at the present time, many general community hospitals have neither a CT scanner nor a neurosurgeon on staff.

Even though experiences in the Korean and Vietnamese wars have led to the development of efficient civilian transport systems for critically injured patients, delay in transfer time still results in significant morbidity and mortality. Studies in the British Isles, where regional medical care has been developed to a very sophisticated degree, have shown that one third of avoidable deaths from head injury were a result of delay in evacuation of an intracranial hematoma.[16] Studies carried out at neurosurgical centers in the United States have shown delays of 1 to 3 hours for treatment of severely head injured patients who are transferred from outlying hospitals.[17] Fortunately, helicopters and mobile intensive care units are becoming more widely available and should increase the efficiency of transfer to a regional neurosurgical center.

Initial Nonoperative Treatment

The importance of early correct management of the head injured patient from the scene of the accident to the emergency department cannot be overemphasized. The first priority is to get oxygen

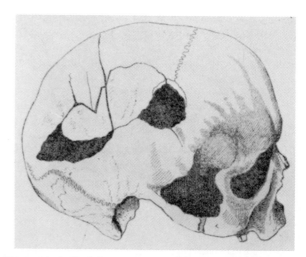

Figure 64–6. Skull from Prunieres' collection, showing a large fracture with defects suggesting surgical removal of bone. (From Walker, A.E.: Clinical Neurosurgery. Baltimore, Williams & Wilkins, 1959. Used by permission.)

to the brain. All unconscious patients should be intubated to provide an unobstructed airway, to facilitate ventilatory support, and to prevent aspiration. One should avoid securing the endotracheal tube with constricting circumferential tapes about the neck, because they can impede venous return. A cricothyroidotomy may be necessary if severe facial fractures are present or if an unstable cervical spine injury is likely. Hyperventilation to a PCO_2 of 30 mm Hg should be routine, because hyperventilation will promote vasoconstriction of intracranial vessels.

The blood pressure must be sufficient to perfuse the brain. Hypotension is not a characteristic feature of severe head injuries and usually indicates an overlooked extracranial injury. Approximately 5 per cent of severe head injuries have associated cervical spine fractures,[18] so great care must be taken to immobilize the spine until adequate radiographs can be obtained. If no cervical fracture is found, the head should be elevated 30 degrees in the neutral position to promote venous drainage and to lower intracranial pressure.

Mannitol, 1 gm per kg, should be administered intravenously only when signs of tentorial herniation have developed. The drug can be lifesaving and will often rapidly reverse neurologic deterioration. Indiscriminate use of mannitol may mask signs of impending herniation and give a false sense of security. Hyperosmolar agents work by extracting fluid from normal brain tissue, thereby decreasing intracranial pressure. As the pressure decreases, the tamponade effect of the blood clot may be lost and further bleeding may occur. Additional improvement, with repeated doses of mannitol, is less likely with acute bleeding. Some centers also routinely administer furosemide (Lasix), 0.5 mg per kg, in addition to mannitol to further dehydrate the brain while preparing for surgery

A CT scan or an angiogram must be promptly carried out on all patients who receive mannitol in order to determine the site of the hematoma. These studies also provide useful diagnostic and anatomic information in patients who do not have progressive herniation. Optimally, hematomas will be discovered prior to the development of brain herniation. CT scan is the procedure of choice for patients with head injuries. Angiography is now used only when a scanner is not available.

Indications for Emergency Cranial Decompression

Emergency decompression should be performed on any patient who demonstrates or has a history of *progressive neurologic deterioration* and signs of brain herniation. Serial neurologic examinations

by the emergency physician are the most reliable indicators of deterioration, but properly trained paramedical personnel can also provide this vital information. Patients who are *immediately* rendered unconscious, who have fixed dilated pupils, and who show absence of eye movements, abnormal posturing (decerebrate), and irregular or absence of breathing from the time of the accident are likely to have sustained a severe generalized brain contusion. The critical damage occurred at the time of injury, and burr holes will generally *not* be of value. A CT scan or an angiogram must nonetheless be performed to confirm this clinical impression.

A history of head trauma in an unconscious patient with a fixed dilated pupil, hemiplegia, and a skull fracture on the side of the dilated pupil strongly suggests *but does not guarantee* an intracranial hematoma on the same side as the dilated pupil. If the pupil remains dilated after initial nonoperative treatment has been completed, one should immediately create a burr hole. There is usually only a brief period of time before the other pupil dilates and irreversible brain damage occurs.

In the absence of other mitigating information, the first burr hole should be made in the temporal area. Frontal and parietal burr holes should be carried out only if the temporal burr hole is negative and if there is a high level of suspicion of a clot in these areas. Epidural hematomas are almost always located under the fracture, whereas subdural hematomas are usually much more extensive and may even develop opposite the site of initial injury. If there is a large acute subdural hematoma, one must consider the possibility of the need for multiple burr holes to evacuate more blood. The reduction in intracranial pressure is directly proportional to the amount of blood removed. A large fronto-temporo-parietal craniotomy is the preferred treatment for acute subdural hematomas, but this may not be feasible until the patient is transferred to a larger medical center. For similar reasons, the burr hole should be expanded to a limited craniectomy if the burr hole is positive for an epidural hematoma, and every effort should be made to identify and to control the bleeding point.

When it is not known which pupil was the first to dilate, emergency *bilateral* burr holes may be necessary as a last resort in the trauma patient who has progressively deteriorated and developed bilateral fixed dilated pupils. In all situations, if burr holes result in negative findings on one side, the other side should always be explored.

Suboccipital burr holes should be considered in any patient who has an occipital skull fracture that extends into the foramen magnum and shows signs of brainstem compression. The burr hole should be placed on the side of the fracture.

There are no absolute contraindications to performing emergency burr holes; however, one subgroup of patients deserves special mention. Prothrombin time (protime) and partial thromboplastin time should be performed with an unconscious patient, and fresh frozen plasma should be administered if a coagulopathy is discovered. Those patients who are on anticoagulants or who are known hemophiliacs are especially susceptible to intracranial hematomas following head injury. If it is known that the patient has been taking anticoagulants, 20 mg of Vitamin K should be given promptly along with fresh frozen plasma after the blood samples for coagulation times have been drawn. Additional doses should be given as needed. Uncontrollable bleeding during the procedure is a definite risk if the patient's coagulopathy has not been reversed completely. In a life-threatening emergency, coumadin–induced bleeding may be immediately reversed with prothrombin complex (konyne or Proplex), but this results in almost a 100 per cent incidence of hepatitis.

Patients who have intracranial hematomas but show no sign of tentorial herniation should *not* be subjected to emergency burr holes. These patients should be taken promptly to the operating room by a neurosurgeon. If a neurosurgeon is not available, arrangements should be made for the patient to be immediately transferred to a medical center with a neurosurgeon on staff. Mannitol should be available to the patient during transfer but should be given only if signs of tentorial herniation develop. The neurosurgical team at the receiving hospital should be alerted by radiotelephone about any change in the patient's condition. After arrival, the patient can then be taken directly to the operating room.

Equipment

Standard Emergency Burr Hole Tray
  Essential Equipment
    No. 4 scalpel handle
    No. 12 blade
    Self-retaining retractor (standard 14.8 cm Wullstein)
    2 hemostats
    Hudson brace
    Cushing perforator and burr attachments for Hudson brace
    Dural hook
    No. 6 scalpel handle and No. 11 blade
    Small cottonoids
  Suture Material
    3-0 silk on spool
    2-0 Vicryl (atraumatic needle)
    2-0 nylon (cutting needle)
  Hemostatic Agents
    Topical thrombin
    Gelfoam
    Bone wax

  Available with Tray but Separately Wrapped
    Kerrison rongeurs (upbiting 5 mm)
    Leksell rongeurs (full curve wide jaw)
    Small perforator and burr attachments for infants and small children
    Dural suction catheter and sterile tubing for attachment to suction 6-ml syringe
    No. 19 needle
    No. 22 needle
Twist Drill Trephination Tray
    Scalpel with No. 11 blade
    15/64-inch-diameter Matthews hand drill

Techniques

TEMPORAL BURR HOLE

The patient is first placed in a supine position with a sandbag or folded towel under one shoulder, and the head is rotated so that the side with the dilated pupil is uppermost. The sandbag prevents kinking of the neck and obstruction of venous return (Fig. 64–7). The hair is shaved from the temporal scalp, and the head is then scrubbed with povidone-iodine scrub. These procedures can be carried out during other resuscitative measures so that critical minutes are not wasted. The area is then painted with povidone-iodine solution and is draped with sterile towels.

A 4-cm vertical skin incision is made, two fingerbreadths anterior and three fingerbreadths above the anterior tragus of the ear (Fig. 64–8). The superficial temporal artery palpable just anterior to the ear should be avoided and the incision should not extend below the zygoma in order to prevent injury to the superior branch of the facial nerve. The zygoma is palpable as a ridge of bone that extends toward the outer canthus of the eye from a point just superior and anterior to the external ear canal.

The incision should first be made through skin and subcutaneous tissues so that bleeding from any branches of the superficial temporal artery can be clamped and ligated. The self-retaining retractor is inserted, and the superficial fascia of the temporalis muscle is exposed. This is divided vertically with a scalpel, and the blunt end of the handle is then scraped back and forth to free the

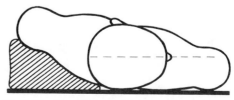

Figure 64–7. The head is turned to the side, and a sandbag is placed under the opposite shoulder. (From Kempe, L.G.: Operative Neurosurgery, vol. 1. Berlin, Springer-Verlag, 1968. Used by permission.)

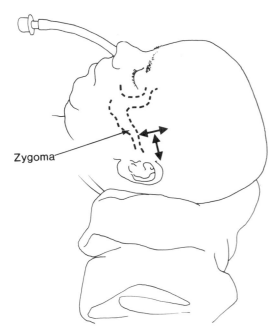

Figure 64–8. The temporal burr hole is placed just above the midpoint of the zygomatic arch and two fingerbreadths anterior to the external auditory canal. (From Simon, R., and Brenner, B.: Procedures and Techniques in Emergency Medicines. Baltimore, Williams & Wilkins, 1983. Used by permission.)

Zygoma

attachments of muscle from the squamosal temporal bone. There is usually some bleeding from the muscle, but this can be controlled by inserting the self-retaining retractor deeper into the wound. The outer surface of the temporal bone should now be visible, and a fracture line can sometimes be identified.

The perforator is connected to the Hudson brace and drilling is begun (Fig. 64–9). A perforating hole is first drilled and then enlarged with a burr. Inserting the tip of the perforator into the fracture line may prevent slippage on the initial turns. It is important to hold the brace perpendicular to the skull so that a clean direct hole is drilled. Firm steady pressure should be used, and frequent checks should be made to assess the depth of the hole. Perforation of the inner table will not be obvious unless an epidural clot is present. The white dura is of a similar color as the surrounding bone. The bone dust must be carefully cleared away with saline irrigation or with the curette to enable one to see the fine line between the inner table and the dura. The soft dura will "give" slightly if gentle pressure is applied with the rounded end of the curette. It is very important not to overdrill with the perforator, because the dura can be torn, or worse, the instrument may plunge into the brain. As soon as the tip of the perforator penetrates the inner table, the perforator bit should be switched to the burr. Drilling is then completed, but it is advisable to leave a thin rim of bone to prevent plunging with the burr.

The rim can be scooped out more safely with a

curette. This can be done by using the edge of the hole as a fulcrum and directing pressure upward while the curette is turned on its axis. Any bleeding from bone is controlled by application of bone wax. The dark clotted blood of an epidural hematoma or the dura should now be clearly visible. If a subdural hematoma is present, the dura will have a dark-bluish tinge. If the burr hole is to be enlarged, a Penfield No. 3 elevator should be inserted between the inner table and the dura all around the burr hole to prevent attached dura from being caught in the jaws of the rongeur. Either a Kerrison or Leksell rongeur can be used (Fig. 64–10). The bone is always removed with upward pressure as the jaws are being closed. An epidural clot should be suctioned cautiously with the dural suction catheter to remove as much of it as possible (Fig. 64–11). In an epidural hematoma, the blood is usually thick and clotted. If liquid, it implies continued bleeding, and a source must be found. The middle meningeal artery lies deep in relation to the clot, its branches being stripped from the inner surface of the bone by the expanding hematoma. Frequently, because of its arterial origin, the bleeding may be profuse. Blood loss must be replaced with adequate transfusion of crystalloid solutions and blood to maintain normal arterial pressure.

Optimally, the patient will soon be taken to the operating room where adequate exposure can be obtained. The bleeding can then be controlled by application of hemoclips on either side of the bleeding point or by cauterization of the vessel with bipolar cautery. If the patient is to be transferred and if specialist care is not immediately available, an attempt should be made to find the bleeding point. If suctioning provides clear visu-

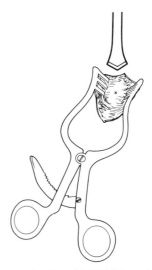

Figure 64–9. The standard hand-held drill introduced through an incision is shown. The drill is centered along the periosteal surface of the outer table. (From Simon, R., and Brenner, B.: Procedures and Techniques in Emergency Medicine. Baltimore, Williams & Wilkins, 1983. Used by permission.)

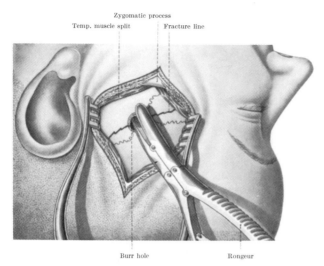

Figure 64–10. Enlarging burr hole for left temporal craniectomy. (From Kempe, L.G.: Operative Neurosurgergy, vol. 1. Berlin, Springer-Verlag, 1968. Used by permission.)

alization, a mosquito hemostat can be applied just proximal to the bleeding point. One must avoid blind grabbing with the hemostat in a pool of blood, because injury to the brain immediately beneath the dura will occur. If bleeding is from the base of the skull where the artery enters through the foramen spinosum, bone must be removed inferiorly toward the zygoma and the opening must be plugged with bone wax. Further bleeding between the dura and the bone can be controlled by inserting thin strips of thrombin-soaked gelfoam around the bony edges.

In the case of a subdural hematoma, the dura is opened by first inserting the dural hook through the outer layer of the dura and pulling upward. The dura is then opened with a No. 11 blade, using gentle stroking motions rather than plunging with the tip of the blade. When the dura is first penetrated, there will often be a sudden gush of bloody fluid if a subdural hematoma is present. When the opening is large enough, a small cottonoid should be inserted to protect the brain beneath and a cruciate opening should be completed. Suctioning a subdural clot is hazardous because of the unprotected brain beneath the clot. The suction should be turned down, and the finger hole on the dural suction catheter should be kept open. Any bleeding points on the surface of the brain can be controlled by applying a small piece of thrombin-soaked gelfoam and holding it in place with a cottonoid.

Prior to closure, a pocket should be created around the burr hole by using the blunt end of the scalpel handle under the temporalis muscle. This will allow further bleeding to accumulate outside the cranial cavity while arrangements are made for more definitive neurosurgical treatment. Under ideal circumstances, the muscle fascia is

closed with running 0-0 Vicryl suture and the skin is closed with a running 2-0 nylon interlocking suture. A quick temporary closure can be performed with a running 2-0 nylon interlocking suture catching skin, subcutaneous tissue, and muscle.

Needling the brain for intracerebral clots is extremely hazardous and should not be carried out in the emergency department. If the brain is bulging out of the initial burr hole, it is likely that a clot is present at some other location, perhaps on the other side. Frontal and parietal burr holes should then be considered, and contralateral burr holes should be contemplated if the initial holes result in negative findings.

FRONTAL AND PARIETAL BURR HOLES

Frontal (anterior) burr holes are made through a 4-cm incision located three fingerbreadths from the midline and three fingerbreadths from the hairline (Fig. 64–12). Parietal (posterior) burr holes are placed four fingerbreadths directly behind the frontal burr hole. The parietal incision should be curved inferiorly so that it may later be incorporated in a skin flap if necessary.

There is no muscle, so skin incisions are made through all layers to the skull. The pericranium is freed by blunt dissection using the scalpel handle. After the self-retaining retractor is inserted, additional cuts may be necessary in the pericranium to create a free surface for the perforator. The

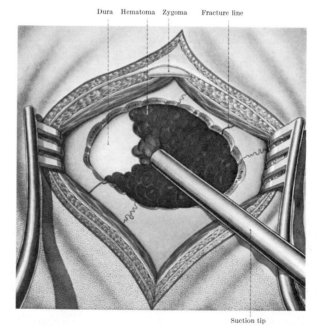

Figure 64–11. Temporal craniectomy for epidural hematoma. Note that the craniectomy reached down to the level of the zygoma. (From Kempe, L.G.: Operative Neurosurgery, vol. 1. Berlin, Springer-Verlag, 1968. Used by permission.)

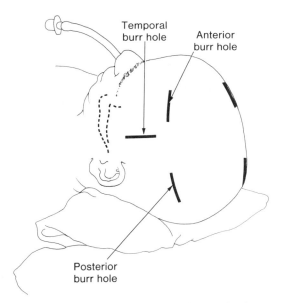

Figure 64–12. The sites of incision and burr hole placement. (From Simon, R., and Brenner, B.: Procedures and Techniques in Emergency Medicine. Baltimore, Williams & Wilkins, 1983. Used by permission.)

convexity of the skull in the frontal and parietal regions makes it more difficult to determine when the brace is perpendicular to the surface, and there is often a tendency to cut the burr hole on a bevel. It is most important that the perforator not bevel toward the midline because of the superior sagittal sinus and large perforating veins in the midline. Arachnoid villi tend to be evident toward the midline, and when a hole is drilled over them, they often bleed profusely. Such hemorrhaging can be controlled by application of thrombin-soaked gelfoam and a cottonoid. If bleeding persists and is uncontrollable, the hole can be plugged with bone wax and another hole can be drilled. Closure of the frontal and parietal burr holes in the emergency department should involve use of one layer of 2-0 nylon through skin and galea if the patient is being taken to the operating room. If not, a two-layer closure with 2-0 inverted Vicryl in the galea and 2-0 nylon in the skin is the preferred technique.

SUBOCCIPITAL BURR HOLES

The patient is best positioned on his side with the head supported on folded towels. The neck must be maximally flexed; therefore, it is mandatory that normal cervical spine radiographs be taken prior to positioning of the patient. The side on which the clot is suspected should be in the uppermost position. The occipital and upper cervical regions must be shaved and scrubbed with povidone-iodine. After infiltration with lidocaine and epinephrine (to control surface bleeding), an incision is made midway between the external

occipital protuberance and the mastoid and is extended 4 cm into the upper cervical region. The posterior fossa is located below the superior nuchal line. The skin and subcutaneous tissues are densely adherent to the underlying tissues and can be undermined with lateral cuts just above the muscle layer. This will allow insertion of the self-retaining retractor. The muscles are then divided vertically. The occipital artery may cause troublesome bleeding and should be ligated. The attachments of the muscles below the superior nuchal line are separated from the occipital bone, and if necessary for better exposure, the attachments along the superior nuchal line may also be divided.

Laterally, it is important to avoid the emissary veins from the epidural venous complex, which penetrate the occipital bone just behind the mastoid. Very profuse venous bleeding may occur if these veins are damaged. If this occurs, bleeding from the bone should be controlled with bone wax and the head should be elevated to collapse the veins. Suture ligature in the muscle may be necessary.

The burr hole should be drilled over the fracture site, if it is evident, and must be either above or below the superior nuchal line to avoid the transverse sinus (Fig. 64–13). If the burr hole is too far lateral, mastoid air cells can be penetrated. If the mastoid air cells are entered, they should be plugged with bacitracin- or neomycin-impregnated bone wax. Also, the transverse sinus curves laterally as the sigmoid sinus, and passes deep to the mastoid. The transverse sinus must also be avoided. Thus, it is important that the burr hole be drilled in the center, midway between the

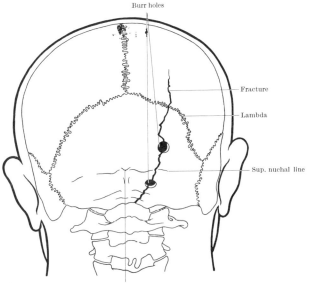

Figure 64–13. Placement of burr holes in extradural hematoma over occipital and suboccipital area. (From Kempe, L. G.: Operative Neurosurgery, vol. 1. Berlin, Springer-Verlag, 1968. Used by permission.)

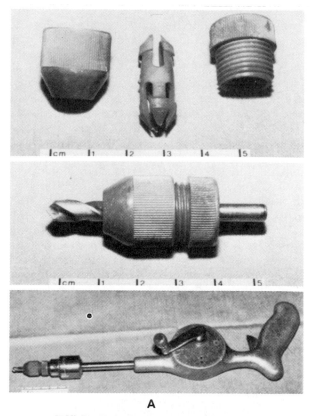

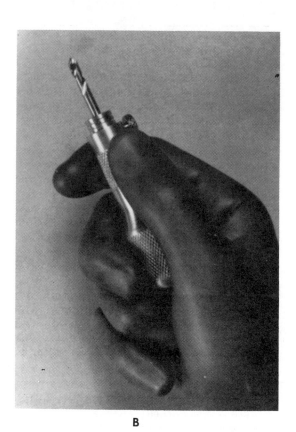

A

B

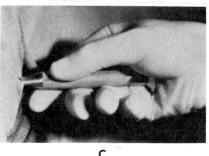

C

Figure 64–14. *A: Top,* Twist drill stop, unassembled. From left to right are the end cap, the central sleeve, and the front cap. *Center,* The twist drill stop in place on the drill bit. *Bottom,* The twist drill with the bit and fully assembled. (From Grode, M.L., and Carton, C.A.: Drill stop for twist drill. Technical note. J. Neurosurg. 52:599, 1980. Used by permission.) *B,* Method of grasping compact hand drill. The bit length can be varied using set screw. (From Burton, C., and Blacker, H.M.: A compact hand drill for emergency brain decompression. J. Trauma 5:643, 1965. Used by permission.) *C.* Trephining the skull. (From Mahoney, B.D., Rockswold, G.L., Ruiz, E., et al.: Emergency twist drill trephination. Neurosurgery 8:552, 1981. Used by permission.)

mastoid and external occipital protuberance and midway between the superior nuchal line and ring of foramen magnum or above the superior nuchal line. If an epidural hematoma is not encountered, the dura should be opened. The muscle fascia is closed with 0-0 Vicryl suture, and the skin is closed with 2-0 nylon interlocking suture.

TEMPORAL TWIST DRILL TREPHINATION

Twist drill trephination uses a 15/64-inch drill bit secured to either a standard surgical drill (Fig. 64–14*A*) or a hand twist drill (Fig. 64–14*B*). The equipment for this technique and the technique itself are simpler than for burr holes, and twist drill trephination can be performed more quickly. The hole, however, is very small, and further decompression by craniectomy is not possible. The procedure is carried out through a small incision

rather than by direct vision as in the case of burr holes. Damage to underlying brain by an inadvertent plunge would be less severe with a twist drill than with the perforator or burr. Unfortunately, only a limited amount of clotted blood can be removed, and there is no way to control recurrent bleeding.

Mahoney and associates[19] have used twist drill trephination for emergency decompression in patients with uncal herniation. Their technique is described in the following paragraph.

After suitable cervical radiographs have been obtained, the patient can be positioned nose up or turned to the side with a sandbag under the shoulder. The hair on the side of the dilated pupil is shaved, and the head is scrubbed with povidone-iodine while other resuscitative measures are taking place. A 2.5-cm vertical incision is made two fingerbreadths anterior and two to three fingerbreadths superior to the tragus of the ear after infiltrating the skin with lidocaine and epinephrine

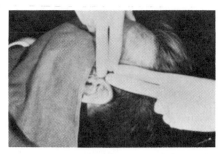

Figure 64–15. Measuring the location of the incision. (From Mahoney, B.D., Rockswold, G.L., Ruiz, E., et al.: Emergency twist drill trephination. Neurosurgery 8:552, 1981. Used by permission.)

(Fig. 64–15). A 15/64-inch-diameter Matthews hand drill (Codman Surgical Instruments, Randolph, MA) is used to trephine the skull (see Fig. 64–14C). Binding of the drill bit can be felt at the diploë and inner table. On penetrating the inner table, the drill is withdrawn and the wound is observed for return of blood. The source of bright red bleeding is likely to be the skin margin or the diploë. Dark clotted blood indicates an epidural hematoma if the dura was not lacerated. If no blood returns, the dura is elevated with a dural hook and a nick is carefully made in the dura with a No. 11 blade. Once again, the wound is observed for the return of dark blood, this time from a subdural hematoma. If dark red blood is obtained, it can sometimes be further evacuated by careful suctioning with a sterile catheter.

INFANT SUBDURAL TAP

The infant is placed supine in the nose-up position. The scalp is then shaved over the lateral margins of the anterior fontanelle. The skin is scrubbed with povidone-iodine, then draped with sterile towels; local anesthetic is not used. A subdural needle is inserted through the skin at the extreme lateral limit of the anterior fontanelle where it meets the coronal suture (Fig. 64–16). A zig-zag puncture is used to prevent later leakage of subdural fluid. The needle is first inserted through the skin, then the skin is moved with the needle in place before the pericranium is penetrated. The needle is then pushed through the pericranium into the subdural space. The subdural fluid is allowed to drain spontaneously, and specimens are collected for Gram stain, culture, cells, sugar, and protein. The fluid is never aspirated for fear of drawing pial vessels into the point of the needle. If a pial vessel is punctured, bleeding will usually cease spontaneously. The procedure is then repeated on the opposite side. A firm sterile occlusive dressing should then be applied. If continued leakage occurs from the puncture site, colodium-impregnated cotton fluff applied over the puncture wound will usually stop it.

VENTRICULAR PUNCTURE

Acute obstruction to the flow of cerebrospinal fluid can produce severe headaches, vomiting, unconsciousness, and death from brain herniation. There are multiple causes for acute hydrocephalus. Most patients with this disorder seen in the emergency department have an obstructed shunt. In certain cases, a small cyst (colloid cyst) acts like a ball valve at the foramen of Monro. Subarachnoid hemorrhage, infection, and various congenital conditions can all cause hydrocephalus. Most often, symptoms progress gradually, and the majority of shunt obstructions can be relieved by tapping the shunt through its reservoir. In certain cases, direct ventricular puncture will be lifesaving.

A needle can be inserted into the lateral ventricle through either a frontal or parietal burr hole (Fig. 64–17). The point of reference for a frontal approach is the inner canthus of the ipsilateral eye, whereas for a parietal approach, the pupil of the ipsilateral eye is the reference point. A maximum of three attempts should be made. The ventricles are usually encountered at a depth of 5.5 cm from the burr hole, but in hydrocephalic patients, they can be encountered at much shallower depths.

Possible complications include ventriculitis, intraventricular hemorrhage, and proencephaly if

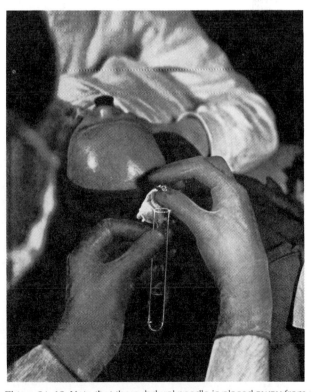

Figure 64–16. Note that the subdural needle is placed away from the midline. The shaft of the needle is held firmly against the scalp so that it will not wiggle. (From Ingraham, F. D., and Matson, D. D.: Neurosurgery of Infancy and Childhood. Springfield, IL, Charles C Thomas, 1954. Used by permission.)

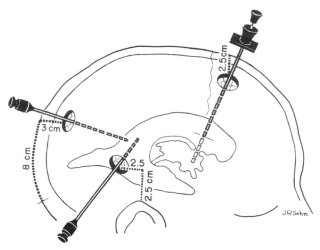

Figure 64–17. The three standard trephination sites used to gain access to the lateral ventricles. The anterior site, or Kocher's point, is 3 cm posterior to the normal hairline and 2.5 cm lateral to the midline. The Keen's point or lateral trephine opening permits tapping of the trigone of the lateral ventricle. Keen's point is 2.5 cm behind and 2.5 cm above the top of the ear. The posterior aspect of the lateral ventricle is approached through a posterior parietal trephine opening that is 8 cm above the inion and 2.5 to 3 cm lateral to the midline. (From Zingesser, L.H., and Schecther, M.M.: Encephalography. In Youmans, J.R.: Neurological Surgery, 2nd ed. vol. 1. Philadelphia, W.B. Saunders Company, 1982. Used by permission.)

the needle is not held steady while it is in the brain.

Complications

The most serious complication of emergency burr hole placement would be an inadvertent plunge with the perforator or burr. Frequent checks of the depth of the hole and controlled pressure are most important to prevent this catastrophe. A plastic drill stop has been designed for twist drills to prevent inadvertent plunge with this instrument (see Fig. 64–14C).[20] If the brain is penetrated, bleeding is usually from superficial vessels in the pial arachnoid. Such bleeding can be controlled with pressure and pieces of thrombin-soaked gelfoam. The patient should be transferred to a neurosurgical center as soon as possible.

Infection is a possible complication. Mahoney and associates reported one death from Pseudomonas meningitis in a patient who had an emergency twist drill trephination.[19] The patient had multiple injuries, including basal skull fractures, and a direct causal relationship to the trephination could not be established. Patients who receive emergency burr holes should be covered with a broad spectrum antibiotic such as ampicillin.

Perforation of major sinuses or other vessels can occur if the burr holes are placed in an improper location.

Conclusions

Emergency trephination was performed by Mahoney and colleagues[19] on 41 patients. Ten patients had bilateral procedures, resulting in a total of 51 trephinations. Twenty-three of these patients had significant extracerebral hematomas, and 18 others had cerebral contusions and intraparenchymal or extraventricular hematomas. Thirty-two of

the patients died (78 per cent) and 9 survived. Of the 23 patients with extracerebral hematomas, 6 of them showed therapeutic efficiency with a rapid decrease in the size of the previously dilated pupil shortly after release of the clotted blood (estimated range 10 to 50 ml; average about 20 ml). Of the 6 patients who showed a therapeutic response, 3 of them later died because of their injuries and 3 recovered to an independent functional state.

Hoff and associates[21] performed exploratory burr holes on 100 patients who had signs of tentorial herniation. In one third of the patients, extracerebral hematomas were shown on the initial burr hole examination. Forty-seven of the patients survived and, of these patients, 22 had removal of a significant hematoma. In 4 of these patients, the burr holes were nondiagnostic and the hematomas were removed after angiography or CT scanning. In the remaining 25 survivors, no further operations for removal of intracranial clot were required. Hoff and coworkers believe that early burr hole exploration was beneficial to one third of their patients.

There is an understandable hesitancy for personnel who do not have formal neurosurgical training to drill holes in the skull and attempt to evacuate intracranial blood. Certain skills are required, but the degree of difficulty should be no greater than insertion of a chest tube. The techniques described should be optional procedures in the emergency physician's management of patients with multiple traumas.

It should be clearly understood that emergency burr holes and trephination are to be considered only as lifesaving procedures. The patient must then have a complete neurodiagnostic work-up, including a CT scan or an angiogram. If the patient is in an outlying hospital, immediate transportation by helicopter or ambulance to a neurosurgical facility must be arranged, regardless of whether the results of the burr hole technique yield blood.

INTRACRANIAL PRESSURE MONITORING

Introduction

Intracranial pressure (ICP) monitoring is critical for the management of patients with intracranial hypertension or for those who have the potential for its development. This vital parameter can warn of potential problems before neurologic deficits develop, thereby leading to earlier diagnostic studies and correction of increased intracranial pressure prior to irreversible brain damage.

ICP monitors are generally inserted by neurosurgical personnel, but more widespread use could significantly decrease morbidity and mortality of unconscious patients by leading to the earlier diagnosis and treatment of intracranial mass lesions.

Insertion of the subarachnoid bolt requires a twist drill trephination, whereas insertion of a fiberoptic pressure transducer requires a burr hole. If the equipment is available, these procedures can be performed without difficulty in the emergency department. They should be carried out if significant intracranial hypertension is suspected or if a prolonged period of resuscitation is necessary to stabilize the patient before obtaining a CT scan. Insertion of the subarachnoid bolt can be accomplished within a few minutes, and insertion of the epidural transducer takes only 10 to 15 minutes. The subarachnoid bolt is inexpensive and requires only a pressure transducer, oscilloscope, and paper recorder. The epidural transducer costs approximately $200 and can be used only four or five times. The sophisticated epidural monitor (Ladd Research Industries, Inc., Burlington, VT), together with paper recorder, is a much more expensive system. There is a hook-up for simultaneous recording of mean arterial blood pressure on the paper recorder, so that the cerebral perfusion pressure can be checked at a glance.

Intracranial pressure can also be monitored by insertion of an intraventricular cannula. This procedure can be difficult and time consuming, especially if the ventricles are collapsed because of edema or an intracranial hematoma. The risk of ventriculitis makes this latter procedure unsuitable to perform in the emergency department. The primary advantage of intraventricular monitoring is the ability to withdraw cerebrospinal fluid periodically and hence to decrease intracranial pressure.

Historical Background

Continuous monitoring of intracranial pressure in clinical practice was first introduced by Guillaume and Janny in 1951.[22]

The development of intracranial pressure monitoring techniques began with intraventricular cannulae. The cannulae were used exclusively until the development of the subarachnoid bolt by Vries, Becker, and Young in 1972.[23] Since that time, a fiberoptic intracranial monitoring system has been developed from the Numoto pressure switch described in 1966.[24, 25] The Ladd monitoring system is composed of a small implantable transducer (1 cm diameter) containing a pressure-sensitive membrane, two fiberoptic columns, and a pneumatic tube (Fig. 64–18). Deflections of light from the reflecting mirror on the pressure-sensitive membrane are corrected by air pumped down the pneumatic tube. The amount of correction required is expressed on a digital display and is recorded simultaneously on paper. This very ingenious device is exceedingly accurate and will detect fluctuations in intracranial pressure caused by just turning the head. Constant adjustment of an external transducer is not required.[26]

Intracranial pressure can be expressed either in centimeters of water or in millimeters of mercury. Intracranial pressure expressed in mm Hg is referred to as *torr*. The upper limit of normal is 15 torr (20 cm H_2O).

In 1960, Lundberg reported that abnormal pressure waves were present in patients with intracranial hypertension.[27] He described two distinct types:

1. "A" waves are ominous episodic elevations in intracranial pressure to 50 to 100 torr, lasting 5 to 20 minutes, and are usually superimposed on an already elevated baseline intracranial pressure (Fig. 64–19). These are known as plateau waves. A terminal wave is a wave during which the intracranial pressure has risen to the level of mean arterial blood pressure, at which point cerebral blood flow has ceased (Fig. 64–20); it often follows a series of plateau waves.

2. "B" waves are short-term oscillations, lower in amplitude than "A" waves, and occur at a rate of one half to two fluctuations per minute. "B" waves are less significant than "A" waves but often precede development of "A" waves (Fig. 64–21).

Both blood pressure and intracranial pressure must be considered in the assessment of cerebral blood flow. Most important is the cerebral perfusion pressure, which is the measure of effective blood flow to the brain. It is calculated by subtracting the intracranial pressure from the mean arterial pressure. Values less than 40 torr are ominous and a cause for them must be sought by CT scanning or angiography. If the studies result in negative findings, the elevated intracranial pressure must

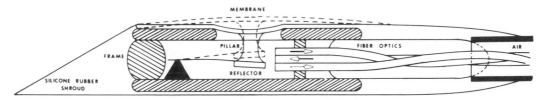

Figure 64–18. Cross section of intracranial portion of pressure transducer. (From Levin, A.B.: The use of a fiberoptic intracranial pressure transducer in the treatment of head injuries. J. Trauma 17:767, 1977. Used by permission.)

be treated aggressively with diuretics, hyperventilation, and elevation of the head. If all other conservative measures have failed, barbiturate coma should be instituted. Elevation of systemic blood pressure to a maximum of 160 mm Hg can effectively increase the perfusion pressure. Above this level, blood pressure and intracranial pressure rise simultaneously and any benefit of further elevation is lost. Conversely, intracranial pressure can be lowered by reducing systemic hypertension to below 160 mm Hg.

Indications

Intracranial pressure monitoring is indicated for any unconscious patient in whom a mass lesion or brain swelling is anticipated. The procedure should become as routine as insertion of an arterial line, central venous pressure line, or Swan-Ganz catheter. An ICP monitor should be left in place in any patient who has an emergency twist drill trephination or in whom an emergency burr hole has been performed. Temporal placement of the epidural monitor would be feasible, but placement of the subarachnoid bolt requires the thicker skull of the frontal region.

Equipment

Subarachnoid Bolt Insertion
  6-ml syringe and No. 27 needle (1½ inch)
  Scalpel with No. 11 blade

Hand twist drill with ¼-inch drill bit
Twist drill stop (optional)
Subarachnoid bolt
Hexagonal screw driver
P-37 Statham transducer
20-ml syringe
Stopcock
Pressure tubing
Manometer with bacteriologic filter
Oscilloscope with paper recorder
2-0 nylon suture with cutting needle
Epidural Pressure Monitor Insertion
  6-ml syringe with No. 27 needle (1½ inch)
  Scalpel with No. 11 blade
  Self-retaining retractor
  Hudson brace
  Perforator and burr attachments
  Penfield No. 3 elevator
  Bone wax
  Thrombin-soaked gelfoam
  2-0 Vicryl suture with atraumatic needle
  2-0 nylon suture with cutting needle
  Fiberoptic pressure transducer
  Ladd fiberoptic monitor and paper recorder
  Beaker of sterile saline

Techniques

INSERTION OF SUBARACHNOID BOLT (Fig. 64–22)

The patient is shaved for a diameter of 4 cm over the right frontal scalp. The area is scrubbed

Figure 64–19. Typical A waves recorded with the fiberoptic intracranial pressure monitoring system. (From Levin, A.B.: The use of a fiberoptic intracranial pressure transducer in the treatment of head injuries. J. Trauma 17:767, 1977. Used by permission.)

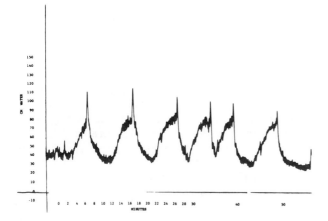

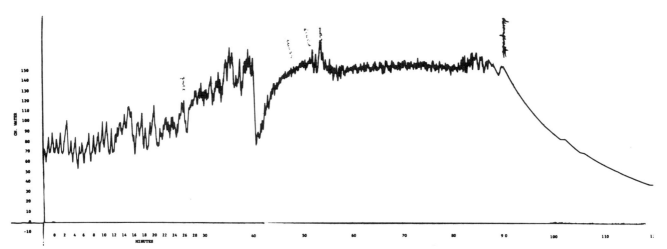

Figure 64–20. Series of progressive A waves culminating in a terminal plateau wave followed by decompensation. (From Levin, A.B.: The use of a fiberoptic intracranial pressure transducer in the treatment of head injuries. J. Trauma 17:767, 1977. Used by permission.)

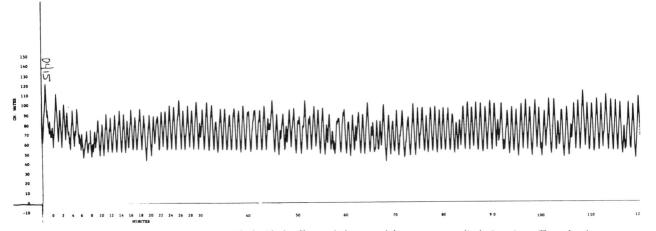

Figure 64–21. Series of B waves recorded with the fiberoptic intracranial pressure monitoring system. (From Levin, A.B.: The use of a fiberoptic intracranial pressure transducer in the treatment of head injuries. J. Trauma 17:767, 1977. Used by permission.)

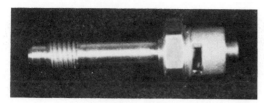

Figure 64–22. Close-up of the subarachnoid screw showing details of the hexagonal collar, tip, and anchoring threads for the skull. (From Vries, J.K., Becker, D.P., and Young, H.F.: A subarachnoid screw for monitoring intracranial pressure. Technical note. J. Neurosurg. 39:416, 1973. Used by permission.)

with povidone-iodine scrub and is then painted with povidone-iodine solution. A 1-cm incision is made 3 cm from the midline and just anterior to the coronal suture in the scalp through to the skull.

A ¼-inch twist drill hole is then made with a hand drill. The drill bit will be felt to bind as it goes through the diploë and the inner table. It is advisable to use a hand drill guard to prevent plunging. After the hole has been drilled, a nick must be made in the dura with a No. 11 blade. Sometimes the dura is penetrated by the drill bit, and a little cerebrospinal fluid (CSF) can be seen issuing from the wound. Alternatively, the dura can be punctured with a No. 18 needle. Use of the needle will also ensure that the inner table has been penetrated. The subarachnoid bolt is then tightened into the hole, using the hexagonal screw driver. The lumen of the subarachnoid bolt should be injected with 2 ml of sterile normal saline to ensure a continuous fluid column from the subarachnoid space to the pressure transducer. A suture can be placed in the incision to close it around the shaft of the bolt.

The bolt is connected to a stopcock assembly via a saline-filled extension tube. The stopcock connections include a P-37 Statham transducer, a saline-filled 20-ml syringe, and a water manometer with a bacteriologic filter. The output of the transducer is displayed on an oscilloscope and written on chart paper.

The system is calibrated by zero balancing the transducer to the water manometer. After matching the height of the water manometer to the level of the end of the screw in the subarachnoid space, the transducer is then opened to the subarachnoid space via the saline-filled extension tube and the calibrated intracranial pressure is recorded. The system can be calibrated by repeating the preceding steps.

When monitoring is to be discontinued, the skin around the shaft is cleansed with hydrogen peroxide and is then prepared with povidone-iodine. The bolt is unscrewed and removed. A couple of nylon sutures can be inserted to close the opening in the skin left by the shaft of the bolt.

INSERTION OF FIBEROPTIC INTRACRANIAL PRESSURE TRANSDUCER (Fig. 64–23)

The fiberoptic pressure transducer is implanted into the epidural space through a burr hole. The right frontal region, 3 cm from the midline and just anterior to the coronal suture, is the usual site.

The technique for drilling the burr hole was described in the first part of this chapter. It is important to free the dura completely around the burr hole with a No. 3 Penfield elevator to prevent an inaccurate reading from "wedging." Prior to insertion, the epidural transducer should always be tested by dipping it into a column of sterile saline. The pressure should sequentially increase as it is lowered into the saline and should decrease as it is removed.

The device is inserted with the pressure-sensitive side toward the dura, and the connecting wire can be brought out through a separate stab wound or through the incision. The skin should be cleaned with alcohol and allowed to dry. The wire is then taped with ¼-inch Steristrips, leaving some slack in the wire.

The device is removed by simply pulling it out through the wound; resuturing the wound is rarely necessary.

Complications

Very few complications have been reported with either the subarachnoid bolt or the fiberoptic transducer. The subarachnoid bolt can clot, and the waveform may be lost. This can usually be corrected by injecting 1 to 2 ml of sterile saline

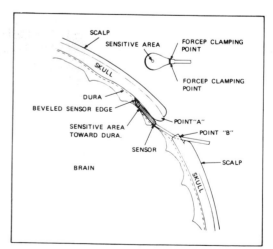

Figure 64–23. Cross-sectional representation of the placement of the pressure sensor. (From Levin, A.B.: The use of a fiberoptic intracranial pressure transducer in the treatment of head injuries. J. Trauma 17:767, 1977. Used by permission.)

through the bolt into the subarachnoid space. The device needs frequent recalibration, and the transducer must be kept at the same level as the head. Infections occurred in 20 of 112 monitored patients in one series.[28] The only other complication was a subdural hematoma in a patient with liver failure and a severe bleeding disorder.[23]

There was no infection in a series involving 86 patients who were monitored with the fiberoptic system.[26] The average length of time of placement of the system was 8 days, the longest being 32 days. In two cases, the transducer head was inadvertently lost. One was retrieved during a subsequent operation, and the other was left without any sequelae.

Conclusions

Both the subarachnoid bolt and the epidural monitor can be inserted by safe simple procedures adaptable to the emergency department. For smaller centers, the subarachnoid bolt may be preferable, because it does not require expensive equipment. The simultaneous recording of arterial and intracranial pressure is very advantageous, and overall, I prefer the Ladd system.

Emergency Drainage of Traumatic Intracranial Hematomas

1. Clifton, G. C.: Head injury incidence and organization of prehospital care. Neurology Clinics IV: 3, 1982.
2. Pitts, L. H., and Martin, N.: Head injuries. Surg. Clin. North Am. 62:47, 1982.
3. Field, J. H.: Epidemiology of head injuries in England and Wales. London: Department of Health and Social Security, Her Majesty's Stationery Office, 1976.
4. Becker, D. P., Miller, J. D., Ward, J. D., Greenberg, R. P., Young, H. F., and Sakalas, R.: The outcome from severe head injury with early diagnosis and intensive management. J. Neurosurg. 47:491, 1977.
5. Bruce, D. A., Gennarelli, T. A., and Langfitt, T. W.: Resuscitation from coma due to head injury. Crit. Care Med. 6:254, 1978.
6. Walker, A. E.: The dawn of neurosurgery. Clin. Neurosurg. 6:3, 16, 1959.
7. Parry, T. W.: Trephination of the living human skull in prehistoric times. Br. Med. J. March 17, 1923.
8. Mumford, J. G.: Narrative of surgery; a historic sketch. *In*

9. Breasted, J. H.: The Edwin Smith Papyrus. Chicago, University of Chicago Press, 1930.
10. Celsus, A. C.: DeMedicina, trans. W. G. Spencer, Vol. 3. London, W. Heineman Ltd., 1938, pp. 294–649.
11. Mettler, C. C.: History of Medicine. York, PA, Maple Press Co., 1947, p. 826.
12. Horrax, H.: Neurosurgery: a historical sketch. Springfield, Charles C Thomas, Publisher, 1952, p. 135.
13. Jamieson, K. G., and Yelland, J. O. N.: Extradural hematoma. Report of 167 cases. J. Neurosurg. 29:13, 1968.
14. Burton, C., and Blacker, H. M.: A compact hand drill for emergency brain decompression. J. Trauma 5:643, 1965.
15. Stone, J. L., Rifai, M. H. S., Sugar, O., Lang, R. G. R., Oldershaw, J. B., and Moody, R. A.: Subdural hematomas: Part I acute subdural hematoma. Progress in definition of clinical pathology and therapy. Surg. Neurol., 19:216, 1983.
16. Jeffreys, R. V., and Jones, J. J.: Avoidable factors contributing to the death of head injury patients in general hospitals in Mersey region. Lancet 2:459, 1981.
17. Rimel, R. W., Jane, J. A., and Edlich, R. F.: An educational training program for the care at the site of injury of trauma to the central nervous system. Resuscitation 9:23, 1981.
18. Saul, T. G., and Ducker, T. B.: Management of severe head injuries. Mo. State Med. J. 45, 1981.
19. Mahoney, B. D., Rockswold, G. L., Ruiz, E., and Clinton, J. E.: Emergency twist drill trephination. Neurosurgery 8:551, 1981.
20. Grode, M. L., and Carton, C. A.: Drill stop for twist drill—technical note. J. Neurosurg. 52:599, 1980.
21. Hoff, J. T., Spetzler, R., and Winestock, D.: Head injury and early signs of tentorial herniation—a management dilemma. West J. Med. 128:112, 1978.

Intracranial Pressure Monitoring

22. Guillaume, J., and Janny, P.: Manométrie intracrânienne continue; Intérêt de la méthodes et premiers résultats. Rev. Neurol. (Par) 84:131, 1951.
23. Vries, J. K., Becker, D. P., and Young, H. F.: A subarachnoid screw for monitoring intracranial pressure. Technical note. J. Neurosurg. 39:416, 1973.
24. Numoto, M., Slater, J. P., and Donaghy, R. M.: An implantable switch for monitoring intracranial pressure. Lancet 1:528, 1966.
25. Numoto, M., Wallman, J. K., and Donaghy, R. M.: Pressure indicating bag for monitoring intracranial pressure. J. Neurosurg. 39:784, 1973.
26. Levin, A. B.: The use of a fiberoptic intracranial pressure transducer in the treatment of head injuries. J. Trauma 17:767, 1977.
27. Lundberg, N.: Continuous recording and control of ventricular fluid pressure in neurosurgical practice. Acta Psychiatr. Scand. (Suppl. 149) 36:1, 1960.
28. Rosner, M. J., and Becker, D. P.: ICP monitoring: Complications and associated factors. Clin. Neurosurg. 23:494, 1976.

65

Spinal Puncture and Cerebrospinal Fluid Examination

JON C. KOOIKER, M.D.

Introduction

Spinal fluid examination is performed in an emergency setting for the purpose of obtaining information that will be relevant to the diagnosis and treatment of specific disease entities. Many urgent and life-threatening conditions require immediate and accurate knowledge of the nature of the cerebrospinal fluid (CSF). Certain harmful consequences may result from a spinal puncture, however, and this procedure should follow a careful neurologic examination with thought given to the risks and merits of the procedure in each given situation.

BACKGROUND

In 1885, Corning punctured the subarachnoid space to introduce cocaine into a living patient.[1] Quincke (1891) first removed CSF in a diagnostic study and introduced the use of a stylet.[2] He studied cellular contents and measured protein and glucose levels. Quincke was also the first to record pressure with a manometer. Subsequently, increasingly sophisticated bacteriologic, biochemical, cytologic, and serologic techniques were introduced. In 1918, Dandy replaced spinal fluid with air to determine normal brain anatomy and changes that would indicate disease.[3] Iodinized oil and, more recently, water-soluble contrast media have been used to delineate the spinal subarachnoid space and cerebral cisterns.[4] Other uses of the spinal puncture include injection of anesthetic agents, chemotherapeutic agents, and antibiotics and drainage of fluids.

ANATOMY OF SPINAL FLUID FORMATION AND CIRCULATION

In the adult, approximately 140 ml of the spinal and cranial cavities is occupied by CSF. This volume is the result of a balance between continuous secretion (primarily by the ventricular choroid plexus) and absorption into the venous system (chiefly by way of the arachnoid villi). After formation, the fluid passes out of the ventricles by way of the foramina of Luschka and Magendie. The fluid then flows into the spinal subarachnoid space, the basilar cisterns, and the cerebral subarachnoid space. Production is approximately 0.35 ml per minute, and CSF ventricular production is such that there is a net flow out of the ventricles of 50 to 100 ml per day.

Spinal fluid may have an embryologic nutritive function; at maturity the CSF most likely acts as a mechanical barrier between the soft brain and the rigid fibrous-osseous dura, skull, and vertebral column. It also appears to support the weight of the brain.[5] Contraction and expansion of the CSF may accommodate changes in brain volume. Additional functions, including intracerebral transport and maintenance of a stable chemical environment of the central nervous system, have been reviewed by Fishman.[6]

INDICATIONS FOR SPINAL PUNCTURE

In recent years, the indications for spinal puncture have been reduced with the introduction of new noninvasive diagnostic procedures—primarily computed transaxial tomography. A few clinical situations require an early, or even an emergent, spinal puncture. The primary indication for an emergent spinal tap is the possibility of central nervous system infection. CSF should be examined in patients with a fever of unknown origin, especially if an alteration of consciousness is present, even in the absence of meningeal irritation. Meningeal signs need not be present in patients who are old, debilitated, or receiving immunosuppressive or anti-inflammatory drugs. In a newborn, even a fever is not a dependable sign; temperatures may be normal or even subnormal. A tense and bulging fontanelle is somewhat more reliable, although this sign may be absent in a dehydrated child. In a child between the ages of 1 month and 3 years, fever, irritability, and vomiting are the most common symptoms of meningitis. Typically, handling is painful for the child, and the child cannot be comforted. In addition, the older child may complain of a headache. In all ages, the patient looks unusually ill and appears drowsy with a dulled sensorium.[7-9] Physical signs become more useful in diagnosing meningitis in children past 3 years of age. These include nuchal rigidity, Kernig's sign (efforts to extend the knee are resisted), and Brudzinski's sign (passive flexion of one hip causes the other leg to rise, and efforts to flex the neck make the knees come up).

A useful aid in distinguishing neck rigidity of meningeal origin from that caused by primary pain in the cervical muscles and the soft tissues is the usual preservation of lateral movement in meningeal irritation.

The second indication for an emergent spinal puncture is a suspected spontaneous subarachnoid hemorrhage. The diagnosis will usually be made by computed tomography or by the finding of blood in the spinal fluid. If computed tomography is available, then this noninvasive radiologic procedure, which has the potential to distinguish between aneurysmal and primary intracerebral bleeding, is preferred over spinal puncture.[10] A normal computed tomogram, however, may not rule out a subarachnoid hemorrhage and in an appropriate clinical setting requires a confirmatory spinal puncture.[11] Failure to detect blood radiographically may indicate a small bleed or a predominant basal accumulation of blood If a patient is seen several days after the hemorrhage, the blood may have become isodense with brain and may no longer be visible.[12, 13] The proper diagnosis would then require spinal puncture.

The usual clinical picture of a subarachnoid hemorrhage is a severe and sudden excruciating headache. The location of the headache is variable and does not give a clue as to the site of hemorrhage. Nausea, vomiting, and prostration are common symptoms, with approximately one third of patients becoming unconscious at the onset. Examination shows an acutely ill patient with an altered mental status. Meningeal signs are commonly present at the time of the initial examination and usually develop in all cases within 2 to 3 days. Meningeal signs may become more severe during the first week after hemorrhage and correspond to the breakdown of blood in the spinal fluid. During the first week, many patients are febrile, reflecting a chemical hemic meningitis.[14, 15] In theory, a small subarachnoid hemorrhage may take several hours to reach the lumbar region. Thus, it is possible that such a patient might have normal lumbar CSF if examined soon after rupture. A second, delayed lumbar puncture may occasionally be required for diagnosis in such a situation. If the neurologic picture demonstrates localizing findings, the presence of a large intracranial hematoma should be suspected, and spinal puncture is contraindicated until computed tomography (or arteriography) delineates the nature of the lesion.

In a patient with suspected cerebral embolus or evolving infarct, either a computed tomogram or clear spinal fluid should be obtained prior to the use of anticoagulants. This seems particularly applicable if persistent neurologic deficits or an altered mental state persists.[16]

Other nonemergent reasons for CSF examination include evaluation of central nervous system syphilis, instillation of chemotherapy and positive contrast agents, evaluation of suspected multiple sclerosis, and treatment of headache from subarachnoid hemorrhage or benign intracranial hypertension.[17]

CONTRAINDICATIONS

Spinal puncture is absolutely contraindicated in the presence of infection in the tissues near the puncture site.[5, 6] Spinal puncture is relatively contraindicated in the presence of increased intracranial pressure from a space-occupying lesion. Caution is particularly advised when lateralizing signs (hemiparesis) or signs of uncal herniation (unilateral third nerve palsy with altered level of consciousness) are present. In such cases, a tentorial or cerebellar pressure cone may be precipitated or aggravated by the spinal puncture. Cardiorespiratory collapse, stupor, seizures, and sudden death may occur when pressure is reduced in the spinal canal.[17] The risk seems to be particularly pronounced in patients with brain abscess.[18, 19] Brain abscesses frequently occur as expanding intracranial lesions with headache, mental disturbances, and focal neurologic signs rather than as infectious processes with signs of meningeal irritation. In 75 per cent of cases, a primary source of chronic suppuration is present.[18] Metastatic hematogenous spread of bacterial infection (from sepsis, intrathoracic infection, or congenital cardiac malformations with endocarditis) and prior otolaryngologic infection are of major importance in the genesis of cerebral abscesses. Although the CSF is usually abnormal (elevated pressure, elevated white blood cell count, and elevated protein concentration), spinal puncture in patients with possible brain abscess should be discouraged. Five of Samson and Clark's 22 patients exhibited signs of midbrain compression within 2 hours of lumbar puncture.[19] Evidence of herniation markedly reduces the patient's chances for survival.

Patients with ruptured brain abscesses, unfortunately, may present with an associated purulent meningitis. If the history suggests possible brain abscess, the computed tomography can rapidly diagnose and localize the lesion.[20–22] Kaufman and Leeds reported rapid and accurate demonstration in nine cases of brain abscesses and in six cases of subdural and epidural empyema with no false-negative studies.[20] Since the appearance of brain abscesses on computed tomograms is similar to that of neoplastic and vascular lesions, however, false positive reports of brain abscess may be encountered.

Spinal epidural hematomas may occur but are rare complications of lumbar puncture in individuals receiving anticoagulant therapy or in patients with disease associated with abnormal clotting mechanisms, especially thrombocytopenia. Edel-

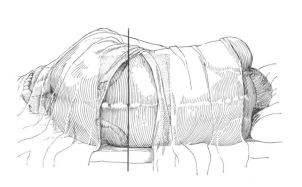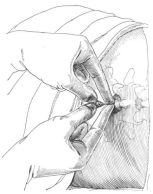

Figure 65–1. When the patient has been correctly positioned for the lumbar tap *(left)*, an imaginary line connecting the iliac crests will be exactly perpendicular to the bed. Insertion sites are marked by "x"; the operative field is draped. The needle should be inserted perpendicularly (or nearly so) to the plane of the back, with the forefingers of both hands guiding it in *(right)*. (From Cole, M.: Pitfalls in cerebrospinal fluid examination. Hosp. Pract. 47, 1969. Illustration by Carol Donner. Used by permission.)

son found over 100 cases of spinal epidural hematoma, approximately one third associated with anticoagulant therapy.[23] Most articles describe isolated cases.[16, 23–25] Spinal subdural hematomas following lumbar puncture are even more rare than epidural hematomas. When a patient is anticoagulated or has a coagulopathy, the tap should be performed by experienced physicians, who are less likely to traumatize the dura. The patient should be carefully followed for progressive back pain, lower extremity motor and sensory deficits, and sphincter impairment after the procedure. *Complaints of motor weakness, sensory loss, or incontinence following lumbar puncture should be thoroughly investigated.* Lumbar puncture may be performed in the presence of a coagulation defect if it is confined to situations in which it may provide essential information, such as in the diagnosis of meningitis. In cases of severe thrombocytopenia, the infusion of platelets prior to the lumbar puncture may be desirable. Similarly, the infusion of clotting factors in the hemophiliac patient and normalization of the prothrombin time with fresh frozen plasma in the anticoagulated patient are desirable if the clinical situation permits such delay.

If the history and picture suggest a treatable illness, such as meningitis, then the physician may perform a spinal puncture after careful consideration of the entire clinical picture. In all cases, the study should be undertaken after careful thought regarding how the results will assist in patient evaluation and treatment. It is unlikely that the spinal puncture will alter management in the presence of a neoplasm, a hematoma, a completed nonembolic infarct or cranial trauma.

Technique

Lumbar puncture is carried out with the patient in the lateral recumbent position. A line connecting the posterior superior iliac crests will intersect the midline at approximately the L-4 spinous process (Fig. 65–1).[26, 27] The adjacent interspace above or below may be used, depending upon which area appears to be most open to palpation. The space between lumbar vertebrae is relatively wide. In the thoracic region, the spinous processes overlap and are directed caudally, and therefore there is no midline area free of overlying bone. In the adult, the spinal cord extends to the lower level of L-1 or the body of L-2, thus eliminating higher levels as sites for puncture. The puncture in adults and in older children may be performed from the L-2 to L-3 interspace to the L-5 to S-1 interspace. Developmentally, the spinal canal and the spinal cord are of equal length in the fetus. Growth of the cord does not keep pace with longitudinal growth of the spinal canal. At birth, the cord ends at the level of the L-3 vertebra. The needle in infants should be placed at the L-4 to L-5 or L-5 to S-1 interspaces. The subarachnoid space extends to an S-2 vertebral level; however, the overlying bony mass prevents entry into this lowermost portion of the subarachnoid space.[26]

Almost all patients are afraid of a spinal puncture because they have heard stories of severe complications. Explaining the procedure in advance and discussing each step during the course of the test aids in reducing patient tension and helps the physician. The physician should inquire about history of allergies to local anesthetic agents and topical antiseptics. A standard informed consent form is available in hospitals. In view of the transient nature of physician-patient relations in emergency departments, this should be used when spinal punctures are performed, providing the patient is competent and of legal majority or an appropriate guardian is present.

The next important step is positioning of the patient. The patient is given a pillow in order to keep his head in the same plane as the vertebral axis. The shoulders and the hips are positioned perpendicularly with the table. A firm table or bed is desirable whenever possible. Flexion of the neck does *not* facilitate the procedure to any great extent, and since severe flexion may add to the patient's discomfort, this step may be omitted. The patient's lower back should be arched toward the physician. Some physicians place the patient in a sitting position, because the midline is more easily identified when the patient is sitting. The higher CSF hydrostatic pressure in a sitting, dehydrated patient may aid CSF flow. Caution regarding orthostatic blood pressure changes and airway maintenance must be observed when the patient is sitting for the procedure. An assistant must also help support the patient during the procedure.

Sterile gloves must be used. The examiner should wash the patient's back with an antiseptic solution applied in a circular motion and should increase the circumference of the pattern during each motion. The patient should be warned that the solution will be cold. The excess fluid is removed with a dry sterile gauze pad. A sterile towel is placed between the patient's hip and the bed. Commercial trays have a second sterile drape with a hole that may be centered over the site selected for the tap (Fig. 65–2).

The skin and deeper subcutaneous tissue are infiltrated with local anesthetic (1 per cent lidocaine). The patient should be warned about transient discomfort from the anesthetic. Anesthetizing the deeper subcutaneous tissue renders the procedure almost painless. Merely raising a skin wheal is insufficient anesthesia. While waiting for the anesthetic to take effect, the physician should attach the stopcock and manometer and see that the valve is working. A 3½-inch, 20 gauge needle should be used in adults, and a 2½-inch, 22 gauge needle should be used in children. (A 1½-inch, 22

gauge needle is available for infants.) A needle of this size has enough rigidity to allow the procedure to be accomplished easily but makes less of a dural tear than do larger instruments. The patient should be told to report any pain and should be informed that he will feel some pressure.

The needle is placed into the skin in the midline parallel to the table. The needle is held between both thumbs and index fingers. After the subcutaneous tissue has been penetrated, the needle is angled toward the umbilicus. The bevel of the needle should be facing laterally. It has been speculated that pointing the bevel laterally may allow the needle to penetrate the transverse fibers of the dura rather than cut through them, allowing for less spinal fluid leakage after the needle has been withdrawn.

The supraspinal ligament connects the spinous process; the interspinal ligaments join the inferior and superior borders of adjacent spinous processes. The ligamentum flavum is a strong, elastic, yellow membrane that may reach a thickness of 1 cm in the lumbar region. The ligamentum flavum covers the interlaminary space between the vertebrae and functions to assist the paraspinous muscles in maintaining an upright posture (Fig. 65–3). The ligaments are stretched in a flexed position and are more easily crossed by the needle. The ligaments offer resistance to the needle, and a "pop" is often felt as they are penetrated. One should remove the stylet frequently to see if the subarachnoid space has been reached. The "pop"

Figure 65–2. Standard lumbar puncture tray. Separate equipment is available for infants, children, and adults. (Courtesy of the American Pharmaseal Company, Glendale, California.)

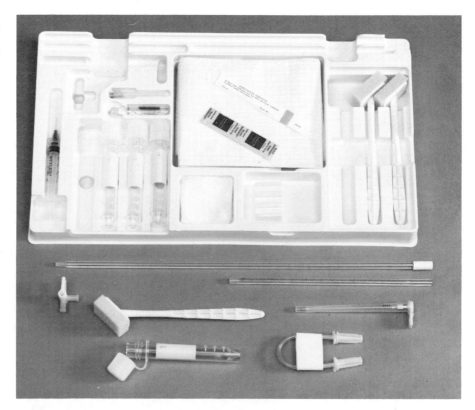

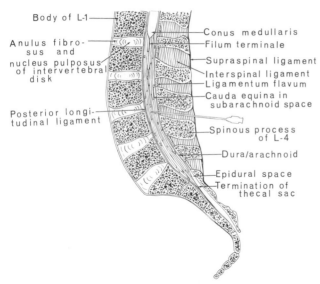

Body of L-1

Anulus fibrosus and nucleus pulposus of intervertebral disk

Posterior longitudinal ligament

Conus medullaris
Filum terminale
Supraspinal ligament
Interspinal ligament
Ligamentum flavum
Cauda equina in subarachnoid space
Spinous process of L-4
Dura/arachnoid
Epidural space
Termination of thecal sac

Figure 65–3. Midsagittal section through lumbar spinal column with spinal puncture needle in place between spinous processes of L-3 and L-4. Note the slightly ascending direction of the needle. The needle has pierced three ligaments and the dura/arachnoid and is in the subarachnoid space. (From Lachman, E.: Anatomy as applied to clinical medicine. New Physician 145, 1968. Used by permission.)

is occasionally not felt with the very sharp needles in disposable trays.

If bone is encountered, the needle must be partially withdrawn to the subcutaneous tissue. The physician should repalpate the back and should ascertain that the needle is in the midline. If bone is again encountered, the needle should be slightly withdrawn and should be reangled, with the point placed so it angles more sharply cephalad. This should avoid hitting the inferior spinous process.

Clear fluid will flow from the needle when the subarachnoid space has been penetrated. The physician should attach the manometer and should record the opening pressure. A three-way stopcock is supplied in disposable trays; this allows both collection and pressure to be measured by a single needle (Fig. 65–4). The patient is then asked to relax and to extend his legs to decrease intra-abdominal pressure. The fluid column is observed

for phasic changes with respirations and arterial pulsations. This ensures placement in the sub-arachnoid space. If the needle is against a nerve root or is only partially within the dura, the pressure may be falsely low, and respiratory excursions will not be seen in the manometer. Minor rotation of the needle may solve these problems. Hyperventilation to relax the patient should not be attempted, since this will reduce the pressure readings owing to hypocapnia and resultant cerebral vasoconstriction.

After measuring the pressure, the physician should turn the stopcock and should collect enough fluid to perform all desired studies. Even if the pressure is elevated, sufficient fluid should be removed for performance of all indicated studies, since the risk of the procedure involves the dural rent and not the amount of fluid removed. Presumably, more fluid will be lost subsequently through the hole in the dura. A dressing is placed over the puncture site. Commercial trays supply four specimen tubes. Tube 1 is used for determining protein and glucose levels and for electrophoretic studies; tube 2 is used for microbiological and cytologic studies; tube 3 is for cell counts and serologic tests for syphilis. In the presence of bloody CSF, cell counts should be performed in tubes 1 and 3 to help differentiate traumatic taps. One may compare water placed in the fourth tube with CSF in tube 3 to detect cloudiness or discoloration.

Traumatic taps can be avoided by proper patient and needle positioning. A traumatic tap most commonly occurs when the subarachnoid space is transfixed at the extrance of the ventral epidural space, where the venous plexus is heavier. A plexus of veins forms a ring around the cord, and these veins may be entered if the needle is advanced too far ventrally or is directed laterally (Fig. 65–5). If blood is encountered and fluid does not clear, the procedure should be repeated at a higher interspace with a fresh needle. A traumatic tap, per se, is not a particularly dangerous problem, and no specific precautions are needed if blood-tinged fluid is obtained. Observation for

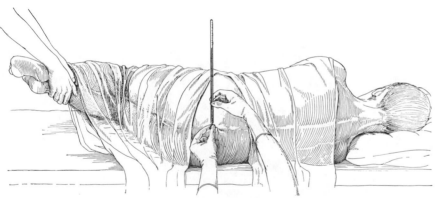

Figure 65–4. Opening pressure should be measured, not estimated, by means of an air-water manometer affixed to the needle by three-way stopcock, thus allowing pressure to be taken and fluid withdrawn through a single needle. If the manometric reading is initially elevated, the assistant or nurse gently extends the patient to see if elevation will subside to normal limits (80 to 180 mm H_2O). (From Cole, M.: Pitfalls in cerebrospinal fluid examination. Hosp. Pract. 47, 1969. Illustration by Carol Donner. Used by permission.)

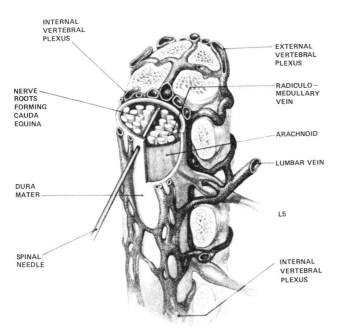

Figure 65–5. Spinal contents at the fourth and fifth lumbar vertebrae to show relationship of a lumbar puncture needle to the major vessels at this level. The major radiculomedullary vein, shown accompanying the L-5 nerve root, is situated far laterally to a needle correctly positioned in the midline of the dural sac. Note the avascular subdural space. (From Edelson, R. N., et al.: Spinal subdural hematomas. Arch. Neurol. 31:136, 1974. Illustration by Lynn McDowell. Used by permission.)

signs of cord or spinal nerve compression from a developing hematoma should be routine for these patients.

LATERAL APPROACH IN LUMBAR PUNCTURE

The supraspinal ligament may be calcified in older people, making a midline perforation difficult. A calcified ligament may deflect the needle. In this case, a slightly lateral approach may be used. As the lower lamina rises upward from the midline, the needle is directed slightly cephalad to miss the lamina and slightly medially to compensate for the lateral approach.[26] The needle passes through the skin, superficial fascia, fat, the dense posterior layer of thoracolumbar fascia, and the erector spinae muscles. The needle then penetrates the ligamentum flavum (bypassing the supraspinal and interspinal ligaments), the epidural space, and the dura before CSF is obtained (Fig. 65–6).

Cisternal Puncture. In situations in which lumbar puncture is contraindicated (such as local infection or acute trauma to the lumbar spine) cisternal, or suboccipital, puncture is the usual alternative. Technical problems, such as morbid obesity, cord tumor, arachnoiditis, bony deformities, or prior spinal surgery (fusion), may make lumbar puncture impossible. Contrast material

may be injected into the cisterna magna to identify the rostral extent of the lesion when lumbar myelography has shown a complete block.

The patient is cleaned and anesthetized in a manner similar to that for a lumbar puncture, after the neck has been shaved from the external occipital protuberance to the mastoid process laterally. The patient is preferably placed in a lateral decubitus position, but a sitting position can be used. A pillow is placed under the head to keep the neck and the vertebral axis in the same plane. The patient's neck is flexed to his chest. The spinal needle is placed in the midline halfway between the spinous process of C-2 and the inferior occiput. The needle is angled cephalad through the subcutaneous tissue until it comes in contact with the bony occiput. The needle is then withdrawn and subsequently advanced at a less acute angle with the horizontal plane of the cervical spine. This is repeated until the dural "pop" is felt. As in the lumbar region, the stylet should be removed frequently, so the dura is not punctured unknowingly. Fluid is removed in the usual manner. Dural veins are less extensive, and bloody taps are less common. Low-pressure headaches are less common, presumably because the subarachnoid pressure is lower and the dural tear can heal faster.

LATERAL CERVICAL PUNCTURE

The patient is placed in a supine position and fully sterilized and anesthetized. A 20 gauge lumbar puncture needle is inserted perpendicularly to the neck and parallel to the bed. The landmark for insertion is a point 1 cm inferiorly and 1 cm dorsally to the mastoid process. The physician frequently removes the stylet to check for fluid return and, as at other sites, advances the needle slowly. If the needle goes too deeply and encounters paraspinous muscles, it is probably too deep

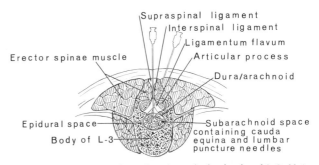

Figure 65–6. Horizontal section through the body of L-3. Note the two puncture needles in the subarachnoid space. The medial one is in the midline corresponding to the position in Figure 65–3. The lateral one exemplifies the lateral approach, which avoids the occasionally calcified supraspinal ligament. Note the lateral needle piercing the intrinsic musculature of the back and only one ligament, the ligamentum flavum. (From Lachman, E.: Anatomy as applied to clinical medicine. New Physician 145, 1968. Used by permission.)

posteriorly and should be repositioned more anteriorly. If bone is encountered, more dorsal placement is needed. Pressure and fluid samples are collected, as in other sites.[28]

The contraindications to cisternal and cervical punctures are the same as those to lumbar puncture. Both techniques are easily mastered, but prior demonstration of the procedure by an experienced neurologist or neurosurgeon is advised. When lumbar puncture cannot be performed for technical reasons and meningitis is suspected, then placement of the needle under fluoroscopy may help obtain spinal fluid.

Lumbar Puncture in Infants. Lumbar puncture in infants in usually performed to exclude meningitis. The sitting position may allow the midline to be more easily identified. Some authors use a nonstyleted needle in small infants, because this device allows the pressure to be estimated as the needle punctures the dura.[29] The failure to use a stylet may be the source of later development of an interspinal epidermoid tumor.[30, 31] A technique of lumbar puncture in the neonate using a butterfly infusion set needle has been described as a simplified procedure that may be useful in the squirming or hyperactive patient.[29]

If the child's neck is very tightly flexed, CSF may not be obtained. If the head is held in midflexion, however, CSF usually flows briskly. Prolonged severe flexion of the neck in an infant may produce dangerous airway obstruction and should be checked if the infant suddenly stops crying. Incorrect positioning usually results in multiple punctures and a bloody tap. If CSF fails to flow, gentle suction with a 1.0-ml syringe may be used to exclude a low-pressure syndrome. Local anesthesia is seldom administered to the neonate, and pressure readings are of little clinical value in the struggling child. Positioning is very important in the infant and is best accomplished by an assistant, who maintains the spine maximally flexed by partially overlying the child and holding him behind the shoulders and the knees. The infant has poor neck control; hence, the assistant must also ensure that the child maintains an open airway.

Complications

POSTSPINAL HEADACHE

A number of complications from lumbar puncture have been reported. By far the most common is the "postspinal headache." This occurs after 5 to 30 per cent of spinal taps.[6, 32, 33] The syndrome starts up to 48 hours after the procedure and usually lasts for 1 to 2 days and occasionally up to 14 days. Exceptional cases lasting months have been described. The headache usually begins within minutes after the patient arises and characteristically ceases as soon as he assumes a recumbent position. The pain is usually cervical and suboccipital in location but may involve the shoulders and the entire cranium. Exceptional cases include autonomic symptoms of nausea, vomiting, and vertigo. The syndrome is caused by leakage of fluid through the dural puncture site. This results in an absolute reduction of cerebrospinal fluid volume below the cisterna magna and a downward movement of the brain with displacement and stretching of pain-sensitive structures, such as meninges and vessels, which in turn causes a traction headache. In the recumbent position there is relief, since the weight of the brain is shifted cephalad. Dural leakage has been confirmed at surgery for disc disease and by at least one isotope myelographic study.[34] The size of the dural rent seems to correlate with the frequency of post–lumbar puncture headaches.[35] Any headaches may be somewhat decreased with the use of a very small spinal needle.

Using normal volunteers, Tourtellotte found the incidence of postural headache to be one case per nine subjects with the use of a 26 gauge needle and one case per three subjects with a 22 gauge needle.[35] The headache was reported to be milder when the smaller needle was used. Practically speaking, a 26 gauge needle is difficult to place and to manipulate into a position in which it does not become intermittently obstructed by nerve roots. In addition, a syringe is needed to withdraw fluid, and pressure cannot be easily recorded. Theoretically, the incidence of headache is greater with an 18 gauge needle.

Other factors that might influence the incidence of postspinal headache have been reviewed by Fishman.[6] The incidence is higher in young patients than in older patients and is also increased in females. Psychological factors, quantity of CSF removed, and position during lumbar puncture have not been found to be relevant in the incidence of headache. Some reports suggest a lower incidence with the lateral approach resulting from the production of holes in the dura and the arachnoid that do not overlap.

The influence of activity on post–spinal puncture headache has been studied with contradicting results, including worsening of, improvement in, and no effect on the incidence of headaches when patients were mobilized.[6, 27, 33, 36, 37] Brocker studied 1094 patients and reported a reduction of headache from 36.5 to 0.5 per cent by having the patients lie prone instead of supine for 3 hours after puncture with an 18 gauge needle.[36] He concluded that the prone position caused hyperextension of the spine and disrupted alignment of the holes in the dura and the arachnoid, making a leak less likely. Others have failed to show a decrease in duration, severity, or incidence of spinal headache with 24 hours of bed rest, although the onset of headache may be delayed if bed rest is enforced.[37]

Many medications have been advocated for treatment of post–spinal puncture headache: barbiturates, codeine, neostigmine, ergots, diphenhydramine hydrochloride (Benadryl), dimenhydrinate (Dramamine), amphetamine sulfate (Benzedrine), caffeine, ephedrine, intravenous fluids, magnesium sulfate, and vitamins.[6] No convincing data exist that any of these agents favorably influence the course of the headache.

Most clinicians generally follow the practice of using a styleted needle that is as small as possible. A 20 gauge needle is often used for adults because of its stiffness and ease of fluid flow. Multiple punctures should be avoided. There is no certainty about activity and position immediately after the procedure, although Brocker's results with the prone position are impressive.[36] Most postspinal headaches can be managed with bed rest with the head in the horizontal position. Dehydration should be avoided, since it lowers CSF pressure and might aggravate the headache. I usually provide simple analgesics but have not been impressed that analgesic medications have any advantage over bed rest and fluid intake.

In cases in which a prolonged low-pressure headache exists, the placing of an epidural patch by experienced anesthesiologists appears to be highly successful.[38] I rarely have had to use this aid.

INFECTION

Spinal puncture is absolutely contraindicated in the presence of local infection at the puncture site (cellulitis, epidural abscess, or furunculosis), because of the danger of inducing meningitis.

The postulation that an association exists between performance of a lumbar puncture during bacteremia and later development of meningitis has been examined by several laboratory and clinical investigators.[39, 40] The meningitis could be coincidental ("spontaneous meningitis") or could result from leakage of blood containing bacteria into the subarachnoid space after lumbar puncture ("lumbar puncture–induced meningitis"). Eng and Seligman reported that 14 per cent of 165 cases of bacteremia caused by *Streptococcus pneumoniae, Haemophilus influenzae,* and *Neisseria meningitidis* had evidence of meningitis at the time of initial lumbar puncture.[41] They argue that one cannot easily differentiate spontaneous meningitis from lumbar puncture–induced meningitis with these organisms because of their ability to invade the meninges spontaneously. Eng and Seligman identified a spontaneous meningitis in 0.8 per cent

of patients (7 of 924) with sepsis due to other organisms, and 2.1 per cent of these patients (3 of 140) had a clinical course consistent with a lumbar puncture–induced meningitis. These differences were not statistically significant, and the investigators concluded that the occurrence was "rare enough to be clinically insignificant." Teele and coworkers, however, reported that 7 of 46 children developed meningitis after an initial normal lumbar puncture in the presence of bacteremia.[40] *Streptococcus pneumoniae, Haemophilus influenzae,* and *Neisseria meningitidis* were recovered in all cases. All cases of "lumbar puncture–induced meningitis" occurred in children under 1 year of age who received no antimicrobial therapy at the time of initial cultures. Teele and associates advise that for children less than 1 year of age, the presence of a high fever and leukocytosis should prompt hospitalization and treatment for bacteremia and meningitis, pending culture results suggestive of infection or development of clinical infection at other sites, such as otitis media or pneumonia. Positive blood cultures would then require a second lumbar puncture to exclude the development of meningitis and to determine the length of antibiotic therapy.

HERNIATION SYNDROMES FOLLOWING LUMBAR PUNCTURE

Lumbar puncture is of value in confirming a diagnosis of meningitis and subarachnoid hemorrhage. Lumbar puncture can be dangerous in patients with intracranial mass lesions, however. Particularly with supratentorial mass lesions, there may be large pressure gradients between the cranial and lumbar compartments. When brain volume is increased because of a mass lesion or edema, rostrocaudal displacement may occur following lumbar puncture if the skull is intact. Lowering the lumbar pressure by removing CSF may increase the gradient, promoting both transtentorial and foramen magnum herniation. The frequency with which a lumbar puncture causes or accelerates transtentorial herniation is difficult to determine, because a patient might have developed herniation spontaneously without the procedure. Conflicting data are present in the literature. Korein and coworkers, in a personal series and literature review of 418 cases, concluded that the risk of an unfavorable response following lumbar puncture is less than 1.2 per cent.[42] Duffy encountered 30 cases referred to a neurosurgical service over a 1-year period because of complications of lumbar puncture:[17] Thirteen patients lost consciousness immediately following lumbar puncture, and another 15 showed a decreased level of consciousness within 12 hours following lumbar puncture. Three patients stopped breathing during the procedure. Twelve died within 10 days of the lumbar puncture. Only 10 of the 30 had papilledema, and in half the lumbar pressure was normal. In each case, clinical deterioration occurred within 12 hours of the lumbar puncture. The use of a small needle and the removal of limited volumes of CSF may not prevent herniation in the presence of increased intracranial pressure, because fluid seepage through the dura may be considerable. This may explain a progressive and worsening herniation syndrome.

A careful neurologic examination should precede all spinal punctures. When there is a history of headache with progressive mental changes and the development of localizing neurologic signs, then spinal puncture should *not* be performed as the initial diagnostic procedure unless there is a suspicion of infection. Papilledema is not a constant feature, even when the history suggests a protracted course. In other situations, a computed tomogram should be performed if available. This should identify hemorrhagic lesions and most neoplasms and should aid in the decision regarding the need for and the risk involved with spinal puncture.

Recognition of Herniation Syndromes

Herniation syndromes are the result of downward displacement of the hemispheres and the basal ganglia, which compress and displace the diencephalon and the midbrain rostrocaudally through the tentorial notch. Etiologic features and pathogenesis are detailed in the monograph by Plum and Posner.[43] Herniations have the potential to initiate vascular and obstructive complications that aggravate the original expanding lesion and can create an irreversible pathologic process. The anterior cerebral artery may be compressed against the falx and may increase ischemia and edema of the herniating hemisphere. Midline displacement posteriorly compresses the deep great cerebral vein and raises pressure in its area of drainage. Compression of the posterior cerebral artery at the tentorial notch can produce occipital infarction and swelling. In addition, kinking of the aqueduct may interfere with CSF circulation. This blockage may produce a normal spinal CSF pressure. Transtentorial herniation displaces the brain stem downward, stretching medial perforating branches of the basilar artery, as the artery is tethered to the circle of Willis. This produces brain stem ischemia and hemorrhages.

In general, pathologic changes with supratentorial mass lesions spread through the hemisphere and move rostrally and caudally in a progressive manner, with progressive dysfunction of the hemisphere and, subsequently, succeeding levels of the brain stem. The infrequent exceptions are seen in patients with acute cerebral-intraventricular hemorrhage and in patients with hemispheral mass lesions with incipient herniation who undergo lumbar puncture. Such conditions may rapidly progress from hemispheral dysfunction to sudden medullary failure.

Central, or *transtentorial*, herniation occurs in response to lesions of the frontal, parietal, and occipital lobes and the extracerebral lesions lying toward the vertex or the fronto-occipital lobes (Fig. 65–7). Frequently, patients are subacutely or

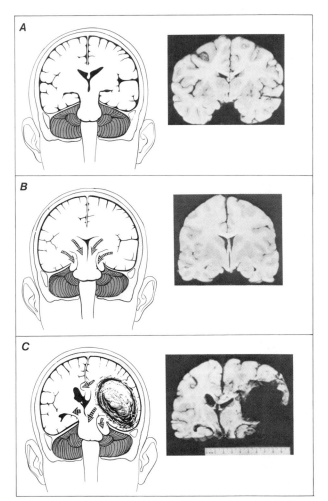

Figure 65–7. Intracranial shifts from supratentorial lesions. *A*, The relationships of the various supratentorial and infratentorial compartments as seen in a coronal section. *B*, Central transtentorial herniation. The photograph is taken from a patient with carcinoma of the lung and multiple cerebral metastases (none are apparent in this section) who died after developing signs and symptoms of the central syndrome of rostral-caudal deterioration. The brain is swollen: The diencephalon is compressed and elongated, and the mammillary bodies lie far caudal to those in the normal brain. Neither the cingulate gyrus nor the uncus is herniated. *C*, Uncal and transtentorial herniation. The photograph is taken from a patient who developed a massive hemorrhagic infarct and who died after developing the syndrome of uncal herniation. The cingulate gyrus is herniated after the falx; there is hemorrhagic infarction of the opposite cerebral peduncle and marked swelling and grooving of the uncus on the side of the lesion. Central downward displacement is also present but is less marked than in the figure above. (From Plum, F., and Posner, J.: The Diagnosis of Stupor and Coma. Philadelphia, F. A. Davis Co., 1980. Used by permission.)

chronically ill with bilateral disease, and the diagnosis may be uncertain. Initially, subjects exhibit a change in alertness or behavior. If the supratentorial lesion enlarges, compressing the diencephalon, stupor and then coma develop. At this point, monitoring of respiratory, ocular, and motor signs helps in diagnosing a supratentorial lesion and in determining the rostrocaudal direction of the disease process. Respirations at this time may be interrupted by deep signs or yawns and periodic breathing of the Cheyne-Stokes type (periods of hyperpnea regularly alternating with apnea). Pupils are small but react briskly. Eye movements may be conjugate or slightly divergent with roving eye movements. Caloric testing with cold water produces a conjugate slow tonic movement to the side of irrigation. Many individuals have a hemiparesis prior to herniation. As the diencephalic stage of the central syndrome evolves, the contralateral hemiplegia may worsen, with the homolateral limbs developing a paratonic resistance to movement, but the individual continues to respond to noxious stimuli appropriately. At this stage both plantar responses are extensor. Decorticate responses appear and consist of flexor muscle hypertonus in the upper extremity with predominantly extensor hypertonus in the leg. Recognition of a diencephalic stage of herniation is important in that it gives warning that a potentially reversible lesion may become irreversible.

Once midbrain signs develop, they will probably reflect infarction rather than reversible ischemia and compression. The chances of successfully removing or alleviating a supratentorial mass are small once a midbrain stage is reached.

Patients who develop midbrain upper pons failure exhibit a sustained tachypnea; pupils dilate to a fixed midposition (3 to 5 mm), and oculovestibular reflexes become difficult to obtain, requiring side-to-side head movements and cold caloric irritation. Dysconjugate eye movements appear with failure to adduction (internuclear ophthalmoplegia). Motor responses give way to extensor hypertonus in all limbs (decerebrate rigidity). Midbrain damage results from ischemia and infarction, and few patients recover.

As the brain stem becomes more ischemic, the pupils maintain a fixed position, eye movements are lost, and decerebration gives way to flaccidity. The medullary stage consists of irregular respirations with long periods of apnea. The pupils dilate and the blood pressure falls, with death being inevitable.

Uncal herniation occurs when expanding lesions in the temporal fossa shift the medial temporal lobe (uncus) and the hippocampal gyrus medially over the incisural edge of the tentorium. This flattens the midbrain, pushing it against the contralateral incisura. The third nerve and the posterior cerebral artery on the side of the lesion are caught between the swollen uncus and the free edge of the tentorium (Figs. 65–8 and 65–9). The earliest sign is a unilaterally sluggish or slightly dilated pupil. Because the diencephalon may not be the first structure encroached upon, impaired consciousness is not consistently present as an early sign of uncal herniation. Other respiratory, ocular, and motor findings may not be appreciably changed from earlier examinations. Pupillary dilation may persist for several hours, but once the patient progresses beyond this stage there is a tendency for midbrain dysfunction to occur rap-

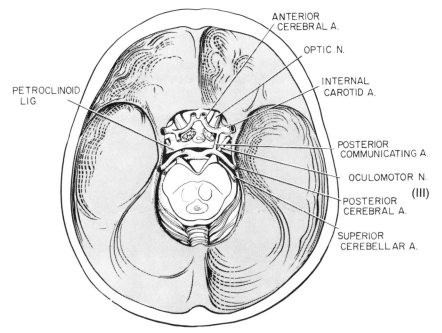

Figure 65–8. The floor of the anterior and middle fossae, illustrating the tentorial notch and the way in which the third nerve passes between the posterior cerebral and superior cerebellar arteries over the petroclinoid ligaments. (From Plum, F., and Posner, J.: The Diagnosis of Stupor and Coma. Philadelphia, F. A. Davis Co., 1980. Used by permission.)

ANTERIOR CEREBRAL A.

OPTIC N.

INTERNAL CAROTID A.

POSTERIOR COMMUNICATING A.

OCULOMOTOR N. (III)

POSTERIOR CEREBRAL A.

SUPERIOR CEREBELLAR A.

PETROCLINOID LIG.

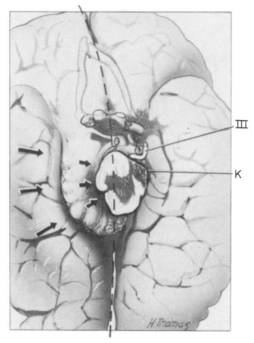

Figure 65–9. The undersurface of the forebrain in transtentorial herniation. Compare the positioning of the III nerve and the adjacent posterior cerebral artery as well as the shape of the midbrain with those in Figure 65–8. Large arrows point to the edge where the hippocampus herniated through the tentorium. Small arrows and the dotted line indicate the lateral shift of the mesencephalon, which produces a hemorrhagic Kernohan's notch at point K. (From Plum, F., and Posner, J.: The Diagnosis of Stupor and Coma. Philadelphia, F. A. Davis Co., 1980. Used by permission.)

idly. Ipsilateral external ophthalmoplegia soon follows pupillary dilation along with stupor and coma. Oculovestibular reflexes disappear as ischemia spreads to the midbrain. As the opposite cerebral peduncle is compressed against the tentorial edge, hemiplegia may appear ipsilaterally to the expanding supratentorial lesion (Kernohan's notch). Decerebrate posturing develops, with the opposite pupil becoming dilated and fixed. Progression then proceeds as described for the central syndrome. As with transtentorial herniation, once midbrain failure occurs, survival is much less likely.

IMPLANTATION OF EPIDERMOID TUMORS

An epidermoid tumor or cyst is a mass of desquamated cells containing keratin within a capsule of well-differentiated stratified squamous epithelium. Congenital lesions are rare and arise from epithelial tissue that becomes sequestrated at the time of closure of the neural groove between the third and fifth weeks of embryonic life. Acquired intraspinal epidermoid tumors result from implantation of epidermoid tissue into the spinal

canal at the time of lumbar puncture performed with needles without stylets or with ill-fitting needles.[30, 31] The clinical syndrome consists of pain in the back and the lower extremities developing years after spinal puncture. Myelography is required for diagnosis and surgery for treatment. Failure to use a stylet may also result in aspiration of a nerve root into the epidural space.

BACKACHE AND RADICULAR SYMPTOMS

Minor backache commonly results from trauma of the spinal needle. Frank disk herniation has been reported from the passing of the needle beyond the subarachnoid space into the anulus fibrosis. Transient sensory symptoms from irritation of the cauda equina are also quite common.

Other reported complications include transient unilateral or bilateral sixth nerve palsies caused by stretching or displacement of the abducens nerve as it crosses the petrous ridge of the temporal bone, subarachnoid hemorrhage, epidural hematoma, anaphylactoid reactions to local anesthetics, and settling of cord tumors. Most of these are rare and are seldom encountered.[6, 23, 25]

Most of the complications of lateral cervical and cisternal puncture are similar to those encountered with a lumbar puncture. In addition, perforation of a large vessel with resultant cisterna magna hematoma or obstruction of vertebral artery flow has been described. Puncture of the medulla oblongata may cause vomiting or apnea, and puncture of the cord may be associated with pain.[28] Long-lasting side effects of cord puncture are probably minor. In addition, traumatic tap and postspinal headache may occur with lateral cervical and cisternal puncture.

Interpretation

PRESSURE

The pressure of the spinal fluid is of great clinical importance. It should be accurately measured whenever possible. Accurate measurement is dependent upon patient cooperation. Normal pressure is between 70 and 180 mm H_2O. In the sitting position, lumbar pressure should not rise above the foramen magnum. Increased intracranial pressure can result from expansion of the brain (edema, hemorrhage, or neoplasm), overproduction of CSF (choroid plexus papilloma), a defect in absorption, or obstruction of flow of CSF through the ventricles. Cerebral edema may be associated with meningitis, carbon dioxide retention, subarachnoid hemorrhage, anoxia, congestive heart failure, or superior vena cava obstruction. Pressure may be falsely elevated in a tense patient, when the head is elevated above the plane of the needle and, possibly, with marked obesity or muscle contraction.[5] Pressure is not usually measured in the neonate, since a struggling or crying child will have a falsely elevated pressure.

Low pressure should suggest obstruction of the needle by meninges. Low pressure can also be seen with spinal block. Rarely, a primary low-pressure syndrome occurs in a setting of trauma, following neurosurgical procedures, secondary to subdural hematomas in elderly patients, with barbiturate intoxication, and in cases of CSF leakage through holes in the arachnoid.[44, 45]

The Queckenstedt test is useful for demonstrating the presence of obstruction in the spinal subarachnoid space.[5, 6, 32] The test is seldom performed today, because myelographic techniques have been refined. This test may be of use in the management of a patient with a myelopathy whose general medical state causes reluctance to perform a myelogram or in whom the need for myelography is uncertain. With the patient in the lateral recumbent position, jugular vein compression causes decreased venous return to the heart. This distends cerebral veins and causes a rise of intracranial pressure, which is transmitted throughout the system and is measured in the manometer. After 10 seconds of bilateral compression, CSF pressure usually rises to 150 mm H_2O over the initial reading and returns to the baseline in 10 to 20 seconds after release. If there is no change in the lumbar pressure or if the rise and fall is delayed, it should be concluded that the spinal subarachnoid space does not communicate with the cranial subarachnoid space. In this situation, Pantopaque should be injected before removal to facilitate subsequent performance of a myelogram. This is necessary because the lumbar dural sac may collapse, making it impossible to re-enter the canal. If cervical cord disease is suspected, the test should be repeated with the neck in the neutral position, hyperextended, and flexed. When lateral sinus obstruction is suspected, unilateral jugular venous compression may be used (Tobey-Ayer test).

APPEARANCE

If the spinal fluid is not crystal clear, a pathologic condition of the central nervous system should be suspected. The examiner should compare the fluid with water, viewing down the long axis of the tube. A glass tube is preferred, because plastic tubes are frequently not clear. The fluid may be clear with as many as 400 cells per mm³.[6]

Xanthochromia is a yellow-orange discoloration of the supernate of centrifuged spinal fluid. Xan-

throchromia is produced by red cell lysis and is caused by one or more of the following pigments: oxyhemoglobin, bilirubin, and methemoglobin. Oxyhemoglobin causes a red color, bilirubin a yellow color, and methemoglobin a brown color. Oxyhemoglobin is seen within 2 hours of subarachnoid bleeding and red cell lysis. Formation reaches a maximum in 24 to 48 hours after hemorrhage and disappears in 3 to 30 days.[5, 32, 46] The appearance of bilirubin in the CSF involves the conversion of oxyhemoglobin by the enzyme hemeoxygenase. The enzyme is found in the choroid plexus, the arachnoid, and the meninges. Enzyme activity appears approximately 12 hours after the bleed.[5, 46] Bilirubin may persist for 2 to 4 weeks. Bilirubin in CSF caused by hepatic or hemolytic disease does not appear until a serum level of 10 to 15 mg total bilirubin per 100 ml is reached, unless underlying disease associated with a high CSF protein is present.

Oxyhemoglobin and bilirubin may be measured chemically or by spectrophotometric analysis. Demonstration of these compounds in CSF may help in the distinction between recent intracranial hemorrhage and a traumatic tap. Oxyhemoglobin may form as a result of red cell lysis if the tube has been allowed to stand for more than 1 hour before testing, however.

Methemoglobin is a reduction product of oxyhemoglobin characteristically found in encapsulated subdural hematomas or in old intracerebral hematomas.

CELLS

The technique involved in cell counts is reviewed in several sources.[5, 6, 32, 46] Cell counts above 5 per mm³ should be taken to indicate the presence of a pathologic condition. In a study of 135 normal university students, Tourtellotte reported almost exclusively lymphocytes and monocytes, and the presence of one to five lymphocytes in the CSF may be normal.[5] It has been stated that polymorphonuclear leukocytes are never seen in normal individuals. With the use of the cytocentrifuge, however, an occasional specimen may show a neutrophil in an otherwise normal individual.[6] Such a finding should routinely prompt culture of the spinal fluid, since the presence of a neutrophilic pleocytosis is commonly associated with bacterial infections or the early stages of viral infections, tuberculosis, meningitis, hematogenous meningitis, and chemical meningitis due to foreign bodies. The use of formulas or calculations to determine if the white blood cell (WBC) count in a traumatic tap is a result of contamination or infection has not been found to be useful.

Small lymphocytes may be seen in normal individuals. Small and large immunocompetent cells are found with a variety of bacterial, fungal, viral, granulomatous, and spirochetal diseases as well as the presence of foreign substances.

Eosinophils are always abnormal and most commonly represent a parasitic infestation of the central nervous system. They may also be seen after myelography and pneumoencephalography and, to a minor degree, in other inflammatory diseases, including tuberculous meningitis and neurosyphilis; CSF eosinophilia has also been reported in cases of subarachnoid hemorrhage, lymphoma, and Hodgkin's disease.[48]

GLUCOSE

The normal range of CSF glucose is between 50 and 80 mg per 100 ml, which is between 60 and 70 per cent of the glucose concentration in the blood. Values below 40 mg per 100 ml are invariably abnormal. Hyperglycemia may mask a depressed CSF level, and the CSF/blood glucose ratio should be measured routinely. Between 90 and 120 minutes are required before the CSF glucose reaches the steady state with blood glucose changes. When CSF glucose is of diagnostic importance, CSF and blood samples should be obtained after a 4-hour fast.

Glucose enters the CSF by way of the choroid plexus as well as by transcapillary movement into the extracellular space of the brain and the cord by carrier-mediated transport. It then equilibrates freely with the CSF subarachnoid space. Fishman concludes that a low CSF glucose concentration indicates increased glucose utilization in the brain and the spinal cord and, to a lesser degree, by polymorphonuclear leukocytes and inhibition of membrane carrier systems.[6]

Low CSF glucose levels may be found in several diseases of the nervous system, as noted in Table 65–1. Elevated CSF glucose levels generally have no significance; elevation usually reflects hyperglycemia.

PROTEIN

The normal range of the lumbar CSF protein level is 15 to 45 mg per 100 ml. The concentration

Table 65–1. LOW CSF GLUCOSE SYNDROMES

Bacterial meningitis	Syphilis
Tuberculous meningitis	Chemical meningitis
Fungal meningitis	Subarachnoid hemorrhage
Sarcoidosis	Mumps meningitis
Meningeal carcinomatosis	Herpes simplex encephalitis
Amebic meningitis	Hypoglycemia
Cysticercosis	
Trichinosis	

is lower in the ventricles and the basilar cisterns. Most of the proteins in CSF normally come from the blood. Protein entry is determined by molecular size and relative impermeability of the blood-CSF barrier. Faulty reabsorption of protein by arachnoid villi may also elevate protein levels. Increases in CSF total protein levels suggest that a disease state may be present. Levels greater than 500 mg per 100 ml are uncommon and are seen mainly in meningitis, in subarachnoid bleeding, and with spinal tumors. The high levels seen with cord tumors result from an increase in local capillary permeability. With high levels (generally 1000 mg per 100 ml), CSF may clot (Froin's syndrome). Protein levels are greatest with lower levels of cord obstruction.

Selective measurement of gamma globulin fractions in CSF has proved to be of diagnostic value in suspected cases of multiple sclerosis; several reviews are available.[49–51] Elevated CSF IgG has been found in many chronic inflammatory conditions, including syphilis, viral encephalitis, subacute sclerosing panencephalitis, progressive rubella encephalitis, tuberculous meningitis, sarcoidosis, cysticercosis, and acute postinfectious polyneuropathy (Guillain-Barré syndrome).

CHLORIDE

CSF chloride was used in diagnosing tuberculous meningitis but has little current application in clinical neurology.

THE TRAUMATIC TAP

It should not be difficult to distinguish between subarachnoid bleeding and bloodshed by the spinal needle if certain steps are taken *at the time of the initial puncture*. In traumatic punctures the fluid generally clears between the first and third tubes as the needle is washed by spinal fluid. Decreasing cell counts on the first and third tubes helps confirm this. In a recent hemorrhage, however, a declining cell count may represent layering of cells in a recumbent patient. The fluid should then be centrifuged. With moderately blood-stained fluid, the supernatant should be clear if the red cells have been present for less than 2 hours (traumatic tap). It should be noted that an early CSF examination may show clear fluid prior to the development of hemolysis, even after spontaneous subarachnoid bleeding. Xanthochromia may be seen after a traumatic tap if the red cell count exceeds 150,000 to 200,000, however. The yellow color may appear if sufficient serum is present.[52] The presence of a clot in one of the tubes strongly favors accidental bleeding. In subarachnoid hemorrhage this does not occur, because blood is defibrinated at the site of the hemorrhage. In states associated with CSF protein greater than 150 mg per dl or if the patient is deeply jaundiced, the fluid can be mildly xanthochromic. Also, any lumbar puncture performed several days after a traumatic tap may yield stained fluid. An immediate repeat puncture at a higher interspace may also help distinguish a traumatic tap.

CSF Analysis with Infections

BACTERIAL

The CSF findings are imperative in establishing the diagnosis of acute bacterial meningitis. CSF analysis establishes the diagnosis, the causative organism, and the choice of antibiotics and helps determine management. CSF must be transported to the laboratory immediately and examined at once. In cases of meningococcal infection, a delay in processing may cause the diagnosis to be missed, since the organism tends to autolyze rapidly. Speed is only slightly less important with other organisms, since early initiation of antibiotic therapy is crucial.

The Gram stain is of great importance, since this often dictates the initial choice of antibiotic therapy. It has been suggested that the physician become expert at examining Gram stains of CSF, and the editors suggest that one should spend 10 minutes personally examining each CSF specimen. Gram-negative intra- or extracellular diplococci are indicative of *N. meningitidis*. Small gram-negative bacilli may indicate *H. influenzae*, especially in children. The presence of gram-positive cocci indicates *S. pneumoniae*, *Streptococcus*, or *Staphylococcus*. Twenty per cent of Gram stains may be falsely negative because too few organisms are present.[46] The Gram stain smear is more likely to be positive in patients who have not received prior antibiotic therapy.

For culture, blood and chocolate agar are required. *N. meningitidis* and *H. influenzae* grow best on chocolate agar. The plates are incubated under 10 per cent carbon dioxide. Thioglycolate medium is used for possible anaerobic organisms. Cultures are examined at 24 and 48 hours, but plates should be kept for at least 7 days.[53]

While the culture is pending, one may suspect a bacterial infection in the presence of an elevated opening pressure and a marked pleocytosis ranging between 500 and 20,000 white cells per mm.[3] The differential count is usually chiefly neutrophils. A count above 1000 cells per mm^3 seldom occurs in viral infections. Occasionally, acellular fluid may be found, and repeat lumbar puncture may be required in febrile patients in whom the clinical features remain compatible with meningitis.[54, 55]

CSF glucose levels less than 40 mg per dl or less than 60 per cent of a simultaneous blood glucose level should raise the question of bacterial meningitis, even in the presence of a negative Gram stain and a low cell count. Glucose levels with bacterial meningitis are occasionally below 10 mg per dl. The CSF protein content in bacterial meningitis ranges from 500 to 1500 mg per dl and usually returns to normal by the end of therapy.

A useful test that can be performed in nearly all laboratories is the measurement of CSF lactate levels. In bacterial and fungal meningitis, levels are increased.[56] Lactic acid may be elevated even in patients who have received antibiotics for 1 or 2 days.[56] Lactic acid levels in viral infections tend to be normal, whereas values in bacterial meningitis are usually two to four times greater than the normal concentration of approximately 1.6 mEq per L.

A recent study by Durack and coworkers questions the use of repeat spinal taps as a test of meningitis cure.[57] Their review of 165 meningitis cases revealed 13 instances in which the repeat tap led to unnecessary intervention and two others in which treatment failure was *not* detected by the repeat spinal tap.

VIRAL

The organisms most commonly isolated in viral meningitis are the enteroviruses (Coxsackie, ECHO) and mumps virus. Enteroviruses are most commonly seen in the summer and fall, and mumps appears most frequently in the winter and spring. Viral cultures in most hospitals are not available and play little role in acute decisions regarding diagnosis and treatment. A tentative diagnosis may be based on analysis of the CSF. The cell count in viral meningitis and encephalitis characteristically shows 10 to 1000 cells per mm^3. The differential cell count is predominantly lymphocytic and mononuclear in type. In the early stages of meningoencephalitis, however, polymorphonuclear cells may predominate, making the distinction between viral and bacterial infections difficult. In such cases, a repeat tap in 12 to 24 hours will assist in clarifying the diagnosis. Protein levels are usually mildly elevated, but normal levels may be seen. The CSF glucose is characteristically normal; however, notable exceptions include some cases of mumps meningoencephalitis and herpes simplex encephalitis.

If the CSF cannot be delivered to the viral laboratory in 24 to 48 hours, it should be refrigerated at 4°C. Members of the enterovirus group are occasionally isolated from CSF. Herpes and arbor viruses are rarely found in CSF. In known viral

CNS disease, the stool is more rewarding (85 per cent positive) than CSF (10 per cent positive).[53] Since CSF is normally sterile, any isolate is significant, whereas a stool isolate does not necessarily indicate that the agent is responsible for central nervous system disease.

NEUROSYPHILIS

The true incidence of this disease is unknown. Approximately 5000 new cases of neurosyphilis are estimated to occur in the United States each year.[58] The natural history and clinical manifestations have been modified in the antibiotic era. The widespread use of oral antibiotics has changed neurosyphilis into a chronic partially treated meningitis. Seizures were considered in the preantibiotic era to complicate general paresis only late in the course of the illness, and then only in untreated patients. Previously, seizures were reported as an early manifestation in less than 5 per cent of symptomatic neurosyphilis. Seizures now occur in 25 per cent of symptomatic cases and may on occasion be the sole manifestation of neurosyphilis.[58] Seizures are usually partial (focal), with one third of patients having no interictal clinical findings. A treponemal serologic test should be obtained in every adult with acquired partial seizures.

Ophthalmologic findings are frequently present in syphilis. These include a slowly progressive optic atrophy, an acute optic neuritis, cranial oculomotor neuropathy, and a chorioretinitis. A more specific sign is a dissociated pupillary response to light and convergence with loss of the light reflex (Argyll Robertson pupil). Meningovascular neurosyphilis involves infection of both the meninges and the cerebral vasculature. The clinical picture is that of a cerebral infarct or an acute meningoencephalitis. Other less common modern syndromes are reviewed in standard texts.[14]

CSF findings suggestive of neurosyphilis include more than five leukocytes per mm³, elevated protein concentration, elevated gamma globulin concentration, and a positive serologic test for syphilis. Glucose is usually normal; the colloidal gold test has largely been replaced by electrophoretic analysis of gamma globulin.

Serologic tests for syphilis are either treponemal or nontreponemal. Nontreponemal tests detect a nonspecific globulin complex called reagin. Reagin tests, such as the Venereal Disease Research Laboratory (VDRL) flocculation test, lack sensitivity and should not be used to exclude the diagnosis of neurosyphilis. One third to one half of patients with neurosyphilis will have a negative VDRL test in the serum, and more than one third will have a negative VDRL test in the CSF.[58]

Treponemal tests provide evidence of a specific immune response to *Treponema pallidum*. Currently, the serum fluorescent treponemal antibody absorption (FTA-ABS) is the test of choice to confirm the diagnosis of neurosyphilis. The serum FTA-ABS test is reactive in 95 to 100 per cent of cases of neurosyphilis. A negative serum FTA-ABS test makes CSF examination unnecessary. Its false positive rate is less than 1 per cent, but the incidence of biological false positive tests may increase in the presence of collagen vascular disorders.

A positive serum treponemal test indicates past infection with syphilis and may be reactive indefinitely, even after treatment. Therefore, CSF is used as a guide to the presence and the activity of neurosyphilis. The VDRL test is currently the test of choice in CSF and, when positive, is strong evidence for neurosyphilis. False positive CSF-VDRL tests are rare. The FTA-ABS test is not currently used in CSF; the false positive rate is between 4 and 6 per cent and is felt possibly to represent antibodies that have passively entered from serum.[59] The CSF-VDRL either may be reactive by contamination with seropositive blood (traumatic tap, subarachnoid hemorrhage) or may occur with entry of serum reagin into CSF during meningitis.

There is some concern that today many patients with parenchymal neurosyphilis have normal CSF. A test has been developed in primates to demonstrate the presence of *T. pallidum* with normal CSF parameters. This finding leads to the recommendation that a patient with signs of progressive neurosyphilis and a positive treponemal serologic test be treated with antibiotics regardless of the CSF findings. A CSF pleocytosis may be provoked after 1 week of therapy and may supply supportive evidence for a diagnosis of neurosyphilis.

Fungal. The most common CNS fungal infection is cryptococcosis. Most patients are found to have elevated intracranial pressure. A lymphocytic pleocytosis with cell counts under 500 cells per mm³ is present. Glucose levels are low in 50 per cent of cases. Most CSF specimens will exhibit an elevated CSF protein. With the India ink preparation, the organisms may be seen in 50 per cent of cases. CSF cultures are positive in approximately 90 per cent of cases. Cisternal punctures for fluid analysis may be helpful in undiagnosed cases of lymphocytic meningitis in which multiple lumbar punctures have not confirmed the diagnosis.[60] Several serologic tests are available and are of value in the diagnosis and prognosis of cryptococcal meningitis and meningoencephalitis. These are based on the detection of cryptococcal polysaccharide capsular antigens in the CSF.[61] Cryptococcal antigens will be positive in more than 90 per cent of proven cases of cryptococcal meningitis. The false positive rate is significant and is reported to be as high as 20 per cent in the CSF.

Many false-positive results are caused by the presence of rheumatoid factor.[60]

Tuberculosis. If tuberculosis is suspected, a large volume of CSF (10 ml) is required for adequate culture. The cell count varies from 100 to 400 cells per mm³, with a lymphocytic predominance. Protein levels are elevated (100 to 500 mg per dl); CSF glucose may be depressed. Acid-fast stains must be examined by experienced observers. Fluid is inoculated onto Löwenstein-Jensen medium and the absence of growth on the medium should not be considered negative until 8 weeks after incubation.[62]

Summary

In a proper clinical setting, a spinal tap should never be performed unless the attending physician has reflected on whether the procedure will be of diagnostic aid. The procedure is often indicated in the diagnosis of meningitis or subarachnoid hemorrhage. Most contraindications are relative and not absolute, particularly if infection is an overriding consideration.

1. Corning, J. L.: Spinal anaesthesia and local medication of the cord. N.Y. State Med. J. 42:483, 1885.
2. Quincke, H.: Die lumbar Punktur des Hydrocephalus. Klin. Wochenschr. 28:929 and 965, 1891.
3. Dandy, W. E.: Experimental hydrocephalus. Ann. Surg. 70:129, 1919.
4. Sackett, J. F., and Scruthe, C. M.: New Techniques in Myelography. Hagerstown, MD, Harper & Row, 1979.
5. Tourtellotte, W. W., and Shorr, R. J.: Cerebrospinal fluid. In Youmans, J. P. (ed.): Neurological Surgery, vol. 1. Philadelphia, W. B. Saunders Co., 1982, pp. 423–486.
6. Fishman, R. A.: Cerebrospinal Fluid in Diseases of the Nervous System. Philadelphia, W. B. Saunders Co., 1980.
7. Smith, D. H.: The challenge of bacterial meningitis. Hosp. Pract. 11:71, 1976.
8. Cramblett, H. G.: Managing the child with bacterial meningitis. Hosp. Pract. 63, Dec. 1969.
9. Mattheis, A. W., and Wehrle, P. F.: Management of bacterial meningitis in children. Pediatr. Clin. North Am. 15:185, 1968.
10. Hayward, R. D., and O'Reilly, G.: Intracerebral hemorrhage, accuracy of computerized transverse axial scanning in predicting the underlying aetiology. Lancet 1:1, 1976.
11. Bouzarth, W. F., and Hedges, J. R.: Computed tomography and lumbar puncture. J. Am. Coll. Emerg. Phys. 8:164, 1979.
12. Bergstrom, M.: Variation with time of the attenuation values of intracranial hematomas. J. Comput. Assist. Tomogr. 1:57, 1977.
13. Bergstrom, M.: Computed tomography of cranial subdural and epidural hematomas: Variation of attenuation related to time and clinical events such as rebleeding. J. Comput. Assist. Tomogr. 1:449, 1977.
14. Vick, N. A.: Grinker's Neurology. Springfield, IL, Charles C Thomas, 1976, pp. 514–524 and 560–576.
15. Sundt, T. M.: Intracranial aneurysms and subarachnoid hemorrhage. In Siekert, R. G. (ed.): Cerebral Vascular Survey Report. Rochester, MN, Whiting Press, 1980, pp. 306–318.
16. Ruff, R. L., and Dougherty, J. L.: Evaluation of acute cerebral ischemia for anticoagulant therapy: Computed tomography or lumbar puncture. Neurology 31:736, 1981.
17. Duffy, G. P.: Lumbar puncture in the presence of raised intracranial pressure. Br. Med. J. 1:407, 1969.
18. Breuer, N. S., MacCarty, C. S., et al.: Brain abscess: A review of recent experience. Ann. Intern. Med. 82:571, 1975.
19. Samson, D. S., and Clark, K.: A current review of brain abscess. Am. J. Med. 54:201, 1973.
20. Kaufman, P., and Leeds, N.: Computed tomography (CT) in the diagnosis of intracranial abscesses. Neurology 27:1069, 1977.
21. Zimmerman, R. A., et al.: Evolution of cerebral abscess: Correlation of clinical features with computed tomography. Neurology 27:14, 1977.
22. Rotheram, E., and Kessler, L.: Use of computerized tomography in nonsurgical management of brain abscess. Arch. Neurol. 36:25, 1979.
23. Edelson, R. N., et al.: Spinal subdural hematomas complicating lumbar puncture. Arch. Neurol. 31:134, 1974.
24. Laglia, A. G., et al.: Spinal epidural hematoma after lumbar puncture. Ann. Intern. Med. 88:515, 1978.
25. Senelich, R. C., et al.: "Painless" spinal epidural hematoma during anticoagulant therapy. Neurology 26:213, 1976.
26. Lachman, E.: Anatomy as applied to clinical medicine. New Phys. 145, June 1968.
27. Cole, M.: Pitfalls in cerebrospinal fluid examination. Hosp. Pract. 47, July 1969.
28. Zivin, J.: Lateral cervical punctures: An alternative to lumbar puncture. Neurology 28:616, 1978.
29. Greensher, J., et al.: Lumbar puncture in the neonate: A simplified technique. J. Pediatr. 78:1034, 1971.
30. Shaywitz, B. D.: Epidermoid spinal cord tumors and previous lumbar puncture. J. Pediatr. 80:638, 1972.
31. Batnitzky, S., et al.: Iatrogenic intraspinal epidermoid tumors. JAMA 237:148, 1977.
32. Cole, M.: Examination of the cerebral spinal fluid. In Toole, J. F. (ed.): Special Techniques for Neurologic Diagnosis. Philadelphia, F. A. Davis Co., 1969, pp. 29–48.
33. Petite, F., and Plum, F.: The lumbar puncture. N. Engl. J. Med. 290:225, 1981.
34. Lieberman, L. M., et al.: Prolonged post–lumbar puncture cerebral spinal fluid leakage demonstrated by radioisotope myelography. Neurology 21:925, 1971.
35. Tourtellotte, W. W., et al.: A randomized double-blind clinical trial comparing the 22 versus the 26 gauge needle in the production of the post–lumbar puncture syndrome in normal individuals. Headache 12:73, 1972.
36. Brocker, R. J.: A technique to avoid post spinal-tap headache. JAMA 168:261, 1958.
37. Carbaat, P. A. T., and van Crevel, H.: Lumbar puncture headache: Controlled study on the preventive effect of 24 hours' bed rest. Lancet 2:1133, 1981.
38. Bradsky, J. B.: Epidural blood patch: A safe effective treatment for post lumbar puncture headaches. West. J. Med. 129:85, 1978.
39. Petersdorf, R. G., et al.: Studies on the pathogenesis of meningitis. II. Development of meningitis during pneumococcal bacteremia. J. Clin. Invest. 41:320, 1962.
40. Teele, D. W., et al.: Meningitis after lumbar puncture in children with bacteremia. N. Engl. J. Med. 305:1079, 1981.
41. Eng, R., and Seligman, S.: Lumbar puncture–induced meningitis. JAMA 245:1456, 1981.
42. Korein, J., et al.: Reevaluation of lumbar puncture. Neurology 9:290, 1954.
43. Plum, F., and Posner, J.: The Diagnosis of Stupor and Coma. Philadelphia, F. A. Davis Co., 1980, pp. 96–112.
44. Shenkin, H. A., and Finneson, B. E.: Clinical significance of low cerebral spinal fluid pressure. Neurology 8:157, 1958.
45. Bell, N. E., et al.: Low spinal fluid pressure syndromes. Neurology 10:512, 1960.
46. Ward, P.: Cerebrospinal fluid data, I. Interpretation in

intracranial hemorrhage and meningitis. Postgrad. Med. 68:181, 1980.

47. Osborne, J. P., and Pizer, B.: Effect on the white cell count of contaminating cerebrospinal fluid with blood. Arch. Dis. Child. 56:400, 1981.

48. Kiberski, T.: Eosinophils in the cerebrospinal fluid. Ann. Intern. Med. 91:70, 1979.

49. Hersey, L. A., and Trotter, J. L.: The use and abuse of the cerebrospinal fluid IgG profile in the adult: A practical evaluation. Ann. Neurol. 8:426, 1980.

50. Laurenzi, M., et al.: Oligoclonal IgG and free light chains in multiple sclerosis demonstrated by thin layer polyacrylamide gel. Ann. Neurol. 8:241, 1980.

51. Johnson, K. A., and Nelson, B. J.: Multiple sclerosis: Diagnostic usefulness of cerebrospinal fluid. Ann. Neurol. 2:425, 1977.

52. McNememey, W. H.: The significance of subarachnoid bleeding. Proc. R. Soc. Med. 47:701, 1954.

53. Schaffer, J. G., and Goldwin, M.: Medical microbiology. In Henry, J. B. (ed.): Todd, Sanford, and Davidson's Clinical Diagnosis and Management by Laboratory Methods. Philadelphia, W. B. Saunders Co., 1974, p. 946.

54. Onorato, I. M., et al.: Normal CSF in bacterial meningitis. JAMA 244:1469, 1981.

55. Vorki, A., et al.: Value of second lumbar puncture in confirming a diagnosis of aseptic meningitis. Arch. Neurol. 36:571, 1979.

56. Beatty, N. H., and Oppenheimer, S.: Cerebrospinal fluid lactic dehydrogenase and its isoenzymes in infections of the central nervous system. N. Engl. J. Med. 297:1197, 1968.

57. Durack, D. T., and Spanos, A.: End-of-treatment spinal tap in bacterial meningitis: Is it worthwhile? JAMA 248:75, 1982.

58. Hanson, J. R.: Modern neurosyphilis: A partially treated chronic meningitis. West. J. Med. 135:191, 1981.

59. Jaffe, H. W.: The laboratory diagnosis of syphilis. Ann. Intern. Med. 83:846, 1975.

60. Yoskikawa, T. T.: Management of central nervous system cryptococcosis. West. J. Med. 132:123, 1980.

61. Goodman, J. S., et al.: Diagnosis of cryptococcal meningitis. N. Engl. J. Med. 285:434, 1971.

62. Kennedy, D. H., and Fallon, R. J.: Tuberculous meningitis. JAMA 241:264, 1979.

66

Caloric Testing

PAUL B. BAKER, M.D.

Introduction

An accurate assessment of the comatose patient requires a thorough neurologic examination, with careful evaluation of the patient's responses to a variety of external stimuli. In an individual with normal brain stem function, stimulation of the vestibular labyrinth will result in compensatory deviation of the eyes. This response is known as the vestibulo-ocular reflex and forms the physiologic basis for the caloric test of the vestibular system. During caloric testing, a thermal stimulus, usually water at a specific temperature, is delivered to the external auditory canal to activate the labyrinth and produce the characteristic ocular movements. Pathologic conditions involving either the vestibular or oculomotor reflex pathways will alter or abolish the response to caloric stimulation.

Caloric tests are performed in both conscious and unconscious patients, depending upon the diagnostic circumstances. Quantitative caloric examination is conducted in the ambulatory patient for evaluation of possible vestibular dysfunction. This type of testing requires precisely controlled irrigation temperatures and specialized recording devices and is best undertaken in a properly equipped laboratory under the supervision of an experienced neurotologist. On the other hand, the neurologist, neurosurgeon, or emergency physician may perform *qualitative* caloric testing in the comatose patient for detection of gross disruption of vestibulo-ocular reflex pathways indicative of structural lesions or metabolic abnormalities involving the brain stem. In this setting, large quantities of ice water provide maximal stimulation of the vestibular apparatus. Such testing needs no special expertise and can be done at the bedside using equipment readily available in the emergency department. This simple procedure can provide valuable diagnostic and prognostic information necessary for management of the comatose patient.

Background

In the middle of the nineteenth century, Brown-Sequard first described the effects of introducing cold water into the ear canal.[1] The clinical importance of the phenomenon was first realized in 1906 by Barany, who developed a caloric procedure using an ice water stimulus.[2] He postulated, correctly, that caloric stimulation of the auditory canal induced formation of convection currents within the semicircular canals of the vestibular labyrinth. Different methods of caloric testing were later proposed by Kobrak and others, but standardization of the procedure awaited the introduction of the Fitzgerald-Hallpike technique in 1942.[3] This technique, which uses both warm and cool water stimuli under rigidly specified conditions, permits quantification of normal and abnormal caloric responses. Today, most formal caloric testing of conscious patients is based on variations of the original Fitzgerald-Hallpike procedure.

The value of caloric testing in the assessment of the comatose patient was emphasized by the work of Klingon[4] and Bender and associates[5] in the 1950's. Vaernet and Ethelberg studied the changes in caloric reactions during transtentorial herniation of the brain stem.[6, 7] Blegvad reported the effects of barbiturate intoxication upon the vestibulo-ocular reflex.[8]

More recent advances include the development of electronystagmography (ENG), which provides a graphic record of reflex eye movements and permits precise determination of the intensity of the caloric response.[9] Researchers have recently investigated the use of heated air as an alternative to traditional water caloric tests.[10]

Physiology and Functional Anatomy

Proper performance and interpretation of the caloric test require a basic understanding of the structure and function of both the vestibular and oculomotor systems. The anatomic pathways underlying the vestibulo-ocular reflex begin in the posterior portion of the labyrinth of the inner ear. The peripheral vestibular apparatus is located within the temporal bone and consists of the utricle, the saccule, and the lateral, anterior, and posterior semicircular canals (Fig. 66–1). Because of its proximity to the external ear canal, the lateral

or horizontal canal is of principal interest in caloric testing. Note that the lateral canal is oriented at a 30 degree angle to the horizontal (Fig. 66–2). Deflections of the cupula due to movement of endolymphatic fluid within the canal results in polarization changes in the underlying hair cell, which in turn are relayed to the afferent limb of the primary vestibular neuron.

Impulses of the primary neuron travel via Scarpa's ganglion and C.N. VIII to the brain stem to synapse with secondary vestibular neurons in the superior and medial vestibular nuclei of the upper medulla and lower pons (Fig. 66–3). Although the connections between the vestibular and oculomotor nuclei in the brain stem are quite complex, two main pathways exist. The direct projection runs from the vestibular complex to the nuclei of C.N. III and C.N. VI via the medial longitudinal fasciculus (MLF) and involves only three neurons: the primary vestibular, secondary vestibular, and oculomotor neurons.[11] The indirect projection between these same nuclei occurs over multisynaptic circuits in the tegmental reticular formation.[12] Another brain stem structure contributing to the vestibulo-ocular interaction is the parapontine reticular formation (PPRF), a poorly characterized group of pontine neurons that coordinate both voluntary and involuntary lateral gaze. The PPRF receives multiple inputs, including projections from the vestibular system and the contralateral frontal cortex, and sends output to oculomotor neurons through both the direct and indirect pathways. Excitatory impulses originating in the lateral canal finally travel via the oculomotor and abducens nerves to the ipsilateral medial rectus and contralateral lateral rectus muscles.

Rotation of the head generates flow of endolymphatic fluid within the semicircular canals. The firing rate of the primary vestibular neuron is

Figure 66–1. Diagram of the external, middle, and inner ear showing the relationship of the semicircular canals to the external auditory canal. (Ossicles have been removed for clarity.) (Modified from Noback, C. R., and Demarest, R. J.: The Human Nervous System. New York, McGraw-Hill, 1981, p. 342.)

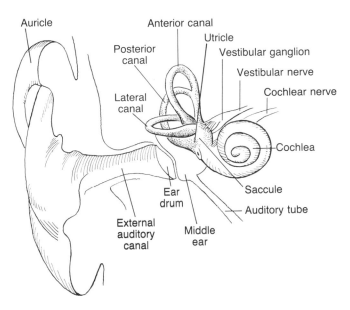

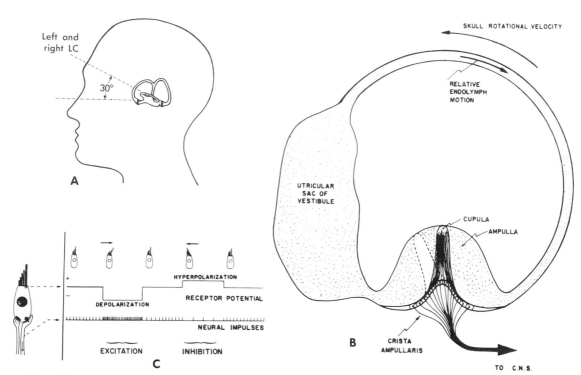

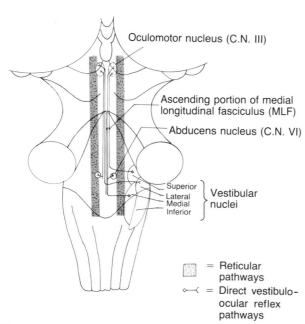

Figure 66–2. *A,* The long axis of the lateral canal forms a 30-degree angle with the horizontal plane. This alignment must be compensated for during caloric testing by proper positioning of the patient. (From Barber, H. O., and Stockwell, C. W.: Manual of Electronystagmography, 2nd ed. St. Louis, C. V. Mosby, 1980. Used by permission.) *B,* Schematic diagram of the semicircular canal showing the relationship between endolymphatic flow and cupular deviation. (From Bach, Y., Rita, P., Collins, C., and Hyde, J. E.: The Control of Eye Movements. New York, Academic Press, 1971. Used by permission.) *C,* Diagram showing effect of deflection on underlying hair cell and its associated primary vestibular neuron. (From Flock, A.: *In* Durrant, J. D., and Lovrinic, J. H.: Bases of Hearing Science. Baltimore, Williams & Wilkins, 1977. Used by permission.)

Figure 66–3. Schematic diagram of the brain stem showing the major elements of the vestibulo-ocular reflex (VOR) pathway. The solid line indicates the direct projection between the vestibular nuclei and the third and sixth nucleus. The stippled area represents the indirect projections between the nuclei. (Modified from Barr, M. L.: The Human Nervous System—An Anatomical Viewpoint, 2nd ed. New York, McGraw-Hill, 1974, p. 316.)

dependent upon the direction of flow. For example, in the lateral canal, flow toward the ampulla (ampullopetal) increases the rate, whereas flow away from the ampulla (ampullofugal) decreases the rate.[13] Increased firing on one side results in conjugate deviation of the eyes toward the opposite side, whereas decreased firing causes deviation to the same side. This principle forms the physiologic basis of caloric testing. When the lateral canal is placed in the vertical position and ice water is infused into the ear, the endolymph nearest the canal will cool and sink, resulting in ampullofugal flow (Fig. 66–4). As the firing rate decreases, the eyes conjugally deviate toward the side of irrigation. Likewise, if warm water were used in the same position or if the canal were inverted 180 degrees, the opposite would occur.

Eye movements induced by caloric stimulation in conscious, neurologically normal individuals are more complex. Ice water infusions will induce a rhythmic jerking of the eyes that includes a slow deviation toward the irrigated side followed by a quick compensatory saccade toward the midline. This is known as *caloric nystagmus.* By convention, *caloric nystagmus is named for the fast component,* thus the popular mnemonic "Fast COWS" (Cold irrigation—Opposite beating nystagmus; Warm ir-

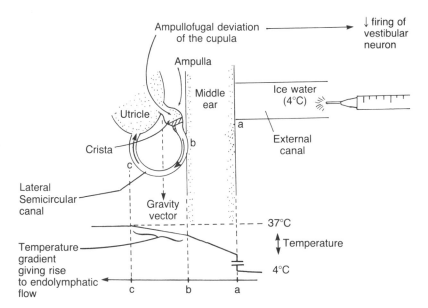

Figure 66–4. The effects of ice water irrigation on the lateral semicircular canal. The cooler endolymph sinks, resulting in ampullofugal flow and decreased neural firing of the primary vestibular neuron. Actual temperature changes within the endolymphatic fluid are on the order of 1° to 2°C. (Modified from Baloh, R. W., and Honrubia, V.: Clinical Neurophysiology of the Vestibular System. Philadelphia, F. A. Davis Co., 1979, p. 133.)

rigation—Same-sided beating nystagmus). Most sources attribute the slow phase of nystagmus to vestibular activity transmitted over the direct pathway, whereas the fast phase is believed to be generated by the PPRF in conjunction with cortical activity and carried over indirect pathways within the reticular formation. Numerous factors, both physiologic and pathologic, can alter caloric-induced eye movements.

Equipment

The equipment needed for performance of the caloric test is minimal and readily available in the emergency department or hospital ward. Although almost any size syringe will suffice, a 12- or 35-ml plastic syringe is ideal for irrigation. The syringe may be used as is or a short length of soft plastic tubing may be attached. A good source of tubing is a butterfly catheter with the needle cut off. Several hundred ml of iced water should be available, although larger quantities of cool (less than 25° C) tap water can be used with similar results if ice is unavailable. Sterile or bacteriostatic saline may be used, although its advantage over tap water has not been shown. A small basin is useful to collect water as it drains from the ear canal.

Additional required equipment includes an otoscope, several sizes of ear speculums, and equipment for removal of cerumen. Towels and a thermometer that reads from 0° to 50° C are also helpful.

Indications and Contraindications

Caloric testing of the comatose patient is indicated when the physician needs information re-

garding the functional integrity of the brain stem. When the cause of the coma is initially unknown, caloric testing will assist in differentiation among structural, metabolic, and psychogenic causes for unresponsiveness. Even when the etiology is clearly known, caloric testing will provide an indication of the depth of coma and the prognosis for eventual recovery.

In conscious patients who complain of vertigo, caloric testing may be indicated for the non-emergency evaluation of possible vestibular disorders. Ice water produces maximal stimulation of the labyrinth and may induce nausea and vomiting in awake, susceptible individuals. These patients are best referred to a qualified neurotologist, who can conduct more accurate testing in the electronystagmography laboratory with much less discomfort to the patient.

There are few contraindications to caloric testing. An absolute contraindication is the presence of a basilar skull fracture, either documented radiologically or suspected by clinical signs, because of the risk of introducing infection into the central nervous system (CNS) through an associated dural tear. If bilateral fracture can be readily excluded, testing of the intact ear with both warm and cold water will yield results similar to those of the standard bilateral examination.

Relative contraindications to water caloric testing include perforations of the tympanic membrane (those not due to temporal fractures), otitis media and externa, and the presence of previous otologic surgery (e.g., mastoidectomy). Although the risk of otitis media is probably small, carrying out the caloric test in the comatose patient under these conditions remains a matter of clinical judgment. When available, auditory evoked potentials provide an alternative source of information when caloric testing is contraindicated.

Procedure

Caloric testing should be deferred until the patient's condition has been stabilized, including protection of the airway and evaluation of the cervical spine in trauma patients. A thorough neurologic assessment should be performed prior to caloric testing, with special attention given to the ocular examination. Pupillary responses, spontaneous ocular movements, and resting eye position should be accurately recorded. The ears should be inspected prior to insertion of the otoscope. If active bleeding or CSF otorrhea/rhinorrhea is noted in the trauma victim, caloric testing and further otoscopic examination should be curtailed and the patient should be treated for a probable basilar skull fracture. If the external ear canal appears normal, the otoscopic examination should be completed. Signs of active ear infection or perforation of the tympanic membrane are contraindications to caloric testing. Tympanic rupture, hemotympanum, and step deformities of the canal may indicate fracture of the temporal bone; caloric testing in this situation is contraindicated (Fig. 66–5). Excess cerumen and foreign material must be removed, and the tympanic membrane must be clearly visualized. The ear speculum may be left in the canal as a guide for irrigation.

The patient should be placed in a supine position, with the head or upper body raised 30 degrees (two pillows will result in the appropriate angle). This angle places the lateral canal in the vertical position and ensures a maximal response. The patient should be draped with a towel, and a small basin should be positioned below the ear to collect the water outflow. A container should be filled with several hundred ml of ice water and placed near the bedside.

The syringe (*minus the needle*) should be filled with 10 ml of ice water, and the irrigation stream should be directed at the upper posterior portion of the tympanic membrane. Because the goal of the qualitative caloric test is to induce a maximum response, the amount and rate of infusion are not critical. As a general guide, 5 to 10 ml of ice water should be initially infused over a period of 5 to 10 seconds; amounts less than 5 ml may be advisable in suspected cases of light coma or psychogenic unresponsiveness. If no response is noted within 1 or 2 minutes, up to several hundred ml should be infused before declaring that there is no response. Testing of the contralateral ear may begin 5 or 10 minutes after the eyes have returned to their original position. At the conclusion of the testing, the otoscopic examination should be repeated to check for blanching of the tympanic membrane, a sign that the irrigation stream was properly directed.

Observation of eye deviation is easier when an

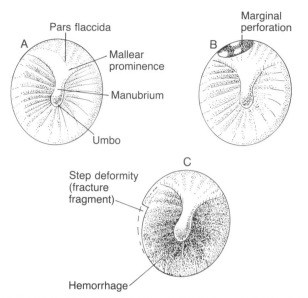

Figure 66–5. Appearance of the tympanic membrane in a normal individual *(A)*, in a patient with a superior marginal perforation and keratoma *(B)*, and in a patient with a step deformity caused by a longitudinal fracture of the temporal bone with associated hemotympanum *(C)*. (Modified from Baloh, R. W., and Honrubia, V.: Clinical Neurophysiology of the Vestibular System. Philadelphia, F. A. Davis Co., 1979, p. 105.)

assistant holds the patient's eyes open. Movement usually occurs after a latency of 10 to 40 seconds, with persistence of the response for as long as 4 or 5 minutes. Small deviations may be detected by focusing on a small scleral vessel. Alternatively, a dermographic pencil may be used to mark the initial position of the pupil with respect to the eyelid.

Variations of the caloric technique may be useful in certain situations. Warm water caloric testing may be performed if no response to bilateral ice water caloric testing is obtained or in cases in which only one ear can be tested. Water temperature should be kept below 50° C. The response elicited will be the opposite of that obtained with ice water. In patients who fail to respond to ice water caloric testing alone, additional stimulation may be obtained by combining irrigation with repeated head turning away from the irrigated side (the "doll's eyes" maneuver). *Obviously, cervical injury must be excluded prior to using this technique.* This combination of techniques may produce eye movements in patients who do not respond to caloric testing alone.[14] Eviatar and Goodhill have described a technique for caloric testing in tympanic perforations using a small latex finger cot placed in the ear canal to prevent water from entering the middle ear.[15]

The technique of bilateral caloric testing is used to evaluate vertical gaze disorders and involves the simultaneous delivery of equal amounts of ice water to both ear canals. A large syringe can be attached to a Y-connector, or two separate syringes can be used. Two people are needed to administer the caloric challenge properly. In normal individuals, upward beating nystagmus is seen after a latency of 1 to 3 minutes (as expected, the opposite is seen with warm water). The mechanism of this phenomenon is not clear, but it may involve stimulation of the remaining two semicircular canals.

Complications

There are few complications with caloric testing, and they can be avoided by carefully selecting those patients who are tested and the equipment and technique used. Using needles or other sharp objects to irrigate the ear may result in laceration or perforation of the tympanic membrane or canal wall if the patient moves unexpectedly. The use of plastic syringes and soft catheter tubing will aid in reducing such occurrences.

Other potential complications of caloric testing include otitis media, meningitis, and the induction of vomiting and subsequent aspiration. Ice water irrigation in the presence of tympanic membrane perforation will increase the chance of middle ear infection; however, the incidence of this complication following caloric testing has not been reported. Meningitis may follow basilar skull fractures with meningeal tears; the additional risk of calorics in such situations is not known. Therefore, caloric testing should be omitted in the head-injured patient if there is any suspicion of temporal fracture. Although ice water irrigation may produce nausea and even emesis in a few awake patients, vomiting or aspiration has not been reported as a complication of caloric testing in the comatose patient. Nevertheless, it is advisable to delay testing until the patient's airway is protected.

Interpretation

The first phase of interpretation of the caloric test involves analysis of initial eye position and spontaneous eye movements prior to irrigation. Comatose patients with intact oculomotor pathways will usually have their eyes directed straight ahead or slightly divergent. Unilateral destructive lesions of the cerebral hemisphere can cause conjugate deviation of the eyes *toward* the side of the lesion, whereas irritative foci, as might be seen in status epilepticus, can cause conjugate deviation *away* from the affected side. Deviations of this type can usually be overcome by caloric stimulation, although combined irrigation and head turning may be required in the first hours following the insult. Lesions in or near the PPRF in the brain stem cause conjugate deviation *away* from the side of the lesion that usually cannot be overcome by calorics. Conjugate downward deviation can be

seen with structural lesions of the brain stem or in the deeper phases of metabolic coma. Dysconjugate gaze either indicates damage at the level of the oculomotor nuclei or below or reflects disruption of the ocular muscles themselves.[16] Dysconjugate gaze may also be seen in drug-induced coma in the presence of a structurally intact brain stem pathway. In the very late stages of brain stem dysfunction, the eyes will usually return to the central position. Spontaneous roving movements of the eyes, either conjugate or dysconjugate, may be seen in supratentorial insults, but these too disappear with brain stem involvement.[14] Ocular "bobbing" is an intermittent, spontaneous downward jerking of the eyes that may occur with massive pontine lesions. There is paralysis of both voluntary and reflex lateral gaze, and caloric stimulation may increase the rate of bobbing without causing lateral deviation of the eyes.[17]

The second phase of interpretation involves analysis of eye movements following caloric irrigation. Reactions to ice water stimuli may be divided into four categories: normal nystagmus, conjugate deviation, dysconjugate deviation, and absent responses (Fig. 66–6). The first reaction, normal nystagmus with the fast component beating away from the side of ice water irrigation, is seen in normal, alert individuals, in cases of psychogenic unresponsiveness, and in those who have very mild organic disturbances of consciousness. The intensity of nystagmus is highly variable in conscious subjects and depends upon the degree of visual fixation and the level of mental alertness. The response is present in more than 90 per cent of children by the age of 6 months and declines in magnitude only after the seventh decade of life.[18, 19] Corneal reflexes and responses to facial pinprick may be abolished by hypnotic suggestion in susceptible individuals; however, caloric nystagmus appears to be immune to similar manipulation.[20]

Normal nystagmus is the usual result of caloric testing in cases of psychogenic unresponsiveness due to catatonia, hysterical conversion, schizophrenia, and malingering. Hyperactive caloric responses result from testing in the presence of tympanic perforation and mastoid disease. Hypoactive responses are recorded in a wide variety of vestibular and neurologic disorders.

Hypoactive responses usually require quantitative caloric testing with electronystagmography for detection. Caloric nystagmus may be *inverted* (beating to the wrong side) or *perverted* (beating in the wrong plane); both responses are seen in brain stem lesions. *Pseudocaloric nystagmus* is a pre-existing latent nystagmus that is brought out by the alerting effects of ice water irrigation and can be distinguished from true nystagmus by its failure to reverse directions with warm water irrigation.

As the level of coma deepens, the fast phase of

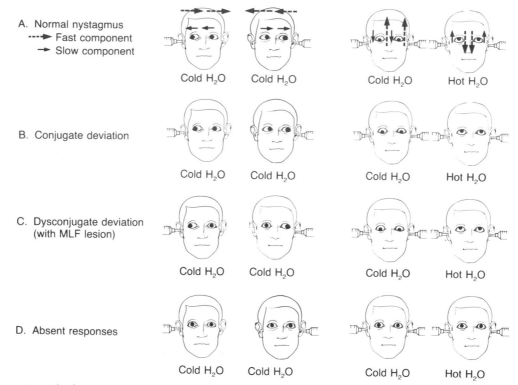

A. Normal nystagmus
- - - → Fast component
→ Slow component

Cold H$_2$O   Cold H$_2$O   Cold H$_2$O   Hot H$_2$O

B. Conjugate deviation

Cold H$_2$O   Cold H$_2$O   Cold H$_2$O   Hot H$_2$O

C. Dysconjugate deviation (with MLF lesion)

Cold H$_2$O   Cold H$_2$O   Cold H$_2$O   Hot H$_2$O

D. Absent responses

Cold H$_2$O   Cold H$_2$O   Cold H$_2$O   Hot H$_2$O

Figure 66–6. The four types of caloric responses seen with unilateral and bilateral irrigations. *A,* Normal nystagmus. *B,* Conjugate deviation. *C,* Dysconjugate deviation. The most common type, internuclear ophthalmoplegia, is shown here. Vertical eye movements usually remain intact in this lesion. *D,* Absent caloric responses. (Modified from Plum, F., and Posner, J. B.: The Diagnosis of Stupor and Coma, 3rd ed. Philadelphia, F. A. Davis Co., 1980, p. 55.)

nystagmus becomes intermittent and finally disappears, probably as a result of decreased activity in the cortex and reticular formation.

In the second type of caloric response, the eyes deviate conjugately toward the side of ice water stimulation (they "look" toward the source of irritation). When present, this reaction indicates intact brain stem function and is seen during general anesthesia, in supratentorial lesions *without brain stem compression,* and in most but not all metabolic and drug-induced comas. In such situations, bilateral simultaneous irrigation with ice water will result in conjugate downward deviation, implying that brain stem centers for vertical gaze are functional.

Dysconjugate reactions constitute the third type of caloric response to ice water stimuli. The most common dysconjugate reaction is intranuclear ophthalmoplegia, in which a lesion of the medial longitudinal fasciculus causes weakness or paralysis of the *adducting* eye following caloric irrigation. Intranuclear ophthalmoplegia may be due to acute damage to the rostral pons or may be seen as a manifestation of multiple sclerosis or previous vascular insult.

In acute supratentorial lesions, the development of dysconjugate caloric responses is a significant sign that may indicate compression of the brain stem and impending herniation. Caloric responses of this type are less common with metabolic and drug-induced coma and, when present in metabolic coma, have less ominous significance. Reversible intranuclear ophthalmoplegia has been reported in hepatic coma and may occur during phenytoin, barbiturate, and amitriptyline toxicities. Forced downward deviation of the eyes, either conjugate or dysconjugate, may be seen in sedative-hypnotic–induced coma when unilateral caloric testing is performed.[21]

Palsies of the oculomotor nerves are another cause of dysconjugate reactions, although most should be apparent before irrigation. Etiologies include diabetic neuropathy (especially C.N. VI), increased intracranial pressure, and Wernicke's encephalopathy. Finally, Plum and Posner report that unusual and poorly characterized caloric responses may be obtained from the testing of comatose patients with long-standing, severe brain injury.[16]

Absent caloric responses are the fourth category of reactions to ice water stimuli. As a general rule, the oculovestibular response is preserved longer than other brain stem reflexes; however, the oculocephalic or "doll's eye" response may persist in the absence of caloric responses due to bilateral labyrinthine disease because of additional input from proprioceptive receptors in the neck. Loss of caloric responses in comatose patients with structural lesions is usually a sign of brain stem damage. In supratentorial lesions, progressive loss of caloric responses may be seen in the final stages of transtentorial herniation. The oculovestibular reflex may also be transiently absent or decreased on the side opposite massive supratentorial damage during the first hours following injury.[22] Absent caloric responses may occur in any subtentorial lesion that affects vestibular reflex pathways, including pontine hemorrhage, basilar artery occlusion, cerebellar hemorrhage or infarction with encroachment upon the brain stem, and any expanding mass lesion within the posterior fossa. Calorics may disappear in deep coma resulting from subarachnoid hemorrhage, perhaps due to pressure upon the brain stem.

The vestibulo-ocular reflex is usually retained until the late stages of metabolic coma. When the reflex does disappear, as in the case of hepatic coma, it is frequently a pre-terminal event.[23] Nevertheless, caloric responses may be transiently absent in certain types of drug-induced coma, with the *eventual complete recovery of the patient.* The vestibulo-ocular reflex seems particularly sensitive to the effects of sedative-hypnotics (barbiturates, glutethimide), antidepressants (amitriptyline, doxepin), and anticonvulsants (phenytoin, carbamazepine).[8, 24, 25] Obviously, neuromuscular blocking agents (e.g., succinylcholine) will abolish caloric-induced ocular movements.

Finally, the caloric response may be absent for reasons other than those responsible for the coma. Inadequate irrigation due to excess cerumen or poor technique and unilateral or bilateral dysfunction of the peripheral vestibular apparatus must be considered. Bilateral loss of caloric response (arreflexia vestibularis) is uncommon in conscious patients, constituting 1.7 and 0.2 per cent of the electronystagmography clinical population in two large series of patients.[26, 27] Some of the causes of unilateral and bilateral loss of oculovestibular reflexes in conscious patients are listed in Table 66–1.

The vestibulo-ocular reflex has prognostic as well as diagnostic significance in the comatose patient. In a study of one hundred patients who were comatose from head trauma, absence of calorics at 1 to 3 days following injury was associated with extremely high mortality.[28] Testing in the immediate post-traumatic period may yield inconsistent responses and is of considerably less prognostic value. Levy and coworkers studied five hundred cases of non-traumatic, non–drug-induced coma in a recent multicenter effort. Absence of the vestibulo-ocular reflex correlated with less than a 5 per cent chance of achieving functional recovery within 1 year when tested within 6 to 24 hours of coma onset.[29] Complete loss of caloric responses is part of the criteria for the legal diagnosis of "brain death" in many localities and correlates with the irreversible cessation of cerebral

Table 66–1. POSSIBLE CAUSES OF ABSENT VESTIBULO-OCULAR REFLEX IN CONSCIOUS PATIENTS

Inadequate Irrigation	**Traumatic**
	Previous temporal
Cerumen Impaction	fracture
	Previous head
Post-Infectious	injury
Meningitis	Post-labyrinthec-
Encephalitis	tomy
Syphilis	
	Labyrinthine
Neoplastic	Vestibular
Acoustic neuroma	neuronitis
Other cerebello-pontine angle	Suppurative
tumors	labyrinthitis
Posterior fossa tumors	
	Congenital
Inflammatory	Congenital
Systemic lupus erythematosus	hydrocephalus
Cogan's syndrome	Hereditary
	spinocerebellar
Drugs	degeneration
Aminoglycoside antibiotics	
Neuromuscular blocking agents	**Idiopathic**
Anticonvulsants*	

*Reported rarely in conscious patients who have taken more than normal therapeutic dosage.

function at least as well as an isoelectric EEG.[30] Excessive reliance on a single clinical sign must be avoided, and decisions regarding neurologic prognosis and future therapy should be based on complete consideration of all evidence available to the physician.

Conclusion

The caloric test is a simple, easily performed procedure that should be a part of the complete neurologic assessment of the comatose patient, unless contraindicated. In the emergency patient, this test should be reserved for the stable patient undergoing secondary assessment. Even when the etiology of the coma is known, the test can provide a baseline for the evaluation of future changes in the patient's status. The examination requires minimal equipment and can be conducted in a few minutes while awaiting laboratory results or during preparation for computed tomographic scanning. Complications are few if patients are properly selected and when correct technique is used. When reliably interpreted, caloric testing furnishes valuable diagnostic and prognostic information necessary for proper care of the comatose individual.

1. Brown-Sequard, C.: Course of Lectures on the Physiology and Pathology of the Central Nervous System. Philadelphia, Collins, 1860, p. 187.
2. Barany, R.: Untersuchungen über den vom Vestibularapparat des Ohres reflektorisch ausgelosten rhythmischen

Nystagmus und seine Begleiterscheinungen Mschr. Ohrenheilk 40:193, 1906.

3. Fitzgerald, G., and Hallpike, C. S.: Studies in human vestibular function: 1. Observations of the directional preponderance ("Nystagmus bereitschaft") of caloric nystagmus resulting from cerebral lesions. Brain 65:115, 1942.

4. Klingon, G. H.: Caloric stimulation in localization of brain stem lesions in a comatose patient. AMA Arch. Neurol. Psychiatr. 68:233, 1952.

5. Bender, M. B., Bergman, P. S., and Nathanson, M.: Ocular movements on passive head turning and caloric stimulation in comatose patients. Trans. Am. Neurol. Assoc. 80:184, 1955.

6. Vaernet, K.: Caloric vestibular reactions in transtentorial herniation of the brainstem. Neurology 7:833, 1957.

7. Ethelberg, S.: Vestibulo-ocular reflex disorders in a case of transtentorial herniation and foraminal impaction of the brainstem. Acta Psychiatr. Scand. 30:187, 1955.

8. Blegvad, B.: Caloric vestibular reaction in unconscious patients. Arch. Otolaryngol. 75:36, 1962.

9. Barber, H., and Stockwell, C.: Manual of Electronystagmography. St. Louis, The C. V. Mosby Co., 1980.

10. Zangemeister, W. H., and Bock, O.: Air vs. water caloric test. Clin. Otolaryngol. 5:379, 1980.

11. Szentagothai, J.: The elementary vestibulo-ocular reflex arc. J. Neurophysiol. 13:395, 1950.

12. Precht, W.: Vestibular mechanisms. Ann. Rev. Neurosci. 2:265, 1979.

13. Baloh, R. W., and Honrubia, V.: Clinical Neurophysiology of the Vestibular System. Philadelphia, F. A. Davis Co., 1979, p. 40.

14. Fischer, C. M.: The neurological exam of the comatose patient. Acta Neurol. Scand. (Suppl. 36) 45:43, 1969.

15. Eviatar, A., and Goodhill, V.: A dry calorization method for vestibular function studies. Laryngoscope 78:1746, 1968.

16. Plum, F., and Posner, J. B.: The Diagnosis of Stupor and Coma, 3rd ed. Philadelphia, F. A. Davis Co., 1980, pp. 57–61.

17. Susac, J. O., Hoyt, W. F., Daroff, R. B., et al.: Clinical spectrum of ocular bobbing. J. Neurol. Neurosurg. Psychiatr. 33:771, 1970.

18. Eviatar, L., Miranda, S., Eviatar, A., et al.: Development of nystagmus in response to vestibular stimulation in infants. Ann. Neurol. 5:508, 1979.

19. Bruner, A., and Norris, T. W.: Age-related changes in caloric nystagmus. Acta Otolaryngol. (Suppl.) 282:1, 1971.

20. Cogan, D. G.: Brain lesions and eye movements in man. In Bender, M. B. (ed.): The Oculomotor System. New York, Harper & Row Publishers, Inc., 1964, p. 487.

21. Simon, R. P.: Forced downward ocular deviation. Arch. Neurol. 35:456, 1978.

22. Posner, J. B., and Plum, F.: Diagnostic significance of vestibulo-ocular responses. J. Neurol. Neurosurg. Psychiatr. 38:727, 1975.

23. Hanid, M. A., Silk, D. B., and Williams, R.: Prognostic value of the oculovestibular reflex in fulminant hepatic failure. Br. Med. J. 1:1029, 1978.

24. Spector, R. H., and Schnapper, R.: Amitriptyline-induced ophthalmoplegia. Neurology 31:1188, 1981.

25. Spector, R. H., Davidoff, R. A., and Schwartzman, R. J.: Phenytoin-induced ophthalmoplegia. Neurology 26:1031, 1976.

26. Simmons, F. B.: Patients with bilateral loss of caloric response. Ann. Otol. Rhinol. Laryngol. 82:175, 1973.

27. Steensen, S. H., Toxman, J., and Zilstorff, K.: Bilateral loss of caloric response in conscious patients (arreflexia vestibularis). Clin. Otolaryngol. 5:373, 1980.

28. Poulsen, J., and Zilstorff, K.: Prognostic value of the caloric vestibular test in the unconscious patient with cranial trauma. Acta. Neurol. Scand. 48:282, 1972.

29. Levy, D. E., Bates, D., Caronna, J. J., et al.: Prognosis in nontraumatic coma. Ann. Intern. Med. 94:293, 1981.

30. Hicks, R. G., and Torada, T. A.: The vestibulo-ocular (caloric) reflex in the diagnosis of cerebral death. Anesth. Intens. Care 7:169, 1979.

11

OPHTHALMOLOGY

67

Ophthalmologic Procedures

DAVID H. BARR, M.D.
JERRIS R. HEDGES, M.D.

Overview. The following sections discuss procedures commonly performed by emergency physicians during the evaluation and treatment of many eye injuries and diseases. The emphasis of these sections will be on the practical application of the techniques and will include cautions to be heeded by the emergency physician.

Dilating the Eye

INTRODUCTION

Dilating the eye is an essential step in the management of common eye emergencies. It is useful for both diagnostic and therapeutic purposes. The correct agent must be chosen, however. In this section the agents will be reviewed and specific recommendations will be made.

BACKGROUND

There are two types of dilators: sympathomimetics, which stimulate the dilator muscle of the iris, and cycloplegics, which block the parasympathetic stimulus that constricts the iris sphincter. Cycloplegics also block the contraction of the ciliary muscles, which control the focusing of the lens of the eye. This second effect of cycloplegics is of great importance in the use of dilators therapeutically for iritis.

Cycloplegics were used cosmetically as early as Galen's time. Beginning in the early 1800s, extracts from the plants *Hyoscyamus* and belladonna were used in ophthalmology. Atropine was first isolated in 1833. Epinephrine was used on eyes in 1900 as the first sympathomimetic.[1]

INDICATIONS AND CONTRAINDICATIONS

Dilation is indicated for diagnosis when the fundus cannot be adequately examined through an undilated pupil. The elderly patient with miotic pupils and cataracts is a common example. Dilation is also indicated therapeutically for all forms of iritis. In the emergency setting, a corneal injury with a secondary traumatic iritis is a common example. Primary iritis, although less common in emergency practice, is also seen. Dilation helps iritis in two ways. First, the dilation of the iris keeps it from sticking to the lens and forming tiny adhesions, called posterior synechiae. If not prevented, such adhesions produce permanent limitation of pupillary function. Second, a cycloplegic agent relaxes the ciliary muscle spasm that accompanies iritis and thus reduces the pain of iritis.

Dilation is contraindicated when the pupillary response needs to be followed as a neurologic sign, such as in head trauma. A second contraindication is in patients with narrow anterior chamber angles; dilation can precipitate an attack of angle-closure glaucoma. One can estimate the depth of the anterior chamber with a penlight by shining the light in from the side and seeing if the nasal side of the iris lights up. Normally it should, but with narrow angles the forward convexity of the iris blocks the light (Fig. 67–1). With a slit lamp, the depth of the anterior chamber can be directly seen.

Systemic effects can develop following the application of eye drops.[3] The reader should review the following sections on agents and complications prior to using these drugs when the patient has a compromised cardiovascular system.

AGENTS (Table 67–1)[4, 5]

Only two dilators are really needed in the emergency department. Phenylephrine (Neo-Synephrine) 2½ per cent is used for diagnostic dilation of the fundus. The drug is short-acting, and since accommodation is not affected, the patient's vision will not be altered. Phenylephrine 10 per cent should not be used, because it can seriously elevate the blood pressure in susceptible adults.[6, 7] For therapeutic cycloplegia in iritis, homatropine 5 per cent works well. Although Table 67–1 indicates a maximum duration of 3 days, 24 hours is a more common duration. Therefore, homatropine 5 per cent is a useful agent for traumatic iritis.

Individuals with lightly pigmented irides tend to have a greater sensitivity to the cycloplegics than do individuals with greater pigmentation; the cycloplegic effect may therefore be more prolonged in people with light eyes. Atropine should not be used for traumatic iritis because the undesirable effects of pupillary dilation and blurred vision persist for a week or longer following healing of associated corneal abrasions. Atropine drops may be prescribed as part of the therapy for

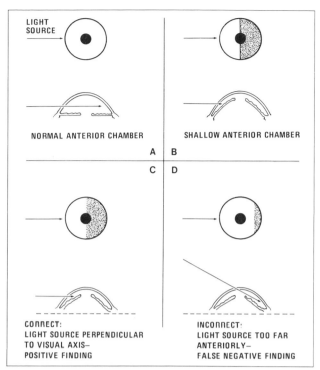

Figure 67–1. Anterior chamber depth and transillumination test. *A,* Normal anterior chamber with negative transillumination test. *B,* Shallow anterior chamber with positive transillumination test. *C,* Shallow anterior chamber with correctly placed light source yielding true positive test result. *D,* Shallow anterior chamber with incorrectly placed light source giving false-negative test result. (From Bresler, M. J., and Hoffman, R. J., Prevention of iatrogenic acute narrow-angle glaucoma. Ann. Emerg. Med. 10:535, 1981. Used by permission.)

nontraumatic iritis following appropriate ophthalmologic consultation.

The physician should be aware that malingerers may use mydriatics to dilate a pupil unilaterally for the purpose of feigning neurologic disease. Normally, a pupillary dilation caused by intracranial third cranial nerve compression will constrict with 2 per cent pilocarpine eye drops. The mydriatic-treated eye can be identified by full motor function of the third cranial nerve and the absence of miosis following pilocarpine instillation. It should be noted that legitimate patients may not recall the name of an eye medicine that they used but will usually recall whether the bottle had a red cap, as is found on all cycloplegic solutions. An unexpected mydriasis in a trusted patient may be the result of such an agent. Medications that constrict the pupil, such as pilocarpine, have a green cap.

PROCEDURE

The instillation of mydriatics is similar to the administration of other eye solutions. For medicolegal purposes, visual acuity should be noted prior to the instillation of the medicine. This will document that any decreased vision is not the result of the mydriatic.

The patient is placed in a supine or a comfortable semirecumbent position. He is instructed to gaze at an object (such as a fixture on the ceiling) in his upper visual field. The physician gently depresses the lower lid using a finger on the epidermis (Fig. 67–2). A *single* drop of the solution is instilled into the lower lid fornix, and the patient is permitted to blink and to spread the medication. More than a single drop is not recommended, since this will produce reflex tearing and will reduce the concentration in contact with the conjunctiva. The patient should be forewarned that the medication will be uncomfortable and that he can blot but *not* rub the closed eye with a tissue after the medicine is used. If the desired effect is not noted in 15 to 20 minutes, a repeat dose may be used but is seldom required.

COMPLICATIONS

As mentioned in the section on contraindications, any dilator can precipitate an attack of angle-closure glaucoma in susceptible patients. In a case of angle-closure glaucoma, the patient will complain of smoky vision with "halos" around lights as well as a severe, aching pain. There may be nausea and vomiting. The affected eye will become injected in association with a hazy cornea, elevated pressure on tonometry, and an oval, fixed pupil. Immediate consultation with an ophthalmologist should be obtained. The treatment will usually include osmotic agents, carbonic anhydrase inhibitors, pilocarpine and, later, definitive laser or surgical procedures.

The practitioner should be aware that the use

Table 67–1. MYDRIATIC AGENTS

Agent	Maximum Mydriasis	Duration of Mydriasis	Common Trade Name
*Sympathomimetics**			
Phenylephrine, 2.5% or 10%‡	20 minutes	3 hours	Neo-Synephrine
Cocaine, 5% or 4%	20 minutes	2 hours	—
Parasympatholytics (Cycloplegics)			
Atropine, 1%	40 minutes	12 days	—
Scopolamine, 0.25%	30 minutes	7 days	—
Homatropine, 5%†	30 minutes	1 to 3 days	—
Cyclopentolate, 1%	30 minutes	6 to 24 hours	Cyclogyl
Tropicamide, 1%	30 minutes	4 hours	Mydriacyl

*Preferred for funduscopic examination
†Preferred for iritis or corneal abrasion therapy
‡10 per cent solution may produce cardiovascular reaction, hence should not be used

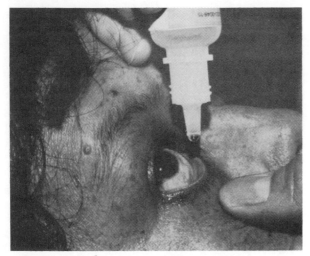

Figure 67–2. Administration of eye drops. The patient should lie in a supine position or with the head tilted back. The patient's gaze should be directed upward. A single drop of medicine is instilled in the lower conjunctival fornix. The patient should be instructed to close the eyelids for 1 minute to increase the contact of the medicine with the globe and to decrease medication outflow down the tear duct and over the lid margin. (From Waring, G. O.: The eye at first sight. Emerg. Med. 15:26, 1979. Used by permission.)

of eye medications may introduce infections. Most solutions contain bactericidal ingredients, although contamination of the tips of the droppers can still occur.[2] Only newly opened bottles of eye medication should be used if the practitioner suspects a deep corneal injury or if the patient has had recent eye surgery.

Any cycloplegic (in contrast with a sympathomimetic) will blur a patient's near vision. Patients should be forewarned of this effect. Vision will be less blurred in adults over 45 years of age, who generally have a reduced ability to focus for near vision. Nonetheless, most adults will be able to drive safely, even with both eyes cyclopleged. Light sensitivity caused by pupillary dilation may also be bothersome; sunglasses are sufficient for this problem.

Systemic reactions can be produced by sympathomimetic and cycloplegic eye drops.[3] Following instillation of eye drops into the conjunctival sac, systemic absorption can occur through the conjunctival capillaries as well as by way of the nasal mucosa, the oral pharynx, and the gastrointestinal tract after passage through the lacrimal drainage system. Mucosal hyperemia enhances absorption. Symptoms can often be avoided by digital pressure on the nasal canthus, thus occluding the puncta.[3]

Thirty-three cases of adverse reactions associated with 10 per cent phenylephrine have been described.[7] These include 15 myocardial infarctions (11 deaths), seven cases of precipitation of angle-closure glaucoma, and development of systemic cardiovascular or neurologic reactions.

The Fluorescein Examination

INTRODUCTION

Fluorescein staining of the eye should be part of the evaluation of all cases of eye trauma and infection. It is a quick and easy technique that is crucial for the proper diagnosis and management of common eye emergencies.

BACKGROUND

Sodium fluorescein is a water-soluble chemical that fluoresces—it absorbs light in the blue wavelengths and emits the energy in the longer green wavelengths. It will fluoresce in an alkaline environment (such as Bowman's membrane, which is located below the corneal epithelium) but not in an acidic environment (such as the tear film over an intact corneal epithelium).[20] Thus, it is very useful in revealing even minute abrasions on the cornea.

Fluorescein was first used in ophthalmology in the 1880s.[21] It was first used as a drop, but when the danger of contamination by bacteria (especially *Pseudomonas*) was recognized in the 1950s,[22] fluorescein was impregnated into paper strips. These now come in individual sterile wrappers and should be used instead of the pre-mixed solution.

INDICATIONS AND CONTRAINDICATIONS

Fluorescein staining is indicated for evaluation of all suspected abrasions, foreign bodies, and infections of the eye.[23] This includes "simple" cases of conjunctivitis, which may actually be herpetic keratitis. In actuality, any red eye should be stained.

The only contraindication to fluorescein staining is in soft contact lens wearers. The stain can permanently tint a soft lens. The lens must be removed and must not be worn for several hours after the stain has been completely removed by thorough irrigation. Topically administered fluorescein is considered nontoxic,[24] although reactions to a fluorescein-containing solution have been described. These reports of vasovagal reactions[25] and a generalized convulsion[26] are rare and are believed to be caused by agents other than fluorescein in the solution. Should the practitioner choose to use one of the fluorescein-containing solutions rather than the fluorescein-impregnated strips, he should be aware of these potential idiosyncratic reactions.

The physician should also be aware that fluorescein dye may enter the anterior chamber of the eye in the presence of deep corneal defects. This form of intraocular fluorescein accumulation is also nontoxic. When the anterior chamber is viewed under the blue filter of the slit lamp, a fluorescein "flare" is visible. This flare reaction should not be confused with the flare reaction noted with iritis.

PROCEDURE

It is best not to use topical anesthetics before fluorescein staining, because some patients will develop a punctate keratitis from the anesthetic,[27] which can confuse the diagnosis. With patients who are profusely tearing and who are squeezing their eyes shut from an abrasion or a foreign body, however, the examination will be impossible if a topical anesthetic is not first used.

The fluorescein strip is grasped by the nonorange end, and the orange end is wetted with *one* drop of saline (most conveniently available as a small bottle of artificial tears) or dextrose solution. The wetted strip is then placed gently onto the inside of the patient's lower lid. The patient's blinking will automatically spread the fluorescein over the eye. The key to a good examination is the application of a *thin* layer of fluorescein over the corneal and conjunctival surfaces. If the strip is heavily wetted prior to application in the lower fornix, the eye may become flooded with the solution, thus making evaluation difficult. On the other hand, use of a dry strip in the unanesthetized eye may be irritating. If too much dye accumulates, the patient can remove the excess by blotting the closed eye with a tissue. The physician uses a Wood's lamp, the blue filter of a slit lamp, or simply a penlight to examine the eye in a darkened room, checking for areas of bright green

fluorescence on the corneal and conjunctival surfaces. Following the completion of the fluorescein examination, excess dye should be irrigated from the eye to minimize damage to the patient's clothing from dye-stained tears.

A special use for fluorescein is in the *Seidel* test[28] for detection of perforation of the eye. To perform this test, the physician instills a large amount of fluorescein onto the eye by profusely wetting the strip. The eye is then examined for a small stream of fluid leaking from the globe. This stream will fluoresce green in contrast with the orange color of the rest of the globe flooded with fluorescein.[29]

INTERPRETATION

Fluorescein is mainly used for evaluation of corneal injuries. Although conjunctival abrasions will pick up the stain, most of the staining on the conjunctiva represents patches of mucus rather than a real pathologic condition. Corneal staining is more specific for injury, and the pattern of injury often reflects the original insult.

The corneal staining will show patterns as illustrated in Figure 67–3. Abrasions usually occur in the central cornea because of the limited protection of the patient's closing eyelids. The margins of the abrasions are usually sharp and linear if seen in the first 24 hours. Circular defects are seen about embedded foreign bodies and may persist for up to 48 hours following removal of a superficial foreign object. Deeply embedded objects may be associated with defects persisting for longer than 48 hours. Objects under the upper lid (including some chalazions) will produce vertical linear lesions on the upper surface of the cornea. Hard contact lens overuse diminishes the nutrient sup-

Figure 67–3. Typical corneal defect patterns for specific injuries. *A,* Typical abrasion. *B,* Abrasion around a corneal foreign body. *C,* Abrasion from a foreign body under the upper lid. *D,* Abrasion from excessive wearing of a contact lens. *E,* Ultraviolet exposure (resulting from sunlamp exposure, welding, or snow blindness). *F,* Herpetic dendritic keratitis.

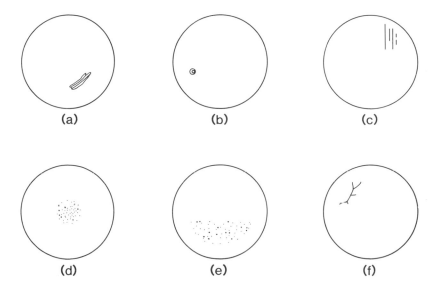

(a)   (b)   (c)

(d)   (e)   (f)

ply to the cornea. The central cornea receives the most injury and thus will fluoresce brightly when stained. Ultraviolet light exposure from sunlamp abuse, snow blindness, or welding flash produces a superficial punctate keratitis, which in its mildest form may not be visible without a slit lamp. The central cornea is the least protected by the lids, and a central horizontal band-like keratitis can result. Herpetic lesions may develop anywhere on the cornea. Classically, these lesions are dendritic, although ulcers may also be punctate or stellate.[30] Other patterns of superficial keratitis have been discussed elsewhere by R.R. Sexton.[31] The interested reader is referred to the work of Sexton for further detail.

Any area of corneal staining with an infiltrate or opacification beneath or around the lesion should alert the practitioner to the possibility of a viral,[30] bacterial,[32] or fungal[33] *keratitis*. Urgent ophthalmologic consultation should be obtained so that cultures of the possible etiologic agents can be procured and treatment initiated.

Frequently, practitioners are unaware that many *Pseudomonas* organisms will fluoresce when exposed to ultraviolet light.[34] The presence of fluorescence prior to the instillation of fluorescein in the red eye should suggest the possibility of a pseudomonal infection.

CONCLUSION

Fluorescein staining is a quick, easy diagnostic procedure that should be part of every eye evaluation. The extra minute that the examination takes provides a wealth of diagnostic information for patients with eye trauma or infection. With the exception of the reactions noted with fluorescein solution, potential discoloration of soft contact lenses, and the potential for infection when the solutions rather than fluorescein-impregnated paper strips are used, no complications are associated with the procedure.

Eye Irrigation

INTRODUCTION

Eye irrigation is the crucial first step in the treatment of chemical injuries to the eye. Ideally, this should be performed immediately at the scene of the injury, *before* the patient is brought to the emergency department.[35] Corneal injury can occur within 10 seconds of contact with an alkaline substance. Eye irrigation must often be continued in the emergency department; methods of irrigation will be discussed here.

INDICATIONS AND CONTRAINDICATIONS

Irrigation is indicated for all acute chemical injuries to the eyes. There is no contraindication to eye irrigation, but if there is also a possible perforating injury to the eye, the irrigation must be performed especially gently and carefully.

EQUIPMENT

The following equipment is necessary for eye irrigation:
1. Topical anesthetic, such as proparacaine 0.5 per cent.
2. Sterile irrigating solution. Usually, intravenous saline in a bag with tubing is the easiest to obtain.
3. A basin to catch the fluid.
4. Applicators.
5. Gauze pads to help hold the patient's lids open.

PROCEDURE

Basic Technique

Topical anesthetic is instilled. Any particulate matter should be swept out of the conjunctival fornices with moistened cotton-tipped applicators.[36] This requires eversion of the upper lid (see the section on foreign body removal and Fig. 67–4). During actual irrigation, the lids must be held open. It is easiest to use the gauze pads to get a grip on the wet, slippery lids. At times the patient will have blepharospasm to such a degree that lid retractors (Desmarres or paper clip retractors—Fig. 67–5) may be necessary (Fig. 67–6). When lid retractors are used, the practitioner must be certain that the eye is well anesthetized, that the retractors do not injure the globe or the lids, and that chemicals are not harbored under the retractors.

Paton and Goldberg recommend an ipsilateral facial nerve block for severe blepharospasm.[37] To avoid swelling of the periorbital tissue, the facial nerve is blocked just anterior to the condyloid process of the ipsilateral mandible. A line of anesthesia (2 per cent lidocaine) is placed subcutaneously to temporarily paralyze the orbicularis muscle. The saline exiting from the intravenous tubing is directed over the globe and into the upper and lower fornices. The choice of fluid is less important than the rapidity of irrigation initiation. Tap water should be readily available at the scene of the injury, and copious immediate irrigation should be encouraged prior to patient transport to the hospital. Prehospital care providers should be taught to irrigate all acid injuries of the eye for at least 5 minutes at the scene and to

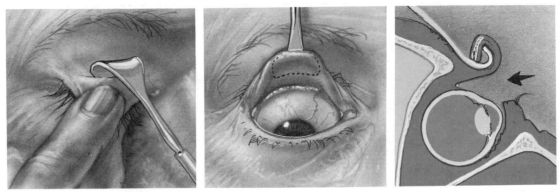

Figure 67–4. Double eversion of upper lid using lid retractor. (From Fogle, J. A., and Spyker, D. A.: Management of chemical and drug injury to the eye. *In* Haddad, L. M., and Winchester, J. F.: Clinical Management of Poisoning and Drug Overdose. Philadelphia, W. B. Saunders Co., 1983. Used by permission.)

irrigate all alkali injuries for at least 15 minutes.[38, 39] Normal saline solution is preferred for eye irrigation, since it is nonirritating and isotonic without dextrose. Dextrose can be quite sticky if spilled and may serve as a nutrient for an opportunistic bacterial infection.

Duration of Irrigation

Although Gombos recommends that a full liter of irrigating solution be used in every case of caustic injury,[40] the duration of the irrigation is best determined by the extent of exposure and the causative agent. Acids are quickly neutralized by the proteins of the eye surface tissues and, once irrigated out, cause no further damage.[41] The only exceptions are hydrofluoric and heavy metal acids, which can penetrate through the cornea. Alkalis can penetrate rapidly and if not removed (because of the slow dissociation of the cation from combination with proteins) will continue to produce damage for days.[42] Therefore, prolonged irrigation

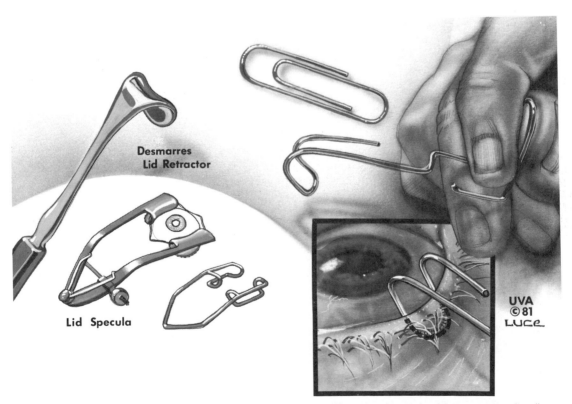

Figure 67–5. Devices for separating eyelids. Desmarres retractor and retractor improvised from a paper clip allow active manipulation of lids. Free-standing specula may require seventh nerve block to reduce blepharospasm. (From Fogle, J. A., and Spyker, D. A.: Management of chemical and drug injury to the eye. *In* Haddad, L. M., and Winchester, J. F.: Clinical Management of Poisoning and Drug Overdose. Philadelphia, W. B. Saunders Co., 1983. Used by permission.)

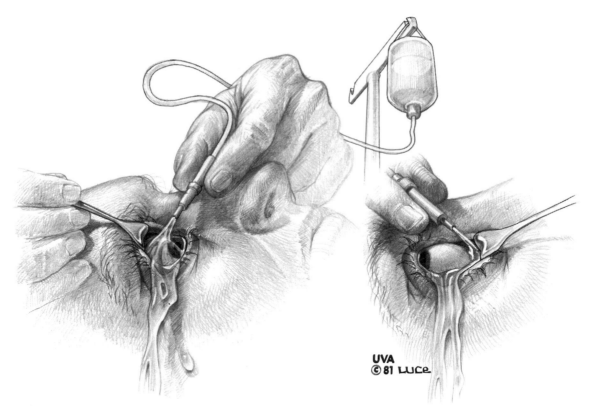

Figure 67–6. Irrigation technique using Desmarres retractor for lid separation. (From Fogle, J. A., and Spyker, D. A.: Management of chemical and drug injury to the eye. *In* Haddad, L. M., and Winchester, J. F.: Clinical Management of Poisoning and Drug Overdose. Philadelphia, W. B. Saunders Co., 1983. Used by permission.)

is indicated; at least 2 liters of solution should be used over 20 minutes for alkaline injury.[43]

Ophthalmologic consultation should be obtained for all alkaline, hydrofluoric acid, and heavy metal acid injuries. Irrigation on an inpatient basis may be required for a period of 24 hours or more. This is especially likely when corneal hazing is present. It should be noted that the magnesium contained in sparklers will combine with water from tears to produce magnesium hydroxide.[44] Such fireworks accidents should be treated as alkaline injuries rather than thermal injuries. Eye damage from hair straighteners[45] and phosphate-free detergents[46] must also be treated as alkaline injuries.

A good method of checking the effectiveness of irrigation is to measure the pH of the conjunctival fornices with a pH paper strip.[47] The pH indicator on urine multi-indicator sticks can also be used. The pH indicator on urine dipsticks is conveniently closest to the handle; all the distal indicator squares can be cut off with scissors. The normal tear film pH is 7.4. If the pH measured in the conjunctival fornices after the initial irrigation is still abnormal, irrigation is to be continued. If the pH is normal after irrigation, one should check it again in 20 minutes to make sure that it remains normal.

Delayed pH changes are usually the result of incomplete irrigation and inadequate swabbing of

the fornices. In anticipation of this deficiency, one should measure the pH deep in the fornices. Often, double-lid eversion with a lid elevator is required to expose the upper fornix for swabbing, irrigation, and pH testing (see Fig. 67–4).

Prolonged Irrigation

Prolonged irrigation may be required with alkali burns. Ophthalmologic consultation is essential in such situations. One technique for prolonged irrigation uses a contact lens–type irrigation device (e.g., Morgan Therapeutic Lens), which allows for continuous irrigation once the more vigorous irrigation described earlier has been used. During use, the device is set on the anesthetized eye, and the lids are allowed to close around the intravenous tubing adaptor. Continuous flow through the device onto the cornea and into the fornices occurs. This contact lens device can become uncomfortable, since local anesthetic agents are washed out during the irrigation process; the anesthetic agent must be reapplied frequently during irrigation for patient comfort. The repeated use of the anesthetic agent may itself inhibit corneal healing.

Another irrigation device can be made for the prolonged irrigation of the fornices by modification of a small-caliber central venous catheter. Multiple perforations are made with a scissors or

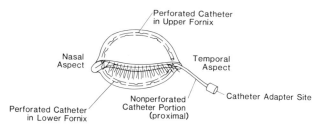

Figure 67–7. Continuous irrigation device. A perforated central venous catheter is looped in the fornices of the anesthetized eye, beginning from the temporal border of the eyelids. The eye is lightly patched after catheter placement.

a scalpel in the distal portion of the catheter. This perforated section is placed in the inferior fornix of the anesthetized eye beginning at the lateral canthus and is then looped back in the upper lid fornix (Fig. 67–7). The patient is instructed to tilt his head toward the side of the tubing to permit drainage into a laterally placed basin. After loosely applying an eye patch, one attaches the catheter to an intravenous setup for continuous irrigation. An anesthetic agent is also needed with this technique, albeit less frequently than with the contact lens–type device.

Lippas described the successful treatment of two alkaline burns using a similar but more invasive continuous irrigation technique for prolonged irrigation following immediate copious irrigation.[48] Continuous irrigation of an alkaline injury with a 10 or 20 per cent acetylcysteine (Mucomyst) solution to inhibit collagenase has been recommended,[49] although one should await ophthalmologic consultation before using this method.

COMPLICATIONS

The only complication from irrigation is abrasion of the cornea or the conjunctiva. This can be a mechanical injury from trying to keep the lids open in an uncooperative patient or a fine punctate keratitis from the irrigation itself.[50] If a superficial corneal defect occurs, it is treated in the usual manner by patching. Deep or penetrating corneal injuries are likely to be the result of the caustic chemical and require emergent ophthalmologic consultation.

In general, the emergency physician should not patch these deeper injuries. They should receive continuous irrigation pending ophthalmologic consultation. Superficial injuries not associated with corneal hazing should be treated in a manner similar to that for corneal abrasions. There is some experimental evidence that massive parenteral or oral ascorbic acid supplementation may prevent the development of deep corneal injury,[51] although this treatment has not gained universal acceptance.

CONCLUSIONS

Eye irrigation is easy, and complications associated with the technique are minimal. At times, the physician may be unsure whether a chemical injury is toxic enough to warrant irrigation. One should irrigate if any doubt exists rather than omit this vital procedure and permit the progression of eye injury.

Ocular Foreign Body Removal

INTRODUCTION

Patients with an external foreign body in the eye are frequently seen in emergency departments. They are often in pain and desperate for help. This section will review the procedures for locating and removing extraocular foreign bodies. A brief discussion covering evaluation for perforation of the globe and for an intraocular foreign body will be presented. Care of the patient following removal of an extraocular foreign body will be reviewed.

INDICATIONS AND CONTRAINDICATIONS

Removal of extraocular foreign bodies is always indicated. The timing of removal and the technique that is required vary according to the patient's clinical status and the type of injury received. For the most part, the emergency physician will be able to proceed directly to removal of the object using the techniques described in this section. When the patient is extremely uncooperative (e.g., a mentally deficient individual or a young child) or when the injury is complicated (e.g., deeply embedded object, multiple foreign objects from a blast injury, or possible globe penetration), immediate ophthalmologic consultation is indicated. A penetrating injury to the cornea is particularly troublesome in that iris tissue may prolapse and may appear to represent a corneal foreign body (Fig. 67–8).

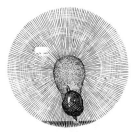

Figure 67–8. Corneal laceration with prolapse of the iris. The extruded iris is dark in appearance, mimicking a corneal foreign body. The pupil is irregular, pointing toward the laceration. Also note the presence of a small hyphema inferiorly. (From Paton, D., and Goldberg, M. F.: Management of Ocular Injuries. Philadelphia, W. B. Saunders Co., 1976. Used by permission.)

EQUIPMENT

The following equipment is necessary for extraocular foreign body removal:

1. Topical anesthetic, such as proparacaine 0.5 per cent.

2. Sterile cotton-tipped applicators.

3. Fluorescein strips.

4. Magnification: loupes plus Wood's lamp or slit lamp.

5. Eye spud or 25 gauge needle attached to a 3-ml syringe or to the tip of a cotton-tipped applicator.

6. Dilator drops, such as Homatropine 5 per cent or Cyclopentolate 1 per cent.

7. Antibiotic ointment, such as sulfacetamide 10 per cent.

8. Eye patches.

9. Tape (nonallergenic paper tape is preferable).

CONSIDERATION OF INTRAOCULAR FOREIGN BODY

The emergency physician should always remain cognizant of the potential for an intraorbital or intraocular foreign body when examining the patient with a "foreign body" sensation. Penetrating injuries represent a greater threat of visual loss than extraocular foreign bodies and can be disastrous if overlooked.

The clinical presentation will be helpful in the determination of which patients are at risk for a penetrating injury to the globe. An individual who complains of a foreign body sensation in the *absence* of trauma or one whose history is simply that something "fell" or "blew" into the eye is at *low* risk for a globe perforation. On the other hand, there is a greater probability of globe penetration in the individual who has sustained a high-velocity wound to the eye (e.g., drilling or grinding metal, blasting rock). The presence of any of the following physical findings should alert the physician to a probable *intra*ocular foreign body: irregular pupil, shallow anterior chamber on slit lamp examination, prolapsed iris, positive Seidel test (see the section on fluorescein examination), focal conjunctival swelling and hemorrhage, hyphema, lens opacification, and reduced intraocular pressure. (It should be noted that *tonometry should not be performed in the presence of other physical findings suggesting penetration of the globe.*) One should be aware that a penetrating injury may *not* be associated with eye pain. Strong historical evidence and physical findings supporting a diagnosis of penetration of the globe should prompt emergent ophthalmologic consultation.

Often, *intraocular* foreign bodies will not be visible on direct ophthalmoscopy. Although or-bital radiographs for radiopaque objects and sonograms of the globe have been used for indirect foreign body localization,[52] computed tomography of the orbit is now considered the most useful technique.[53, 54] Therapy of intraocular and intraorbital foreign bodies must be individualized. Often, an ophthalmologist can localize an intraocular foreign body (if the vitreous is clear) using indirect ophthalmoscopy. The role of the emergency physician is to suspect the diagnosis, to protect the eye from further harm, and to obtain ophthalmologic consultation. The remainder of this section will address the problem of extraocular foreign bodies.

PROCEDURE

Foreign Body Location

The first step is to locate the foreign body. A drop of both topical anesthetic and fluorescein is applied to the inside of the lower lid (see the section on the fluorescein examination). Vertical corneal abrasions from foreign bodies under the lids are helpful for localizing these hidden foreign objects (see Fig. 67–3C). One should use a penlight and loupes or a slit lamp to examine the bulbar conjunctiva by having the patient look in all directions. The physician examines the inside of the lower lid by pulling it down with the thumb while the patient looks up. One everts the upper lid by having the patient look down as the end of an applicator stick is pressed against the superior edge of the tarsal plate of the upper lid. Meanwhile, the physician grasps the lashes and pulls down and then up to flip the lid over (Fig. 67–9).

Minute foreign bodies under the lid will be missed with simple visual inspection. Ideally, the everted lid should be examined under magnification with loupes or a slit lamp. With simple lid eversion it is still not possible to see the far recesses of the upper conjunctival fornix. Al-

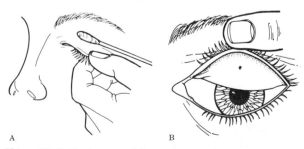

Figure 67–9. Single upper lid eversion. *A*, The end of a cotton-tipped applicator is placed above the tarsal plate while the lashes and the lid margin are pulled down and out. *B*, One everts the lid and holds it by pressing the lashes against the superior orbital rim. (From Pavan-Langston, D.: Manual of Ocular Diagnosis and Therapy. Boston, Little-Brown, 1980. Used by permission.)

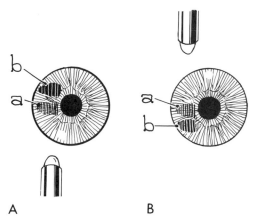

Figure 67–10. An "invisible" corneal abrasion casts an obvious shadow on the iris. The relative positions of (a) the corneal abrasion and (b) the iris shadow depend on the direction of the incident light (as in A and B). (From Paton, D. and Goldberg, M. F.: Management of Ocular Injuries. Philadelphia, W. B. Saunders Co., 1976. Used by permission.)

though double eversion of the upper lid (Fig. 67–4) is helpful, the best way to rule out a foreign body in the upper fornix is to sweep the anesthetized fornix with a wetted applicator as the upper lid is held everted. The applicator tip should be examined for removed foreign material. Small conjunctival foreign bodies not hidden by the lids are often best removed with a wetted nasopharyngeal swab (e.g., nasopharyngeal Calgi-Swab).

The cornea is then re-examined. Most corneal foreign bodies will have an area of fluorescein staining around them. A slit lamp makes the examination easy. If the physician is limited to loupes and a penlight, the light is shined diagonally on the cornea. One then finds a foreign body directly or indirectly by noting a shadow on the cornea or the iris (Fig. 67–10).[55]

With a history of a high-speed projectile hitting the eye, one must rule out an intraocular foreign body. Except in the case of a blast injury, if one foreign body is found on the surface of the globe, it is highly unlikely that there is a second foreign body inside the eye. If a foreign body cannot be found on the surface despite a suggestive history, the eye should be examined for physical evidence of penetration as discussed earlier. The fundus is dilated and examined. If in doubt regarding an intraocular foreign body, one should consider computed tomography and ophthalmologic consultation.

Foreign Body Removal

Once an extraocular foreign body is located, the technique of removal depends on whether it is embedded. If the foreign body is lying on the surface, a stream of water ejected from a syringe through a plastic catheter will usually wash the object onto the bulbar conjunctiva. Once the for-

eign body is on the conjunctiva, a wetted cotton-tipped applicator can be gently touched to the conjunctiva, and the object will adhere to the applicator tip. Overzealous use of an applicator for corneal foreign body removal can lead to extensive corneal epithelial injury. A spud device is required for removal of objects that cannot be irrigated off the cornea.

Embedded corneal foreign bodies are best removed with a commercial spud device or a 25 or 27 gauge needle on a small-diameter syringe or a cotton-tipped applicator. The applicator or the syringe serves as a handle for the attached needle. Contrary to what one might expect, it is very difficult to penetrate the sclera or the cornea with a needle.[56] As with removal of conjunctival foreign bodies, the eye must be well anesthetized. The patient should be positioned such that his head is well secured (preferably in a slit lamp frame). The patient must be instructed to gaze at an object in the distance (e.g., the practitioner's ear when a slit lamp is used) to stabilize the eye further. The spud device is held *tangentially* to the globe, and the foreign object is picked or scooped out (Fig. 67–11). During removal, the physician should brace his hand against the patient's face. The right-handed physician should place his lower hand against the left maxillary bone when removing a foreign object from the left eye and against the bridge of the patient's nose or infranasal area when removing an object from the right eye. These positions should be reversed by the left-handed physician. The use of loupes or a slit lamp for magnification is recommended to minimize further injury during removal. In particular, corneal contact with the spud device is more readily discerned when magnification is used. Only topical anesthesia is required to remove foreign bodies from the cornea. Although the patient may feel pressure during foreign body removal, pain should not be felt after the eye is anesthetized.

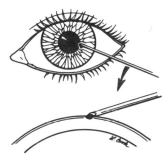

Figure 67–11. Removal of a superficial corneal foreign body. Side view illustrates the thickness of the cornea relative to the beveled needle edge. The needle or eye spud should be tangential to the cornea, and the object should be gently scraped off the cornea. (From Pavan-Langston, D.: Manual of Ocular Diagnosis and Therapy. Boston, Little-Brown, 1980. Used by permission.)

Rust Rings

A common problem with metallic foreign bodies is rust rings. These can develop within hours because of oxidation of the iron in the foreign body. There are two preferred techniques for removal of a rust ring. The most direct method is to remove it at the same time as the foreign body, either with repeated picking away with a spud device or with a rotating burr. The second approach is to let the iron of the rust ring poison and kill the surrounding epithelial cells during a 24- to 48-hour patching period. At that time, the rust ring will be soft and often comes out in one solid plug.[57] Following rust ring removal, the eye must be patched again for another 24 hours to allow the residual corneal defect time to heal. Generally, a small rust ring produces little visual difficulty unless it is directly in the line of sight. The rust ring, if large, may delay corneal healing.

Multiple Foreign Bodies

The patient with multiple foreign bodies in the eye, such as from an explosion, should be referred to an ophthalmologist. A technique that may be chosen by the ophthalmologist is to denude the entire epithelium with alcohol and remove the superficial foreign bodies. The deeper ones will gradually work their way to the surface, sometimes years later.[58]

Aftercare

After removing the foreign body, one should patch the eye if there is any corneal abrasion (see the section on patching). An antibiotic ointment is frequently instilled prior to patching, but the value of the ointment for very *superficial* corneal defects following foreign body removal is unknown. Conjunctival abrasions do not need patching. If the eye is patched, the patient should be re-examined in 24 hours. An antibiotic ointment is applied prior to placement of the patch. If the patient sustains a *superficial* injury from the foreign body and an eye patch is applied primarily for comfort, the physician may wish to instruct the patient to return only if the eye does *not* feel completely normal *or* if there is any blurred vision. The majority of superficial injuries heal without difficulty. The patient should be warned that the foreign body sensation may return temporarily prior to patch removal when the anesthetic agent has worn off.

Use of Ophthalmic Anesthetic Agents

Application of topical anesthetic agents can be both diagnostic and therapeutic. Relief of discomfort with topical anesthetic use suggests a conjunctival or corneal injury. An ocular irritant may also be masked by the use of these agents. Classic teaching is that the anesthetic preparations should not be self-administered by patients. The absence of protective reflexes while the patient is under the effect of the medicine may encourage him to use the eye while a foreign body or a corneal infection inflicts further corneal injury.

As evident from Table 67–2, the anesthetic solutions that are commonly used have a duration of action of less than 20 minutes. The patient requiring patching may need a more extended period of pain relief. The discomfort associated with a healing corneal lesion is usually made tolerable by a pressure patch, bed rest, analgesics, and sedatives (e.g., secobarbital or chloral hydrate). Patients with large corneal defects may occasionally benefit from the use of an ophthalmic anesthetic *ointment* (e.g., 0.5 per cent tetracaine [Pontocaine] ointment). The ointment form maintains anesthesia for several hours more than the anesthetic solution. In the absence of infection or a retained foreign body, the *repeated* use of ophthalmic anesthetic ointments may still be detrimental to corneal healing. The frequent removal of a pressure patch to anesthetize the cornea may lead to disruption of migrating corneal epithelial cells and may thus prolong corneal repair.

A final word of caution should be added regarding the use of ophthalmic solutions. Guaiac solutions are commonly supplied in dropper bottles similar in size and appearance to those containing ophthalmic solutions. Well-intentioned emergency

Table 67–2. OPHTHALMIC ANESTHETIC AGENTS

Generic name	Tetracaine	Proparacaine	Benoxinate
Trade name	Pontocaine	Ophthaine, Ophthetic	Dorsacaine
Concentration	0.5 to 1.0%	0.5%	0.4%
Onset of anesthesia	Less than 1 minute	Less than 20 seconds	1 to 2 minutes
Duration of anesthesia	15 to 20 minutes	10 to 15 minutes	10 to 15 minutes
Comments	Marked stinging; also available in ointment	Least irritating; no cross-sensitization with other agents	Only anesthetic compatible with fluorescein in solution

department personnel may store the guaiac reagent bottles with the ophthalmic bottles. One should encourage both color coding of the bottles and examination of the bottle prior to each use to avoid corneal injury from the guaiac reagent.

COMPLICATIONS

Complications associated with ocular foreign body removal are rare. The most frequent problem is incomplete removal of the foreign body. In such cases the epithelium has difficulty healing over the affected area, and thus the eye stays inflamed. Eventually, the diseased epithelium either will slough off and heal or will heal over the foreign body remnants, which will be gradually absorbed. In either case, the adverse effects on the eye are minimal; a minute scar on the cornea, even directly in the center, will rarely affect the vision. Nonetheless, incomplete removal of a corneal foreign object warrants ophthalmologic follow-up.

Conjunctivitis may develop following removal of an extraocular foreign body. In most cases, the bacteria producing the infection are introduced by the patient through rubbing of the irritated eye.

Although perforation of the globe by the physician's spud device is theoretically possible, this complication is exceedingly rare. To our knowledge, only one anecdotal case occurred some 20 years ago. Treatment of such a minor corneal puncture wound would consist of antibiotics, eye shield placement, and ophthalmologic consultation. Permanent sequelae are unlikely to develop.

It should be mentioned again that much epithelial injury can occur when cotton-tipped applicators are vigorously used to remove corneal foreign bodies. Indeed, we condemn the use of cotton-tipped applicators for *corneal* foreign body removal.

CONCLUSIONS

Ocular foreign bodies are one of the most common eye emergencies. Searching for and removing the foreign body is usually straightforward. The only real trap is missing an intraocular foreign body. This must be ruled out if there is a history of a high-speed projectile hitting the eye or if physical findings suggestive of globe penetration are present.

Eye Patching

INTRODUCTION

Patching the lids shut is the last step in treatment of a number of common eye emergencies. Many physicians, however, have only a vague idea of what the purpose of patching is, how to do it, and how to follow up. Even this simple procedure can be performed incorrectly. This section will provide a complete discussion of patching.

INDICATIONS AND CONTRAINDICATIONS

Patching is indicated whenever the surface of the cornea has been injured. This can occur following a mechanical abrasion, such as a fingernail scratch, or after the removal of a foreign body. Chemical damage, damage from prolonged contact lens use, and ultraviolet light injuries, which are commonly seen in the emergency department, also require patching. With each of these forms of injury, the purpose of the patch is to keep the lids from moving over the cornea and to keep light out. After patching, the patient immediately experiences less pain and tearing and the epithelium heals faster.

Patching is contraindicated when the corneal epithelial loss results from an active infection— such as a corneal ulcer—rather than from an abrasion. The first consideration in the differentiation between ulcer and abrasion is the history of the injury (how recently it occurred and how clean the offending object was). The second determining factor is the appearance of the cornea (that is, an ulcer will have an infiltrate of white cells beneath the area of epithelial loss and will be accompanied by a purulent discharge). A pressure patch should never be applied to an eye with a penetrating injury. A protective cup is the preferred covering pending ophthalmologic consultation.

EQUIPMENT

The following equipment is necessary for patching the eye: two gauze eye patches, tape (e.g., 1-inch paper tape, preferably nonallergenic), an antibiotic ointment (e.g., sulfacetamide 10 per cent), and a dilator drop (cyclopentolate [Cyclogel] 1 per cent or homatropine 5 per cent). The tape should be pre-cut into 4-inch strips and should be kept within reach.

PROCEDURE

Before patching a corneal abrasion, one should apply both a dilator drop and an antibiotic ointment.[59] The dilator must be a cycloplegic in order to relax the ciliary muscle spasm that accompanies corneal abrasions. Both cyclopentolate 1 per cent and homatropine 5 per cent will last approximately 24 hours. The patient should be checked for a narrow anterior chamber before the drop is applied (see Fig. 67–1). Antibiotic ointment is used prophylactically, although it is rare for abrasions to become infected. In the past it was thought that the ointment vehicle would slow epithelial healing, but the vehicles that are currently used do not have this effect.[61-63]

An effective patch must be put on tightly enough to keep the lids shut. The physician should have the patient shut both eyes and should remind him to keep them shut throughout the entire procedure. Two patches are used. The vertically positioned first patch is doubly folded and placed over the closed lids. The unfolded second patch is then put horizontally over the first (Fig. 67–12). The tape strips are stretched diagonally from the center of the forehead to the cheekbone. The physician can pull up the skin of the cheek; when he lets go, the tape will be even tighter. If the tape completely covers the patch, slippage of the patch and resultant eye movement will be avoided (Fig. 67–13). The tape should not extend onto the angle of the mandible, since mastication will loosen the tape in such a situation. Some physicians will paint the skin about the eye with tincture of benzoin to help secure the tape. Care must be taken not to introduce the benzoin into the eye. The presence of extensive facial hairs may prevent tight taping of the patch. If the patient refuses shaving of the facial hairs, a gauze wrap using Kerlex or Kling to encircle the head and hold the patch in place may be used (Fig. 67–14).

COMPLICATIONS

There are few complications involved in patching. It is possible to patch the patient's lashes in between the lids so that they abrade the cornea. This can occur if the patient partially opens his eye during the procedure. You can avoid this by insisting that both eyes stay closed during the entire patching.

Most problems develop when the eye is not securely patched and excessive lid motion occurs. In this situation the corneal epithelial cells are not permitted to migrate over and close the epithelial defect. This leads to increased pain and delayed healing. Some corneal defects will be extensive and may require 3 to 5 days for healing. Patients with extensive injuries should be followed frequently and treated with cycloplegics, pain medication, and (if clinically indicated) sedatives for sleep. The practitioner should document the size of the corneal defect at each visit. If healing does not occur in a progressive fashion, ophthalmologic consultation should be obtained. As mentioned earlier, patching when a corneal ulcer is present is contraindicated. A corneal "abrasion" that does not heal could very well be a herpetic ulcer.

All patients whose eyes have been patched for a corneal abrasion should be warned about possible *recurrent erosions* that might occur in the future as a complication of the original injury. The original abrasion may appear to have healed perfectly, but days, weeks, or even months later a small area

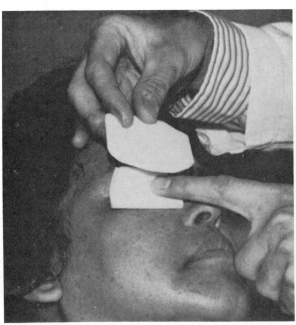
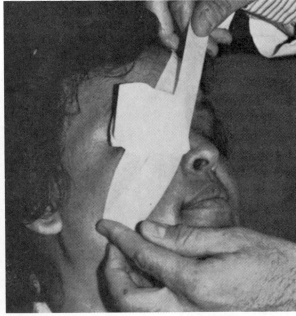

Figure 67–12. Application of eye patch. A, Vertically folded first patch in orbital recess. B, Horizontally oriented second patch with forehead to cheek taping. (Courtesy of Waring, G. O.: Emergency Medicine, November 1979, p. 39.)

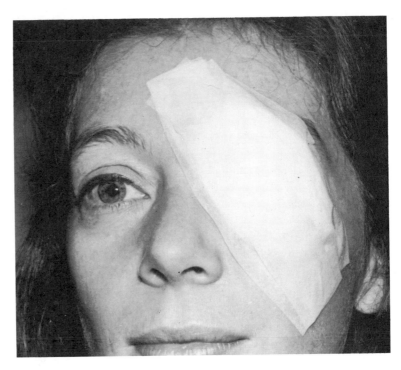

Figure 67–13. Final appearance of pressure eye patch. (From Paton, D., and Goldberg, M. F.: Management of Ocular Injuries. Philadelphia, W. B. Saunders Co., 1976. Used by permission.)

of corneal epithelium can come off, re-creating the symptoms of the original abrasion. This usually occurs in the mornings as the patient opens his eyes. These erosions may heal before the patient is re-examined and can be very puzzling. The cause is a failure of bonding of the corneal epithelium to its basement membrane.[64] Patients who develop this syndrome are given 5 per cent sodium chloride ointment to use nightly to prevent the erosions; some require bandage-soft contact lenses.[65]

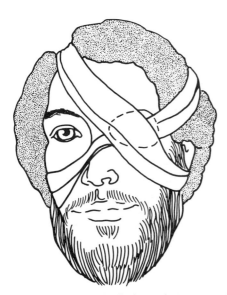

Figure 67–14. Alternative method of securing an eye patch in a bearded individual. Gauze wrap holds the patch in place.

CONCLUSION

Patching should be an easy, straightforward procedure. A common problem is the lack of follow-up instructions given to the patient after the patching. Too often, the patient is given a bottle of antibiotic to be used every 4 hours and only vague recommendations for a follow-up check. When the patient removes the patch to put in an antibiotic drop, he will never be able to replace the patch properly again. Instead, he should be told to keep the patch on for 24 hours and to return to have his abrasion checked by a physician after that time. This is the only safe way of ensuring that the abrasion has healed properly. As discussed earlier, trustworthy patients with very *superficial* corneal injuries may be given more responsibility (and instruction) for their own subsequent care. The physician should, however, make a follow-up telephone call to these individuals if they choose not to return in order to ascertain their compliance with the instructions.

The patient with an eye patch should be instructed to rest the uninjured eye. Reading should be discouraged, since involuntary movement of the patched eye will result. Watching television from a distance of 10 feet or more promotes eye fixation and is acceptable. Distant vision is unaffected by patching, although a small degree of peripheral vision is lost on the patched side. Driving after a patch is placed is generally safe, although not advisable. The patient should be driven home from the hospital to minimize the medicolegal risk to both patient and physician if the patient becomes involved in an accident. An elderly patient may require assistance with routine ambulation after eye patching.

Contact Lens Procedures

INTRODUCTION

An estimated 15 million Americans wear a form of contact lenses.[66] Removal of these lenses in the emergency department may be required to permit further evaluation of the eye or to prevent injury from prolonged wear. Emergency physicians also evaluate patients for "lost" contacts, which may be trapped under the upper lid. At times, the patient may request that the physician remove a lens that he has failed to extract from the cornea.

This section on contact lens procedures will address these concerns and will discuss injuries associated with removal attempts, the mechanism of injury from prolonged wear, and instructions to be given to patients at discharge.

BACKGROUND

The first "contact" lenses were scleral lenses made of glass. These lenses, covering the cornea as well as much of the surrounding sclera, are reported to have been in use from 1888 to 1948.[67] Glass corneal lenses (sitting entirely on the cornea) made by the Carl Zeiss Optical Works of Jena were first described in 1912. A practical synthetic scleral lens using methyl methacrylate rather than glass was discussed by Mullen and Obrig in 1938.[68, 69] In 1947, Tuohy redeveloped the corneal lens using methyl methacrylate. This was the forerunner of the current hard contact lens.[70] The development in Czechoslovakia of lenses made of soft gas-permeable polymers was reported in 1960.[71] These hydrogel (hydrophilic gelatinous-like) lenses have evolved into today's soft contact lenses.

MECHANISM OF CORNEAL INJURY FROM CONTACT LENS WEAR

Hard Contact[72]

The oxygenation of the cornea is dependent upon movement of oxygen-rich tears under the hard contact lens during blinking. During the "adaptation" phase of early wear, the wearer of hard contacts produces hypotonic tears as a result of mechanical irritation from the lens. This results in corneal edema, which reduces subsequent tear flow under the lens during blinking. Extended wear at this time leads to corneal ischemia with superficial epithelial defects predominantly in the

central corneal area (see Fig. 67–3D), where the least tear flow occurs. With adaptation, the tears become isotonic and the blinking rate normalizes, permitting extended wear. It should be noted that during early adaptation blinking is more rapid than normal and then slows to a subnormal rate during late adaptation. Mucus delivery to the cornea in the tear film may also play an important role in maintaining corneal lubrication. Tight-fitting contacts may never permit good tear flow despite an adaptation phase; individuals with tightly fitted lenses may never be able to wear their original contacts for longer than 6 to 8 hours. Lenses that are excessively loose can also cause corneal injury by moving during blinking. Rough or cracked edges can compound these injuries.

In the emergency department, the patient who presents with irritation caused by prolonged wear may be either a new or an "adapted" wearer. The adapted wearer may have been exposed to chemical irritants (e.g., smoke), which reduce the tonicity of tears and lead to corneal edema and decreased tear flow. Alternatively, the adapted wearer with irritation may have ingested sedatives (e.g., alcohol) or may have fallen asleep wearing the contacts, thus decreasing blinking and tear flow. Another possibility is that the patient may actually be wearing tight-fitting contacts that have never allowed true adaptation despite many months of wear.

The patient with the overwear syndrome usually awakens 3 hours after removing the lenses. The patient experiences intense pain and tearing similar to that caused by a foreign body. The delay in the onset of symptoms until after removal of the lenses is caused by a temporary corneal anesthesia produced by the anoxic metabolic by-products that build up during extended lens wear.[73] A second factor is the slow passage of microcysts of edema, which are pushed up to the corneal surface by mitosis of the underlying cells. When the cysts break open on the surface, the corneal nerve endings are exposed.[74]

Most patients with the overwear syndrome can be managed with reassurance, frequent administration of artificial tears, oral analgesics, and advice to "wait it out" in a darkened room. Some patients require patching for comfort. If the patient has experienced no problems with contact lenses prior to an overwear episode, he can return to using his lenses after 2 or 3 days in glasses but should be advised to build up his wearing time gradually. If the patient was having chronic problems with lens comfort prior to the episode, he should check with his ophthalmologist before using the contacts again.

Soft Contact[75]

Although there is also oxygenation of the cornea by way of the tear film with soft contact lenses, only approximately one tenth of the flow behind the lens that occurs with a hard lens is present during soft contact wear. The high degree of lens gas permeability permits the majority of oxygenation to occur directly through the lens. The hydrogel lens is more comfortable than the hard contact because lid motion over the lens is smooth. The minimization of lid and corneal irritation allows a more rapid adaptation phase because the initial reflex-induced tearing and blinking changes are reduced. Nonetheless, the lenses may still lead to corneal edema and secondary hypoxic epithelial changes if worn for an excessive period when blinking is inhibited. Some individuals can tolerate the lenses for extended periods and may on occasion sleep with the contacts in place, although this practice is not encouraged. Newer extended wear hydrogel lenses (e.g., Permalenses) permit wear for several weeks without injury. These lenses are not discernible from standard soft lenses on examination.

Although the acute overwear syndrome that occurs with hard contacts can also occur with soft lenses, it is very infrequent. More commonly, ocular damage from soft contact lenses falls into one of the three following categories:

1. Corneal neovascularization. Often the patient is asymptomatic, but on slit lamp examination fine vessels are seen invading the peripheral cornea. The treatment is to have an ophthalmologist refit the patient with looser or thinner lenses or with contacts that are more gas-permeable.

2. Giant papillary conjunctivitis.[79] The patient notes decreased lens tolerance and increased mucus production. On examination of the tarsal conjunctiva (best seen on eversion of the upper lid), large papillae are seen. These grossly appear as a cobblestoned surface. The treatment is to discontinue wearing the lenses until the process reverses and then have the lenses refitted.

3. A sensitivity reaction to the contact lens solutions (usually Thimerosol or Chlorhexidine).[80, 81] There is diffuse conjunctival injection and sometimes a superficial keratitis. The treatment is to switch to preservative-free saline with the use of heat sterilization.

All three of the aforementioned problems with soft lenses have bilateral, subacute onsets and do not require emergency treatment. The only form of ocular damage associated with soft contact lenses that is a true emergency is a bacterial or fungal corneal ulcer.[82–84] Because the nature of soft contact lenses is to absorb water, they can also absorb pathogens, which then can invade the cornea. This is especially true if the soft lens is worn continuously during both day and night. The patient will present with a painful, red eye associated with discharge and a white infiltrate on the cornea. Immediate ophthalmologic consultation is required for appropriate culturing and antimicrobial treatment.

INDICATIONS FOR REMOVAL

Removal of a contact lens is recommended in the following situations:

1. Contact lens wearer with an altered state of consciousness. The emergency physician should always be aware that the patient with a depressed or acutely agitated sensorium may be unable to express the need to have his contact lenses removed. Furthermore, it is likely that patients with a depressed sensorium will have decreased lid motion. During the secondary survey of these patients, the emergency physician should identify the presence of the lenses and should arrange for their removal and storage to prevent harm from excessive wear or possible accidental dislodgement at a later time. Without magnification, soft contacts may be difficult to see. Examination with an obliquely directed penlight should reveal the edge of the soft lens a few millimeters from the limbus on the bulbar conjunctiva.

2. Eye trauma with lens in place. Following measurement of visual acuity with the patient's lenses in place, the contacts should be removed to permit more detailed examination of the cornea. It should be noted that fluorescein may discolor hydrogel lenses; when possible, extended wear lenses should be removed prior to the use of this chemical. After the dye is instilled, the eyes should be flushed with normal saline; at least 1 hour should pass prior to reinsertion.[76] The recent availability of single-use droppers of 0.35 per cent fluorexon (Fluresoft) has permitted the safe staining of eyes when soft lenses are to be worn immediately following the examination. A limited eye irrigation following the use of fluorexon drops is still recommended prior to the reinsertion of soft contacts.

3. Inability of the patient to remove the contact lens. A patient may present with a hard contact that cannot be removed because of corneal edema from prolonged wear. Alternatively, the patient may present with a "lost contact" that he believes to be behind the upper lid. It should be noted that there is no urgency for contact removal in the prehospital setting; hence, removal can wait until the patient has been evaluated by a physician.

CONTRAINDICATION TO REMOVAL

The only major problem with contact lens removal occurs when the cornea may have been perforated. In this case, the suction cup technique of removal described later is preferred.

PROCEDURE

Hard Contact Lens Removal

A number of maneuvers have been devised for removal of the corneal lens. One technique is to first lean the patient's face over a table or a collecting cloth. The physician pulls the lids temporally from the lateral palpebral margin to lock the lids against the contact lens edges. The patient should look toward his nose and then downward toward his chin. This movement works the lower eyelid under the lower lens edge and flips the lens off the eye. The technique requires a cooperative patient, since the physician must pull the patient's lids tightly against the edge of the contact lens. The movement of the patient's eye then flips the contact free.

In the unresponsive patient, a modification of the technique can be used while the patient is supine. The physician takes a more active role in lid movement using the following procedure: One thumb is placed on the upper eyelid and the other on the lower eyelid near the margin of each lid. With the lens centered over the cornea, the eyelids are opened until the lid margins are beyond the edges of the lens (Fig. 67–15A). The physician then presses both eyelids gently but firmly on the globe of the eye and moves the lids so that they are barely touching the edges of the lens (Fig. 67–15B). One presses slightly harder on the lower lid to move it under the bottom edge of the lens. As the lower edge of the lens begins to tip away from the eye, the lids are moved together, allowing the lens to slide out to where it can be grasped (Fig. 67–15C). The physician should remember to use clean hands when removing the lens.

Alternatively, one can move the lens gently off the cornea using a cotton-tipped applicator to guide the lens onto the sclera, where the applicator tip can be forced under an edge of the lens to flip the contact loose. Topical anesthesia is indicated when using an applicator and the patient is awake. Care must be taken with this technique to avoid contact of the applicator with the cornea when the lens is moved off the eye. Perhaps the easiest technique is to use a moistened suction-tipped device and simply lift the lens off the cornea (Fig. 67–16). A drop of honey on the fingertip can be used by the patient or the physician to remove a hard contact lens if a suction-tipped device is not available. The honey is easily washed off a hard lens.

Scleral lenses (those hard contact lenses that cover both the cornea and an amount of the sclera) can be removed by an exaggeration of the manual technique described earlier (Fig. 67–17). Elevation of the lens with a cotton-tipped applicator or a suction-tipped device is also an effective technique.

Soft Contact Lens Removal

With clean hands, the physician pulls down the lower eyelid using the middle finger. The tip of the index finger is placed on the lower edge of the lens. The lens is slid down onto the sclera and is compressed slightly between the thumb and the index finger. This pinching motion folds the lens and allows removal from the eye (Fig. 67–18).

LENS STORAGE

After a contact lens has been removed, it should be stored in sterile normal saline solution. It is best to use the patient's own storage container and, if available, a buffer solution. A variety of alternative sterile containers are available for use in the emergency department. One should be

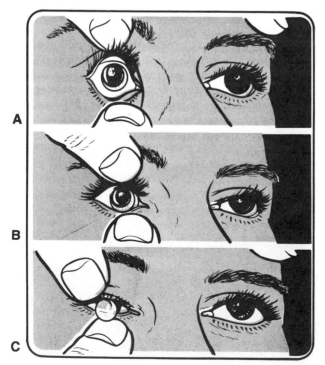

Figure 67–15. Manual technique for removing a hard contact lens. A, Separation of lids. B, Entrapment of lens edges with lids. C, Expulsion of lens by forcing of lower lid under inferior edge of lens. (From Grant, H. D., et al.: Emergency Care, 3rd ed. Bowie, MD, Robert J. Brady Co., 1982. Used by permission.)

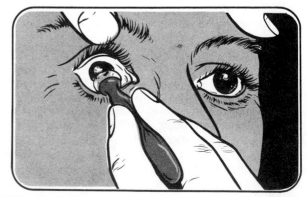

Figure 67–16. Use of a moistened suction cup to remove a hard contact lens. (From Grant, H. D., et al.: Emergency Care, 3rd ed. Bowie, MD, Robert J. Brady Co., 1982. Used by permission.)

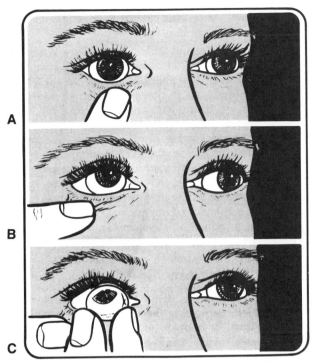

Figure 67–17. Removal of a hard scleral lens. A, Separation of lids. B, Forcing of lower lid beneath edge of scleral lens by temporal traction on lower lid. C, Lifting of lens off eye. (From Grant, H. D., et al.: Emergency Care, 3rd ed. Bowie, MD, Robert J. Brady Co., 1982. Used by permission.)

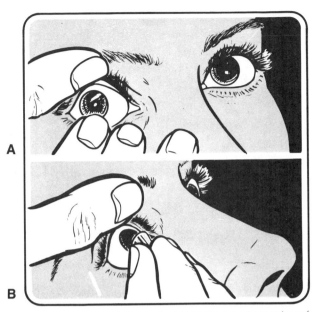

Figure 67–18. Removal of a soft contact lens. A, Separation of lids and movement of contact onto sclera using index finger. B, Pinching of lens between thumb and index finger. (From Grant, H. D., et al.: Emergency Care, 3rd ed. Bowie, MD, Robert J. Brady Co., 1982. Used by permission.)

certain that right and left lenses are kept separate and in appropriately labeled containers. The containers should be kept with the patient until a friend or family member can procure them or should be locked with the patient's valuables.

EVALUATION OF THE "LOST CONTACT"

A patient may present with a request to be examined for a "lost" contact lens. The patient may be unsure if the lens is hidden under a lid, remains on the cornea, or is truly outside the eye.

The evaluation of the patient with a "lost" contact should begin, as should all eye examinations, with the measurement of visual acuity. Visual acuity is preferably measured using a 20-foot eye chart. A diminished visual acuity in the eye in which a patient "just can't seem to take out" a soft contact lens may be the most convincing evidence that the lens is missing. Although transparent, soft contacts in proper position are usually seen easily when viewed closely with loupes or on slit lamp examination. The lens forms a fine line where it ends on the sclera several millimeters peripherally to the limbus. Hard contact lenses are even more evident as they change in position on the cornea. (Hard scleral lenses appear similar to the soft contacts when in proper location and in general are too large to be lost in the upper fornix).

If the contact is not evident on initial inspection, the lids are everted as discussed in the section on foreign body removal (double eversion of the upper lid). If the lens is still not visible, a drop of topical anesthetic is placed in the eye. The upper fornix is gently swept with a wetted cotton-tipped applicator while the patient looks toward his chin. If the lens is still not evident although the patient remains insistent that it is in the eye, one may perform a fluorescein examination after explaining that the dye will color the lens (permanently). The upper lid should again be doubly everted and visualized using an ultraviolet light source.

If the lens remains elusive, the patient should be reassured that a thorough examination has been performed and that no object has been located under the eyelids or on the cornea. The cornea should then be examined for defects that warrant antibiotic ointment and a pressure patch (as discussed in the section on patching). Follow-up with the patient's eye specialist for a replacement lens and further reassurance is encouraged. One should also ask the patient to retrace his movements at the time the contact began to give him trouble or was missed and to check his clothing for the presence of the lens. A final possibility is that the patient may have accidentally placed the two lenses together in the same side of his carrying case, causing them to stick together. In fact, patients have inadvertently placed one contact over the other—both in the same eye! One should note that hard contacts have been found embedded in conjunctival tissue under the upper lid (Fig. 67–19), at times for over a year.[77, 78]

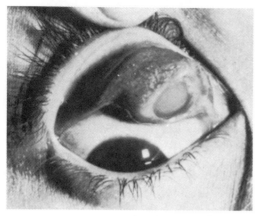

Figure 67–19. Hard contact lens embedded in conjunctival tissue of upper lid. (From Mandell, R. B.: Contact Lens Practice, 3rd ed. Springfield, IL, Charles C Thomas, 1981. Used by permission.)

COMPLICATIONS OF LENS REMOVAL

Unless care is used during lens removal, a corneal abrasion can occur. It may be difficult at times to determine whether the injury was produced by the patient or was a result of the physician's technique. Fortunately, the corneal injury is usually of a superficial nature and responds well to eye patching.

CONCLUSIONS

Contact lens removal is seldom a difficult task. More challenging situations are the identification of emergency patients at risk of overuse corneal injury, the evaluation of patients who cannot locate a soft lens, and the instruction of patients with contact lens–related problems concerning aftercare.

Tonometry

INTRODUCTION

Tonometry is the indirect estimation of intraocular pressure obtained by measurement of the resistance of the eyeball to indentation by an applied force. Tonometry is important to the emergency physician for several reasons. Elevated ocular pressure has been associated with loss of visual field and even blindness. The elevation of intraocular pressure can occur gradually or suddenly. Sudden ocular pressure increases can follow trauma or can occur with primary angle-closure glaucoma. Often, affected patients come to the emergency department with systemic complaints (e.g., nausea, vomiting, headache), and the emergency physician must determine the ocular pressure and its relationship to the systemic symp-

toms. Furthermore, patients with elevated intraocular pressures may be at risk for retinal hypoperfusion when their systemic pressure is suddenly lowered. The emergency physician who treats patients who are in shock or in need of antihypertensive therapy must be cognizant of the patient's intraocular pressure and its potential adverse effect on retinal perfusion.

BACKGROUND

Ophthalmologists depended upon tactile estimation of eye pressure until the 1860s, when von Graefe developed the first mechanical tonometer.[85] Applanation tonometry was introduced in 1885 by Maklakoff[86] but was not popularized until Goldmann improved the instrument in the 1930s.[87] Schiötz developed an impression tonometer in 1905 and modified it in the 1920s; this form is still in use today.[88] Aside from modifications in configuration, current tonometers closely resemble the devices popularized by Schiötz and Goldmann. The most dramatic variations are the Mackay-Marg tonometer,[89] which permits a continuous tonographic recording, and the noncontact tonometer, which is a pneumatic applanation tonometer.[90]

TONOMETRIC PRINCIPLES

There are two tonometric techniques that are reliable and clinically useful for estimating intraocular pressure:

1. The impression method, whereby a plunger 3 mm in diameter deforms the cornea and the "indentation" is measured. This technique was popularized by Schiötz and commonly bears his name.

2. The applanation method, whereby a plane surface is pressed against the cornea. One can either measure the pressure necessary to flatten a defined area or determine the size of a flattened area produced by the defined pressure.

Both tonometric principles are based on the Imbert-Fick law, which states: If a plane surface is applied with force (F) to a thin, spheric membrane within which a pressure (P_t) exists, at equilibrium the expression $P_t = F/A$ is valid if A is the area of the applied surface (Fig. 67–20). It should be noted that the Schiötz tonometer (Fig. 67–21) actually measures the total intraocular pressure (initial pressure plus the pressure added by the weight of the tonometer and the plunger). Friedenwald[91] empirically found that a "rigidity coefficient" could be introduced to allow an estimation of the true intraocular eye pressure. One must be aware, however, that calculated conversion tables for Schiötz tonometers use an average estimate of the rigidity coefficient and hence are not accurate

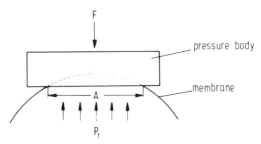

Figure 67–20. Principle of tonometry. At equilibrium: $P_t = F/A$. (From Draeger, J., and Jessen, K.: Tonometry and tonography. *In* Bellows, J. G.: Glaucoma: Contemporary International Concepts. New York, Masson Publishing USA, 1979. Used by permission.)

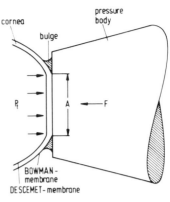

Figure 67–22. Principle of applanation tonometry. The effect of surface tension counters the pressure rise produced by application of the instrument. (From Draeger, J., and Jessen, K.: Tonometry and tonography. *In* Bellows, J. G.: Glaucoma: Contemporary International Concepts. Masson Publishing USA, 1979. Used by permission.)

when eye rigidity is altered (e.g., after scleral buckle procedures for retinal detachment). Although the applanation tonometer (Fig. 67–22) also increases the intraocular pressure during eye measurement, the applied pressure is much smaller and is partially countered by the surface tension of the eye tear film. Studies have shown the applanation tonometer measurements to be within 2 per cent of the true intraocular pressure.[92]

The noncontact tonometer is a pneumatic applanation tonometer that permits intraocular pressure measurement without eye contact. A pulsed air jet is used to deform the cornea. The technique is also dependent upon ocular rigidity. Although readings taken by different examiners correlate well, the measurements are altered by the use of local anesthetics and show a wide standard deviation of measurements for patients with pathologic elevation of ocular pressure (when standard applanation tonometry is used as a reference).[93] Furthermore, the technique is not useful with corneal surface irregularities (e.g., corneal edema, keratoconus, corneal perforation) or when medications in viscous preparations have been used.

INDICATIONS FOR TONOMETRY

Measurement of intraocular pressure in the emergency department is part of any complete eye

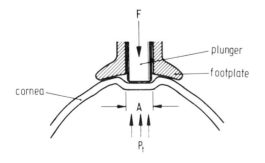

Figure 67–21. Principle of impression tonometry. In reality, P_t is increased slightly by the weight of the instrument. (From Draeger, J., and Jessen, K.: Tonometry and tonography. *In* Bellows, J. G.: Glaucoma: Contemporary International Concepts. New York, Masson Publishing USA, 1979. Used by permission.)

examination. Special situations in which tonometry is required are as follows:

1. *Confirmation of a clinical diagnosis of acute angle-closure glaucoma.* The middle-aged or elderly patient who presents with acute aching pain in one eye, blurred vision (including "halos" around lights), and a red eye with a smoky cornea and a fixed midposition pupil will obviously need a pressure reading. Sometimes the findings are less dramatic, and sometimes the patient will complain mostly of nausea and vomiting that suggest a "flu" rather than an eye disorder.

2. *Determination of a baseline ocular pressure following blunt ocular injury.* Patients with hyphema will often have acute rises in intraocular pressure because of blood obstructing the trabecular meshwork.[94] Later, angle recession can cause a permanent form of open-angle glaucoma.

3. *Determination of a baseline ocular pressure in a patient with iritis.* Patients with iritis can develop both open- and closed-angle glaucoma as well as steroid-induced glaucoma.

4. *Documentation of ocular pressure in the patient at risk for open-angle glaucoma.* All patients over age 40 with a familial history of open-angle glaucoma, optic disk changes, visual field defects, and pressures over 21 mm Hg should be referred to an ophthalmologist for further workup. Referral should also be made for those patients with suspiciously cupped disks who have normal pressures; some of these patients may have "low-pressure" glaucoma associated with visual field defects.

5. *Measurement of ocular pressure in patients with glaucoma and hypertension.* There is conflicting evidence[96–102] concerning the relationship between acute reductions in systemic blood pressure and further visual field loss in glaucoma patients. Progressive or rapid visual field loss is a rare but reported phenomenon in association with sys-

temic blood pressure reduction. The prudent physician will measure the intraocular pressure and will consult with the glaucoma patient's ophthalmologist prior to instigating treatment for systemic hypertension. Consideration should also be given to the use of a beta-blocking agent to lower intraocular and systemic pressures simultaneously.

CONTRAINDICATIONS TO TONOMETRY

Tonometry is relatively contraindicated in eyes that are infected.[103] One should sterilize a tonometer after applying it to a potentially infected eye. The contact portions are to be swabbed with alcohol and allowed to dry prior to use on another eye. Viruses may not be destroyed by alcohol cleansing. Ultraviolet sterilization, cold-sterilizer bathing of the footplate and plunger, and ethylene oxide sterilization have been advocated as alternatives. The Schiötz tonometer may also be used with sterile disposable coverings (marketed as Tonofilm), although these are seldom available in emergency practice. Nonetheless, measurement of intraocular pressure can be deferred until a subsequent visit to the emergency department or private physician unless the red eye demands an immediate determination of intraocular pressure. Examples of a need for immediate tonometry are suspected angle-closure glaucoma (acute onset of redness and pain in the eye with smoky vision, a cloudy cornea, and a fixed pupil in mid-dilation) and iritis (ciliary injection with photophobia), in which secondary angle-closure or steroid-induced pressure changes may occur. Reported cases of conjunctivitis spread by tonometry predominantly tend to be viral infections. Particular efforts should be made to avoid use of the instrument on patients with active facial or ocular herpetic lesions.

The presence of corneal defects also represents a relative contraindication to tonometry.[21] The use of a tonometer on an abraded cornea may lead to further injury and is best deferred until a subsequent visit. Patients who cannot maintain a relaxed position (e.g., because of significant apprehension, blepharospasm, uncontrolled coughing, nystagmus, or uncontrolled singultus) are unlikely to permit an adequate examination and can receive corneal injury when sudden movements occur during an examination. Furthermore, tonometric examination, with the exception of the palpation technique (through the lids) and the noncontact method, should not be performed on a cornea without complete anesthesia.

The major contraindication to tonometry is suspected penetrating ocular injury.[103] Globe perforation may be exacerbated by pressure on the globe with resultant extrusion of intraocular contents. Slit lamp examination as discussed subsequently can be used to compare anterior chamber depth and hence to detect the possibility of perforation.

PROCEDURE

Palpation Technique

All forms of tonometry are essentially ways of determining the ease of deforming the eye; an eye that can easily be deformed has a low pressure. The most direct way to do this is simply to press on the sclera through the lids and grossly compare one eye with the other. One can easily distinguish the rock-hard eye of acute glaucoma from the normal opposite eye by this method. Another method is to anesthetize the eyes topically and press a wetted applicator on the sclera of each eye. Again, eye deformation is inversely related to ocular pressure. Rigidity of the globe also is a factor in this crude method of tonometry.

Impression (Schiötz) Technique

Use of the Schiötz tonometer requires relaxation on the part of the patient and steadiness on the part of the physician. The patient is placed in either a supine or a semi-recumbent position and is instructed to gaze at a spot directly above the eyes. A spot on the ceiling should suffice; alternatively, the patient can stretch his arm up over his head and gaze at his thumb. A drop of topical anesthetic is placed in each eye. The patient is allowed to blink while the physician blots the tears away with a tissue. Rubbing the eyes will lower intraocular pressure.

The patient *keeps both eyes wide open and fixed on an object*, and the physician separates the eyelids on the side to which he is standing. Care must be taken to direct pressure onto the orbital rims rather than into the orbit, since pressure directed into the orbit falsely raises the reading (Fig. 67–23). The tonometer is momentarily held over the open eye, and the patient is informed that the instrument will block vision in the one eye. The patient is instructed to continue to gaze at the fixation point as though the instrument were not there. After the patient relaxes the involuntary muscle contraction that occurs when the instrument is first placed in the line of sight, the instrument is gently lowered onto the middle portion of the cornea. The instrument should be vertically aligned with the footplate resting on the cornea; the reading should be in midscale. Should the reading be on the low end of the scale (less than 5 units), additional weight should be added to the plunger after the instrument has been removed. The process should be repeated as before with the additional weight.

The opposite eye should be measured in the same fashion. A converted scale reading (Table

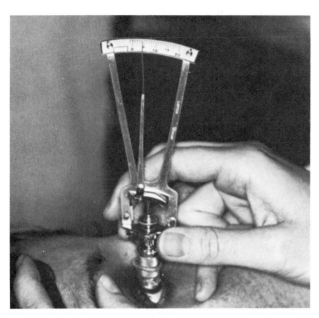

Figure 67–23. One technique of lid separation and Schiötz' tonometer placement. Lid separation pressure is applied to the bony orbital rims. The tonometer is held vertically during use, and the physician's hand is established against the patient's facial bones. (From Keeney, A. H.: Ocular Examination, 2nd ed. St. Louis, C. V. Mosby Co., 1976. Used by permission.)

Table 67–3. SCHIÖTZ TONOMETRY

Tonometer Scale Reading (units)	Tonometer Weights (grams)		
	5.5 (mm Hg)	7.5 (mm Hg)	10 (mm Hg)
2.50	27	39	55
3.00	24	36	51
3.50	22	33	47
4.00	21	30	43
4.50	19	28	40
5.00	17	26	37
5.50	16	24	34
6.00	15	22	32
6.50	13	20	29
7.00	12	18	27
7.50	11	17	25
8.00	10	16	23
8.50	9	14	21
9.00	8	13	20
9.50	8	12	18
10.00	7	11	16

The table provides estimates of the intraocular pressure to the nearest mm Hg for the different weight of the Schiötz tonometer. Accuracy is most dependable with scale readings larger than 5. If the scale reading is less than 5, use the next highest weight that will give a reading of 5 or more.

67–3) giving an intraocular pressure of greater than 21 mm Hg requires ophthalmologic consultation. Associated symptoms or signs of angle-closure glaucoma (primary or secondary) represent an ophthalmologic emergency.[104]

Errors with Impression Tonometry Inaccurate readings can occur with the Schiötz tonometer for a variety of reasons. If the plunger is sticky, falsely low readings may be obtained. Plunger motion and the zero point of the tonometer should be checked on a firm test button prior to use. A sticky plunger can be cleaned with isopropyl alcohol and dried with tissue. When the lids are held open, pressure directed into the orbit will elevate the intraocular pressure and will provide a falsely elevated reading. The following eye movements have been found to elevate the intraocular pressure: closure of the lids (increase by 5 mm Hg), blinking (increase by 5 to 10 mm Hg), accommodation (increase by 2 mm Hg), and looking toward the nose (increase by 5 to 10 mm Hg).[105] Repeated measurements or prolonged measurements have been found to lower the intraocular pressure approximately 2 mm Hg and may also lower the pressure in the opposite eye.[106] As mentioned in the introduction to this section, the calibration of the Schiötz tonometer is based upon a mean rigidity coefficient. Factors that produce a reduction in ocular rigidity falsely lower the measured pressure. These factors include high myopia, anticholinesterase drugs, overhydration (4 cups of coffee or 6 cans of beer), and scleral buccal operations.[105, 107]

Ocular pressure measurements can vary with ocular perfusion. When measured after a premature ventricular contraction, the intraocular pressure may be reduced as much as 8 mm Hg.[108] Similarly, decreased venous return as produced by breath holding, the Valsalva maneuver, or a tight collar can increase the intraocular pressure.[105]

Applanation Technique[109, 110]

One can perform this technique using a slit lamp attachment for an applanation tonometer with the patient's head stabilized in the headrest of the slit lamp (see the following section on the slit lamp examination) (Fig. 67–24). A portable device is also available and is similar in principle. The portable device will not be specifically discussed.

The patient must be comfortable and relaxed. The physician should anesthetize the eye as discussed previously, avoiding ocular pressure, which can lower the subsequent measurements. Fluorescein should be applied to each eye. Excess fluorescein should be blotted from the eye. The patient's head should be in the slit lamp with the forehead firmly against the headrest, and the physician should direct the patient to gaze straight ahead. One can use a light for fixation or can ask the patient to focus on the physician's ear on the side opposite the eye being examined.

The cobalt blue light filter is placed in the light beam, and the slit diaphragm is opened fully. The light arm is angulated to shine on the applanation prism in the region of the encircling black line near the anterior prism tip at an angle of 45 to 60

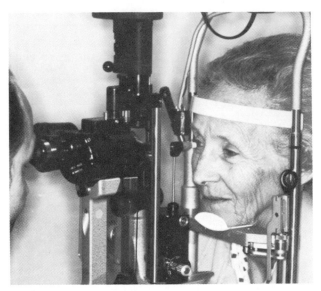

Figure 67–24. Goldmann applanation tonometer with biprism in contact with patient's right cornea. (From Keeney, A. H.: Ocular Examination, 2nd ed. St. Louis, C. V. Mosby Co., 1976. Used by permission.)

degrees to the line of observation. The voltage is turned to the maximum setting, and the low-power microscopic system is focused through the plastic prism so that the front face is clearly seen through the chosen eyepiece. The pressure knob of the tonometer is turned to 1 gm (10 mm Hg), bringing the prism arm to its forward stop. Thus, when corneal contact is made, the prism will be exerting only light pressure. The room lights are dimmed.

The patient's eye that is being examined and the applanation prism are watched from the side (or with the eye not sighting through the microscope) as the instrument is brought forward by the "joy stick" control until gentle contact is made between the prism face and the corneal center. Contact is evidenced by an immediate bluish glow throughout the limbus. The patient's lids must be wide open and unblinking. Contact with the lid margins will produce reflex blinking, and the lids may require separation by the physician's fingers. Pressure during lid separation must be exerted only against the orbital rims. Through the microscope, the physician will see two blue semicircles (surrounding the flattened area of cornea). Each semicircle is bordered by an arc of green light and pulses synchronously with the cardiac rate (Fig. 67–25).

The semicircles should be of equal size; their width should be approximately one tenth the diameter of the flattened surface contained within each arc. If the semicircles are grossly widened, either excessive tears are present or the prism was probably wet before contact. A wet prism must be withdrawn, dried, and reapplied. If the semicircles are grossly narrowed, the tear film has dried excessively. In this case, the prism must be withdrawn and the patient instructed to blink several times before contact with the cornea is attempted again. If the semicircles are so broad that they extend beyond the illuminated field, there is excessive flattening, and the slit lamp must be drawn back. If the semicircles suddenly shrink, either the patient has moved back or the instrument has been backed away from the eye. The semicircles should be of equal extent above and below a horizontal dividing line. If the dividing line is not horizontal, the applanation prism assembly should be rotated on its holder until the line is horizontal. If the semicircles are not equally divided above and below the line, vertical adjustments of the slit lamp should be made.

Readings should be taken at approximately the midpoint between systole and diastole, when the inner (concave) boundaries of each semicircle rhythmically glide past each other through excursions of equal distance (see Fig. 67–25C). One finalizes adjustments to the end point of properly located and sized semicircles by rotating the pressure knob back and forth. When applanation pres-

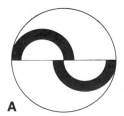
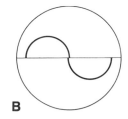
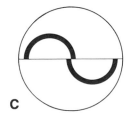
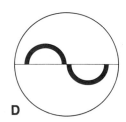

A B C D

Figure 67–25. Schematic representation of semicircles seen through contact applanation prism of Goldmann tonometer. A, Semicircles are too wide, suggesting excessive moistening of the prism or cornea. The prism must be withdrawn and dried. B, Semicircles are too narrow, suggesting that the lacrimal fluid has dried out, as during a prolonged measurement. The prism must be withdrawn so that the patient may blink a few times. The measurement is then repeated. C, Semicircles are of appropriate width, and their inner borders just touch. Cardiac pulsations transmitted through the globe cause rhythmic or pulsating movement of the semicircles over each other through a small amplitude. D, Semicircles are slightly separated, indicating applied pressure below that of the eye. The measuring drum must be turned to increase applanation pressure until the end point is reached. (From Keeney, A. H.: Ocular Examination, 2nd ed. St. Louis, C. V. Mosby Co., 1976. Used by permission.)

sure exceeds intraocular pressure, the semicircles are too small to intersect.

At the end point is a flattened disk area 3.06 mm in diameter within the 7-mm diameter of the prism face. Here the attractive surface tension of the tears toward the prism is counterbalanced by the elasticity, or springiness, of the cornea; at this point the grams of force applied through the prism (indicated on the pressure knob) are directly convertible (when multiplied by 10 into millimeters of mercury) to express intraocular pressure. With an applanation tonometer, the average intraocular pressure in a seated adult is 14 to 17 mm Hg.

After use, the tonometer should be wiped dry and removed for storage if used infrequently in the emergency department. One should verify the pressure adjustment periodically using the test weight or metal balance bar supplied with the instrument.

Potential sources of error with the applanation tonometer are similar to those mentioned for the impression tonometer, with the exception that ocular rigidity is not a factor. Inaccuracies primarily result from ocular motion or tensing of the lids.

COMPLICATIONS

When tonometric instruments are used properly and reasonable precautions are taken, complications are unusual. The eye with pre-existing corneal injury should be spared the additional trauma of tonometer placement. Corneal abrasions can be produced by ocular movement during testing. In particular, patients with uncontrollable nystagmus, singultus, or coughing or those who are extremely apprehensive should not be subjected to tonometry. Infection can be transmitted by the use of the instrument. Careful cleansing of the device and avoidance of tonometry in patients with obvious conjunctivitis, corneal ulcers, or active herpetic lesions should minimize the risk of spreading the infection to the unaffected eye or to subsequent patients. Although protective coverings can be placed over the tonometer contact, tonometry can usually be postponed in the aforementioned individuals until the risk of infection is minimal. Extrusion of ocular contents with penetrating injuries is a potential but rare complication.

CONCLUSIONS

Tonometry is an easily learned technique that should be used by the emergency physician for the detection of elevated intraocular pressure. An elevated intraocular pressure in conjunction with physical findings suggestive of acute angle-closure glaucoma is an indication for therapy and consultation with an ophthalmologist. Baseline evalua-

tion of intraocular pressure for conditions associated with a secondary glaucoma (e.g., hyphema and iritis) will aid the ophthalmologist during subsequent evaluation. In addition, the emergency physician can serve as a referral source for patients with elevated intraocular pressure who are suspected of having open-angle glaucoma. In particular, future drug therapy for systemic hypertension may be altered by the presence of concomitant intraocular hypertension. The emergency physician who aggressively manages patients with hypertensive crises must also be aware of potential visual field defects when systemic pressures are vigorously lowered without concurrently lowered intraocular pressures.

Slit Lamp Examination

INTRODUCTION

The slit lamp is an extremely useful instrument; it makes the examination of the anterior segment of the eye a pleasure. The instrument can reveal pathologic conditions that would otherwise be invisible. The slit lamp permits detailed evaluation of external eye injury and is the definitive tool for diagnosing anterior chamber hemorrhage and inflammation. The emergency physician should not attempt to diagnose any but the simplest of eye problems without the aid of a slit lamp.

BACKGROUND[111]

Since the 1800s, physicians have searched for a better way both to magnify and to illuminate the anterior segment of the eye. In 1891, Aubert developed the first true binocular stereoscopic microscope. Then, in 1911, Gullstrand introduced a slit illuminator device. The microscope and the illuminator were combined by Henker in 1916; the result was the first true slit lamp. Goldmann improved the mechanical supports for the microscope and the illuminator and in 1937 marketed a slit lamp that resembles closely the device that is used today.

INDICATIONS AND CONTRAINDICATIONS

The slit lamp can be used in every eye examination. It is especially useful in the emergency department for the diagnosis of abrasions, foreign bodies, and iritis.[112] The slit lamp facilitates foreign body removal and is also used in conjunction with most applanation tonometers. Although portable slit lamp instruments exist, emergency physicians generally have access only to a stationary, upright device. Therefore, a slit lamp examination is contraindicated in patients who cannot tolerate an upright sitting position (e.g., those in profound shock).

EQUIPMENT

The slit lamp has three components: a binocular microscope mounted horizontally, a light source that can create a beam of variable width, and a mechanical assembly to immobilize the patient's head and to manipulate the microscope and the light source. The location and arrangement of the knobs that control these components will vary in devices made by different manufacturers, but all slit lamps are basically alike. By simply turning each knob and watching the results, one can quickly master a new machine. Figure 67–26 illustrates the location of the functional controls on one particular instrument.

The first knob that one should locate is the on/off switch for the entire machine. Often this switch will provide two or three different power settings. The lowest setting is adequate for routine examination and will preserve bulb life. One can use a high-intensity setting when examining the anterior chamber with a narrow slit beam. The second knob that one should find is the locking nut for the mechanical assembly. This must be loosened in order for the assembly to be focused.

The patient should be comfortable while sitting with his head in the device. The patient's forehead should be firmly against the headrest, and his chin should be in the chin rest. By varying the table height, one should be able to maximize the comfort of the patient's neck and back. The headrest has control knobs for raising and lowering the chin rest. The chin rest should be adjusted to align the patient's eye level with the mark on the headrest support rods.

The binocular microscope has a control for varying the magnification. Usually low powers, such as $10\times$ or $16\times$, are the most useful. A higher power is helpful when the anterior chamber is examined for cells and flare. The binocular interpupillary distance should be adjusted to match that of the examiner. One can focus the eye pieces by moving the instrument forward and backward until the narrowed vertical beam is sharpest on the patient's cornea when viewed with the unaided eye. Then, while viewing through each eye piece individually, the physician adjusts the focus of each to produce a sharp image of the anterior cornea.

The light source is mounted on a swinging arm. There are knobs to vary the width and the height of the light beam. There are also filters that can be "clicked" in; only white and blue are needed.

The angle of the slit beam can be varied from vertical to horizontal. The vertical alignment is preferred for routine examinations in the emergency department.

Both the microscope and the light source are mounted on swivel arms, linked at their base to a movable table. One can change the position of this table by pushing on any part of it. For finer movements, the physician uses a "joy stick." One can vary the height of the microscope and the light source by twisting either the "joy stick" or a separate knob at the base, depending on the design of the instrument.

PROCEDURE[113, 114]

There are three setups that every slit lamp operator must know. The first (and most helpful) is for an overall screening of the anterior segment of the eye. For examination of the patient's right eye, the light source is swung to the examiner's left at a 45-degree angle while the microscope is directly in front of the eye. The slit beam is set at the maximum height and the minimum width using the white light. To scan across the patient's cornea, one first focuses the beam on the cornea by moving the entire base of the slit lamp forward and backward. One then moves the whole base left and right to scan across. The 45-degree angle between the microscope and the light source should not be varied. The most common mistake is to try to scan by swinging the arm of the light source in an arc; this will not work because the light beam will remain centered on the same point of the patient's eye. The examiner scans across at the level of the conjunctiva and the cornea and then pushes slightly forward on the base and scans at the level of the iris. The depth of the anterior chamber is determined with this setup. The depth of the chamber may be reduced with corneal perforation or in individuals predisposed to angle-closure glaucoma.

This basic setup can also be used to examine the conjunctiva for traumatic lesions, inflammation, mucus secretions, and foreign bodies. The lids can be examined for hordeolum, blepharitis, or trichiasis. A cotton-tipped applicator can be placed in the fossa above the tarsal plate of the upper lid and rotated to evert the upper lid partially. Complete lid eversion (as described in the section on foreign body removal) can be performed in conjunction with the slit lamp examination to permit evaluation of the undersurface of the upper lid for foreign body retention.

Corneal foreign body removal can be enhanced by use of the slit lamp. In particular, the instrument allows stabilization of the patient's head. Magnification will also minimize corneal injury

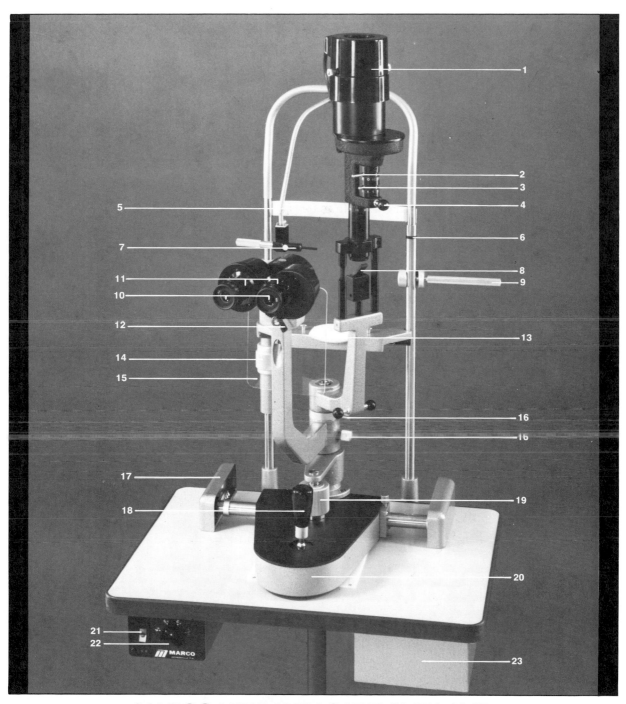

MARCO I PRIMARY CARE SLIT LAMP

NOMENCLATURE

1. Cover for Lamp Bulb
2. Slit Width Controls (Red-Free Filter)
3. Slit Height Control (Cobalt Blue Filter)
4. Control of the Rotation of Slit
5. Headrest
6. Eye Level Marker
7. Fixation Lighthead
8. Mirror

9. Examiner's Handrest
10. Eyepieces
11. Knurled Rings for Refractive Error Adjustment
12. High-Low Magnification Lever
13. Patient's Chinrest
14. Headrest Elevation Control
15. Breath Shield

16. Fixing Screws for Arm
17. Rail Covers
18. Joystick
19. Elevation Control
20. Slit Lamp Base
21. On-Off Switch
22. Intensity Control
23. Accessory Storage Drawer

Figure 67–26. Slit lamp controls. (From Marco Equipment, Inc.: Operating Instructions for Slit Lamp Microscopes. Jacksonville, FL, Marco Equipment, Inc. Used by permission.)

during foreign body or rust ring removal. The upper eyelid is best immobilized by a cotton-tipped applicator, as discussed previously. The physician's hand can be steadied against the patient's nose, cheek, or forehead or against the support rods of the headrest. The patient should be instructed to stare straight ahead at a fixed light or at the physician's ear during removal of the foreign body.

The second setup is essentially the same as the first but uses the blue filter. The purpose is to pick up any areas of fluorescein staining. After fluorescein is applied, the blue filter is "clicked" into position, and the beam is widened to 3 or 4 mm. It should be noted that a patient can tolerate a wider beam if it is blue. Corneal defects (as discussed in the section on the fluorescein examination) are sought with this setup. The blue filter is also used with applanation tonometry, as discussed in the section on tonometry.

The purpose of the third setup is to search for cells in the anterior chamber—either the white cells of iritis or the red cells of a microscopic hyphema. The height of the beam should be shortened to 3 or 4 mm and should be as narrow as possible. The microscope should be switched to high power. The beam is first focused on the center of the cornea and is then pushed forward slightly so that it is focused on the anterior surface of the lens. When the "joy stick" is again pulled back to a focus point midway between the cornea and the lens, it will be focused on the anterior chamber. One should keep the beam centered over the pupil so that there is a black background. Normally, the aqueous of the anterior chamber is totally clear. If small particles are visible floating up or down through the beam, the examiner is seeing cells in the aqueous. If the beam lights up the aqueous like a searchlight in the fog, then the examiner has found the protein flare that accompanies iritis. Note should be made of the fact that fluorescein can penetrate an abraded cornea, producing a fluorescing flare by slit-lamp evaluation. In order to avoid confusion, some physicians prefer to examine for anterior chamber flare before the stain is used.

CONCLUSIONS

In practice, the three setups described here take only one minute per eye. Experience with the instrument enhances future use. The device is helpful for the evaluation of ocular infections and corneal lesions, the removal of corneal foreign bodies, the measurement of intraocular pressure by applanation tonometry, and the diagnosis of iritis.

Dilating the Eye

1. Duke-Elder, S.: System of Ophthalmology, vol. III. St. Louis, C. V. Mosby, 1962, pp. 542, 571.
2. Hovding, G., et al.: Bacterial contamination of drops and dropper tips of in-use multidose bottles. Acta Ophthalmol. 60:213, 1982.
3. Adler, A. G., McElwain, G. E., Merli, G. J., et al.: Systemic effects of eye drops. Arch. Intern. Med. 142:2293, 1982.
4. American Academy of Ophthalmology: Ophthalmology Basic and Clinical Science Course. Rochester, MN, American Academy of Ophthalmology, 1977, p. 127.
5. Physicians' Desk Reference for Ophthalmology. Oradell. NJ, Medical Economics Co., 1982, p. 2.
6. Lanscke, R. K.: Systemic reactions to topical epinephrine and phenylephrine. Am. J. Ophthalmol. 61:95, 1966.
7. Fraunfelder, F. T., and Scafidi, A. F.: Possible adverse effects from topical ocular 10% phenylephrine. Am. J. Ophthalmol. 85:447, 1978.
8. Bresler, M. J., and Hoffman, T. L. S.: Prevention of iatrogenic acute narrow-angle glaucoma. Ann. Emerg. Med. 10:535, 1981.
9. Solosko, D., and Smith, R. B.: Hypertension following 10% phenylephrine ophthalmic. Anesthesiology 36:187, 1972.
10. McReynolds, W. V., Havener, W. H., and Henderson, J. W.: Hazards of the use of sympathomimetic drugs in ophthalmology. Arch. Ophthalmol. 56:176, 1956.
11. Kim, M. K., Stevenson, C. E., and Mathewson, M. D.: Hypertensive reactions to phenylephrine eye drops in patients with sympathetic denervation. Am. J. Ophthalmol. 85:862, 1978.
12. Adler, A. G., McElwain, G. E., Martin, J. H., et al.: Coronary artery spasm induced by phenylephrine eye drops. Arch. Intern. Med. 141:1384, 1981.
13. Fraunfelder, F. T.: Interim report: National registry of possible drug induced ocular side effects. Ophthalmology 86:126, 1979.
14. Hoefnagel, D.: Toxic effects of atropine and homatropine eye drops in children. N. Engl. J. Med. 264:168, 1961.
15. Heath, W. E.: Death from atropine poisoning. Br. Med. J. 2:608, 1950.
16. Freund, M., and Meun, S.: Toxic effects of scopolamine eye drops. Am. J. Ophthalmol. 70:637, 1970.
17. Beswick, J. A.: Psychosis from cyclopentolate. Am. J. Ophthalmol. 53:879, 1962.
18. Binkharst, R. D., Weinstein, G. W., Borety, R. M., et al.: Psychotic reaction induced by cyclopentolate: Results of pilot study and double-blind study. Am. J. Ophthalmol. 55:1243, 1963.
19. Carpenter, W. T., Jr.: Precipitous mental deterioration following cycloplegia with 0.2% cyclopentolate HCl. Arch. Ophthalmol. 18:445, 1967.

The Fluorescein Examination

20. Havener, W. A.: Ocular Pharmacology. St. Louis, C. V. Mosby, 1978, p. 413.
21. Duke-Elder, S.: System of Ophthalmology, vol. VII. St. Louis, C. V. Mosby, 1962, p. 243.
22. Vaughn, D. G.: The contamination of fluorescein solutions. Am. J. Ophthalmol. 39:55, 1955.
23. Paton, D., and Goldberg, M. F.: Management of Ocular Injuries. Philadelphia, W. B. Saunders Co., 1976, p. 194.
24. Grant, M. W.: Toxicology of the Eye. Springfield, IL, Charles C Thomas, 1974, p. 495
25. National Registry of Drug Induced Ocular Side Effects, Case Reports 404a, 404b, 421. Portland, OR, University of Oregon Health Sciences Center, 1979:
26. Cohn, H. C., et al.: A unique case of grand mal seizures after Fluress. Ann. Ophthalmol. 13:1379, 1981.

27. Havener, W. A.: op. cit., pp. 70–74.
28. Cain, W., et al.: Detection of anterior chamber leakage with Seidel's test. Arch. Ophthalmol. 99:2013, 1981.
29. Havener, W. A.: op. cit., p. 419.
30. Sexton, R. R.: Herpes simplex keratitis. In Wilson, L. A. (ed.): External Diseases of the Eye. Hagerstown, MD, Harper & Row, 1979, pp. 235–260.
31. Sexton, R. R.: Superficial keratitis. In Wilson, L. A. (ed.): External Diseases of the Eye. Hagerstown, MD, Harper & Row, 1979, pp. 203–213.
32. Wilson, L. A.: Bacterial corneal ulcers. In Wilson, L. A. (ed.): External Diseases of the Eye. Hagerstown, MD, Harper & Row, 1979, pp. 215–233.
33. Jones, D. B.: Fungal keratitis. In Wilson, L. A. (ed.): External Diseases of the Eye. Hagerstown, MD, Harper & Row, 1979, pp. 265–277.
34. Weiss, J. N., Kreter, J. K., Dalton, H. P., et al.: Detection of Pseudomonas aeruginosa eye infections by ultraviolet light. Ann. Ophthalmol. 14:242, 1982.

Eye Irrigation

35. Paton, D., and Goldberg, M. F.: op. cit., p. 166.
36. Ibid., p. 167.
37. Ibid., p. 168.
38. American Academy of Orthopedic Surgeons: Emergency Care and Transportation of the Sick and Injured, 3rd ed. Menasha, WI, George Banta Co., Inc., 1981, p. 298.
39. Grant, H. D., Murray, R. H., and Bergeron, J. F.: Emergency Care, 3rd ed. Bowie, MD, R. J. Brady Co., 1982, pp. 166–167.
40. Gombos, G. M.: Handbook of Ophthalmologic Emergencies. Flushing, NY, Medical Examination Publishing Co., 1973, p. 90.
41. Paton, D., and Goldberg, M. F.: op. cit., p. 163.
42. Ibid., p. 164.
43. Pavan-Langston, D.: Manual of Ocular Diagnosis and Therapy. Boston, Little, Brown & Co., 1980, p. 32.
44. Harris, L. S., et al.: Alkali injury from fireworks. Ann. Ophthalmol. 3:49, 1971.
45. Smith, R. S., and Shear, G.: Corneal alkali burns arising from accidental instillation of a hair straightener. Am. J. Ophthalmol. 79:602, 1975.
46. Scharpf, L. G., et al.: Relative eye-injury potential of heavy-duty phosphate and non-phosphate laundry detergents. Food Cosmet. Toxicol. 10:829, 1972.
47. Havener, W. A.: op. cit., p. 573.
48. Lippas, J.: Continuous irrigation in the treatment of external ocular diseases. Am. J. Ophthalmol. 57:298, 1964.
49. Vaugn, D., and Asbury, J.: General Ophthalmology, 8th ed. Los Altos, CA, Lange Medical Publishers, 1977, p. 40.
50. Rost, K. M., et al.: Eye contamination: A poison center protocol for management. Clin. Toxicol., 14:295, 1979.
51. Levinson, R. A.: Ascorbic acid prevents corneal ulceration and perforation following experimental alkali burns. Invest. Ophthalmol. 15:992, 1976.

Ocular Foreign Body Removal

52. Paton, D., and Goldberg, M. F.: op. cit., pp. 111–129.
53. Grove, A. S., New, P. F. J., and Momose, K. J.: Computerized tomographic (CT) scanning for orbital evaluation. Trans. Am. Acad. Ophthalmol. Otolaryngol. 79:137, 1975.
54. Lobes, L. A., Jr., Grand, M. G., Reece, J., et al.: Computerized axial tomography in the detection of intraocular foreign bodies. Ophthalmology 88:26, 1981.
55. Paton, D., and Goldberg, M. F.: op. cit., p. 195.
56. Pavan-Langston, D.: op. cit., p. 37.
57. Newell, F. W.: Ophthalmology Principles and Concepts. St. Louis, C. V. Mosby, 1978, p. 186.
58. Paton, D., and Goldberg, M. F.: op. cit., pp. 200, 203.

Eye Patching

59. Paton, D., and Goldberg, M. F.: op. cit., p. 202.
60. Gombos, G. M.: op. cit., p. 88.
61. Havener, W. A.: op. cit., p. 119.
62. Hanna, C., et al.: The effect of ophthalmic ointment on corneal wound healing. Am. J. Ophthalmol. 76:193, 1973.
63. Fraunfelder, F. T., et al.: Entrapment of ophthalmic ointment in the cornea. Am. J. Ophthalmol. 76:475, 1973.
64. Sexton, R. R.: Superficial keratitis, op. cit., pp. 208–210.
65. Laibson, P. R.: Epithelial basement membrane dystrophy and recurrent corneal erosion. In Fraunfelder, F. T., and Roy, F. H. (eds.): Current Ocular Therapy. Philadelphia, W. B. Saunders Co., 1980, pp. 362–363.

Contact Lens Procedures

66. Forstot, S. L., and Ellis, P. P.: Identifying and managing contact lens emergencies. E. R. Reports 3:35, 1982.
67. Mandell, R. B.: Contact Lens Practice. Springfield, IL, Charles C Thomas, 1981, p. 11.
68. Obrig, T., and Salvatori, P.: Contact Lenses, 3rd ed. New York, Obrig Laboratories, 1957, p. 188.
69. Mullen, J. E.: Contact Lens. U.S. Patent 2,237,744.
70. Nugent, M. W.: The corneal lens, a preliminary report. Ann. West. Med. Surg. 2:241, 1948.
71. Dreifus, M., Wichtenle, O., and Lim, D.: Intercameral lenses of hydrocolloid acrylates. Cesk. Oftalmol. 16:154, 1960.
72. Mandell, R. B.: op. cit., pp. 142–168.
73. Krezanoski, J. Z.: Physiology and biochemistry of contact lens wearing, In Encyclopedia of Contact Lens Practice, vol. 4. South Bend, IN, International Optic, 1959, pp. 18–26.
74. Cogger, T. J.: Correction with hard contact lenses, In Duane, T. D. (ed.): Clinical Ophthalmology. New York, Harper & Row, 1982, p. 17.
75. Mandell, R. B.: op cit., pp. 496–513.
76. Ibid., p. 574.
77. Long, J. C.: Retention of contact lens in upper fornix. Am. J. Ophthalmol. 56:309, 1963.
78. Michaels, D. D., and Zugsmith, G. S.: An unusual contact lens complication. Am. J. Ophthalmol. 55:1057, 1963.
79. Fowler, S. A., and Allansmith, M. R.: Evolution of soft contact lens coatings. Arch. Ophthalmol. 98:95, 1980.
80. Mondino, B. J., and Gorden, L. R.: Conjunctival hyperemia and corneal infiltrates with chemically disinfected soft contact lenses. Arch. Ophthalmol. 98:1767, 1980.
81. Shaw, E. L.: Allergies induced by contact lens solutions. Contact Intraocular Lens Med. J. 6:273, 1980.
82. Krachmer, J. H., and Purcell, J. J., Jr.: Bacterial corneal ulcers in cosmetic soft contact lens wearers. Arch. Ophthalmol. 96:57, 1978.
83. Bohigian, G. M.: Management of infections associated with soft contact lenses. Ophthalmology 86:1138, 1979.
84. Binder, P. S.: Complications associated with extended wear of soft contact lenses. Ophthalmology 86:1093, 1979.

Tonometry

85. Duke-Elder, S.: System of Ophthalmology, vol. VII. St. Louis, C. V. Mosby, 1962, pp. 349–350.
86. Maklakoff, C.: L'ophthalmotonometrie. Arch. Ophthalmol. (Paris) 5:159, 1885.
87. Goldmann, H.: Un nouveau tonometre à applanation. Bull. Soc. Franc. Ophthalmol. 67:474, 1955.
88. Schiötz, H.: Tonometry. Br. J. Ophthalmol. 4:201, 1920.
89. Mackay, R. S., and Marg, E.: Fast automatic electronic tonometers based on an exact theory. Acta Ophthalmol. 37:495, 1959.
90. Grolman, B.: A new tonometer system. Am. J. Ophthalmol. 49:646, 1972.
91. Friedenwald, J. S.: Tonometer calibration: an attempt to

remove discrepancies found in the 1954 calibration used for the Schiötz tonometers. Trans. Am. Acad. Ophthal. Otolaryngol., 61:108, 1957.

92. Goldmann, H., and Schmidt, T. H.: Uber Applanation stonometrie. Ophthalmologica 134:221, 1957.

93. Longham, M. E., and McCarthy, E.: A rapid pneumatic applanation tonometer. Arch. Ophthalmol. 79:389, 1968.

94. Wilensky, J. T.: Blood induced secondary glaucomas. Ann. Ophthalmol. 11:1659, 1979.

95. Krakan, C. E. T.: Intraocular pressure elevation—cause or effect in chronic glaucoma? Ophthalmologica 182:141, 1981.

96. Bouzas, A., Kampitsopoulos, G., and Kalliterakis, E.: La decoloration paillaire dans les hemorragies gastrointestinales. Bull. Soc. Ophthalmol. Fr. 87:296, 1975.

97. Jampol, L. M., Board, R. J., Manmenu, A. E.: Systemic hypotension and glaucomatous changes. Am. J. Ophthalmol. 85:154, 1978.

98. Drance, S. M., Sweeney, V. P., Morgan, R. W., et al.: Factors involved in the production of low tension glaucoma. Can. J. Ophthalmol. 9:399, 1974.

99. Harrington, D. O.: The pathogenesis of the glaucoma field. Clinical evidence that circulatory insufficiency in the optic nerve is the primary cause of visual field loss in glaucoma. Am. J. Ophthalmol. 47:177, 1959.

100. Francois, J., and Neetans, A.: The deterioration of the visual fields in glaucoma and the blood pressure. Doc. Ophthalmol. 28:70, 1970.

101. Jonasson, F.: Dangerous antihypertensive treatment. Br. Med. J. 2:1218, 1979.

102. Phelps, G. K., and Phelps, C. D.: Blood pressure and pressure amaurosis. Invest. Ophthalmol. 14:237, 1975.

103. Keeney, A. H.: Ocular Examination. St. Louis, C. V. Mosby, 1970, pp. 120–123.

104. Hillman, J. S.: Acute closed-angle glaucoma: An investigation into the effect of delay in treatment. Br. J. Ophthalmol. 63:817, 1979.

105. Gorin, G.: Clinical Glaucoma. New York, Marcel Dekker, 1977, p. 76.

106. Wilke, K.: Effects of repeated tonometry. Genuine and sham measurements. Acta Ophthalmol. 50:574, 1972.

107. Harbin, T. S., Laikam, S. E., Lipsitt, K., et al.: Applanation—Schiötz disparity after retinal detachment surgery utilizing cryopexy. Ophth. AAO 86:1609, 1979.

108. Lichter, P. R., and Bergstrom, T. J.: Premature ventricular systole detection by applanation tonometry. Am. J. Ophthalmol. 81:797, 1976.

109. Keeney, A. H.: Ocular examination, Basis and Technique. St. Louis, C. V. Mosby, 1976, pp. 141–147.

110. Chandler, P. A., and Grant, W. M.: Glaucoma, 2nd ed. Philadelphia, Lea & Febiger, 1979, p. 11.

Slit Lamp Examination

111. Tate, G. W., and Safir, A.: The slit lamp: History, principles, and practice. In Duane, T. D. (ed.): Clinical Ophthalmology, vol. I. New York, Harper & Row, 1981, Chapter 59.

112. Pavan-Langston, D.: op. cit., p. 9.

113. Cogger, T. J.: Correction with hard contact lenses. In Duane, T. D. (ed.): Clinical Ophthalmology, vol. I. New York, Harper & Row, 1981, Chapter 54.

114. Keeney, A. H.: op. cit., pp. 85–90.

12

OTOLARYNGOLOGY

68

Otolaryngologic Procedures*

TOM I. ABELSON, M.D.
WILLIAM J. WITT, M.D.

Physical Examination of the Larynx

The ability to perform a thorough and accurate physical examination is critical in all areas of medical evaluation and diagnosis. All physicians have the ability to visually examine the larynx. To do so requires only a knowledge of several techniques, including indirect laryngoscopy, telescopic examination of the larynx, and flexible laryngoscopy, and practice in their use.

INDICATIONS

In an emergency department setting, laryngoscopy is indicated when visualization of the hypopharynx and larynx might enhance the ability to diagnose and treat the patient's problem. Unexplained hoarseness, dysphagia, odynophagia, recurrent aspiration, and a feeling of a lump in the throat are all indications for laryngoscopy. Foreign bodies such as fish bones and other small, sharp objects that may become lodged in the pharynx or hypopharynx can often be visualized by laryngoscopy.

There are some situations in which laryngoscopy should be avoided or should be performed only under very controlled circumstances. In children with epiglottitis, in patients with foreign bodies that are partially obstructing the airway, and in patients with severe neck trauma (including possible laryngotracheal separation or crush injuries of the larynx), all examinations should be performed in an operating room or in a specially prepared room in the emergency department. In these situations, the examining physician and team must be prepared to perform *any* procedure necessary to secure an airway under *any* circumstance. The team must be able to immediately intubate the patient, even under difficult circumstances. If attempts at intubation are unsuccessful, the ability to pass a rigid bronchoscope and/or perform an emergency tracheotomy or cricothyrotomy is critical. Any manipulation or examination of the larynx in these situations may precipitate complete airway obstruction.

It should also be stressed that patients who have laryngeal symptoms but normal results from emergency department laryngoscopic examination should have close otolaryngologic follow-up and repeat examination. When laryngeal findings are evident on examination, repeat examination to document complete resolution of these findings is indicated.

INDIRECT LARYNGOSCOPY

The oldest technique for examination of the larynx and the one used most commonly by otolaryngologists is indirect laryngoscopy, using a headlight or head mirror with an angled laryngeal mirror. Using this technique, most larynges are visualized with the excellent and undistorted optics of a flat reflecting mirror. The few cooperative patients who cannot be examined with the indirect mirror technique include those with severe psychological gag reflex that cannot be overcome with topical anesthesia, those with uncontrollable coughing, and those with cervical spine, pharyngeal, or oral conditions that prevent appropriate positioning or visualization.

Procedure. The patient is seated in an upright position with the legs uncrossed, the upper torso leaning slightly forward, and the head slightly extended in the "sniffing" position. If the head mirror is placed over the physician's left eye, the light bulb is placed to the patient's right or vice versa. It does not matter which side is used. The light bulb is placed just behind and to the side of the patient's head at a slightly higher level than the patient's eyes. This placement prevents the physician's hands from interfering with the light shining on the head mirror. An unfrosted 150-watt light bulb provides excellent illumination. Some otolaryngologists place this light in a silver or white reflector. Use of a headlight precludes the need for the reflecting light. The examination can be performed with the physician either sitting or standing.

The keys to satisfactory examination of the larynx are practice, a reassured patient, and avoidance of contact with the *posterior pharyngeal wall* and the *posterior tongue*. Touching either of these areas will elicit a gag reflex, but contact with the soft palate or uvula will usually be tolerated. During the examination, the patient is advised to relax and to continuously breathe in and out through the mouth. It is important that he not

*Acknowledgments: The authors would like to thank Kathy Jung, medical illustrator, and Jeri Kay, typist.

hold his breath, because in doing so, he will often constrict the pharyngeal inlet, initiating contact with the mirror and precipitating a gag reflex. The patient is asked to protrude the tongue, which is grasped with a gauze sponge between the thumb and forefinger, pulling it outward and downward. This movement tends to raise the larynx and pull the epiglottis forward, opening the laryngeal inlet. The patient is instructed to keep his eyes open and to gaze at an object over the physician's shoulder. This maneuver minimizes supratentorial input to the gag reflex. The laryngeal mirror is slightly warmed, either in a flame or other type of warmer, and is tested for excess heat on the physician's hand or cheek prior to introduction into the patient's mouth. Warming the mirror inhibits fogging. Commercial solutions (Clear-dip) may also be used. While encouraging the patient to relax and to continue inhalation and exhalation, the mirror is passed into the mouth and over the back of the tongue where it can be gently placed against the soft palate and uvula if necessary (Fig. 68–1).

By reflecting the light off the mirror and by rotating the mirror, the base of the tongue, vallecula, epiglottis, pyriform sinus, post-cricoid area, arytenoids, aryepiglottic folds, false vocal cords, ventricles, true vocal cords, supraglottic area, and the upper part of the trachea can be examined. The anterior commissure of the vocal cords is the most difficult area to examine, because the epiglottis tends to overhang it. By asking the patient to phonate a high-pitched sound such as "Eeeeee," the larynx is further raised and tilted to permit more complete examination of the anterior larynx. Vocal cord mobility can also be observed through this maneuver.

In patients who are unable to control their gag reflex or in those in whom it is difficult to avoid touching sensitive areas, a topical anesthetic, gargle, or spray can be used. Those agents containing benzocaine (Cetacaine or Hurricaine) are most commonly used. If, despite adequate anesthesia, the patient is still unable to be examined, one of the two techniques described below can be used.

RIGHT-ANGLE TELESCOPES

In the second method for visually examining the larynx, one of several right-angle telescopes is used. One popular telescope is the LarynxVue II (Fig. 68–2A). This type of telescope obtains its energy from a wall plug or light-weight battery pack that can be carried on the physician's belt.

Procedure. The patient is positioned in a manner identical to that used for indirect laryngoscopy (Fig. 68–2B). Topical anesthesia is used, if necessary. As the instrument is passed into the oral cavity, it is rested on either a guide attached to the hand that is holding the tongue or rested on

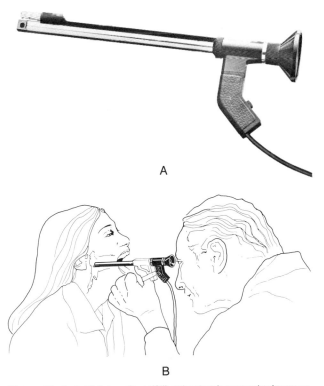

A

B

Figure 68–2. A, Right-angle self-illuminating laryngeal telescope. This one is called the LarynxVue II. It can be used as pictured or with a guide strapped to the examiner's thumb. (Courtesy of Astralite Corp., 4378 East LaPalma Avenue, Anaheim, California 92807). B, The laryngeal telescope is held in the same hand that holds the patient's tongue, leaving the other hand free to use instruments.

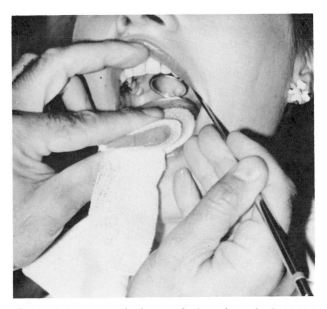

Figure 68–1. To insert the laryngeal mirror, the patient's tongue is grasped between the thumb and first or second finger with a gauze pad. The other finger is used to retract the upper lip. The indirect laryngeal mirror is passed into the mouth, avoiding contact with the tongue. It can touch the palate and uvula without creating a gag reflex. Contact with the posterior pharynx should also be avoided.

the fingers of that hand. It is important to place the instrument in a position very close to that needed for examination of the larynx under direct vision before beginning to look through the eyepiece. Again, by asking the patient to breathe quietly, to phonate, or to take a deep breath, the larynx can be examined for mucosal lesions and for function.

FLEXIBLE LARYNGOSCOPY

In patients who have a psychological gag reflex that cannot be controlled by reassurance or topical anesthesia or in those with anatomic abnormalities that preclude examination of the larynx via the oral cavity, a flexible fiberoptic laryngoscope or bronchoscope passed through the nose permits examination of the larynx. Several companies, including Machida and Olympus, manufacture flexible scopes specifically designed for examination of the nasopharynx and larynx. These scopes are very small and do not have suction channels. They are shorter than bronchoscopes and can be attached to light-weight, portable light sources.

Procedure. The physician must carry out a thorough examination of the nose to determine the side of the nasal cavity through which he will pass the instrument. After this decision has been made, topical anesthetic and vasoconstrictor medications are applied to the nasal mucosa. This step greatly enhances the patient's comfort and cooperation during the procedure and permits a more leisurely evaluation. Four per cent topical lidocaine can be applied by spray or on cotton pledgets as described in the section on epistaxis in this chapter. The author prefers to use several drops of topical epinephrine mixed with a few ml of 4 per cent lidocaine. This mixture is applied to self-made rolled pledgets of cotton, which are placed in the floor of the nose and along the inferior turbinate on the side to be examined (see Fig. 68–16). After waiting several minutes, the nose is re-examined. It is often useful to place another larger pledget farther into the nose to anesthetize the nasal cavity posteriorly. After the nose is adequately vasoconstricted, a small amount of 4 per cent lidocaine is sprayed through that nostril to partially anesthetize the nasopharynx and posterior pharyngeal wall. The patient is again positioned in the "sniffing" position, and, under direct vision, the flexible endoscope (prelubricated with water soluble jelly) is passed through the nasal cavity and turned downward into the nasopharynx. The larynx is examined for lesions and function. The scope should not be passed below the level of the tip of the epiglottis unless the larynx itself has been anesthetized.

WHICH PROCEDURE SHOULD BE USED?

Indirect laryngoscopy using an angled mirror requires the least expensive equipment and provides the best optics, because there is minimal distortion from a good mirror. This technique requires practice to become proficient. Therefore, it is valuable to practice indirect laryngoscopy on normal patients to gain confidence in the technique and to become familiar with normal anatomy. Many physicians who infrequently examine the larynx find the right-angle telescope easier to use. Although the optics in these telescopes are not as good as those provided by a mirror, they *are* excellent and the laryngeal view may be better. The fiberoptic flexible laryngoscope is generally reserved for use when the other techniques are not successful. It must be stressed that no examination will yield adequate results unless the physician has experience using the technique and is thoroughly comfortable with the normal anatomy and variations thereof that he will observe.

USE OF THE HEAD LAMP

As discussed in several sections of this chapter, direct "through the eye" illumination is necessary to accomplish many of the procedures required for treatment of head and neck diseases. Although the head mirror and separate light bulb provide the most traditional, least expensive method of illumination, frequent practice is needed to become proficient in its use. Many physicians find that a headlight is more convenient to use and provides more flexibility. There are many types of headlights, but the principles involved in using them essentially are the same. The light source must emanate from directly between the eyes rather than from the forehead or the side in order to provide enough direct light into the depths of the nasal or oral cavities.

Procedure. As with all techniques in medicine, practice is necessary to improve proficiency in the use of the headlight. The key to success is to line up the direction of the light beam with a comfortable head position. First, place the head gear in position and tighten it enough to prevent slippage but not so tight as to cause pressure or pain over the length of a procedure. Next, gaze comfortably at a spot on the patient or on your outstretched hand at a comfortable working distance. Finally, without moving your eyes or head, move the headlight into position, so that the light beam is focused on the spot where you would like to work while not obstructing the view of either eye. If you find, as you begin working, that your head must constantly turn in order to bring the light into the appropriate position, these steps must be repeated. With the equipment in the appropriate position, the light will automatically be shining where the operator is comfortably looking.

Procedures in the External Auditory Canal

ANATOMY

The external auditory canal, or meatus, is S-shaped and is approximately 2.5 cm long. The lateral one third is cartilaginous, and the medial two thirds is bony. The medial margin of the canal is the tympanic membrane, which lies in an oblique position with its anterior edge deeper than its posterior edge. (This oblique position permits a larger tympanic membrane to fit into the restricted size of the ear canal, resulting in greater mechanical advantage for carrying sound energy to the inner ear.) The bony canal is directed slightly downward and forward in relation to the cartilaginous canal; thus, pulling the pinna upward, backward, and outward tends to straighten the canal and permits a better view of the tympanic membrane. The external canal is intimately related to the temporomandibular joint, the parotid gland, and the mastoid air cells.

The skin of the osseous canal is very thin, with few cutaneous organs. The skin of the cartilaginous canal is thicker, with hair follicles, sebaceous glands, and apocrine glands. Cerumen is formed by these glands and from exfoliated cells of the skin. Cerumen is bacteriostatic and water-repellent, not waterproof. Under positive pressure or after repeated douching with water or after mild trauma (e.g., by cotton-tipped applicators), the protection offered the skin by the cerumen may be breached. Water, debris and bacteria can then enter the follicular space and precipitate an infection.[1]

EXAMINATION

A thorough examination with good illumination and a gentle but effective touch is required to evaluate the external ear canal. Illumination can be provided in several ways. The hand-held otoscope can be equipped with fiberoptic heads, which provide excellent illumination. The operating head otoscope may not be quite as bright as the fiberoptic otoscope but permits the passage of instruments through the earpiece for the removal of debris while still providing magnification (Fig. 68–3).

The headlight or head mirror and light bulb can serve to illuminate the ear canal through a separate metal or plastic speculum. This method maximizes

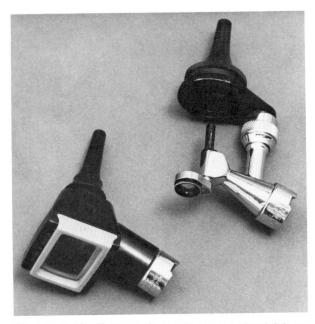

Figure 68–3. The fiberoptic diagnostic otoscope head (*left*) provides the best lighting for examination of the ear canal but is more difficult to use with instruments. The operating head (*right*) provides both magnification and access to the ear canal for instrumentation.

the ability to use instruments but provides no magnification unless loupes are used (Fig. 68–4). The best illumination is provided by the operating microscope, which also permits binocular vision and frees both hands for manipulation.

CERUMEN IMPACTION

Cerumen and squamous debris normally migrate out of the healthy ear canal, but impaction of cerumen may occur for various reasons. An unusually tortuous canal, a small meatus, or a large number of vibrissae may impede removal of cerum. Cotton-tipped applicators are frequently used by patients for self-cleaning. Although some earwax may be removed by the sides of an applicator, the tip often pushes the wax deeper into the canal. It is not unusual to find a deep cerumen impaction with a concavity the size and shape of the tip of a cotton-tipped applicator. Earwax is frequently brown, and its visible presence in the ear canal is considered poor hygiene by many people. It is not unusual for parents to be embarrassed by or apologetic for the presence of wax in their children's ears during routine examination. The old adage "don't put anything smaller than your elbow in your ear" is one of the best known and most frequently ignored rules of hygiene.

The most common complaint of the patient with cerumen occlusion is of a blocked ear. Slight unsteadiness and even dizziness and mild pain are often reported. A superimposed external otitis

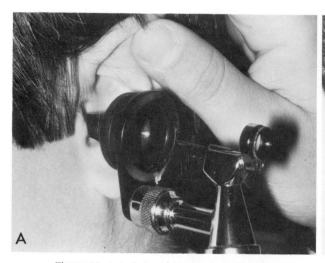
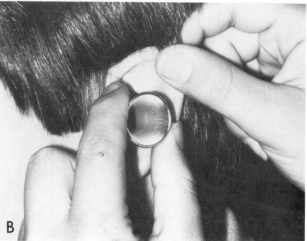

Figure 68–4. *A*, Patient being examined using an otoscope with an operating head. Note that the pinna is pulled upward and backward. *B*, Patient being examined using a metal speculum. Light is supplied with a head mirror or a headlight. This method of examination provides the most flexibility when instrumentation is needed.

may be present from the patient's attempts to remove the cerumen. Hearing loss frequently occurs suddenly. Hearing is not affected by cerumen as long as a tiny air passage exists through it. If water or manipulation blocks that passageway, a significant conductive hearing loss results. Removal of the impaction results in a most grateful and relieved patient.

Removal

Procedure. Cerumen can be removed by irrigation, suction, or metal probe curettage. Irrigation should be the initial procedure of choice if there is no history of a perforated tympanic membrane. Irrigation is best accomplished with a DeVillbiss irrigator activated by compressed air (Fig. 68–5). Alternatively, a metal ear syringe or Waterpik can

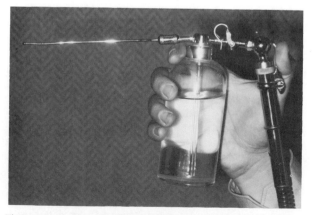

Figure 68–5. This DeVillbiss irrigator uses compressed air to eject the irrigant, which should be at or near body temperature to avoid caloric stimulation of the inner ear. The more conventional metal ear syringe can be equally effective and does not require a source of compressed air to function.

be used. One can also use a 20-ml syringe and a butterfly infusion catheter. The metal tip and plastic butterfly are cut off, and the plastic catheter is placed in the external canal. Irrigation fluid is then inserted through the syringe. An 18 gauge Teflon intravenous catheter can likewise be used with a 20-ml syringe for irrigation. The patient or an assistant holds a kidney basin or an ear basin to catch the irrigating fluid. The irrigator is *inserted only into the cartilaginous canal and is directed along the superior canal wall* (Fig. 68–6). The irrigant is tap water, at or near body temperature, to prevent caloric stimulation of the inner ear and resultant pain or vertigo. There is no advantage to irrigating with peroxide or other solutions. Most cerumen can be removed with persistent irrigation. Irrigation is a safe and easy method that rarely fails. Tympanic membrane perforation is a theoretical complication but occurs very rarely when the above methods have been properly used. Irrigation, however, should not be performed if there is a history of a perforated tympanic membrane, because water within the middle ear space will inevitably result in infection and pain.

Occasionally, irrigation will loosen but not remove debris, and it may be necessary to alternate between irrigation and manual removal. After irrigation, the ear canal should be dried with a cotton-tipped applicator or a few drops of 70 per cent alcohol. If irrigation is not successful and if external otitis is not present, a cerumen-softening solution such as Cerumenex may be placed in the ear for 15 to 30 minutes and the irrigation should be repeated. Occasionally, 2 to 3 days of softening at home is required. The disadvantage of this procedure is that some patients develop a contact dermatitis to the softening agent.

The consistency of cerumen varies. A soft, semi-

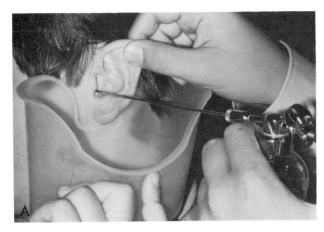

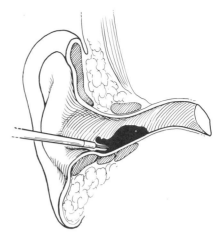

Figure 68–7. Removal of impacted cerumen using a small wire loop or cerumen spoon. This procedure is done under direct vision through a speculum or otoscope (not pictured in the drawing). The key is to separate the cerumen from the skin of the ear canal and to move it toward the center of the canal before attempting to extract it.

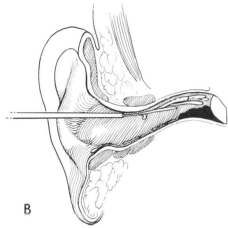

Figure 68–6. A, Patient is positioned for irrigation of the external auditory canal. The patient is holding a specially shaped ear basin to catch the irrigating fluid. The auricle is pulled upward, backward, and outward in order to straighten the ear canal, and the irrigation is directed along the posterior superior canal wall. Water warmed to approximately body temperature should be used to avoid caloric stimulation of the semi-circular canals. B, The tip of the irrigator is passed only into the cartilaginous section of the external ear canal.

liquid wax is best removed with irrigation. More firm cerumen can be removed mechanically. A wire loop or blunt right-angle hook is introduced under direct vision along, but not touching, the skin of the ear canal. Cerumen is gently teased away from the skin into the center of the canal (Fig. 68–7). The instrument is then passed just beyond the bolus, turned 90 degrees to engage the cerumen, and withdrawn. At all times, both hands should be supported against the head of the patient so that they will move with the head, preventing aural injury. *A confident, gentle touch is critical*, because a loop or hook improperly used may be very painful and traumatic to the patient. It is not uncommon to precipitate bleeding of the canal, because the skin is quite fragile. It is imprudent to persist in removal techniques if the pain caused by the procedure is significant. Patients can be prepared by warning them and then deliberately but gently touching the canal skin so they will be less startled when manipulation begins. An anxious patient may not tolerate the procedure

after the first perception of pain. It is impossible to safely remove cerumen from a screaming or agitated child; irrigation is the method of choice for pediatric patients.

EXTERNAL OTITIS

External otitis or swimmer's ear presents with varied symptoms, including itching, fullness, hearing loss, drainage, burning and pain. These symptoms may occur in any combination and from mild to severe degrees. As previously suggested, humidity, high temperatures, local trauma, and the introduction of an exogenous material are the conditions most often associated with external otitis. Senturia divides the disease into three stages.[1]

1. Pre-inflammatory
2. Acute inflammatory
   Mild
   Moderate
   Severe
3. Chronic inflammatory

The pre-inflammatory stage manifests with mild edema and itching and can easily lead to the mild-acute stage, with erythema, edema, and some debris. In the moderate-acute stage, pain and edema are more severe with partial blockage of the ear canal with debris. In the severe stage, pain is intense. Manipulation of the pinna and tragus causes pain. The ear canal may be completely occluded by tissue edema and debris. Pain may radiate to the jaw or neck. Infra-auricular or cervical lymph adenopathy is often evident. Pseudomonas is most often identified in cultures, but the associated cellulitis is usually caused by Gram-positive organisms. The chronic stage is identical to any chronic dermatitis with exfolliative debris, scaling, and Gram-negative or fungal contamination.

Treatment

Procedure. The techniques used in the treatment of external otitis are designed 1) to remove debris from the canal so that medication can come in contact with the skin, 2) to provide antimicrobial or antifungal action, and 3) to decrease the inflammatory response.

Treatment of the pre-inflammatory stage involves removal of debris and the use of ear drops. Debris may be removed by irrigation with 3 per cent hypertonic saline, by suction, or by swabbing the canal under otoscopic vision with self-made cotton-tipped applicators (Figs. 68–8 and 68–9). Note that commercial *flexible* urethral or nasopharyngeal swabs (Calgi-Swab) can be used for this purpose. The cotton of the applicator is soaked with the medicated solution that the patient will use as drops for several days. Solutions with

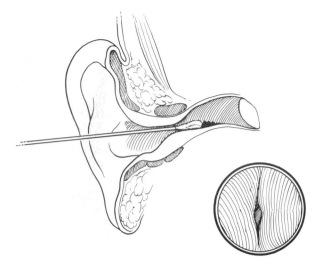

Figure 68–8. Diagram showing a severe stage of external otitis with edema almost closing the external canal. A self-made cotton-tipped applicator is represented cleaning debris from the ear canal so as to permit medicated ear drops to come in contact with the skin. This applicator is used under direct vision through an otoscope (not pictured here).

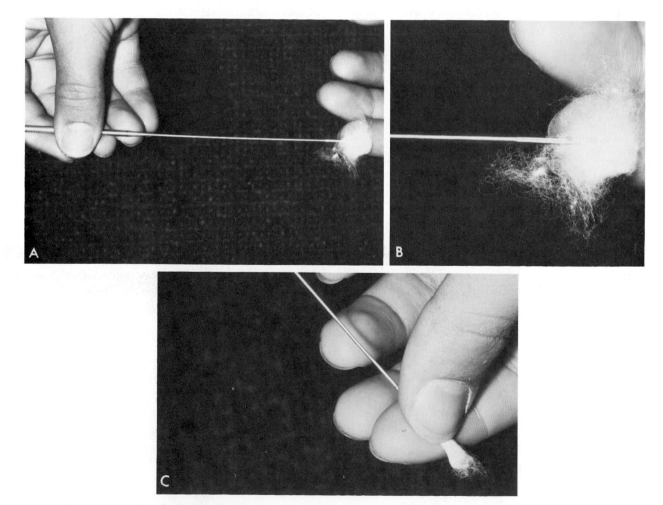

Figure 68–9. A–C, Individual applicators are made by applying a small tuft of cotton to a wire applicator and rotating it. The size of the tuft of cotton can be varied as needed. These applicators are used to clean the external ear canal and to apply topical medications.

polymyxin, neomycin, and hydrocortisone (Cortisporin Otic Suspension or Solution, Coly-Mycin S Otic) are most commonly used. Note that Cortisporin Otic Solution contains preservatives that can irritate the middle ear if the tympanic membrane is perforated. Therefore the cloudy *suspension* and not the clear *solution* should be used if a tympanic membrane defect is suspected. Solutions that acidify the ear canal are also effective microbials. Acetic acid and hydrocortisone (VoSol HC) or a saturated solution of boric acid in alcohol (made by the pharmacist) may be useful. Allergy to neomycin is common. However, if medication is changed because of sensitivity and the reaction persists, remember that propylene glycol may also cause skin reactions and is a carrier in many of these medications. If the ear canal is patent, it is easy for the patient to apply the ear drops at home. The patient is instructed to place four to six drops of medication in the affected ear while lying down with the affected ear up. The tragus and pinna are manipulated to work the drops into the canal. The patient should remain in that position for about 5 minutes. A wad of cotton is placed in the concha to catch the extra medication that will drain out when the patient sits up. The drops are placed two to four times per day, depending upon the severity of the disease. When eczema of the skin of the concha or pinna is present, a corticosteroid cream is also used.

The mild acute inflammatory stage is treated in a similar manner; however, *irrigation is avoided* because the irritation may cause increased swelling of the canal. The moderate acute inflammatory stage may be associated with significant edema of soft tissue and debris, hence antibiotic drops may be impeded from entering the canal easily. The canal must first be cleared of debris using cotton-tipped applicators and suction if necessary. Occasionally, a short-acting intravenous narcotic may be helpful with this painful procedure. Bleeding may be easily precipitated, and one should not be overzealous in attempting to remove every bit of debris. If pain is intolerable, one should treat for 24 to 48 hours before proceeding with further débridement of the canal. A wick is then inserted into the ear canal to draw the medication drops into the ear. This can be done in many ways. One-quarter inch Nu-Gauze (Johnson & Johnson) impregnated with an antibiotic and corticosteroid cream (Cortisporin Cream) can be packed into the ear canal. This is done through the otoscope using a small alligator forceps, and the leading edge of the gauze is placed as deeply into the canal as possible. The deeper parts of the canal are carefully packed through the otoscope. The otoscope is removed, and the rest of the lateral part of the external canal is packed.

A second method is to place just one thickness of Nu-Gauze into the ear canal without packing it tightly. The patient can then apply ear drops, which will be drawn into the canal by the gauze. A cotton wick may be fashioned by wrapping cotton around a forceps. The cotton is dipped into the antibiotic solution and gently placed into the canal. If the wick is thin enough, it will reach deeply into the canal. The cotton is then kept moist with repeated antibiotic drops. Commercially made wicks are available as well. With any method, the patient keeps the gauze moistened with applications of ear drops, which are allowed to soak in. The patient or physician removes the wick or pack 24 to 36 hours later and continues using the drops as previously indicated. In most cases, it is desirable to see the patient 24 to 36 hours later to ensure that a re-accumulation of debris has not occurred. Patients with this amount of edema are placed on an oral antibiotic as well. A reasonable choice is cloxacillin or erythromycin. Oral analgesics are frequently required for this painful condition.

In the severe acute inflammatory state of external otitis, pain and diffuse inflammation are most prominent. Temporomandibular motion may be quite painful, resulting in poor oral intake. Nausea and vomiting secondary to pain may complicate the syndrome. Strong pain medication is indicated, as well as some sedation to permit sleep. A gauze wick is again used; however, because of severe edema and pain, the wick can only be inserted a short distance. The patient should be started on a broad-spectrum oral antibiotic. The patient is seen again in 24 hours, at which time the gauze wick can be changed and most likely can be more deeply inserted. Within 48 hours, marked improvement is generally seen.

During the entire course of treatment for any stage of external otitis, the patient must be advised to keep his ears dry. When bathing, cotton impregnated with Vaseline can be placed in the concha and care should be taken to prevent water from seeping into the ear canal. If the canal does get wet, drops should be applied immediately. Following resolution of the infection, the canal is kept dry after swimming or bathing with a few drops of isopropyl (rubbing) alcohol or by drying the canal with a hair dryer.

It should be noted that although cultures are not routinely taken for uncomplicated otitis externa, Pseudomonas or Proteus may frequently be isolated. The cellulitis, however, may be due to other organisms. Therefore, the local antibiotic drops will be sufficient for Gram-negative organisms, whereas oral cloxacillin or erythromycin seem to hasten the resolution of the surrounding cellulitis. Patients do not need to be admitted to the hospital for intravenous antibiotics to treat Pseudomonas or Proteus infections unless they fail to respond to the previous course of therapy.[1] The only time when this advice does not hold true is in the case of malignant external otitis, which is also discussed in this chapter.

OTOMYCOSIS

Fungi can cause external otitis of any degree. The mycelia and spores are visible as a fuzzy coating on the skin of the ear canal. The most common fungus to cause this type of infection is *Aspergillus niger*. If fungi are observed, corticosteroids are avoided. Effective anti-fungal agents to use in this situation are M-Cresyl Acetate or a saturated solution of boric acid in alcohol.

Treatment

The critical aspect of treatment is complete manual removal of the organism. This is accomplished using cotton-tipped applicators impregnated with the treatment solution. Care must be taken to avoid depositing the medication, which can be quite irritating, on the external skin. A complete swabbing of the ear canal and removal of all debris is usually sufficient to control this disease.

A follow-up visit in 3 to 7 days is indicated to permit re-application of medication and re-cleaning of the canal if the infection recurs. Otomycosis can also complicate chronic bacterial external otitis and may not be obvious. In recurrent cases, it is useful to culture for fungus. Because special media are required, the bacteriology laboratory should be consulted about the techniques of culturing the specimen. In chronic cases, any one of several anti-mycotic agents can be used, including Halotex, Lotrimin, MicaTin, Tinactin, and Nilstat. These agents can be used as drops in the ear canal or applied to the ear canal using cotton-tipped applicators. It must be stressed that cleansing of the ear canal is the most critical aspect of the treatment of fungal disease.

MALIGNANT EXTERNAL OTITIS

Malignant external otitis is misnamed, because it does not represent a neoplastic process. However, it certainly is malignant in relation to its progressive and often life-threatening characteristics. The disease presents in diabetics, in immunosuppressed patients, or in patients who are taking systemic steroids. It manifests as an external otitis due to Pseudomonas, resulting in extensive necrosis and osteomyelitis that may progress to the base of the skull, resulting in cranial nerve deficits.

The disease is recognized by its severity and poor response to usual treatment. A severe external otitis in such patients warrants immediate otolaryngologic evaluation. Treatment requires hospitalization, varying degrees of débridement and long-term high-dose intravenous antibiotics. It is presumed that the severity of the disease is related to compromised local defense mechanisms.

FOREIGN BODY OF THE EAR

The techniques for examining the ear and removing cerumen were described earlier in the chapter. The presence of a foreign body is a different challenge to the emergency physician, although many of the techniques for removal of a foreign body are similar to those used for the removal of cerumen. The junction of the cartilaginous and bony sections of the external auditory canal is both the narrowest point of the canal and the location of a curve in the canal. Thus, most foreign bodies lodge in the outer two thirds of the canal and are relatively easy to remove. Those lying more medial are in a more sensitive portion of the canal and may be lying on the tympanic membrane. The nature of the foreign body is determined by history and direct examination.

Removal

Procedure. When a foreign body has been identified, all the necessary equipment is readied and the patient is positioned comfortably. The first attempt at removal is the best chance for success. The ear canal may be irrigated with water to remove small, hard objects in the same manner in which cerumen is removed (see Fig. 68–6). Irrigation should not be used when the foreign body is a seed or bean, because these organic objects may swell, rendering removal more difficult.

Illumination for the removal of foreign bodies of the ear canal is critical. An operating microscope should be used, if available. Binocular vision provides depth of field perception and permits more accurate placement of instruments. An operating head on an otoscope or a head mirror with separate speculum can be used. Wire loops, blunt hooks of various sizes, suction heads (Nos. 3 and 5), and alligator forceps should be available (Fig. 68–10).

A frequent foreign body found in children is a bead or the eye from a stuffed toy. These polished, smooth materials can be exceedingly difficult to grasp. If there is a space between the object and the skin of the ear canal, a right-angle hook can be passed beyond it, turned 90 degrees, and withdrawn with the bead (Fig. 68–11). The Richard's Manufacturing Company manufactures a plastic

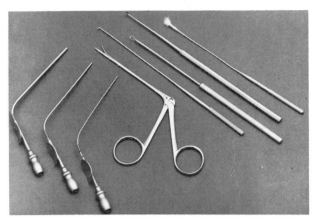

Figure 68–10. Left to right, suction tips (No. 7, 5, and 3), alligator forceps, right-angle blunt hook, wire loop, ear curette, and self-made cotton-tipped applicators. All these instruments are used when working within the ear canal. All can cause damage unless used in a controlled manner under direct vision.

suction catheter with a soft funnel tip. The suction catheter can often grasp and easily withdraw a smooth foreign body, making a difficult task both easy and safe (Fig. 68–12). A Fogarty catheter may be passed beyond the foreign body, the balloon inflated, and the catheter withdrawn to force the object from the canal. Care must be taken in this situation, however, to avoid puncturing the eardrum.

Living insects present a special challenge when lodged in the ear. Their movement can be exceed-

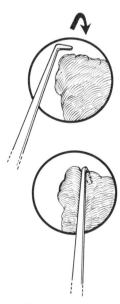

Figure 68–11. This technique may be used to remove hard, smooth foreign bodies or firm concretions of cerumen. A small blunt right-angle hook (available in various sizes) is passed between the foreign body and canal skin under direct vision. After its tip is medial to the foreign body, it is rotated 90 degrees and withdrawn.

ingly irritating, and the insect itself or the patient's attempts to remove the insect may excoriate the canal skin. The insect is first suffocated by filling the ear canal with mineral oil, ether, or alcohol. The insect can then be removed by irrigation or other mechanical means. An insect often fragments, making irrigation the most useful technique.

Alligator forceps are useful when the object has an easily grasped edge or protrusion. When not using binocular vision, special care must be taken to prevent the open jaws from touching the canal skin.

The keys to successful removal of a foreign body in the ear are good lighting and equipment and a cooperative patient. Even the most cooperative patient may become difficult after the first inadvertent twinge of pain. It is impossible for anyone to lie still while someone touches an unanesthetized tympanic membrane. It is also impossible for an assistant to hold the head of an uncooperative patient still enough for delicate instrumentation of the ear canal. Instrumentation of the ear canal may also produce a reflex cough in older children and adults.

The removal of foreign bodies can be facilitated by local anesthesia, but children may require general anesthesia for removal of foreign bodies for which there may be complications. The injection of local anesthetic in the ear canal is quite painful and should not be given to compensate for poor illumination or faulty techniques. The hand-held speculum, with either an operating microscope, headlight, or head mirror, permits the mobility necessary to give these injections. A 1½-inch or 2-inch needle (25 or 27 gauge) is used, and a three-finger syringe provides the best control. One per cent lidocaine, with or without epinephrine (1:100,000), is used.

The subcutaneous injections are made in four quadrants to encircle the ear canal. This field block is placed laterally, near the opening of the meatus. The largest speculum permitting a good view of the canal is used. The speculum is then withdrawn slightly, and the injection is made just under the skin. Less than 0.5 ml is used in each quadrant, just enough to slightly bulge the skin forward (Fig. 68–13). After waiting 2 to 3 minutes, the speculum can be re-introduced. If more anesthesia is necessary, a very small injection can be made in the anterior and posterior canal walls, just under the skin at the junction of the bony and cartilaginous canals. The skin is very thin in this area; thus, care must be taken to avoid lacerations. If placed correctly, a small bleb of anesthesia will dissect down toward the tympanic membrane. As mentioned previously, the placement of local anesthetic should not change the care with which

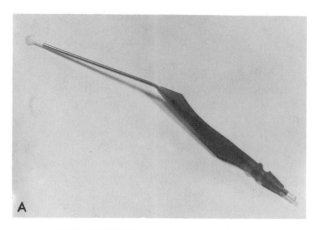

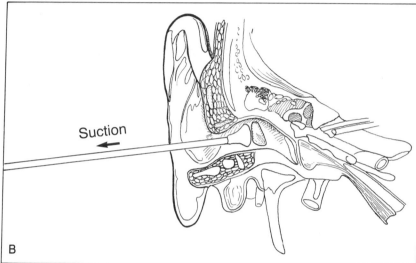

Figure 68–12. *A* and *B*, This suction catheter has a soft, flexible funnel-shaped tip, which is able to grasp some foreign bodies of the ear or nose and provide a mechanism for easy removal. (Courtesy of Richards Manufacturing Co.)

Figure 68–13. Four-quadrant field block anesthesia of the external auditory canal. Local anesthetic is injected subcutaneously in the four quadrants of the lateral portion of the ear canal. The largest speculum that will fit is used to guide the injections. The speculum is withdrawn slightly, tilted toward each of the four quadrants, and the needle is inserted subcutaneously (x). A very small amount of anesthetic (¼ to ½ ml) is injected to produce a slight bulge in the soft tissue. A total of 1½ to 2 ml of anesthetic is usually sufficient to anesthetize the ear canal and permit painless removal of a foreign body.

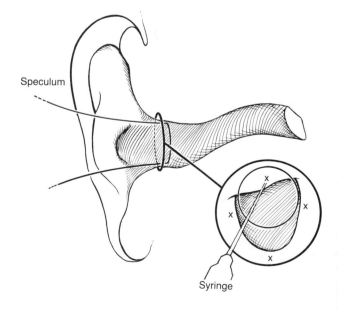

objects are removed, because lacerations of the canal, skin, or tympanic membrane are to be avoided.

Epistaxis

Nasal hemorrhage is one of the most common otolaryngologic emergencies confronting the emergency physician. Most episodes of epistaxis are controlled by patients outside the hospital setting, despite the fact that many commonly used methods of control are based on folk remedies. Lying with the head hanging over the edge of a bed allows the blood to run posteriorly to be swallowed but increases venous pressure and can prolong bleeding. Although holding ice behind the neck is innocuous, it is also ineffective in controlling bleeding. Epistaxis is frequently terrifying to the patient and to the physician who is not comfortable with all aspects of treatment. An anterior septal bleed is a minor inconvenience, whereas massive posterior bleeding may be disastrous.

ANATOMY AND PHYSIOLOGY

The nasal mucosa serves to warm and humidify inspired air. To this end, it is supplied with freely anastomosing blood vessels from the internal and external carotid systems. The external carotid provides the major blood supply via the internal maxillary artery (leading to the greater palatine and sphenopalatine arteries) and the facial artery. The internal carotid artery supplies the nose via the ophthalmic artery (leading to the anterior ethmoid artery) and the posterior ethmoid artery. The sphenopalatine artery is the site of bleeding in most posterior bleeds. Bleeding from the upper recesses of the nasal chamber originates mainly from the ethmoid arteries. Terminal branches of the internal and external carotid systems supply the nasal septum. Knowledge about the detailed anatomy of these vessels becomes critically important when dealing with the surgical ligation of vessels for uncontrolled nasal hemorrhage. In the usual emergency department situation, the important distinctions are knowing which side is bleeding and whether it is anterior or posterior.

ETIOLOGY

Most nose bleeds occur in the anterior or caudal septum in an area of anastomosing vessels called *Little's area* (Fig. 68–14). The relatively exposed position of this area accounts for the most common cause of bleeding, mucosal disruption. It is very

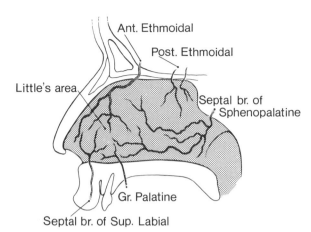

Figure 68–14. Little's area contains Kiesselbach's plexus of arterioles and is the most common site of epistaxis.

common for bleeding to occur spontaneously, without identifying precipitating factors. Although local mucosal trauma is most often involved, patients are reluctant to admit to nose-picking or the use of cocaine.

Mucosal problems can be caused by digital or external trauma, simple drying of the mucosa, upper respiratory infection (URI), irritants (over-the-counter medications such as nose sprays and chemicals such as cocaine), or foreign bodies. The use of aspirin can prolong any minor bleed. Vascular abnormalities, including superficial vasculature, varices, and hereditary hemorrhagic telangiectasia account for a small percentage of epistaxis cases. Platelet and coagulation disorders are also uncommon but cause a significant percentage of severe and difficult-to-control bleeds. Benign and malignant tumors are always included in the differential diagnosis, especially in patients with recurrent posterior bleeds and increasing nasal obstruction. Hypertension is frequently encountered in the patient with epistaxis. In the past, it has been thought to be a major cause of epistaxis, but hypertension is probably more often the result of fear or a reflection of arteriosclerosis, rather than a cause of bleeding.

HISTORY

As in every aspect of medical care, an accurate, concise history of the patient is critical. One should always inquire about the following specifics: From which nostril did the bleeding start? Did it run out of the nose or drain posteriorly? Is there a past history of similar bleeding? If so, how was it controlled? If the patient attempted to squeeze the nostrils closed, did the bleeding stop or drain into the pharynx? Was there an inciting incident or was the bleed spontaneous? Did the blood clot? Is the patient taking anticoagulants or aspirin? Is there bleeding in the bowels, urine, or gums? Are there skin ecchymoses? The answers to many of these questions will help indicate the anterior or posterior location of the bleeding. In anterior epistaxis, blood tends to flow out of the nostril and tends to stop with external pressure. When external pressure causes the bleeding to flow into the nasopharynx, it is apparent that the source of bleeding may be more posterior. Trauma results in anterior epistaxis more often than posterior epistaxis. The patient's past medical history and medication list should always be obtained. All pertinent information can be gathered while preparation is being made for the physical examination and treatment.

It is not uncommon to encounter patients who have stopped bleeding by the time they reach the emergency department. In such cases, one is tempted to do nothing, because the problem appears to have been solved. Once the patient returns home, however, the bleeding often recurs. *It is prudent to attempt to identify the bleeding site in all patients*, and one should not be reticent to provoke bleeding by stroking the septum with a cotton-tipped applicator or by having the patient blow his nose, so that definitive steps may be taken to prevent re-bleeding.

TREATMENT

Because physical examination and treatment are so intertwined, they will be discussed together. Throughout the entire encounter, the physician must provide reassurance. As mentioned previously, many epistaxis patients are terrified. They have blood coming from within their head, and they may have heard that epistaxis precedes stroke or that it serves to prevent a stroke. Although epistaxis is messy and scary, it is rarely life-threatening.

The patient should be told that every step in the treatment will be explained before it is carried out and that the bleeding *will* be controlled. A hospital gown or other cover is provided for both the patient and the doctor, but the patient should be asked not to worry about or be embarrassed by soiling of clothes or instruments with blood. After the bleeding has been stopped, everything can be cleaned up. An emesis basin is kept handy, because swallowed blood often induces nausea, and the patient may vomit large quantities of clot or coffee-ground material.

Obviously, a patient with a minor or recurrent bleed may not be fearful, but careful and complete reassurance is still indicated. Such reassurance is most easily given by a physician who has confidence in himself, based on knowledge and experience.

General Approach

If the patient has been bleeding for a few days, the physician should send blood for determination of hemoglobin and hematocrit. *If the patient is taking anticoagulants, clotting studies are mandatory*, even in cases of the most minor bleeding. The persistence of epistaxis in the patient on aspirin should also suggest a possible von Willebrand's syndrome associated with a prolonged partial thromboplastin time. If the patient is hypotensive, an intravenous infusion should be started for volume replacement and blood should be sent for typing and possible crossmatching. Treating hypertension will not stop most nose bleeds. Moderate hypertension is best left untreated, because it will usually subside following successful treatment of the bleeding. Most physicians prefer to sedate hypertensive and extremely anxious patients with diazepam or morphine intramuscularly before attempting to manipulate the nose. Patients who remain hypertensive after bleeding has been controlled may require medication to control the blood pressure. Laboratory studies are not required for most nose bleeds, but it should be noted that significant blood loss may occur in patients with chronic epistaxis.

Equipment

Chair with headrest
Headlight, or head mirror and light bulb
Suction and several suction tips (8- to 10-French catheter)
Clothing protection
Nasal speculum
Bayonet forceps
Topical anesthetic and vasoconstrictor
Cotton
Kidney basin
Cautery material [silver nitrate or heat cautery]
1/2-inch × 72-inch Vaseline gauze packing
Tongue depressors
2 small red rubber catheters
No. 2 silk surgical thread
2- × 2-inch gauze pads
Tonsil clamp or hemostat
Balloon tampons (pediatric Foley catheters are adequate) for posterior bleeds

Examination

The patient is seated in an upright position, leaning slightly forward in the "sniffing" position. Remember that the floor of the nose is parallel to the palate and only a small part of the nasal cavity can be seen with the patient's head tilted backward (Fig. 68–15). The physician may either sit or stand. A nasal speculum is always used to properly visualize the anterior nasal mucosa. The head

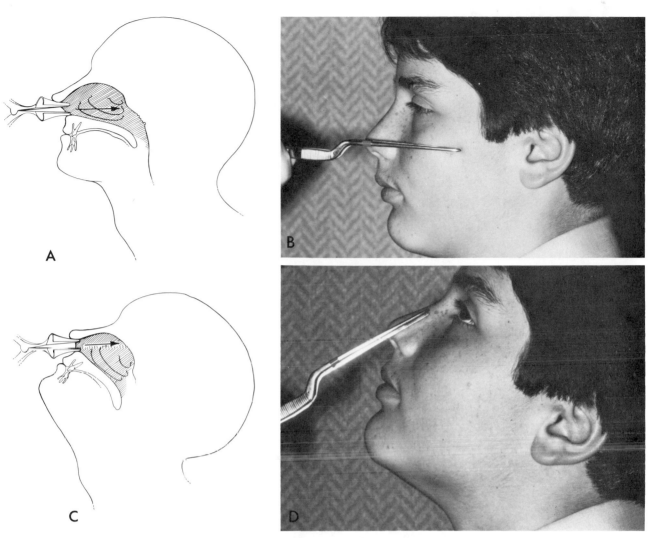

Figure 68–15. *A* and *B*, Photograph showing the correct position for examining and treating disease of the nasal cavity. The patient is in the "sniffing position," sitting upright or leaning slightly forward with the head only slightly extended. When the nasal tip is raised with the nasal speculum, the view is parallel to the floor of the nose and allows visualization of the entire nasal cavity. *C and D*, When told that their nose will be examined, most patients extend the neck and look toward the ceiling. In this position, only the most anterior portions of the nasal cavity are visible.

mirror and light are the simplest way to provide direct "from the eye" illumination; however, for those not experienced in the use of the mirror, a headlight may be easier to use. A hand-held flashlight or other light source does *not* provide an adequately directed light beam, will not permit visualization of the nasal cavities, and makes treatment difficult.

With all the necessary or potentially necessary equipment available, with the patient reassured and positioned, and with an assistant standing by, the examination can begin. Blood clots must be expelled from the nasal cavities before the nose can be properly examined. This can be accomplished with suction or by asking the patient to vigorously blow his nose. Often, the expulsion of clots results in a marked diminution of the rate of bleeding. Careful search for the bleeding site is

then made, followed by the placement of topical anesthetic and vasoconstrictors in the side from which there was bleeding. Four per cent cocaine provides the optimal combination of local anesthesia and vasoconstriction. Because of cocaine's low therapeutic-to-toxicity ratio and its strictly controlled status, it is often simpler, safer, and more convenient to use a combination of 4 per cent lidocaine and topical epinephrine. One can inadvertently cause a patient to be cocaine toxic if the 10 per cent cocaine solution is used or if the nose is repeatedly packed. A maximum of 4 ml of 4 per cent cocaine solution or 2 ml of 10 per cent solution should be used in adults.

If an anterior bleeding site is easily seen, one may simply place a ball of cotton soaked with anesthetic in the nasal cavity and have the patient squeeze the nostrils together. Often, cotton pledgets are required for adequate anesthesia or vasoconstriction.

The technique for placing local anesthesia pledgets is illustrated in Figure 68–16. The cotton pledgets are left in place for 5 minutes. After they are removed, if bleeding has not significantly diminished, new cotton pledgets can be placed for another 5 minutes to ensure adequate vasoconstriction and anesthetic effect (some of the anesthetic may have been washed away with the bleeding). The patient is told that the topical anesthetic may drain into the throat and produce a sensation of not being able to swallow. Reassurance of the temporary nature of this condition and of the fact that they actually can swallow when they make the attempt will calm most patients. The pledgets are then removed, and the nose is examined. With the nasal speculum in one hand and the 8- or 10-French suction tip in the other, the nose can be examined while gently suctioning blood away in order to see the spot that is bleeding. *The key to successful treatment of epistaxis is identification of the site of bleeding!*

Anterior Epistaxis

As mentioned previously, the most common site of bleeding is from the easily visualized part of the nasal septum. The exact spot of bleeding can be identified using gentle suction if the bleeding is brisk or diffuse. If the hemorrhage has stopped with vasoconstriction but the bleeding site is not apparent, bleeding may be provoked by gentle stroking with a cotton-tipped applicator. If a prominent blood vessel or excoriated area is visible, cauterization can be used. Silver nitrate sticks are most commonly used to control this type of bleeding when a definite bleeding site has been identified. The mucosa is cauterized by firmly touching the area around the bleeding site for 10 to 15 seconds and turning the end of the silver nitrate stick. Cautery should begin in concentric circles, starting away from the bleeding site itself so as to cauterize the vessels feeding the site of injury. When approaching the site itself, it is often helpful to begin just above it and come down on it so that the silver nitrate does not become coated with blood before touching the area that is bleed-

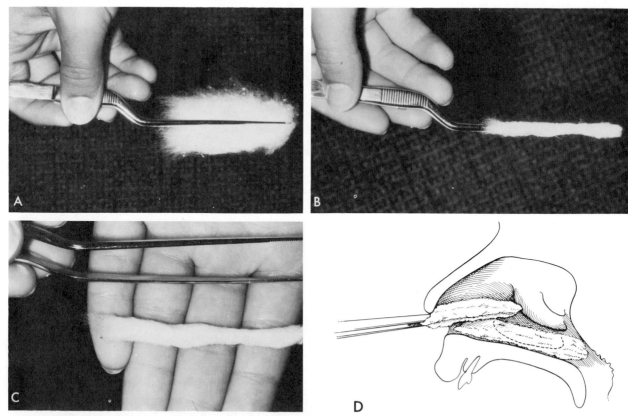

Figure 68–16. Topical anesthetic and vasoconstrictors are applied on individually made cotton pledgets. The size of the pledget may be changed according to the extent of the nasal cavity to be anesthetized and the size of the patient. *A,* An appropriately sized cotton pledget is grasped in a bayonette forceps. *B,* The cotton is then grasped with the opposite hand, and the forcep is rotated. *C,* The pledget is then removed and is ready for insertion. *D,* To completely anesthetize the nasal cavity, three pledgets are necessary. The first is placed on the floor of the nose, the second in the middle meatus between the inferior and middle turbinates, and the third in the roof of the nasal cavity and the anterior nasal vestibule.

Note: This pledget technique can be used to make a cotton wick for the treatment of otitis externa.

ing. One cannot cauterize an actively bleeding vessel with silver nitrate; hemostasis before cautery is required. Frequently repeated, overly aggressive, or bilateral cautery with silver nitrate can produce septal perforation.

The patient should be informed that he might feel some pressure during cauterization but that he should not feel pain if the mucosa is anesthetized properly. If any burning results, the nose should be re-anesthetized. At times, mucus draining over the cauterized area can carry silver nitrate into the floor of the nose and unanesthetized areas. Therefore, after controlling bleeding, it helps to wipe the area with a cotton pledget impregnated with local anesthetic. There should be no concern about causing bleeding while wiping the area, because this would indicate inadequate cauterization. It is common for patients to sneeze soon after the silver nitrate is applied.

Nasal packing is not usually necessary for a first time bleed. Patients should be advised not to place anything inside the nose and to be careful not to insert fingers into the nostrils when wiping the nose with tissues. They should be advised not to blow the nose and to open the mouth in order to relieve pressure when sneezing. The patient should be observed for 30 minutes in the emergency department to be certain that bleeding does not recur.

Aspirin should not be used for the next 3 to 4 days. Antibiotics or decongestants are not required. Patients are advised to avoid strenuous activity for a few days. Minor re-bleeding should be treated at home with rest and by pinching the nose continuously for 20 minutes. Vaseline or antibiotic ointment may be applied to the cauterized area to prevent dryness; however, this should not be done for more than several days. A crust usually forms and should be permitted to release itself.

Should bleeding recur from the same spot within several days, the procedure should be repeated and the nose packed according to the following directions. The purpose of the packing is not only to control bleeding with pressure but also to protect the cauterized area from drying and trauma and to permit healing. Generally, packing alone without cautery should not be used for control of anterior epistaxis, especially if it is done as a blind procedure without identifying the bleeding point. Movement of the packing may continue to abrade the mucosa and actually prolong bleeding or permit it to recur as soon as the packing is removed. The physician should note that nasal packing is quite uncomfortable and sometimes painful and try to avoid packing the nose unless the bleeding cannot be controlled with cautery alone. Bilateral anterior packs should also be avoided when possible.

The technique for placing an anterior pack is critical. A poorly placed pack will not control bleeding, may fall out sooner than is desired, or may fall backward into the nasopharynx, causing discomfort and a feeling of choking in an already fearful patient. Blind packing with large amounts of loose gauze should not be attempted. The key to placement of packing is adequate visualization and the placement of packing in an "accordion" manner, so that part of each layer of packing is near the front of the nose (Fig. 68–17). As each layer is placed, the nasal speculum is removed and replaced above it and the packing is gently pushed down to the floor of the nose. It should not be necessary to force the packing tightly into the nose. In a difficult-to-control nose bleed, 6 feet of 1/2-inch × 72-inch Vaseline gauze packing can be placed fairly easily and gently, if done correctly. When just covering a cauterized area, it is not necessary to place this much packing, but it should be remembered that a very small amount may easily become dislodged. The anterior pack is removed in 2 to 4 days.

An anterior pack is an intranasal foreign body. As such, it stimulates nasal mucous production and may block normal drainage of the paranasal sinuses. Occasionally, one will see blood from the ocular puncta, because blood may be forced back through the lacrimal duct. If mucous production is excessive, a decongestant/antihistamine may be given orally. Antibiotics are not routinely used, but coating the packing gauze with antibiotic ointment is often suggested. The value of antibiotic ointment is unproven.

Posterior Epistaxis

Posterior epistaxis is identified by nasal hemorrhage that tends to flow posteriorly into the nasopharynx and pharynx. Posterior bleeding is also suggested when an anterior bleed appears to be bilateral. If an anterior pack has already been placed, hemorrhage continues posteriorly. Anterior nasal packing is unsuccessful in controlling posterior epistaxis, because the packing material cannot exert direct pressure on a posterior bleeding site. Although humidification and vasoconstrictor sprays may be effective for controlling many cases of posterior epistaxis, recalcitrant cases may require placement of a posterior pack. The purpose of the posterior pack is two-fold. The pack may actually compress the bleeding point and stop hemorrhage. More often, it simply forms a buttress against which an anterior pack is placed to tamponade the bleeding site.

There are two major types of postnasal packs. The classic posterior nasal pack (Fig. 68–18A) consists of a gauze tampon placed transorally into the nasopharynx and held in place by silk strings or

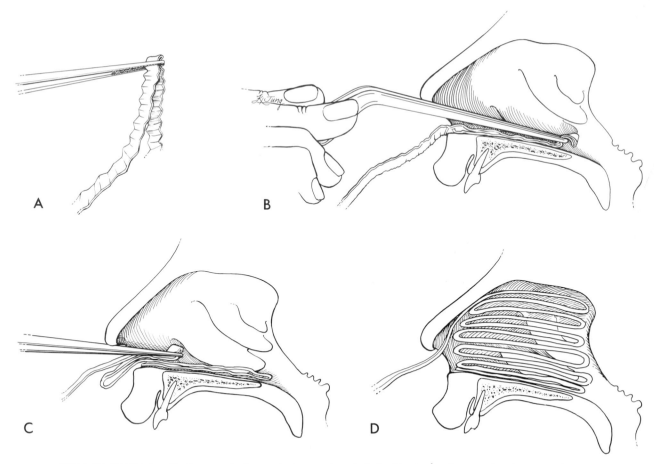

Figure 68–17. The key to placement of an anterior nasal pack that will adequately control epistaxis and stay in place is to lay the packing into the nasal cavity in an "accordion" manner, so that part of each layer of packing lies anteriorly, preventing the gauze from falling posteriorly into the nasopharynx. *A,* The first layer of ¼-inch Vaseline gauze strip is grasped approximately 2 to 3 cm from its end. *B,* This first layer is then placed on the floor of the nose through the nasal speculum (not pictured here). The bayonet forceps and nasal speculum are then withdrawn. *C,* The nasal speculum is reintroduced on top of the first layer of packing, and a second layer is placed in an identical manner. After several layers have been placed, it is often useful to reintroduce the bayonet forceps to push the previously placed packing down onto the floor of the nose, making it tighter and more secure. *D,* A complete anterior nasal pack can tamponade a bleeding point anywhere in the anterior nasal cavities and will stay in place until removed by the physician or patient.

umbilical tape brought out through the nostril. The second type of posterior pack consists of an inflatable balloon, which is placed transnasally, blown up in the nasopharynx, and retracted into the posterior nasal cavity. Because they are more convenient to use and less uncomfortable to the patient during placement, balloon devices have become more popular. Both methods will be described here.

The classic gauze nasal pack is formed of rolled gauze or a cotton-filled gauze pad (Fig. 68–18B). The end of the pack or the middle of the gauze roll is tied twice with No. 2 silk ties or umbilical tapes. All strands are left long. After anesthetizing the patient's nose and posterior pharyngeal wall, a small No. 10-French red rubber catheter is placed through the bleeding nostril and brought out through the mouth. A catheter placed in the nonbleeding side can be used to retract the palate

anteriorly while positioning the pack (Fig. 68–18C). Two of the silk ties secure the pack to the end of the catheter. This catheter is then pulled back through the nose, bringing the ties out with it. The sutures themselves are then grasped, and the pack is pulled into the nasopharynx.

Placement of the pack is facilitated by directing the pack into the patient's oral cavity and nasopharynx with a finger (Fig. 68–18D). This uncomfortable step must be accomplished as smoothly and efficiently as possible. A silk tie is left protruding from the mouth and can be used later for removal of the pack. The string can be taped to the patient's cheek. An assistant then holds mild tension on the ties in order to hold the posterior pack in position *while anterior nasal packing is placed* as previously described.

The silk sutures are tied over a large gauze pad or a dental roll to hold the posterior pack in

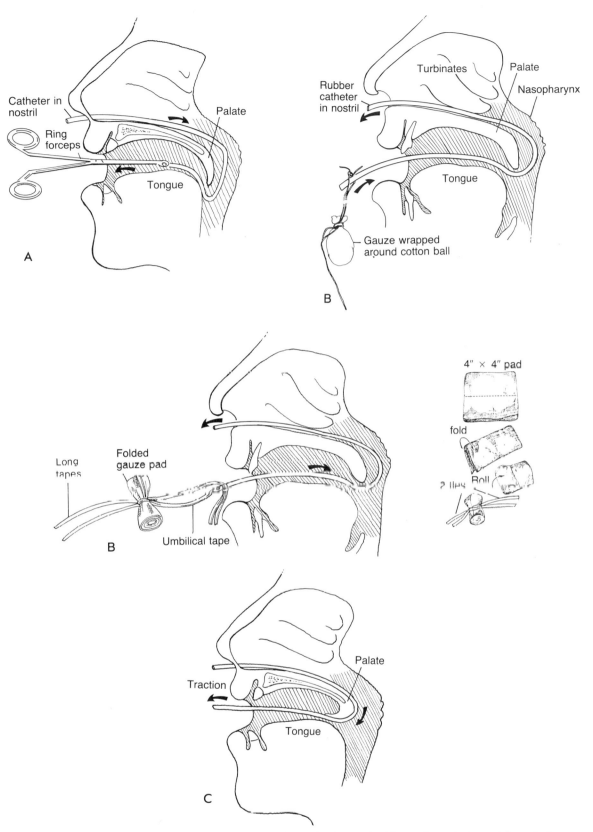

Figure 68–18. Posterior nasal pack. *A,* Following topical anesthesia, a red rubber catheter is passed through the nose and carefully grasped in the oral pharynx with ringed forceps and brought out through the mouth. *B, Upper,* A posterior nasal pack, made by wrapping a cotton ball in a 4- × 4-inch gauze pad and tying two long silk sutures or umbilical tapes around the neck of the pack. *Lower,* Alternatively, a gauze pad can be folded and rolled into a cylinder and tied with two strings. Two of the strings are used to tie the pack to the tip of the catheter. *C,* As an option, a second catheter, which has been passed through the non-bleeding side and brought out the mouth, can be used to retract the palate forward to aid in the placement of the pack (not shown). The optional catheter is removed after the pack is in the proper position.

Illustration continued on following page.

933

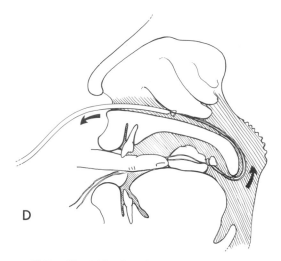

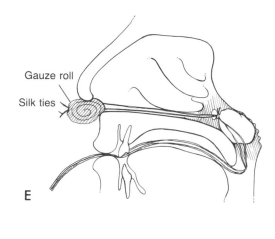

Figure 68–18 *(Continued)*. *D,* The finger is used to guide the pack through the mouth and into the proper position as traction on the catheter pulls the pack from above. This uncomfortable step is the most difficult of the procedure and must be performed deliberately and smoothly. If the patient has teeth, a dental roll or bite block is placed to prevent the patient from biting the physician's finger. *E,* Proper position of the posterior pack, wedged in the posterior portion of the nose. A long strand attached to the pack exits from the mouth and is taped to the cheek. If the pack slips posteriorly, the mouth string is pulled to avoid suffocation. A large gauze pad or roll is used to keep slight tension on the pack (after the anterior pack has been placed). A large roll is used to prevent pressure necrosis on the nasal ala and columella.

position. This pad can cause alar or columellar necrosis if it is too small or too tight. The postnasal pack is left in place for 3 to 5 days, and the patient is hospitalized and carefully observed as described below. The entire procedure is obviously uncomfortable for the patient; however, if it is explained in advance and accomplished rapidly, a very effective, custom-made tampon can be placed.

As previously mentioned, inflatable balloon packs are the most convenient packs to use and are successful in controlling most cases of posterior epistaxis. There are two general types of balloon tampons. The first is a Foley catheter with a 30-ml balloon (Fig. 68–19). Some physicians prefer to use a 10-French pediatric Foley catheter with a smaller balloon. The tip of the catheter is cut off so that it will not push against the posterior pharyngeal wall and cause necrosis or gagging. After clearing the nose of clots, determining the site of bleeding, and applying topical anesthesia, a 12- to 16-French Foley catheter is placed along the floor of the nose until the balloon is seen in the nasopharynx. The balloon is then slowly filled with 5 to 15 ml of water, and the Foley catheter is retracted anteriorly to wedge the balloon snugly in the posterior nasal cavity. If the soft palate is grossly displaced inferiorly or if there is significant pain, the balloon is slightly deflated. An anterior pack is then placed as previously described. The catheter is held in position with slight tension by padding the alar and nasal columella with gauze and applying a nasogastric tube clamp or plastic umbilical clamp.

Several companies manufacture balloon tamponade devices specifically designed for the temporary control of epistaxis. These devices are often effective for the control of bleeding in the emergency department and are more easily placed than the conventional posterior gauze packs.

A balloon tamponade device is a double balloon system that serves as both an anterior and posterior pack, eliminating the need to place an additional pack after the posterior pack has been positioned. Two such devices are the Nasostat balloon and the Exomed Epistat.

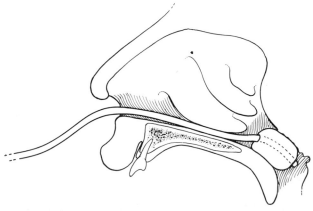

Figure 68–19. Foley catheter placed into the nasopharynx, inflated with water, and retracted into position. The distal tip of the catheter has been cut off. An anterior pack (not shown) is then placed around the catheter. The ala and columella are protected with gauze padding, and a plastic umbilical clamp or nasogastric clamp is applied to the catheter to maintain slight tension on the balloon.

The device (22-French Foley catheter) resembles a nasal airway with a double-lumened, independently inflatable, low-pressure double balloon system (Fig. 68–20). To use the balloon, the nose is cleared of clots, the device is lubricated with an anesthetic ointment, and the deflated system is slowly passed along the floor of the nose. The device is fully advanced so that the posterior balloon extends into the nasopharynx. The posterior balloon is inflated with 4 to 8 ml of water, and slight forward traction is applied. The anterior balloon is then *slowly* inflated with 10 to 25 ml of air or saline, securing the anterior pack.

The device is constructed of soft, pliable silicone rubber, which allows atraumatic expansion of the balloon into the entire nasal cavity. If the patient complains of excessive pain, the anterior balloon is slightly deflated.

If the balloon tampons are unsuccessful in controlling epistaxis, they should be replaced with conventional packs before more complicated techniques are attempted. Patients with the balloon devices are treated similarly to those with conventional posterior packs.

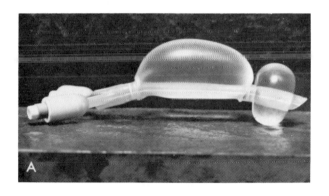

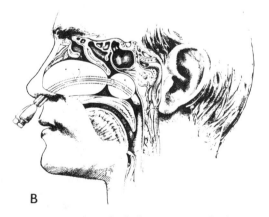

Figure 68–20. *A* and *B*. The balloon tamponade device serves as both an anterior and posterior pack. It is easily inserted and is often successful for the temporary control of posterior epistaxis in the emergency department. The balloon shown here is the Epistat balloon. (Courtesy of Exomed Inc., Jacksonville, Florida).

CARE OF THE PATIENT WITH A POSTERIOR NASAL PACK

All patients with posterior nasal packs should be admitted to the hospital. Posterior packs are uncomfortable when being placed and annoying when in place. Mild sedation is often required for packs to be tolerated. Posterior nasal packs are associated with a significant incidence of morbidity and even mortality. Complications include hypoventilation with hypoxia and hypercarbia, infection, pain, and dysphagia.

Because many patients with severe posterior epistaxis are elderly and have some manifestations of arteriosclerosis or chronic lung disease, they are susceptible to life-threatening complications from even mild hypoxia. Cook and Komorn noted a statistically significant decrease in PO_2 [average 7.5 to 11 mm Hg] and an increase in PCO_2 [average 7 to 13 mm Hg] in patients with anterior and posterior nasal packs who were treated with sedation and bed rest.[2] The changes were most pronounced in patients with pre-existing chronic obstructive pulmonary disease. Recent studies have not confirmed the presence of a previously reported reflex increase in pulmonary vascular resistance (the so-called *nasopulmonary reflex*).[3] There is, however, no question that hypoxia, hypercarbia, and death can follow the placement of these packs. Therefore, patients with posterior packs must be closely monitored, preferably in an intensive care setting for at least the first night.

The accidental dislodgement of a posterior pack into the airway could be disastrous. The emergency removal of the classic pack by pulling the mouth string should be familiar to all nursing personnel. Patients should be routinely provided with humidification and oxygen as indicated by blood gas determinations. Sedation should be used with extreme caution. Broad-spectrum antibiotics are given routinely to help prevent complications of bacterial nasopharyngitis and sinusitis caused by blockage of the sinus ostea and poor drainage. Oral intake may be compromised because of discomfort, and fluid balance must be carefully monitored. Other complications include necrosis of the nasal ala or columella from improper padding, necrosis of the palate, or nasal mucosa. Complications increase with the length of packing, and the posterior pack should be removed within 3 to 5 days.

UNCONTROLLED EPISTAXIS

There are a few patients whose epistaxis cannot be controlled by the methods previously described. In some, the bleeding site can be identified and cauterized by examination under anesthesia. In others, ligation of vessels is necessary. The anterior and posterior ethmoid arteries can be ligated through an external incision medial to the medial canthus of the eye. The sphenopalatine artery and other branches from the external carotid system are approached through the maxillary sinus and lie just posterior to its posterior wall.

More recently, epistaxis has been controlled by embolization of the internal maxillary artery [usually with Gelfoam] after catheterization under radiologic control. Each of these methods of treating epistaxis has risks and potential complications, but the details are beyond the scope of this book.

SUMMARY

Most cases of epistaxis can be readily controlled in the emergency department with a minimum of complications. One should not, however, underestimate the amount of blood that can be lost in chronic epistaxis. Significant hemorrhage may not be appreciated until the patient faints in the waiting room during his third visit within 1 week for seemingly minor bleeding. Elderly patients are especially prone to complications and require thorough investigation and definitive measures to stop the bleeding. Finally, persistent bleeding should always raise the possibility of a bleeding disorder or an occult nasopharyngeal carcinoma. All but the most straightforward cases of epistaxis require follow-up evaluation.

Septal Hematoma

The portion of the nasal septum that provides support to the tip of the nose consists of a thin section of cartilage enveloped by a layer of muco-perichondrium on each side. When nasal trauma occurs, with or without fracture, the bending and shearing forces can cause separation of the perichondrium from the cartilage. The resultant potential space may fill with blood, resulting in a septal hematoma. Failure to recognize and appropriately treat a septal hematoma can have disastrous cosmetic and even life-threatening consequences. If the hematoma becomes infected, cartilage destruction with a saddle nose deformity can result. Meningitis or cavernous sinus thrombosis can complicate inadequately treated septal abscess. Posterior septal hematomas also occur and may be more difficult to recognize.

DIAGNOSIS

A thorough nasal examination is indicated after any degree of nasal trauma. Suspicion of septal hematoma is heightened if nasal obstruction has resulted, but an adequate nasal airway does not rule out hematoma. As discussed in the section entitled Epistaxis, good "from the eye" illumination is required. The nasal mucosa is anesthetized and vasoconstricted as previously described. A fresh septal hematoma is often the same color as the nasal mucosa and may not be ecchymotic. Therefore, it may easily be missed unless the septal is palpated with a blunt instrument. On palpation, one finds a baggy, slightly fluctuant septum that is tender to the touch. A septal hematoma can occur on one or both sides (Fig. 68–21). The patient with a septal hematoma or abscess may complain of nasal pain out of proportion to other findings.

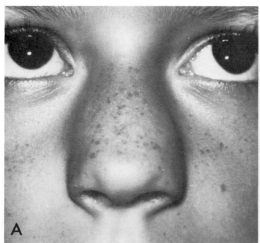 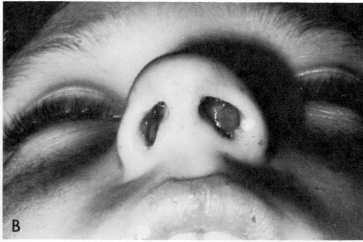

Figure 68–21. Photograph of a left septal abscess in a 7-year-old boy who sustained blunt nasal trauma 1 week previously. He had immediate nasal obstruction that persisted, and he presented with fever, widening of the nasal dorsum (A), and a visible mass in the nose (B). Early diagnosis and treatment of septal hematoma would have prevented this complication.

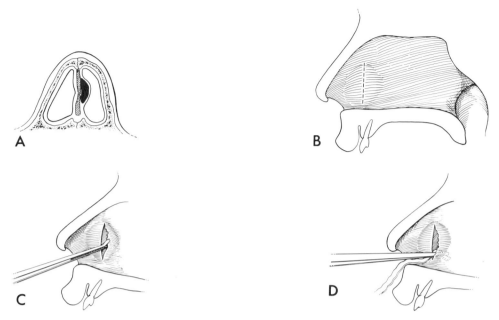

Figure 68–22. *A*, A small left-sided septal hematoma. *B*, After applying appropriate topical anesthesia, supplemented with local infiltrative anesthesia if necessary, an incision is made through the mucosa and perichondrium covering the hematoma. *C*, A small cup forceps or scissor is used to remove enough mucosa to help prevent premature closure of the wound and re-accumulation of hematoma. *D*, A sterile rubber band is then placed as a drain, and the wound is packed as described in the section entitled Epistaxis.

TREATMENT

Because the cartilage receives its nutrient supply via the perichondrium and because devitalized septal cartilage will inevitably become infected and "melt away," the key to treatment is to re-establish close approximation of the perichondrium and cartilage. A long vertical incision is made through the mucosa overlying the hematoma (Fig. 68–22). A small cup forceps or punch forceps is used to remove a small area of mucosa to allow constant drainage. All clots are removed with suction or irrigation (normal saline). A small drain such as a sterile rubber band is placed, and the nose is packed with an anterior pack as described in the section entitled Epistaxis. The packing is removed daily, and recurrent hematoma is re-aspirated. When no recurrence is seen, the drain is removed. The following day the packing is discontinued. The patient is advised to avoid blowing his nose and to open his mouth when sneezing to avoid large intranasal pressure changes. Continued observation is indicated until healing is completed.

Bilateral hematomas can be handled in one of two ways. After one side has been incised and drained as previously described, a piece of septal cartilage can be removed to permit drainage through the septum from the opposite side. Extreme care must be taken to avoid a mucosal laceration on the second side; otherwise, a septal perforation is likely to occur. The second method is to incise the mucosa on each side, leaving the cartilage intact. Here, it is critical that the two incisions be staggered so that they are not directly opposite one another; otherwise, septal perforation is likely to occur. Septal perforation often results in recurrent epistaxis and nasal stuffiness or even saddle deformity.

At the first sign of suppuration, hospital admission, wide drainage, irrigation, and intravenous antibiotics are indicated to avoid both saddle deformity and infectious complications such as meningitis or cavernous sinus thrombosis.

Nasal Foreign Bodies

The examination of the nose is discussed in the section entitled Epistaxis. Nasal foreign bodies are most commonly found in children and include objects such as buttons, beads, cotton, beans, and other appropriately sized objects. Vegetable foreign bodies will absorb water from the nasal mucosa and swell with time, making removal much more difficult than insertion. A child with a retained nasal foreign body often presents with a foul odor, unilateral purulent rhinorrhea, or persistent epistaxis.

The key to removal of a nasal foreign body is reassurance and immobilization of the child, good lighting, and appropriate instrumentation.[4] In a very young or uncooperative patient, general anesthesia is indicated. Topical anesthesia and vasoconstriction can be applied as a spray or by drops, using 4 per cent topical lidocaine and 0.25 per cent phenylephrine hydrochloride or 1 ml of 4 per cent cocaine solution. The nose is then carefully examined, and a determination is made as to which instrument provides the best chance for removal of the foreign body. A smooth, round object can be removed using the suction instrument pictured in Figure 68–12 or using right-angle hooks as described in Figure 68–11. An alligator forceps or bayonet forceps can be used to grasp an object that has a small leading edge. Unlike foreign bodies of the ear, foreign bodies in the nasal cavity cannot be removed by irrigation, because the nasal cavity is open posteriorly. One should not push a nasal foreign body back into the pharynx hoping that the object will be swallowed, because aspiration may occur.

Fox describes the successful use of a No. 4-Fogarty vascular catheter for the removal of blunt nasal foreign bodies in children.[4] The catheter is passed beyond the foreign body, and the balloon is inflated. Slow, gentle traction is maintained on the catheter while the object is carefully extricated. This technique may be less traumatic than manual removal with forceps.

The Fogarty catheter balloon may also be used to stabilize the foreign body from behind while it is removed with forceps, because attempts to remove a foreign body may result in the object being forced into the oral pharynx, with subsequent aspiration. Aspiration is especially likely in the struggling child. A balloon inflated behind the foreign body will help to prevent this.

Auricular Hematoma

The anatomy of the pinna of the ear correlates in many ways with that of the nasal septum. It consists of cartilage enveloped on each side by perichondrium covered closely by skin. As previously noted, cartilage is avascular and receives its nutrients and oxygenation through the perichondrium. Any process that disrupts the close approximation of perichondrium to cartilage can threaten its integrity.

Auricular hematoma may occur after any blunt trauma, but it occurs most commonly in wrestlers as a result of a shearing force that separates the perichondrium from the cartilage. If left untreated, such a hematoma tends to become infected and the resultant chondritis produces a cosmetic auricular deformity called *cauliflower ear* (Fig. 68–23).

TREATMENT

The first step in treatment of an auricular hematoma consists of sterile needle aspiration of the

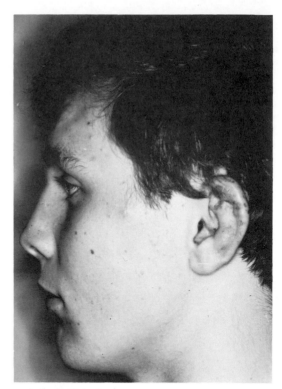

Figure 68–23. High-school wrestler with a cosmetic auricular deformity known as *cauliflower ear*, resulting from inadequate removal of blood from an auricular hematoma.

hematoma (Fig. 68–24).[5] If aspiration is successful, a pressure dressing is applied as described in Figure 68–25.

The ear must be re-examined daily for re-accumulation of the hematoma, because recurrence is common. The ear must be examined sooner if pain increases or if there is fever, because these findings indicate possible infection.

Re-aspiration may be required at the patient's return visit, but if the hematoma recurs after re-aspiration, it should be incised and drained, using strict sterile technique. A sterile rubber band or small Penrose drain can be used as a drain (Fig. 68–26) and a pressure dressing is re-applied. The ear should be re-examined daily, and the patient should be kept on a broad-spectrum antibiotic. If the hematoma does not reform, the drain can be removed in 2 to 3 days and a pressure dressing is left in place for one more day.

An alternative technique for applying a pressure dressing consists of a tie-over stent (Fig. 68–27).[6] A sterile dental roll is cut to the size of the hematoma and placed over it. A second dental roll is placed in the postauricular sulcus. A 3-0 or 4-0 monofilament suture on a straight needle is placed through the center of one dental roll, through the ear, back through the posterior dental roll, and through the ear again, where the two ends are tied. Additional tie-over sutures are used as necessary. Care must be taken to ensure that

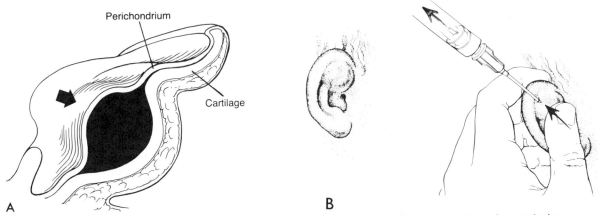

Figure 68–24. A, Sub-perichondrial hematoma within the concha of the ear. B, Needle aspiration of an auricular hematoma. A topical antiseptic is used to clean the ear, but local anesthesia is seldom required. While stabilizing the pinna with the thumb and fingers, the most fluctuant part of the hematoma is punctured with a 20 gauge needle. The thumb "milks" the hematoma into the syringe until the entire hematoma has been evacuated. The thumb maintains continued pressure on the ear for 3 minutes after the needle has been withdrawn. A pressure dressing is then applied, and the ear is checked for re-accumulation of blood in 24 hours. Re-aspiration may be required, and persistent accumulations require incision and drainage. (B Redrawn from Fleisher et al.: Textbook of Pediatric Emergency Medicine. Baltimore, Williams & Wilkins, 1983.)

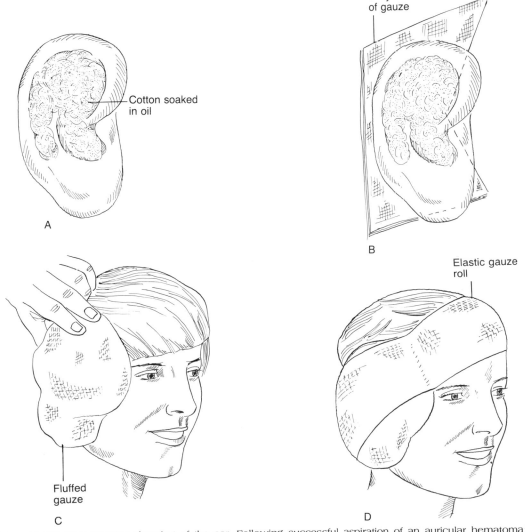

Figure 68–25. Compression dressing of the ear. Following successful aspiration of an auricular hematoma a compression dressing is used to prevent re-accumulation of the hematoma or fluid. A, Dry cotton is first placed into the ear canal. A conforming material is then carefully molded into all the convolutions of the auricle. One may use Vaseline gauze or cotton soaked in mineral oil or saline. B, When the convolutions are fully packed, a posterior gauze pack is placed behind the ear. A V-shaped section has been cut from the gauze to allow it to easily fit behind the ear. C, Multiple layers of fluffed gauze are placed over the packed ear, and the entire dressing is held in place with Kling or an elastic gauze roll (D). The ear is thus compressed between two layers of gauze, and the packing assures even distribution of pressure to all parts of the auricle.

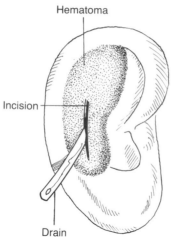

Figure 68–26. If repeated aspiration of an auricular hematoma is unsuccessful, the hematoma is incised and drained, as shown. The drainage incision must go through the perichondrium in order to be successful. Following placement of the drain beneath the perichondrium, a compression ear dressing is placed, as shown in Figure 68–25.

the vascular supply to the auricle is not compromised by sutures tied too tightly. The patient and his family are advised to observe the auricle frequently and to return to the doctor if discoloration occurs. Again, the ear is examined daily and if there is no re-accumulation of hematoma and no compromise of the skin, this type of pressure dressing is left in place for 3 to 5 days, with the patient on a broad-spectrum antibiotic. As in the case of septal hematoma, any sign of abscess or chondritis is treated with aggressive surgical drainage and intravenous antibiotics in the hospital.

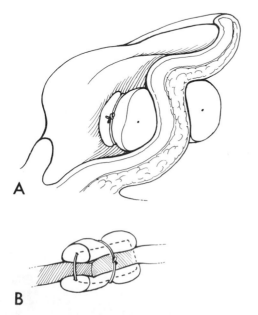

Figure 68–27. A, After aspiration by needle or incision and drainage, sterile dental rolls are used as a tie-over stent. B, One suture has been placed through the center of each roll, and the other is perpendicular to it and surrounds both dental rolls. The sutures are tied firmly but must not be so tight that pressure necrosis is risked.

Transillumination of the Sinuses

"I have sinus" is a common complaint of patients who present to family practitioners, otolaryngologists, and emergency physicians. Most patients have been educated about problems related to the sinuses by commercial advertisements for common cold remedies. In these advertisements, no distinction is made between nasal symptoms and sinus symptoms; thus, anything that causes a stuffy or runny nose is thought to be "sinus."

Bacterial sinusitis most frequently occurs as a complication of a viral upper respiratory infection. The maxillary sinuses are those most commonly infected. Maxillary sinusitis is characterized by partial or complete nasal obstruction; purulent nasal discharge; pain located in the cheek, teeth, or palate; and tenderness to palpation of the cheek on the affected side. Ethmoid sinusitis, with tenderness and pain in the area of the medial canthus and lateral wall of the nose, frequently accompanies maxillary sinusitis in adults. Complicated ethmoid sinusitis is more common in children than adults and can lead to periorbital cellulitis and periorbital abscess, both of which require aggressive hospital treatment and possibly a surgical drainage procedure. Frontal sinusitis presents with frontal headache, pain, and tenderness, with soft-tissue swelling and possibly periorbital edema in severe cases. Complications of frontal sinusitis include meningitis, brain abscess, and cavernous sinus thrombosis. Therefore, this entity must be treated aggressively, and otolaryngologic consultation is indicated. Although sphenoid sinusitis may occur, it is unusual as an isolated entity. The patient with sphenoid sinusitis complains primarily of headache, which is frequently occipital.

The diagnosis of sinusitis and the determination of which sinuses are involved can be *suspected* by the patient's medical history and physical examination, but an exact and certain diagnosis is best made by sinus radiographs. Transillumination of the sinuses can identify unilateral frontal or maxillary sinusitis. However, false-positives and false-negatives occur frequently enough so that transillumination should probably be used primarily as a tool for following and evaluating the resolution of sinusitis that has previously been documented by radiographic evaluation. Radiographic examination is necessary for any complicated or recurrent sinus infection. After treatment, follow-up films are indicated in order to confirm re-aeration of the affected sinuses or to identify continued opacification and thus indicate the need for further treatment.

ETIOLOGY

The paranasal sinuses communicate with the nasal cavity through relatively small ostea. Any

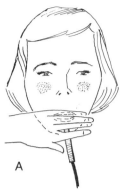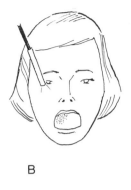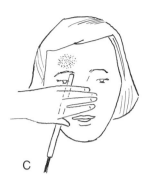

Figure 68–28. Transillumination of the maxillary (A and B) and frontal sinuses (C). This is an inexact test that should be confirmed with radiographs. The key to success is a totally dark room and a bright light source.

process that interferes with aeration of the sinuses may eventually result in bacterial sinusitis. The most common pathogens include pneumococcus, *Hemophilus influenzae* and streptococcus.

PROCEDURE

Many types of transilluminators can be found in most medical equipment catalogues. Transillumination must be done in a completely darkened room. Incomplete exclusion of light is probably the most common reason for inaccurate transillumination.

The sphenoid and ethmoid sinuses are not amenable to evaluation by transillumination. For evaluation of the maxillary sinuses, the transillumination light is placed into the patient's mouth, and his lips are closed around the light source (Fig. 68–28A). Normal sinuses will transmit the light through the cheeks, which will glow in the darkened room. If one sinus is opacified, it will appear dark. Alternatively, the light source may be placed on each infraorbital rim and the roof of the mouth can be examined for symmetry of transillumination (Fig. 68–28B). For evaluation of the frontal sinuses, the transilluminator is placed under the medial aspect of the supraorbital ridge (Fig. 68–28C). The clear frontal sinus will transmit this light.

Care must be taken in evaluating asymmetrical frontal sinuses, because there may be great differences in the size of the right and left frontal sinuses in normal patients. Thus, in any patient in whom a false-positive or a false-negative test is possible, sinus films should be obtained to confirm the findings.

Peritonsillar Abscess

Peritonsillar abscess, also called *quincy*, is the most common head and neck abscess in adults. It most frequently occurs in teen-agers and young adults and rarely occurs in children younger than 10 years old. Over the past decade, the treatment for peritonsillar abscess has undergone controversial changes.

ANATOMY

The palatine tonsils are aggregations of lymphatic tissue covered by mucous membrane. They are located in the tonsillar fossa, between the glossopalatine arch (anterior tonsillar pillar) and the pharyngopalatine arch (posterior tonsillar pillar). The lateral or deep surface of the tonsil is adherent to a fibrous capsule, which is separated from the inner surface of the superior pharyngeal constrictor muscle by loose connective tissue. This muscle lies between the tonsil and the external maxillary artery. The internal carotid artery lies 2.0 to 2.5 cm behind and lateral to the tonsil.

PATHOPHYSIOLOGY

A peritonsillar abscess begins as a tonsil infection that extends through the capsule into the soft connective tissue between the tonsil and the superior constrictor muscle. Here the infection suppurates and extends superiorly into the soft palate, where the median raphe limits its medial extent. Usually, the abscess will form over the superior lateral aspect of the tonsil, but it can form in the mid-posterior portion, and more uncommonly, along the inferior tonsillar pole.

The abscess can spontaneously rupture into the oropharynx, followed by resolution of the process. If rupture occurs during sleep, pyogenic aspiration may occur. A breakthrough can also occur through the superior pharyngeal constrictor muscle into the parapharyngeal space, resulting in a deep neck space infection and its potential complications. Occasionally, edema of the larynx may follow if the abscess extends down the lateral pharyngeal wall. Deep cervical vessel thrombosis and septicemia are also possible complications.

The bacteria most commonly associated with peritonsillar abscess is group A streptococcus. However, Gram-negative and mixed anaerobic infections are common. Because of the frequency of prior antibiotic coverage, cultures taken during incision and drainage may be sterile.

Although peritonsillar abscess usually follows untreated or inappropriately treated tonsillitis, we have seen several cases that followed treatment of tonsillitis with intramuscular long-acting penicillin or other, appropriate oral antibiotics.

DIAGNOSIS

The typical patient with a peritonsillar abscess gives a history of a generalized sore throat in the recent past (2 days to 2 weeks), which was either not treated or partially treated with antibiotics. Prior to seeking medical attention, the pain localizes to one side, frequently with ipsilateral otalgia. The patient becomes toxic with temperature elevations between 101° and 103° F. Trismus develops because of pterygoid muscle irritation, making intraoral examination difficult. As the abscess expands, swallowing becomes more painful, eventually resulting in drooling and possibly dehydration if the process lasts long enough. The patient develops so-called "hot potato" muffled speech, and halitosis may be severe. Tender ipsilateral cervical lymph adenopathy is usual, and secondary torticollis may develop, with the head tilted toward the affected side.

Physical examination is difficult, secondary to trismus; however, an accurate assessment and treatment can usually be accomplished. It is important to reassure the patient and to encourage him to relax and open his mouth as wide as possible. Depress the tongue with a tongue depressor, preferably the L-shaped metal depressor, which gives greater leverage and keeps the examiner's hand out of the field of vision. Placing the depressor at the level of the tonsil gives the best visualization. Positioning the depressor too far posteriorly will cause reflex gagging, whereas positioning it too far anteriorly will result in inadequate exposure.

The affected tonsil usually appears larger than its counterpart, is hyperemic, and may be covered with exudate (Fig. 68–29). The tonsil is displaced downward, forward, and medially by the inflamed

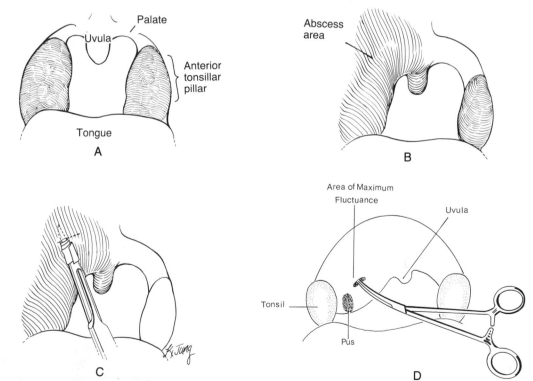

Figure 68–29. A, In tonsillitis, the tonsils are enlarged. They may be covered by white exudate. The margin between the tonsil and the anterior tonsillar pillar and palate is well defined. B, In peritonsillar abscess, the tonsil, palate, and anterior tonsillar pillar may be bulging medially in one unit. The margin between the tonsil, palate, and anterior tonsillar pillar is somewhat effaced. The uvula is usually edematous and may be pointing toward the opposite tonsil. C, The safest area to incise and drain a peritonsillar abscess is usually just above the tonsil in the soft palate. This location, with tape wrapped around the knife blade to prevent deep penetration, will serve to guard the deep vessels of the neck from inadvertent injury. D, Following mucosa incision, a hemostat is placed in the incision and gently spread to break up loculations and enhance drainage.

and edematous palate. The uvula is usually edematous and may seem to point toward the unaffected side. A useful sign is that the normally sharp cufflike border of the anterior tonsillar pillar is obliterated by bulging edema.

Digital palpation is not recommended unless carotid aneurysm is suspected, as secondary spasm may cause injury to the examining finger. Fluctuation is not needed to make the diagnosis or to initiate treatment, because the abscess may not yet have "headed."

The differential diagnosis includes severe unilateral tonsillitis, acute leukemia, chancre, gumma, carcinoma, carotid artery aneurysm, and tumor of the parapharyngeal space. These diagnoses can usually be ruled out because the peritonsillar abscess is an acute process, associated with toxicity and surrounding tissue edema, especially of the uvula. It is often more difficult to rule out peritonsillar cellulitis, because the history and physical findings can be almost identical to those of an abscess. Differentiation between peritonsillar abscess and cellulitis can be made during the course of treatment.

TREATMENT

The treatment for peritonsillar abscess has undergone change over the past 5 years. If a true abscess has formed, some type of incision and drainage is necessary to prevent the complications previously described.

If the suspected diagnosis is peritonsillar *cellulitis*, the patient is treated with high-dose oral penicillin (500 mg q.i.d. orally) and analgesics. With a responsible nontoxic patient who can maintain close contact with the physician, this treatment can be done on an outpatient basis, provided that the patient is advised to call the physician if the symptoms become more severe with increasing fever, trismus, or pain. The patient should be seen again within 24 hours unless there is marked improvement in the symptoms. If there is any question about being able to maintain close followup or if the patient is unable to adequately take oral antibiotics and fluids, hospitalization with intravenous antibiotics and fluids is indicated. Penicillin has been the mainstay of treatment in the past, pending cultures from the abscess fluid; however, broad-spectrum antibiotics such as the new cephalosporins are probably more commonly used today. If symptoms worsen and if the situation does not improve in 24 hours, the diagnosis of peritonsillar abscess becomes evident.

The classic treatment of a peritonsillar *abscess* stresses that a peritonsillar abscess should be incised and drained, followed by an interval tonsillectomy in 4 to 8 weeks. Tonsillectomy was suggested to prevent recurrence of peritonsillar

abscess, and the time period of 4 to 8 weeks was decided on so that inflammation would have subsided but dense scarring would not yet have occurred.

During the mid to late 1970's, emergency tonsillectomy gained some popularity for the treatment of peritonsillar abscess.[7] Removing the tonsil completely unroofs the abscess cavity and serves to prevent future infections. The fear of operative bleeding and septicemia is unfounded, because all these patients are treated with pre-operative intravenous antibiotics, and the surgery is performed under endotracheal anesthesia to control the airway. It is now apparent that this procedure is safe; however, emergency tonsillectomy is based on the premise that peritonsillar abscesses are recurrent and that tonsillectomy will eventually be necessary.

Recent studies indicate that this premise may be incorrect. Retrospective studies indicate that recurrence rates for abscesses may be as low as 7 per cent in children, suggesting that the need for tonsillectomy is doubtful.[8] Tonsillectomy is probably only indicated for patients with recurrent abscesses; those who have complications of an abscess, such as airway compromise or parapharyngeal space infection; or those who have other indications for tonsillectomy, notwithstanding the present abscess.

There has been some suggestion that needle aspiration can be used as curative treatment, along with antibiotics for peritonsillar abscess. Because controlled studies have not been carried out, it is suggested that a positive needle aspiration be used to confirm a diagnosis of peritonsillar abscess and that incision and drainage then be accomplished. *A negative needle aspiration does not necessarily rule out abscess.*

Once peritonsillar abscess has been diagnosed based on the patient's history and physical examination or on a lack of response to oral or intravenous antibiotics, an incision and drainage is indicated. Toxic or unreliable patients should be admitted to the hospital. With appropriate reassurance and encouragement and with the prospect of both immediate and great relief of the worst of their symptoms, most patients are able to cooperate with an incision and drainage carried out under local anesthesia in an outpatient setting.

Procedure. Again, good "through the eye" lighting with a head mirror or headlight is necessary. The patient is seated upright with his head supported by a headrest. The mouth is anesthetized with topical anesthesia such as 4 to 10 per cent lidocaine or Cetacaine spray. The area in which the incision will be made is then infiltrated with approximately 1 ml of 1 to 2 per cent lidocaine combined with epinephrine in a concentration of 1:100,000, using a fine needle (25 or 27 gauge). Lidocaine is used to anesthetize the overlying oropharyngeal mucosa where the incision is made, not the underlying abscess wall. It is our impression that, with careful infiltration, there is much less discomfort during the actual incision and drainage.

The incision is made in the soft palate in the area that is bulging most prominently. This is usually just superior and lateral to the tonsil. Some physicians prefer to localize the incision site with a 20 gauge needle on a syringe. A needle guard can be made by amputating the distal 0.5 cm of the plastic needle cover provided with individually packaged needles. With the needle cover (guard) over the needle, the needle protrudes only a short distance past the tip of the cylindrical guard. This minimizes the risk of major vessel injury when aspirating for purulence. Once purulence has been found, the incision can be made with greater certainty. The incision is 1 to 2 cm long and can be made with a No. 15 or No. 11 blade. It is useful to place tape around the blade as pictured in Figure 68–29C, leaving approximately 0.5 cm of the blade exposed in order to prevent an uncontrolled deeper incision. It must be remembered that the major vessels of the neck travel within the parapharyngeal space lateral to the tonsil. The patient is advised to expectorate the pus, which is forthcoming. Suctioning with a tonsil suction tip or a No. 9 to No. 10 Frazier suction tip will aid in the removal of pus. A closed Kelly clamp is then cautiously placed through the incision and gently opened in order to open up loculated abscess spaces (see Fig. 68–29D). A culture of the abscess wall, preferably for aerobic and anaerobic bacteria, is taken at this time. The patient's mouth can then be rinsed with hydrogen peroxide. The small amount of bleeding that invariably occurs with this procedure will spontaneously stop. Drains are never placed in peritonsillar abscesses.

After incision and drainage, antibiotics are continued for a total of 3 weeks. The lengthy postoperative course of antibiotics empirically seems to decrease the incidence of recurrence. The postoperative treatment may be performed on an outpatient basis or started while the patient is still in the hospital if there is a question of the ability for adequate oral intake and follow-up. The patient is seen routinely midway through the course of treatment, as well as 1 week after the cessation of all antibiotics. Recurrence of symptoms always requires *prompt* re-evaluation.

1. Senturia, B.H., Marcus, M.D., and Lucente, F.E.: Diseases of the External Ear. An Otologic-Dermatologic Manual. 2nd ed. New York, Grune & Stratton, Inc., 1980.
2. Cook, T.A., and Komorn, R.M.: Statistical analysis of the alterations of blood gases produced by nasal packing. Laryngoscope 83:1802, 1973.
3. Larsen, K.: Arterial blood gases and pneumatic nasal packing in epistaxis. Laryngoscope 92:586, 1982.
4. Fox, J.R.: Fogarty catheter removal of nasal foreign bodies. Ann. Emerg. Med. 9:37, 1980.
5. Potsic, W.P.: Management of trauma of the external ear. *In* English, G.M. (ed.), Otolaryngology: A Textbook. New York, Harper & Row Publishers, 1981, Chapter 14.
6. Scarcella, J.V.: Tie-over dressing to prevent recurrence of a hematoma of the ear. Plast. Reconstr. Surg. 61(4):610, 1978.
7. Templer, J.W., Holinger, L.D., Wood, R.P., 2nd, et al.: Immediate tonsillectomy for the treatment of peritonsillar abscess. Am. J. Surg. 134:596, 1977.
8. Holt, G.R., and Tinsley, P.: Peritonsillar abscess in children. Laryngoscope 91:1226, 1981.

13

DENTISTRY

69

Emergency Dental Procedures

JAMES T. AMSTERDAM, D.M.D., M.D.

BARRY H. HENDLER, D.D.S., M.D.

LOUIS F. ROSE, D.D.S., M.D.

Introduction

Patients with a variety of general dental, oral, and maxillofacial emergencies may present to any emergency unit. Emergencies may range from an agonizing toothache to massive maxillofacial trauma or infection. Most general dental emergencies can be evaluated and managed initially by the emergency physician; however, pediatric dental emergencies and dentoalveolar trauma may require immediate dental consultation and early follow-up. In addition, consultation is essential in maxillofacial trauma or in certain dental infections in which a seemingly minor problem may have potential life-threatening implications, including airway compromise, septicemia, and dehydration. The management of oral and facial pain, dentoalveolar trauma, dental infection, and maxillofacial trauma requires an understanding of the anatomy of the stomatognathic system; the relevant anatomy will therefore be discussed. This chapter will conclude with an overview of the oral manifestations of systemic disease that are of particular importance to the emergency physician.

Anatomy of the Stomatognathic System

The muscles of mastication are divided into two groups: the supramandibular muscles, or elevators of the mandible, and the inframandibular muscles, or depressors. The most important elevating muscles are the masseters, the medial pterygoids, and the temporalis. The bilateral simultaneous function of this group is to move the condyle of the mandible superiorly and posteriorly. The muscles involved in the depressor function of the mandible are the lateral pterygoids, the digastric muscles, the geniohyoid, and the mylohyoid. The unilateral contraction of the lateral pterygoid muscle will cause movement of the mandible to the opposite side. If both lateral pterygoids contract simultaneously, the mandible will be depressed, causing the jaw to open in a downward and forward movement.

The mandible is essentially formed bilaterally by two rami—the horizontal portion and the ascending portion (Fig. 69–1). The ascending ramus of the mandible extends up to form two processes: the coronoid process, which extends anteriorly, and the more important condylar process, which extends posteriorly. The temporomandibular articulation is a diarthrosis joining the mandibular fossa and the articular tubercle of the temporal bone with the condyle of the mandible. A fibrous connective-tissue articular disk or meniscus intervenes between the articulating bones. A joint capsule surrounds the temporomandibular joint. The capsule consists of an outer fibrous layer, which is strengthened on its lateral surface to form the temporomandibular joint and the capsular ligaments. The capsular ligaments reinforce the capsule and function to limit mandibular movement. A small amount of synovial fluid may be found in the articulatory spaces. Frequently, trauma to the mandibular condyle produces pain resulting from extension or torquing of these ligaments, which should be distinguished from pain caused by a fracture in this area.

Anatomy of the Teeth

A tooth has been described as a homogeneous body of dentin surrounding a central pulp—the neurovascular supply—from which the microporous dentin is nourished and was initially derived. The pulp continuously lays down additional dentin throughout life. The tooth may also be divided into coronal and root portions. The enamel-covered coronal portion is the part that is normally seen in the mouth. The root portion of the tooth, which serves to anchor it, is covered with cementum, a substance that is much softer than enamel (Fig. 69–2).

There are numerous classifications for the teeth. The permanent dentition generally consists of 32 teeth, which comprise four types—incisors, canines, premolars, and molars (Fig. 69–3). If one begins from the midline and counts backward one will find one central incisor, one lateral incisor, one canine, two premolars, and three permanent molars in the normal dental anatomy. The third molar is commonly referred to as the wisdom tooth. Agenesis, or absence, of any of these teeth can occur occasionally. In addition, a patient can have extra, or supernumerary, teeth, which are somewhat small and unusually shaped. There are many methods of notation in the literature for numbering or classifying teeth. Although some

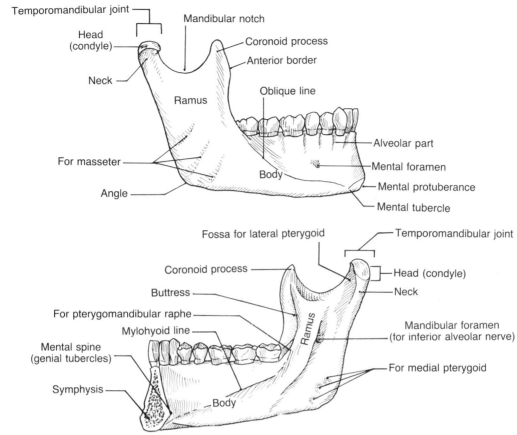

Figure 69–1. Anatomy of the mandible. (Redrawn from Grant, J. C.: Grant's Atlas of Anatomy, 5th ed. Baltimore, Williams & Wilkins, 1962.)

systems are more universal than others, it is perhaps best for the emergency physician simply to describe the type of tooth and the location involved in a particular emergency, e.g., an upper right second premolar or a lower left canine. Dental nomenclature that may be of use to the emergency physician includes the following terms:

Facial: That part of a tooth that faces the oral vestibule, or the cheek and the lips. In the area of incisors to canines this surface is called the *labial* surface; for premolars and molars it is referred to as the *buccal* surface.

Oral: That part of a tooth that faces the tongue or the palate, usually referred to as the *lingual* surface of the tooth.

Approximal: The contacting areas of adjacent teeth. The area closest to the midline is called the *mesial* surface, and the area toward the posterior aspect of the mouth is referred to as the *distal* surface.

Occlusal: Biting surfaces of the premolars and the molars.

Incisal: Biting surface of the canines and incisors.

Apical: The tip of the root.

Coronal: Toward the biting surface of the tooth.

The Normal Periodontium

The normal periodontium can be divided into two major components, the gingival unit and the attachment apparatus. The *gingival unit* is composed of the soft tissues investing the teeth and the alveolar bone. The *gingiva* is covered by a keratinized, stratified squamous epithelium. It extends from the free gingival margin to the mucogingival junction. In a position apical to the mu-

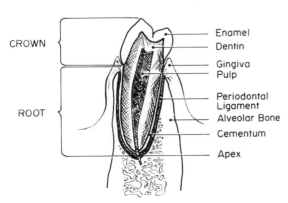

Figure 69–2. The dental anatomic unit.

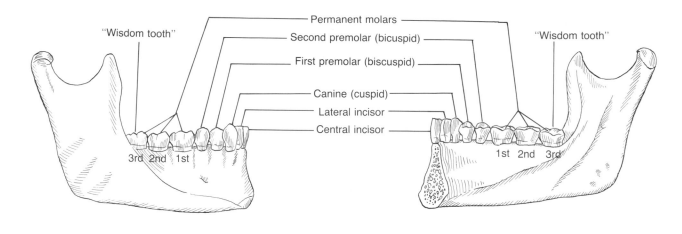

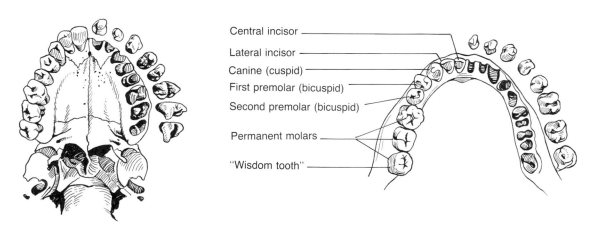

Figure 69–3. Classification of teeth. (Redrawn from Grant, J., and Basmajian, J.: Grant's Method of Anatomy, 7th ed. Baltimore, Williams & Wilkins, 1965.)

cogingival junction is the *alveolar mucosa,* which is covered by a nonkeratinized, stratified squamous epithelium and is continuous with the mucosa of the lip and the cheek.

In healthy individuals, the gingiva is attached tightly to the tooth. From a level that is coronal to the margin of the alveolar bone to the level of the cementoenamel junction, connective tissue fibers from the gingiva insert into the cementum of the root.

Coronally to the epithelial attachment is a space bounded on one side by enamel and on the other by a continuation of the gingival epithelium. This space is called the *gingival sulcus.* It is the cuff that is formed around the necks of the teeth by the gingival tissues. The gingiva lining this space is not attached to the tooth and is therefore called

free gingiva. The gingiva apical to the base of the gingival sulcus is called *attached gingiva.* In the healthy periodontium, the gingival sulcus is rarely greater than 2 to 3 mm in depth.

The *attachment apparatus* is, as the name implies, the group of structures that attach the teeth to the jaws. It consists of the cementum covering the root, the alveolar bone surrounding the root, and the periodontal ligament. The periodontal ligament is composed of collagen fibers that insert on one end in the alveolar bone and on the other end in the cementum. It is important to note that the union of the tooth to the alveolar bone is not a direct calcific union but a fibrous attachment. The anatomy of the dental unit (crown and root) and the periodontium is illustrated in cross section in Figure 69–2.

Dental Alveolar Trauma

FRACTURES OF TEETH

The simplest type of dental trauma involves the fracture of anterior teeth. The management of dental fractures is based on (1) the extent of the fracture in relation to the pulp of the tooth and (2) the age of the patient. A classification system, the Ellis system, was developed to describe the anatomy of fractures of teeth. The emergency physician may alternatively use a descriptive classification of traumatic injuries to teeth and supporting structures, as advocated by Johnson.[1]

The Ellis class I fracture involves only the enamel portion of the tooth (Fig. 69–4). This is generally a minor problem and requires immediate intervention only if a sharp piece of tooth is causing trauma to soft tissues. In such situations, the rough edge may be smoothed with something as simple as an emery board, or the patient may be referred at his convenience to a general dentist for more definitive management. What is perhaps most important is that the emergency physician can reassure anxious parents that with the new plastic enamel bonding materials, a cosmetic restoration of the tooth is possible. It would be inappropriate for the emergency physician to attempt the immediate restoration of these teeth; however, no irreversible damage would occur from the smoothing of rough edges. These fractures are not painful and do not result in sensitivity to heat or cold.

The Ellis class II fracture is a more complicated fracture in that it involves not only the enamel but also the exposure of dentin. On inspection, dentin is identified by its pinkish or yellow appearance as opposed to the white hue of enamel. The patient with exposed dentin may frequently complain of sensitivity to hot or cold or even air. The immediate treatment of the Ellis class II fracture is dictated by the age of the patient (Table 69–1). Since as the tooth matures the pulp continues to produce a larger amount of dentin and the pulp itself shrinks in size, the dentin that is exposed in

Table 69–1. ERUPTION OF DECIDUOUS AND PERMANENT ANTERIOR TEETH

Deciduous Teeth	Eruption (Months)	Root Completed (Years)
Central incisor	6–9	½–2
Lateral incisor	7–10	1½–2
Cuspid	16–20	2½–3
Permanent Teeth	Eruption (Years)	Root Completed (Years)
Maxillary central incisor	7–8	10
Maxillary lateral incisor	8–9	11
Maxillary cuspid	11–12	13–15
Mandibular central incisor	6–7	9
Mandibular lateral incisor	7–8	10
Mandibular cuspid	9–11	12–14

Adapted from Wheeler R: Dental Anatomy and Physiology. Philadelphia, W. B. Saunders Company, 1969, p. 30.

the Ellis class II fractures in patients less than 12 years of age is closer to pulpal tissue.

Because dentin is a microtubular structure that can permit the passage of microorganisms from the oral environment directly to the pulp, contamination and resulting inflammation to the pulp can be anticipated in affected patients if dentin is exposed to the oral environment for more than 24 hours. Therefore, because of the possibility of damage to the pulp, the management of Ellis class II fractures in younger patients (under 12 years of age) requires the immediate placement of a dressing on the exposed dentin. The dressing not only provides pain relief but also helps prevent infection.

A simple dressing that the emergency physician can apply consists of a calcium hydroxide resin paste (Dycal), which is available from dental supply companies (Fig. 69–5). One prepares calcium

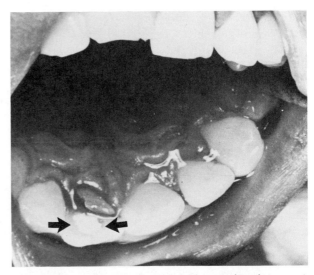

Figure 69–5. Temporary dressing for fractured tooth (*arrows*).

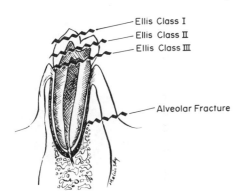

Figure 69–4. Ellis classification for fractured alveolar teeth.

hydroxide paste by mixing a small amount of base and accelerator from two tubes with an applicator. The exposed dentin is dried with a piece of gauze, and a small amount of calcium hydroxide is placed on the exposed area with a cleansed applicator instrument; the tooth surface must be perfectly dry or the Dycal will not adhere. The tooth is then covered with a small piece of tin foil or dental "dry" foil. Dycal will set in approximately 2 minutes and will set more quickly if exposed to humidity. Dycal is easily removed by the dentist. Patients are advised not to eat to prevent dislodging of the Dycal dressing.

More sophisticated techniques involve covering the tooth with the plastic bonding materials described previously; an aesthetic restoration will then result. The patient treated by the emergency physician requires referral within 24 hours. In simple class II fractures, older patients (12 to 14 years), who have a greater dentin-to-pulp ratio, may be advised to avoid extremes in temperature and to seek dental care the following day. A protective dressing need not be routinely applied. Patients with severe Ellis class II fractures (which may usually be recognized because of their larger exposed areas of pinkish- or yellowish-tinged dentin) should be treated with a dressing in a manner similar to that for younger patients. Analgesics may also be required, depending on the degree of sensitivity of the patient. It should be noted that the correct management of Ellis class II fractures may obviate the need for root canal therapy. The emergency physician, however, should warn any patient who has sustained trauma to the anterior teeth, no matter how minor, that disruption of the neurovascular supply to the tooth may have occurred. The long-term complication of the initial trauma may be necrosis of the pulp or resorption (dissolving) of the root.

Ellis class III fractures of the teeth involve, in addition to fracture of enamel and exposure of dentin, the actual exposure of the pulp. One may differentiate the Ellis class III fracture from the Ellis class II fracture by gently wiping a tooth clean with a piece of gauze to remove any blood that may be present from soft tissue trauma. The tooth is then examined for any red blush of dentin or frank drops of blood that may be extruded from the pulp. A patient may complain of exquisite pain; however, on occasion the tooth may be in "shock," in which case the patient will feel little sensitivity in the tooth.

Ellis class III fractures are true dental emergencies and require immediate attention from a general dentist or endodontist (root canal specialist) (Fig. 69–6). Ultimate treatment will consist of the total removal of pulpal tissue (pulpectomy). Alternatively, in the case of primary teeth, partial amputation of pulpal tissue (pulpotomy) may be performed. Delaying either of these procedures will result in significant pain and, probably, abscess formation. If a dentist is not immediately available, the tooth may be temporarily covered with tin foil so as to minimize pulpal irritation and pain. Because of bleeding or other sources of moisture, it may be difficult to apply Dycal to these fractures effectively. Analgesics should be prescribed, and the patient should be told to see a dentist as soon as possible. It should be noted that one should neither prescribe nor apply any of the over-the-counter topical dental analgesic preparations. Although these agents may give the patient temporary relief from pulpal pain, they often cause severe soft tissue damage because of

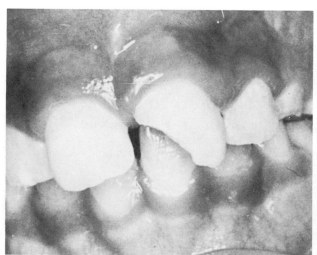 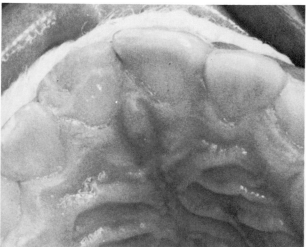

Figure 69–6. Recognition of the Ellis III fracture. (From Johnson, R.: The treatment of the child patient. *In* University of Pennsylvania School of Dental Medicine: Continuing Dental Education, vol. 2, no. 2. Philadelphia, University of Pennsylvania, Oct. 1978. Used by permission.)

their irritant effects. Use of these agents has been known to result in sterile abscesses. In all cases of tooth fracture, the soft tissue should be palpated for tooth fragments and radiographed if swelling limits the examination and if one has not accounted for tooth fragments.

SUBLUXATION AND AVULSED TEETH

The same force that may have resulted in the fracture of anterior teeth may also result in actual loosening of the tooth in its socket. This is called subluxation. Traumatized teeth should always be examined for subluxation by pressure applied with the fingers or with two tongue blades on each side of the tooth. The tooth is wiggled in a back-and-forth motion. A more subtle indication that teeth have been traumatized is the appearance of blood in the gingival crevice of the tooth. Teeth that are minimally mobile usually heal well if the patient is kept on a soft diet for 1 to 2 weeks. Teeth that appear grossly mobile to the eye require stabilization as soon as possible. The techniques for stabilization will be described later. Although stabilization procedures are usually performed by the general dentist or the oral and maxillofacial surgeon, the techniques that will be described can be used by the emergency physician who is trained in such procedures. As a temporary measure for teeth that are very loose, it is often useful to have the patient bite gently on a piece of gauze to keep the tooth in place pending examination by a dentist or an oral surgeon.

Avulsed and Intruded Teeth

Teeth that have been completely avulsed from the socket constitute a true dental emergency. If the patient is unaware of the location of the missing tooth, a complete *intrusion* of the tooth below the level of the gingiva must be ruled out with a radiograph (Fig. 69–7). An intruded tooth has been forced back into the alveolar bone, implying disruption of the supporting structures and possible fracture of the alveolar bone. Intrusion may be missed by a superficial examination, and one should not automatically conclude that all spaces in dentition following trauma represent avulsed teeth. Dice and coworkers[2] have reported a case in which an intruded tooth was initially thought to be a fractured tooth; a facial cellulitis and subsequent periodontal infection developed as a result of the misdiagnosis. Intruded primary teeth ("baby teeth") in the absence of infection are allowed to erupt for 6 weeks prior to considering repositioning. Intruded permanent teeth are surgically repositioned with a forcep and are then stabilized. Failure to diagnose intruded teeth may also result in cosmetic deformity.

As in other cases of dental alveolar trauma, the management of an avulsed tooth depends upon the age of the patient and the length of time that the tooth has been absent from the oral cavity. Avulsed primary anterior teeth in the pediatric patient (aged 6 months to 5 years) *are not replaced into their sockets.* Loss of these primary anterior teeth poses no threat to normal development and alignment of permanent teeth. Reimplanted primary teeth have a high tendency to ankylose, or fuse to the bone itself. The most serious consequence of an ankylosed primary tooth is facial deformity in the child. As growth continues, it may hinder the eruption of the permanent tooth, and as time progresses ankylosed teeth are surgically more difficult to remove. Temporary prosthetic replacement of avulsed primary teeth is easily accomplished if a cosmetic effect is desired.

In general, *permanent* teeth should be replaced in their sockets as soon as possible. It must be

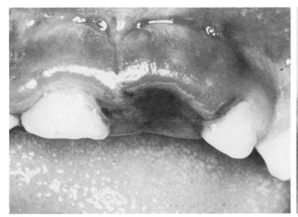
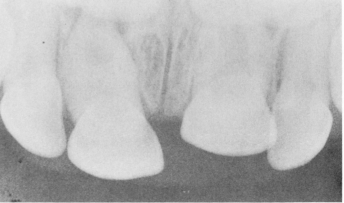

Figure 69–7. Intruded tooth secondary to trauma. A dental radiograph is necessary to determine intrusion or avulsion. (From Johnson, R.: The treatment of the traumatized incisor in the child patient. *In* University of Pennsylvania School of Dental Medicine: Continuing Dental Education, vol. 2, no. 2. Philadelphia, University of Pennsylvania, Oct. 1978. Used by permission.)

remembered that a percentage point for successful reimplantation is lost every minute that the tooth is absent from the oral cavity. Therefore, when a call is received about an avulsed tooth, the first question that should be asked is the age of the patient. If it has been determined that the tooth is permanent, the parent or patient should be instructed to rinse the tooth under running tap water quickly and to reimplant the tooth in its socket immediately. If actual reimplantation is not possible, the patient should be advised to bring the tooth to the emergency unit as quickly as possible in moist gauze or a cup of water or milk. Ideally, the patient may be allowed to place the tooth in his own mouth to bathe in saliva. In all cases, one should attempt to prevent dehydration of the avulsed tooth, since teeth that become dehydrated have the poorest prognosis for healing.

The procedure for the reimplantation of permanent teeth in the emergency unit is illustrated in Figure 69–8. The avulsed tooth is held by the crown at all times. It is rinsed under saline or under running water but is *not* scrubbed in order to conserve as much of the remaining periodontal ligament fibers as possible, since these fibers ultimately play a role in reattachment. The socket is then inspected. Blood clots or bone fragments, which may prevent reimplantation, should be irrigated or removed by gentle suction. When reimplantation is delayed (½ hour or more), local anesthesia is suggested (see later). The socket is suctioned and debrided of foreign matter, and the tooth is immediately reimplanted. The socket should not be sharply scraped, since this may damage the periodontal ligament or the attachment fibers. If the tooth will not fully sit in the socket as compared with the alignment of the adjacent teeth or if there is confusion as to the position of the tooth after reimplantation, the procedure should stop at this point. The patient should then gently bite on a piece of gauze until seen by a general dentist or an oral and maxillofacial surgeon.

Prognosis of Avulsed Teeth. When a tooth is avulsed, the neurovascular supply to the tooth is completely disrupted. If the tooth is reimplanted within a few minutes, there may be some restoration of the neurovascular supply, but most avulsions result in hypoxia and ultimate necrosis of the pulp. Therefore, almost all reimplanted teeth will require subsequent root canal therapy within a short period. The purpose of root canal therapy is to debride the pulp, to render the tooth insensitive to pain, and to fill and seal the pulp chamber with an inert material. This inert material prevents infection or chronic inflammation, which may interfere with stabilization of the tooth by the periodontal ligament.

The object of immediate reimplantation is not necessarily to keep the tooth alive but to keep the periodontal ligament alive, thus assuring a retained functional tooth. Healing of the periodontal ligament is variable following reimplantation. In addition, some resorption of the root surface always follows replantation. The degree of resorption varies and may even result in ankylosis of the tooth with surrounding bone. Although the long-term prognosis favors retaining an avulsed tooth if timely treatment is available, the patient should always be advised of the possibility of losing the tooth in a few months to a number of years following replantation. In general, immature permanent teeth have a better prognosis for survival than do older teeth.

Stabilization Techniques. Avulsed teeth require immediate stabilization so that they will not exfoliate. Although stabilization is normally performed by the general dentist or the oral and maxillofacial surgeon, there are situations in which it may be performed by the emergency physician. Stabilization is indicated in the case of a single avulsed tooth that has been placed back into the socket with satisfactory alignment. Satisfactory alignment of the tooth is judged both by visual inspection and by a report from the patient that there is no prematurity of occlusion when the jaw is closed. Even a millimeter of extrusion of a reimplanted tooth may cause occlusal disharmony in some patients, and we believe that finite occlusal adjustment should not be performed by the emergency physician.

Any tooth stabilized by the emergency physician should be evaluated by the general dentist or the oral and maxillofacial surgeon within 24 hours. Several techniques are available to the emergency physician for the stabilization of a single avulsed tooth. The application of Erich arch bars is perhaps the oldest technique used for stabilization of avulsed teeth. These arch bars are also used for the stabilization of mandibular and maxillofacial fractures. Figure 69–9 shows the application of the Erich-type arch bar. The application of the arch bar is not a simple technique and consequently is not recommended for application by the nondentist. A temporary measure to stabilize avulsed or subluxated teeth in the emergency unit by nondentists has been described by Medford.[3] A temporary splint that has been accepted by the Council on Dental Therapeutics of the American Dental Association[4] is the commercially available Coe-Pak (Coe Laboratories, Inc., Chicago, Illinois). Coe-Pak is a zinc oxide preparation that sets to semihardness. It is prepared from tubes that contain a base and a catalyst (Fig. 69–10). Following reimplantation of the tooth, the splint material is applied in a soft, clay-like consistency and is molded

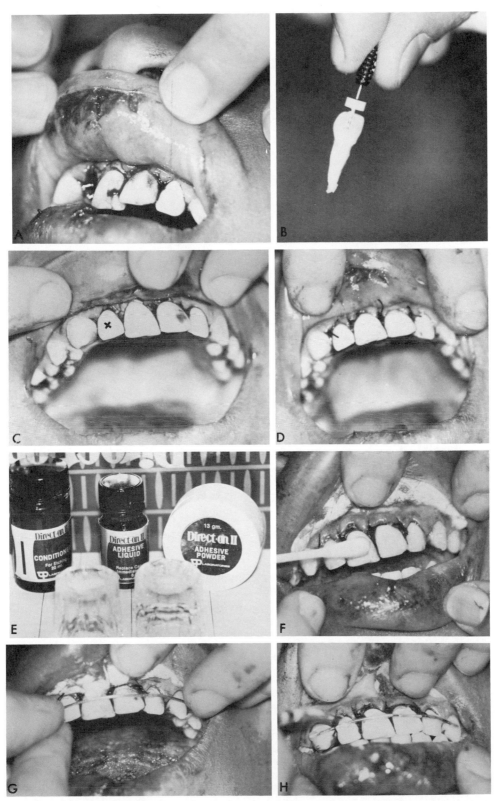

Figure 69–8. Procedure for reimplantation and stabilization of avulsed permanent teeth. *A* and *B*, The tooth is held in gauze and rinsed; root canal therapy is performed, if indicated. *C*, The tooth is reimplanted (marked with an *x*). *D*, Gingival lacerations are closed. The tooth is then acid-etched and bonded to the arch wire. *E*, Direct-on system. *F*, Acid etching. *G*, Wire application. *H*, Wire bonding.

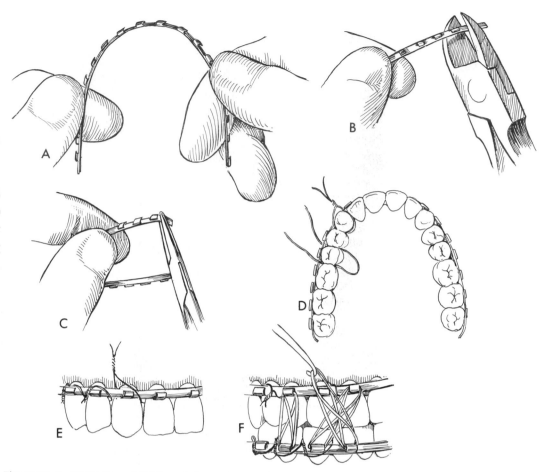

Figure 69–9. Application of Erich arch bars. *A, B,* and *C,* Commercially available arch bar is shaped to fit the maxillary and mandibular arches. *D* and *E,* Stainless steel wire secures the bar to the necks of the teeth. *F,* The maxilla and the mandible are brought into occlusion and are held in place with rubber bands. (From Converse, J. M.: Reconstructive Plastic Surgery, 2nd ed., vol. 2. Philadelphia, W. B. Saunders Co., 1977. Used by permission.)

over the gingival line and into the spaces between the teeth. A liquid diet is possible with the splint in place, and the patient should be directed to see a dentist within 24 hours.

Another system is available for stabilization of teeth. The avulsed teeth are first stabilized with light ligature wire (Fig. 69–11). Light ligature wire

is approximately 28 gauge. A band of wire is looped circumferentially around the avulsed tooth. The area encompassed by the wire should also include at least one to two teeth adjacent to the avulsed tooth. For example, in the case of an avulsed upper left central incisor, the wire would include the upper right lateral incisor and the

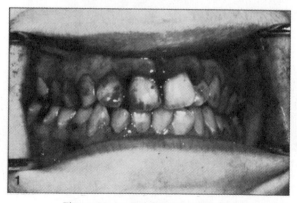

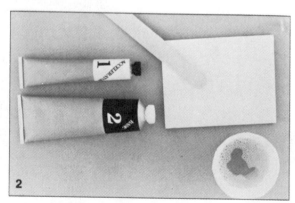

Figure 69–10. Stabilization of teeth with Coe-Pak. *1,* Dental trauma on examination. *2,* Armamentarium.

Illustration continued on opposite page.

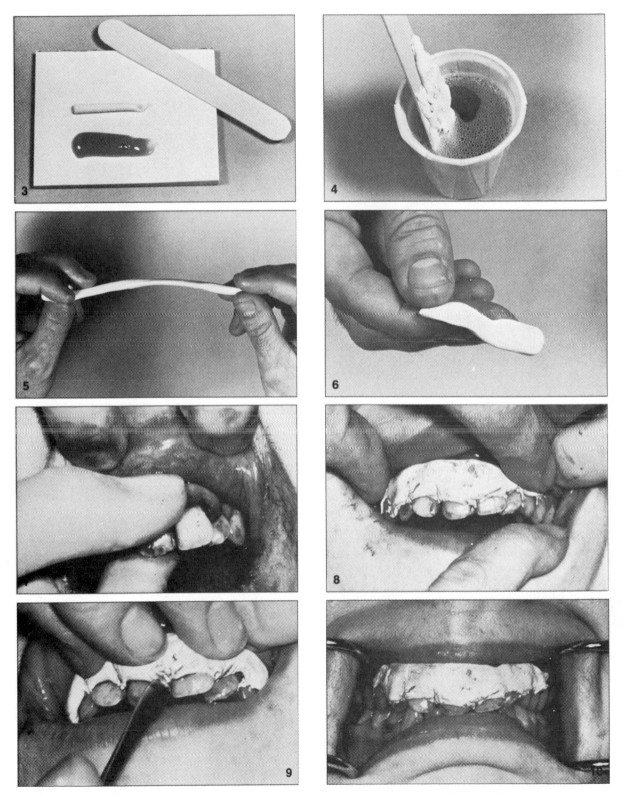

Figure 69–10 *(Continued)*. *3*, Dispensation of ingredients. *4*, Storage of spatulated splint material. *5*, Shaping the splint material into rope form. *6*, The splint material ready for application. *7*, Repositioning the traumatized teeth. *8*, Applying the splint to the cervical line and embrasures. *9*, Adapting the splint to the embrasures with a blunt instrument. *10*, Patient in full closure to check for interferences. (From Medford, H. M.: Temporary stabilization of avulsed or luxated teeth. Ann. Emerg. Med. 11:490, 1982. Used by permission.)

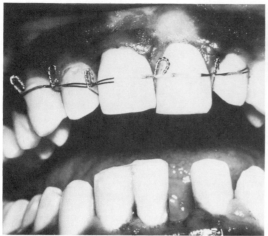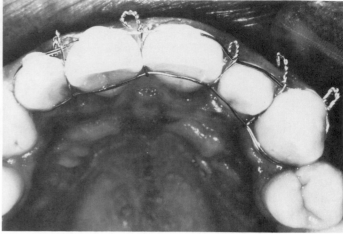

Figure 69–11. Stabilization of teeth with ligature wire.

upper left lateral incisor or canine tooth. The wire is gently wrapped at the area of the canine tooth. This wire is further stabilized interdentally with small sections of wire. These are passed labially above the light ligature wire and interdentally over both sections of it in a lingual direction. They are then brought anteriorly under both sections of the wire and are finally tied on the anterior side. The interdental sections are secured, and the initial wire is tightened at the area of the canine. Care must be taken at this point not to break the wire; if this occurs, the entire procedure must be redone. Light ligature wire has poor tensile strength and will loosen rapidly. Therefore, this wire is secured with bonding material made of beads of acid-etched resin. In addition to the acid etching, a material called "Direct-on," consisting of a powder and liquid, is used with a brush. Small beads of material are placed on the wire, bonding it to each individual tooth. This procedure may be performed in a matter of minutes.

Avulsed teeth are stabilized for approximately 10 days to 2 weeks and are then brought back into function. General precautions to be taken in order to avoid long-term complications are explained to the patient, as in any type of dentoalveolar trauma. When there are concomitant alveolar fractures, the stabilization of avulsed or subluxated teeth serves to stabilize not only the teeth but also their alveolar bone. In this situation, therapy is directed toward the conservation and healing of bone, and therefore stabilization is left for a minimum of 6 weeks, recognizing the risk of possible ankylosis of the teeth. The indiscriminate loss of alveolar bone will lead to much more difficult prosthetic restoration of this area than with the removal of an ankylosed tooth. Generally, prophylactic antibiotics (phenoxymethyl penicillin, 250 to 500 mg qid) are used when avulsed teeth are reimplanted in the oral cavity. Tetanus prophylaxis should also be instituted when needed.

LACERATIONS ASSOCIATED WITH DENTOALVEOLAR TRAUMA

Subluxated or avulsed teeth are frequently accompanied by associated lacerations of the gingiva, the mucosa, the lips, and other facial soft tissues. Emergency physicians must remember that the stabilization procedures described previously should always precede the definitive closure of any soft tissue laceration. The lips and the oral mucosa undergo constant manipulation during the stabilization procedures for teeth; therefore, carefully placed sutures may be torn and may increase the existing soft tissue injury, making aesthetic closure more difficult. Plastic closure, once dental stabilization has been first performed, may then be left undisturbed.

Gingival avulsions should be placed in approximately their original position with fine silk sutures. Gingiva is very friable, and suturing may be difficult. The suture may be passed between teeth and may be anchored to the mucosa on the other side of the teeth. When appropriate, patients with large gingival avulsions should be referred to the oral surgeon.

A frequently encountered problem is that of the through-and-through laceration resulting in an open communication between the skin and the oral cavity. This may result from a tooth being forced through the upper or lower lip. Occasionally, pieces of a fractured tooth are found imbedded in the soft tissue. Devitalized tissue should be removed by sharp debridement, and the area should be irrigated under pressure. After appropriate debridement and irrigation, it is best to close mucosal lacerations larger than 0.5 cm with sutures. Mucosal lacerations can be closed with 4-0 chromic or 3-0–4-0 black silk sutures; gingival lacerations are closed with 4-0 black silk. The cut ends of nylon sutures are very irritating and should not be used. Large, open intraoral mucosal lacerations result in much discomfort for the patient and frequently become infected from the accumulation of debris.

Patients with sutured intraoral lacerations are advised to keep the area clean by rinsing with warm saline and swabbing locally with hydrogen peroxide. Lip sutures may be covered with a thick coating of petrolleum jelly or antibiotic ointment. Patients are given the usual wound precautions and are checked within 24 to 48 hours. A certain amount of edema may be found when the wound is checked; in addition, a whitish granulation tissue, resembling pus, may have developed. The emergency physician should not immediately assume that this means that the area is infected. Significant pain usually signifies infection, however. If there is any suspicion of infection, the patient should be rechecked at 24-hour intervals until the edema has resolved. Frank infection should be treated with penicillin and hot compresses. Occasionally, sutures may need to be removed to promote drainage. Like patients with reimplanted avulsed teeth, individuals with through-and-through lacerations should be given tetanus prophylaxis; antibiotic coverage is often prescribed. Penicillin or erythromycin is advocated by many. It should be noted that there are few clinical studies to support the routine use of prophylactic antibiotics in intraoral lacerations. Skin sutures are frequently removed in 3 to 5 days to minimize scar formation. Intraoral sutures are removed in 5 to 7 days.

Hemorrhage

Oral hemorrhage may be spontaneous from the gingiva or, more commonly, may be the result of dental treatment, especially the surgical extraction of teeth. Patients with this complaint will frequently present at night, when their dentist or oral surgeon is not immediately available. A patient presenting with a bleeding gingiva should be questioned about any recent dental scaling, curettage, or prophylaxis. Such bleeding usually responds to peroxide mouth rinses and local pressure with gauze. In patients with advanced periodontal disease, small remnants of missed granulation tissue may ooze continously for hours. Spontaneous gingival hemorrhage without a history of recent dental therapy may be the initial presentation of a systemic process, e.g., leukemia or coagulopathy. A decision to investigate such hemorrhage with laboratory testing is based on the extent of the hemorrhage, the age of the patient, and other information obtained from the history and physical examination.

Most commonly, patients present with bleeding following dental extraction. Postextraction bleed-ing most often responds to sustained pressure, which can be produced by having the patient bite on gauze. Patients will frequently report that they have already been doing this for hours. One should then ask whether the patient has been spitting excessively, smoking cigarettes, or using straws, each of which may create a negative intraoral pressure. A negative intraoral pressure removes blood clots from sockets and aggravates postextraction bleeding.

The procedure for the management of postextraction bleeding is a very systematic one. If clots are present, they should be removed with suction or wiped with gauze. Patients are then instructed to bite on gauze for 15 to 20 minutes. If bleeding continues after 15 to 20 minutes, local anesthesia consisting of 2 per cent lidocaine (Xylocaine) with 1:100,000 or 1:50,000 epinephrine is infiltrated in the area of the socket to a point at which the tissue blanches (turns white). Gauze pressure is then reapplied. The epinephrine reduces bleeding, and the lidocaine allows the patient to bite without pain. Continued bleeding after 20 minutes may respond to the placement of a small piece of Surgicel or Gelfoam in the socket. This is then secured with a 3-0 black silk suture.

Sustained vigorous oozing after all the aforementioned procedures have been performed warrants a screening coagulation profile, consisting of a complete blood count with differential, prothrombin time and partial thromboplastin time and a platelet count. Postextraction bleeding is often caused by aspirin use. The patient must be questioned about all medication that may contain aspirin. Postextraction bleeding may also be the initial manifestation of a coagulopathy, such as hemophilia, especially in younger individuals. In some instances, postextraction bleeding results from improper surgical technique or flap design or lack of a sufficient number of sutures. Such flaps may need to be revised and resutured.

Following treatment, the emergency physician should warn the patient to avoid all liquids and solid foods for 2 hours and to avoid extremes in temperature, excessive spitting, smoking, or the use of straws or aspirin. If bleeding occurs at home, gauze pressure should be used.

The patient should be advised of the possibility that a *dry socket* will develop in 2 to 3 days. The patient becomes aware of a dry socket when excruciating pain develops in the area of the socket and a foul odor or taste occurs in the mouth after a day or two of no pain. Patients should know that the pain of a dry socket is easily managed by their dentist or an emergency physician. Application of local anesthesia to the area of the involved tooth, gentle irrigation of the socket, and application of an iodoform pack dipped in eugenol or Campho-Phenique or a commercial sedative dressing will relieve the pain. The packing is placed gently in the socket while avoiding manipulation of the walls of the socket. A dry socket is a localized alveolar osteitis. Because of the high incidence of osteomeylitis secondary to scraping of a dry socket to initiate bleeding, aggressive débridement of the dry socket is contraindicated.

Patients with dry sockets are frequently given oral antibiotics (penicillin or erythromycin is preferred). The use of topically applied antibiotics is not indicated because of the increased incidence of sensitivity reactions. The dressing is replaced at 24-hour intervals until the patient is pain-free.

In addition to dental extractions, bleeding is frequently seen after periodontal (gingival) surgery. The tissue involved in the surgical site is usually covered with a surgical dressing, which may be dislodged by bleeding. Bleeding following periodontal surgery will generally respond to gauze pressure. It should be noted, however, that the periodontal surgical dressings are extremely important for wound healing, and the incorrect placement of the pack can result in treatment failure. Therefore, the periodontist should be informed immediately that bleeding has occurred and should see the patient as soon as possible.

Drainage of Infection of Dental Origin

Acute infection of the oral cavity and the jaws can be minor or life-threatening. The most common dental infection is the periapical abscess, or the acute alveolar abscess, which usually begins in the periapical region of the tooth as a result of nonvitality or degeneration of the pulp. One can usually easily manage these infections by treating the tooth with endodontics or extraction.

Periodontal and pericoronal infections are generally more difficult to manage. Most intraoral infection will form an abscess and drain intraorally. When the infection is well contained, drainage of these areas is generally easy. Extension of this same infection to the fascial planes of the head and neck, however, may result in much more serious infection in the parapharyngeal space or may track exteriorly to drain at the surface of the skin (Fig. 69–12). Drainage of an infection of dental origin by the emergency physician should be limited to well-confined intraoral abscesses requiring intraoral drainage and fluctuant extraoral swellings that require drainage externally by an incision on the face.

PULPAL INFECTION (ABSCESSED TOOTH)

Although physical and chemical injuries to teeth result in pulpal necrosis and infection, dental infection most frequently is the result of a carious (decay) exposure of the pulp. Destruction of the enamel and the dentin by caries opens a portal to the pulp for oral microorganisms. Before invasion of the pulp by microorganisms, the affected tooth usually becomes sensitive. Invasion of the pulp produces either a localized or a generalized pulpal infection. If the portal of entry into the pulp is adequate to allow spontaneous drainage, the patient may be asymptomatic. If drainage is obstructed, rapid involvement of the entire pulp results in pulpal necrosis. The patient can experience moderate to severe pain that has been ranked second only to that of renal colic. Untreated inflammation progresses through the teeth and extends into the periapical region; irritation in this area by inflammatory products in the necrotic pulp may result in the formation of periapical granuloma. This process may be asymptomatic and will persist as long as drainage through the tooth continues.

Treatment consists of removing the infected pulp and obliterating the pulp chamber, allowing the tooth to remain (root canal therapy) or extracting the infected tooth and draining the periapical region. Antibiotic therapy is indicated if drainage cannot be established when the infection has perforated the cortex and has spread into the surrounding soft tissue. Frequently, physical examination will reveal a grossly decayed tooth. Alternatively, no apparent pathologic condition may be seen, or many teeth may appear decayed. One may localize the offending tooth by percussing individual teeth with a tongue blade; in most cases, tapping the involved tooth will elicit a sharp pain.

In most minor dental infections, oral phenoxymethyl penicillin in doses of 250 to 500 mg four times a day is the drug of choice. Erythromycin, 250 to 500 mg four times a day, and cephalexine (Keflex) are alternatives. Analgesics can be prescribed. If the infection has broken through the cortex and there is subperiosteal extension of the infection with swelling, incision and drainage is the treatment of choice, as in any abscess.

PERIODONTAL INFECTION

Periodontal disease is a progressively destructive bacterial process involving the supporting structures of the teeth, which include the gingiva, the periodontal ligament, and the alveolar bone. Unlike the relatively confined pulp chamber, inflammatory exudate produced in periodontal infection usually drains freely, and the patient experiences little, if any, discomfort. Significant symptoms may not be apparent for many years. If for any reason drainage from the infected area is interrupted, the inflammation will become acute

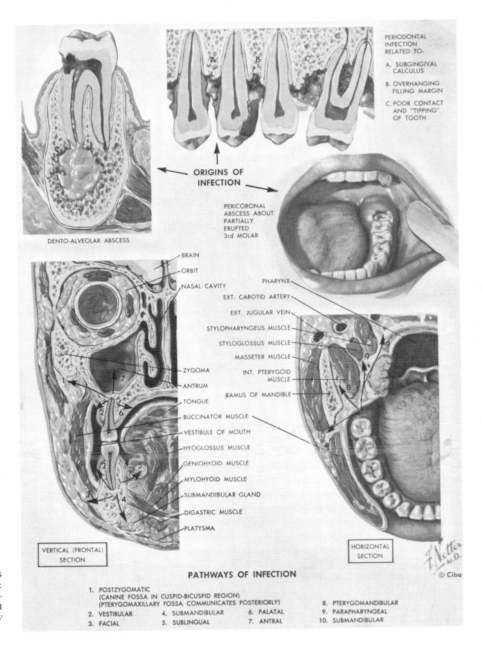

Figure 69–12. Origin and pathways of dental infection. (From Netter, F.: CIBA collection of medical illustrations, vol. 3: Digestive System, part I, section V, plate no. 6. Used by permission.)

and will be similar to an acute periapical infection that spreads to the soft tissue. The lack of a carious lesion in the involved tooth and a dental radiograph will help in distinguishing between these two processes. In most cases, acute periodontal infections will tend to remain in the intraoral soft tissues rather than spread to the face and the neck.

Immediate treatment of periodontal infections includes drainage of the infected tissue (see later), which may require removal of the involved tooth. Antibiotic therapy is usually instituted only if drainage cannot be achieved or if spread to tissues of the face and the neck has occurred. Follow-up periodontal therapy is needed to prevent recurrence. Warm saline rinses frequently promote drainage in periodontal areas, and antibiotics are

prescribed if there are systemic manifestations. The condition usually does not require urgent referral. Frequently, a scaling and curettage of the area will relieve the abscess. In the emergency unit, however, incision and drainage of the abscess is generally preferred.

PERICORONAL INFECTION

Pericoronitis occurs when debris and microorganisms become trapped under soft tissues that partially overlie the crown of a tooth, usually in an erupting or partially impacted third molar (wisdom tooth). A localized infection that drains from under the tissue becomes established. If drainage is interrupted by sudden swelling of the overlying

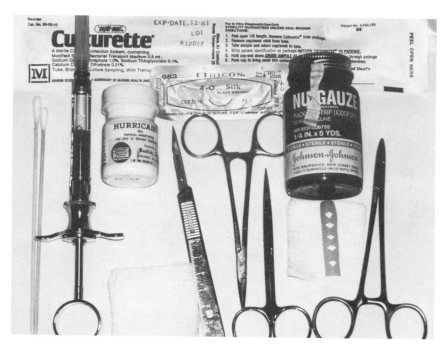

Figure 69–13. Equipment for incision and drainage of dental infection.

tissue, caused either by trauma from an impacted third molar or by the inflammatory process itself, the entrapped exudate will spread through other pathways, usually into the pterygomandibular or submasseteric spaces (see Fig. 69–12). The underlying bone is generally not involved. Clinically, marked trismus secondary to irritation of the masseter or the medial pterygoid muscles predominates. The pericoronal tissues are erythematous and swollen. Digital pressure in the area will often elicit pain and will produce a small amount of exudate under the infected flap.

Treatment includes antibiotics in virtually all cases. Removal of the impacted tooth or the infected tissue ensures good drainage. Frequent irrigations with warm saline during this period are beneficial and should be instituted immediately. An oral and maxillofacial surgeon should be consulted in 24 to 48 hours. Fluctuant swelling is amenable to incision and drainage. Soft tissue dissection should be performed with caution, since the space extends posteriorly in the retropharyngeal area. Incisions are made with great care in this region because of the possible proximity of the internal carotid artery, which may have been moved anteriorly with tissue swelling.

In many instances, progression of oral infection may cause acute facial cellulitis. The extent of the cellulitis, of course, is dependent upon the virulence of the organism and the resistance of the host. In general, cellulitis from odontogenic infections arising from the maxillary teeth will involve the lower half of the face and the neck. This pertains only to the earlier stages of infection, since in many instances the entire side of the face may be involved, regardless of the origin of infec-

tion. In the nondebilitated host, most untreated odontogenic infections tend to localize and drain spontaneously (usually extraorally).

TECHNIQUE OF INCISION AND DRAINAGE

Intraoral Technique

Before attempting incision and drainage of an intraoral abscess, the emergency physician should first determine whether the infection or abscess is a simple one. The patient should have minimal trismus and should be able to open the mouth widely to allow inspection of the pharynx. The area of maximal fluctuance is anesthetized superficially with either a topical anesthetic spray, such as Cetacaine, or (better) 2 per cent lidocaine (Xylocaine) with 1:50,000 epinephrine by injection until tissue blanching occurs. One should always remember that attainment of profound anesthesia in an infected site is often difficult. Superficial anesthetic techniques are used so as not to track infection more distally with a long needle.

The required equipment for incision and drainage consists of the instruments found in a standard incision and drainage tray (Fig. 69–13). A number 11 scalpel blade is recommended, as are a mosquito hemostat and drain material (such as ¼-inch iodoform gauze or a small 3-cm fenestrated Penrose drain). Antiseptic cleansing of the area to be drained is generally not necessary. A small 1-cm incision is made superficially over the area of fluctuance, with the point of the scalpel blade always facing toward the alveolar bone (Fig. 69–

14). Blunt dissection is then carried out with a mosquito hemostat to avoid any vascular structures. Cultures of draining pus may or may not be obtained. The drained area is copiously irrigated. If possible, one places the iodoform or the Penrose drain by packing the site and securing one end of the drain with a black silk suture (4-0) to prevent aspiration of the drain. The patient is instructed to continue warm salt water rinses hourly for the next 24 to 48 hours and to rinse several times during the night. The drain is removed in 24 to 48 hours, and intraoral rinsing is continued every 4 hours for another day. Patients generally begin taking oral antibiotics during the course of this therapy. Although the emergency physician may manage the initial phase of the dental infection, referral to a dentist or an oral and maxillofacial surgeon is required for definitive therapy of the infection.

Extraoral Technique

If the dental infections described in the preceding section do not drain intraorally, they may spread to the face. Again, the emergency physician must determine that the infection, although it has an extraoral spread, is a simple one. The patient should have no trismus, and the retropharynx should be adequately visualized. Drainage of an infection of dental origin on the face requires more attention and care because of the cosmetic consequences of the procedure (Fig. 69–15). The patient is placed in a reclining position and is externally draped well so as to prevent drainage of purulence on the patient's clothing, the stretcher, and other materials in the treatment area. The skin is cleansed with a scrub, prepared with povidone-iodine solution, and draped in an appropriate manner. The skin is anesthetized superficially with 2 per cent lidocaine (Xylocaine) and 1:100,000 epinephrine.

It is important to note that the incision in this case will not be made over the area of maximal fluctuance but inferiorly to the area of infection in a zone of *healthy* skin. A 1- to 1½-cm incision that follows the natural tissue line as closely as possible is made through skin and subcutaneous tissue; blunt dissection with a mosquito hemostat is then carried out toward the area of infection to establish drainage. A culture should be taken, and the area should be gently irrigated with saline. Again, a Penrose drain should be placed. The area is covered with a gauze dressing, and the patient is instructed to remove the dressing four times a day and to apply heat in order to promote drainage in this zone. It is important to note that this is one of the few indications for the application of warm compresses to the face in the presence of dental infection. In general, all attempts should be made to establish drainage intraorally, but this procedure is used when extraoral drainage is inevitable. Any facial infection of dental origin that would require 24 hours of heat to obtain maximal fluctuance for drainage extraorally could probably be managed at that time with intraoral drainage. Obviously, scarring will result from any extraoral drainage. Therefore, the procedure should be avoided if possible, but if it is necessary, the incision is made over healthy tissue.

Complicated Head and Neck Infections

The emergency physician is often responsible for the actual incision and drainage of simple dental infections. When the infections described previously extend to the fascial compartments of the head and the neck, they immediately fall into the serious and complicated category (Fig. 69–16). The spread of dental infection through fascial

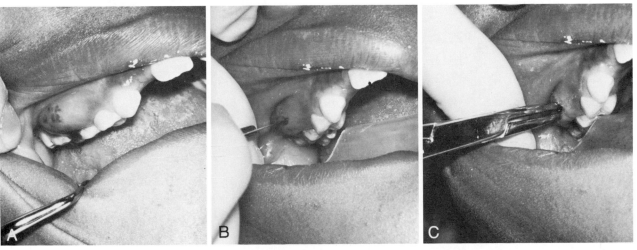

Figure 69–14. A, Drainage of localized dental infection. B, Incision. C, Blunt dissection.

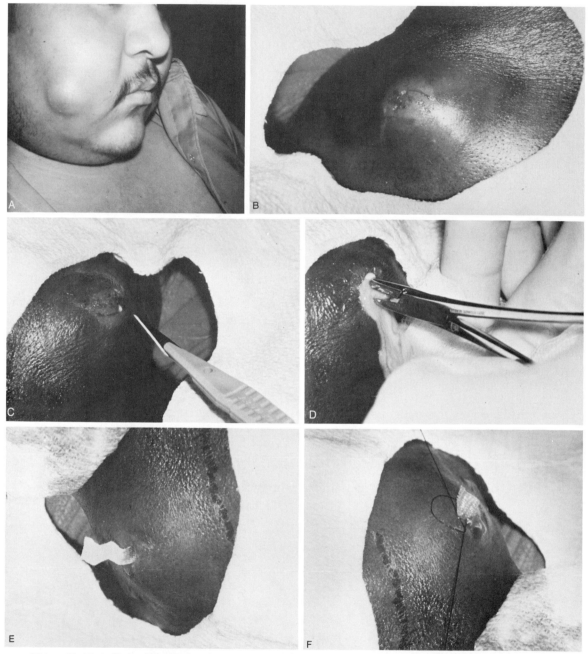

Figure 69–15. *A*, Illustration of a facial abscess that points extraorally. *B–F*, Technique of cutaneous drainage in a second patient. *B*, Anesthetic infiltrated below abscessed area. *C*, Incision. *D*, Drainage with blunt dissection. *E*, Gauze packing. *F*, Gauze sutured in place.

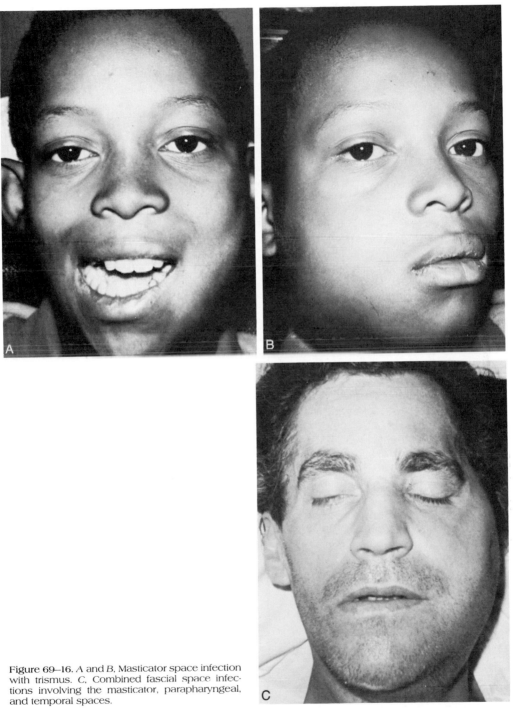

Figure 69–16. *A* and *B*, Masticator space infection with trismus. *C*, Combined fascial space infections involving the masticator, parapharyngeal, and temporal spaces.

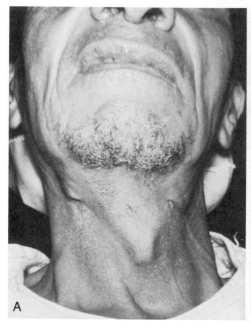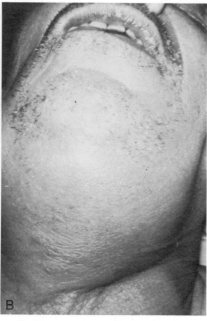

Figure 69–17. *A*, Ludwig's angina may initially appear benign. *B*, In Ludwig's angina, rapid progression may compromise the airway in a few hours.

planes of the head and the neck is particularly serious. Toxic febrile patients with marked trismus require immediate attention to airway and the early institution of intravenous antibiotics. The patient should immediately be referred to the oral and maxillofacial service for admission.

A common complicated infection of dental origin seen by the emergency physician is Ludwig's angina. This infection is a bilateral, board-like swelling involving the submandibular, submental, and sublingual spaces with elevation of the tongue. Emergency physicians frequently see affected patients prior to elevation of the tongue, during the initial manifestations of the infection. In the early stages, Ludwig's angina may appear deceptively benign (Fig. 69–17*A*). Brawny induration is characteristic, and there is no fluctuance present for incision and drainage. Infection is commonly caused by hemolytic *Streptococcus* organisms, although it may be a *Staphylococcus/Streptococcus* mixed infection or a combination of aerobic or anaerobic organisms. The presence of anaerobes commonly accounts for the presence of gas in the tissues. Chills, fever, difficulty in swallowing, stiffness of tongue movements, and trismus are common presenting signs. Respiration becomes increasingly difficult as the tongue is elevated, and the oral pharynx becomes edematous (Fig. 69–17*B*). Progression to airway obstruction may be rapid—over only a few hours.

Treatment consists of high-dose intravenous antibiotic therapy. Intubation or tracheostomy should be considered in the acute stage to maintain the airway if respiration becomes embarrassed. Constant observation is important, since the airway may become obstructed without much warning. Although hospital admission (preferably in a surgical intensive care setting) is mandatory, surgical intervention may be required only if antibiotic therapy is not successful. The most common locations of dental infection in this condition are the lower second and third molar teeth; pus formation usually occurs medially or on the lingual aspect of the mandible. In Ludwig's angina as in any parapharyngeal space infection, mediastinal descent can occur because of the communication of the parapharyngeal space with the visceral space.

THERAPEUTIC CONSIDERATIONS

The most important therapeutic modality for pyogenic orofacial infections of odontogenic origin is surgical drainage and removal of necrotic tissue. The need for definitive restoration or extraction of the infected teeth, the primary source of infection, is readily apparent. Antibiotic therapy, although important in halting local spread of infection and preventing hematogenous dissemination, cannot substitute for evacuation of pus.

Penicillin remains the antibiotic of choice for treating orofacial infections of odontogenic origin. *Bacteroides fragilis*, which is highly resistant to penicillin, is not normally a resident in the oral cavity; however, this organism has been recovered in 15 to 20 per cent of anaerobic pleuropulmonary infections and is presumably related to aspiration of oropharyngeal flora. It is interesting to note that penicillin has remained effective in such cases despite recovery of this organism as part of the mixed flora.

Cephalosporins, particularly cefoxitin (Mefoxin), may be excellent alternatives for penicillin-allergic patients, since the action of these agents against oral-obligate anaerobes is comparable with that of penicillin and they also are effective against certain aerobic bacteria. The usual dosage of a cephalosporin is 1 to 2 gm intramuscularly or intravenously every 6 hours. Clindamycin (600 mg intramuscularly or intravenously every 8 hours) is also highly effective, especially against anaerobes, when used in a controlled fashion and when possible side effects are monitored. Erythromycin is generally active against most indigenous oral bacteria but is compartively less active against anaerobic and microaerophilic streptococci, *Fusobacterium*, and anaerobic gram-negative cocci. Chloramphenicol, although highly active against obligate anaerobes, is potentially toxic and should be reserved for situations in which the pathogenic role of *B. fragilis* is of prime importance or for use as an alternative agent in patients allergic to penicillin, cephalosporins, or clindamycin.

Intra- and Extraoral Local Anesthesia

The use of intraoral and extraoral regional anesthesia is both simple and convenient. Nerve blocks are used to attain anesthesia in areas of broad distribution in the face with a minimal amount of anesthetic and tissue distortion. Local anesthetic blocks are effective for closing facial lacerations, especially those of the lips, the forehead, and the mid-face, where the swelling caused by local infiltration is undesirable. Local anesthetic blocks are also effective for the relief of pain, for anesthesia in debridement, and for diagnostic purposes.

The procedures and techniques described here generally carry a low morbidity. The supraperiosteal and mental infiltrations can generally be learned through reading and experimentation; more sophisticated blocks are best learned under the instruction of an experienced physician, a dentist, or an oral and maxillofacial surgeon.

ANATOMY OF THE FIFTH, OR TRIGEMINAL, NERVE

The fifth cranial nerve (the trigeminal nerve) is the sensory nerve to the face (Fig. 69–18*A*) and is the largest of the cranial nerves. It takes its origin from the midbrain and enlarges into the gasserian, or semilunar, ganglion. One gasserian ganglion supplies each side of the face. The gasserian ganglion is a flat, crescent-shaped structure approximately 10 mm long and 20 mm wide that divides into three branches: the ophthalmic, maxillary, and mandibular nerves (Fig. 69–18*B*).

The first division, the ophthalmic nerve (V-1), is the smallest branch in the gasserian ganglion. It leaves the cranium through the superior orbital fissure and has five cutaneous branches. These branches are:

1. The medial and lateral branches of the supraorbital nerve, which emerge on the face through the supraorbital notch. These two sensory nerves pierce the frontalis muscle and extend to the lambdoid suture on the back of the skull.

2. The supratrochlear nerve, which is sensory to the medial aspect of the forehead just above the glabella.

3. The infratrochlear nerve.

4. The lacrimal nerve.

5. The external nasal nerve.

In addition to being sensory to the forehead, branches of the ophthalmic nerve are sensory to the cornea, the upper eyelid, structures in the orbit, and the frontal sinuses.

The second division, the maxillary nerve (V-2), is sensory to the maxilla and associated structures, such as the teeth, the periosteum and the mucous membranes of the maxillary sinus and the nasal cavity, the soft and hard palate, the lower eyelids, the upper lip, and the side of the nose. The second division exits the cranium from the foramen rotundum and ultimately enters the face through the infraorbital canal; it terminates as the infraorbital nerve. The infraorbital nerve gives sensory branches to the lower eyelids, the side of the nose, and the upper lip.

The detailed anatomy of the maxillary nerve is rather complicated, consisting of a number of branches. The first branch comprises two short sphenopalatine nerves to the pterygopalatine ganglion, also called Meckel's ganglion or the sphenopalatine ganglion. The next two branches of clinical importance are the nasopalatine and the greater (anterior) palatine nerves. The nasopalatine nerve arises from the pterygopalatine ganglion, courses down along the nasal septum, and is transmitted through the anterior portion of the hard palate by way of the anterior palatine canal. This canal is located in the median line approximately 10 mm palatally to the maxillary central teeth and immediately behind the incisors. The nasopalatine nerve is sensory to the most anterior portion of the hard palate and the adjacent gum margins of the upper incisors. This nerve is rarely blocked in clinical practice, except in dental operations (Fig. 69–19*A*). The anterior, or great palatine, nerve arises from the pterygopalatine ganglion and passes down through the posterior palatine foramen. The posterior palatine foramen is located 10 mm palatally to the third molar and the bicuspid teeth and intermingles with the nasopalatine nerve opposite the cuspid tooth. The greater palatine nerve is sensory to most of the

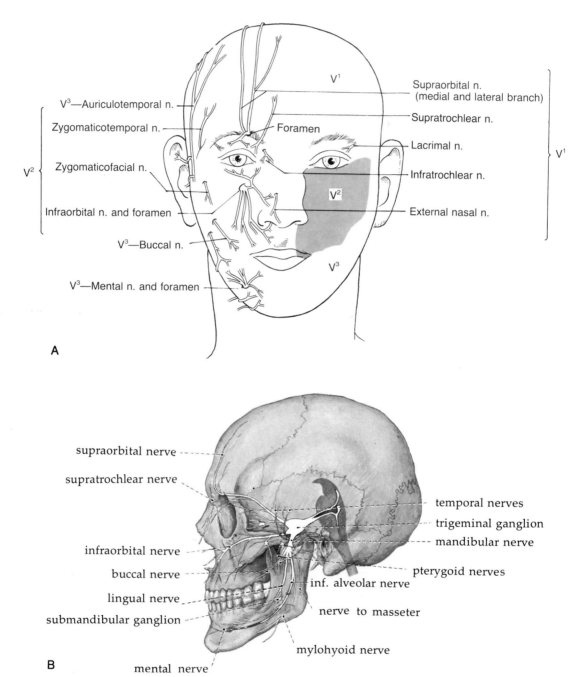

Figure 69–18. *A*, Cutaneous distribution of the trigeminal nerve. Note that the supraorbital, infraorbital, and mental foramina are all in line with the pupil when the patient looks straight ahead. *B*, Branches of the trigeminal nerve. (From Langman, J., and Woerdeman, M. W.: Atlas of Medical Anatomy. Philadelphia, W. B. Saunders Company, 1978. Used by permission.)

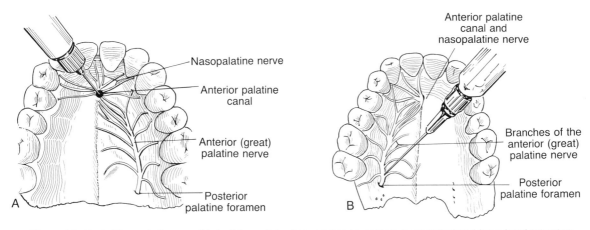

Figure 69-19. *A,* The anterior one third of the palate, from canine to canine, is anesthetized by a local injection near the anterior palatine canal. There may be some overlapping branches of the anterior palatine nerve. *B,* Anesthesia of the posterior two thirds of the palate is obtained by a local injection in the area of the posterior palatine foramen. Note: *Do not enter the foramen itself, since the anesthetic may reach the middle palatine nerve and produce anesthesia of the soft palate, resulting in gagging.*

hard palate as well as the palatal aspect of the gingiva. It is rarely blocked in the emergency department (Fig. 69-19B).

The next branch consists of the posterior superior alveolar nerve, which courses down the posterior surface of the maxilla for approximately 20 mm, at which point it enters one or several small posterior superior dental foramina. This nerve supplies all the roots of the third and second molar teeth and two roots of the first molar tooth. A third branch consists of the middle superior alveolar nerve, which branches off about midway within the infraorbital canal and then courses downward in the outer wall of the maxillary sinus. This nerve supplies the maxilliary first and second bicuspid teeth and the mesiobuccal root of the first molar. The last branch consists of the anterior superior alveolar nerve, which branches off into the infraorbital canal approximately 5 mm behind the infraorbital foramen, just before the terminal branches of the infraorbital nerve emerge. This nerve descends in the anterior wall of the maxilla to supply the maxillary central, lateral, and cuspid teeth; the labial mucous membrane; the periosteum, and the alveoli on one side of the median line. There is an intercommunication between the anterior, middle, and posterior superior alveolar nerves.

The third division, the mandibular nerve (V-3), is the largest branch of the trigeminal nerve. It exists from the cranium through the foramen ovale and divides into three principal branches.

1. The long buccal nerve branches off just outside the foramen ovale. It passes between the two heads of the external pterygoid muscle and crosses in front of the ramus to enter the cheek through the buccinator muscle, buccally to the maxillary third molar. The buccal nerve supplies sensory branches to the buccal mucous membrane and the mucoperiosteum over the maxillary and mandi-

bular teeth. The cutaneous branch is the sensory nerve to the cheek.

2. The lingual nerve courses forward toward the median line. The nerve courses downward superfically to the internal pterygoid muscle to pass lingually to the apex of the mandibular third molar. It enters the base of the tongue at this point through the floor of the mouth and supplies the anterior two thirds of the tongue, the lingual mucous membrane, and the mucoperiosteum.

3. The largest of the branches is the inferior alveolar nerve. It is sensory to all of the lower teeth, although the central and lateral incisors and the buccal aspect of the molar teeth may receive additional sensory innervation. The nerve descends, covered by the external pterygoid muscle, and passes between the ramus of the mandible and the sphenomandibular ligament to enter the mandibular canal. It is accompanied by the inferior alveolar artery and vein and proceeds along the mandibular canal, innervating the teeth. At the mental foramen, the nerve bifurcates into an incisive branch, which continues forward to supply the anterior teeth. It gives off a side branch, the mental nerve, which exits from the mental foramen to supply the skin. The mental foramen is located approximately between the apices of the lower first and second bicuspids, or premolar teeth. This is a very useful site, because it is sensory to the integument of the chin and the skin and the mucous membrane of the lower lip.

EQUIPMENT FOR DENTAL NERVE BLOCKS

One may easily give extraoral injections with standard injection equipment. Intraoral local anesthesia is conveniently administered with a monojet aspirating dental syringe, which uses carpules of

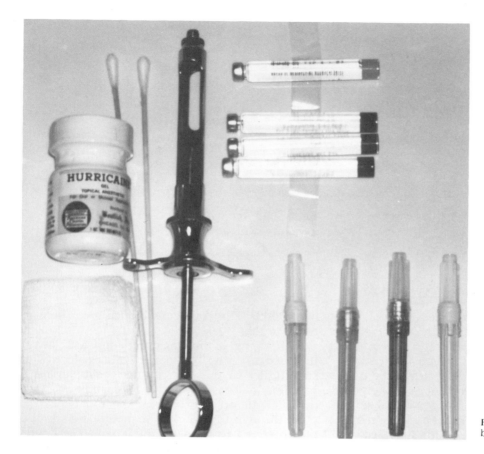

Figure 69–20. Local anesthesia—basic set-up for intraoral application.

anesthetic and disposable needles (Fig. 69–20). A needle not smaller than 27 gauge is recommended for deep block techniques. Generally, a long needle is used for block techniques and a short needle is used for infiltrations. The needle is screwed to the hub of the monojet syringe, which in turn is attached to an adaptor; the adaptor may be removed for cleaning. When removing the disposable needle, one must take care not to remove and discard the adaptor as well; this would render the syringe functionless (Fig. 69–21). One pulls back the end of the syringe on its spring, allowing room for the carpule of anesthetic to be

inserted (Fig. 69–22A). The metal end of the carpule is inserted, which engages the needle (Fig. 69–22B). The handle of the syringe is then released and tapped to engage a barb into the rubber stopper of the carpule (Fig. 69–22C). One now may perform simple aspiration by retracting the handle, pulling on the rubber stopper within the carpule.

To discard a carpule, one should leave the needle in place on the syringe. One withdraws the handle of the syringe rapidly, disengaging the barb. If the needle has been removed, great care must be taken, because the negative pressure

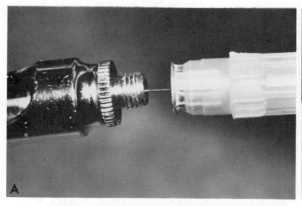
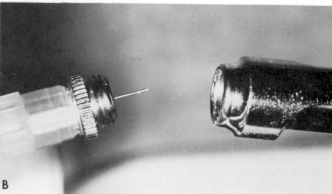

Figure 69–21. A, Proper technique for removal of the disposable hypodermic from the monojet syringe. B, Incorrect technique involves removal of the adapter.

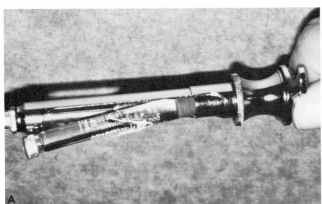

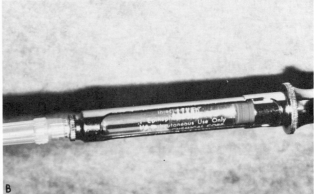

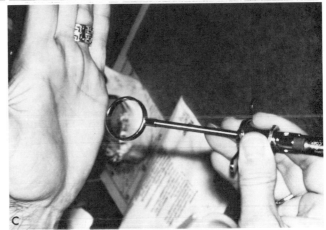

Figure 69–22. Loading the dental aspirating syringe. A, The end of the syringe is pulled back. B, The carpule engages the needle. C, The barb is snapped into place.

created in the carpule upon withdrawal of the barb may cause shattering. Other adjuncts that are helpful in the administration of intraoral anesthesia include topical local anesthetic agents, such as gels or sprays. It should be noted that dental syringes are not mandatory for intraoral local anesthesia but do make the procedure more simple. Reusable glass and disposable plastic aspirating syringes that do not use dental carpules are also available.

The anesthetic agent most frequently used is 2 per cent lidocaine with a vasoconstrictor, such as 1:100,000 or 1:50,000 epinephrine. Many other anesthetic agents, such as mepivacaine (Carbocaine) and Cetacaine with or without vasoconstrictor agents, are also available. Although available, bupivacaine (Marcaine) is frequently not found in dental carpules. A carpule of a different anesthetic may be emptied, however, and bupivacaine may be drawn up in the evacuated carpule. Because of the rich vascularity of the oral cavity, vasoconstrictors are important in sustaining the duration of anesthesia and should be used wherever possible when no medical contraindications exist.

GENERAL PRECAUTIONS

Needles no smaller than 27 gauge should be used for block techniques, because a higher gauge makes aspiration difficult and may lead to inadvertent intravascular injection. When an intraoral block procedure is performed, the needle should never be inserted to its full length at the hub. Should inadvertent breakage occur in such a situation, needle retrieval may be difficult. Furthermore, the direction of a needle should not be changed while the needle is deep in the tissue. Topical anesthetics can be placed on mucous membranes to make needle puncture painless. One should inject slowly to minimize pain and should always aspirate before injection.

An important precaution for intraoral local anesthesia is that the injection should not be made into or through an infected area. This is especially important in inferior alveolar nerve blocks, in which tracking of an infection can be serious and difficult to treat. Trismus, lack of access, and direct extension to parapharyngeal spaces can result. Therefore, local anesthesia should be only superficial prior to incision and drainage, unless a block can be performed far proximal to the site of infections.

OPHTHALMIC NERVE BLOCK

The lateral and medial branches of the supraorbital nerve, the supratrochlear nerve, and the infratrochlear nerve may be blocked as the nerves

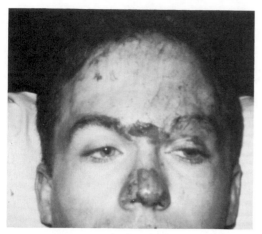

Figure 69–23. This patient had multiple small pieces of glass imbedded in the forehead from a windshield injury. Removal was accomplished painlessly with bilateral supraorbital and supratrochlear nerve blocks.

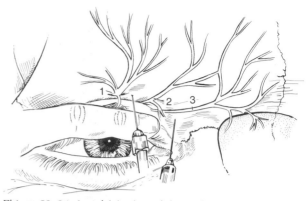

Figure 69–24. Local injection of the (1) lateral and (2) medial branch of the supraorbital nerve and the (3) supratrochlear nerve. It should be noted that a finger is placed on the inferior rim of the infraorbital rim to avoid swelling of the eyelid. (From Eriksson, E.: Illustrated Handbook in Local Anesthesia. Philadelphia, W. B. Saunders Co., 1980.)

emerge from the superior aspect of the orbit by a percutaneous local injection. Anesthesia of the forehead and the scalp is achieved as far posteriorly as the lambdoid suture. Although anesthesia is easily obtained for suturing lacerations of the forehead and the scalp, the nerve block may also be used for debridement or topical treatment of burns or abrasions and for delicate lacerations of the upper eyelid. Such anesthesia is ideal for removing small pieces of glass that are imbedded in the forehead from a windshield injury (Fig. 69–23).

The subtle supraorbital notch, which is in line with the pupil, may be palpated along the superior orbital rim. This landmark is the site of injection for blockage of the supraorbital nerves. The supratrochlear nerve is found 0.5 to 1.0 cm medially to the notch. The infratrochlear nerve is not usually blocked but is found in the most medial aspect of the superior orbital rim. If the anesthetic is placed on the forehead proper, this block may not produce complete anesthesia of the skin of the upper eyelid if the sensory branches to the eyelid are given off before the supraorbital nerve transverses the forehead.

With the patient in the supine position, a skin wheal is raised. Paresthesias in the form of an electric shock sensation over the forehead are sought; these ensure a successful nerve block. One to 3 ml of the anesthetic is placed in the area of the supraorbital notch. A finger or a roll of gauze should be held firmly under the orbital rim to avoid ballooning of anesthetic into the upper eyelid (Fig. 69–24).

If paresthesias cannot be elicted or if the nerve block is unsuccessful, a line of anesthetic solution placed along the orbital rim from the lateral to the medial aspect will ensure block of all of the branches of the ophthalmic nerve (Fig. 69–25).

Hematoma formation or swelling of the eyelid may occur but requires only local pressure. Occasionally, ecchymosis of the periorbital region will appear the next day, and the patient should be warned of this possibility.

Although this block is infrequently used, it is easily performed and is not associated with serious side effects. Its use should be considered when anesthesia of the forehead or the anterior scalp is desired.

INFRAORBITAL NERVE BLOCK

Intraoral and Extraoral Approach

The infraorbital nerve block injection can be used to anesthetize the mid-face (Fig. 69–26). A solution of local anesthetic deposited at the infraorbital foramen will anesthetize not only the middle and superior alveolar nerves but also the main trunk of the infraorbital nerve that in-

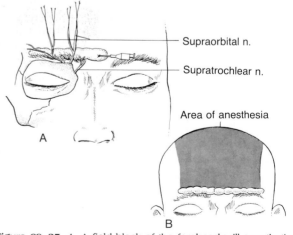

—— Supraorbital n.

—— Supratrochlear n.

Area of anesthesia

A

B

Figure 69–25. A, A field block of the forehead will anesthetize the supraorbital and supratrochlear nerves. B, Area of anesthesia with a bilateral field block. (From Moore, D.: Regional Block. 4th ed., Springfield, Ill., Charles C Thomas, 1975.)

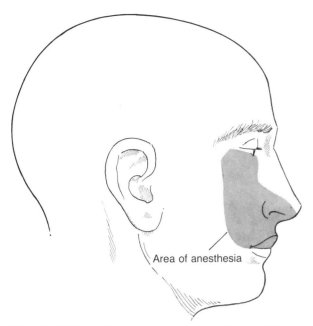

Figure 69–26. Area of anesthesia of a unilateral infraorbital nerve block. Anesthesia includes the lower eyelid and the upper lip. (From Moore, D.: Regional Block. 4th ed., Springfield, Ill., Charles C. Thomas, 1975.)

nervates the skin of the upper lip, the nose, and the lower eyelid. The infraorbital foramen is difficult to palpate. It is found on the inferior border of the infraorbital ridge on a vertical line with the pupil when the patient stares straight ahead.

When performing the intraoral approach, one keeps the palpating finger in place. The cheek is retracted, as in the supraperiosteal injection, and puncture is made in the mucosa opposite the upper second bicuspid (premolar tooth) approximately 0.5 cm from the buccal surface (Fig. 69–27 A and B). The needle should be directed parallel with the long axis of the second bicuspid until it is palpated at the foramen, a depth of approximately 2.5 cm. If the entry is too acute initially, one will encounter the malar eminence prior to approaching the infraorbital foramen. In addition, if the needle is extended too far posteriorly and superiorly, the orbit may be entered (Fig. 69–27C). Therefore, the procedure should be halted if the physician is unsure of the location of the needle or if patient cooperation is unsatisfactory. When the location has been determined and aspiration has been performed, 1 to 2 ml of solution is

Figure 69–27. A, Intraoral approach for infraorbital nerve block. B, Note the position of the infraorbital foramen (arrow) on the inferior portion of the infraorbital ridge. C, Incorrect infraorbital injection technique may result in needle entry into the orbit.

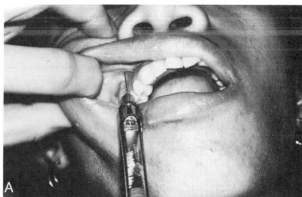
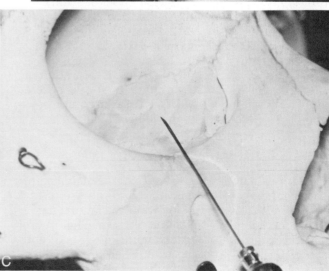
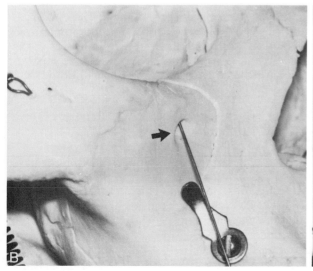

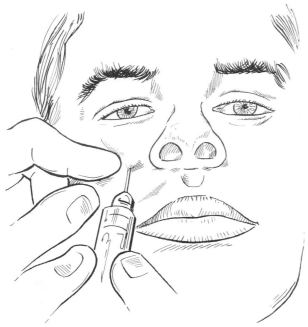

Figure 69–28. Extraoral approach to the infraorbital nerve. This procedure is more difficult than the intraoral approach, especially when attempting to obtain anesthesia of the upper lip. (From Eriksson, E.: Illustrated Handbook in Local Anesthesia. Philadelphia, W. B. Saunders Co., 1980.)

injected. A finger should be held firmly on the inferior orbital rim to avoid ballooning of the lower eyelid with anesthetic solution. If one is not certain of the exact location of the infraorbital foramen, one may obtain anesthesia by performing a field block. Five ml of the anesthetic solution is infiltrated in a fan-like direction in the upper buccal fold. This technique is not as precise as a discrete nerve block but will usually produce the same effect.

The infraorbital foramen may also be approached from an extraoral route (Fig. 69–28). In the extraoral approach, similar landmarks are used to locate the infraorbital foramen. The needle can be felt to pass through the skin, the subcutaneous tissue, and the quadratus labii superioris muscle. Care must be taken not to anesthetize the facial artery and vein, since these may lie on either side of the needle. Vasoconstrictors should not be used in this technique if possible. The extraoral approach, of course, requires external preparation of the skin. If vasoconstrictors are used and severe blanching of the face occurs, warm compresses should be immediately applied to the face.

INFERIOR ALVEOLAR NERVE BLOCK

In some situations, such as extreme dental pain, the emergency physician may find the use of the inferior alveolar nerve block and the lingual nerve block useful. This injection is somewhat more difficult than the other techniques described, and the emergency physician is advised to view demonstrations of this procedure prior to attempting

it. The inferior alveolar nerve block will provide anesthesia of all of the teeth on that side of the mandible and will desensitize the lower lip and the chin along the distribution of the mental nerve. This technique is primarily useful for anesthetizing patients who have sustained severe dentoalveolar trauma; those with complaints of postextraction pain, dry socket, or pulpitis (toothache); or those with periapical abscess.

The technique involves palpation of the retromolar fossa with the index finger so that the convexity of the mandibular ramus can be palpated (Fig. 69–29 A and B). The tissues are then retracted toward the buccal (cheek) side, and the pterygomandibular triangle is visualized. The syringe should be held parallel to the occlusal surfaces of the teeth and should be angled so that the barrel of the syringe is in line between the first and second premolars on the opposite side of the mandible. Puncture is made in the triangle, and the needle should be felt to pass through the ligaments and the muscles covering the internal surface of the mandible. One should stop when the needle has reached the posterior wall of the mandibular sulcus. The needle should then be withdrawn slightly and aspirated, and approximately 1 to 2 ml of solution should be deposited. In children, the angulation is not parallel to the occlusal surfaces of the teeth; the barrel of the syringe must be held slightly higher, since the mandibular foramen is lower. One may anesthetize the lingual nerve by placing several drops of anesthetic solution in the path while withdrawing the syringe. Half of the tongue can thus be anesthetized.

Complications include inadvertent administration of anesthetic posteriorly in the region of the parotid gland, which will anesthetize the facial nerves (Fig. 69–29C). This will cause temporary facial paralysis affecting the orbicularis oculi muscle and will result in inability to close the eyelid. The eye must be protected until the local anesthetic has worn off (approximately 2 to 3 hours), and the patient must be reassured. Anesthesia with bupivacaine (Marcaine) presents a serious problem if this complication occurs, since bupivacaine anesthesia will last from 10 to 18 hours.

SUPRAPERIOSTEAL INFILTRATIONS

The most common technique for intraoral local anesthesia of individual teeth is the supraperiosteal infiltration injection. This technique may supply complete relief of a toothache and is a useful emergency department procedure that can provide non-narcotic analgesia in the middle of the night. The area to be anesthetized is selected and dried with gauze. A topical anesthetic, such as cocaine

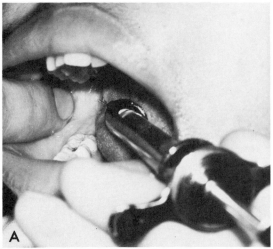

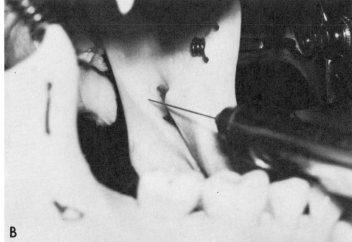

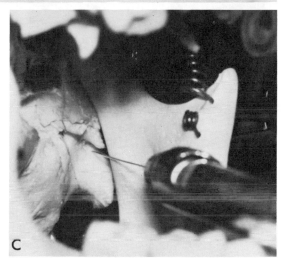

Figure 69–29. *A* and *B,* Infraorbital nerve block injection technique (see text). *C,* Directing the needle too far posteriorly during the inferior alveolar nerve block technique will result in entry into the area of the parotid gland. Anesthesia of the seventh nerve may result.

or lidocaine, renders the needle puncture painless. The mucous membrane of the area is grasped with a piece of gauze; it is pulled downward in the maxilla and upward in the mandible to extend the mucosa fully and to delineate the mucobuccal fold. The mucobuccal fold is then punctured with the bevel of the needle facing the bone. The area is aspirated, and approximately 1 to 2 ml of local anesthetic is deposited at the apex (area of the root tip) of the tooth involved (Fig. 69–30).

The purpose of the injection is to deposit the anesthetic near the bone that supports the tooth. Since the anesthetic must be absorbed by the bone in order to reach the nerve of the individual tooth, the injection may fail if the solution is deposited too far from the periosteum, if the needle is passed too far above the roots of the teeth, or if the bone in the area is unusually thick or dense. If anesthesia is unsuccessful, one may also inject the palatal side. It may take 5 to 10 minutes to achieve full anesthesia with this technique, and the procedure may not be as effective for the posterior molars. Infiltration of the area around the maxil-

lary canine and the first premolars will anesthetize the middle and anterior superior alveolar nerves; lacerations of the upper lip can be treated by bilateral injection in the canine fossa areas.

Similarly, infiltration around the mandible and the apices of the first and second premolars provides sufficient anesthesia to block mental nerves that supply the lower lip. This technique is referred to as a *mental nerve infiltration,* as opposed to a mental nerve block (Fig. 69–31). A true mental nerve block would involve the introduction of the needle in the mental foramen; this can cause neurovascular damage. Placement of anesthetic only in the region of the mental foramen is required for anesthesia of the lower lip. Lacerations of the midline of the lips require administration of anesthetic to the side of the midline opposite the site of the attempted block; this location reaches crossing-over fibers. This technique is useful for administering intraoral local anesthesia, especially in children. These blocks are relatively painless if performed after application of a topical anesthetic and if a slow injection technique is used.

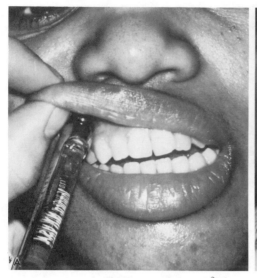

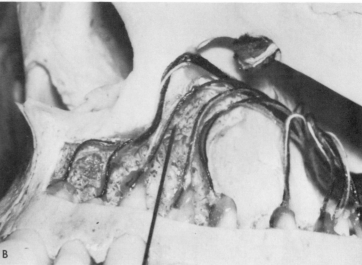

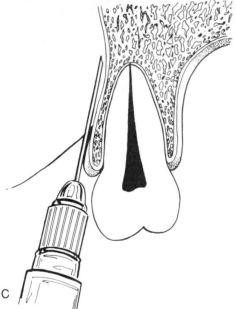

Figure 69–30. *A* and *B*, Supraperiosteal injection technique in maxillary canine fossa for anesthesia of the upper lip or individual teeth. *C*, Schematic illustration of supraperiosteal injection. (From Manual of Local Anesthesia in Dentistry. New York, N.Y.: Cook-Waite Laboratories, Inc.)

Disorders of the Temporomandibular Joint (TMJ) and Related Structures

MANDIBULAR DISLOCATION

In acute dislocation of the mandible, the condyle moves too far anteriorly in relation to the eminence and becomes locked (Fig. 69–32). Subsequent muscular trismus prevents the condyle from moving back into the temporal fossa. The spasm of the external pterygoid, masseter, and internal pterygoid muscles as well as associated edema result in extreme discomfort and anxiety for the patient. It is difficult for the patient to verbalize a complaint because he cannot close the mouth. Predisposing factors include anatomic disharmonies between the fossa and the interior articular eminence, weakness of the capsule forming the temporomandibular ligaments, and torn ligaments. Dislocation is likely to occur during maximum opening, such as occurs during yawning, laughing, or "popping" of the mandible in an open position. Although the temporomandibular joint is a double joint, dislocation may occur bilaterally or unilaterally. The jaw may be locked open symmetrically or may deviate to the side opposite the side of dislocation. Palpation of the temporomandibular joints may reveal them to be anterior to the articular eminence. In the face of trauma, radiographs should be taken to rule out fracture, since the clinical picture of both these conditions is similar and similar occlusal disturbances are produced. Radiographs may not be necessary on an emergent basis

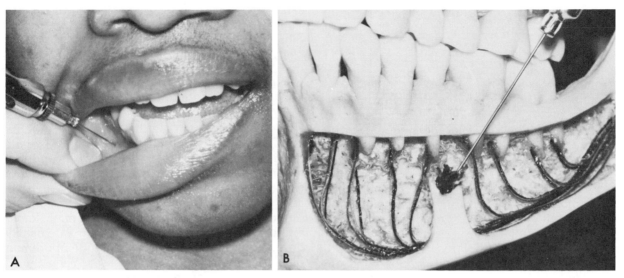

Figure 69–31. Mental infiltration technique. *A,* The correct supraperiosteal approach is an *infiltration* technique; this is all that is required for anesthesia of the lower lip or individual teeth. *B,* Mental nerve *block* technique involves actual introduction of the needle into the mental foramen. Obvious neurovascular damage may result; therefore, this technique is not recommended.

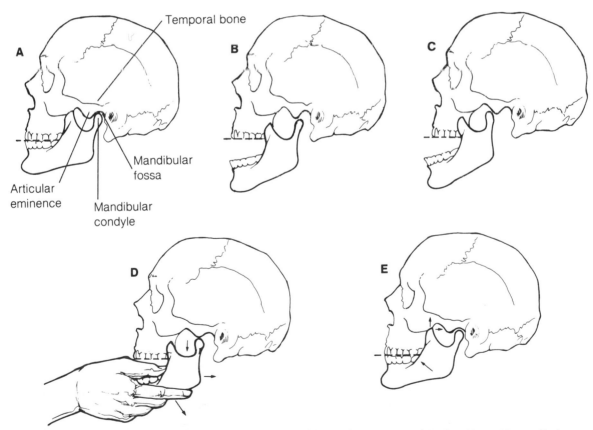

Figure 69–32. The temporomandibular joint, in normal and dislocated positions. *A,* Closed position, with mandibular condyle resting in the mandibular fossa, behind the articular eminence. *B,* In maximally open position, the condyle is just under and slightly behind the eminence. *C,* The dislocated jaw traps the condyle forward of and slightly above the eminence. *D,* To reduce the dislocation, pressure is applied to the lower molars near the jaw angle in a downward and backward direction (with well-padded thumbs!). As soon as the condyle is past the articular eminence, the muscles will cause the jaw to return to the normal closed position (*E*), usually with a swift snap. (From Amsterdam, J. T., Hendler, B. H., and Rose, L. F.: Temporomandibular joint dislocation. Consultant, 23:151, 1982. Used by permission.)

if there is no history of trauma of if the condition is recurrent.

Technique for Reduction

If one appreciates the anatomy of the temporomandibular joint, the proper sequence for manual manipulation to reduce the dislocation is clear (see Fig. 69–32D). Following dislocation, the powerful masseter muscles may be in tremendous spasm. For a smooth reduction, it is mandatory to relieve the patient's pain and tense muscle spasm with diazepam or a narcotic by slow intravenous injection. Some advocate direct injection of the condylar area with a local anesthetic. When the patient is sufficiently relaxed and analgesia is obtained, the physician faces the patient and grasps the mandible with both hands—one on each side with the thumbs (which have been wrapped with gauze or tongue blades) facing the occlusal surfaces of the posterior teeth. The fingertips are placed around the inferior border of the mandible in the region of the angles. Some prefer to have the patient seated in a chair or on the floor with the patient's back against the wall. Downward pressure is slowly and steadily applied to free the condyles from their anterior position to the eminence. The chin is then pressed backward after the jaw has been forced downward, and the mouth is closed while the condyle returns to its position in the fossa. In cases of severe muscle spasm, the jaw may snap back quickly. Therefore, protection of the thumbs is essential.

Following the procedure, the patient should be instructed to stay on a soft diet for 1 week, to avoid wide opening of the mandible, and to take analgesics and muscle relaxants. Local heat may also provide relief. Chronic dislocators or patients who suffer acute recurrences may be helped by a Barton bandage applied around the head for 2 weeks to prevent maximum opening, but this is rarely used. Very severe cases may require intermaxillary wiring and fixation for complete control with the use of Erich arch bars (described in the section on dentoalveolar trauma). Patients who have suffered dislocation of the temporomandibular joint should be referred to an oral and maxillofacial surgeon for follow-up, since chronic dislocation may require a surgical alteration of the eminence for relief.

TEMPOROMANDIBULAR MYOFASCIAL PAIN DYSFUNCTION SYNDROME

The temporomandibular myofascial pain dysfunction syndrome, or simply the TMJ syndrome, is a complex neuromuscular disturbance possibly resulting from and definitely aggravated by occlusal disturbances and disharmonies between occlusal relations and the anatomy of the temporomandibular joint. Other entities, such as trauma, psychological tension, and neuromuscular habits (e.g., bruxism and clenching), contribute to the problem. Patients who present to the emergency unit will frequently complain of unilateral facial pain. The pain is fairly nonspecific and is generalized to the region of the temporomandibular joint. The pain is of a dull nature in most patients and increases throughout the day with continued jaw motion. Clinical examination will frequently reveal spasm of the masseter muscle externally and the internal pterygoid muscle intraorally. There is usually limitation of opening. Radiographs of the temporomandibular joint are usually normal unless there is an associated temporomandibular joint degenerative disease. When the diagnosis of TMJ syndrome is suspected, it is important for the emergency physician to rule out acute otalgia or pain of odontogenic origin.

Treatment

Severe trismus associated with TMJ syndrome may be treated by the emergency physician locally with the application of a refrigerant anesthetic spray, such as ethyl chloride. The skin of the patient's face around the masseter muscle at the angle of the mandible is covered with a light coating of petroleum jelly. A towel is placed over the midline of the face to protect the region of the eye, and ethyl chloride is gently sprayed at the angle of the mandible in a rotary fashion from a distance of approximately 10 inches. The physician should take care not to produce frostbite of the tissues. The patient is instructed to open and close the mouth gently as the refrigerant spray is being applied. Frequently, this will break the muscle spasm. Diazepam may also be of use. Physiotherapy is continued at home and consists of the application of moist heat for 15 minutes four times a day. The patient should stay on a soft diet for approximately 2 weeks. Analgesics, such as aspirin or aspirin-codeine combinations, are effective, as are muscle relaxants and tranquilizers.

Patients should be referred to a general dentist, a periodontist, or a periodontal prosthodontist for follow-up and a course of therapy consisting of occlusal adjustment, if indicated. It is possible that some patients may have to be referred to an oral and maxillofacial surgeon for an intra-articular injection of cortisone or, rarely (in the most intractable cases), surgery (high intracapsular condylectomy). The various modalities described here should always be attempted by a dentist before intra-articular injection of steroids is considered. Although useful, the intra-articular injection of steroids in the temporomandibular joint is associated with a high incidence of subsequent fibrosis.

Conclusion

Although patients having dental complaints do not represent a high percentage of emergency visits, individuals with dental emergencies frequently do present to the emergency unit. The most common procedures available to the emergency physician in the management of general dental emergencies have been described in detail in this chapter. Although many procedures, such as the stabilization of a reimplanted avulsed tooth, are more easily and perhaps better performed by a dentist or an oral and maxillofacial surgeon, in some cases this type of consultation may not be readily available for several days. Emergency physicians can render a great service to the patient in these cases by performing whatever stabilization is possible for the reimplanted tooth. The majority of procedures described in this chapter are useful for the emergency physician and should be performed whenever indicated. The emergency physician should feel free to call on dental colleagues for further demonstration and explanation when necessary.

1. Johnson, R.: Descriptive classification of trauma—the injuries to the teeth and supporting structures. J. Am. Dent. Assoc. 102:195, 1981.
2. Dice, W. H., Pryor, G. J., and Kilpatrick, W. R.: Facial cellulitis following dental injury in a child. Ann. Emerg. Med. 11:541, 1982.
3. Medford, H. M.: Temporary stabilization of avulsed or luxated teeth. Ann. Emerg. Med. 11:490, 1982.
4. American Dental Association Council on Dental Therapeutics: Accepted Dental Therapeutics, 38th ed. Chicago, American Dental Association, 1979.

General References

5. Alderman, M.: Disorders of the temporomandibular joint and related structures. In Lynch, M. (ed.): Burket's Oral Medicine. Philadelphia, J. B. Lippincott Co., 1977, pp. 235–274.
6. Akamine, R. N.: Diagnosis of traumatic injuries of the face and jaws. Oral Surgery 8:349, 1955.
7. Amsterdam, J.: General Dental Emergencies, A Study Guide in Emergency Medicine. Dallas, TX, American College of Emergency Physicians, 1980.
8. Amsterdam, J., Wagner, D., and Rose, L.: Interdisciplinary training hospital dental general practice/emergency medicine. Ann. Emerg. Med. 9:310, 1980.
9. Amsterdam, J., and Rose, L. F.: Dental alveolar trauma. Curr. Top. Emerg. Med. II, Vol 2(9):1, 1981.
10. Amsterdam, J., and Hendler, B.: Approach to oral and facial pain. Curr. Top. Emerg. Med. II, Vol 2(10):1, 1981.
11. Bennett, C. R.: Manheim's Local Anesthesia and Pain Control in Dental Practice. St. Louis, C. V. Mosby Co., 1978.
12. Brightman, V. J.: Chronic oral sensory disorders—pain and dysgeusia. In Lynch, M. (ed.): Burket's Oral Medicine. Philadelphia, J. B. Lippincott Co., 1977, pp. 302–342.
13. Buzzard, E. M., Smith, H. C., and Hayton-Williams, D. S.: Symposium: Medical and surgical considerations in the treatment of maxillofacial injuries. Br. Dent. J. 116:63, 1964.
13b. Braham, R., Roberts, M., and Morris, M.: Management of dental trauma in children and adolescents. J. Trauma 17:857, 1977.
14. Committee on Trauma, American College of Surgeons: The Management of Fractures and Soft Tissue Injuries, 2nd ed. Philadelphia, W. B. Saunders Co., 1965, pp. 16–20, 247–264.
15. Converse, J. M., and Smith, B.: Blowout fractures of the floor of the orbit. In Converse, J. M. (ed.): Reconstructive Plastic Surgery, 2nd ed., vol. 2. Philadelphia, W. B. Saunders Co., 1977, pp. 752–775.
16. Dingman, R. O., and Natvig, P.: Surgery of Facial Fractures. Philadelphia, W. B. Saunders Co., 1964.
17. Hagan, E. H., and Huelke, D. F.: An analysis of 319 case reports of mandibular factures. J. Oral Surg. 19:93, 1961.
18. Hendler, B. H.: Maxillofacial fractures—Spread of Infection of Odontogenic Origin, A Study Guide in Emergency Medicine. Dallas, TX, American College of Emergency Physicians, 1980.
19. Hendler, B. H., and Quinn, P. D.: Fatal mediastinitis secondary to odontogenic infection. J. Oral Surg. 36:308, 1978.
20. Hendler, B., and Amsterdam, J.: Infection of dental origin. Curr. Top. Emerg. Med. II, Vol 2 (8):1, 1981.
21. Hendler, B. H., and Wagner, D.: Problem—blow to the jaw, Trauma Rounds. Emerg. Med. 5:60, 1973.
22. Hendler, B. H., and Wagner, D.: Injury to the lip and oral mucosa, Trauma Rounds. Emerg. Med. 6:278, 1974.
23. Huelke, D. F., and Harger, J. H.: Maxillofacial injuries: Their nature and mechanisms of productions. J. Oral Surg. 27:451, 1969.
24. Kruger, G. O.: Textbook of Oral and Maxillofacial Surgery, 5th ed. St. Louis, C. V. Mosby Co., 1979.
25. Laskin, D.: The role of the dentist in the emergency room. Dent. Clin. North Am., 19:675, 1975.
26. LeFort, R.: Etude experimentale sur les fractures de la machoire superieure. Rev. Chir. (Paris) 23:360, 1901.
27. Lynch, M. (ed.): Burket's Oral Medicine, 7th ed. Philadelphia, J. B. Lippincott Co., 1977, Chapters 1–12.
28. Manual of Local Anesthesia and General Dentistry. New York, Cook-Waite Laboratories, Inc., 1947.
29. McCarthy, F.: Emergencies in Dental Practice: Prevention and Treatment. Philadelphia, W. B. Saunders Co., 1979.
30. Osbon, D. B.: Facial trauma. In Irby, W. B. (ed.): Current Advances in Oral Surgery, vol. 1. St. Louis, C. V. Mosby Co., 1974, pp. 214–241.
31. Rose, L. F.: General health affecting periodontal disease and therapeutic response. In Goldman, H. M., and Cohen, D. W.: Periodontal Therapy, 6th ed. St. Louis, C. V. Mosby Co., 1979.
32. Shafer, W. G., Hine, M. K., and Levy, B. M.: Oral Pathology, 3rd ed. Philadelphia, W. B. Saunders Co., 1974, pp. 308–365.
33. Ship, I., and Lynch, M.: General health status affecting periodontal disease and therapeutic response. In Goldman, H. M., and Cohen, D. W. (eds.): Peridontal Therapy, 5th ed. St. Louis, C. V. Mosby Co., 1973.
34. Sicher, H.: Structural and functional basis for disorders of the temporomandibular articulation. J. Oral Surg. 13:275, 1955.
35. Sicher, H.: The Propagation of Dental Infections in Oral Anatomy. St. Louis, C. V. Mosby Co., 1965, pp. 470–482.
36. Solinitzky, O.: The fascial compartments of the head and neck in relation to dental infections. Bull. Georgetown U. Med. Ctr. 7:86, 1954.
37. Smith, B., and Converse, J. M.: Early treatment of orbital floor fractures. Trans. Am. Acad. Ophthalmol. Otolaryngol. 61:602, 1957.
38. Thoma, K. H.: Oral Surgery, 5th ed. St. Louis, C. V. Mosby Co., 1969.
39. Thompson, C. W.: Primary care of the acute trauma patient. In Irby, W. B. (ed.): Current Advances in Oral Surgery. St. Louis, C. V. Mosby Co., 1977.
40. Weisgold, A., Baumgarten, H., Rose, L., Amsterdam, J., and Brown. S.: Dental medicine. In Kaye, D., and Rose, L. (eds.): Fundamentals of Internal Medicine. St. Louis, C. V. Mosby Co., 1983, pp. 1228–1251.
41. Wise, R. A., and Baker, H. W.: Surgery of the Head and Neck, 3rd ed., Chicago, Year Book Medical Publishers, 1968, pp. 80–122.

14

DERMATOLOGY

70

Incision and Drainage of Cutaneous Abscesses and Soft Tissue Infections

TODD M. WARDEN, M.D.

General Considerations

Cutaneous abscesses are among the soft tissue infections most frequently encountered in the emergency department. In contrast with most bacterial diseases, which are usually described in terms of their etiologic agent, cutaneous abscesses are more conveniently described in terms of their location. There has been little systematic investigation into the bacteriology of simple cutaneous abscesses, and there have been few new recommendations for improved management over the years. The probable reason for this is the predictable and striking recovery of the patient once a mature abscess is incised and drained. The exact reasons for this amelioration of local and constitutional symptoms are unknown, but it is clear that the specific bacteriology of abscesses in the vast majority of cases is unimportant to the outcome.[1]

Etiology and Pathogenesis

Localized pyogenic infections may develop in any region of the body and usually are initiated by a breakdown in the normal epidermal defense mechanisms, with subsequent tissue invasion by normal resident flora. Thus, infection in most areas is likely to be caused by the flora that are indigenous to that area. Staphylococcal strains, which are normally found on the skin, produce rapid necrosis, early suppuration, and localized infections with large amounts of creamy yellow pus. This is the presentation of a typical abscess. Group A beta-hemolytic streptococcal infections, on the other hand, tend to spread through tissues, causing a more generalized infection characterized by erythema and edema, a serous exudate, and little or no necrosis. This is the presentation of a typical cellulitis. Anaerobic bacteria proliferate in the oral and perineal regions, produce necrosis with profuse brownish, foul-smelling pus,[1] and may cause both abscess and cellulitis formation.

Normal skin is extremely resistant to bacterial invasion, and few organisms are capable of penetrating the intact epidermis. In the normal host with intact skin, the topical application of even very high concentrations of pathogenic bacteria will not result in infection. The requirements for infection include a high concentration of pathogenic organisms, such as occurs in the hair follicles and their adnexa; occlusion, which prevents desquamation and normal drainage, creating a moist environment; adequate nutrients; and trauma to the corneal layer, which allows organisms to penetrate.[2] This trauma may be the result of abrasions, hematoma, injection of chemical irritants, incision, or occlusive dressings that cause maceration of the skin. Foreign bodies can also potentiate these infections and decrease the number of bacteria necessary for infection. An example of this is the ubiquitous suture abscess, which frequently develops in wounds closed by suture material. When favorable factors are present, the normal flora of the cutaneous areas can then colonize and infect the skin. The bodily area involved depends primarily on host factors. Persons performing manual labor with the arms and the hands are infected most frequently. In women, the axilla and submammary regions are frequently infected because of minor trauma from shaving and garments and because of the abundance of bacteria in these areas. In addition, areas with compromised blood supply will be more prone to infection, because normal host cell–mediated immunity is not as available.[2] Septic emboli from endocarditis may cause abscess formation by bacteremic migration of infected material into subcutaneous tissue.

Cutaneous abscesses do not develop de novo. Infection in the soft tissue usually begins as a cellulitis. Some organisms will eventually cause necrosis, liquefaction, and accumulation of leukocytes and debris, followed by loculation and walling off of pus, which results in the formation of one or more abscesses. There may be involvement of the lymph tissues, producing lymphangitis and subsequent bacteremia. As the process progresses, the area of erythema lessens and the area of liquefaction increases until it "points" and eventually ruptures into the area of least resistance. This may be toward the skin or the mucous membrane, into surrounding tissue, or into a body cavity. If the abscess is particularly deep-seated, spontaneous drainage may occur with persistence of a fistulous tract and the formation of a chronic draining sinus. This development or the recurrence of an abscess that has been previously drained should always suggest the possibility of osteomyelitis, a retained foreign body, or the presence of unusual organisms, such as *Myocobacterium* or *Actinomyces*.[1]

Bacteriology of Cutaneous Abscesses

Recent studies have investigated the bacteriology of abscesses of different areas of the body and have added to the general knowledge of cutaneous abscess formation and treatment.

Meislin and coworkers[3] cultured abscesses in 135 patients. This study yielded data that may be applicable to abscess treatment in general. The treatment involved simple incision and drainage, and all subjects were followed as outpatients. Both aerobic and anaerobic cultures were taken. Ninety-six per cent of cultures were positive for bacteria. Four per cent were sterile (Table 70–1).

In this series predominantly mixed aerobic bacteria were isolated in abscesses of the trunk, the axilla, the extremities, and the hand. In the pure cultures, *Staphylococcus aureus* was found in 72 per cent of cases. One third of the cultures from the perianal region contained only anaerobes. Mixed cultures of both aerobic and anaerobic bacteria were obtained from all sites of the body, but there was a 67 per cent incidence of such mixed cultures from the perirectal area. Commonly isolated anaerobes included various *Bacteroides* species, peptococci, peptostreptococci, *Clostridium* species, *Lactobacillus* species, and *Fusobacterium* species.

Bacteria from abscesses in areas remote from the rectum were generally aerobic strains and were primarily indigenous microflora of the skin. *Staphylococcus aureus* was the most prevalent aerobic organism; it was isolated in 24 per cent of all abscesses.

Gram-negative aerobes were isolated infrequently from cutaneous abscesses. *Escherichia coli*, *Neisseria gonorrhoeae*, and *Pseudomonas* species were rarely found. The most commonly isolated gram-negative organism was *Proteus mirabilis*, and this organism was found almost exclusively in the axilla. This may be related to the use of underarm deodorants.[4]

Brooks and associates[5] studied the bacteriology of cutaneous abscesses in children. Their results closely correlate with those of Meislin.[3] They found aerobes (staphylococci and group A beta-hemolytic streptococci) to be the most common isolates from abscesses of the head, the neck, the extremities, and the trunk, with anaerobes predominating in abscesses of the buttocks and the perirectal sites. Mixed aerobic and anaerobic flora were found in the perirectal area, the head, and the finger and nail bed area. This study found an unexpectedly high incidence of anaerobes in non-perineal abscesses. Anaerobes were found primarily either in areas adjacent to mucosal membranes, where these organisms tend to thrive (e.g., the mouth), or in areas that are easily contaminated (e.g., by sucking fingers, which causes nail bed and finger infections or bite injuries).

Special Considerations

Parenteral drug abusers, insulin-dependent diabetics, hemodialysis patients, cancer patients, and individuals with acute leukemias have an increased frequency of abscess formation. Local symptoms may not be the primary complaint, and indeed the patient may present only with an exacerbation of the underlying disease process. These abscesses tend to have exotic or uncommon bacteriologic causes and typically respond poorly to therapy. The diabetic patient in diabetic ketoacidosis should be evaluated extensively for an infectious process; a rectal examination should be included with the physical examination to rule out a perirectal abscess. This also holds true for the

Table 70–1. CHARACTERIZATION OF 135 OUTPATIENT ABSCESSES*

Anatomic Areas	Abscesses	Per Cent of Total Cultures	Type of Bacterial Growth (Per Cent from Each Area)				Bacterial Species per Abscess†	
			No Growth	Aerobes Only	Anaerobes Only	Aerobes and Anaerobes	Aerobes	Anaerobes
	No.						*Average no.*	
Head and neck	25	19	4	28	20	48	1	2
Trunk	11	8	0	45	18	36	1	2
Axilla	22	16	0	55	5	41	1	1
Extremity	16	12	19	44	13	25	1	1
Hand	8	6	25	63	0	13	2	0
Inguinal	7	5	0	29	57	14	0	3
Vulvovaginal	13	10	0	15	46	38	1	3
Buttock	12	9	0	33	33	33	1	3
Perirectal	21	16	0	0	33	67	1	5

*From Meislin, H. W., et al.: Bacterial characterization profile of 135 outpatient abscesses. Ann. Intern. Med. 87:146, 1977. Used by permission.
†Cultures with no growth were excluded.

septic leukemic individual or the dialysis patient. The increased frequency of abscess formation in these patients and in the parenteral drug abuser is multifactorial. There may be intrinsic immune deficiencies in all these patients; they have an increased incidence of *Staphylococcus* carriage, and they have frequent needle punctures, which allow access of pathogenic bacteria.[6]

It is important to note that a substantial percentage of abscesses in parenteral drug abusers are sterile and are the result of the injection of necrotizing chemical irritants.[7] Drug abusers frequently use veins of the neck and the femoral areas, producing abscesses and other infectious complications at these sites.[8] Any abscess of the antecubital fossa or the dorsum of the hand should alert the physician to possible intravenous drug abuse.

Manifestations of Abscess Formation

The diagnosis of cutaneous abscess formation is relatively straightforward. The presence of a fluctuant mass in an area of induration, erythema, and tenderness is clinical evidence that an abscess exists. An abscess may appear initially as a definite tender soft tissue mass, but in some cases of obvious soft tissue infection, the presence of a distinct abscess may not be readily evident. Most abscesses have an area of surrounding cellulitis, but in borderline cases one may aspirate the area with a needle and syringe to confirm the presence of pus. If the abscess is quite deep, as is true of many perirectal or breast abscesses, the clinician may be misled by the presence of only a firm, tender, indurated area without a definite mass. Although a localized abscess is present, the uninitiated will frequently diagnose cellulitis in such cases. Occasionally, one will be misled by a mycotic aneurysm or an inflamed lymph node simulating an abscess. A specific entity that is commonly mistaken for a discrete abscess is the sublingual cellulitis of Ludwig's angina.

If there is a significant area of surrounding cellulitis or vascular seeding of bacteria, the patient may appear quite toxic. Bacteremia from simple abscess formation is quite rare.

Laboratory Findings

The patient may demonstrate a leukocytosis, depending on the severity and duration of the abscess process; however, the majority of patients with an uncomplicated cutaneous abscess will have a normal complete blood count (CBC) and will not experience fever, chills, or malaise. The Gram stain of the pus is usually diagnostic for bacteria, but the Gram stain is generally not indicated or helpful in the management of routine cases. The Gram stain should be used, however, in the patient who is immunocompromised to help in the selection of adjunctive antibiotic treatment. In uncomplicated abscesses, *routine culture is unnecessary* because of the expected prompt response to surgical therapy, but in complicated cases or in immunosuppressed patients, the pus from an abscess should be cultured. The information obtained from a culture may later be useful if there is poor response to the initial surgical drainage, secondary spread of the infection, or the occurrence of bacteremia.[1] If one takes a culture, it is best to aspirate the pus with a needle and syringe *before* incision and drainage. Material is cultured for aerobic and anaerobic bacteria. The finding of a "sterile" culture in an abscess that has been cultured with a standard cotton swab *after* incision is frequently the result of improper anaerobic culture techniques. As a side note, there is a general misconception that foul-smelling pus is a result of *E. coli*. This foul odor is actually caused by the presence of anaerobes; the pus of *E. coli* is odorless.

Therapeutic Considerations

Surgical incision and drainage is the only *definitive treatment* of a soft tissue abscess. Antibiotics alone are generally *ineffective* in the face of a localized collection of pus. The drainage of a suppurative focus results in a marked improvement in symptoms and a rapid resolution of the infection in uncomplicated cases. Premature incision before localization of pus will not be curative and may be deleterious, since extension of the infectious process and bacteremia from manipulation can result. In some cases, the application of heat to an area of inflammation may ease pain, speed resolution of the cellulitis, and facilitate the localization and accumulation of pus. It must be stressed that nonsurgical methods are not a substitute for surgical drainage and should not be continued for more than 24 to 36 hours before the patient is re-evaluated for surgical therapy. Diagnostic needle aspiration is recommended if one is unsure of pus localization.

Antibiotics may be indicated *before* incision and drainage and for a few days afterward if the patient is significantly toxic or if the cellulitis surrounding the abscess is extensive, but the benefit of preoperative antibiotics in such cases has not been well studied. In general, if pus can be drained, foreign matter can be removed, and the patient has a normal immune system, antibiotics will have little effect on the success of the procedure and will add only expense and possible side effects.

Antibiotics are of limited value in the treatment of most abscesses because of inadequate penetration of the antibiotic into the abscess cavity. The low metabolic activity of bacteria in the abscess cavity also limits the effectiveness of antibiotics, and phagocytosis of cells in the abscess cavity is decreased.[1]

High-Risk Patients. There are four general categories of high-risk patients with cutaneous abscesses who may benefit from antibiotic coverage. The first subgroup consists of previously healthy patients who develop signs of significant *systemic toxicity* secondary to the infectious process, with signs of an extension of the inflammation into deeper structures. These patients are best admitted to the hospital for continued antibiotic treatment or drainage under general anesthesia.

The second category of high-risk patients includes immunosuppressed patients, or those with serious underlying disease, such as diabetes, renal failure, cancer, or cirrhosis. The third category consists of patients with valvular heart disease. There is controversy as to the need for antibiotic administration prior to incision and drainage in patients with mitral valve prolapse or in drug addicts who have heart murmurs without documented valvular disease. General consensus is that such patients should probably receive antibiotics before *and* after incision and drainage. The last category includes patients with abscesses or cellulitis in the region of the face drained by the cavernous sinus. These patients must be considered for hospital admission and antibiotic therapy while preparations for surgical intervention are made. The decision to admit patients to the hospital is based on the clinical condition of the patient (e.g., the degree of toxicity), the ability to drain infected foci, and the potential for poor response to therapy or noncompliance. The majority of patients who undergo simple incision and drainage in the emergency department will do quite well with home care and careful follow-up.

If one opts for antibiotics before incision and drainage, a single intravenous dose 1 hour before surgery is advised. There are few data on the value of this procedure, but one should select antibiotics that cover a broad spectrum.[9] A reasonable choice is a semisynthetic penicillin, clindamycin with an aminoglycoside, or one of the cephalosporins alone such as cefoxitin (Mefoxin) or cefazolin (Ancef). Coverage should be directed against *Staphylococcus aureus* and anaerobes. Coverage of anaerobes should include *Bacteroides* species if the perirectal area is involved.

Incision and Drainage Procedure

Definitive incision and drainage of a simple soft tissue abscess is easily performed in the emergency department. Some centers prefer to drain all abscesses in a special area of the emergency departments, which can subsequently be decontaminated. A standard suture tray provides the adequate instruments if a scalpel and packing material are added. Although sterility is impossible during the procedure, one should avoid contamination of surrounding tissue. Some physicians prefer to use an obligatory skin scrub with an antiseptic solution, but the value of this step is unproved.

It is often quite difficult to obtain local anesthesia in infected tissue because of the poor function of the local anesthetic agents in the low pH of the infected areas. Furthermore, the distention of sensitive structures by a local injection is quite painful and hence poorly tolerated by most patients. Skin anesthesia is usually possible, but total anesthesia of the abscess cavity itself generally cannot be achieved. If a regional block can be performed in the area, this type of anesthesia is preferred. A field block may be used if there is no area of cellulitis surrounding the abscess. It should be noted that infected tissue is very vascular, and local anesthetics are quickly absorbed. Strict adherence to maximum safe doses of a local anesthetic is required.

The skin over the dome of an abscess is often quite thin, making skin anesthesia difficult. If a 25-gauge needle is carefully used, one can often inject the dome of the abscess subcutaneously. The anesthetic solution spreads over the dome through the subcutaneous layers and provides excellent skin anesthesia. If the needle is in the proper plane, the skin blanches during infiltration. In the extremely anxious or uncomfortable patient, the judicious use of preoperative intravenous narcotics (such as meperidine), sedatives (such as diazepam) or nitrous oxide makes the procedure easier for both patient and physician. If adequate anesthesia cannot be obtained and pain limits the procedure, the patient should be admitted and treated under general anesthesia.

Some authors recommend the use of topical ethyl chloride spray for the initial skin incision, but the pain relief offered by this agent is variable and fleeting. Ethyl chloride spray is occasionally useful to provide momentary anesthesia for the initial skin incision if the incision is made while the ethyl chloride is being sprayed.

One should make all incisions conform with skin creases or natural folds to minimize visible scar formation (Fig. 70–1). Extreme care should be taken in such areas as the groin, the posterior knee, the antecubital fossa, and the neck, so that vascular and neural structures are not damaged.

A number 11 scalpel blade is used to nick the skin over the fluctuant area, and then a simple linear incision is carried the total length of the abscess cavity (Fig. 70–2A). This will afford more

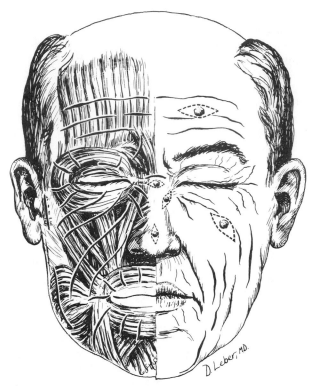

Figure 70–1. The relation of the elective lines of tension in the face to the underlying mimetic musculature. Only in the lower eyelid are these lines not perpendicular to the muscles. The left side of the drawing shows the use of this principle when common facial lesions are excised or a facial abscess is drained. (From Schwartz, S. I., et al.: Principles of Surgery, 2nd ed. New York, McGraw-Hill, 1974. Used by permission.)

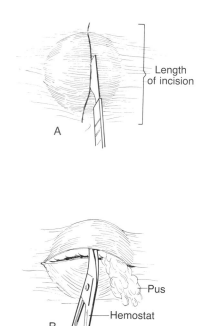

Figure 70–2. *A*, The skin over the abscess is incised the full length of the abscess. A small stab incision does not allow for proper drainage. *B*, A hemostat or a finger is inserted into the abscess cavity to spread the skin, to drain the pus, and to break up loculations.

complete drainage and will facilitate subsequent break-up of loculations. A cruciate incision or an ellipitic skin *excision* is to be avoided in the routine treatment of cutaneous abscess. The tips of the flaps of a cruciate incision may necrose, resulting in an unsightly scar. A timid stab incision (the so-called "medical incision") is not adequate for proper drainage. An exception to this rule is an abscess in a cosmetic area, where a stab incision may be initially tried to limit scar formation. It should be emphasized that the scalpel is used only to make the skin incision and is never used deep in the abscess cavity.

The physician should probe the depth of an abscess with a gloved finger or a hemostat to assess the extent of the abscess and to ensure proper drainage by breaking open loculations (Fig. 70–2B). One is often surprised at the depth of an abscess during probing. Sharp curettage of the abscess cavity is usually not required and may produce bacteremia.[9] Although tissue probing is usually the most painful aspect of the technique and total local anesthesia is difficult to obtain, this portion of the procedure should not be abbreviated. If the procedure is limited because of pain, the patient should be drained under general anesthesia.

Following the break-up of loculations, copious irrigation with normal saline should be performed to ensure adequate removal of excess debris from the wound cavity. The hyperemic tissue may bleed profusely, but bleeding usually stops in a few minutes if packing is used. Abscesses of the extremities should be drained with the use of a tourniquet to provide a bloodless field. After irrigation, a loose packing of gauze or other material is placed gently into the abscess cavity to prevent the wound margins from closing and to afford continued drainage of any exudative material that may otherwise be trapped. One need not force excessive amounts of packing material tightly into the incision. The purpose of the packing is primarily to promote drainage by keeping the skin edges apart. Packing also serves to hasten the formation of granulation tissue at the depths of the wound and thus hastens ultimate wound closure. Some prefer to use plain gauze, some use gauze soaked in povidone-iodine, and some use gauze impregnated with iodine (iodoform). The iodoform gauze will sting the patient for a few minutes after it is inserted. The value of antibiotic-impregnated gauze is uncertain. Absorbent gauze dressing should be placed over the packed abscess or, if an extremity is involved, a lightly wrapped circumferential dressing should be used. Generous amounts of dry gauze are used over the packing to soak up any drainage or blood. The affected part should be splinted if possible, and elevation should be routine. Drainage relieves most of the pain of an abscess, but postoperative analgesics may be required.

The patient should return within 48 hours for a wound check and packing removal. The abscess may be gently irrigated after removal of the packing if there is extensive purulent drainage. The decision to start warm soaks or to replace the bulky packing with one that is less substantial depends on the cosmetics of the site and the amount of drainage. If it appears that the wound margins are gaping enough to allow continued drainage, no further packing is required. If, on the other hand, it appears that there is an excessive amount of debris or exudate or if the skin edges are opposed, the wound is repacked accordingly, and ultimate removal is deferred. Patients should not be expected to change their own packing. Large abscesses, such as pilonidal abscesses, may require packing for extended periods.

A number of other options for packing material are available. An old but reliable method consists of daily packing with simple table sugar mixed with povidone-iodine.[10] Large wounds may also be packed with a standard gauze sponge measuring 4 inches × 4 inches. A simple but effective pack is the "wet-to-dry" pack. Saline-soaked gauze is used to pack the wound, and dry gauze is fluffed over it; this acts as a wick to promote drainage. Many authors believe that packing should be discontinued after the acute infection subsides and suggest that repeated packing delays healing. At the first recheck, an assessment of the degree of resolution of the inflammatory process should be made, and treatment should be guided accordingly. In most cases, once the abscess begins to fill with granulation tissue, no further packing is required.

An effective alternative to packing the abscess is the catheter system of drainage.[11-13] In selected cases in which extensive or prolonged drainage occurs or in patients who are unable to return for proper follow-up care, the catheter system of drainage may be preferred. Following incision, a balloon-tipped or flared-tip catheter is placed into the abscess cavity, and pus is allowed to drain continuously through the catheter lumen. This technique has been most successful in pilonidal and in Bartholin gland abscesses, but the technique is applicable to any abscess *not* on the face.

Following the discontinuation of packing, the patient should begin warm soaks. The procedure should be explained carefully to the patient. Plain warm tap water soaks are adequate, and sterile water or expensive additives are generally unnecessary. If a splint is in place, removal and replacement of the splint should be demonstrated. Time should be taken to impress upon the patient the importance of soaking the affected part at least four times per day for 20 minutes at a time.

Following the soaks, a light bandage should be applied and the splint should be replaced. If the abscess is in the perineal area, the patient should be instructed on how to take sitz baths. The use of a feminine napkin may control the drainage from a perirectal abscess more conveniently than attempts at bandaging. If the abscess is in an area that is difficult to soak, one may advise warm compresses or the use of warm water from a shower. The gentle force from a shower faucet may be directed into the abscess cavity to promote healing by mild mechanical debridement. Some physicians instruct the patient to clean the base of the abscess cavity daily with a cotton-tipped applicator dipped in hydrogen peroxide. This ensures the removal of blood and debris and also ensures that the skin edges will remain apart.

The abscess cavity is generally not sutured closed. Once granulation tissue fills the cavity, healing is rapid, and the incision often heals with surprising cosmesis. The possibility of later revision of an unsightly scar should be explained to the patient. After all infection has been cleared, some physicians will consider secondary suture closure of large abscess cavities. This should not be considered if continued serous drainage is excessive. If the abscess cavity is to be sutured, the skin edges are "freshened" by sharp debridement and a standard secondary closure is performed. The abscess is treated like a previously infected wound with delayed closure.

Facial abscesses should be handled carefully and checked frequently. Any abscess above the upper lip and below the brow may drain into the cavernous sinus, and thus manipulation may predispose to septic thrombophlebitis of this system. Treatment should include antistaphylococcal antibiotics and warm soaks until resolution of the process. Areas *not* in this zone of the face can be treated in a manner similar to that for other cutaneous abscesses. In all facial abscesses, note should be made of the direction of the natural lines of the skin, and the incision over the abscess should be directed along these lines in order to maximize the cosmetic effect (see Fig. 70–1). Since cosmesis is important on the face, the packing should be removed after only 24 hours, at which time warm soaks should be started.

Specific Abscess Therapy

STAPHYLOCOCCAL DISEASES

The *Staphylococcus* is a ubiquitous parasite that frequently colonizes the nose, the skin, the perineum, and the gut. The umbilicus of neonates is also commonly colonized. It grows on the skin and thrives particularly well in hair follicles, causing boils (furuncles), wound infections, and occasionally carbuncles. The pathogenesis of staphylococcal disease is a complex host-bacteria interaction. *Staphylococcus aureus* invades the skin by way of the hair follicles or an open wound and produces local tissue destruction followed by hyperemia of vessels. Subsequently, an exudative reaction occurs, during which polymorphonuclear cells invade. The process then extends along the path of least resistance. The abscess may "point," or form sinus tracts. The process can disseminate by invasion of vessels and thus can infect other organs. Most cases of staphylococcal osteomyelitis, meningitis, and endocarditis occur by this mechanism.[14, 15]

When a small abscess occurs at the root of a hair, the condition is termed *folliculitis*. Local measures, including warm compresses and antibacterial soaps and ointments, are the usual treatment. Furuncles, or boils, are acute circumscribed abscesses of the skin and subcutaneous tissue that most commonly occur on the face, the neck, the buttocks, the thigh, the perineum, or the breast or in the axilla. The local application of heat and bacitracin ointment is usually adequate until spontaneous drainage occurs,[14, 15] but incision and drainage are occasionally required.

Recurrent *suppurativa*, furuncles involving sweat glands produce a condition termed *hydradenitis* to be discussed later. Furuncles of the face above the upper lip are more dangerous because of the possibility of extension into the cavernous venous sinus. In these cases, treatment consists of warm soaks and oral antistaphylococcal drugs. Manipulation of facial abscesses should be avoided.[16]

Carbuncles are aggregates of interconnected furuncles that frequently occur on the back of the neck. In this area the skin is thick, and extension therefore occurs laterally rather than toward the skin surface. Carbuncles may attain large size and can cause systemic symptoms and complications. They are found in increased frequency in diabetics. Treatment should consist of surgical drainage and occasionally, the administration of systemic antibiotics.[14, 15] Large carbuncles are impossible to drain adequately in the emergency department. Occasionally, wide excision and skin grafting are required.

Most cases of recurrent staphylococcal skin infections are caused by autoinfection from existing skin lesions or nasal reservoirs. Management is directed at eliminating the organism. This is accomplished by the application of bacitracin to the nares and good hygiene, including frequent cleansing with antibacterial soap. If these measures are unsuccessful, then systemic antistaphylococcal treatment is instituted for 2 to 3 weeks. Detection and treatment of infection in family members may be necessary.[14, 15]

BREAST ABSCESS

The most common type of breast infection, post partum mastitis, occurs in 1 to 3 per cent of nursing mothers within the first 2 to 6 weeks after delivery. The infection is usually precipitated by milk stasis following weaning or missed feedings. The cause is usually the invasion through a cracked or abraded nipple by *S. aureus* or streptococci originating from the nursing child. Initially, a cellulitis occurs; this may progress to frank abscess formation. The patient may be quite ill and may appear toxic. Manifestations are redness, heat, pain, fever, and chills. Treatment consists of antistaphylococcal antibiotics, continued breast emptying with a breast pump, and the application of heat. It is important to encourage continued breast emptying to promote drainage. Nursing can be continued with the noninfected breast, although the passage of the antibiotics through the breast milk may result in some infant diarrhea. These abscesses rarely require surgical drainage. Strict adherence to nipple hygiene to avoid cracks or inflammation is helpful in prophylaxis.

Staphylococcal breast abscesses may also occur in the absence of nursing. Superficial abscesses in the subcutaneous tissue may be drained under local anesthesia by means of an incision that radiates from the nipple (Fig. 70–3A).

The deeper and more extensive intramammary abscess appears as a generalized swollen, tender breast (Fig. 70–3B). Fluctuance is not always obvious, since the abscess is located in the mammary tissue itself. These intramammary infections are complex and require incision and drainage under general anesthesia. They do not lend themselves to outpatient treatment.

A retromammary abscess lies in the undersurface of the breast between the breast and the chest wall (Fig. 70–3C). Fluctuance may be difficult to appreciate because of the depth of the infection. Drainage under general anesthesia is required.

It may be difficult to diagnose a breast abscess in the early stages, when cellulitis predominates. In equivocal cases, antibiotics may be curative, but when pus is present, incision and drainage must be performed.

BARTHOLIN GLAND ABSCESS

The Bartholin glands (vestibular glands) are secretory organs located at 5 and 7 o'clock on each side of the vestibule of the vagina. Asymptomatic cysts frequently occur from duct blockage and retention of secretions. Chronic low-grade inflammation from gonococcal infections has been implicated as an etiologic factor in cyst formation, but

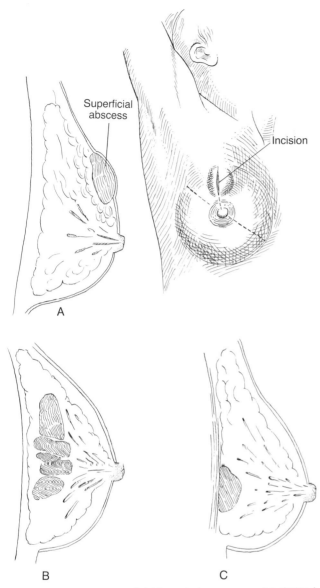

Figure 70–3. A, A superficial breast abscess may be drained with a linear incision that radiates from the nipple. B and C. Diagrams of intramammary abscess (B) and retromammary abscess (C). Both require drainage under general anesthesia. The abscess itself may not be fully appreciated if it is deep-seated, and the mistaken diagnosis of cellulitis may be made. (Redrawn from Wolcott, M. W.: Ferguson's Surgery of the Ambulatory Patient, 5th ed. Philadelphia, J. B. Lippincott Co., 1974.)

occasionally frank abscess formation results. Such patients present with swollen and tender labia and a fluctuant, grape-sized mass that may be palpated between the thumb and the index finger. *Neisseria gonorrheae* organisms are infrequently cultured from the abscess cavity, and various anaerobes, especially *Bacteroides* species and other colonic bacteria, are usually found. It is reasonable to take cervical and anal cultures for gonorrhea from patients with Bartholin gland abscesses because of the association of these infections with venereal disease, but one need not routinely treat patients for gonorrhea.

The initial treatment of a Bartholin gland abscess is simple incision and drainage. The abscess is packed for 24 to 48 hours, and sitz baths are started after the first revisit. Broad-spectrum antibiotics are helpful if there is significant cellulitis or if actual abscess formation has not yet occurred, but these agents are not required following routine incision and drainage.

It is preferable to make the drainage incision on the mucosal surface rather than on the skin surface. The incision is made over the medial surface of the introitus on a line parallel to the posterior margin of the hymenal ring (Fig. 70–4A). The abscess cavity is slightly deeper than most cutaneous abscesses, and one must be certain to enter the actual abscess cavity to achieve complete drainage. This is most easily accomplished if one inserts a hemostat through the mucosal incision and spreads the tips of the instrument in the deeper soft tissue. If the abscess recurs, more definitive therapy in the form of marsupialization (Fig. 70–4B) or complete excision of the gland may be required, but these procedures are not performed initially. Since recurrence is common with simple incision and drainage, some authorities suggest definitive surgery routinely following the first infection, whereas others prefer to wait until a recurrence is documented.

Word[13] has described a very effective treatment of Bartholin gland abscess with a balloon-tipped catheter that may obviate the need for marsupialization (Fig. 70–5). The procedure involves fistulization of the duct cavity by a catheter, which acts as a foreign body. Following a stab incision, the catheter is placed in the abscess cavity. The balloon is filled with 2 to 4 ml of water (not air) and is left in place for 6 to 8 weeks. This is an interesting technique that even allows for sexual intercourse with the catheter in place. Word's original description should be read carefully if this technique is to be used.

HYDRADENITIS SUPPURATIVA

This is a very troublesome, chronic, suppurative disease of the apocrine glands that occurs primarily in the axillae, although the genital and perineal areas may also be involved. The condition is more common in women. It is thought to be secondary to keratinous plugging of the ducts of the apocrine glands, which produces dilation and rupture of the gland into surrounding tissues. The disorder may be manifested in the initial lesion as reddish purple nodules that become fluctuant and drain. Irregular sinus tracts are formed, producing

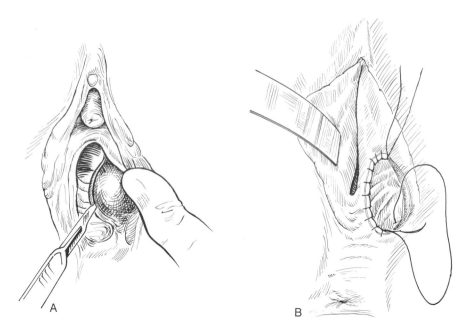

Figure 70–4. A, Incision for a Bartholin gland cyst or abscess. The incision should be made over the medial surface of the introitus on a line parallel with the posterior margin of the hymenal ring. At this point, a Bartholin gland cyst or abscess is most superficial. One exposes the incision area by displacing the cyst outward. B, Marsupialization of a Bartholin gland cyst. The skin edge is joined to the cyst wall with a continuous locking suture or with interrupted sutures. A number 3–0 absorbable suture is highly suitable. Exposure is aided if traction is made on a continuous locking suture.

groups of interconnected abscess cavities. These lesions eventually become infected with staphylococci, nonhemolytic streptococci, *Escherichia coli*, *Proteus mirabilis*, and *Pseudomonas aeruginosa*. Anaerobes have also been isolated. In the chronic form, there are multiple nodules and extensive fibrous tissue reaction.

Curative treatment of hydradenitis suppurativa is difficult because of the complications involved with providing adequate drainage of all the deep-seated foci that are present. Antimicrobial therapy and local moist heat to promote drainage are helpful adjunctive measures when frank abscess formation cannot be identified. Chronic cases have been treated with long-term continuous broad-spectrum antibiotic therapy; results have varied. Surgical drainage is usually necessary for large lesions, and every attempt should be made to incise and drain the area widely. Drainage of discrete abscesses can be accomplished as an outpatient procedure in the usual fashion. As many of the extensive loculations as possible should be broken down. In some very resistant cases, radical excision of the area may be necessary, followed by skin grafting.[14, 16] Patients with this disorder will have recurring problems with abscesses, and follow-up care is required.

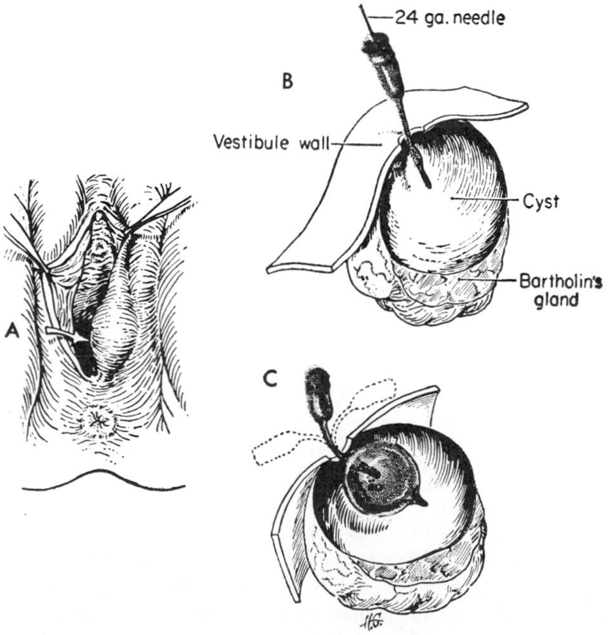

PILONIDAL ABSCESS

Pilonidal sinuses are common malformations that occur in the sacrococcygeal area. The etiology of the sinus formation is unclear, but the malformation may occur during embryogenesis. Pilonidal cyst formation is thought to be secondary to blockage of a pilonidal sinus. The result of pilonidal sinus obstruction is repeated soft tissue infection followed by drainage and partial resolution with eventual reaccumulation. The blockage is most commonly the result of hairs in the region, and the lesion may in part be a foreign body (hair) granuloma. Although pilonidal sinuses are present from birth, they usually are not manifested clinically until adolescence or the early adult years. The sinuses and cysts are lined with stratified squamous epithelium and may contain wads of hair and debris when excised.

Figure 70–5. Use of the Word catheter for outpatient drainage of a Bartholin gland abscess. A stab incision is made on the mucosal surface (A). A catheter is inserted into the cyst cavity (B) and filled with 3 to 4 ml of water (C). (From Word, B.: Office treatment of cyst and abscess of Bartholin gland. JAMA 190:777, 1964. Used by permission.)

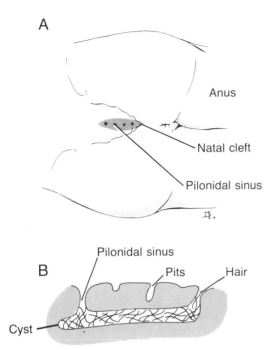

Figure 70–6. Pilonidal sinus. A, Sinuses occur in midline some 2 inches above the anus in the natal cleft. B, Longitudinal section showing sinuses and pits. (From Hill, G. J., II: Outpatient Surgery, 2nd ed. Philadelphia, W. B. Saunders Co., 1980. Used by permission.)

The patient with a pilonidal abscess will seek care for back pain and local tenderness. On physical examination the area is indurated, but frank abscess formation may not be appreciated. One will usually see barely perceptible dimples or tiny openings at the rostral end of the gluteal crease (Fig. 70–6). A hair or a slight discharge may be noticed at the opening. One may find a more caudal cyst or abscess, possibly with a palpable sinus tract connecting the two. The sinus and cyst may be chronically draining or they may become infected as the size increases and blockage occurs.[17]

Treatment of the acutely infected cyst is the same as previously discussed for any fluctuant abscess; all hair and pus should be removed, and the lesion should be packed. Antibiotic therapy is not usually required. It may take many weeks for the initial incision to heal. The area may be repacked at 2- to 4-day intervals as an outpatient procedure, although some prefer to discontinue packing after the first week. Since simple incision and drainage is often not curative, secondary removal of both the cyst and the sinus should be planned after the inflammatory process has resolved. The elective surgical procedure should be complete and should involve all of the possible arborizations of the sinus.

In a very few cases, recurrence will not take place following simple incision and drainage, especially if the incision is wide and adequate drainage is obtained. More commonly, recurrence can be expected unless excision of the sinus tract is performed. Small abscesses may be incised and drained as an outpatient procedure performed under local anesthesia, but the disease process is often extensive, and general anesthesia may be required to complete drainage. One is often surprised by the extent of the cyst cavity and the volume of pus that is encountered when the area is probed during initial incision; because of the degree of these abscesses, only localized infection lends itself to outpatient therapy. A method of catheter drainage for pilonidal abscesses has been described[11, 12] in which a flared-end Pezzer catheter is used for extended periods in the abscess cavity. The catheter allows the patient more freedom from local care and provides continual drainage (Fig. 70–7).

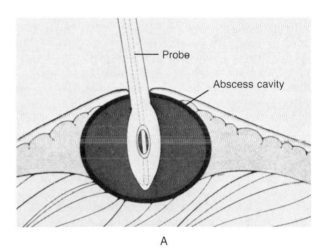

A

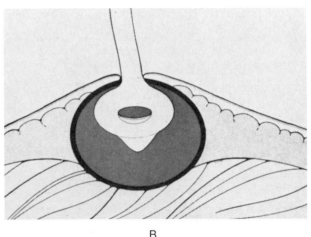

B

Figure 70–7. A method of prolonged drainage of a pilonidal abscess with a flared-end Pezzer catheter. Following a stab incision, a stretched catheter (probe inside lumen) is inserted into the abscess cavity (A). When the probe is removed, the head of the catheter expands and remains in the abscess cavity (B). Drainage is continuous through the lumen of the catheter. (From Phillip, R. S.: A simplified method for the incision and drainage of abscesses. Am. J. Surg. 135:721, 1978. Used by permission.)

PERIRECTAL ABSCESSES

Perirectal infections can range from minor irritations to fatal illnesses. Successful management depends on early recognition of the disease process and adequate surgical therapy. Because of the morbidity and mortality associated with inadequate treatment of these conditions, patients with all but the most localized abscesses should be promptly admitted to the hospital for evaluation and treatment under general or spinal anesthesia.

It is important to understand the anatomy of the anal canal and the rectum in order to appreciate the pathophysiology of these abscesses and their treatment (Fig. 70–8). The mucosa of the anal canal is loosely attached to the muscle wall. At the dentate line, where columnar epithelium gives way to squamous epithelium, there are vertical folds of tissue, called the rectal *columns of Morgagni,* which are connected at their lower ends by small semilunar folds, called *anal valves.* Under these valves are invaginations, called *anal crypts.* Within these crypts are collections of ducts from anal glands. These glands are believed to be responsible for the genesis of most, if not all, perirectal abscesses. These glands often pass through the internal sphincter but do not penetrate the external sphincter.

The muscular anatomy divides the perirectal area into compartments that may house an abscess, depending on the direction of spread of the foci of the infection (Fig. 70–9).[17, 18] The circular fibers of the intestinal coat thicken at the rectalanal junction to become the internal anal sphincter. The muscle fibers of the levator ani fuse with those of the outer longitudinal fibers of the intestinal coat as it passes through the pelvic floor. These conjoined fibers then are connected by fibrous tissue to the external sphincter system, which consists of three circular muscle groups.

Pathophysiology

As described previously, the anal glands are mucus-secreting structures that terminate in the area between the internal and external sphincters. It is believed that most perirectal infections begin in the *intersphincteric* space secondary to blockage and subsequent infection of the anal glands. Normal host defense mechanisms then break down, followed by invasion and overgrowth by bowel flora.[19]

If the infection spreads across the external sphincter laterally, an *ischiorectal abscess* is formed. If the infection dissects rostrally, it may continue between the internal and external sphincters, causing a *high intramuscular abscess.* The infection may dissect through the external sphincter over the levator ani to form the *pelvirectal abscess.*[17]

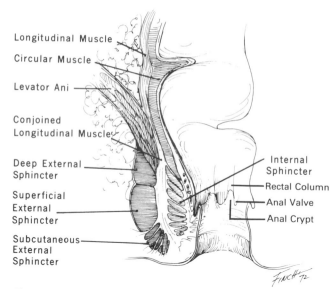

Figure 70–8. Schematic coronal section of the anal canal and the rectum. (From Schwartz, S. I., et al.: Principles of Surgery, 2nd ed. New York, McGraw-Hill, 1974. Used by permission.)

When the infection of an anal crypt extends by way of the perianal lymphatics and continues between the mucous membrane and the anal muscles, a *perianal abscess* forms at the anal orifice. The perianal abscess is the most common variety of perirectal infection. The abscess lies immediately beneath the skin in the perianal region at the lowermost part of the anal canal. It is separated from the ischiorectal space by a fascial septum that extends from the external sphincter and is continuous with the subcutaneous tissue of the buttocks. The infection may be small and localized or may be very large with a wall of necrotic tissue and a surrounding zone of cellulitis.[14] Perianal abscesses may be associated with fistula in ano. The *fistula in ano* is an inflammatory tract with an external opening in the skin of the perianal area and an internal opening in the mucosa of the anal canal.

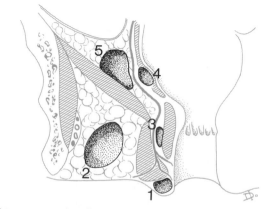

Figure 70–9. Classification of perirectal abscesses: *1.* Perianal. *2.* Ischiorectal. *3.* Intersphincteric. *4.* High intramuscular. *5.* Pelvirectal. (From Hill, G. J., II: Outpatient Surgery, 2nd ed. Philadelphia, W. B. Saunders Co., 1980. Used by permission.)

The fistula in ano is usually formed after partial resolution of a perianal abscess, and its presence is suggested by recurrence of these abscesses with intermittent drainage. The external opening of the fissure is usually a red elevated piece of granulation tissue that may have purulent or serosanguineous drainage on compression. Many times the tract may be palpated as a cord. Patients with anal fistulas should be referred for definitive surgical excision.[17]

Ischiorectal abscesses are fairly common. They are bounded superiorly by the levator ani, inferiorly by the fascia over the perianal space, medially by the anal sphincter muscles, and laterally by the obturator internus muscle. These abscesses may commonly be bilateral and, if so, the two cavities communicate by way of a deep postanal space to form a "horseshoe" abscess.[14]

Intersphincteric abscesses are less common. They are bounded by the internal and external sphincters and may extend rostrally into the rectum, thereby separating the circular and longitudinal muscle layers.

The *pelvirectal*, or *supralevator*, *abscess* lies above the levator ani muscle in proximity to the rectal wall and remains extraperitoneal. The etiology of this abscess is controversial.[7] Kovalcik and colleagues[19] suggest that supralevator abscesses are primarily an extension of an intra-abdominal process, such as diverticulitis or pelvic inflammatory disease. Read and associates[20] evaluated 474 patients with perirectal abscesses in a prospective study. They found that of the 36 supralevator abscesses, none was caused by an intra-abdominal or pelvic pathologic condition. They determined that supralevator abscesses were most commonly associated with ischiorectal abscesses and suggested that these conditions may be an extension of the ischiorectal abscesses through the floor of the levator ani. Nonetheless, the investigators found rare isolated pelvirectal abscesses without intra-abdominal, pelvic, ischiorectal, or perianal infection.

Causes of perirectal abscesses other than the so-called cystoglandular process have been documented but are fairly rare. It is believed that hemorrhoids, anorectal surgery, episiotomies, or local trauma cause abscess formation by altering local anatomy and thus destroy natural tissue barriers to infections.[19–21]

Epidemiology

Anorectal abscesses occur most commonly in healthy adults; they occur more frequently in males, in greater than a 2 to 1 ratio.[19, 20] These abscesses commonly appear during the fourth decade of life. Possible predisposing medical conditions are diabetes mellitus, inflammatory bowel disease, and other immunocompromised states.

Thirty per cent of patients have a history of previous perirectal abscess, and 75 per cent of anorectal abscesses occur in the same location as the prior abscesses.[19] Of perirectal abscesses, usually greater than 45 per cent are perianal, 20 per cent are ischiorectal, 12 per cent are intersphincteric, and 7 per cent are pelvirectal.[20]

Physical and Laboratory Findings

The diagnosis of a *perianal abscess* is generally not difficult. The throbbing pain in the perianal region is acute and is aggravated by sitting, coughing, sneezing, and straining. There is swelling, induration, and tenderness, and a small area of cellulitis is present in proximity to the anus. Rectal examination of the patient with a perianal abscess reveals that most of the tenderness and induration is below the level of the anal ring.

Patients with *ischiorectal abscesses* present with fever, chills, and malaise, but at first there is less pain than with the perianal abscess. Initially on physical examination, one will see an asymmetry of the perianal tissues, and later erythema and induration become apparent. Digital examination reveals a large, tense, tender swelling along the anal canal that extends above the anorectal ring. If both ischiorectal spaces are involved, the findings are bilateral.

Patients with *intersphincteric abscesses* usually present with dull, aching pain in the rectum rather than in the perianal region. No external aberrations of the perianal tissues are noted, but tenderness may be present. On digital examination one frequently palpates a soft, tender, sausage-shaped mass above the anorectal ring; if the mass has already ruptured, the patient may give a history of passage of purulent material during defecation.[17, 19, 20]

Diagnosis of the *pelvirectal abscesses* may be very difficult. Usually fever, chills, and malaise are present, but because the abscess is so deeply seated, there are few or no signs or symptoms in the perianal region. Rectal or vaginal examination may reveal a tender swelling that is adherent to the rectal mucosa above the anorectal ring.

Laboratory findings usually do not aid in the diagnosis. Kovalcik[19] found that less than 50 per cent of his patients had a white blood count of greater than 10,000 per cubic millimeter. Cultures of perirectal abscesses usually show mixed infections involving anaerobic bacteria, most commonly *Bacteroides fragilis* and Gram-negative enteric bacilli.

Treatment

Successful management of perirectal abscesses depends on adequate surgical drainage. Complications from these infections may necessitate multiple surgical procedures, may prolong hospital stay, and may result in sepsis and death. Bevans and associates[21] retrospectively studied the charts of 184 patients who were surgically treated over a 10-year period. These patients were evaluated primarily to identify the factors that contributed to morbidity and mortality. Initial drainage was performed under local anesthesia in 38 per cent of the patients and under spinal or general anesthesia in 62 per cent. The authors identified three key factors in excessive morbidity and mortality: (1) a delay in diagnosis and treatment, (2) inadequate initial examination or treatment, and (3) associated systemic disease. It was their belief that the only way to examine effectively and drain adequately all but the most superficial perirectal abscesses was under spinal or general anesthesia. This was supported by evidence of an increased incidence of recurrence in patients treated with local anesthesia and an increased incidence of sepsis and death. Drainage under local anesthesia simply does not allow drainage of all hidden loculations. In addition, local anesthesia is not adequate for treatment of associated pathologic conditions.

Small, well-defined perianal abscesses are the only perirectal infections that lend themselves to outpatient therapy. The result of incision and drainage is almost immediate relief of pain and rapid resolution of infection. Indications for inpatient drainage are failure to obtain adequate anesthesia, systemic toxicity, extension of the abscess beyond a localized area, or a recurrence of a perianal abscess. Recurrence may be caused by the presence of a *fistula in ano*.

A perianal abscess is drained through a single linear incision over the most fluctuant portion of the abscess in a manner previously described for other cutaneous abscesses. It is extremely painful to probe a perianal abscess and to break up loculations, and liberal analgesia is advised. The patient may begin sitz baths at home 24 hours following surgery. Packing is replaced at 48-hour intervals until the infection has cleared and granulation tissue has appeared. This usually occurs within 4 to 6 days. Antibiotics are generally not required. All other perirectal abscesses require hospitalization for definitive therapy.

Perirectal abscesses are now recognized as a fairly common cause of fever in the granulocytopenic patient. These abscesses have a different bacteriologic profile: *P. aeruginosa* organisms are isolated more frequently. These patients present later because pain develops later in the course, and fever may be the first manifestation. Therefore, any patients who are granulocytopenic with vague anorectal complaints, especially those with fever, should be examined carefully for perirectal abscesses. Any abscess that is found should be drained immediately under appropriate anesthesia, and extensive intravenous antibiotic coverage should be initiated.

INFECTED SEBACEOUS CYST

A very common entity that appears as a cutaneous abscess is the infected sebaceous cyst. Sebaceous cysts may occur throughout the body and result from obstruction of sebaceous gland ducts. The cyst becomes filled with a thick, cheesy sebaceous material, and the contents frequently become infected. Sebaceous cysts may be quite large and may persist for many years before they become infected. When infected, they clinically appear as tender, fluctuant subcutaneous masses, often with overlying erythema.

The initial treatment of an infected sebaceous cyst is simple incision and drainage. The thick sebaceous material must be expressed, since it is too thick to drain spontaneously (Fig. 70–10). A very important difference exists between infected sebaceous cysts and other abscesses. A sebaceous cyst has a definite pearly white capsule that must be excised to prevent recurrence. It is preferable to drain the infection initially and to remove the shiny capsule on the first follow-up visit, when it may be more easily identified. At the time of capsule removal, the edges are grasped with clamps or hemostats, and the core is removed by sharp dissection with a scalpel or scissors. Following excision of the capsule, the area is treated in the same manner as a healing abscess cavity. Simple drainage without excision of the capsule will often lead to recurrence.

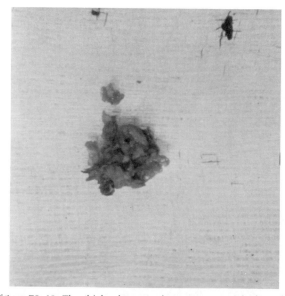

Figure 70–10. The thick, cheesy sebaceous material of a sebaceous cyst must be expressed after incision.

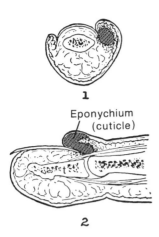

Eponychium
(cuticle)

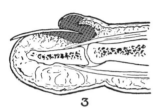

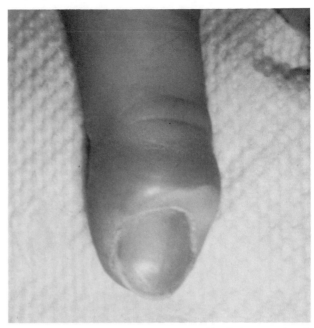

Figure 70–12. A paronychia may occur with obvious pus localization.

Figure 70–11. Paronychia. *1*, The site of the abscess at the side of the nail. *2*, The infection has extended around the base of the nail. It has raised the eponychium but has not penetrated under the nail. *3*, End stage of paronychia with a subeponychial and subungual abscess. (From Wolcott, M. W.: Ferguson's Surgery of the Ambulatory Patient, 5th ed. Philadelphia, J. B. Lippincott Co., 1974. Used by permission.)

PARONYCHIA

A paronychia is an infection localized to the area around the nail root (Fig. 70–11). Paronychias are common infections probably caused by frequent trauma to the delicate skin around the fingernail and the cuticle. When a minor infection begins, the nail itself may act like a foreign body. Usually the infectious process is limited to the area above the nail base and underneath the eponychium (cuticle), but occasionally it may spread to include some area under the nail as well, forming a subungual abscess. Lymphadenitis and lymphadenopathy are usually not seen. Generally, a paronychia is a mixed infection. *Staphylococcus* is commonly cultured from these lesions; however, anaerobes and numerous gram-negative organisms may be isolated. Paronychias in children are often caused by anaerobes, and it is believed that this is the result of finger sucking and nail biting. Occasionally, a group A beta-hemolytic infection will develop in a paronychia if the child with a strep throat puts his fingers in his mouth.

A paronychia appears as a swelling and tenderness of the soft tissue along the base or the side of a fingernail (Fig. 70–12). Pain, often around a hangnail, usually prompts a visit to the emergency department. The infection begins as a cellulitis, and may form a frank abscess. If the nail bed is mobile, the infectious process has extended under the nail, and a more extensive drainage procedure should be performed.[22] If soft tissue swelling is present without fluctuance, remission may be obtained from frequent hot soaks (6 to 8 times a day). Incision will be of no value at this early cellulitic phase. The value of antibiotics in this early stage is unproved, but if a significant cellulitis is present, a broad-spectrum antistaphylococcal antibiotic (cephalosporin or semisynthetic penicillin) may be tried. One should never rely solely on antibiotic therapy once frank pus has formed.

Technique

When a definite abscess has formed, incision and drainage is usually quickly curative. A number of invasive operative approaches have been suggested, but actual skin incision or removal of the nail is rarely required and *need not be the initial form of treatment*. One can obtain adequate drainage by simply lifting the skin edge off the nail to allow the pus to drain. This may be accomplished without anesthesia in selected patients, but it frequently requires a digital nerve block. A number 11 blade or an 18 gauge needle is advanced parallel to the nail and under the eponychium at the site of maximal swelling (Fig. 70–13). Pus rapidly escapes with immediate relief of pain.

If more than a tiny pocket of pus is present, one should fan the knife tip or needle under the eponychium, keeping the instrument parallel to

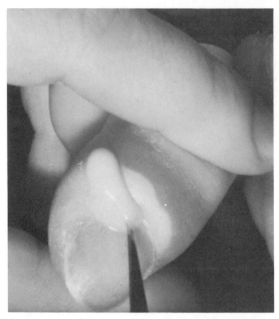

Figure 70–13. An initial treatment method for a well-localized paronychia. The eponychium (cuticle) is elevated at the area of fluctuance. Actual incision or removal of the nail is generally reserved for complicated or resistant infections.

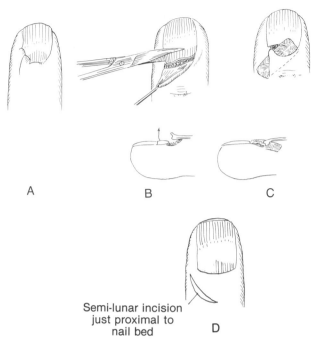

Semi-lunar incision just proximal to nail bed

Figure 70–14. A–C, Aggressive treatment of recurrent paronychia or subungual abscess includes removal of a portion of the proximal nail and incision of the eponychium. D, Some physicians prefer to use a semi-lunar incision proximal to the eponychium rather than directly incising and potentially injuring the cuticle permanently. These aggressive therapies are seldom required.

the plane of the fingernail. When a large amount of pus is drained, a small piece of packing gauze is slipped under the eponychium for 24 hours to provide continual drainage. Cultures are generally not indicated, and antibiotics are not useful if drainage is complete or if the surrounding area of cellulitis is minimal. In 24 hours the patient may be started on frequent soaks in hot tap water at home. The patient may easily remove the packing after the first soak, and the area is covered by a dry, absorbent dressing. An antibiotic ointment may be used on the site for a few days. The benefit of antibiotic ointments in reducing infection is unproved, but instructing the patient concerning the use of the ointment may prompt soaking. In addition, the ointment helps to keep the bandage from sticking.

If the initial assessment suggests that there is subungual involvement, a hole may be placed in the proximal nail with a hot paper clip. A large hole should be placed to ensure continued drainage. If the subungual involvement is extensive, one may lift a flap of tissue to expose the nail bed and then lift and excise the affected portion of the nail (Fig. 70–14). Most paronychias will resolve in 5 to 10 days, and one or two postoperative visits should be scheduled to evaluate healing and to reinforce soaking and proper home care.

Occasionally, patients will develop chronic paronychias that do not respond to standard therapy. These infections are generally fungal or viral. A particular viral infection that may puzzle the physician is a herpes paronychia, termed a "herpetic whitlow." It may be recognized by the presence of herpetic vesicles, the absence of frank pus, the slow response to treatment, and the tendency to recur. Herpetic lesions are generally quite painful but are self-limited (2 to 3 weeks) and require no specific therapy. Occasionally, secondary bacterial infection may occur and require drainage. In persistent fungal infections, the nails should probably be avulsed, and long-term treatment with topical antifungal agents should be initiated. Fungal cultures should be taken to guide therapy, since both *Candida* and dermatophytic (tinea) infections may occur. Referral to a dermatologist is suggested.

FELON

A felon is an infection of the pulp of the distal finger (Fig. 70–15). The usual cause is trauma with secondary invasion by bacteria. A felon may develop in the presence of a foreign body, such as a thorn or a splinter, but often a precipitating trauma cannot be identified. An important anatomic characteristic of this area is that there are many fibrous septa extending from the volar skin of the fat pad to the periosteum of the phalanx; these subdivide and compartmentalize the pulp area. When an infection occurs in the pulp, these same structures make it a closed space infection. The septa limit swelling, delay pointing of the abscess, and inhibit drainage after incomplete surgical decompression. Pressure may increase in the closed space, initiat-

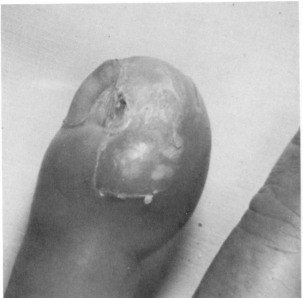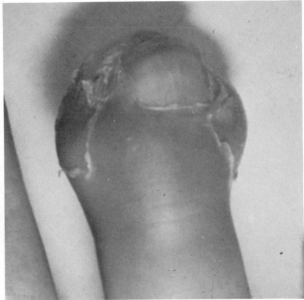

Figure 70–15. A well-developed felon. This advanced case had little pain at the time of presentation, and the distal phalanx was almost completely resorbed owing to the extensive pressure and inflammation.

ing an ischemic process that compounds the infection. The infection can progress readily to osteomyelitis of the distal phalanx. Although the septa may facilitate an infection in the pulp, they provide a barrier that protects the joint space and the tendon sheath by limiting the proximal spread of infection.

The offending organisms are usually *Staphylococcus* or *Streptococcus*, although mixed infections and gram-negative infection may occur. A felon is one of the few soft tissue infections in which a culture should be routinely obtained, since osteomyelitis and prolonged infection may occur. Culture will aid in the subsequent choice of antibiotics for complicated infections.

The patient developing a felon will describe the gradual onset of pain and tenderness of the fingertip. In a few days the pain may be constant and throbbing and gradually becomes severe. In the initial stages, physical examination may be quite unimpressive, because the fibrous septa limit swelling in the closed pulp space. As the infection progresses, swelling and redness may become obvious. Occasionally, one may elicit point tenderness, but frequently the entire pulp space is extremely tender. The patient characteristically arrives in the emergency department with the hand elevated over the head because pain is so intense in the dependent position. The cessation of pain indicates extensive necrosis and nerve degeneration.

Proper treatment of a well-developed felon consists of early and complete incision and drainage. Antibiotics alone are not curative once suppuration has occurred. Broad-spectrum antibiotics in high doses may be tried for 24 to 48 hours in early

cases with minimal swelling, but surgical incision is usually required. Delaying surgery may result in permanent disability and deformity. Most surgeons will routinely administer broad-spectrum antibiotics to the patients for 5 to 7 days following surgical incision.

Technique

A number of surgical approaches have been suggested. Three incisions have been advocated: "hockey stick," "through-and-through," and "fishmouth" or "horseshoe" incisions. All three incisions have their advocates, but most authors agree that a simple stab incision is inadequate. The surgery can usually be performed as an outpatient procedure using a digital nerve block. A long-acting solution (bupivacaine) will prolong anesthesia. A tourniquet (½-inch Penrose drain) should be used to allow digital incision in a bloodless field.

The hockey stick incision is a well-accepted drainage procedure (Fig. 70–16). This incision is advantageous if the infection points to one side of the finger, but it can be used for generalized infections. The incision begins in the midline of the tip of the fat pad just under the distal edge of the fingernail. It is extended to the lateral tip of the finger and proximally along the side of the distal phalanx (at the junction of the volar and dorsal skin markings) to a few millimeters distal to the distal interphalangeal joint. The tip of the knife blade is inserted just under the bone to a depth corresponding to the opposite edge of the distal phalanx—slightly more than halfway across the volar surface of the finger. A hemostat is

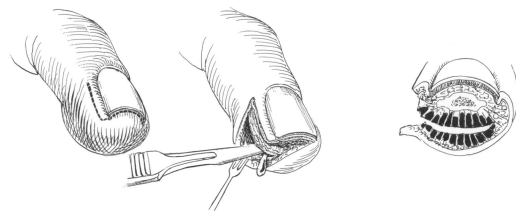

Figure 70–16. Hockey stick incision for the drainage of a felon. This is a preferred initial incision because it does not leave a scar on the working surface of the fingertip. *Note:* An incision on the ulnar side of the index, middle, and ring fingers is appropriate. The little finger is best incised on the radial side. The site of the incision on the thumb is also preferably on the radial side but may depend on the occupation of the patient. (From Chase, R. A.: Atlas of Hand Surgery. Philadelphia, W. B. Saunders Co., 1973. Used by permission.)

inserted into the incision and is spread in the plane of the fingernail (perpendicular to the septa) to break open remaining septa and loculations. Necrotic tissue or any foreign matter is excised under direct vision and the wound irrigated. A small gauze pack is placed in the incision. Because the incision may produce partial numbness of the fingertip by associated digital nerve injury the incision should *not* be made on the radial aspect of the index finger or the ulnar aspect of the thumb or little finger.

An acceptable alternative to the hockey stick, or median, incision is the through-and-through incision (Fig. 70–17). This is basically a hockey stick–type incision (without the curved distal portion of the hockey stick) that is carried through to opposite side of the finger. A hemostat is used to break up loculations, and a rubber drain (Penrose) is placed through the incision for continual drainage. The through-and-through incision is probably the easiest procedure for most felons.

The fishmouth, or horseshoe, incision is basically two hockey stick incisions that meet at the tip of the finger. A gauze pack is placed between the flaps and should be removed in a few days. This is a rather radical procedure but allows complete visualization and debridement of necrotic tissue (Fig. 70–18). Some physicians advise against this incision because it is extensive and may take a long time to heal. In addition, it produces a

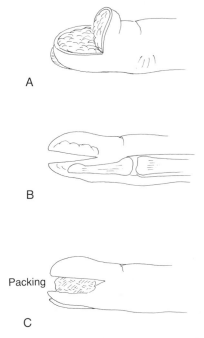

Figure 70–18. Fishmouth incision. This is a rather radical incision that is best reserved for resistant cases. Its advantage is that it allows for complete drainage and visualization of the infection in complicated cases. This incision takes longer to heal than others and may leave a large and sensitive scar. The incision is seldom used on an outpatient basis for these reasons.

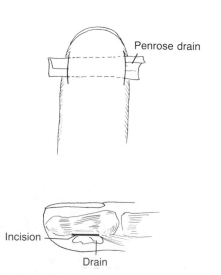

Figure 70–17. Through-and-through incision for a felon. A Penrose drain is placed for a few days to promote the withdrawal of fluid. This is an alternative to the hockey stick incision.

sizable scar. The fishmouth incision may be used if more conservative incisions are not successful, but it is not recommended for use initially.

No matter which incision is made, it must not be carried proximal to the closed pulp space because of the danger of entrance into the tendon sheath or the joint capsule. The patient should be rechecked in 2 to 3 days. A snug dressing, splinting and elevation, and adequate narcotic analgesics are prerequisites for a successful outcome and a happy patient.

On the first postoperative visit, a digital block is again performed, and the packing is removed. The incision is irrigated copiously with saline, and any additional necrotic tissue is removed. At this time, the drain may be replaced for 24 to 48 hours if there is continued drainage, but usually it can be removed and a snug dressing reapplied. Soaking may be advised, but it is not as helpful in felon therapy as it is with other soft tissue infections. At the first revisit the sensitivities of the bacterial cultures are checked and a decision to continue or change antibiotics is made. Most felons are empirically treated with antibiotics for at least 5 days. A broad-spectrum cephalosporin is a reasonable choice, pending cultures.

A few additional points should be emphasized at this time. Frank pus may be encountered during incision, but usually only a few drops are expressed. One more often drains a combination of necrotic tissue and interstitial fluid. A careful search for a foreign body should be made even if the history is not known. Some physicians advocate radiographic evaluation for retained foreign bodies and a baseline evaluation of the bone for subsequent evaluation of osteomyelitis at the initial visit. Other physicians will reserve radiographs for wounds not showing significant improvement in 5 to 7 days. Evidence of osteomyelitis, however, may not be found radiographically for several weeks after the appearance of the lesion. More radical incision and drainage may be required in persistent infections. Following adequate drainage, osteomyelitis may respond surprisingly well to outpatient antibiotic therapy with almost complete regeneration of bone if incision and drainage have been adequate. Persistent cases may require intravenous antibiotics.

SUBUNGUAL HEMATOMA

Subungual hematoma is an injury that is frequently seen in the emergency department. Any digit may be affected. The hematoma often results from hitting the fingertip with a hammer. The main concern of the patient is relief of the terrible throbbing pain that accompanies the condition as the pressure of the hematoma increases. Pain relief can be accomplished quickly with nail trephina-

tion. Trephination may be performed with a large paper clip that has been heated until red hot. The instrument is applied to burn a hole at the base of the nail (Fig. 70–19). Blood rapidly exits, and the blackened nail regains its normal color (Fig. 70–20). The blood usually remains fluid for 24 to 36 hours and is easily expressed with slight pressure. Care should be taken to make a hole large enough to allow continued drainage. An oversized paper clip is the simplist apparatus. Although a portable hot-wire electrocautery unit is available and is frequently recommended, it is difficult to obtain an adequate drainage hole without adapting the instrument and its use. One can modify the electrocautery device to burn a larger hole by "fattening" the end of the wire loop and rotating the device slowly as the nail is penetrated. In addition to being convenient, the cautery device is desirable because the wire stays hotter longer, thus enhancing nail penetration. In the stoic patient no anesthesia may be necessary, but a digital block affords painless trephination, and its routine use is suggested with the anxious patient.

The majority of subungual hematomas are painful but minor injuries. Complicated cases involve fractures of the distal phalanx. When the fingertip is unstable or the mechanism of injury suggests a significant distal phalanx fracture, a radiograph should be obtained. If a significant fracture is present, the digit should be splinted. A distal

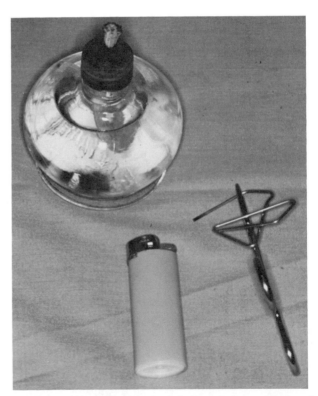

Figure 70–19. An adequately sized drainage hole may be placed in the nail with a heated paper clamp. Small holes, which tend to clog and inhibit drainage, should not be used.

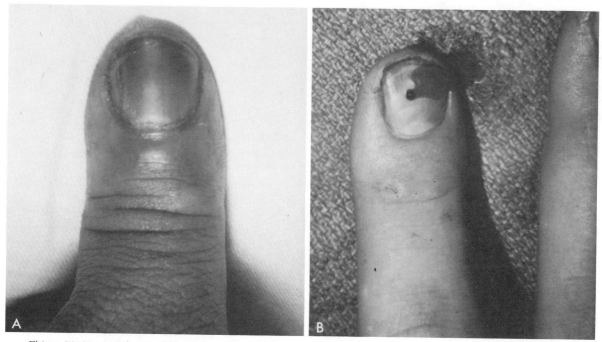

Figure 70–20. *A*, Subungual hematoma with a blackened nail bed. *B*, Following trephination, blood flows freely from the puncture site.

phalangeal fracture with a subungual hematoma is technically an open (compound) fracture. Such injuries usually heal without problems, although osteomyelitis of the tuft is a theoretical complication. The value of routine antibiotic prophylaxis in such cases is unproved. It is difficult to predict the fate of the fingernail following drainage of a subungual hematoma. Many patients with subungual hematomas will lose the nail. They should be informed of this and should be advised to protect the loosely adherent nail from further trauma. A fractured distal phalanx or a lacerated nail often signifies an underlying nail bed laceration. Although a controlled study has not been conducted, one report[24] recommends complete removal of injured nails to permit nail bed repair (6-0 absorbable sutures) to reduce the incidence of subsequent nail deformities. If the nail is removed, care must be taken to maintain an open nail fold with a nonadherent packing for a few weeks to promote normal growth of a new fingernail.

INGROWN TOENAILS

The ingrown toenail appears to be a disease of a civilization forced to wear shoes. An ingrown toenail is a common, painful, and recurrent condition that is most frequently seen in young adults. It occurs most commonly on the lateral side of the big toe. No totally effective treatment has been devised; therefore, there is a plethora of approaches and no real consensus among specialists on how to manage this entity.[23–30]

Tight-fitting nonventilated footwear has a tendency to direct the growing toenails into the soft tissue of the lateral nail fold. Normally there is a free space between the nail margin and the adjacent soft tissues (Fig. 70–21). The inherent moisture and constant motion of the toes in the shoe cause maceration of tissue, an increase in inflammatory tissue in the normally free space, and subsequent bacterial invasion. As more granulation tissue heaps up, the lateral nail margin is directed more into the toe itself. This cycle may

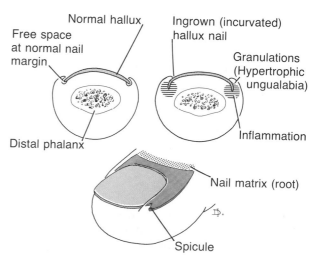

Figure 70–21. Pathology of an ingrown toenail. The normal free space at the nail margin is obliterated by inflammation and granulation tissue, which is caused by improper nail trimming, trauma to the matrix, and faulty foot gear. (From Hill, G. J., II: Outpatient Surgery, 2nd ed. Philadelphia, W. B. Saunders Co., 1980. Used by permission.)

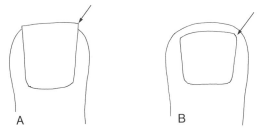

Figure 70–22. The proper way to trim a toenail to avoid an ingrown toenail is to trim the end at a right angle to the long axis and to leave the nail longer than usual (A). Trimming the lateral distal edge close to the skin in a rounded fashion predisposes the nail to become ingrown (B).

be initiated by improper care of the toenail, usually from attempts to trim it very close to the skin. It has been suggested that a straight edge be maintained on the toenail so that the lateral nail margins are not cut back near the skin edge (Fig. 70–22).

Nail-Bed Sparing Techniques. Nail-bed sparing techniques are performed in the very early stages of the condition or when the patient does not desire the loss of a portion of the nail. Complete avulsion of the nail has been one of the most frequent means of treatment over the years. This technique, although curative initially, has a high recurrence rate (approximately 60 to 70 per cent) if the avulsed nail is allowed to regrow. Unless the nail matrix is destroyed, a new toenail will grow in 4 to 6 months. With simple nail removal the problem is recurrent because, if the ingrown toenail has been present for any length of time, the lateral nail fold has become fibrosed and enlarged from chronic irritation. As the new nail grows, it is unable to depress this tissue. After the nail has been avulsed, the nail pulp rises up dorsally. The new nail may subsequently grow

into it, and the problem returns. In addition, the new nail is often thicker and less pliant and tends to invade the hypertrophied tissue rather than grow over it.

Another nail-bed sparing technique involves local care of the distal nail groove. This approach should be used only in the early stages of the ingrown toenail, when there is no significant infection and little granulation tissue. Therapy includes frequent soaks in warm antiseptic solutions. Antibiotic ointments or occlusive dressings that may increase maceration should be avoided. Following proper trimming of the nail, a twist of cotton or a small piece of dry gauze is placed under the lateral margin of the distal nail to lift it out of the nail groove. This procedure should be repeated daily by the patient until healing has occurred and the nail edge has grown beyond the danger zone. This treatment requires a motivated patient but may obviate the need for more aggressive surgical therapies.

Nail-Bed Ablating Technique. A more curative procedure involves avulsion of a portion of the nail, excision of inflammatory tissue, and excision and cautery of the nail matrix.[29] This procedure keeps the patient out of work for a few days, but with this more aggressive approach, one should expect a recurrence rate of less than 5 per cent.

The procedure is easily performed on an outpatient basis under digital block anesthesia. Following anesthesia, a tourniquet is placed at the base of the toe to allow the physician to operate in a bloodless field. A number 11 scalpel blade is used to cut the lateral one third of the toenail from the tip to its base (Fig. 70–23). Scissors are run under the nail parallel to the nail bed to loosen the nail from its bed. Once the nail is loosened, the tip is grasped with a needle holder or a

Figure 70–23. The nail ablation technique for the treatment of an ingrown toenail. The lateral portion of the nail is cut and removed (A), exposing the nail bed. The matrix is excised. Granulation tissue is excised in a V-shaped wedge (B and C), and the nail matrix is cauterized with absolute phenol for 10 minutes (D).

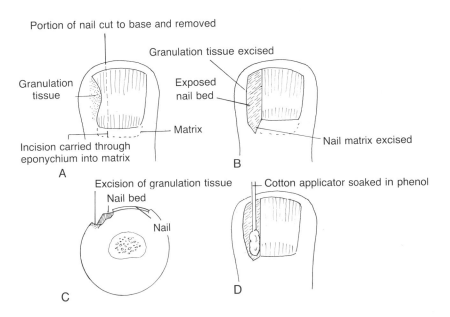

hemostat and is pulled in a longitudinal direction to avulse the nail from its base. One then removes the lateral nail matrix by making an incision into the eponychium and directly excising the pale white matrix under direct vision. When the outer portion of the nail and the matrix has been removed, a V-shaped section of hypertrophied lateral nail fold and granulation tissue is sharply excised. To avoid regrowth of the avulsed portion of the nail and subsequent recurrence of the problem, the nail matrix area is ablated with an 80 per cent phenol solution. A cotton-tipped applicator soaked in the phenol is inserted deeply into the nail fold under the cuticle of the area where the matrix was excised. The applicator should remain in place for 10 minutes to ensure ablation of the matrix. Alternatively, silver nitrate sticks may be used to destroy the remaining matrix. The silver nitrate sticks should be left in place for only 1 minute.

The nail bed is covered with a nonadherent dressing and is bandaged. The patient should avoid walking and should elevate the foot for the first 24 hours. Elevation relieves pain and decreases bleeding. Pain is usually mild and can be easily controlled with oral analgesics. At 48 hours the patient may remove the dressing and may begin warm soaks 2 to 3 times per day. In approximately 1 week the nail bed becomes dry and hard and pain ceases. A follow-up visit is scheduled for 1 week. At this point healing is evaluated, and excessive granulation tissue may be treated with silver nitrate application. Antibiotics are not required unless the patient is at high risk (diabetic) or if there is significant cellulitis.

1. Thorn, G. W., Adams, R. D., Braunwald, E., et al.: Harrison's Principles of Internal Medicine, 8th ed. New York, McGraw-Hill Book Co., 1977.
2. Peterson, P. K., James, E. C., and Ronald, A. R.: The Management of Infectious Diseases in Clinical Practice. New York, Academic Press, 1982.
3. Meislin, H. W., Lerner, S. A., Graves, M. H., et al.: Cutaneous abscesses: Anaerobic and aerobic bacteriology and outpatient management. Ann. Intern. Med. 87:145, 1977.
4. Cutaneous abscesses. (Editorial). Br. Med. J. 2:1499, 1977.
5. Brook, I., and Finegold, S. M.: Aerobic and anaerobic bacteriology of cutaneous abscesses in children. Pediatrics 67:891, 1981.
6. Floyd, J. L., and Goodman, E. L.: Soft-tissue abscesses in a diabetic patient. JAMA 246:675, 1981.
7. Mehar, G. L., Colley, D. P., Clark, R. A., et al.: Computed tomographic demonstration of cervical abscess and jugular vein thrombosis. Arch. Otolaryngol. 107:313, 1981.
8. Lewis, J. W., Groux, N., Elliott, J. P., et al.: Complications of attempted central venous injections performed by drug abusers. Chest 78:613, 1980.
9. Blick, P. W. H., Flowers, M. W., Marsden, A. K., et al.: Antibiotics in surgical treatment of acute abscesses. Br. Med. J. 280:111, 1980.
10. Knutson, R. A., Merbitz, L. A., Creekmore, M. A., et al.: Use of sugar and povidone-iodine to enhance wound healing: Five years experience. South. Med. J. 74:1329, 1981.
11. Crile, G. C.: A definitive ambulatory treatment for infected pilonidal cysts. Surgery 24:677, 1948.
12. Phillip, R. S.: A simplified method for the incision and drainage of abscesses. Am. J. Surg. 135:721, 1978.
13. Word, B.: Office treatment of cysts and abscess of Bartholin's gland duct. South. Med. J. 61:514, 1968.
14. Mandell, G. L., Douglas, G. R., and Bennett, J. E.: Principles and Practice of Infectious Disease. New York, John Wiley & Sons, 1979.
15. Wherle, P. F., and Top, F. H.: Communicable and Infectious Diseases, 9th ed. St. Louis, C. V. Mosby Co., 1981.
16. Santoro, J.: Staphylococcal and streptococcal infections in office practice. Current Topics in Emerg. Med. 1(4):1, 1978.
17. Schwartz, S. I., Lillehei, R. C., and Shires, T. G., et al.: Principles of Surgery, 2nd ed. New York, McGraw-Hill Book Co., 1974.
18. Arko, F. R.: Anorectal disorders. Am. Fam. Phys. 22:121, 1980.
19. Kovalcik, P. F., Perriston, R. L., and Cross, G. H.: Anorectal abscess. Surg. Gynecol. Obstet. 149:884, 1979.
20. Read, D. R., and Abcarian, H.: A prospective surgery of 474 patients with anorectal abscess. Dis. Colon Rectum 22:566, 1979.
21. Bevans, D. W., Westbrook, K. C., Thompson, B. W., et al.: Perirectal abscesses: A potentially fatal illness. Am. J. Surg. 126:765, 1975.
22. Schwartz, G. R., Safar, P., Stone, J. H., et al.: Principles and Practice of Emergency Medicine. Philadelphia, W. B. Saunders Co., 1978.
23. Palmer, B. V., and Jones, A.: Ingrowing toenails: The results of treatment. Br. J. Surg. 66:575, 1979.
24. Ashbell, T. S., and Kleinhert, H. E.: The deformed fingernail: A frequent result of failure to repair nailbed injuries. J. Trauma 7:177, 1967.
25. Care of the ingrowing toenail: Guidelines in technique. Hosp. Med. 72BB, Feb. 1982.
26. Cameron, P. F.: Ingrowing toenails: An evaluation of two treatments. Br. Med. J. 283:821, 1981.
27. Wallace, W. A., Milne, D. D., and Andrew, T.: Gutter treatment for ingrowing toenails. Br. Med. J. 2:168, 1979.
28. Brown, F. O.: Chemocautery for ingrowing toenails. J. Dermatol. Surg. Oncol. 7:331, 1981.
29. Lathrup, R.: Ingrown toenails: Cause and treatment. Cutis 20:119, 1977.
30. Murray, W. R., and Robb, J. E.: Soft-tissue resection for ingrowing toenails. J. Dermatol. Surg. Oncol. 7:157, 1981.

71

Soft-Tissue Needle Aspiration

EDWARD J. OTTEN, M.D.

Introduction

Soft-tissue infections, cellulitis and abscesses, are frequent problems in emergency medicine. The management of abscesses is discussed in Chapter 70. Once the diagnosis of abscess has been made, the treatment is surgical incision and drainage. Antibiotics are often used in conjunction with surgical drainage of an abscess but are not a substitute for it. The management of cellulitis is quite different. Although the diagnosis of cellulitis is often obvious, the correct antibiotic treatment may not be as obvious. The goal of treatment is to prevent abscess formation, sepsis, and other serious complications. Classically, the treatment consists of local wound care, such as elevation of an extremity and warm compresses. Antibiotics are prescribed, and the choice of antibiotic should ideally be based on knowledge of the causative organism. Determination of the causative organism, unfortunately, is often difficult in most cases of simple cellulitis.[1, 2] In addition, it is often difficult to distinguish other inflammatory soft-tissue conditions, such as insect bites, tenosynovitis, contusion, or contact dermatitis, from bacterial cellulitis.

The site of entry for cellulitis is found in only about 50 per cent of clinical cases, and when found, the source is usually a wound, ulcer, injection site, or bite. Although drug addiction, diabetes, alcoholism, and peripheral vascular disease are frequently associated with cellulitis, many patients are healthy, with no obvious underlying diseases.

Cellulitis in children is often an indication of an underlying osteomyelitis. Many patients with cellulitis have no elevated white blood count and are afebrile.

Culture isolation of the causative organism using needle aspiration of cellulitis has resulted in varying degrees of success depending upon the area of the body involved and the organism present. The current indications and accepted technique for aspiration of cellulitis will be discussed.

Historical Background

Hughes, in 1912, described a method for diagnosing and treating the offending organism in cellulitis by incising the infected area, inoculating an agar plate with whatever exuded from the incision, and preparing a vaccine against the organism that grew on the agar.[3] Drinker and associates, in 1935, found that tissue fluid aspirated from dogs with chronic lymphedema and acute cellulitis was positive for streptococcus if obtained early in the disease (less than 12 hours).[4] He also noted that blood cultures were negative on all occasions when drawn concomitantly with cellulitis cultures. In 1972, Minnefor and Murray found that aspiration of cellulitis in a pediatric patient grew *Hemophilus influenzae*, even though the blood culture was negative.[5] Goetz and colleagues, in 1974, found that cultures of facial cellulitis were positive in two of three patients with *Hemophilus influenzae* bacteremia.[6] Table 71–1 summarizes several recent studies that examined the value of aspiration of cellulitis and its correlation with blood cultures.[3–5]

From these results, it can be concluded that aspiration of cellulitis, a procedure with practically zero morbidity, may be helpful in identifying the organism causing the cellulitis, even when blood cultures are negative. *Hemophilus influenzae* is the predominant organism cultured from facial cellulitis, whereas *Staphylococcus aureus* and *Streptococcus pyogenes* are the most common extremity pathogens isolated. Although only the predominant organism is listed in Table 71–1, other organisms were occasionally cultured, and mixed infections do occur.

Indications

Because potentially valuable information can be obtained from this procedure with little cost or harm to the patient, it is recommended that needle aspiration be performed on all patients with facial or extensive soft-tissue infections where cellulitis is present. At times, one may be uncertain as to whether the soft-tissue infection represents an abscess or cellulitis. Needle aspiration of the central core of the infection should identify abscesses by the aspiration of purulent material. Note that with *cellulitis* though, tissue fluid from the *central* portion of the infection is undesirable for microbiologic evaluation. The peripheral margin of an area of cellulitis is the location for sampling with the best chance of a positive culture.

There are no absolute contraindications to needle aspiration of cellulitis.[7–9] Aspiration can be

Table 71–1. VALUE OF ASPIRATION OF CELLULITIS AND ITS CORRELATION WITH BLOOD CULTURES

Author	Number of Patients	Location of Cellulitis	Positive Growth from Tissue	Positive Growth from Blood Cultures	No Organism Isolated	Predominant Organism
Fleisher, G., et al., 1980	8	face	1	3	4	*Hemophilus influenzae*
	42	extremities	20	1	22	Staphylococcus/ Streptococcus
Fleisher, G., et al., 1981	5	face	2	2	2	*H. influenzae*
	23	extremities	10	1*	11	Staphylococcus/ Streptococcus
Ginsberg, M. B., 1981	16†	extremities	2	0	41†	Staphylococcus/ Streptococcus
Ho, R. W. L., et al., 1979	76	various	64	1	12	Staphylococcus Streptococcus
Rudoy, R. C., et al., 1979	5	extremities	3	4	1	*H. influenzae*
Szilagyi, A., et al., 1982	28	face extremities	12	–‡	16	Staphylococcus/ Streptococcus

*Blood cultures were drawn on only 16 patients.
†Only 16 patients had aspiration, 27 had blood cultures.
‡No blood cultures were done.

performed in a patient with a coagulopathy. One should carefully avoid introducing infection into a joint, tendon sheath, or blood vessel during aspiration.

Technique

The technique for aspiration of cellulitis is straightforward. An 18 gauge needle (22 gauge is preferred for the face) attached to a 5-ml syringe should be used. The skin should be prepared by wiping with isopropyl alcohol or povidone-iodine solution and allowed to dry. The *leading edge of the cellulitis* should then be entered to a depth of 1 cm, with the needle bevel pointing downward and the syringe angled approximately 10 to 15 degrees to the skin (Fig. 71–1). The cellulitic area should then be aspirated by pulling back on the plunger. Previous studies have shown that aspiration of the central area of the cellulitis does not produce positive cultures.[2] Only a few drops of fluid will usually be aspirated. If the initial aspiration fails to produce any material, 0.5 ml of *nonbacteriostatic* normal saline should be injected and immediately aspirated. Any material obtained by either method should be inoculated onto sheep blood agar and chocolate agar. If no material is obtained, the needle tip may be used to inoculate the agar or the needle itself cultured by rinsing it in beef infusion broth. Gram stain of aspirated material may be helpful if sufficient material is obtained on initial aspiration; however, in many cases, positive cultures are obtained when gram stains have not shown organisms. After aspiration, the puncture site can be covered with a sterile dressing.[6, 7, 10, 11]

Complications

Complications of needle aspiration are unusual. The theoretical possibility of extending the cellu-

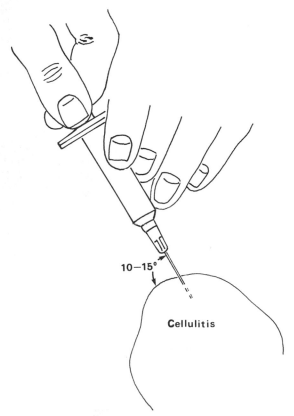

Figure 71–1. The leading edge of an area of advancing cellulitis is aspirated. The injection of 1 ml of nonbacteriostatic normal saline prior to aspiration will often enhance tissue fluid recovery.

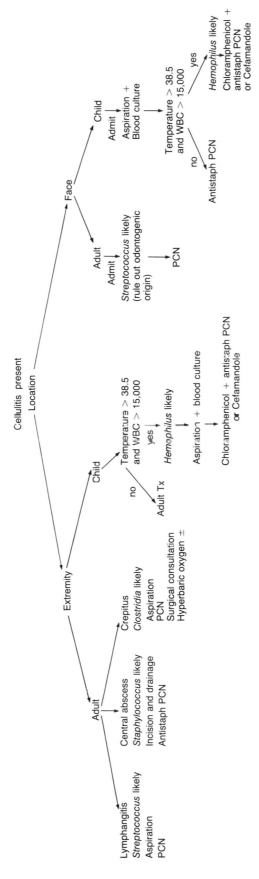

Figure 71–2. Management of cellulitis.

litis to deeper structures exists, but the added morbidity associated with this is small. Fistula formation and the possibility of continued bleeding in selected individuals are extremely rare.[9]

Conclusions

Needle aspiration of areas of suspected cellulitis is helpful for microbial isolation and for guiding therapy (Fig. 71–2). The technique described here is rapid and rarely associated with morbidity.

1. Ginsberg, M. B.: Cellulitis: analysis of 101 cases and review of the literature. South Med. J. 74:530, 1981.
2. Szilagyi, A., Mendelson, J., and Portnoy, J.: Cellulitis of the skin: clinical observations of 50 cases. Can. Fam. Phys. 28:1399, 1982.
3. Hughes, B.: The treatment of cellulitis with special reference to the hand and arm. Practitioner 89:142, 1912.
4. Drinker, C. K., Field, M. E., Ward, H. K., and Lyons, D.: Increased susceptibility to local infection following blockage of lymph drainage. Am. J. Physiol. 112:74, 1935.
5. Minnefor, A. B., and Murray, J. J.: Hemophilus influenzae cellulitis of the lower extremity. Am. J. Dis. Child 124:920, 1972.
6. Goetz, J. P., Tafari, N., and Boxerbaum, B.: Needle aspiration in Hemophilus influenzae Type B cellulitis. Pediatrics 54:504, 1974.
7. Fleisher, G., Ludwig, S., and Campos, J.: Cellulitis: bacterial etiology, clinical features, and laboratory findings. J. Pediatr. 97:591, 1980.
8. Fleisher, G., Ludwig, S., Henretig, F., et al.: Cellulitis: initial management. Ann. Emerg. Med. 10:356, 1981.
9. Uman, S. J., and Kunin, C. M.: Needle aspiration in the diagnosis of soft-tissue infections. Arch Intern. Med. 135:959, 1975.
10. Fleisher, G., and Ludwig, S.: Cellulitis: a prospective study. Ann. Emerg. Med. 9:246, 1980.
11. Rudoy, R. C., and Nakashima, G.: Diagnostic value of needle aspiration in Hemophilus influenzae Type B cellulitis. J. Pediatr. 94:924, 1979.
12. Ho, P. W. L., Pien, F. D., and Hamburg, D.: Value of cultures in patients with acute cellulitis. South Med. J. 72:1402, 1979.
13. Middleton, D. B., and Ferrante, J. A.: Periorbital and facial cellulitis. Am. Fam. Phys. 21:98, 1980.

15

MICROBIOLOGY

72

Microbiological Procedures

FRANK P. BRANCATO, PH.D.

DIRECT PREPARATIONS OF CLINICAL MATERIALS, STAINED AND UNSTAINED, IN EMERGENCY MEDICAL CARE*

Introduction

EVOLVEMENT OF STAINED SMEARS

Histologists have used organic dyes to stain tissues since 1856. In 1869, Hoffman used these dyes to stain bacteria. In 1875, Weigert stained cocciform bacteria in tissue with methyl violet. Three years later, Koch introduced dried bacterial films on glass and stained these films with various dyes. Early in the next decade, Ehrlich (1882) developed a method for acid-fast staining of bacteria, followed 2 years later by Gram's accidental discovery of a very important differential staining technique that now bears his name. One of the numerous modifications of the Gram stain is in use in clinical laboratories over most of the world.

Interest in the physiology and method of disease production by bacteria, however, took precedence over the microscopic examination of these organisms in clinical materials. Apparently it was not appreciated that both the infectious pathophysiology and microscopic examination of pathogens have a place in providing optimal patient care. Although the isolation of a pathogen is a delayed process, the information that is learned from microscopic evaluation of clinical materials is of immediate value to the emergency physician.

For the first half of the twentieth century, there was scant attention in the literature regarding the direct microscopic examination of clinical material either as a wet mount or as a Gram-stained film on a glass slide. This is not to imply that microscopic examinations of Gram-stained smears were not being done. These smears were being done in all medical bacteriology courses; however, they

were of colonies from cultures or of growth in broth.

In 1958, Newman[1] and, in 1959, Blenden[2] emphasized the importance of the initial microscopic examination in selecting the proper culture medium and in evaluating the culture results. Brancato and Parker,[3] in 1966, provided their direct smear data based on experience compiled from 1954 to 1964 at the Seattle U.S. Public Health Service Hospital. Their data documented the benefit of this tool to the patient, to the physician, and to the microbiologist. Path Capsule 26, published and copyrighted in 1965 by the College of American Pathologists,[4] very succinctly pointed out the value of direct smear results. In the 1970's, Provine and Gardner[5] and, a few years later, others,[6–12] reaffirmed their conclusions. As Washington[13] wrote about the Gram-stained smear in 1979: "Curiously this test is *vastly* underused, sometimes misused, and *often* misinterpreted." (My emphasis)

Indication

A direct preparation is indicated when the practitioner concludes after physical examination of the patient that an infection may be present or must, at least, be ruled out. This conclusion can be supported rapidly and accurately, in most instances, by microscopic examination of a direct smear of appropriate clinical material. The direct smear can also aid in the choice of antibiotic therapy, provided the bacterial morphology and staining properties are correlated with the associated cellular reaction and clinical picture to suggest a specific infecting organism or category of organisms.

The importance of the collection of the clinical material, which forms the base from which an accurate smear and, if necessary, a culture can be prepared, has been emphasized but never often enough. In the following section, primary attention is directed toward the collection of clinical material from various body areas.

Collection Technique (General Principles)

BODY FLUIDS AND TRANSUDATES

The vascular network is accessed via venipuncture and the central nervous system via lumbar tap. Body cavities are accessed via pleural, peritoneal or joint tap.

Collection
1. Sterilize the skin surface selected for penetration (alcohol rub, povidone iodine rub followed by alcohol rub; allow to dry).

---

*A procedural atlas is provided at the end of this section.

2. Administer local anesthetic when clinically indicated, using sterile technique.

3. Penetrate with a sterile needle and syringe.

4. After aspiration of specimen, remove trapped air from syringe and replace needle guard.

Direct Examinations

1. Gram-stained smear (except blood).

2. India ink mount (spinal fluid).

3. Wright-Giemsa-stained smear (blood when blood parasites are a consideration).

4. Acid-fast-stained smear.

5. Acridine orange-stained smear (if fluorescent microscope is available).

Discussion

These fluids and transudates are sterile and, other than blood, normally are free of host-reactive cells, such as leukocytes. The presence of a host reaction strongly points to a microbial infection. Organisms are also uncommonly seen in direct smears from these body fluids. In order to see at least one organism per oil immersion field, there must be at least 100,000 organisms per ml (conservatively). Rarely will organisms be seen when the count is under 10,000 per ml.[14-16] Consequently, materials should be forwarded to the laboratory for culture when a host reaction is present, even though no organisms are seen on the smear.

EXUDATES FROM SITES WITH RESIDENT FLORA

Primary sites with resident flora include the upper respiratory tract, the female urogenital tract, draining cutaneous lesions, and anorectal lesions.

Collection

1. Rinse and gently cleanse the site free of contamination from earlier exudation.

2. Touch two sterile swabs (cotton, calcium alginate) to fresh exudate.

3. Make thin smear by rolling one swab over a 1-sq cm area of a clean glass slide. Several slides may be made.

4. Insert the other swab into sterile tube (dry or with suitable carrying fluid, such as 1 to 2 ml of physiological saline or broth).

Direct Examinations

1. Gram-stained smear.

2. Acid-fast-stained smear.

Discussion

The existence of a resident flora presents two problems. First, because collection is affected, the lowest possible level of contamination by the resident flora must be sought. Second, interpretation of the smear microscopically and, if cultured, of the culture findings in the presence of resident flora may be difficult.

It is immediately obvious that a knowledge of the resident flora and their levels at the aforementioned body sites is necessary.[17] Not as obvious is the need for knowledge about the host reaction in the form of inflammation and phagocytic cells at these sites. In normal individuals or in immunosuppressed individuals, such host reactions are generally reduced or lacking.

STERILE FLUIDS GENERALLY COLLECTED BY PASSAGE THROUGH AREA HAVING RESIDENT FLORA

Lower Respiratory Tract

Collection

1. The patient rinses the oral cavity and throat by gargling with tap water; then the patient expectorates a *deep* cough sputum into a sterile container (quality, not quantity, of the specimen is the goal).

Alternatives

2. Nasotracheal aspiration. Sterile tubing is passed through the nasal passage into the trachea.

3. Transtracheal aspiration (as per needle cricothyroidotomy discussed in Chapter 4).

Direct Examinations

1. Gram-stained smear.

2. Acid-fast-stained smear.

3. Wright-Giemsa-stained smear (for quantitation of eosinophiles).

4. Acridine orange-stained smear (if fluorescent microscope is available).

Upper Urinary Tract

Collection

1. The patient voids a clean catch (midstream) specimen. The external genitalia are first cleansed front to back, and the patient is encouraged to void approximately 20 ml of urine before collecting 1 to 2 ml in a sterile container for smear and culture (if indicated).

Alternatives

2. An in and out catheterized specimen collected in a sterile container.

3. Patients with indwelling catheters should have a new sterile catheter placed before collection of the specimen.

4. Suprapubic tap, best obtained from hyperdistended bladder. Cleanse and anesthetize the skin (see genitourinary procedures for complete discussion), then aspirate.

Direct Examinations

1. Gram-stained smear.
2. Acridine orange-stained smear (if fluorescent microscope is available).

Male Urogenital Tract

Collection

1. If penile discharge is present, the external genitalia are washed and the discharge is expressed by gentle massage, and collected with a sterile swab. Place discharge in plugged or capped tube.

2. If no penile discharge is present, the external genitalia are washed and a thin alginate swab (may or may not be moistened with sterile water) is inserted approximately 2 cm into the distal urethra and rotated gently. The swab is then placed in a plugged or capped tube.[18]

Direct Examination

1. Gram-stained smear.

Closed Cutaneous Lesions Such As Furuncles, Vesicles

Collection

1. Swollen lesion (pooled exudate). Sterilize the surface (e.g., povidone iodine rub followed by alcohol rub) and aspirate exudate with a sterile needle and syringe. Alternatively, one can incise and drain the lesion, collecting a sample with a sterile swab from the inner wall of the lesion.

2. Inflammation with no obvious exudate accumulating. After sterilizing the surface, insert and withdraw approximately 0.5 ml of sterile physiological saline from the margin of the lesion with a sterile needle and syringe (see Chapter 71).

Direct Examination

1. Gram-stained smear.

Discussion

Exudates derived from closed lesions represent a significant proportion of the clinical materials submitted to the laboratory, and, if the specimen has been properly collected, a direct smear evaluation can result in highly accurate and rapid guidance to the requestor.

EXCRETION WITH RESIDENT FLORA (FECES)

Collection

1. Fluid feces. Have the patient defecate directly into a waterproof container with secure lid.

2. Formed feces. Have the patient provide a sample as above. Examine the entire surface for adhering helminths or parts thereof; then take small portions from different areas, especially those with mucus or blood, with a disposable wood spatula (tongue blade), and place them in a waterproof container.

Direct Examinations

1. Place a drop of freshly passed (warm) fluid feces on a slightly warmed slide. Immediately seal it with a petrolatum-rimmed coverslip.

2. Gram-stained smear of thin film of fluid feces or of mucus or blood adhering to formed feces.

3. Wright-Giemsa-stained smear of thin film of fluid feces or of mucus or blood adhering to formed feces.

Primary Staining Methods

Procedural steps for popular staining methods are listed in Table 72–1. Additional comments regarding the methods are provided in the following sections.

GRAM STAIN

The Gram stain allows one to see the morphologic differences among bacteria and separates bacteria into two broad groups. The ability of bacteria to retain the primary crystal violet dye and to resist decolorization is termed *gram-positive*. *Gram-negative* denotes that the primary dye stain taken up by the organism is susceptible to decolorization.

Although gram-positive bacterial cell walls resist decolorization, some decolorization is possible with errors in technique,[19] and gram-positive organisms may be incorrectly perceived as gram-negative. The following procedural points, which may influence the degree of decolorization, should be noted. A thick smear is more resistant to decolorization than a thin smear; thus, it is important to spread the specimen evenly over the slide so that individual cells may be separated from one another. Air drying a smear may be an inadequate method for fixation of the specimen. Gentle heating of the slide with an alcohol lamp or Bunsen burner allows for better fixation. Heat fixation should not be excessive and, optimally, when time permits, should be done *after* the specimen has been allowed to air dry. A few quick passes over an open flame is usually sufficient for heat fixation. The flame should not be used to dry the specimen. Excessive heating may damage cell walls and may cause a gram-positive organism to stain negatively. Some authorities prefer to fix the specimen with methanol.[19]

The leukocytes may serve as a guide to decolorization. Normally, the crystal violet is completely

Table 72–1. COMMON STAINING METHODS

Gram Stain

Fixation

Prepare a thin smear by spreading material from swab (or 0.01 ml calibrated loop in the case of unspun urine) evenly onto a glass slide over a 2-cm^2 area. Allow the slide to air dry then *briefly* heat fix.

Primary Stain

Flood the slide with crystal violet, or methyl violet, 6B for several seconds. Rinse the slide with tap water immediately, and drain off the water. During drainage, the slide should be held vertically with the frosted end up and the unfrosted end resting on blotting paper.

Mordant

Flood the slide with Gram's iodine for at least 10 seconds. Rinse with tap water and drain again, as previously.

Decolorization

Flood the slide with acetone-alcohol (1:1), drain, and repeat the acetone-alcohol flood. Rinse the slide with tap water, and drain. Note that at the end of this step the slide should be similar in appearance to the original unstained smear. Some authors recommend either 95 per cent ethanol or acetone alone rather than the combination (1:1) used here.

Counterstain

Flood the slide with 0.1 per cent aqueous basic fuchsin, and rinse with tap water. Drain the slide, and allow it to air dry. Note that many laboratories use safranin rather than basic fuchsin for counterstaining. Basic fuchsin tends to produce a darker counterstain.

Kinyoun-Tergitol Acid-Fast Stain

Fixation

A thin smear is preapared on a glass slide. The smear is air dried and briefly heat fixed.

Primary Stain

Flood the slide with carbol-fuchsin, and allow the slide to stand for at least 1 minute.

Decolorization

Decolorize the slide with acid alcohol until the washing is no longer red.

Counterstain

Counterstain the slide with methylene blue for 30 seconds. Rinse the slide with tap water, and allow it to air dry. Acid-fast organisms retain the carbol-fuchsin red stain.

Wright-Giemsa Stain

Fixation

A thin smear is fixed by flooding the slide with methanol for 1 minute. A thick smear, if blood is studied, is allowed to dry for at least 1 hour but less than 8 hours. The thick smear is subsequently immersed in distilled water for 5 minutes.

Primary Stain

The smear is flooded with filtered Wright-Giemsa stain for 10 to 30 minutes.

Rinse

The stain is washed off with buffered water. The slide is held vertically over blotting paper and allowed to drain, then it is allowed to air dry.

Methylene Blue Wet Mount

Preparation

A drop of specimen is placed beside a drop of methylene blue on a glass slide. The drops are allowed to mix.

Cover Slip and Seal

A cover slip is placed over the specimen stain mixture. Vaseline is used to seal the edges of the cover slip. The specimen is allowed to stand 5 to 10 minutes to permit complete staining prior to examination. Overstaining can occur after 30 minutes.

Acridine Orange Stain

Fixation

A thin smear is prepared in the standard manner. The smear is allowed to air dry and is then briefly heat fixed.

Stain

The slide is flooded with 0.5 per cent acridine orange solution (0.15 M acetate buffer, pH 4.0) for 2 minutes.

Rinse

The slide is rinsed with tap water and allowed to air dry. The slide is examined under high-dry and oil immersion magnification with a fluorescent microscope. Microbes will stain orange against a faint green background with this method.

---

removed from the leukocyte with the decolorizer, and the leukocyte assumes the red color of the counterstain. Retention of the violet stain by the leukocyte is presumptive evidence of insufficient decolorization. As a general guide to the use of the decolorizer, one should use the decolorizer until the solution flows colorlessly from the edge of the slide.

Gram's iodine, a mordant composed of aqueous iodine with potassium iodide (I_2-KI), forms a stable complex with the crystal violet, which limits the degree of decolorization of the organism. The solution has a relatively short half-life. Gram's iodine may be somewhat unstable if it is stored for long periods of time, and the iodine may be lost from the solution. The available iodine concentration of an open bottle stored at 25° C decreases to 10 per cent of its original concentration at 30 days. As the concentration of iodine decreases, the smear may become more susceptible to decolorization. The problem of iodine loss may be remedied by using iodophor as the mordant.

Host cells, epithelial and reactive, thin organisms (spirochetes), and protozoan appendages (flagella of the Mastigophora) are distinctly stained by the use of basic fuchsin as the counterstain.

ACID-FAST STAIN

The Kinyoun-tergitol modification is a rapid, cold method for staining those organisms with cell walls resistant to decolorization with a dilute acid solution. With careful timing, the acid-fastness of all mycobacteria and nocardias can be demonstrated. The acid-fast stain can be modified to detect *Pneumocystis carinii*, cytomegalovirus inclusion bodies, and Legionella.[20] Rather than decolorizing as in step 3 of the procedure (Table 72–1), the slide is washed with tap water. The counterstain (methylene blue) is allowed to sit a full 5 minutes prior to again being rinsed with tap water.

WRIGHT-GIEMSA STAIN

This commonly used hematologic tool is effective in differentially staining leukocytes, blood parasites, and some fecal protozoa.

METHYLENE BLUE WET MOUNT

This stain provides a rapid demonstration of the presence of fecal leukocytes and also emphasizes nuclear details of intestinal protozoa.[21] The technique is also helpful in the rapid analysis of cerebral spinal fluid.

ACRIDINE ORANGE STAIN

This stain is useful in staining certain body fluids in which there may be a paucity of microbes, making them difficult to discern among the host cells and debris.[22, 23] The disadvantage of this staining method is that a fluorescent microscope must be available.

Direct Smear Evaluation

GENERAL

The routine evaluation of a direct smear can be done at all hospitals, and the equipment should be available in the emergency department for use by the physician when time allows. The stained specimens are best evaluated with the low-dry and the high-power oil immersion lenses without a coverslip. The most frequent errors are improper collection and improper preparation of the material and a hasty evaluation of the slide under the microscope. At least 5 minutes of uninterrupted examination of a slide is necessary for optimal evaluation. Although it is time consuming to look at all smears and although most laboratories have

Table 72–2. SMEAR-CULTURE CORRELATION (Seattle U.S. Public Health Service Hospital, 1964–1979)

	Number	Percentage
Postive smear-culture agreement Either positive smear with positive culture or negative smear with negative culture	199,336	98.1
Negative smear-culture agreement Either positive smear with negative culture or negative smear with positive culture	3,783	1.9
Total smears and cultures reported	203,119	100

personnel with these skills, in such critical illnesses as suspected meningitis, all smears should be viewed personally by the physician in charge.

Table 72–2 contains data compiled over 15 years at the Seattle U.S. Public Health Service Hospital. A review of more than 200,000 cases in this study indicates an impressive 98 per cent correlation of smear and culture results. Certainly, the degree to which a slide is helpful greatly depends upon the skill of the physician in collecting and interpreting that specimen.

Individuals not completely at ease with the microscopic examination of direct smears of clinical materials will find Charts 72–1 through 72–5, Microbiology Algorithms, of help. Some of the algorithms have corresponding illustrations of a diagnostic field to further aid the neophyte. Because an infecting organism and the host-reactive cells will not differ markedly from one clinical material to another, repetition is avoided by presenting descriptive algorithms and illustrations of their presence in only one clinical material.

UPPER RESPIRATORY TRACT

Various anatomic areas of the upper respiratory tract may manifest signs of infection (e.g., pharynx, tonsils, sinuses, gingiva, and epiglottis). Because these areas can be visualized relatively easily, a thin smear made from a swab of the inflamed site or the purulent area will quickly reveal the presence and type of host reaction and the associated probable etiologic agent.

Keitel,[24] Provine and Gardner,[5] and Bannatyne and associates[25] stated that the abundant upper respiratory mixed flora, including numerous streptococci, rendered the Gram-stained pharyngeal smear difficult to interpret and generally worthless

Chart 72–1. MICROBIOLOGY ALGORITHM: UPPER RESPIRATORY TRACT INFECTIONS
GRAM-STAINED SMEAR EVALUATION*

1. No inflammatory cells, only squamous epithelial cells (SEC) and mixed resident flora (see Fig. 72–1).
   Impression: no pathology evident; normal.
2. Intact mixed leukocytes. Foamy macrophages may be present; ciliocytophthoria (disrupted ciliated columnar epithelial cells) may be present. Mixed resident flora (see Fig. 72–2).
   Impression: presumptive viral infection.
3. Host reaction as in No. 2, but mixed resident flora is present in overwhelming numbers.
   Impression: presumptive viral infection, with abundant microbial overgrowth (bacterial component).
4. Host reaction as in No. 2, but elongated, encapsulated, gram-positive diplococci are very prominent and associated with leukocytes.
   Impression: presumptive viral infection, with presumptive *Streptococcus pneumoniae* (bacterial component) infection.
5. Host reaction as in No. 2, but small, gram-negative coccobacilli are very prominent and associated with leukocytes.
   Impression: presumptive viral infection, with presumptive *Haemophilus* (bacterial component) infection.
6. Host reaction as in No. 2, with neutrophils prominent and numerous gram-negative diplococci, often phagocytized.
   Impression: presumptive viral infections with presumptive *Neisseria* (bacterial component) infection.
7. Host reaction as in No. 2, but large, plump, gram-negative diplobacilli (*Moraxella*) are very numerous.
   Impression: presumptive viral infection, with postnasal drainage.
8. Host reaction as in No. 2, but with marked numbers of spherical, gram-positive cocci in clusters with diphtheroids.
   Impression: presumptive viral infection; pharyngeal aspiration from "runny" nose (*Staphylococcus* and *Corynebacterium*)
9. Many leukocytes generally disrupted; spherical, single, and paired. Gram-positive cocci associated with leukocytic remnants (see Fig. 72–3).
   Impression: presumptive group A beta-hemolytic Streptococcus infection.
10. Many neutrophils generally disrupted; numerous fusobacteria and treponemes (see Fig. 72–4).
    Impression: Vincent's infection.
11. Many leukocytes, generally neutrophils, intact and disrupted; slender pleomorphic, gram-positive bacilli are prominent and associated with the leukocytes (see Fig. 72–5).
    Impression: presumptive *Corynebacterium diphtheriae* vs. *C. haemolyticum* infection.

*At least five different portions of the smear must be examined with lower-power and oil immersion lens.

in diagnosing the cause of pharyngitis. In these publications, there was no mention of attention being given to the host's cellular reaction in interpreting the significance of the organisms present. The data in Table 72–3 reveal the considerable degree of accuracy of the direct Gram-stained smear in the presumptive diagnosis of streptococcal pharyngitis. These data have been affirmed in studies published in 1978,[7] 1979,[10] and 1981[11] as well as in clinical practice.[12]

Chart 72–1 (Microbiology Algorithm for Upper Respiratory Tract Infections) presents the evaluation of Gram-stained smears for upper respiratory

infections. The importance of correlating the bacterial and host cell reaction is emphasized in this chart. Illustrative examples are shown in Figs. 72–1 through 72–5.

The emergency physician can use the Gram-stained smear as a screening tool to limit the number of throat cultures or fluorescent antibody studies carried out in his practice. A positive direct smear is strong, presumptive evidence of a group A beta-hemolytic streptococcal pharyngitis.[7, 10, 12, 13] Because of a small but definite number of false-negative pharyngeal direct smears for group A beta-hemolytic streptococcal pharyngitis, the phy-

Chart 72–2. MICROBIOLOGY ALGORITHM: LOWER RESPIRATORY TRACT INFECTIONS
GRAM-STAINED SMEAR EVALUATION*

1. 25 or more squamous epithelial cells (SEC) per low-power field (LPF); resident flora of upper respiratory tract (URT).
   Impression: gross URT contamination; poor collection.
2. 11–25 SEC/LPF; resident flora of URT; few scattered leukocytes.
   Impression: moderate URT contamination; fair collection.
3. 4–10 SEC/LPF; scant resident flora of URT; leukocytes present.
   Impression: slight URT contamination; good collection.
4. 0–3 SEC/LPF; many leukocytes present, generally neutrophils.
   Impression: good collection, most microbial pneumonias; etiologic agent generally abundant and associated with neutrophils (*Streptococcus pneumoniae* (see Fig. 72–7), *Haemophilus influenzae* (see Fig. 72–6), *Staphylococcus aureus, Klebsiella*).
5. 0–3 SEC/LPF; mixed intact leukocytes; foamy macrophages often abundant; some URT flora may be present with minimal cellular association.
   Impression: good collection; presumptive viral or mycoplasma pneumonia.†
6. 0–3 SEC/LPF; few to many intact, mixed leukocytes; ciliated columnar epithelial cells may be prominent (if fragmented, they are called *ciliocytophthoria*).
   Impression: Good collection; presumptive viral bronchial entity (see Fig. 72–2).

*At least five different portions of the smear must be examined with low-power and oil immersion lens.
†Mycoplasma pneumonias generally present with a nonproductive cough.

Chart 72–3. MICROBIOLOGY ALGORITHM: URINARY TRACT INFECTIONS
GRAM-STAINED SMEAR EVALUATION*

1. No inflammatory cells; no organisms.
   Impression: normal (no infection).
2. No inflammatory cells; squamous epithelial cells (SEC); resident urogenital flora (varies with gender).
   Impression: poor collection.
3. Male: 1–3 WBC/LPF†; no organisms, or there may be urogenital meatal flora such as diphtheroids and staphylococci.
   Impression: not an infection of the urinary tract.
4. Female: 5–10 WBC/LPF; varying numbers of SEC; no organisms, or there may be urogenital flora such as lactobacilli, streptococci, etc.
   Impression: not an infection of the urinary tract.
5. Male: 4 or more WBC/LPF; female: 10 or more WBC/LPF; no organisms seen (bacterial count may be under 10,000//ml).
   Impression: should be cultured; may represent a urethral syndrome patient.[45-47]
6. Rare–many WBC/LPF; gram-negative bacilli generally plump.‡
   Impression: presumptive acute infection; obtain culture (see Fig. 72–21).
7. Rare–many WBC/LPF, and SEC often present; mixed gram-negative bacilli; chaining or clumping gram-positive cocci may also be present.
   Impression: presumptive chronic infection often precipitated by instrumentation; obtain culture.
8. Male: generally older than 45 years; WBC and Gardnerella-type bacilli (often in clumps).
   Impression: prostatism with a microbial component and not a cystitis.

*Entire film (0.01 ml of unspun urine) screened under low-power magnification and at least 10 oil immersion fields examined.
†WBC (white blood cells)/LPF (low-power field)
  rare: 1–3 few: 4–10 moderate: 11–25 many: more than 25
‡organisms/OIF(oil immersion field)
10^5/ml: averages 1/OIF for 10 OIF
6×10^4/ml to 9×10^4/ml: 5–9 in 10 OIF
10^4/ml to 5×10^4/ml: 1–5 in 10 OIF

sician must use clinical judgment in determining how to work-up symptomatic patients with a negative smear.[26]

Other infections with characteristic Gram-stained direct smears that require antibiotic therapy include *Corynebacterium diphtheriae* or *hemolyticum* pharyngitis (see Fig. 72–5), and Vincent's infection (see Fig. 72–4). The presence of several species of Neisseria (*N. sicca*, *N. subflava*, *N. flavescens*, and *N. lactamica* and *Branhamella catarrhalis* (formerly *N. catarrhalis*) as endogenous flora minimizes the usefulness of the direct smear in diagnosing *Neisseria gonorrhoeae* pharyngitis.[27] Nonetheless, the presence of gram-negative intracellular diplococci (see Fig. 72–20) together with a sugges-

tive case history should prompt culture for *N. gonorrhoeae*.

LOWER RESPIRATORY TRACT

Expectorated sputum often containing varying amounts of cellular and microbial contamination from the upper respiratory tract is the most common sputum specimen submitted to the laboratory. Endotracheal tube collections are the second most often submitted. Specimens from endotracheal tubes generally reveal upper respiratory contamination but often to a lesser degree than that found in deep cough specimens. Less often re-

Chart 72–4. MICROBIOLOGY ALGORITHM: MALE UROGENITAL TRACT INFECTIONS
GRAM-STAINED SMEAR EVALUATION*

1. Many neutrophils; gram-negative diplococci; "key" cells (at least three pairs of cocci intracellular and no other oganisms).
   Impression: neisserial, presumptive *N. gonorrhoeae* infection (see Fig. 72–20).
2. Many leukocytes and squamous epithelial cells (SEC) may be present; many phagocytized microbes.
   Impression: microbial (could be *Gardnerella*, *Escherichia*, *Streptococcus*, *Candida*, *Haemophilus*); may be secondary to viral or chlamydial urethritis.
3. At least 10 WBC/high-power field(HPF); scattered round-to-cuboidal epithelial cells; no organisms or meatal "skin" flora (diphtheroids, micrococci).
   Impression: non-gonococcal urethritis.
4. Many intact mixed WBC's; foamy macrophages; no specific microbial agent seen in Gram stain.
   Impression: non-gonococcal urethritis; possible viral or chlamydial urethritis.
5. Many WBC's; no specific microbial agent seen Gram stain.
   Impression: non-gonococcal urethritis; rule out trichomoniasis.
6. Chancres
   soft: chancroid—*Haemophilus ducreyi*: Gram stain of chancre exudate not of much value because of microbial contamination.
   hard: syphilis—*Treponema pallidum*; darkfield microscopic examination and/or serologic tests necessary as organism does not take the Gram stain as does *Treponema genitalis*.

*At least five different portions of the smear must be examined with low-power and oil immersion lens.

Chart 72–5. MICROBIOLOGY ALGORITHM: FEMALE UROGENITAL TRACT INFECTIONS
GRAM-STAINED SMEAR EVALUATION*

General Statement:

Normal vaginal-cervical secretions vary among women and in each woman throughout the menstrual cycle. Lactobacilli are the normal resident flora, but occasionally other acidophilic organisms such as *Escherichia* and streptococci may be present. Leukocytes (WBC) and erythrocytes (RBC) are also found periodically, often in large numbers.

1. Many squamous epithelial cells (SEC); WBC's, few to many, may be present; normal flora are numerous.
   Impression: normal flora (Fig. 72–17).
2. Cellular aspect as in No. 1: lactobacilli and yeast-type fungal elements are prominent.
   Impression: if pseudomycelium and budding yeast cells are present, candidiasis; specific diagnosis of *Candida albicans* if germ tube is seen in the smear (see Fig. 72–18).
   Impression: if only budding yeast cells are seen, may be *Torulopsis* glabrata (Candida glabrata).
3. Many WBC's; SEC's may or may not be present; abnormal bacterial flora are generally abundant and mixed.
   Impression: *Trichomonas vaginalis* may be present; discernible with low-power scanning (see Fig. 72–19).
   Impression: *Neisseria gonorrhoeae* may be present; diagnosis is established if "key" cell (at least three pairs of intracellular gram-negative diplococci and no other organisms are seen) is present.
4. Many WBC's and SEC's; many small, gram-variable, pleomorphic bacilli; these may be phagocytized and/or the SEC's may be completely covered by adhering organisms ("clue" cells).
   Impression: *Gardnerella vaginalis.*
5. Many WBC's; SEC's may or may not be prominent; many, small, slightly curved, slender, gram-negative bacilli with pointed ends.
   Impression: Campylobacter- or Vibrio-type bacilli.
6. Mixed WBC's and SEC's in variable numbers; one of the following organisms may be predominant in a mixed flora (*Escherichia, Clostridium, Bacillus, Staphylococcus*).
   Impression: Some strains of these organisms produce enzymes, such as lecithinase, which may act as a mucosal irritant.
7. Many cervical epithelial cells; sometimes their nuclei are naked; few other cellular components are present; resident flora are generally few in number.
   Impression: chronic cervicitis; postmenopausal.

*At least five different portions of the smear must be examined with low-power and oil immersion lens.
†Special stains, serological tests, and possibly cultural procedures are necessary to rule out chlamydia, viruses, mycoplasma, etc.

ceived are transtracheal specimens that require a surgical procedure and, consequently, added trauma to a patient who is already seriously ill.

The quality of the material submitted as sputum should be ascertained by careful macroscopic and microscopic scrutiny. Macroscopic examination not only will reveal the presence of food, tobacco, or other contamination, which would render the specimen less than satisfactory, but also may disclose the presence of mucopurulent patches, which would reverse the earlier opinion.

Table 72–3. INCIDENCE OF GROUP A BETA-HEMOLYTIC PHARYNGITIS WITH SMEAR-CULTURE CORRELATION
(Seattle U.S. Public Health Service Hospital, 1964–1979)

	Number	Percentage
Positive smear with positive culture	3,610	91.4
Negative smear with positive culture	338	8.6
Total streptococcal isolates with smears	3,948	
Total pharyngeal cultures with smears	42,035*	100

*Most cultures had a negative smear and a negative culture for streptococci. Unfortunately no count was kept of the very small number of cases with positive smears with negative cultures, which were considered culture failures.

In addition to the rapid Gram stain, a wet mount of sputum has been advocated by Epstein[28] as a faster method by which structures such as eosinophiles, Charcot-Leyden crystals (see Fig. 72–27), Curschmann's spirals (see Fig. 72–10), and alveolar macrophages would be revealed, which are likely to be missed or inadequately distinguished by the Gram stain. The addition of buffered crystal violet to a wet sputum mount has also been proposed as a method of enhancing cellular differentiation.[29] Although more time consuming, the use of a Wright-Giemsa-stained thin sputum film is helpful in differentiating and quantifying eosinophiles and polymorphonuclear leukocytes. A 10 per cent sodium hydroxide, NaOH, wet mount of expectorated sputum can establish the diagnosis of *Coccidioides immitis* pneumonitis (see Fig. 72–9).

Bartlett[30] and Heinemann and coworkers[8] found smear and culture correlation more than 50 per cent of the time. Yet, in a survey by Heinemann and associates,[8] only 13 of 38 hospitals in the Philadelphia area included a Gram stain routinely in the evaluation of sputum.

Interestingly, the microbiological significance of clinical material from the lower respiratory tract, specifically expectorated sputum, has been under adverse criticism in recent years.[31] What may appear to be a good collection of sputum as evidenced by the direct Gram-stained smear, revealing many neutrophils, numerous bacteria of one morphologic type, and only rare or no squamous epithelial cells, may sometimes be at odds with physical and radiologic findings. Although a positive Gram stain for gram-positive diplococci will correlate with a positive sputum growth of *S. pneumoniae* (pneumococcus) in 60 to 90 per cent of cases of community-acquired pneumonias, a Gram stain may miss up to 38 per cent of specimens ultimately growing pneumococcus. Exudative upper respiratory tract infection must be ruled out, because aspiration of upper respiratory exudate may be coughed up and, mistakenly, assumed to be sputum. Aspiration of potential pathogens into the lower respiratory tract may or may not produce tracheitis, bronchitis, bronchiolitis, or pneumonitis. Without the direct microscopic examination, the value of the sputum culture has been questioned, and rightly so, by various investigators.[8, 9, 32] It appears that in the clinical analysis of materials from the respiratory tract, both upper and lower, the Gram-stained smear and other direct microscopic procedures should be guides to culture interpretation and arbiters of the accuracy and quantification of the culture.

The emergency physician can best use the direct sputum smear (wet mount as discussed by Epstein[28] or Gram stain) to support a clinical and radiological diagnosis of pneumonia. The absence of a chest film abnormality in a normally hydrated patient should make one suspicious of the diagnosis of pneumonitis even in the presence of a productive cough. The examination of such a patient's sputum should suggest whether the illness is allergic, viral, bacterial, or a combination of pathogens (see Chart 72–2: Microbiology Algorithm for Lower Respiratory Tract Infections) (see also Figs. 72–6 through 72–10). The Kinyoun-tergitol acid-fast stain can be used to identify presumptive *Mycobacterium tuberculosis* in expectorated sputum (see Fig. 72–8). This rapid stain is relatively easy to perform and should be considered by the emergency physician for high-risk patients with pulmonary symptoms.

Microscopic examination of sputum should also suggest the origin of the specimen, whether it be upper or lower respiratory tract, because more than 25 squamous epithelial cells per low-power field[33] are indicative of gross upper respiratory tract contamination and culture is not warranted. In a recent publication, Wong and colleagues[34] compared six different criteria, including the one just mentioned,[33] in determining the quality of sputum. The other criteria included a complicated scoring system of pluses for leukocytes and minuses for epithelial cells;[35, 36] averaging the number of epithelial cells per low-power field, with 10 being the cutoff point for an acceptable sample;[37] averaging the number of leukocytes per low-power field, with 25 being the cutoff point;[38] and averaging the ratio of leukocytes to epithelial cells,

with 10 being the cutoff point.[39] These different screening criteria yielded similar results.

URINARY TRACT

Urinary tract excretions represent a large proportion of the clinical materials submitted for microbiologic analysis. Urine will be sterile and practically acellular unless an infection is present. Most specimens are ordered as clean catch (midstream) voided urine for culture, however, and all voided specimens must pass through the urogenital tract. Only a scrupulous collection technique will prevent contamination of the urine with resident flora or with infectious organisms and host-reactive cells of the urogenital tract (especially in the female). The difficulty in securing a suitable collection is greatly magnified in debilitated, obese, aged, very young, or certain types of handicapped individuals. Catheterization may be resorted to in some female patients, with the knowledge that there is a risk of an infection being initiated where there was none initially.[40, 41] Kaye[42] estimates the incidence of infection after single catheterization in the female under the following circumstances: if the patient is ambulatory/nonpregnant (1 per cent), hospitalized/nonpregnant (4 per cent), bedridden/nonpregnant (13 per cent), or pregnant and catheterized at delivery (20 per cent).

The data in Table 72–4 illustrate the smear-culture correlation of urines submitted to the laboratory of the Seattle U.S. Public Health Service Hospital over an 11-year period. These data are slightly more accurate than those of Barbin and associates,[43] who had an 8 per cent negative microscopy culture result. They used a technique developed by Kunin[44] in which a drop of manually agitated, uncentrifuged urine was used for a wet reading under a cover slip using oil immersion.

Table 72–4. URINE SMEAR-CULTURE CORRELATION (Seattle U.S. Public Health Service Hospital, 1969–1979)

	Number	Percentage
Positive smear-culture agreement Either positive smear with positive culture or negative smear with negative culture	64, 279	98.8
Negative smear culture agreement Either positive smear with negative culture or negative smear with positive culture	761	1.2
Total urine specimens	65,079	100

The sample was considered positive if there was at least one bacterium per oil field in each of the five fields *and* if the bacteria had smooth surfaces without adherent material.

The Gram-stained direct smear of properly handled, uncentrifuged voided or catheterized urines has a value that cannot be overstated. The following features of the specimen are immediately revealed: contamination or lack of contamination; if contamination is present, its degree and origin; presence or absence of inflammatory cells; and suggestion of a particular etiologic agent. It is important to emphasize that the unspun urine sample is the sample of choice.

The number of leukocytes and bacteria in the centrifuged specimen will vary greatly, depending upon the force and length of centrifugation. In an obviously infected urine, spinning down a sample may concentrate pathogens and facilitate identification but the sediment should not be quantitated for purposes of determining or ruling out infection. The Gram-stained direct smear provides useful clinical information and avoids needless cultures (see Chart 72–3: Microbiology Algorithm for Urinary Tract Infections) (see also Figs. 72–21 and 72–22). The emergency physician may prefer the wet mount technique described previously[43] to the technique of reading the Gram-stained smear. Certainly, the speed with which the wet mount technique can be performed lends itself well to emergency care. The practitioner should be aware, however, that the wet mount technique has a 4 per cent false-positive and a 4 per cent false-negative potential when compared with the standard urine culture (positive culture: colony count greater than 10^5 per ml).

UROGENITAL TRACT

The normal male urogenital tract mucosa and secretions are considered sterile, whereas in the normal female (approximately 12 to 45 years of age), the presence of a resident flora of acidophilic, facultative to anaerobic microbes (essentially lactobacilli) results in a varying degree of protection from pathogens. In Table 72–5, the incidence of gonorrhea diagnosed at the Seattle U.S. Public Health Service Hospital and the smear-culture correlation attained are tabulated.

Wald[48] found that a 10-minute examination of a cervical Gram-stained smear for at least eight or more pairs of gram-negative, kidney bean-shaped diplococci in polymorphonuclear leukocytes was specific for gonorrhea in the female adolescent (see Fig. 72–20). He found that when the smear was positive, the culture was positive in 96 per cent of the cases. The test is faulty primarily in its sensitivity; if the culture were positive, the smear was positive 63 per cent of the time. This correlates with the 38 to 69 per cent sensitivity rate reported elsewhere in the literature for older women.[49–52]

Most recently, Lossick and colleagues[53] found the cervical Gram stain to be 97 per cent specific. Use of the Gram stain, combined with epidemiologic treatment of potentially exposed patients, permitted treatment of 91 per cent of the infected women at the initial clinic visit. Of patients with positive cultures who were not treated initially, 7.3 per cent developed salpingitis between visits. This stresses the value of the cervical smear Gram stain in the evaluation and treatment of gonorrhea. The presence of a vaginal discharge in the pre-adolescent female should alert the practitioner to the possibilities of a vaginal foreign body or sexual abuse.[54] Smear and culture evaluation of the vaginal discharge is warranted.[55, 56]

In the symptomatic male with a urethral discharge, the finding of typical gram-negative, intracellular diplococci within pus cells has a 93 to 99 per cent sensitivity rate.[49] The smear has also been found to detect 70 per cent of the subsequently culture-proven cases of gonorrhea in asymptomatic males.[57] Chart 72–4 (Microbiology Algorithm for Male Urogenital Tract Infections) describes an approach to evaluating the urethral Gram-stained

Table 72–5. INCIDENCE AND SMEAR-CULTURE CORRELATION OF GONORRHEA
(Seattle U.S. Public Health Service Hospital 1964–1979)

	Number	Percentage
Positive gonorrhea patients	1,698 (male) 1,040 (female) 658	
Positive smear, positive culture	1,528	94.6
Negative smear, positive culture	87	5.4
No smear made, positive culture	83 (all females)	
Total	1,698	
Positive smear, negative culture	51*	
Positive smear, no culture done	33 (all males)	

*Data for total number of urogenital tract specimens smeared and cultured are not available.
†During the same time period, *Trichomonas vaginalis* was diagnosed 903 times and *Candida albicans* was diagnosed 644 times by the Gram-stained smear.

smear of male patients. One should be aware that in the male, the distal portion of the urethral meatus harbors a "skin" flora that consists of micrococci and diphtheroids that could conceivably contaminate a deeper collection. The long urethra prevents contamination by anorectal flora.

In Chart 72–5 (Microbiology Algorithm for Female Urogenital Tract Infections), the author's approach to evaluating vaginal smears is described (see also Figs. 72–17 through 72–19). Note that in the female, the proximity of the anorectal opening to the vulva is an ever-present source of contamination. *Gardnerella vaginalis* (formerly *Haemophilus vaginalis* and *Corynebacterium vaginale*) vaginitis is suggested on Gram stain by the large numbers of gram-variable, small coccobacilli (salt and pepper appearance) and "clue" cells (vaginal epithelial cells stippled with small coccobacilli).[58] The wet preparation will reveal many coccobacilli, often in clumps, floating between the epithelial cells and, at times, the "clue" cells.[59] Recent studies have indicated that this form of vaginitis is susceptible to metronidazole.[59, 60] Action against symbiotic anaerobic bacteria may be the mechanism of response.[61]

The wet preparation (a drop of vaginal secretion mixed with a drop of saline) examined under high-dry power is also useful for diagnosing trichomoniasis.[62, 63] The motile, pear-shaped organisms are slightly larger than polymorphonuclear leukocytes (see Fig. 72–19). Because the organisms "round up" when they die and are difficult to differentiate from white blood cells, the wet preparation should be examined immediately. The sensitivity of the wet preparation has been estimated at approximately 76 per cent.[62, 63]

Candidiasis can also be diagnosed by wet mount with a sensitivity ranging from 40 to 80 per cent.[59, 61] Mixing the discharge with 10 per cent potassium hydroxide (KOH) or sodium hydroxide (NaOH) solution and briefly heating the slide will lyse the other cellular elements, thus aiding in the visualization of the fungi. The hydroxide wet mount is not suitable for determining the presence of trichomonads. The sensitivity of the Gram stain for candidiasis (see Fig. 72–18) has been estimated to approach 100 per cent.[64]

EXUDATES (Other Than Respiratory or Urogenital)

Cutaneous exudates represent a significant portion of the clinical materials submitted to the microbiology laboratory (see Figs. 72–11 through 72–15). Smear correlation with culture result is rarely a problem, but this information does not always contribute to the immediate care of the patient. Unopened abscesses, furuncles, and vesicles are excellent sources of diagnostic smears when sampled immediately upon incision and drainage, and yield approximately 100 per cent accuracy. Spontaneously draining abscesses, abrasions, ulcers, and wounds, however, are not adequate sources of smears.

After gentle cleansing with saline-soaked gauze, the extending edge of shallow ulcers generally supplies stained films accurately portraying host-reactive cells with probable specific etiologic associated microbes. In Fig. 72–16, a 10 per cent NaOH or KOH wet mount of skin scrapings from a shallow, slightly raised, discolored lesion confirms the clinical diagnosis of tinea versicolor due to *Pityrosporum obiculare*. The acid-fast stain of an ulcer-like lesion may reveal acid-fast organisms that could be *Mycobacterium marinum*, *M. ulcerans*, or *M. leprae*.

In deep lesions, such as osteomyelitis, it is necessary to penetrate more deeply to obtain exudate. Too often, surface exudate will yield a potentially pathogenic microbe mistakenly considered the causative agent, which is located much deeper in the lesion.

A knowledge of the location of the lesion is essential to the microscopist. Proximity to the various body apertures increases the risk of transposed resident flora contaminating lesions or aggravating infections initiated by another microbe or actually initiating lesions.

INTESTINAL TRACT

Commonly, a smear of a freshly passed portion of feces and, less commonly, smears of fecal exudate secured by proctoscopy or sigmoidoscopy may be subjected to microscopic examination. In recent years, swabs of the distal 2 to 3 cm of the anal mucosa with attendant stained smears have been studied with promising results (see Figs. 72–23 through 72–27). Multiple smears should be prepared so that a Gram stain and a Wright-Giemsa stain can be done. Methylene blue staining of wet mounts for leukocytes and microbes may be desired.[21]

Exudate from the anorectal or sigmoid mucosa has been important in various instances, reducing the problem of determining the etiologic agent from the abundant resident flora. A report of a *Streptococcus pyogenes* epidemic due to an anal mucosa carrier was published by McIntyre.[65] Schroeter and Reynolds[66] reported that 30 per cent of the failures in the treatment of gonorrhea in 908 female patients would have been missed if rectal mucosa cultures had not been done concurrently with cultures of the cervical site. Unfortunately, direct smears were not done in either of the aforementioned studies. Other studies have reported a 30 to 48 per cent sensitivity rate of the rectal smear in detecting the presence of gonorrhea.[49, 67]

In another report, direct Gram-stained smears of anal mucosa exudate from a homosexual male revealed the presence of numerous treponemes.[68] Therapeutic clearing of the organisms and exudate with antibiotics occurred, suggesting a treponemal etiology. In another patient undergoing sigmoidoscopy, the author's microscopic examination of exudate from numerous bleeding petechiae revealed an overwhelming number of treponemes, accounting in all probability for the positive fecal occult blood. Using the Gram stain, Quinn and associates[69] reported the presence of anorectal leukocytic exudate in 42 of 52 male homosexuals. In 28 of these men and in 2 of 10 men without an exudate, one or more probable etiologic agents were identified. Despite the purulent exudates, the etiologic agents, including *Neisseria gonorrhoeae* in 7 men, were not always seen by Gram stain.

Gram-stained and Wright-Giemsa-stained thin smears of fluid feces can aid in the diagnosis of giardiasis, cryptosporidiosis, and other diarrhea-causing agents.[70, 71] Ho and colleagues[72] found that the Gram stain of stool was greater than 43 per cent sensitive and greater than 99 per cent specific for *Campylobacter* enteritis. An "s"-shaped (equivalent sign) or "seagull"-shaped gram-negative curved rod was found to be diagnostic of *Campylobacter jejuni*. False-positive smears were rare. Direct wet mount smears of fluid feces that are examined when they are freshly passed and warm may be more rapid aids in establishing an early diagnosis of strongyloidiasis (larva), of amebiasis (trophozoite), giardiasis (trophozoite), cryptosporidiosis (oocyst), and other parasitic infections. Immunocompromised patients are at high risk for superinfection with various protozoan parasites and with the helminth, *Strongyloides stercoralis*.[70, 71, 73, 74]

The macroscopic examination of formed feces may frequently reveal the clearly visible (2 × 1 cm or larger) proglottids of Taenia, especially *Taenia saginata*, the beef tapeworm, or the less visible (about 1 cm × 0.5 mm) female gravid *Enterobius vermicularis*, the pinworm.[75] Even when the macroscopic examination is negative, the modified Graham's cellulose tape technique, in which the adhesive side of the tape is first applied to the perianal folds and then placed adhesive side down on a glass slide,[76, 77] is a microscopic examination that can be easily and rapidly carried out and is very effective.[78] The characteristic spherical ova of Taenia (35 micron diameter), containing a hexacanth embryo (six hooklets), or the characteristic egg-shaped ova of Enterobius (about 60 × 26 microns), containing a motile embryo, are easily

recognized and identified using the low-power (100×) and the high-dry power (450×) microscope lens. A single negative examination does not rule out either of these parasites because of variables that can alter the findings, such as bathing just before the examination, the time of the day that the collection is made, and so on. Consequently, multiple examinations may be necessary. One text suggests that seven examinations be carried out on different days before a negative diagnosis is reported.[79] Brugmans and coworkers[80] pointed out that analysis of a placebo treatment group yielded a false-negative rate (13 per cent [children] to 24 per cent [adults]) with either one or two examinations in the group that was negative before receiving the placebo but positive afterwards. The rate was 6 per cent (adults) to 14 per cent (children) in the group that was positive before receiving the placebo but negative afterwards.

Conclusion

In the last few years, there have been increasing numbers of publications stressing the value of the direct analysis of clinical materials. This direct analysis may vary from an unstained wet mount (in saline or 10 per cent hydroxide) to variously stained wet mounts and dried thin smears. The microscope used may be compound, phase, darkfield, or fluorescent. The Gram-stained thin smear viewed through the compound microscope is the most familiar approach.

The expression that "An immediate Gram stain of a specimen often provides proof of good-will; . . . "[81] is woefully inadequate. Although the patient is the primary beneficiary of this rapid and accurate tool, it must be stressed that the requestor is the recipient of the confidence factor. This may be defined as the laboratory-physical examination correlation. Moreover, the microbiologist also benefits because the direct analysis provides a very basic type of quality control by delineating the quality of the submitted specimen, the degree and type of host reaction, if any, and the probable etiologic agent. With this information, the microbiologist can determine whether to proceed with culture of the specimen, what substrates to use in culturing it, and what results to expect.

In this text, special emphasis is placed on the fact that equal value can be obtained from direct analysis of materials from the upper respiratory tract as from other areas or tracts of the body. In any area in which there is an abundant resident flora, knowledge of the components of such a flora and a careful collection technique will eliminate any hesitancy in "reading" such smears and producing a rapid, highly accurate smear report.

Text continued on page 1028

DESCRIPTION OF PHOTOMICROGRAPHS IN FIGURES 72–1 THROUGH 72–6

Figure Number	Source	Preparation	Chart Index	Description	Interpretation	Comment
72–1	Throat	Gram	Chart 72–1 (#1)	Squamous epithelial cells; resident flora	Normal	
72–2	Throat	Gram	Chart 72–1 (#2)	*Ciliocytophthoria* (cough cells); resident flora	Viral	Coughing is a primary symptom of viral upper respiratory tract infection
72–3	Throat	Gram	Chart 72–1 (#9)	Disrupted leukocytes; associated spherical gram-positive cocci	Streptococcal (*Streptococcus pyogenes*)	Generally in pairs or singly; rarely very short chains
72–4	Throat	Gram	Chart 72–1 (#10)	Disrupted leukocytes; gram-negative bacilli (slightly curved and pointed ends) and undulating fine filaments	Vincent's disease (*Fusobacterium* and *Treponema*)	Anaerobic entity; generally secondary infection; other bacteria often present
72–5	Throat	Gram	Chart 72–1 (#11)	Leukocytes generally intact; associated slender, pleomorphic, gram-positive bacilli	Corynebacterial (*Corynebacterium haemolyticum*)	Often mimic streptococcal infection, even including rash
72–6	Sputum	Gram	Chart 72–2 (#4)	Leukocytes; "foamy" macrophages; many small gram-negative coccobacilli	Viral with *Haemophilus*	Part of resident flora; this bacillus is often very numerous in viral infections

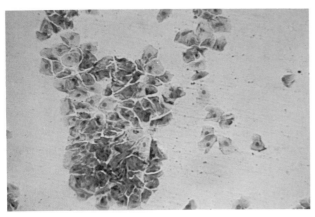

Figure 72–1.

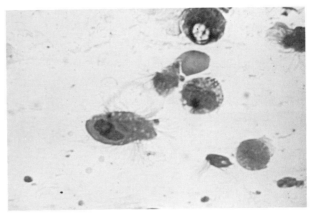

Figure 72–2.

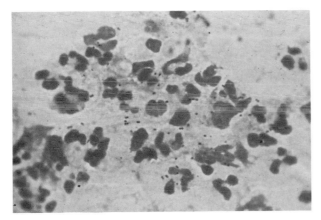

Figure 72–3.

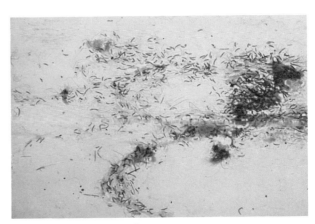

Figure 72–4.

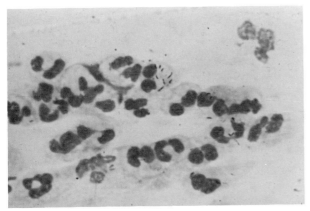

Figure 72–5.

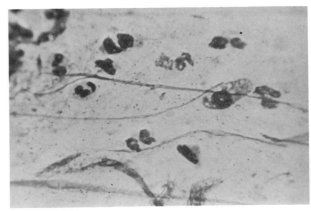

Figure 72–6.

DESCRIPTION OF PHOTOMICROGRAPHS IN FIGURES 72–7 THROUGH 72–12

Figure Number	Source	Preparation	Chart Index	Description	Interpretation	Comment
72–7	Sputum	Gram	Chart 72–2 (#4)	Leukocytes; macrophages; numerous encapsulated elongated, gram-positive diplococci (short chains)	Viral with *Streptococcus pneumoniae*	As with *Haemophilus*
72–8	Sputum	Kinyoun		Slender, beaded, acid-fast bacilli	*Mycobacterium tuberculosis*	Specimen digested and concentrated
72–9	Sputum	Sodium hydroxide (10 per cent)		Two thick-walled spherules; squamous epithelial debris; resident flora	*Coccidioides immitis*	Easily seen on low power (100×) with controlled lighting
72–10	Sputum	Gram		Coiled, snake-like mucus strands	Curschmann's spirals characteristic of bronchial asthma but may be encountered in other catarrhal conditions	Sometimes eosinophils and Charcot-Leyden crystals enveloped
72–11	Eye drainage	Gram		Fibrinoleukocytic debris; plump gram-negative diplobacilli	*Moraxella*	Resident flora of nasopharyngeal mucosa; reflects eye contamination by nasal discharge
72–12	Ear discharge	Gram		Cellular debris (leukocytes and epithelial cells); conidia and gram-variable fungal hypha	*Aspergillus* most likely	Slender gram-negative bacilli; pleomorphic gram-positive bacilli; gram-positive cocci present

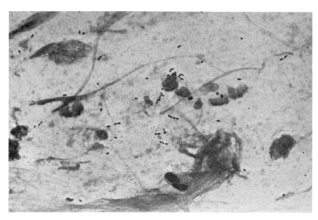

Figure 72–7.

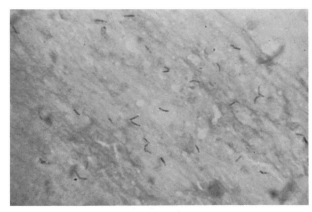

Figure 72–8.

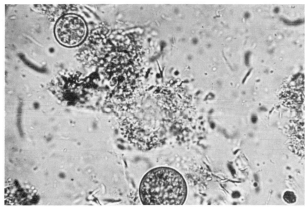

Figure 72–9.

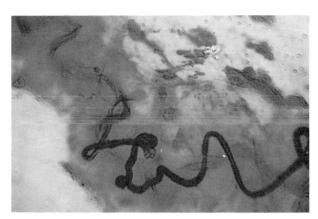

Figure 72–10.

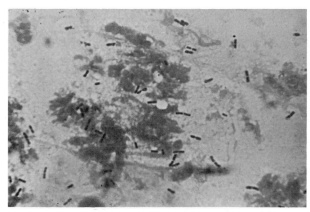

Figure 72–11.

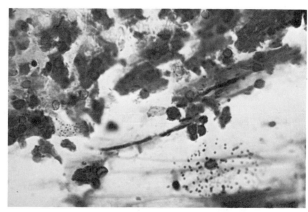

Figure 72–12.

DESCRIPTION OF PHOTOMICROGRAPHS IN FIGURES 72–13 THROUGH 72–18

Figure Number	Source	Preparation	Chart Index	Description	Interpretation	Comment
72–13	Cheek abscess	Gram		Many neutrophils; fragmented slender gram-positive filaments	Actinomycosis (*Actinomyces israelii*)	Resident flora of dentiginous crevices and tonsillar crypts—"sulfur" granule
72–14	Foot lesion	Gram		Many neutrophils; associated spherical gram-positive cocci in clumps	Staphylococcal (*Staphylococcus aureus*)	Often resident flora of skin and mucosa
72–15	Gangrene ankle	Gram		Large gram-positive bacilli in seroerythrocytic matrix; rare neutrophils	Gas gangrene (*Clostridium perfringens*)	Host reaction appears mild relative to the dangerous nature of the lesion
72–16	Skin scrapings from chest	Sodium hydroxide (10 per cent)		Squamous epithelial cells; clusters of spherules and short filaments	*Pityrosporum furfur* (formally *Malassezia furfur*)	Easly seen on low power; diagnostic of tinea versicolor
72–17	Vagina	Gram	Chart 72–5 (#1)	Squamous epithelial cells; uniform, moderately thick gram-positive bacilli; spermatozoa	Normal (*Lactobacillus*)	
72–18	Vagina	Gram	Chart 72–5 (#2)	Squamous epithelial cells and leukocytes; budding yeast cells and filaments; germ tube present	*Candida albicans*	The presence of germ tube is diagnostic

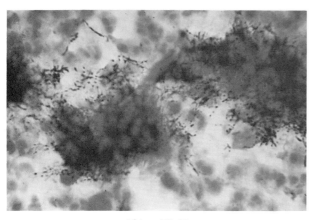

Figure 72–13.

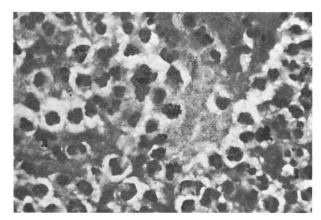

Figure 72–14.

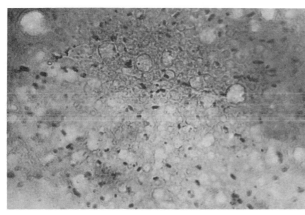

Figure 72–15.

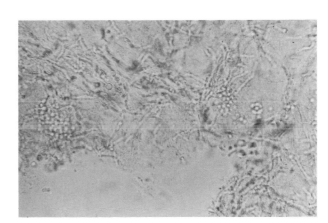

Figure 72–16.

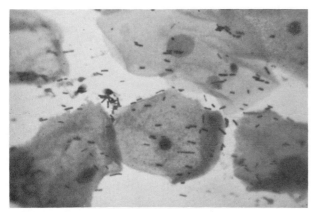

Figure 72–17.

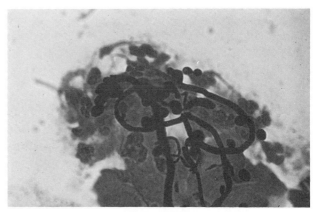

Figure 72–18.

DESCRIPTION OF PHOTOMICROGRAPHS IN FIGURES 72–19 THROUGH 72–24

Figure Number	Source	Preparation	Chart Index	Description	Interpretation	Comment
72–19	Vagina	Gram	Chart 72–5 (#3)	Neutrophils; four trichomonads	*Trichomonas vaginalis*	Flagella seen in two lenticular nuclei; small relative to cell size
72–20	Urethra	Gram	Chart 72–4 (#1)	Neutrophils; associated gram-negative diplococci (often intracellular)	Neisserial (*Neisseria gonorrhoeae*)	"Key" cells = only gram-negative diplococci within neutrophils
72–21	Urine	Gram	Chart 72–3 (#6)	Neutrophils; associated plump gram-negative bacilli	Coliforms (*Escherichia coli*)	Most common cause of acute bacterial urinary tract infection
72–22	Urine	Gram		Neutrophils; associated slender gram-negative bacilli	Pseudomonad (*Pseudomonas aeruginosa*)	Generally in chronic infections, especially after instrumentation
72–23	Fluid feces	Wright-Giemsa		Mucus shreds; leukocytes; fecal flora; protozoa	*Cryptosporidium* (approximately 4 microns in diameter)	Internal content took stain, but electron microscopy used for detail
72–24	Mucoid feces	Wright-Giemsa		Pear-shaped, binucleated protozoa; some fecal flora	*Giardia lamblia* trophozoites	

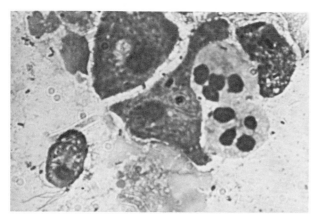

Figure 72–19.

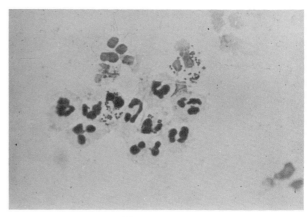

Figure 72–20.

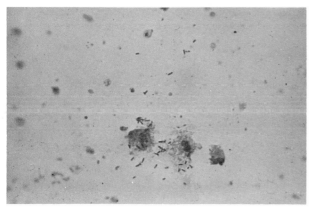

Figure 72–21.

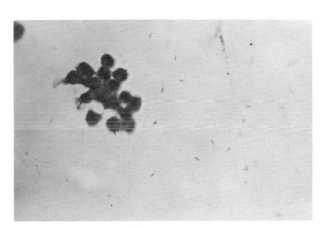

Figure 72–22.

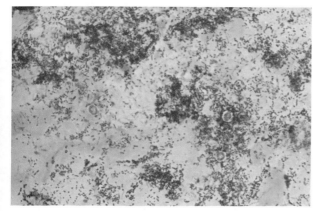

Figure 72–23.

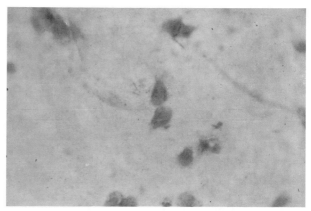

Figure 72–24.

DESCRIPTION OF PHOTOMICROGRAPHS IN FIGURES 72–25 THROUGH 72–27

Figure Number	Source	Preparation	Chart Index	Description	Interpretation	Comment
72–25	Anal folds	Cellulose tape		Multiple ovoid bodies	Ova of *Enterobius vermicularis*	Easily seen on low power
72–26	Fluid feces	Direct		*Amoeba* trophozoite with ingested yeast cells	Presumptive *Entamoeba histolytica*	Rapid directional mobility on warm mount
72–27	Fluid feces	Direct		Elongated, diamond-shaped crystals	Charcot-Leyden crystals in mucosal secretions following foreign body irritation; associated with elevated eosinophil levels	Exact nature unknown; generally in bronchial asthma and in amebic colitis

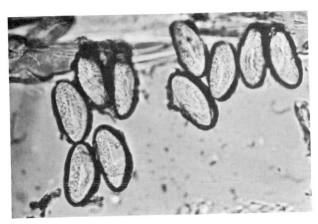

Figure 72–25.

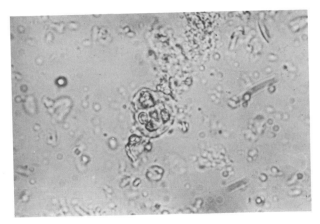

Figure 72–26.

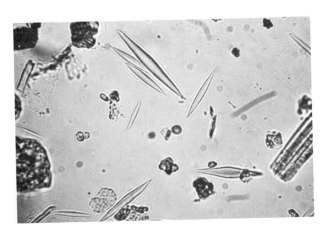

Figure 72–27.

BLOOD CULTURE TECHNIQUE

Introduction

Hippocrates considered blood one of four humors in the body, the proper balance of which results in the body's good health. Today, it is recognized that blood plays an essential role in infectious disease. As Bennett and Beeson[82] state, "Of all tissues which display defensive powers, the blood stands at the top." In addition to the importance of blood as a carrier of antibodies and phagocytic cells, it is also important as a disseminator of disease-causing microbes and toxins throughout the body. Detection and identification of micro-organisms in the blood are two of the most important functions of a clinical microbiology laboratory.

Studies have shown that blood is rarely *directly* invaded by micro-organisms.[82] Bacteria usually enter the circulation through the lymphatic system, and bacteremias follow increased lymph flow from infected foci. Exceptions to this are intravascular infections, such as endocarditis, suppurative thrombophlebitis, and mycotic aneurysm or uncontrolled infections such as typhoid fever and brucellosis. Although entrance into the blood stream by microbes or microbial toxins is considered by some investigators to be a relatively benign event in itself compared with focal tissue invasion, systemic manifestations such as fever, chills, and malaise can be important causes of clinical concern, especially when no tissue foci are immediately obvious.

The likelihood of bacteremia is related to local conditions that favor drainage of lymph from infected areas. Nodes throughout the body usually function as microbial filters as lymph enters the blood stream. Nonetheless, nodes may malfunction and hence increase the likelihood of bacteremia in the following situations: when an extensive number of microbes reach the node, early in the infection when there may be a deficiency of phagocytic cells in the nodes, when the perfusion pressure of the lymph is high, when the microbes are unusually virulent or survive ingestion to be egested later in the blood stream, or when the node is manipulated.[82]

Indications for Blood Culture

The culturing of blood has become a major component of the clinical microbiology laboratory. A patient who presents with a fever of unknown origin is a prime candidate for blood culture because bacteremia with sepsis is a likely possibility. The blood culture may provide the only positive isolation of an organism that is causing a hidden focal infection somewhere in the body.

Clinically, bacteremia may be transient, intermittent, or continuous. Transient bacteremias are common and may occur from manipulation of infected or contaminated tissues, such as gastrointestinal procedures, dental procedures, instrumentation of the genitourinary tract, or surgical incision of an abscess. Sigmoidoscopy-associated bacteremias have been reported to occur in as many as 9.5 per cent of patients, and the rate associated with barium enema has ranged as high as 40 per cent.[83] Also, transient bacteremia may occur in the early phases of other infections such as pneumococcal pneumonia. The significance of a transient bacteremia varies with host resistance and the recurrence of the precipitating cause.

Bacteremia and septicemia are not synonymous. Bacteremia represents the presence of *bacteria* in the blood stream, whereas septicemia refers to the presence of *bacterial toxins* in the blood stream. Bacteremia usually results in chills and fever, but bacteremias can be present without detectable systemic symptoms.[84] Septicemia, on the other hand, can result from bacterial toxins disseminating into the blood stream from an infected focus (toxemia). Furthermore, a bacteremia of a low order of magnitude may lead to a septicemia with negative cultures because of the paucity of organisms.

Indications for blood culturing in the emergency department include the following: 1) Evaluation of the toxic-appearing patient with normal immune defenses and a fever, 2) Evaluation of the toxic-appearing patient with immune dysfunction with or without a fever (immunosuppressed, elderly, neonate), 3) Documentation of the infection and determination of the sensitivity of the organism in the patient with suspected endocarditis or other infectious focus with bacteremia. In general, blood cultures have been of little value in the *outpatient* work-up of *adults* with fever and are rarely indicated.[85] Blood cultures may have an important role, however, in the outpatient work-up of nontoxic children with fever and no obvious source of infection as a means of identifying bacteremia.[86] Pneumococcal bacteremia may occur in young children who appear only minimally ill and have unexplained fever with no localizing signs or symptoms. Blood cultures may be the only means of detecting bacteremia in these patients.

Collection Technique

Venous blood is usually drawn for culture. Collection of venous blood is less hazardous than that of arterial blood and it has been shown, at least in patients with subacute bacterial endocarditis, that arterial blood is no more likely to contain organisms than is venous blood.[87] To minimize contamination with skin flora, antisepsis must be obtained at the site of proposed venipuncture. Because it may be difficult to disinfect the skin of the groin, it is best to avoid femoral vein puncture when obtaining blood for culture.

Many reports cite iodine as superior to other materials for producing skin antisepsis.[88-93] Story[94] and Lee and associates,[95] however, reported studies that indicate that two washes with 70 per cent isopropyl alcohol compare favorably with an iodine wash followed by an alcohol wash. Coulthard and Sykes[96] found isopropyl alcohol to be more effective than ethyl alcohol.

The optimal method is a three-step procedure.[97, 98] First, the site is cleansed with 70 per cent isopropyl alcohol. Second, a 2 per cent tincture of iodine or 10 per cent povidone-iodine is applied concentrically. Many authorities advise using a soaked sponge to keep the puncture site wet with the solution for a full 2 minutes before venipuncture. Third, after venipuncture, the residual iodine is removed with an alcohol sponge in order to prevent burns or sensitization. Eisenberg and colleagues[85] reversed the order, using tincture of iodine first and then scrubbing with alcohol prior to venipuncture, without increasing the rate of contamination. A common procedural error is to contaminate the skin with a finger, which is used to palpate a vein before venipuncture.

Scott[99] found that the use of two needles significantly reduced the number of contaminated cultures. This is supported by the work of Eisenberg and coworkers,[85] who had a low contamination rate using two needles. The first needle is used to draw the sample; it is then discarded, and a second sterile needle is used to inject the collected blood into the culture media. Today, many commercially packaged blood culture kits provide a two needle setup in which the needles are joined by sterile tubing. One needle is for the venipuncture, and the other side punctures the culture bottle or collection container, thereby allowing the blood to flow directly from the patient's vein into the culture media. If two collection bottles (broth media) are used with the double needle and tubing apparatus, the anaerobic bottle is filled first (5 to 10 ml blood added). The aerobic bottle is then "filled" and allowed to vent by removing the venipuncture needle from the arm. If a single collection bottle is used, the bottle is "filled" as for an anaerobic culture and the specimen is subsequently split in the laboratory, with venting of the aerobic portion at that time. Hoffman and associates[100] warn that if blood is drawn for multiple purposes in a single syringe, the blood culture bottles should be inoculated before entering other collection tubes. They reported that reflux of blood introduced into EDTA (ethylenediamine tetra-acetic acid)-containing tubes resulted in false-positive blood cultures with *Serratia marcescens*.

Tonnesen and colleagues[101] reported obtaining promising results using blood drawn from indwelling venous catheters compared with venipuncture. Handsfield[102] pointed out that the false-positive rate of 37 per cent in the data of Tonnesen and coworkers[101] was not acceptable. Although it is tempting to aspirate blood from indwelling venous catheters such as a central venous pressure line, such practice results in a higher level of contamination and does not improve detection rates.

It should be noted that clotted blood or citrated blood are generally unsuitable for culture, because the isolation rate from these samples is substantially decreased.[103]

Smears

Unless the bacteremia is overwhelming, direct Wright-Giemsa or Gram-stained blood smears or buffy-coat smears are generally of no value.[104, 105] This opinion may be reversed if an acridine orange stain is done as early as 6 hours after incubation of the blood culture.[106] Mirrett and associates demonstrated that this stain was more sensitive than methylene blue or Gram stains when small numbers of organisms are involved.[106]

Cultures

It is standard practice to vent one bottle of culture medium, thus replacing the partial vacuum in the bottle with air to enhance the growth of aerobes. This is done by puncturing the diaphragm of the collection bottle with a cotton-plugged needle to allow equilibration. One bottle is left unvented to facilitate recovery of anaerobes. This may be done in the laboratory or at the patient's bedside.

In recent years, many substrates for culturing blood have been devised. These have varied from fluid to fluid-agar slant bottles with additives, which not only serve as anticoagulants but also are capable of neutralizing some antibiotics, complement, lysozyme activity, and phagocytosis. If a patient has previously been treated with penicillin, for example, one may add penicillinase directly to the culture to inactivate the antibiotic remaining in the blood sample. Although this practice is controversial, it may be of value in some instances. If a patient is currently taking antibiotics, the laboratory should be informed so that appropriate steps may be taken to maximize the culture yield. It has become obvious that no specific substrate will suffice to isolate all microbes that might be found in the blood stream. Most laboratories use a two-bottle system to cover aerobic and anaerobic flora and incubate these at 37° C for 7 days. The time period may be extended to 14 days if the patient has been partially treated. Approximately two thirds of blood cultures from bacteremic patients who have not been treated with antibiotics will be positive within 24 hours, and 90 per cent will be positive within 3 days.

VOLUME

The volume of blood cultured is important. Various investigators have shown that increasing the inoculum from 2 ml to as high as 40 ml yielded corresponding increased numbers of positive cultures.[107-109] Most commercial and laboratory-prepared systems are suitable only for between 2 and 10 ml of inocula. The 10-ml inoculum, which is preferable for adults, is not suitable for children. Generally, in children, 1 to 5 ml of blood is recommended for culture, and the younger the child, the smaller the amount.[110] A minimum ratio of blood to broth, 1:10, will usually suffice if one is in doubt as to the volume of blood required. Because fresh human serum has inherent bactericidal properties, it is important to quickly dilute or neutralize this effect with culture media.

TIMING

The timing of the blood culture is important, especially in instances in which the bacteremia may be transient (occurring after insult to infected tissues) or intermittent (undrained abscesses sporadically seeding). The classic teaching method suggests that blood for culture should be drawn just before a chill or febrile episode, but in practice, the onset of such episodes results in blood cultures being initiated after the chill or temperature spikes. Musher and coworkers[111] reported on fever patterns in 102 patients and concluded that in most infectious states, the release of pyrogenic substances into the blood stream is continuous. Exaggeration of the normal variation probably results because of reactivity of the hypothalamus to these stimuli and varies in accordance with circadian rhythm. These findings do not support the recommendation to draw blood cultures just before fever spikes in infected patients unless one were to presume that bacteremia also has a diurnal variation.

The timing of blood culture is even more complicated when one considers the fact that the influx of bacteria into the blood stream will produce a shaking chill or fever only when following a lag period of 30 to 90 minutes. If the host's defenses are active, bacteria may be rapidly removed from the blood by phagocytosis and the blood culture taken at the time of the rigor may be negative. The ideal time for obtaining a blood culture may be determined only retrospectively.

In most adult infections, 2 or 3 cultures, taken at 1-hour intervals, are recommended, but if immediate antimicrobial therapy is planned, the interval should be reduced appropriately.[110] In critically ill patients, it is best to draw all blood samples simultaneously from different anatomic sites and to begin antibiotic therapy promptly. If three separate blood cultures are taken over 24 hours in the nontoxic bacteremic patient, the cumulative yield has been shown to be 99 per cent in the bacteremic adult. A single blood culture has been shown to be frequently satisfactory in the bacteremic neonate.[112]

CONTAMINATION AND FALSE-POSITIVE CULTURES

Gross contamination of blood cultures may occur, resulting in pseudobacteremia.[113] Contamination with skin bacteria often produces blood cultures that are positive for diphtheroids, micrococcus species, bacillus, and staphylococcus epidermidis. It should be noted that these organisms can occasionally be true pathogens, especially in immunosuppressed patients.

Contamination can be kept to a minimum if proper attention is focused on technique. Generally "false-positive" blood cultures can be identified by the clinical course of the patient and the failure of repeat cultures to grow the same organism. In contaminated specimens, growth in the broth generally does not appear earlier than the third or fourth day of incubation and the organism will often not grow in more than one sample.

Ideally, contamination should occur in less than 3 per cent of all blood cultures performed.[114] To attain this goal, it is preferable to have blood drawn directly from the patient into the blood culture media using a double-ended needle. After the needle has been withdrawn, the culture is a closed system, and it should not be re-opened unless it is necessary to check growth. A diphasic or triphasic[115] fluid-agar slant or similar modification[116] would eliminate the need for blind subcultures (required when broth type substrates are used). Even the proposed use of acridine orange–stained smears as an alternative to early routine subcultures[110] would require entry into a closed system. Consequently, to reduce the risk of contamination, these procedures should be performed in laminar air-flow facilities, with aseptic technique.

Most of the additives in blood culturing have potential disadvantages that must be considered.[117-121] There have been false-positive diag-

Table 72-6. BLOOD CULTURES (Seattle U.S. Public Health Service Hospital)

Year	Average Daily Patient Load	%	Blood Cultures	No Growth	%	Significant Growth	%	Contaminated	%
1962			289	263	91.0	26	9.0	17	4.4
1963	235	1.8	388	319	82.2	52	13.4	14	3.4
1964	226	2.0	417	363	87.0	40	9.6	36	8.0
1965*	235	2.3	451	352	78.0	63	14.0	18	3.4
1966	213	2.7	530	463	87.4	49	9.2	15	2.6
1967†	208	4.4	572	506	88.5	51	8.9	38	4.1
1968	198	5.0	922	785	85.2	99	10.7	55	5.6
1969	180	6.6	984	872	88.6	57	5.8	40	3.4
1970	165	7.3	1189	1088	91.5	61	5.1	47	3.9
1971	154	6.4	1206	1095	90.8	64	5.3	18	1.8
1972	136	8.7	991	917	92.5	56	5.7	11	0.9
1973			1179	1086	92.1	82	7.0	12	0.9
1974			1261	1176	93.3	73	5.8	43	3.0
1975			1443	1309	90.7	91	6.3	31	2.2
1976	122	11.5	1400	1297	92.6	72	5.1	25	1.5
1977	133	12.4	1646	1536	93.3	85	5.2	23	1.2
1978	133	14.8	1974	1820	92.2	131	6.6	42	2.0
1979	130	15.9	2070	1916	92.6	112	5.4		
Totals %			18912	17163	90.7	1264	6.7	485	2.6

*Diaphragm caps on culture bottles introduced.
†Full integration with the University of Washington Medical School teaching program.

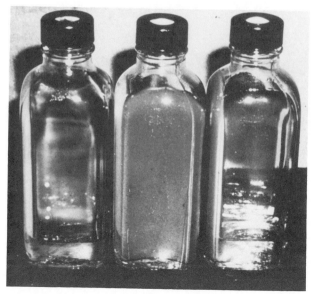

Figure 72–28. Three views of the trisubstrate blood culture medium used at the U.S. Public Health Service Hospital during the years 1962 to 1979. There was a trypticase soy agar slant, an enriched chocolate agar slant, and a trypticase soy broth with heparin. These were incubated in a special rack so that fluid with inoculum made contact with agar only once a day.

must be weighed against their high initial cost, continuing operating costs, and performance efficiency. It is interesting to note that Carlson and Plorde,[124] using the BACTEC radiometric system, cultured 4690 samples over a 2-year period. Their significant positive culture rate of 6.7 per cent is identical to the result of blood cultures done at the Seattle U.S. Public Health Service Hospital (Table 72–6). Carlson and Plorde's contamination rate, however, was 4.2 per cent compared with 2.6 per cent in the Seattle series. The U.S. Public Health Service Hospital data were collected using a triphasic bottle (Fig. 72–28), together with a bottle containing 50 ml of fluid thioglycolate medium without an indicator. Neither of these bottles, prepared in the laboratory, was very expensive or difficult to prepare. Most positive cultures were detected after 12 to 24 hours of incubation. Results of controlled evaluation studies of radiometric methods are not encouraging.[113]

FUNGAL CULTURES

Generally, fungi are very difficult to isolate in blood cultures, and it may take 4 to 6 weeks to obtain a positive yield. If a fungemia is suspected, it is best to discuss culture media and technique with the laboratory before cultures are taken. Cultures of bone marrow are occasionally positive in deep mycoses when blood cultures are negative.

Occasionally, blood cultures are positive in cases of disseminated histoplasmosis or candidiasis, but other fungi, such as Cryptococcus and Aspergillus or fungi-like bacteria such as Nocardia and Actinomycosis, are rarely isolated from the blood.

noses of bacteremias with Escherichia[122] and with Moraxella[123] owing to the addition of contaminated penicillinase when the blood cultures were initiated. There is no definitive evidence that penicillinase enhances isolation of bacteria from blood, but its use does enhance the risk of contamination.

Various radiometric methods of assaying blood for bacteria are available commercially. The degree of information produced by these instruments

ANAEROBIC CULTURE TECHNIQUES

Introduction

Pure anaerobic infections are rarely encountered. The presence of anaerobes, as a microbial component of an infection in which facultative microbes are also prominent, however, is not rare. Unfortunately, the presence of the anaerobes in such an infection may often be overlooked. Because anaerobic infections are often polymicrobic in nature, it is common to find numerous different strains of anaerobic bacteria associated with a single localized necrotic infection, such as an ab-

scess. Anaerobes are the predominant normal flora of the skin and mucous membranes. The resident flora of the various mucosal tracts and epithelial glandular areas of the body consist of a mixed microbial population, including surface aerobes and deep anaerobes with facultative organisms throughout. Often the synergistic interaction of the organisms is required for pathogenicity. Given a suitable environment in an immunocompromised or otherwise weakened host or when local tissue redox potentials are reduced by ischemia, necrosis, or infection, the anaerobes can cause an infection or compound the seriousness of an existing infection. A relatively common example of such an anaerobic disease entity is Vincent's oral mucosal disease (fusospirochetal necrotizing lesions). Anaerobes indigenous to the tonsillar crypts (actinomycetes, fusobacteria, spirochetes, peptostreptococci) that are introduced into other anatomic sites (Table 72–7) such as the lungs can

Table 72–7. ANAEROBES ISOLATED FROM SELECTED CLINICAL MATERIALS (Seattle U.S. Public Health Service Hospital)

Throat Cultures 1967–1979: 34,856	
Vincent's angina	357
Vincent's angina and *Streptococcus pyogenes*	2
Vincent's angina and *Corynebacterium hemolyticum*	1
Peptostreptococcus	2
Peptostreptococcus and *Haemophilus influenzae*	1
Bacteroides	1
Blood Cultures 1962–1979: 18,912	
Clostridium	2(2)*
C. perfringens	4(3)
C. histolyticum	2(1)
C. lentoputrescens	1(1)
C. cochlearum	1(1)
Propionibacterium acnes	125(125)
Peptococcus	4(4)
Peptostreptococcus	23(17)
Bacteroides	29(22)
Fusobacterium	1(1)
Bacteroides and *Peptostreptococcus*	9(2)
Bacteroides and enteric *Streptococcus*	2(2)
Mixed anaerobes	2(2)
Pleural Fluid	
C. difficile	1

*Isolates (patients).

cause life-threatening, often slowly resolving disease in the form of an aspiration pneumonia or a lung abscess.

Certain clinical findings are often associated with the presence of anaerobic bacterial disease. The presence of a foul-smelling discharge, infection located in or adjacent to a mucous membrane, or the presence of crepitus (subcutaneous emphysema) or gangrene suggest infection by anaerobes. Some common primary anaerobic infections include dental abscess, infected human bites, infections developing in patients with malignancies where necrotic tissue is seen, septic thrombophlebitis, pelvic inflammatory disease, perirectal abscess, lung abscess, and those developing in patients who are on aminoglycoside antibiotics.

Indications for Anaerobic Culture

The isolation and identification of anaerobic bacteria are often expensive and time consuming. Not all infections require highly specialized anaerobic culture techniques, and only certain specimens should be cultured for anaerobic bacteria. Potential specimens for anaerobic culture include all cutaneous lesions and fluid aseptically aspirated from sites that are sterile under normal conditions. Such fluids include blood, spinal fluid, pleural fluid, transtracheal aspirate, and pus obtained directly from an abscess cavity or by culdocentesis. Upper respiratory tract collections, expectorated sputum, feces, urogenital collections, and voided urine are generally cultured only aerobically or under increased carbon dioxide–reduced oxygen tensions. Certainly, when there has been suspected or obvious soil and/or foreign body contamination of wounds, direct smears (generally Gram-stained) and anaerobic cultures should be performed. Likewise, when there has been penetration through a mucosal area harboring anaerobes or a suspected pulmonary aspiration of fluids from similar mucosal areas, direct smears and anaerobic cultures should be done.

It is common to obtain a report of "no growth" in foul-smelling abscess cultures. Such cultures are often anaerobic strains that would have been positive if careful anaerobic cultures had been performed.

Collection Technique

Classically, collection and culture techniques stress speed as an essential element. It has been shown that this process may not be that urgent.[126] Thirty-seven strains of anaerobes previously considered to be oxygen-sensitive were actually aerotolerant, surviving in purulent exudate exposed to air at room temperature up to 24 hours before processing.[126] Not all clinical materials are as dense as purulent exudate, however, so that a careful collection technique and expeditious transport to the laboratory are essential for maximum yield.[127]

Generally, ordinary cotton swabs or applicators are unsatisfactory for collecting anaerobic organisms. If the specimen is fluid, it is best to collect the specimen with a sterile needle and syringe. Once the fluid is aspirated, air should be expelled from the syringe and the needle capped to minimize exposure to atmospheric oxygen. If an abscess is to be cultured, percutaneous aspiration of pus for culture and Gram stain before incision and drainage is preferred. When a swab is used to make the collection, the swab should be inserted deeply in a thioglycolate (without indicator) or other suitable reduced broth tube immediately. Oxygen-free tubes that contain swabs are available for obtaining anaerobic cultures. Such tubes should not be opened until the culture is taken. The tube is then sealed promptly, and the specimen is quickly transported to the laboratory.

Smears

In the hands of an experienced clinical microscopist, direct smears of clinical material often will be interpreted as consisting of anaerobic bacteria with a significant host–cell relationship and may establish the microbiologic diagnosis. The direct smear of a possible clostridial-caused gangrenous infection is essential and can be lifesaving, because time is extremely important.

Because the initial incubation period for anaerobes is usually 48 hours, the immediate examination of a Gram-stained smear of clinical material for anaerobes is more urgent than when aerobes or facultative organisms are suspected to be the etiologic agent.[125] Note that the highly toxic *Clostridium perfringens* organism is present in approximately 50 per cent of gangrenous lesions[125] (see Fig. 72–15).

Cultures

The same nutritionally enriched broths that are available commercially for the isolation of aerobic and facultative microbes can be used for the isolation of anaerobic microbes. *Unvented* vacuum bottles of commercially produced media have a sufficiently low redox potential to support the growth of anaerobic bacteria.[128] Therefore, thioglycolate broths and other specially prepared anaerobic broths are not needed initially.

Conclusion

Because such a large proportion of the resident flora of the upper respiratory mucosa, the female urogenital mucosa, cutaneous glands, and the colon are anaerobes (reported as 10:1 for the first three cited areas and at least 1000:1 for the colon),[125] smears and cultures of drainage from these areas or from lesions near these areas must be interpreted very cautiously. Certainly, clinical findings have an even more important role in these instances. The foul odor of expectorated sputum from a patient with aspiration pneumonia and probable lung abscess, fetid breath of persons with sore throats or sinusitis, and stench and/or crepitation at a wound site[129] suggest the presence and significance of anaerobes such as species of *Bacteroides*, *Peptostreptococcus*, *Actinomyces*, and *Clostridium*.

Direct Preparations of Clinical Materials, Stained and Unstained, in Emergency Medical Care

1. Newman, J. P.: Diagnostic bacteriological procedures and the practitioner. M.S.U. Veterinarian Fall, 1958, p. 11.
2. Blenden, D. C.: Bacteriology in the veterinarian's office. Vet. Scope. 9:7, 1959.
3. Brancato, F. P., and Parker, M. J.: The stained direct smear of clinical material. Health Lab. Sci. 3:69, 1966.
4. Path Capsule 26. The routine throat culture. College of American Pathologists, 1965.
5. Provine, H., and Gardner, P.: The Gram-stained smear and its interpretation. Hosp. Prac. 85, 1974.
6. Baker, L. H., and Hodges, G. R.: Examination of pharyngeal secretions to determine the etiology of pharyngitis. Am. J. Med. Sci. 272:89, 1976.
7. Hedges, J. R., and Wagner, D. K.: Pharyngeal gram stains in the treatment of sore throats. JACEP 7:229, 1978.
8. Heinemann, H. S., Chawla, J. K., and Lofton, W. M.: Misinformation from sputum cultures without microscopic examination. J. Clin. Microbiol. 6:518, 1977.
9. Bartlett, R. C., Tetreault, J., Evers, J., et al.: Quality assurance of Gram-stained direct smears. Am. J. Clin. Pathol. 72:984, 1979.
10. Crawford, G., Brancato, F., and Holmes, K.: Streptococcal pharyngitis: diagnosis by Gram stain. Ann. Int. Med. 90:293, 1979.
11. Sharma, S. C., and Subbukrishnan, P.: Streptococcal pharyngitis—rapid diagnosis by Gram stain. Postgrad. Med. J. 57:13, 1981.
12. McGovern, J. J., Jr. Personal communication. May, 1978.
13. Washington, J. A., II: Use and abuse of the Gram-stained smear. Clin. Microbiol. Newsletter 1:4, 1979.
14. Willis, H. H., and Cummings, M. M.: Diagnostic and Experimental Methods in Tuberculosis. 2nd ed. Springfield, Illinois, Charles C Thomas Publishing Co., Chapter IV, 1952, p. 95.
15. Barry, A. L., Smith, P. B., and Turck, M.: Laboratory diagnosis of urinary tract infections. Cumitech 2. American Society of Microbiologists, Washington, D.C., April, 1975.
16. Isenberg, H. D., Schoenknecht, F. D., and von Graenitz, A.: Collection and processing of bacteriological specimens. Cumitech 9. American Society of Microbiologists, Washington, D.C., August, 1979.
17. Rosebury, T.: Life on Man. New York, Berkley Publishing Group, 1952.
18. Kellogg, D. S., Jr., Holmes, K. K., and Hill, G. A.: Laboratory diagnosis of gonorrhea. Cumitech 4. American Society of Microbiologists, Washington, D.C., October, 1976.
19. Magee, C. M., Rodehaever, G. T., Edgerton, M. T., et al.: A more reliable gram staining technique for diagnosis of surgical infections. Am. J. Surg. 130:341, 1975.
20. Macher, A. M.: Presented at 22nd Interscience Conference on Antimicrobial Agents and Chemotherapy. 1982.
21. Nair, C. P.: Rapid staining of intestinal amoeba on wet mounts. Nature 172:1051, 1953.
22. Kronvall, G., and Myhre, E.: Differential staining of bacteria in clinical specimens using acridine orange buffered at low pH. Acta Pathol. Microbiol. Scand. (B) 85:249, 1977.
23. Murray, P. R.: Principles and uses of bacterial stains. API Species 6:1, 1982.
24. Keitel, H. G.: Pitfalls in laboratory tests. Pediatr. Clin. North Am. 12:17, 1965.
25. Bannatyne, R. M., Clausen, C., and McCarthy, L. R.: Laboratory diagnosis of upper respiratory tract infections. Cumitech 10. American Society of Microbiologists, Washington, D.C., December, 1979.
26. Wood, R. W., Tomkins, R. K., and Wolcott, B. W.: An efficient strategy for managing acute respiratory illness in adults. Ann. Intern. Med. 93:757, 1980.
27. Rein, M. F.: Gonorrhea. *In* Practice of Medicine. New York, Harper & Row, Publishers Inc., 1975, Vol. III, Chapter 19, pp. 1–18.
28. Epstein, R. L.: Constituent of sputum: a simple method. Ann. Intern. Med. 77:259, 1972.
29. Chodosh, S.: Examination of sputum cells. N. Engl. J. Med. 282:854, 1970.
30. Bartlett, R. C.: How fast to go—how far to go. *In* Lorian, V. (ed.): Significance of Medical Microbiology in the Care of Patients. Baltimore, Williams & Wilkins, 1977, pp. 15–35.

31. Quintiliani, R.: Complete abandonment urged for expectorated sputum tests. Clinical Lab Forum July, 1971.
32. Barrett-Connor, E.: Nonvalue of sputum culture in the diagnosis of pneumococcal pneumonia. Am. Rev. Respir. Dis. 103:845, 1971.
33. Geckler, R. W., Gremillion, D. H., McAllister, C. K., et al.: Microscopic and bacteriological comparison of paired sputa and transtracheal aspirates. J. Clin. Microbiol. 6:396, 1977.
34. Wong, L. K., Barry, A. L., and Horgan, S. M.: Comparison of six different criteria for judging the acceptability of sputum specimens. J. Clin. Microbiol. 16:627, 1982.
35. Bartlett, R. C.: Medical Microbiology: Quality, Cost, and Clinical Relevance. New York, John Wiley & Sons Inc., 1974, pp. 24–31.
36. Barry, A. L.: Clinical specimens for microbiologic examination. In Hoeprich, P. D. (ed.): Infectious Diseases, 2nd ed. New York, Harper & Row, Publishers Inc., 1978, pp. 92–96.
37. Murray, P. R., and Washington, J. A., II: Microscopic and bacteriologic analysis of expectorated sputum. Mayo Clin. Proc. 50:339, 1975.
38. Van Scoy, R. E.: Bacterial sputum cultures, a clinician's viewpoint. Mayo Clin. Proc. 52:39, 1977.
39. Heinemann, H. S., and Radano, R. R.: Acceptability and cost savings of selective sputum microbiology in a community teaching hospital. J. Clin. Microbiol. 10:567, 1979.
40. Beeson, P. B.: Editorial: the case against the catheter. Am. J. Med. 24:1, 1958.
41. Kimmelstiel, P., Kim, O. J., Beres, J., et al.: Chronic pyelonephritis. Am. J. Med. 30:589, 1961.
42. Kaye, D.: Host defense mechanisms in the urinary tract. Urol. Clin. North Am. 2:407, 1975.
43. Barbin, G. K., Thorley, J. D., and Reinarz, J. A.: Simplified microscopy for rapid detection of significant bacteriuria in random urine specimens. J. Clin. Microbiol 7:286, 1978
44. Kunin, C. M.: The quantitative significance of bacteria visualized in the unstained urinary sediment. N. Engl. J. Med. 265:589, 1961.
45. Paavonen, J.: Chlamydia trachomatis-induced urethritis in female partners of men with nongonococcal urethritis. Sex. Transm. Dis. 6:69, 1979.
46. Stamm, W. E., Wagner, K. F., Amsel, R., et al.: Etiology of acute urethral syndrome, abstracted. Clin. Res. 1:79, 1980.
47. Greenberg, R. N., Rein, M. F., Sanders, C. V., et al.: Urethral syndrome in women. JAMA 245:923, 1981.
48. Wald, E. R.: Gonorrhea: diagnosis by Gram stain in the female adolescent. Am. J. Dis. Child 131:1094, 1977.
49. Rothenberg, R. B., Simon, R., Chipperfield, E., et al.: Efficacy of selected diagnostic tests for sexually transmitted disease. JAMA 235:49, 1976.
50. Caldwell, J. G., Price, E. U., Pagin, G. J., et al.: Sensitivity and reproductivity of Thayer-Martin culture medium in diagnosing gonorrhea in women. Am. J. Obstet. Gynecol. 109:463, 1971.
51. Parisen, H., and Farmer, A. D.: Diagnosis of gonorrhea in the asymptomatic female. South. Med. J. 61:505, 1968.
52. Thin, R. N. T., Williams, I. A., and Nicol, C. S.: Direct and delayed methods of immunofluorescent diagnosis of gonorrhea in women. Br. J. Vener. Dis. 47:27, 1970.
53. Lossick, J. G., Smeltzer, M. P., and Curran, J. W.: The value of the cervical Gram stain in the diagnosis and treatment of gonorrhea in women in a venereal disease clinic. Sex. Transm. Dis. 9:124, 1982.
54. Tokarski, P. A.: Sexual abuse of the child. Top. Emerg. Med. 3:15–21, 1982.
55. Folland, D. S., Burke, R. E., Hinman, A. R., et al.: Gonorrhea in preadolescent children: an inquiry into source of infection and mode of transmission. Pediatrics 60:153, 1977.
56. Farrell, M. K., Billmire, M. E., Shamroy, J. A., et al.: Prepubertal gonorrhea: a multidisciplinary approach. Pediatrics 67:151, 1981.
57. Handsfield, H. H., Lipman, T. D., Harnish, J. P., et al.: Asymptomatic gonorrhea in men: diagnosis, natural course, prevalence, and significance. N. Engl. J. Med. 209:117, 1974.
58. Smith, R. F., Rodgers, H. A., Hines, P. A., et al.: Comparisons between direct microscopic and cultural methods for recognition of Corynebacterium vaginale in women with vaginitis. J. Clin. Microbiol. 5:268, 1977.
59. Balsdon, M. J., Taylor, G. E., Pead, L., et al.: Corynebacterium vaginale and vaginitis: a controlled trial of treatment. Lancet 1:501, 1980.
60. Pheifer, T. A., Forsyth, P. S., Durfee, M. A., et al.: Nonspecific vaginitis role of Haemophilus vaginalis and treatment with metronidazole. N. Engl. J. Med. 298:1429, 1978.
61. Spiegal, C. A., Amsel, R., Eschenbach, D., et al.: Anaerobic bacteria in nonspecific vaginitis. N. Engl. J. Med. 303:601, 1980.
62. McClennon, M. T., Smith, J. M., and McClennon, C. E.: Diagnosis of vaginal mycosis and trichomoniasis. Reliability of cytologic smear, wet smear, and culture. Obstet. Gynecol. 40:231, 1972.
63. Nagesha, C. N., Ananthakrishna, W. L., and Sulochana, P.: Clinical and laboratory studies on vaginal trichomoniasis. Am. J. Obstet. Gynecol. 106:933, 1970.
64. Eddie, D. A. S.: The laboratory diagnosis of vaginal infection caused by Trichomonas and Candida (Monilia) species. J. Med. Microbiol. 1:153, 1968.
65. McIntyre, D. M.: An epidemic of Streptococcus pyogenes puerperal and postoperative sepsis with an unusual carrier site–the anus. Am. J. Obstet. Gynecol. 101:308, 1968.
66. Schroeter, A. L., and Reynolds, G.: The rectal culture as a test of cure of gonorrhea in the female. J. Infect. Dis. 125:499, 1972.
67. Bhattacharyya, M. N., and Jephcott, A. E.: Diagnosis of gonorrhoea in women. Role of the rectal sample. Br. J. Vener. Dis. 50:109, 1974.
68. Kaplan, L. R., and Takeuchi, A.: Purulent rectal discharge associated with a nontreponemal spirochete. JAMA 241:52, 1979.
69. Quinn, T. C., Corey, L., Chaffee, R. G., et al.: The etiology of anorectal infections in homosexual men. Am. J. Med. 71:395, 1981.
70. Tzipori, S., Angus, K. W., Gray, E. W., et al.: Vomiting and diarrhea associated with cryptosporidial infection (letter). N. Engl. J. Med. 303:818, 1980.
71. Garcia, L. S., et al.: Clinical laboratory diagnosis of Cryptosporidium from human fecal specimens. Clin. Microbiol. Newsletter 4:136, 1982.
72. Ho, D. D., Ault, M. J., Ault, M. A., et al.: Campylobacter enteritis: early diagnosis with Gram's stain. Arch. Intern. Med. 142:1858, 1982.
73. Parasite causes death in immunodeficient patients. JAMA (Medical News) 224:581, 1973.
74. Bradley, S. L., Dines, D. E., and Brewer, N. S.: Disseminated Strongyloides stercoralis in an immunosuppressed host. Mayo Clin. Proc. 53:332, 1978.
75. Markell, E. K., and Voge, M.: Medical Parasitology, 5th ed. Philadelphia, W. B. Saunders Company, 1981.
76. Graham, C. F.: A device for the diagnosis of Enterobius vermicularis. Am. J. Trop. Med. 21:159, 1941.
77. Brooke, M. M., Donaldson, A. W., and Mitchell, R. B.: A method of supplying cellulose tape to physicians for diagnosis of enterobiasis. Public Health Rep. 64:897, 1949.
78. Mazzotti, L., and Osorio, M. T.: The diagnosis of enterobiasis. Comparative study of the Graham and Hall techniques in the diagnosis of enterobiasis. J. Lab. Clin. Med. 30:1046, 1945.
79. Kolmer, J. A., and Boerner, F.: Approved Laboratory

Technic, 4th ed. East Norwalk, Conn., D. Appleton-Century Co., Inc., 1945, p. 571.

80. Brugmans, J. P., Thienpont, D. C., van Wijngaarden, I., et al.: Mebendazole in enterobiasis: radiochemical and pilot clinical study in 1,278 subjects. JAMA 217:313, 1971.

81. Isenberg, H. D.: The role of clinical microbiology in health care. American Society of Microbiologists Newsletter 48:101, 1982.

Blood Culture Technique

82. Bennett, I. L., Jr., and Beeson, P. B.: Bacteremia: consideration of some experimental and clinical aspects. Yale J. Biol. & Med. 26:241, 1954.

83. Everett, E. D., and Hirschmann, J. V.: Transient bacteremia and endocarditis prophylaxis. A review. Medicine 56:61, 1977.

84. Gleckman, R., and Hibert, D.: Afebrile bacteremia: a phenomenon in geriatric patients. JAMA 248:1478, 1982.

85. Eisenberg, J. M., Rose, J. D., and Weinstein, A. J.: Routine blood cultures from febrile outpatients: use in detecting bacteremia. JAMA 236:2863, 1976.

86. Rosenberg, N. R., and Cohen, S. N.: Pneumococcal bacteremia in pediatric patients. Ann. Emerg. Med. 11:2, 1982.

87. Mallen, M. S., Hube, E. L., and Brenes, M.: Comparative study of blood cultures made from artery, vein, and bone marrow in patients with subacute bacterial endocarditis. Am. Heart J. 33:692, 1947.

88. Braude, A. I., Sanford, J. P., Bartlett, J. E., and Mallery, O. T.: Effects and clinical significance of bacterial contaminants in transfused blood. J. Lab. Clin. Med. 39:902, 1952.

89. Gardner, A. D.: Rapid disinfection of clean unwashed skin. Lancet 255:760, 1952.

90. Gershenfeld, L.: Iodine. In Reddish, G. F. (ed.): Antiseptics, Disinfectants, Fungicides, and Chemical and Physical Sterilization. Philadelphia, Lea & Febiger, 1954.

91. Lovell, D. L.: Preoperative skin preparation with reference to surface bacteria contaminants and resident flora. Surg. Clin. North Am. 26:1053, 1946.

92. Scurr, C. F.: Emergencies in general practice: accidents with injections. Br. Med. J. 1:1289, 1956.

93. Zintel, H. A.: Asepsis and antisepsis. Surg. Clin. North Am. 36:257, 1956.

94. Story, P.: Testing of skin disinfectants. Br. Med. J. 2:1128, 1952.

95. Lee, S., Schoen, I., and Malkin, A.: Comparison of use of alcohol with that of iodine for skin antisepsis in obtaining blood cultures. Am. J. Clin. Pathol. 47:646, 1967.

96. Coulthard, C. E., and Sykes, G.: Germicidal effect of alcohol. Pharm. J. 137:79, 1936.

97. Washington, J. A., II: Blood cultures: principles and techniques. Mayo Clin. Proc. 50:91, 1975.

98. Tandberg, D., and Reed, W. P.: Blood cultures following rectal examination. JAMA 239:1789, 1978.

99. Scott, A. C.: Blood-culture technique: two needles or one (letter). Lancet 1:1414, 1979.

100. Hoffman, P. C., Arnow, P. M., Goldman, D. A., et al.: False-positive blood cultures: association with nonsterile blood collection tubes. JAMA 236:2073, 1976.

101. Tonnesen, A., Peuler, M., and Lockwood, W. R.: Cultures of blood drawn by catheters vs venipuncture. JAMA 235:1877, 1976.

102. Handsfield, H. H.: Blood cultures drawn through catheters (letter). JAMA 236:2944, 1976.

103. Ellner, P. D., and Stoessel, C. J.: The role of temperature and anticoagulant in the in vitro survival of bacteria in blood. J. Infect. Dis. 116:238, 1966.

104. Bartlett, R. C., and McCarthy, L.: Edited transcript, Pfizer Diagnostics "Dialogue." (Annual Meeting) American Society of Microbiologists, Chicago, Illinois, 1974.

105. Reik, H., and Rubin, S. J.: Evaluation of the buffy-coat smear for rapid detection of bacteremia. JAMA 245:357, 1981.

106. Mirrett, S., Lauer, B. A., Miller, G. A., et al.: Comparison of acridine orange, methylene blue, and Gram stains for blood culture. J. Clin. Microbiol. 15:562, 1982.

107. Hall, M. M., Ilstrup, D. M., and Washington, J. A., 2d: Effect of volume of blood cultured on detection of bacteremia. J. Clin. Microbiol. 3:643, 1976.

108. Tenney, J. H., Reller, L. B., Mirrett, S., et al.: Controlled evaluation of the volume of blood cultured in detection of bacteremia and fungemia. J. Clin. Microbiol. 15:558, 1982.

109. Washington, J. A., 2d: Conventional approaches to blood culture. In The Detection of Septicemia. Boca Raton, Florida, CRC Press, Inc., 1978, pp. 41–88.

110. Reller, L. B., Murray, P. R., and MacLowery, J. D.: Blood cultures II. Cumitech 1. Washington, J. A., 2d (coordinating ed.). American Society of Microbiologists, Washington, D.C., June, 1982.

111. Muscher, D. M., Fainstein, V., Young, E. J., et al.: Fever patterns: their lack of clinical significance. Arch. Intern. Med. 139:1225, 1979.

112. Franciosi, R. A., and Favara, B. E.: A single blood culture for confirmation of the diagnosis of neonatal sepsis. Am. J. Clin. Pathol. 57:215, 1972.

113. Griffin, M. R., Miller, A. D., and Davis, A. C.: Blood culture cross contamination associated with a radiometric analyzer. J. Clin. Microbiol. 15:567, 1982.

114. Wilson, W. R., Van Scoy, R. E., and Washington, J. A., 2d: Incidence of bacteremia in adults without infection. J. Clin. Microbiol. 2:94, 1975.

115. Brancato, F. P.: Unpublished data.

116. Pfaller, M. A., Sibley, T. K., Westfall, L. M., et al.: Clinical laboratory comparison of a slide-blood culture system with a conventional broth system. J. Clin. Microbiol 16:525, 1982.

117. Bartlett, R. C., Ellner, P. D., and Washington, J. A., 2d: Blood cultures. Cumitech 1. Sherris, J. C. (coordinating ed.). American Society of Microbiologists, Washington, D.C., October, 1974.

118. Rosner, R.: Effect of various anticoagulants and no anticoagulant on ability to isolate bacteria directly from parallel clinical blood specimens. Am. J. Clin. Pathol. 49:216, 1968.

119. Evans, G. L., Cekoric, T., Jr., and Searcy, R. L.: Comparative effects of anticoagulants on bacterial growth in experimental blood cultures. Am. J. Med. Tech. 34:1, 1968.

120. Pai, C. H., and Sorger, S.: Enhancement of recovery of Neisseria meningitidis by gelatin in blood culture media. J. Clin. Microbiol. 14:20, 1981.

121. Hall, M. M., Warren, E., et al.: Comparison of sodium amylosulfate and sodium polyanetholsulfonate in blood culture media. J. Clin. Microbiol. 3:212, 1967.

122. Norden, C. W.: Pseudo-septicemia. Ann. Intern. Med. 71:789, 1969.

123. Faris, H. M., and Sparling, F. F.: Mima polymorpha bacteremia. JAMA 219:76, 1972.

124. Carlson, L. G., and Plorde, J. J.: Influence of a blood culture inoculation technique on detection of bacteremia by the BACTEC system. J. Clin. Microbiol. 16:590, 1982.

Anaerobic Culture Techniques

125. Finegold, S. M., Shepherd, W. E., and Spaulding, E. H.: Practical anaerobic bacteriology. Cumitech 5. American Society of Microbiologists, Washington, DC, April, 1977.

126. Bartlett, J. G., Sullivan-Sigler, N., et al.: Anaerobes sur-

vive in clinical specimens despite delayed processing. J. Clin. Microbiol. 3:133, 1976.

127. Holdeman, L. V., Cato, E. P., Moore, W. E. C. (eds.): Anaerobe Laboratory Manual, 4th ed. Virginia Polytechnic Institute and State University, Blacksburg, Virginia, 1977.

128. Reller, L. B., Murray, P. R., and MacLowry, J. D.: Blood cultures II. Cumitech 1. Washington, J. A., 2d (coordinating ed.). American Society of Microbiologists, Washington, D.C., June, 1982.

129. Pulaski, E. J.: Common Bacterial Infections. Philadelphia and London, W. B. Saunders Company, 1964, Chapter 3, pp. 76–80.

16

SPECIAL PROCEDURES

73

Treatment of Accidental Hypothermia and Rewarming Techniques

KEVIN M. O'KEEFFE, M.D.

Introduction

There is growing interest in accidental hypothermia (AH). Fortunately, the recent surge in the medical literature has gone beyond mere anecdotal case reports to careful analysis of larger series of patients in urban settings.[1, 2] The publishing of such retrospective series, which involve a cohesive approach to treatment, and the promise of comparative prospective studies is heartening, because although much information has been presented on AH in the past few decades, it has also resulted in some disagreement among authorities and no general consensus about specific aspects of therapy. This has caused confusion for practitioners who attempt to treat victims of this uncommon, but certainly not rare, entity. In this chapter, I undoubtedly display my own bias, but I have tried to make a conscious effort to refer to the work and conclusions of others. Hopefully, the reader will adopt a consensus approach that is rational, practical, safe, and, above all, beneficial to the patient.

Before considering the various techniques that may be used in rewarming patients, it is essential that the condition that is being treated is understood. Although a core temperature of less than 35° C is sufficient for the diagnosis of hypothermia, it must not be the sole stimulus for reflexly launching into a singular type of therapy. AH is a potentially serious condition, with definite associated mortality; however, it is now known that of itself, AH is not as lethal as was previously believed.

Most deaths occur in those victims with serious associated (and possibly precipitating) medical conditions, and those deaths generally occur *after* the patient's temperature has been restored to a normal core temperature.[1, 3] Complications do occur from AH alone, but often the most significant complications occur as a result of therapy.[2, 4, 5]

Note that throughout this chapter, temperatures will be given in Celsius (centigrade) degrees. A temperature conversion scale is provided in Fig. 73–1.

Historical Background

It is disconcerting to note that the origin of investigation into AH can largely be traced to the inhuman experimentation performed in Block 5 of Dachau by Nazi physicians during World War II.[6] Perhaps the impossibility of reproducing such a study, which was as loosely designed as it was heinous, has given that work undue credence as "science." The often-cited conclusions that the target lethal effect of AH is "inevitably" ventricular fibrillation and that the "necessary" therapy is rapid external rewarming are largely based on the Dachau data.

More credibility should be given to carefully designed studies that expanded this data, including that carried out on experimental animals, the attempted therapeutic use of hypothermia in cancer patients, and, most importantly, the widespread use of controlled hypothermia in thoracic surgery.[2, 7, 8] The initial reports of treatment of actual AH victims were primarily single case observations. A compilation of these individual cases led to the early conviction that AH was "highly lethal," with mortality rates ranging from 60 to 100 per cent in studies done from 1958 to 1970, despite varying methods of treatment (overall combined mortality rate for 131 victims was 79.2

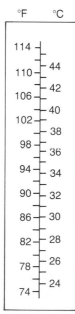

Figure 73–1. Temperature conversion scale. To change Celsius (centigrade) to Fahrenheit, multiply the Celsius temperature by 9/5 and add 32. To change Fahrenheit to Celsius, subtract 32 from the Fahrenheit number and multiply by 5/9.

per cent).[3] Yet, scattered among all the reported cases were several sequential claimants that "record" low core temperatures and full recovery without aggressive treatment were achieved.[8] Likewise, there are reports of successful treatment with very aggressive therapy. Southwick and Dalglish report a 40-year-old patient with hypothermia-induced asystole that reverted to a cardiac rhythm after 2¼ hours of cardiopulmonary resuscitation (CPR), extensive drug therapy, heated lavage of the stomach and peritoneum, and heated IV fluids.[4] This patient left the hospital neurologically intact.

In the past decade, there has been increasing evidence that mortality in AH victims is closely, if not totally, related to the presence of serious associated conditions. Two authors simultaneously introduced this observation in January 1974.[3, 9] Subsequent larger series involving 62 and 135 cases managed at one institution with a cohesive therapeutic approach confirmed this.[1, 2]

The remaining step in the evolution of the literature is the controlled comparison of techniques used in treating AH. Table 73–1 is a summary of the more salient of recent reports on animal experiments, human volunteers, and actual victims. Specific conclusions from these and other reports will be incorporated in the discussion of the selection and performance of the various rewarming techniques.

Types of Accidental Hypothermia

As previously noted, one cannot reflexly begin rewarming therapy (that is, that beyond supportive care) once the diagnosis of AH has been made.

The following questions must first be addressed: What was the rapidity of onset and the duration of the hypothermia? What is the physiologic "age" of the victim? Only when one knows the answers to these questions should one focus on the actual extent of decrease in core temperature.

At one extreme, a young healthy victim with acute immersion hypothermia can seemingly be safely and very quickly rewarmed by warm water reimmersion. (One cannot conclude, however, that such a therapy was essential for a favorable outcome.) In contrast, an elderly (or otherwise debilitated) victim who has slowly become hypothermic over a period of many hours or even days may not tolerate such aggressive treatment. More important, *it has not been shown that more conservative passive treatment, even with its slower rewarming rate, is associated with a poorer outcome.*[2, 10, 11]

As previously noted, if serious disease or injury is present, it is likely to be of higher priority than the AH, and, ironically, the AH may have somewhat of a protective effect on the associated dis-

order.[12] Some conditions not only may be causal to AH but also may in turn be masked by the hypothermic state. These disorders include pneumonia and other infectious disorders, head and spinal cord injuries, stroke, myocardial infarction, diabetes (with either insulin shock or ketoacidosis), hypothyroidism and other endocrine deficiencies, and numerous endogenous and exogenous intoxications, especially alcohol intoxication.[1, 3, 10, 11, 13] The current physiologic state of the victim should be assessed with due allowance for the apparent appropriateness of any measurable deviations from "normal" values for an individual with significantly reduced cellular temperature.[2, 10, 14]

MILD HYPOTHERMIA

Mild (32° to 35°C)* to moderate hypothermia may easily be overlooked in the emergency department, because the signs and symptoms may be misleading. A common error is failure to routinely obtain a core temperature on all patients. Presenting symptoms such as confusion in the elderly and combativeness in the intoxicated patient may not initially be recognized as symptoms of hypothermia. *Hypothermic patients frequently will not feel cold* or shiver, and a "paradoxical undressing" has been described in confused patients who apparently have the sensation of heat at lowered body temperatures.

In mildly hypothermic patients, the AH itself poses no significant danger and requires only what I consider to be baseline hypothermia care (BLHC). First and foremost, BLHC consists of preventing further heat loss by counteracting the hypothermia-favoring triad of "cold–wind–wet." The victim should be placed in an ambient setting of at least 23° to 25°C. Wet clothing should be removed and the skin should be dried. Some form of insulation is then provided; this can be as simple as one or two tightly woven blankets or a sleeping bag. The main value of blankets is to create a trapped air layer that is protected from removal by air currents. Some authors stress that there is a theoretical advantage to covering the head and neck, because it is known that at colder ambient temperatures much heat is lost from these areas. However, I believe that this modification has no significant advantage in patients who have a significant drop in core and skin temperatures and who are now located at higher ambient temperatures.

---

*Obviously, the temperature limits for *mild, moderate,* and *severe* are somewhat arbitrary, and patients at "overlap" temperatures should be treated based on their overall status and not on core temperature alone.

Table 73–1. SUMMARY OF RECENT STUDIES ON ACCIDENTAL
HYPOTHERMIA/REWARMING TECHNIQUES

Reference	Clinical Material	Techniques	Results	Conclusion	Comments
Animal Studies					
Norman 1979	20 dogs Cooled to 29°C by immersion	a) Drying insulation plus shivering b) Drying insulation *and* airway heating by intubation c) Airway heating alone (shivering prevented) d) Water immersion	Shivering caused considerable heat output. Airway heating only constituted 10% of metabolic production and did not accelerate rewarming beyond treatment (a)	Limited heat transfer by airway heating which may have been affected by loss of nasopharyngeal heat transfer	Questionable relevance to human victims
Human Volunteers					
Collis et al 1980[33]	7 subjects Lowered to 35°C by immersion	a) Warmed mist inhalation b) Local heating pad c) Warmed-mist inhalation and local heating pad d) Whirlpool bath e) Shivering	a) Did not demonstrate any A/D* difference from (d) b) Increased A/D c) Largest A/D d) Fastest rewarming rate e) Significantly increased core A/D	1) Warmed mist avoids danger of and provides safe rewarming. 2) Shivering among some of the volunteers had considerable impact on A/D. 3) Tympanic temperature monitoring correlated well with rectal values.	The applicability of findings from a few healthy volunteers who were barely made hypothermic is questioned. Too much emphasis is placed on parameter of A/D alone. Also, shivering in AH is uncommon, but as this study suggests, it is also possibly deleterious.
Hasnett et al 1980[32]	16 subjects 72 runs Cooled only to 35°C	a) Trunk immersion at 43.5°C b) Warmed mist inhalation by mask c) Heating pads and plumbed garment d) Body-to-body contact e) Spontaneous rewarming	a) Smallest A/D and most rapid rewarming b) Small A/D c) Large A/D d) Surprisingly high A/D, but rewarming rate was increased	1) Recommended inhalation as sole "safe and practical" measure for treating profound AH in the field. Did increase in rewarming rate over spontaneous rewarming. 2) True AH victims might have impaired respiratory volumes and, thus, reduced heat transfer. 3) Possible role of shivering in altering rates.	Authors of article based their conclusions principally on minimizing afterdrop because of fear of shock owing to rewarming. Limited applicability to victims with significant hypothermia.
Actual Victims					
Miller et al 1980[1]	135 episodes (114 patients)	a) Passive external (64 cases) b) Active external (14 cases) c) Heated mist by mask (13 cases) d) Heated mist by ET tube† (40 cases)	a) Rewarmed at 0.71°C per hr with 5% mortality rate b) Rewarmed at 0.90°C per hr with 64% mortality rate c) Rewarmed at 0.74°C per hr with 7% mortality rate d) Rewarmed at 1.22°C per hr with 5% mortality rate	1) Use of heated mist, even with intubation, is safe and effective. 2) Confirmed role of underlying disease in determining prognosis	Authors did not (and could not) conclude the preferability of inhalation over the passive method based on their series or the review of literature but offer it as a practical alternative.

Table 73–1. SUMMARY OF RECENT STUDIES ON ACCIDENTAL HYPOTHERMIA/REWARMING TECHNIQUES (*Continued*)

Reference	Clinical Material	Techniques	Results	Conclusion	Comments
O'Keeffe 1977[2]	63 episodes	a) Simple passive (56 cases) b) Cardiopulmonary bypass (7 cases)	a) All 56 cases treated survived. Rewarming rate at >1°C per hour b) 7 cases (3 in study) with successful defibrillation and rewarming, but 4 subsequent deaths	1) Mild to moderately severe victims in *stable* states can be effectively treated without active measures. 2) Victims in arrest need direct *cor* rewarming for survival. 3) Confirmed role of serious underlying disease in prognosis.	No comment!
Ledingham and More 1980[28]	44 patients	a) External Radiant Heat Cradle (42 cases) b) Mediastinal lavage (2 cases)	No complications from rewarming itself Overall rate 1.13°C per hour	Suggested simple surface rewarming is sufficient for all but profound cases or arrested victims.	Used supplemental warm mist where indicated for oxygenation and/or ventilation without inducing complications.
Hudson and Conn 1974[9]	16 patients	Simple passive rewarming (1 patient had augmentation by warmed mist)	55% survival rate is totally related to presence of serious disease.	The possibility of underlying serious disease is the overriding determinant in prognosis, cautioned against overaggressive treatment of AH itself.	Even the deaths occurred late, after recovery of core temperature to normal in all but 1 patient (35.5°C)
Weyman et al 1974[3]	39 patients	a) "Active" rewarming with K-Therma blanket (32 patients) b) Passive rewarming with cloth blanket	8 deaths (all but 1 with serious U/L‡ disease) in active group. Rewarming rate correlated more with presence of U/L disease than with method.	Underlying serious disease is the main correlate with lethality above fibrillatory threshold. Any method of rewarming is OK.	Use of a K-Thermal blanket and simple passive rewarming should be in the same classification.

*A/D = Afterdrop
†ET = Endotracheal tube
‡U/L = underlying

Most mild AH victims do not require actual augmentation of heat delivery to their body, provided that they have relatively intact metabolic and circulatory capabilities. Restoration of their body temperature *is* likely to be facilitated by providing supplemental glucose and oxygen, as well as by correcting any apparent hypovolemia. Warm oral fluids are of little value in augmentation of heat and could result in aspiration, and alcohol and tobacco are specifically to be avoided.[15]

As with all levels of AH, a careful delineation of physiologic status must be done. Oral temperature is an *inappropriate* determinant in evaluating significant hypothermia. Core temperature can be accurately and safely obtained and monitored via an electronic rectal probe (esophageal and tympanic probes have also been used) inserted at least 5 to 10 cm beyond the anal sphincter (Fig. 73–2). Standard glass/mercury thermometers are not adequate for the evaluation of hypothermia, because they generally cannot record reductions in temperature less than 34.4°C.* Blood pressure measurement may require the use of a Doppler device for accurate blood pressure determination; intra-arterial transducers have also been used.[16] EKG monitoring provides rate and rhythm status. All patients who have more than minimal impairment require frequent determination of their oxygenation, ventilation, and acid/base status via arterial blood gases. Hypothermia may significantly alter arterial blood gas analysis.[17] The laboratory can correct arterial blood gas values for temperature automatically on most machines if personnel are properly informed of the patient's hypothermic state. If uncorrected for hypothermia, the pH of the blood will be falsely low by approximately 0.015 unit for each change of 1°C and the P_{O_2} and P_{CO_2} will be falsely high (Table 73–2). A metabolic acidosis is invariably present in patients with severe hypothermia. The acidosis is partly protective, because it shifts the oxygen-dissociation curve to the right. Vigorous correction of the acidosis may be detrimental.

All patients should have an adequate-bore IV line established for fluid, glucose, and possible drug administration. Most hypothermic patients are *dehydrated*, because fluid intake is reduced and cold causes a diuresis; maintenance IV fluids should be given routinely. Warming of all IV fluids to 40° to 42°C is reasonable, but the usual volumes administered will not contribute many calories of heat.[18] If the patient is significantly hypotensive or his ability to tolerate fluid infusion is uncertain, a CVP line may be justified, but a central line should *never* be allowed to infuse *unwarmed* fluid.

Overall, one must realize that with the reduction of core and cellular temperature, it is not suprising

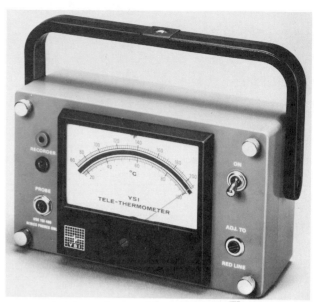

Figure 73–2. Electric thermometer (without probe). This is model 43TA with Fahrenheit and Celsius scales. (Courtesy of Yellow Springs Instrument Company, Yellow Springs, Ohio.)

to find a parallel reduction in all parameters of vital activity, because the enzymatic rate of metabolism itself decreases two to three times with each 10°C drop[7] and cerebral blood flow decreases 6 to 7 per cent per 1°C drop. Profound hypothermia results in coma, hyporeflexia, fixed and dilated pupils, severe bradycardia, and often unobtainable blood pressure.

Table 73–2. CHANGES IN pH, P_{O_2}, AND P_{CO_2} IN HYPOTHERMIA*

Temperature		Correction†		
F	C	P_{CO_2}	P_{O_2}	pH
108	42.2	1.25	1.35	− .08
106	41.1	1.19	1.26	− .06
104	40.0	1.14	1.19	− .04
102	38.9	1.08	1.11	− .03
98.6	37.0	1.00	1.00	0
95	35.0	0.92	0.89	+ .03
90	32.2	0.82	0.76	+ .07
88	31.1	0.78	0.72	+ .09
86	30.0	0.74	0.67	+ .10
84	28.9	0.71	0.63	+ .12
82	27.8	0.68	0.59	+ .14
80	26.7	0.64	0.56	+ .15
78	25.6	0.61	0.52	+ .17
76	24.4	0.59	0.49	+ .18
74	23.3	0.56	0.46	+ .20
72	22.2	0.53	0.43	+ .22

*pH increases 0.008 unit per degree F fall in temperature; P_{O_2} decreases 3.3% per degree F fall in temperature; and P_{CO_2} decreases 2.4% per degree F fall in temperature

†This table gives corrections for blood gas analysis that have not been already corrected by the laboratory for hypothermic patients. Note that to obtain the corrected P_{O_2} and P_{CO_2}, one *multiplies* the reported value by the appropriate factor but the pH factor is *added* to the reported value.

From Ann. Emerg. Med. 8(6):247, 1979.

---

*Glass thermometers that read down to 23.8°C are available from Dynamed, Inc., Carlsbad, California 92008.

When one considers that in the most extreme situation, an AH victim might appear to be *dead* yet be totally recoverable, one can more readily understand progressive decreases in mentation, muscular response, respiration, and circulation with progressive decreases in temperature. There are no absolute values for "acceptable" deviations of these parameters from normal at a given level of core temperature. However, it is clear that it is the *stability* of such values and their expected rapid resolution with the return toward normal core temperatures that are useful prognostic guides. Such an improvement is to be contrasted with any observed degeneration to even more agonal states of rhythm or worsening neurologic signs.

With a mild to moderate reduction in core temperature, the level of mentation correlates with the severity of the AH or associated illness or both. In alcoholics in particular, coma at higher core temperatures may be due to unsuspected hypoglycemia and a trial of glucose by bolus infusion is justified. In the 22 cases of AH reviewed by Fitzgerald, all except two were alcoholics.[19] The serum glucose was less than 50 mg/dl in 41 per cent (9 patients). This study noted glycosuria in two patients, even when low serum glucose values were evident, and described a renal tubular glycosuria in AH. Such glycosuria may worsen or cause hypoglycemia; *glycosuria in AH is no guarantee of adequate serum glucose.* This supports the routine use of supplemental intravenous glucose unless a normal serum glucose can be quickly assured. Intravenous thiamine (100 mg) and a trial dose of 2 mg intravenous naloxone (Narcan) should also be given to *all obtunded victims* to treat thiamine deficiency and narcotic overdose, respectively. Although failure to rewarm spontaneously has been noted in victims with hypothyroidism and other endocrine deficiencies, the use of thyroid hormones in relevant cases did not improve rewarming; steroids have also been found to be of no value in this situation.[14]

Antibiotics are not routinely indicated in uncomplicated mild hypothermia. Although there is no consensus on the value of routine antibiotic therapy in severe AH, the inaccuracy of historical, laboratory, and clinical data in distinguishing the infected from the noninfected hypothermic patient has prompted some authors to advocate the routine initiation of broad spectrum antibiotics upon admission of severely hypothermic patients.[20]

Most victims with mild AH will respond readily to the above outlined BLHC approach alone. Need for further care or admission to the hospital will be based only on associated conditions, including psychosocial problems.*

---

*For the purpose of maximum understanding, at this time we will skip from this generally noncontroversial care of mild hypothermia to an "almost" equal consensus regarding care of severe AH before considering cases with intermediate decreases in core temperature.

SEVERE HYPOTHERMIA

Patients who appear dead after prolonged exposure to cold temperature should not be considered so until they are at near normal core temperature and are still unresponsive to cardiopulmonary resuscitation. It may require as much as 1 or 2 minutes to fully assess the vital signs in severely hypothermic patients. The absence of a palpable pulse or the presence of apnea does not necessarily signify that the patient is unsalvageable. Whereas it is reasonable to exercise a gentle and cautious approach to the stable patient with severe hypothermia, cardiac arrest mandates the immediate institution of heart and core rewarming techniques. Considerable experience indicates that severe AH is actually protective to victims in danger of, or actually in, cardiac arrest. This effect is distinguishable from the element of the "dive" reflex seen in young victims of cold water near-drowning.[21] Victims have fully recovered from cardiac arrest with CPR of periods up to 3½ hours.[8] This consolation is, however, offset by the equal experience that victims of AH in cardiac arrest have not been resuscitated by the usual measures of advanced cardiac life support when core temperature was below approximately 28°C. Basic CPR, defibrillation, and initial courses of drugs can be used, but if they are not successful, such efforts represent only a "holding action" until the myocardium can be rewarmed to a level at which the arrest can be terminated. In severe hypothermia, it is common to encounter ventricular fibrillation, which is resistant to all standard forms of therapy, and *core rewarming* offers the only chance for reverting to a cardiac rhythm.

There is at least theoretical objection to repeated courses of drugs during a resuscitation because of reduced cellular metabolism. Drugs injected into a hypothermic patient may accumulate in peripheral tissues and may cause toxicity when vasodilatation occurs during rewarming. Recently, it has been suggested that bretylium might be successful in reversing ventricular fibrillation when countershock has been successful, thus avoiding the need for more aggressive rewarming therapy.[22] *Prophylactic* bretylium has been advocated by some for use in moderate to severe hypothermia when a viable rhythm is present.

Core rewarming requires rewarming of the blood and viscera, and external warming measures are not successful in victims without peripheral blood flow. Literally, one may need to provide *cor* (heart) rewarming in addition to *core* rewarming. Intermediate measures such as warmed mist inhalation may not provide enough heat transfer to the heart for resuscitation from cardiac arrest. Direct lavage of the heart muscle with warmed fluid and partial extracorporeal bypass have been shown to be effective for core rewarming.

The critical aspect in treating severe AH is

whether *all* patients with core temperatures below 28°C (a "fibrillatory threshold" based on Dachau, animal studies, and cardiac surgery) should have cor rewarming to a level beyond the critical temperature value or *only* those who have already arrested. (Note that although fibrillation has been used as the indicator of cardiac arrest, some investigators have reported the occurrence of asystole in AH victims;[4] the technique of rewarming would be performed in a similar manner regardless of the dysrhythmia.) Observations indicate that the heart itself is not always the target organ for lethality from AH, with reports of respiratory arrest and noncardiogenic pulmonary edema in some victims.[23, 24]

Evidence indicates that fibrillation is most likely to occur in AH victims at temperatures far below 28°C (i.e., 20° to 23°C).[1, 25, 26] More important, it seems particularly likely to occur when victims are handled roughly or when invasive procedures are conducted.[2, 4, 5, 10, 11, 25, 27] Other investigators have carried out similar procedures (carefully and with attention to adequate patient oxygenation) without initiating arrest in victims with severe AH.[1, 28] Consequently, the practitioner must decide whether to prophylactically respond to the risk of arrest or to cautiously warm the victim by less aggressive means beyond this critical temperature and to carefully use only those invasive measures that are required for support of the other vital parameters. Significant rhythms other than ventricular fibrillation or asystole, such as marked bradycardias and slow atrial fibrillation, will almost invariably resolve spontaneously with rewarming.[2] For these reasons, caution is suggested *against* using the overaggressive medical or procedure-directed therapy of hypotension, bradycardia, hypoventilation, and coma in the *non–cardiac arrest situation.* In the *stable and recovering patient,* the routine use of tracheal intubation, nasogastric tubes, esophageal probes, prophylactic cardiac pacing, and central vascular cannulation should be avoided unless the patient manifests a definite indication for the use of these procedures. A Foley catheter and peripheral intravenous line are indicated. Urine should be monitored for total output and the possibility of myoglobinuria.

MODERATE HYPOTHERMIA

In the midrange of core temperatures, there can be significant physiologic impairment caused by the hypothermic state or associated conditions. Several studies have shown that victims in this range can also be successfully treated by the same measures of BLHC as those used for mild cases.[2, 3, 11] Other investigators have reported that the use of more active rewarming measures has somewhat increased the rewarming rate and has

yielded an equally successful outcome without complications.[1, 3, 9, 29] I question whether there is adequate proof that any real benefit is obtained by using the more aggressive techniques.

At this time, such therapy as rewarming via inhalation mist, peritoneal lavage, gastric lavage and hemodialysis is theoretically justifiable, with the underlying rationale that prolonged hypothermia may increase tissue injury and that the risk of complications from AH would be minimized. Some of the concern can be assuaged by studies that indicate, for example, that although cardiac output and coronary flow are reduced in AH, they have been shown to be adequate to the metabolic needs of the organism.[30, 31]

The current research project of The University Study Group on Hypothermia, comparing passive rewarming with the least invasive of the more active measures, namely, warmed mist inhalation, will hopefully allow for a more decisive basis for choosing either approach.

Rewarming Techniques

The techniques described in this section include the assumption that BLHC, as previously described, is used, that any recognized associated condition should receive appropriate care, and that any sudden alteration in the status of the victim may require a change in approach.

PASSIVE REWARMING

At its simplest, passive rewarming is synonomous with BLHC (Table 73–3).[2, 11] Some investigators, including myself, have slightly modified BLHC to supplement heat recovery with the use of frequent blanket exchanges, with the blankets being warmed in a dryer or, if available, a blanket warmer. Theoretically, peripheral rewarming may

Table 73–3. PASSIVE EXTERNAL REWARMING

Advantages
Minimal harm from method
Proven successful outcome for mild to moderate AH
Adaptable to field care or limited facilities
Low-cost technology

Disadvantages
Slower return to normal core temperature
Inadequate for arrested victims
Insufficient for patients with hypothyroidism or other metabolic impairments

Complications
None reported

From O'Keeffe, K. M.: Accidental hypothermia: a review of 62 cases. JACEP 6:491, 1977; and Goldfrank, L., and Kirstein, R.: Emergency management of hypothermia. Hosp. Phys. Jan., 1979, p. 47.

result in vasodilatation, leading to the phenomenon of core temperature afterdrop. The increased circulation to the cold extremities causes warmer core blood to be further cooled and then returned to the central circulation, causing an increased drop in core temperature and possibly initiating cardiac dysrhythmias. Although some investigators believe that afterdrop may be minimized by uncovering the extremities during passive external rewarming or by relying on core rewarming methods, the exact mechanism of afterdrop is as yet unclear.[32, 33] My approach to passive rewarming is to also cover the arms and legs, because only a gradual peripheral rewarming is effected with blanket exchanges and afterdrop is minimized. Any uncovered skin could predispose to shivering. Although shivering can (at least in normal subjects) increase heat production up to three to four times, shivering should be avoided, because it has been shown to increase core temperature afterdrop.[32] Any calories generated by passive rewarming occur in the skin and musculature and do not enhance the core. Interestingly, AH victims usually do not shiver if they are covered.[2, 32]

In mild to moderate hypothermia, the approach of passive rewarming with blankets has resulted in rewarming rates of up to about 1°C per hour (in my series, the only patient unable to achieve that rate with passive techniques died).[2] Other investigators have reported rewarming rates from 0.3 to 2.0°C per hour.[1] Possible modifications to this therapy include use of a commercial warming mattress (Fig. 73–3). In the field, some investigators have used air mattresses, modified to allow warm fluid flow, or warmed rocks. Others have developed special "piped" suits for thoracic and groin rewarming. I have no objection to the use of common electric blankets in the emergency department if they do not interfere with monitoring or pose an electrical shock hazard. All techniques of active, or augmented, external rewarming have the potential risk of causing burns if contact temperatures are high enough. Also, if external rewarming is pursued aggressively, as per tub rewarming, it can possibly cause rewarming shock by inducing peripheral vasodilatation and increased circulation of peripheral blood to the core, which is still cooler than the core temperature.

ACTIVE EXTERNAL REWARMING

Warm Water Immersion

The immersion technique is the fastest noninvasive way to rewarm the core (Table 73–4).[34, 35] The technique is *not* recommended by the editors for the treatment of hypothermia. The technique does have its advocates and is included here for completeness.

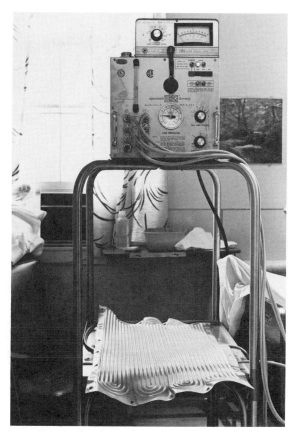

Figure 73–3. K-Thermia rewarming mattress. An automated unit such as this one can be used to augment simple passive rewarming.

One may be tempted to place hypothermic patients in a tub of warm water to quickly raise the core temperature, but this technique should be used only for those who approach the ideal of a young, healthy victim of acute immersion or other "wet" hypothermia. Patients immersed in a tub are difficult to monitor and resuscitate, and there must be standby CPR capability. Any large tub is

Table 73–4. ACTIVE EXTERNAL REWARMING (WARM WATER IMMERSION)

Advantages
Fastest return to normal temperatures of external measures
Generally available

Disadvantages
May not have suitable facility
Feasible for selected cases only
Difficulty of monitoring and, if needed, resuscitation of victims

Complications
Rewarming shock
Cardiac arrest

From Ledingham, I. M., and Moore, J. G.: Treatment after exposure to cold. Lancet 1:534, 1972; and Meriwether, W. D., and Goodman, R. M.: Severe accidental hypothermia with survival after rapid rewarding. Am. J. Med. 53:505, 1972; and other individual cases.

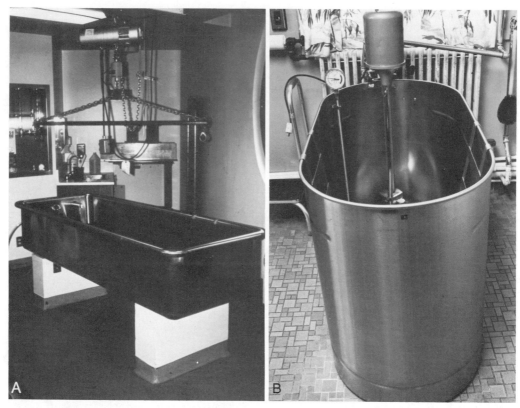

Figure 73–4. Warm water immersion is a rapid technique for active rewarming but should be used only for selected patients. A large burn care tub or other physical therapy devices may be used (A). If the patient can sit upright, a standard whirlpool tub can be used (B), or a standard bathtub will suffice.

satisfactory if a sling harness is available for non-mobile patients (Fig. 73–4).

An intravenous line and oxygen supplementation and monitoring leads are recommended, although the latter should be disconnected unless there is no chance of current leakage. There is no undisputed setting for water temperature; however, the setting for frostbite treatment is generally used (40° to 42°C), with a recommendation that the bath be gradually brought to that temperature.

Authorities vary as to whether the arms and legs should be left exposed during tub immersion. Because this aggressive rewarming therapy should be used only for suitable candidates, I doubt whether extremity immersion is a significant factor, but patients with actual frostbitten extremities might warrant this and will require additional separate, rapid rewarming of their affected extremities *after* correction of core temperature. Myers calculates that a normal-sized patient with a core temperature of 28°C and a water bath at 45°C could possibly receive up to 2400 kcal per hour, whereas the estimated basal metabolic rate at 28°C is only 30 kcal per hour and the normothermic metabolic generation is 70 kcal per hr.[18] This calculation illustrates the tremendous heat potential of warm water immersion. The victim should be rewarmed to above the hypothermia level of 35°C, because there is often a slight fall after removal

from the bath. The most significant complication from immersion rewarming is induced arrest, which is often difficult to respond to because of the immersed patient's location. Inducement of cardiac arrest is minimized by using this technique only on low-risk victims. Even in low-risk cases, there are reports of the rewarming shock phenomenon or a relative hypovolemia with significant hypotension requiring fluid administration, resulting from the vasodilatation of rewarming. Recent studies have shown that this phenomenon and the associated incidence of core temperature afterdrop can be explained by a noncirculatory thermodynamic gradients model.[32, 33]

External Radiant Heat Cradle

The external radiant heat cradle method has had limited use, but it was reported as being successful in one large series, although it was used in conjunction with other measures. A rewarming rate of 1.13°C per hour was achieved. For further details about this method, the Ledingham and Moore article is an excellent source.[28] I see no practical advantage to this method, which produced significant hypotension in 14 of 44 patients. Further investigation of the external radiant heat cradle may be merited, particularly in its potential use for infants and small children.

INDIRECT CORE REWARMING

Warmed Mist Inhalation

The warmed mist inhalation technique is receiving considerable attention and has been safely and successfully used on a large number of victims. It is virtually universally applicable, because it uses standard equipment that is available even in ambulance transport and potentially in the field as well (Table 73–5).[1, 29, 36]

Baseline hypothermia and other supportive care measures are established first. An arterial gas specimen should be obtained, and clinical assessment of the ventilatory volume of the victim should be carried out. If these parameters are adequate for the metabolic needs of the victim, intubation can then be avoided. If intubation is required, ventilator settings that provide a partial oxygen pressure (P_{O_2}) that gives 90 per cent hemoglobin saturation and nonretention of carbon dioxide should be selected.

A conventional ventilator such as the Bennet MA–1 can be used with the attached Cascade humidifer (Fig. 73–5). Some units have an existing heater for the humidifier; for those that do not,

Table 73–5. INHALATION OR MIST REWARMING

Advantages
Can be instituted in the field
Readily available equipment
Minimizes potential hazards of peripheral rewarming
Allows support of oxygenation/ventilation

Disadvantages
Limited heat transfer capability for severe AH and arrested victims

Complications
Potential risk of inducing arrest
Possible impairment of cilia and surfactant action

From Miller, J. W., Danzl, D. F., and Thomas, D. M.: Urban accidental hypothermia: 135 cases. Ann. Emerg. Med. 9:456, 1980; Lloyd, E. L.: Accidental hypothermia—treatment by central rewarming through the airway. Br. J. Anaesth. 45:41, 1974; and Shanks, C. A.: Heat gain in the treatment of accidental hypothermia. Med. J. Aust. 2:346, 1975.

an attachable electrical heating jacket such as the Bard–Parker nebrilizer heater Model 5292 is attached. The water or saline (although some investigators believe that saline causes membrane irritability and affects ciliary action, other recent

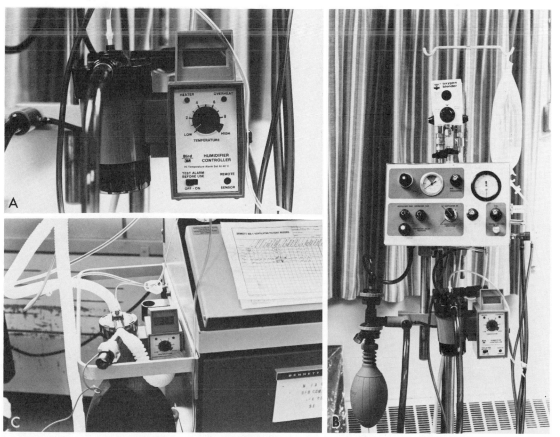

Figure 73–5. *A,* Humidifier-heater. These units provide full humidification at a set temperature for mist or inhalation rewarming. These units can be attached to standard respirators, such as the Bird or the Bennett MA-1. *B,* Bird respirator with attached humidifier-heater. *C,* Humidifier-heater attached to a Bennett MA-1 respirator.

studies have shown that water might damage surfactant)[45] used in humidification is heated to about 50°C, giving a desired entrance gas temperature of about 45°C. The tubing used should be as short as possible, and the entrance gas temperature should be prevented from exceeding 46°C.

Heated humidified gas can also be administered by a tight mask (Fig. 73–6). In patients with inadequate oxygenation or ventilation, intubation is required.[1] Ventilator settings are selected in the normal manner, based on the individual characteristics of the patient (see Chapter 3). Some authors have expressed doubt about the extent of possible heat transfer using this technique, even with normal tidal volumes.[18, 37] Myers and associates estimated that warmed mist may afford a doubling of basal heat production from 30 to 60 kcal per hour at 28°C.[18] There does not seem to be any increased afterdrop in core temperature with this technique.[32, 33, 38] As noted, only with intubation was there an increase in the rewarming rate beyond that of passive rewarming (1.22°C per hour vs 0.71°C).

Lloyd estimated that a portable mask apparatus that he developed could provide up to 30 per cent of the heat production of a victim.[40] The device that he developed for use in the field uses the heat generated from CO_2 absorption by soda lime

in a closed circuit system. Although I do not believe that this device offers any practical advantage for most urban practices, those investigators who work in the prehospital field or those involved with patients requiring long transport times are referred to Lloyd's article for details.

The slight improvement in core rewarming by inhalation does not clearly, in my opinion, mandate its use over simple passive rewarming unless there are other gains in oxygenation and ventilation for which intubation is warranted. The bottom line is that although no complications have ensued due to warmed mist inhalation, there has also been no proven benefit to the patient except for a slight increase in the rewarming rate.

Peritoneal Lavage/Dialysis

Although not as widely used as inhalation mist therapy, peritoneal lavage/dialysis has been favorably used in treating AH and is cited for completeness (Table 73–6).[39] Only those features related to its use for AH are discussed here; the general technique is the same as that described in Chapter 46. Isotonic dialysate (potassium-free and with glucose) is heated by an external bath (at about 50° to 54°C) or a blood-warming coil to about 40° to 43°C. For adults, a run of about 2 L retained for 20 to 30 minutes, repeated to a total volume of 10 to 20 L, has yielded rewarming rates of 1° to 2°C per hour. Few complications have been reported, but electrolyte monitoring and resultant modification of dialysate are warranted. There has even been a report of two successful resuscitations from apparent asystole with this technique.[39] The heat transfer with this technique is not significantly greater than that with the less invasive method of mist inhalation, and for patients in critical condition, it is far less than that achievable by hemodialysis or partial cardiac bypass rewarming.

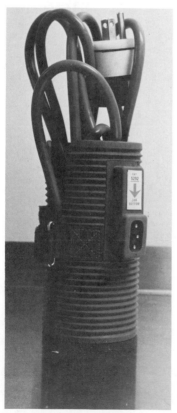

Figure 73–6. If the patient does not require a respirator, a nebulizer heater (Bard-Parker) may be used to warm a wall oxygen bottle.

Table 73–6. PERITONEAL DIALYSIS/LAVAGE

Advantages
Generally available
Can be simultaneously used for other indications for dialysis

Disadvantages
Relatively slow rewarming rates
Requires experienced personnel

Complications
Mechanical injury from catheter
Sepsis
Electrolyte derangements

From Davis, F. M., and Judson, J. A.: Warm peritoneal dialysis in the management of accidental hypothermia: report of 5 cases. N. Z. Med. J.: 94:207, 1981.

MYOCARDIAL LAVAGE

In situations in which alternative techniques are not available for rapid core rewarming in an arrested AH victim, direct myocardial lavage has proved to be successful (Table 73–7).[41, 42] Certainly it is the most direct method of rewarming the heart to a temperature past the fibrillatory threshold. In controlled hypothermia in surgery, this method has commonly been used to rewarm hearts that were directly cooled with chilled saline.

The thoracotomy is conducted as for any emergency left thoracotomy (see Chapter 6). Only the features pertinent to care of AH victims are mentioned here.

CPR is maintained while preparations are made to carry out the procedure. A balanced salt solution is warmed in a water bath to about 40°C. After the chest is opened, the heart is bathed with 1 to 2 L of warmed isotonic electrolyte fluid. Coughlin used large quantities of warmed tap water.[41] An exchange period of 3 to 5 minutes is allowed before suctioning and replacement with new fluid. I find no basis for actually opening the pericardium. When the myocardial temperature is above 26°C, it is possible to try internal or external defibrillation. If defibrillation is not successful, lavage and CPR should be continued and defibrillation should be tried again at 1° to 2°C intervals. When the fibrillation is terminated (which can occur spontaneously), the overall core temperature will often start to rise quickly with the restoration of cardiac output, but it is prudent to continue lavage until the myocardial temperature is above 32°C or until the core temperature is above 28°C. The chest should not be closed until the core temperature is above 32°C.

Although there are few reported cases in which this technique was used, it is reasonable to infer that complications should be similar to those observed when the technique is used for acute trauma (assuming appropriate surgical skills and technique). It should thus be expected that wound infections will be uncommon.[43] Interestingly, the standard post-procedure placement of a left chest tube could afford a unique means of further rewarming and raises the possibility for future investigation of its primary use, even without thoracotomy, in patients receiving positive pressure ventilation.

PARTIAL CARDIAC BYPASS

As I have reported, partial cardiac bypass has been used with good restoration of normal core temperatures in AH victims at Denver General Hospital (Table 73–8).[8, 27] At that institution, there is an experienced team, which performed frequent bypass surgery. During the period reported, partial cardiac bypass was used for all arrested victims and in several other patients with core temperatures below 28°C. The only complications involved minor controllable bleeding.

During preparation for the technique, CPR is maintained while the AH victim is transported to surgery, or the bypass machine is brought to the emergency department. The actual technique of conducting bypass surgery is beyond the scope of this book and should be performed only by experienced personnel. In an adult victim, a groin cutdown is done. The common femoral artery and femoral vein are cannulated; in children, they may not be of adequate caliber, requiring access to the iliac vessels. The pump does not require priming with blood, but the patient must be anticoagulated (dose of 3000 to 5000 units heparin IV for an average adult).

Flow rates used for an adult have been approximately 3.5 L per minute. The external warmer is set at 37° to 39°C (with a reported venoarterial gradient noted at 5°C).

Partial cardiac bypass causes rapid reversal of core temperature, with temperatures reportedly rising more than 10°C per hour. Spontaneous

---

Table 73–7. DIRECT MYOCARDIAL WARMING

Advantages
Proven successful in arrested AH victims
Uses available procedures and skills

Disadvantages
Requires special training and experience
Creates need for prolonged post-procedure care and monitoring

Complications
Similar to those seen with emergency thoracotomy for trauma

From Coughlin, F.: A heart-warming procedure (letter). N. Engl. J. Med. 288:326, 1973; and Linton, A. L., and Ledingham, I. M.: Severe hypothermia with barbiturate intoxication. Lancet 1:24, 1966.

Table 73–8. PARTIAL CARDIOPULMONARY BYPASS

Advantages
Proven successful for arrested AH victims
Rapid method
Allows support of oxygenation and blood flow in seriously impaired/arrested victims

Disadvantages
Requires high-cost technology that is of limited availability
More difficult to use in children

Complications
Hemorrhage related to heparinization
Thrombosis of cutdown vessels

From Kugelberg, J., Schuller, H., Berg, B., et al.: Treatment of accidental hypothermia. Scand. J. Thorac. Cardiovasc. Surg. 1:142, 1967; Wickstrom, P., et al.: Accidental hypothermia: core rewarming with partial bypass. Am. J. Surg., 131:622, 1976.

resolution of rhythm disturbances has occurred, but generally defibrillation is carried out after the core temperature is at about 26°C and re-tried, if necessary, at 1° to 2°C intervals. After the patient has been resuscitated, it is advisable to continue to restore core temperature to above 32°C before removing the patient from the machine, but it is also preferable to keep the time allotted for bypass surgery to under 1 hour in order to minimize damage to the blood elements. Even with this very central rewarming technique, evidence of rewarming shock has been reported.[8]

HEMODIALYSIS

The use of hemodialysis has been reported for the treatment of AH. There has been a significant technical advance that may make this method a worthwhile alternative treatment for victims of moderate to severe AH. This advance is the development of a two-way flow catheter that allows cannulation of a single vessel. The catheter is placed regularly in some institutions via a subclavian vein approach for ambulatory dialysis. A standard hemodialysis machine, including the available external warmer, is used. To this device, a Drake-Willock SND (single-needle dialysis) Controller, which allows cycling of the blood pump, is added. The SND Controller allows variable setting of cycle times and pressure limits. The problem is that in order to allow adequate admixture time for the inflow and outflow, the dialysis exchange cycle volumes are generally set at about 200 ml per minute, which in comparison with the volume of two-vessel cardiac bypass or standard hemodialysis, mandates a more limited heat exchange. Nonetheless, it is a readily usable alternative technique, and because of its central venous location, this technique may be more effective on a calorie-delivered basis than those with a more peripheral delivery.

In conventional two-vessel hemodialysis, a different apparatus is used for warming; the device has rewarming capabilities similar to those of partial cardiopulmonary bypass but requires an available, experienced dialysis facility. Myers noted that, along with bypass, hemodialysis would seem to afford the most efficient means of rewarming. With dialysis rates of 18 to 30 L per hour, the victim on conventional two-vessel hemodialysis with bypass, with 45°C dialysate, would receive 300 to 500 kcal per hour or 10 times the caloric load of other methods.[18]

Emergency Response to Critical Patients: A Scenario

In most cases of AH, the hypothermic state itself is not immediately life threatening and the emer-gency physician has time to consider and choose among the various options for care. Nevertheless, the emergency department staff must be able to respond to critical situations quickly, almost reflexively, without the luxury of a leisurely mental or literary review. The following case is theoretical but illustrates a reasonable scenario.

Case History

B. R. is a 38-year-old white man who was found lying in an alley next to an empty wine bottle in the early morning hours. It had been a night of near-freezing rain and the victim's clothing was soaked.

The emergency medical team (EMT) ambulance crew could not clearly detect any vital activity in the victim other than the possibility of a faint, slow pulse. With this uncertainty, they elected to institute basic CPR along with bagging with O_2 after insertion of a plastic airway and brief suctioning. There was no sign of trauma, but they protected the cervical spine and initiated quick transport to the emergency department while maintaining CPR.

Upon arrival at the emergency department, quick-look paddles established that the patient was in ventricular fibrillation. With the cervical spine still protected, B. R.'s wet clothing was quickly removed and a full cardiac arrest protocol with continued closed chest CPR was begun. Blind nasotracheal intubation was successful by auscultation, and a large bore IV was established in an antecubital vein, which was narrow in caliber but not collapsed. An external jugular vein was visible and considered as an alternative route. Because the patient was young, the veins were not distended and dextrose in 1000 ml normal saline was started intravenously and set to infuse in 30 minutes, both for rehydration and as a route for drugs.

An electronic rectal probe temperature gave a reading of 24°C, even cooler than had been expected from the history and the extreme coolness of the skin. A blood warmer was used for the IV fluid and set at 42°C. The patient was placed in a ventilator with heated humidifier (set at 50°C). Arterial blood gases drawn on arrival (before intubation) and corrected for the core temperature were Po_2 of 112 (on 3 to 4 L/min of O_2), pH of 7.16, and Pco_2 of 30.

Bloods were also drawn for alcohol and other toxicologic studies, CBC (complete blood count), electrolytes and blood sugar, clotting studies, amylase and liver/cardiac enzymes. Extra tubes of blood were drawn for possible endocrine studies and for type and hold. A rapid blood dipstick test for glucose showed less than 90 mg/dl, so a 50-ml bolus containing 50 per cent glucose and 100 mg of thiamine were given after the bloods were drawn. Five ampules of naloxone were also given intravenously, although narcotic overdose was considered unlikely.

The patient did not respond to an initial series of two 200-watt second attempts at defibrillation nor was there any change in the monitor pattern with 2 ampules of bicarbonate and 1 mg of epinephrine IV. It was then decided to try bretylium at an initial dose of 10 mg per kg, which, when unsuccessful, was repeated with an additional 5 mg per kg; this was also unsuccessful. Repeated defibrillation was also interposed at 320 joules.

It was decided that while good CPR was being maintained it would be unlikely that continued Advanced

Cardiac Life Support (ACLS) techniques would be fruitful as long as myocardial temperatures were so low (the rectal temperature actually dropped to 23.2°C after 40 minutes of CPR). The pupils were mid range but not reactive. The second blood gas analysis corrected for temperature was PO_2 of 284, PCO_2 of 26, and pH of 7.32.

This hospital had neither a cardiac bypass device nor a hemodialysis machine to effect high-flow external blood warming. It was decided that rather than prolong the time that B. R. would be in cardiac arrest by attempting intermediate rewarming measures with peritoneal dialysis, the heart muscle would be directly rewarmed.

Fortunately, a general surgeon and an operating room crew were readily available. The emergency department physician had had experience in emergency thoracotomy and would have contemplated performing the procedure if he had been at a less well-staffed facility.

CPR was continued during transit to the operating room, where the patient was quickly prepped and the left chest was opened. Internal cardiac massage was performed while the heart was lavaged with normal saline (warmed to 40°C). When 14 L had been used, with 3 to 5 minutes of exchange time between aliquots, the epicardial temperature had risen to 29°C and the first attempt at internal defibrillation (50 joules after suction of almost all the saline) resulted in a ventricular rate of 60, with peripheral pulses. Lavage continued while an additional 8 L were administered, at which time the epicardial temperature was 32.6°C and the rectal temperature 30.8°C. The chest was closed and a chest tube was placed.

In the recovery room, the torso of the patient was covered with a thermal blanket set at 42°C and the rest of the patient was covered with blankets.

Initially, the rhythm was atrial fibrillation, but at 1 hour, it had converted to a normal sinus rhythm, at which time the core temperature was 34.0°C. The patient had an uneventful recovery thereafter, with resumption of spontaneous respiration and rapid clearing of consciousness, despite the 1½ hours of known cardiac arrest. The only associated finding was a blood alcohol of 320 mg/dl.

Although this patient had a relatively smooth response, it is not necessarily an unrealistic depiction. Even patients with serious associated conditions to which they may eventually succumb can regularly be initially resuscitated and returned to a normal core temperature with appropriate treatment, reflecting once again that AH is both potentially lethal and potentially treatable.

Conclusions

At one time I heard an aphorism that I have long endeavored to use in both my practice and my teaching. Embarrassingly, although I can quote the aphorism, I cannot locate its source. With full credit to that unnamed person, the aphorism is as follows:

Learn principles, not techniques. For the mind that grasps the underlying principles will develop its own techniques.

This philosophy is applicable to most medical practice, particularly to AH care. Modern medicine has gone beyond preoccupation with the core temperature itself and the overstated lethality that was once implied. Although the literature has recently begun to compare the value of different

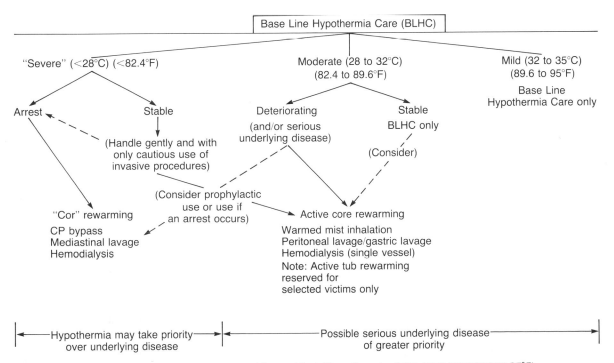

Figure 73–7. Algorithm for treatment of the accidental hypothermia victim (core temperature 35°C).

techniques, the *need* for active rewarming in non-arrested victims has yet to be validated.

If one studies the early history of AH treatment, one sees that in the 201 cases collected between 1951 and 1972, the overall mortality rate for external passive rewarming was one third lower than that for active external rewarming.[44] At present, we are eager to use invasive "central" measures but still have no evidence of improved outcome. Therefore, the problem is in determining the optimal therapy for use by practitioners who will infrequently encounter victims of AH, some of whom will be severe, with even a rare case of actual arrest. Hopefully, the material presented in this chapter will assist physicians in responding to the needs of their patients.

Figure 73–7 is an algorithm, which provides a "quick shorthand" for approaching AH. After categorizing the victim, the physician can determine appropriate therapy.

Overall, the physician should recall the following fundamental "truths":

1. The elements of BLHC are always warranted.

2. Certain techniques are not practical because of the particular skills or resources available.

3. *Aggressive techniques are essential to the care of arrested victims.*

4. With mild to moderate cases, it is the victim's tolerance of the hypothermic state and any associated diseases that determine the urgency of the rewarming care needed.

5. One must do not merely what can be done but what is necessary to help the patient.

1. Miller, J. W., Danzl, D. F., and Thomas, D. M.: Urban accidental hypothermia: 135 cases. Ann. Emerg. Med. 9:456, 1980.
2. O'Keeffe, K. M.: Accidental hypothermia: a review of 62 cases. JACEP 6:491, 1977.
3. Weyman, A., Greenbaum, D. M., and Grace, W. J.: Accidental hypothermia in an alcoholic population. Am. J. Med. 56:13, 1974.
4. Southwick, F. S., and Dalglish, P. H.: Recovery after prolonged asystolic cardiac arrest in profound hypothermia. JAMA 243:1250, 1980.
5. Lloyd, E. L., and Mitchell, B.: Factors affecting the onset of ventricular fibrillation in hypothermia. Lancet 2:1294, 1975.
6. Alexander, L.: The Treatment of Shock from Prolonged Exposure to Cold, Especially in Water. Report No. 250, Office of the Publication Board, Dept. of Commerce, Washington, D.C., 1945.
7. Swan, H., et al.: Hypothermia in surgery analysis of 100 clinical cases. Ann. Surg. 142:383, 1955.
8. Kugelberg, J., Schuller, H., Berg, B., et al.: Treatment of accidental hypothermia. Scand. J. Thorac. Cardiovasc. Surg. 1:142, 1967.
9. Hudson, L. H., and Conn, R. D.: Accidental hypothermia—associated diagnoses and prognosis in a common problem. JAMA 227:37, 1974.
10. Maclean, D.: Accidental Hypothermia. London, Blackwell Scientific Publications, 1977.
11. Goldfrank, L., and Kirstein, R.: Emergency management of hypothermia. Hosp. Phys. Jan. 1979, p. 47.
12. Carlsson, C., Magerdal, M., and Shesjo, B. K.: Protective effect of hypothermia in cerebral oxygen deficiency caused by arterial hypoxia. Anaesthesiology 44:27, 1976.
13. Stine, R. J.: Accidental hypothermia. JACEP 6:413, 1977.
14. Maclean, P. D., et al.: Metabolic aspects of spontaneous rewarming in accidental hypothermia and hypothermic myxoedema. Q. J. Med. 171:371, 1974.
15. Goldman, R. F., Newman, R. W., and Wilson, O.: Effects of alcohol, hot drinks, and smoking on hand and foot heat loss. Acta Physiol. Scand. 87:498, 1973.
16. O'Keeffe, K., and Bookman, L.: The portable Doppler; practical applications in EMS care. JACEP, 5:987, 1976.
17. Severinghaus, J. W.: Oxyhemoglobin dissociation-curve correction for temperature and pH variations in human blood. J. Appl. Psychol. 9:201, 1956.
18. Myers, R. A., Britten, J. S., and Cowley, R. A.: Hypothermia: quantitative aspects of therapy. JACEP 8:523, 1979.
19. Fitzgerald, F. T.: Hypoglycemia and accidental hypothermia in an alcoholic population. West. J. Med. 133:105, 1981.
20. Lewin, S., Brettman, L. R., and Holzman, R. S.: Infections in hypothermia. Arch. Intern. Med. 141:920, 1981.
21. Nugent, S. K., and Rogers, M. C.: Resuscitation and intensive care monitoring following immersion hypothermia. J. Trauma 20:814, 1980.
22. Dronen, S., Nowak, R. M., and Tomlanovich, M. C.: Bretolyl tosylate and hypothermia ventricular fibrillation (letter). Ann. Emerg. Med. 9:336, 1980.
23. Bristow, G., et al.: Resuscitation from cardiopulmonary arrest during accidental hypothermia due to exhaustion and exposure. Can. Med. Assoc. J. 117:247, 1977.
24. O'Keeffe, K. M.: Noncardiogenic pulmonary edema from accidental hypoteria. Colorado Med. J. 77:580, 1980.
25. Golden, F. St.: (*In*) Wright Hanson (ed.): Medical Management of the Critically Ill. New York, Grune & Stratton, 1978, p. 130.
26. Glenn, et al.: In Thoracic and Cardiovascular Surgery. Norwalk, Connecticut, Appleton-Century-Crofts, p. 1178.
27. Wickstrom, P., et al.: Accidental hypothermia: core rewarming with partial bypass. Am. J. Surg. 131:622, 1976.
28. Ledingham, I. M., and Moore, J. G.: Treatment of accidental hypothermia: a prospective clinical study. Br. Med. J. 280:1102, 1980.
29. Lloyd, E. L.: Accidental hypothermia—treatment by central rewarming through the airway. Br. J. Anaesth. 45:41, 1974.
30. Penrod, K. E.: Cardiac oxygenation during severe hypothermia in dogs. Am. J. Physiol. 164:79, 1951.
31. Berne, R. M.: Cardiodynamics and the coronary circulation in hypothermia. Ann. Acad. N.Y. Sci. 80:365, 1959.
32. Hasnett, R. M., et al.: Initial treatment of profound hypothermia. Aviat. Space Environ. Med. 51:680, 1980.
33. Collis, M. L., Steinman, A. M., and Chaney, R. D.: Accidental hypothermia: an experimental study of practical rewarming methods. Aviat. Space Environ. Med. 48:625, 1980.
34. Ledingham, I. M., Moore, J. G.: Treatment after exposure to cold. Lancet, 1:534, 1972.
35. Meriwether, W. D., Goodman, R. M.: Severe accidental hypothermia with survival after rapid rewarming. Am. J. Med. 53:505, 1972.
36. Shanks, C. A.: Heat gain in the treatment of accidental hypothermia. Med. J. Aust. 2:346, 1975.
37. Hudson, M. D., and Robinson, G. J.: Treatment of accidental hypothermia. Med. J. Aust. 1:410, 1973.
38. Hayward, J. S., and Steinman, A. M.: Accidental hypothermia: an experimental study of inhalation rewarming. Aviat. Space Environ. Med. 46:1236, 1975.
39. Davis, F. M., and Judson, J. A.: Warm peritoneal dialysis in the management of accidental hypothermia: report of 5 cases. N.Z. Med. J. 94:207, 1981.
40. Lloyd, E. L., et al.: Accidental hypothermia—an apparatus for central rewarming as a first-aid measure. Scott. Med. J. 17:83, 1972.

41. Coughlin, F.: A heart-warming procedure (letter). N. Engl. J. Med. 288:326, 1973.
42. Linton, A. L., and Ledingham, I. M.: Severe hypothermia with barbiturate intoxication. Lancet 1:24, 1966.
43. Mattox, K. L., and Jordan, G. L.: The emergency center as a site for major surgery. JACEP 3:372, 1974.
44. Gregory, R. T., and Doolittle, W. H.: Accidental hypothermia: clinical implications of experimental studies. Alaska Med. 15:48, 1973.
45. Greenberg, M. I., et al.: Effects of endotracheally administered distilled water and normal saline on the arterial blood gases of dogs. Ann. Emerg. Med. 11:600, 1982.

74

The Amobarbital Interview

KENNETH V. ISERSON, M.D.

Introduction

Emergency physicians occasionally encounter patients presenting with complaints of sudden, nontraumatic paresis or paralysis of the extremities, as well as those presenting in catatonia-like states.[1] Although an underlying primary psychiatric etiology is usually suspected by the experienced emergency physician, nagging questions about the presence of exotic or rare organic etiologies usually remain.[2] This dilemma, as well as the physician's frequent inability to alleviate acute symptoms, often causes difficulty and confusion in the patient's initial disposition and treatment. The use of sodium amobarbital (Amytal) interviews in these patients quickly resolves such problems.[3, 4] The procedure can be easily accomplished in either the emergency department or the physician's office in about 20 minutes.

Background

Amobarbital (sodium iso-amyl ethyl barbiturate) was first synthesized by the Lilly Company in the late 1920's. It is a moderately long-acting barbiturate with a moderately rapid induction time.[5] In 1930, W. J. Bleckwenn began using amobarbital to produce a drug-induced narcosis for the treatment of neuropsychiatric disorders.[6-8] The technique was quickly picked up and expanded by much of the psychiatric community under the general term narcoanalysis.[9, 10] It was generally used in institutionalized or long-term patients. World War II brought a resurgent interest in the amobarbital interview. At this time, it was introduced for use in acute paralysis, amnesia, aphonia, or pseudocatatonic states on the front lines. Grinker and colleagues used the technique successfully for both diagnostic and therapeutic purposes.[11, 12] Since World War II, however, the psychiatric community has lost interest in narcoanalysis. Current textbooks of psychiatry give little space to narcoanalysis, and many practicing psychiatrists have little familiarity with the technique.[13]

Recently, the emergency medicine community has developed an interest in narcoanalysis for symptoms similar to the "war neuroses."[14] A series of actual emergency department cases of catatonic-like symptoms and conversion reactions has also been reported.[15]

Indications

The amobarbital interview is a rapid and safe method for distinguishing and treating the functional factors that contribute to several types of symptom complexes presenting to the emergency department.

Over the years, a variety of indications have been developed for acute outpatient use of the amobarbital interview. These indications include the following:

1. Resolve conversion symptoms so that their crystallization and permanence may be avoided.

2. Treat acute panic states following such traumatic events as rape, catastrophic loss, or disaster.

3. Diagnose and treat mute and unresponsive patients (benign stupor) or patients with acute hysterical amnesia.

4. Diagnose malingering.

5. Reveal suicidal ideations.

6. Gain information in criminal cases (of dubious merit or legal worth).[16]

7. Differentiate between organic illness or organic psychosis and functional psychosis.

The use of the test to differentiate an organic from a functional illness can be of considerable concern and of life-threatening importance to those involved with the care of catatonic-like patients. Because many patients choose the emergency department as their first access into the medical system, an organic etiology for such complaints must be considered by the emergency physician. Many psychiatrists have lost sight of this possibility[1] or have come to rely heavily on "medical clearance", which is at times done hastily in a busy emergency department by psychiatrically inexperienced physicians. Patients who appear to be catatonic or in benign stupor have been reported to have such conditions as intracranial infections[17, 18] and hemorrhage,[19] endocrine abnormalities,[20] liver failure,[21] atrioventricular (AV) malformations, tumors, and drug ingestions.[22] Delay in diagnosis and therapy has led to deaths in patients with these conditions as well as in those with acute lethal catatonia.[23] Either an admission protocol (vital signs, history, and physical examination) or the amobarbital interview should suggest an organic etiology for these patients.[1]

Most emergency department experience with the amobarbital interview has been with adults presenting with one of two specific syndromes, either hysterical conversion reactions that significantly impair the patient's functions or a catatonic-like state. The catatonic-like state is different from the common condition that Plum and Posner describe as psychogenic unresponsiveness.[24] Patients with psychogenic unresponsiveness are usually hysterical, with symptoms lasting for several minutes. They lie with their eyes closed and actively resist opening the lids. When opened, the eyelids flutter or close rapidly rather than with the smooth motion seen in coma. These patients normally will respond quickly to noxious stimuli and a firm approach by the emergency department staff.

Patients in a catatonic-like state, however, often present either in a state of mute wakefulness without response to verbal or tactile stimuli or in a mildly stuporus condition. Patients in a state of mute wakefulness will often track the observer with their eyes (coma vigil, akinetic mutism) and may show a waxy flexibility of the extremities.[22] Those in stupor are sometimes mistakenly assumed to have either a neurologic condition or drug ingestion.

Contraindications

Contraindications to the amobarbital interview fall into two categories: psychiatric and medical (Table 74–1). From the psychiatric standpoint, most contraindications are relative ones. That is, potential benefit from the procedure must be weighed against the potential harm under the circumstances. Patients presenting with an overt paranoid reaction or those patients unwilling to passively submit to the procedure are unlikely to gain maximum benefit and may incur additional psychiatric trauma by undergoing the interview. Likewise, the patient who is overeager may be describing a condition from which secondary gain is involved in having the procedure performed. Using this technique on such patients may be both dangerous and unnecessary.

Medical contraindications are both absolute (i.e., porphyria and barbiturate allergy) and relative. Relative contraindications include already being under the influence of depressant drugs and having a history of barbiturate addiction, although the interview can also be used as a test of current addiction. However, even when there is concomitant drug ingestion, the interview may still be performed if the dose of amobarbital is very carefully titrated. Relative contraindications also include the presence of severe liver, cardiac, or renal disease. Severe hyper- or hypotension may suggest an organic cause, but use of the drug in these states poses a medical risk only if more than the maximum safe dose (500 mg amobarbital sodium IV) is given. The presence of mild pulmonary infection, pulmonary edema, or laryngitis poses only the theoretical risk of increasing the chance of laryngospasm. Generally, in the presence of significant concomitant medical diseases, it is best to forgo the amobarbital interview and concentrate on stabilizing the patient in the emergency de-

Table 74–1. CONTRAINDICATIONS TO USE OF AMOBARBITAL INTERVIEW

	Medical Contraindications	Psychiatric Contraindications
Absolute	Porphyria Allergy to barbiturates	None
Relative	History of barbiturate addiction Under influence of depressant drugs Severe liver, cardiac, or renal disease Severe hyper- or hypotension (only if more than 500 mg is used) Pulmonary infection or edema	Paranoid reaction Unwilling patient Overeager patient

partment. The interview may be performed later in the hospital stay.

Equipment

One should never attempt the amobarbital interview unless one has the proper time, space, equipment, and ancillary personnel available. A relatively quiet room, stretcher, or table with side rails up and basic resuscitation equipment (airway, intubation equipment, Ambu bag) are the primary requirements. IV equipment (generally 0.9 NS or D_5NS) with an injection port should be used. Amobarbital sodium (Amytal sodium, Lilly) is supplied as a dry powder, which must be reconstituted with sterile water. In reconstituting the amobarbital, it is important to rotate, not shake, the ampule. Five hundred mg of amobarbital sodium should be prepared as a 5 per cent by weight solution by diluting 500 mg of the powder in 10 ml of sterile water.

Sodium amobarbital is not the only drug that has been used in this manner. Some psychiatrists now use thiopental and mixtures of thiopental and amobarbital.[25] Others have used chloroform, cannabis indica, paraldehyde, scopalomine, chloral hydrate, and most modern barbiturates for the same purpose.[26] Amobarbital, however, seems to be the best choice for emergency department use. (The editors recommend that the procedure be done only with amobarbital.) Aside from the wealth of clinical experience with amobarbital in this setting and its theoretical superiority to thiopental for interviewing,[27] it is already familiar to most emergency physicians and is stocked as a second-line anticonvulsant in many departments.

Procedure

A medical history emphasizing prior psychiatric problems, drug overdose and abuse, allergies, medications, and contraindications to the procedure must be obtained from the patient, relatives, or friends. A complete physical examination must be performed to identify any obvious organic problems. Glucose, blood urea nitrogen (BUN), electrolytes, and a complete blood count (CBC) are obtained in cases of stupor. Samples for toxicology should be obtained, and glucose, naloxone, and thiamine should be administered. Prior records, when obtainable, should be reviewed. If a proper history, physical examination, or laboratory analysis is not possible, the procedure should not be performed. *The physician's zeal to try the procedure should not tempt him to take short cuts or to hastily examine the patient.*

After deciding that the symptoms are possibly of a nonorganic psychiatric etiology, the procedure

of the amobarbital interview is explained to the patient and/or his relatives. Reassurance should be given that Amytal is not, in fact, "truth serum." The patient should be placed in a relatively quiet room with the patient's relative or a chaperone in attendance. It may be extremely helpful for relatives to observe the interview, because it is often difficult for them to comprehend that certain symptoms, such as paralysis, have a psychogenic basis. Successful results may further reinforce the need for the family to arrange for follow-up psychiatric care.

An IV line should be secured in a large peripheral vein. Sodium amobarbital (10 per cent solution) is administered at a rate of 50 mg (0.5 ml) per minute. A conversation (or monologue in the stupor cases) about benign, non-threatening topics should be held with the patient during induction. A calm, reassuring attitude and suggestions similar to hypnotic inductions are useful, because the effect of the interview may be as great as that of the medication.[28, 29]

There is a close similarity between the state produced with Amytal and the light stages of hypnosis.[30] Some investigators have, in fact, considered it just another hypnotic medium that allows simple, direct psychotherapy with little or no analysis.[31] If a psychiatrist is present during the interview, some of the information obtained can be beneficial in future analysis. We suggest that whenever possible, the interview should be performed in consultation with a psychiatrist who will be involved in the subsequent care of the patient.

The levels of narcosis are staged using the criteria developed by Lorenz.[32] The interview is conducted during Stage II narcosis. In the responsive patient, Stage I narcosis is reached when the patient describes his first symptoms: fatigue, light-headedness or dizziness, or blurring or double vision. Stage II occurs when the responsive patient becomes euphoric or drowzy and when the unresponsive patient begins answering questions. Stage III, absence of corneal reflexes, should be avoided.

When Stage II is reached, the actual interview is begun. It usually requires 250 to 500 mg of amobarbital to reach this stage, although some investigators report success with as little as 100 mg.[14] The patient is initially questioned with such non-threatening topics as identification data, his current personal situation, predisposing factors, and further medical history (including drug ingestion).

The next stage of the interview is tailored to the specific problem. For example, if the patient has paralysis of an arm or leg, the interviewer suggests that the patient try to move and use the affected part. Once the paralysis is overcome, the interviewer reinforces the fact that the extremity is now back to normal and that it will continue to be normal after the patient leaves the hospital. It is not advisable to confront the patient with a psychiatric diagnosis at this time, even though such a diagnosis is now obvious to the family. If the patient is catatonic or unresponsive, spontaneous speech or movement will return and it is emphasized to the patient that such a responsive state is normal and desirable. Patients with organic/toxic psychoses will not respond verbally and will merely fall asleep or become more sedated during the interview. If this occurs during the interview process, the interview can be terminated with the knowledge that the patient should be presumed to have an organic etiology. Patients who have an organic basis for paresis or paralysis will still show this deficit during the interview.

Near the end of the interview, it is suggested to the patient that he remember a pleasant occurrence. This helps to improve the patient's emergence from the interview. A few patients may become slightly upset during the interview. They can be given an extra 50 to 100 mg of amobarbital at the conclusion of the interview to obtain a slightly longer sleep period.[33] Respirations are the only vital sign monitored after the procedure begins. As long as sodium amobarbital is given by this protocol, there are no significant effects on blood pressure, pulse, or respiratory rate.[32] A cardiac monitor is not required routinely but is advised in any patient with cardiovascular disease and in the elderly. Patients who are not hospitalized should be observed for 2 to 4 hours after the interview has been completed. Patients usually fall asleep for 2 to 3 hours following the conclusion of the interview, and when the patient is awakened, the proper disposition should be made.

Catatonic and pseudocatatonic patients who now have established psychiatric diagnoses should be admitted to a psychiatric service. Patients with resolved conversion reactions can be discharged with follow-up. When a psychiatric basis cannot be proven, the patient requires further evaluation for a presumed organic etiology.

Complications

Many thousands of amobarbital interviews have been conducted, usually in settings that are not conducive to advanced life support, with few complications.[9, 32, 34, 35] Nevertheless, the editors believe that resuscitation facilities must be readily available if this procedure is undertaken. The few complications reported have been primarily respiratory depression or apnea and were associated with too rapid administration (greater than 50 mg per minute) or occasionally too much (greater than 500 mg) of the drug.[35] Vasomotor collapse and laryngospasm have also been reported on rare occasions. The latter complications are reported to occur only in Stage III (usually greater than 700 mg) or anesthetic levels of narcosis, and they are not reported at all in most series. Most complications are probably related to physician error or inaccurate calculation of drug doses.

Interpretation

The patient with a supposed psychiatric symptom who does not initially respond to the amobarbital interview warrants intensive investigation for an anatomic/physiologic basis for the deficit. Failure to alleviate symptoms with the amobarbital interview is often due to the failure of the physician to make the proper pre-interview diagnosis. This is usually the result of an inadequate physical examination or incomplete laboratory or radiographic evaluation prior to the technique being used. If the patient has a firm belief or delusion, such as a feeling that he is God or that he is from outer space, the amobarbital interview will not abolish that belief. Likewise, it obviously will not render a schizophrenic normal while under the influence of the drug.

Some cases of catatonia may not respond to this technique. It must be emphasized, however, that if a psychiatric diagnosis is not firmly made from the results of the interview, it is mandatory that the patient receive intensive medical care and evaluation before he is referred to a psychiatric facility.

Conclusion

The amobarbital interview has been shown to be a rapid and safe technique that can be readily performed by the emergency physician. It is useful for the confirmation of the psychiatric basis of stupor in catatonic-like patients and for diagnosis and resolution of similarly based nontraumatic paresis and paralysis. When possible, we suggest that the procedure be carried out in conjunction with a psychiatric colleague to obtain the maximum clinical benefit.

1. Belfer, M. L., and d'Autremont, C. C.: Catatonia-like symptomatology: an interesting case. Arch. Gen. Psychiatry 24:119, 1971.
2. Slater, E.: Diagnosis of "hysteria." Br. Med. J. 1:827, 1922.
3. Mann, J.: The use of sodium amobarbital in psychiatry. Ohio State Med. J. 65:700, 1969.
4. Stevens, H.: Conversion hysteria: a neurologic emergency. Mayo Clin. Proc. 43:54, 1968.
5. Churchill-Davidson, H. C.: A Practice of Anaesthesia. Philadelphia, W. B. Saunders Company, 1978.
6. Bleckwenn, W. J.: Narcosis as therapy in neuropsychiatric conditions. JAMA 95:1168, 1930.
7. Bleckwenn, W. J.: Sodium amytal in certain nervous and mental conditions. Wis. Med. J. 29:693, 1930.
8. Bleckwenn, W. J.: The use of sodium amytal in catatonia.

Association for Research in Mental Diseases. 10:224, 1931.

9. Horsley, J. S.: Narco-analysis. J. Ment. Sci. 82:416, 1936.
10. Lindemann, E.: Psychological changes in normal and abnormal individuals under the influence of sodium amytal. Am. J. Psychiatry 88:1038, 1932.
11. Grinker, R. R., and Spiegel, J. P.: War Neuroses. Philadelphia, Blakiston, 1945.
12. Grinker, R. R., and Spiegel, J. P.: Men Under Stress. Philadelphia, Blakiston, 1945.
13. Cole, J. O., Davis, J. M., Freedman, A. M., et al.: Comprehensive Textbook of Psychiatry, 2nd ed. Baltimore, Williams & Wilkins, 1975, pp. 1968–1969.
14. Wettstein, R. M., and Fauman, B. J.: The amobarbital interview. JACEP 8:272, 1979.
15. Iserson, K. V.: The emergency amobarbital interview. Ann. Emerg. Med. 9:513, 1980.
16. Redlich, F. C., Ravitz, L. J., and Dession, G. H.: Narcoanalysis and truth. Am. J. Psychiatry 107:586, 1951.
17. Raskin, D. E., and Frank, S. W.: Herpes encephalitis with catatonic stupor. Arch. Gen. Psychiatry 31:544, 1974.
18. Penn, H., Racy, J., Lapham, L., et al.: Catatonic behavior, viral encephalopathy, and death. Arch. Gen. Psychiatry 27:758, 1972.
19. Michaels, L. J.: Catatonic syndrome in a case of subdural hematoma. J. Nerv. Ment. Dis. 117:123, 1953.
20. Hockaday, T. D. R., Keynes, W. M., and McKenzie, J. K.: Catatonic stupor in elderly woman with hyperparathyroidism. Br. Med. J. 1:85, 1966.
21. Jaffe, N.: Catatonia and hepatic dysfunction. Dis. Nerv. Syst. 28:606, 1976.
22. Morrison, J. R.: Catatonia: diagnosis and management. Hosp. Commun. Psychiatry 26:91, 1975.
23. Regestein, Q. R., Alpert, J. S., and Reich, P.: Sudden catatonic stupor with disastrous outcome. JAMA 238:618, 1977.
24. Plum, F., and Posner, J. B.: The Diagnosis of Stupor and Coma. Philadelphia, F. A. Davis Co., 1972, pp. 217–221.
25. Smith, J. W., Lemere, F., and Dunn, R. B.: Pentothal interviews in the treatment of alcoholism. Psychosomatics 12:330, 1971.
26. Hart, W. L., Ebaugh, F. G., and Morgan, D. W.: The amytal interview. Am. J. Med. Sci. 210:125, 1945.
27. Naples, M., and Hackett, T. P.: The amytal interview: history and current uses. Psychosomatics 19:98, 1978.
28. Stevenson, I., Buckman, J., Smith, B. M., et al.: The use of drugs in psychiatric interviews: some interpretations based on controlled experiments. Am. J. Psychiatry 131:707, 1974.
29. Smith, B. M., Hain, J. D., and Stevenson, I.: Controlled interviews using drugs. Arch. Gen. Psychiatry 22:2, 1970.
30. Burnett, W. E.: A critique of intravenous barbiturate usage in psychiatric practice. Psychiatr. Q. 22:45, 1948.
31. Morris, D. P.: Intravenous barbiturates: an aid in the diagnosis and treatment of conversion hysteria and malingering. Milit. Surg. 96:509, 1945.
32. Lorenz, W. F., Reese, H. H., and Washburne, A. C.: Physiological observations during intravenous sodium amytal medications. Am. J. Psychiatry 13:1205, 1934.
33. Marcos, L. R., Goldberg, E., Feazell, D., et al.: The use of sodium amytal interviews in a short-term community-oriented inpatient unit. Dis. Nerv. Ssyt. 38:283, 1977.
34. Kameneva, E. N., and Yagodka, P. K.: Sodium amytal: its therapeutic and diagnostic uses. Neuropathologiya Psykhatriya 12:44, 1943.
35. Lambert, C., and Rees, W. L.: Intravenous barbiturates in the treatment of hysteria. Br. Med. J. 2:70, 1944.
36. Sullivan, D. J.: Psychiatric uses of intravenous sodium amytal. Am. J. Psychiatry 99:411, 1942.

75

Compartmental Syndrome

DAVID E. VAN RYN, M.D.

Introduction

A compartmental syndrome requres prompt recognition and treatment. The syndrome may be defined as a condition of increased tissue pressure within an enclosing envelope, resulting in compromised local circulation and subsequent dysfunction of contained myoneural elements. Despite this specific definition, the syndrome is poorly understood. The point at which significant microcirculatory compromise occurs remains a matter of conjecture. Though the syndrome is still relatively uncommon, its incidence is increasing as we become more aware of the problem. Recognized etiologies include an increasing number of traumatic, surgical, and ischemic conditions.[1] If muscle ischemia is extensive enough acutely, a progression to myoglobinuric renal failure and shock may occur.[2] If the syndrome is not treated, the long-term sequelae of loss of function of the involved myoneural elements can be devastating. Because clinical signs are easily misinterpreted, the diagnosis is often unclear even to physicians experienced with the problem. In this potentially disastrous condition with its complicated clinical picture, any tool that aids in the early recognition of the problem is invaluable. Compartmental pressure measurement can serve as that tool. The purpose of this chapter is to describe the various techniques for compartmental pressure measurement and discuss their usefulness to the practitioner.

Background

Postischemic myoneural dysfunction and contractures were first described in the 1870's by Von Volkmann.[3] In 1935, Henderson and associates developed an open-needle technique for measuring "muscle tonus."[4] Their method consisted of the three-way connection of a syringe, a manometer, and a needle placed into the muscle itself. In the 1960's, the technique was applied to muscle compartmental pressure measurement. In 1975, Whitesides and colleagues refined the technique and described its ability to accurately reflect muscle compartmental pressures.[5] They also related elevated pressures to a need for fasciotomy to relieve a compartmental syndrome.

Other investigators were less comfortable with the reproducibility of the intermittent readings. In 1976, Matsen and coworkers modified the technique to include a constant infusion pump that allowed for prolonged, continuous monitoring.[6] Mubarek and associates objected to Matsen and coworker's modification, because the continuous infusion method injected more fluid into a compartment with increased pressure.[7] Modifying a technique developed by Scholander[8] for fluid monitoring in plants, Mubarek and associates showed that a "wick" catheter accurately reflected compartmental pressures in humans.[7, 9] This method proved as reproducible as the infusion technique. Objections subsequently arose to the degeneration of the biodegradable wick as a source of error and to the potential for retained wick upon removal of the catheter. Rorabeck and colleagues developed a "slit" catheter to replace the wick.[10] Accuracy and reproducibility of the wick and the slit catheters have been very similar in recent studies.[11, 12]

Pathophysiology of Compartmental Syndrome

Pressure studies clearly show a linear relationship between increased tissue pressure and decreased blood flow.[1] These data are against a "critical closure" pressure of compartmental vessels or a microvascular occlusion mechanism. The most acceptable theory for the reduced perfusion relates local blood flow to the arteriovenous (AV) pressure gradient: the greater the gradient, the greater the blood flow.[1, 13] In this model, veins are easily collapsed and therefore venous pressure can be no lower than tissue pressure. As tissue pressure increases, venous pressure increases. Without a concomitant increase in arterial pressure, the AV gradient and, hence, local blood flow decreases. When local blood flow fails to meet metabolic needs, ischemia causes tissue dysfunction and a compartmental syndrome follows. This the-ory accounts for observed exacerbations of compartmental syndromes by decreased arterial pressure such as with systemic hypotension or elevation of a limb. These relationships have been explored and upheld in several pressure studies.[14-16] Early in the syndrome, the dysfunction is reversible if conditions are changed. Histologic studies have shown that as ischemia continues, degeneration and necrosis occur.[17] As cell death occurs, edema may further exacerbate the pressure problem and the entire process may become worse. If the situation has progressed to this point, some permanent dysfunction is inevitable. Early attention to ischemic symptoms coupled with pressure measurements will help to avoid these sequelae.

Clinical Presentation

Even experienced personnel may find it difficult to evaluate a potential compartment sydrome, because the time of onset is extremely variable. Matsen and Clawson have found the onset of symptoms to range from 2 hours to 6 days post-insult.[18] The peak time seems to be 15 to 30 hours.

The limiting envelope required to produce a compartmental syndrome may include fascia, skin, casts, external dressings, or even epimysium alone.[1] General categories for the many etiologies of increased pressure within these envelopes include decreased compartmental volume, increased compartmental contents, and externally applied pressure. Table 75–1 lists the reported etiologies in each category. Because of the nature of the limiting envelopes and the acknowledged etiologies, compartmental syndromes are primarily restricted to the extremities. The lower leg is at high risk because of its propensity for injury and the existence of several low-volume compartments.

Clinical examination is the first step in the evaluation of an injury at risk for a compartmental syndrome. Signs and symptoms resulting from locally decreased tissue perfusion are pain and neurologic dysfunction. Evidence of dysfunction forms the basis for the physical diagnosis.

Often the first symptom described by the patient is pain greater than expected for a given clinical situation. There is often increased pain with the passive stretching of muscles in the involved compartment. The muscles may also be weak in comparison to normal. There may be hypesthesia in the distribution of nerves and palpable tenseness in the involved compartment. These findings usually progress during a period of observation. As a rule, *the presence or absence of arterial pulsation is not an accurate indicator of increased pressure;* pulses may be present in a severely compromised compartment.[19] When pulses are obliterated distally, irre-

Table 75–1. ETIOLOGIES OF COMPARTMENTAL SYNDROME

Decreased Compartmental Volume
  Closure of fascial defects
  Application of excessive traction to fractured limbs

Increased Compartmental Content
  Bleeding
    Major vascular injury
    Coagulation defect
      Bleeding disorder
      Anticoagulation therapy
    Post-arterial line placement
  Increased capillary filtration
    Increased capillary permeability
      Reperfusion after ischemia
        Arterial bypass grafting
        Embolectomy
        Ergotamine ingestion
        Cardiac catheterization
        Lying on limb
      Trauma
        Fracture
        Contusion
      Intensive use of muscles
        Exercise
        Seizures
        Eclampsia
        Tetany
      Burns
        Thermal
        Electric
      Intra-arterial drug injection
      Cold
      Orthopedic surgery
        Tibial osteotomy
        Hauser procedure
        Reduction and internal fixation of fractures
      Snakebite
    Increased capillary pressure
      Intensive use of muscles
      Venous obstruction
        Phlegmasia cerulea dolens
        Ill-fitting leg brace
        Venous ligation
    Diminished serum osmolarity, nephrotic syndrome
  Other causes of increased compartmental content
    Infiltrated infusion
    Pressure transfusion
    Leaky dialysis cannula
    Muscle hypertrophy
    Popliteal cyst

Externally Applied Pressure
  Tight casts, dressings, or air splints
  Lying on limb
  Pneumatic anti-shock garment
  Congenital bands

Modified from Matsen, F. A.: Compartmental syndromes. New York, Grune & Stratton, Inc., 1980.

versible damage has often occurred. Table 75–2 provides a summary of the signs and symptoms of compartmental syndrome according to compartment.

Patients who have an altered mental status and younger, uncooperative patients may make the interpretation of neuromuscular signs difficult. In addition, casts or bulky dressings may make care-ful examination impossible. Attributing the signs and symptoms to other pathologic entities is also a problem. Primary nerve and muscle injuries can produce similar finding, but the deficit should be maximal initially and should not progress. Arterial injuries and subsequent ischemia may produce pain and dysfunction, although neurologic changes may be less pronounced unless secondary edema produces a compartmental syndrome. Thrombophlebitis[21] and cellulitis[18] must also be considered in the differential diagnosis.

Indications for Monitoring

The diagnosis of compartmental syndrome must be made early if serious sequelae are to be avoided. Permanent damage may occur within 6 to 12 hours of the onset of elevated pressure. In cases of high clinical suspicion or when bulky dressings or poor cooperation make evaluation difficult, pressure measurement is warranted. Furthermore, in high-risk injuries, such as severe lower leg fractures, long-term prophylactic monitoring may be desired.

Pressure Measurement Techniques

The pressure measuring techniques described in this chapter include the needle technique, the wick catheter technique, and the slit catheter technique. All three methods provide rapid pressure measurement with acceptable accuracy. The needle technique is the easiest to perform.[5] The required equipment for the needle technique is the most readily available and the least expensive, although the needle technique is also the least accurate and the least reproducible.[1, 7, 12] After they have been properly set up, the wick and slit methods allow automatic pressure reading. Because these techniques are mechanized, they are the most accurate and the most reproducible. They also allow for continuous and prolonged monitoring.

Prior to attempts at compartmental pressure measurement, the physician should review the regional anatomy. In order to accurately reflect compartmental pressure, the probe must be in the correct compartment. Published investigations provide little specific advice for probe placement. Reference to a gross anatomy text will help one identify landmarks and permit entry into the desired compartment while avoiding penetration of neurovascular structures. Most compartments are superficial. The deep posterior compartment of the leg and the gluteal compartments of the hip may require deeper placement. The open needle is generally placed perpendicular to the skin, whereas wick and slit catheters are placed and

Table 75–2. COMPARTMENTAL SYNDROMES AND ASSOCIATED PHYSICAL SIGNS

Compartment	Sensory Loss	Muscles Weakened	Painful Passive Motion	Tenseness Location
Forearm				
Dorsal	—	Digital extensors	Digital flexion	Dorsal forearm
Volar	Ulnar/median nerves	Digital flexors	Digital extension	Volar forearm
Hand				
Interosseus		Interosseus	Abduct/adduct (metacarpo-phalangeal joints)	Dorsum hand between metacarpals
Leg				
Anterior	Deep peroneal nerve	Toe extensors Tibialis anterior	Toe flexion	Anterior aspect leg
Lateral	Superficial and deep peroneal nerves	Peroneal muscles	Foot inversion	Lateral aspect leg over fibula
Superficial posterior	—	Soleus and gastrocnemius	Foot dorsiflexion	Calf
Deep posterior	Posterior tibial nerve	Toe flexors Tibialis posterior	Toe extension	Distal medial leg between Achilles tendon and tibia
Gluteal	(Rarely sciatic)	Gluteals, piriformis, or tensor fascia lata	Hip flexion	Buttock

*Adapted from Matsen, F. A.: Compartmental syndrome; a unified concept. Clin. Orthop. 113:8, 1975, and Owen, C. A., Moody, P. R., Mubarek, S. J., et al.: Gluteal compartment syndromes. Clin. Orthop. 132:57, 1978.

anchored at an angle. Adequate sterile prep and anesthesia are common to all methods and should be meticulously observed. Equipment listings that follow are suggestions only; alternatives are listed wherever possible.

NEEDLE TECHNIQUE [5]

Equipment

Intavenous extension tubing (2)
18 gauge needles (2)
20-ml syringe
Three-way stopcock
Bacteriostatic normal saline
Column-type mercury manometer
Prep equipment
Anesthetic equipment
Dressing equipment

Procedure

The needle technique is based on the premise that pressures are equal in an open system. Therefore, the pressure required to inject a small amount of saline into a compartment should be equal to the pressure of the compartment. This pressure is quantified by elevation of a mercury column that is also open to the system.

Assemble the syringe, stopcock, extension tubing, and an 18 gauge needle as shown in Figure 75–1. Insert the needle into the vented vail of saline. Carefully aspirate a column of saline into

the tubing approximately halfway to the stopcock. Avoid bubbles if possible. Close the stopcock to avoid loss of saline during transfer.

The compartment to be entered is selected by testing for paresthesias and pain (during passive or active muscle stressing), representing myoneuronal dysfunction within the compartment. An area overlying the compartment to be entered is prepared as for any sterile procedure. When an

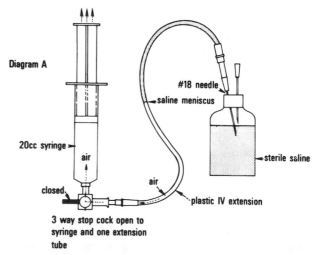

Figure 75–1. Needle technique for measurement of compartmental pressure. The syringe is used to aspirate a column of saline approximately halfway up the tubing. The stopcock is then closed to the tubing to avoid loss of saline during transfer of the needle to the tissue compartment. (From Whitesides, T. E., Haney, T. C., Morimoto, K., et al.: Tissue pressure measurements as a determinant for the need of fasciotomy. Clin. Orthop. 113:43, 1975. Used by permission.)

overlying cast is present, it can be windowed. The skin may be anesthetized with a small amount of local anesthetic. During placement of the anesthetic, care should be taken to avoid deep injection into the muscle or surrounding fascia, which could elevate the pressure obtained. The needle is carefully inserted into the compartment. Entry into *deep* compartments may require an 18 gauge spinal needle. A second extension tubing is connected between the third port of the stopcock and the manometer. The stopcock is turned to create an open system as shown in Figure 75–2. The syringe plunger is slowly depressed to increase the pressure in the system. When the system pressure just equals the tissue pressure, a small amount of saline will be injected into the compartment and the saline column will move toward the patient. Just as the air-fluid meniscus moves toward the needle, the pressure is read from the manometer. At least two readings should be made. A third reading may be required to get two that are in agreement. Rapid depression of the syringe may cause rapid fluctuations of the mercury column and less accurate readings. The needle should be checked between readings for tissue plugs or blood clots.

WICK CATHETER TECHNIQUE.[7]

Equipment

Wick catheter
Low-pressure transducer (e.g., Statham P-23 transducer)
Low-pressure monitor/recorder
High-pressure connector tubing (intravenous connector tubing can also be used)
Three-way stopcock
20-cm epidural catheter
1-0 Dexon suture
6-0 Nylon suture
20-ml syringe
Heparinized sterile saline (20 units/ml)
Prep equipment
Anesthetic equipment
Dressing equipment
16 gauge intravenous catheter

Procedure

The wick catheter technique is also based on the equilibration of pressures in an open system. The method uses a wick in the tissue catheter orifice to prevent blockage of the catheter tip. A low-pressure transducer is coupled to an electronic monitor to read equilibrium compartmental pressures. Essentially, any pressure monitor available for measuring arterial pressure can be connected to a wick catheter with saline-filled connector tubing for the determination of compartmental **pressure**.

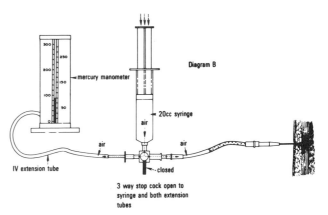

Figure 75–2. Needle technique for measurement of compartmental pressure. The stopcock is turned to create an open system. The syringe is depressed to slowly increase the pressure in the system. When the system pressure equals the tissue pressure, the saline column will begin to move and the pressure may be read from the manometer. (From Whitesides, T. E., Haney, T. C., Morimoto, K., et al.: Tissue pressure measurements as a determinant for the need of fasciotomy. Clin. Orthop. 113:43, 1975. Used by permission.)

The wick catheter may be constructed by tying two 3.5-cm lengths of 1-0 Dexon at their midpoint to a 25-cm length of 6-0 nylon. The nylon suture is passed through the distal end of the epidural catheter until it protrudes from the other end. The nylon suture is used to pull the Dexon suture pieces about 1 cm into the end of the catheter. The nylon is then cut off inside the Luer-Lok adaptor on the epidural catheter (see Fig. 75–3). This entire assembly is sterilized by the ethylene oxide technique.

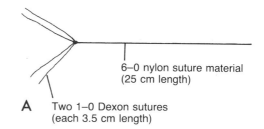

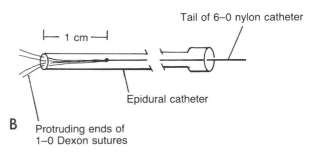

Figure 75–3. Assembly of wick catheter for pressure measurement. A, Nylon suture is used to tie two Dexon sutures at their midpoint. B, Nylon suture is drawn through the epidural catheter so that the knotted end extends approximately 1 cm into the distal end of the catheter. The Nylon suture is then cut off inside the Luer-Lok adapter.

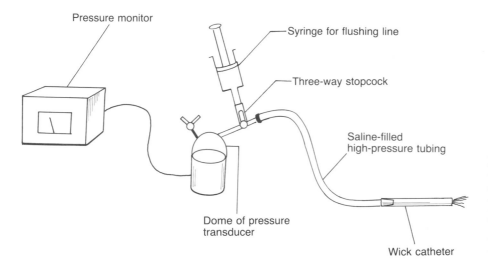

Figure 75–4. Arrangement of equipment for use of wick catheter. Note that the dome of the pressure transducer is zeroed at the same elevation as the compartment is entered with the wick catheter. The equipment is arranged similarly for the slit catheter with the substitution of the slit catheter for the wick catheter.

The catheter, high-pressure connector tubing, transducer, and monitor are assembled as shown in Figure 75–4. The entire system is filled with heparinized saline, expelling any residual air in the system. The transducer and catheter are immobilized at the level of the compartment to be measured. The catheter is wiped of excess saline, and the monitor is set to zero.

The overlying skin is prepared and anesthetized as in the needle technique. The 16 gauge intravenous catheter is introduced into the compartment at an angle (30 to 45 degrees) to the skin. The introducer needle is removed, and the wick catheter is inserted through the 16 gauge catheter until resistance is met. The catheter is secured, and a dressing is placed over the site. Pressure readings may begin after a 5-minute equilibration period. Confirmation of catheter position may be obtained by digital pressure over the compartment or muscular motion, which should produce transient pressure elevations.

SLIT CATHETER TECHNIQUE [10]

Equipment

Slit catheter (PE-60 tubing)
Low-pressure transducer
Low-pressure monitor
14 gauge intravenous catheter
20 gauge blunt-tipped needle
High-pressure connector tubing (intravenous connector tubing can be substituted)
Three-way stopcock
Prep equipment
Anesthetic equipment
Heparinized normal saline (20 U/ml)

Procedure

The slit catheter technique is also based on equilibrated pressures in an open system. The modified catheter is slit several times up the end to help prevent tissue obstruction. An electronic transducer–monitor system detects changes in pressure through a continuous saline column, without repeated infusion.

The slit catheter is constructed from a 20-cm length of PE-60 tubing slit five times approximately 2 mm up the end as shown in Figure 75–5. A 20 gauge needle is inserted into the opposite end of the tubing to provide an adapter for the pressure tubing. Prior to clinical use, the slit catheter is gas sterilized. The high-pressure connector tubing is connected between the catheter and the transducer. The transducer is connected to the monitor as in the wick catheter technique. The syringe is filled with saline and connected to the other transducer port by the stopcock. The setup is depicted in Figure 75–4. Using the 20-ml syringe, the transducer, pressure tubing, and catheter are filled with saline. Care must be taken to avoid bubbles. The monitor is zeroed by holding the catheter tip at the level of the transducer and adjusting the monitor to zero.

The overlying skin is prepared and anesthetized as in the previously described techniques. The limb is immobilized at the level of the transducer. A 14 gauge intravenous catheter is inserted at an angle (30 to 45 degrees) to the skin. The needle is withdrawn, and the slit catheter is inserted into the catheter until resistance is met. The catheter sheath is removed. Care must be taken not to

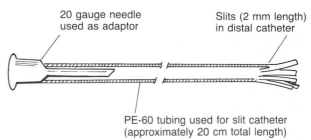

20 gauge needle used as adaptor

Slits (2 mm length) in distal catheter

PE-60 tubing used for slit catheter (approximately 20 cm total length)

Figure 75–5. Assembly of slit catheter.

move the slit catheter. A small amount of saline should be injected with the syringe to expel any air at the tip of the catheter. Pressure introduced in the system can be removed by temporarily decompressing the transducer dome. The catheter is secured, and a dressing is placed. Readings may begin after a 5-minute equilibration period. The system is checked by direct digital pressure over the comparment or by muscular motion, as described previously.

When continuous monitoring is not desired, a standard 16 gauge intravenous catheter can be substituted for the slit catheter. Prior to catheter placement a syringe filled with heparinized saline is attached to the needle stylet of the catheter. After flushing the stylet with saline, the catheter–stylet unit is advanced into the compartment. Then as the stylet is slowly withdrawn from the catheter, the catheter itself is slowly filled with saline from the syringe. After removal of the stylet with attached syringe, the saline-filled catheter is attached to the saline-filled connector tubing. The system is then cleared of air bubbles as before. The advantage of the slit catheter is that the slits prevent occlusion of the catheter tip.

Complications

All the procedures have a similar risk of infection, both local and systemic; exact risk figures are unavailable. Strict adherence to aseptic technique, careful sterilization of catheters, and use of sterile, disposable components wherever possible will help to minimize this risk.

All monitoring procedures cause some pain. The pain associated with the actual insertion of needles and catheters may be reduced by local anesthesia. Caution is advised to avoid intracompartmental injections, which might result in inaccurate readings or actually increase tissue pressure. Once inserted and secured, the wick or slit catheters should produce only minimal discomfort. The needle technique may cause increased pain by injection of saline into an already tense compartment. Reassurance and systemic analgesia may be required to gain the cooperation necessary for accurate readings. Technically, the injection of fluid may actually exacerbate a compartmental syndrome. Whitesides and colleagues found an increase in compartmental pressure of 1 mm Hg for each 1 ml of saline infused into human anterior compartments. It is difficult to assess the relevance of this problem, but recognition of the potential is important.

The wick catheter also has the potential for retained wick on removal. Wick and slit catheters require the use of a 14 to 16 gauge needle for placement. Combined with the use of heparinized saline for these techniques, there may be some

increased risk of bleeding. These larger needles may also cause slightly more pain on insertion.

Interpretation

When properly performed, each method has an acceptable accuracy in the clinical setting. Investigators report standard deviations from 2 to 6 mm Hg with any of the techniques.[1, 7, 11, 12] It is generally agreed that the needle method is the least accurate. For research, the infusion (described elsewhere[1, 6]), wick, or slit techniques offer increased accuracy and continuous readings. Normal human compartmental pressures vary in the literature. In comparing several techniques, Shakespeare and associates found an average pressure of 8.5 mm Hg.[11] Other investigators have found similar pressures with a range from 0 to 16.[1, 7, 17, 21] Shakespeare and associates found higher pressures in individuals who were physically fit.

Hargens and coworkers found dog muscle capillary pressures to be 20 to 30 mm Hg.[14] Whitesides and associates showed a significant decrease in tissue perfusion when compartmental pressures rose to 10 to 30 mm Hg below diastolic blood pressure.[5] Mubarek and colleagues showed that tissue pressures of 30 mm Hg closely corresponded to the onset of pain and paresthesias.[9] Therefore, a tissue pressure of 25 to 30 mm Hg is abnormal but would not necessarily precipitate a compartmental syndrome in the absence of other factors.

There seems to be some variability among patients for tolerance of increased pressures. Matsen found that no patients with pressures of less than 45 mm Hg had symptoms of compartmental syndrome, whereas all patients with pressures greater than 60 mm Hg had symptoms.[1] Factors other than compartmental pressure alone are important. Systemic hypotension or pre-existing vascular disease may compromise a patient's ability to tolerate even mildly elevated pressures. Zweifach and associates showed that there is significant muscle damage with tissue pressure at 20 mm Hg in the presence of a systemic blood pressure at 65 mm Hg.[15] Duration of increased pressure is also important. Matsen found that 12 hours of increased pressure reliably produces deficits.[1] One series showed that none of the patients undergoing fasciotomy for compartmental syndrome prior to 12 hours had residual deficits. In another Matsen series, 3 of 18 compartments decompresed prior to 12 hours and 22 of 24 of those decompressed after 12 hours had residual deficits.

As always, all data, including symptoms, physical examinations, and pressures must be considered before a decision to treat can be made. Falsely elevated pressures may be a result of needles placed into tendons or fascia, plugged catheters, or faulty electronic systems. Falsely low readings may result from bubbles in the lines or transducer, plugged catheters, or faulty electronic systems. One must carefully troubleshoot the system prior to making a decision to treat a presumed compartmental syndrome.

Actual treatment consists of alleviating the limiting envelope, if possible. This initially requires removing a pneumatic anti-shock garment or loosening casts or dressings. If noninvasive therapies fail, fasciotomy, which involves opening the fascia at key points overlying the involved compartments, should be considered. The escape of enclosed muscles causes a decrease in compartmental pressure, thereby improving blood flow to the tissues. This procedure is best left to personnel who are experienced in the problem and who will subsequently manage the patient. Details of fasciotomy technique may be found in surgical or orthopedic texts.

Conclusions

Compartmental syndrome is a challenging problem for all physicians. If untreated, the sequelae can be devastating. There are a myriad of potential causes. Appropriate management requires rapid assessment and treatment. Due to a variety of factors, clinical examination may be equivocal. Pressure readings can be an objective aid to prompt recognition of this problem. All the techniques outlined in this chapter are clinically acceptable. The needle technique is simple, inexpensive, and fast. For these reasons, it may be the technique best suited to emergency department use in the evaluation of acute compartmental syndrome. For more prolonged in-hospital monitoring or research, a technique with reliable serial measurement capability is needed. For these applications, the wick or slit catheter techniques (or the continuous infusion technique, discussed elsewhere[1]) may be preferable. The complications from all these procedures are negliglible.

The information presented in this chapter should aid in the evaluation of a patient with a potential compartmental syndrome. Once the decision is made to measure compartmental pressures, these techniques should provide sufficient information to guide decisions regarding treatment management.

1. Matsen, F. A.: Compartmental syndromes. New York, Grune & Stratton, Inc., 1980.
2. Mubarek, S. J., and Owen, C. A.: Compartment syndrome and its relation to the crush syndrome: a spectrum of disease. *Clin. Orthop.* 113:81, 1975.
3. VonVolkmann, R.: Verletzingon und Krankheiten der Beuengungsorgane. Hanbude der Allgeemeinen und Speciellen Chirugie, 1872.
4. Henderson, Y., Oughterson, A. W. Greenberg, L. A., et al.: Muscle tonus, intramuscular pressure, and the venopressor mechanism. Am. J. Physiol. 114:261, 1935–1936.
5. Whitesides, T. E., Haney, T. C., Morimoto, K., et al.: Tissue pressure measurements. A determinant for the need of fasciotomy. Clin. Orthop. 113:43, 1975.
6. Matsen, F. A., Mayo, K. A., Sheriden, G. W., et al.: Monitoring of intramuscular pressure. Surgery 79–702, 1976.
7. Mubarek, S. J., Hargens, A. R., Owen, C. A. et al.: The wick catheter technique for meaurement of intramuscular pressure. A new research and clinical tool. J. Bone Joint Surg. 58:1016, 1976.
8. Scholander, P. F., Hargens, A. R., and Miller, S. C.: Negative pressure in the interstitial fluid of animals. Science 161:321, 1968.
9. Mubarek, S. J., et al.: Acute compartment syndromes: diagnosis and treatment with the aid of a wick catheter. J. Bone Joint Surg. 60(A):1091, 1978.
10. Rorabeck, C. H., Castle, G. S., Hardie, R., et al.:The slit catheter: a new device for measuring intracompartmental pressure. Am. Coll. Surg. Surgical Forum 31:513, 1980.
11. Shakespeare, D. T., Henderson, N. J., and Clough, G.: The slit catheter: a comparison with the wick catheter in the measurement of compartment pressures. Injury 13:404, 1981.
12. Rorabeck, C. H., Castle, G. S., Hardie, R., et al.: Compartmental pressure measurements: an exerimental investigation using the slit catheter. J. Trauma 21:446, 1981.
13. Matsen, F. A.: Compartmental syndrome. a unified concept. Clin. Orthop. 113:8, 1975.
14. Matsen, F. A., Krugmire, R. B., and King, R. U.: Increased tissue pressure and its effects on muscle oxygenation in level and elevated human limbs. Clin. Orthop. 144:311, 1979.
15. Zweifach, S. S., Mubarek, S. J., et al.: Skeletal muscle necrosis in pressurized compartments associated with hemorrhagic hypotension. J. Trauma 20(11):941, 1980.
16. Hargens, A. R., et al.: Fluid balance within canine anterolateral compartment and its relationship to compartment syndomes. J. Bone Joint Surg. 60(A):499, 1978.
17. Sanderson, R. A., et al.: Histological response of skeletal muscle to ischemia. Clin. Orthop. 113:27, 1975.
18. Matsen, F. A., and Clawson, D. K.: The deep posterior compartmental syndrome of the leg. J. Bone Joint Surg. 57A:34, 1975.
19. Matsen, F. A., Mayo K. A., et al.: A model compartmental syndrome in man with particular reference to quantification of nerve function. J. Bone Joint Surg. 59:648, 1977.
20. Owen, C. A., Moody, P. R., Mubarek, S. J., et al.: Gluteal compartment syndromes. Clin. Orthop. 132:57, 1978.
21. Gelberman, R. H., Garfin, S. R., et al.: Compartment syndromes of the forearm: diagnosis and treatment. Clin. Orthop. 161:252, 1981.

APPENDIX
Commonly Used Infusion Rates

MARY ANN HOWLAND, PHARM. D.
ELAENA QUATTROCCHI RPh

Aminophylline

DOSAGE

Aminophylline is given as a loading dose of 5.6 mg per kg, followed by a continuous infusion to maintain the serum theophylline level between 10 and 20 mcg/ml. There is considerable variation in theophylline metabolism, and serum levels must be carefully monitored.

AVAILABLE PREPARATIONS

Each 10-ml ampule contains 250 mg of aminophylline; each 20-ml ampule contains 500 mg aminophylline. The concentration of aminophylline in each ampule is 25 mg/ml.

AMINOPHYLLINE—LOADING DOSE (5.6 mg/kg*, based on a zero theophylline level to start)

Weight									
10 kg	20 kg	30 kg	40 kg	50 kg	60 kg	70 kg	80 kg	90 kg	100 kg
56 mg	112 mg	168 mg	224 mg	280 mg	336 mg	392 mg	448 mg	504 mg	560 mg

*Diluted in 50 to 100 ml and infused over a period of 20–30 minutes

AMINOPHYLLINE—MAINTENANCE DOSE* (250 mg diluted in 250 ml; concentration of 1 mg per ml)

Age Group and Dose	Infusion Rate in Microdrops Per Minute									
	10 kg	20 kg	30 kg	40 kg	50 kg	60 kg	70 kg	80 kg	90 kg	100 kg
Children, ages 1–9 yrs 1 mg/kg/hr	10	20	30	40	—	—	—	—	—	—
Children, older than 9 yrs, healthy adult smokers 0.75 mg/kg/hr					37	45	52	60	67	75
Healthy adults, nonsmokers 0.5 mg/kg/hr					25	30	35	40	45	50
Adults with cardiac failure or liver disease 0.25 mg/kg/hr					12	15	17	20	22	25

*Frequent monitoring of serum theophylline levels is required.

Intravenous Nitroglycerin

Note: Filters and plastic bottles and tubing (especially polyvinyl chloride tubing) may absorb nitroglycerin. Glass infusion bottles, special tubing (supplied by manufacturer), and the avoidance of in-line filters are recommended.

DOSAGE

There is no fixed optimum dose. The usual starting dose is 3–5 mcg/minute, with increases of 5–10 mcg/minute every 5 minutes depending upon clinical response.

AVAILABLE PREPARATIONS

Several preparations, which differ in concentration and/or volume per ampule, are available.

Nitro-Bid (Marion Laboratories)

Each 1-ml ampule contains 5 mg nitroglycerin.
Each 5-ml ampule contains 25 mg nitroglycerin.
Each 10-ml ampule contains 50 mg nitroglycerin.

Nitrostat (Parke-Davis)

Each 10-ml ampule contains 8 mg nitroglycerin

Tridil (American Critical Care)

Each 10-ml ampule contains either 5 or 50 mg nitroglycerin.
Each 5-ml ampule contains 25 mg nitroglycerin.

NITROBID or TRIDIL (50 mg diluted in 1000 ml; concentration 50 mcg/ml)

Dose (mcg/min)*	Infusion Rate (microdrops/min)
2.5	3
5	6
10	12
15	18
20	24
30	36
40	48
50	60
60	72
80	96
100	120

*Note: This is *not* a dose/weight calculation.

For 25 mg/500 ml (50 mcg/ml), use same infusion rate as in chart.

For 50 mg/500 ml (100 mcg/ml), divide the infusion rate by 2 for desired microdrops/min.

For 25 mg/1000 ml (25 mcg/ml), multiply the infusion rate by 2 for desired microdrops/min.

NITROSTAT (8 mg diluted in 250 ml; concentration 32 mcg/ml)*

Dose (mcg/min)*	Infusion Rate (microdrops/min)
5	9
10	18
15	27
20	36
30	54
40	72
50	90†
60	108†
80	144†
100	180†

*Note: This is *not* a dose/weight calculation.
†It may be more reasonable to increase concentration to limit volume.

For 16 mg/250 ml (64 mcg/ml), divide the infusion rate by 2 for desired microdrops/min.

For 24 mg/250 ml (96 mcg/ml), divide the infusion rate by 3 for desired microdrops/min.

For 16 mg/500 ml (32 mcg/ml), use same infusion rate.

Dobutamine (Dobutrex)

DOSAGE

There is no fixed optimum dose. The infusion rate may be started at 2.5 mcg/kg/min and increased every 5–10 minutes based on clinical response. Doses up to 40 mcg/kg/min have been used.

AVAILABLE PREPARATION

Dobutrex (Lilly Pharmaceutical Company)

Each 20-ml ampule contains 250 mg dobutamine.

DOBUTAMINE (250 mg diluted in 250 ml; concentration 1000 mcg/ml)

Dose (mcg/kg/min)	Infusion Rate (microdrops/min for various weights)		
	50 kg	70 kg	100 kg
2.5	7.5	10.5	15
5	15	21	30
10	30	42	60
15	45	63	90
20	60	84	120*
30	90	126*	180*
40	120	168*	240*

*It may be more reasonable to double concentration to reduce volume.

For 250 mg/500 ml (500 mcg/ml), multiply the infusion rate by 2 for desired microdrops/min.

For 250 mg/1000 ml (250 mcg/ml), multiply the infusion rate by 4 for desired microdrops/min.

For 500 mg/250 ml (2000 mcg/ml), divide the infusion rate by 2 for desired microdrops/min.

For 500 mg/500 ml (1000 mcg/ml), use same dose schedule as in chart.

For 500 mg/1000 ml (500 mcg/ml), multiply the infusion rate by 2 for desired microdrops/min.

For 1000 mg/250 ml (4000 mcg/ml), divide the infusion rate by 4 for desired microdrops/min.

Dopamine

DOSAGE

There is no fixed optimum dose. An infusion rate of 2–5 mcg/kg/min is considered to be low and is a reasonable starting dose. Rates of 5–10 mcg/kg/min are moderate, and rates of 10–20 mcg/kg/min are large. Doses up to 50 mcg/kg/min have been used.

AVAILABLE PREPARATIONS

Intropin (American Critical Care)

Each 5-ml vial, ampule, or syringe may contain *either* 200 mg, 400 mg, or 800 mg dopamine HCl.

Dopamine HCl (Elkins-Sinn)

Each 5-ml ampule may contain *either* 200 mg or 400 mg dopamine HCl.

Dopastat (Parke-Davis)

Each 5-ml ampule contains 200 mg dopamine HCl.

DOPAMINE (800 mg diluted in 500 ml; concentration
1600 mcg/ml)

Dose (mcg/kg/ min)	Infusion Rate (microdrops/min for various weights)		
	50 kg	70 kg	100 kg
5	9.4	13	19
10	19	26	37.5
15	28	39	56
20	37.5	52.5	75
30	56	79	112.5

For 800 mg/250 ml (3200 mcg/ml), divide the infusion rate by 2 for desired microdrops/min.

For 800 mg/1000 ml (800 mcg/ml), multiply the infusion rate by 2 for desired microdrops/min.

For 400 mg/250 ml (1600 mcg/ml), use same dose schedule as in chart.

For 200 mg/250 ml (800 mcg/ml), multiply the infusion rate by 2 for desired microdrops/min.

For 200 mg/500 ml (400 mcg/ml), multiply the infusion rate by 4 for desired microdrops/min.

Isoproterenol (Isuprel)

DOSAGE

There is no fixed optimum dose. The usual starting dose is 1–2 mcg/min, with increases of 1–2 mcg/min every 5–10 minutes depending upon clinical response.

AVAILABLE PREPARATIONS

Each 5-ml ampule contains 1 mg isoproterenol. The concentration is 0.2 mg/ml as a 1:5000 solution. It is also available as 1-ml ampules containing 0.2 mg of isoproterenol.

ISOPROTERENOL (ISUPREL) (2 mg diluted in 250 ml;
concentration of 8 mcg/ml)

Dose* (mcg/min)	Infusion Rate (microdrops/min)
1	7.5
2	15
4	30
6	45
8	60
10	75
12	90
14	105†
16	120†
20	150†

*Note that this is *not* a dose/weight calculation.
†It may be more reasonable to increase concentration to limit volume.

For 2 mg/500 ml (4 mcg/ml), multiply the infusion rate by 2 to obtain desired microdrops/min.

For 1 mg/250 ml (4 mcg/ml), multiply the infusion rate by 2 to obtain desired microdrops/min.

For 1 mg/500 ml (2 mcg/ml), multiply the infusion rate by 4 to obtain desired microdrops/min.

For 4 mg/250 ml (16 mcg/ml), divide the infusion rate by 2 to obtain desired microdrops/min.

Norepinephrine (Levophed)

Note: Norepinephrine should be administered with a solution containing dextrose as opposed to a plain saline solution to protect the drug from loss of potency owing to oxidation.

DOSAGE

There is no fixed optimum dose. The usual starting dose is 2–4 mcg/min, with increases of 2–4 mcg/min every 5–10 minutes depending upon clinical response.

AVAILABLE PREPARATIONS

Each 4-ml ampule contains 4 mg norepinephrine, at a concentration of 1 mg/ml.

NOREPINEPHRINE (LEVOPHED)
(8 mg diluted in 500 ml; concentration of 16 mcg/ml)

Dose (mcg/min)*	Infusion Rate (microdrops/min)
1	3.75
2	7.5
4	15
6	22.5
8	30
10	37.5
12	45
16	60
20	75

*Note that this is *not* a dose/weight calculation.
For 16 mg/500 ml (32 mcg/ml), divide the infusion rate by 2 to obtain desired microdrops/min.
For 4 mg/500 ml (8 mcg/ml), multiply the infusion rate by 2 to obtain desired microdrops/min.

Procainamide (Pronestyl)

DOSAGE

A loading dose may be given by intermittent intravenous injection (slow push not to exceed 50 mg/min) at a dose of 100 mg every 5 minutes or as a continuous intravenous infusion at 20 mg/min. The loading dose should not exceed 1 g. A constant maintenance infusion of 1–4 mg/min may be started following the loading dose.

AVAILABLE PREPARATIONS

Each 10-ml ampule provides 1 g of procainamide at a concentration of 100 mg/ml. It is also available as 2-ml ampules providing 500 mg/ml.

PROCAINAMIDE MAINTENANCE DOSE
(PRONESTYL)
(2 g diluted in 500 ml; Concentration of 4 mg/ml)

Dose (mg/min)*		Infusion Rate (microdrops/min)
Low	1	15
	2	30
	3	45
High	4	60

*Note that this is *not* a dose/weight calculation (see following table).

PROCAINAMIDE MAINTENANCE DOSE
(PRONESTYL)
(2 g diluted in 500 ml)

Maintenance Dose (calculated by weight)	Infusion Rate (microdrops/min for Various Weights)		
	50 kg	70 kg	100 kg
1.4 mg/kg/hr (low)	17.5	24.5	35
2.8 mg/kg/hr (average)	35	49	70

Lidocaine HCl

Note: Lidocaine should be administered as a bolus followed by a continuous infusion.

DOSAGE

The average bolus over the first 20 minutes is 150–225 mg, *in divided doses*. The first bolus should not exceed 100 mg. Immediately following the first bolus, an infusion of 1–4 mg/min is begun, depending upon the clinical condition and the response to therapy. A reasonable regimen for lidocaine loading is to give an initial 75–100 mg bolus, followed by 50 mg every 5 minutes to a total of 200–225 mg. The infusion rate should not exceed 300 mg/hour.

AVAILABLE PREPARATIONS

Although many preparations for intravenous infusion are available, it is most reasonable to use 1 g/5 ml- or 2 g/10 ml-vials (such as the Inject-all syringe safety vial by Bristol).

LIDOCAINE HCl (2 g diluted in 500 ml; concentration of 4 mg/ml)

Dose (mg/min)*		Infusion Rate (microdrops/min for average 70 kg adult)
Low	1	15
	2	30
	3	45
High	4	60

*Note: This is *not* a dose/weight calculation (see following table).

For 1 g/500 ml (2 mg/ml), multiply the infusion rate by 2 to obtain desired microdrops/min.

LIDOCAINE HCl (2 g diluted in 500 ml; concentration of 4 mg/ml)

Dose	Infusion Rate (microdrops/min for various weights)		
	50 kg	70 kg	100 kg
10 mcg/kg/min (hepatic insufficiency or older than 70 years)	7.5	10.5	15
20 mcg/kg/min (hepatic insufficiency or older than 70 years)	15	21	30
30 mcg/kg/min	22.5	31.5	45
40 mcg/kg/min	30	42	60
50 mcg/kg/min (high dose)	37.5	52.5	75

For 1 g/500 ml (2 mg/ml), multiply the infusion rate by 2 to obtain desired microdrops/min.

Metaraminol (Aramine)

DOSAGE

There is no fixed optimum dose. An intravenous infusion is titrated according to clinical response.

AVAILABLE PREPARATIONS

Aramine (Merck Sharp and Dome)

Each 10-ml ampule contains 100 mg metaraminol (10 mg/ml).

INFUSION

Mix 1–4 vials in 250–1000 ml and begin as a slow infusion, changing the rate every 5–10 minutes depending upon clinical response.

Suggested starting dose: dilute 100 mg/250 ml and begin at 10 microdrops/min. Wait at least 5 minutes before increasing the dose.

Intravenous Ethanol (in the treatment of poisoning by methanol or ethylene glycol)

Note: Concentrations above 10 per cent are not recommended for intravenous administration. Concentrations above 30 per cent are not recommended for oral administration.

The dose schedule is based on the premise that the patient initially has a *zero* ethanol level. The aim of therapy is to maintain a serum ethanol level of 100–150 mg/dl, but constant monitoring of the ethanol level is required because of wide variations in endogenous metabolic capacity. Activated charcoal will adsorb oral ethanol. Ethanol will be removed by dialysis, and the infusion rate of ethanol must be increased during dialysis. Prolonged ethanol administration may lead to *hypoglycemia*.

INTRAVENOUS ETHANOL: LOADING DOSE
(A 10% volume/volume concentration yields approximately 100 mg/ml)

	Volume of loading dose (given over 1–2 hours as tolerated)					
	10 kg	15 kg	30 kg	50 kg	70 kg	100 kg
Loading dose of 1000 mg/kg of 10% ethanol (infused over 1–2 hours as tolerated) *Assumes a zero ethanol level to start.* Aim is to produce a serum ethanol level of 100–150 mg/dl.	100 ml	150 ml	300 ml	500 ml	700 ml	1000 ml

ORAL ETHANOL: LOADING DOSE
(A 20% volume/volume concentration yields approximately 200 mg/ml)

	Volume of loading dose					
	10 kg	15 kg	30 kg	50 kg	70 kg	100 kg
Loading dose of 1000 mg/kg of 20% ethanol, diluted in juice. May be administered orally or via nasogastric tube. *Assumes a zero ethanol level to start.* Aim is to produce a serum ethanol level of 100–150 mg/dl.	50 ml	75 ml	150 ml	250 ml	350 ml	500 ml

INTRAVENOUS ETHANOL: MAINTENANCE DOSE
(A 10% volume/volume concentration yields approximately 100 mg/ml. Infusion to be started immediately following the loading dose. Aim is to maintain serum ethanol level of 100–150 mg/dl)*

Normal Maintenance Range	Infusion Rate (microdrops/min for various weights)†					
	10 kg	15 kg	30 kg	50 kg	70 kg	100 kg
80 mg/kg/hr	8	12	24	40	56	80
110 mg/kg/hr	11	16	33	55	77	110
130 mg/kg/hr	13	19	39	65	91	130
Approximate maintenance dose for chronic alcoholic 150 mg/kg/hr‡	15	22	45	75	105	150
Range required during hemodialysis 250 mg/kg/hr‡	25	38	75	125	175	250
300 mg/kg/hr‡	30	45	90	150	210	300
350 mg/kg/hr‡	35	53	105	175	245	350

*Serum ethanol levels should be monitored closely.

†Rounded off to nearest drop.

‡At higher infusion rates, it may be necessary to administer by volume rather than by microdrops/min. Because microdrops/min equal ml/hr, the infusion rate in the chart may be used to calculate both microdrops/min and ml/hr.

ORAL ETHANOL: MAINTENANCE DOSE
(A 20% volume/volume concentration yields approximately 200 mg/ml. Infusion to be given each hour immediately following a loading dose. Aim is to maintain serum ethanol level of 100–150 mg/dl.* Each dose may be diluted in juice and given orally or via nasogastric tube)

	Infusion Rate (ml/hr† for various weights‡)					
	10 kg	15 kg	30 kg	50 kg	70 kg	100 kg
Normal maintenance ranges						
80 mg/kg/hr	4 ml	6	12	20	28	40
110 mg/kg/hr	6	8	17	27	39	55
130 mg/kg/hr	7	10	20	33	46	66
Approximate range for chronic alcoholic or for patient receiving continuous oral activated charcoal						
150 mg/kg/hr	8	11	22	38	53	75
Range required during hemodialysis						
250 mg/kg/hr	13	19	38	63	88	125
300 mg/kg/hr	15	23	46	75	105	150
350 mg/kg/hr	18	26	52	88	123	175

*Serum ethanol levels should be monitored closely.
†For a 30% concentration, divide the amount by 1.5.
‡Rounded off to nearest ml.

Sodium Nitroprusside

DOSAGE

There is no fixed optimum dose. Infusion rates range from 0.5–10 mcg/kg/min. The dose is titrated to clinical response.

AVAILABLE PREPARATIONS

Nipride (Roche)

Nitropress (Abbott)

Sodium Nitroprusside (Elkins-Sinn)

Each 5 ml vial contains 50 mg sodium nitroprusside.
Mix only in D5W, and wrap bottle in aluminum foil.

SODIUM NITROPRUSSIDE
(50 mg diluted in 250 ml; concentration 200 mcg/ml)

Dose (mcg/kg/min)	Infusion Rate (microdrops/min for various weights)		
	50 kg	70 kg	100 kg
0.5	7.5	10.5	15
3	45	63	90
6	90	126*	180*
8	120*	168*	240*
10	150*	210*	300*

*It may be more reasonable to increase concentration to limit volume.
For 50 mg in 500 ml (100 mcg/ml), multiply the infusion rate by 2 for desired microdrops/min.
For 100 mg in 250 ml (400 mcg/ml), divide the infusion rate by 2 for desired microdrops/min.
For 100 mg in 500 ml (200 mcg/ml), use same dose schedule as in chart.
For 200 mg in 250 ml (800 mcg/ml), divide the infusion rate by 4 for desired microdrops/min.

INDEX

Page numbers in *italics* refer to illustrations; page numbers followed by (t) refer to tables.